Complimentary Access

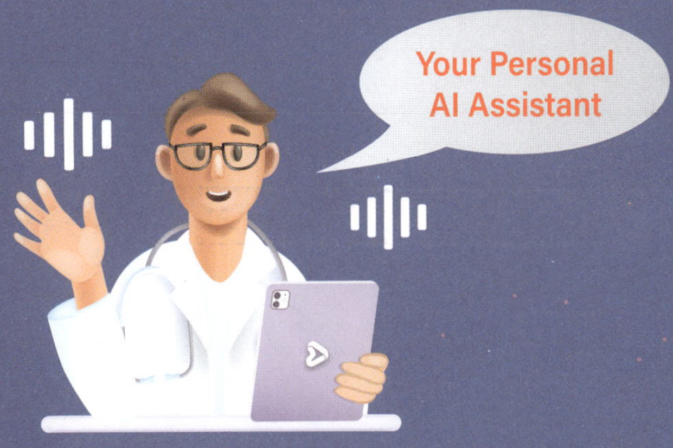

Dr. Wise

Be Wise, Ask Dr. Wise!

You can search Anything, Anywhere, Anytime

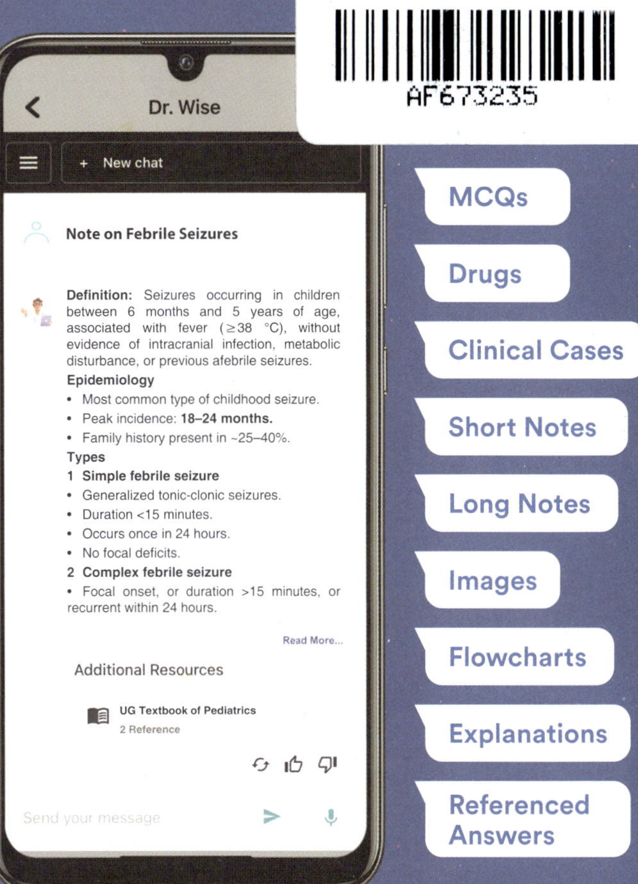

- MCQs
- Drugs
- Clinical Cases
- Short Notes
- Long Notes
- Images
- Flowcharts
- Explanations
- Referenced Answers

Precisely Crafted Answers with References!

Concepts with Detailed Explanation

Easy Steps to Access Dr. Wise Features

New User:

1. Scan the QR code to Install App
2. Click redeem and enter the redemption code
3. Create account to access Dr. Wise
4. If you are an existing user of learn.Ejaypee, login with same email & password and follow point 2 below

Existing User/Add New Book in Dr. Wise App:

1. Login with Dr. Wise email & password
2. In more options, redeem code to add new book

DOWNLOAD APP

Download on the App Store

GET IT ON Google Play

UG Textbook of

PEDIATRICS

As per the Revised Competency-based Medical Education Curriculum (NMC)

Second Edition

Piyush Gupta
MD FAMS FRCPCH
Former Professor of Pediatrics and Principal
University College of Medical Sciences
New Delhi, India
President, Indian Academy of Pediatrics (2021)

Assistant Editor

Nidhi Bedi
MD
Professor
Department of Pediatrics
Faculty of Medicine and Health Sciences and SGT Hospital
Gurugram, Haryana, India

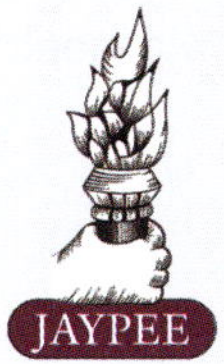

JAYPEE BROTHERS MEDICAL PUBLISHERS
The Health Sciences Publisher
New Delhi | London

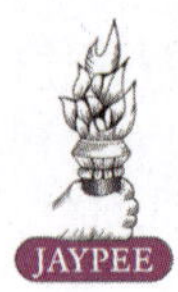

Jaypee Brothers Medical Publishers (P) Ltd

Headquarters

EMCA House, 23/23-B
Ansari Road, Daryaganj
New Delhi 110 002, India
Landline: +91-11-23272143, +91-11-23272703
+91-11-23282021, +91-11-23245672
E-mail: jaypee@jaypeebrothers.com

Corporate Office

4838/24, Ansari Road, Daryaganj
New Delhi 110 002, India
Phone: +91-11-43574357
Fax: +91-11-43574314
E-mail: jaypee@jaypeebrothers.com

Overseas Office

J.P. Medical Ltd
83 Victoria Street, London
SW1H 0HW (UK)
Phone: +44 20 3170 8910
E-mail: info@jpmedpub.com

EU GPSR Authorised Representative
Logos Europe, 9 rue Nicolas Poussin
17000, La Rochelle, France
Phone: +33 (0) 6 67 93 73 78
E-mail: contact@logoseurope.eu

Website: www.jaypeebrothers.com
Website: www.jaypeedigital.com

Inquiries for bulk sales may be solicited at: jaypee@jaypeebrothers.com

UG Textbook of Pediatrics

First Edition: 2023
Reprint: 2024
Second Edition: **2026**

ISBN: 978-93-6616-479-3

Printed in India

Dedicated to

Children of India
and
Those who Care for them

Contributing Authors

Aaradhana MD
Professor
Department of Pediatrics
University College of Medical Sciences and
Guru Teg Bahadur Hospital
Delhi, India
Email: *draaradhanasingh@gmail.com*

Aashima Dabas MD
Professor
Department of Pediatrics
Maulana Azad Medical College and
Associated Lok Nayak Hospital
New Delhi, India
Email: *dr.aashimagupta@gmail.com*

Ajay Gaur MD PhD FIAP FRCPCH
Professor and Head
Department of Pediatrics
GR Medical College, Gwalior MP, India
Email: *drajaygaur@gmail.com*

Anju Gupta MD
Professor
Division of Pediatric Allergy Immunology
Department of Pediatrics
Post Graduate Institute of Medical Education and
Research
Chandigarh, India
Email: *anjupgi@gmail.com*

Ankur Bhardwaj M Ch
Assistant Professor
Department of Pediatric Surgery
Lady Hardinge Medical College
New Delhi, India
Email: *ankur.sprout@gmail.com*

Anup Mohta MS MCh FAMS
Former Director-Professor and Head
Department of Surgery
Lady Harding Medical College and
Associated Hospitals, New Delhi, India
Email: *mohtaanup@gmail.com*

Arpita Gupta MD
Associate Professor
Department of Pediatrics
Vardhman Mahavir Medical College
and Safdarjung Hospital
New Delhi, India
Email: *arpita1517@gmail.com*

Arvind Shah MD FRCPCH FRCP DCH
Consultant
Department of Pediatrics
Royal Free North Middlesex Hospital
London, United Kingdom.
Email: *arvindshah55@hotmail.com*

Atul Kulkarni MD
Associate Professor
Ashwini Rural Medical College
Solapur, Maharashtra, India
Email: *dratulkulkarni@rediffmail.com*

Bobbity Deepthi MD
Associate Professor
Department of Pediatrics
Jawaharlal Institute of Postgraduate Medical
Education and Research
Puducherry, India
Email: *deepu.reddy222@gmail.com*

Chabungbam Smilie MD
Assistant Professor
Department of Pediatrics
Regional Institute of Medical Sciences
Imphal, Manipur, India
Email: *smiliecha55@gmail.com*

Chander Grover MD DNB FAMS
Director-Professor
Department of Dermatology and STD
University College of Medical Sciences and
Guru Teg Bahadur Hospital
Delhi, India
Email: *chandergroverkubba76@gmail.com*

Devendra Mishra MD
Director-Professor
Department of Pediatrics
Maulana Azad Medical College
New Delhi, India
Email: *drdmishra@gmail.com*

Dheeraj Shah MD DNB FAMS
Principal and Director-Professor
Department of Pediatrics
University College of Medical Sciences and
Guru Teg Bahadur Hospital
Delhi, India
Email: *dshah@ucms.ac.in*

DK Singh MD
Professor
Department of Pediatrics
Postgraduate Institute of Child Health
Noida, Uttar Pradesh, India
Email: *drdksingh1999@gmail.com*

Hema Gupta Mittal MD
Professor and In-Charge
Division of Pediatric Pulmonology
Department of Pediatrics
Atal Bihari Vajpayee Institute of Medical Sciences
and Dr Ram Manohar Lohia Hospital
New Delhi, India
Email: *hema_g10@hotmail.com*

Jagdish P Goyal MD MAMS
Professor, Department of Pediatrics
All India Institute of Medical Sciences
Jodhpur, Rajasthan, India
Email: *goyal.drjagdish@gmail.com*

Kanika Kapoor MD Fellow IPNA
Professor
Department of Pediatrics
Vardhman Mahavir Medical College and
Safdarjung Hospital
New Delhi, India
Email: *kanikataurus84@gmail.com*

Kirtisudha Mishra MD DNB ISPN FIPNA
Associate Professor
Department of Pediatrics
Chacha Nehru Bal Chikitsalaya
(Affiliated with Guru Gobind Singh Indraprastha
University)
New Delhi, India
Email: *kirtisen@gmail.com*

Manish Kumar MD
Professor
Department of Pediatrics
Chacha Nehru Bal Chikitsalaya
Affiliated with Guru Gobind Singh Indraprastha
University
New Delhi, India
Email: *manishkp75@yahoo.com*

Mukta Mantan MD DNB
Director-Professor
Department of Pediatrics
Maulana Azad Medical College and
Associated Lok Nayak Hospital
New Delhi, India
Email: *muktamantan@hotmail.com*

Munesh Tomar MD FNB FACC
Associate Professor
Department of Pediatrics
Unit In-Charge, Pediatric Cardiology
Lala Lajpat Rai Memorial Medical College
Meerut, Uttar Pradesh, India
Email: *drmuneshtomar@gmail.com*

Narayan Prasad Modi MD DAA FIAP ICPP
Professor and Head
PG Department of Pediatrics, MKCG MCH
Brahmapur, Odisha, India
Email: *npm234@gmail.com*

Neetu Sharma MD
Associate Professor
Department of Pediatrics
Gajra Raja Medical College
Gwalior, Madhya Pradesh, India
Email: *drneetuagarwal@gmail.com*

Nidhi Bedi MD
Professor
Department of Pediatrics
Faculty of Medicine and Health Sciences
and SGT Hospital
Gurugram, Haryana, India
Email: *drnidhibedi@gmail.com*

Nihar Ranjan Mishra MD FACI
Additional Professor
Department of Pediatrics
All India Institute of Medical Sciences
Kalyani, West Bengal, India
Email: *drnihar.mishra@gmail.com*

Niranjan Shendurnikar MD FIAP
Consultant Pediatrician
Ankur Maternity Hospital
Vadodara, Gujarat, India
Email: *drniranjan@rediffmail.com*

Nitin Dhochak MD DM
Clinical Fellow
Great Ormond Street Hospital for Children
London, UK
Email: *nitind.aiims@gmail.com*

OP Mishra MD FIAP FAMS
Professor and Head
Department of Pediatrics
Heritage Institute of Medical Sciences
Varanasi, Uttar Pradesh, India
Email: *opmpedia2@gmail.com*

Pallab Chatterjee DCH MD DNB FIAP
European Diplomate of Pediatric Pulmonology
Visiting Consultant
Apollo Multispeciality Hospital
Fortis Hospital and Manipal Hospital
Kolkata, West Bengal, India
Email: *pallabchatterjee@gmail.com*

Paresh A Thakkar MD DNB DCH
Professor
Department of Pediatrics
Govt Medical College
Baroda, Gujarat, India
Email: *pareshthakkar@yahoo.com*

Payal Gupta DNB, FCO & FPOS (SNC)
Pediatric Ophthalmologist and Phacosurgeon
Consultant
Department of Ophthalmology
Fortis Hospital
Greater Noida, Uttar Pradesh, India
Email: *drpayal.pg@gmail.com*

Piyush Gupta MD FAMS FRCPCH
Former Principal and Professor
Department of Pediatrics
University College of Medical Sciences and
Guru Teg Bahadur Hospital
Delhi, India
Email: *prof.piyush.gupta@gmail.com*

Pooja Dewan MD MNAMS
Director-Professor
Department of Pediatrics
University College of Medical Sciences and
Guru Teg Bahadur Hospital
Delhi, India
Email: *poojadewan@hotmail.com*

Poonam Singh MD DNB
Additional Professor
Department of Neonatology
All India Institute of Medical Sciences
Rishikesh, Uttarakhand, India
Email: *drpoonamujn@gmail.com*

Prawin Kumar MD
Associate Professor
Department of Pediatrics
All India Institute of Medical Sciences
Jodhpur, Rajasthan, India
Email: *drprawin484@gmail.com*

R Ganesh DNB FRCPCH PhD
Senior Consultant and Head
Department of Pediatrics
Rainbow Children's Hospital
Chennai, Tamil Nadu, India
Email: *ganeped@gmail.com*

Rajesh Kumar Meena MD
Associate Professor
Department of Pediatrics
Vardhman Mahavir Medical College and
Safdarjung Hospital
New Delhi, India
Email: *raj.mamc@gmail.com*

Rajniti Prasad MD FIAP FAMS
Professor
Department of Pediatrics
Institute of Medical Sciences
Banaras Hindu University
Varanasi, Uttar Pradesh, India
Email: *rajnitip@gmail.com*

Rakesh Lodha MD
Professor
Department of Pediatrics
All India Institute of Medical Sciences
New Delhi, India
Email: *rakesh_lodha@hotmail.com*

Ranjana Mishra DGO DNB (Obs & Gynae) DNB (Medical Genetics)
Senior Consultant
Yashoda Super Speciality Hospital and Research
Centre, Ghaziabad
BLK-MAX Hospital
Delhi, India
Email: *mishraranjana312@gmail.com*

Richa Jain MD DM
Additional Professor
Pediatric Hematology and Oncology Unit
Advanced Pediatrics Centre
Postgraduate Institute of Medical Education and
Research
Chandigarh, India
Email: *docrichajain@gmail.com*

Romit Saxena MD DNB MNAMS
Professor
Department of Pediatrics
Maulana Azad Medical College and
Associated Lok Nayak Hospital
New Delhi, India
Email: *drromit@gmail.com*

Ruchi Rai MD
Professor and Head
Department of Neonatology
Postgraduate Institute of Child Health
Noida, Uttar Pradesh, India
Email: *ruchiraialld@gmail.com*

Sakshi Sachdeva MD DNB FNB DM
Associate Professor
Division of Pediatric Cardiology
Department of Pediatrics
Atal Bihari Vajpayee Institute of Medical Sciences
and Dr Ram Manohar Lohia Hospital
New Delhi, India
Email: *sakshisachdeva21@gmail.com*

Sarika Gupta MD PhD FRCPCH FICS
Professor
Department of Pediatrics and Medical Education
King George's Medical University
Lucknow, Uttar Pradesh, India
Email: *sgguptasarika@gmail.com*

Satnam Kaur MD
Professor
Department of Pediatrics
Vardhman Mahavir Medical College and
Safdarjung Hospital
New Delhi, India
Email: *sk_doc@yahoo.co.in*

Satvik C Bansal MBBS MD
Associate Professor
Department of Pediatrics
Gajra Raja Medical College
Gwalior, Madhya Pradesh. India
Email: *drsatvikbansal@gmail.com*

Sejal Saglani MD FRCPCH
Professor of Pediatric Respiratory Medicine
Head of Inflammation
Repair and Development Section
National Heart and Lung Institute
Imperial College
London, United Kingdom.
Email: *s.saglani@imperial.ac.uk*

Shetanshu Srivastava MD MNAMS DPAA
Additional Professor
Department of Pediatrics
Dr Ram Manohar Lohia Institute
of Medical Sciences
Lucknow, Uttar Pradesh, India
Email: *drsitanshu@yahoo.co.in*

Shilpa Sharma MS MCh PhD FAMS
Professor
Department of Pediatric Surgery
All India Institute of Medical Sciences
New Delhi, India
Email: *drshilpas@gmail.com*

Shubha R Phadke MD, DM
Professor
Department of Medical Genetics
Bharati Vidyapeeth
Pune, Maharashtra, India
Email: *shubharaophadke@gmail.com*

Sidharth Totadri
MD DM (Pediatric Hematology Oncology)
Associate Professor
Department of Pediatric Hematology Oncology
St. Johns Medical College and Hospital
Bengaluru, Karnataka, India
Email: *totadri86@yahoo.com*

Srikanta Basu MD MNAMS FIAP
Director-Professor
Department of Pediatrics
Lady Hardinge Medical College and
Kalawati Saran Children's Hospital
New Delhi, India
Email: *srikantabasu@gmail.com*

Sriparna Basu MD DCH FRCPCH
Professor and Head
Department of Neonatology
All India Institute of Medical Sciences
Rishikesh, Uttarakhand, India
Email: *sriparna.neonat@aiimsrishikesh.edu.in*

Sriram Krishnamurthy MD FIAP
Professor
Pediatric Nephrology Services
Department of Pediatrics
Jawaharlal Institute of Postgraduate Medical
Education and Research
Puducherry, India
Email: *drsriramk@yahoo.com*; *drsriramkris@gmail.com*

Sudarsan Krishnasamy MD DM
Assistant Professor
Department of Pediatrics
Jawaharlal Institute of Postgraduate Medical
Education and Research
Puducherry, India
Email: *sudarsanjipmer@gmail.com*

Sumaira Khalil DNB
Associate Professor
Department of Pediatrics
University College of Medical Sciences and
Guru Teg Bahadur Hospital
New Delhi, India
Email: *sumairakhalil@yahoo.com*

Sunil Kumar Rao MD
Professor and In-Charge
Pediatric Intensive Care and Pulmonology
Institute of Medical Sciences
Banaras Hindu University
Varanasi, Uttar Pradesh, India
Email: *drsunilrao21@gmail.com*

Vidushi Mahajan DNB
Associate Professor
Department of Pediatrics
Government Medical College
Chandigarh, India
Email: *vidushimahajan2003@gmail.com*

Vikram Bhaskar MD
Associate Professor
Department of Pediatrics
University College of Medical Sciences and
Guru Teg Bahadur Hospital
Delhi, India
Email: *vikrambhaskar8884@gmail.com*

Vinod Kumar MD DNB MNAMS
Associate Professor
Department of Pediatrics
King George's Medical University
Lucknow, Uttar Pradesh, India
Email: *vinodmbbs52@gmail.com*

Vishal Sondhi MD DM
Professor of Pediatrics and Pediatric Neurology
Department of Pediatrics
Armed Forces Medical College
Pune, Maharashtra, India
Email: vishalsondhi@gmail.com

Preface to the Second Edition

We extend our heartfelt gratitude to the thousands of students, educators, and clinicians across India who embraced the first edition of the *UG Textbook of Pediatrics* with such overwhelming appreciation. Your feedback, enthusiasm, and trust have been the driving force behind this second edition—released within just 3 years of the original, a testament to its impact in undergraduate pediatric education.

This revised edition has been meticulously restructured to align with the *2024 Revised Competency List* issued by the *National Medical Commission (NMC), India*. Every *"Must Know"* competency is now comprehensively covered in the print version, ensuring that students are equipped with the essential knowledge and clinical understanding expected at the undergraduate level. To complement the core curriculum, we have introduced a *dedicated online section* featuring *"Good to Know"* topics—curated to broaden perspectives, spark curiosity, and deepen understanding of pediatric practice beyond the mandated competencies. These topics, while not compulsory, are invaluable for those who wish to explore the subject more holistically.

We have retained and refined the features that made the first edition so student-friendly and pedagogically sound:

- *Case Studies* that bring clinical scenarios to life
- *"In A Nutshell"* boxes for quick revision and clarity
- *Color Coding* for intuitive navigation and emphasis
- *Figures, Tables, and Photographs* to enhance visual learning
- *Easy-to-read Text* that simplifies complex concepts without diluting depth

A special mention must be made of the completely rewritten chapter on Neurological Disorders, which now reflects current clinical practices and pedagogical clarity, making it more accessible and relevant for learners.

Our hope is that this edition will not only serve as a *primary textbook for undergraduate students in India* but also foster a deeper appreciation for pediatrics as a dynamic and compassionate discipline. We remain committed to making pediatric education engaging, evidence-based, and aligned with the evolving needs of medical learners.

September 2025 **Piyush Gupta**

Preface to the First Edition

Medical education in India is evolving fast and has achieved a new landmark by adapting a competency-based curriculum. This book is specifically designed to cater to the requirement of undergraduate students pursuing the competency-based pediatric curriculum in India and abroad. In an era where the existing textbooks of pediatrics have become largely theoretical, needlessly bulky, and specialty-based; this tome focuses precisely on the 35 Topics and 406 core Competencies as outlined by the National Medical Commission (NMC). Salient unique points of the book are highlighted below:

- *Competency Index:* An index of NMC Competencies is provided in the preliminary pages to locate every prescribed competency. Additionally, every chapter begins with a list of Competencies covered in that particular chapter.
- *Figures, flowcharts, and clinical photographs:* The text is replete with fully colored figures and photographs, to facilitate easy retention. In fact, they form the bulk of the book.
- *Text:* The focus remains on the core pediatric topics; the text is to-the-point, concise and yet complete; and interspersed with multiple Tables and Boxes, wherever essential. Every chapter is thoroughly updated.
- *Case scenarios:* The text is supplemented by a sprinkling of Case Studies highlighting the common scenarios of common illnesses in children. Case studies are a unique feature of this textbook in keeping with the requirement of competency-based curriculum. These are intended to help students visualize the presentation in the true clinical context.
- *Revision points:* Every important topic is followed by a summary of take-home messages in a revision box as "In A Nutshell." The entire book thus, can be revised in a matter of hours by just reading these boxes.
- *Writing style:* The language is simple, the paragraphs short, and the jargon simplified to have a flow in readability. The editing style facilitates understanding. All chapters have been kept on an even keel.
- *The layout:* Entire book is in full color, with color-coding to highlight treatment, case studies, revision points, tables, boxes, and suggested reading.
- *Faculty:* Contributed by more than 60 teachers of pediatrics from all over the country and from premier institutions.
- *Target readership:* This is a complete book on Pediatrics for the undergraduate medical students. At the same time, this treatise has the potential to serve as a foundation text for those pursuing specialization in Pediatrics.

All the above points together make this book an invaluable asset for understanding pediatrics, practicing pediatrics, and taking the examinations. I welcome comments concerning omissions and errors; constructive reviews regarding content, critical thoughts; and suggestions for further editions.

Enjoy reading!

Piyush Gupta

Acknowledgments

I express my thanks to M/s Jaypee Brothers Medical Publishers (P) Ltd, New Delhi, India, for publishing this book so well. I sincerely thanks Shri Jitendar P Vij (Group Chairman), Mr Ankit Vij (Managing Director), Mr MS Mani (Group President), Dr Madhu Choudhary (Director-Educational Publishing), Ms Pooja Bhandari [Director-Production (Books and Journals)], Mr Ajay Kumar Sharma [Deputy General Manager (Books and Journals)], Dr Aditya Tayal (Senior Editorial Manager-Content Strategy), Mr Vijay Kumar Bhatia (Manager-Production), Mr Bishan Singh (Production Manager-Press), Ms Neha Verma (Graphic Designer-Cover), Mr Laxmidhar Padhiary (Team Lead-Production), Mr Dinesh Bhardwaj (Typesetter), Mr Mahesh Joshi (Typesetter), Mr Nitesh Jain (Team Lead-Graphic Designer), for their help, guidance and timely active intervention in composing, designing and editing of the book.

I also like to acknowledge the help of Ms Anju Kumari for Secretarial Services to the Editor.

Contents

(For Online content, scan QR code given in the begining of the respective chapters)

CHAPTER 14 Infections and Infestations 261

Piyush Gupta, and Aaradhana; with Pooja Dewan (HIV; online only) and Atul Kulkarni (Rickettsial Diseases; online only)

CHAPTER 15 Care of the Normal Newborn 346

Ruchi Rai and DK Singh

CHAPTER 16 Care of the High-risk Newborn 381

Sriparna Basu and Poonam Singh

CHAPTER 17 Disorders of Kidneys and Urinary Tract 440

OP Mishra, Rajniti Prasad [Anatomy and Physiology of Kidney (Online Only), Edema, HUS, AKI, CKD]; Bobbity Deepthi, Sriram Krishnamurthy (Evaluation of Genitourinary System); Shilpa Sharma, Ankur Bhardwaj (Cystic Kidney Disease) (Online Only); Kirtisudha Mishra (UTI); R Ganesh (Hematuria); Kanika Kapoor (Glomerulonephritis); Sudarsan Krishnasamy, Sriram Krishnamurthy (Proteinuria); Sriram Krishnamurthy, Sudarsan Krishnasamy (Nephrotic Syndrome); Richa Jain (Wilms Tumor); Anup Mohta (Genitourinary Malformations) (Online Only); and Manish Kumar (Referral and Parent Education for Kidney Disease)

CHAPTER 18 Rheumatological and Immune System Disorders 493

Anju Gupta

CHAPTER 19 Cardiovascular Disorders 519

Sakshi Sachdeva, Munesh Tomar, Piyush Gupta; and Mukta Mantan (Hypertension)

CHAPTER 20 Diarrheal Diseases 575

Dheeraj Shah and Rajesh Kumar Meena

CHAPTER 21 Gastrointestinal and Hepatobiliary Disorders 590

Rajesh Kumar Meena and Dheeraj Shah

CHAPTER 22 Respiratory Disorders 626

Satvik C Bansal (Anatomy and Physiology of the Respiratory Tract); Vinod Kumar (Examination of ENT, Approach to Child with Upper Respiratory Symptoms, Making a Diagnosis in a Child with ENT Symptoms, Approach to Stridor); Satnam Kaur (Examination of ENT, AOM); Hema Gupta Mittal, Sarika Gupta (Nasopharyngitis and Tonsillopharyngitis); Nihar Ranjan Mishra, Narayan Prasad Modi (Allergic Rhinitis, Approach to Child with Wheeze); Romit Saxena {Acute Epiglottitis, Acute Laryngotracheobronchitis (Croup)}; Pallab Chatterjee (FB Aspiration); Vikram Bhaskar (Approach to a Child with Fast Breathing, Approach to a Child with Wheeze); Jagdish P Goyal (Pneumonia); Sunil Kumar Rao (Empyema Thoracis); Sejal Saglani, Arvind Shah (Bronchiolitis); Prawin Kumar (Bronchial Asthma); Nitin Dhochak, Rakesh Lodha (Imaging in Respiratory Disorders); Shetanshu Srivastava (Parental Counseling for Prevention of Respiratory Disorders)

CHAPTER 23 Hematological Disorders 684

Sidharth Totadri and Pooja Dewan

CHAPTER 24 Neurological Disorders 737

Vishal Sondhi

CHAPTER 25 Genetic and Metabolic Disorders 811

Shubha R Phadke and Ranjana Mishra

CHAPTER 26 Endocrine Disorders 841

Aashima Dabas

CHAPTER 27 Common Emergencies and Poisonings 864

Chabungbam Smilie and Piyush Gupta

CHAPTER 28 National Health Programs Related to Children 929

Piyush Gupta and Chabungbam Smilie

CHAPTER 29 Skin Disorders 959 (Chapter Available Online Only)

Chander Grover

CHAPTER 30 Ophthalmic Disorders 959 (Chapter Available Online Only)

Payal Gupta

CHAPTER 31 Drug Therapy 959 (Chapter Available Online Only)

Nidhi Bedi and Pooja Dewan

Annexures 961

Case Studies

18. Rheumatological and Immune System Disorders

19. Cardiovascular Disorders

20. Diarrheal Diseases

21. Gastrointestinal and Hepatobiliary Disorders

22. Respiratory Disorders

23. Hematological Disorders

25. Genetic and Metabolic Disorders

27. Common Emergencies and Poisonings

NMC Competencies as per CBME Curriculum 2024

Number	COMPETENCY The student should be able to	Core Y/N	Suggested teaching learning methods	Chapter number	Page number
Topic 1: Normal Growth and Development					
PE1.1	Define the terminologies growth and development and describe the factors affecting normal growth	Y	LGT, SGT	1.1, 1.2, 1.3	1, 3, 5
PE1.2	Describe the methods of assessment of growth including use of WHO and Indian national standards. Enumerate the parameters used for assessment of physical growth in infants, children and adolescents and perform anthropometric measurements, document in growth charts and interpret	Y	LGT, SGT	1.4, 1.5, 1.6, 1.7	8, 10, 14, 15
PE1.3	Define development and describe the normal developmental milestones with respect to motor, behavior, social, adaptive and language. Discuss the factors affecting development and describe the assessment methods of development	Y	LGT, SGT	1.8, 1.9	27, 33
Topic 2: Common Problems Related to Growth					
PE2.1	Discuss the etiopathogenesis, clinical features, assessment and management of a child who fails to thrive.	Y	LGT, SGT	2.1	41
PE2.2	Counselling the parent of a child with failure to thrive.	Y	OSPE	2.1	41
PE2.3	Discuss the etiopathogenesis, clinical features and management of a child with short stature. Assessment of a child with short stature.	Y	LGT, SGT	2.2	45
Topic 3: Common Problems Related to Development-1					
PE3.1	Define developmental delay. Describe the causes of developmental delay and disability including intellectual disability in children.	Y	LGT, SGT	3.1	54
PE3.2	Explain the approach to a child with developmental delay.	Y	Bedside clinics, Skills lab	3.1	54
PE3.3	Counsel a parent of a child with developmental delay.	Y	DOAP	3.1	54
PE3.4	Visit a Child Developmental Unit and observe its functioning.	Y	LGT, SGT	3.1	54
Topic 4: Common Problems Related to Development-2					
PE4.1	Describe the etiology, clinical features, diagnosis and management of a child with attention deficit hyperactivity disorder (ADHD).	N	LGT, SGT	3.2	66
PE4.2	Describe the etiology, clinical features, diagnosis and management of a child with autism.	N	LGT, SGT	3.3	68
Topic 5: Common Problems Related to Behavior					
PE5.1	Describe the clinical features, diagnosis and management of feeding problems	N	LGT, SGT	4.2, 4.3, 4.4	71, 72, 73
PE5.2	Describe the clinical features, diagnosis and management of breath holding spells	N	LGT, SGT	4.5	74
PE5.3	Describe the clinical features, diagnosis and management of temper tantrums and Pica	N	LGT, SGT	4.6, 4.7	75, 76
PE5.4	Explain the etiology, clinical features and management of enuresis	N	LGT, SGT	4.8	77
Topic 6: Adolescent Health and Common Problems Related to Adolescent Health					
PE6.1	Define adolescence and describe the stages of adolescence	Y	LGT, SGT	5.1, 5.2	82, 83
PE6.2	Describe the physical, physiological and psychological changes during adolescence (puberty)	Y	LGT, SGT	5.2	83

PE6.3	Describe the general health problems during adolescence	Y	LGT, SGT	5.3	86
PE6.4	Describe adolescent sexuality and common problems related to it	N	LGT, SGT	5.4	87
PE6.5	Describe the common adolescent eating disorders (anorexia nervosa, bulimia)	N	LGT, SGT	5.5	88
PE6.6	Describe the common mental health problems during adolescence	Y	LGT, SGT	5.6, 5.7	90, 92
PE6.7	Respecting patient privacy and maintaining confidentiality while dealing with adolescence	Y	Bedside clinics	5.8	93
PE6.8	Perform routine adolescent health check-up including eliciting history, performing examination including SMR (sex maturity rating), growth assessments (using growth charts) and systemic exam including thyroid and breast examination and the HEADSS screening	Y	Bedside clinics	5.2, 5.8	83, 93
PE6.9	Explain the objectives and functions of AFHS (Adolescent Friendly Health Services) and the referral criteria	N	LGT, SGT	5.9	95
PE6.10	Visit to the adolescent clinic	Y	DOAP	5.9	95
PE6.11	Enumerate the importance of obesity and other NCD in adolescents	Y	LGT, SGT	5.7	92
PE6.12	Enumerate the prevalence and the importance of recognition of sexual abuse and drug abuse in adolescents and children	N	LGT, SGT	5.4, 5.6	87, 90
Topic 7: To Promote and Support Optimal Breastfeeding for Infants					
PE7.1	Awareness on the cultural beliefs and practices of breastfeeding and explain physiology of lactation	N	LGT, SGT	6.2, 6.4	98, 101
PE7.2	Describe the composition and types of breast milk and discuss the differences between cow's milk and human milk	Y	LGT, debate	6.3	100
PE7.3	Describe the advantages of breast milk	Y	LGT, SGT	6.4	101
PE7.4	Observe the correct technique of breastfeeding and distinguish right from wrong techniques	Y	Bedside clinics, Skills lab	6.5, 6.6	103, 105
PE7.5	Enumerate the baby friendly hospital initiatives	Y	LGT, SGT	6.9	108
PE7.6	Describe the principles of IYCF (Infant and Young Child Feeding)	N	SGT	6.10	108
PE7.7	Participate in World Breastfeeding Week (WBW) celebration at your institute	N	Outreach activities	6.11	109
PE7.8	Describe the structure and functioning of human milk bank and visit the nearest human bilk bank	N	SGT	6.12	110
Topic 8: Complementary Feeding					
PE8.1	Define the term complementary feeding	Y	LGT, SGT	7.1	111
PE8.2	Explain the principles, the initiation, attributes, frequency, techniques and hygiene related to complementary feeding	Y	LGT, SGT	7.1	111
PE8.3	Enumerate the common complementary foods	Y	LGT, SGT	7.2	116
PE8.4	Elicit history on the complementary feeding habits	Y	Bedside clinics, Skills lab	7.3	118
PE8.5	Counsel and educate mother son the best practices in complementary feeding	Y	DOAP	7.4	119
Topic 9: Normal Nutrition, Assessment and Monitoring					
PE9.1	Describe the age-related nutritional needs of infants, children and adolescents including micronutrients and vitamins	Y	LGT, SGT	8.1	121
PE9.2	Describe the tools and methods for assessment and classification of nutritional status of infants, children and adolescents	Y	LGT, SGT	8.3	130
PE9.3	Explain the calorific value of common Indian foods	Y	LGT, SGT	8.2	125
PE9.4	Elicit document and present an appropriate nutritional history and perform a dietary recall	Y	Bedside clinic, Skills lab	8.3	130

PE9.5	Calculate the age-related calorie requirement in health and disease and identify gap	Y	Bedside clinics, SGT	8.3	130
PE9.6	Assess and classify the nutrition status of infants, children and adolescents and recognize deviations	Y	Bedside clinic, SGT	8.3	130
PE9.7	Plan an appropriate diet in health and disease	N	Bedside clinic, SGT	8.4	133
Topic 10: Provide Nutritional Support, Assessment and Monitoring for Common Nutritional Problems					
PE10.1	Define and describe the etiopathogenesis, classify including WHO classification, clinical features, complication and management of severe acute malnutrition (SAM) and moderate acute malnutrition (MAM)	Y	LGT, SGT	9.1, 9.2, 9.3, 9.4, 9.5	137, 139, 141, 143, 153
PE10.2	Outline the clinical approach to a child with SAM and MAM	Y	LGT, SGT	9.4, 9.5, 9.8	143, 153, 158
PE10.3	Assessment of a patient with SAM and MAM, diagnosis, classification and planning management including hospital and community-based intervention, rehabilitation and prevention	Y	Bedside clinics, Skills lab	9.2, 9.4, 9.5, 9.8	139, 143, 153, 158
PE10.4	Counsel parents of children with SAM and MAM	Y	Bedside clinic, Skills Station	9.4, 9.5, 9.7	143, 153, 156
PE10.5	Enumerate the role of locally prepared therapeutic diets and ready to use therapeutic diets	N	LGT, SGT	9.6	155
PE10.6	Explain the adolescent nutrition and common nutritional problems	Y	LGT, SGT	9.9	161
Topic 11: Obesity in Children					
PE11.1	Describe the etiology, clinical features and management of obesity in children	Y	LGT, SGT	9.10	162
PE11.2	Describe the risk approach for obesity and discuss the prevention strategies	Y	LGT, SGT	9.10	162
PE11.3	Assessment of a child with obesity with regard to eliciting history including physical activity, charting and dietary recall	Y	Bedside clinics, Standardized patients	9.10	162
PE11.4	Examination including calculation of BMI, measurement of waist-hip ratio, identifying external markers like acanthosis, striae, pseudogynecomastia, etc.	Y	Bedside clinics, Standardized patients, Videos	9.10	162
Topic 12: Micronutrients in Health and Disease-1 (Vitamins ADEK, B Complex and C)					
PE12.1	Describe the RDA, dietary sources of vitamin A, its metabolism	Y	LGT, SGT	10.2	171
PE12.2	Describe the causes, clinical features, classification, diagnosis and management of deficiency/excess of vitamin A	Y	LGT, SGT	10.2	171
PE12.3	Describe the causes, clinical features, diagnosis and management of deficiency/excess of vitamin D (rickets and hypervitaminosis D)	Y	LGT, SGT	10.3	175
PE12.4	Describe the causes, clinical features, diagnosis and management of deficiency of vitamin E	N	LGT, SGT	10.4	180
PE12.5	Describe the RDA, dietary sources of vitamin K and their role in health and disease	N	LGT, SGT	10.5	181
PE12.6	Describe the causes, clinical features, diagnosis management and prevention of deficiency of vitamin K	N	LGT, SGT	10.5	181
PE12.7	Describe the causes, clinical features, diagnosis and management of deficiency of B complex vitamins	Y	LGT, SGT	10.6	182
PE12.8	Describe the RDA, dietary sources of vitamin C and their role in health and disease, clinical features of deficiency and management	N	LGT, SGT	10.7	191
Topic 13: Micronutrients in Health and Disease-2: Iron, Iodine, Calcium, Magnesium					
PE13.1	Describe the RDA, dietary sources of iron and their role in health and disease, clinical features of iron deficiency, and management	Y	LGT, SGT	11.2	195

PE13.2	Describe the national anemia control program and its recommendations	Y	LGT, SGT	11.3	197
PE13.3	Describe the RDA, dietary sources of iodine and their role in health and disease, deficiency, and goiter control program	Y	LGT, SGT	11.4	198
PE13.4	Describe the RDA, dietary sources of calcium and magnesium and their role in health and disease, clinical features and management of deficiency states	Y	LGT, SGT	11.6	205
Topic 14: Poisoning					
PE14.1	Explain the risk factors, clinical features, diagnosis and management of kerosene ingestion	N	LGT, SGT	27.13	918
PE14.2	Explain the risk factors, clinical features, diagnosis and management of organophosphorus poisoning	N	LGT, SGT	27.14	918
PE14.3	Describe the risk factors, clinical features, diagnosis and management of paracetamol poisoning	N	LGT, SGT	27.15	921
Topic 15: Fluid and Electrolyte Balance					
PE15.1	Describe the fluid and electrolyte requirement in health and disease	Y	LGT, SGT	12.1, 12.2	209, 211
PE15.2	Interpret electrolyte report and describe the management of sodium and potassium imbalance	Y	Bedside clinics, SGT	12.3, 12.4, 12.5, 12.6	215, 217, 219, 220
PE15.3	Demonstrate the steps of inserting an IV cannula in a model	Y	Skills Lab	12.7	223
PE15.4	Demonstrate the steps of inserting an interosseous line in a mannequin	Y	Skills Lab	12.8	224
Topic 16: Integrated Management of Neonatal and Childhood Illnesses (IMNCI) Guideline					
PE16.1	Explain the components of Integrated Management of Neonatal and Childhood Illnesses (IMNCI) guidelines and method of risk stratification	Y	LGT, SGT	28.7	950
PE16.2	Assess children <2 months using IMNCI guidelines	Y	DOAP	28.7	950
PE16.3	Assess children 2 months to 5 years using IMNCI guidelines and stratify risk	Y	DOAP	28.7	950
PE16.4	Identify children with undernutrition as per IMNCI criteria and plan referral	Y	DOAP	28.7	950
PE16.5	Identify and stratify risk in a sick neonate using IMNCI guidelines	Y	DOAP	28.7	950
PE16.6	Apply the IMNCI guidelines in risk stratification of children with diarrheal dehydration and refer	Y	Bedside clinics, Skills lab	28.7	950
Topic 17: The National Health Programs, NHM					
PE17.1	Describe the vision and outline the goals, strategies and plan of action of NHM and other important national programs pertaining to maternal and child health including RCH, RMNCHA+, RBSK, RKSK, JSSK, mission Indradhanush and ICDS	Y	LGT, SGT	28.3, 28.4, 28.5, 28.6	937, 940, 941, 944
Topic 18: National Programs, RCH-Universal Immunizations Program					
PE18.1	Explain the components of the universal immunization program and the national immunization program	Y	LGT, SGT	13.2	229
PE18.2	Explain the epidemiology of vaccine preventable diseases	Y	LGT, SGT	13.1	227
PE18.3	Describe vaccine with regards to classification of vaccines, strain used, dose, route, schedule, risks, benefits and side effects, indications and contraindications	Y	LGT, SGT	13.3	231
PE18.4	Define cold chain and discuss the methods of safe storage and handling of vaccines	Y	LGT, SGT	13.4	246
PE18.5	Describe immunization in special situations—HIV positive children, immunodeficiency, preterm, organ transplants, those who received blood and blood products, splenectomised children, adolescents, travellers	Y	LGT, SGT	13.5	249

PE18.6	Assess patient for fitness for immunization and prescribe an age appropriate immunization schedule	Y	Outpatient clinics, Skills lab	13.2	229
PE18.7	Educate and counsel a parent for immunization	Y	DOAP	13.6	252
PE18.8	Describe the components of safe vaccine practice—patient education/counselling; adverse events following immunization, safe injection practices, documentation and medicolegal implications	Y	LGT, SGT	13.6, 13.7, 13.8	252, 253, 256
PE18.9	Observe the handling and storing of vaccines	Y	DOAP	13.4	246
PE18.10	Document immunization in an immunization record	Y	Outpatient clinics, Skills lab	13.9	257
PE18.11	Observe the administration of UIP vaccines	Y	DOAP	13.7	253
PE18.12	Demonstrate the correct administration of different vaccines in a mannequin	Y	DOAP	13.7	253
PE18.13	Explain the term implied consent in immunization services	Y	SGT	13.9	257
PE18.14	Enumerate available newer vaccines and their indications including pentavalent pneumococcal, rotavirus, JE, hepatitis A, influenza, COVID, typhoid, IPV and HPV	N	LGT, SGT	13.10	258
Topic 19: Care of the Normal Newborn, and High-risk Newborn					
PE19.1	Define the common neonatal nomenclatures including the classification newborn and describe the characteristics of a normal term neonate and high-risk neonates, explain the care of a normal neonate	Y	LGT, SGT	15.1, 15.3, 15.6, 15.7	346, 354, 364, 370
PE19.2	Perform neonatal resuscitation on a manikin	Y	DOAP	15.2, 15.6	347, 364
PE19.3	Assessment of a normal neonate. Explain the follow up care for neonates including breastfeeding, temperature maintenance, immunization, importance of growth monitoring and red flags	Y	Bedside clinics, Skills lab	15.3, 15.4, 15.5, 15.6, 15.7, 15.9, 15.10, 15.11	354, 357, 359, 364, 370, 373, 377, 378, 378
PE19.4	Describe the etiology, clinical features and management of birth asphyxia	Y	LGT, SGT	16.3	390
PE19.5	Describe the etiology, clinical features and management of respiratory distress in newborn including meconium aspiration and transient tachypnoea of newborn	Y	LGT, SGT	16.5	396
PE19.6	Explain the etiology, clinical features and management of birth injuries	Y	LGT, SGT	16.4	395
PE19.7	Explain the etiology, clinical features and management of hemorrhagic disease of newborn	Y	LGT, SGT	16.12	419
PE19.8	Describe the clinical characteristics, complications and management of low birth weight (preterm and small for gestation)	Y	LGT, SGT	16.2	385
PE19.9	Describe the temperature regulation in neonates, clinical features and management of neonatal hypothermia	Y	LGT, SGT	15.8	373
PE19.10	Describe the temperature regulation in neonates, clinical features and management of neonatal hypoglycemia	Y	LGT, SGT	16.8, 16.9	410, 411
PE19.11	Explain the etiology, clinical features and management of neonatal hypocalcemia	Y	LGT, SGT	16.10	412
PE19.12	Describe the etiology, clinical features and management of neonatal seizures	Y	LGT, SGT	16.7	406
PE19.13	Explain the etiology, clinical features and management of neonatal sepsis	Y	LGT, SGT	16.11	413
PE19.14	Describe the etiology, clinical features and management of perinatal infections	Y	LGT, SGT	16.14	429
PE19.15	Describe the etiology, clinical features and management of neonatal hyperbilirubinemia	Y	LGT, SGT	16.13	421

PE19.16	Identify clinical presentations of common surgical conditions in the newborn including TEF, esophageal atresia, anal atresia, cleft lip and palate, congenital diaphragmatic hernia and causes of acute abdomen	Y	LGT, SGT	16.16	432
PE19.17	Describe the risk factors, clinical features, diagnosis and management of oxygen toxicity	N	LGT, SGT	16.15	431
Topic 20: Genitourinary System					
PE20.1	Enumerate the etiopathogenesis, clinical features, complications and management of urinary tract infection in children	Y	LGT, SGT	17.2	445
PE20.2	Enumerate the etiopathogenesis, clinical features, complications and management of acute post-streptococcal glomerular nephritis in children	Y	LGT, SGT	17.5	457
PE20.3	Describe the approach and referral criteria to a child with proteinuria	Y	LGT, SGT	17.6 17.7	464, 468
PE20.4	Describe the approach and referral criteria to a child with hematuria	Y	LGT, SGT	17.4, 17.5	453, 457
PE20.5	Enumerate the etiopathogenesis, clinical features, complications and management of acute renal failure in children	Y	LGT, SGT	17.8, 17.9	473, 479
PE20.6	Enumerate the etiopathogenesis, clinical features, complications and management of chronic renal failure in children	Y	LGT, SGT	17.10	481
PE20.7	Enumerate the etiopathogenesis, clinical features, complications and management of Wilms tumor	Y	LGT, SGT	17.11	485
PE20.8	Perform and interpret the common analytes in a urine examination	Y	Bedside clinics, Skills lab	17.1	440
PE20.9	Interpret report of plain X-ray of KUB	Y	Bedside clinics, Skills lab	17.1	440
Topic 21: Approach to and Recognition of a Child with Possible Rheumatologic Problem					
PE21.1	Enumerate the common rheumatological problems in children. Discuss the clinical approach to recognition and referral of a child with rheumatological problem	Y	LGT, SGT	18.1	493
PE21.2	Describe the etiopathogenesis, diagnosis and management of Henoch-schoenlein purpura	N	LGT, SGT	18.4, 18.6	503, 507
PE21.3	Describe the etiopathogenesis, diagnosis and management of Kawasaki disease	N	LGT, SGT	18.4, 18.5	503, 504
PE21.4	Describe the etiopathogenesis, diagnosis and management of SLE	N	LGT, SGT	18.3	500
PE21.5	Describe the etiopathogenesis, diagnosis and management of JIA	N	LGT, SGT	18.2	496
Topic 22: Cardiovascular System—Heart Diseases					
PE22.1	Describe the hemodynamic changes, clinical presentation, complications and management of acyanotic heart disease	Y	LGT, SGT	19.6, 19.7, 19.9, 19.10, 19.11	541, 543, 548, 551, 554
PE22.2	Describe the hemodynamic changes, clinical presentation, complications and management of cyanotic heart diseases	Y	LGT, SGT	19.6, 19.8, 19.12, 19.13	541, 547, 556, 559
PE22.3	Explain the etiopathogenesis, clinical presentation and management of cardiac failure in infant and children	Y	LGT, SGT	19.5	537
PE22.4	Explain the etiopathogenesis, clinical presentation and management of acute rheumatic fever in children	Y	LGT, SGT	19.14	561
PE22.5	Describe the etiopathogenesis, clinical features and management of Infective endocarditis in children	Y	LGT, SGT	19.15	566
PE22.6	Describe the etiopathogenesis, grading, clinical features and management of hypertension in children	Y	LGT, SGT	19.16	568
PE22.7	Record pulse, blood pressure, temperature and respiratory rate and interpret as per the age	Y	Bedside clinics, Skills lab	19.3	522

PE22.8	Perform independently examination of the cardiovascular system—look for precordial bulge, pulsations in the precordium, JVP and its significance in children and infants, relevance of percussion in pediatric examination, auscultation and other system examination and document	Y	Bedside clinics, Skills lab	19.3	522
PE22.9	Interpret a chest X-ray and recognize cardiomegaly	Y	Bedside clinics, Skills lab	19.4	531
PE22.10	Interpret pediatric ECG	Y	Bedside clinics, Skills lab	19.4	531
PE22.11	Demonstrate empathy while dealing with children with cardiac diseases in every patient encounter	Y	SGT	19.17	573
Topic 23: GIT and Hepatobiliary System					
PE 23.1	Define vomiting, discuss causes, evaluation and management of vomiting in children	Y	LGT, SGT	21.1	590
PE23.2	Define constipation discuss causes, evaluation and management of constipation in children	Y	LGT, SGT	21.1	590
PE23.3	Discuss the causes, evaluation and management of abdominal pain in children	Y	LGT, SGT	21.1	590
PE23.4	Define diarrhea (acute diarrhea, chronic diarrhea, persistent diarrhea). Discuss etiology, risk factors, clinical features, complications, investigations and treatment (according to WHO guidelines) of acute gastroenteritis	Y	LGT, SGT	20.1, 20.7, 20.8	575, 586, 588
PE23.5	Discuss the causes, clinical presentation and management of dysentery in children	Y	LGT, SGT	20.5	583
PE23.6	Discuss the physiological basis of ORT, types of ORS and the composition of various types of ORS. Discuss composition of fluids used in management of diarrhea. Discuss the role of antibiotics, antispasmodics, anti-secretory drugs, probiotics, antiemetics in acute diarrheal diseases	Y	LGT, SGT	20.3, 20.4	579, 580
PE23.7	Elicit history pertaining to diarrheal diseases. Assess for signs and symptoms of dehydration, shock, prerenal AKI, electrolyte disturbances, document and present	Y	Bedside clinics, Skills lab	20.2, 20.6	577, 584
PE23.8	Perform and interpret stool examination including hanging drop, interpret RFT and electrolyte report in the context of diarrhea	N	Bedside clinics, Skills	20.6	584
PE23.9	Perform NG tube insertion in a manikin	Y	DOAP	20.3	579
PE23.12	Discuss the etiopathogenesis, clinical presentation and management of malabsorption in children and its causes including celiac disease	N	LGT, SGT	21.3, 21.4, 21.5	607, 608, 610
PE23.13	Discuss the etiopathogenesis, clinical features and management of acute hepatitis in children	Y	LGT, SGT activity	21.6, 21.10	613, 625
PE23.14	Discuss the etiopathogenesis, clinical features and management of fulminant hepatic failure in children	Y	LGT, SGT activity	21.7, 21.10	615, 625
PE23.15	Discuss the etiopathogenesis, clinical features and management of chronic liver diseases in children	Y	LGT, SGT activity	21.8	616
PE23.16	Discuss the etiopathogenesis, clinical features and management of portal hypertension in children	Y	LGT, SGT activity	21.9	621
PE23.17	Elicit document and present the history related to diseases of gastrointestinal system	Y	Bedside clinics, Skills lab	21.1	590
PE23.18	Identify external markers for GI and Liver disorders, e.g., jaundice, pallor, gynecomastia, spider angioma, palmar erythema, Ichthyosis, caput medusa, clubbing, failing to thrive, vitamin A and D deficiency	Y	Bedside clinics, Skills lab	21.2	603

PE23.19	Perform examination of the abdomen, demonstrate organomegaly, ascites, etc.	Y	Bedside clinics, Skills lab	21.2	603
PE23.20	Interpret liver function tests, viral markers, ultrasonogram report	Y	Bedside clinics, Skills lab	21.1	590
PE23.21	Enumerate the indications for upper GI endoscopy	N	SGT	21.9	621
Topic 24: Pediatric Emergencies—Common Pediatric Emergencies					
PE24.1	Describe the etiopathogenesis, clinical approach and management of cardiorespiratory arrest in children	Y	LGT, SGT	27.2	868
PE24.2	Describe the etiopathogenesis and management of respiratory distress in children	Y	LGT, SGT	27.5	879
PE24.3	Describe the etiopathogenesis, clinical approach and management of shock in children	Y	LGT, SGT	27.7	885
PE24.4	Describe the etiopathogenesis, clinical approach and management of status epilepticus	Y	LGT, SGT	27.8	895
PE24.5	Describe the etiopathogenesis, clinical approach and management of an unconscious child	Y	LGT, SGT	27.9	898
PE24.6	Explain oxygen therapy, in pediatric emergencies and modes of administration	Y	LGT, SGT	27.6	882
PE24.7	Observe the various methods of administering oxygen	Y	Demonstration	27.6	882
PE24.8	Assess airway and breathing: recognise signs of severe respiratory distress. Check for cyanosis, severe chest in drawing, grunting	Y	DOAP, Skills lab	27.1, 27.3, 27.8	865, 869, 895
PE24.9	Assess airway and breathing. Demonstrate the method of positioning of an infant and child to open airway in a simulated environment	Y	DOAP, Skills Lab	27.1, 27.3	865, 869
PE24.10	Assess airway and breathing: administer oxygen using correct technique and appropriate flow rate	Y	DOAP, Skills Lab	27.1, 27.4, 27.6	865, 873, 882
PE24.11	Assess airway and breathing perform assisted ventilation by bag and mask in a simulated environment	Y	DOAP, Skills lab	27.1, 27.4	865, 873
PE24.12	Check for signs of shock, i.e., pulse, blood pressure, CRT	Y	DOAP, Skills Lab	27.7	885
PE24.13	Secure an IV access in a simulated environment	Y	DOAP, Skills Lab	27.4, 27.7	873, 885
PE24.14	Choose the type of fluid and calculate the fluid requirement in shock	Y	DOAP, SGT activity	27.4, 27.7	873, 885
PE24.15	Assess level of consciousness and provide emergency treatment to a child with convulsions/coma: - Position an unconscious child - Position a child with suspected trauma Administer IV/per rectal diazepam for a convulsing child in a simulated environment	Y	DOAP, Skills Lab	27.9	898
PE24.16	Assess for signs of severe dehydration	Y	Bedside clinics, Skills lab	27.3, 27.7	869, 885
PE24.17	Monitoring and maintaining temperature: define hypothermia. Describe the clinical features, complications and management of hypothermia	Y	LGT, SGT	27.10	903
PE24.18	Describe the advantages and correct method of keeping an infant warm by skin to skin contact	Y	LGT, SGT	27.10	903
PE24.19	Describe the environmental measures to maintain temperature	Y	LGT, SGT	27.10	903
PE24.20	Assess for hypothermia and maintain temperature	Y	Skills lab	27.10	903
PE24.21	Provide BLS for children in manikin	Y	Skills lab	27.3	869
PE24.22	Counsel parents of dangerously ill/terminally ill child to break the bad news	Y	DOAP	27.17	925
PE24.23	Obtain informed consent	Y	DOAP	27.17	925

Topic 25: Respiratory System					
PE25.1	Describe the etiopathogenesis, clinical features and management of acute otitis media (AOM)	Y	LGT, SGT	22.2	630
PE25.2	Describe the etiopathogenesis, clinical features and management of epiglottitis	Y	LGT, SGT	22.7	645
PE25.3	Explain the etiopathogenesis, clinical features and management of acute laryngotracheobronchitis	Y	LGT, SGT	22.8	647
PE25.4	Describe the etiology, clinical features and management of stridor in children	Y	LGT, SGT	22.6	643
PE25.5	Describe the types, clinical presentation, and management of foreign body aspiration in infants and children	Y	LGT, SGT	22.9	651
PE25.6	Describe the etiopathogenesis, diagnosis, clinical features, management and prevention of lower respiratory infections including bronchiolitis, wheeze associated LRTI pneumonia and empyema	Y	Bedside clinics, SGT, LGT	22.10, 22.11, 22.12, 22.13, 22.14	654, 656, 660, 665, 668
Topic 26: Anemia and Other Hemato-oncologic Disorders in Children					
PE26.1	Explain the etiopathogenesis, clinical features, classification and approach to a child with anemia	Y	LGT, SGT	23.3	690
PE26.2	Describe the etiopathogenesis, clinical features and management of iron deficiency anemia	Y	LGT, SGT	23.4	695
PE26.3	Describe the etiopathogenesis, clinical features and management of Vitamin B12, folate deficiency anemia	Y	LGT, SGT	23.5	699
PE26.4	Explain the etiopathogenesis, clinical features and management of hemolytic anemia, thalassemia major, sickle cell anemia, hereditary spherocytosis, autoimmune hemolytic anaemia and hemolytic uremic syndrome	Y	LGT, SGT	17.9, 23.6, 23.7, 23.8, 23.9, 23.10, 23.11	479, 703, 707, 709, 713, 716, 717
PE26.5	Describe the National Anemia Control Program	Y	LGT, SGT	11.3	197
PE26.6	Describe the cause of thrombocytopenia in children: describe the clinical features and management of idiopathic thrombocytopenic purpura (ITP)	N	LGT, SGT	23.13	721
PE26.7	Explain the etiology, classification, pathogenesis and clinical features of hemophilia in children	N	LGT, SGT	23.12, 23.14	718, 723
PE26.8	Explain the etiology, clinical presentation and management of acute lymphoblastic leukemia in children	N	LGT, SGT	23.15	728
PE26.9	Explain the etiology, clinical presentation and management of lymphoma in children	N	LGT, SGT	23.16	729
PE26.10	Perform examination of the abdomen, demonstrate organomegaly	Y	Bedside clinics, Skills lab	23.2	686
PE26.11	Interpret CBC, LFT	Y	Bedside clinics, Skills lab	23.2	686
PE26.12	Perform and interpret peripheral smear	Y	DOAP	23.2	686
PE26.13	Explain the indications for hemoglobin electrophoresis and interpret report	N	SGT	23.7, 23.8	707, 709
PE26.14	Demonstrate performance of bone marrow aspiration in manikin	Y	Skills lab	23.18	734
PE26.15	Enumerate the referral criteria for hematological conditions	Y	Bedside clinics, SGT	23.17	734
PE26.16	Counsel and educate patients about prevention and treatment of anemia	Y	Bedside clinics, Skills lab	23.19	735
PE26.17	Enumerate the indications for splenectomy and precautions	N	SGT activity	23.9	713

Topic 27: Systemic Pediatrics: Central Nervous System					
PE27.1	Explain the etiopathogenesis, clinical features, complications, management, and prevention of acute bacterial meningitis in children	Y	LGT, SGT	24.3	749
PE27.2	Describe the etiopathogenesis, clinical features, complications, management and prevention of tuberculous meningitis	Y	LGT, SGT	24.4, 24.5	756, 763
PE27.3	Distinguish bacterial, viral and tuberculous meningitis	Y	LGT, SGT	24.2, 24.3, 24.4, 24.5	744, 749, 756, 763
PE27.4	Explain the etiopathogenesis, classification, clinical features, complication and management of hydrocephalus in children	Y	LGT, SGT	24.7	770
PE27.5	Explain the etiopathogenesis, clinical features, and management of Infantile hemiplegia	Y	LGT, SGT	24.8	773
PE27.6	Explain the etiopathogenesis, clinical features, complications and management of febrile seizures in children	Y	LGT, SGT	24.9	778
PE27.7	Define epilepsy. Discuss the pathogenesis, clinical types, presentation and management of Epilepsy in children	Y	LGT, SGT	24.10	781
PE27.8	Define status epilepticus. Discuss the clinical presentation and management	Y	LGT, SGT	27.8	895
PE27.9	Describe the etiopathogenesis, clinical features and management of mental retardation in children	Y	LGT, SGT	3.1	54
PE27.10	Describe the etiopathogenesis, clinical features and management of children with cerebral palsy	Y	LGT, SGT	24.11	786
PE27.11	Enumerate the causes of floppiness in an infant and discuss the clinical features, differential diagnosis and management	Y	LGT, SGT	24.12, 24.13	791, 794
PE27.12	Explain the etiopathogenesis, clinical features and management of Duchene muscular dystrophy	Y	LGT, SGT	24.14, 24.15	802, 806
PE27.13	Interpret and explain the findings in a CSF analysis	Y	SGT	24.2	744
PE27.14	Perform in a mannequin lumbar puncture. Discuss the indications, contraindication of the procedure	Y	Bedside clinics, Skills lab	24.2	744
Topic 28: Allergic Rhinitis, Atopic Dermatitis, Bronchial Asthma					
PE28.1	Describe the etiopathogenesis, clinical signs, management and prevention of allergic rhinitis in children	Y	LGT, SGT	22.5	638
PE28.2	Explain the etiopathogenesis, clinical types, presentations, management and prevention of childhood asthma	Y		22.15	670
PE28.3	Develop a treatment plan for asthma appropriate to clinical presentation and severity	Y		22.15	670
PE28.4	Enumerate the indications for PFT	N		22.15	670
PE28.5	Observe administration of nebulization	Y		22.15	670
Topic 29: Chromosomal Abnormalities					
PE29.1	Describe the genetic basis, risk factors, clinical features, complications, prenatal diagnosis, management and genetic counselling in Down syndrome.	Y		25.3, 25.4, 25.5, 25.6	824, 831, 834, 835
PE29.2	Interpret normal karyotype and recognize Trisomy 21	Y	Bedside clinics, Skills lab	25.1, 25.2	811, 815
PE29.3	Counsel parents regarding (1) Present child, (2) Risk in the next pregnancy	N	Bedside clinics, Skills lab	25.3, 25.6, 25.7	824, 835, 839
PE29.4	Describe the genetic basis, risk factors, clinical features, complications, prenatal diagnosis, management and genetic counselling in Turner's syndrome	N	LGT, SGT	25.3, 25.4, 25.5, 25.6	824, 831, 834, 835

PE29.5	Describe the genetic basis, risk factors, clinical features, complications, prenatal diagnosis, management and genetic counselling in Klinefelter syndrome	Y	LGT, SGT	25.3, 25.4, 25.5, 25.6	824, 831, 834, 835
Topic 30: Endocrinology					
PE30.1	Describe the etiology (congenital and acquired), clinical features, management of hypothyroidism in children	Y	LGT, SGT	26.3, 26.4, 26.5	844, 845, 847
PE30.2	Interpret and explain neonatal thyroid screening report	Y	Bedside clinics, SGT	26.4	845
PE30.3	Describe the etiology, clinical types, clinical features, diagnostic criteria, complications and management of diabetes mellitus in children	Y	LGT, SGTs	26.6	849
PE30.4	Recognize clinical features DKA, perform and interpret urine dipstick for sugar and ketone bodies and refer	Y	DOAP	26.7, 26.8	854, 856
PE30.5	Perform genital examination and recognize ambiguous genitalia, counsel and refer	Y	Bedside clinic, Skills lab	26.9	856
PE30.6	Define precocious and delayed puberty, perform sexual maturity rating (SMR), recognize precocious and delayed puberty and refer	Y	LGT, SGT	26.10, 26.11, 26.12, 26.13	858, 858, 861, 862
PE30.7	Identify deviations in growth and plan appropriate referral	Y	Bedside clinics, Skills lab	26.2	842
Topic 31: Vaccine Preventable Diseases: Tuberculosis					
PE31.1	Describe the epidemiology, clinical features, clinical types, complications of tuberculosis in children and adolescents	Y	LGT, SGT	14.3	270
PE31.2	Describe the various diagnostic tools for childhood tuberculosis	Y	LGT, SGT	14.3	270
PE31.3	Describe the various regimens for management of tuberculosis as per national guidelines	Y	LGT, SGT	14.3	270
PE31.4	Describe the preventive strategies adopted and the objectives and outcomes of the National Tuberculosis Control Program	Y	LGT, SGT	14.3	270
PE31.5	Elicit, document and present history of contact with tuberculosis in every patient encounter, identify BCG scar and interpret a Mantoux test	Y	Bedside clinics, Skill lab	14.3	270
PE31.6	Interpret blood tests in the context of laboratory evidence for tuberculosis	N	Bedside clinics, SGT	14.3	270
PE31.7	Describe the various samples for demonstrating the organism, e.g., gastric aspirate, sputum, CSF, FNAC	Y	Bedside clinics, SGT	14.3	270
PE31.8	Enumerate the indications, discuss the limitations of methods of culturing *M. tuberculosis* and the newer diagnostic tools for tuberculosis including BACTEC CBNAAT and their indications	Y	SGT	14.3	270
PE31.9	Enumerate the common causes of fever and describe the etiopathogenesis, clinical features, complications and management of fever in children	Y	LGT, SGT	14.1, 14.2	262, 267
PE31.10	Enumerate the common causes of fever and describe the etiopathogenesis, clinical features, complications and management of child with exanthematous illnesses like measles, mumps, rubella and chicken pox	Y	LGT, SGT	14.4, 14.5, 14.6, 14.7	279, 282, 285, 287
PE31.11	Enumerate the common causes of fever and discuss the etiopathogenesis, clinical features, complications and management of child with diphtheria, pertussis, tetanus	Y	LGT, SGT	14.8, 14.9, 14.10	290, 293, 296
PE31.12	Enumerate the common causes of fever and discuss the etiopathogenesis, clinical features, complications and management of child with typhoid	Y	LGT, SGT	14.11	299

PE31.13	Enumerate the common causes of fever and discuss the etiopathogenesis, clinical features, complications and management of child with dengue, chikungunya and other vector-borne diseases	Y	LGT, SGT	14.12, 14.13	303, 313
PE31.14	Enumerate the common causes of fever and discuss the etiopathogenesis, clinical features, complications and management of children with common parasitic infections, malaria, leishmaniasis, filariasis, helminthic infestations, amebiasis, giardiasis	Y	LGT, SGT	14.14, 14.15, 14.16, 14.17, 14.18, 14.19, 14.20, 14.21, 14.22, 14.23, 14.24	314, 324, 327, 333, 335, 337, 337, 339, 340, 341, 342, 343, 344
Topic 32: The Role of the Physician in the Community					
PE32.1	Identify, describe and defend medicolegal, sociocultural and ethical issues as they pertain to health care in children (including parental rights and right to refuse treatment)	Y	SGT	28.8	956

1 CHAPTER

Normal Growth and Development

AS PER NMC COMPETENCIES

PE 1.1	Define the terminologies growth and development. Discuss the factors affecting normal growth and development.	*Ch 1.1, Ch 1.2, Ch 1.3*
PE 1.2	Discuss and describe the methods of assessment of growth including use of WHO and Indian national standards. Enumerate the parameters used for assessment of physical growth in infants, children and adolescents and perform anthropometric measurements, document in growth charts and interpret.	*Ch 1.4, Ch 1.5, Ch 1.6, Ch 1.7*
PE 1.3	Define development and discuss the normal developmental milestones with respect to motor, behavior, social, adaptive and language. Discuss the factors affecting development and methods of assessment of development.	*Ch 1.8, Ch 1.9*

1.1 Definitions *PE 1.1*

GROWTH

Growth is defined as an increase in body size in terms of weight, height, and other measurable domains. It is also defined as a measurable change in physical size of body and its parts. It is used to designate all the quantitative changes brought about in structure and function of human anatomy and physiology. Growth reflects an increase in body dimensions and a resultant change in mass of body tissue like fat, muscle, and bone. Examples of growth include change in weight, height, bone density, and dental structure.

During the growth of a child, there is increase in both cell numbers (hyperplasia) and cell size (hypertrophy). The growth is not a steady process; the rate of growth varies with periods of rapid growth and slow growth. For instance, infancy and adolescence are characterized by periods of rapid growth.

DEVELOPMENT

Development is defined as a progressive series of orderly coherent changes that occur as a result of maturity and experience. It may also be defined as behavioral changes in skills and functional abilities. Development refers to gaining of skills in all aspects of child's life like physical development, social and emotional development, intellectual development, communication, and speech development. Hence, the development is not easily measurable. The terms "maturation" and "learning" are often used along with development.

- ***Maturation*** refers to process of become fully developed in terms of physiological and behavioral aspects toward attainment of his or her best physical, emotional, intellectual, and social potential.
- ***Learning*** refers to assimilation of information once the child is mature for a particular learning experience resulting in behavioral change.

The terms "growth" and "development" are conceptually different, and denote two altogether different aspects of the change, i.e., growth is quantitative while development is qualitative. However, both are interdependent. For instance, to learn to open a door, the child must be able to reach the doorknob (physical growth) and also must have a sufficient learning as to how to open the doorknob (development).

CONCEPT OF EARLY CHILDHOOD DEVELOPMENT

Contrary to the traditional definitions as discussed above, it is now being recognized that the terms "Growth" and "Development" are inseparable and cannot be seen in isolation from each other. Realizing that the ultimate functional potential of humans is primarily dependent on brain growth that occurs in the first 2–3 years of life, the emphasis has shifted to growth and development in early childhood period.

Definition: Early childhood development (ECD) is a generic term that refers to a child's cognitive, social, emotional, langu-

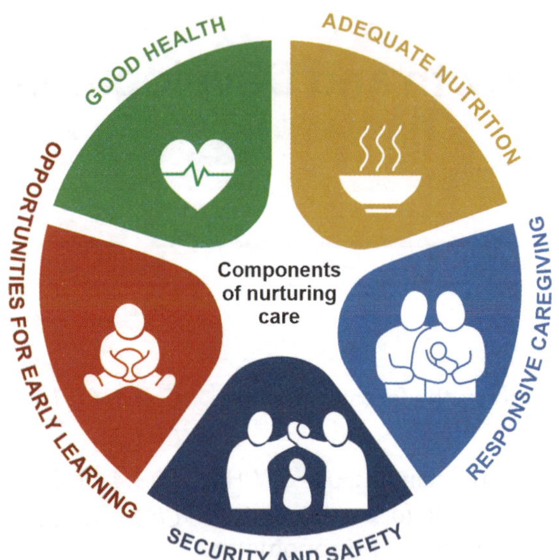

Fig. 1.1: Components of nurturing care for early childhood development

Source: World Health Organization, United Nations Children's Fund, World Bank Group. Nurturing care for early childhood development: a framework for helping children survive and thrive to transform health and human potential. Geneva: World Health Organization; 2018

age, and physical development. Implying that it includes both growth and development as per definitions given above. The early childhood starts from the time of conception and may span up to first 8 years of life.

Early childhood development is a relatively new term that represents the thrive agenda of the global strategy for women, children, and adolescent health and is also included in WHO agenda for action. Lancet, in 2017, reported that 250 million under-5 children (43%) are not able to achieve their optimal development potential. In India, 45% children under 5 years (70 million) are at risk.

Nurturing Care for Early Childhood Development (NC-ECD)

Nurturing care is the key to children in their formative years, i.e., between 0 and 3 years (because maximum brain growth occurs in this period) to achieve optimal development. The domains of nurturing care include: (1) good health, (2) appropriate nutrition, (3) ensuring safety and security, (4) promotion of responsive parenting, and (5) facilitating early learning opportunities (**Fig. 1.1**).

WHY STUDY GROWTH AND DEVELOPMENT?

It is important to study growth and development because of the following reasons:

- ***To know what is expected*** of a child at a given age, in terms of physical and mental ability, especially in high-risk babies.
- ***To identify children who may not look apparently*** sick but are having a disease process that is affecting growth. For example, a child with celiac disease may remain asymptomatic except for faltering of linear growth. This initial clue for diagnosis can prevent the long-term physical and emotional consequences of the disease (both for the child and the family). Growth charting also helps to monitor the effect of treatment/intervention modalities on the pattern of growth.
- ***Early identification of handicaps:*** Developmental assessment helps in early diagnosis of global developmental delay, intellectual disability, cerebral palsy, hearing and visual handicaps, neurological and metabolic disorders, disorders of muscle tone, and physical handicaps.
- ***To assess the general health and nutrition status of the community:*** Prevalence of wasting, underweight, and stunting in under-5 children serve as indirect indicators of health and nutritional status of the entire community, and may provide a launching pad for advocacy, and planning the most appropriate intervention.
- ***Evaluation of social action:*** Effectiveness of medical or social actions for promoting health of the community can be evaluated by comparing the growth data before and after the intervention, such as midday meal or preschool children feeding programs.
- ***To assess suitability of a baby for adoption:*** Parents may approach pediatrician before adopting a child to assess whether the child has a normal growth and to exclude developmental disabilities.

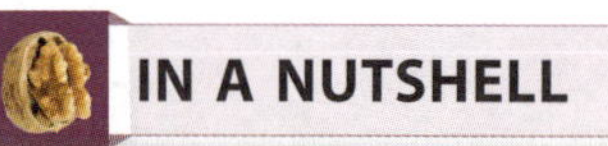

IN A NUTSHELL

Definitions

1. ***Growth:*** *Quantitative increase* in structure of body (e.g., gain in weight or height).
2. ***Development:*** *Qualitative changes* in body function leading to acquisition of skills in all aspects of child's life such as physical development, social and emotional development, intellectual development, communication, and speech development.
3. ***Early childhood development:*** A holistic term that encompasses both growth and development. Starts from conception, continuing till 8 years of age. Of these, the antenatal period and up to 3 years are the most crucial as 90% of neuronal connections are formed in this period.
4. ***Nurturing care:*** Caregivers need to provide nurturing care to their children to achieve ECD. Nurturing care has five components: good health, adequate nutrition, safety and security, responsive parenting, and early learning opportunities.

Countdown to 2030. (2021). Women, Children and Adolescents health. India Country Profile. [online] Available from www.nurturing-care.org. [Last accessed August, 2025].

Gupta P. President's Page. IAP Commitment to Nurturing Care for Early Childhood Development. Indian Pediatr. 2021;58(Suppl 1):S3.

Mukherjee SB, Agrawal D, Mishra D, Shastri D, Dalwai SH, Chattopadhyay N, et al. Indian Academy of Pediatrics Position Paper on Nurturing Care for Early Childhood Development. Indian Pediatr. 2021;58(10):962-9.

World Health Organization. Operationalizing Nurturing Care for Early Childhood Development. Geneva: WHO; 2019.

1.2 Factors Affecting Growth and Development

PE 1.1

INTRODUCTION

- Growth at birth is dependent on *intrauterine factors* that include various maternal, fetal, and placental factors.
- Postnatal growth is controlled by various genetic, environmental, and endocrine factors. These are broadly classified as *intrinsic factors* (genetic and endocrinal factors) and *extrinsic factors* (nutritional, sociocultural, psychological, and environmental factors).
- Poverty, broken homes, nutritional insults, and parental education mainly affect ECD. Imbalance between protective factors and triggers affects brain growth, physical health, and psychological development.

Box 1.1 summarizes the factors affecting growth and development.

FACTORS AFFECTING FETAL GROWTH

Maternal malnutrition: Undernutrition of the mother is identified with intrauterine growth retardation and consequently small size of the fetus. Fetal nutrition involves three stages: (1) intake of food by the pregnant woman, (2) placental transfer to fetus, (3) and utilization and metabolism of nutrients by the fetus. The fetal nutrition is affected when any of the maternal, placental, or fetal factors are affected. Adequacy of maternal nutrition is predicted by gestational weight gain and her past nutritional intake (reflected by her weight, height, body mass index, and hemoglobin).

Substance abuse: Maternal smoking, alcohol, and tobacco consumption leads to direct neurotoxic effect as well as resultant decreased placental blood flow which can adversely affect the fetal growth.

Box 1.1 Factors Affecting Growth

A. ***Factors predicting fetal growth:***
- *Demographic factors:* Ethnicity/race, infant sex, parity, maternal age, socioeconomic status, and history of prior low birthweight
- *Nutritional factors:* Prepregnancy maternal weight, maternal gestational weight gain, maternal height, and maternal caloric intake
- *Substance abuse:* Maternal alcohol/tobacco consumption
- Maternal infections (toxoplasmosis, rubella, and syphilis)
- Maternal medications (thalidomide, ethanol, and antiepileptic medications)
- Maternal illness (preeclampsia, anemia, and malnutrition)

B. ***Factors affecting postnatal growth:***
- *Genetic factors:* Race, heredity, sex, and genetic disorders
- *Hormonal factors:* Growth hormone, thyroid and gonadal hormones
- *Nutritional factors:* Malnutrition
- *Sociocultural factors:* Socioeconomic status, cultural beliefs, and family size and structure
- *Environmental factors:* Secular trends, geographic factors, physical environment, access to health care
- *Health factors:* Chronic ailments
- Psychological factors

Teratogens: Maternal infections (e.g., toxoplasmosis, rubella, and syphilis), maternal medications (e.g., antiepileptic drugs, thalidomide, and ethanol) and maternal radiation exposure can adversely affect the fetal growth especially in early gestation which is the period of maximum growth and differentiation.

Maternal illness and obstetric disorders (preeclampsia, anemia, malnutrition, and heart disease): These could adversely affect the fetal growth leading to intrauterine growth retardation.

FACTORS AFFECTING POSTNATAL GROWTH

Genetic Factors

- ***Race:*** Genetic influences are responsible for marked variation in body size and structure among different races across the globe. Americans and Europeans are taller while Japanese and Chinese are shorter.
- ***Heredity:*** Genetic makeup of an individual is primarily determined by what has been inherited from previous generation. Final height of a child is influenced by paternal and maternal height. Daughters often reach menarche at a similar age as their mother.
- ***Sex:*** On an average, girls are lighter and shorter than boys. Boys tend to be ahead of girls in terms of weight and height till puberty. Girls achieve puberty earlier than boys hence in 12–14 years age group girls may become taller than boys. Shoulders are wider in boys while hips are broader in girls.
- ***Genetic disorders:*** Defect in chromosomes (e.g., Down syndrome), single gene, a group of gene or a defect in product of a gene can result in short stature (e.g., Turner syndrome) or failure to thrive (inborn errors of metabolism).

Hormonal Factors

Prenatal growth is primarily influenced by insulin and insulin-like growth factors (IGF); while growth hormone and thyroxine are the most important hormones responsible for postnatal growth.

- ***Growth hormone:*** It is secreted by anterior pituitary and induces production of IGF-1 in the liver and skeletal tissues. IGF-1 acts as the final mediator of growth. Thyroxine and cortisol may also influence the IGF plasma levels. The GH–IGF axis is also influenced by nutritional, systemic, and endocrine disorders.
- ***Thyroid hormones:*** These are crucial for epiphyseal development and growth.
- ***Gonadal hormones:*** They play an important role in inducing pubertal growth spurt. Gonadal steroids are responsible for pubertal growth, calcium accretion, and skeletal growth. Estrogens are responsible for epiphyseal closure in both boys and girls.

Nutritional Factors

Nutrition is the most important environmental factor influencing growth. Any imbalance in diet might result in either undernutrition or obesity.

- ***Undernutrition:*** Appropriate macronutrient (calorie, protein, fat, etc.) and micronutrient (vitamins and minerals) intake is essential for adequate growth. Indian Council of Medical Research (ICMR) has outlined estimated average requirement (EAR) of all nutrients for sustenance and maintenance of growth. Undernourished children lag in attainment of age-appropriate weight, height, head circumference, and intellectual scoring.
- ***Obesity:*** Introduction of JUNCS (Junk food high in fat, salt, sugar; Ultraprocessed, nutritionally inappropriate, colored/caffeinated/carbonated foods, and sugar sweetened beverages), lack of physical activity, excessive and inappropriate dietary choices, and food fads could lead to inappropriately high body weight.

Sociocultural Factors

- ***Socioeconomic status:*** Children belonging to high socioeconomic status tend to be taller and heavier. Adolescents belonging to families of higher socioeconomic status are predisposed to developing obesity.
- ***Cultural beliefs:*** Culture influences every aspect of child rearing, nutrition, hygiene, health, and development. The culture, in turn, is influenced by ethnicity, religion, lifestyle, social class, and geographic location.
- ***Family size and structure:*** Number of children in a family and birth order might impact the food distribution in underprivileged households. Poverty, broken homes, nutritional insults, parental education, separated or divorced parents, family quarrels/conflicts, unemployment, and moving homes might deprive the emotional component to child's growth and development.

Environmental Factors

- ***Secular trends:*** India is following a secular trend of growth and puberty with subsequent generations having better height and early puberty, due to increasing industrialization and changing lifestyle.
- ***Geographic factors:*** Growth patterns differ between countries and climates. Iodine deficiency disorder, a widespread nutritional deficiency prevalent in children from mountainous Himalayan regions, may predispose to growth retardation.
- ***Environmental factors:*** Both indoor and outdoor air pollutants such as smoke, carbon monoxide, sulfur dioxide, and chlorofluorocarbons (CFCs) might influence the respiratory system and hence indirectly influence the growth and well-being. Similarly, sanitation, sewage treatment, waste disposal, and provision of safe water have impact on health.
- ***Access to healthcare:*** Ease of access to healthcare along with appropriate healthcare seeking behavior including well child visits during early childhood influence the growth in a positive direction.

Health Factors

Chronic ailments like congenital malformations and chronic infections; progressive renal, cardiac, gastrointestinal, and neurological illness; or malignancy could adversely affect the growth of child either directly or indirectly by interfering with the child's nutritional intake and metabolism.

Psychological Factors

Health and growth can be affected by the way the individuals feel about themselves (self-esteem and self-image). Stress may lead to decline of growth hormone levels leading to psychosocial dwarfism.

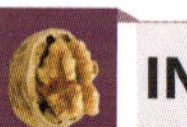

IN A NUTSHELL

Factors Affecting Growth and Development

1. Growth at birth is mainly dependent on intrauterine factors.
2. Postnatal growth is influenced by both genetic and environmental factors.
3. Maternal malnutrition, illness, and teratogens are the main factors controlling size at birth.
4. Race, heredity, and genetic disorders determine the basic framework of growth.
5. Prenatal growth is primarily influenced by IGF-1, while thyroid and gonadal hormones are important for postnatal growth.
6. Nutrition is the most important limiting or facilitating factor for postnatal growth.
7. Early childhood development is hampered by poverty, broken, parental illiteracy, and nutritional insults.

Ahmed SF, Phillip M, Grimberg A. The physiology and mechanism of growth. World Rev Nutr Diet. 2016;114:1-20.

Cavallera V, Tomlinson M, Radner J, Coetzee B, Daelmans B, Hughes R, et al. Scaling early child development: what are the barriers and enablers? Arch Dis Child. 2019;104(Suppl 1):S43-S50.

Hellström A, Ley D, Hansen-Pupp I, Hallberg B, Ramenghi LA, Löfqvist C, et al. Role of insulin like growth factor 1 in fetal development and in the early postnatal life of premature infants. Am J Perinatol. 2016;33(11):1067-71.

Prentice AM. Environmental and physiological barriers to child growth and development. Nestle Nutr Inst Workshop Ser. 2020;93:125-32.

1.3 Principles and Phases of Growth

PE 1.1

PRINCIPLES OF GROWTH

- Growth and development are orderly and predictable. Every child goes through the same process. The growth is considered *sequential* with one stage leading to next stage.
- Growth progresses in a *cephalocaudal* and *proximodistal* manner. The process starts from the head to toe. Axial functions develop before functions of extremities. For *example*: Arm growth occurs before the finger growth.
- Growth is considered cyclic in the sense that the rate of *growth is not constant*. From birth to 2 years, there is a period of rapid growth. This is followed by a period of slow growth till puberty (10–12 years). This phase is followed by a phase of rapid growth again till 15–16 years of age. Periods of rapid growth are called *critical periods* and are most vulnerable to an external insult.
- ***Rate of growth is not similar for all children.*** Growth shows wide individual variation and is unique for every child. All children do not grow at same pace. Some children at the age of 1 year weigh 11 kg and a few might weigh 9 kg. Similarly, children reach puberty at different ages.
- ***Different tissues of body grow at different rates.*** Somatic growth follows a sigmoid curve with periods of rapid growth during infancy and puberty. The postnatal brain growth primarily occurs in the first year of life so that at 1 year infant has 90% adult brain size. In contrast to brain growth, *lymphoid growth* starts after 5 years of age. It peaks during 6–9 years of age and declines steadily, thereafter. *Gonadal development* resulting an increase in the size and function of reproductive organs starts after the onset of puberty (10–14 years) **(Fig. 1.2)**.
- Growth is measurable both in terms of distance and velocity.
  - ***Linear (distance) growth*** refers to overall growth at one point of time. Linear growth of a child can be compared to growth standards, and it can be interpreted whether the growth at the time of examination is within the normal range or not. But linear growth does not predict the growth pattern in the recent past.
  - ***Growth velocity or rate of growth*** is used to determine the growth pattern in recent past and it refers to increment of growth in a unit of time. Growth velocity can predict the ultimate growth potential and helps in early assessment of factors leading to growth retardation.

PHASES OF GROWTH

It is amazing to realize the transformation of a fertilized egg to develop into an embryo and then into fetus and finally a complete human being. These phases of the growth can be classified into embryonic growth, fetal growth, somatic growth in infancy, preschool years, middle childhood, and adolescent **(Table 1.1)**. A few authors have classified the phases of growth into two broad categories: Prenatal growth (before the birth) and postnatal growth (after birth).

1. ***The prenatal period is characterized by three phases:*** Fertilized ovum or zygote (first 2 weeks), embryo (2–8 weeks), and fetus (9 weeks to birth).
2. ***Postnatal growth also has three phases:*** Infancy, childhood, and adolescence.

Age of viability refers to the earliest age at which a fetus could survive, if they were born at that time, generally accepted as 23 weeks, or fetal weight of >400 g.

Conceptus is reserved for growing embryo or fetus and placental structure, throughout the pregnancy.

Puberty refers to that period of life when the ability to reproduce sexually begins. It is characterized by maturation of the genital organs, development of the secondary sex characteristics, and the onset of menstruation (menarche) in girls.

Prenatal Growth

Embryonic Period (0–8 Weeks)

Egg is fertilized by sperm to form a fertilized egg which gets transformed into a blastocyst and gets implanted in uterus with establishment of uteroplacental blood flow by 2 weeks of gestation. By 3 weeks of gestation, all the three germ layers are formed—endoderm, ectoderm, and mesoderm along with formation of primitive neural tube and blood vessels. By the end of embryonic period, rudiments of all major organs are formed. Times of intense development and rapid cell divisions are called critical period with development of each organ and tissue being

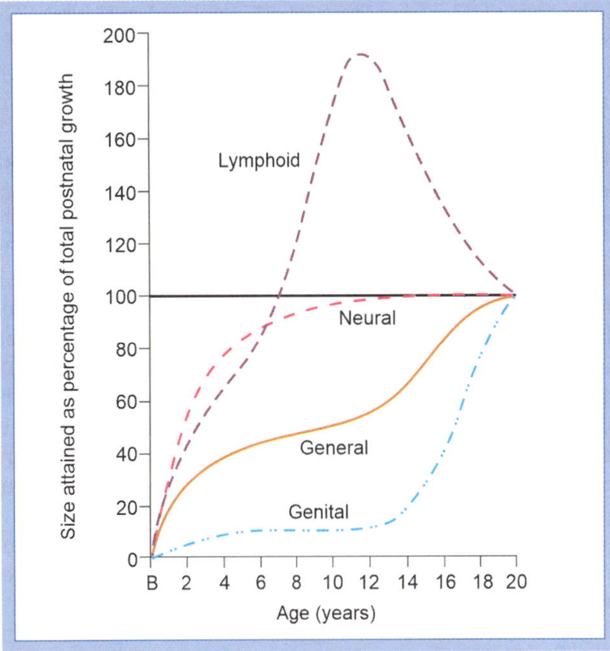

Fig. 1.2: Scammon's curves of systemic growth. Figure depicts the differential growth of body, brain, lymphoid organs, and genital organs, as the child passes through different phases of growth

Table 1.1 Phases of Growth	
Embryo	0–8 weeks
Fetus	9 weeks–birth
Early neonatal period	0–7 days
Late neonatal period	7–28 days
Infancy	Birth–1 year
Toddler	1–2 years
Preschool	2–5 years
Middle childhood	5–11 years
Adolescent	11–19 years

most vulnerable to adverse influences during these periods. For example, critical period for neural tube development is 17-30 days; folate deficiency during this period could predispose to a neural tube defect.

Fetal Growth (9 Weeks to Birth)

During the fetal period starting from 9th week, there is consistent increase in cell number and cell size and differentiation of cells into tissues, organs, and systems. There is a rapid increase in fetal weight, length, and head circumference in the last half of gestation. Intrauterine fetal growth can be assessed by ultrasonography in terms of fetal weight, femur length, and biparietal diameter.

In human fetus in the early half of pregnancy, only 10-12% of body weight gain occurs. Early pregnancy is characterized by tissue differentiation, organ formation, and further development of fetal structures. However, there is a steady increase in weight at the rate of 15 g/day from 24-37 weeks of gestation. The weight gain declines in the last 2-3 weeks to 6 g/day. When the pregnancy proceeds beyond 42 weeks of gestation, the weight starts to decline. Similar reduction occurs in growth velocity for length, chest circumference, and head circumference after 37 weeks of gestation. The intrauterine growth curve for fetal body weight is S shaped or sigmoid in shape (*See* **Annexures** for fetal growth curves).

Fetal length (crown heel length) reaches to half of term length by 20 weeks of gestation. Rate of growth in fetal length reaches a peak of 1 cm/4 weeks by 20 weeks of gestation, and then it decreases. The growth curves for head and chest circumference resemble the fetal weight growth curve, but after 35 weeks of gestation, chest circumference appears to grow more rapidly reducing the difference between chest and head circumference. The normative curves for intrauterine growth have been constructed and any deviation or reduction in expected fetal growth pattern can result in intrauterine growth retardation (IUGR). These normative curves vary with ethnicity, socioeconomic status, parity, and multiple pregnancies. Hence, a caution needs to be exercised before labeling a fetus to be having IUGR.

Fetal Proportions

The embryo has gross anatomical features of human form. There is differential growth of body segments including the head, trunk, and lower extremity. At 2 months of gestation, the fetus has enormous head in proportion to body. By mid-gestation, growth of trunk and extremities occurs but still head looks proportionally larger. This differential growth continues in the postnatal period **(Fig. 1.3)**.

Fetal Differentiation

Early weeks of pregnancy are characterized by differentiation and development of neurons and glial cells with neuronal migration. Major part of "brain growth spurt" is characterized by rapid multiplication of glial cells in early stages, followed by myelination of nerve fibers, extending from mid-gestation to 18 months of age. Normal pattern of fetal growth is determined by genetic potential, maternal nutrition, ability of placenta to transfer the nutrients, intrauterine hormones, and growth factors.

Fetal Growth Factors

Fetal growth in contrast to postnatal growth is not governed by growth hormones although the growth hormone levels in fetus are high. Hormones such as insulin, insulin-like growth factor (IGF), and thyroid hormones have an important role in late gestation for tissue differentiation and growth. Their growth promoting effect is primarily attributed to their anabolic effect on fetal metabolism. Glucocorticoids play an important role near term gestation for initiation and control of maturational events that occur in organs such as lung, liver, and gut.

POSTNATAL GROWTH

Normal growth pattern in children is shown in **Figure 1.4**.

Infancy (birth to 1 year): Infancy comprises of first year of life with maximum rate of growth. Physical, cognitive, and emotional development occurs in the first year of life. There is a rapid growth in most of the body systems and development of neuromuscular system.

Childhood (1-11 years): It consists of three broad groups: Toddler (1-2 years), Preschool (2-5 years), and school-going age group (5-11 years). This period is marked by steady progress in growth and maturation with a rapid progress in motor development. The phase of rapid growth in infancy is followed by slower growth rate after 1 year of age. Child attains to twice his birth length at the end of 2 years. Toddlers have relatively short leg, long torso, and exaggerated lumbar lordosis resulting in a protuberant abdomen. Growth at this stage depends on growth hormone and thyroid hormone. The deficiencies of growth hormone or thyroid hormone will typically present during this period with short stature.

Adolescence: The period of adolescence extends from the age of 11-19 years. It is marked by hormonal influences leading to attainment of sexual maturity and adolescent growth spurt. This growth spurt differs by gender, with girls attaining it around 2 years prior to boys. Average age of adolescent growth spurt is 12-15 years in boys. This period is marked by alteration in relative proportion of muscle, fat, and bone resulting in change in body size and shape.

There is marked evolution of reproductive organs during adolescence. Sexual maturity is characterized by development

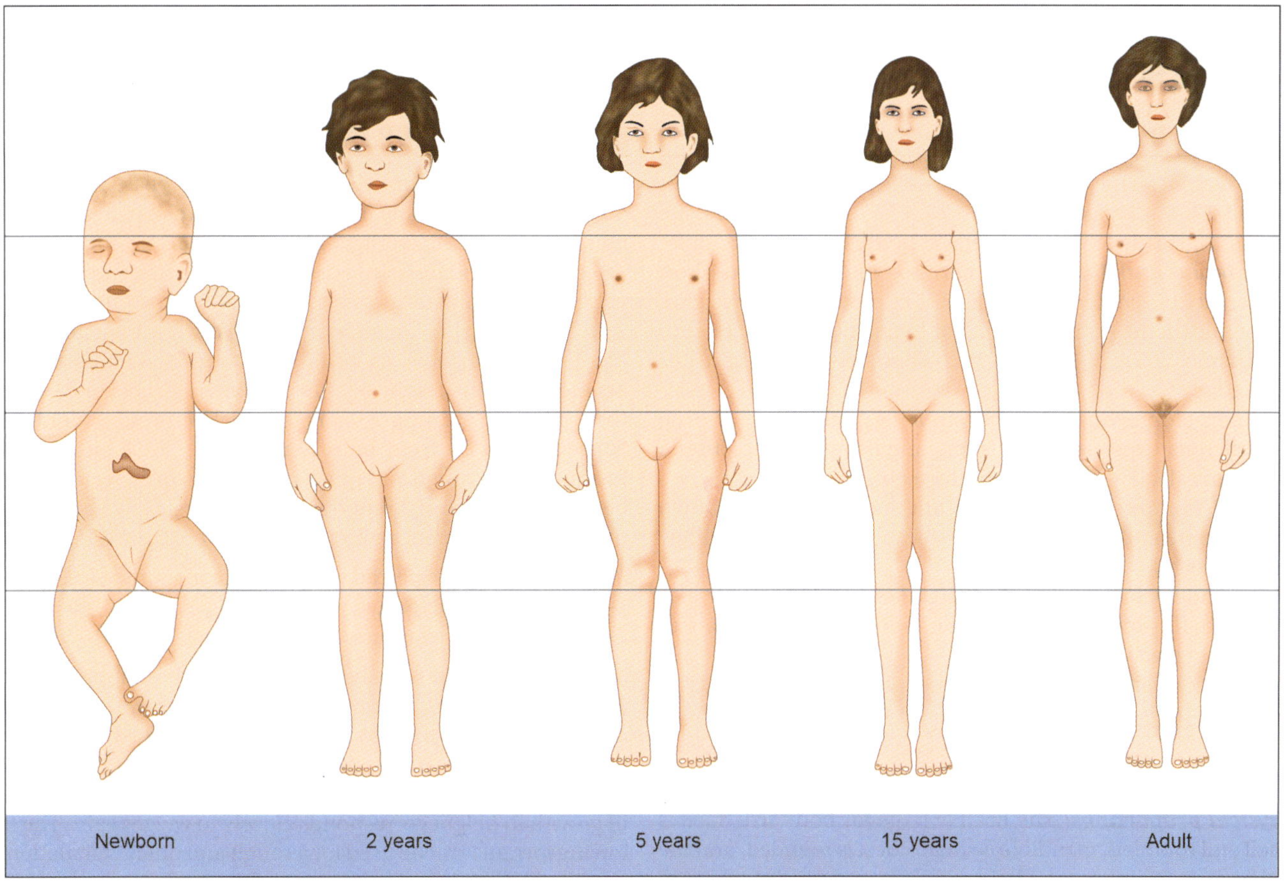

Fig. 1.3: Body proportions as the child grows through different phases of growth

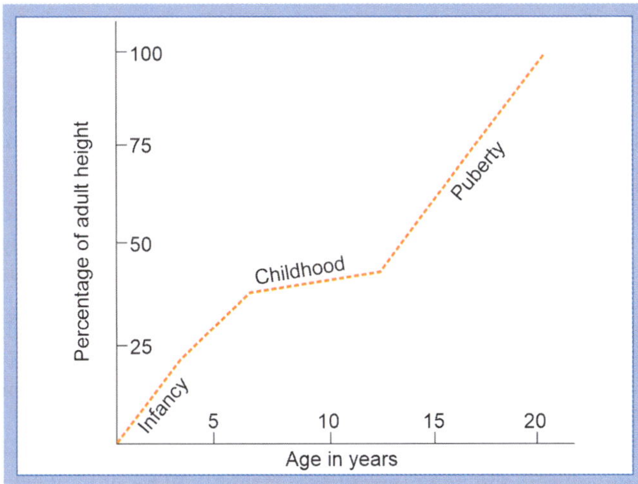

Fig. 1.4: Normal growth pattern in children

of primary followed by secondary sexual characteristics. By the end of adolescence, boys acquire broader shoulder with deepening of voice, whereas girls acquire a broader pelvis and fat accumulation in buttock and breast region. During puberty, the child achieves almost 40% of peak bone mass. The average gain in height during adolescent period in boys is around 20–35 cm and in girls is around 15–25 cm.

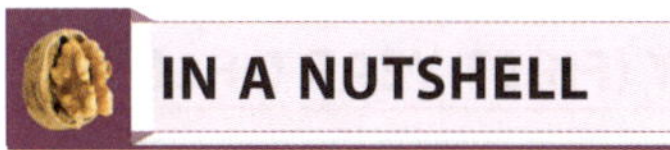

IN A NUTSHELL

Principles and Phases of Growth

1. Different tissues of the body grow at different rates. Maximum brain growth occurs in the first year of life.
2. Growth is described in two categories: Prenatal and postnatal.
3. Prenatal growth is characterized by three phases (ovum, embryo, and fetus 9 weeks to birth).
4. Postnatal growth is characterized by three phases (infancy 0–1 year, childhood 1–11 years, adolescence 11–19 years).

Bernstein RM, O'Connor GK, Vance EA, Affara N, Drammeh S, Dunger DB, et al. Timing of the infancy-childhood growth transition in rural Gambia. Front Endocrinol (Lausanne). 2020;11:142.

Giglione E, Lapolla R, Cianfarani S, Faienza MF, Fintini D, Weber G, et al. Linear growth and puberty in childhood obesity: what is new? Minerva Pediatr (Torino). 2021;73(6):563-71.

Hansen-Pupp I, Löfqvist C, Polberger S, Niklasson A, Fellman V, Hellström A, et al. Influence of insulin-like growth factor I and nutrition during phases of postnatal growth in very preterm infants. Pediatr Res. 2011;69(5 Pt 1):448-53.

Rossavik IK, Brandenburg MA, Venkataraman PS. Understanding the different phases of fetal growth. Horm Res. 1992;38(5-6):203-7.

1.4 Normal Growth

PE 1.2

SIZE AT BIRTH

Birth weight: The average birthweight of Indian infants is around 2.8–2.9 kg as compared to 3.4 kg in White Caucasian infants. The birthweight is influenced by the following factors:

- ***Maternal nutrition:*** Infants born to mothers who are short (height <145 cm), underweight (<45 kg prepregnancy weight), anemic (hemoglobin <8 g/dL), or hypoalbuminemic (serum albumin <2.5 g/dL) are likely to be born low birthweight, i.e., <2.5 kg.
- Maternal infection, cigarette smoking, alcoholism or drug addiction, exposure to radiation, and living at high altitude also may lead to decreased birthweight.
- ***Fetal factors:*** Chromosomal anomalies, such as Down syndrome and gonadal dysgenesis, are associated with low birthweight.
- Singleton babies are heavier than infants of multiple births.
- Maternal toxemia, hypertension, and cardiac disease can result in low birthweight.
- Infants of diabetic mothers are generally heavier than average.

Length of a normal full-term male infant is around 50 cm.

Head circumference at birth is 35–37 cm.

Physical proportions: The head is large for body size, face is small and rounded, mandible is small, chest is rounded, and the abdomen is protuberant. Limbs are short and ratio of upper to lower segment is high (1.7:1).

GROWTH IN INFANCY (FIRST YEAR OF LIFE)

Weight: A term child loses 10% of his weight during first 3 days of life because of excretion of excess extravascular fluid and possibly poor intake. The birthweight is regained by 10 days of life. Subsequently, the weight gain occurs at a rate of 25–30 g/day for the first 3 months of life. Thereafter, about 400 g of weight gain occurs every month, for the remaining part of the first year. The consistent gain of weight during infancy provides a useful guide to nutritional status and health of the infant; it is not as sensitive a guide in the older child. Usually, the infant doubles his birthweight by 5 months and triples the birthweight by 1 year of age. The weight at 5 months, 1 year, and 2 years is approximately 6, 9, and 12 kg, respectively.

Length: The most dynamic linear growth spreads over during the first 2 years of life. A term newborn measures 50 cm at birth, 60 cm at 3 months, 70 cm at 9 months, and 75 cm at 1 year of age.

Head growth: It occurs in parallel to the rapid brain growth during this period. There is a 5–6 cm increase in head size during the first 3 months after birth and an additional 5–6 cm during the rest 9 months in the first year. Head circumference at 1 year of age is 45–47 cm. If the head growth exceeds 1 cm in 2 weeks during the first 3 months, hydrocephalus should be suspected.

Chest circumference: This is less than the head circumference at birth. The two equalizes by 6 months of age.

GROWTH AFTER INFANCY

Weight: The weight of a child at the age of 2 years is four times and at 3 years is usually five times that of the birthweight. The child gains, on an average, about 1.5–2.5 kg/year, from the age of 2 years till onset of adolescence. During the preschool years, between 2 and 5 years, the child gains on an average 2 kg (1.5–2.5 kg) in weight per year. Weight for age at a given age is more for boys as compared to girls. The adolescent acceleration in weight occurs earlier in girls (10–12 years) than boys (beginning 2 years later). The rapid weight gain is greatest in the year before menarche. Find below some formulae for a rough and quick calculation of expected weight between the ages of 3 months and 12 years. However, refer to the standard reference growth charts for exact values.

3–12 months	expected weight = (age in months + 9)/2
1–6 years	expected weight = 2 (age in years) + 8
7–12 years	expected weight = [7 (age in years) – 5]/2

Stature: The child usually reaches a length of approximately 88–90 cm by 2 years. Height at 4 years of age is 100 cm (which is double the length at birth). The child gains on an average about 4–5 cm/year from the age of 2 years till the onset of puberty. By 13 years of age, a child triples the birth length. Adolescent spurt of growth in height corresponds closely to weight gain. The following formula can be used for a rough and quick calculation of expected height between the ages of 2–12 years.

Expected height = (age in years × 6) + 77

Head circumference: It increases less rapidly during the second year of life in accordance with the decreased growth of the brain. The head circumference increases by 2 cm in the second year of life (47–49 cm by 2 year) and then at a rate of 1 cm per year from 2–5 years of age. At 12 years of age, the average head size is 52 cm.

Mid-upper arm circumference: Normal mid-upper arm circumference of a term newborn is 9–11 cm. By 1 year of age, it grows to 16 cm. Mid-upper arm circumference (MUAC) increases by only 1.0 cm between the ages of 6 months and 5 years, therefore, it is also called an age-independent criterion between these ages. A child between 6 months and 5 years is termed undernourished, if the mid-arm circumference is <12.5 cm. Severe acute malnutrition is characterized by mid-arm circumference <11.5 cm (between 6 months and 5 years of age).

Velocity of growth in terms of both height and weight is most rapid during the first year of life and then falls rapidly. Weight velocity is 6 kg in the first year of life, and 2 kg/year in the preschool child, and 3 kg/year till puberty. Height velocity is 25 cm in the first year of life, 12 cm in the second year, followed by around 5–6 cm per year till puberty.

Body proportion: The ratio of upper segment (crown to pubic symphysis) and the lower segment (pubic symphysis to heel) is 1.7 at birth. Thus, sitting height represents 65–70% of total length in the newborn infant. After birth, limbs grow much faster than the trunk resulting in reduction of sitting height percentage. The ratio is 1.3 at 3 years of age. The upper segment equalizes the lower segment by 8–10 years of age (ratio 1:1).

Arm span is less than the stature by 1–2 cm by 10 years of age. Thereafter, arm span exceeds the height, but the difference always stays <3–5 cm.

ERUPTION OF TEETH

The deciduous teeth start erupting at 6 months of age and the permanent teeth at about 6 years of age. All the deciduous teeth are replaced by the permanent teeth by the age of 12 years. A child between the age of 6 and 12 years has a mixed dentition. Ages of eruption and shedding of primary (deciduous) teeth are provided in **Table 1.2**.

Primary dentition: The lower central incisors appear between the ages of 5 and 8 months. The upper central incisors appear a month later and the lateral incisors usually within the next 3 months. The first molar teeth appear around the age of 12–15 months, preceding the eruption of canine teeth by 6 months, which appear between the age of 18 and 21 months. The second molars are out at the age of 21–24 months.

Table 1.2 Eruption and Shedding of Primary (Deciduous) Teeth

Primary (deciduous) teeth		
	Eruption	*Shedding*
Maxillary		
Central incisor	7½ months	7–8 years
Lateral incisor	9 months	8–9 years
Canine	18 months	11–12 years
First molar	14 months	10–11 years
Second molar	24 months	10–12 years
Mandibular		
Central incisor	6½ months	6–7 years
Lateral incisor	7 months	7–8 years
Canine	16 months	9–11 years
First molar	12 months	10–12 years
Second molar	20 months	11–13 years

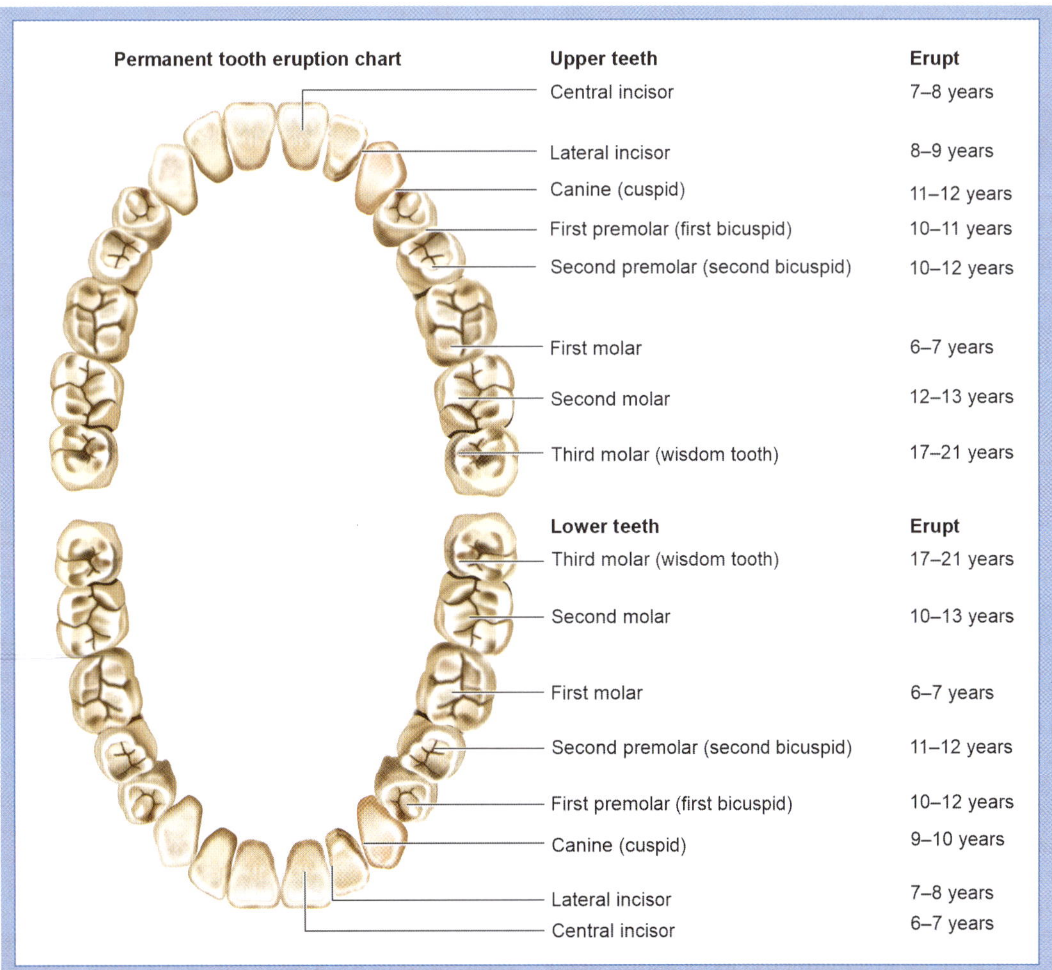

Fig. 1.5: Timing of permanent tooth eruption

Source: Adapted from ADA Division of Communications; Journal of the American Dental Association; ADA Council on Scientific Affairs. For the dental patient. Tooth eruption: the permanent teeth. J Am Dent Assoc. 2006;137(1):127

Permanent teeth erupt in the following order. 1st molar—6 years; central and lateral incisors—6-8 years; canines and premolars—9-12 years; second molars—12 years; third molars—18 years or later **(Fig. 1.5)**.

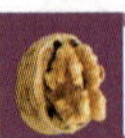

IN A NUTSHELL

Normal Growth

1. *Average size at birth:*
   - *Weight 2.8 kg; Length 50 cm; Head circumference 35–37 cm.*
2. *Average size at 1 year:*
   - *Weight 8–10 kg; Length 75 cm; Head circumference 45–47 cm.*
3. After 2 years, weight increases by 1.5–2.5 kg/year and height increases by 4–5 cm/year, till puberty.
4. Mid-arm circumference is 9–11 cm at birth, increases to about 16 cm at 1 year. After 1 year, it increases @only 0.25 cm/year; thus, called age-independent between 1 and 5 years of age.
5. Deciduous teeth start erupting by 6 months, and permanent teeth by 6 years of age.

ADA Division of Communications; Journal of the American Dental Association; ADA Council on Scientific Affairs. For the dental patient. Tooth eruption: The primary teeth. J Am Dent Assoc. 2005;136(11):1619.

Cameron N. The biology of growth. Nestle Nutr Workshop Ser Pediatr Program. 2008;61:1-19.

Fernández MA, Delchevalerie P, Van Herp M. Accuracy of MUAC in the detection of severe wasting with the new WHO growth standards. Pediatrics. 2010;126:e195-201.

Rogol AD, Roemmich JN, Clark PA. Growth at puberty. J Adolesc Health. 2002;31:192-200.

1.5 Assessment of Physical Growth: Anthropometry *PE 1.2*

INTRODUCTION

Anthropometry (Greek *anthropos*—man and *metron*—measure) refers to the measurement of the human. Measurements that can be made on the body are almost limitless but weight and stature (height/length) are the most widely taken growth measurements. Commonly measured parameters are discussed below.

WEIGHT

Before the advent of digital electronic scales, two types of weighing scales were commonly used: Beam balance scales (with moving weights) and the spring balance scales. Of these, beam-balancing scales were more accurate.

The basket/pan type scale for infants can be used to weigh children up to 10.0 kg. Infants can be placed on the tray, which is supported on a reading frame calibrated for measuring a minimum of 10 g increment. The platform scale is for older children who can climb and stand up on the scale.

- Weigh the child in bare minimum of clothes and without shoes. Infants should be weighed naked (without diapers) and older children can be weighed with a vest and brief.
- Ensure that the scale is resting on firm, stable and even surface, or uncarpeted floor.
- Check the zero of the scale before weighing. Calibrate the weight scale at the beginning and at the end of each measurement.
- ***Infants:*** Place the infant in a manner so as to distribute the weight evenly about the center of the pan. If a diaper is worn, its weight should be subtracted from the observed weight, because the reference data for infants is based on nude weight.
- ***Children:*** Ask them to stand in the center of the platform, with bodyweight evenly distributed on both feet. Ensure that the child is not holding onto anything.
- A child on follow-up should preferably be weighed on the same scale.
- Read the weight by standing in front of the scale and not from the side.

STATURE

Stature is ascertained by measuring the length (in children <2 years old) or height (in older children).

Harpenden infantometer: It is used to measure the length of a newborn and infant. The tool consists of a horizontal wooden board limited by two vertical planks perpendicular to the two ends **(Fig. 1.6)**. At one end, plank is fixed to the wooden board (headpiece); the other end has a movable vertical plank to adjust to the infant's length (foot piece). There is a calibrated reading strip in the middle of the board on which the length of the baby can be read directly. The infantometer is designed to measure lengths between 0 and 100 cm, with a precision of 1 mm.

Stadiometer: It is used for measuring standing height. The child stands on a wooden plank with his back against a wooden board that is calibrated in cm/inches. A flat board (wooden, metallic or cardboard) is placed at head end of the

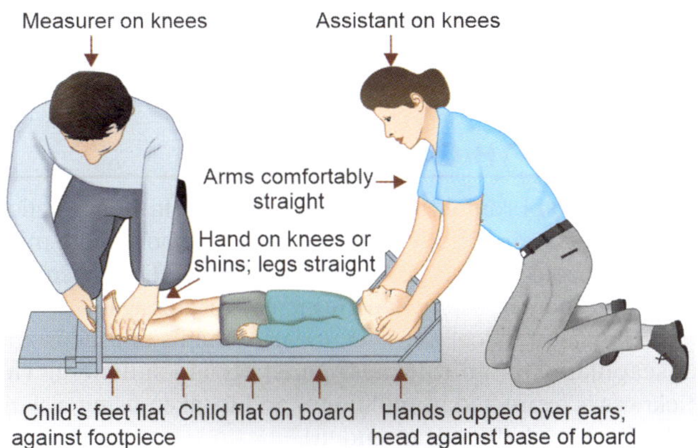

Fig. 1.6: Taking length on an infantometer

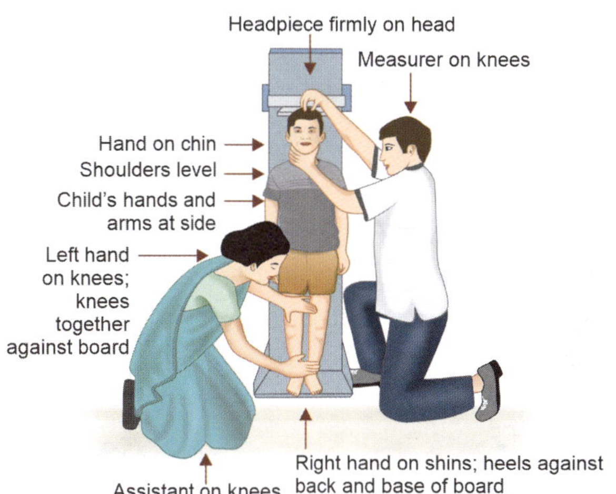

Fig. 1.7: Measurement of standing height

child to level off the height. Alternatively, the height can also be measured against a flat wall.

Length

- Place the child supine on the infant measuring board.
- Ask the assistant to hold the child's head in the Frankfort plane, while you steady the legs. The head is positioned in the Frankfort plane when the crown touches the headpiece and a vertical line from the ear canal to the lower border of the eye socket is perpendicular to the horizontal board (i.e., positioned vertically). Apply gentle traction to bring the head into contact with the fixed headpiece.
- Position the child's shoulders and hips at right angles to the long axis of the body. Apply gentle pressure on the knees to straighten the legs and prevent the knees from flexing.
- Bring the movable footboard to rest firmly against the child's feet with the soles flat on the board and the toes pointing directly upward.
- Record the measurement to the nearest 0.1 cm from the counter on the measuring board.

Height

- Remove the hair ornaments, undo the buns and braids, and take off the footwear.
- Ask the child to stand on the stadiometer with feet slightly apart at a 60° angle and confirm that the weight is evenly distributed on both feet. The arms hang freely by the sides of the trunk with palms facing the thighs.
- Ensure that the back of the head, shoulder blades, buttocks, calves, and heels are touching the vertical board/wall. This can be done by trying to insert a plastic rule at places where these points touch the wall. Inability to insert the rule implies good contact.
- Ask the child to look straight. Position the child's head so that a horizontal line drawn from the external auditory meatus to the lower edge of the eye socket runs parallel to the baseboard (i.e., the Frankfort plane positioned horizontally) **(Fig. 1.7)**.
- The headpiece is moved down to rest firmly on top of the child's head, compressing the hair; keeping it perpendicular to the wall.
- Record the reading to the last completed 0.1 cm.

BODY CIRCUMFERENCES

Circumferences are measured to nearest 0.1 cm with a tape made up of a soft and nonshrinkable material.

Head Circumference

The head circumference is recorded between birth and 6 years of age (the period of brain growth) as the maximum circumference of the head with measuring tape overlying the occiput at back and supraorbital ridges in front.

- Anchor the tape just above the eyebrows.
- Ensure that the tape overlies the most prominent part of the occipital prominence at the back of the head.
- The tape should be perpendicular to the long axis of the face and should be pulled firmly to compress the hair, skin, and underlying soft tissues.
- Record measurement over the parietal eminence by cross-over technique **(Fig. 1.8)**.

Chest Circumference

- Place the infant in the lap of the mother and stand in front. The chest should be bare.

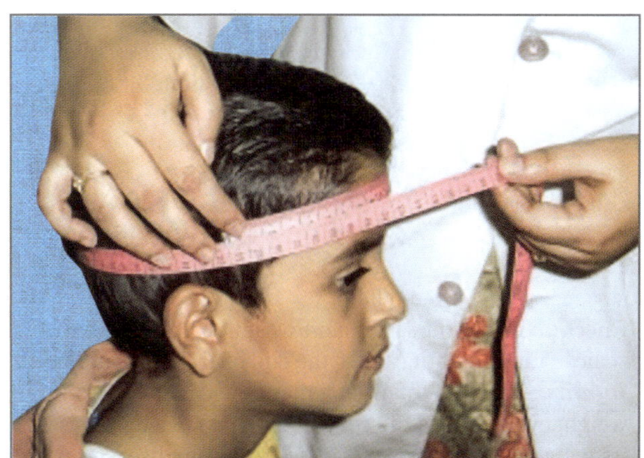

Fig. 1.8: Measurement of head circumference

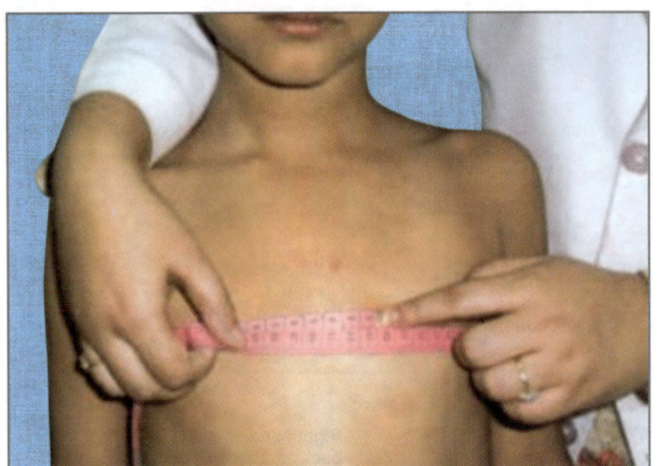

Fig. 1.9: Measurement of chest circumference

- Abduct the arms of the infant slightly to permit passage of the tape around the chest.
- Pass the tape around the chest of the infant, at the level of nipples or 4th costosternal joints.
- Lower the arm to their natural position, once the tape is snugly in place.
- Record the circumference in a horizontal plane, midway between inspiration and expiration **(Fig. 1.9)**.

Mid-upper Arm Circumference

Mid-upper arm circumference (MUAC) is recorded for children between 6 months and 5 years of age to nearest of 0.1 cm. A mid-upper arm circumference of <12.5 cm indicates malnutrition.

- Palpate and mark the two important bony landmarks, i.e., the acromion process and the olecranon. Forearm should be flexed while marking these points.
- Mark the mid-upper arm point. It is half the distance between the acromion process and the olecranon.
- Encircle the tape around the arm, over the marked midpoint, perpendicular to the long axis of the upper arm, with arm hanging freely in a relaxed position **(Figs. 1.10A to C)**.
- Ensure that the tape lies flat around the arm, without compressing the skin or underlying tissue; there should be no gap or compression on the inner part of the arm.

SKINFOLD THICKNESS

Measurements of skinfold thickness may be useful in the estimation of muscle mass or of body fat content. The proportionate mass of subcutaneous tissue is greatest at about 9 months. It decreases steadily till about 6 years, when the increase begins again.

In clinical practice, however, measurements of triceps and subscapular skinfold thickness generally are sufficient. The thickness is expressed in millimeter and is taken using a skinfold caliper (Holtain or Harpenden).

BODY PROPORTIONS

Useful body proportions that may help in understanding various growth disturbances include body mass index (BMI), sitting height for upper segment/lower segment ratio, and arm span.

Body mass index: It is calculated as weight in kg/(height in m^2) and considered as the most important parameter used for assessment of growth in adolescents and adults. For Asian adults, the normal BMI lies between 18.5 and 23. Those having a BMI of between 23 and 28 are called overweight. Obesity is defined as a BMI of >28. Adults with BMI of <18.5 are termed to be having "chronic energy deficiency".

Absolute cut-off values for defining chronic energy deficiency, overweight, and obesity are not applicable for children and adolescents. Therefore, evaluation of BMI in these age groups is carried out by comparison with age-related standard percentile charts. Obesity is defined as BMI greater than the 95th percentile for age whereas overweight refers to BMI between 85th and 95th percentile.

Sitting height: It denotes the upper segment length and represents 65–70% of total length in the newborn infant. After birth, limbs grow much faster than the trunk resulting in reduction of sitting height percentage. By the time of adolescence, the upper

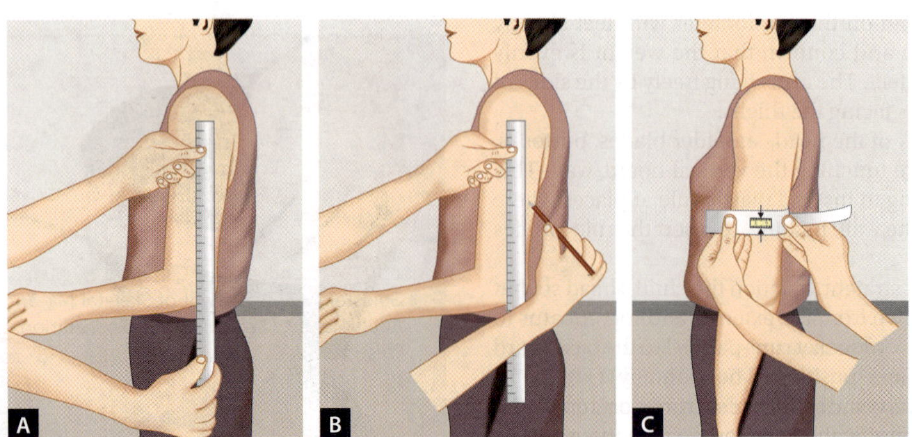

Figs. 1.10A to C: (A and B) The mid-upper arm point; (C) Measuring mid-arm circumference

segment almost equals with the lower segment. High upper/ lower segment ratio indicates short limb dwarfism.

Arm span: It is the physical measurement of the length from one end of an arm (measured at the fingertips) to the other when raised parallel to the ground at shoulder height at 180° angle. The arm span as compared to the total stature is a useful index. Usually, the difference between the two is not >3 cm. Longer arm span is seen in Marfan syndrome. For detailed description of methods of anthropometry and its interpretation, refer to "Clinical Methods in Pediatrics" by Piyush Gupta.

VELOCITY OF PHYSICAL GROWTH

Measurement of the velocity of growth or increment in a unit of time is a better tool for early identification of factors affecting growth. Velocity of growth can also help in predicting the ultimate adult height. The normal growth velocity curve for height is shown in **Figure 1.11**. The growth velocity is maximum during the first year of life. A second growth spurt occurs during puberty. This is known as the peak height/weight velocity. Maximum growth velocity occurs at sexual maturity rate (SMR) stage 3–4 in girls and SMR stage 4–5 in boys. Girls achieve pubertal growth spurt about 2 years prior to boys.

BONE AGE ASSESSMENT

Bone age is a tool to evaluate skeletal maturation which in turn depends on hormonal influences. Assessment of bone age is thus used for diagnostic evaluation of children with growth failure, and advanced or delayed puberty. In healthy children, bone age corresponds to chronological age. A discrepancy between the two suggests a defect of the endocrine system. Characteristically, hypothyroidism slows the skeletal growth; ossification is delayed and bone age is less than the chronological age.

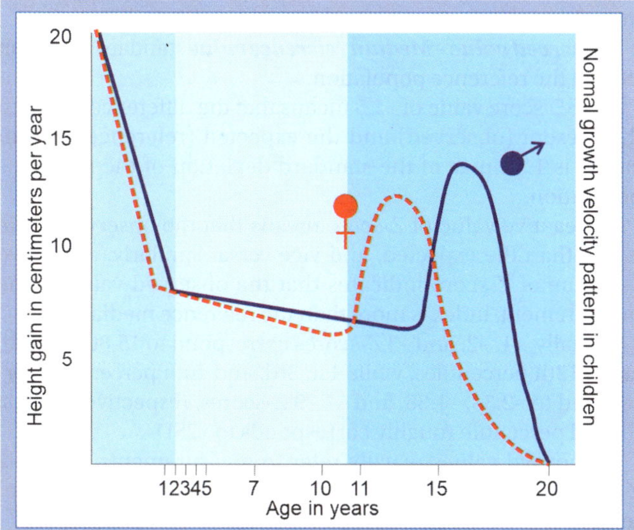

Fig. 1.11: Normal growth velocity in children (boys and girls). The figure shows that girls achieve pubertal growth spurt about 2 years prior to boys

Ossification of skeleton begins in the intrauterine period—starting first in the clavicles followed by skull, long bones, and spine. Shaft ossifies earlier than the ends of the bone. The earliest epiphyseal centers to appear are those for os calcis and talus (22–26 weeks of gestation). At the time of birth in a full term newborn, the distal epiphyses of femur (age of appearance: 31–39 weeks of gestation) and the proximal epiphyses of tibia (age of appearance: 34 weeks of gestation to 5th postnatal week) are usually present. Two carpal bones are present at 1 year, and by 6 years, epiphyses of 7 carpal bones are present except pisiform, which ossifies later during puberty.

By convention, radiograph of the left limb is taken for computing bone age. At different chronological ages, radiographs of different parts of the body are required for correct assessment. For example, in the newborn period, radiographs of foot and knee are helpful. Between 3 and 9 months, radiographs of the shoulder is taken. X-ray of hands and wrists should be obtained between 1 and 12 years of age. For children between 12 and 14 years, radiographs of elbow and hip are helpful. A serial evaluation is always much more helpful than a single radiograph. Girls are more advanced than boys in skeletal development at all ages. Bone age corresponds more closely to SMR staging than to chronological age during puberty.

The two most widely used tools to assess bone age are the Greulich–Pyle Atlas method and the Tanner–Whitehouse 2 Individual Bones method (TW2 method). It is important to note that these methods are not always comparable and cannot be considered an advanced text interchangeable. Readers are advised to refer to advanced text for more details.

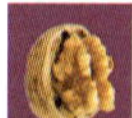

IN A NUTSHELL

Assessment of Physical Growth: Anthropometry

1. Commonly measured anthropometric parameters include weight, length, height, head and chest circumference, and mid-arm circumference.
2. Weight and height/length are to be measured throughout childhood while body circumferences are important to be measured between birth and 5 years.
3. Body mass index (BMI) is calculated as [weight in kg/height in m^2] and considered as most important parameter to assess growth in older children and adolescents.
4. Bone age is a tool to evaluate children with growth failure or those with advanced/delayed puberty.

Greulich WW, Pyle SI. Radiographic Atlas of Skeletal Development of Hand and Wrist. Stanford, CA: Stanford University Press; 1959.

Gupta P. Clinical Methods in Pediatrics, 5th edition. New Delhi: CBS Publishers; 2022.

Tanner JM, Whitehouse RH, Cameron N, Marshall WA, Healy MJR, Goldstein H. Assessment of Skeletal Maturity and Prediction of Adult Height (TW2 Method), 2nd edition. London: Academic Press; 1983.

1.6 Statistical Principles in Assessment of Growth *PE 1.2*

GAUSSIAN DISTRIBUTION

If measurements of any of the growth parameters (e.g., weight and height) are obtained in a large population of normal children and then arranged in a regular order starting from the lowest to the highest, a bell-shaped curve is formed **(Fig. 1.12)**. This symmetrical curve illustrates a typical Gaussian (Normal) distribution, in which maximum values lie around the middle of the curve. The curve tapers off on the either side, with fewer observations at both the ends of the curve. Mean and median are equal in a Gaussian distribution.

MEAN AND STANDARD DEVIATION

Measurement of a parameter in a sample and its recording in a continuous numerical manner generates several measurements, the most important of them being mean and standard deviation (SD).

- ***Mean:*** It is obtained by dividing the sum of all observations by the number of observations. In a Gaussian distribution, the maximum number of values cluster around the average or mean.
- ***Standard deviation:*** It denotes the degree of dispersion or the scatter of observations away from the mean. It is estimated that 68.3% (approximately two-thirds) of the observations lie within 1 SD above or below the mean value of the observations. Values within the range of ±2 SD include 95.4% of all values. Values beyond 2 SD are unusual in a normal population. 3 SD around the mean includes 99.7% of all values.

MEDIAN AND PERCENT MEDIAN

When data are arranged in ascending or descending order of magnitude, half of the observations are above and the other half below a certain point. This point or value is known as the median. The median thus indicates that 50% of observations are above and 50% are below this point. In a typical Gaussian distribution, the median is expected to be equivalent to the arithmetic mean. Median, rather than the mean, is considered as the central value for most of the anthropometric parameters since the population data has a non-Gaussian (skewed) distribution.

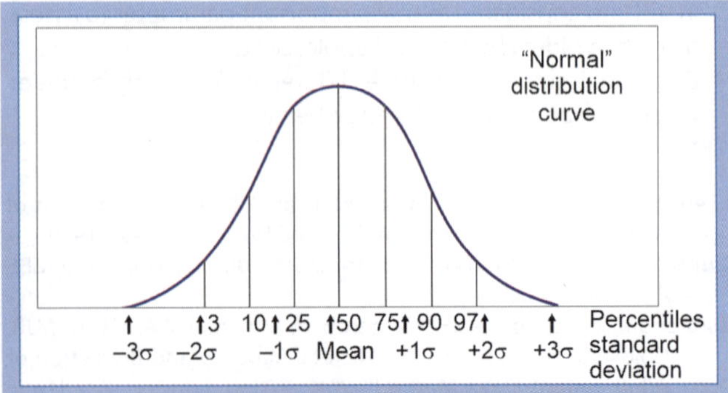

Fig. 1.12: Normal bell-shaped distribution curve

PERCENTILES

Percentile indicates the position that a measurement would hold in a typical series of 100 arranged in ascending order. The median lies at the 50th percentile, on either side of which lie half the observations. Another example is the 85th percentile curve, which denotes that 15% of observations are expected to be above and 84% below it.

Percentile location is used to designate where an individual stands with respect to other members of the population. The WHO growth standards show curves at 3rd, 15th, 50th, 85th and 97th percentiles, corresponding to distances from the average values. One standard deviation above or below the mean coincides with the 84th or 16th percentile curve, respectively.

Eighty percent of the weight/height measurements of healthy children at a given age are expected to lie between 10th and 90th percentiles. Further, 95% of the weight/height measurements of healthy children at a given age are expected to lie between 3rd and 97th percentile values. Thus, allowable normal range of variation in observations is between 3rd and 97th percentiles, which roughly corresponds to ±2 SD.

A healthy child normally remains and follows the same percentile curve during the entire period of his/her growth.

Z (SD)-SCORE

It represents the deviation of anthropometric measurement from the reference median and is calculated as follows:

Observed value - Median reference value standard deviation (SD) of the reference population.

An SD score value of +1.5 means that the difference between the present (observed) and the expected (reference median value) is 1.5 times of the standard deviation of the reference population.

A negative value of *Z*-score means that the observed value is less than the expected, and vice versa. Similarly, a positive (+) value of *Z*-score indicates that the observed value of the measurement/index is more than the reference median.

Usually, -1, -2, and -3 *Z*-scores correspond to 15.8th, 2.28th, and 0.13th percentiles, while 1st, 3rd, and 10th percentiles correspond to -2.33, -1.88, and -1.29 *Z*-scores, respectively. Thus, the 3rd percentile roughly corresponds to -2SD.

Abnormal values usually refer to measurements below -2 *Z*-score (2.3rd percentile) or above +2 *Z*-score (97.7th percentile) relative to the reference median.

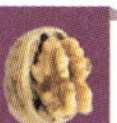

IN A NUTSHELL

Statistical Principles in Assessment of Growth

1. Median, rather than mean, is considered as the central value for most anthropometric parameters.
2. Percentile indicates the position that a value will hold, arranged chronologically in a series of 100 values. Median is thus the 50th percentile.
3. Most normal children are expected to have their anthropometric measurements between 3rd and 97th percentiles.
4. *Z*-score (also known as SD score) represents deviation from the central value.
5. Usually, values between ±2 *Z*-scores are considered normal.

Curtis AE, Smith TA, Ziganshin BA, Elefteriades JA. The Mystery of the *Z*-Score. Aorta (Stamford). 2016;4(4):124-30.

1.7 Growth Charts, Growth References, and Growth Standards

PE 1.2

GROWTH CHARTS

The growth charts comprise an X-axis that corresponds to the age in months or years; and Y-axis denoting the value of the anthropometric parameter, for example, weight (kg), height (cm), body mass index (kg/m^2), etc. WHO growth charts are available for both percentiles and *Z*-score, separately.

- The WHO percentile charts depict 5 percentiles lines corresponding to 3rd, 15th, 50th, 85th, and 97th percentiles (from below to above) **(Fig. 1.13A)**. Any child who is below the 3rd or above the 97th centile is likely to be abnormal.
- The WHO *Z*-score charts display curves for median, –2*Z*, –3*Z*, 2*Z*, and 3*Z*-scores **(Fig. 1.13B)**. Abnormal is defined as any

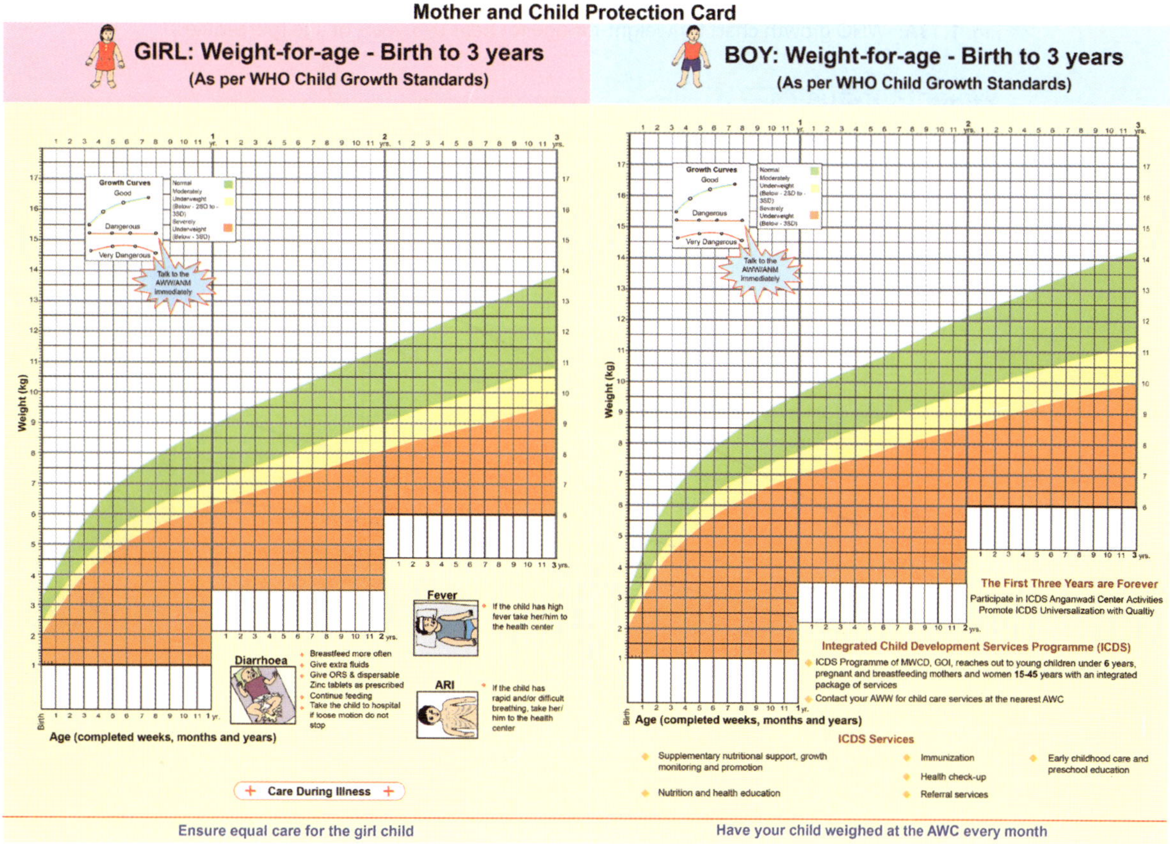

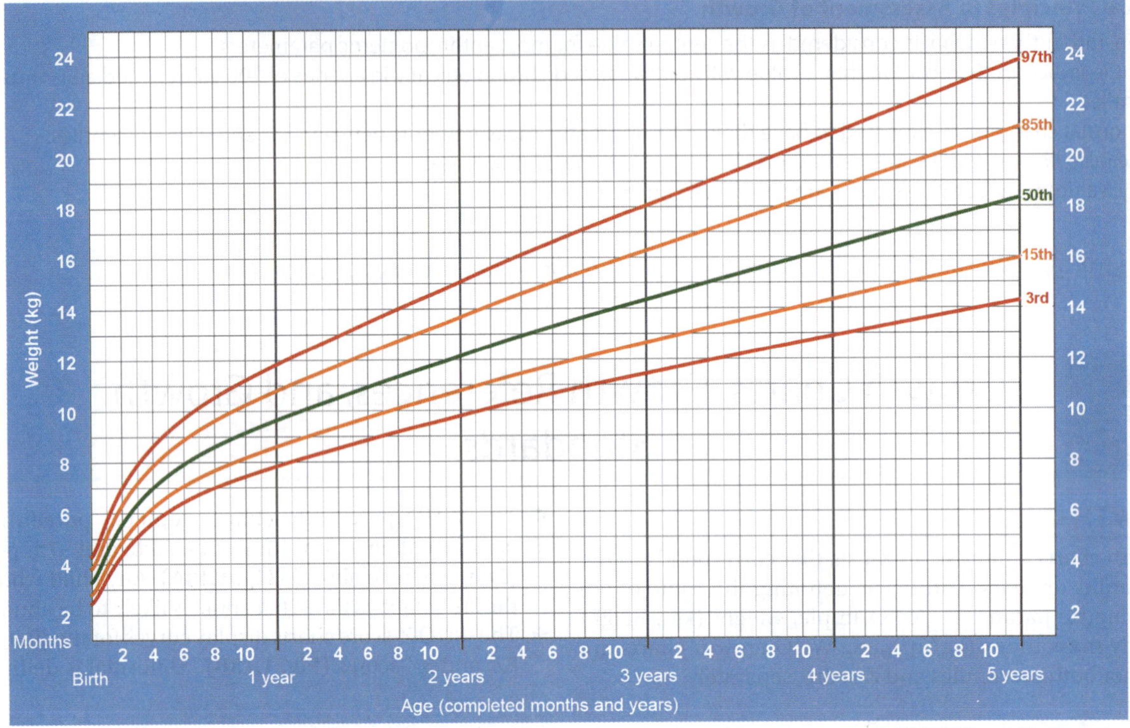

Fig. 1.13A: WHO growth chart for weight-for-age for boys 0–5 years of age (percentiles)

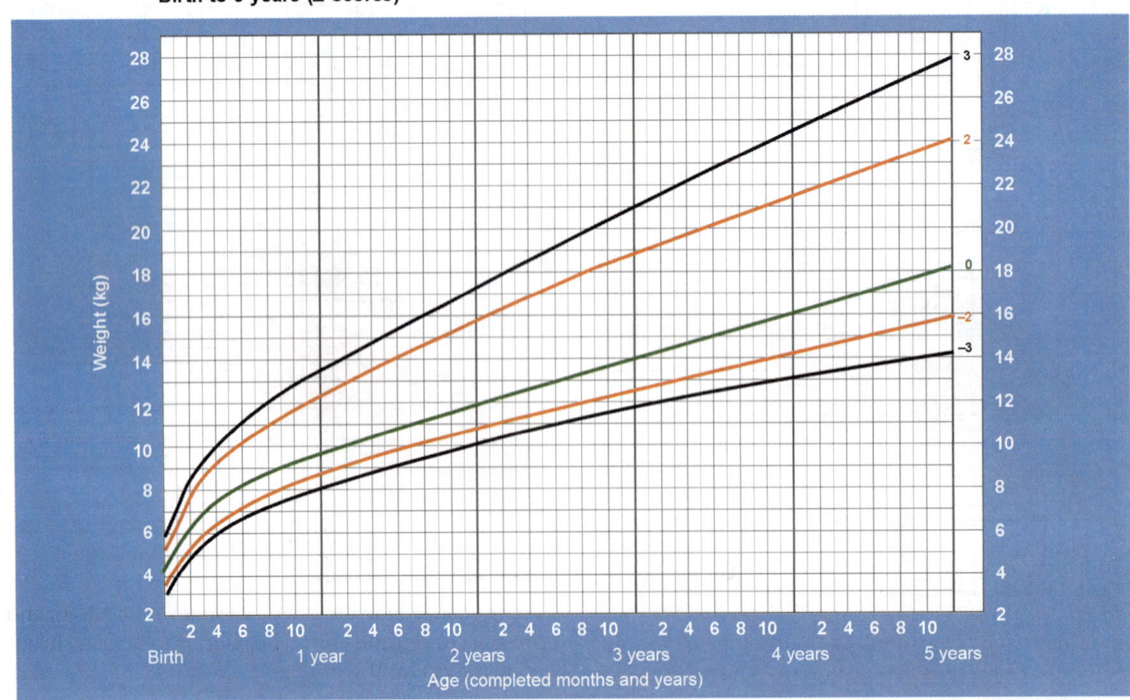

Fig. 1.13B: WHO growth chart for weight-for-age for boys 0–5 years of age (*Z*-scores)

discrepancy of more than -2*Z*-scores. A deviation by more than -3*Z*-score denotes severe malnutrition. On the charts of growth velocity, the cut-off line for defining low-height velocity is below the 25th centile.

WHO growth standards for children <5 years have been adopted in many countries including India as the universal global standard, for monitoring growth in under-5 children. In 2015, Indian Academy of Pediatrics published new revised growth charts for Indian children 5–18 years of age in view of the changing trend in nutritional status of older children.

GROWTH REFERENCES VERSUS GROWTH STANDARDS

- ***Growth standards:*** These represent data on how a population of children should grow, under the given optimal nutritional and health conditions.
- ***Growth references:*** These are descriptive data that define how children in the population are growing under the best possible state of nutrition and health in a given community. They represent how children are actually growing rather than how they should be growing.

The WHO growth charts published in 2006, based on the WHO Multicenter Growth Reference Study (MGRS) for children under the age of 5 years, are an example of growth standards. Whereas the 2015 IAP growth charts are growth references which describe how children in India were actually growing at that point of time.

WHO GROWTH STANDARDS

The 2006 growth curves and charts developed by the World Health Organization (WHO) provide a single international standard that represents the best description of physiological growth for all children from birth to 5 years of age. These charts are based on the growth of exclusively breastfed infants. The second unique feature of these standards is that it is based on growth of children from many of the world's major regions: Brazil (South America), Ghana (Africa), India (Asia), Norway (Europe), Oman (the Middle East), and the USA (North America).

These standards show that all children of the world grow similarly till 5 years of age, provided the optimal environment, regardless of ethnicity and socioeconomic status. The standards show that nutrition, environment, and healthcare are stronger factors in determining growth and development than gender or ethnic background. The WHO standards differ from other existing growth charts in a number of innovative ways.

- WHO standards are based on longitudinally collected data as opposed to cross-sectional data in erstwhile NCHS reference (based on growth of North American Children). This is particularly useful in development of growth velocity standards.
- WHO standards describe "how children should grow," as compared to earlier NCHS references which simply stated "how children are growing."
- WHO standards make breastfeeding the biological "norm" and establishes the breastfed infant as the normative growth model. NCHS reference was based on the growth of artificially-fed children.
- WHO standards also include other growth indicators such as the skinfold thickness and body mass index. These are useful to define obesity and overweight.
- MGRS also provide the Windows of Achievement standards for six motor development milestones including sitting, standing, and walking.

WHO charts have now replaced the National Center for Health Statistics (NCHS)/Centers for Disease Control and Prevention (CDC) Growth Charts for assessing the growth of children up to 5 years of age. The WHO growth charts are provided for weight-for-age (birth–5 years) **(Figs. 1.13A to D)**; length/height-for-age (birth–5 years) **(Figs. 1.14A to D)**; weight-for-length (birth–2 years) **(Figs. 1.15A to D)**; and weight-for-height (2–5 years) **(Figs. 1.16A to D)**. Corresponding tables are reproduced in the Annexures.

GROWTH REFERENCE FOR INDIAN CHILDREN 5–18 YEARS

Even though growth occurs in a similar manner among under-5 children throughout the world, but there do exist some regional variations among the pattern of growth of older children. The average adult weight and height are also different in different regions of the world because of the same reason. Thus, for Indian children older than 5 years, the ideal reference standards would be the ones derived from Indian population itself.

In 2015, Indian Academy of Pediatrics (IAP) published the revised growth charts based on data collected from published studies on apparently healthy Indian children and adolescents in the past one decade. IAP recommends use of these charts as reference values for Indian children between 5 and 18 years of age. These reference curves are provided as **Figures 1.17 and 1.18**. We suggest using these charts as reference values for children above 5 years of age. Corresponding tables are reproduced in the Annexures.

GROWTH MONITORING

Growth monitoring is a screening tool used to diagnose nutritional discrepancies, chronic systemic illnesses, and endocrine disorders. Growth monitoring involves taking the same and multiple anthropometric measurements at regular intervals, approximately at the same time of the day and to see their changing trend. A single value only denotes the measurement at that point of time.

National Health Mission encourages growth monitoring of children <3 years of age. Children are monitored monthly in the Mother and Child Protection (MCP) Card *(See below)*. The chart can detect whether a child is growing normally or having faltering in growth. A rising curve denotes "good" growth; a flattening curve is dangerous; and a downward curve calls for immediate management/referral. Green zone in the chart represents normally growing child; Yellow should be viewed with caution; and Orange represents undernutrition. The chart is to be used by all Anganwadi workers (AWWs) and auxiliary nurse midwife (ANM).

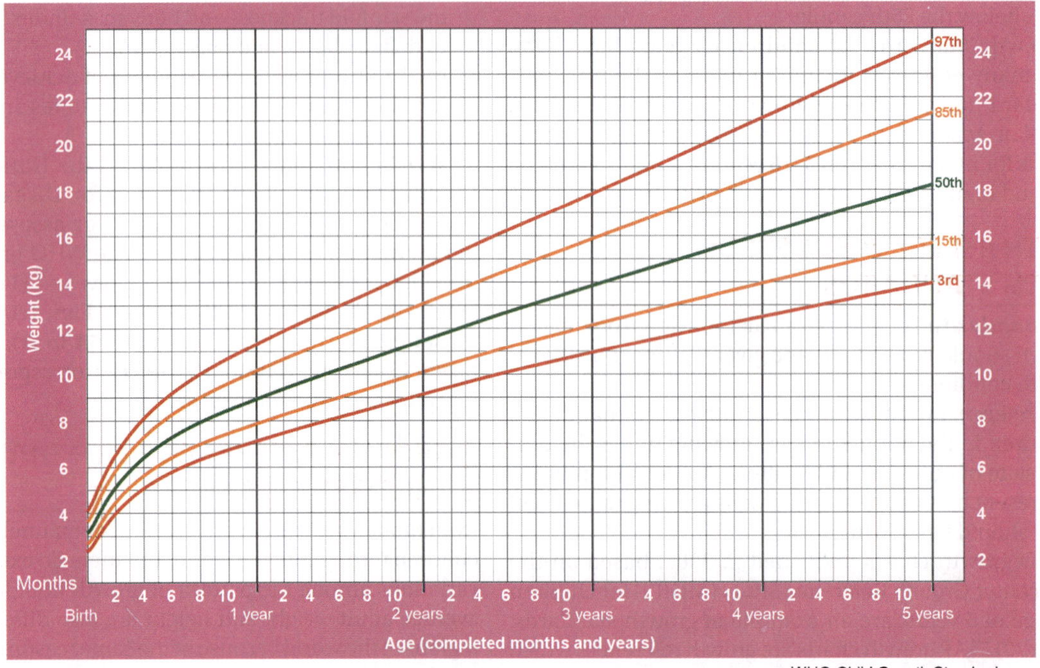

Fig. 1.13C: WHO growth chart for weight-for-age for girls 0–5 years of age (percentiles)

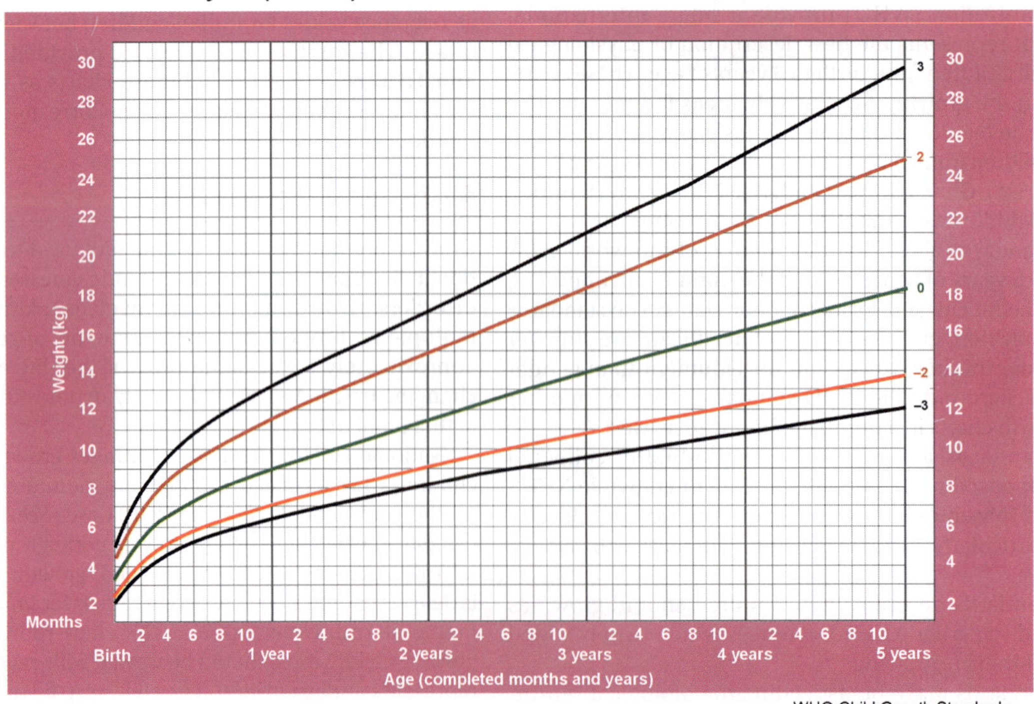

Fig. 1.13D: WHO growth chart for weight-for-age for girls 0–5 years of age (*Z*-scores)

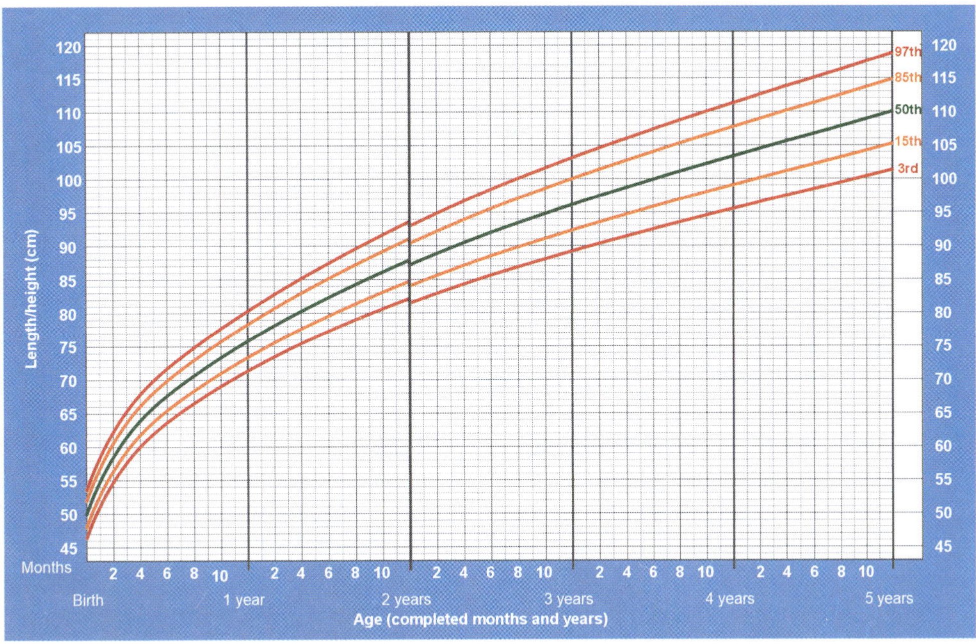

Fig. 1.14A: WHO growth chart for length/height-for-age for boys 0–5 years of age (percentiles)

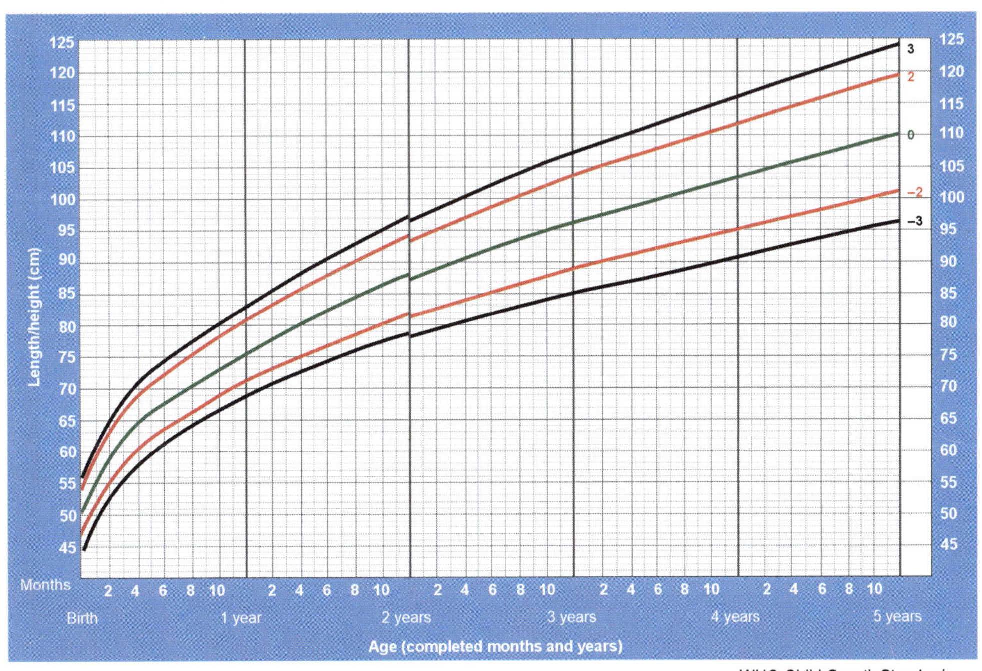

Fig. 1.14B: WHO growth chart for length/height-for-age for boys 0–5 years of age (*Z*-scores)

Length/height-for-age GIRLS

Birth to 5 years (percentiles)

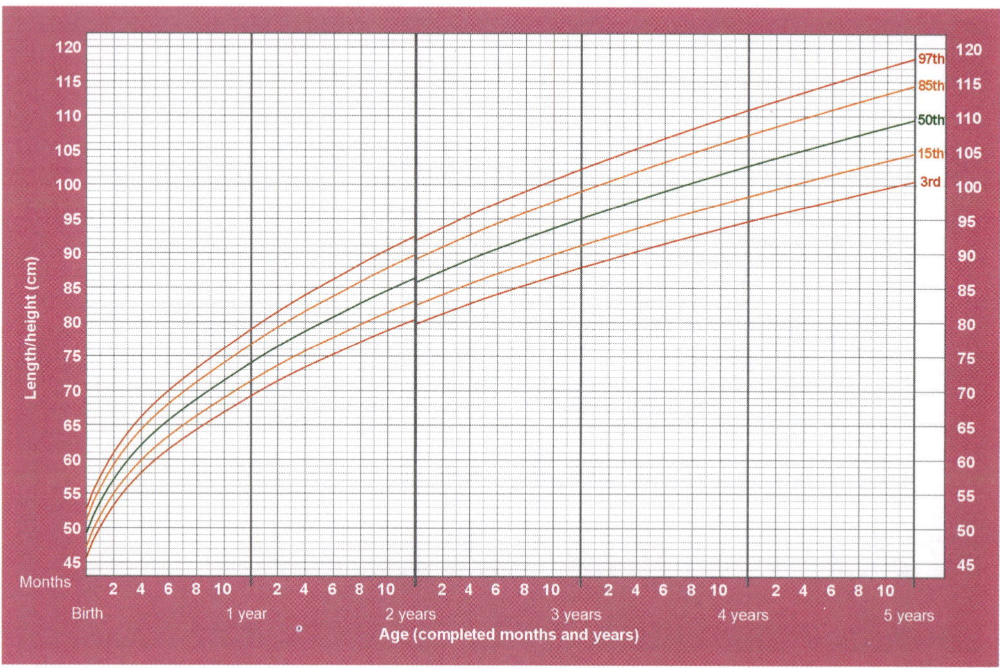

WHO Child Growth Standards

Fig. 1.14C: WHO growth chart for length/height-for-age for girls 0–5 years of age (percentiles)

Length/height-for-age GIRLS

Birth to 5 years (Z-scores)

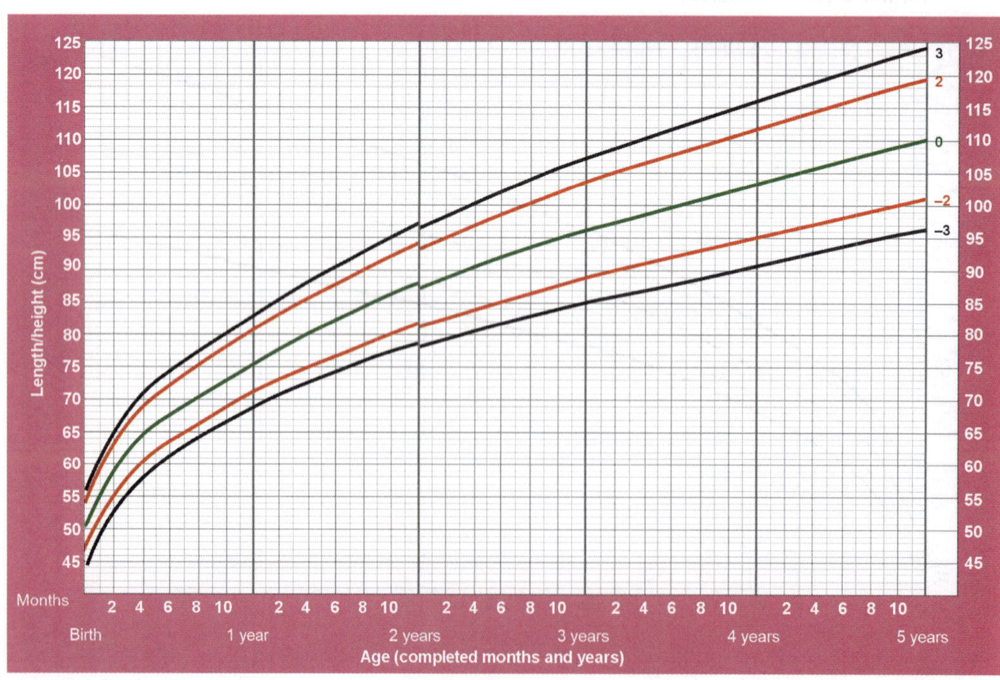

WHO Child Growth Standards

Fig. 1.14D: WHO growth chart for length/height-for-age for girls 0–5 years of age (*Z*-scores)

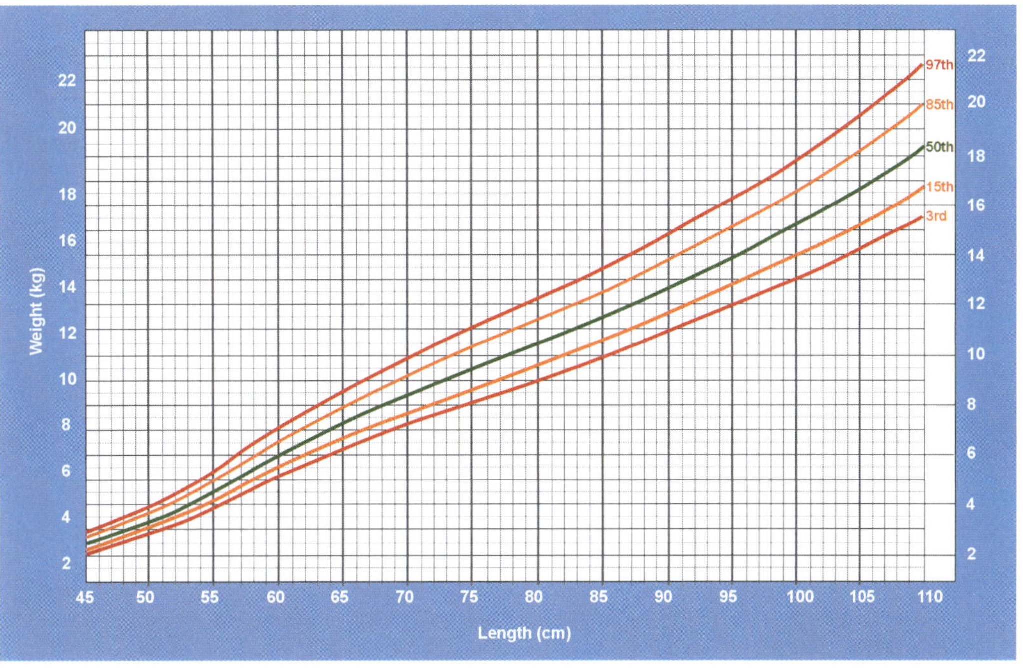

Fig. 1.15A: WHO growth chart for weight-for-length for boys 0–2 years of age (percentiles)

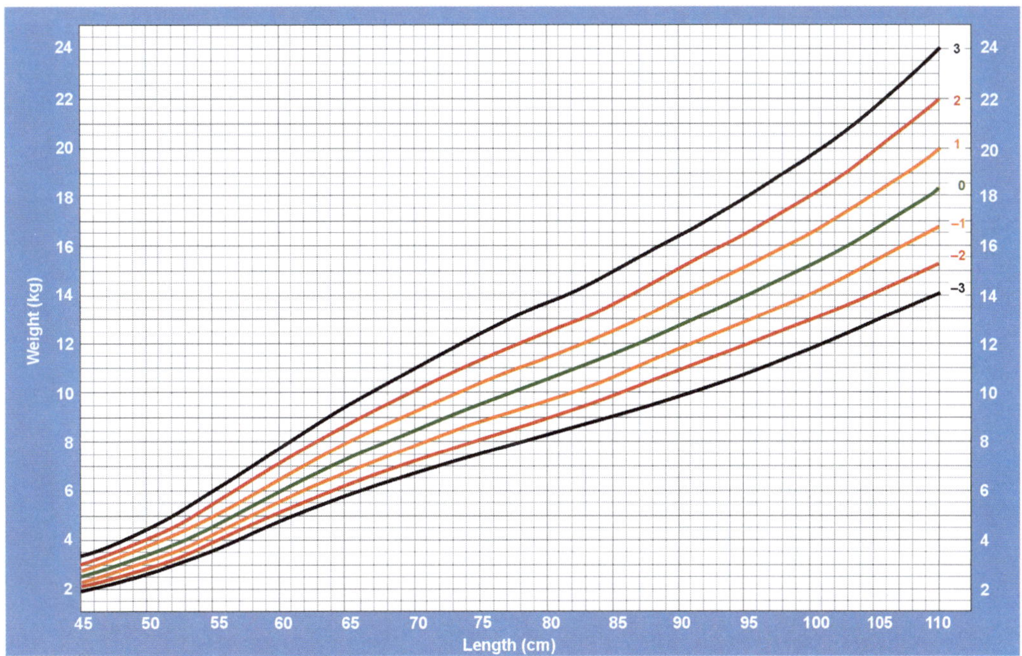

Fig. 1.15B: WHO growth chart for weight-for-length for boys 0–2 years of age (*Z*-scores)

Weight-for-length GIRLS

Birth to 2 years (percentiles)

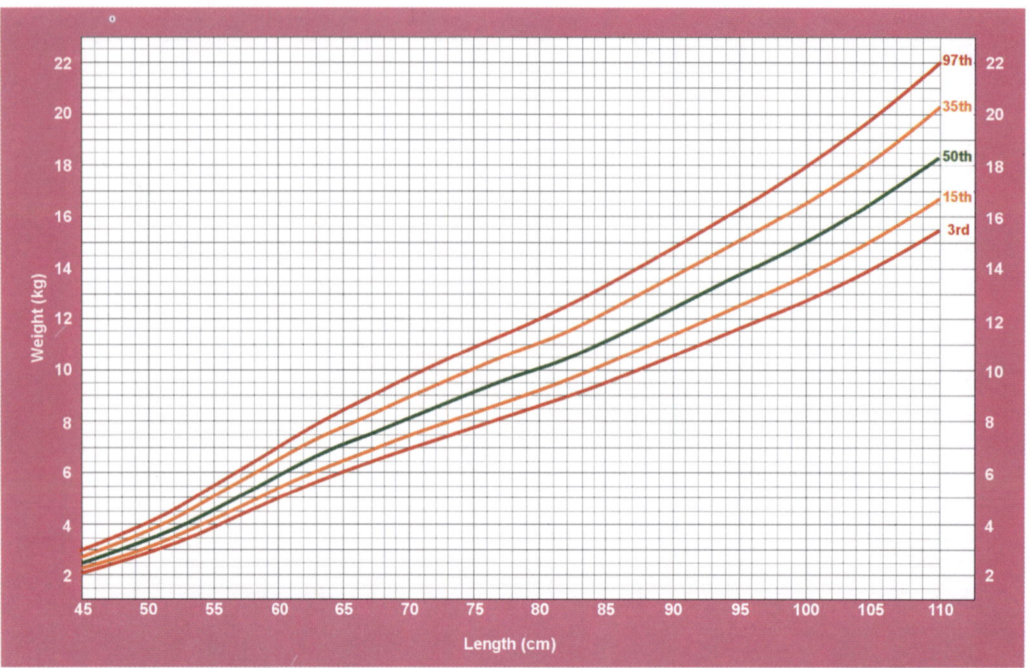

WHO Child Growth Standards

Fig. 1.15C: WHO growth chart for weight-for-length for girls 0–2 years of age (percentiles)

Weight-for-length GIRLS

Birth to 2 years (Z-scores)

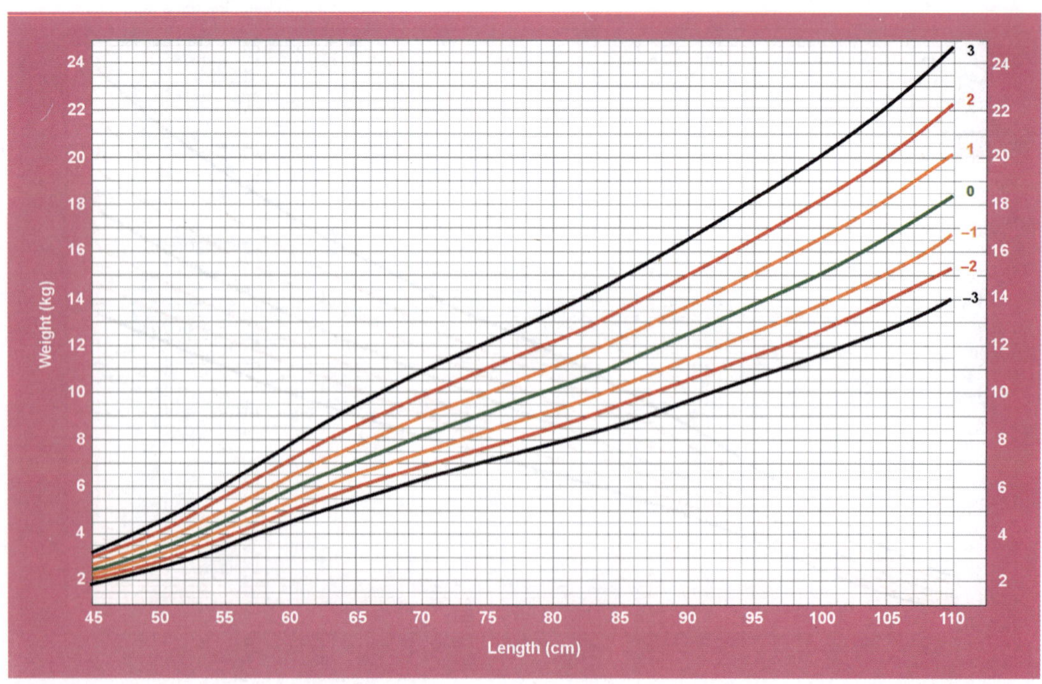

WHO Child Growth Standards

Fig. 1.15D: WHO growth chart for weight-for-length for girls 0–2 years of age (*Z*-scores)

Weight-for-height BOYS

2 to 5 years (percentiles)

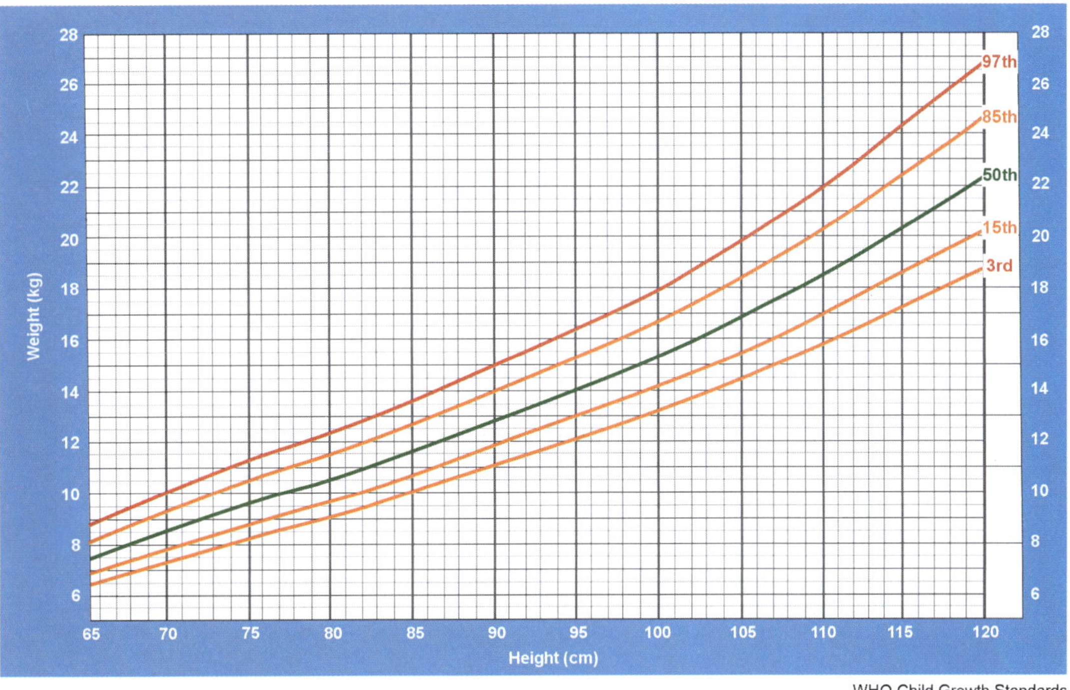

Fig. 1.16A: WHO growth chart for weight-for-height for boys 2–5 years of age (percentiles)

Weight-for-height BOYS

2 to 5 years (*Z*-scores)

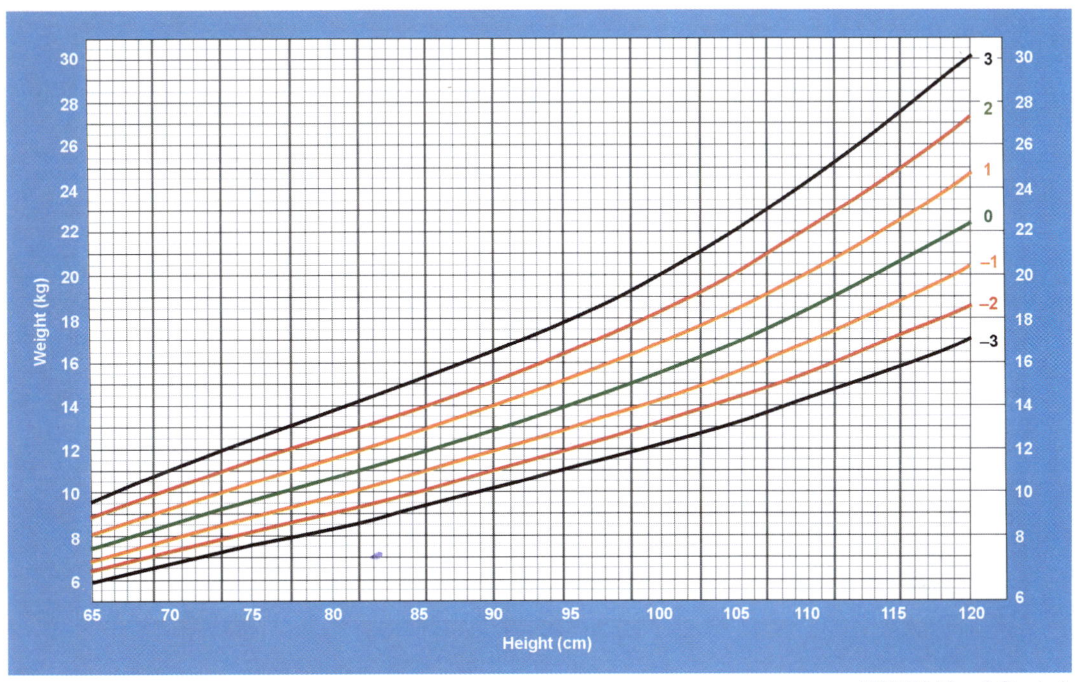

Fig. 1.16B: WHO growth chart for weight-for-height for boys 2–5 years of age (*Z*-scores)

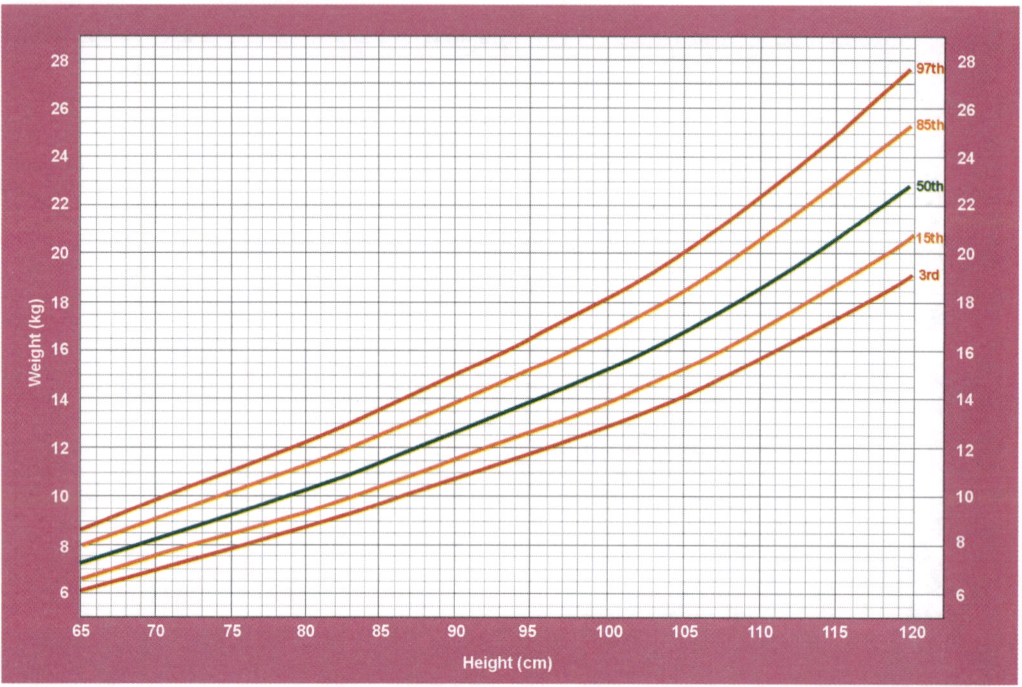

Fig. 1.16C: WHO growth chart for weight-for-height for girls 2–5 years of age (percentiles)

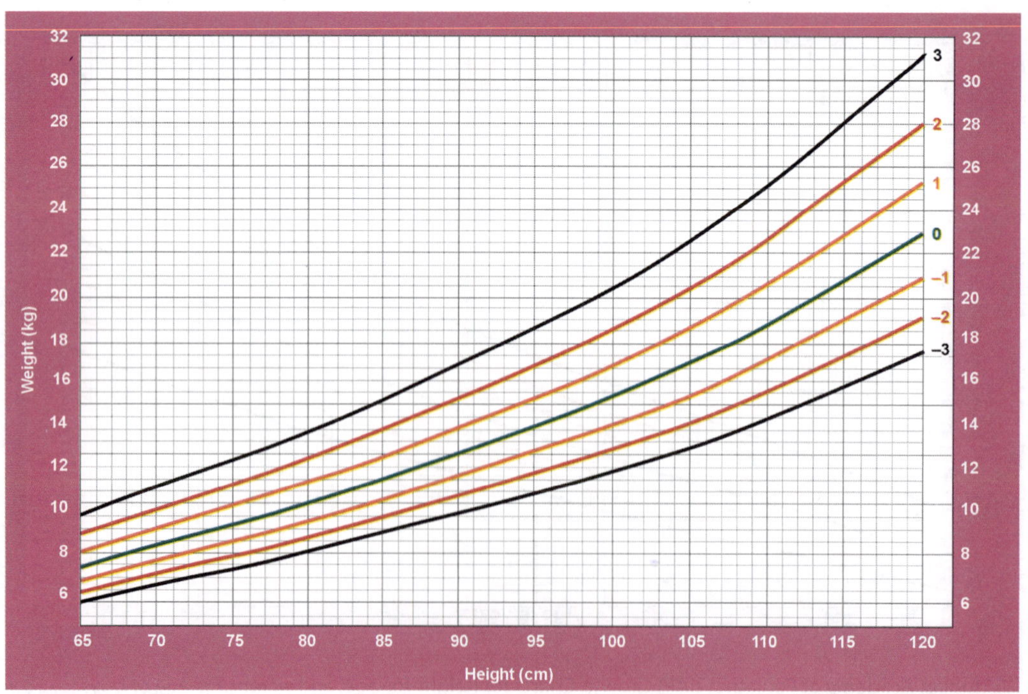

Fig. 1.16D: WHO growth chart for weight-for-height for girls 2–5 years of age (*Z*-scores)

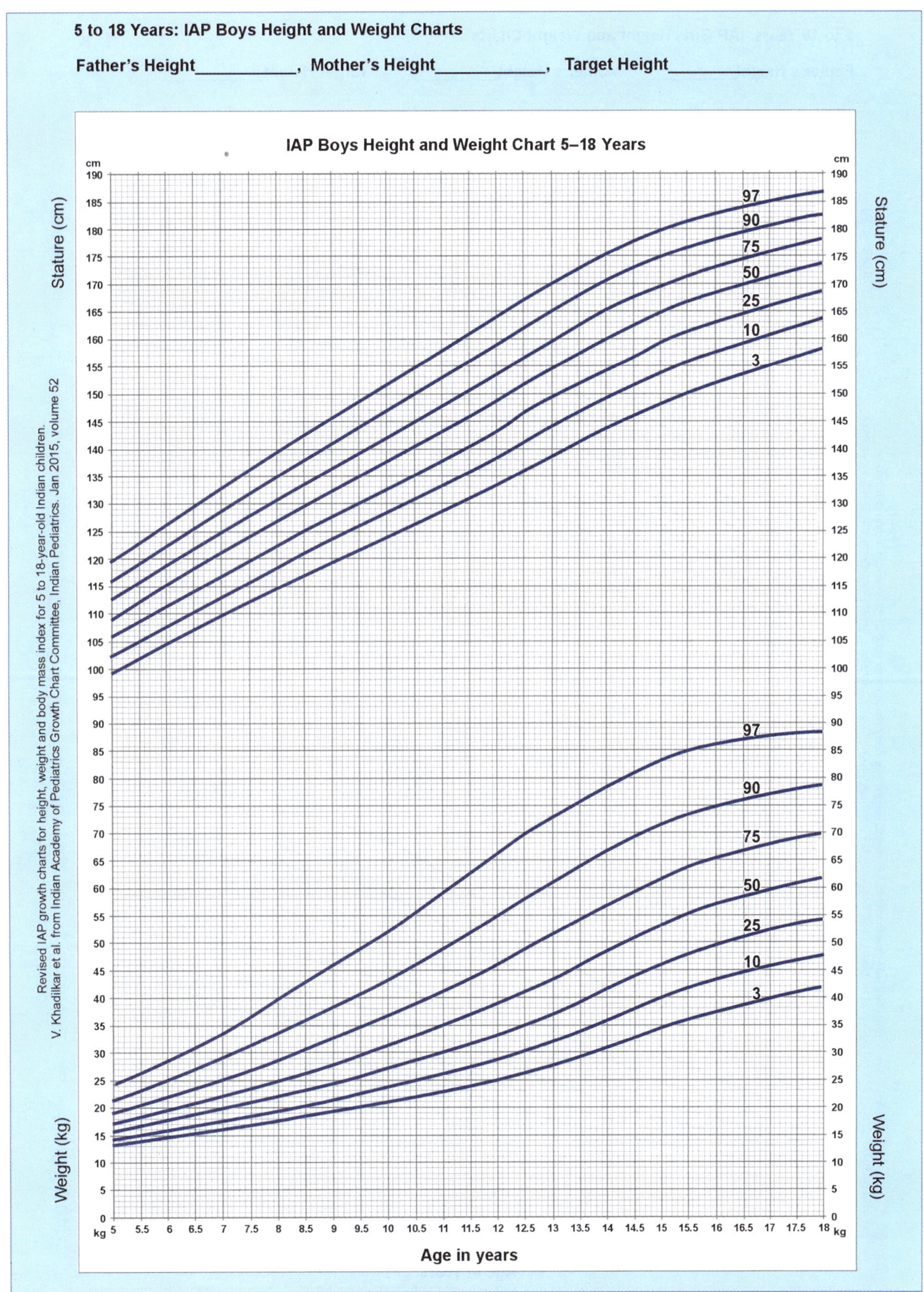

Fig. 1.17: Indian Academy of Pediatrics (IAP) Growth Charts for height-for-age, and weight-for-age of boys (5–18 years)

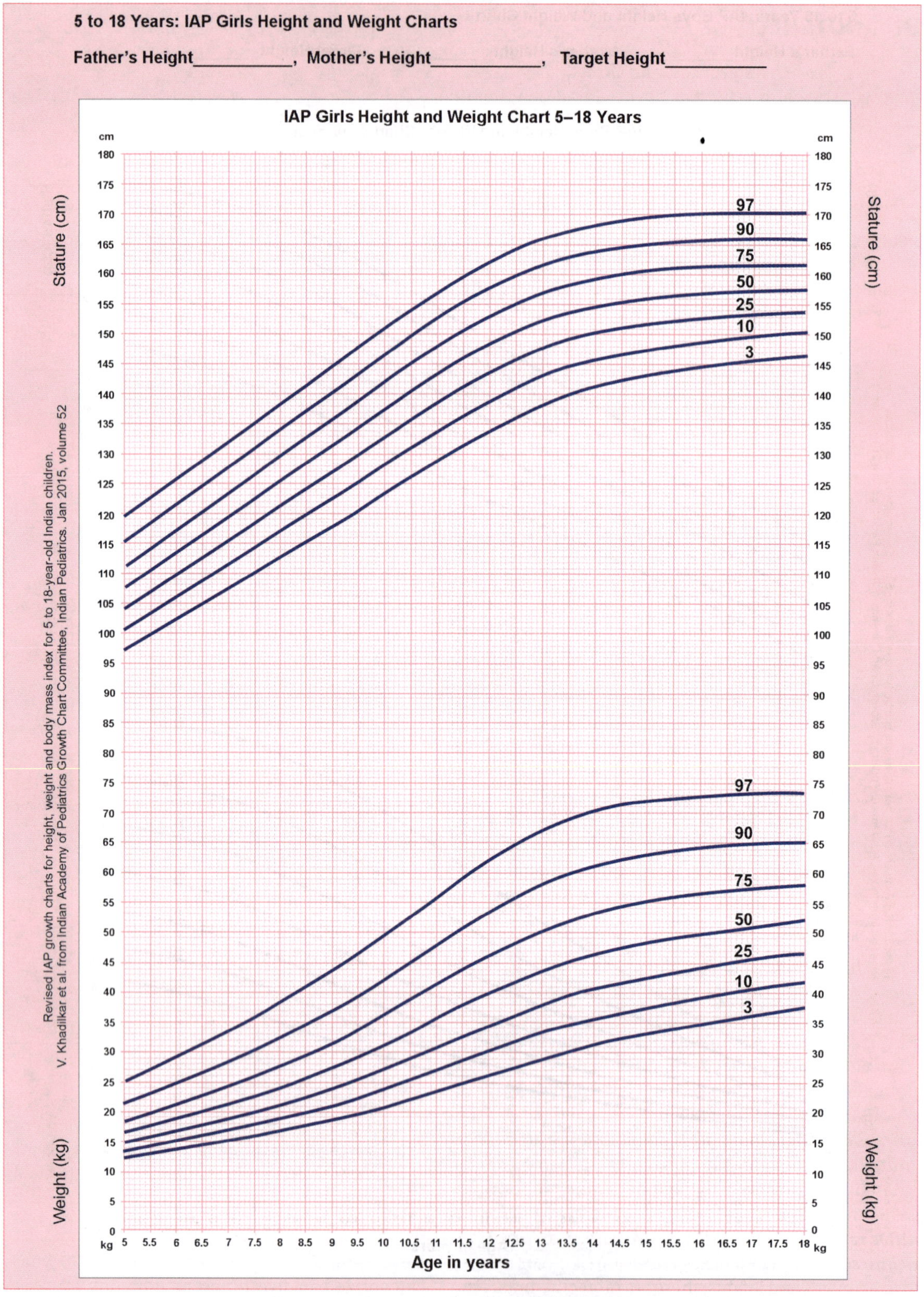

Fig. 1.18: Indian Academy of Pediatrics (IAP) Growth Charts for height-for-age and weight-for-age of girls (5–18 years)

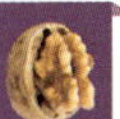

IN A NUTSHELL

Growth Charts, Growth References, and Growth Standards

1. WHO growth standards represent how children between 0 and 5 years should grow and show that all children of the world grow similarly till 5 years of age.
2. WHO growth charts are available as (a) percentile curves (corresponding to 3rd, 15th, 50th, 85th, and 97th percentiles); and (b) *Z*-score curves (corresponding to 3*Z*, −2*Z*, median, +2*Z*, and +3*Z* scores).
3. Indian Academy of Pediatrics (IAP) growth charts (for weight, height, and BMI) are used as references for evaluating growth of children between 5 and 18 years of age.

de Onis M, Garza C, Onyango AW, Borghi E. Comparison of the WHO child growth standards and the CDC 2000 growth charts. J Nutr. 2007;137:144-8.

de Onis M. 4.1 The WHO Child Growth Standards. World Rev Nutr Diet. 2015;113:278-94.

Indian Academy of Pediatrics Growth Charts Committee. Revised IAP growth charts for height, weight and body mass index for 5- to 18-year-old Indian children. Indian Pediatr. 2015;52(1):47-55.

Ong KK. WHO Growth standards: suitable for everyone? Yes. Paediatr Perinat Epidemiol. 2017;31(5):463-4.

Singh P, Gandhi S, Malhotra RK, Seth A. Impact of using different growth references on interpretation of anthropometric parameters of children aged 8–15 Years. Indian Pediatr. 2020;57(2):124-8.

van Dommelen P, van Buuren S. Methods to obtain referral criteria in growth monitoring. Stat Methods Med Res. 2014;23(4):369-89.

WHO Multicentre Growth Reference Study Group. Relationship between physical growth and motor development in the WHO Child Growth Standards. Acta Paediatr Suppl. 2006;450:96-101.

WHO Multicentre Growth Reference Study Group. WHO Child Growth Standards based on length/height, weight and age. Acta Paediatr Suppl. 2006;450:76-85.

Ziegler EE, Nelson SE. The WHO growth standards: strengths and limitations. Curr Opin Clin Nutr Metab Care. 2012;15(3):298-302.

1.8 Normal Development

PE 1.3

LAWS OF DEVELOPMENT

- ***Development is a continuous process from conception to maturity, and implies maturation of function,*** interaction with environment, communication, and independence in day-to-day activity. For example, at birth, a neonate is not able to roll over, sit, approach objects voluntarily, laugh, or interact with the help of language. In due course of time, sequentially, the infant acquires all such functions.
- ***Normal development requires an anatomically and functionally normal central nervous system***, peripheral nervous system, musculoskeletal system, hearing and vision, supported by a suitable environment. A child with a morphologically abnormal central nervous system (e.g., anencephaly and meningomyelocele) or damaged neurons and pathways (e.g., following hypoxic or ischemic insult) is unlikely to have a normal development.

  Abnormal development may result from intrauterine and perinatal insults (perinatal asphyxia, kernicterus, etc., resulting in delayed development right from birth), or disease affecting neuronal pathways and myelination in later life (trauma, meningitis, CNS hemorrhage, etc. during first 6 years of life, while the brain is still growing).
- ***The sequence of development is same and predictable in all children, but the rate may vary,*** e.g., head control always precedes sitting; however, the age of acquisition of these milestones may vary.
- ***Primitive reflexes are to be lost before voluntary functions are acquired.*** Primitive reflexes are group of motor reflexes found in neonates and infants; these are protective brainstem reflexes, which develop sequentially during late fetal life. These reflexes are essential for survival, feeding and movement while neonatal CNS is immature. For example, the grasp reflex should be lost (by 3–4 months) before the infant can learn to reach for objects and to grasp them voluntarily (by 4–5 months). Similarly, asymmetric tonic neck reflex should be lost before a child learns to turn over in bed (think, why?). Persistence of a primitive reflex, beyond the age at which it should have disappeared, indicates and predicts abnormal development. For example, Moro reflex should disappear by 4–6 months of age. A 6-month-old child with a positive Moro reflex is suggestive of abnormal development.
- ***Development always proceeds in a cephalocaudal manner,*** i.e., from head to toe. Thus, a child will learn to hold his head, followed by ability to sit and then be able to walk. This sequence will always remain the same; though, the age at which each function is achieved may differ within physiological range.

  The fine motor function of upper extremity develops in proximodistal manner, i.e., beginning at the shoulder girdle and progressing to fine movement of hands and fingers attaining important milestone of pincer grasp.
- ***Generalized mass activity is usually replaced by specific individual response,*** e.g., nonspecific, symmetric movements of arms and legs in infants are replaced by asymmetric precise grasping in older children, when presented with a toy.

DOMAINS OF DEVELOPMENT

Developmental milestones in the first 5 years of life are categorized in five different domains for assessment and screening purpose:

1. ***Motor development:***
   - ***Gross motor:*** Pertaining to development of locomotion, general body control and specific motor skills.
   - ***Fine motor:*** Pertaining to development of finer limb movements and coordination, i.e., grasping, fine hand movements, hand-eye co-ordination.
2. ***Cognition/problem solving:*** Refers to mental abilities of the child and includes imitation, simple problem solving, puzzles, drawings that eventually transform into reading, writing, and academic skills.
3. ***Personal-social development:*** Child's reaction to other persons and his adjustment to domestic life, social groups, and community conventions. This includes social behavior, feeding, sphincter control, general understanding, play activity, and dressing.
4. ***Language and speech development:*** Ability to communicate; including comprehension (receptive language) as well as expression of language (expressive language includes gestures, speech, and written language).
5. ***Adaptive/activity of daily living:*** Development of skills needed by the child to initiate new experiences and to profit by past experiences. This adaptivity includes alertness, intelligence, and various forms of constructiveness and exploration. This subset majorly decides for self-help activities transforming into independent living in society in later life.

DEVELOPMENTAL MILESTONES

Children accomplish maturation of different biological functions (level of development or milestone) at an anticipated age, with a margin of a few months on either side. Milestones are like guideposts for various stages of development, through which every child passes in the normal trajectory at a particular age.

Motor Milestones

Gross motor development: It involves control of the child over his body and locomotion, i.e., head control, sitting, standing, walking, jumping, etc. Motor development depends on the maturation of muscular, skeletal, and nervous systems **(Figs. 1.19 to 1.24)**. Ages of attainment of important gross motor milestones are provided in **Table 1.3**.

Fine motor development: It assesses the finer upper limb movements and coordination. This includes coordination of eyes, hand-eye coordination, hand-mouth coordination, and skills for manipulation with hands, i.e., grasping, fine hand movements **(Figs. 1.25 to 1.29)**, making a tower, writing, etc. Ages of attainment of important fine motor milestones are provided in **Table 1.4**.

Adaptive/Cognitive Milestones

Adaptive/cognitive development is the ability to learn or deal with new situations. In initial few weeks of life, infant explores the environment visually. Initially, he follows faces and then objects. After gaining better control of arms and hands, he starts batting at and then reaching for objects. At first, objects

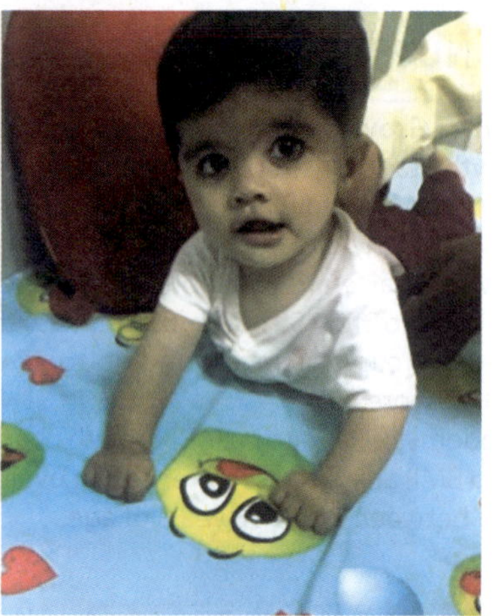

Fig. 1.19: A 12-week-old infant. The child can lift the chin and shoulders bearing weight on forearms. Plane of face reaches 90° to couch, also can be noted here social smile and connect

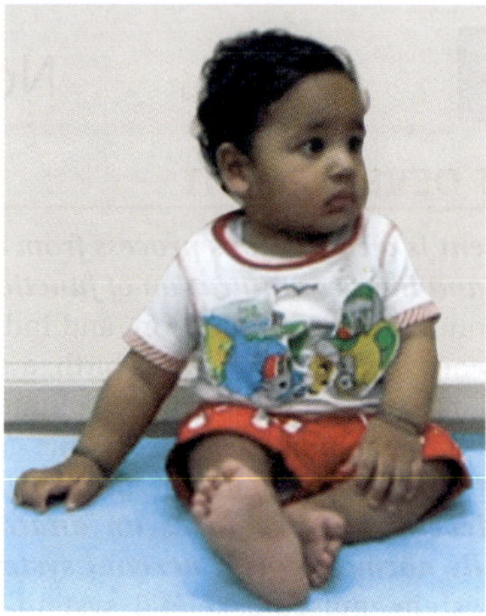

Fig. 1.20: A 6-month-old child sitting supported by hands in front or side

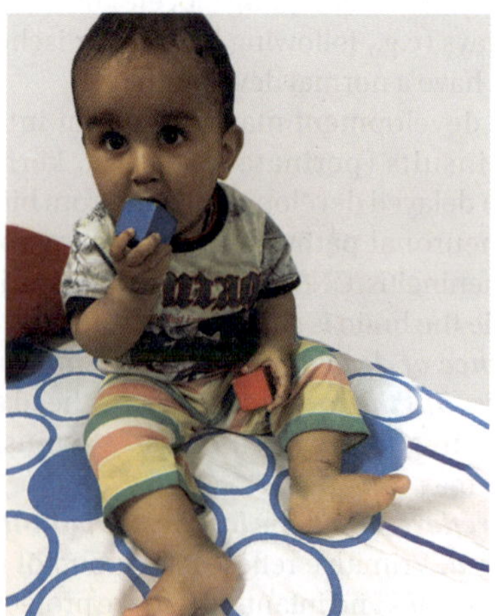

Fig. 1.21: A 9-month-old infant with stable independent sitting, mouthing from right hand and radial digital grasp on left hand

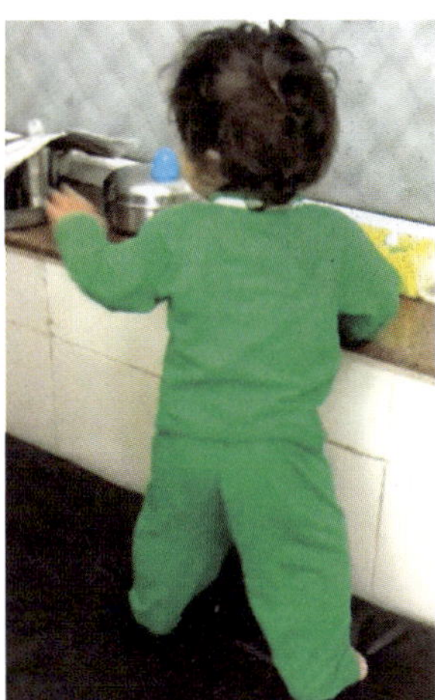

Fig. 1.22: An 11-month-old-child walking with support (cruising) able to free hands intermittently

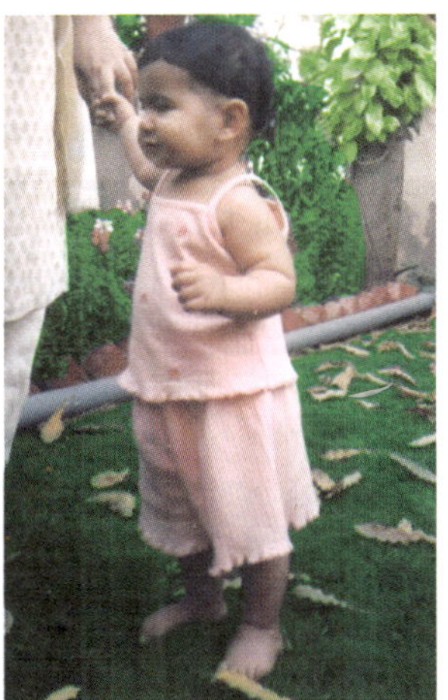

Fig. 1.23: A 12-month-old child walking with one handheld

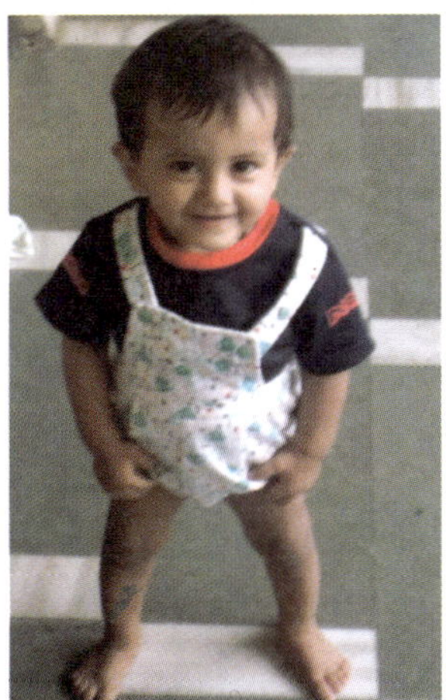

Fig. 1.24: A 13-month-old child walking independently

Table 1.3	Gross Motor Milestones: Age of Achievement
1 month	Lifts up chin momentarily in prone position
1–3 months	Lifts and controls head in the horizontal plane and then above the horizontal plane when held in ventral suspension
3 months	Neck holding, infant lifts his head and upper part of chest on forearms in prone position
5 months	Sitting with support, head control is complete
6 months	Rolling over prone to supine, sits with support
7 months	Rolling over supine to prone
8 months	Commando crawling, sits without support
9 months	Pulls to stand, begins creeping (on four)
10 months	Walking with support, creeps well
11 months	Pivots, cruises
12 months	Walks with one handheld, stands well
13 months	Walking without support
18 months	Runs stiffly, walks backward
2 years	Climbing upstairs (2 feet per step)
30 months	Jumps on both feet
3 years	Climbing upstairs (1 foot per step), riding tricycle
4 years	Comes downstairs (1 foot per step), hops on one foot
5 years	Skips with both feet

are brought to the mouth for oral exploration. Later, the infant visually examines an object held in one hand while manipulating it with the other.

With maturation of vision, infant can focus on small objects by about 5 months of age. By 1 year, the child explores objects by poking and discovering how they work. The child learns to shift attention between two objects, learns how his actions produce certain effects, and how to repeat these actions to get the same effects, and later, how to vary the action to produce a

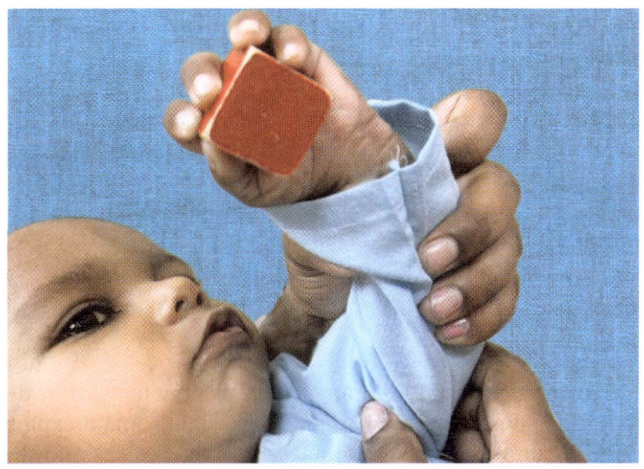

Fig. 1.25: A 6-month-old infant holding a block with ulnar palmar grasp

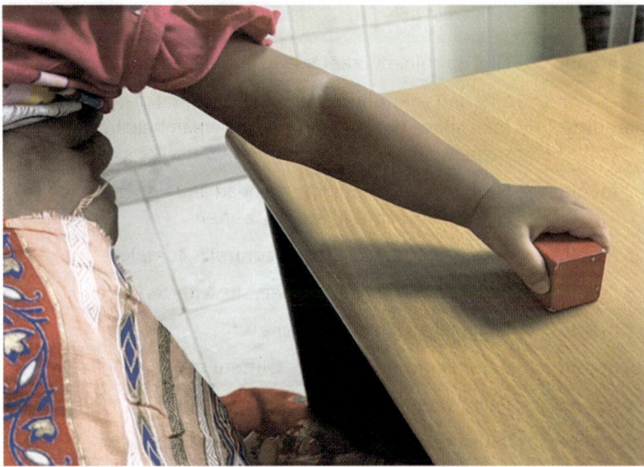

Fig. 1.26: A 9-month-old baby. Holds cube steady with index finger and thumb (radial digital grasp)

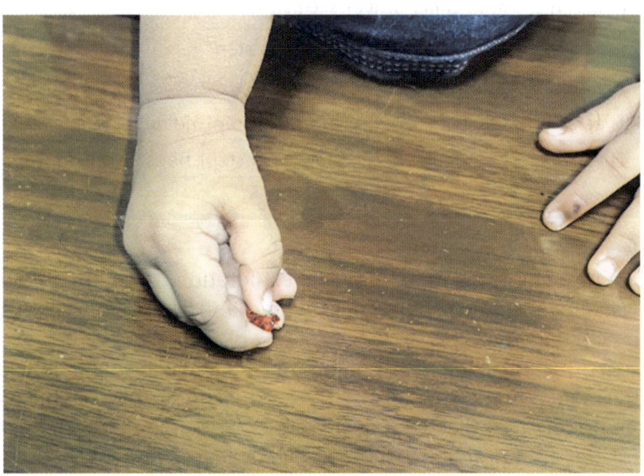

Fig. 1.27: An 11-month-old baby with mature pincer grasp

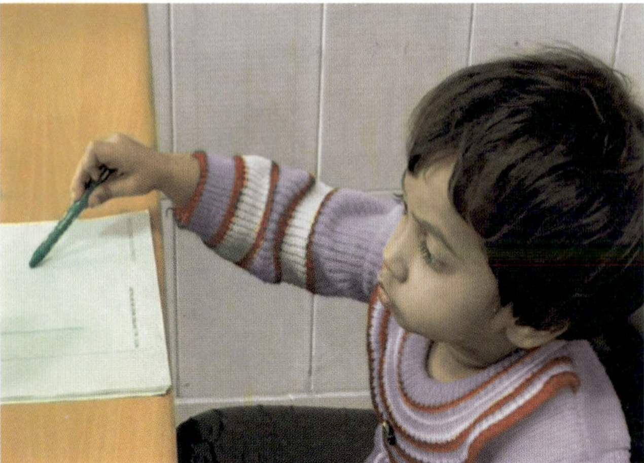

Fig. 1.28: A 20-month-old child holding color pen with digital pronate grasp

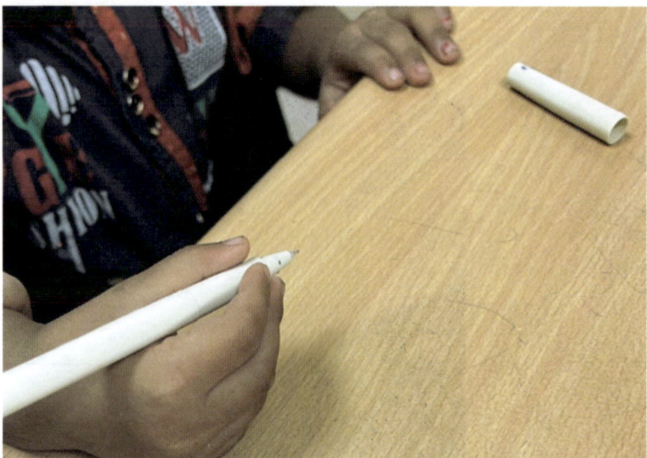

Fig. 1.29: A 3.5-year-old child holding pen in tripod grasp

Table 1.4	Fine Motor Milestones: Age of Achievement
3 months	Opens hand spontaneously, holds objects when given in hand, inspects fingers (hand regards)
4 months	Tries to reach for objects (red ring), overshoots
5 months	Reaches (bidextrous approach) for a red cube held within reach; holds it with both hands
6 months	Unidextrous approach, transfers objects from one hand to another hand
7 months	Radial palmar grasp
8 months	Finger-thumb scissors grasp
9–10 months	Pincer grasp (holding between index finger and thumb), voluntary release (mature)
10–11 months	Mature pincer grasp (can pick a pellet neatly, using ends of his thumb and index fingers)
1 year	Tower of 2 cubes, casting, imitates scribbling
13 months	Can turn two or three pages of a book at a time
15 months	Tower of 3 cubes
18 months	Tower of 4 cubes, imitates vertical line
2 years	Tower of 6 cubes, imitates a horizontal line, imitates train, no chimney
2½ years	Tower of 8 cubes, imitates train, adds chimney
3 years	Tower of 9–10 cubes, copies a circle, imitates bridge
4 years	Copies a cross (plus sign), imitates gate
5 years	Copies multiplication sign, triangle, gate

novel effect. These skills need combined efforts of motor skills, normal vision, hearing, coordination, and cognitive skills. Ages of attainment of important adaptive/cognitive milestones are provided in **Table 1.5**.

Personal Social Milestones

Personal social development is a very broad area that includes intellectual, moral, emotional, social, and spiritual development.

Table 1.5	Adaptive/Cognitive Milestones: Age of Achievement
4 weeks	Follows red ring by 45°
6 weeks	Follows up to 90°
8 weeks	Follows moving person
3 months	Hand regards, follows to 180°
4 months	Excited on seeing food, toys; shows pleasure by massive response
5 months	Mouthing, no hand regards
6 months	Looks for dropped toy
7 months	Observes cubes in each hand, finds partially hidden objects
8 months	Reaches for out of reach toys
10 months	Responds to "No"
11 months	Looks at picture in book, finds toys under the cup
15 months	Turns 2–3 pages at a time
18 months	Turns 1 page at a time, names one common object
2 years	Points at 4–6 body parts, sorts objects
30 months	Names 1 color, matches shape/colors
3 years	Names 2 colors, knows gender and age
4 years	Names 5–6 colors, right-left discrimination
5 years	Counts till 10, names 10 colors, identifies coins

Ages of attainment of important personal social milestones are provided in **Table 1.6**.

Table 1.6	Personal Social Milestones: Age of Achievement
2 months	Social smile **(Fig. 1.29)**
3 months	Recognizing mother
5–6 months	Smiles at mirror image
6–7 months	Enjoys peek-a-boo
8–9 months	Stranger anxiety
10 months	Waves "bye-bye"
1 year	Helps in dressing, plays a simple ball game
18 months	Engages in domestic mimicry
2 years	Dry by day
30 months	Washes hands, brushes teeth
3 years	Dry at night, can withhold bowel movement, dresses, undresses fully if helped with buttons
4 years	Goes to toilet alone
5 years	Dressing and bathing independently

Table 1.7	Language Milestones: Age of Achievement
1 month	Turns head to sound
3 months	Cooing
4 months	Laughs aloud, says Ah-goo
6–7 months	Speaks monosyllables (ma, ba)
8–9 months	Speaks bisyllables (mama, baba)
1 year	Speaks 2–3 words with meaning
18 months	Speaks 10 words with meaning
2 years	Can form simple sentence using 2 words
3 years	3 words sentence, 250 words vocabulary
4 years	4 words sentence, tells stories
5 years	5–8 words sentence, knows telephone number

Language Milestones

Language is the expression of communication through which knowledge, belief, and behavior can be experienced, explained, and shared with others. *Receptive language* is the ability to understand what is being said. *Expressive language* refers to the ability to make thoughts, ideas known to others through speech, gestures, and facial expressions. Ages of attainment of important language milestones are provided in **Table 1.7**.

Table 1.8 provides a bird's eye view of achievement of various milestones at key ages.

Variations in Normal Development

There is no set age at which all children must acquire a particular milestone. One particular aspect, e.g., motor development or speech, may be delayed in the child without being abnormal or retarded. Due to wide variability in the ages of attainment of different milestones, it may be difficult to draw a strict line between normal and abnormal on single assessment.

Children who are at borderline may ultimately turn out to be abnormal or just a variant of the normal. For correct diagnosis, one should follow these children regularly with a screening test as described in the next section.

Children who are ideal in all fields are not that common. Some are slow starters in a field and then catch up after a time-lag. Some children start well but may have a temporary cessation in development due to illness, protein energy malnutrition or other factors. Some may deteriorate after a point referred to as to neurological or developmental regression. A few children with development delay due to lack of stimulation may show unexpected improvement when placed in appropriate environment.

Table 1.8 A Guide to Developmental Assessment of the Child

Age	Gross motor	Fine motor/vision	Adaptive/cognitive	Language/hearing	Personal/social
6 weeks	Body straight on ventral suspension	Turns to light	Follows red ring up to 90°	Startles to loud sound	Social smile
3 months	Neck holding	Tries to reach for objects, overshoots	Follows up to 180°, hand regards	Vocalization, cooing	Recognizing mother
6 months	Rolls prone to supine, sits with support	Unidextrous approach, transfers objects from hand to hand	Looks for dropped toy	Monosyllables (ma)	Smiles/vocalizes at mirror image (5–6 months), peek-a-boo (6–7 months)
9 months	Sits unsupported (8 months) standing with support	Assisted pincer grasp	Responds to "no" (10 months)	Bisyllables (mama)	Stranger anxiety (8–9 months)
12 months	Walks with one handheld	2 cubes tower	Puts objects in/out of container	Speaks 2–3 words with meaning	Plays simple ball game, helps in dressing
15 months	Walks alone (13 months)	3 cubes tower	Turns 2–3 pages at a time	Speaks 3–5 words	Indicates desire by pointing at objects
18 months	Running, walks backward	4 cubes tower, imitates (vertical line)	Turns 1 page at a time, names 1 object	Speaks 10–15 words	Symbolic play alone, feeds independently
2 years	Climbs upstairs (2 feet per step)	6–7 cubes tower, imitates (horizontal line)	Points at 4–6 body parts	2 words sentence, use 50+ words	Dry by day, parallel play
3 years	Climbs upstairs (1 foot per step), walks downstairs (2 feet per step), rides tricycle	10 cubes tower, copies ○ (circle)	Names 2 colors, knows gender/age	3 words sentence, 250+ words vocabulary	Dry by night
4 years	Walks downstairs (1 foot per step), hops on one foot	Copies bridge and + (plus sign)	Names 5–6 colors, discriminates right-left	4 words sentence, 250+ words vocabulary	Goes to toilet alone, plays with up to 3 other kids
5 years	Skips with both feet	Copies gate, ×, Δ (cross and triangle)	Names 10 colors, identifies coins	5–8 words sentence, grammatical speech	Independent dressing and bathing

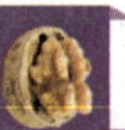

IN A NUTSHELL

Normal Development

1. At birth, a child's sensory, motor, and neurologic capacities attribute to organizing experiences and interacting with the environment, resulting in development.
2. The laws of development are universal, and every child goes through the same sequence although rate and character may vary.
3. Development depends upon various mutually interactive factors which can be broadly divided into biological, social, and psychological factors.
4. Development is usually defined and measured under five domains namely: (1) Motor development (Gross motor and Fine motor), (2) Cognition/problem solving, (3) Personal-social development, (4) Language and speech development, and (5) Adaptive functioning/activity of daily living.
5. There may be variations in normal development which could manifest as developmental dissociation, developmental delay, and developmental deviance, and therefore development should be monitored over time.

Berk LE. Child Development, 9th edition. Boston, MA: Pearson; 2013.
Bridgman A. Child Development. Child Dev. 2015;86(2):337-41.
Cioni G, Sgandurra G. Normal psychomotor development. Handb Clin Neurol. 2013;111:3-15.
Gupta P. Clinical Methods in Pediatrics, 5th edition. New Delhi: CBS Publishers; 2022.
Illingworth RS. Child care in general practice. Normal development. Br Med J. 1964;2(5419):1245-8.
Machado LR, da Silva CFR, Hadders-Algra M, et al. Psychometric properties of the Infant Motor Profile (IMP): A scoping review protocol. PLoS One. 2022;17(11):e0277755.
Misirliyan SS, Huynh AP. Development Milestones. In: StatPearls [Internet]. Treasure Island (FL): Stat Pearls Publishing; 2022.
Sadaka Y, Sudry T, Zimmerman DR, et al. Assessing the Attainment Rates of Updated CDC Milestones Using a New Israeli Developmental Scale. Pediatrics. 2022:e2022057499.
Scharf RJ, Scharf GJ, Stroustrup A. Developmental milestones. Pediatr Rev. 2016;37(1):25-47.
Thompson RA. Development in the first year of life. Future Child. 2001;11(1):20-33.
Wilks T, Gerber RJ, Erdie-Lalena C. Developmental milestones: cognitive development. Pediatr Rev. 2010;31(9):364-7.

1.9 Developmental Assessment

PE 1.3

TIMING OF ASSESSMENT

Developmental surveillance (an informal, more flexible, and ongoing assessment of development) should be a part of all well-baby clinic visits like immunization. During each visit the clinician should observe the normal milestones and presence of any red flags. Presence of any developmental red flag warrants an immediate referral and a detailed assessment. The list of developmental red flags are given in **Table 1.9**.

Developmental screening: Supported with culturally accepted tools, developmental screening is considered superior to developmental surveillance. Indian Academy of Pediatrics (IAP) recommends routine developmental screening using standardized screening tools at 9–12 months, 18–24 months of age, and at school entry and additionally at 4–6 months of age for high-risk infants. The age of routine screening coincides with the immunization visits. For autism, IAP recommends, children should be screened by standardized autism screening tools like Modified Checklist for Autism in Toddlers M-CHAT, and Trivandrum Autism Behavior Checklist (TABC) at 18 and 24 months of age.

DEVELOPMENTAL HISTORY

A detailed history is vital part of developmental assessment. History of prenatal and perinatal risk factors is highly relevant to mental and physical development. Additionally, history of important genetic conditions, degenerative disorders, and environmental factors (child abuse, parent child relations, etc.) that may lead to delayed development are important. Relevant illnesses such as rickets, malnutrition, and systemic disorders that may adversely affect development should be inquired about.

Assessment of chronology of development and age of achievement of milestones is the next step. This history should preferably be taken from the mother. There may be a family history of early or late motor, social, or language development. The developmental history should be asked in simple language and a precise manner. During inquiry about developing a new skill, the following questions should be asked: (i) when did it develop; (ii) how often it is practiced; and (iii) what is the degree of maturity with which this skill is performed.

Table 1.9 Developmental Red Flags

Motor development:	
• 1–2 months	• Early rolling/log rolling
• 3 months	• Persistent fisting
• 4 months	• Poor head control in prone or supported sitting/no purposeful hand use
• 9 months	• No independent sitting/not bearing weight on feet
• 18 months	• Not walking independently
• <18 months	• Hand dominance
• Any age	• Parental concern on rate of development or unusual postures (e.g., scissoring, frog leg posture, w-sitting, bunny hopping)
Language development:	
• 6 months	• No cooing responsively
• 9 months	• No babbling
• 18 months	• No meaningful use of single words like mama, papa, dada • No understanding of simple commands • Not pointing to need based objects
• 24 months	• No 2 words phrases, <50% intelligibility of speech
• 36 months	• No 3 words sentences, <75% intelligibility of speech
• 4–5 years	• Not able to tell a simple story
Personal-social development:	
• 6 months	• Lack of smile or other joyful expression
• 9 months	• Lack of reciprocal vocalizations/responsive smiling
• 12 months	• Failure to respond to name (with intact hearing), lack of gestures (showing, reaching, and waving)
• 15 months	• Lack of pointing to need based objects (protoimperative)
• 18 months	• Lack of pointing to show interest (protodeclarative) or no joint attention
• 24 months	• Lack of simple pretend play
Adaptive/cognitive development:	*In the presence of normal vision and hearing:*
• 2 months	• Lack of fixation
• 4 months	• Lack of visual tracking
• 6 months	• Failure to turn to sound or voice
At any age	Loss of previously attained milestones

DEVELOPMENTAL EXAMINATION

Prerequisites: Developmental examination in a young child is difficult. Therefore, it should preferably be performed before systemic examination and should be done when the child is well fed, not sleepy, happy and in a playful mood. The assessment should be performed in front of mother or primary caregiver and care should be taken to keep only relevant toys and objects so as not to distract the child. No rigid pattern should be followed while doing the assessment. Before performing the developmental assessment, the vision and hearing of the child should be checked as it may affect development and interpretation of assessment.

Tools for developmental assessment: For a good developmental assessment, examiner should observe the child during free play and child's interaction with peers. For children till 5 years of age, tools required for developmental assessment include:

- A red ring (for visual fixation and tracking and reaching for objects)
- A small bell (for testing hearing; held 30 cm away from ear and away from the sight)
- Pellets made of cardboard, wool or paper; 8 mm size (pincer grasp)
- 10 cubes of 1 inch each (transfer of objects, different types of grasp, imitating/building tower/bridge)
- Crayon and paper (scribbling, imitating, and copying strokes/shapes, naming colors)
- A picture book of common objects (pointing, naming objects, fine motor skills of turning paper, joint interest)
- Doll (pretend play)
- Simple form board
- Colored and uncolored geometric forms
- Goddard's form board (for children >3 years of age)

PROCESS OF ASSESSMENT

Between 1 and 3 Months

- Observe the baby in the mother's lap; observe for any obvious abnormality such as fisting, tightness of body, etc.
- Notice, if the child watches the mother, smiles or produces sound. The child starts smiling at the mother from 6 to 8 weeks onward in response to visual/verbal contact.
- Note the shape and size of the head. Palpate sutures and anterior fontanel.
- Assess resistance to passive movement for tone. Loose limbs indicate *hypotonia* while stiff limbs indicate *hypertonia*.
- Place the child supine on the surface and observe the posture:
  - ***Up to 8–10 weeks:*** Generally, flexed posture with symmetrical writhing. Arm extends on the same side, to which the head is turned (asymmetric tonic neck reflex) **(Fig. 1.30)**.
  - ***12 weeks:*** No more appearance of asymmetric tonic neck reflex.
- Observe the hands:
  - ***4 weeks:*** Closed hands, presence of grasp reflex.
  - ***8 weeks:*** Opens hands frequently, slight grasp reflex.
  - ***12 weeks:*** Hands loosely open, may hold a rattle for a minute, if placed in hand. No grasp reflex.

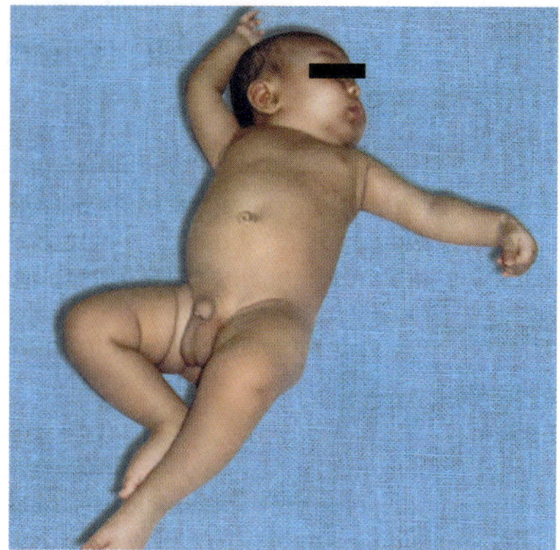

Fig. 1.30: Asymmetric tonic neck reflex

- Pull the child from supine position. Observe head lag and back:
  - ***4 weeks:*** Complete head lag, back completely rounded **(Fig. 1.31A)**.
  - ***8 weeks:*** Able to hold up head momentarily, less rounding of back **(Fig. 1.31B)**.
  - ***12 weeks:*** Head held up most of the time.
- Hold the child in standing position:
  - Child should have some flexion at hips and knees and able to place sole on the surface **(Fig. 1.32)**.
  - In a hypotonic child, the arms and legs hang loosely; while in a spastic child, the two legs may cross each other in a scissoring position.
- Hold the child in ventral suspension as shown in **Figures 1.33A to C** by placing the child prone in air with hand under the abdomen. Watch for position of limbs and head control:
  - ***0–2 weeks:*** Curled up on ventral suspension. Note flexion of elbows, knees with some extension at hips **(Fig. 1.33A)**.
  - ***4 weeks:*** The child holds up the head momentarily. There is some flexion at the knees and hip. Back is rounded **(Fig. 1.33B)**.
  - ***6 weeks:*** Head held momentarily in plane of body.
  - ***8 weeks:*** Maintains head in the same plane as rest of the body **(Fig. 1.33C)**.
  - ***12 weeks:*** The child holds the head up and above the plane of the body for considerable time.
- Keep the child prone on an even surface. Observe the posture; especially chin, pelvis, and thighs **(Figs. 1.34A to C)**:
  - ***0–2 weeks:*** The pelvis is high and the knees are drawn under the abdomen. Back is rounded, head remains on one side **(Fig. 1.34A)**.
  - ***6 weeks:*** Knees are not under abdomen. Hips extended. Chin raised from the couch intermittently.
  - ***8 weeks:*** Head mostly in midline. Lifts chin off the couch up to 45°C **(Fig. 1.34B)**.
  - ***12 weeks:*** Child can lift the chin as well as the shoulders off the surface or couch, up to 90°, bearing weight on the forearms. Pelvis is flat on the surface **(Fig. 1.34C)**.

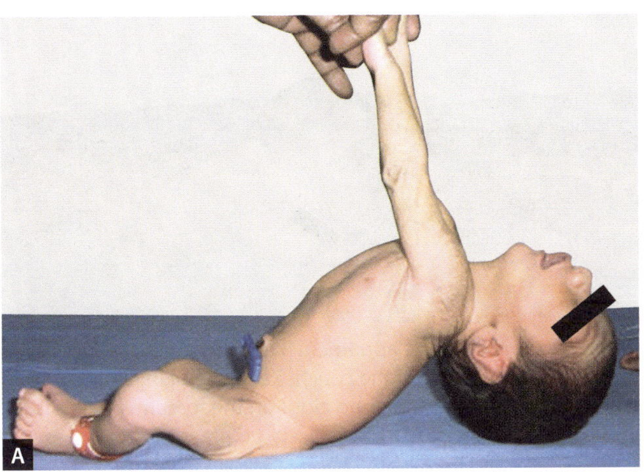

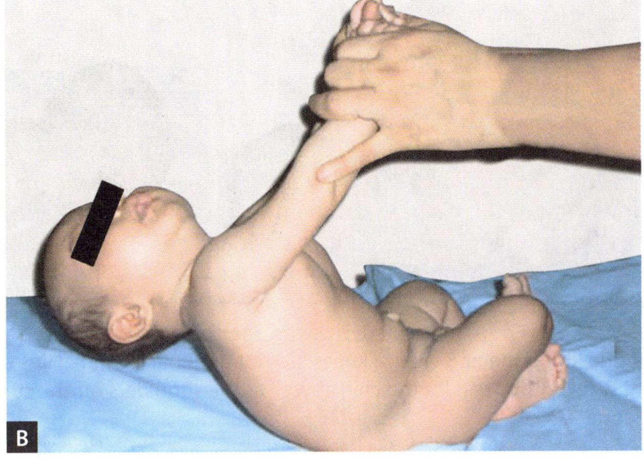

Figs. 1.31A and B: Pull from supine: (A) Complete head lag, back completely rounded at 4 weeks; (B) Able to hold up head momentarily at 8 weeks; back is less rounded

Between 4 and 6 Months

- ***Observe the child:*** Note facial expressions, vocalization, altertness, and interest in surroundings. Check vision and hearing.
- Place a rattle in the hand of the child. Observe, how he plays with it? At 4 months, the child plays with rattle placed in hand for long period; but cannot pick it up, if he drops it. At 5 months, he recovers the rattle, if dropped; and at 6 months, he looks for the dropped rattle.
- Place a 1-inch cube in front of the child. Observe whether he gets it (5 months) and if yes, whether he transfers it from one hand to the other (6 months).
- Watch for hand regards (normal between 3 and 5 months of age). It should disappear by 5 months of age.
- Place the child in prone position and observe:
  - ***4–5 months:*** Can lift the head and chest off the surface, bearing weight on forearms **(Fig. 1.35)**.
  - ***5–6 months:*** Can lift the head and chest off the surface with weight bearing only on hands, may roll from prone to supine.
- ***Place the child supine and observe:*** The child lifts the head off the surface when about to be pulled up (6 months).

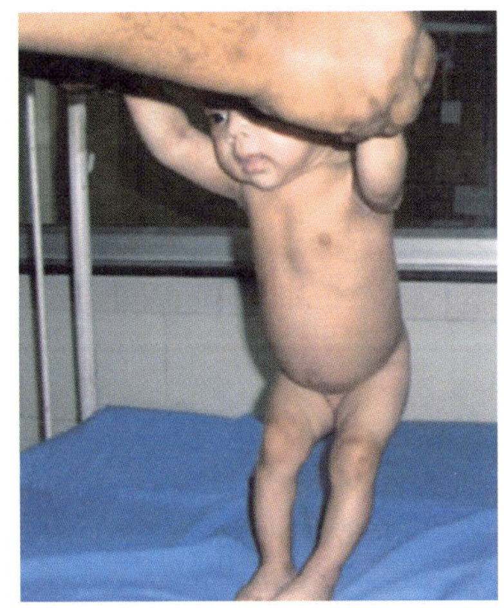

Fig. 1.32: Child <12-week-old is able to place sole on surface while held in stand position. No weight bearing

- Pull the child to sitting position. Look for head lag:
  - If head lag is present, the development is <5 months. There may be a slight head lag at beginning of 4 months.

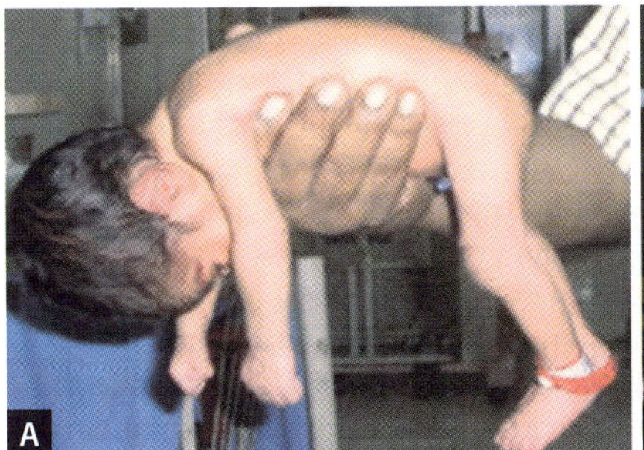

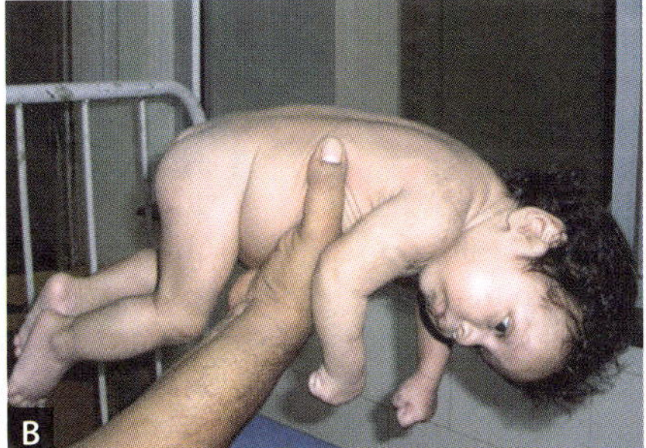

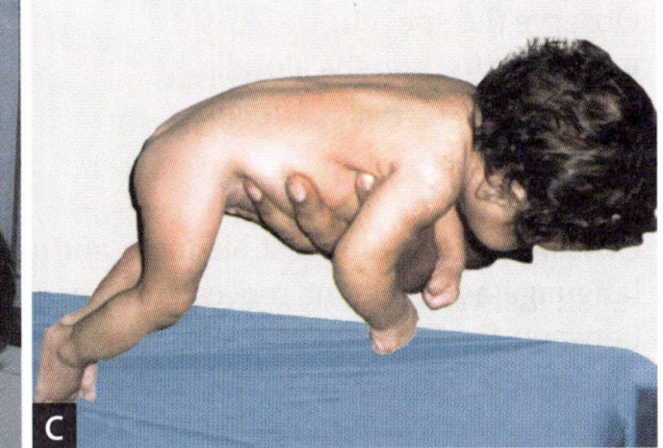

Figs. 1.33A to C: (A) Ventral suspension at 0–2 weeks. Child curled up; flexion of elbows and knees with some extension at hips; (B) Ventral suspension at 4 weeks. Child holds up the head momentarily. There is some flexion at the knees and hip. Back is rounded; (C) Ventral suspension at 8 weeks. Head is maintained in the same plane as rest of the body

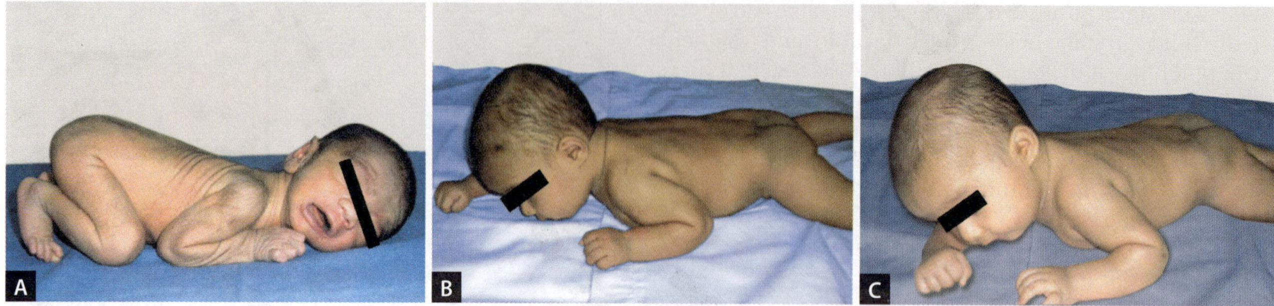

Figs. 1.34A to C: (A) Prone at 0–2 weeks: The pelvis is high and the knees are drawn under the abdomen. Back is rounded, head remains on one side; (B) Prone at 8 weeks: Knees are not under abdomen. Hips extended. Chin raised from the couch. Keeps head in midline; (C) Prone at 12 weeks: Child can lift the chin as well as the shoulders off the surface or couch, up to 90°, bearing eight on the forearms. Pelvis is flat on the surface

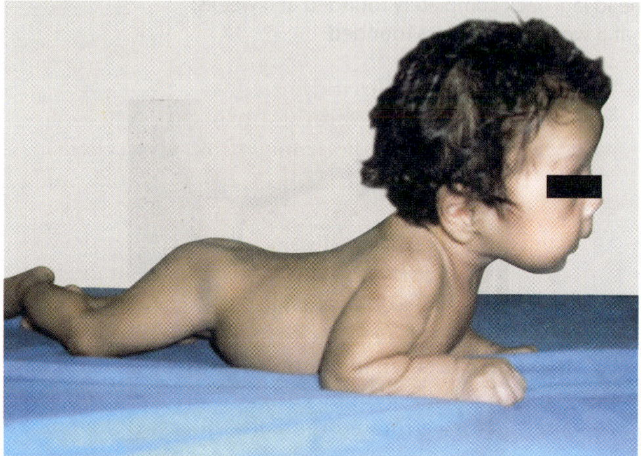

Fig. 1.35: Prone: A 4–5-month-old child can lift the head and chest off the surface, bearing weight on forearms

- If there is no head lag, watch for the support required for sitting:
  - ***4 months:*** Sits with both hands held **(Fig. 1.36A)**.
  - ***5 months:*** Sits supported in a high chair or mother's lap.
  - ***6 months:*** Sits with his own hands on surface for support **(Fig. 1.36B)**.
- Hold the child in standing position. By 5-6 months, the child is able to bear most of the weight on legs.
- ***Show a mirror:*** Smiles at mirror image by 6 months.
- Observe the speech:
  - ***4 months:*** Laughs aloud.
  - ***5 months:*** Speaks *Ah-goo*.

Between 6 and 12 Months

- Observe the child's interest, alertness, and quality of vocalization/language as he sits or moves around. Does he differentiate between family and strangers? Also, notice interaction with mother, e.g., in peek-a-boo and pat-a-cake games.
- ***Offer a cube:*** With the child sitting in the mother's lap, place a cube on the table in front of the child. Observe, how the child approaches the cube and also observe what the child does with it:

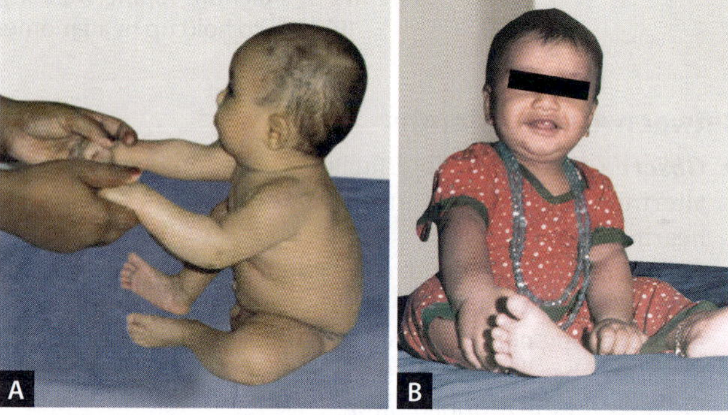

Figs. 1.36A and B: Pull the child to sitting position: (A) Sits with both hands held at 4 months; (B) Sits with hands on surface for support

  - ***6 months:*** Approaches cube with fingers and holds cube with the palm on the ulnar side **(Fig. 1.25)**. *Unidextrous approach*.
  - ***7 months:*** Radial *palmar grasp* of cube.
  - ***8 months:*** *Scissor grasp* (using all four fingers against the thumb).
  - ***9–12 months:*** Approaches cube by index finger and holds cube steady with index finger and thumb **(Fig. 1.26)**. This is *mature grasp*.
- As soon as the child takes one cube, offer the second cube:
  - ***5 months:*** Drops first cube when second is offered.
  - ***6 months:*** Retains the first cube in hand and takes the second cube also. Transfers from one hand to another.
  - ***9 months:*** Compares two cubes by bringing them together.
- Offer a pellet. Watch the approach and the grasp:
  - ***7–9 months:*** Approaches with all the fingers/hand (rakes). Not able to pick it up.
  - ***9–12 months:*** Able to pick up the pellet between tip of thumb and forefinger **(Fig. 1.27)**.
- Place the child in the sitting posture and observe:
  - ***7 months:*** Can sit unsupported, momentarily.
  - ***8 months:*** Can sit steadily on floor without support.
  - ***10 months:*** Sits steadily without risk of imbalancing. Can pivot around to pick a toy from back/side.
- Place in the prone position and observe for creeping (9–10 months).

- Pull to the stand position, offer support of a table and observe. If the child can stand holding on to furniture and whether he can pull himself to standing position. Also watch, if he can walk around holding on to furniture.
  - ***9–10 months:*** Stands holding on to furniture, pulls to stand.
  - ***10–11 months:*** Can walk around holding onto the furniture.
  - ***12–13 months:*** Stands independently, takes a few independent steps.

Between 1 and 2 Years

- If child comes walking into the room, watch his gait and assess its maturity. Observe his interest in toys or pictures hanging in the room. Does he point at things to ask for them or show something interesting to parents?
- ***Offer 10 cubes:*** Show him how to build a tower and then let him do the same. This process is known as *imitating*. See how many cubes he can utilize in building a tower **(Fig. 1.37)**.
  - ***15 months:*** Tower of 2 cubes.
  - ***18 months:*** Tower of 3–4 cubes.
  - ***2 years:*** Tower of 6–7 cubes.

  Warning signs: The child should not take the cube to his mouth after the age of 15 months. Similarly, he should not be throwing cubes on the floor, one after another, after 18 months.
- ***Train and chimney:*** Demonstrate how to make a train of 9 cubes and place the 10th one on top of the first one (chimney). Ask him to do the same. A 2-year-old child can make the train, but fails to put the chimney.
- ***Picture identification and naming:*** Show picture cards or book, and ask to identify them in the following format "where is the cat"? At a later age, you may ask "what is that"? This is known as *picture naming* and more difficult **(Fig. 1.38)**.
  - ***18 months:*** Identifies 1 object and names 1 object.
  - ***2 years:*** Identifies 5 objects; can name 3 objects.
- ***Give a picture book:*** See, how many pages of a book, he can turn at one time.
  - ***15 months:*** Turns 2–3 pages at a time.
  - ***18 months:*** Turns 1 page at a time.
- ***Offer pen and paper and notice any spontaneous scribbling.*** Ask to *imitate* (by showing how to do it by drawing in his/her sight) the drawing of a vertical stroke (|), horizontal stroke (—), and a circle. Interpret as follows:
  - ***12 months:*** Imitates scribbling.

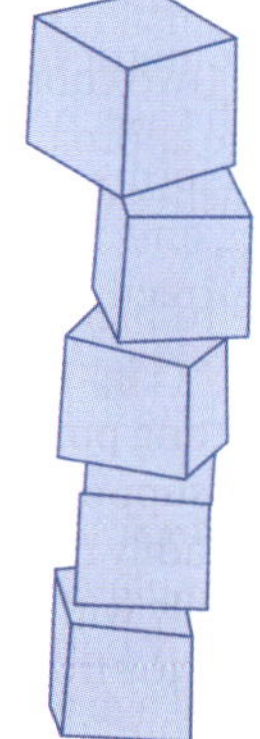

Fig. 1.37: Tower of cubes

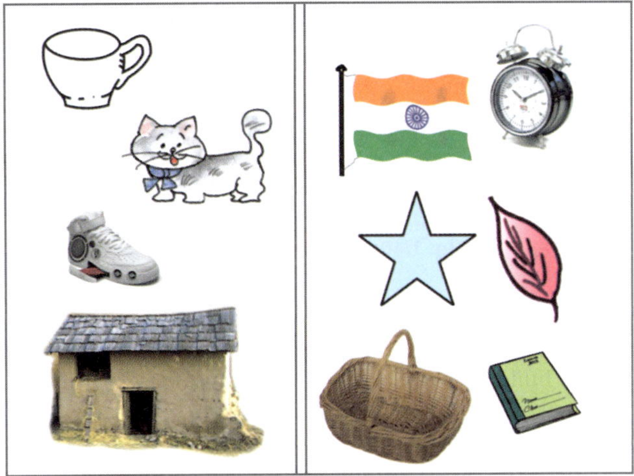

Fig. 1.38: Common pictures for identification

  - ***15 months:*** Scribbles haphazardly.
  - ***18 months:*** Imitates vertical stroke.
  - ***2 years:*** Can imitate horizontal stroke and a circle.
- ***Offer simple form board*** **(Fig. 1.39)**. First, offer only the round block.
  - If the child puts the round block in the correct slot without error, rotate the form board by 180°, take out the inserted block and ask the child to do it again. The child can do this by 15 months.
  - If a child can put in the round block, offer all three blocks. If the child puts all three correctly then ask to do it again, after you have rotated the Form board. If the child can correctly put in the blocks two to three times, he/she is at least 2 years of age.

Between 2 and 5 Years

- ***Notice the gait.*** At the end of the session, see how he climbs stairs, jumps/hops/skips.
- Can he throw a ball overhead? Undressing/buttoning-unbuttoning can be observed before the physical examination.

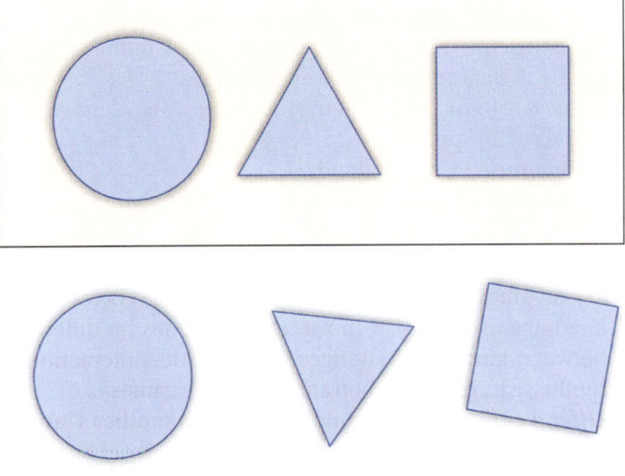

Fig. 1.39: Simple form board

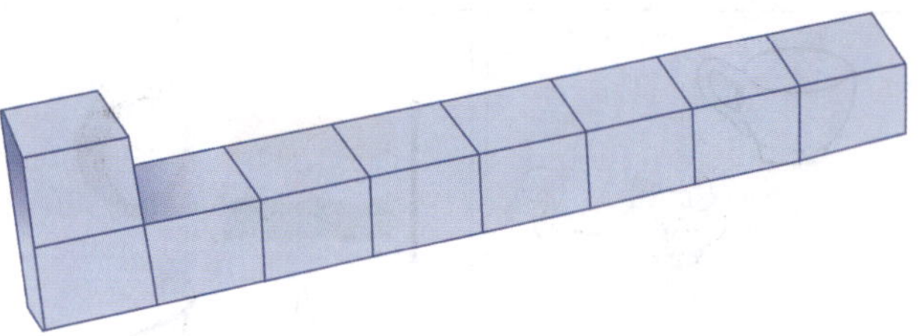

Fig. 1.40: Train with a chimney

Offer 10 cubes:

- Usually, a child in this age group spontaneously begins to build a tower. Notice how many cubes he utilizes in making the tower.
- Ask the child to imitate/copy (depending on expected maturity level) a train, bridge, gate, and steps, one by one **(Figs. 1.40 to 1.43)**. (Note: *Imitation* means building the model while the child is watching and then asking him to build the same; while *Copying* means building the model out of sight of child, shielding with a paper, and then showing him the final model and asking him to build the same.)
  - ***2½ years:*** Tower of eight cubes; imitates train with chimney.
  - ***3 years:*** Tower of 9–10 cubes, imitates bridge.

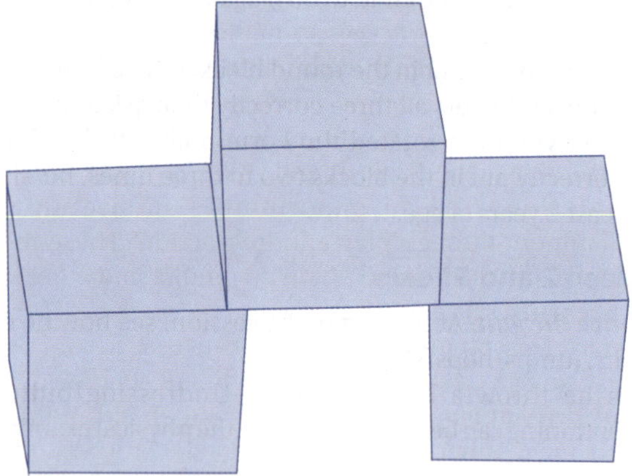

Fig. 1.41: Bridge of cubes

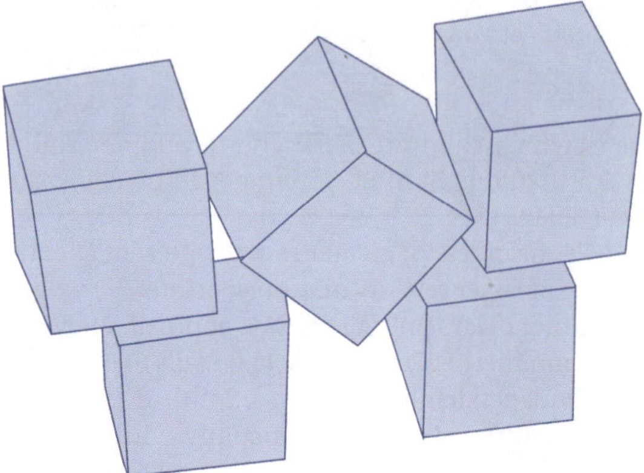

Fig. 1.42: Gate of cubes

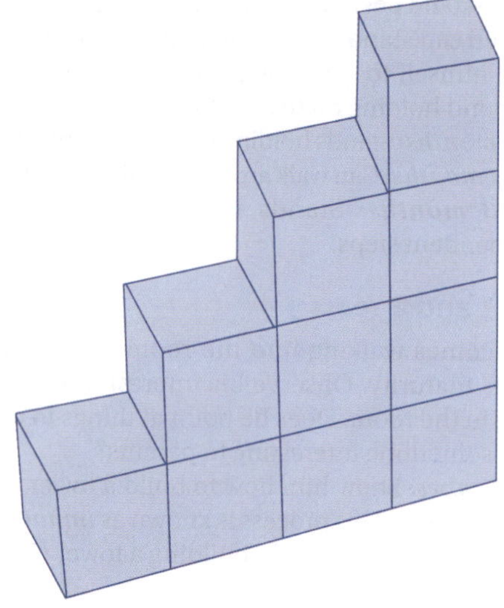

Fig. 1.43: Steps of cubes

  - ***3½ years:*** Copies bridge.
  - ***4 years:*** Imitates gate.
  - ***5 years:*** Copies gate.
  - ***6 years:*** May copy steps.

While the child is handling cubes, observe minutely for any abnormal hand movements or disability.

- ***Give a pencil and paper:*** Ask to imitate vertical and horizontal stroke, circle, cross, square, triangle, and diamond, in that order. If the child is able to imitate a task, ask to copy the same.
  - ***2 years:*** Imitates horizontal/circular stroke.
  - ***3 years:*** Copies circle and horizontal stroke. Imitates cross.
  - ***4 years:*** Copies cross.
  - ***4½ years:*** Copies square.
  - ***5 years:*** Copies triangle.
  - ***6 years:*** Copies diamond.
- ***Show the picture cards*** and ask to *identify* or *name* the objects
  - ***2½ years:*** Identifies seven objects; names up to 5.
  - ***3 years:*** Names 8–10 objects.
- Offer simple form board and observe the ability of the child to insert the blocks and the accuracy with which he does that.
- If the child is successful with simple form board, he should be tried with the colored geometric forms followed by uncolored geometric forms. In each case, he is asked where the shapes fit, being given different forms one after the other. He is not told about his mistakes and is given another chance with those he has placed incorrectly.
- After developmental age (DA) of 3½ years, time his performance in Goddard Form board, the score being based on the best of 3 trials.
- ***Goodenough draw-a-man test:*** After DA of 3 years, ask the child to draw a man as completely as he knows. Child is given 1 point for each of the body parts added. For each 4 points, 1 year is added to the basal age which is 3 years. The test has 51 items, details of which can be found in textbooks. This test

Box 1.2 Identifiable Risk Factors for Developmental Delay on Physical Examination

1. Abnormal growth (e.g., height or weight less than 3rd percentile or head circumference less than –3 SD or >2 SD)
2. Major congenital anomalies (e.g., spina bifida or midline defects)
3. Minor congenital anomalies (e.g., hypertelorism, hirsutism, or micrognathia)
4. Neurocutaneous skin lesions (e.g., neurofibromatosis or *café au lait* spots)
5. Abnormal optical findings (e.g., esotropia, exotropia, cataracts, or poor visual tracking)
6. Abnormal findings in ears (e.g., unusual shape or placement or recurrent acute or serous otitis media)
7. Visceral abnormalities (e.g., hepatosplenomegaly)
8. Skeletal abnormalities (e.g., brittle bones or dwarfism)
9. Neurologic abnormalities (e.g., lack of alertness, abnormal reflexes, hypertonia or hypotonia, or asymmetric findings)

can be used for developmental assessment *between 3 and 10 years of age.*

- ***Gessel "Incomplete Man" test:*** In this test, picture of a man which is halfway complete is given to the child. The picture consists of a small circle for a head and below it a larger incomplete circle representing the trunk with one stick arm and one stick leg protruding. The head has one ear, half hair, a mouth and a nose but is missing eyes, one ear, half hair, one arm and one leg and various connecting elements. Child is asked to complete the man. Depending on how many and in what way the child adds the parts, DA is deciphered.
- ***Digit repetition:*** Child is asked to repeat digits, e.g., six, five, and seven. Initially, he is given two digits. If he can repeat them, ask him to repeat three and then four digits followed by five. In each case, he is given three trials with different numbers.
- Ask the child to identify colors in pictures.

Perform Relevant Physical Examination

Box 1.2 provides a list of risk factors that you need to look for. If present, they place the child at a higher risk of having abnormal development. Note that you have to take anthropometric measurements; look for major and minor congenital anomalies; examine carefully the skin, eye, ear, extremities in detail; and conduct a thorough neurological examination. Also look for the presence of hepatosplenomegaly. A few warning signs of developmental delay are listed in **Box 1.3**.

Box 1.3 Warning Signs of Delay in Development

1. Shrill/high-pitched cry
2. Excessive sleepiness/irritability
3. Frog-legged positioning/opisthotonus
4. Tremors/convulsions
5. Small/large head size for age
6. Poor eye following/poor response to sound
7. Asymmetrical/increased/absent/persistent neonatal reflexes
8. Hypotonia/hypertonia/dystonia
9. Delayed developmental milestones

INTERPRETATION OF DEVELOPMENTAL ASSESSMENT

Based on the performance on developmental assessment a functional/developmental age (DA) is assigned to the child, on the basis of which developmental quotient (DQ) is obtained.

Development Quotient

Development quotient (DQ) is the numeric expression of a child's developmental level as measured by dividing the DA by the chronologic age (CA) and multiplying by 100. Ideally, CA should be equal to DA and the DQ should, therefore, be 100. A DQ of <70 is considered as delay. DQ should be estimated separately for each area of development, viz., motor, adaptive/cognitive, language, and personal/social. For preterm children till 2 years of age, corrected gestational age should be used instead of chronological age.

Factors Affecting Development

A number of factors affecting development have been identified. The following factors may be easily identified and can be addressed by already available interventions:

- ***Nutrition:*** Lack of adequate maternal and baby nutrition, including breastfeeding and complementary feeding. Additionally, deficiencies of key nutrients, especially iron, affects development significantly.
- ***Healthcare:*** Lack of access to quality healthcare services during pregnancy and early childhood. These include care during pregnancy and birth, immunizations services, and management of infections, especially prevention and management of tuberculosis and HIV.
- ***Stimulation:*** Lack of opportunities for learning and development through play and interaction. These include reciprocal interaction and play with mother and other family members in a safe environment.
- ***Support:*** Lack of emotional support and resources for parents and caregivers. Lack of a safe environment at home or in the society, which may predispose to child abuse and neglect (CAN), may further hinder developmental progression.

Birth defects, especially affecting the special senses, hindering mobility or affecting the brain.

Inadequate WASH (water, sanitation and hygiene) facilities are associated with poor developmental outcome.

Presentation of Developmental Disorders

The age at which child presents with developmental delays varies with the domain of development in question and the severity of delay.

- Generally, disorders of greater severity present at early ages and those of lesser severity may present later.
- Severe motor delays present earliest, approximately between 6 and 12 months of life when the child fails to hold head, sit, or stand independently.
- Sensory deficits also present usually within the first 6 months when the child does not respond to sound or fails to fixate.

- Language and cognitive delays usually present after 24 months, when the child fails to demonstrate the expected expressive language.
- Social and behavioral delays present over wide range of ages depending upon the extent to which it is affecting the functioning of child or life of caregivers. Adaptive skill delays are usually not the presenting complaints but may be noted during the developmental history and examination of children who present with other concerns.

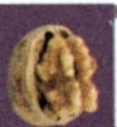

IN A NUTSHELL

Developmental Assessment

1. Developmental surveillance is an informal and ongoing method of assessing development whereas developmental screening and assessment use standardized tools at recommended age groups for diagnosing developmental delays.
2. A good history and examination are the cornerstone for developmental assessment. Developmental examination should be performed with the age-appropriate toys in a comfortable and amiable setting.
3. While assessing development of the child, care should be taken as not to miss any red flag which usually indicates an abnormal development and warrants immediate attention.
4. Developmental quotient (DQ) is the numeric expression of a child's developmental level as measured by dividing the developmental age (DA) by the chronologic age (CA) multiplied by 100. DQ should be calculated for each domain separately. DQ < 70 is considered delay.
5. For preterm children till 2 years of age, corrected gestational age should be used instead of chronological age for calculating DQ.

Berk LE. Child Development, 9th edition. Boston, MA: Pearson; 2013.

Cairney DG, Kazmi A, Delahunty L, Marryat L, Wood R. The predictive value of universal preschool developmental assessment in identifying children with later educational difficulties: a systematic review. PLoS One. 2021;16(3):e0247299.

Cheung YB, Gladstone M, Maleta K, Duan X, Ashorn P. Comparison of four statistical approaches to score child development: a study of Malawian children. Trop Med Int Health. 2008;13(8):987-93.

Del Rosario C, Slevin M, Molloy EJ, Quigley J, Nixon E. How to use the Bayley scales of infant and toddler development. Arch Dis Child Educ Pract Ed. 2021;106(2):108-12.

Gupta P. Clinical Methods in Pediatrics, 6th edition. New Delhi: CBS Publishers; 2025.

Hadders-Algra M, Tacke U, Pietz J, Rupp A, Philippi H. Standardized infant neurodevelopmental assessment developmental and socio-emotional scales: reliability and predictive value in an at-risk population. Dev Med Child Neurol. 2020;62(7):845-53.

Lipkin PH, Macias MM; Council on Children with Disabilities, Section on Developmental and Behavioral Pediatrics. Promoting Optimal Development: Identifying Infants and Young Children with Developmental Disorders Through Developmental Surveillance and Screening. Pediatrics. 2020;145(1):e20193449.

2 CHAPTER

Common Problems Related to Growth

AS PER NMC COMPETENCIES

PE2.1	Discuss the etiopathogenesis, clinical features and management of a child who fails to thrive.	*Ch 2.1*
PE2.2	Counselling the parent of a child with failure to thrive.	*Ch 2.1*
PE2.3	Discuss the etiopathogenesis, clinical features and management of a child with short stature. Assessment of a child with short stature.	*Ch 2.2*

Topics available online: ***Abnormalities of Head Size and Shape***

2.1 Failure to Thrive *PE 2.1, PE 2.2*

INTRODUCTION

The term "failure to thrive" (FTT) is assigned to a child whose weight-for-age is below 5th percentile or a downward change in growth that has crossed two major growth percentiles (i.e., downward shifting from 75th percentile to below 25th percentile) in a short time. FTT objectively denotes growth failure on serial monitoring. Criteria used to define FTT are listed in **Box 2.1**. Weight remains the most common and simplest parameter to define FTT as is affected first during any illness, much before stunting manifests.

This term should not be confused with short stature as FTT describes retarded growth in height and weight, whereas short stature is diagnosed in comparison to a reference height-for-age or to one's own height over time.

Besides growth deficit, FTT also results in alteration in immunity (predisposing to infections) and dysfunction in intellect, development, and behavior. Other associated complications with FTT are listed in **Box 2.2**. FTT should never be considered as a primary disease. It is always a manifestation of an underlying cause which should be investigated through proper clinical examination and relevant investigations.

ETIOLOGY

The adequacy of growth is dependent on various physiological processes in the body. The chief determinant is food intake measured in terms of both quality and quantity. FTT can result, if the child is taking less food, the food is not being properly absorbed, or nutrients and fluids are being lost excessively.

Box 2.1 Diagnostic Criteria of Failure to Thrive*

1. Weight-for-age below 5th percentile
2. Weight deceleration—serial weight monitoring shows downward trend and has crossed two major growth percentiles (i.e., 75th percentile to below 25th percentile) in a short time
3. Weight-for-age <75% of the median
4. Weight-for-length <75% of the median
5. Length-for-age <5th percentile
6. Body mass index <5th percentile

**On Serial Growth Monitoring*

Box 2.2 Systemic Complications of Failure to Thrive

- *Short-term:*
  - Hypothermia
  - Hypoproteinemia
  - Predisposition to infections
  - Nutritional deficiencies and electrolyte imbalance
- *Long-term:*
  - Neurocognitive delay
  - Behavioral problems
  - Short stature
  - Adult onset metabolic diseases

Table 2.1 Major Organic Causes of Failure to Thrive

System	*Cause*
Gastrointestinal	Recurrent diarrhea (poor sanitation), gastroesophageal reflux disease, celiac disease, pyloric stenosis, cleft palate/cleft lip, lactose intolerance, Hirschsprung disease, milk protein intolerance, hepatitis, cirrhosis, pancreatic insufficiency, biliary disease, inflammatory bowel disease, and malabsorption
Renal	Urinary tract infection, renal tubular acidosis, diabetes insipidus, and chronic renal insufficiency
Cardiopulmonary	Cardiac diseases leading to congestive heart failure, asthma, bronchopulmonary dysplasia, cystic fibrosis, anatomic abnormalities of upper airway, and obstructive sleep apnea (snoring)
Endocrine	Hypothyroidism, diabetes mellitus, adrenal insufficiency or excess, parathyroid disorders, pituitary disorders, and growth hormone deficiency
Neurological	Global developmental delay, cerebral hemorrhage, and degenerative disorders
Infectious	Parasitic or bacterial infections of the gastrointestinal tract and human immunodeficiency virus disease
Metabolic	Inborn errors of metabolism
Congenital	Chromosomal infections, congenital syndromes (fetal alcohol syndrome), and perinatal infections
Miscellaneous	Psychosocial/environmental neglect, lead poisoning, malignancy, and collagen vascular disease

The second process which can result in FTT is an underlying organic disease (renal, cardiac, gastrointestinal, and respiratory) or a metabolic cause which causes increased energy expenditure, thereby creating an energy deficit. Apart from these biological causes, psychosocial or environmental deprivation, child abuse and neglect, can also result in growth failure in childhood. Major organic causes of FTT are listed in **Table 2.1**. The causes of FTT based on energy balance are categorized in **Table 2.2**.

APPROACH TO DIAGNOSIS

A child with FTT should have a detailed evaluation of the following aspects:
- Dietary assessment
- Medical assessment
- Psychosocial assessment
- Developmental assessment

History

Ask the parents about the onset of growth failure to differentiate between congenital and acquired causes. Ask for common symptoms of possible organic disorders. An assessment of dietary intake and dietary habits is essential part of clinical history. The amount of food offered and consumed should be separately measured. Details of milk preparation, dilution, and reconstitution should be checked in an infant. Growth failure due to energy deficit is commonly seen during late infancy when the baby is shifted from breastfeeding to complementary feeding. Feeding habits should be enquired for both home and outside home settings (day-care and school). Sociocultural environment of the child should be assessed. Family dynamics, parental education, employment, substance abuse, and cultural factors should also be assessed.

Table 2.2 Causes of Failure to Thrive Based on Energy Balance

Inadequate caloric intake	*Inadequate caloric absorption*	*Excessive caloric expenditure*
Infancy • Inadequate breastmilk • Inadequate amount or improper dilution of top/formula milk • Inadequate complementary feeding • Gastroesophageal reflux disease • Cleft palate/cleft lip • Maternal factors—low education and younger age	*Infancy* • Congenital gastrointestinal anomalies such as duodenal atresia and malrotation of gut • Cow milk protein allergy • Gastrointestinal parasitic infections • Chronic liver disease • Short gut syndrome (ileal resection postsurgery)	*Infancy* • Chronic systemic diseases—congenital heart disease, lung disease, renal disease, cystic fibrosis and endocrinal causes • Chronic infection such as intrauterine infections and tuberculosis • Immunodeficiency—congenital or acquired (HIV) • Genetic syndromes • Inborn errors of metabolism • Malignancy
Childhood • Food scarcity • Neurodevelopmental disorders which affect swallowing coordination like cerebral palsy • Gastroesophageal reflux disease • Behavioral disorders and eating disorders	*Childhood* • Food allergy • Malabsorption—celiac disease and chronic diarrhea • Inflammatory bowel disease • Inborn errors of metabolism	*Childhood* • Chronic systemic illness • Chronic systemic infections • Malignancy • Inborn errors of metabolism

(HIV: human immunodeficiency virus)

Psychosocial assessment should include evaluation of socioeconomic status, family dysfunction, and feeding problems. Child's drive for autonomy, attention seeking, gaining independence, and expressing anger or dislike by refusing food are also important causes for creating a feeding disorder. Physical or mental abuse, though seen in small percentage of cases, is an important cause of FTT. Developmental assessment should include assessment for developmental delay, and abnormalities of posture, tone, and attention and language domains. Standardized developmental assessment may be required. Any delay in two or more domains is abnormal. Mild degree of motor delay is commonly seen in children with FTT due to poor skeletal mass and muscle tone.

Clinical Examination (Medical Assessment)

A detailed medical history should be elicited for an underlying medical disorder. Obtain complete and accurate anthropometry. Serially measured values rather than a single observation are mainstay for diagnosing FTT. Anthropometry should be interpreted on age and gender specific population reference growth charts. Separate charts for preterm babies should be used to monitor their growth during infancy. Besides this, a thorough general and systemic examination should be done to search for:

- ❖ Any clue to organic disorders (facial dysmorphism, neurocutaneous markers, and clubbing).
- ❖ Physical abuse (fractures, bruises, hematomas, and cigarette marks).
- ❖ Markers of severe malnutrition and associated deficiencies (loss of buccal fat, edema, mucositis, and corneal ulcers).
- ❖ A detailed neurological and developmental assessment using appropriate tests.
- ❖ Any abnormal behavioral pattern, response to external stimulus, etc.

The red flag signs that should alert the physician toward an underlying systemic cause of FTT are highlighted in **Table 2.3**.

Laboratory Evaluation

The FTT is a clinical diagnosis and most children do not need investigations. Tests are of prime importance when an organic etiology is suspected or in the presence of a red flag sign.

- ❖ Some minimal initial tests which may be performed are: hemoglobin, blood counts, urea, electrolytes, creatinine, liver function tests, total proteins, antiendomysial antibodies (to screen for celiac disease), and urinalysis.
- ❖ Other tests include sweat chloride test for cystic fibrosis in genetically predisposed population; blood pH, anion gap, and urine pH for renal tubular acidosis; and stool examination in children with diarrhea or suspected malabsorption.
- ❖ Radiological assessment may be useful for determining bone age or fractures, if physical abuse is suspected.
- ❖ A karyotype may be ordered in suspected chromosomal disorder.

An algorithmic approach to management of FTT is shown in **Flowchart 2.1**.

Table 2.3 Red Flag Signs in a Child with Failure to Thrive with Probable Etiology

Clinical symptoms/signs	*Probable etiology*
Failure to show catch up growth after calorie deficit has been corrected	Underlying systemic disorders
Global developmental delay	Syndromic causes and chromosomal disorders
Family history of unexplained sibling deaths or abortions	Chromosomal disorders and inborn errors of metabolism
Seizures	Inborn errors of metabolism, brain malformations and intrauterine infections
Jaundice	Chronic liver disease and storage disorders
Nondiarrheal dehydration	Diabetes and adrenal insufficiency
Dysmorphic features	Chromosomal disorders
Skeletal deformities	Child abuse, distal renal tubular acidosis, and metabolic bone disease
Lymphadenopathy	Tuberculosis and lymphoreticular malignancies
Clubbing	Chronic disease of liver and lung
Skin lesions	Specific patterns seen in different diseases

Flowchart 2.1: Approach to a child with failure to thrive

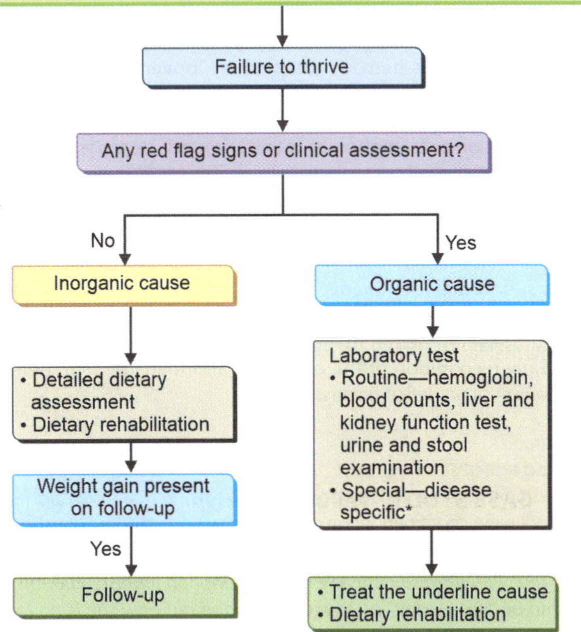

*Investigation specific for an underlying systemic disorder

TREATMENT Failure to Thrive

Studies have shown that there is no difference in the outcome of children who are hospitalized or managed at home. Indications of hospitalization are as follows:
- Severe malnutrition especially with life-threatening complications.
- As a part of diagnostic work-up, if organic cause is suspected.
- Child unresponsive to initial management.
- Where parent neglect, abuse, or maltreatment is suspected.

The FTT resolves with medical interventions. However, the management should be comprehensive and long-term. A multidisciplinary and stepwise approach is most effective.

Dietary management: Nutritional rehabilitation aims at—achievement of ideal weight for height and correction of nutritional deficits, allowing catch up growth, restoration of optimal body composition, and parental education regarding nutritional requirements and feeding of the child. Diet management of a child with FTT is similar to that of a child with severe acute malnutrition (see details in Chapter 9).

Parental counseling and education: Parents should be involved in feeding actively. They should be told about their child's requirements and how they can be met. They should be counseled about calorie content of different food items, how to make calorie rich, simple, and appealing food preparations, right techniques of feeding, and how to inculcate good feeding habits in their children. Misconceptions and food fads should be addressed carefully. Counseling a parent/caregiver for need of their active participation in continued rehabilitation and psychosocial care is important.

Medical management: Several medical issues may be identified in children with FTT which may be primary or secondary and require specialized interventions. Special diets may be required lifelong, e.g., celiac disease or special enzyme supplements for cystic fibrosis. Drugs may be required (e.g., for gastroesophageal reflux disease) or special training in neuromotor dysfunction (e.g., cerebral palsy).

Psychosocial management: The psychosocial aspects differ widely and hence the management cannot be generalized. A good rapport is essential for both diagnosing and managing such issues. The need of a psychiatrist in cases of depression, substance abuse, and behavioral problems is unavoidable. Behavioral modifications in feeding disorders, psychotherapy, and counseling are of tremendous help. In cases where poverty is the cause of malnutrition, social relief organizations can be approached. In cases where there is severe abuse, neglect, and maltreatment, hospitalization or foster homes may be essential temporarily before the parental issues are resolved.

Developmental management: This is the most challenging aspect that requires long-term care. Studies have shown that even after aggressive nutritional rehabilitation, minor deficits such as language skills, subnormal intelligence quotient (IQ) scores, and decreased head circumference, can be detected on follow-up. Thus, the key to neurodevelopmental management lies in prevention of severe FTT, early recognition of the condition, and management, before a permanent brain deficit occurs.

CASE STUDY Failure to Thrive

A 30-month-old girl was brought with complaints of not gaining weight for 1 year. Parents also noticed excessive urination for last 3 months. She used to be "dry by day" at 24 months of age but now she is no longer continent. Recently, her mother has noted a soft swelling over her scalp for last 1 month. Her dietary intake does not reveal any major deficit in intake of protein or calories.

She now weighs 9.2 kg. Her present height is 85 cm. Her birth weight was 2.8 kg. She weighed 9 kg at 18 months as recorded on her immunization chart. Examination revealed mild anemia, dry skin, and loss of subcutaneous fat. There was a 2 × 3 cm soft swelling over occipital region of scalp. Systemic examination was normal.

Interpret the anthropometry

Her weight at birth (2.8 kg) was at 15th centile (WHO charts). She continued to follow her centile for weight till 18 months of age. Her present weight is 9.2 kg which is below the 3rd centile. Her weight has crossed two major centiles and shown a downward trend which is pathological. Her current height is just above 3rd centile. According to these measurements, she has FTT or growth failure.

What is the cause of FTT? Justify.

The likely case is organic. Her dietary assessment seems normal which rules out nutritional etiology.

Clinical clues in this case which suggest an organic cause are:
- Growth faltering in a previously normal growing child.
- Urinary incontinence and excessive urination (other systemic symptoms).
- Positive systemic findings—scalp swelling and anemia.

The case was further worked up to find an underlying organic cause. Polyuria was documented and confirmed. Laboratory tests showed anemia (hemoglobin 9.5 g%) and high serum sodium (149 mEq/L). Needle aspirate from the scalp swelling was positive for malignant cells which were confirmed to be Langerhans cells on special stains (S-100 and CD1A). X-ray of the skull showed a bony defect. Bone marrow examination was normal. She was diagnosed with central diabetes insipidus with underlying Langerhans cell histiocytosis.

How will you counsel the family for management of failure to thrive?

The child requires treatment of the underlying medical condition (chemotherapy for Langerhans cell histiocytosis and oral desmopressin for diabetes insipidus). The child also requires a detailed assessment for nutritional requirements, developmental and psychosocial needs. The parents need to be counseled about the nature of underlying disease and options of treatment. The importance of maintaining a good diet and compliance to the medical instructions during hospital visits should be reiterated. Counseling should be done in a nonthreatening and nonjudgmental manner. This child gradually improved and achieved a catch up in her growth on follow-up.

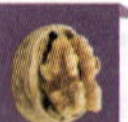

IN A NUTSHELL

Failure to Thrive

1. Failure to thrive is a term to denote the overall nutritional status of a child with respect to less energy intake or more energy expenditure.
2. Weight for age remains the most common parameter to monitor growth.
3. Serial weight monitoring if showing downward trend and crossing two major growth percentiles defines FTT.
4. The approach to clinical diagnosis should include detailed history and examination clues of underlying organic causes.
5. The management should be based on nutritional rehabilitation, parental counseling, development supportive practices, and appropriate medical therapy, as appropriate.

Becker P, Carney LN, Corkins MR, et al. Consensus statement of the Academy of Nutrition and Dietetics/American Society for Parenteral and Enteral Nutrition: indicators recommended for the identification and documentation of pediatric malnutrition (undernutrition). Nutr Clin Pract. 2015;30(1):147-61.

Bouma S. Diagnosing Pediatric Malnutrition: Paradigm Shifts of Etiology-Related Definitions and Appraisal of the Indicators. Nutr Clin Pract. 2017;32(1):52-67.

Kristjansson E, Francis DK, Liberato S, et al. Food supplementation for improving the physical and psychosocial health of socioeconomically disadvantaged children aged three months to five years. Cochrane Database Syst Rev. 2015;2015(3):CD009924.

2.2 Short Stature

PE 2.3

DEFINITION

Short stature is defined as height below -2 *Z*-score or below 3rd percentile. Height below -3 *Z*-score or below the first percentile indicates severe short stature with a high likelihood of pathological cause. Growth velocity below 10th percentile over a year or crossing of two percentile lines between the age of 2 years and puberty are also indicative of growth failure.

It is essential to use gender specific growth reference charts/ values to interpret growth patterns. The growth of Indian children is plotted on world health organization (WHO) growth charts from 0 to 5 years of age, and on revised Indian Academy of Pediatrics (IAP) 2015 growth charts from 5 to 18 years of age. A combined WHO and IAP growth chart is also available from *https://iapindia.org/iap-growth-charts/*.

DETERMINANTS OF GROWTH

Genetic growth potential [midparental height (MPH)]: Height shows a marked variability between children which is dependent on their age, gender, nutrition, genetics, ethnicity, and racial differences. One of the important determinants of height in children is their genetic potential which is determined by their parents' heights and is calculated as MPH. A child may remain short, if he is born to shorter parents and diagnosed as familial short stature.

Box 2.3 shows the formula to calculate MPH for boys and girls. MPH is marked at gender appropriate chart at 18/20 years. In normally growing child, height at any given age corresponds to lie within 2 standard deviations of the MPH when it is extrapolated till adult height on a growth chart (target height range).

Nutrition: The effect of nutrition during fetal period affects the final height, e.g., babies who experience intrauterine growth retardation and are born as small for gestational age, gain weight and length rapidly after birth to catch-up to the normal growth centiles. A few fail to achieve catch-up growth and do not attain normal height in childhood. Deficiency of both macronutrients and micronutrients such as zinc and iron during growing years adversely impacts attainment of height. Malnutrition has been reported as one of the most common causes of short stature in Indian settings. Such children show growth faltering for both weight and height which can be easily discerned on a growth chart.

Systemic disease: Chronic diseases, syndromic genetic disorders, diseases of musculoskeletal system, and those affecting the hypothalamic-pituitary axis [affecting growth hormone (GH), etc.], are other causes of short stature.

Box 2.3 Calculation of Midparental Height (MPH)

MPH (boy) = (Father's height + Mother's height + 13)/2, or
= [(Father's height + Mother's height)/2] + 6.5
MPH (girls) = (Father's height + Mother's height – 13)/2, or
= [(Father's height + Mother's height)/2] – 6.5

ETIOLOGY

Physiological variants account for over two-thirds of all cases of short stature. Pathological short stature can be caused by a variety of factors related to genetics or nutrition, systemic diseases, and endocrine imbalance **(Box 2.4)**. Short stature may

Box 2.4 Causes of Short Stature

Normal variants

- Familial short stature
- Constitutional growth delay

Pathological short stature

- *Malnutrition:* Macronutrient or micronutrient deficiencies and small for gestational age
- *Chronic systemic diseases:*
  - *Gastrointestinal:* Celiac disease and chronic liver disease
  - *Cardiopulmonary:* Acyanotic and cyanotic heart disease and congestive heart failure
  - *Infections:* Tuberculosis, giardiasis, and human immunodeficiency virus (HIV)
  - *Renal:* Chronic kidney disease, renal tubular acidosis, and chronic pyelonephritis
  - *Hematological:* Nutritional anemia, leukemia, and thalassemia
  - *Pulmonary:* Chronic asthma and bronchiectasis
  - *Storage disorders:* Mucopolysaccharidosis and glycogen storage disorders
  - *Neurological:* Cerebral palsy
- Metabolic bone disease—rickets
- *Endocrine causes:*
  - *Hypothalamic-pituitary axis:* Growth hormone deficiency, growth hormone receptor defect (Laron dwarfism)
  - *Other endocrine organs:* Hypothyroidism, Cushing syndrome, diabetes, and precocious puberty
- *Genetic syndromes:* Turner syndrome, Prader–Willi syndrome, Russell–Silver syndrome, and Noonan syndrome
- *Skeletal dysplasia:* Achondroplasia and osteogenesis imperfecta
- Psychosocial dwarfism
- *Drugs:* Systemic steroids and substance abuse

be proportionate or disproportionate as assessed by the ratio of upper and lower segment length.

Disproportionate Short Stature

Disproportionate short stature occurs because of abnormal skeletal growth. Either the limbs or the trunk is short. Short limb dwarfism can be further classified into *rhizomelic* (shortening of proximal limb segment), *mesomelic* (shortening of middle segments), and *acromelic* (shortening of the distal segments) short stature. These disorders present with severe short stature, disproportionate development of spine and limbs, and abnormal facies.

- In *short limb dysplasia*, e.g., achondroplasia **(Fig. 2.1)**, chondrodysplasia, arm span is less than height and upper segment (US)/lower segment (LS) ratio is high.
- In *short trunk anomalies*, e.g., mucopolysaccharidosis, spondyloepiphyseal dysplasia, US/LS ratio is decreased, and arm span exceeds the height.

Proportionate Short Stature

This is more common, all the body proportions are equally shortened. This may occur secondary to constitutional delay in growth, chronic infections, malabsorption, congenital heart disease, renal failure, or endocrine disorders, except hypothyroidism which has disproportionate short stature. A child with proportionate short stature may be thin or fat. Thin and short children usually have an underlying systemic disorder, while fat and short children are likely to have an endocrine etiology.

Constitutional delay: This represents a group of children with delayed maturation but preserved growth potential. This is particularly common in boys. Family history of delayed puberty is common in father or elder brothers. These children grow at a normal rate in childhood, show a late height spurt and pubertal onset, and continue to grow beyond the normal stage of growth to achieve a normal final adult height. They have a mild delay in bone age.

Children with familial short stature on the other hand have normal bone age, normal pubertal onset, and usually end up short.

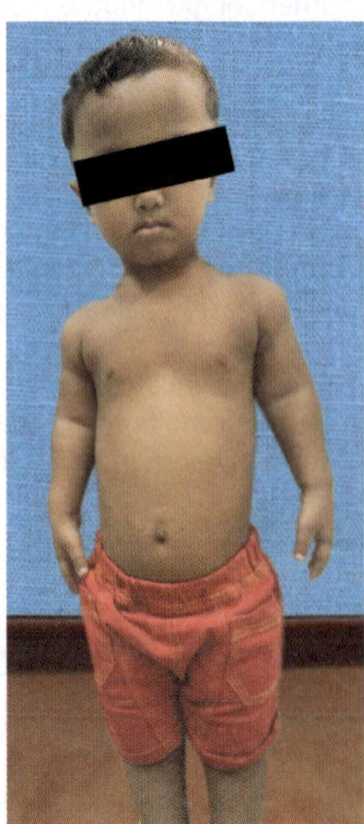

Fig. 2.1: A 6-year-old boy with achondroplasia. Note the short stature with apparent increased upper segment than lower segment (short limbs)

Malnutrition: It is the most common pathological cause of short stature. Growth failure is preceded by poor weight gain. This contrasts endocrine short stature where weight is usually normal. Zinc deficiency is an important rare but treatable cause of short stature.

Intrauterine growth retardation (IUGR): This might be due to genetic disorders, intrauterine infections, maternal malnutrition, and placental disorders. Most of these children achieve catch-up growth in the first 2 years of life and have final height in the target height range. Around 15%, however, fail to grow normally and have short stature.

Systemic disease: Short stature occurs in all chronic systemic disorders and infections. Most of these conditions are readily identifiable on a detailed clinical examination, celiac disease, renal failure, and renal tubular acidosis, however, a few might be asymptomatic and be missed.

Chromosomal/genetic syndrome: Down syndrome is the most common chromosomal disorder associated with growth retardation. Turner syndrome is an important cause of short stature in girls. While classical features are easily identified, girls with mosaic forms of Turner syndrome might appear normal and may present with short stature and delayed puberty later in adolescence. Turner syndrome should be investigated in all short girls.

Endocrine causes: Disorders of the GH are important causes of short stature and discussed in Chapter on Endocrine Disorders. These children have normal growth at birth, retardation becomes apparent around 1 year of age. Hypothyroidism, growth hormone deficiency (GHD), type 1 diabetes mellitus, pseudohypoparathyroidism, and rickets are also associated with growth retardation.

Table 2.4 shows the differentiating features between various causes of short stature in children.

EVALUATION

A child with height above –2 *Z*-score (third percentile) or growth velocity above 25th percentile (or at least 5 cm per year in prepubertal years) is essentially growing normal. On the other hand, immediate evaluation is warranted, if height is below –3 *Z*-score (first percentile). Children with height *Z*-score between –2 and –3 should be followed up. Work-up is required if growth velocity is below 25th percentile.

A summary of clinical clues to ascertain the etiology of short stature is provided in **Table 2.5**.

Step 1: History Taking

Perinatal history and birth weight should be recorded. Nutritional assessment is crucial part of evaluation of short stature.

Table 2.4 Differences Between Various Causes of Short Stature

	Familial short stature	*CDGP*	*Hypothyroidism*	*Growth hormone deficiency*	*Malnutrition/chronic systemic illness*
Age of onset	Short since birth	Short after infancy	Short since birth	Short since late infancy	Short since onset of disease/ nutrient deficiency
Birth weight	Low	Normal	High or normal	Normal	Normal
Family history	Present—parents are short	Present—parents have history of delay in growth	Normal	Normal	Normal
Pubertal onset	Normal	Delayed	Delayed	Delayed	Delayed
Clinical examination	Normal	Normal	Coarse facies and delayed developmental milestones	Infantile facies	Stigmata of chronic disease or vitamin deficiencies
Body proportion	Normal	Normal	Disproportionate	Normal	Normal
Height velocity	Normal	Normal	Delayed	Delayed	Delayed
Bone age (relation with CA and HA)	Normal (CA = BA > HA)	Delayed (CA > BA = HA)	Delayed (CA > HA > BA)	Delayed (CA > HA > BA)	Delayed— CA > HA > BA (BA delay is lesser than in endocrine causes)
Management	Reassurance	Reassurance	Thyroid hormone	Growth hormone	Treatment of underlying cause

(BA: bone age; CA: chronological age; CDGP; constitutional delay in growth and puberty; HA: height age)

Table 2.5 Clinical Clues to Etiology of Short Stature

	History
Present history	• Age of onset of growth faltering • Prior growth record • Any other associated symptoms
Specific symptoms:	
• Polyuria	• Renal tubular acidosis, chronic kidney disease
• Chronic diarrhea, greasy stools	• Malabsorption, celiac disease
• Lethargy, constipation, weight gain	• Hypothyroidism
• Headache, visual disturbance, seizures	• Intracranial tumor affecting pituitary or hypothalamus
Past history disease:	Known disorder—history of chronic systemic disorder like asthma, chronic liver chronic kidney disease, congenital heart disease
• Birth and antenatal history	• Birth weight—whether born small for gestational age • Maternal symptoms of intrauterine infections • Maternal ill-health, maternal alcohol or tobacco use • Neonatal hypoglycemia or prolonged jaundice—growth hormone (GH) deficiency
• Dietary history	Evaluation of daily protein and calorie consumption. Also evaluate for micronutrients
• Family history	Chronic systemic disorder and history of pubertal delay in parents
• Social history	Psychosocial environment
	Examination
Anthropometry	Weight, height, height velocity, body proportions, head circumference
Face including skull	• Facies—syndromic or dysmorphic facies in genetic syndromes, infantile facies in growth hormone deficiency, coarse in hypothyroidism or mucopolysaccharidosis • Skull—microcephaly, craniotabes in rickets, large fontanelle in achondroplasia • Eyes—anemia, cataract in intrauterine infections, blue sclera in osteogenesis imperfecta • Ears, nose, and palate—for any congenital defects in genetic syndromes • Teeth—delayed dentition in hypothyroidism and rickets, dental caries in rickets
Musculoskeletal	Limbs for deformities seen in rickets, skeletal dysplasia
Genitalia	Assess for pubertal maturation (delayed or advanced), any abnormalities in structure
Systemic	Evaluate for any underlying systemic disorder
Miscellaneous	Clubbing, skin for striae (Cushing syndrome), stigmata of Turner syndrome, and goiter

Family history of short stature or delayed puberty suggests familial short stature or constitutional short stature.

- Features of chronic infections, malabsorption, raised intracranial tension, and cardiopulmonary disorders should be enquired.
- Polyuria and polydipsia suggest diabetes insipidus, diabetes mellitus and/or renal tubular acidosis.
- Constipation, delayed milestones, lethargy, and cold intolerance pinpoint hypothyroidism.
- History of birth asphyxia, breech presentation, neonatal hypoglycemia, and prolonged jaundice are indicative of hypopituitarism.

Step 2: Growth Assessment

It involves comparison of height with population standards and parental height along with monitoring of longitudinal growth.

- Growth velocity should be measured over at least 12 months. Growth velocity <6 cm/year from the age of 1–3 years, below 5 cm/year during prepubertal growth years is suggestive of growth retardation.
- Midparental height should be plotted on the growth curve at around 18–20 years and the percentiles compared with current height percentiles. Plot this value of adult height prediction on the reference growth chart of height-for-age. The percentile line nearest to this point is known as the midparental 50th percentile. The child's own percentile curve is expected to be between 10th and 90th percentiles (MPH ± 8.5 cm, target height range) on the MPH percentile chart.
- ***Height age (HA):*** The HA of the child is the age at which his/her current height would match the 50th percentile or median for that age and sex. It can be assessed on a growth chart by drawing a horizontal line from the child's current height to intersect the growth curve at 50th percentile. Likewise, weight age can be plotted as the age at which his/her current weight would match the 50th percentile or median for that age and sex. In children with systemic disease, the weight age is usually more affected than HA, unlike endocrinal disorders where HA is more affected than weight age.
- Body mass index (BMI) can be calculated as weight/(height)^2 in kg/m^2. The reverse side of IAP growth charts shows the BMI chart that can be used to classify the nutritional status of the child (further details in section on obesity).

Detailed anthropometric measurements (weight, weight for height, and head circumference) should be taken. Reduced weight is suggestive of nutritional growth retardation (malnutrition, systemic illness, and malabsorption) while weight is generally preserved in endocrine causes. Body proportions are helpful in identifying skeletal dysplasia.

- Increased upper segment to lower segment ratio is indicative of hypothyroidism, achondroplasia, and Turner syndrome.
- Decreased upper segment to lower segment ratio is characteristic of Morquio syndrome and spondyloepiphyseal dysplasia.
- Body proportions are normal in GHD.

Specific features of GHD, hypothyroidism, and Turner syndrome should be looked for. Rickets and anemia should prompt evaluation for malnutrition, celiac disease, or renal failure. Shortening of fourth metacarpal is present in children with Turner syndrome and pseudohypoparathyroidism. Evaluation for dysmorphism, skeletal deformities, and sexual maturity rating is essential part of examination of children with short stature.

Referral Criteria for Growth-related Problems

The following criteria should be investigated for short stature in childhood:

- ***Severe short stature:*** Height <–3 *Z*-score.
- ***Short stature:*** Height *Z*-score <–2.25 with poor growth.
- Downward crossing of growth centiles.
- Prepubertal growth velocity below 5 cm/year.
- Difference between target height *Z*-score and current height *Z*-score >2

Children who are short and require referral should be offered further investigations as mentioned underneath.

Step 3: Investigations

Skeletal Age

Estimation of skeletal age or bone age (BA) is the first investigation to be ordered in a child with short stature. It is estimated by evaluating the skeletal maturity of bones of the left hand and wrist using standard bone atlas (Greulich–Pyle atlas or Tanner–Whitehouse method). Normally, the bone age matches the chronological age (CA) of the child. In case the BA shows a delay of >2 standard deviations than the CA, it is called delayed BA as seen in pathological short stature. An understanding of the BA can help us understand the normal variant growth patterns.

- ***Familial short stature (FSS):*** This variation is seen as short stature in a child who is born to short parents, thereby implying the role of genetic potential for growth. These children are short but their extrapolated height falls within the range of MPH. The general and systemic examination is normal. They have normal skeletal maturation and thus their BA matches their CA. However, as they are short, the HA is lesser than both CA and BA (BA = CA > HA). This entity does not need any further investigation or treatment. It is essential to reassure and monitor their growth annually. The growth pattern of FSS is shown in **Figure 2.2**.
- ***Constitutional delay in growth and puberty (CDGP):*** Another variant of growth which is considered normal is "constitutional short stature" or constitutional delay in growth and puberty. These children have normal growth potential but show poor growth in late childhood. The height velocity is normal. There is usually associated delay in puberty which makes poor height more discernible in peripubertal years. They need close monitoring of growth as they catch up subsequently on their height to attain final height within their MPH range. Usually, there is history of similar delay in puberty in their parents. These children have delayed BA which matches their HA. Both are less for their CA (HA = BA < CA). The growth pattern of CDGP is shown in **Figure 2.2.**

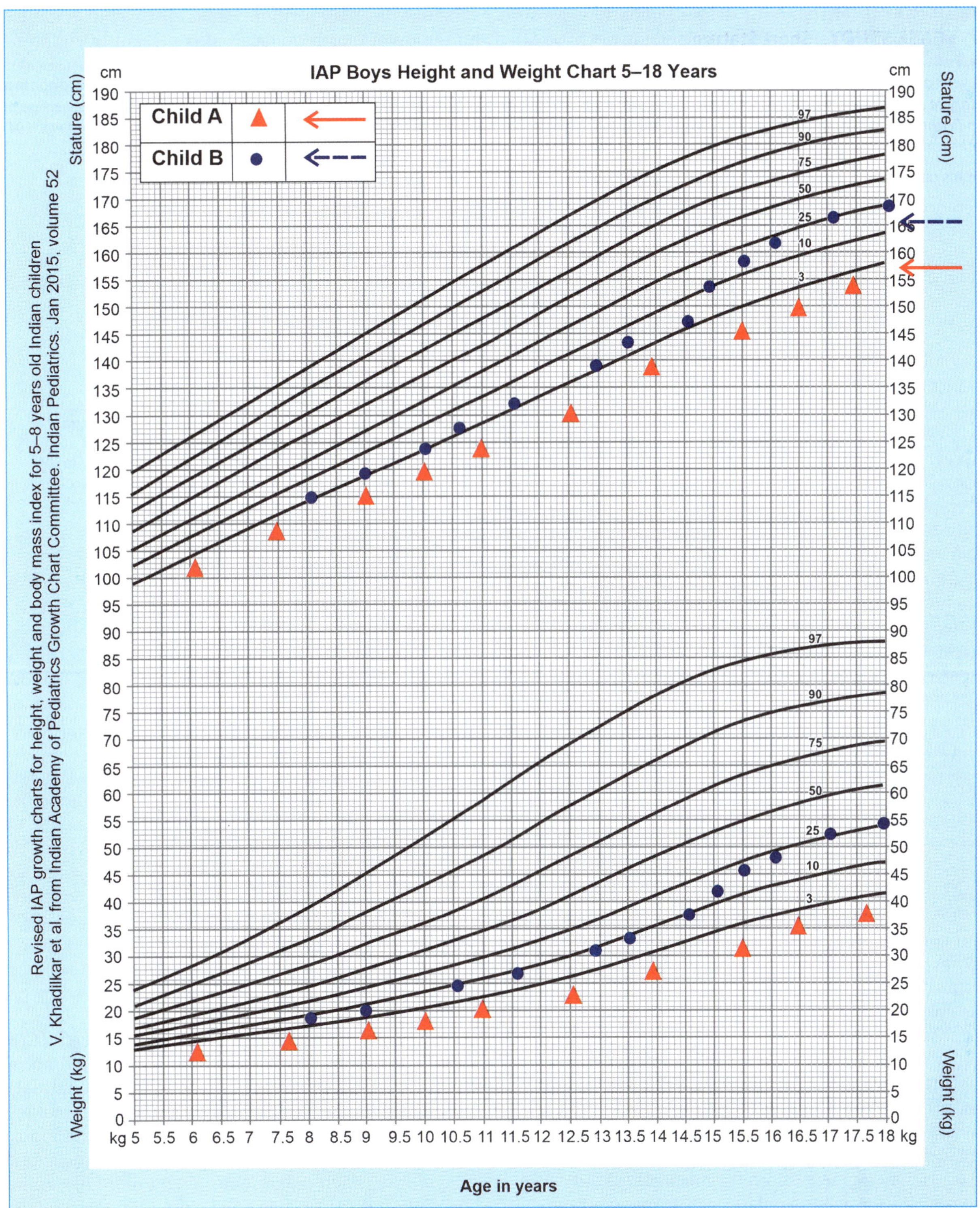

Fig. 2.2: Growth patterns in short stature. The figure above shows growth monitoring of two boys with their respective midparental heights marked as arrows on right. Child A has familial short stature and child B has constitutional delay in growth and puberty. (Weight and height should be marked as small dots on growth chart; magnification and use of shapes is for better depiction only. Use a single chart for a single child)

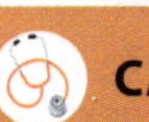

CASE STUDY Short Stature

A 9-year-old boy was brought with complaints of not growing well since early childhood. His birth weight was 2.5 kg. Mother gave some nonspecific history of abdominal discomfort and frequent loose stools in early childhood, but the child was never investigated for the same. There were no other significant systemic complaints. Family history was normal, his elder brother was tall. On examination, his weight was 15 kg and height was 104 cm. Mother and father height were 153 and 158 cm, respectively.

Plot his growth on a growth chart. How will you proceed?

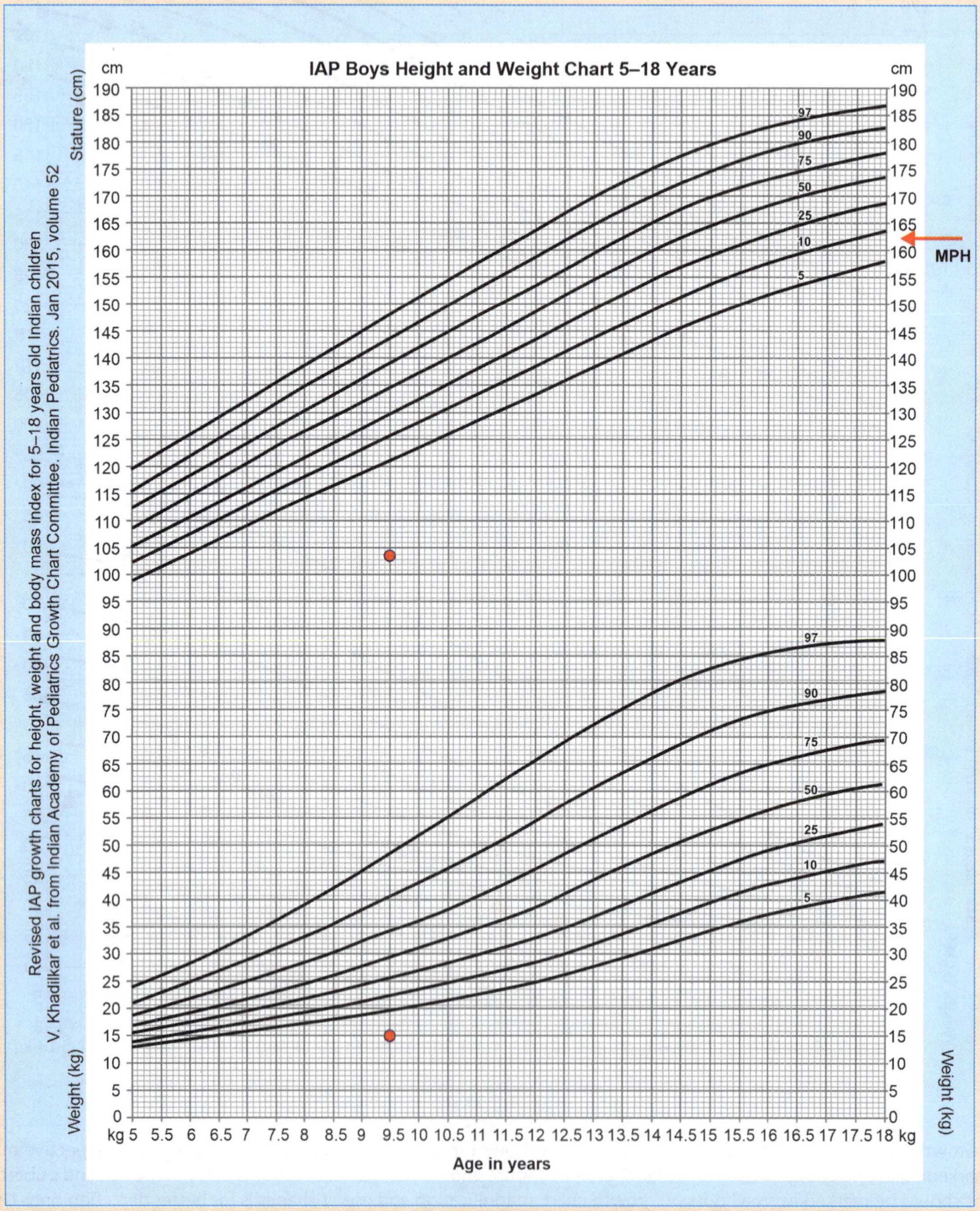

IAP Boys Height and Weight Chart 5–18 Years

Revised IAP growth charts for height, weight and body mass index for 5–18 years old Indian children
V. Khadilkar et al. from Indian Academy of Pediatrics Growth Chart Committee. Indian Pediatrics. Jan 2015, volume 52

Stature (cm)

Weight (kg)

MPH

Age in years

His height is grossly below his MPH (162 cm). There are no prior height records available. But with a corresponding low weight against a low height, a systemic disorder should be looked for. Next investigation to be ordered is a bone age.

His bone age was 5 years. Examination revealed clubbing, anemia, and signs of vitamin B deficiency. How will you proceed now?
Bone age is grossly delayed. Height age was 5.5 years. Therefore, diagnosis of pathological short stature is made. We will like to order the next line of screening investigations.

The investigations were suggestive of celiac disease (serum tissue transglutaminase was raised). This is a malabsorption disorder which was confirmed by duodenal biopsy. The micronutrient deficiencies were a result of malabsorption. The child was shifted on gluten-free diet and started on micronutrient supplements after which he showed improvement in growth (chart shown below).

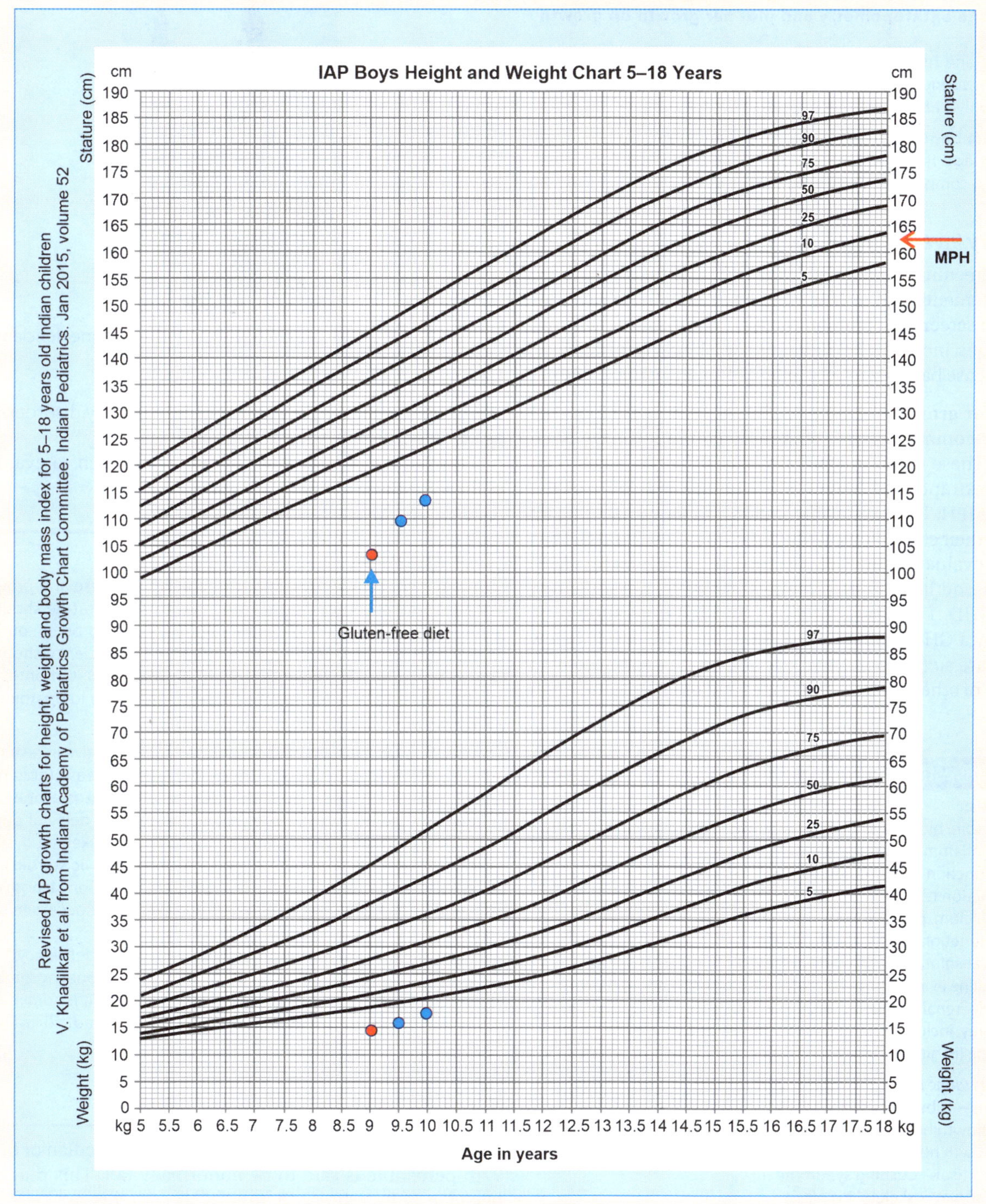

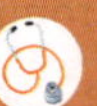

CASE STUDY Exercise

An 8-year-old girl (birth weight—2.3 kg), brought with poor growth since 2 years of age. There is history of blood transfusion 1 year back (hemoglobin—7.2 g%). She is diagnosed with celiac disease. Present weight is 14.2 kg, height is 110.3 cm, MPH is 154 cm. Bone age is 6 years.

Interpret the anthropometry and plot her growth on growth charts.
Her weight and height *Z*-scores on IAP charts are –3.03 and –2.4, respectively, suggesting more severe impact on weight than height. The BMI is only 11.57 kg/m^2, that suggests poor nutrition.

Interpret her bone age with relation to height age.
Her height age is approximately 5.5 years, bone age is 6 years suggesting a comparative delay in both.

Laboratory Investigations

A simple screening set of investigations which should be ordered initially are mentioned in **Box 2.5**. The screening set includes tests which screen for common causes of short stature. Further investigations, including hormonal assays, should be ordered on individual case basis according to historical and clinical cues.

Evaluate for growth hormone deficiency: Evaluate for GHD after other common causes of growth retardation have been excluded. These children generally have infantile facies **(Fig. 2.3)**. The extrapolated height falls significantly short of the respective MPH. The skeletal maturation also shows a significant delay than their chronological age (BA < HA < CA). Basal GH has no role in evaluating the GH-insulin-like growth factor (IGF) axis. IGF-1 and its binding protein-3 (IGFBP-3) are screening tests for GHD. Low levels of IGF-1 and IGF-BP3 should be followed by a GH stimulation test. Stimulated GH levels below 10 ng/mL are suggestive of GHD. This should be followed with evaluation of other pituitary hormones and brain imaging. High GH levels are suggestive of rare GH insensitivity disorders such as Laron syndrome.

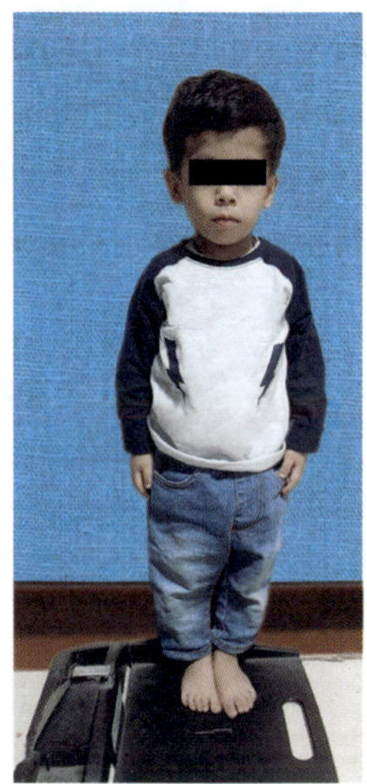

Fig. 2.3: A 6-year-old child with growth hormone deficiency

Flowchart 2.2 shows a schematic approach to evaluate a child with short stature.

Box 2.5 Investigations in Pathological Short Stature

First line tests:
- Hemoglobin, blood counts, ESR—anemia, hematological disorders, chronic inflammatory diseases
- Kidney function tests—chronic kidney disease
- Liver function tests—chronic liver disease
- Serum calcium, phosphorus—rickets
- Thyroid function test—hypothyroidism
- Serum transglutaminase—celiac disease
- Urine routine examination—diabetes mellitus, nephrotic syndrome
- Urine pH—renal tubular acidosis
- Chest X-ray, including hand X-ray for bone age assessment
- Karyotype (in girls)—Turner syndrome

Specific tests (done on case-to-case basis):
- Infections—tuberculosis, HIV
- Serum growth hormone (GH), IGF-1 levels and GH stimulation test—growth hormone deficiency (GHD)
- Serum cortisol—Cushing syndrome
- Skeletal survey—skeletal dysplasia
- Imaging of brain including pituitary fossa—GHD
- Genetic mutations—*POU1F1, PIT1, PROP1, HESX1, SHOX*

TREATMENT Short Stature

Management includes treatment of underlying cause and provision of adequate nutrition intake. Patients with short stature should be advised high protein and calorie diet. They should be encouraged to increase physical activity. Iron and vitamin deficiency should be corrected. Zinc supplementation (10 mg/day for 3–6 months) has been shown to be effective in improving growth in idiopathic short stature.

Specific therapy: Initiation of specific treatment is effective in restoration of growth in hypothyroidism (thyroxine), celiac disease (gluten-free diet), and renal tubular acidosis (bicarbonate). Testosterone (short course) should be given in boys with constitutional delay of puberty and growth. Treatment of genetic syndromes and skeletal dysplasia is difficult. Recombinant GH, androgen, and anabolic steroids have been tried with success in some of these conditions. Bone lengthening (Ilizarov technique) has been used with variable success in a few children.

Recombinant GH therapy is highly effective in GH deficiency, Turner syndrome, chronic renal failure, small for gestational age infants, Prader–Willi syndrome, and idiopathic short stature. It is administered as a daily subcutaneous injection and continued till the child completes linear growth.

TALL STATURE

A child with a height of >2 *Z*-score above the median or beyond 97th percentile is said to be abnormally tall. This may occur because of hereditary factors (if the parents are tall), cerebral gigantism, acromegaly, and chromosomal abnormality (Klinefelter syndrome). Tall stature associated with dispro-

Flowchart 2.2: Algorithmic approach for clinical evaluation of short stature

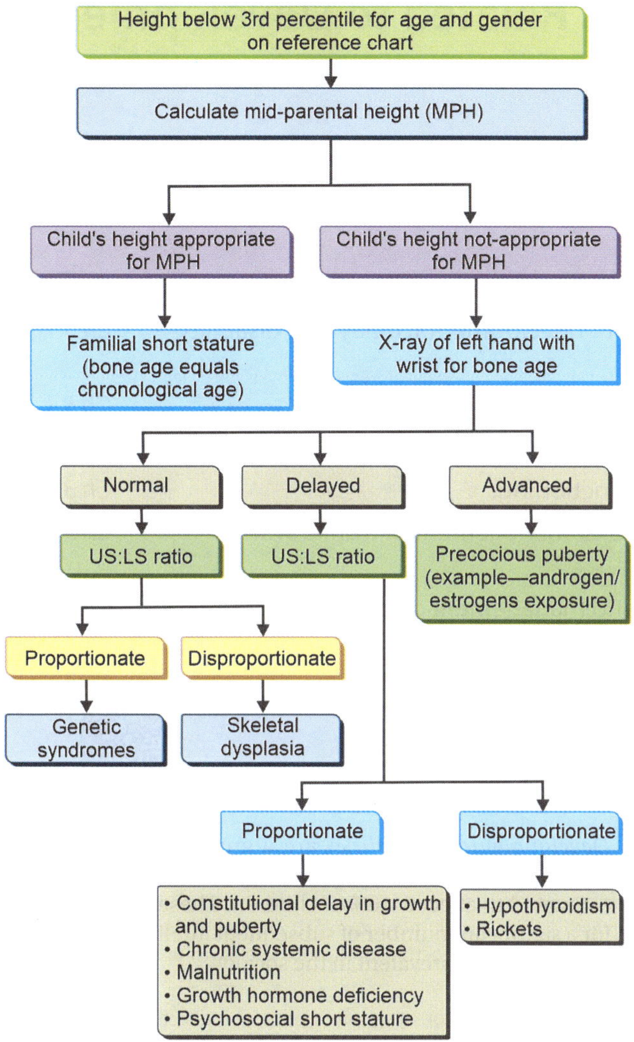

(LS: lower segment; SD: standard deviation: US: upper segment)

portionately long limbs is characteristic of Marfan syndrome and homocystinuria.

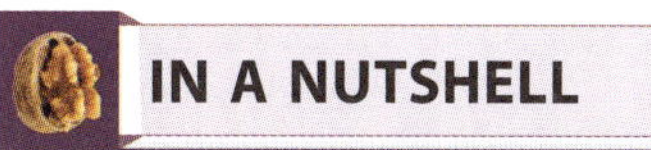

IN A NUTSHELL

Short Stature

1. Correct measurement and interpretation of anthropometry is the most important step in assessment of short stature.
2. Growth charts are the most important tool to interpret the growth patterns. Growth velocity is a better indicator than single-point value.
3. Systemic causes, familial short stature, and constitutional delay in growth are common causes of poor growth than endocrinal causes of short stature.
4. Assessment of growth should be in accordance with the pubertal growth pattern (in children of peripubertal age) and skeletal age (assessed on plain radiograph of left hand with wrist and fingers).

Chiarelli F, Primavera M, Mastromauro C. Evaluation and management of a child with short stature. Minerva Pediatr. 2020;72(6):452-61.

Grigoletto V, Occhipinti AA, Pellegrin MC, et al. Definition and prevalence of familial short stature. Ital J Pediatr. 2021;47(1):56.

Grunauer M, Jorge AAL. Genetic short stature. Growth Horm IGF Res. 2018;38:29-33.

Jee YH, Baron J, Nilsson O. New developments in the genetic diagnosis of short stature. Curr Opin Pediatr. 2018;30(4):541-7.

Patel R, Bajpai A. Evaluation of short stature in children and adolescents. Indian J Pediatr. 2021;88(12):1196-202.

Şıklar Z, Berberoğlu M. Syndromic disorders with short stature. J Clin Res Pediatr Endocrinol. 2014;6(1):1-8.

Singh K, Puri RD, Bijarnia-Mahay S, et al. Clinical and genetic profile of children with short stature presenting to a genetic clinic in Northern India. Indian Pediatr. 2022;59(6):463-6.

Yadav S, Dabas A. Approach to short stature. Indian J Pediatr. 2015;82(5):462-70.

3 CHAPTER Common Problems Related to Development

AS PER NMC COMPETENCIES

PE3.1	Define developmental delay. Describe the causes of developmental delay and disability including intellectual disability in children.	*Ch 3.1*
PE3.2	Explain the approach to a child with developmental delay.	*Ch 3.1*
PE3.3	Counsel a parent of a child with developmental delay.	*Ch 3.1*
PE3.4	Visit a child developmental unit and observe its functioning.	*Ch 3.1*
PE4.1	Describe the etiology, clinical features, diagnosis and management of a child with attention deficit hyperactivity disorder (ADHD).	*Ch 3.2*
PE4.2	Describe the etiology, clinical features, diagnosis and management of a child with autism.	*Ch 3.3*

Topics available online: ***Scholastic Backwardness and Learning Disorders***

Having read about the principles of development, and the normal developmental milestones, the natural question is, what if the development does not happen as per the normal milestones.

- *Disorders of development* are the result of an aberrant development sequence in one or more domains.
- *Developmental disabilities* are a group of related neurodevelopmental disorders with onset in early age and are estimated to affect 5–10% of children. These are responsible for a significant number of subsequent intellectual disability and handicaps prevalent in the society.

3.1 Developmental Delay *PE 3.1, PE 3.2, PE 3.3, PE 3.4*

DEFINITIONS

Development Delay

Developmental delay refers to significant delay in the acquisition of milestones in one or more developmental domains as compared to the peers. It is defined as a performance two standard deviations or more below the mean (–2SD) on age-appropriate, standardized norm referenced testing, in one or more of the domains of development (gross/fine motor, speech/language, cognition, and personal/social).

This term is used in children less than 6 years, as formal tools for assessing IQ in this age-group are not available, and also because quite a few children with developmental delay may not have any intellectual disability subsequently.

Developmental Quotient

It is the numeric expression of a child's developmental level, measured by dividing the developmental age by the chronologic age and multiplying by 100. Ideally, chronological age should be equal to that of developmental age and the developmental quotient (DQ) should, therefore, be 100. A DQ of <70 is labeled as delay. DQ should be estimated separately for each area of development, viz., motor, adaptive/cognitive, language, and personal/social.

Global Developmental Delay

It is defined as a significant delay in two or more (≥2) of the following developmental domains: (1) Gross/fine motor, (2) speech/language, (3) cognition, (4) social/personal, and (5) activities of daily living. Significant delay means performance being two or more standard deviations lower than the mean, on age-appropriate, standardized norm-referenced testing. Usually children with global developmental delay have delay across all the domains. This term is reserved for children below 5 years of age.

Intellectual disability is the term used for children older than 5 years in whom formal intelligence quotient (IQ) testing is possible.

Developmental Dissociation

Development in one domain may not necessarily run parallel to that in the other spheres. Developmental dissociation occurs when the rates of development differ in different domains. For example, a child with autism is grossly delayed in language and personal social spheres but may have a normal gross motor development.

Developmental Deviance

There is non-sequential unevenness in the achievement of milestones within one or more streams of development. It is considered normal variant. For example, some infants are bottom shufflers and never attain creeping; still walking will be achieved within physiological period.

Developmental Regression

It refers to the loss of previously acquired skills or milestones and should alert to a possibility of a degenerative brain disorder.

ETIOLOGY

There are many conditions underlying developmental delay (**Box 3.1**). The more common ones reported among children in India are genetic conditions, hypoxic ischemic encephalopathy (HIE) following perinatal asphyxia, and hypothyroidism.

Box 3.1 Common Causes of Abnormal Development

- ***Genetic:*** One of the common causes of developmental delay. There may be copy number variants (CNVs), insertions, deletions, and duplications.
  Some of the important syndromes associated with developmental delay:
  - Down syndrome
  - Fragile X syndrome
  - Prader-Willi syndrome
  - Rett syndrome
- ***Acquired:***
  - *Antenatal:*
    - *Maternal factors:* Exposure to teratogens (alcohol, drugs, radiation, etc.) in pregnancy, infections such as cytomegalovirus, rubella, toxoplasma, HIV, placental dysfunction, toxemia, antepartum hemorrhage, etc.
    - *Fetal factors:* Congenital CNS malformations, extreme prematurity, metabolic disorders (hypoglycemia, galactosemia, mucopolysaccharidosis, phenylketonuria), etc.
  - *Natal:* Hypoxic-ischemic insult and birth injuries, intracranial hemorrhage.
  - *Postnatal:* Meningitis, encephalitis, hypoxia, kernicterus, stroke.
  - *Others:*
    - Hypothyroidism is the most important preventable cause of intellectual disability.
    - *CNS disorders:* Cerebral palsy, neurocutaneous syndromes (neurofibromatosis, tuberous sclerosis) and degenerative brain diseases.
- ***Psychosocial factors:***
  - Maternal stress such as depression, anxiety, etc.
  - Maltreatment and/or domestic violence
  - Poverty
  - Malnutrition, especially multivitamins and minerals deficiency, such as iron, folate, vitamin D, calcium

EARLY DETECTION OF DEVELOPMENTAL DELAY

Developmental Surveillance

Surveillance refers to the informal, more flexible and ongoing assessment of development and includes process of identification of potential risk factors for abnormal development. It goes hand-in-hand with developmental screening and is achieved by eliciting a good history, observing the child by a close follow-up, keeping a continuous record of these findings, and attending to parents' concerns. Close continuous contact with the parents is the key for good developmental surveillance.

Developmental Screening

Developmental screening refers to administration of standard and validated norm-referenced tests that help in early identification of children at risk for a developmental disorder. Developmental screening supported with culturally acceptable tools is considered superior to developmental surveillance. It is desirable for a developmental screening tool to have a specificity and sensitivity of at least 70–80%. Children who fail a screening test need close follow-up and additional diagnostic assessment.

Time of Screening

Indian Academy of Pediatrics (IAP) recommends routine developmental screening using standardized screening tools at 9–12 months, 18–24 months of age, and at school entry and additionally at 4–6 months of age for high-risk infants. The age of routine screening coincides with the immunization visits. American Academy of Pediatrics (AAP) recommends routine developmental screening at 9, 18, and 24–30 months of age.

Tools for Screening

American Academy of Pediatrics uses Parents' Evaluation of Developmental Status (PEDS) or Ages and Stages Questionnaire (ASQ) tests for developmental screening. Indian adaptations and versions of development screening tests available include the Phatak Baroda Screening Test (for children up to 30 months) and Trivandrum Development Screening Chart (TDSC) (till 6 years of age). Both these tests have been developed from the Bayley scales of infant development. It takes around 5 minutes to administer the TDSC. *Rashtriya Bal Swasthya Karyakram* (RBSK) screening tool is a newer test developed by the Government of India, which assesses vision, hearing, speech, motor, cognition, and social milestones in children up to 6 years of age, and requires 10 minutes to be administered.

Other Screening Tools

- ***Ages and Stages Questionnaire (ASQ)*** is an internationally validated developmental screening tool with a good sensitivity/specificity. It takes just 15 minutes to administer and can be used to screen children between 1 month and 5.5 years of age.
- ***Development Profile-3rd edition*** (DP-3) is a commonly used screening tool used in children up to 12 years age and provides age equivalent and norm based standard scores in each domain and an overall DQ.
- ***Denver-II (DDST-II)***, is the newer version of Denver Development Screening Test (DDST). It is designed to be used with apparently well children till 6 years of age and takes around 10–15 minutes.
- ***Parents' Evaluation of Developmental Status (PEDS)*** is another screening tool that can be used to screen children up to 8 years of age.

MOTHER AND CHILD PROTECTION CARD

Mother and Child Protection (MCP) card is a simple, community-based, culturally appropriate tool used by accredited social health activists (ASHA)/anganwadi workers (AWW) throughout India for monitoring maternal and child health, educate families regarding positive health practices, and provide information regarding available healthcare services for women and children under the age of 3 years.

- It gives information regarding the neonatal care, immunization, infant and young child feeding, and growth and development of the child.
- The development component is meant for children between 2 and 36 months across seven age groups, and includes a guide for monitoring, giving parenting tips for stimulation and identifying presence of warning signs for timely referrals.
- Each age group is divided into three color zones containing age-specific textual and pictorial information (**Figs. 3.1A to G**):
    1. The *green zone* comprises age-appropriate developmental skills that the mother ticks/checks, once attained, or alternatively, the health worker does it at any contact with family.
    2. The *blue zone* contains parenting tips pertaining to age-appropriate developmental stimulation.
    3. The *red zone* of MCP card depicts clinical indicators of possible atypical development and intends to link the family members to RBSK through which they can: (1) understand and identify any development faltering in their child at the right time, and (2) avail free management and treatment at tertiary level.

DEFINITIVE TESTS FOR DIAGNOSIS OF DEVELOPMENTAL DELAY

- Children suspected to be abnormal on a screening test should undergo definitive intelligence tests. These tests are based on evaluation of gross motor, fine motor, language, behavior, and visual problem-solving skills. *Bayley Scale of Infant Development (BSID-IV)* is the most used intelligence scale for children 16 days to 3½ years of age.
- The Indian counterpart of this test is known as *Developmental Assessment Scale for Indian Infants (DASII)* and is the most widely applied tool for definitive diagnosis of developmental delay in Indian children.
- Wechsler Intelligence Scale for Children (WISC) is used to assess intelligence in children above 6 years.
- In India, Malin Intelligence Scale for Indian Children (MISIC) is used for assessment in children older more than 5 years; this test is an adaptation of WISC.

For developmental evaluation of preterm babies, corrected gestational age is used till 2 years of chronological age.

APPROACH TO DEVELOPMENTAL DELAY

It is difficult to diagnose developmental delay in the early weeks of life. A correct diagnosis is mainly based on a detailed history. History of prenatal and perinatal risk factors is highly relevant to mental and physical development. Also obtain history of important genetic conditions, degenerative disorders, and environmental factors (child abuse, parent child relations, etc.) that may lead to delayed development. Inquire about relevant illnesses such as rickets, malnutrition, and systemic disorders. Results of newborn screening, if done, are essential.

Assessment of chronology of development and age of achievement of milestones is the next step. Ask this history from the mother or caregiver. There may be a family history of early or late motor, sphincter, or language development. Be careful to ask the developmental history in simple language and in a precise manner. When inquiring about developing a new skill, ask: (1) when did it develop; (2) how often it is practiced; and (3) what is the degree of maturity with which this skill is performed.

Additionally, the child should be subjected to a complete developmental examination.

Early Diagnosis of Global Developmental Delay and Intellectual Disability

The degree of intellectual disability (mild, moderate, or severe) usually modulates the age of diagnosis.

- Infants with *severe disability* are markedly delayed with their psychomotor skills in the first year of life.
- A severely disabled child exhibits global developmental delay from early infancy and may exhibit one or more of the following features:
    - Sleeps excessively, is lethargic, and has feeding difficulties.
    - Does not take notice of surroundings, and social smile is delayed.

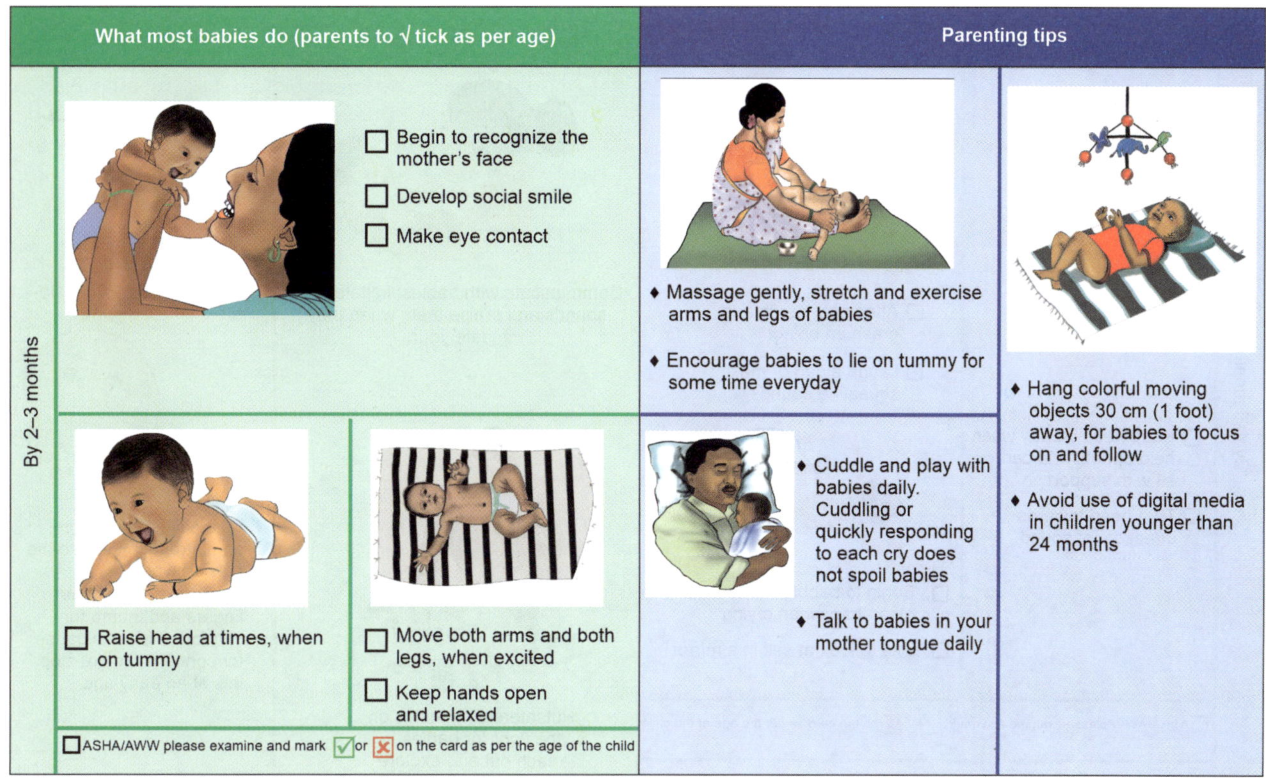

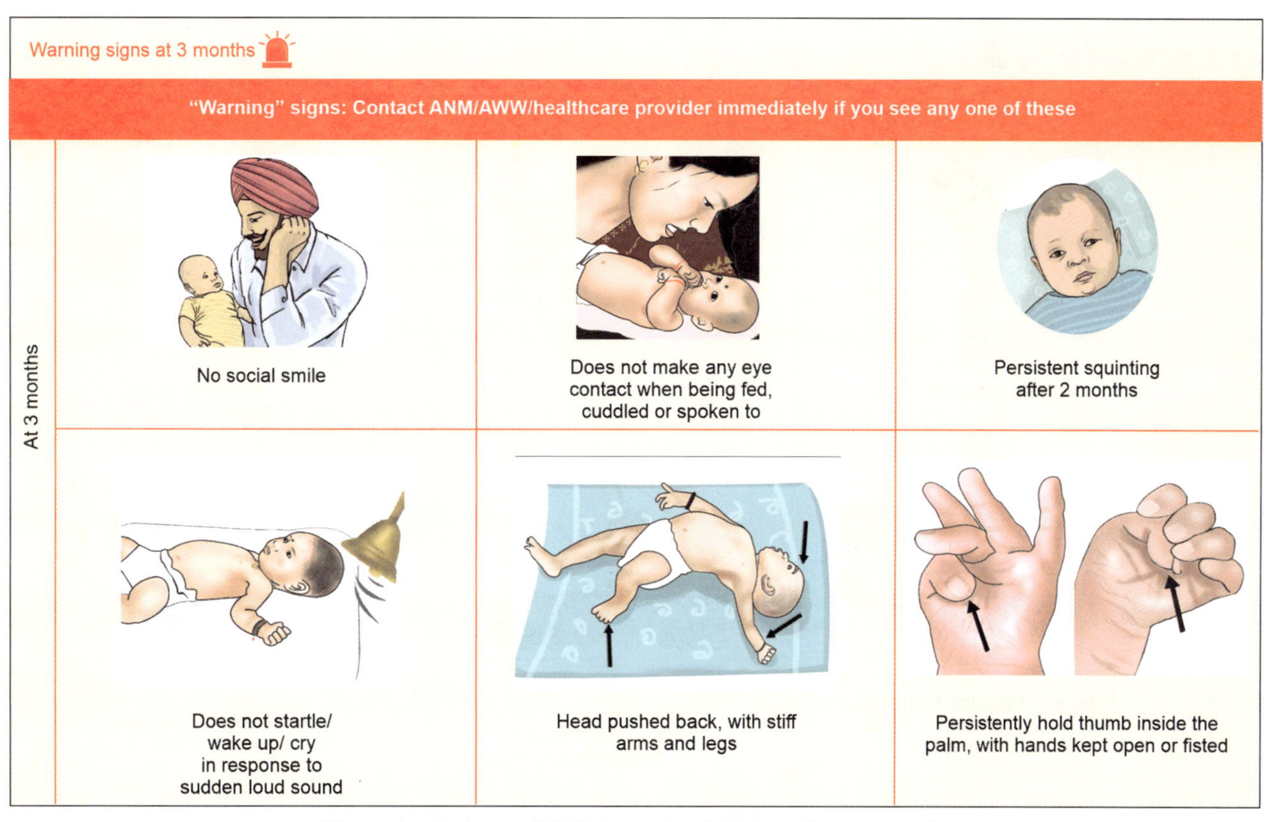

Fig. 3.1A: Mother and Child Protection (MCP) card for 2–3 months

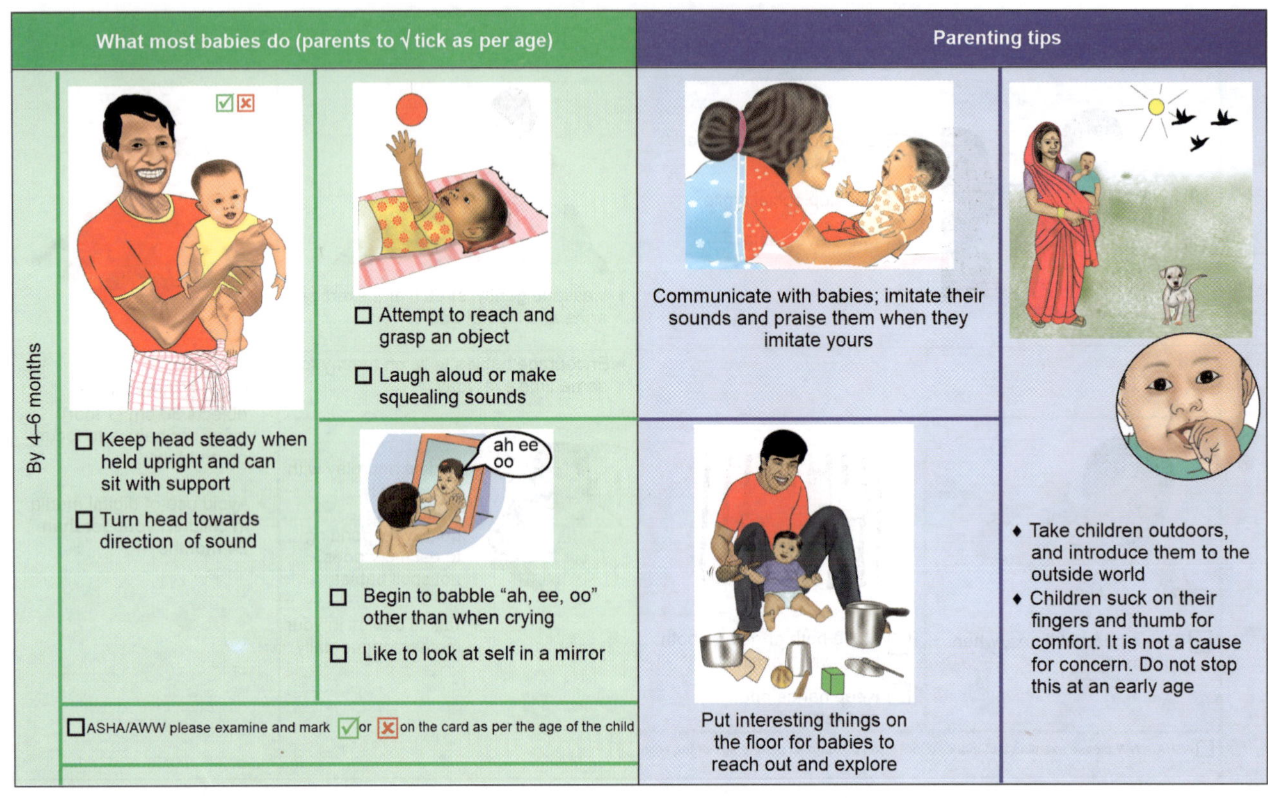

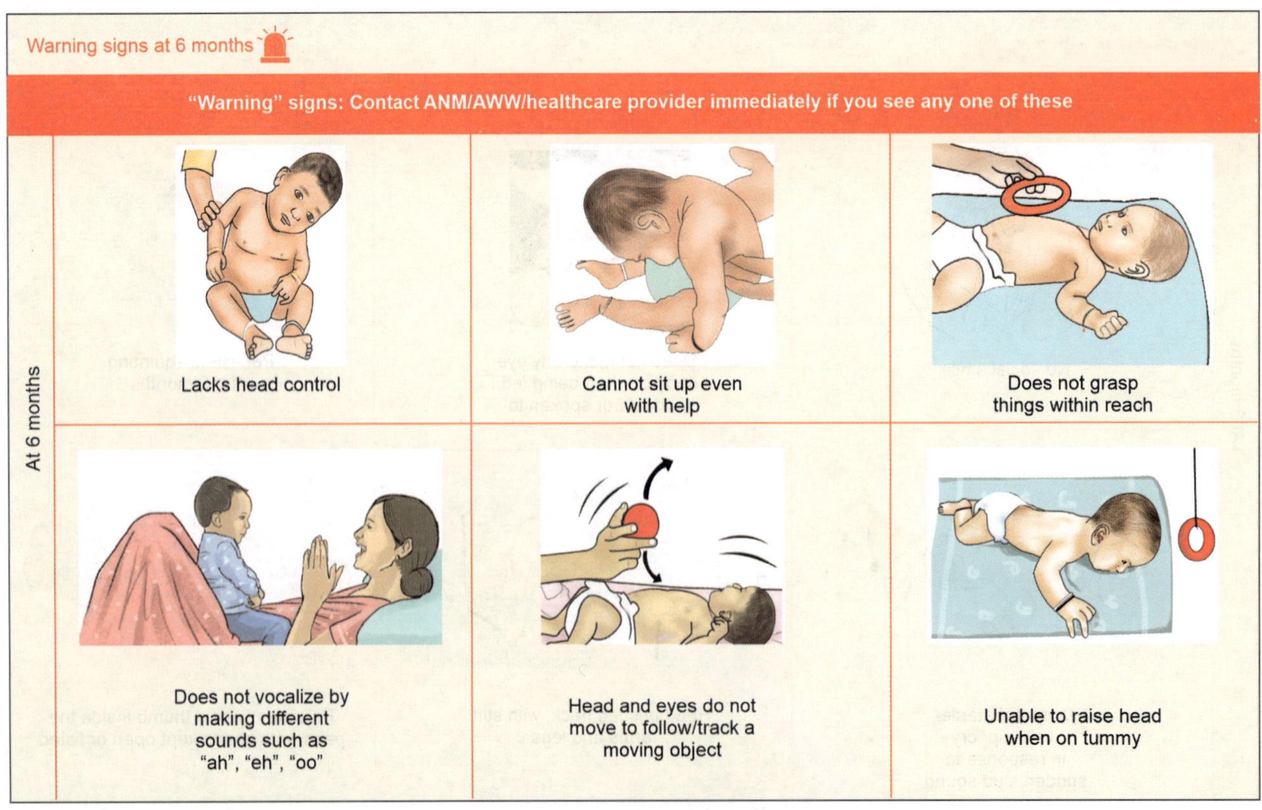

Fig. 3.1B: Mother and Child Protection (MCP) card for 4–6 months

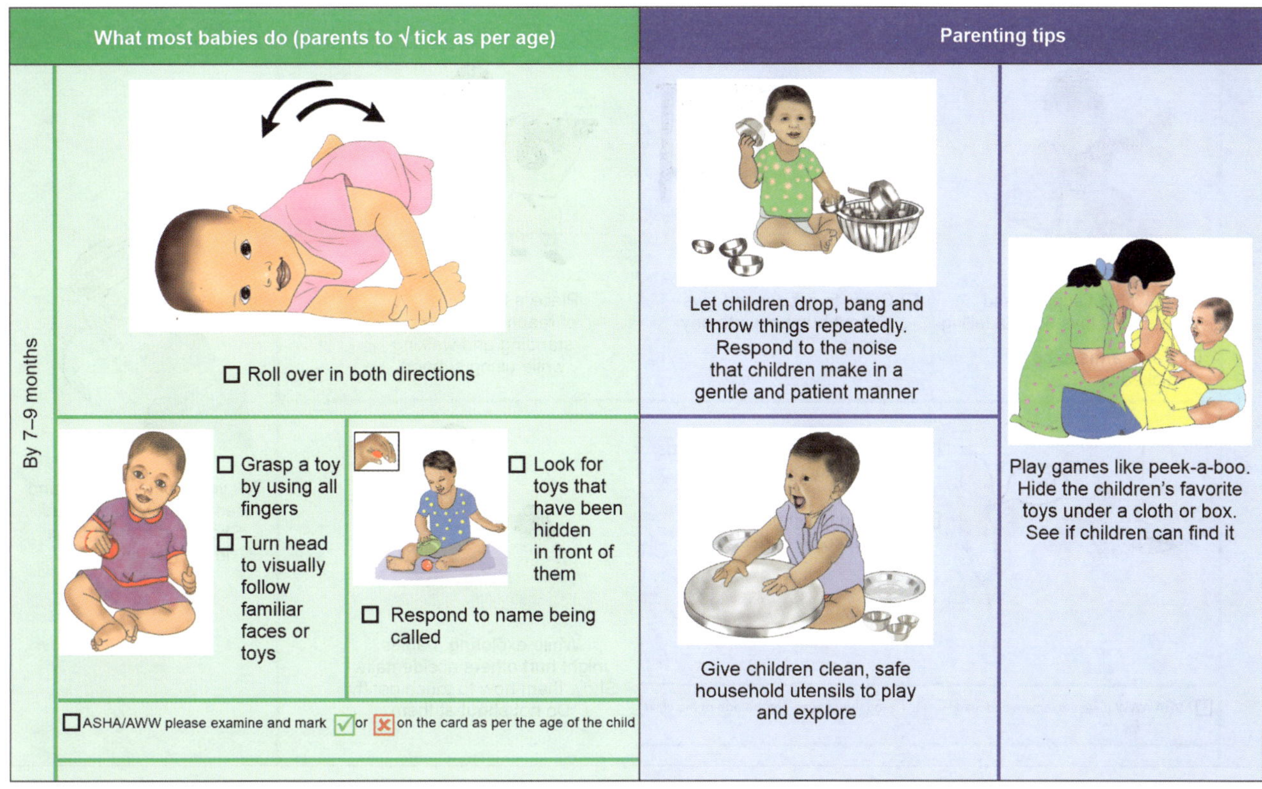

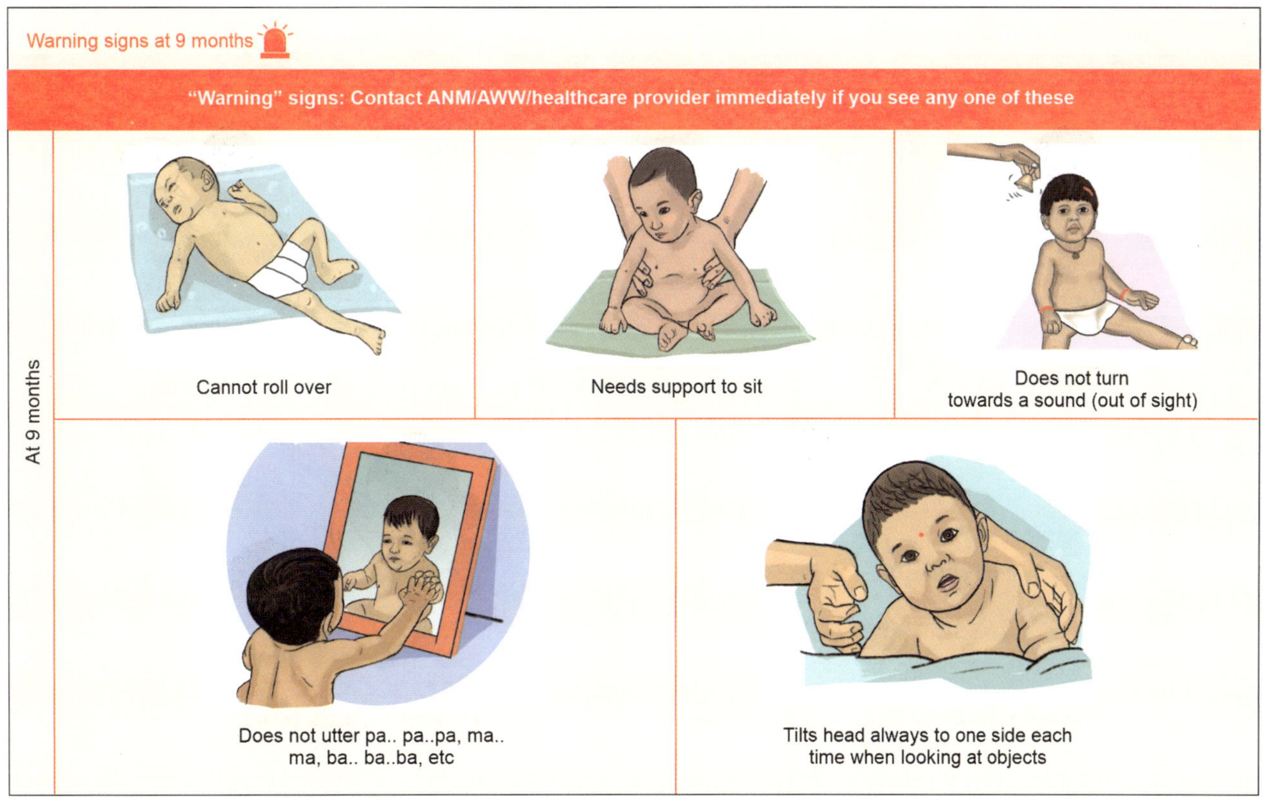

Fig. 3.1C: Mother and Child Protection (MCP) card for 7–9 months

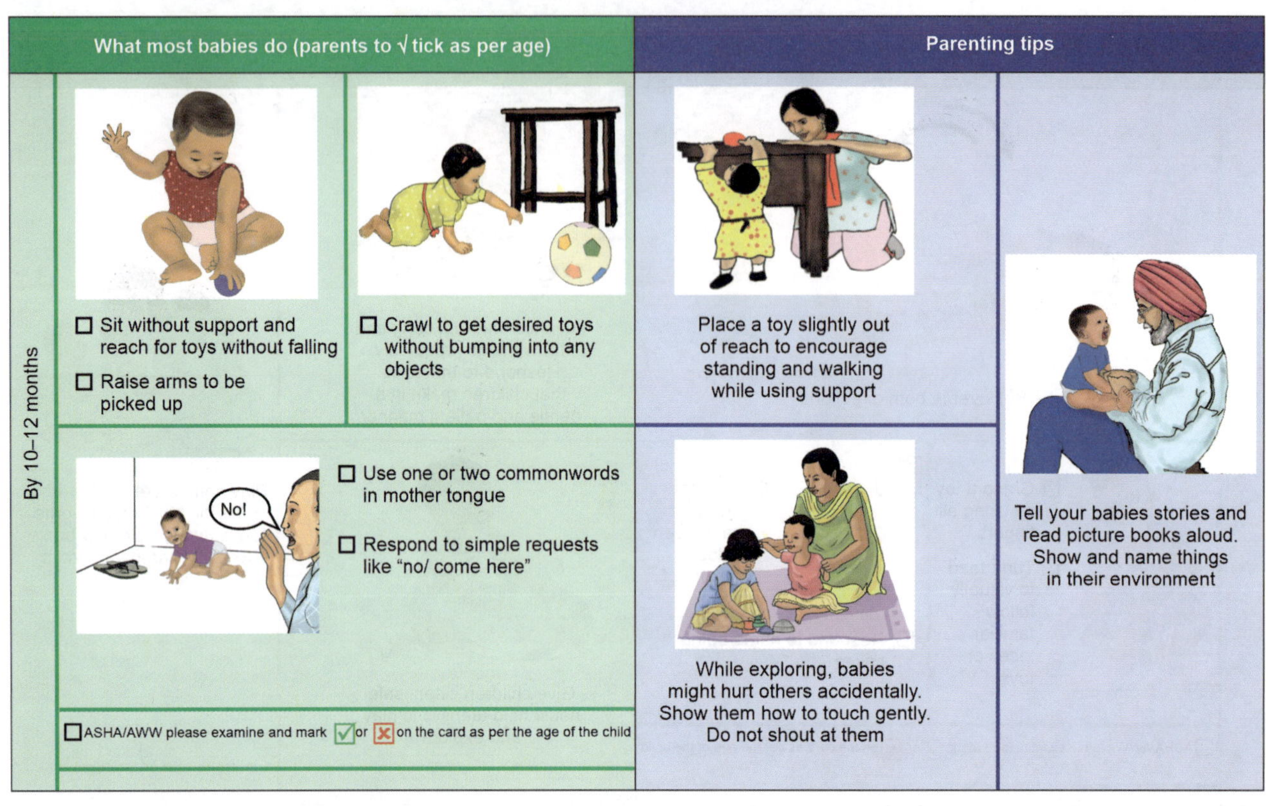

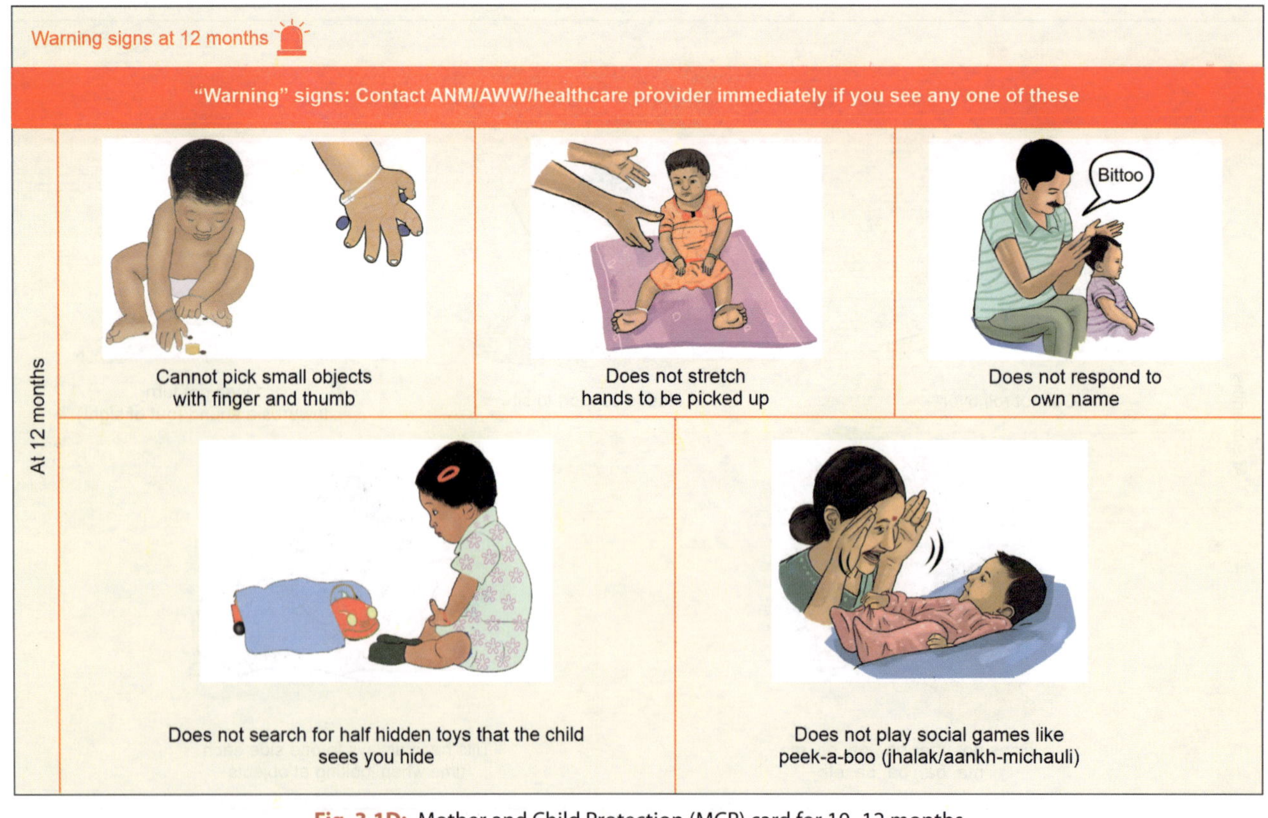

Fig. 3.1D: Mother and Child Protection (MCP) card for 10–12 months

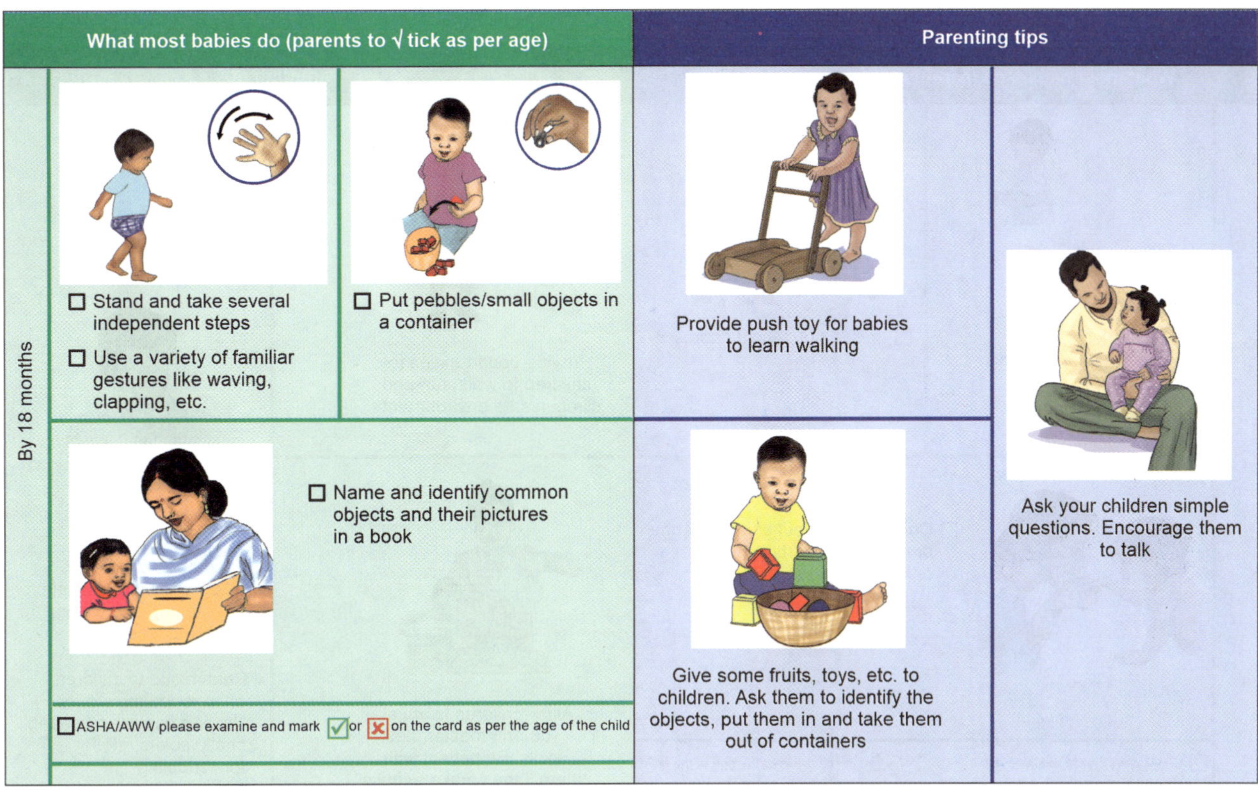

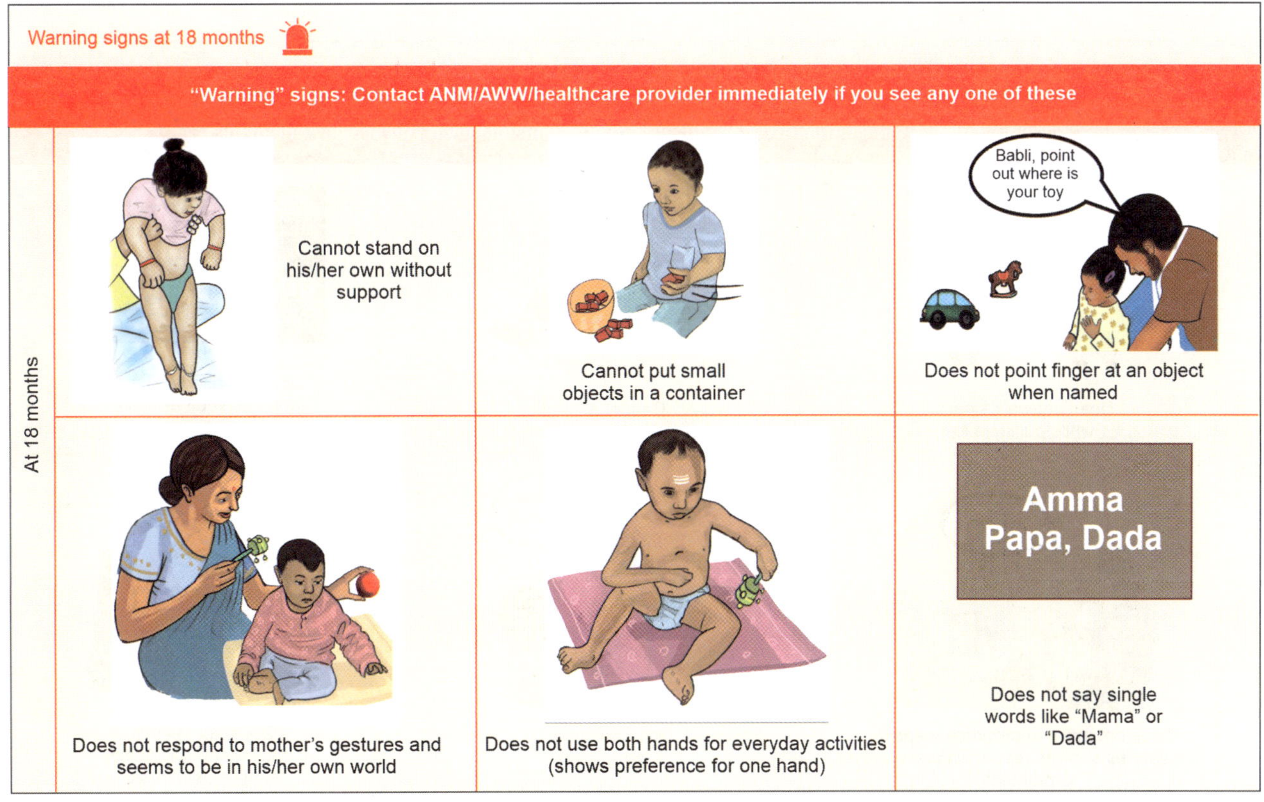

Fig. 3.1E: Mother and Child Protection (MCP) card for 18 months

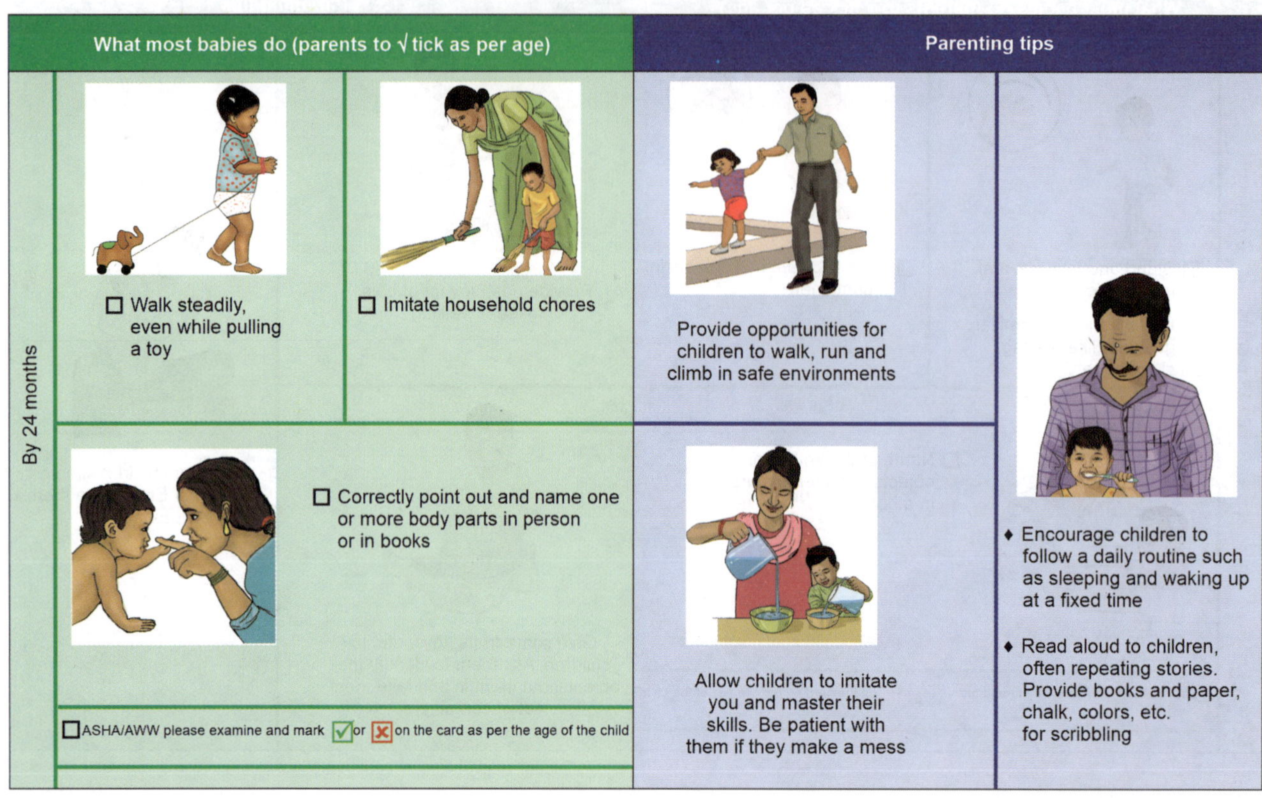

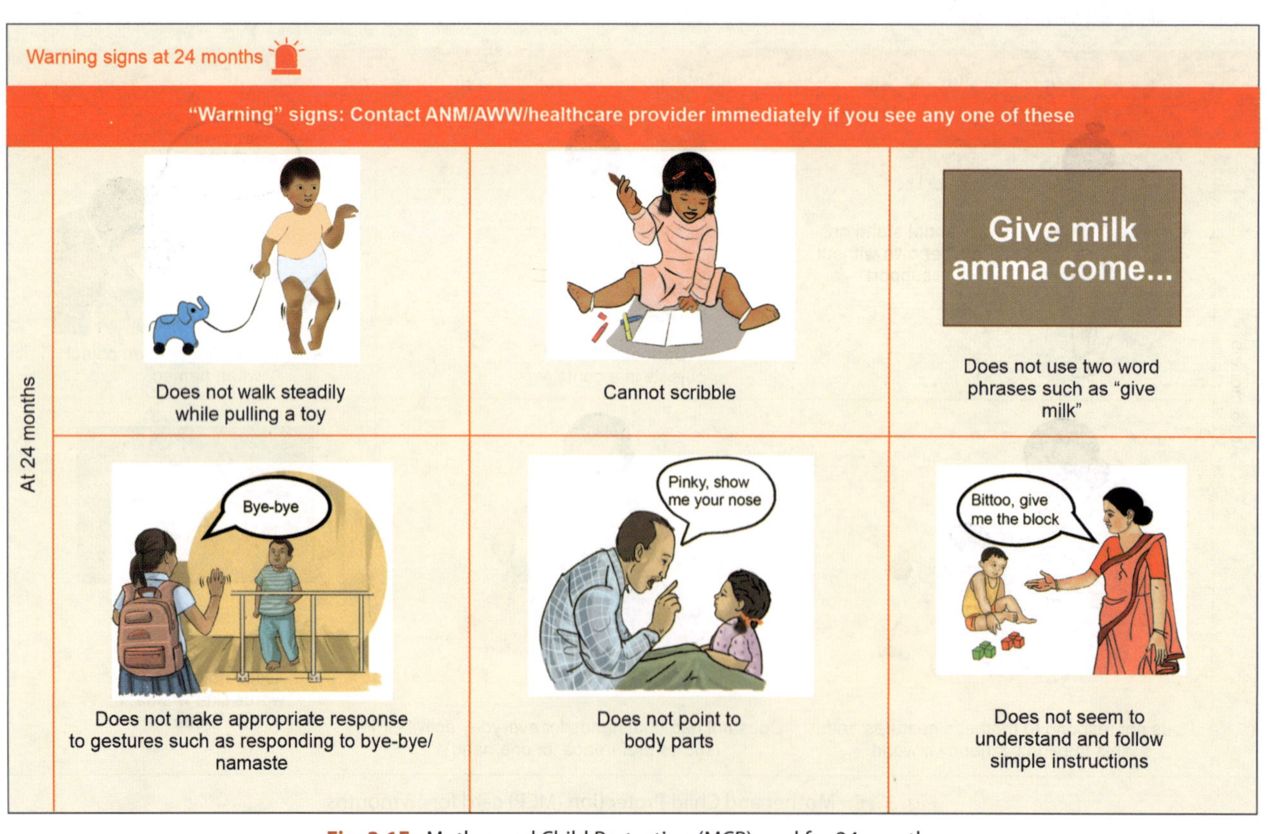

Fig. 3.1F: Mother and Child Protection (MCP) card for 24 months

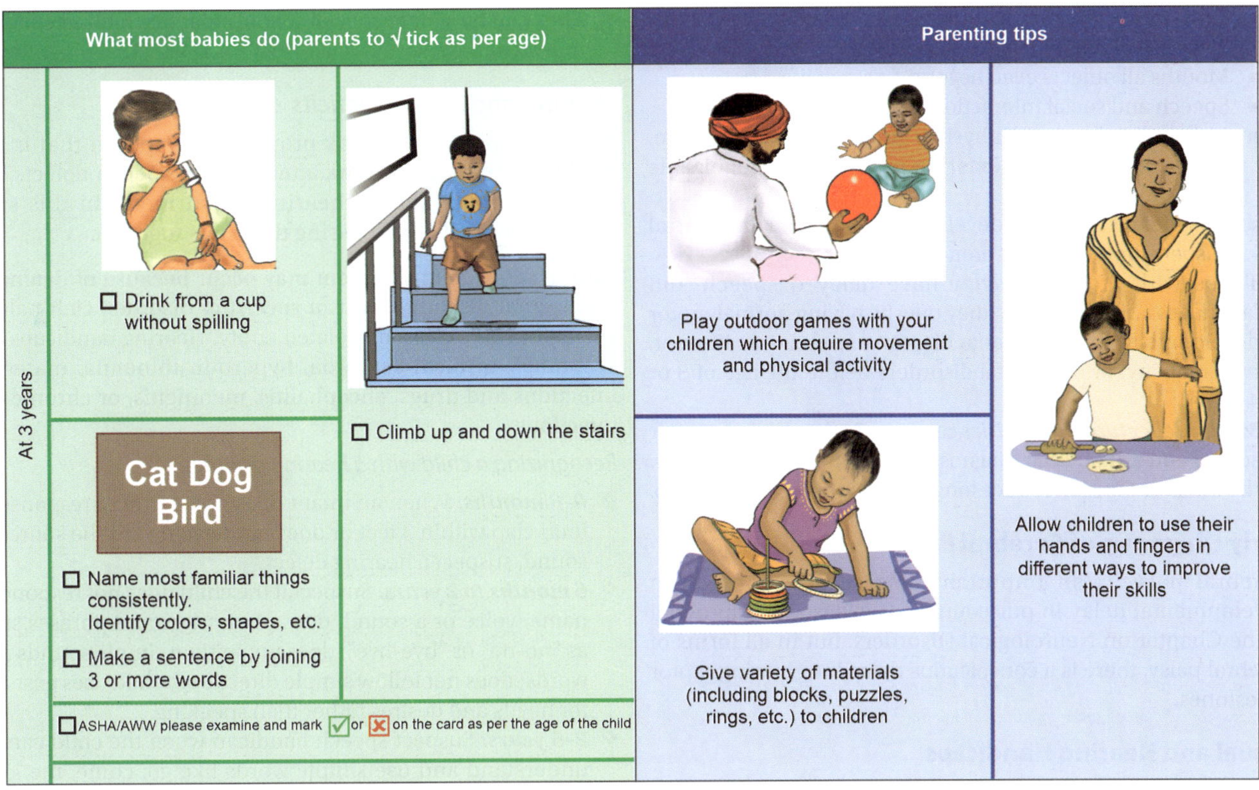

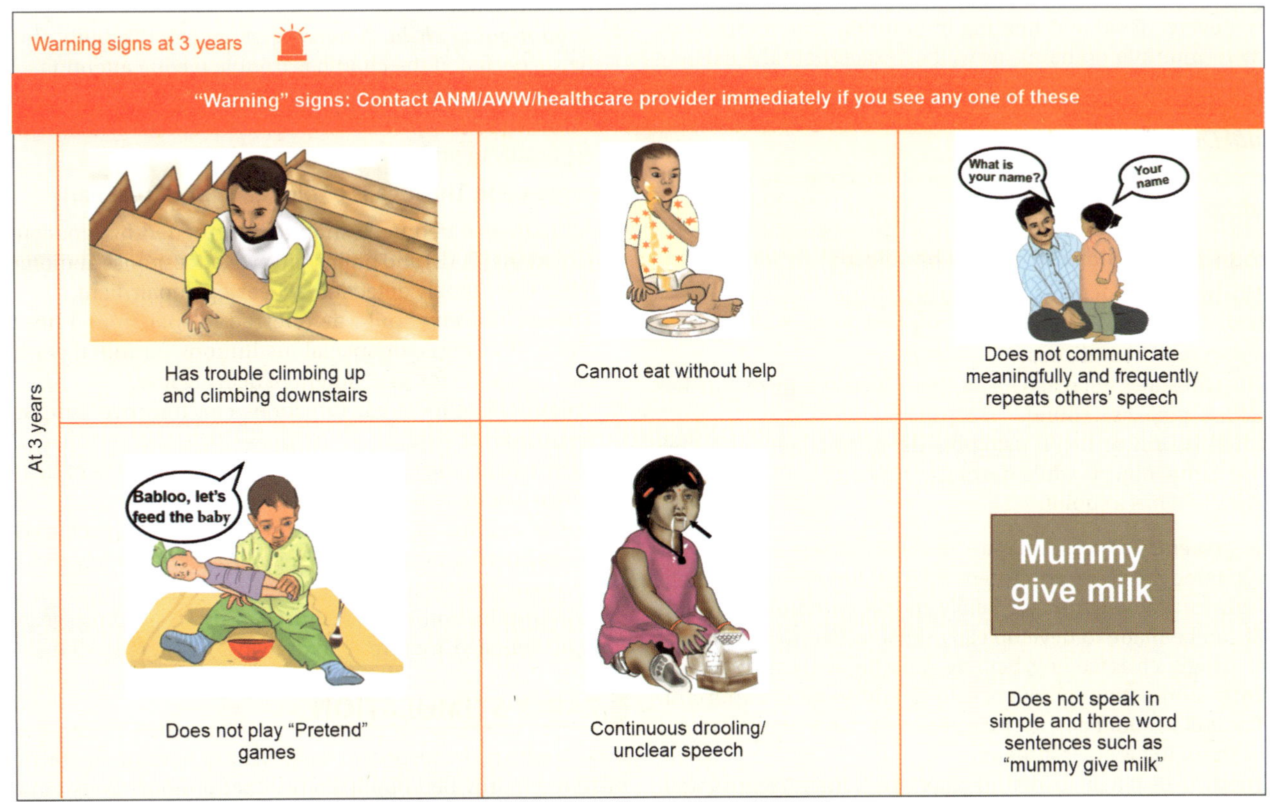

Fig. 3.1G: Mother and Child Protection (MCP) card for 3 years

Figs. 3.1A to G: Mother Child Protection cards for different ages of child

- Constantly keeps watching his hands even after 20 weeks of life (persistent hand regard).
- Mouths all objects even beyond 1 year of life.
- Speech and social interaction are delayed.
- May have abnormal physical findings (dysmorphism, congenital malformations) suggestive of a recognizable syndrome.
- Has delayed motor development as seen in ventral suspension, supine, or prone position.

❖ Those with *moderate delay* have delayed speech and languages abilities though they may be having normal motor development. It is unusual to diagnose speech impairment, hyperactivity, or emotional disorders before the age of 3 or 4 years.

❖ ***Mild intellectual disabilities*** can be only detected at or after school entry. If one can diagnose developmental delay early, the intervention can reduce long-term sequelae or handicap.

Early Diagnosis of Cerebral Palsy

Cerebral palsy is an important disease presenting with developmental delay in our country. It is described in detail in the Chapter on Neurological Disorders, but in all forms of cerebral palsy, there is a conspicuous delay in achieving motor milestones.

Visual and Hearing Handicaps

Sensory handicaps include visual and hearing defects. They may be isolated or associated with mental or physical handicaps. Severe visual and hearing impairment can manifest as delay in multiple domains, as well as exacerbate the existing developmental problems.

Visual Deficits

The severity of visual handicaps varies from complete blindness to not being able to see clearly.

Recognizing a child with a visual handicap:

❖ The infant may have a white or a gray pupil.

❖ If by 3 months, the child does not look at mother's face or object or light and does not follow them.

❖ The child does not reach for an object held in front of him/her unless it makes a sound.

❖ Child is slow to begin using hands, move about, and may bump into objects while moving around.

❖ The child has a squint.

Management: Early referral must be made to an eye specialist for ascertaining the cause and extent of visual handicap. With help and encouragement from the family and the community, a blind child can be made to develop early skills related to activities of daily living such as feeding, bathing, dressing, and caring for self.

❖ Early stimulation by touch, sound, and smell is important. The child should be informed about each activity and sound to orient to his environment.

❖ They can be taught to identify places and landmarks and walk with the help of a stick.

❖ They can be sent to special schools that teach blind children to read and write.

Hearing and Speech Deficits

A child's inability to speak properly or a speech that is not easily understood or draws attention is a speech defect. The most common cause is hearing impairment. In this subsection, we shall be discussing these two together.

Causes: Speech impairment may occur because of deafness, intellectual disability, autism spectrum disorder, cleft palate, voice disorders or as an isolated entity. Hearing handicaps are secondary to birth asphyxia, hyperbilirubinemia, maternal infections and drugs, encephalitis, meningitis, or chronic ear infections.

Recognizing a child with a hearing disorder:

❖ ***0–6 months:*** When an infant does not startle in response to loud clap within 3 feet or does not turn toward the source of sound, suspect a hearing defect.

❖ ***6 months to 2 years:*** Suspect if the child does not respond to name, voice or a sound, does not understand phrases such as "no-no" or "bye-bye"; does not initiate simple sounds and words; does not follow simple directions; child uses gestures for needs and desires rather than speaking.

❖ ***2–5 years:*** Suspect speech handicap when the child cannot understand and use simple words like go, come, me, etc., cannot carry on a simple conversation and speech is difficult to understand.

❖ ***School-going child:*** A hearing or speech disability should be suspected, if the child has trouble paying attention, does not answer when called, gets confused about directions or questions, appears slow and does not do well in school, especially in oral tests.

Management: The idea is to pick early and treat early

❖ All high-risk neonates should be screened by otoacoustic emissions (OAE) and brainstem evoked response audiometry (BERA) for timely detection of hearing impairment.

❖ These children should be referred to speech and hearing clinic, ENT clinic or special institutions for initial work up and guidance for assessment of hearing loss.

❖ Treatment of local ear infections can improve temporary hearing loss.

❖ Hearing aids may be needed to improve the level of hearing which would help in speech therapy.

❖ Cochlear implant, done as early as possible, is preferred for sensorineural hearing loss in children and widely used for secondary prevention of hearing handicap.

❖ Communication can be improved by lip reading, gesture, sign language, pictures and drawing, or finger spelling.

EARLY STIMULATION

Infants who show suspect or early signs of developmental delay need to be provided opportunities that promote body control, acquisition of motor skills, language development, and psychosocial maturity. These inputs, termed early stimulation, include measures such as making additional efforts to make the child sit and walk, giving toys to manipulate, playing with the child, showing objects, speaking to the child, and encouraging him to speak, and prompting the child to interact with others, so as to stimulate all sensory and motor faculties.

CHILD DEVELOPMENT UNIT

A child development unit is the cornerstone of management of children with development delay, and other development and behavioral problems. It usually comprises a multidisciplinary team of experts consisting of pediatrician/pediatric neurologists, psychologists, occupational therapists, physiotherapists, special educators, and speech therapists.

The team is specialized in assessing child's development, behavioral problems, assessment and diagnosis of various developmental disorders, planning the relevant investigations, management of associated comorbidities, providing the intervention, and caregiver counseling. The team works in collaboration to provide a comprehensive assessment and management tailored to the specific needs of children and families. Services of the pediatrician are usually required to coordinate various therapies and medications.

Box 3.2 provides an overview of what all you should observe when visiting a child development unit.

Counseling of the Parent of a Child with Developmental Delay

Counseling is an important aspect of the composite management of a child with development delay. The professional guidance is given to the parent/family of the child to understand nature of the developmental delay, etiology, anticipated comorbidities, requisite investigations, prognosis, therapy goals and follow-up schedule. The counseling should be done in a clear, direct and compassionate manner, preferably in the family's local language, emphasizing equally on child's strengths as well as deficits, and the potential for improvement with interventions.

It is important to reiterate on the possibility of improvement with consistent intervention, even in a severely delayed child of any age, especially if younger than 5 years.

Box 3.2 | Visit to a Child Development Unit (CDU)

When visiting a child development unit, students should at least note the following:

1. How is the building/room designed—is it disabled-friendly? Does it have a child friendly color to interior decoration? Are there any areas which may be dangerous to a young child? Is there a separate area for parents to wait?
2. What are the professionals working there?
3. What are the diagnostic tools being used there? Conners/MCHAT/ INDT-ASD/ISAA/DASII/ GLAD/NIMHANS Index, etc.
4. Are there any specialized instruments/machines there? Look for BERA/OAE, sensory room, occupational therapy, and physiotherapy equipment.

Write in your notebook on above points. Close with your impression about the role of CDU, and importance of these para-professionals in the care of children with developmental problems.

Referral Criteria for Global Developmental Delay

Presence of certain red flags may be indicative of an alternate disease process such as neurodegenerative disorders and children with these features should be referred for further evaluation. Referral criteria/red flag signs have also been marked with red colored sections in the MCP card, and should be referred to at each immunization visit.

Red Flags on History

- Positive family history of global developmental delay (GDD) in other family members
- Progressive neurological symptoms
- Paroxysmal worsening of symptoms in relation with illness/ diet/time of the day
- ***Regression of milestones:*** History of normal development followed by regression

Red Flags on Examination

- Dysmorphic features/neurocutaneous stigmata
- ***Involvement of other organ systems:*** Cardiomyopathy, hepatosplenomegaly, etc.
- Isolated motor dysfunction such as severe hypotonia, isolated ataxia
- ***Peripheral nervous system abnormalities:*** Absent reflexes, sensory abnormalities
- ***Abnormal eye movements:*** Oculogyria, paroxysmal saccadic eye head movements
- ***Abnormal eye/fundus examination:*** Cataract, lens dislocation, cherry red spot, retinopathy
- ***Neuroimaging:*** Suggestive of findings of specific neurometabolic or genetic disorders

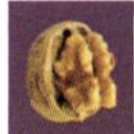

IN A NUTSHELL

Developmental Delay

1. *Global developmental delay* is significant delay in two or more of the five developmental domains and is used for children <5 years, whereas *intellectual disability* is used for children ≥5 years when formal testing of intelligence is possible.
2. Features of global developmental delay in early life depends upon the degree of severity. It usually manifests as motor delay, language delay, excessive lethargy, poor muscle tone or spasticity, feeding issues, etc.
3. Concomitant visual and hearing handicaps should be identified and addressed early as they can exacerbate the existing developmental problems.
4. Regular developmental surveillance and screening are the key to the early diagnosis and should be performed regularly according to the recommendations.
5. Child development unit consisting of a multidisciplinary team of experts is the cornerstone for management of global developmental delay.
6. Neurodegenerative disorders may mimic global developmental delay and should be carefully looked for if history or examination is suggestive.

Desmond P, Kelly MJN. Neurodevelopment and Executive function and dysfunction. In: M. Kliegman, Richard E. Behrman HBJ (Eds). Nelson Textbook of Pediatrics, 21st edition. New York: Elsevier Inc.; 2020. pp. 1690-1.
Juneja M, Gupta A, Sairam S, et al. Diagnosis and Management of Global Development Delay: Consensus Guidelines of Growth, Development and Behavioral Pediatrics Chapter, Neurology Chapter and Neurodevelopment Pediatrics Chapter of the Indian Academy of Pediatrics. Indian Pediatr. 2022;59(5):401-15.
Shekhawat DS, Gupta T, Singh P, et al. Monitoring tools for early identification of children with developmental delay in India: an update. Child Neuropsychol. 2022;28(6):814-30.

3.2 Attention Deficit Hyperactivity Disorder

PE 4.1

INTRODUCTION

Attention deficit hyperactivity disorder (ADHD) is characterized by persistent inattention, hyperactivity, and impulsivity, for at least a consecutive period of 6 months, starting in a child prior to 12 years of age.

EPIDEMIOLOGY

The recent worldwide prevalence of ADHD is reported to be in the range of 3–13% in children and adolescents between 2 and 17 years of age. Boys are affected three times more often as compared to girls. In India, approximately 11% primary school children are affected, and the prevalence ranges from 2–17% in children and adolescents.

ETIOLOGY

Attention deficit hyperactivity disorder is attributable to abnormal dopamine transmission in the frontal lobes and the frontostriatal circuitry. Some children with symptoms suggestive of ADHD may have neurologic or psychiatric conditions that are the cause of those symptoms such as sleep disorders, epilepsy, and learning disorders; although, in others, these may be coexistent with ADHD.

CLINICAL FEATURES

The diagnosis of ADHD is based on specific clinical criteria, as per the Diagnostic and Statistical Manual of Mental Disorders-Fifth Edition (DSM-5), given by American Psychiatric Association in 2013, and using diagnostic tools to elicit these criteria. The criteria provide list of symptoms for inattention and for hyperactive-impulsive behavior (**Box 3.3**).

Subtypes: Depending upon the predominant symptoms, ADHD can be categorized into one of the three subtypes; although, the subtype of ADHD in a given patient can change over time.

1. ***Predominantly inattentive:*** ≥6 symptoms of inattention for children and <6 symptoms of hyperactivity-impulsivity
2. ***Predominantly hyperactive-impulsive:*** ≥6 symptoms of hyperactivity-impulsivity for children and <6 symptoms of inattention
3. ***Combined:*** ≥6 symptoms each of both inattention and hyperactivity-impulsivity for children

The course of ADHD is highly variable. Symptoms may persist into adolescence or adult life, they may remit at puberty, or the hyperactivity may disappear, but the decreased attention span and impulse-control problem may persist.

Box 3.3 Diagnosis Criteria of Inattention, Hyperactivity and Impulsivity

- *Six or more of the following symptoms of inattention for at least 6 months:*
  1. Makes careless mistakes in schoolwork, work, or other activities.
  2. Has difficulty in keeping attention on tasks or play activities.
  3. Does not seem to listen when spoken to directly.
  4. Does not follow instructions and fails to finish schoolwork, chores, or duties in the workplace
  5. Has trouble organizing activities.
  6. Avoids, dislikes, or does not want to do things that take a lot of mental effort
  7. Loses things needed for tasks and activities (e.g., toys, school assignments, pencils, books, or tools).
  8. Easily distracted
  9. Forgetful in daily activities
- *Six or more of the following symptoms of hyperactivity-impulsivity have been present for at least 6 months to an extent that is disruptive and inappropriate for developmental level.*

  Hyperactivity:
  1. Fidgets with hands or feet or squirms in seat.
  2. Gets up from seat when remaining seat is expected.
  3. Runs about or climbs when and where it is not appropriate (adolescents or adults may feel very restless).
  4. Has trouble playing or enjoying leisure activities quietly.
  5. Acts as if "driven by a motor" and is often "on the go"
  6. Talks excessively.

  Impulsivity:
  1. Blurts out answers before questions have been finished.
  2. Has trouble waiting one's turn.
  3. Interrupts or intrudes on others (e.g., butts into conversations or games).

The symptoms should be persistent for at least 6 months in more than one setting (e.g., home and school) and should be causing an impairment of function in academic, social, or occupational activities

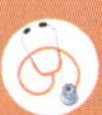

CASE STUDY Hyperactive Child

A 7-year-old male is brought to the OPD with complaints of acute respiratory infections (ARIs). While entering the OPD, the child is noticed pushing other children out of the way. The physician had previously noted that the child was repeatedly jumping from the bench to the ground. However, on entering the doctor's room, he is an alert, quiet child who, however, keeps getting distracted by outside noises. On enquiry, the parents agreed that the child is always very active at home and frequently engages in dangerous activities such as jumping from walls, breaking household objects, running on the road among heavy traffic, etc. They also informed about similar complaints from teachers. There is a history of changing three schools due to the educational problems and taking opinion from multiple doctors, all of whom advised that child is "hyperactive" and would grow out of the problem.

Learning Points

- As the parents have consulted many doctors previously, they did not even complain of the behavioral problem. The physician noted the child's over activity and lack of inhibition and probed further.
- In an unfamiliar situation, the child may in fact be not hyperactive; as in the doctor's chamber.
- "Growing out of hyperactivity", and not "coping with studies" are common misconceptions among parents, educationists, and sometimes, even health workers.

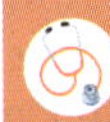

CASE STUDY Inattentive Child

A 9-year-old boy is a class 4 student, brought by the parents with complaints of poor school performance and forgetfulness. He experiences difficulties with schoolwork completion, inattentiveness, and distractibility. His teachers describe him as a cooperative student, but reports that the child will do better academically if he starts paying attention as he often requires reminders to help him stay on task. Also, he can do complex mathematical calculations and spelling are usually spot on when paying attention, however, commits silly mistakes frequently. He starts nicely but almost always leaves his schoolwork, artwork unfinished. He often blurts out answers and interrupts other students in the classroom. His mother reports difficulties at home with following routines and remembering instructions and has to sit with him for completion of homework. Mother remembers he was always a difficult child and at the age of 4–5 years, he was constantly running around. He was very difficult to manage when visiting relatives/friends/ attending any social functions.

Learning Points

- In school-aged children, there are more features of inattention and relatively lesser complaints of hyperactivity; however, there may be history of hyperactivity during early childhood.
- School-aged children with ADHD usually present with complaints of poor scholastic performance, therefore a detailed history and assessment is required to differentiate it from other causes of scholastic backwardness.
- Presence of comorbidities (e.g., SLD), should always be looked for, which may further hamper functioning of the child.

DIAGNOSIS

Routine diagnostic testing is not needed in the evaluation of a child for ADHD. Hearing and vision screening, and evaluation for learning disability (especially when problems are specifically restricted to the school or during studies) should be undertaken. Hypothyroidism, hyperthyroidism, phenylketonuria, and lead toxicity have all been reported to manifest with ADHD. Investigations for these disorders may be carried out depending on the clinical setting. Imaging studies for a stable child with ADHD (without any coexisting conditions) are not indicated.

INCLEN Diagnostic Tool for ADHD (INDT-ADHD) is an Indian diagnostic tool based on DSM-IV and available in multiple Indian languages. Other diagnostic tools include Conners-3 parent and teacher rating scales, and Vanderbilt parent scale.

TREATMENT Attention Deficit Hyperactivity Disorder

Treatment of ADHD is multidisciplinary, involving parents, teachers, behavioral therapist, clinical psychologist, pediatrician, and social worker.

- ***Pharmacotherapy*** involves the use of *stimulant* medications (methylphenidate, amphetamine, dextroamphetamine, etc.), and nonstimulant medications (norepinephrine-specific reuptake inhibitors, e.g., atomoxetine, guanfacine, clonidine). For severe irritability and aggression, atypical antipsychotics such as risperidone and aripiprazole may be added.
- ***Behavioral and psychological treatment*** involves reinforcing positive behaviors by praise or by using daily consistency charts ("star" or "happy face" charts), providing a distraction-free environment, social skills training, and adapting tasks to ensure ease of completion (simple clear commands, addressing tasks one at a time, etc.).
- ***Nonpharmacologic therapies*** such as biofeedback programs are less effective than stimulants but when used with drugs, may improve social skills. Nutritional supplements or exclusion diets are not of any use.

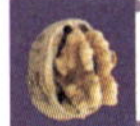

IN A NUTSHELL

Attention Deficit Hyperactivity Disorder

1. Persistent inattention, hyperactivity, and impulsivity for at least 6 months should alert to a possibility of attention deficit hyperactivity disorder (ADHD), starting in children before 12 years of age.
2. The diagnosis should be considered, if the problem behavior is present in at least two different settings, e.g., home, school, play, social situations, tuition, etc.
3. Behavioral management is the initial treatment modality.
4. Methylphenidate and atomoxetine are the most commonly used drugs for therapy.
5. Best success rate is achieved with a combination of behavioral and drug therapy.

American Psychiatric Association. Diagnostic and statistical manual of mental disorders: DSM-5, 5th edition. Virginia: American Psychiatric Association; 2013.

Chauhan A, Sahu JK, Singh M, et al. Burden of attention deficit hyperactivity disorder (ADHD) in Indian children: a systematic review and meta-analysis. Indian J Pediatr. 2022;89(6):570-8.

Cortese S. Pharmacologic Treatment of Attention Deficit–Hyperactivity Disorder. N Engl J Med. 2020;383:1050-6.

National Consultation Meeting for Developing IAP Guidelines on Neuro Developmental Disorders under the aegis of IAP Childhood Disability Group and the Committee on Child Development and Neurodevelopmental Disorders, Dalwai S, Unni J, Kalra V, et al. Consensus Statement of the Indian Academy of Pediatrics on Evaluation and Management of Attention Deficit Hyperactivity Disorder. Indian Pediatr. 2017;54(6):481-8.

3.3 Autism *PE 4.2*

INTRODUCTION

Autism spectrum disorders (ASDs), previously also known as pervasive developmental disorders (PDD), are a continuum of associated cognitive and neurobehavioral disorders, with the following core defining features: Deficits in social communication, and restricted and repetitive patterns of behaviors, interests (verbal and/or non-verbal), and activities. Childhood autism is the most common disorder in this spectrum.

EPIDEMIOLOGY

The recent worldwide prevalence of autism spectrum disorder is reported to be around 1 per 100. In India the prevalence is reported to be 1 in 65 in 2–9 year old children. Cognitive functions can range from profound mental retardation to above average on IQ tests in ASD. Male to female ratio is 4:1 for milder forms and 1.3:1 with severe cognitive impairment.

ETIOLOGY

The precise etiology of ASD is precisely unknown and is likely to be multifactorial, with the role of both genetic and nongenetic factors. These risk factors may be attributed alone or in combination, in the development of ASD. Some pathological mechanisms such as alteration in brain development and function, and synaptic defects are proposed to be responsible for the core features of ASD. Also, certain extracerebral processes such as gastrointestinal (GI) disturbances are contemplated to be the reason of problem behaviors in children with ASD.

Autism spectrum disorders may be associated with certain known syndromes (syndromic ASD), which can be chromosomal alterations or monogenic abnormalities. *Examples:* Fragile-X syndrome, Rett syndrome, Prader-Willi syndrome, Angelman syndrome. The genetic heterogeneity such as de-novo mutations, epigenetics and environmental factors are thought to play a role in the occurrence of nonsyndromic ASD.

CLINICAL FEATURES

- The average age of diagnosis of autism is 3–6 years, but it can be reliably diagnosed in children as young as 18–24 months.
- The correct diagnosis is often delayed or missed altogether with many children diagnosed as hearing deficient, learning disabled, ADHD, or with global developmental delay.
- Autism characteristics observable in children younger than 3 years include: *Decreased use of nonverbal behavior* (eye-to-eye gaze, facial expressions, body postures, gestures); *lack of social or emotional reciprocity*—lack of seeking to share enjoyment, interests or achievements with other people (absent showing or pointing); and *delayed or absent language skills.*

SCREENING AND DIAGNOSIS

Since autism features may be missed in early childhood, Indian Academy of Pediatrics (IAP) recommends that all children should be screened by a standardized autism screening tool at 18 and 24 months of age. The Modified checklist for autism in toddlers (M-CHAT), Pervasive developmental disorders screening test-II (PDDST-II), and Social communication questionnaire (for children older than 4 years) are some of the *screening instruments.*

Additionally, for a child with concerns in personal-social and/or speech/language domains, proceed as follows:

- ***If the child is above 18 months:*** Administer the ASD-specific screening tool
- ***If the child is below 18 months:*** Evaluate social communication skills, commence parental education and reschedule next visit after 3 months (if child's age <12 months) or after 1 month (if child's age >12 months). If concerns persist, then administer the ASD-specific screening tool.
- ***If screening results are positive or concerning:*** Continue parental education, refer the child for comprehensive ASD evaluation, initiate an early intervention program, evaluate hearing status, and schedule next follow-up visit after a month.

Diagnosis of ASD is made as per the Diagnostic and Statistical Manual of Mental disorders-fifth edition (DSM-5). Independent checklists are used to elicit the diagnostic features as per DSM-5, e.g., *INCLEN Diagnostic Tool for Autism Spectrum Disorders (INDT-ASD)* and *Indian Scale for Assessment of Autism (ISAA)* are the two DSM-based tools for diagnosis of autism in India. Both can be used for the diagnosis of ASD, ISAA is used by the Government of India for certification of the disease severity for disability benefits. INDT-ASD tool is available in many Indian languages, as compared to ISAA, which is available only in English.

Childhood Autism Rating Scale II (CARS-II), Autism Diagnostic Interview-Revised (ADI-R), and Autism Diagnostic Observation Schedule-General (ADOS-G) are the other *diagnostic instruments* for ASD. Hearing evaluation is essential both to guard against misdiagnosis, and to rule out associated significant hearing loss.

TREATMENT Autism Spectrum Disorders

Management of ASD is a life-long process and requires a multidisciplinary team. It involves speech and language therapy, special education, parent education, and pharmacotherapy for comorbid conditions or symptoms such as ADHD, anxiety, epilepsy, sleep problems, etc.

Stimulants for hyperactivity, risperidone for maladaptive behaviors, and SSRIs for rigidity/repetitive behaviors are the commonly used drugs for ASD.

Outcomes are encouraging with early diagnosis and intervention.

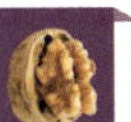

IN A NUTSHELL

Autism

1. Autism spectrum disorders (ASD) are characterized by deficits in social communications, repetitive behavior, and lack in interest and activities. The IQ is usually normal.
2. Average age of diagnosis is 3–6 years. It is important to screen for autism at 18 months for early recognition.
3. Delay in verbal/nonverbal communication is the most important early pointer to autism.
4. Management of autism is life-long, consisting of individualized multiple disciplinary approach.

Global Burden of Disease Study 2021 Autism Spectrum Collaborators. The global epidemiology and health burden of the autism spectrum: findings from the Global Burden of Disease Study 2021. Lancet Psychiatry. 2025;12(2):111-21.

Dalwai S, Ahmed S, Udani V, et al. Consensus Statement of the Indian Academy of Pediatrics on Evaluation and Management of Autism Spectrum Disorder. Indian Pediatr. 2017;54(5):385-93.

4 CHAPTER Common Problems Related to Behavior

AS PER NMC COMPETENCIES

PE5.1	Describe the clinical features, diagnosis and management of feeding problems.	*Ch 4.2, Ch 4.3 Ch 4.4*
PE5.2	Describe the clinical features, diagnosis and management of breath holding spells.	*Ch 4.5*
PE5.3	Describe the clinical features, diagnosis and management of temper tantrums and pica.	*Ch 4.6, Ch 4.7*
PE5.4	Explain the etiology, clinical features and management of enuresis.	*Ch 4.8*

Topics available online: ***Stranger Anxiety; Encopresis; Stuttering, Tics, and Nail Biting; Masturbation; and Sleep Disorders***

4.1 Introduction

Behavioral disorders represent significant departures or deviations from the accepted "normal" behavior. Common behavioral disorders include thumb-sucking, pica, breath-holding spells, and nocturnal enuresis. Up to 20% of children presenting to primary care are estimated to have behavioral and psychosocial problems. Common behavioral problems are:

- ***Habit problems:*** Thumb-sucking, nail-biting, bruxism, tics, enuresis, encopresis, breath-holding spells, trichotillomania, and aerophagia.
- ***Feeding problems:*** Pica, food fads, food refusal/overeating, vomiting, and anorexia.
- ***Personality problems:*** Shyness, timidity, fears, anger, and jealousy.
- ***Sleep problems:*** Night terrors, nightmares, somnambulism, insomnia, sleep-talking, and narcolepsy.
- ***Speech problems:*** Stuttering, mutism, phonation, and articulation disorders.
- ***Scholastic problems:*** Reading, writing or mathematical disorders, repeated failures, absenteeism, truancy, and school phobia.

ETIOLOGY

Behavioral problems are usually caused by maladjustment at home or school, in a child with precipitating factors operating during pregnancy, during delivery and in neonatal period. Faulty emotional environment, constituted by parental attitudes, siblings, neighborhood, school and mass media, play a major role. Faulty parental attitudes resulting in behavioral difficulties include rejection, overprotection, unrealistic expectations, discrimination, over criticism, over discipline, and unfavorable comparisons with siblings and peers.

TREATMENT Behavioral Disorders

Behavioral assessment is used to determine the precipitating events and consequences that maintain the behavioral problem. The antecedent-behavior-consequence (ABC) model and the principles of reinforcement and punishment are used for assessment and management of behavioral problem. Behavioral assessment guides *behavioral intervention*, which is designed to modify variables that trigger, maintain, or mediate problem behavior.

Psychopharmacology can play some role in children with behavioral disorders. The main classes of drugs used are typical and atypical antipsychotic drugs, tricyclic antidepressants, selective serotonin reuptake inhibitors (SSRIs), stimulants, and antianxiety drugs. The choice of drug depends on the predominant behavior and/or the underlying disorder.

Mukherjee SB, Kaushik JS. Psychopharmacology for behavior problems in children. Indian Pediatr. 2019;56(8):683-4.

Vaidyanathan S, Kuppili PP, Menon V. Eating disorders: An overview of Indian research. Indian J Psychol Med. 2019;41(4):311-7.

Problems During Infancy

4.2 Infantile Colic

PE 5.1

INTRODUCTION

Evening colic is characterized by the *rule of three*. Infantile colic is defined as crying for no apparent cause in children younger than 3 months of age, who presents with intermittent episodes of abdominal pain and excessive crying lasting >3 hours per day, for >3 days per week, in an otherwise well fed and healthy child. Colic is a diagnosis of exclusion after ruling out less common organic causes of incessant and repetitive crying. Around 5–25% of infants in the community have colic.

ETIOLOGY

Exact cause of colic is not known. Gastrointestinal (increased gas production from colon, milk allergy, hyperperistalsis), psychosocial, and neurodevelopmental disorders have been suggested as the possible etiology. Infantile colic is more likely to occur if the child is overactive and the parents are overanxious. These episodes could also be a manifestation of hunger, aerophagia, or overfeeding. It appears unrelated to environmental events.

CLINICAL FEATURES

Infant colic usually begins suddenly with a bout of screaming in the evening. Crying is associated with motor behaviors such as flushed face, furrowed brow, and clenched fists. The legs are pulled up to the abdomen, and the infant emits a piercing, high-pitched scream. Crying is concentrated in the late afternoon and evening, occurs in prolonged bouts, and is unpredictable and spontaneous. These episodes are associated with hypertonia, facial flushing, circumoral pallor, tense or distended abdomen, drawing up of the legs, clenching of the fingers, stiffening and tightening of the arms, or arching of the back. The child cannot be soothed, even by feeding. Attacks may terminate after the infant is exhausted or passes feces or flatus.

Typically, the paroxysms of colic start within a few weeks after birth, reach a peak by 4–6 weeks, and subside by 3–4 months of age. Differential diagnosis includes a neurological abnormality or infection, gastroesophageal reflux (GER), otitis media, urinary tract infection, fractured bone/dislocated joint, and child abuse.

DIAGNOSIS

The diagnosis depends on a good and detailed clinical history, describing the entire episode and a thorough physical examination for identifiable causes of crying/fussiness. Laboratory or imaging studies generally are not necessary. The thoroughness of the history and examination is reassuring to parents and may strengthen the clinician-family relationship.

TREATMENT Infantile Colic

Treatment is limited. The physician's role is to ensure that there is no organic cause for the crying, offer balanced advice on treatments, and provide support to the family. Long-term follow-up studies have shown no difference in behavior among colicky and noncolicky infants. Above all, parents need reassurance that their baby is healthy, and that colic is self-limited with no long-term adverse effects.

During an episode, hold the child erect or prone in the lap or on a hot water bottle. There is not much role of carminatives, suppositories, or enema. Avoid drugs to reduce intestinal motility. Sedate the child, if attacks do not respond to above measures. Anticholinergic drugs have shown some benefit for the acute episode but should be used with caution.

Feeding technique should be explained. Feed in erect position. Practice proper burping and place the child on right lateral position for about half an hour after feeding. Possible allergenic food should be identified and removed. Selected probiotics have demonstrated efficacy in infantile colic, especially in the breastfed group.

They should be nurtured in emotionally stable environment. Try to calm the anxious parents and clear their self-doubts regarding child rearing. Reduce the parental anxiety by counseling them about the nature of the problem, lack of effect of soothing, and self-remission by about 4–6 months. Encourage exclusive breastfeeding.

IN A NUTSHELL

Infantile Colic

1. Infantile colic is characterized by the "rule of 3", i.e., excessive cry for >3 hours/day for >3 times/week and lasting for >3 weeks; in a child younger than 3 months.
2. Etiology is not known. Infantile colic is a diagnosis of exclusion after ruling out other common causes of incessant cry.
3. There is no effective medication.
4. Child needs to be comforted and parents need counseling.
5. Infantile colic is self-remitting and subsides spontaneously by 4–6 months of age.

Gordon M, Biagioli E, Sorrenti M, et al. Dietary modifications for infantile colic. Cochrane Database Syst Rev. 2018;10(10):CD011029.
Sarasu JM, Narang M, Shah D. Infantile colic: An update. Indian Pediatr. 2018;55(11):979-87.

4.3 Feeding Problems

PE 5.1

INTRODUCTION

Feeding problems in the first year of life occur because of erratic feeding, oversensitive infant and parents' ignorance regarding feeding. Other parental problems leading to feeding difficulties include anxiety, depression, unwillingness to nurture, substance abuse, psychosocial stress, or other serious mental illness. Usual manifestations are underfeeding, overfeeding, spitting, regurgitation, and constipation.

UNDERFEEDING

Underfeeding occurs when either (1) infant is not offered enough feed; or (2) the infant is not able to take a sufficient quantity of food even when offered. This can be caused by improper feeding techniques such as decreased frequency or duration of feeding, inadequate quantity and quality of feeding, early introduction of top feeding, nipple confusion, breast problems, improper burping, abnormal mother–infant bonding and chronic systemic illness in the infant.

Clinical Features

These depend upon the extent and duration of underfeeding. Initially, there might be constipation, failure to sleep, irritability, and excessive crying. If underfeeding continues for prolonged period, the child fails to gain weight and may progress to have failure to thrive.

Diagnosis

Detailed clinical evaluation with anthropometry and physical examination helps in making a diagnosis.

TREATMENT Underfeeding

It depends upon the condition of the child. If severe malnutrition is present, it is of utmost importance to manage fluid and electrolyte, associated infection, hypoglycemia, hypothermia, and anemia. Following this, the child should be provided adequate calories and supplemented with appropriate minerals and vitamins. Treat the underlying systemic infection and diseases, if any. Identify and treat associated psychological problems such as child abuse or neglect. Counsel the parents about feeding techniques.

OVERFEEDING

Overfeeding can be qualitative or quantitative. It is usually caused by parents' ignorance about nutritional requirement of their infants. Psychosocial problems in parents may also result in overfeeding. Unwillingness of mother to breastfeed and reliance on bottle feeding may be associated.

Clinical Features

The most common clinical manifestation of overfeeding is regurgitation and vomiting. Infant may present with abdominal distention and discomfort due to delayed gastric emptying if the diet contains too much fat or carbohydrates. It may be associated with abdominal distention or passage of excessive flatulence. Overfeeding leads to rapid and excessive weight gain, resulting in childhood obesity.

Diagnosis

Patients presenting with a change in weight combined with intense exercise; or maintained with laxatives and vomiting; or binge eating should raise a high suspicion of eating disorder. Weight and height monitoring on growth charts are important to quickly capture weight loss or failure to achieve expected weight gain. Rapid weight gain or weight fluctuations may cue pediatrician to question binge eating. The communication between a patient and healthcare providers is very important, as well as the documentation on the prevalence of eating disorders.

TREATMENT Overfeeding

Proper nutritional assessment including dietary history and intake should be taken. This is to be followed by a detailed physical examination and anthropometry. On this basis, one can determine the infant's status by calculating appropriate nutritional value of the food and comparing them with actual required recommended dietary allowances. Parents should be counseled regarding daily dietary allowance, feeding technique, and types of food to be used. They should be told that healthy child does not mean obese child. Adequate and exclusive breastfeeding can overcome the problem of overfeeding.

EXCESSIVE SPITTING

It is normal in 15% of infants. It can also be associated with GER and overfeeding. Clinical manifestations depend upon severity of the problem. Failure to thrive occurs in extreme cases.

TREATMENT Excessive Spitting

Reassure the parents, if their infant is gaining weight adequately and there are no underlying factors such as overfeeding, psychosocial stress and GER. Determine whether stress is present during feeding. If yes, identify its cause and manage appropriately. Provide proper counseling.

RUMINATION

This is habitual regurgitation and reswallowing of stomach contents by increasing intra-abdominal pressure by putting finger or fist in the mouth. This occurs secondary to unconscious but voluntary contraction of abdominal wall muscles leading to increasing intragastric pressure with reflux of gastric contents into mouth and esophagus. Therefore, this disorder may be associated with GER, esophagitis, or developmental delay. There is increased association of rumination with other gastrointestinal symptoms such as abdominal pain, constipation, and nausea. Diaphragmatic breathing is the mainstay of management in

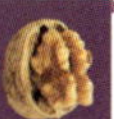

IN A NUTSHELL

Feeding Problems

1. Underfeeding occurs when infant is not offered sufficient quantity of feed or the infant is not able to take a sufficient quantity of food even when offered.
2. Nutritional rehabilitation, treating underlying systemic infection and associated psychological problems are the mainstay of management of underfeeding.
3. Overfeeding occurs usually due to ignorance about nutritional requirement of their infants.
4. The most common clinical manifestation of overfeeding is regurgitation and vomiting.
5. Parental counseling regarding exclusive breastfeeding, feeding technique, daily dietary allowance, and type of food to be given are the mainstay of management.

children with rumination. Infants with psychogenic rumination respond well if they are held 15 minutes before and after feeding. Child without intellectual disability or global developmental delay may respond to behavioral modification technique such as "time out."

Forsum E, Flinke E. Premature birth did not have a pronounced impact on eating behaviour of four-year-old children, but some effects were observed in girls. Acta Paediatr. 2022;111(12):2331-6.

Galai T, Friedman G, Moses M, et al. Demographic and clinical parameters are comparable across different types of pediatric feeding disorder. Sci Rep. 2022;12(1):8596.

Hornberger LL, Lane MA; Committee on Adolescence. Identification and Management of Eating Disorders in Children and Adolescents. Pediatrics. 2021;147(1):e2020040279.

Mandera-Grygierzec A, Kostrzewska P, Szuster E, et al. Eating disorders in children and adolescents: the current state of knowledge. J Educ Health and Sport. 2022;12(7):906-11.

Martinez M, Rathod S, Friesen HJ, et al. Rumination syndrome in children and adolescents: A mini review. Front Pediatr. 2021;19(9):709326.

Mudholkar A, Korostenski L, Blackwell D, Lane AE. Factors associated with the early emergence of atypical feeding behaviours in infants and young children: A scoping review. Child Care Health Dev. 2022.

Early Childhood Problems

4.4 Thumb Sucking *PE 5.1*

INTRODUCTION

It is a common, generally harmless, behavior of infancy and early childhood, and appears to be a way of securing extra self-nurturance. Usually, most children stop thumb sucking by 2 years of age. It is considered as a marker of insecurity and loneliness if it persists till late childhood or adolescents.

CLINICAL FEATURES

When persisting after age 4, it is a mild to moderate health risk as it may occasionally lead to dental, dermatological, orthopedic, and psychological problems. It poses risk of malocclusion of developing dentition, malocclusion of jaw and digital deformity. Some children may develop speech difficulty for consonants like D and T. If it persists in later childhood, it can affect permanent teeth eruption, teeth alignment and shape of the mouth.

DIAGNOSIS

An oral examination is imperative for evaluation for possible complications of thumb sucking. The first oral evaluation for all children is recommended no later than 12 months. Examining the oral soft tissues, palate, alveolar ridges, and any erupted/erupting teeth is essential. Once dental care is established, monitoring the developing primary dentition and occlusion should be done at regular clinic visits. A child who discards this habit initially and resumes at 7–8 years, needs to be evaluated for associated psychological problems. Resumption of this habit suggests that the child is suffering from stress or insecurity.

TREATMENT Thumb Sucking

Indications

Persistent thumb sucking after 4 years age should be treated when it is associated with presence of dental problems due to the behavior. Treatment is not indicated when thumb-sucking is infrequent or it has an important function in alleviation of stress due to substantial loss (e.g., parent, pet), fear (e.g., surgery), or pain (e.g., injury, illness), when it acts as a temporary adaptive coping strategy.

Strategies

Management options are—(1) planned ignoring; (2) giving attention to more positive aspects of the child's behavior; and (3) monitoring followed by rewards or incentives for sucking-free days *(positive reinforcement)*. Use of bitter agents on thumbs or tying a cloth on thumb should not be considered as a first-line approach.

Parental Counseling

Parents should be counseled regarding the self-remitting nature. Children with thumb-sucking should not be punished for this act. Punishment would only reinforce this habit. A positive feedback is helpful when the child is not sucking. Child who looks depressed should be referred for detailed psychological evaluation and management. The child should be praised and encouraged if he tries to indulge in activities other than thumb-sucking.

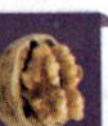

IN A NUTSHELL

Thumb Sucking

1. Thumb sucking is a harmless, behavior of infancy and early childhood, usually children overgrow it by 2 years of age.
2. It leads to dental, psychological, orthopedic, and dermatological problems.
3. Positive reinforcement and detailed psychological evaluation and management are the cornerstone of treatment.

Bryce C, Liddell T, Gideon G. Early Childhood Concerns: Counseling on Sleep Issues, Thumb-Sucking, Picky Eating, School Readiness, and Oral Health. Am Fam Physician. 2025;111(1):31-6.

Sadoun C, Templier L, Alloul L, et al. Effects of non-nutritive sucking habits on malocclusions: a systematic review. J Clin Pediatr Dent. 2024;48(2):4-18.

Staufert Gutierrez D, Carugno P. Thumb Sucking. Treasure Island (FL): StatPearls Publishing; 2022.

4.5 Breath-holding Spells

PE 5.2

INTRODUCTION

Breath-holding spells are paroxysmal self-limiting events usually consisting of multiple (three or more) episodes of the following sequence: provocation, followed by crying to a point of noiselessness and accompanying change of color, and ultimately, a loss of consciousness with an associated alteration in body tone. These episodes occur in up to 10% of healthy children between the age of 6 months and 6 years.

The episodes are involuntary in nature and occur during expiration, contrary to the terminology, which implies that the child voluntarily holds the breath in inspiration.

EPIDEMIOLOGY

Breath-holding spells constitute 4–18% of all the psychosomatic disorders seen in the pediatric age group, with a male-to-female ratio of 3:1. A community survey in India among 0–3 years old children reported breath-holding spells to be the most common psychiatric disorder in this age group, with a prevalence of 5.9%. There was no difference in prevalence among rural, urban, and slum children. Among an Indian general hospital psychiatry clinic, 11% of the preschoolers had breath-holding spells.

ETIOLOGY

Breath-holding spell is a neurobehavioral problem and categorized as a nonepileptic paroxysmal disorder. Recent research indicates that a genetically-mediated dysregulation of autonomic nervous system reflexes is responsible for the spells. As no difference has been found in prevalence of behavioral problems in children with breath-holding spells and controls; the time-honored belief that these spells result from frustration due to a disciplinary conflict between parents and the child stands discounted.

CLASSIFICATION

The spells are classified according to skin color change of the child during the episode, as cyanotic, pallid, and mixed. Cyanotic episodes are more common than pallid episodes.

- ***Cyanotic*** type in which the face turns blue; this is precipitated by anger or frustration.
- ***Pallid*** type where face is pale; usually provoked by sudden fright or pain.
- ***Mixed***—there is no clear distinction between cyanosis or pallor, or a conflicting history is given by the parents.

CLINICAL FEATURES

The typical age of onset is between 6 and 18 months. The frequency ranges from multiple episodes daily to as few as one per year, and gradually increases in frequency during the second year of life followed by gradual decrease to nil by 6 years.

The spell usually occurs at the initiation of a tantrum. The child holds his breath in expiration after a bout of crying. The child becomes rigid and attains opisthotonic posture. This is followed by limpness. Normal breathing and alertness is resumed within a minute.

DIFFERENTIAL DIAGNOSIS

Breath-holding spell should be differentiated from *epilepsy* and *hypercyanotic spell*.

- ***Epilepsy:*** A breath-holding spell is predisposed by anger, frustration, or fright. The child becomes completely normal after the attack. An epileptic seizure has no such predisposing factor and the child remains in a postictal state, with short-lasting altered sensorium or drowsiness after the attack. Electroencephalogram (EEG) is likely to be normal in majority of children with breath-holding spell.
- ***Hypercyanotic spell (Tet spells):*** Differentiation from hypercyanotic spells associated with cyanotic congenital heart disease can be done by the presence of physical findings (clubbing, auscultation findings, cyanosis of mucosa persisting for a long time, and no spontaneous resolution) and presence of baseline cyanosis since early infancy. In a hypercyanotic spell, the cyanosis is also present before and after the attack, while there is no cyanosis before or after a breath-holding spell.
- Child never develops neurological deficits after the breath-holding spells.

DIAGNOSIS

The diagnosis of breath-holding spell depends on a good and detailed clinical history, describing the entire episode. It should also include presence of any precipitating event like emotional stimuli or trauma. Other important clues from the history that could help in diagnosis include the presence or urinary incontinence, uprolling of eyeballs, and deviation of mouth, (which are more commonly seen with seizures), especially if not preceded by a cry. If feasible, parents may be encouraged to make a video recording of a typical episode that could further help in confirming the diagnosis.

A complete physical examination including growth and development is essential, especially cardiovascular examination for any rhythm disturbances or murmurs. No imaging or specific laboratory test is needed to make the diagnosis. An EEG is usually not indicated unless when clear description of attacks is not available, history of painful stimulus/crying is not present in some episodes, risk factors for epilepsy are present, or there is associated status epilepticus. Workup for iron deficiency must be done.

TREATMENT Breath-holding Spells

- ***Immediate measures:*** Prevent injury during the episode. Help the child to floor and have him lie flat. If loss of consciousness occurs, place the child on the side to protect against aspiration. Maintain patent oral airway but do not start CPR. Do not shake the baby, splash water or put anything in the mouth.
- ***Long-term measures:*** There are no prophylactic medications. Iron deficiency has been reported to be associated with breath-holding spells, and treatment with oral iron (4–6 mg/kg/day) for 6–8 weeks is recommended, if documented. Such attacks can be averted by behavioral modification and strong physical stimuli before the onset of attack. Parents should also be advised to divert the attention of the child when a precipitating factor occurs.
- ***Parental education:*** Parents should be reassured that breath-holding spell does not cause irreversible hypoxia, brain injury, epilepsy, and subsequent impairment in cognitive development. Avoid precipitating factors such as exhaustion, hunger, or injury. Do not give toys or tasks beyond the child's abilities. Avoid excessive rules and restrictions. Try to remove unnecessary frustrations.
- *Refer* if the child is <3 months, unconsciousness lasts for more than 1 minute, attacks are too frequent, or seizure disorder or hypercyanotic spell is suspected.

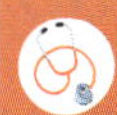

CASE STUDY Breath-holding Spells

A 2½-year-old girl is brought with complaints of poorly controlled seizures since 8 months. There is 1 year history of sudden cry following any sudden painful stimulus, followed by cessation of respiration and fall. This is followed by tonic-clonic activity that lasts for 1–2 minutes. There is no clear-cut history of any color change during the episode. After the episode is over, the child usually gets up and is alert, though she goes off to sleep after some episodes. These episodes occur up to 3–4 times per day, though may not occur for up to a week also. An initial diagnosis of breath-holding spells had been made. However, her episode was observed by her local physician, who advised an EEG. The child was started on valproate by the physician, after the EEG was reported as abnormal (showed occasional sharp waves). The frequency of attacks is the same but tonic-clonic movements rarely occur. The parents were not satisfied with the response and wanted a second opinion. History and course were consistent with a diagnosis of breath-holding spells. The parents were counseled and anticonvulsants stopped. Investigations revealed iron deficiency that was managed by oral iron therapy. The frequency of the attacks gradually decreased and stopped completely over the next 2 years.

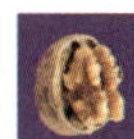

IN A NUTSHELL

Breath-holding Spells

1. Breath-holding spells are characterized by multiple episodes of cry followed by cessation of breath following some provocation. They typically occur between 6 months and 5 years of age.
2. Breath-holding spells should be differentiated from hypercyanotic spells which are characteristic of congenital cyanotic heart disease.
3. Breath-holding spell is a clinical diagnosis and does not require EEG or neuroimaging.
4. Iron therapy is effective in management.

Dai AI, Demiryürek AT. Effectiveness oral theophylline, piracetam, and iron treatments in children with simple breath-holding spells. J Child Neurol. 2020;35(1):25-30.

Hecht EM, Layton MR, Abrams GA. Iron supplementation for the treatment of breath-holding spells: a systematic review and meta-analysis. Clin Pediatr (Phila). 2020;59(8):819-22.

Sharawat IK, Dawman L, Panda P, et al. Efficacy of piracetam in children with breath-holding spells: a systematic review and meta-analysis. Eur J Pediatr. 2025;184:89.

4.6 Temper Tantrum

PE 5.3

INTRODUCTION

From the age of 18 months to 3 years, the child begins to develop autonomy and starts separating from primary caregivers. At this age, they also develop negativism, i.e., they do things opposite to what has been requested or opposite of their own desire (oppositionalism). As and when they cannot express their autonomy, they become frustrated and angry. Some of them show their frustration and defiance with physical aggression or resistance such as biting, crying, kicking, throwing objects, hitting, and head banging. This type of physical aggressive behavior is known as temper tantrum.

This behavior reaches its peak point during second and third year of life and gradually subsides between 3 and 6 years as the child learns to control his negativism and complies with the requests of others.

ETIOLOGY

Noncompliant or defiant behavior is a normal part of the developmental process, particularly in the preschool-age child (and also at adolescence). The most likely function of noncompliant behavior is access to positive attention and escape/avoidance of undesirable tasks, commands or activities. Continuation of temper tantrums depends on parental response to this behavior. Inconsistent and indiscriminate use of behavioral management strategies by parents is one of the main predisposing factors of temper tantrums. Parental anger and frustration may reinforce the defiance of the noncompliant child and aggravate the problem further.

CLINICAL FEATURES

Toddlers present with screaming, head banging, crying, going limp, hitting, pushing, and biting. The temper tantrums are benign and do not lead to developmental and cognitive abnormalities. The behavior sometimes could be disruptive especially in classrooms, leading to complaints from school and increased anxiety amongst parents and caregivers.

DIAGNOSIS

There is no specific laboratory investigation that can help in making a diagnosis of temper tantrum. A detailed clinical history and physical examination helps you to differentiate from developmental disorders, and psychiatric disorders. The history should include when do the tantrum occurs, what are the triggering factors, how does the child behave during the tantrum, how long it lasts and how it is stopped. A detailed assessment of family dynamics is also essential along with how the caregiver handles and reacts to the tantrum. Characteristics such as aggression, prolonged duration, and frequent occurrences may indicate an underlying organic disease.

MANAGEMENT STRATEGY

Management depends on prevention of extreme and recurrent attacks of temper tantrums by preventing common triggers like hunger, fatigue, injury, and illness. *RIDD* is a strategy that can help in managing tantrums.

- ***R:*** Remain calm during the attack, and redirecting and distracting the child
- ***I:*** Ignore the tantrum
- ***D:*** Distract the child, you can leave the room and let the child settle down by keeping a distant eye on the child to ensure safety
- ***D:*** Do say "yes" to acknowledge the physical demands of the child but do not give into the demands.

TREATMENT Temper Tantrum

- At the time of the tantrum, parents should turn away briefly (to give the child time and space to recover). The child can later be explained that such behavior is not acceptable.
- For noncompliant behavior, consequences should be provided immediately after every occurrence, and should be constant across all time periods and settings. Diverting his attention from the immediate cause and changing the environment can reduce the tantrum.
- Parents should provide ample amount of praise for positive behavior. Clear communication and consistent limit setting regarding what is acceptable and not acceptable, and frequent approval are helpful strategies.
- Parents should be calm, loving, firm and consistent; and such behavior should not allow the child to take advantage of gaining things.
- Time-out may be used (1 minute/year of age), if the behavior continues, but requires detailed instructions for effective use.

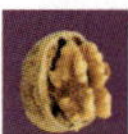

IN A NUTSHELL

Temper Tantrum

1. It occurs with lack of expression of their autonomy causing frustration and anger.
2. A detailed clinical history and physical examination helps you to differentiate from developmental disorders.
3. Management depends on prevention of extreme and recurrent attacks of temper tantrums by preventing common triggers such as hunger, fatigue, injury and illness.
4. *RIDD* is a strategy that can help in managing tantrums.

Sisterhen LL, Wy PAW. Temper Tantrums. Treasure Island (FL): StatPearls Publishing; 2025.

4.7 Pica

PE 5.3

INTRODUCTION

Pica is an eating disorder defined as "the repeated and chronic ingestion of non-nutritive substances including mud, plaster, charcoal, chalk, paint, earth, clay, etc., for a period of at least 1 month. This should be inappropriate to the developmental level of the child (age <24 months) and should not be a part of culturally acceptable practices" (DSM-5).

ETIOLOGY

The cause of pica remains unknown, and a variety of nutritional, neuropsychiatric, cultural, and psychological theories are proposed. Pica is a physiological phenomenon during oral phase. Children between 18 and 24 months often try to eat nonfood items and it is not considered abnormal. Persistence after 2 years of age needs attention and workup for lead toxicity, iron-deficiency anemia, parasitic infections, and lead toxicity. Although it has been thought of as a symptom of iron-deficiency, it is more commonly found in patients who are not anemic. Pica is more prevalent among children with intellectual disabilities, and those with lack of parental supervision.

CLINICAL FEATURES

Children with pica can present with inherent toxicity; intestinal obstruction (such as that occurring with trichophagia, or hair eating); excessive caloric intake (such as that occurring with starch); nutritional deprivation; parasitic infestations; and dental injury. In many cases, complications do not occur or are not recognized. It usually remits with age.

DIAGNOSIS

As per DSM-5, pica is diagnosed by the presence of:

- Repeated eating of non-nutritional and nonfood substances, e.g., gum, hair, dirt, paint, chalk, clay, paper, soap, wool, strings, for at least a month
- The eating behavior is not culturally supported or socially normal and is inappropriate to the patient's development
- The severity of eating behavior warrants additional clinical attention if it occurs in presence of another medical illness or mental disorder, e.g., intellectual disability, schizophrenia, or autism.

TREATMENT Pica

- Pica below 2 years does not need any intervention.
- Children with pica are at increased risk of lead poisoning, iron-deficiency, bezoars, and parasitic infections. They should be investigated for these problems and if present, treated suitably. Deworming needs to be done, as worm infection is generally associated.
- Education, guidance and counseling of the family. The reason for lack of supervision needs to be looked into, if present.
- Child should be given more affection and attention. The child has to be kept occupied in other tasks and provided with environmental stimulation.
- Prevent unsupervised access to mud/chalk/paint, etc.

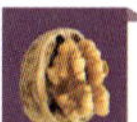

IN A NUTSHELL

Pica

1. Pica is an eating disorder defined as "the repeated and chronic ingestion of non-nutritive substances including mud, plaster, charcoal, chalk, paint, earth, clay for a period of at least 1 month.
2. Persistence of pica after 2 years of age needs attention and workup for lead toxicity, iron-deficiency anemia, and parasitic infections, and lead toxicity.
3. Parental education, guidance and counseling are the mainstay of management.

Ellwanger JH, Ziliotto M, Kulmann-Leal B, et al. Iron deficiency and soil-transmitted helminth infection: classic and neglected connections. Parasitol Res. 2022;121(12):3381-92.

Rajput N, Kumar K, Moudgil K. Pica an eating disorder: an overview. Pharmacophore. 2020;11(4):9.

Problems of the Young Child

4.8 Enuresis

PE 5.4

INTRODUCTION

Voluntary or involuntary repeated discharge of urine into clothes or bed, after a developmental age when bladder control should be established (usually 5 years), is labeled as enuresis. Bedwetting or urinary incontinence is labeled as enuresis, only if urine is being voided twice a week for at least 3 consecutive months, or if it is causing clinically significant distress in the child's life. Around 15% of the 5-year-old have primary enuresis; approximately 15% enuretics resolve their symptoms each year, and about 5% of 10-year-old and 1% of the adolescents remain enuretic. Enuresis is divided into monosymptomatic and nonmonosymptomatic forms. Monosymptomatic is defined as enuresis without any lower urinary tract symptoms or bladder dysfunction. Nonmonosymptomatic enuresis is associated with other lower urinary tract symptoms such as weak stream, daytime incontinence, hesitancy, postmicturition dribble and urgency. Monosymptomatic enuresis is further classified into primary and secondary enuresis.

CLASSIFICATION

Enuresis may be primary or secondary; or nocturnal/diurnal.

- ***Primary enuresis:*** This is defined as repeated (at least twice a week for at least three consecutive months) passage of urine into clothes/bed during night in a child >5 years, who has never been dry in night. This is three times more common in boys.
- ***Secondary enuresis:*** The child had been dry for several (at least 6) months and again starts bedwetting. In such cases, look for the underlying causes. Too enthusiastic and immature toilet training can result in secondary enuresis. Other causes include emotional stress, parent-child maladjustment, urinary tract infections, diabetes mellitus or diabetes

insipidus. Secondary enuresis is frequently associated with stressful or traumatic events.

- ***Nocturnal and diurnal enuresis:*** Nocturnal and diurnal enuresis refers to voiding of urine during night-time and while awake, respectively. Diurnal enuresis is more common in girls, is usually due to micturition deferral (waiting till the last moment to pass urine, and then being unable to hold any longer) in the preschool child, and usually settles by age 9 years. Stress incontinence, urinary tract infection, and diabetes are the other causes of diurnal enuresis. When both diurnal and nocturnal enuresis are present, abnormalities of the urinary tract or voiding disorders are likely.

Chronic constipation is an important risk factor for enuresis and associated encopresis is found in about 15% children with enuresis.

ETIOLOGY

The pathogenesis is multifactorial and could be related to sleep disorder, genetic, psychological causes, or reduced nocturnal secretion of antidiuretic hormone.

- Less than 3% cases have organic etiology such as obstructive uropathy or urinary tract infections.
- There might be a delay in neurological maturation to control bladder sphincter; associated with mental retardation or spinal cord abnormalities.
- Children who undergo training late (after 24 months) are prone to develop late nocturnal bladder control; recommended age to begin toilet training is around 12–18 months.
- Physiologic factors have been studied the most. These include hyposecretion of arginine vasopressin (AVP), decreased responsiveness to low urine osmolality, loss of circadian rhythm of ADH secretion, altered AVP receptor function in the tubule, diminished capacity to be aroused, and altered sleep architecture.
- *Genetic factors:* There is a strong association between nocturnal enuresis and genetic predisposition. If both parents have nocturnal enuresis, children have a 75% chance of being affected.

CLINICAL FEATURES

Clinical features depend on the underlying cause. Common symptoms are wetting of clothes, hesitancy, poor urinary stream, burning while passing urine, applying excessive pressure during micturition, interrupted micturition, and presence of associated constipation.

DIAGNOSIS

History and examination should be able to rule out the possibility of any underlying neurological disorder, polyuric conditions (diabetes mellitus, diabetes insipidus, chronic renal failure) and bacterial cystitis.

- Evaluation in case of primary nocturnal enuresis involves routine urine examination including osmolality, microscopy, sugar, and culture.
- A *frequency void chart* often helps to differentiate primary nocturnal enuresis from voiding dysfunction. The normal frequency of daytime void in a child is 4–7 times per day. A frequency of >8 times or at duration <2 hours is considered abnormal.
- A good *ultrasonogram* (USG) on full bladder can also give a rough estimate of bladder capacity. A full bladder and post-void USG is an essential part of evaluation.
- *Urodynamic study* is needed to assess bladder capacity and detrusor pressures in a child who has an abnormal frequency void chart.

TREATMENT Enuresis

Treatment should be aimed at completely stopping the enuresis. After establishing the diagnosis of primary nocturnal enuresis, a treatment plan should be discussed. The child's cooperation in the management plan is essential. Any serious attempt to treat the condition should begin only beyond 7–8 years of age as enuresis interferes with socialization and behavior in older children.

Nonpharmacological Methods

Nonpharmacological management is effective in 30% cases and consists of behavior modification, bladder strengthening exercises and alarm systems.

- ***Behavioral treatment:*** Behavioral treatment is the first mode of therapy for a child with enuresis without any disorder of the genitourinary tract.
  - Counseling and reassurance to the family is the most essential step. They need to be assured of the benign nature of the condition, and high spontaneous resolution rate.
  - Ask the parents to maintain a diary record of dry nights; reward the child for such nights.
  - Parents should provide emotional support to the child, avoid criticism, and change the bed sheets without child's notice.
  - Avoid punitive measures. Positive reinforcement has been shown to have a success rate of >85%.
  - Children should have an early dinner and appropriate fluids with dinner. It is recommended to avoid any form of fluid at least 2–3 hours prior to sleep. Ask the child to void before going to sleep.
  - Repeated waking to void is not helpful, though using an alarm clock to wake the child once 2–3 hours after falling asleep is indicated. Child should be fully aroused and walk unaided to the toilet to urinate.
- ***Behavior conditioning:*** Behavior conditioning with use of alarms is extremely effective. The alarm is either a sound or a vibratory device and rings as soon as voiding starts. It is helpful in training the child to improve bladder capacity and avoid enuresis. It requires long-term use and approximately 50–70% improve on this therapy. Relapse rates are lower than that with pharmacotherapy.
- ***Bladder training exercises:*** Daytime bladder exercises are useful, especially in those with low functional bladder capacity—(a) hold urine as long as possible during the day; (b) practice repeated starting and stopping the stream at the toilet bowl; and (c) practice getting up from bed and going to the bathroom at bedtime before sleep.
- ***Caffeine reduction:*** Some dietary products like soft drinks, cocoa and chocolates have significant amount of caffeine, which is known to have a diuretic action. Excessive consumption of these items can result in enuresis and should be avoided.

Drug Therapy

Medications are indicated only in children older than 6 years who fail behavioral treatment. Drugs used are: (1) desmopressin; (2) oxybutynin; and (3) imipramine.

- ***Desmopressin acetate*** (DDAVP) is the first modality of treatment in children with monosymptomatic enuresis and is advised in combination with alarm therapy. It is given orally or intranasally (nasal spray, 10 µg per spray) at bedtime. It acts by reducing the nocturnal urine output to a volume less than the functional bladder capacity. Start with 10 µg given at bedtime daily and increase gradually by 10 µg/per week to a maximum of 40 µg per day. If effective, it should be used for 3–6 months. Success rate is 40–60%, relapse rate 90%. It is a costly drug, but has a fast onset of action, and may be helpful for specific events, e.g., camping and stayovers.
- ***Oxybutynin*** is an anticholinergic agent that can be used in those above 6 years of age in enuresis nonresponsive to desmopressin therapy. It is considered in combination with desmopressin as it reduces uninhibited bladder contractions and useful in children manifesting with urgency and urge incontinence during daytime.
- ***Tablet imipramine (25, 50 mg tablets):*** Imipramine is a tricyclic antidepressant which alters the arousal-sleep mechanism, and is used as follows: 6–8 years (25 mg), 9–12 years (50 mg), >12 years (75 mg) once a day at bedtime. It is a tricyclic antidepressant which alters the arousal-sleep mechanism. It should be used as a third-line treatment modality once desmopressin, alarm therapy and anticholinergics have been unsuccessful. Success rate 30–60%, and this proportion increases once desmopressin is added, relapse rate 90%. Common side effects are drowsiness, lethargy, and sleep disturbances.

The various treatment modalities available are not used exclusive of each other and often a combination works best. Failure of one form of therapy should result in substitution or addition of another. The best treatment option, if behavioral therapy fails, is the use of combination therapy with alarms and drugs simultaneously.

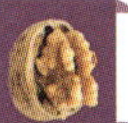

IN A NUTSHELL

Enuresis (Bedwetting)

1. Primary nocturnal enuresis is defined as repeated passage of urine in clothes/bed during night in a child >5 years of age.
2. Primary enuresis needs to be differentiated from secondary enuresis, where the child had been dry for at least 6 months, before starting bedwetting.
3. Behavioral modification, bladder training exercises, use of alarm systems, and desmopressin (DDAVP) either singly or in combination are the treatment modalities.
4. Relapse rate after any treatment is high.

Nevéus T, Fonseca E, Franco I, et al. Management and treatment of nocturnal enuresis: an updated standardization document from the International Children's Continence Society. J Pediatr Urol. 2020;16:10-9.

Roth EB, Austin PF. Evaluation and treatment of nonmonosymptomatic enuresis. Pediatr Rev. 2014;35:430-6.

Traisman ES. Enuresis: evaluation and treatment. Pediatr Ann. 2015;44:133-7.

4.9 Digital Media Exposure

INTRODUCTION

Digital media is defined as a source that allows the creation of user generated content by using encoded numeric data formats. Devices used to access digital media are laptops, computers, smartphones, and tablets. The World Health Organization in its global action plan in 2019 recommended no screen time in children <1 year and <1 hour/day in children 2–5 years old. Indian Academy of Pediatrics (IAP) guidelines on screen time are depicted in **Box 4.1**.

Box 4.1 Indian Academy of Pediatrics (IAP) Guidelines for Screen Exposure in Children

1. Children below the age of 2 years should not be exposed to any type of screen except for occasional video call with relatives
2. Screen time for children between the age of 2 and 5 years should not exceed 1 hour; the lesser, the better
3. For older children and adolescents, it is important to balance screen time with other activities that are required for overall development
4. These activities include an hour of physical activity (play time), adequate duration of sleep (recommended sleep time varies with age, for example, adolescents require 8–9 hours of uninterrupted sleep at night), and time for schoolwork, meals, hobbies, and family time
5. If any of these activities is displaced due to screen use, then it is called excessive screen time and it should be reduced

HARMFUL EFFECTS OF SCREEN TIME EXPOSURE

- ***Obesity:*** Screen time exposure of >2 hours/day is known to be associated with development of obesity. Snacking and meals while watching screen, food advertisement of processed and junk food, lack of physical activity are all predisposing factors leading to obesity.
- ***Cognitive development:*** Excessive screen exposure is known to cause language delay, learning disabilities, and reading difficulties. In older children anxiety, aggressive behavior can be precipitated due to watching adult directed media. Excessive exposure to violent video games also acts as triggers of aggressive behavior.
- ***Sleep disturbances:*** Watching screen just before bedtime is known to precipitate sleep disorders.
- Excessive screen exposure leads to attention problems and depressive symptoms.

- Visual abnormalities such as astigmatism, refractive errors, and excessive watering of eye with discomfort are all ill effects of excess screen exposure.

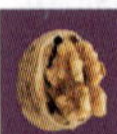

IN A NUTSHELL

Digital Media Exposure

1. Indian Academy of Pediatrics recommends no screen exposure in children <2 years and <1 hour/day in children 2–5 years old.
2. Excess exposure can lead to obesity, learning disabilities, sleep disorders, depressive symptoms, and visual abnormalities.
3. An hour of physical activity, adequate duration of sleep and time for schoolwork, meals, hobbies, and family time are the mainstay of management.

Gupta P, Shah D, Bedi N, et al. Indian Academy of Pediatrics Guidelines on Screen Time and Digital Wellness in Infants, Children and Adolescents. Indian Pediatr. 2022;59(3):235-44.

4.10 Approach to a Child with Suspected Behavioral Disorders

INTRODUCTION

Childhood behavior is typically considered a problem when the child's behavior or developmental stage does not match with parental expectations. Inconsistent expectations are most frequent with children under age 3, because some parents are not prepared for the frequent crying, negativism and high energy levels of normal infants and small children. An important aspect of the physician's role is to educate parents about the normal phases and behavior problems that tend to occur at each age.

EVALUATION

- ***Background history:*** Child's early development of the personality and behavior depends upon the environment in which he is raised. Children raised in emotionally supportive, caring and responsive environment are well adjusted. The type of family, school, community and society has a lot of influence on the overall development of behavior. Hence, it is important to take a detailed history about the place, family and society when dealing with children having behavior problem. History of high screen exposure, poor sleep hygiene, speech delay, nutritional deficiencies are all triggers of behavioral problems and must be dealt in history. A detailed assessment of family social structure including parental stress, bereavement, parental separation, household stress, child abuse must be a part of detailed history.
- Detailed development examination is mandatory while doing an assessment. It includes evaluation of the nutritional assessment, a developmental assessment, general behavior of the child, behavior of the child when you are interacting with the parents and child's interaction with the physician and the family members.
- ***Severity assessment:*** It is important to find out day-to-day activity of the child and influence on day-to-day activity by this problem. It is also important to assess severity of the problem.
- ***Identify triggers:*** In order to classify the severity of the problem, it is important to find out the events, nature, duration, frequency and situations that trigger the problem.

ACTION

When problem behaviors arise in children, three approaches can be considered by the physician: (1) identify the behavior as age-appropriate and reassure the parents; (2) advise the parents to attempt to stop the unacceptable behavior and/or (3) introduce a new, preferred behavior. Parents need to avoid power struggles and "no-win" situations.

Some principles related to behavioral modification are: People tend to continue a behavior when it is rewarded; they tend to stop a behavior when it is consistently ignored (extinguished) or punished; alternately rewarding and ignoring the same behavior (intermittent reinforcement) is known to prolong a behavior and make it very difficult to suppress. This is one reason; consistency is so important in changing behavior. When change is desired, parents are encouraged to limit their focus to one or two related behaviors. If too many behaviors are addressed simultaneously, the effort will be less effective.

Increase Appropriate Behavior

Interventions that are intended to increase the appropriate behaviors use principle of reinforcement and intervention. The reinforcement techniques are: (1) social reinforcement (attention, praise), (2) tangible reinforcement (material objects of personal value), and (3) token economy.

Decrease Inappropriate Behavior

Those used to decrease inappropriate behavior use the principle of punishment. The punishment techniques are: (1) extension, (2) time out for positive reinforcement, (3) response cost, and (4) overcorrection.

Skill Development

Children are helped to develop particular skills. Skill training is encouraged in prosocial activities of children such as sharing toys, waiting for turn, asking for helps. This helps the children for joining in-group activities and resolving conflicts. The areas of skill training are: (1) problem solving skill, (2) social skills, and (3) anger coping skills.

Loving Attitude

Provide supportive, tender, and loving care to children with behavior problems. Parents should also be great listeners to understand the exact nature of their problems. Physician should counsel the parents and family members appropriately. Children who are taught that inappropriate behavior is not going to be tolerated and that appropriate behavior will be consistently rewarded and praised, are learning skills that will lead to lifelong discipline.

On evaluation, presence of red flag signs is the indicators of referral to child guidance clinics (CGC). Children should be referred if:

- Suspicion of a neurodevelopmental disorder, e.g., autism spectrum disorder, attention deficit hyperactive disorder
- There is risk of self-physical harm
- Signs of conduct or defiant disorders
- Presence of anxiety or depression
- Behavioral problems are affecting quality of life
- Behavioral issues are affecting family functioning
- Family history of parental health issues or difficult familial structure

CHILD GUIDANCE CLINICS

Child guidance clinics are specialized clinics catering to children with normal and delayed development or those with behavioral and psychological problems. These CGCs ensure annual examination and developmental evaluation of each child and help in early detection and prevention of a large number of disabilities. Child guidance clinics were started for the prevention of juvenile delinquency sponsored by "Commonwealth Fund's Program" in the year 1920. The first CGC was established in TATA Institute, Mumbai in the year 1939.

Objectives of Child Guidance Clinic

- To identify children between 0 and 12 years having difficulties in learning and behavior.
- To provide professional assessment services for children with difficulties.
- To provide guidance and counseling services to children and parents.
- To refer children to institutions for specialized services and help.

Services Available at Child Guidance Clinic

- Educational assessment
- Remedial education
- IQ and other psychological assessment
- Medicinal intervention
- Counseling and guidance to children and parents
- Play observation and therapy
- Referral services

The team comprises child development professional, child counselors, psychiatrist, psychologist and speech therapist. It offers specialized screening and diagnosis of children suspected of, at risk of or showing learning, behavior, attention, and developmental difficulties. Comprehensive assessments are carried out of the child by multidisciplinary team in 8–10 assessment sessions with the child and the family.

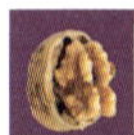

IN A NUTSHELL

Child Guidance Clinics

1. Child guidance clinics are specialized clinics catering to children with normal and delayed development or those with behavioral and psychological problems.
2. The objective is to identify children with learning and behavioral difficulties, to provide professional assessment and guidance and counseling services.

National Institute of Public Cooperation and Child Development. Child Guidance Center. [online] Available from https://www.nipccd.nic.in/hn/schemes/child-guidance-centre-21#gsc.tab=0. [Last accessed August, 2025].

5 CHAPTER

Adolescent Health and Common Problems Related to Adolescent Health

AS PER NMC COMPETENCIES

PE6.1	Define adolescence and describe the stages of adolescence.	*Ch 5.1, Ch 5.2*
PE6.2	Describe the physical, physiological and psychological changes during adolescence (puberty).	*Ch 5.2*
PE6.3	Describe the general health problems during adolescence.	*Ch 5.3*
PE6.4	Describe adolescent sexuality, diversity in sexual orientation, and gender identity.	*Ch 5.4*
PE6.5	Describe the common adolescent eating disorders (anorexia nervosa, bulimia).	*Ch 5.5*
PE6.6	Describe the common mental health problems during adolescence.	*Ch 5.6, Ch 5.7*
PE6.7	Respecting patient privacy and maintaining confidentiality while dealing with adolescence.	*Ch 5.8*
PE6.8	Perform routine adolescent health checkup including eliciting history, performing examination including SMR (sex maturity rating), growth assessments (using growth charts) and systemic examination including thyroid and breast examination and the HEADSS screening.	*Ch 5.2, Ch 5.8*
PE6.9	Explain the objectives and functions of AFHS (Adolescent Friendly Health Services) and the referral criteria.	*Ch 5.9*
PE6.10	Visit to the adolescent clinic.	*Ch 5.9*
PE6.11	Enumerate the importance of obesity and other NCD in adolescents.	*Ch 5.7*
PE6.12	Enumerate the prevalence and importance of recognition of sexual abuse and drug abuse in adolescents and children.	*Ch 5.4, Ch 5.6*

5.1 Definition and Importance of Adolescent Health *PE 6.1*

Adolescence is a period of transition between childhood and adulthood—a time of rapid physical, cognitive, social, and emotional maturing as the boy prepares for manhood and girl prepares for womanhood. The term adolescence is derived from Latin word "*adolescere*" meaning "to grow and to mature." UNICEF defines adolescent as "the sequence of events by which the individual is transformed into a young adult by a series of biological changes".

The precise boundaries are difficult to define, but this period is customarily viewed as a lifespan beginning with the gradual appearance of secondary sex characteristics at about 10–11 years of age and ending with cessation of body growth at 18–20 years of age. Commonly used definitions for adolescence age are shown in **Box 5.1**.

Apart from physical, emotional, and psychological changes, adolescence is also characterized by spiritual changes, desire for exploration, identity formation, and evolving personal relationships. This is also a time of behavioral changes when the reproductive capacity is established. It is a time when children psychologically move from areas of relative comfort and emotional security to places and situations that are far more complex and often much more challenging. The adolescence

Box 5.1 Definition of Adolescence

- WHO defines "adolescence" as age between 10 and 19 years
- Government of India in the National Youth Policy defines adolescence as 13–19 years
- "Youth" refers to ages 15–24 years. Government of India defines this age group as 15–35 years
- "Young people" refers to ages 10–24 years
- "Young adults" refers to ages 20–24 years

is divided into three phases: (1) early, (2) middle, and (3) late adolescence. Early adolescence refers to age 10–13 years, middle adolescence refers to age 14–16 years and late adolescence refers to age 17–19 years.

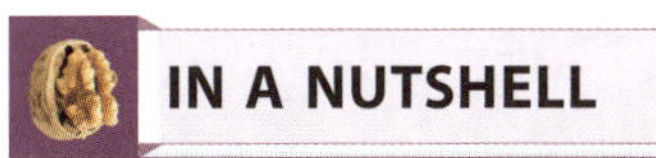

Adolescence

1. Adolescent is the period of transition between childhood and adulthood.
2. The most accepted age range is 10–19 years as defined by World Health Organization (WHO).

World Health Organization. (2013). Adolescent health. [online] Available from https://www.who.int/health-topics/adolescent-health [Last accessed September, 2025].

5.2 Changes During Adolescence *PE 6.1, PE 6.2, PE 6.8*

INTRODUCTION

Except for the newborn and early infancy, no period of the human lifespan encompasses more dramatic changes than does adolescence. Biologic and cognitive changes that occur, their interrelatedness, and their potential impact on adolescent health are discussed here.

Biological Development

Puberty primarily refers to the maturational, hormonal, and growth process that occurs when the reproductive organs begin to function, and secondary sexual characters develop. It is primarily due to hormonal activity under the influence of central nervous system. The orderly appearance of secondary sexual characteristics is depicted in **Table 5.1**.

Marshall and Tanner have described the appearance of secondary sexual characteristics as sexual maturity rating (SMR). SMR stages are assigned numbers from 1 to 5, with 1 representing no pubertal development and 5 signifying full adult development (**Tables 5.2 and 5.3**).

Typically, girls develop breast buds as the first sign of puberty (although about 15% develop pubic hair first). Approximately 1 year after breast budding, girls reach their peak height velocity, and 1 year later menarche ensues. After menarche, a girl usually grows only an additional 4–5 cm.

Onset of puberty in boys is heralded by an increase in testicular volume, followed by pubic hair growth, then enlargement (length and circumference) of the penis. Peak height velocity occurs 2 years after the onset of testicular enlargement. Adolescents gain about 15–25% of their final adult height during their pubertal growth spurt.

Pubertal development starts 1–2 years earlier in girls as compared to boys. There is a wide variation in age and velocity with which growth and development proceeds. In a group of adolescents who are growing together this wide variation leads to development of anxiety—"Am I normal?" and needs a lot of reassurance.

Appearance of secondary sexual characters before the age of 8 years in girls and 9 years in boys, and nonappearance of secondary sexual characters by the age of 13 years in girls and 14 years in boys is considered abnormal. A girl who does not menstruate by 16 years should be thoroughly evaluated for the presence of chronic illness, malnutrition, or other conditions that may affect physical development.

Table 5.1 Usual Sequence of Maturational Changes

Girls	*Boys*
1. Breast changes	1. Enlargement of testes
2. Rapid increase in height and weight	2. Growth of pubic hair, upper lip, facial hair
3. Growth of pubic hair	3. Rapid increase in height
4. Appearance of axillary hairs	4. Changes in larynx and voice
5. Menstruation (usually begins 2 years after first sign)	5. Nocturnal emission
6. Abrupt deceleration of linear growth	6. Abrupt deceleration of linear growth

Cognitive and Developmental Changes

Adolescents must cope, not only with changes in their physical appearance, but also with associated emotional changes and emerging and compelling sex urges.

- ❖ Bodily changes cause emotional stress and strain as well as abrupt and rapid mood swings. Hormonal changes are likely to result in thoughts pertaining to sex, irritability, restlessness, anger, and tension.
- ❖ Sexual attraction leads to a desire to mix freely and interact with each other.

Adolescence is characterized by an emerging capacity to reason in an increasingly more sophisticated manner. Younger teens are relatively concrete in their thinking and have difficulty with abstract concepts. During middle and late adolescence, the ability to reason abstractly, to handle multiple concepts

Table 5.2 Tanner Staging for Sexual Maturity Rating (SMR) in Girls

Tanner stage	*Breast (B)*	*Pubic hair (P)*
Stage 1	Prepubertal—no breast tissue	Same as abdominal hair
Stage 2	Breast bud appears, enlargement of areola	Sparse hair along labia, minimally pigmented
Stage 3	Further enlargement of breast and areola but contour separation between the two	Darker and coarser hair on mons pubis
Stage 4	A secondary mound is formed by areola and papilla above the level of the breast	Adult type, but limited to mons and labia
Stage 5	Adult breast contour with projection of papilla alone	Adult type, spreads to medial thigh

Table 5.3: Tanner Staging for Sexual Maturity Rating (SMR) in Boys

Tanner stage	*Genitalia (G)*	*Testicular volume*	*Pubic hair (P)*	
Stage 1	Prepubertal	<4 mL	Same as abdominal hair	<3 mL; <2.5 cm
Stage 2	Early penile growth, thinning and reddening of scrotal skin	4–10 mL	Sparse growth at the base of penis	4 mL; 2.5–3.2 cm
Stage 3	Increase in penile length, scrotal thickening and darkening	10–15 m	Darker, coarser, curled hair: spreads to mons pubis	10 mL; 3.3–4.0 cm
Stage 4	Increase in penile length and breadth, pigmentation of scrotum	15–20 mL	Adult type, not on thighs	18 mL; 4.1–4.5 cm
Stage 5	Adult genitalia	>20 mL	Adult type, spreads to medial thigh	25 mL; >4.5 cm

simultaneously, and to use a "what if" approach emerges. Older teens can take another person's perspective and are better able to project themselves into the future and reflect about events that may be remote in time.

These differences have significant implications for healthcare encounters. For example, counseling younger teens about smoking is more likely to have an impact if the focus is on the immediate consequences of smoking (bad breath, yellow teeth, and decreased exercise performance) rather than on long-term (and fairly abstract) conditions (lung cancer or emphysema). Terms such as cancer or emphysema may be too abstract to have an impact on their decision regarding smoking.

Because of their developmental level, adolescents have a sense of uniqueness and personal invulnerability. Negative health outcomes, such as unintended pregnancy, a serious injury, or a sexually transmitted disease, happen to other teenagers but not to them. This sense of personal invulnerability, coupled with a desire to test and master and their newly emerging physical and mental capabilities, may also explain the risk-taking behaviors observed during this age.

PHASES OF ADOLESCENCE

Adolescence is customarily divided into the stages: (1) early (age 11–14 years), (2) middle (age 14–17 years) and (3) late (age 17–21 years) (**Table 5.4**).

- ***Early adolescence*** is characterized by a focus on the physical changes that accompany puberty and by concrete thinking. Separation from parents and the rise in peer group influence begins during this stage but is not prominent.
- ***Middle adolescence:*** Peer group influence and conflicts with parents peak. Risk-taking behaviors, such as cigarette smoking, drinking, and sexual intercourse become common. Concerns about one's developing sense of self and autonomy become increasingly important.
- ***Late adolescence:*** The focus shifts to developing the capacity for intimacy in relationships and defining one's career goals and place in society. Generally, peer group influence lessens, and a rapprochement with parents occurs. Older adolescents are often idealistic and may be highly critical of traditional institutions.

The adolescent age group is relatively healthy phase of their lifespan but there are few health implications which arise due to all the changes that are taking place in this age group. **Table 5.5** summarizes the possible health implications of adolescent development and various influencing factors.

Adolescents are vulnerable by virtue of the normal development process, family/peer/environmental influences that may be protective or negative (e.g., broken family, drug use in family members or peers) and lifestyle pattern they choose and certain "At risk" behaviors.

Table 5.4 Stages of Adolescence

Developmental parameters	*Early adolescence*	*Middle adolescence*	*Late adolescence*
Age	10–13 years	14–17 years	17 years upward
SMR stage	1 and 2	3 and 4	5
Physical development	• Rapidly occurring changes, body image issues • Interest about anatomy and physiology of sex organs increases	• Peaks in growth in height and weight occurs • They focus on making themselves more attractive to others	The body develops like an adult, and they have a realistic body image
Cognitive development	• Concrete thinkers • There is lack of control of impulsive actions that this may result in risk taking behavior	• Abstract reasoning and formal operational thinking begins • Feeling of supremacy and immortality increase and this may lead to risk taking behavior	Establishment of abstract reasoning is achieved. Ability to weigh different options develops and decision making become more rational and realistic
Family	• Desire for autonomy begins • Find flaws in home rules and traditions • Increased tension with parents • Mood swings are common	• More autonomous • Spend more time with friends • Acquire rules and roles of their friendship group. This may lead to conflict between parents and adolescents	• Reconcile the relationship with parents and the conflicts with parents are less • Begin to have faith in moral, religious, and sexual values of family and community
Peers	Friends of same sex become more important than family	• Friendship with both sexes is common now • Experimental and exploitative relationships develop	• Relationship becomes less exploitative • Committed relationship with opposite sex partner can begin at this level
Scholastic competence	• Conceptual comprehension of the material begins • Learning disabilities can be identified	Higher order thinking begins	Able to make realistic decisions about education and carrier

Table 5.5: Possible Health Implications of Adolescent Growth and Development

Changes during adolescence	*Health implications in adolescence*
Physical changes	
Normal growing-up	Undue anxiety and tension
Increase in height and weight	Increase nutrition requirement— if inadequate, under nutrition and anemia
Breast development	Stooping of shoulders, poor posture, back pain
Skin becomes oily	Acne
Desire to be thin, have a good figure	Malnutrition, anemia, stunting
Sexual development	
Desire to have sex	Unsafe sex leading to unwanted pregnancy, STIs and HIV
Ejaculation	Fear, guilt, myths—emotional problems
Menstruation	Dysmenorrhea, menorrhagia—anemia, poor menstrual hygiene may lead to RTIs
Emotional changes and social development	
Development of identity	Confusion, moodiness, irritation
Very curious	Experimentation, risk taking behavior
Peer pressure	*Effect on lifestyles:* • Unhealthy eating habits leading to obesity • Smoking and alcohol • Speed driving, accidents

(HIV: human immunodeficiency virus; RTIs: reproductive tract infections; STIs: sexually transmitted infections)

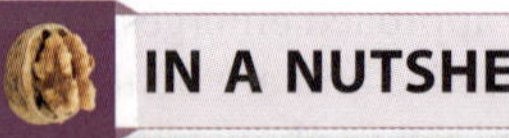

IN A NUTSHELL

Changes in Adolescence

1. Adolescence is accompanied by physical, cognitive, emotional, social and behavioral changes due to interplay of various hormones during puberty.
2. Physically, an individual gains the final 15–20% of adult height; 50% of the adult body weight; and 40% of the adult skeletal mass in adolescence.
3. Marshall and Tanner have described the appearance of secondary sexual characteristics as sexual maturity ratings (SMR).
4. Adolescence is customarily divided into the three stages: early (11–14 years), middle (14–17 years) and late (17–21 years).

Katsantonis I, McLellan R, Marquez J. Development of subjective well-being and its relationship with self-esteem in early adolescence. British Journal of Developmental Psychology. 2023;41(2):157-71.

National Health Mission. Orientation program for Medical Officers to provide Adolescent-Friendly Health Services: Handouts. [online] Available from https://nhm.gov.in/images/pdf/programmes/RKSK/Medical_Officer_Training_Manual/Resource_Book_Medical_Officer.pdf. [Last accessed August, 2025].

Sabiston CM, Doré I, Lucibello KM, et al. Body image self-conscious emotions get worse throughout adolescence and relate to physical activity behavior in girls and boys. Soc Sci Med. 2022;315:115543.

Vasilenko SA. Sexual behavior and health from adolescence to adulthood: Illustrative examples of 25 years of research. J Adolesc Health. 2022;71(6S):S24-S31.

5.3 General Health Problems

PE 6.3

INTRODUCTION

Adolescence is considered a healthy period, however, >33% of the disease burden and almost 60% of premature deaths among adults can be associated with behaviors or conditions that began or occurred during adolescence, for example, tobacco and alcohol use, poor eating habits and physical activity, sexual abuse, and risky sex.

Health problems in the adolescents can be grouped under medical and nonmedical problems (**Box 5.2**). It is interesting to note that the major cause of mortality in this age group is not due to medical illnesses rather condition arising out of their "risk taking behavior".

A list of "priority" health problems affecting adolescents is based on data from around the world is provided in **Box 5.3**. Each of these items meets the following three criteria:

Box 5.2 Adolescent Health Problems

1. ***Medical diseases:*** Asthma, respiratory infections, tuberculosis, precocious or delayed puberty short stature, and chronic disorders such as diabetes, celiac diseases, heart diseases, etc., diabetes mellitus (DM), celiac, malignancies, renal disorders, thalassemia
2. ***Consequences of risk-taking behavior:*** Accidents and injuries, violence, homicide, suicide, substance abuse
3. ***Nutritional problems:*** Undernutrition, micronutrient deficiencies such as iron deficiency, obesity, and eating disorders—anorexia nervosa, bulimia
4. ***Reproductive health problems:*** Teenage pregnancy, abortion, menstrual problems, and reproductive tract infections
5. ***Mental health problems:*** Substance abuse, violence, depression and suicide, learning disorders, and other psychiatric disorders

Box 5.3 Priority Health Problems Affecting Adolescents

1. Nutritional problems
2. Sexual and reproductive health problems (including HIV/AIDS)
3. Noncommunicable diseases
4. Mental health problems
5. Substance use and abuse (tobacco, alcohol, and other substances)
6. Injuries and violence (including gender-based violence)
7. *Endemic and chronic diseases:* TB, malaria, asthma

Box 5.4 Priority Health Problems Affecting Adolescents

1. Behavior contributing to unintentional violent injuries
2. Tobacco use
3. Alcohol and other drug use
4. Sexual behaviors contributing to unintended pregnancy, STD and HIV
5. Unhealthy dietary behavior
6. Physical inactivity

1. Firstly, they cause mortality or morbidity either during the adolescent period, or in later life because of behaviors initiated during this period.
2. Secondly, they cause significant levels of mortality and morbidity.
3. Thirdly, many of these health problems and problem behaviors are interrelated. For instance, substance use is associated with depressive states, and alcohol use is associated with road traffic accidents.

Box 5.4 lists the 6 priority health-risk behaviors in youth as identified by Center for Disease Control (CDC), Atlanta. Based on these six priority areas, CDC has developed the Youth Risk Behavior Surveillance System (YRBSS) to monitor the health risk behaviors. The YRBSS data can be used to describe risk behaviors, create awareness, set program goals, develop programs and seek program resources for adolescents and young people.

PROTECTIVE FACTORS

These factors increase the likelihood of adolescents making decisions that contribute positively to their health and development and decrease the likelihood of engaging in risky behavior. Protective factors include: (1) caring and meaningful relationships; (2) positive school environment; (3) structure and boundaries for behaviors; (4) having spiritual beliefs; (5) encouragement of self-expression; and (6) opportunities for participation and contribution.

Protective factors work in three ways: (1) they encourage and sustain positive behavior, (2) they reduce the risk of negative health behavior and outcomes; and (3) they diminish the effect of, and support recovery from, negative health outcomes.

It is important to understand that the most significant aspect of providing health care to adolescents lies in reaching them effectively. Establishing and maintaining rapport with young people is as important as the timely intervention or the provision of knowledge, skills, supplies and services.

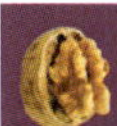

IN A NUTSHELL

Health Issues in Adolescence

1. Though adolescence is considered relatively a healthy period, but many health risk behaviors such as smoking, alcohol consumption, sedentary lifestyle are formed in this age, which are responsible for significant morbidity and mortality in the adult life.
2. Health problems encountered in adolescence can be broadly grouped as medical and nonmedical.
3. Apart from medical issues, mental health issues, drugs, and injuries and violence are the major causes of morbidity and mortality in adolescents.
4. Protective factors increase the likelihood of adolescents making decisions that contribute positively to their health and development, and decrease the likelihood of engaging in risky behavior.

Neinstein LS, Katzman DK, Callahan T, et al. Neinstein's Adolescent and Young Adult Health Care: A Practical Guide, 6th edition. Netherlands: Wolters Kluwer; 2016.

5.4 Adolescent Sexuality

PE 6.4, PE 6.12

DEFINITIONS AND IMPLICATIONS

Sex and Sexuality

The terms sex and sexuality often confuse the adolescents.

- The term ***sex*** is often used for the intercourse whereas it denotes the biological difference between women and men. The goal of sex drive is biological sexual maturity, i.e., capacity to love, mate, reproduce and care for the young ones.
- ***Sexuality*** is broad term, which includes the sum of person's personality, thinking and behavior toward sex. It includes the identity, emotions, thoughts, actions, relationships, affection, love, feelings, caring, sharing, and the intimacy the person has and displays. The negative aspect of sexuality includes sexual coercion, eve teasing, sexual harassment, rape, and prostitution.

Adolescents develop and become aware of their sexual drives and feelings. They also tend to explore the various aspects/dimensions of being sexual. They are likely to be curious and try to experiment. Many adolescents adopt high-risk behavior due to the numerous myths and lack of skills—especially the ability to negotiate and to deal with peer pressure effectively. Consequences of unsafe sexual behaviors include adolescent pregnancy, unsafe abortions, and sexually transmitted infections (STIs).

Adolescent Pregnancy

Globally, 15% of all births are to women 15–19 years old. Nineteen percent of total fertility in India is contributed by girls in the 15–19 age group.

- Adolescent pregnancy and breastfeeding puts both mother and child at higher risks of morbidity and mortality.
- Early pregnancy exposes both the mother and her baby to risk owing to the potential competition for dietary energy and nutrients.
- Because adolescent girls (below 17 years) have not reached physical maturity and their pelvis are not fully developed; pregnancy could lead to obstructed or prolonged labor, hemorrhage, and even death for both mother and child.
- Young adolescent girls are also likely to experience premature labor, spontaneous abortion, and stillbirths.
- Pregnancy-related illnesses such as hypertension and anemia are also more common among adolescents.
- Young mothers are also likely to have a higher incidence of poor childcare and poor child feeding practices and they are less likely to breastfeed their babies. Thus, the intergenerational consequences of poor nutrition are perpetuated.

Adolescent marriage, high fertility, and early childbearing (leading to maternal mortality) contribute to a wide difference in mortality rates in adolescent females and males, especially in the older adolescent age group. About 13% of deaths of females below the age of 24 years are related to pregnancy and childbirth causes. Similar trends also prevail in the rural and urban age groups.

Unsafe Abortion

Adolescents often resort to abortion at a later stage of pregnancy. Unsafe abortion could result in complications such as hemorrhage, septicemia, injuries, infertility, and death. Abortion also has psychological consequences such as depression. Adolescent abortions are estimated globally at 2.5 million per year, representing 14% of all unsafe abortions. Most of them are performed illegally or under hazardous circumstances.

Sexually Transmitted Infections

Each year, >1 out of 20 adolescents contract a curable STI. At least one-third of total estimated new STI cases occur in young people. More than half of all new HIV infections reported globally are from the age group of 15–24 years.

PROMOTING THE SEXUAL AND REPRODUCTIVE HEALTH

To function as effective and well-adjusted adults, adolescents need to have clear, accurate and precise information to understand the various aspects of human sexuality, sexual roles and responsibilities. They also need to possess skills to negotiate sexual demands that may be put on them or that they may put on others. Promoting the sexual and reproductive health of adolescents involves the implementation of the following:

- ***Proper information*** that will help adolescents understand how their bodies work and what the consequences of their actions are likely to be.
- ***Social skills*** that will enable them to say no to sex with confidence and to negotiate safer sex.
- ***Counseling*** to make informed choices.
- ***Health services*** can help adolescents to stay well, and ill adolescents get back to good health.

Adolescents are a diverse group, thus their needs are correspondingly heterogeneous. Adolescents who are not yet sexually active have different needs from those who are sexually active; adolescents in stable, monogamous relationships may have different needs from those in more casual relationships. Quite different needs characterize those faced with unwanted pregnancies or infection, or those who have been coerced into sex. It is important, therefore, to be aware of the diversity of sexual and reproductive health needs of adolescents, and to tailor our responses to their specific needs.

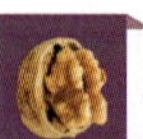

IN A NUTSHELL

Adolescent Sexuality

1. Sexuality is broad term, which includes the sum of person's personality, thinking and behavior toward sex.
2. Nineteen percent of total fertility in India is contributed by girls in the 15–19 age group.
3. Adolescent pregnancy and breastfeeding puts both mother and child at higher risks of morbidity and mortality.
4. To function as effective and well-adjusted adults, adolescents need to have clear, accurate and precise information to understand the various aspects of human sexuality, sexual roles, and responsibilities.

World Health Organization. WHO recommendations on adolescent health: guidelines approved by the WHO Guidelines Review Committee. Geneva: World Health Organization; 2017

5.5 Eating Disorders: Anorexia and Bulimia *PE 6.5*

INTRODUCTION

Eating disorders are psychological disorders that typically start during preadolescence or adolescence and are often due to extreme disturbance in eating behavior. Three most prevalent disorders are: anorexia nervosa, bulimia nervosa, and binge eating disorder.

The teen is often preoccupied with having a thin body and suffers from low self-esteem. However, many adolescents go undiagnosed as they often try to hide this behavior or are in denial mode and even their weight is normal and consequently do not receive treatment until their eating disorders are at an advanced stage.

Symptoms of eating disorders may include the following: a distorted body image, skipping most meals, unusual eating habits (such as eating many calories at one meal or skipping meals), frequent weighing, extreme weight change, insomnia, constipation, skin rash, dental cavities, loss of hair or nail quality, hyperactivity, and high interest in exercise.

ANOREXIA NERVOSA

This is an eating disorder occurring more commonly in adolescent girls and young women shortly after completion of puberty. The male to female ratio is 1:10 with a bimodal age distribution with one peak at 14.5 years and other at 18 years. In western countries, it occurs in 1% of all adolescent girls. The disorder is characterized by deliberate weight loss induced by the adolescent by reducing food intake, in relentless pursuit of thinness.

Etiology

Anorexia nervosa is more common in girls with excessive dependence, low self-esteem, high anxiety, and affective disorder. Their families are overprotective. It is now thought to be a disorder of mood or problem in identity development.

Hypothalamic abnormalities are noted in them prior to onset of weight loss. Although the fundamental cause is not clear, a complex interaction between sociocultural, biological and psychological factors contributes to its causation.

Diagnostic Criteria

1. Persistent restriction of energy intake leading to significantly low body weight.
2. Either an intense fear of gaining weight or of becoming fat, or persistent behavior that interferes with weight gain.
3. Disturbance in the way one's body weight or shape is experienced.

Clinical Manifestations

- Young females begin to eat less and less food, leading to profound weight loss and emaciation. Typically, there is avoidance of "fattening foods" with or without self-induced vomiting or purging. There may be a history of excessive exercise, use of appetite suppressants, or diuretics. Physical profile of starvation is present.
- Affected girl will complain of abdominal pain and bloating of abdomen even with ingestion of small amounts of food.
- There is disorder of hypothalamic-pituitary axis, manifesting as amenorrhea.
- Weight loss >30% leads to lethargy, cachexia, and generalized weakness.
- There is undernutrition of varying severity, with resulting secondary endocrine and metabolic changes and disturbance of bodily functions.
- The mortality is 10% and is due to electrolyte imbalance, cardiac arrhythmias or congestive heart failure, hypothermia, and hypotension. Bone marrow hypoplasia, constipation, esophagitis, hypophosphatemia, potassium depletion, hypochloremic alkalosis, and elevation of BUN may also be present.

TREATMENT Anorexia Nervosa

Treatment involves a combined approach of (1) individual and family psychotherapy, (2) behavioral modification, and (3) nutritional rehabilitation. Those with associated depression may require antidepressants.

Role of parents is very important and they should be fully involved in their child's therapy. Psychotherapy helps children improve their self-esteem, peer relationship, and resolving parental conflicts.

The adolescent needs to be hospitalized, if there is severe malnutrition or danger of suicide is present, otherwise they can be treated in outpatient setting. Diet therapy should be instituted after explaining the problems related with starvation. Diet should be increased slowly, and weight gain is monitored. The ultimate target should be to achieve the weight and height appropriate for age.

BULIMIA NERVOSA

Bulimia nervosa is predominantly seen in adolescent females, characterized by recurrent episodes of binge eating accompanied by purging through vomiting, overuse of laxatives, enemas, diuretics, fasting, or excessive exercise. Eating binges may occur as often as several times a day but are most common in the evening and night hours.

Clinical Features

These episodes must occur at least once a week for 3 months to meet the diagnostic criteria for DSM-V classification. Some of the salient features of this condition are as follows:

- Rapid consumption of large amounts of high calorie food with no apparent change in weight.
- Binging is often followed by purging, which is often done secretly.
- ***Evidence of binge eating:*** Hiding food or discarded food containers and wrappers, stealing, hoarding food.
- ***Evidence of purging:*** Frequent trips to bathroom, especially after meals, signs and/or smells of vomiting, presence of empty containers or packages of drugs such as laxatives or diuretics.
- Excessive exercise or fasting, frequent weighing, peculiar eating habits or rituals, preoccupation with food, body weight and image.
- Overachieving and impulsive behaviors.

Physical signs of bulimia nervosa include dental enamel erosion, odor on the breath, skin changes such as calluses/scarring on the dorsum of hands caused by self-inducing vomiting, enlargement of salivary glands, and edema.

TREATMENT Bulimia Nervosa

Early diagnosis and management are the mainstay, requires a multidisciplinary team approach comprising of physician, therapist and a nutritionist with very good communication skills. Broadly it includes medical and nutritional intervention with the aim of restoring weight, nutritional rehabilitation, and treatment of complications. Family-based treatment is often the mainstay of psychological intervention. Coexisting mental illness such as anxiety and depression are also treated. Selective serotonin uptake inhibitors (fluoxetine, sertraline, etc.) are used in resistant cases.

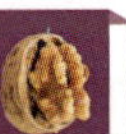

IN A NUTSHELL

Eating Disorders in Adolescence

1. Eating disorders are psychological disorders that typically start during preadolescence or adolescence and are often due to extreme disturbance in eating behavior.
2. Three most prevalent disorders are—anorexia nervosa, bulimia nervosa, and binge eating disorder.
3. Early diagnosis and management are the mainstay of these disorders and require a multidisciplinary team approach comprising of physician, therapist and a nutritionist with very good communication skills.

Neinstein LS, Katzman DK, Callahan T, et al. Neinstein's Adolescent and Young Adult Health Care: A Practical Guide, 6th edition. Netherlands: Wolters Kluwer; 2016.

Silén Y, Keski-Rahkonen A. Worldwide prevalence of DSM-5 eating disorders among young people. Curr Opin Psychiatry. 2022;35(6):362-71.

5.6 Mental Health Problems

PE 6.6, PE 6.12

PREVALENCE

As per WHO "globally, one in seven 10–19-year-old experiences a mental disorder, accounting for 13% of the global burden of disease in this age group" and is considered most common non-communicable disease (NCD) in this age group.

In any given year, about 20% of adolescents will experience a mental health problem, most commonly depression, anxiety, or behavioral disorders. In India, it is documented that the prevalence of psychiatric disorders among adolescents under 16 years is 12.5%. In addition, almost half of the mental illnesses diagnosed in adults have their onset in the adolescent period and those with onset in childhood are invariably found to persist into adolescence. Depressive disorders, along with some behavioral disturbances, such as suicidality, eating disorders, and substance abuse, begin to emerge in these years. Approximately 40–90% of adolescents with depression have a comorbid psychiatric disorder such as anxiety disorder, conduct disorder, substance abuse, and personality disorder.

ETIOLOGY

Risky behavior (such as unsafe sex, hazardous/drunk driving, smoking), self-harm, physical inactivity, educational failure, and school dropout are associated with mental health problems. Strong emphasis placed on educational achievement. This causes a lot of stress among adolescents, which could cause headaches, eyestrain, difficulty in concentrating, and sleep problems.

ASSESSMENT

Mental illness can present in a variety of ways. Changes in mood and behaviors can provide important indicators of an adolescent's mental well-being, but these observations alone are not conclusive. The HEEADSSS approach (**Table 5.6**) can help the clinicians assess whether an adolescent is mentally well or ill and, if they are ill, to assess the severity of the illness.

Table 5.6	HEEADSSS Approach: Warning Signs for Screening Mental Health Issues
Home	Adolescent has no support at home or anywhere else
Education	• Adolescent is having trouble at school or work, e.g., problems with school or work, bullying, or problems with teachers or bosses • Adolescent frequently misses school or work
Eating	• Adolescent is overweight and has poor eating habits • Adolescent believes he or she is very overweight, when it is evident that this is not the case • Adolescent is absorbed or obsessive about food, exercise, body weight or shape • Adolescent is underweight, and from the discussion it appears that financial constraints are contributing to this
Exercise	• Adolescent participates in no or very little physical activity • Adolescent is overweight and unfit (e.g., breathless, tires easily walking upstairs) • Adolescent is absorbed or obsessive about exercise and body weight • Adolescent is undernourished or engages in excessive physical labor
Activities	• Adolescent has no friends and spends most of their time alone • Adolescent spends most of their time with people who are 4–5 years older, who affect their behaviors negatively
Drugs	• Adolescent regularly uses legal or illegal substances • Adolescent has tried illegal substances or has friends who do so • Substance use is having a negative impact on adolescent's health or ability to function • Other people have expressed concern about adolescent's substance use

Contd...

Contd...

Sex	• Adolescent is being or has been pressured to have sex • Adolescent seems at risk for early sexual activity • Adolescent has had unsafe sex or has had a number of sexual partners • Adolescent seems upset or worried about his or her sexual orientation
Safety	• Adolescent is experiencing bullying, violence, sexual harassment, or abuse • Adolescent is withdrawn and unable to talk of experiences, or examination reveals signs of violence
Suicide and depression	• Adolescent is sad or anxious or feels hopeless most of the time • Sleep disturbances • Adolescent talks about hurting or killing themselves, or has tried to hurt or kill themselves • Adolescent frequently uses alcohol or drugs to escape negative feelings • Adolescent has poor self-esteem and no sense of self-worth

Unexplained aches and pains, inability to concentrate, disruptions in sleep habits, changes in appetite and eating, heightened irritability, agitation, and moodiness should alert to presence of a mental illness. Persistence of symptoms for >2 weeks are important "Red flags" for depression.

Stress and Related Symptoms

Multiple changes occurring in adolescents potentially result in great stress (**Box 5.5**). The adolescent is faced with pressures from peers to conform, which often involve flaunting adult authority and even serious health risks. Then they must meet parental expectations and expectations from the society. Today's youth experience both normative stressors (e.g., physical changes) as well as unforeseen stressful life (e.g., breakup in relationship) and at times lack the requisite coping and adaptive skills for negotiation. Occasionally these may result in variety of bodily reactions which is often perceived or reported as pain or discomfort (psychosomatic symptoms).

Common psychosomatic symptoms include *recurrent abdominal pain, headaches, chest pain, and chronic fatigue.* Other nonspecific symptoms include dizziness, syncope and/or tiredness are often found associated with family problems, stress, school problems, and depression.

Box 5.5 Areas of Stress in Adolescents

1. Body image
2. Sexuality conflicts
3. Scholastic pressures
4. Competitive pressures
5. Relationship with parents
6. Relationship with siblings and peers
7. Finances
8. Decision about present and future roles
9. Career planning
10. Ideological conflicts

Suicidal Behavior

Teenagers may attempt suicide more commonly than we realize. So we should ask this question rather directly and without any hesitation, e.g., "Have you ever felt so bad that you felt like committing a suicide?" Remember, asking about suicidal behavior does not precipitate or trigger it. Any suicidal ideation should prompt a more careful assessment of the patient's suicide risk and must include a referral to a mental health expert. Previous suicide attempts are often a strong risk factor for future attempts and completed suicides. Ensure that adolescents have access to quality and affordable mental health services.

SUBSTANCE ABUSE

Illiteracy, economic background, unemployment, and family disharmony increase vulnerability to drug abuse. Worldwide data shows that harmful substance (tobacco, alcohol, and illicit substances) use among adolescents is rising. It increases the risk of cancer, cardiovascular disease, and respiratory illness later in life.

Tobacco

Globally, 300 million young people (10–24 years) smoke. The use of tobacco by adolescents in India is alarming. Half of these, who would smoke all their life, are likely to die of tobacco-related diseases. Adolescents are beginning to start smoking at increasingly younger ages some begin as early as 10-year-old. The earlier adolescents start using tobacco, the more likely that they will get addicted, and the less likely they are to quit.

Alcohol

Alcohol is the most common element in substance use related death of young people. Alcohol and substance abuse are further associated with poor scholastic attainment, increased drop out from school, drink and drug driving delinquency, early pregnancy and family difficulties. The comorbidity of substance use and other mental health disorders is particularly important, with positive correlation between suicide, depression, and conduct disorder. There is growing evidence of "clustering" of behaviors risky to health. A recent review by WHO has shown that that the use of substance by adolescents is associated with greater likelihood of early sexual initiation.

Drugs

Drug abuse is a sensitive issue and must be discussed frankly with the adolescents in detail. More often they do not admit doing drugs when directly asked but are willing to tell about their friends. If you ask "Do any of your friends use drugs or alcohol (or get drunk or high)?", they might be more forthcoming (**Box 5.6**: CRAFT questionnaire).

PROMOTING MENTAL HEALTH

Mental health promotion has the potential to improve the overall development of adolescents and reduce the impact of risk factors for mental health problems and disorders.

Box 5.6 The CRAFT Questionnaire to Detect Substance Abuse

1. Have you ever ridden in a Car driven by someone who was high or had been using drugs or alcohol?
2. Do you ever use alcohol or drugs to Relax, feel better about yourself, or fit in?
3. Do you ever use drugs or alcohol when you are Alone?
4. Do you Forget things you did while using drugs or alcohol?
5. Do your family or Friends ever tell you that you should cut down your drinking or drug use?
6. Have you ever gotten into Trouble while using drugs or alcohol?

Two or more "Yes" answers suggest high risk of a serious substance-use problem or a substance-use disorder

- Promote positive, caring and supportive relationships between adolescents and their families and peers, teachers, and other adults.
- Ensure that adolescents' lives are free from neglect, trauma, excessive stress, violence, abuse, and discrimination.
- Ensure good living conditions including access to sporting facilities.
- Accept diversity among adolescents.
- Help adolescents to develop life skills including communication, decision making, negotiation, critical thinking, stress management skills to help them cope with the demands of daily life.
- Ensure that adolescents have access to educational and vocational training to enhance their abilities and employment opportunities.
- Integrate mental health promotion and life skills development in the school curriculum.

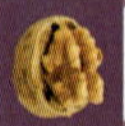

IN A NUTSHELL

Mental Health in Adolescence

1. In India, the prevalence of psychiatric disorders among adolescents under 16 years is 12.5%.
2. Nearly 50% of mental health issues diagnosed in adults have their onset in the adolescent period.
3. HEEADSSS approach related to mental health can help the clinicians to assess mental well-being and their severity in adolescents.
4. Some of the common mental health problems prevalent in this age group are substance abuse, violence, depression, suicide, learning disorders, and other psychiatric disorders.

National Health Mission. Orientation programme for Medical Officers to provide Adolescent-Friendly Health Services: Handouts. [online] Available from https://nhm.gov.in/images/pdf/programmes/RKSK/Medical_Officer_Training_Manual/Resource_Book_Medical_Officer.pdf. [Last accessed May 2025].

World Health Organization. Adolescent mental health. [online] Available from https://www.who.int/news-room/fact-sheets/detail/adolescent-mental-health. [Last accessed May, 2025].

Mehra D, et al. Mental Health Interventions among Adolescents in India: A Scoping Review. Healthcare (Basel). 2022;10(2):337.

5.7 Noncommunicable Diseases in Adolescents *PE 6.6, PE 6.11*

INTRODUCTION

In 2019, globally, one in five deaths among adolescents were caused by NCDs and estimated to cause over half of the disability-affected life years (DALYs). Behaviors, responsible for the majority of NCDs in adulthood, have their origin in adolescence; and include physical inactivity, unhealthy diet, tobacco use and harmful use of alcohol. **Box 5.7** enlists major NCDs in adolescents.

Box 5.7 Major Noncommunicable Diseases in Adolescents

1. Injuries and violence
2. Mental health disorders and substance abuse disorders (major depressive, conduct and anxiety disorders, drug use disorders)
3. Chronic respiratory disorders (asthma)
4. Musculoskeletal disorders (low back pain, neck pain)
5. Neurological disorders (epilepsy, migraine)
6. Dermatological disorders (dermatitis, acne vulgaris)
7. Endocrine disorders (diabetes)
8. Hematological disorders including malignancies
9. Urogenital and digestive disorders
10. *Nutritional disorders:* Iron deficiency anemia and micronutrient deficiencies (iodine, zinc, vitamin B_{12}), overweight, obesity

Tobacco, alcohol, and processed food and beverage industries influence consumption of products related to poor diets, smoking, and alcohol use, which in turn impact adolescent NCD burden are known as commercial determinants of health. For example, the global food industry has been identified as the leading driver of NCD epidemics related to diet. The commercial determinants of health fall under the larger macro, societal and political social determinants of NCDs in adolescents, and they modify the behaviors of individuals in meaningful ways. Mental health issues are the leading causes of NCDs in this age group.

INJURIES AND VIOLENCE

Overall rates of injury and death increase dramatically from childhood to late adolescence, as adolescents are more likely to engage in risk-taking behaviors than younger children or adults. Nearly 50% of the morbidity and mortality in adolescents stems from four behaviors: *sexual activity, substance use and abuse, motor vehicle use, and interpersonal violence.* These behaviors have their origin in adolescence, and are common among all age, socioeconomic and ethnic groups. However, these behaviors are largely preventable.

Interpersonal violence is also increasing among young people, with girls especially being victimized. Although boys are far more likely than girls to be the perpetrators of violence, research is now showing that boys are also victim of violence.

Maltreatment and abuse including *sexual abuse* is a significant, though usually "invisible" cause of injuries among adolescents. Apart from physical injuries child and adolescent maltreatment is associated with several other consequences, including: (1) alcohol and drug abuse; (2) delinquent, violent and other risk-taking behaviors; (3) eating and sleep disorders; (4) reproductive health problems; (5) post-traumatic stress disorder (PTSD); (6) depression and anxiety; and (7) suicidal behavior and self-harm.

Sexual Violence

A high proportion of rape victims in many developing countries are under 15 years of age and that most perpetrators are known to their victims. *Sexual violence* is associated with several health consequences, including unwanted pregnancy, vaginal bleeding, fibroids, chronic pelvic pain and urinary tract infections, sexually transmitted diseases, including HIV/AIDS, depression, PTSD, and suicidal thoughts and behavior. Victims of sexual abuse may also face ostracism from family, friends, and their communities. *Suicide* in young people is increasing and is a major cause of death; especially of adolescent males. India and China present a paradox where female suicide rates are higher.

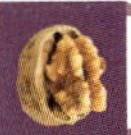

IN A NUTSHELL

Noncommunicable Diseases in Adolescence

1. Behaviors responsible for the majority of NCDs in adulthood have their origin in adolescence.
2. Physical inactivity, unhealthy diet, tobacco use, harmful use of alcohol, and indicators of metabolic syndrome (high blood pressure, high cholesterol, diabetes) are some of the important behaviors responsible for the majority of NCDs of adult life.
3. Injuries and violence including sexual violence is an important cause of morbidity and mortality among adolescents.

Akseer N, Mehta S, Wigle J, et al. Non-communicable diseases among adolescents: current status, determinants, interventions and policies. BMC Public Health. 2020;1908:20.

Bennett JE, Stevens GA, Mathers CD, et al. NCD countdown 2030: worldwide trends in non-communicable disease mortality and progress towards sustainable development goal target 3.4. Lancet. 2018;392(10152):1072-88.

5.8 Adolescent Health Checkup

PE 6.7, PE 6.8

COMMUNICATION AND COUNSELING

Communication and counseling are very important and integral part of managing adolescent health issues. Communication is an exchange of information, knowledge, ideas, or feelings. In a face-to-face situation, communication is not just exchange of information. It also conveys one's feelings, by use of gestures, facial expressions, language, and the manner of tone. It is both a tool and vehicle to reach out to adolescents. It helps in building bridges with the client and positive communication is a skill that requires practice. Counseling is not simple advising rather it is helping people to identify problem, make decisions, and giving them confidence to put their decision into practice. A very useful mnemonic to remember the steps of counseling is given in **Box 5.8**.

Some of the important techniques of good communication while counseling are: creating a good, friendly first impression, rapport building during the first session; nonjudgmental, active listening; asking nonthreatening issues in the beginning; providing information in the simple way; ask appropriate and effective question; and recognizing and taking advantage of the teachable moment. Maintain confidentiality and involve parents in care of adolescents.

Box 5.8 Steps of Counseling: "GATHER"

- *G:* Greet the person
- *A:* Ask how can I help you
- *T:* Tell them any relevant information
- *H:* Help them to make decisions
- *E:* Explain any misunderstanding
- *R:* Return to follow-up for referral

Privacy and Confidentiality

- ***Privacy*** is discussing the issues in a clinic in a friendly manner, free from any kind of disturbance.
- ***Confidentiality*** is defined as an agreement between the patient and provider whereby information discussed during or after the encounter is not shared with other parties without the explicit permission of the patient. The only exception is—if the person himself or herself has been physically harmed or is about to be physically harmed (homicide, suicide, physical or sexual abuse) or can cause harms to others. But clinicians must determine the limits of confidentiality based on the specific laws of the state he or she practices. So, if it is clearly spelled in the first meeting itself with the adolescent in front of parents and the caregivers, it becomes very reassuring for the adolescents to trust the doctor and the system and makes future interactions very congenial and fruitful.

HISTORY TAKING: PSYCHOSOCIAL SCREENING

Obtaining a history from the adolescents is very challenging. Once you have obtained the history of presenting complaints it is often advised to go beyond the problem and explore whether

Box 5.9	HEEADSSS Tool for Psychosocial Assessment

- ***H:*** *Home* (Consider—living arrangements, relationships with carers/ significant others, supervision, childhood experiences, family cultural background/s)
- ***E:*** *Education, Employment* (Consider—school/work retention and relationships, bullying, belonging, study/career progress and goals, change in grades/performance)
- ***E:*** *Eating, Exercise* (Consider—diet, eating patterns including recent changes, weight gain/loss, physical activity, fitness, energy, preoccupation with weight or body image, attempts to lose or control weight or bulk up including restricting, purging, supplements)
- ***A:*** *Activities, Hobbies, and Peer Relationships* (Consider—free time, hobbies including screen time and use of technology, culture, belonging to peer group, peer activities and venues, involvement in organized sport, religion, lifestyle factors, risk-taking, including managing chronic illness and adjustments in adolescence, injury avoidance)
- ***D:*** *Drug Use* (Consider—alcohol, cigarettes, caffeine, prescription/ illicit drugs and type, quantity, frequency, administration, interactions, access, increases/decreases with treatments, education)
- ***S:*** *Sexual Activity and Sexuality* (Consider—knowledge, sexual activity, age onset, safe sex practices, same sex attraction ± activity, sexual identity, STI screening, unwanted sex ± sexual abuse, pregnancy)
- ***S:*** *Suicide, Depression, Anxiety, and Mental Health* (Consider—normal vs. clinical, mood, anxiety symptoms vs. stress, change in sleep patterns, self-harm, suicidal thoughts/ideation/intent/method/ past attempts/treatment, depression screen and mental state examination)
- ***S:*** *Safety, Spirituality* (Consider—bullying, abuse, traumatic experiences, risky behavior, belief, religion; What helps them relax, escape? What gives them a sense of meaning?)

the adolescent has some other issues to discuss. There are three important factors in the adolescent's environment which play a very important part during their growing up years: (1) parents and family, (2) peers, and (3) the school. Enquire about them.

Psychosocial history is a must know area for all the clinicians dealing with adolescents. HEEADSSS tool (**Box 5.9**), is a very useful tool used globally that captures almost all the domains affecting the psychosocial development of the adolescent.

This interview is a practical, time-tested, strategy that helps clinicians to explore into the details of the presenting problems and uncover some issues or factors, which are affecting his behavior directly or indirectly (home, school, peer pressure, etc.). It often starts with less threatening issues to more personal and intrusive issues and often helps to build up the trust and rapport. As described under communication, do not strive to get all the information in the first interview, with time and building of trust further sessions can be arranged and then one can go deeper and develop intervention plan. You can make a "problem list" which can be explored over time and can be tackled by counseling or therapeutic intervention, the only exception if you suspect a crisis or impending crisis wherein you intervene early.

Physical Examination

Examining the adolescents is a tactful issue and one must be aware of certain legal implications as well. There are certain examinations (e.g., SMRs) which are sensitive in nature and certain routine precautions are necessary before carrying these examinations in an adolescent.

- ❖ Inform and explain the adolescent about nature and the purpose of the examination. Especially before the SMR staging and genital examination, explain the procedure in detail.
- ❖ Obtain the consent of the adolescent. (If the adolescent is below the legal age of being able to give consent, you will need to obtain consent from a parent or guardian. However, even if you have obtained consent from a parent or guardian, you should not proceed with the examination unless the adolescent agrees).
- ❖ Ideally same sex doctor is preferable; if not available, a chaperone (preferably a same gender nurse) should be made available.
- ❖ The examination should be done in a room designated for adolescents and ensure privacy, i.e., doors are shut, curtain drawn and no one enters during the examination.
- ❖ Watch for any signs of discomfort or pain during the examination and if necessary, stop the examination.
- ❖ Once the history has been taken in detail and rapport and trust has been established one should proceed with the examination.
- ❖ After doing the examination properly explain the findings and its implications.

The physical examination is almost same that we do in older children but few pertinent areas which are specific for this age group are given in **Box 5.10**.

HEALTH PROMOTION IN ADOLESCENTS

At the end of the visit physician counseling should focus on encouraging the adolescents to adopt health promoting behaviors and to reduce identified risk behaviors.

The adolescents should be encouraged *to participate in regular sport activities* and remain fit as it provides exercise for growing muscles, interaction with peers, and a socially enjoyable stimulation and conflict. In addition, competitive activities help the teenager in the process of self-appraisal, development of self-respect, and concern for others.

Promoting abstinence or ***use of condoms*** for sexually active adolescents is important for prevention of sexually transmitted

Box 5.10	Physical Examination of Adolescent

1. ***Anthropometry:*** Calculate and plot the BMI on IAP standard growth charts
2. Measure the blood pressure and plot on the nomogram
3. Vision and hearing screening
4. ***Skin:*** Inspect for acne, acanthosis nigricans, tattoos, signs of abuse or self-inflicted injury
5. Inspect breast and genitalia
   - *Breast:* Assess for SMR and examine for breast disorders, including gynecomastia versus in boys
   - *Genitalia:* Inspect for SMR, anatomic and skin abnormalities and signs of STIs (warts, vesicles and abnormal penile or vaginal discharge), pelvic examination in girls, and testes examination in boys (for hydrocele, hernias, varicoceles, and mass)

diseases. Discussions about effective means of contraception should be done with sexually active adolescents at risk for pregnancy. Sexually active girls should routinely be counseled about emergency contraception also.

Reduction of risky behaviors includes smoking cessation, avoiding drinking and driving, limiting number of sexual partners, and not swimming while intoxicated. The ideal method for promoting a reduction in risk behaviors has not been established. Motivational interviewing, used widely in the field of substance abuse treatment, may be an effective means. This approach relies on direct feedback to the adolescent, based on information gathered during the interview, regarding the negative health consequences he or she has experienced because of health-risking behaviors. For example, an adolescent smoker can be reminded that the frequent colds he or she has had over the last year are due to the deleterious effects cigarette smoke has on the protective mechanisms of the lungs. Reminding an adolescent that he or she has occasionally thought about quitting smoking or needing to cut down on drinking may be enough motivation for the adolescent to try a period of abstinence. The motivational interviewing approach avoids physicians and patients from being locked in discussions about whether risky behaviors are good or bad.

After the interview is complete, the clinicians must summarize their conclusion from the gathered responses. She must highlight the strengths of the teenager and should explain them and their parents (ensuring confidentiality) the line of treatment. Remember, it may take more than one session to reach a definitive treatment plan.

Efforts to update immunizations should occur at each visit. Adolescents 11-year-old and older should receive an adult booster dose of diphtheria and tetanus toxoids (Td), depending on the time elapsed since their last one, and a second dose of measles-mumps-rubella vaccine if they have not previously had one. Three doses of hepatitis B vaccine should be administered over a 6-month period. Adolescents without a clinical history of varicella should receive one (if younger than age 13) or two (if age 13 or older) doses of varicella vaccine. Adolescent girls should be offered rubella vaccine unless they are planning to conceive.

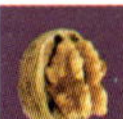

IN A NUTSHELL

Adolescent Health Checkup

1. Communication and counseling are the integral part of managing adolescent health issues.
2. Privacy and confidentiality are the important pillars of counseling in adolescents.
3. "HEEADSSS" is a psychosocial screening tool used globally that captures almost all the domains affecting the psychosocial development of the adolescents.
4. The counseling process should focus on encouraging the adolescents to adopt health promoting behaviors and to reduce identified risk behaviors.
5. All adolescents should undergo physical examination according to the prescribed norms.

Goldenring, JM, Cohen E. Getting into adolescent heads. Contemp Pediatr. 1998;5:75-90.

Gupta P. Clinical Methods in Pediatrics, 6th edition. New Delhi: CBS Publishers and Distributors; 2025.

5.9 Adolescent Friendly Health Services

PE 6.9, PE 6.10

INTRODUCTION

Health services can play an important role in helping adolescents to stay healthy and to complete their journey to adulthood; supporting young people who are looking for a route to good health, treating those who are ill, injured, or troubled and reaching out to those who are at risk. Often in numerous surveys, adolescents expressed their views about what they want from health services. They want a friendly and welcoming facility, where they can "drop in" at convenient time without being seen and can be attended quickly. They want privacy and confidentiality, and do not want to have to seek parental permission to attend. They want a service which is affordable for them. They want to be treated nonjudgmentally and with respect at the facility. They want a range of services under one window and with minimal referral. The basic principles of adolescent health care are 6 "As"—*availability, accessibility, approachability, acceptability, appropriateness, affordability.* The important attributes of a good and effective adolescent health service should provide most of these services:

- Screening for health issues (including problem behaviors)
- Manage and treat illness including other health concerns
- Prevent and respond to health issues that can endanger young lives or result in ill health or disability
- Support young people to lead healthy life, by monitoring progress and addressing concerns
- Interact with adolescents at times of concern or crisis, when they are looking for a way out of their problems
- Provide counseling services on wide range of issues, which can support adolescents
- Provide health promotional and preventive services such as immunization, contraception, etc.
- Early referral for conditions not manageable at the clinic

This is far from being the case in many countries. Health services often regard adolescents as a healthy group who do not need priority action, and so provide a minimum subset of adult or pediatric services with no adjustments for their special needs. There is evidence that many young people regard such health services as irrelevant to their needs and distrust them. They avoid such services altogether or seek help from them

Box 5.11 Barriers to Health Seeking Behavior by Adolescents

- ***Barrier related to adolescents:***
  - Discomfort with perceived clinic condition or attitudes (hostile, judgmental) of the providers
  - Concern over lack of privacy and confidentiality
  - Fear of medical procedure
  - Embarrassment or shame at needing reproductive health services
- ***Barrier related to health facility:***
  - Lack of designated space for adolescents
  - Unfriendly environment, lack of privacy and confidentiality
  - Unsuitable timing
  - Nonavailability of adolescent health specific services
  - Location and distance
- ***Barrier related to health providers and policies:***
  - Untrained providers
  - Providers not sensitive to adolescent's needs
  - Unempathetic and judgmental attitude of providers and staff
  - Discriminatory policies
  - Unclear laws and policies
  - Unaffordable and costly services

only when they are desperate. There are barriers (**Box 5.11**) related to healthcare provider or policy, health facility or even the adolescents themselves which prevents them from best utilization of the services.

Globally, adolescent specific health services and centers are existent in many western countries but in developing countries it is a upcoming specialty. In last few years, WHO along with other global partners have taken big steps to guide the setting of adolescent health services in many countries. India has taken a lead in providing countrywide adolescent friendly health services. In 2014, National Adolescent Health Strategy and a new national health program for adolescents named *Rashtriya Kishor Swasthya Karyakram (RKSK)* were announced. The strategy is a paradigm shift as it realigns existing approaches to focus on community-based health promotion and prevention along with strengthening of clinic-based preventive, diagnostic and curative services across levels of care.

ROLE OF HEALTHCARE PROVIDER AT THE ADOLESCENT HEALTH CENTER

While dealing with adolescents, the role of health provider is threefold: (1) to reassure the adolescent that his or her development is normal or identify problems that may require further evaluation or treatment; (2) to assess the adolescent and his or her family for factors that may predispose to or protect against the adolescent's pursuit of health-risking behavior, and (3) to promote a healthy lifestyle that will continue throughout adulthood.

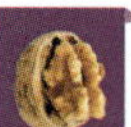

IN A NUTSHELL

Adolescent Friendly Health Services

1. Adolescent friendly health service is a form of service delivery system that plays an important role in helping adolescents to stay healthy and to complete their journey to adulthood.
2. The basic principles of adolescent health care are 6 "As"—availability, accessibility, approachability, acceptability, appropriateness, affordability.

MoHFW. Strategic Approach to Reproductive, Maternal, Newborn Child and Adolescent Health (RMNCH +A) in India – For Healthy Mother and Child. New Delhi: Ministry of Health and Family Welfare, Government of India; 2013.

National Health Mission. Orientation programme for Medical Officers to provide Adolescent-Friendly Health Services: Handouts. [online] Available from https://nhm.gov.in/images/pdf/programmes/RKSK/Medical_Officer_Training_Manual/Resource_Book_Medical_Officer.pdf. [Last accessed April, 2025].

6 CHAPTER

Breastfeeding and Lactation

AS PER NMC COMPETENCIES

PE7.1	Awareness on the cultural beliefs and practices of breastfeeding and explain physiology of lactation.	*Ch 6.2, Ch 6.4*
PE7.2	Describe the composition and types of breast milk and discuss the differences between cow's milk and human milk.	*Ch 6.3*
PE7.3	Describe the advantages of breastmilk.	*Ch 6.4*
PE7.4	Observe the correct technique of breastfeeding and distinguish right from wrong techniques.	*Ch 6.5, Ch 6.6*
PE7.5	Enumerate the baby friendly hospital initiatives.	*Ch 6.9*
PE7.6	Describe the principles of IYCF (Infant and Young Child Feeding).	*Ch 6.10*
PE7.7	Participate in World Breastfeeding Week (WBW) celebration at your institute.	*Ch 6.11*
PE7.8	Describe the structure and functioning of human milk bank and visit the nearest human milk bank.	*Ch 6.12*

Topics available online: ***Problems in Breastfeeding, Breastfeeding in Special Situations and National Programs on Breastfeeding***

6.1 Importance and Terminology

INTRODUCTION

Breastmilk is ideal for the newborn baby as it is tailormade to suit all the requirements of the baby. *Exclusive breastfeeding* is the single most important and simple intervention that can prevent a significant proportion of neonatal morbidity and mortality. All healthcare personnel should be dedicated and motivated toward helping mothers to breastfeed their babies and identify and rectify any problems faced by them. The apprehensions of the mother should be addressed, and the mother should be confident in breastfeeding. It must be ensured that breastfeeding is established before the mother and the baby are discharged from the health facility.

TERMINOLOGY

Exclusive Breastfeeding

All babies should receive exclusive breastfeeding from birth up till 6 months of completed age.

- ***Exclusive breastfeeding*** implies that the baby should receive only mother's milk. Anything else such as water, animal milk, and ghutti, should not be given; only oral medications, if needed, can be given.
- Breastfeeding should start within 1 hour of birth, known as the golden hour, irrespective of the mode of delivery. Most mothers are able to breastfeed their babies soon after a cesarean section also, in lying down position but they need support and help.

Prelacteal Feeds

Prelacteal feeds include anything which is given to the baby before breastfeeds are given. Common prelacteal feeds include sugar water, honey, or any other milk. Prelacteal feeds should not be given as it satisfies the baby's hunger and then the baby may not suck well at the mother's breast and interferes in successful breastfeeding. This can also lead to infection in the baby.

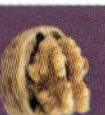

IN A NUTSHELL

Importance and Terminology

1. Exclusive breastfeeding is giving only breastmilk to a baby and no water, animal/formula milk, honey, ghutti, etc.
2. Exclusive breastfeeding should be done till the baby is 6 months old.
3. Prelacteal feeds, such as honey and sugar water should also not be given before starting breastfeeding.
4. Exclusive breastfeeding till 6 months of life is the most effective way of preventing malnutrition in these babies.

BPNI. (2025). Breast Feeding Promotion Network of India. [online] Available from https://bpni.org [Last accessed August, 2025].

WHO. Session 2, The physiological basis of breastfeeding. Infant and Young Child Feeding: Model Chapter for Textbooks for Medical Students and Allied Health Professionals. Geneva: World Health Organization; 2009.

6.2 Anatomy and Physiology of Lactation *PE 7.1*

BREAST ANATOMY

The female breast has many lobes, lobules, ducts and also fat, glandular and connective tissue, lymph nodes, blood vessels, nerves and ligaments **(Fig. 6.1)**. Each lobe has many lobules; each lobule has many sac like structures known as alveoli. These alveoli have milk secreting cells which secrete milk, the alveoli also store milk in between feeds. Numerous small ducts combine to form larger ducts in the areola which the carry the milk to the nipples. There are tiny pores in the nipple through which the milk is ejected when the baby sucks at the mother's breast. There are also many nerve endings present in the areola and the nipple which carry the sensation to the brain when the baby sucks at the breast.

Nipple and Areola

The nipple has an average of nine milk ducts passing to the outside, and also muscle fibers and nerves. The nipple is surrounded by the circular pigmented areola, in which are located Montgomery glands. These glands secrete an oily fluid that protects the skin of the nipple and areola during lactation, and produce the mother's individual scent that attracts her baby to the breast.

During pregnancy, the breast tissues undergo hypertrophy and hyperplasia under the influence of maternal and placental hormones. Milk synthesis is inhibited by estrogens and progesterone at this stage. At delivery, the inhibiting influence is removed and milk production is stimulated by prolactin released in response to suckling. The ducts beneath the areola fill with milk and become wider during a feed, when the oxytocin reflex is active.

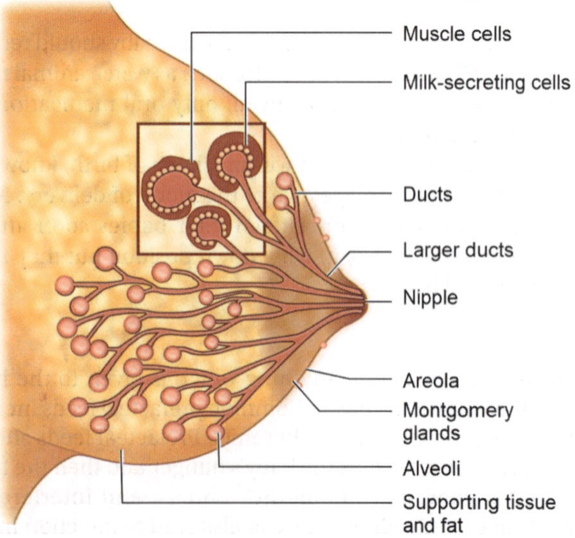

Fig. 6.1: Anatomy of the breast

PHYSIOLOGY OF MILK PRODUCTION

Two hormones play a crucial role in lactation: (1) Prolactin and (2) Oxytocin. When the baby suckles at the breast the nerve endings on the nipple and areola transmit the impulses to the brain. The anterior lobe of the pituitary gland in response secretes prolactin and the posterior lobe of pituitary secretes oxytocin. Prolactin helps in production of milk and oxytocin is responsible for ejection of milk.

Prolactin Reflex (Milk Secretion Reflex) (Fig. 6.2)

Anterior pituitary gland in the brain releases prolactin hormone, which is necessary to produce milk by the alveolar cells of the breast. After the birth of the baby, milk secretion begins and every time the baby suckles at the breast, the nerve endings at the nipple get stimulated and the level of prolactin increases leading to secretion of milk. Thus, frequent sucking by the baby at the breast is the single most important factor determining the milk production in the mother. More prolactin is produced at night, therefore, night-time feeding is very important to maintain good milk output in the mother.

Oxytocin Reflex (Milk Ejection Reflex/ Let-down Reflex) (Fig. 6.3)

After the milk is produced, it should be available to the baby when the baby needs it. This is facilitated by another hormone,

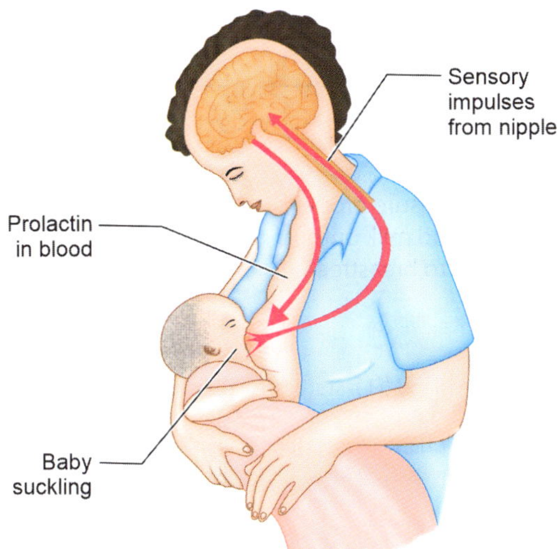

Fig. 6.2: Prolactin reflex

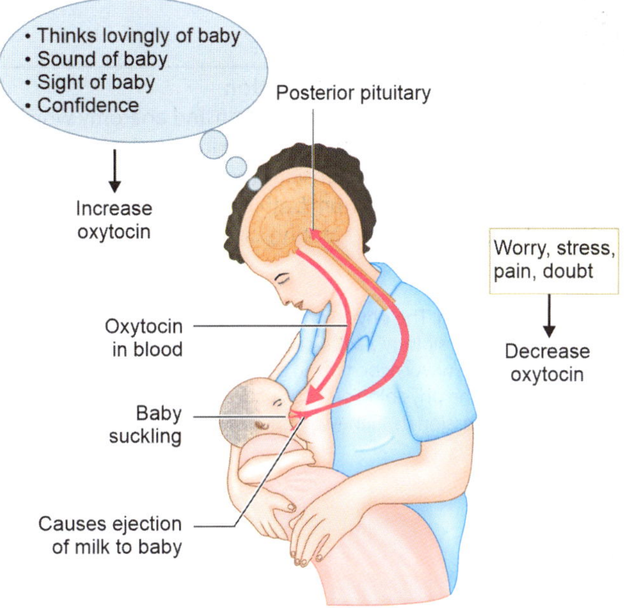

Fig. 6.3: Oxytocin reflex

oxytocin which is secreted by the posterior lobe of the pituitary gland in the brain. The production of this hormone is stimulated by suckling by the baby at the breast leading to stimulation of the nerve endings near the nipple which in turn lead to release of oxytocin. Oxytocin leads to contraction of the muscle cells (myoepithelial cells) around the alveoli in the breast leading to ejection of the milk. Oxytocin release is facilitated by a confident, tension-free mental state of the mother. In situations, when the mother has worries or is in stress or pain, the release of oxytocin may be affected leading to poor ejection of milk and ultimately decrease in milk output.

Feeding Reflexes in the Baby

A healthy, term baby is born with certain reflexes, which help in breastfeeding soon after birth:

- ***Rooting reflex:*** When the mother's breast or nipple touches the baby's cheek/lips, the baby opens its mouth and turns toward the breast **(Fig. 6.4A)**.
- ***Suckling reflex:*** This reflex is essential for successful lactation. A baby reflexly suckles at the nipple and areola placed in his mouth. The tongue presses the nipple and areola against the palate squeezing the underlying sinuses by compressing and stretching the nipple between the tongue and palate, thus, milking the lactiferous sinuses. Hence, for effective suckling not only the nipple but a part of the areola should also be in the baby's mouth. If the baby suckles only at the nipple, milk is not ejected, baby does not get sufficient milk, suckles more vigorously resulting in sore nipples **(Fig. 6.4B)**.
- ***Swallowing reflex:*** When the baby's mouth is filled with milk, it starts swallowing. It develops earlier than sucking reflex, thus, a baby who can suckle well, will always be able to swallow.

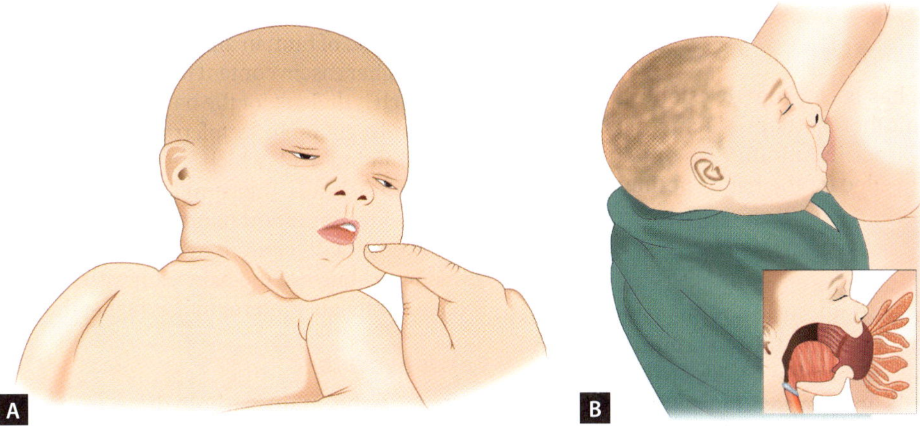

Figs. 6.4A and B: (A) Rooting reflex; (B) Suckling reflex

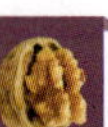

IN A NUTSHELL

Anatomy and Physiology of Lactation

1. Female breast has specialized function and anatomy which helps in lactation soon after birth.
2. Two hormones play an important role in lactation: prolactin and oxytocin.
3. A relaxed, confident, and tension-free state of mind of the mother are essential to ensure proper breastfeeding.
4. Frequent breastfeeding from both breasts is the most important way to ensure good milk output.
5. Neonatal reflexes such as rooting, suckling and swallowing reflexes help the baby to breastfeed.

Akre J. Infant feeding. The physiological basis. Bull World Health Organ. 1989;67(Suppl):1-108.

Pillay J, Davis TJ. Physiology, Lactation. [Updated 2023 Jul 17]. In: StatPearls [Internet]. Treasure Island (FL): StatPearls Publishing; 2025 Jan-. Available from: https://www.ncbi.nlm.nih.gov/books/NBK499981/. Accessed Aug, 2025.

WHO. Session 2, The physiological basis of breastfeeding. Infant and Young Child Feeding: Model Chapter for Textbooks for Medical Students and Allied Health Professionals. Geneva: World Health Organization; 2009.

6.3 Composition of Breastmilk

PE 7.2

TYPES OF MILK

Colostrum

This is the milk that the mother produces in the first 2–3 days after delivery. This is thick, sticky, yellow, and energy dense. The colostrum is secreted in small quantities but is sufficient to fulfill the baby's needs. It is rich in vitamin A, anti-infective factors such as immunoglobulin (Ig) A, white blood cells, and lactoferrins and growth factors. It also has larger proportion of proteins, and fat-soluble vitamins. It is the first immunization of the baby as it protects the baby against many infections. Colostrum is available to the baby only for the first few days and all newborns must receive it.

Transitional Milk

This is secreted from day 4–5 till the 2nd week after the birth of the baby. The volume of milk significantly increases and breast starts feeling full. The fat and carbohydrate content now increase as compared to the colostrum, and immunoglobulin and protein content decrease.

Mature Milk

Once the breastfeeding has been properly established by the end of 2nd week, the mother starts producing mature milk which is thinner and larger in amount. It contains all the necessary constituents needed for the baby's optimum growth and development.

Preterm Milk

Preterm milk is the breastmilk of a mother who delivers prematurely. It contains more proteins, sodium, iron, and immunoglobulins that are needed by her preterm baby. It approaches term milk in composition after 4–6 weeks. Term milk is produced by mothers who deliver at term gestation.

Foremilk and Hindmilk

The milk which is ejected when the baby starts feeding is the *foremilk* which is watery to quench the thirst of the baby and fulfill the fluid requirement. It is poor in fat and rich in sugar, proteins, vitamins, minerals, and water. Later, toward the end the milk becomes more energy dense and has more fat, to fulfill the energy requirement and satisfy its hunger, this is known as the *hindmilk*. A feeding session must last for a minimum of 15–20 minutes so that the baby gets both the foremilk and also the hindmilk.

HUMAN BREASTMILK

The composition of human breastmilk is shown in **Table 6.1**.

Proteins

The breastmilk contains all the proteins which are most essential and beneficial for the baby. The main proteins present in the breastmilk are whey and casein, the ratio of whey-to-casein being 60:40. This is the ideal ratio for easy digestibility, whey being more easily digestible of the two. The ratio gets almost reversed in animal milk, casein being more in content than whey protein. A comparison of human and cow's milk is given in **Table 6.1**.

The higher casein content in animal milk leads to formation of curd which is difficult for the baby to digest. The human milk also has alpha-lactalbumin, lactoferrin, and IgA. The breastmilk has the essential amino-acids which are very crucial for the development of the baby's brain. Breastmilk is also a rich source of taurine and cysteine, important neurotransmitters, in brain and retina. The lower protein content of breastmilk does not overload the immature kidneys of the baby with waste nitrogenous products. Protein content of preterm milk is higher than term milk.

Carbohydrate

Lactose is the main carbohydrate in breastmilk and is an important source of energy. The lactose content in breastmilk is higher than other animal milk.

Table 6.1 Differences Between Human Milk and Cow's Milk

	Human milk	*Cow's milk*
Protein (g/dL)	1.1	3.3
Fat (g/dL)	4.2	3.8
Carbohydrate (g/dL)	7.4	4.8
Energy (kcal/dL)	67.0	67.0
Water (g/dL)	87.0	87.0
Calcium (mg/dL)	35.0	120.0
Phosphorus (mg/dL)	15.0	90.0

Fats

Nearly 50% of energy in human milk is derived from fat. Fat is the most variable constituent of human milk. Maternal diet influences the fat content of milk. Fat content becomes higher in the latter portion of the breastfeeding (hindmilk) which may help to satiate the infant at the end of feeding. Human milk is rich in long chain fatty acids including essential fatty acids and medium chain triglycerides. Long chain fatty acids (e.g., docosahexaenoic acid) present in human milk may influence brain structure and function. This may partly help explain better cognitive functioning of breastfed babies. Fat in human milk is better absorbed than in cow's milk.

Vitamins and Minerals

The breastmilk contains all vitamins and minerals needed for the baby except vitamin D and K. The content of iron and zinc is less than animal milk but the bioavailability is much higher, the calcium and phosphorus are also present in sufficient amount and the ratio of calcium-to-phosphorus is 2:1, which is ideal for their absorption.

Others

Bile salt-stimulated lipase facilitates the complete digestion of fat once the milk has reached the small intestine. Epidermal growth factor stimulates maturation of the infant's intestine, so that it is better able to digest and absorb nutrients, and is less easily infected or sensitized to foreign proteins.

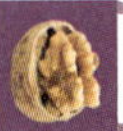

IN A NUTSHELL

Composition of Breastmilk

1. Breastmilk is tailored to suit the nutritional requirement of the baby and provides wholesome nutrition to the baby.
2. Colostrum is the milk produced in first 2–3 days after delivery and is rich in anti-infective factors. It is the first vaccination for the baby.
3. Baby must get the hindmilk to have good weight gain.
4. Breastmilk is easy to digest for the baby.
5. Breastmilk contains essential amino acids and long chain polyunsaturated fatty acids for the development of brain.

Hasen. In: Eichenwald EC, Hansen AR, Martin CR, Stark AR, Jain N (Eds). Cloherty and Stark's Manual of Neonatal Care, 2nd South Asian edition, Gurugram, Haryana: Wolters Kluwer; 2023.

6.4 Advantages of Breastfeeding *PE 7.1, PE 7.3*

BENEFITS TO THE BABY

Right Nutrients

- The breastmilk contains the right nutrients (proteins, carbohydrates, fats, vitamins, and minerals) in right amount, which is optimum for the baby.
- The nutrients in breastmilk are better absorbed than from any other source, especially iron.

Protection from Infections

It has anti-infective factors and growth factors like *Lactobacillus bifidus* which help the baby fight infections and grow well. Infants who are breastfed are 15 times less likely to die from pneumonia and 11 times less likely to die from diarrhea. The anti-infective factors present in breastmilk are listed in **Box 6.1**.

Intelligence

Studies show improved scores of cognitive function on average 8 points higher among children who were breastfed compared

Box 6.1 Anti-infective Factors in Human Milk

1. ***Immunoglobulins:*** IgA, IgG, and IgM
2. ***Cells:*** Macrophages and lymphocytes
3. ***Complements:*** C3 and C4
4. Lysozymes
5. Lactoperoxidase
6. Lipids (antiviral and antistaphylococcal)
7. ***Iron-binding proteins:*** Lactoferrin
8. Bile salt-stimulated lipase (antiprotozoal)
9. Interferon
10. Growth factor for *Lactobacillus bifidus*

with those who were formula fed. This may be due to unique composition of breastmilk, better mother-infant bonding, and lower infectious morbidity and thus better brain growth in these children.

Economic Benefits

Breastmilk is much cheaper than animal milk or powdered milk. All it costs is the extra food needed by the lactating mother. In a way, breastfeeding contributes to national economy as in its absence, young infants would require alternative resources for feeding.

Psychological Benefits

Breastfeeding helps form a close, loving relationship between the mother and the baby. Close contact soon after birth helps this relationship to develop. This process is called bonding. There is better parent-child adjustment and fewer behavior disorders in these children. Child abuse is also less common.

Miscellaneous

Breastfeeding provides some protection against allergic disorders such as atopic eczema and asthma. The incidence of sudden infant death syndrome (SIDS) is less in breastfed children. Human milk reduces the incidence of necrotizing enterocolitis (NEC) in preterm babies.

The beneficial effects of breastfeeding may extend to later life. There is compelling evidence to suggest that breastfeeding reduces the incidence of atherosclerosis, non-insulin dependent diabetes mellitus, obesity, hypertension, and certain cancers later in life.

BENEFITS TO THE MOTHER

- It reduces postpartum bleeding and hence anemia in mothers.
- The mother is less likely to conceive till the time she breastfeeds her baby. This is called lactational amenorrhea.
- It helps the mother shed extra weight which is gained during pregnancy.
- Breastfeeding protects the mother from breast and ovarian cancers.
- It saves the mother a lot of time and effort, as the breastmilk is readily available and needs no preparation.

BENEFITS TO THE SOCIETY

- The cost involved in breastfeeding is negligible as compared to the expenditure that the society has to make toward procuring and feeding with animal or formula milk.
- As breastfeeding prevents infection, it also reduces the healthcare cost.
- It is eco-friendly and does no harm to the environment.

DISADVANTAGES OF ARTIFICIAL/ ANIMAL FEEDING

- It is not suited to the nutritional requirements of the baby.
- The babies are at high risk of infections such as diarrhea and respiratory tract infections.
- It is the most important factor behind malnutrition especially in young infants.
- Some newborns on top feeds especially those on predominantly formula feeds tend to become overweight and obese.
- The mortality rates are much higher in babies who are on artificial feeds.

DESIRABLE PRACTICES WHICH PROMOTE BREASTFEEDING

- Antenatal counseling of the mother regarding breastfeeding and its importance and benefits to the baby.
- Rooming in should be practiced, i.e., the mother and the baby should be kept together close to each other. The trend of keeping babies in the crib has, therefore, been done away with.
- The baby is allowed to suck at the mother's breast as early as within 1 hour after birth.
- Prelacteal feeds or pacifiers are not recommended.
- Letting the baby suck frequently at the breast is the single most important factor which enhances milk output in mothers and hence promotes breastfeeding.
- No artificial feeds should be given to the baby by bottle or by any other method.
- The mother should be tension-free and relaxed.
- The mother should receive proper privacy to breastfeed her baby in the hospital and at home.

FACTORS HINDERING BREASTFEEDING

- Separation of the mother and the baby especially immediately after birth.
- Delayed and infrequent feeding, no night feeds.
- Unconfident and stressed mother.
- Painful breast conditions such as cracked nipples, engorged breasts, and breast abscess.
- Improper positioning and attachment of the baby to the breast.
- Mixed feeding, i.e., feeding with animal or formula milk along with breastfeeds.
- Maternal illness.

CONTRAINDICATIONS OF BREASTFEEDING

In extremely rare circumstances, the mother is advised not to breastfeed her baby. Some contraindications to breastfeeding are:

- If the mother is on antithyroid drugs, such as carbimazole or methimazole, or anticancer drugs.
- Intake of drugs, such as radioactive compounds, lithium and gold salts.
- If the baby is suffering from a disorder, such as galactosemia or phenylketonuria.

If the mother who is breastfeeding is on any medication, a doctor must be consulted regarding the safety of the drug to the baby. Infections such as human immunodeficiency virus (HIV), hepatitis B, and tuberculosis in the mother are not contraindications to breastfeeding.

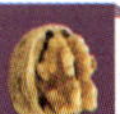

IN A NUTSHELL

Advantages of Breastfeeding

1. Exclusive breastfeeding is giving only breastfeeds to the baby till 6 months of age, water, honey, ghutti or top feeding should not be given.
2. Exclusive breastfeeding protects the baby from all kinds of infection and reduces morbidity and mortality in neonates and infants.
3. Growth and development is optimum in baby's receiving exclusive breastfeeding.
4. Breastfeeding has benefits for the mother and society at large.
5. Practices promoting breastfeeding must be adopted.
6. Top/animal feeding is very harmful for the baby.

Belfort MB. The Science of Breastfeeding and Brain Development. Breastfeed Med. 2017;12(8):459-61.

Ministry of Health and Family Welfare Government of India. (2016). Programme for Promotion of Breastfeeding. [online] Available from https://nhm.gov.in/MAA/Operational_Guidelines.pdf [Last accessed August, 2025].

WHO. Session 2, The physiological basis of breastfeeding. Infant and Young Child Feeding: Model Chapter for Textbooks for Medical Students and Allied Health Professionals. Geneva: World Health Organization; 2009.

6.5 Technique of Breastfeeding *PE 7.4*

INTRODUCTION

The right technique of breastfeeding is important to stimulate the nipple and ensure adequate milk output. Proper positioning and attachment would help the baby suck well and it can be an enjoyable experience for the mother and the baby.

POSITIONING

Any position which is comfortable to the mother and the baby is good for breastfeeding. The mother should sit with her back being supported or may even breastfeed in lying posture. The following points indicate a good position of the baby with respect to the mother **(Fig. 6.5)**:

- The baby is held close to the mother.
- The body of the baby, i.e., the head, neck, and trunk, should be in straight line or the head bent slightly backwards.
- Baby's whole body should be supported.
- Baby should be facing the breast and its nose should be opposite the nipple.

ATTACHMENT

To ensure successful breastfeeding, it is important that the baby sucks effectively at the breast so as to express milk. For this, the baby should be attached well to the breast. Points of good attachment are as follows **(Figs. 6.6A and B)**:

- The baby's chin should touch the breast.
- Baby's mouth should be wide open.
- The lower lip should be turned outward.
- More areola should be visible above the baby's mouth than below it.

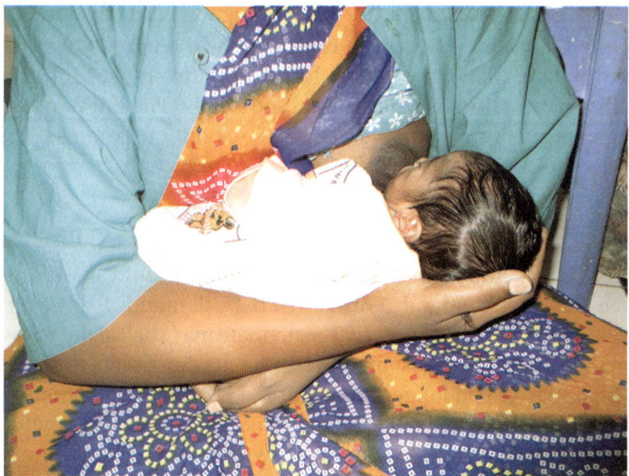

Fig. 6.5: Proper positioning of the baby while breastfeeding

The baby should take deep and slow sucks with pauses in between. The sound of swallowing should be audible in between sucking.

Inappropriate positioning and attachment leads to ineffective suckling by the baby and therefore decrease in milk output. This is also the most common cause of sore nipples and may cause pain and discomfort to the mother.

Causes of Poor Attachment

- Inexperienced mother.
- A mother who is not confident about feeding her baby and its right technique.

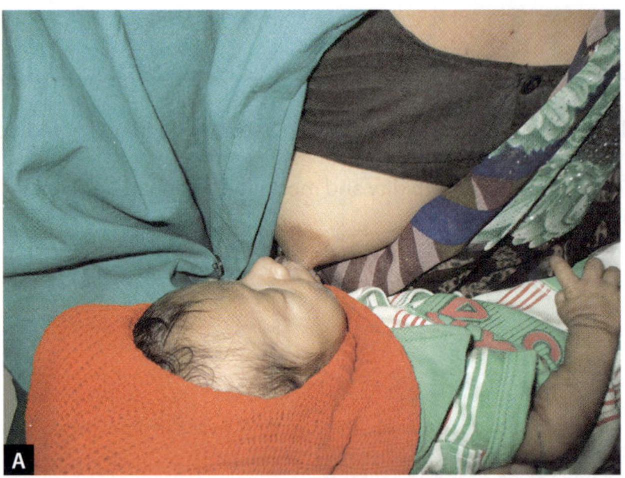

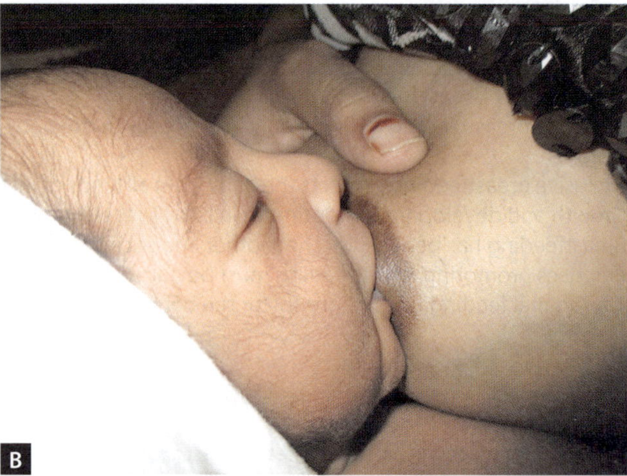

Figs. 6.6A and B: (A) Poor attachment; (B) Good attachment

- Flat/inverted nipple.
- Lack of support from healthcare workers.
- Use of a bottle to feed the baby.
- Cleft palate.

MECHANISM OF SUCKLING

As the baby sucks the areola is pressed by the tongue over the hard palate, making the milk flow out of the sinuses into the baby's mouth through the pores in the nipple. The baby applies negative suction not only to express milk out of the breast but also to hold a large part of the breast into its mouth.

DEMAND FEEDING

After timely initiation of feeding, the baby should be offered breastfeeds on demand. Normally, a baby demands feeds every 1½–2 hours but this may vary. The neonate may suck at the breast for 15 minutes to almost an hour. Some newborns like to suckle even if they are no longer hungry. It is a pleasant experience for them as they are close to their mothers. The mother must allow the baby to leave the breast on its own rather than forcing the baby to stop sucking.

BREAST MANAGEMENT

It is not necessary to breastfeed from both breasts in one session. One breast must be emptied fully before the other breast is offered. This also prevents engorgement of the breasts. If one breast is being offered at one time, then care should be taken that feeding is done from the alternate breast in the next feed to ensure emptying of each breast. If a baby is feeding for a short duration at one time this deprives the baby of the hindmilk which is essential for proper growth of the baby.

FREQUENCY OF FEEDING

The baby must be breastfed frequently, a minimum of 8–10 times in 24 hours to maintain adequate milk supply. Night feeds are very important as the baby is usually more active in the night. The secretion of prolactin, which is the hormone responsible for increasing the milk output in the mother, is also secreted more during the night. The importance of feeding during the night must be explained to the mother otherwise she may be tired and reluctant to feed at night.

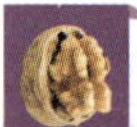

IN A NUTSHELL

Technique of Breastfeeding

1. Proper technique of breastfeeding will promote exclusive breastfeeding.
2. Proper positioning and attachment are essential for the baby to suck well at the mother's breast.
3. This also ensures good milk output by the mother.
4. Night-time feeding is very important and promotes milk output and growth in the baby.

Ministry of Health and Family Welfare Government of India. Operational Guidelines for Facility Based Integrated Management of Neonatal and Childhood Illness (F-IMNCI). [online] Available from http://nhm.gov.in/images/pdf/programmes/child-health/guidelines/operational_guidelines_for_fimnci.pdf [Last accessed August, 2025].

Ministry of Health and Family Welfare Government of India. Facility based Integrated Management of Neonatal and childhood illnesses (F-IMNCI) IMNCI Chart Booklet. [online] Available from https://nhm.gov.in/images/pdf/programmes/child-health/guidelines/imnci_chart_booklet.pdf [Last accessed August, 2025].

UNICEF. (2018). Breastfeeding, A Mother's Gift, for Every Child. [online] Available fromwww.unicef.org/media/48046/file/UNICEF_Breastfeeding_A_Mothers_Gift_for_Every_Child.pdf [Last accessed August, 2025].

WHO. (2021). Infant and young child feeding. [online] Available from www.who.int/news-room/fact-sheets/detail/infant-and-young-child-feeding [Last accessed August 2025].

6.6 Observing a Breastfeed

PE 7.4

INTRODUCTION

Box 6.2 depicts feeding assessment form for an infant <6 months old and **Box 6.3** reproduces a breastfeeding observation form.

WHEN TO OBSERVE A BREASTFEED

You need to observe breastfeeding in following situations:

Outpatient Settings, e.g., Outpatient Department or Well-baby Clinic

- If infant's weight is ≤2 SD for that age.
- Baby is taking any other feed/drink (other than breastmilk).
- If the frequency of breastfeeding is <8 times/day.
- If mother reports any problem with breast or difficulty in feeding (pain, fissure, or not enough milk).

Inpatient Setting, e.g., Postnatal Ward or Neonatal Units

- All primipara mothers.
- Mothers having lower (uterine) segment cesarean section (LSCS).
- If baby birth weight <2.5 kg.
- Mothers who were separated from babies due to sickness.
- Any mother reporting any problem in feeding.
- History of not able to breastfeed exclusively for 6 months in previous pregnancy.

Remember the following when you decide to observe breastfeeding:

- Take mother's consent to examine baby's feeding.
- Make sure the mother is sitting in a comfortable and relaxed position.
- Then ask her to feed and observe.

DECISION

Based on your assessment of form (Part A and B) **(Boxes 6.2 and 6.3)**, *decide* whether feeding problem is present or not. You will

Box 6.3 Feeding Assessment Form (Part B) Recording Form for Observing Breastfeeding in <6 Months

Feeding Assessment Form (Part B)

Observe breastfeeding for 4 minutes:

1. *Well attached/poorly attached:*
   To check attachment look for:
   - Chin touching breast
   - Mouth wide open
   - Lower lip turned outward, and
   - More areola visible above than below the mouth.

   (All of these signs should be present, if the attachment is good.)
2. *Check position:*
   - Whether infant's head and body is straight or not?
   - Whether the baby is facing breast with infant's nose opposite her nipple or not?
   - Whether infant's body is close to mother's body or not?
   - Whether mother supporting infant's whole body or not?

   (The answer to all these questions should be yes, if the positioning is correct.)
3. Is the infant suckling effectively (i.e., slow deep sucks, sometimes pausing)?
   Not suckling at all   Not suckling effectively   Suckling effectively
4. *If baby not suckling effectively or mother complains pain during feeding:*
   - Check the baby for ulcer in mouth.
   - Check mother's breast for:
   - Flat or inverted nipple;
   - Engorged breasts; and
   - Breast abscess

Box 6.2 Feeding Assessment Form (Part A) Recording Form for Infants <6 Months

Feeding Assessment Form (Part A)

Name of Mother .... Name of Baby ....

Age (weeks) .... Weight (in grams) .... SD score

1. When was the first feed given? ....
2. Whether baby received any prelacteal fees? .... Yes/No
3. How many times breastfeed was given in last 24 hours? ....
4. How many night feeds were given? ....
5. Does the child receive any other food or drink in addition to breastfeeds?
   .... Yes/No
6. If yes, which food and drink? ....
7. If animal milk/formula milk—how many times in last 24 hours? .... /dilution
8. What is being used to feed the child, if baby is receiving feed other than breastfeeds? Cup/spoon/bottle ....
   ....
9. How feeding bottle/cup is prepared—washing .... Yes/No, Boiling .... Yes/No
10. How many times baby is passing urine in 24 hours? ....
11. What is the color of urine? ....
12. Ask mother is she has any pain during breastfeeding (for sore nipples/breast abscess)?
    .... Yes/No

classify it as feeding problem, if one or more of the following five situations are present:

1. If the baby is not exclusively breastfed.
2. If the baby is on animal or formula feeds which is diluted.
3. If the mother is using the bottle for feeding.
4. If the mother is having breast or nipple problem.
5. If the baby is suckling poorly.

ACTION: COUNSELING

If you have identified feeding problem, you will need to counsel the mother for breastfeeding.

Adhere to the following rules of "nonverbal communication," while you are counseling the mother:

- Keep yourself at the same head level as that of the mother.
- Maintain an appropriate distance from her.
- Maintain eye contact and pay attention.
- Take time while talking.
- Remove barriers and use touch appropriately.
- Give her information according to your specific case.

RESPECT MOTHER'S PRIVACY

Mother's privacy must be always respected. Every time the mother is examined whether during the antenatal period or while observing breastfeeding or examining the breast for any problems, one must be sensitive to the mother's need of privacy. Whenever a male doctor examines the mother, it should always be done in the presence of another female.

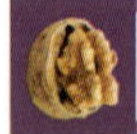

IN A NUTSHELL

Observing a Breastfeed

1. Breastfeeding must be observed whenever a problem in breastfeeding is identified.
2. Breastfeeding problems are more common in primi mothers, LSCS deliveries, preterm babies, and low birth weight babies.
3. Problems in breastfeeding can be managed by counseling the mother.

Ministry of Health and Family Welfare Government of India. Operational Guidelines for Facility Based Integrated Management of Neonatal and Childhood Illness (F-IMNCI). [online] Available from http://nhm.gov.in/images/pdf/programmes/child-health/guidelines/operational_guidelines_for_fimnci.pdf [Last accessed August 2025].

Ministry of Health and Family Welfare Government of India. Facility based Integrated Management of Neonatal and childhood illnesses (F-IMNCI) IMNCI Chart Booklet. [online] Available from https://nhm.gov.in/images/pdf/programmes/child-health/guidelines/imnci_chart_booklet.pdf [Last accessed August, 2025].

6.7 Counseling for Breastfeeding

INTRODUCTION

Breastfeeding plays a crucial role in growth and development of the baby, builds up the immunity and is beneficial to the mother also. The mother needs support and guidance for initiation of breastfeeding, allay her anxiety, and continue to exclusively breastfeed her baby. She needs counseling right from the antenatal period to after the birth of the baby, till breastfeeding has been properly established and the mother is confident and knows about different aspects of breastfeeding. The father and other family members must also be counseled, as they also a play an important role in supporting the mother and decision making. Breastfeeding, though a natural phenomenon, may be quite demanding for the mother, and she may need to learn the skill, especially if she is a first-time mother. Following points need to be emphasized while counseling.

- The mother must be explained about the advantages of exclusive breastfeeding, duration of exclusive breastfeeding, and harms of giving animal or top milk.
- She must be prepared from the antenatal period.
- Breastfeeding must be initiated, within 1 hour of birth.
- She should be told about the right technique of breastfeeding, basic science behind breastfeeding, and also anticipated problems she may face.
- Skill development needs to be done not only by giving her the information but also demonstrating the correct method of breastfeeding.
- A mother will need a lot of encouragement from the family members and healthcare workers.
- Provide her support and help during the first week after birth when breastfeeding is being established.
- She will also need support in proper positioning and attachment of the baby to the breast. The counseling of the mother regarding breastfeeding should also include the points listed in **Box 6.4**.

Box 6.4 Counseling the Mother on Breastfeeding

1. Breastfeeding should be started within 1 hour of birth of the baby
2. Technique of breastfeeding
3. Baby must be breastfed frequently on demand and night feeds are important
4. Advantages of exclusive breastfeeding
5. Disadvantages of bottle feeding/feeding of top/animal milk
6. Anticipated problems, she may face while breastfeeding
7. Breastmilk is sufficient for her baby
8. Exclusive breastfeeding needs to be done for 6 months
9. Complimentary feeding should be started after the 6th month of life

Educate Mothers on Antenatal Breast Care and Prepare Mothers for Lactation

The first and the foremost step for successful exclusive breastfeeding is counseling of the mothers. This counseling must start right from the antenatal period. Antenatal counseling helps in motivating the mothers for initiation of breastfeeding immediately after birth and practicing exclusive breastfeeding for first 6 months. The aim is to prepare the expectant mother for breastfeeding, so that it is a natural and pleasant experience for the mother rather than a painful and stressful one.

All pregnant women should be informed about the benefits and management of breastfeeding on a priority basis during antenatal visits. Breast care during pregnancy is often neglected and if done properly, will take care of any breast or nipple problems that may be experienced during or after pregnancy.

Breast examination should be an integral part of the examination done during antenatal visits. A thorough breast examination should be performed and followed by appropriate recommendations for hygiene and correction of existing defects. She may be assured that a daily bath, omitting soap on the nipples (soap tends to dry and crack the nipples), will provide adequate cleanliness. Flat or depressed nipples sometimes correct themselves during pregnancy, but the corrective process can be greatly helped by a regular regimen of care directed toward toughening and erecting them. A manipulative procedure may have some benefit in women who have retracted or flat nipples. The maneuver is done by placing the thumb and the forefingers, close to the inverted nipple. The nipple is grasped between thumb and forefinger and pill-rolled for about 1 minute. The procedure is repeated five times in the horizontal plane and then five times in the vertical plane.

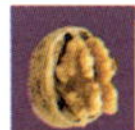

IN A NUTSHELL

Counseling for Breastfeeding

1. Counseling for breastfeeding should start from the antenatal period.
2. Mother needs support, encouragement, and guidance while breastfeeding her baby.
3. Breastfeeding can be exhausting for the mother.
4. Father of the baby and other family members should also be counseled regarding breastfeeding.

WHO. The optimal duration of exclusive breastfeeding report of an expert consultation. [online] Available from https://apps.who.int/iris/bitstream/10665/67219/1/WHO_NHD_01.09.pdf [Last accessed August, 2025].

WHO. 13, Breastfeeding. Counselling for Maternal and Newborn Health Care: A Handbook for Building Skills. Geneva: World Health Organization; 2013.

6.8 Successful Breastfeeding

Successful breastfeeding motivation and support to the mother are the most important factors for successful breastfeeding. The following steps must be practiced for initiation and continuation of successful breastfeeding:

1. ***Motivate:*** Mother should be motivated right from the antenatal period. Her breasts should be examined and she should be informed about the benefits of breastfeeding.
2. ***Start early:*** The baby must be put to the breast within 1 hour of birth irrespective of the route of delivery.
3. ***Rooming in:*** Since suckling is the best stimulus for milk production, babies should be roomed-in with mother and fed on demand till the baby is satisfied. One breast must be emptied out fully before the second is offered, so that the baby receives both foremilk and hindmilk.
4. ***Frequency:*** Frequent suckling helps to stimulate milk production. It also prevents engorgement of breasts. The baby should be fed whenever hungry. Initially, some babies feed at short intervals of 1–2 hours. Later the babies settle into a more relaxed routine of feeding every 2–3 hours.
5. ***Prelacteal feeds:*** This refers to giving small quantities of fluids such as water, glucose water, tea, and honey, as the first feed to the baby. This harmful practice must be condemned as it deprives baby of colostrum, delays initiation of breastfeeding, and also exposes the baby to the risk of infection.
6. ***Avoid bottle feeds:*** No bottle feed should ever be given. It causes nipple confusion and interferes with suckling at the breast. It is also a potent source of infection. Bottle feeding also undermines mother's confidence in breastfeeding.
7. ***Feeding from both breasts:*** When the baby releases one breast the other breast is offered. If the baby is still hungry, he/she will feed on the other breast. Alternate breasts should be offered first at each feed. This ensures complete emptying of both the breasts. The baby should be allowed to feed till satisfied.
8. ***Duration/continuation of breastfeeding:*** A baby should be exclusively breastfed for the first 6 months. Supplementary feeds given to the baby before 6 months reduce milk production and also lead to infection and poor weight gain in the baby.
9. ***Cost of lactation:*** Nursing mother needs only 600 calories extra for maintaining her lactation, which amounts to additional home-made food and fluids.
10. ***Cleaning the breasts:*** There is no need to wash the breasts before or after a feed as frequent washing removes the natural oil from the nipple and predisposes to fissures in the nipple. The mother should wash her breasts during her daily bath.
11. ***Complementary feeds:*** A baby should be given additional food after 6 months. Breastfeeding should be continued for at least 2 years; and also beyond, if feasible.

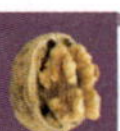

IN A NUTSHELL

Successful Breastfeeding

1. Motivation and support are the most important factors to promote breastfeeding.
2. Babies should be breastfed on demand.
3. Babies should be breastfed exclusively for first 6 months of life.
4. After 6 months, complimentary feeding should be started. Mother can continue to breastfeed her baby till 2 years and beyond.

Ministry of Health and Family Welfare, Government of India. (2013). Facility based care of severe acute malnutrition. [online] Available from www.nhm.gov.in/images/pdf/programmes/child-health/IEC-materials/PARTICIPANT-MANUAL_FBCSA-Malnutrition.pdf [Last accessed August, 2025].

6.9 Baby Friendly Hospital Initiative *PE 7.5*

INTRODUCTION

This initiative was started by the World Health Organization (WHO) and the United Nations International Children's Emergency Fund (UNICEF) to primarily promote breastfeeding in health facilities providing maternity and newborn care services. Under this, the hospital must adopt a breastfeeding policy and follow the 10 steps to successful breastfeeding.

10 STEPS TO SUCCESSFUL BREASTFEEDING

1. Have a written breastfeeding policy that is routinely communicated to all health staff.
2. Train all healthcare staff in skills necessary to implement this policy.
3. Inform all pregnant women about benefits and management of breastfeeding.
4. Help mothers initiate breastfeeding within 1 hour of birth.
5. Show mothers how to breastfeed and how to maintain lactation even if they are separated from their infants.
6. Give newborns no food or drink other than breastmilk, unless medically indicated.
7. Practice rooming in, allow mothers and infants to remain together all 24 hours of the day.
8. Encourage breastfeeding on demand.
9. Give no artificial teats or pacifiers to breastfeeding infants.
10. Foster the establishment of breastfeeding support groups and refer mothers to them on discharge from the hospital or clinic.

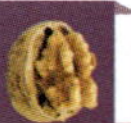

IN A NUTSHELL

Baby Friendly Hospital Initiative

1. All hospital catering to young infants must have a written breastfeeding policy.
2. Training of the healthcare workers is the first and the most important step to promote exclusive breastfeeding.
3. Babies must be breastfed within 1 hour of birth.

UNICEF. Baby-Friendly Hospital Initiative, Ten steps to successful breastfeeding, from UNICEF and the World Health Organization. [online] Available from https://www.unicef.org/documents/baby-friendly-hospital-initiative [Last accessed August 2025].

WHO. Promoting baby-friendly hospitals. [online] Available from www.who.int/activities/promoting-baby-friendly-hospitals [Last accessed August 2025].

6.10 Principles of Infant and Young Child Feeding (IYCF) *PE 7.6*

The World Health Organization (WHO) and the Ministry of Health and Family Welfare (MOHFW) have laid down certain guidelines for infant and young child feeding (IYCF). All the healthcare professionals including doctors, nurses and paramedical staff and community volunteers like ASHA and Anganwadi workers should be aware of the correct practices. The guidelines cover feeding of newborn babies and children up to the age of 2 years. The feeding of children 6 months to 2 years have been covered in the next chapter on complementary feeding. The main principles of breastfeeding, the details of which have been covered in this chapter as follows:

1. Early initiation of breastfeeding; immediately after birth, preferably within one hour.
2. Exclusive breastfeeding for the first 6 months of life, i.e., 180 days (no other foods or fluids, not even water; but allows infant to receive ORS, drops, syrups of vitamins, minerals and medicines when required).

STATUS OF BREASTFEEDING IN INDIA

Breastfeeding rates in India are very low contributing to high neonatal and infant mortality and malnutrition. As per the National Family Health Survey (NFHS)-5 conducted in 2019-2021, only 41.8% of children less than 3 years of age were breastfed within one hour of birth. Babies under 6 months of age who were exclusively breastfed were only 63.7%.

6.11 World Breastfeeding Week

PE 7.7

World Breastfeeding Week (WBW) is celebrated each year from 1st to 7th August. It is a global campaign to raise awareness and galvanize action on themes related to breastfeeding. This was started in 1992 with each year having a different theme **(Fig. 6.7)** related to breastfeeding, women and their problems, community mobilization, ecology, economy, science and education. In 2018, the World Health Assembly endorsed the WBW as an important strategy to promote breastfeeding. This week is celebrated in all healthcare facilities and various programs are organized to increase awareness about the importance of breastfeeding.

The programs that can be held during the week include:

1. Public awareness campaigns **(Fig. 6.8)**.
2. Health check-ups for breastfeeding mothers and their infants.
3. Creating support groups for breastfeeding mothers to share their experiences, challenges, and solutions.
4. Use of online forums and social media platforms to foster a sense of community and provide support.
5. Organize public events like walks, marathons, street plays **(Fig. 6.9)**, or picnics to raise awareness about breastfeeding; and invite local celebrities and influencers to participate and endorse the cause.

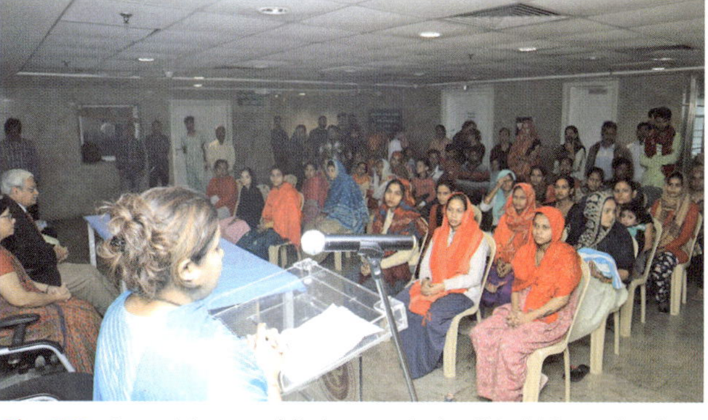

Fig. 6.8: Organizing a public lecture during World Breastfeeding Week

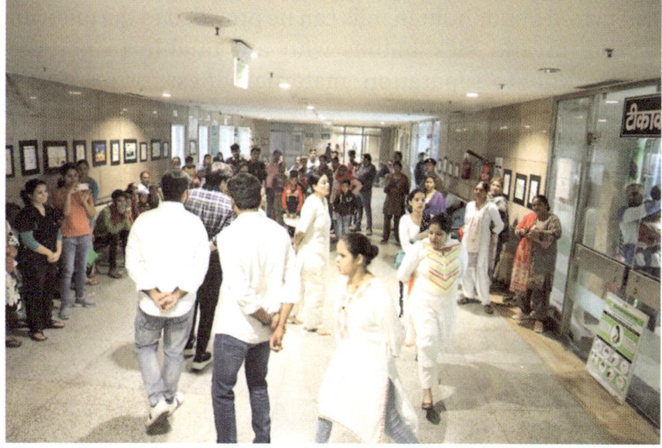

Fig. 6.9: Organizing a street play during World Breastfeeding Week

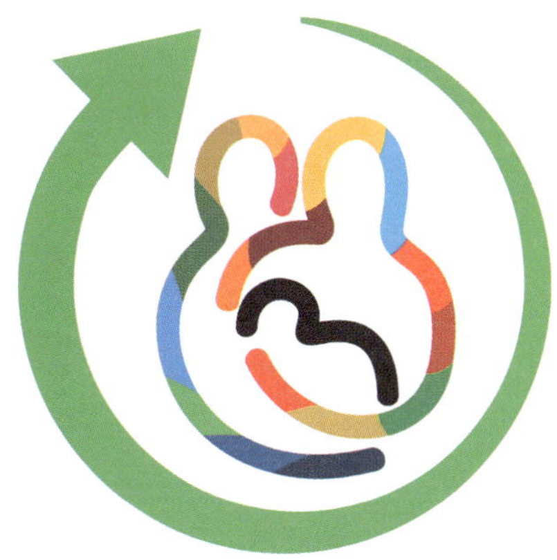

Fig. 6.7: Logo of World Breastfeeding Week

6. Training programs for healthcare professionals and community workers.
7. Media campaigns on TV, radio, and social media.
8. Advocacy for policies supporting breastfeeding in workplaces and public spaces.
9. Community meetings and events to promote breastfeeding-friendly environments.
10. Contests like essay writing, poster designing, and photography competitions.

Students and teachers should participate in WBW celebrations at their college and raise awareness about breastfeeding.

6.12 Human Milk Banking

PE 7.8

INTRODUCTION

Feeding a baby with the mother's own milk (MOM) is the best way of feeding, but in certain circumstances, this may be difficult or impossible. Providing breastmilk to some babies, especially those who are preterm or with very low birth weight (VLBW) is a challenge. When MOM is not available then the alternatives are either formula milk or pasteurized donor human milk. Evidence suggests that donor milk when compared to formula milk is associated with lower incidence of severe gut disorders, necrotizing enterocolitis, and other infections during hospital stay. Therefore, donor human milk is the next best option for newborns when their MOM is not available.

Human milk banks collect, screen, and process the donated human milk, ensure milk safety and quality and make it available for newborns, who need it. The primary aim of these milk banks is to provide donor milk to high-risk newborns admitted in a neonatal intensive care unit (NICU). The facility of a donor human milk banking is not available very widely in our country but more and more of these banks are coming up.

PASTEURIZED DONOR HUMAN MILK

Pasteurized donor human milk can be provided to the following:

- Preterm and sick babies who are unable to get their MOM due to separation, maternal illness, or insufficient lactation.
- Babies of mothers who are temporarily unable to provide breastmilk due to illness/hospitalization.
- Babies of mothers who are unable to offer breastmilk to their infants due to health risk (like a mother on a certain drug in which breastfeeding may be contraindicated).
- Adopted babies.
- Babies whose mothers are unable to secrete sufficient milk initially in the first few days, especially those with multiple births.
- Babies whose mothers have died in the postpartum period.

The donor human milk is collected from healthy mothers who volunteer to donate their breastmilk without compromising the breastfeeding of their own baby. The milk is pasteurized and stored in deep freezers. The donor milk is then dispensed after informed consent of the parents and prescription of the physician.

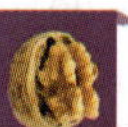

IN A NUTSHELL

Human Milk Banking

1. Human milk banks are comprehensive lactation management centers where donor milk is collected, stored, and processed.
2. Pasteurized donor human milk may be used in special circumstances when the MOM is not available.
3. Healthy mothers can voluntarily donate their breastmilk without compromising breastfeeding of their own baby.

Indian Academy of Pediatrics (IAP). Guidelines on Breastfeeding. [online] Available from https://iapindia.org/guidelines-on-breastfeeding/ [Last accessed August, 2025].

Ministry of Health and Family Welfare Government of India. (2017). National Guidelines on Lactation Management Centres in Public Health facilities. [online] Available from http://nhm.gov.in/images/pdf/programmes/IYCF/National_Guidelines_Lactation_Management_Centres.pdf [Last accessed August, 2025].

Ruchi Rai and Piyush Gupta

7 CHAPTER

Complementary Feeding

AS PER NMC COMPETENCIES

PE8.1	Define the term complementary feeding.	*Ch 7.1*
PE8.2	Explain the principles, the initiation, attributes, frequency, techniques and hygiene related to complementary feeding.	*Ch 7.1*
PE8.3	Enumerate the common complementary foods.	*Ch 7.2*
PE8.4	Elicit history on the complementary feeding habits.	*Ch 7.3*
PE8.5	Counsel and educate mothers on the best practices in complementary feeding.	*Ch 7.4*

7.1 Principles and Attributes of Complementary Feeding

PE 8.1, PE 8.2

DEFINITION

Complementary feeding implies giving the child other nutritious foods in addition to breast milk (WHO, 2000). The literal meaning of the term *weaning* is taking the infant away from the breast and nourishment by other means. As breastmilk continues to be an important source of good quality proteins, vitamin A and C even for older infants, the use of this term has now been discarded in favor of *complementary feeding*.

Optimal nutrition during first 2 years of life is important to lay down a strong foundation for growth and development of children. Recently, the focus has been drawn to the first 1,000 days of nutrition that include both intrauterine period (270 days of pregnancy) plus first 2 years of life. Infant should receive nutritionally adequate and safe complementary foods while breastfeeding continues for up to 2 years of age or beyond.

Breastmilk alone is sufficient food for first 6 months. Thereafter, concentrated energy dense complementary foods are essential to maintain an adequate velocity of growth for the infant. Adequate complementary feeding has been recognized as an important preventive strategy for child deaths, preventing 6% of child deaths, and child undernutrition. Introduction of diverse foods during infancy might have a protective effect on asthma, food allergy, and food sensitization with increased expression for regulatory T-cells marker.

CHALLENGES IN COMPLEMENTARY FEEDING

Some challenges to complementary feeding at 6 months of age are (4T's):

- ***Teeth:*** No teeth to chew the food
- ***Taste:*** Not familiar with the food taste
- ***Tongue movements:*** Baby moves tongue in a manner to swallow liquid. In the process solids are spit out. This is often perceived as 'not liking the food',
- ***Texture of food:*** Too thin food is swallowed as liquid, too thick is difficult to swallow as baby is unable to chew food.

These challenges should be met by providing appropriate food and technique of feeding.

STATUS OF COMPLEMENTARY FEEDING IN INDIA

Complementary feeding (CF) practices in our country are dismal and require interventions in the form of (1) counseling in food secure situations and (2) counseling along with provision of foods in food insecure situations. The proportion of children in India, who are not fed with appropriate complementary feeding practices like timely initiation at 6–8 months; and not getting adequate diet in the form of food quantity, frequency and diversity, is very large. The National Family Health Survey-5 (NFHS-5) (2019–2021) provides details on two indicators of appropriate CF: (1) timely introduction of CF at 6–8 months, and (2) adequacy of CF.

Complementary feeding is not initiated in more than half of infants aged 6–8 months. A substantial decreasing trend of timely introduction of CF was observed in Bihar. The NFHS-5 reported that 24% of breastfed children had an adequately diverse diet, while 31% had been fed the minimum number of times appropriate for their age. Only 11% of all children aged 6–23 months received the minimum acceptable diet.

PRINCIPLES OF COMPLEMENTARY FEEDING

The following principles are for directing policy and programs at global, national and community levels:

1. ***Duration of exclusive breastfeeding and age of introduction of complementary foods:*** Practice exclusive breastfeeding from birth to 6 months of age and introduce complementary foods at 6 months of age (180 days) while continuing to breastfeed.
2. ***Maintenance of breastfeeding:*** Continue frequent, on-demand breastfeeding until 2 years of age or beyond.
3. ***Responsive feeding practices:***
   - Feed infants directly and assist older children when they feed themselves, being sensitive to their hunger and satiety cues.
   - Feed slowly and patiently, and encourage children to eat, but do not force them.
   - If child refuse many foods, experiment with different food combinations, tastes, textures and methods of encouragement.
   - Minimize distractions during meals if the child loses interest easily.
   - Remember that feeding times are periods of learning and love. Talk to children during feeding, with eye-to-eye contact.
   - Do not engage the child in screen while feeding.
4. ***Safe preparation and storage of complementary foods:*** Practice good hygiene and proper food handling by:
   - Washing caregivers' and child's hands before food preparation and eating
   - Storing foods safely and serving foods immediately after preparation
   - Using clean utensils to prepare and serve food
   - Using clean cups and bowls when feeding children
   - Avoiding the use of feeding bottles, which are difficult to keep clean.
5. ***Amount of complementary food needed:*** Start at 6 months of age with small quantity of food and increase the quantity as the child gets older, while maintaining frequent breastfeeding. Complementary foods should provide at least 200 kcal per day at 6–8 months of age, 300 kcal per day at 9–11 months and 550 kcal per day at 12–23 months of age.
6. ***Food consistency:*** Gradually increase food consistency and variety as the infant gets older, adapting to the infant's requirements and abilities.
   - Infants can eat pureed, mashed, and semisolid foods beginning at 6 months.
   - By 8 months most infants can also eat "finger foods" (snacks that can be eaten by children alone).
   - By 1 years, most children can eat the same types of foods as consumed by the rest of the family

   Avoid foods that may cause choking, i.e., items that have a shape or consistency that may cause them to become lodged in the trachea, such as nuts, grapes, or raw carrots.
7. ***Meal frequency and energy density:*** Increase the number of times that the child is fed complementary foods as he/she gets older. The adequate number of feedings depends on the energy density of the foods and the amounts consumed at each feeding. For the average healthy breastfed infant, complementary foods should be provided 2–3 times per day at 6–8 months of age and 3–4 times per day at 9–11 and 12–24 months of age, with additional nutritious snacks (such as a piece of fruit or bread or *chapatti* with nut paste) offered once or twice a day, as desired. Snacks are defined as foods eaten between meals, usually self-fed, convenient and easy to prepare. If energy density or amount of food per meal is less, or the child is no longer breastfed, more frequent meals may be required.
8. ***Nutrient content of complementary foods:*** Feed a variety of foods to ensure that nutrient needs are met. Complementary foods should have diet diversity of the seven major food groups, i.e., (1) cereals, tubers, roots; (2) legumes and pulses; (3) vitamin A rich fruit and vegetables; (4) other fruit/vegetables; (5) milk, cheese, etc., (6) eggs; and (7) flesh foods (meat, fish, etc.); of which *at least 4 groups should be included in diet daily*. This is known as *minimal dietary diversification*. Tea, coffee, and sugary drinks are *not* to be given at all. Fruit juices are not recommended below 2 years of age (IAP, 2019).
9. ***Use of vitamin-mineral supplements:*** Iron supplementation is routinely recommended after 6 months of age. Vitamin D supplementation (400 IU/day) is recommended between birth and 1 year.
10. ***Feeding during and after illness:*** Increase fluid intake during illness, including more frequent breastfeeding, and encourage the child to eat soft, varied, appetizing, favorite foods. During recovery, give food more often than usual and encourage the child to eat more. Avoid giving fruit juices in illness or during recovery.

WHEN TO START?

National Nutrition Institute-Indian Council of Medical Research (NIN-ICMR) recommends home-based semisolid foods to the infant after 6 months of age. Breastmilk is sufficient to promote growth and development till 6 months of age. Thereafter, there is a gap between the total energy needs and the energy provided by breast milk **(Fig. 7.1)**. The gap increases as the child grows. Also, around this age, infant's development and behavior makes him or her ready for foods other than breastmilk.

Gradually, infant's tendency to push solids out of mouth decreases; infant starts showing interest in other people eating and reaches for food; holds objects and likes to put things in his or her mouth; and starts moving the food around the mouth with better control of tongue; teeth begin to erupt, and the biting movements begins so child starts chewing the food. Also, the digestive system is mature enough to digest a range of foods. Therefore, 6 months is considered the best time to begin complementary feeding as the child is ready to eat soft and starchy foods. Care must be taken to ensure that these foods complement, and not replace the breastmilk.

ATTRIBUTES OF COMPLEMENTARY FEEDING

Attributes of appropriate complementary foods include: (1) timely start; (2) adequate in amount, variety, and frequency; and (3) proper and safe feeding.

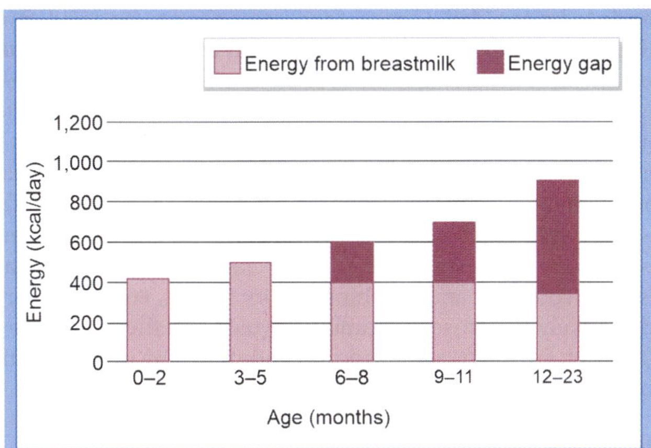

Fig. 7.1: Energy gap to be filled by complementary foods after 6 months of age

Source: World Health Organization. Infant and young child feeding. In: textbooks for medical students and allied health professionals. Geneva: WHO; 2009

Timely Start

Complementary foods should be introduced after 6 months of age along with continued breastfeeding when need for energy and nutrients exceeds that can be provided through exclusive breastfeeding. This is called *timely complementary feeding.*

Introduction of complementary foods before 6 months of age may decrease the intake of breastmilk, making it difficult to meet the child's nutritional needs as other foods are nutritionally inferior to the breast milk. Also, it exposes the child to risks of diarrhea and other infections at an earlier age.

Addition of complementary foods in formula fed infants before 4 months of age has been found to increase the risk of developing childhood obesity.

Adding complementary foods too late may lead to suboptimal growth and development, and risk of nutritional deficiencies, and malnutrition.

Adequate in Amount, Variety, and Frequency

Amount and Texture

All foods provide some energy. However, the taste, consistency and the texture of foods have important bearing on successful complementary feeding. Complementary foods should be of right consistency, soft, easy to digest, inexpensive, locally available, culturally acceptable ingredients; and easy to prepare at home. The stomach of a young child is small. Thin foods and liquids fill it quickly. To address the issue of a small stomach size which can accommodate limited quantity at a time, each meal must be made energy dense by adding sugar/jaggery and ghee/butter/oil.

The consistency or thickness of foods makes a big difference to how well that food meets the young child's energy needs. Foods of a thick consistency help to fill the energy gap. To provide more calories from smaller volumes, food must be thick in consistency—thick enough to stay on the spoon without running off, when the spoon is tilted **(Fig. 7.2)**.

- The first food a child eats should be soft, homogeneous (mashed or strained) and bland in taste.
- When the infant has accepted soft food, different tastes should be gradually introduced with increasing thickness and varying texture.
- Consistency of foods should be appropriate to the developmental readiness of the child in munching, chewing, and swallowing. Foods which can pose choking hazard are to be avoided. You can start with mashed and semisolid foods (e.g., porridge).
- Gradually, food consistency, amount, and variety are increased with age. Introduction of lumpy or granular foods should be done by about 9-10 months. Small, chopped pieces of food can also be mixed. Infant can be fed with finger foods by 8-9 months of age and by 12 months, family foods can be eaten. Missing this age may lead to feeding fussiness later.

A food that stays easily on the spoon is just the right consistency.

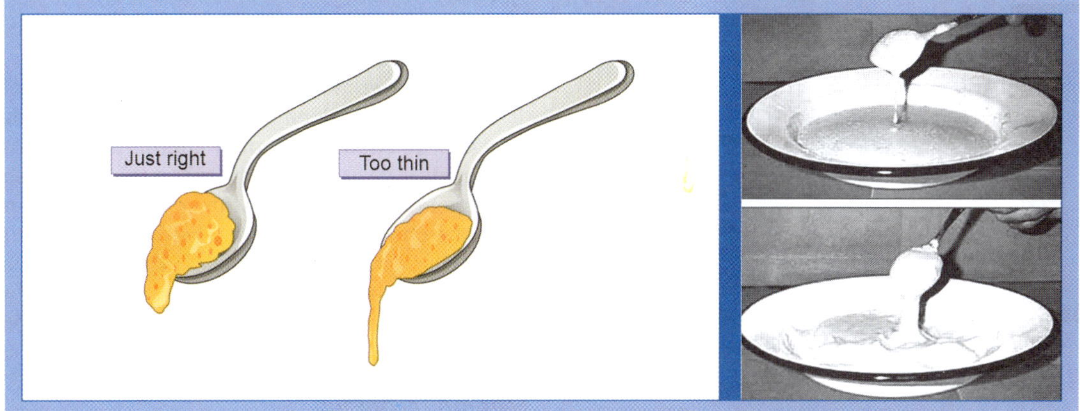

Fig. 7.2: Consistency of complementary food (6–8 months)

Source: World Health Organization. Complementary feeding—family foods for breastfed children. Geneva: WHO; 2000

Variety: Adequate in all Food Groups

Dietary diversity: Complementary foods should be containing various food groups to provide sufficient calories, protein, and micronutrients to meet a growing child's nutritional needs. While deciding the menu for complementary feeding *dietary diversity* should be taken in account. Dietary diversity means feeding a child different types of foods so that his/her nutrient requirements are adequately met.

As also discussed earlier a diverse diet should include foods from at least 4 out of 7 groups each day: (1) grains, roots and tubers; (2) legumes, nuts and seeds; (3) dairy (milk, yoghurt, cheese); (4) flesh foods (meat, fish, poultry, and liver or organ meats); (5) eggs; (6) vitamin A-rich fruits and vegetables (carrots, mangoes, dark green leafy vegetables, pumpkins, orange sweet potato); and (7) other fruits and vegetables. Providing children diverse range of foods ensures fulfillment of their micronutrient requirements, including the need for vitamin A, iron, calcium, thiamine, folate, zinc, vitamins B_6 and B_{12}.

Minimum dietary diversity is consumption of 4 or more food groups from the 7 food groups to meet daily energy and nutrient requirements. This ensures that the child has a high likelihood of consuming at least one animal-source food and one fruit or vegetable that day, in addition to a staple food (grain, root, or tuber).

Iron gap: Full-term infants are born with adequate iron store and get some iron in breastmilk, thus do not require additional iron for first 6 months of life. After 6 months of life, breastmilk iron is grossly inadequate and most of iron demand needs to be met with complementary foods. It is important to provide iron rich foods to children during this period to fill iron gap. Iron rich foods include green leafy vegetables, legumes, dried fruits, meat, fish, and poultry products. Bioavailability of iron from plant foods is not optimum, addition of fruits rich in vitamin C increases the absorption of iron from plant foods. It is important to note that with increasing age (6–24 months), requirement for iron decreases **(Fig. 7.3)**.

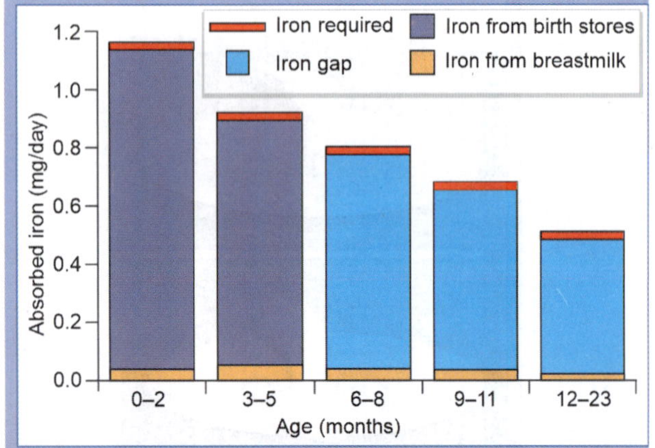

Fig. 7.3: Iron need and supply in infants and young children

Source: World Health Organization. Complementary feeding—family foods for breastfed children. Geneva: WHO; 2000

Foods to be avoided: Certain food items need to be avoided in infants and young children, e.g., tea and coffee (interfere with iron absorption), aerated beverages (no nutritional value), too much sugary drinks and fruit juices (cause decreased appetite for other nutritious foods and also may cause loose stools), and nuts (may cause choking). Consumption of commercial complementary foods in comparison to home-made foods early in life is associated with lower intake of fruit and vegetables. Use of ultra-processed and commercial snack foods such as biscuits, cookies, candies, chips, savory snacks, etc., which are aggressively advertised, should be avoided as these foods are often rich in sugar, salt, and fats and deficient in important nutrients.

Frequency

Frequency of complementary feeding should also increase with age. When food is first introduced, a small amount should be given 1–2 times a day and slowly increased to 3–4 times daily. The frequency of complementary foods required by young children in addition to breastmilk is given in **Table 7.1**. If a child is not breastfed, complementary foods should be given more frequently. If baby is not breastfed, give in addition: 1–2 cups of milk per day, and 1–2 extra meals per day.

In between snacking: Adequate total energy intake can also be ensured by addition of one to two nutritious snacks between the three main meals. Snacks are in addition to the meals and should not replace meals. They should not be confused with foods such as sweets, chips or other processed foods. Junk food and commercial food, readymade, processed food from the market, e.g., tinned foods/juices, cold-drinks, chocolates, crisps, health drinks, bakery products, etc., should be avoided. Giving drinks with low nutritive value, such as tea, coffee and sugary drinks should also be strictly avoided.

Responsive and Safe Feeding

Responsive feeding means the reciprocity between child and caregiver. It is important to make feeding a pleasurable experience for the infant. It also helps in ensuring intake of adequate amount of variety of foods. Responsive feeding is a three steps process:

1. The child signals requests through motor actions, facial expressions, or vocalizations.
2. The caregiver recognizes the signals and responds promptly in a manner that is emotionally supportive, contingent on the signal, and developmentally appropriate **(Fig. 7.4)**.
3. The child experiences a predictable response to signals. Responding to the child with smiles and eye contact; talking to the child while feeding; feeding the child slowly with patience increase food intake; experimenting with different food combinations, tastes, and textures; and minimizing distractions during meals are few practices, which helps in achieving responsive feeding.

Feeding Technique

As a general principle, a single complementary food is added at a time, in small quantities. This is followed by introduction

Table 7.1 Practical Guidance on the Quality, Frequency, and Amount of Food to Offer Children 6–23 Months of Age Who are Breastfed on Demand

Age	*Energy needed per day in addition to breast milk*	*Texture*	*Frequency*	*Amount of food an average child will usually eat at each meal*
6–8 months[1]	200 kcal	• Start with thick porridge and well mashed foods • Continue with mashed family foods	• 2–3 meals per day • Depending on child's appetite, 1–2 snacks may be offered	Start with 2–3 tablespoonful per feed and increase gradually to ½ of a 250 mL cup
9–11 months	300 kcal	Finely chopped or mashed foods and foods that baby can pick up	• 3–4 meals per day • Depending on child's appetite, 1–2 snacks may be offered	½ of a 250 mL cup/bowl
12–23 months	550 kcal	Family foods, chopped or mashed if necessary	• 3–4 meals per day • Depending on child's appetite, 1–2 snacks may be offered	¾ to 1 of a 250 mL cup

[1]The age ranges should be interpreted as follows: a child 6–8 months is 6 months or older (>180 days) but not yet 9-month-old (<270 days)
Source: Reproduce with permission from World Health Organization. Infant and young child feeding model. In: Textbooks for medical students and allied health professionals. Geneva: WHO; 2009

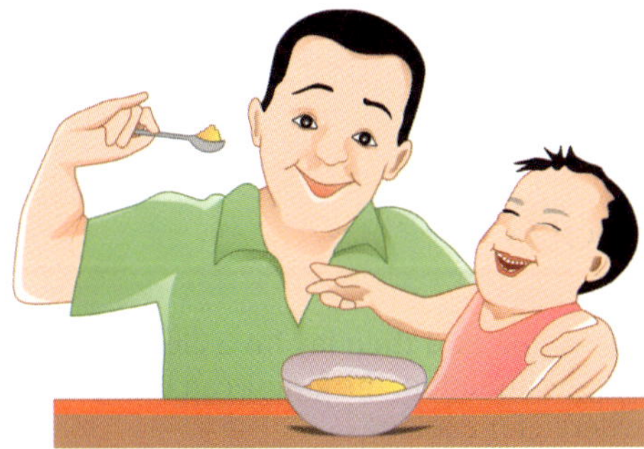

Fig. 7.4: Responsive feeding. Both (the caregiver and the child) should enjoy the experience and be part of it without any external distractions

of the second complementary food after some days. The child should be fed slowly and patiently. Force feeding and bribing should be avoided. Forced feeding, threatening and punishment interfere with development of good/proper feeding habits.

As the child grows older, he should be encouraged to feed by self with fingers or spoon. Self-feeding should be encouraged despite spillage. Each child should be fed under supervision in a separate plate to develop an individual identity. Along with feeding, mother and caregivers should provide psychosocial stimulation to the child through ordinary age-appropriate play and communication activities to ensure early childhood development. Young children should be actively encouraged to take feed by praising them and their foods, paying attention, talking, playing with him, and showing pleasure.

Hygiene Related to Complementary Feeding

Careful preparation and storage of the complementary food is essential to prevent contamination. Unhygienic feeding practices result in infections like diarrhea which may further compromise the child's nutritional state. Complementary foods should be hygienically prepared and stored, and fed. This can be achieved by:

- Washing caregiver's and child's hands before preparing, handling, eating food, and after using toilet.
- Using clean water and raw materials to cook food
- *Storing foods safely:* Keeping food covered and serving shortly after preparation
- Using clean utensils to prepare and serve food
- Using clean bowls and cups when feeding the child and not using bottles and teats.

NATIONAL GUIDELINES ON INFANT AND YOUNG CHILD FEEDING

Infant and Young Child Feeding (IYCF) practices are a set of recommendations to achieve appropriate feeding of newborn and children under 2 years of age to achieve optimal nutritional outcomes in populations.

Recommendations

- Early initiation of breastfeeding; immediately after birth, preferably within 1 hour.
- Exclusive breastfeeding for the first 6 months of life, i.e., 180 days (no other foods or fluids like honey, *ghutti*, animal or powdered milk, tea, or glucose water, not even water since these are potentially harmful; but allows infant to receive ORS, and drops or syrup of vitamins, minerals and medicines when required).
- Breastfeed should be given as often as the baby desires and each feed should continue for as long as the infant wants to suckle.
- Timely introduction of nutritionally adequate and safe complementary foods (solid, semisolid, or soft foods) after the age of 6 months, i.e., 180 days, to meet their growing nutritional requirements.

- Continued breastfeeding for 2 years or beyond.
- Expectant mothers should be motivated and prepared for early initiation of breastfeeding, within first hour after birth, and exclusive breastfeeding.
- Age-appropriate complementary feeding for children 6–23 months, while continuing breastfeeding. Children should receive diversity from 4 or more food groups [(1) Grains, roots and tubers; (2) legumes, and nuts; (3) dairy products; (4) flesh foods (meat fish, poultry); (5) eggs; (6) vitamin A rich fruits and vegetables; (7) other fruits and vegetables] and fed for at least a minimum number of recommended times as per age (two times for breasted infants 6–8 months; three times for breastfed children 9–23 months; four times for nonbreastfed children 6–23 months).
- Active feeding for children during and after illness.
- All HIV infected mothers should receive counseling, which should include provision of general information about meeting their own nutritional requirements, and about the risks and benefits of various feeding options, and specific guidance in selecting the option most likely to be suitable for their situation. The aim of the counseling for feeding infants in maternal HIV should be to avoid mixed feeding. Mothers opting for breastfeeding should be supported for exclusive breastfeeding up to 6 months. If the woman chooses not to breastfeed, she should be provided support for artificial feeding to make it safe.

WHO (2023) GUIDELINES FOR COMPLEMENTARY FEEDING OF INFANT AND YOUNG CHILDREN 6–23 MONTHS OF AGE

1. Breastfeeding should continue up to 2 years or beyond.
2. For infants 6–11 months of age who are fed milk other than breastmilk, either formula milk or animal milk can be fed.
3. For young children 12–23 months of age who are fed milk other than breastmilk, animal milk should be fed.
4. Food higher in sugar, salt and trans-fat should not consumed.
5. Sugar sweetened beverages should not be consumed.
6. Non-sugar sweeteners should not be consumed.
7. Consumption of 100% fruit juice should be limited.
8. ***Responsive feeding:*** Children 6–23 months of age should be responsively fed, defined as "feeding practice that encourage the child to eat autonomously and in response to physiological and developmental needs, which may encourage self-regulation in eating and support cognitive, emotional and social development."

7.2 Complementary Foods

PE 8.3

The complementary foods should be well balanced nutritionally and at least 8–10% of the energy should be obtained from proteins of good quality. Complementary foods should be prepared from cereals such as rice, wheat or maize, pulses, milk, and root staples like potato. Deficiency of lysine, an essential amino acid in the protein of wheat, can be compensated, if both wheat and legumes (rich in lysine) are consumed simultaneously.

Complementary foods based on vegetable protein alone may not always provide essential amino acids in a balanced proportion, comparable to the egg or milk protein. Therefore, addition of small quantities of proteins of animal origin such as milk, egg, or meat is usually sufficient to make up the deficiency of limiting amino acids, in a diet based on a mixture of a staple cereal and a legume.

Oils, fats, and sugars increase dietary energy levels and improve taste of the food. Addition of vegetables and fruits will further enhance the nutritional quality of food by providing minerals such as iron and vitamins.

Additional tips for improving quality of feeds are given below:

- Complementary feeds containing a cereal pulse combination of rice/rice flakes (*poha*)/wheat and roasted Bengal gram dhal/soybean/green gram dhal would increase intakes of iron, compared to other cereal: pulse combinations due to either higher absorption and/or higher iron content.
- Soaking, germination/sprouting of cereals and pulses will reduce their phytate content by about half. To do this, soak grains overnight, and then lay on a clean wet cloth for 1–2 days. After germination, the grains can be lightly dry roasted and powdered for cooking.
- If locally available fruits such as guava (in children over 1 year of age), papaya, *musambi* (sweet lime), orange, and lime rich in ascorbic acid are provided as a freshly made mash along with the food, it will increase absorption of iron.
- If an iron supplement is to be given, it is best provided after meals. This will reduce the risk of adverse events. To improve bioavailability of iron taken after the meal, use grains that are less inhibitory for iron absorption. For this purpose, rice is most neutral, followed by wheat and lastly millets. Examples of rice-based complementary foods with lower iron inhibitory effect are a cereal: pulse combination of rice with roasted Bengal gram or sprouted and roasted green gram. These combinations can be made into local recipes such as rice *khichdi* or rice *pongal* or *idlis* for younger children. For older children, *poha* with crushed groundnuts can also be given.

AGE-WISE COMPLEMENTARY FOODS

A good regimen of complementary feeding is to start with mashed bananas, as it is easily accepted. Within a week or two the infant can be put on semolina (*suji*) cooked in milk. Both of these provide additional calories. Shortly thereafter, well-cooked and mashed lentils or peas, followed by *khichri* (*kanji*) are added. By 8–9 months of age, the child should be consuming

Table 7.2 Age-wise Complementary Foods

Age	*Type of supplement*	*Examples of food to be given*
7–8th months	Semisolid	Well-blended porridge, *kheer*, well mashed lentil with a boiled vegetable, potato and spinach puree, blended rice khichri, vermicelli khichri, and dalia
9–12th months	Semisolid-solid	Poha with curd, potato with curd, millet khichri, upma, idli, and moong dal mixture
Above 1 year	Solid	Roti, cheela, paratha, laddoo, biscuits, rice and dal (family food)

Source: IBFAN Asia, Navdanya, IHES, BPNI. Complementary foods for children and young children (recipe for the people by the people). Washington DC: World Bank; 2009

most of foods (after appropriate modification) cooked in the house for adults.

Delayed complementary feeding and undue dependence on milk as food result in iron deficiency anemia. Hence iron-fortified foods, iodized salt, vitamin A enriched food, etc., are to be encouraged. Soup or purees of dark green leafy vegetables are good source of iron for infants and should be added to complementary foods. Addition of vegetables and fruits will further enhance the nutritional quality of food by providing minerals such as iron and vitamins. Animal milk is also a poor source of iron.

Foods can be enriched by making a fermented porridge, use of germinated or sprouted flour and toasting of grains before grinding.

- In most parts of India, a well-cooked gruel (*khichri*, *kanji*) prepared from rice (3 parts), legume (1 part), green leafy vegetable, and some milk curd is a satisfactory complementary food.
- Another good complementary food is wheat gruel (*dalia*) made in milk with added sugar. Oil should be added to these foods to make them energy dense.
- Local variations of the complementary food may be made according to the availability of food in the region **(Table 7.2)**.
- Commercially available complementary foods are convenient but expensive and offer no distinct advantages over the home-made complementary foods.

A few recipes for complementary foods are given in **Boxes 7.1** and **7.2**.

Box 7.1 Recipes for Home-Made Instant Food for Complementary Feeding

Wheat food

Ingredient: Wheat 100 g, roasted Bengal gram dal 30 g, groundnut 20 g and sugar 50 g

Method of preparation:

- Clean and roast wheat and groundnut separately (remove the outer skin of groundnut)
- Grind roast Bengal gram dal and roasted groundnut and wheat separately to a fine powder. Mix all the ingredients thoroughly and add powdered sugar
- Fill in dry airtight container and store

Nutritive value per 100 g: Calories 386, protein 11.64 g, iron 3.75 mg, and carotene 51.5

Chivda mix

Ingredient: Chivda (rice flakes) mix 100 g, Bengal gram 30 g (roasted and dehusked), and groundnut 20 g (roasted)

Method of preparation:

- Roast chivda and grind
- Grind roasted groundnut (without skin) and Bengal gram separately
- Mix all thoroughly. Store in a dry airtight container

Nutritive value per 100 g: Calories 381, protein 12.39 g, iron 15.63 mg, and carotene 22.6 µg

Box 7.2 Recipes for Fresh Complementary Foods

Suji halwa

Ingredients: Suji (roasted) 200 g, groundnut (roasted) 40 g, jaggery 100 g, oil 10 mL, and water 800 mL

Method of preparation:

- Grind groundnuts coarsely after removal of skin
- Heat oil in a pan, add *Suji*, and fry till light brown
- Add groundnuts to *Suji* and mix well
- Add jaggery and water to the above and cook till it leaves sides

Nutritive values per 100 g: Calories 408, protein 9.05 g, and iron 2.02 mg

Dalia porridge

Ingredients: Dalia (broken wheat) 25 g, *moong dal* 20 g, milk 60 mL, sugar 30 g, and *ghee* or oil 15 g

Method of preparation:

- Roast broken wheat in a pan
- When half-done add *dal* and continue roasting till light brown
- Add water to the above, cook till soft, and slightly thick (semisolid)
- Remove from fire. Add milk, sugar, and oil. Boil for a few minutes and serve

Nutritive value per 100 g: Calories 310, protein 6.5 g, iron 1.5 mg, and carotene 497 µg

7.3 History Taking for Complementary Feeding

PE 8.4

Table 7.3 details how to assess the practices of complementary feeding, and counsel on ideal feeding practices.

Table 7.3 Assessing the Practices of Complementary Feeding and Counsel on Ideal Feeding Practices

Reference tool: Food intake—6 up to 24 months		
Feeding practice	*Ideal feeding practice*	*Key messages to help counsel mothers*
Growth appropriate?		*Look at the shape of the growth curve of the child: is the child growing?*
Child received breast milk?	Yes	Breastfeeding for 2 years or longer helps a child to develop and grow strong and healthy
How many meals of a thick consistency did the child eat yesterday? (use *food consistency pictures* as needed)	3 meals	Foods that are thick enough to stay on the spoon give more energy to the child
Child ate an animal-source food yesterday (meat/fish/offal/bird/eggs)?	Animal-source foods should be eaten daily if culturally appropriate	Animal-source foods are especially good for children, to help them grow strong and lively
Child ate a dairy product yesterday?	Try to give dairy products daily	Animal-source foods are especially good for children, to help them grow strong and lively
Child ate pulses, nuts or seeds yesterday?	If meat is not eaten, pulses or nuts should be eaten daily, with an iron enhancer such as a vitamin C-rich food	Peas, beans, lentils, nuts and seeds are good for children
Reference tool: Food intake—6 up to 24 months		
Feeding practice	*Ideal feeding practice*	*Key messages to help counsel mothers*
Child ate a dark-green or yellow vegetable or yellow fruit yesterday?	A dark-green or yellow vegetable or yellow fruit should be eaten daily	Dark-green leaves and yellow-colored fruits and vegetables help the child to have healthy eyes and fewer infections
Child ate sufficient number of meals and snacks yesterday, for their age?	• *Child 6–8 months:* 2–3 meals plus 1–2 snacks if hungry • *Child 9–24 months:* 3–4 meals plus 1–2 snacks if hungry	A growing child needs 2–4 meals a day, plus 1–2 snacks if hungry: give a variety of foods
Quantity of food eaten at main meal yesterday appropriate for child's age?	• *Child 6–8 months:* Gradually increased to approx. 1/2 cup at each meal • *Child 9–11 months:* Approx. 1/2 cup at each meal • *Child 12–24 months:* Approx. ¾–1 cup at each meal	A growing child needs increasing amounts of food
Caregiver assisted the child at mealtimes?	Yes, assists with learning to eat	A young child needs to learn to eat: encourage and give help with lots of patience
Child took any vitamin or mineral supplements?	Vitamin and mineral supplements may be needed if child's needs are not met by food intake	*Explain how to use vitamin and mineral supplements if they are needed*
Child ill or recovering from an illness?	Continue to eat and drink during illness and recovery	Encourage the child to drink and eat during illness, and provide extra food after illness to help them recover quickly

Source: Infant and Young Child Feeding Counselling: an integrated course. Trainer's Guide, 2nd edition. Geneva: World Health Organization; 2021

7.4 Counseling and Education for Complementary Feeding

PE 8.5

Comprehensive message for *balanced food* should be given to the mother during complementary feeding counseling (**Table 7.4**). The food should consist of various (as diverse as possible) food groups/components in different combinations. As the babies start showing interest in complementary feeds, the variety should be increased by adding new foods in the staple food one by one. Easily available, cost-effective seasonal uncooked fruits, green and other dark-colored vegetables, milk and milk products, pulses/legumes, animal foods, oil/butter, sugar/jaggery may be added in the staples gradually.

Table 7.4 Comprehensive Message of Counseling to the Mother: Recommendation During Health

Up to 6 months of age	*6 months up to 12 months (200–300 kcal)*	*12 months up to 2 years (550 kcal)*	*2 years and older*
• Breastfeed as often as the child wants (day and night). At least 8 times in 24 hours • Do not give any other food or fluids not even water **Remember** Continue breastfeeding even if the child is sick	• Breastfeed as often as the child wants • Give at least 1 *katori* serving (150 mL) at a time, of: ▪ Mashed *roti*/rice/ bread mixed in thick dal with added ghee/oil or khichdi with added oil/ghee. Add cooked vegetables also in the servings or mashed roti/ bread/biscuit mixed in sweetened undiluted milk; or ▪ *Sevian/dalia/halwa/kheer* prepared in milk or any cereal porridge cooked in milk, or	• Breastfeed as often as the child wants • Offer food from the family pot • Give at least 1 and a half *katori* serving at a time, of: ▪ Mashed *roti*/rice /bread mixed in thick dal with added ghee/oil or *khichdi* with added oil/ ghee. Add cooked vegetables also in the servings or ▪ Mashed *roti*/rice/bread mixed in sweetened milk or	• Give family foods as 3 meals each day • Also, give nutritious food between meals, twice daily Such as: Banana/biscuit/cheeko/ mango/papaya as snacks **Remember** • Ensure that the child finishes the serving
	▪ Mashed boiled potatoes ▪ Offer banana/biscuit/cheeko/mango/ papaya as snacks in between the serving **Frequency** • Three times per day if breastfed • Five times per day if not breastfed and 1–2 snacks **Remember** • Keep the child in your lap and feed with your own • Wash your own and child's hand with soap and water every time before feeding	▪ *Sevian/dalia/halwa/kheer* prepared in milk or ▪ Offer banana/biscuit/cheeko/ mango/papaya as snacks **Frequency** Give 5 times per day if "not breastfeed" and 3–4 times if breastfed and 1–2 snacks **Remember** • Sit by the side of child and help him to finish the serving • Wash your own and child's hand with soap and water every time before feeding	• Teach your child to wash his hands with soap and water every time before feeding

1 katori = 150 mL

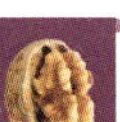

IN A NUTSHELL

Counseling and Education for Complementary Feeding

1. Start complementary feeds after 6 months.
2. Continue breastfeeding up to 2 years of age along with appropriate complementary feeding.
3. Give semi-solid food (Avoid watery food such as soups, fruit juices, and animal milk). Prefer home-made food (clean, fresh, cheap, and easily available)
4. Prefer balanced food (Cereal + pulse + vegetables) using locally available ingredients preparations.
5. Introduce one food at one time; once child starts accepting it, introduce another preparation.
6. Addition of ghee, oil, and fats adds to energy, and palatability of food.
7. Child's choice and preferences shall be respected. Avoid force feeding.
8. Avoid ultra-processed, refined, packaged, commercial and Junk foods.
9. Avoid foods with excess of sugar, salt, and transfatty acids.
10. Avoid feeding while watching television or mobile.

Arikpo D, Edet ES, Chibuzor MT, et al. Educational interventions for improving primary caregiver complementary feeding practices for children aged 24 months and under. Cochrane Database Syst Rev. 2018;5(5):CD011768.

Foterek K, Hilbig A, Alexy U. Associations between commercial complementary food consumption and fruit and vegetable intake in children. Results of the DONALD study. Appetite. 2015;85:84-90.

Guiding Principles for Complementary Feeding of the Breastfed Child. PAHO/WHO, Division of Health Promotion and Protection/Food and Nutrition Program. Washington, DC: PAHO/WHO; 2003.

IAP Parental Guideline on Complementary Feeding. https://iapindia.org/pdf/Ch-040-IAP-Parental-Guideline-Complementary-Feeding.pdf. Accessed 27 Feb, 2025.

Ministry of Health and Family Welfare (MoHFW), Government of India, UNICEF and Population Council. 2019. Comprehensive National Nutrition Survey (CNNS) National Report. New Delhi: MoHFW; 2019.

Shah D, Singh M, Gupta P, et al. Effect of sequencing of complementary feeding in relation to breastfeeding on total intake in infants. J Pediatr Gastroenterol Nutr. 2014;58(3):339-43.

United Nations Children's Fund (UNICEF). Improving Young Children's Diets during the Complementary Feeding Period. UNICEF Programming Guidance. New York: UNICEF; 2020

WHO, WHO Guideline for complementary feeding of infants and young children 6-23 months of age. World Health Organization; 2023 Oct 13. https://www.who.int. Accessed 27 Feb, 2025.

WHO. Infant and young child feeding counselling: an integrated course. Trainer's Guide, 2nd edition. Geneva: World Health Organization; 2021.

8 CHAPTER

Normal Nutrition, Assessment, and Monitoring

AS PER NMC COMPETENCIES

PE9.1	Describe age-related nutritional needs of infants, children and adolescents including micronutrients and vitamins.	*Ch 8.1*
PE9.2	Describe the tools and methods for assessment and classification of nutritional status of infants, children and adolescents.	*Ch 8.3*
PE9.3	Explain the calorific value of common Indian foods.	*Ch 8.2*
PE9.4	Elicit document and present an appropriate nutritional history and perform a dietary recall.	*Ch 8.3*
PE9.5	Calculate the age-related calorie requirement in health and disease, and identify gap.	*Ch 8.3*
PE9.6	Assess and classify the nutrition status of infants, children and adolescents and recognize deviations.	*Ch 8.3*
PE9.7	Plan an appropriate diet in health and diseases.	*Ch 8.4*

Topics available online: ***Unhealthy Foods, National Nutritional Initiatives, Nutritional Surveillance, Education, and Rehabilitation***

8.1 Nutrients and Nutritional Requirements *PE 9.1*

INTRODUCTION

Nutrients are the chemical substances in the food that the body uses for functions that support growth, tissue maintenance, and repair. There are six categories of nutrients: (1) carbohydrates, (2) proteins, (3) fats, (4) vitamins, (5) minerals, and (6) fibers.

- Carbohydrates, fats, and proteins are the chief sources of energy for man, and therefore, are also known as, *macronutrients*.
- ***Micronutrients*** are the nutrients required in tiny amounts, may be a few micrograms per day, and include various minerals and vitamins.

Nutrients, which are not synthesized in the body or not synthesized adequately by the body, are known as *essential nutrients*. They need to be provided by the diet and include carbohydrates, essential amino acids, essential fatty acids (EFAs), vitamins, minerals, and water. Nonessential nutrients can be synthesized by the body (e.g., glucose and cholesterol).

ENERGY

Energy is required for growth, metabolism, maintenance of body temperature, and physical activities. The factors that affect energy requirements are age, sex, type, and extent of physical activity, climate, body size and composition, and physiological status such as pregnancy and lactation. Children require energy for growth, whereas pregnant and lactating mothers need additional energy for the growth of fetus, and maintaining milk secretion, respectively. Even when an individual is in a state of complete rest, energy is spent for basal metabolism.

Sources of Energy

Carbohydrates, fats, and proteins are the chief sources of energy for man. Of the total energy, at least 10–15% should be provided by proteins, 20–30% by fats, and 50–60% by carbohydrates. The energy obtained from food is usually expressed in terms of thermochemical kilocalories (103 calories), also referred to as kilocalories (kcal) or simply calories (Cal). As per the International system of units, energy requirement of the body is mentioned in Joules [1 Cal = 4.184 Joules, 1 thermochemical kilocalorie (kcal or Cal) = 4184 Joules (J) or 4.184 kJ]. One gram of carbohydrate or protein provides 4 kcal or 16.7 kJ, while 1 gram of fat releases 9 kcal or 37.7 kJ of energy.

Table 8.1 Recommended Dietary Allowances (RDA) of Energy and Nutrients

	Energy (kcal) (EAR)	*Protein (g)*	*Dietary fiber (g)*
Infants 0–6 months (adequate intake)	530	5.8	–
Infants 6–12 months	660	8.5	–
Children 1–3 years	1,110	12.5	15
Children 4–6 years	1,360	16	20
Children 7–9 years	1,700	23	26
Boys 10–12 years	2,220	32	33
Girls 10–12 years	2,060	33	31
Boys 13–15 years	2,860	45	43
Girls 13–15 years	2,400	43	36
Boys 16–18 years	3,320	55	50
Girls 16–18 years	2,500	46	38

There is no RDA for energy, estimated average requirement (EAR) for energy is equivalent to estimated energy requirement

Source: Indian Council of Medical Research (ICMR), National Institute of Nutrition (NIN); 2020

Energy Requirement for Different Ages and Groups

The energy requirement of infants, older children, and adults as recommended by Indian Council of Medical research (ICMR) in 2020 is presented in **Table 8.1**.

Pregnant women require additional supplements of energy giving foods for the growth of the fetus and the deposition of fat, which is used during lactation to meet the additional energy needs for milk secretion. The optimal additional needs are estimated as 70–85 kcal/day during the first trimester and 350 kcal/day during the second and third trimesters. Even though malnourished mothers continue to produce good quantity of milk during lactation, additional energy is required for maintaining mother's own nutritional status so that this additional input could be utilized for breastmilk production.

During the period of lactation, additional energy requirement is 600 kcal/day during first 6 months of exclusive breastfeeding and 520 kcal/day for continued breastfeeding from 7-12 months.

CARBOHYDRATES

Carbohydrates provide energy, contribute to taste and texture of foods, preserve foods, and are essential for digestion and assimilation of other foods. They also protect the proteins from being used for energy. Monosaccharides (glucose, fructose, galactose, ribose, and deoxyribose) and disaccharides (sucrose, lactose, and maltose) are known as *simple carbohydrates* while polysaccharides (starch, glycogen, and fiber) are referred to as *complex carbohydrates.*

Starch is a complex carbohydrate made up of thousands of glucose molecules linked together. Grains are the richest food source of starch. Other important sources of starch are legumes (beans and peas) and tubers (potato, cassava, etc.). Body converts all carbohydrates (except those coming from fiber) to glucose. Glucose is used as a fuel by brain and muscle tissue or converted to glycogen and stored by liver and muscles. Excess carbohydrates are converted to fat.

Carbohydrates are the major source of energy. Carbohydrates provide 4 Cal/g. Indian Council of Medical Research, 2020 guideline recommends a minimum intake of 100–130 gram of carbohydrates per day in all groups >1 year of age. This is the minimum level required for brain glucose utilization. Carbohydrates should contribute to 45–65% of total energy intake; and preferably obtained from grains, legumes, vegetables, and fruits. Such a diet is lower in fat and energy and higher in fiber, vitamin, and minerals. These diets also contribute to lower rates of undernutrition, obesity, tooth decay, cardiovascular disease, and diabetes.

WHO, in its 2023 recommendations, states that carbohydrate intake for everyone 2 years of age and older should come primarily from whole grains, vegetables, fruits and pulses. The intake of fruits and vegetables age-wise has been recommended as: 2–5 years old, at least 250 g per day; 6–9 years old, at least 350 g per day; 10 years or older, at least 400 g per day.

Excessive carbohydrate consumption in form of concentrated sweets is associated with dental caries, obesity, and ischemic heart disease. Added sugar should constitute not >5% of total caloric intake. Regular consumption of high-fructose diet may lead to obesity and metabolic syndrome. Lack of carbohydrates may produce ketosis, loss of energy, depression, and breakdown of body proteins.

PROTEINS

Protein is the second most abundant substance in the body, next to water. These are made up of 24 different amino acids. The proteins differ in their arrangement and quantity of amino acids. A few amino acids can be adequately synthesized in the body (*nonessential amino acids*), while others must be supplied in the diet (*essential amino acids*). Human body cannot synthesize these indispensable amino acids (essential amino acids) in adequate amounts. They are valine, leucine, isoleucine, lysine, tryptophan, methionine, threonine, and phenylalanine. Histidine is indispensable in infants. Arginine, cysteine, tyrosine, and taurine are also indispensable for low-birth-weight babies.

Functions of Protein

Protein helps the child to grow, as the constituent amino acids are necessary for the synthesis of tissues in the body. Proteins are needed for growth and tissue repair. They form structural proteins, immunoglobulins, and help in transporting other nutrients. Protein is essential for the formation of digestive juices, hormones, plasma proteins, enzymes, vitamins, and hemoglobin. Proteins also act as buffers to maintain acid-base equilibrium in the body. They are also a source of energy for the body.

Excess protein, not used for building tissues or providing energy, is converted by the liver into fat and stored in body tissues. The amino acids, which can be converted to glucose, are called glucogenic amino acids. Lysine and threonine are the only two glucogenic amino acids.

Requirements

Protein requirements of children are given in **Table 8.1**. Indian estimates are higher as these are calculated in terms of the proteins present in Indian diets (cereals + legumes + milk).

- An adult eating a standard Indian predominantly vegetarian diet requires 1.0 g/kg body weight of protein daily. If the protein in the diet is obtained from animal sources such as egg, meat, fish, or milk; lower intake of protein may be sufficient.
- During pregnancy (assuming 10 kg gestational weight gain), additional requirements are 8 and 18 grams/day of high-quality protein in 2nd and 3rd trimesters, respectively.
- During lactation, an additional daily intake of 13.6 g of high-quality protein during the first 6 months and 10 g during 6–12 months is required.

Complete Protein

A complete protein contains all the essential amino acids in relatively the same amount as humans require for maintenance of good health and optimal growth. The proteins of animal origin generally have a higher content of essential amino acids. These are, therefore, classified as biologically complete protein. Proteins from vegetable sources are often biologically incomplete, as these usually lack one or more of the essential amino acids. However, proteins of vegetable origin may be used together in a judicious combination so that limiting essential amino acid in one of these is compensated for by an excess of that amino acid in the complementing protein.

Biological Value

A high-quality protein should be complete as well as digestible. This is measured best by the biological value (BV) of the protein. BV is calculated as the fraction of absorbed nitrogen retained in the body for growth or maintenance. Egg protein is considered a *reference protein* in this context as it is complete and well digested. The BV of egg protein is 100. The BVs of milk, rice, and fish are 75, 67, and 75, respectively. The quality of protein depends on the extent to which the amino acid pattern resembles the reference protein. The combination of vegetable proteins may provide all the essential amino acids as in the reference protein. Limiting amino acid is the one found in lowest quantity in that protein compared to the reference protein. For example, protein from legumes is deficient in methionine whereas cereals are poor in lysine; both taken together in the diet compensate for each other.

FATS (LIPIDS)

Lipids are a concentrated source of energy and provide insulation to the body. One gram of long chain fat provides 9 Cal. They help in digestion, absorption, and transport of fat-soluble vitamins, and are precursors of sex hormones and long chain polyunsaturated fatty acids (PUFAs). Fats improve the palatability of diet and delay gastric emptying. Lipids include triglycerides (fats and oils), phospholipids (lecithin), and sterols (cholesterol); each important to nutrition.

Triglycerides

Triglycerides are the most abundant lipids. Food lipids are 95% triglycerides. Lipids stored in the body are 99% triglycerides. These are esters of 3 molecules of fatty acids attached to glycerol. Glycerol molecule is thus similar in all triglycerides while fatty acids differ in the (*i*) length of carbon chain (short chain, medium chain, and long chain); and (*ii*) degree of unsaturation (saturated, monounsaturated, and polyunsaturated).

- ***Medium chain triglycerides (MCTs):*** These are fatty acids containing 8–14 carbon atoms. They can be absorbed directly into the portal veins without the help of lipase or bile salts. Hence, MCTs will be absorbed even in conditions with fat malabsorption. Coconut oil and cotton seed oil are rich sources of MCTs.
- ***Saturated fatty acids:*** These are primarily derived from animal sources (except coconut oil) and remain solid at 20–30°C. Palmitic and stearic acids are saturated fatty acids. These can be synthesized in the body from the acetate residues following catabolism of carbohydrates and protein.
- ***Unsaturated fatty acids:*** These are usually liquid at room temperature, and obtained from vegetables, nut, or seed sources. Unsaturated fats may be converted to solid fats by hydrogenation. *Monounsaturated fatty acids* (MUFAs), such as oleic acid, have only one point of unsaturation while PUFAs have two or more points of unsaturation. Fatty acids with one unsaturated link can also be synthesized in the body, but PUFAs cannot be adequately synthesized in the body.

Two families of PUFA are important: (*a*) *omega-6 fatty acids* [linoleic acid (LA: 18:2 omega-6) and arachidonic acid (AA: 20:4 omega-6)] and (*b*) *omega-3 fatty acids* [alpha-linolenic acid (ALA: 18:3 omega-3), eicosapentaenoic acid (EPA: 20:5 omega-3), and docosahexaenoic acid (DHA: 22:6 omega-3)].

Hydrogenation of vegetable oils will convert the unsaturated fats in them to saturated fats. Hydrogenation increases the storage life and baking quality of the oils. But saturated fat increases the blood level of low-density lipoprotein (LDL) cholesterol.

Essential Fatty Acids

The EFAs are omega-6 or omega-3 PUFAs. PUFAs are important components of cell membrane, besides being involved as inflammatory mediator precursors for prostaglandin (PG). These EFAs constitute a major component of the phospholipids of central nervous system. They are also needed to produce prostaglandins and thromboxanes. EFAs are essential for normal fetal and infant growth, brain growth, and visual acuity. These should be available in the diet for maintaining good health and are referred to as EFAs. At least 3% of energy requirement of an individual should be derived from linoleic and linolenic acids. Important EFAs include linoleic acid, arachidonic acid, linolenic acid, EPA, and DHA. Linoleic acid is present in vegetable oils and human milk. ALA is present in fish oil and flax seed.

Eicosapentaenoic acid and DHA lower blood cholesterol and triglyceride concentrations—these may also serve as raw materials for synthesis of eicosanoids (prostaglandins, thromboxane, and leukotrienes). Eicosanoids play an important role in regulation of lipid concentration, blood pressure, immune response, and inflammatory response to injury and infection. EPA produces the series-3 prostanoids, e.g., PG_3, thromboxane-3 (Tx3), and PGI3. PG3 and Tx3 inhibit formation of series-2 prostanoids (PG2 and Tx2), which favor atherogenesis. DHA is especially active in retina and cerebral cortex.

Body can synthesize very small amounts of (*i*) arachidonic acid from ingested linoleic acid; and (*ii*) EPA and DHA from linolenic acid. But the endogenous synthesis is not enough to sustain the body demands, therefore, omega lipids have to be supplied in diet.

Normal diet with vegetable oils is usually sufficient in omega-6 lipids but may lack optimal quantity of omega-3 lipids. Omega-3, especially DHA and EPA are plentiful in fish. Conventional formula milk may contain linoleic acid and linolenic acid but is low in arachidonic acid. Arachidonic acid is plentiful in meat. Mustard oil, safflower oil, corn oil, and sunflower oil are rich in polyunsaturated EFAs.

Deficiency of EFAs in the diet may result in growth retardation, reproductive failure, skin disorders, increased susceptibility to infections, decreased myocardial contractility, renal hypertension, and hemolysis. Selective deficiency of omega-6 fatty acids leads to skin changes while lack of omega-3 results in neurological and visual symptoms. Omega-6: omega-3 ratio of 5:1 or less is ideal for cardiovascular health. High omega-6 and low omega-3 content as in ground nut and sunflower oil, respectively can lead on to free radical injury, angiotoxicity, and impaired immune function.

Recommended Intake of Fats

Total fat intake (beyond infancy) should provide no >30% of daily energy intake. Saturated fats should not exceed 10% and *trans* fatty acids should not exceed 1% of total energy intake from fats. A minimum of 3% energy from n-6 PUFA and 0.6–1.2% energy from n-3 PUFA for a 2,000 Kcal diet is required. Approximately, 6% energy should be derived from PUFA (with at least 2.5% from linoleic acid and 0.5% from linolenic acid).

Excess fat contributes to obesity, type-2 diabetes, cancer, hypertension, and atherosclerosis. It is better to avoid excess of total fats, *trans* fats, saturated fats, and cholesterol, in that order of priority.

DIETARY FIBER

Dietary fiber refers to the edible components in plant materials that are not digested in the small intestine. Instead, they are digested and absorbed in the large intestine. Fiber components include polysaccharides such as cellulose, hemicellulose, pectins, gums, mucilages, and nonpolysaccharide lignins. Organic acids (butyric acid) and polyols (sorbitol) are also considered as part of fiber. Gums, pectin, and mucilage are examples of water-soluble fibers and hemicelluloses, cellulose, lignin are water insoluble fibers. Fibers insoluble in water result in softening of stools and acceleration of intestinal transit time. This property helps in preventing constipation, hemorrhoids and diverticulitis. The large water-holding capacity of soluble dietary fiber allows it to bind to bile acids, helps to reduce blood cholesterol levels, and limit glucose absorption. Bacteria in the large intestine ferment soluble fiber, generating short-chain fatty acids (SCFAs) that contributes to favorable composition of the gastrointestinal tract flora.

Whole grains, cereals, pulses, legumes, vegetables, and fruits are excellent sources of dietary fiber. Fruits and vegetables contain more water-soluble fiber. An adequate fiber consumption can be achieved by having at least two servings of fruits, three servings of vegetables, and six servings of grain products per day after the age of 2 years. Consumption of 30 g/2,000 kcal is recommended for fibers based on energy intake, by ICMR in 2020 (**Table 8.1**). World Health Organization (WHO) recommends intake of >25 g of total dietary fiber in children >10 years or older, 21 g/day in 6–9 years, and >15 g/day in 2–5 years old. However, consumption of >60 g a day can reduce the absorption of nutrients and may cause bowel irritation or diarrhea and can lead to flatulence, diarrhea, and decreased appetite.

High-fiber diet decreases the rate of glucose absorption and may prevent cardiovascular disease and colonic cancer. High fiber diet is advocated for chronic constipation, diabetes, obesity, and hypercholesterolemia. Low fiber diet is particularly useful in irritable bowel syndrome, chronic colitis, and partial chronic gastrointestinal obstruction.

Traditionally, fiber was considered a non-nutrient food component, but soluble fiber fermenting in the colon provides 2 kcal/g of fiber. Staple foods such as wheat and rice with about 13 g of digested fiber can contribute around 50 kcal to the calorie intake. Fiber intake is not calculated for infants up to 12 months of age who are breastfed.

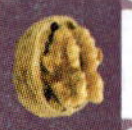

IN A NUTSHELL

Nutrients and Nutritional Requirements

1. Of the total energy, at least 10–15% should be provided by proteins, 20–30% by fats, and 50–60% by carbohydrates.
2. Free sugar intake should not be >5% of total calorie intake.
3. As per standard Indian predominantly vegetarian diet, a person requires 1.0 g/kg body weight of protein daily.
4. Saturated fats should not exceed 10% and *trans* fatty acids should not exceed 1% of total energy intake from fats.

Indian Council of Medical Research. Dietary Guidelines for Indians: A Manual, 2nd edition. Hyderabad: National Institute of Nutrition, ICMR; 2011 and 2024.

ICMR. Nutrient requirements for Indians: a report of the expert group. ICMR, National Institute of Nutrition; 2024.

Dietary Guidelines for Indians. https://www.nin.res.in/downloads/DietaryGuidelinesforNINwebsite.pdf [Last accessed August, 2025].

WHO: WHO updates guidelines on fats and carbohydrates [2023, online]. Available from https://www.who.int/news/item/17-07-2023-who-updates-guidelines-on-fats-and-carbohydrates. [Last accessed August, 2025]

8.2 Nutritional Value of Foods

PE 9.3

INTRODUCTION

Indian Council of Medical Research-National Institute of Nutrition (ICMR-NIN) 2024 classifies food into 10 groups based on their nutritive value namely (1) Cereals and millets, (2) Pulses, (3) Vegetables, (4) Nuts, oil seeds and fats, (5) Green leafy vegetables (GLVs), (6) Fruits, (7) Dairy, (8) Root and tuber, (9) Flesh foods, (10) Spices and herbs. To fulfill the nutritional requirement of the body, it is important to include each group in daily diet, in the recommended proportion. Nutritive values of common food items in these groups are provided in **Tables 8.2 to 8.10.** Foods can also be categorized according to their functions:

- ***Energy-rich food:*** Carbohydrate-rich foods such as cereals, millets, sugar, starchy vegetables, and the fat-rich foods such as oil, ghee, butter, nuts, and oilseeds are rich in calories. Intake of these foods is must for physical activity and maintenance of overall health, growth, and recovery from illness.
- ***Body building food:*** Protein rich foods, e.g., pulses, legumes, and nuts; milk and other dairy products, egg, meat, and fish, belong to this group. This category is vital for growth spurt, maturation, and bone development.
- ***Protective food:*** Protective food comprises of vitamin and mineral rich food sources such as fruits and vegetables, eggs, milk, and milk products. Food material from this group is required to fight infections in children and prevent oxidative damage.

CEREALS AND MILLETS

Cereals (e.g., wheat, rice, corn, oats, and barley) form the major staple food in most parts of the world. They furnish generous amounts of energy and nutrients at low-cost. Rice and wheat are the most widely consumed cereals. Cereals are an economical source of energy, mainly contributed by starch and fat, and a significant source of protein (6–12%), although of low BV (incomplete protein). Cereals are better utilized when supplemented by the more complete proteins of milk, meat, and eggs as they supply the amino acids lacking in cereals. Nearly 20% of cereals (raw weight) should be consumed in form of millets in children <10 years and 20–30% in children >10 years.

Whole grain cereals are considerable sources of iron, phosphorus, thiamine, zinc, manganese, folate, magnesium, copper, niacin, vitamin B_6, selenium, vitamin A, and dietary fiber. Cereals are easily digestible, supply roughage, and have a laxative property. Incorrect cooking practices lead to loss of water-soluble vitamins, i.e., by cooking in large volume of water and draining away the excess of it.

PULSES AND LEGUMES

Pulses and legumes are the essential components of vegetarian diets due to their high protein content (20–40%). Groundnut and soybean are rich in oils. They are also good sources of Ca, Mg, Zn, Fe, K, and P, and are rich in niacin, but poor in riboflavin and contain small amounts of carotene. Legumes are excellent sources of dietary fiber and folate.

Germination improves the nutritive value of pulses. The ascorbic acid riboflavin, niacin, choline, and biotin content increase considerably, and antinutritional factors (phytates and tannins) and toxic factors are eliminated. Fermentation increases digestibility, palatability, and improves availability of essential amino acids.

VEGETABLES, GLVs, TUBERS, AND ROOTS

Vegetables vary widely in their composition and nutritive value, depending on the part of the plant, which is used as a vegetable. Water is the major constituent of vegetables (about 99%). Vegetables contribute to the bulk of the diet and are low in calories, proteins, and fats. Green leafy vegetables (GLV) such

Table 8.2 Nutritive Value of Common Cereals (per 100 g of Edible Portion)

Name of foodstuff	*Energy (kcal)*	*Protein (g)*	*Fat (g)*	*CHO (g)*	*Crude fibers (g)*	*Zinc (mg)*	*Iron (mg)*	*Calcium (mg)*
Bajra (*Pennisetum typhoideum*)	347	11.0	5.4	61.8	11.5	2.8	6.4	27.4
Maize, dry (*Zea mays*)	333	8.8	3.8	64.8	12.2	2.3	2.5	8.9
Ragi (*Eleusine coracana*)	320	7.2	1.9	66.8	11.2	2.5	4.6	364.0
Rice, raw, milled (*Oryza sativa*)	355	7.9	0.5	78.2	2.8	1.2	0.7	7.5
Rice, puffed (*Oryza sativa*)	360	7.5	1.6	77.7	2.6	1.5	4.6	15.1
Wheat, whole (*Triticum aestivum*)	321	10.6	1.5	64.7	11.2	2.9	4.0	39.4
Wheat, flour, refined (*Triticum aestivum*)	350	10.4	0.8	74.3	2.8	0.9	1.8	20.5
Jowar (*Sorghum vulgare*)	333	10.0	1.7	67.7	10.2	2.0	4.0	27.6

(CHO: carbohydrate)

Source: Indian Food Composition Tables. National Institute of Nutrition, Indian Council of Medical Research; 2017

Table 8.3 Nutritive Value of Commonly Consumed Pulses (per 100 g of Edible Portion)

Name of foodstuff	*Energy (kcal)*	*Protein (g)*	*Fat (g)*	*CHO (g)*	*Crude fibers (g)*	*Zinc (mg)*	*Iron (mg)*	*Calcium (mg)*
Bengal gram, dal (*Cicer arietinum*)	328	21.6	5.3	46.7	15.2	3.7	6.1	46.4
Black gram, dal (*Phaseolus mungo*)	323	23.1	1.7	51.0	11.9	3.0	4.7	55.7
Green gram, whole (*Phaseolus aureus*)	293	22.5	1.5	46.1	17.0	2.7	6.8	150.0
Green gram, dal (*Phaseolus aureus*)	325	23.9	1.4	52.6	9.4	2.5	3.9	43.1
Moth beans (*Vigna aconitifolia*)	307	19.8	1.8	52.1	15.1	1.9	7.9	154.0
Rajma, red (*Phaseolus vulgaris*)	298	19.9	1.8	48.6	16.6	2.7	6.1	126.0
Soybean, white (*Glycine max*)	376	37.8	19.4	10.2	22.6	3.5	8.2	195.0

(CHO: carbohydrate)

Source: Indian Food Composition Tables. National Institute of Nutrition, Indian Council of Medical Research; 2017

Table 8.4 Nutritive Value of Common Vegetables (per 100 g of Edible Portion)

Name of foodstuff	*Energy (kcal)*	*Protein (g)*	*Fat (g)*	*CHO (g)*	*Crude fibers (g)*	*Zinc (mg)*	*Iron (mg)*	*Calcium (mg)*
Roots and tubers								
Carrot, red (*Daucus carota*)	38	1.0	0.5	6.7	4.5	0.3	0.7	41.1
Colocasia (*Colocasia antiquorum*)	89	3.3	0.2	17.9	3.2	0.4	0.7	30.2
Onion big (*Allium cepa*)	48	1.5	0.2	9.6	2.5	0.4	0.4	21.0
Potato (brown skin big) (*Solanum tuberosum*)	70	1.5	0.2	14.9	1.7	0.3	0.6	9.5
Radish, round white skin (*Raphanus sativus*)	31	0.8	0.1	6.1	2.4	0.2	0.4	30.2
Leafy vegetables								
Bathua leaves (*Chenopodium album*)	27.6	2.5	0.4	2.6	4.0	1.0	2.7	211.0
Cabbage, green (*Brassica oleracea var. capitata f. alba*)	21.4	1.4	0.1	3.3	2.8	0.2	0.4	51.8
Fenugreek leaves (*Trigonella foenum-graecum*)	34.3	3.7	0.8	2.2	4.9	0.5	5.7	0.00
Lettuce (*Lactuca sativa*)	21.6	1.5	0.3	3.0	1.8	0.5	2.7	0.00
Mustard leaves (*Brassica juncea*)	30.2	3.5	0.5	2.4	3.9	0.7	2.8	0.00
Spinach (*Spinacia oleracea*)	24.2	2.1	0.6	2.1	2.4	0.5	3.0	82.3
Other vegetables								
Bitter gourd, jagged, teeth ridges, elongate (*Momordica charantia*)	20.7	1.4	0.24	2.8	3.8	0.3	1.2	21.4
Brinjal-all varieties (*Solanum melongena*)	25.2	1.5	0.32	3.5	4.0	0.2	0.4	16.6
Cauliflower (*Brassica oleracea*)	22.8	2.2	0.44	2.0	3.2	0.3	1.0	25.2
Cucumber, green elongalo (*Cucumis sativus*)	19.5	0.7	0.16	3.5	2.1	0.2	0.5	16.4
French beans, country (*Phaseolus vulgaris*)	24.2	2.5	0.26	2.7	4.4	0.5	1.3	56.0
Jackfruit, raw (*Artocarpus heterophyllus*)	26.2	2.0	0.35	3.5	7.7	0.2	0.3	45.7
Ladies fingers (*Abelmoschus esculentus*)	27.3	2.1	0.22	3.6	4.1	0.5	0.8	86.1
Pumpkin fruit, orange, round (*Cucurbita maxima*)	23.0	0.8	0.16	4.00	2.6	0.1	0.4	23.1
Tinda, tender (*Praecitrullus fistulosus*)	13.8	1.0	0.17	1.9	2.0	0.2	0.4	19.7

(CHO: carbohydrate)

Source: Indian Food Composition Tables. National Institute of Nutrition, Indian Council of Medical Research; 2017

Table 8.5 Nutritive Value of Common Fruits (per 100 g of Edible Portion)

Name of foodstuff	Energy (kcal)	Protein (g)	Fat (g)	CHO (g)	Crude fibers (g)	Zinc (mg)	Iron (mg)	Calcium (mg)
Apple, big (*Malus domestica*)	62.1	0.3	0.64	13.1	2.6	0.1	0.3	13.7
Banana, ripe (*Musa x paradisiaca*)	110.2	1.3	0.32	30.0	2.2	0.2	0.4	6.8
Grapes, seeded, round, green (*Vitis vinifera*)	56.0	0.8	0.29	12.2	1.3	0.1	0.2	11.2
Guava, white flesh (*Psidium guajava*)	32.1	1.4	0.32	5.1	8.6	0.2	0.3	18.5
Jambu fruit, ripe (*Syzygium cumini*)	56.0	0.8	0.17	12.3	3.1	0.1	0.3	25.4
Lemon, juice (*Citrus limon*)	36.4	0.4	0.75	7.0	0	0.1	0.1	22.7
Litchi (*Nephelium litchi*)	53.5	1.0	0.26	11.4	1.3	0.2	0.8	5.8
Mango, ripe, kesar (*Mangifera indica*)	55	0.5	0.57	11.4	2.0	0.1	0.0	15.7
Watermelon, dark green (Sugar baby) (*Citrullus vulgaris*)	287	2.9	0.15	67.4	5.3	0.1	0.2	5.3
Orange, pulp (*Citrus aurantium*)	37	0.7	0.1	7.9	1.3	0.0	0.8	19.5
Papaya, ripe (*Carica papaya*)	24	0.42	0.2	4.6	2.8	0.1	0.2	15.0
Pineapple (*Ananas comosus*)	43	0.52	0.2	9.4	3.5	0.1	0.3	10.9
Pomegranate, maroon seeds (*Punica granatum*)	55	1.33	0.2	11.6	2.8	0.2	0.3	10.7
Tomato, ripe, hybrid (*Lycopersicon esculentum*)	19	0.8	0.3	3.2	1.6	0.1	0.2	8.9

(CHO: carbohydrate)

Source: Indian Food Composition Tables. National Institute of Nutrition, Indian Council of Medical Research; 2017

Table 8.6 Nutritive Value of Milk (per 100 mL)

Name of foodstuff	Energy (kcal)	Protein (g)	Fat (g)	CHO (g)	Zinc (mg)	Iron (mg)	Calcium (mg)
Milk, whole, buffalo	107	3.7	6.6	8.4	0.3	0.2	121.0
Milk, whole, cow	73	3.3	4.5	4.9	0.3	0.2	118.0
Paneer	257	18.9	14.8	12.4	2.7	0.9	476.0
Khoa	315	16.3	20.6	16.5	2.3	2.3	602.0

(CHO: carbohydrate)

Source: Indian Food Composition Tables. National Institute of Nutrition, Indian Council of Medical Research; 2017

Table 8.7 Nutritive Value of Egg, Meat, Fish (per 100 g of Edible Portion)

Name of foodstuff	Energy (kcal)	Protein (g)	Fat (g)	Zinc (mg)	Iron (mg)	Calcium (g)
Fish and other sea foods						
Catfish (*Tandanus tandanus*)	123	15.9	6.2	0.7	0.8	22.0
Catla (*Catla catla*)	94	17.9	2.2	0.7	1.1	43.5
Crab (*Menippe mercenaria*)	82	10.2	1.4	0.8	1.1	128.0
Crab (*Pachygrapsus sp.*)	102	19.7	2.4	2.5	1.1	199.0
Hilsa (*Tenualosa ilisha*)	258	21.8	18.5	0.6	1.2	19.8
Lobster, brown (*Thenus orientalis*)	70	16.0	0.6	1.2	0.7	73.1
Oyster (*Crassostrea sp.*)	60	9.5	2.4	7.4	0.9	126.0
Pomfret, white (*Pampus argenteus*)	122	19.0	5.1	0.5	0.3	13.6
Prawns, Big (*Macrobrachium rosenbergii*)	73	13.2	0.9	1.4	0.8	48.6
Rohu (*Labeo rohita*)	203	17.1	16.8	0.8	1.0	39.4
Salmon (*Salmo salar*)	172	21.0	9.9	0.5	1.0	24.3
Sardine (*Sardinella longiceps*)	152	17.9	9.0	0.9	0.8	42.3
Tuna (*Euthynnus affinis*)	112	24.5	1.4	0.7	1.6	9.8

Contd...

Contd...

Name of foodstuff	Energy (kcal)	Protein (g)	Fat (g)	Zinc (mg)	Iron (mg)	Calcium (g)
Meat and poultry						
Chicken, poultry, leg, skinless	382	19.4	12.6	1.8	1.3	20.5
Egg, country hen, whole, raw	168	13.1	13	1.1	1.6	50.1
Egg, poultry, whole, raw	134	13.3	9.2	1.2	1.8	49.4
Goat, chops	135	20.4	6.0	4.6	1.9	7.4
Goat, shoulder	187	20.3	11.9	4.2	1.5	6.2
Pork, shoulder	236	17.4	18.8	2.1	0.9	10.0
Turkey, breast, with skin	160	22.0	8.0	1.3	1.0	14.4

Source: Indian Food Composition Tables. National Institute of Nutrition, Indian Council of Medical Research; 2017

Table 8.8 Nutritive Value of Nuts and Oilseeds (per 100 g of Edible Portion)

Name of foodstuff	Energy (kcal)	Protein (g)	Fat (g)	CHO (g)	Crude fibers (g)	Zinc (mg)	Iron (mg)	Calcium (mg)
Almond (*Prunus amygdalus*)	607	18.4	58.5	3.0	13.1	3.5	4.6	228.0
Cashew nut (*Anacardium occidentale*)	580	18.8	45.2	25.5	3.9	5.3	6.0	34.0
Coconut, kernel, dry (*Cocos nucifera*)	622	7.3	63.3	8.0	15.9	1.4	3.1	32.0
Coconut, kernel, fresh (Cocos nucifera)	407	3.8	41.4	6.3	10.4	0.6	1.3	8.0
Groundnut (*Arachis hypogea*)	518	23.7	39.6	17.3	10.4	3.2	3.4	54.0
Pistachio nut (*Pistacia vera*)	537	23.4	42.5	15.8	10.6	2.4	4.5	135.0
Walnut (*Juglans regia*)	669	14.9	64.3	10.1	5.4	2.9	3.2	105.0

(CHO: carbohydrate)

Source: Indian Food Composition Tables. National Institute of Nutrition, Indian Council of Medical Research; 2017

Table 8.9 Nutritive Value of Sugar and Jaggery (per 100 g of Edible Portion)

Name of foodstuff	Energy (kcal)	Protein (g)	Fat (g)	CHO (g)	Zinc (mg)	Iron (mg)	Calcium (mg)
Honey							
Jaggery, cane (*Saccharum officinarum*)	352	1.9	0.2	84.9	0.5	4.6	107.0
Sugarcane, juice (*Saccharum officinarum*)	58	0.2	0.4	13.1	0.1	1.1	18.0

(CHO: carbohydrate)

Source: Indian Food Composition Tables. National Institute of Nutrition, Indian Council of Medical Research; 2017

as spinach (*palak*), fenugreek (*methi*), *chaulai*, cabbage are good sources of vitamin A, iron, ascorbic acid, calcium, and B-group vitamins. Tuberous vegetables such as potato, sweet potato, and yam (*garadu* or *ratalu*) are good sources of carbohydrates, but are poor in proteins, vitamins, and minerals. Carrots have rich amounts of beta carotene.

FRUITS

Fruits are valued for their minerals, vitamins, and digestible fiber. Citrus fruits and guava are rich in ascorbic acid, whereas yellow fruits contain carotenoids (precursors of vitamin A). Bananas provide calories in a nonresidue diet. They act as a mild laxative in constipation. Fruits are not good sources of calcium, phosphorus, and iron. However, dried apricots, dates, and grapefruit are fair sources of iron and calcium.

Vegetables and fruits are also rich sources of phytonutrients, which act as natural antioxidants. Eating a wide variety of fruits and vegetables is recommended as a preventive measure against various free-radical mediated diseases.

MILK AND MILK PRODUCTS (DAIRY PRODUCTS)

Milk and milk products are rich sources of calcium, protein, and riboflavin, good sources of vitamin A, phosphorus, and

Table 8.10 Nutritive Value of Condiments and Spices (per 100 g of Edible Portion)

Name of foodstuff	Energy (kcal)	Protein (g)	Fat (g)	CHO (g)	Crude fibers (g)	Zinc (mg)	Iron (mg)	Calcium (mg)
Asafoetida (*Ferula assa-foetida*)	330	6.3	10.3	72.0	5.1	1.0	15.7	266.0
Cardamom, green (*Elettaria cardamomum*)	254	8.1	2.6	47.8	23.1	3.7	8.3	378.0
Chilies, red (*Capsicum annuum*)	236	12.7	6.4	29.5	31.2	1.7	6.2	99.8
Cloves dry (*Syzygium aromaticum*)	186	5.9	8.4	18.7	34.5	1.1	9.4	567.0
Coriander, seeds (*Coriandrum sativum*)	268	10.7	17.5	13.0	44.8	3.9	17.6	718.0
Cumin seeds (*Cuminum cyminum*)	303	13.9	16.6	22.6	30.4	4.3	8.5	135.0
Fenugreek seeds (*Trigonella foenum-graecum*)	234	25.4	5.7	10.6	47.6	3.8	8.5	135.0
Ginger fresh (*Zingiber officinale*)	55	2.2	0.9	9.0	5.4	0.4	1.9	18.9
Pepper, black (*Piper nigrum*)	217	10.1	2.7	36.2	33.2	1.2	11.9	405.0
Turmeric powder (*Curcuma domestica*)	280	7.7	5.0	49.2	21.4	2.6	46.1	122.0

(CHO: carbohydrate)

Source: Indian Food Composition Tables. National Institute of Nutrition, Indian Council of Medical Research; 2017

thiamine; and poor sources of iron and ascorbic acid. Milk is the only sources of vitamin B_{12} for strict vegetarians and the only natural source of lactose.

EGG, MEAT, AND FISH (FLESH FOODS)

- ***Egg:*** It consists of approximately 11% shell, 58% white, and 31% yolk. Egg protein is considered a standard or reference protein. It supplies generous amounts of both fat- and water-soluble vitamins. Vitamin C is present in small quantity. Calcium, phosphorus, iron, and zinc are also present in egg. Iron and vitamin A are contained only in the yolk. Egg is easily digestible and low in fiber hence, suited for convalescing.
- ***Meat:*** Meats contain about 15–20% proteins of high-nutritive value, with good amounts of essential amino acids. Fat content of meat varies between 5–40%. Organ meats (liver and kidney) are iron rich, especially heme iron, which is more bioavailable than the nonheme iron found in plant sources. Meat also provides zinc and B-vitamins. It is a poor source of calcium. Liver is a rich source of vitamin A.
- ***Fish:*** It is an excellent source of proteins (16–20%) of good BV, and of unsaturated fats especially omega-3 fats. Vitamin A and D are plenty in fish liver oils. B-vitamins and ascorbic acid present in raw fish are heat labile. Fish is also rich in calcium and phosphorus.

NUTS, OIL AND SEEDS

Nuts and oil seeds: These are good sources of energy and contain good quality proteins in small amounts. Nuts contain appreciable amounts of carbohydrates, B-group vitamins, vitamin E, and some minerals such as calcium, phosphorus, and iron. Oilseed proteins are of inferior quality as they lack methionine. But, being rich in lysine, they can be used to supplement cereals for development of weaning foods.

SPICES AND HERBS

- ***Condiments and spices:*** These are used as flavoring substances. Chilies and coriander (dhania) have little amounts of bcarotene. Most of them contain tannin, which interferes with absorption of iron. Garlic is considered to have antibacterial property. Turmeric, ginger, garlic, cumin, and cloves are rich in antioxidants. Excessive amounts of condiments cause gastritis peptic ulcers.
- ***Salt:*** Sodium is vital to nerve conduction and fluid balance in the body. High intake of salt (sodium chloride) is associated with high blood pressure, and reduction in bone density due to increased calcium excretion. Preserved foods such as pickles, papads, sauces, ketchup, and canned foods contribute to higher intakes of salt. The intake of sodium chloride should not exceed 4–5 g/day.

OTHERS

- ***Sugar and jaggery:*** They contribute calories and palatability to the diet. Some amount of iron is also obtained from jaggery. However, excessive amounts of sugar should be avoided as it might cause dental caries in small children. Intake of free sugar should be <5% of total energy. Sugar sweetened beverage mostly supplies empty calories without nutritional value.
- ***Tea and coffee:*** Caffeinated drinks, in any form should not be given at all to children <5 years [Indian Academy of Pediatrics (IAP), 2019]. Older children should not consume >100 mg of caffeine per day. Higher intake of caffeine can lead to anxiety, nervousness, higher blood pressure, arrhythmia, and insomnia.
- ***Soft beverages:*** Synthetic drinks are best avoided as they contain artificial colors, flavors, and preservatives, but no nutrients. Carbonated beverages also affect appetite adversely and damage teeth enamel due to the phosphoric acid content.

Packaged fruit juices are high in sugar. Whole fruit is always better than even fresh juice. IAP does not recommend any fruit juices in children <2 years. Natural drinks such as *lassi*, coconut water, and buttermilk are healthier options.

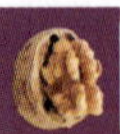

IN A NUTSHELL

Nutritional Value of Foods

1. Ten main food groups are: (1) Cereals and millets, (2) Pulses, (3) Vegetables, (4) Nuts, oil seeds and fats, (5) Green leafy vegetables, (6) Fruits, (7) Dairy, (8) Root and tuber, (9) Flesh foods, (10) Spices and herbs.
2. Carbohydrates are classified as energy rich food, proteins as body building food, and vitamins and minerals as protective food.
3. Milk is the only source of vitamin B_{12} for strict vegetarians and the only natural source of lactose.
4. Caffeinated drinks or caffeine in any form should not be given to children <5 years.

Centre for Disease Control (CDC). (2022). Childhood Nutrition Facts. [online] Available from https://www.cdc.gov/school-nutrition/facts/?CDC_AAref_Val=https://www.cdc.gov/healthyschools/nutrition/facts.html [Last accessed August, 2025].

Gupta P, Shah D, Kumar P, et al. Indian Academy of Pediatrics Guidelines on the fast and junk foods, sugar sweetened beverages, fruit juices, and energy drinks. Indian Pediatr. 2019;56(10):849-63.

Indian Council of Medical Research. Dietary Guidelines for Indians—A Manual. Hyderabad: National Institute of Nutrition, ICMR; 2024.

8.3 Nutritional Assessment

PE 9.2, PE 9.4, PE 9.5, PE 9.6

INTRODUCTION

Nutritional status is the condition of health of an individual or population as influenced by utilization of the nutrients. It can be determined with the help of nutritional assessment, which includes the interpretation of anthropometric, biochemical, clinical, and dietary data. Nutritional assessment can be done by both direct and indirect methods.

- ***Direct methods:*** It include elicitation of clinical signs, nutritional anthropometry, and various biochemical tests and field surveys.
- ***Indirect nutritional assessment:*** Based on vital statistics, mortality and morbidity rates, and the study of ecological factors. We will discuss each of the methods in brief.

NUTRITIONAL ANTHROPOMETRY

Nutritional anthropometry is based on the fact that physical state and gross composition of body are influenced by diet and nutrition, especially in the rapidly growing period of early childhood, and adolescence.

Depending on the anthropometric indicators selected, it can be used for various purposes such as screening at-risk children and measuring short-term or long-term changes in nutritional status. However, there are inherent limitations in using anthropometry as a tool for nutritional assessment. Changes in anthropometry may take some time after nutritional deprivation to set in and for linear growth retardation the deprivation may be long standing. Also, simple anthropometry in the context of overnutrition may cause difficulty in distinguishing lean from adipose tissue thus failing to distinguish well-built from obese people. Despite these limitations, anthropometry is the most practical way of measuring nutritional status of individuals or populations.

Anthropometric Tools

The four measures used to undertake anthropometric assessment are: (i) age, (ii) sex, (iii) weight, and (iv) height or length. Each of these variables provides one piece of information about a person. When they are used together, they can provide important information about a person's nutritional status. When two of these measurements are used together, they are called an *index*. The indices commonly used in assessing the nutritional status of children are "weight-for-age", "length-for-age or height-for-age", "weight-for-length or weight-for-height" and body mass index. There are many other anthropometric measures including mid-upper arm circumference (MUAC), waist-hip ratio, and skinfold thickness.

Anthro-based Nutritional Assessment

World Health Organization classification of undernutrition is based on comparing the growth of children from birth to 5 years with the WHO Child Growth Standards. These standards were derived from children who were raised in environments that minimized constraints to growth. Their mothers followed healthy practices such as exclusive breastfeeding and not smoking during and after pregnancy. WHO standards can be used to assess children (0–5 years) everywhere, regardless of ethnicity, socioeconomic status, and type of feeding.

World Health Organization has prepared reference percentiles and *Z*-score curves (and Tables) for weight-for-age, length/height-for-age, weight-for-length/height and body mass index-for-age for children <5 years of age (separately for boys and girls). WHO has also developed a software for ease of growth monitoring using computers. This Anthro software is available for free download and use from WHO website. It automatically calculates the *Z*-scores as well as prepares the required graphs.

Three standard indices of physical growth that describe the nutritional status of children are described here:

1. ***Wasting:*** It is measured by weight for length/height (WFL or WFH). It indicates a deficit in tissue and fat mass and may result either from failure to gain weight or from weight loss. Wasting represents the failure to receive adequate nutrition in the period immediately preceding the measurement may be the result of inadequate food intake or a recent episode of illness causing loss of weight and the acute onset of malnutrition. Children whose WFL/WFH *Z*-score is below minus two standard deviations (–2 SD) from the median of the reference population are considered thin (*wasted*) for their height and are acutely malnourished. Children whose weight-for-height is below minus three standard deviations (–3 SD) from the median of the reference population are considered to be *severely wasted.*
2. ***Stunting:*** It reflects failure to receive adequate nutrition over a long period of time and is also affected by recurrent and chronic illness. *Height-for-age* represents stunting. Children whose height-for-age *Z*-score is below minus two standard deviations (–2 SD) from the median of the reference population are considered short for their age (*stunted*) and are chronically malnourished. Children below minus three standard deviations (–3 SD) from the median of the reference population are considered to be *severely stunted.* Stunting may also be a residue of past malnutrition or could be due to non-nutritional disorders like genetic short stature or endocrinal disorders.
3. ***Underweight:*** It is measured by *weight-for-age* and is a composite index of height-for-age and weight-for-height. It considers both acute and chronic malnutrition. Children whose weight-for-age is below minus two standard deviations from the median of the reference population are classified as *underweight.* Children whose weight-for-age is below minus three standard deviations (–3 SD) from the median of the reference population are *severely underweight.*

Wasting and stunting are frequently coexistent and a greater and disproportionate reduction in weight as compared to reduction in height indicates acute or chronic undernutrition. The WHO recommends the use of SD classification to categorize the children in different grades of nutritional status (**Table 8.11**). This classification is also used for assessing the magnitude of malnutrition amongst under-five children in national health programs.

Another age independent growth parameter often used for determining the severity of undernutrition is 'mid-upper arm circumference (MUAC). A MUAC of <11.5 cm and 11.5–12.5 cm for children between 6–59 months years is considered as a marker of severe wasting and wasting respectively.

In children <6 months, anthropometric criteria to identify those at risk of poor growth and development include WAZ <–2 SD, WLZ <–3 SD, MUAC <110 mm for infants between 6 weeks and less than 6 months of age and failure to gain weight based on two consecutive measurements.

Table 8.11 WHO Classification for Undernutrition

	Moderate undernutrition	*Severe undernutrition*
Symmetrical edema	No	Yes* *Edematous malnutrition*
Weight for height (measure of wasting)	SD score† –2 to –3 (70–79% of expected‡) *Moderate Wasting*	SD score† <–3 (<70% of expected) *Severe Wasting*
Height for age (measure of stunting)	SD score† –2 to –3 (85–89% of expected‡) *Moderate Stunting*	SD score† < –3 (<85% of expected) *Severe Stunting*

*This includes kwashiorkor and marasmic kwashiorkor

†SD score = observed value – expected value standard deviation of reference population

‡Median (50th percentile of WHO standards)

BIOCHEMICAL ASSESSMENT

Biochemical tests can identify specific nutrition related abnormalities. These may help to indicate nutritional abnormality (marginal malnutrition) even prior to clinical or anthropometric changes. Most of the biochemical tests are carried out on serum/blood and urine as they are easily obtainable in the field. The ideal criteria for these tests in the field are that:

- The sample should be easily collectable—for instance, blood sample should be taken either by finger prick or from forearm;
- The test should not be affected by recent meal or water load; and
- It should be easy to conduct and provide additional information not available by nonbiochemical techniques.

The tests most used in surveys are measurement of hemoglobin, thiamine and riboflavin in urine, vitamin A, carotene, ascorbic acid in blood. Micro methods that require only a few drops of blood obtained by finger prick and are sensitive have been developed and applied in survey studies.

CLINICAL ASSESSMENT

This method examines the changes, which are believed to be due to inadequate nutrition that can be felt or seen in the superficial epithelial cells—skin, hair, buccal mucosa, or in the thyroid gland.

Clinical examination has some drawbacks: (a) Sometimes non-nutritional factors can also be the cause for similar clinical appearance. For instance, dry appearance of skin—a sign of xerosis due to vitamin A deficiency can also be a result of hot, dry or windy conditions. (b) Many deficiency states have similar signs and symptoms—glossitis may be observed in riboflavin, niacin, folic acid, and vitamin B_{12} deficiencies leading to lack of specificity and subjectivity of some of the physical signs. (c) Malnutrition cannot be quantified on the basis of clinical signs. (d) Many deficiencies are unaccompanied by physical signs.

Despite all these drawbacks, the method has many advantages. It is cheap and does not require elaborate equipment or expensive laboratory tools. Other members of the community can be taught to recognize these clinical signs with training and supervision. It gives quick results and is easy to use.

Diagnosis of anemia by looking at the palmar creases is the most common employed method of clinical assessment. Presence of goiter, Bitot spots, and visible severe wasting are used to assess hypothyroidism, vitamin A deficiency, and severe acute malnutrition, respectively. A few signs used to assess undernutrition clinically are listed in **Table 8.12**.

Table 8.12 Clinical Signs of Undernutrition

Organ	*Signs*	*Cause*
Hair	• Lack of luster • Thinness and sparseness • Straightness • Dyspigmentation • Flag sign • Easy pluckability	Protein and micronutrient deficiency
Face	• Diffuse depigmentation • Nasolabial dyssebacia • Moon face	Riboflavin or multiple deficiency
Eyes	Pale conjunctiva	Iron, folate or vitamin B_{12} deficiency
	• Bitot spots • Conjunctival xerosis • Corneal xerosis • Keratomalacia • Angular palpebritis	Vitamin A deficiency
Lips	• Angular stomatitis • Angular scars • Cheilosis	Riboflavin and iron deficiency
Tongue	• Edema • Scarlet and raw tongue • Atrophic papillae	Riboflavin and iron deficiency
Teeth	Mottled enamel	Calcium and vitamin D deficiency
Gums	Spongy and bleeding gums	Vitamin C deficiency
Glands	• Thyroid enlargement • Parotid enlargement	Iodine deficiency
Skin	• Xerosis • Follicular hyperkeratosis	Vitamin A, essential fatty acid deficiency
	Petechiae	Vitamin C deficiency
	Pellagrous dermatosis	Niacin deficiency
	• Flaky paint dermatosis • Scrotal and vulval dermatosis	Multiple deficiency
Nails	Koilonychia	
Subcutaneous tissue	• Edema • Amount of subcutaneous fat reduced	Protein and vanadium deficiency
Muscular and skeletal systems	• Muscle wasting • Craniotabes	Protein deficiency
	Frontal and parietal bossing	Vitamin D deficiency
	• Epiphyseal enlargement • Beading of ribs (tender/nontender) • Wide open anterior fontanel • Knock-knees or bow legs • Diffuse or local skeletal deformities • Deformities of thorax	Vitamins D and C deficiency
	Musculoskeletal hemorrhages	Vitamins C and K deficiency
Gastro-intestinal tract	Hepatomegaly	Lipoprotein deficiency
Nervous system	Psychomotor change	Iron and multiple deficiency
	Mental confusion	Vitamin B_6 and B_{12} deficiency
	Sensory loss	Protein, potassium, and vitamin D deficiency
	Motor weakness	Vitamin B_6 and B_{12} deficiency
	Loss of position sense	Vitamin B_6 and B_{12} deficiency
	• Loss of ankle and knee jerks • Calf tenderness	Vitamins B and E deficiency
Cardiovascular system	• Cardiomegaly • Microcardia • Tachycardia	• Thiamine and selenium deficiency • Iron deficiency

DIETARY SURVEY

Nutritional History

Breastfeeding, complementary feeding, and family pot feeding history is taken. Feeding practices are also taken in account.

- ***An average food intake*** (prior falling ill) detail is obtained by a 24-hour recall method. During the mid-week average of a 3-day recall (not including a festival day) is recommended.
- A ***food frequency table*** is used to record the frequency of intake of each food item, i.e., thrice a day, once a week, etc. It is interpreted as daily, frequently (4–6 days/week), occasional (1–3 days/week), or never.
- ***Weighing*** the uncooked as well as the cooked food and then assessing the nutritive value of food eaten are the other methods, but often not practical.

The calculated intake should be finally compared with the recommended dietary allowances for the age.

Group Methods

- ***Food balance sheet:*** On the basis of food availability 'Food balance sheet' for the entire population is prepared. The mean annual amount per person is obtained by dividing the total amount of different foods with the total population of the area.
- ***Household food consumption:*** It is an estimate of the total amount of food used by an entire household for a fixed duration. The most commonly used methods are *food account* (by checking the food inventory), *food list* (by recall), and *food record* (by recording).

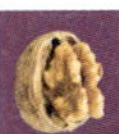

IN A NUTSHELL

Nutritional Assessment

1. Nutritional assessment is done by four methods namely nutritional anthropometry, biochemical assessment, clinical assessment, and dietary survey.
2. Wasting represents acute malnutrition, stunting reflects chronic malnutrition whereas underweight is a composite index of acute and chronic malnutrition.
3. Biochemical tests help to indicate nutritional abnormality prior to clinical or anthropometric changes.

Food and Nutrition Technical Assistance III Project (FANTA). (2016). Module 2. Nutritional Assessment and Classification. [online] Available from https://www.fhi360.org/projects/food-and-nutrition-technical-assistance-iii-fanta-project/ [Last accessed August 2025].

World Health Organization. (2017). Guideline: assessing and managing children at primary health-care facilities to prevent overweight and obesity in the context of the double burden of malnutrition. Updates for the Integrated Management of Childhood Illness (IMCI). [online] Available from https://apps.who.int/iris/handle/10665/259133 [Last accessed August, 2025].

8.4 Diet in Health and Disease

PE 9.7

DIET IN HEALTH

Balanced Diet

A diet can be termed as "balanced" if it contains all nutrients in right quantity and required proportion offering diversity of belonging to the four basic good groups. Though, these quantities and proportions would differ as per age, physical activity, gender, and physiological status, normally in a balanced diet, around 50–60% of total calories would come from carbohydrates, preferably complex carbohydrates, 20–30% from visible and invisible fats, and 10–15% from proteins. Besides, several nonnutrients such as antioxidants, phytochemicals, and dietary fiber should also be the parts of a balanced diet. While phytochemical such as polyphenols, flavones save from oxidant damage, antioxidants such as vitamins C and E, betacarotene, riboflavin, and selenium save from free radical damages. Some of the best sources of antioxidants in our everyday food are garlic, ginger, clove, cumin, and turmeric.

Food Pyramid

The food pyramid, a valuable roadmap for healthy diet planning, rests on the concept of energy density, which combines nutritional values with portion sizes to cater to different needs or situations. Since no single food offers all essential nutrients in sufficient amount, a diet can be balanced only if it consists of food from all different food groups. Not all foods in a food group contain the same nutrients. So, within each food group, the food selection should be assorted, or diverse rather than one to fulfill the requirements of essential ingredients. Lastly, ensuring a proportionate intake of each selected food is as vital as is the assortment or balance itself. As illustrated in **Figure 8.1**, in each of the food groups, a specific number of servings is recommended, and healthy choices are emphasized.

Vegetables and fruits are at the *first layer of the pyramid.* Vegetables and fruits are rich sources of minerals, vitamins, and phytonutrients. Fruits and vegetables are also rich in complex carbohydrates and fiber. Dietary fiber is important for proper bowel function, to reduce chronic constipation, and reduce plasma cholesterol. Some vegetables and fruits provide very low calories, whereas some others such as potato, sweet potato, tapioca and yam, and banana are rich in starch, which provides energy in good amount. Therefore, vegetables and fruits can be used to increase or decrease calories in our diet.

In the *second layer of the pyramid* (at the bottom) are the cereals, advised to be taken in adequate amount, as cereals or millets are used as staple food and are major sources of most nutrients, At least 50% cereal intake should be as whole grains.

The third layer of *pyramid*, including milk, pulses, legumes/flesh food, are about the use of protein which dictates that it should be used in moderation. Consumption of fish, beans, and low-fat dairy products are encouraged from this layer. Higher amount of protein is needed for growing and ill children. At

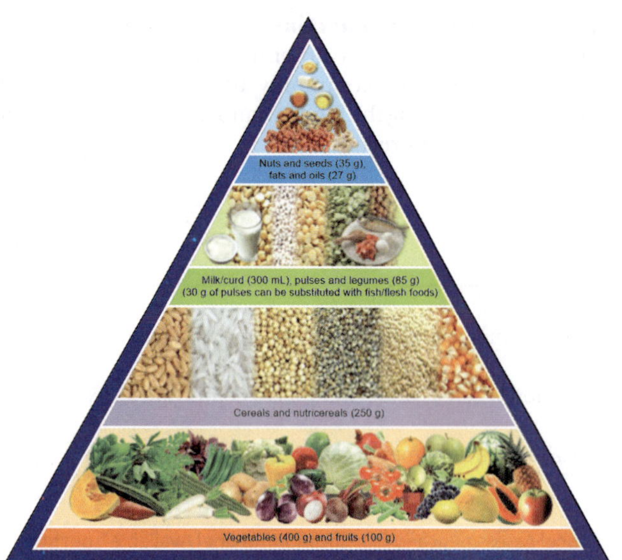

Fig. 8.1: Food pyramid

Source: Dietary Guidelines for Indians; Revised edition. National Institute of Nutrition, Indian Council of Medical Research; 2024

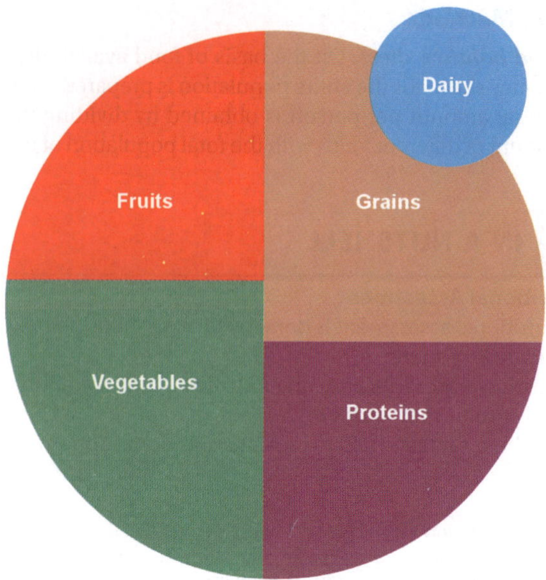

Fig. 8.2: My plate-ensures balanced diet

least 10–15% of total calories per day should be obtained from proteins. Animal proteins are considered superior due to better availability and presence of all amino acids.

The *top (fourth) layer* consists of fats, oils and nuts. The intake of PUFA should be 8–10% of energy intake. Ideally, a ratio of polyunsaturated to saturated (PUFA to SFA) of 0.8–1.0 and linoleic to α-linolenic (n-6/n-3) of 5–10 is required. The intake of TFA's should not exceed 1% of energy intake. A combination of oils like *soybean*, sesame, mustard, and sunflower should be used to achieve minor components in the diet. The use of *ghee*, butter, *vanaspati*, animal food, and processed food should be minimized. Prefer fish over meat and poultry. Use of reheated oil and fat should be avoided. Ill effects of excess dietary fats are initiated early in life. Use of skimmed milk is advocated beyond 2 years of age.

My Plate

The concept of "my plate" **(Fig. 8.2)** originally populated by the US Department of Agriculture (USDA), provides a visual concept of the proportion of different food groups needed for ensuring a balanced diet. Variety is encouraged within the different food groups. This is an easy-to-follow food guide and helps in nutritional education of parents and children.

Food for Preschool and School Children

Young children between 1–5 years should be given food items, which are rich in energy and protein and low in bulk (examples are: legumes, pulses, nuts, edible oil or ghee, sugar, milk, and eggs). Young children will consume more calories if small frequent feeds are given. The energy gap could be corrected by adding vegetable oil, ghee, or sugar to the food. Food items, which do not swell much on cooking such as potato and banana are also energy dense. Vegetables including green leafy vegetables and locally available seasonal fruits should be part of their daily menu. Majority of children eat more than three meals per day.

Snacks make a useful contribution to nutrient requirements, particularly in older children and adolescents. Snacks should be carefully chosen so that they are nutrient rich. Frequent changes in the menu are often liked by children. Older children and adolescents should consume plenty of milk to fulfill the high calcium requirements. Excessive salt intake should be avoided particularly by children having a family history of hypertension. Schoolchildren should be encouraged not to miss breakfast and practice healthy eating using the food guide my plate.

Food for Adolescents

Adolescence is a period of rapid growth and is spread over a decade. This is a transitional stage in human development. It is characterized by rapid increase in height and weight, hormonal changes, sexual maturation, and wide swings in emotion. Adolescent growth spurt starts at about 10–12 years in girls and 2 years later in boys. Development of critical bone mass is essential during this period as this forms the ground for maintaining mineral integrity of the bone in later life. The pattern and proportion of various body components such as body water, muscle mass, bone, and fat increase during the entire childhood and adolescence to reach adult values by about 18 years. Adolescent girls are at greater physiological stress than boys because of menstruation. Their nutritional needs are of particular importance, as they have to prepare for motherhood. All these rapid anabolic changes require more nutrients per unit body weight.

An adolescent boy is expected to consume 2,200–3,300 kcal/day, as equivalent to the requirement of an adult sedentary male. Adolescent girl requires 2,000–2,500 kcal/day, which is more than the requirement of an adult sedentary female. Carbohydrates should make up 45–65% of energy intake; protein 10–30%; and fat 25–35%. Dietary fat should come primarily from sources of polyunsaturated and MUFAs, such as fish, nuts, and vegetable oils. Trans fats, found in hydrogenated oils used primarily in bakery products, should be avoided altogether because they increase serum levels of LDL. Dietary intake of total cholesterol, found in animal products, should be limited to 300 mg/day. Growing children and adolescents particularly require more calcium to achieve high peak bone mass. Adolescents are also at risk of vitamin D deficiency due to inadequate exposure to sunlight. Adequate intake of iron should be ensured, as iron is needed to build up the muscle mass and to prevent the development of anemia due to menstrual loss in girls.

DIET IN DISEASE

Nutrition can have a powerful impact on maintaining health and preventing disease. Diet in chronic diseases such as diabetes, hypertension, obesity, kidney, liver, and heart disorders should be appropriately modified.

Diabetes

Lifestyle, and particularly dietary habits, plays an important role in the management of diabetes. Apart from regular physical activity and maintaining a normal body weight, a diet high in fiber and low in glycemic index can delay the onset of type 2 diabetes and help maintain the sugar values in type 1 diabetes. Adherence to a healthy dietary pattern, exerts a beneficial role control of diabetes.

There is no universal dietary strategy to prevent diabetes or delay its onset. Together with the maintenance of ideal body weight, the promotion of the so called prudent diet (characterized by a higher intake of food groups that are generally recommended for health promotion, particularly plantbased foods, and a lower intake of red meat, meat products, sweets, high fat dairy, and refined grains) or a diet rich in olive oil, fruits and vegetables, including whole grains, pulses and nuts, low-fat dairy, appears as the best strategy to decrease diabetes risk.

Some basic tips for a diabetic diet include eating whole grain foods and avoiding sugar, salt, and saturated fat. Intake of vegetables and low fructose fruits should be increased to increase the fiber content.

Hypertension

In children and adolescents who are overweight, weight loss and physical activity are the most effective strategies for lowering blood pressure. Salt restriction to not >5 g/day should be recommended, lesser with lower age. Dietary intake of many servings of vegetables and fruits daily, a modest decrease in meat consumption and substitution of low fat for high fat dairy products is an effective preventive strategy against hypertension. The DASH (Dietary Approaches to Stop Hypertension) diet too recommends high intake of fruits, vegetables, whole grain, low-fat dairy products and high protein foods and avoidance of red meat, sugar, salt, and saturated fats.

Obesity

The prevalence of obesity is increasing in almost all parts of the world including developing countries where it once used to be rare. Imbalance of energy intake being greater than energy expenditure is the major factor leading to weight gain.

Nutrition interventions have the most important role in prevention and treatment of obesity. There are many different methods to decrease total intake of calories. Limiting the consumption of specific high-calorie foods, the portion size, or the number of servings from food groups are methods of decreasing total caloric intake and can be effective in individual patients. Whatever the method, a key point is that dietary changes should be approached as a sustained lifestyle change, as opposed to "going on a diet". The key points include reducing free sugars to <5% of total energy intake, decrease saturated fat intake to <10% and transfat to nil, increase consumption of vegetables and fruits and avoid consumption of sugar sweetened beverages and juices.

Celiac Disease

Diet in celiac disease aims at avoiding any intake of food containing even traces of gluten. Gluten is found in wheat, barley, rye, and any derivatives of these grains. Eating gluten free diet helps these children to live near normal life. Fruits, vegetables, dairy products, meat, poultry, fish, dals, and certain flours such as amaranth, buckwheat, corn, millet, and coconut are all gluten-free options, which the affected children can consume in good amounts. If the diet is gluten-free, the energy (from carbohydrates, fats, and proteins), vitamins, and mineral requirements remain the same as in other children.

Kidney and Liver Diseases

Children with chronic liver disease have higher energy requirement than normal children. The total energy requirement is almost 130% of the requirement as for the age of which 30–50% should be provided by fats, mainly MCTs, and 40–60% by carbohydrates. The protein requirement is also increased many times due to poor intake and absorption. Small feeds given more frequently are advocated. A bedtime snack can be added in older children. There is also increased requirements of vitamins, especially fat soluble, due to poor absorption.

Children with chronic kidney disease also have a high energy requirement. The protein intake should be balanced so as to exceed to put burden on kidney and not too low to compromise the nutrition. The protein requirement increases in children on dialysis. Food high in sodium such as ultraprocessed food, canned food, and some of the frozen foods should be avoided. The amount of sodium requirement varies on the stage of kidney disease, requirement decreasing as the disease stage worsens. Foods high in potassium and phosphorous, such as some fruits (banana, dried fruits) and vegetables (GLV) should be avoided.

Diet in Malignancies

Children with malignancies generally need more calories and proteins to ensure adequate growth and healing. High calories, high protein food in form of small frequent feeds is advised. These children often have associated problems due to ongoing chemotherapy such as oral ulcers, poor taste, dry mouth, diarrhea, gastritis, and infections. These lead to poor oral intake and increased catabolism, thereby leading to weight loss. Children with poor oral intake may need tube feeding to support adequate nutrition.

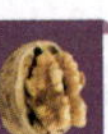

IN A NUTSHELL

Diet in Health and Disease

1. A balanced diet has 50–60% of total calories from carbohydrates, 20–30% from fats, and 10–15% from proteins along with antioxidants, phytochemicals, and dietary fibers.
2. Young children between 1–5 years should be given energy and protein-rich food but low in bulk.
3. Chronic illnesses often have higher energy requirements to overcome the ongoing catabolic losses due to poor oral intake, malabsorption, and cell breakdown.

ICMR. Dietary Guidelines for Indians; Revised edition. National Institute of Nutrition, Indian Council of Medical Research; 2024.

ICMR. Nutrient requirements for Indians: a report of the expert group. ICMR, National Institute of Nutrition; 2020.

Milton Keynes University Hospital NHS Foundation Trust. Dietary Advice for Children Newly Diagnosed with Type 1 Diabetes. [online] Available from https://www.mkuh.nhs.uk/patient-information-leaflet/paediatric-diabetes-clinic-brochure [Last accessed August, 2025].

Mouzaki M, Bronsky J, Gupte G, et al. Nutrition support of children with chronic liver diseases: a joint position paper of the North American society for pediatric gastroenterology, hepatology, and nutrition and the European society for pediatric gastroenterology, hepatology, and nutrition. J Pediatr Gastroenterol Nutr. 2019;69(4):498-511.

Nidhi Bedi, Neetu Sharma, and Piyush Gupta

9 CHAPTER

Undernutrition and Obesity

AS PER NMC COMPETENCIES

PE10.1	Define and describe the etiopathogenesis, classify including WHO classification, clinical features, complication and management of severe acute malnutrition (SAM) and moderate acute malnutrition (MAM).	*Ch 9.1, Ch 9.2 Ch 9.3, Ch 9.4 Ch 9.5*
PE10.2	Outline the clinical approach to a child with SAM and MAM.	*Ch 9.4, Ch 9.5 Ch 9.8*
PE10.3	Assessment of a patient with SAM and MAM, diagnosis, classification and planning management including hospital and community-based intervention, rehabilitation and prevention.	*Ch 9.2, Ch 9.4 Ch 9.5, Ch 9.8*
PE10.4	Counsel parents of children with SAM and MAM.	*Ch 9.4, Ch 9.5 Ch 9.7*
PE10.5	Enumerate the role of locally prepared therapeutic diets and ready to use therapeutic diets.	*Ch 9.6*
PE10.6	Explain the adolescent nutrition and common nutritional problems.	*Ch 9.9*
PE11.1	Describe the etiology, clinical features and management of obesity in children.	*Ch 9.10*
PE11.2	Describe the risk approach for obesity and discuss the prevention strategies.	*Ch 9.10*
PE11.3	Assessment of a child with obesity with regard to eliciting history including physical activity, charting and dietary recall.	*Ch 9.10*
PE11.4	Examination including calculation of BMI, measurement of waist-hip ratio, identifying external markers like acanthosis, striae, pseudogynecomastia, etc.	*Ch 9.10*

Topics available online: ***Obesity: Waist Circumference Charts***

9.1 Undernutrition: Prevalence and Classification *PE 10.1*

INTRODUCTION

Adequate food and nutrition are essential for proper growth and physical development to ensure optimal work capacity, normal reproductive performance, adequate immune mechanism, and resistance to infections. Undernutrition can be categorized as macronutrient (protein, fat, and carbohydrates) and micronutrient (vitamins and minerals) deficiency. Nutritional deficiency of macronutrients is a major health problem in the developing countries. Severe acute malnutrition (SAM), the most severe and life-threatening form of undernutrition, is often associated with infection; and contributes to high child mortality. Early onset of undernutrition can also have lasting effects on growth and long-term functional status. Children with mild-to-moderate undernutrition are likely to remain unrecognized because clinical criteria for their diagnosis are imprecise and difficult to interpret accurately.

Undernutrition (including intrauterine growth restriction, stunting, wasting, severe acute malnutrition, and various micronutrient deficiencies) is the major underlying factor contributing to the deaths of about 45% of the total children below 5 years of age (WHO 2020). Data from the India State-Level Disease Burden (ISLDB) Initiative indicate that undernutrition is the predominant risk factor for loss of health in all age groups, and responsible for 17.3% of total disability-adjusted life years (DALYs). Undernutrition was also the main risk factor, accounting for around 68.2% of under-5 deaths in India in 2017.

BURDEN OF UNDERNUTRITION

Prevalence

Global Situation

As per the Joint Child Malnutrition reports, in year 2022, 148.1 million (22.3% of under 5 population) were stunted, 37 million overweight, and 45 million wasted **(Fig. 9.1)**. Amongst these, 52% of stunted, 48% of overweight and 70% of wasted children were from Asia alone. **Figure 9.2** depicts the global lag in projected 2030 global targets.

India

Burden of undernutrition in India, as per the National Family Health Survey (NFHS)-5 (2019-2021), is depicted in **Figure 9.3**. The trends over last 15 years are shown in **Figure 9.4**. Almost 35.5% of under-5 children are stunted, 32.1% are underweight and 19.3% wasted.

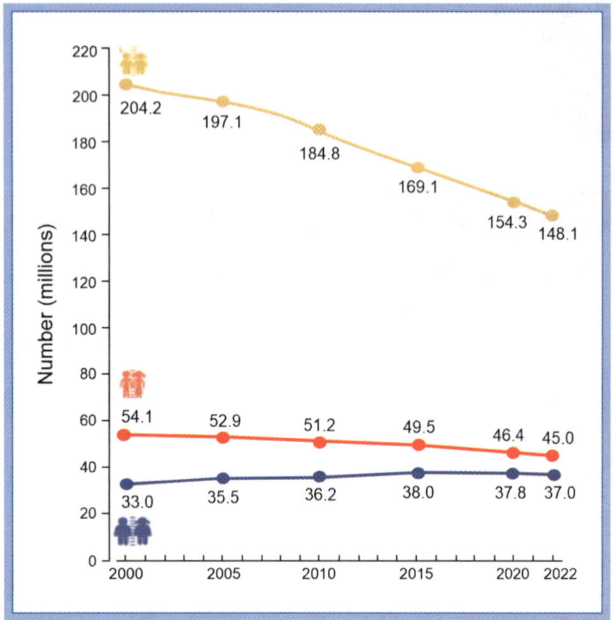

Fig. 9.1: Number (millions) of children under-5 affected by stunting, wasting, and overweight

Source: UNICEF/WHO/World Bank group Joint Malnutrition Estimates, 2023 edition.

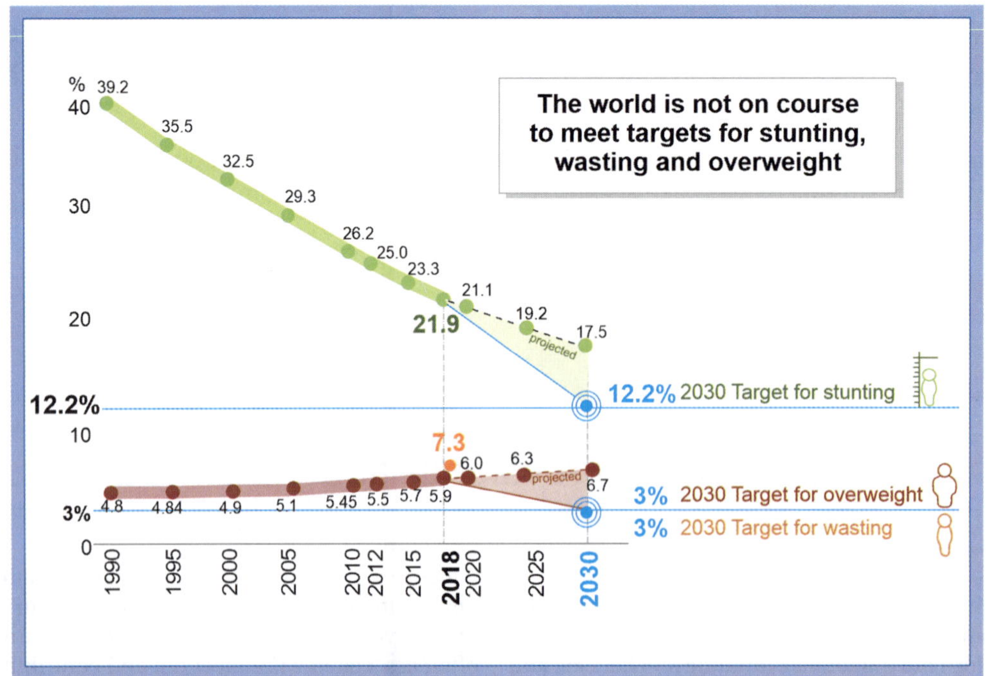

Fig. 9.2: Projection of undernutrition in children under-5 compared to 2030 global targets

Source: UNICEF/WHO/World Bank group Joint Undernutrition Estimates, 2019 edition

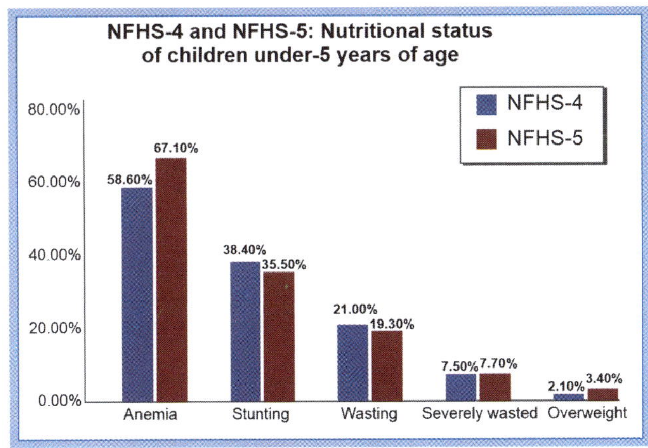

Fig. 9.3: Nutritional status of children under 5 years of age. NFHS-4 and NFHS-5 (NFHS: National Family Health Survey)

Stunting is higher in rural areas (37%) than urban areas (30%). In a state-wise assessment according to NFHS-5, Sikkim (22.3%) and Puducherry (20%) have the lowest while Meghalaya (46.5%), Bihar (42.9%), Uttar Pradesh (39.7%), and Jharkhand (39.6%) have the highest rates of stunting. Two states, Goa (from 20.1 to 25.8%) and Kerala (from 19.7 to 23.4%) that had the lowest stunting rates in children in NFHS-4 showed a substantial rise as per the NFHS-5.

It appears that despite a significant decrease in low birth weight, wasting, and underweight the downward trend is far below that required to achieve the National Nutrition Mission (NNM) 2022 target. If, based on the current trends, projection of the prevalence of undernutrition is done until 2030, it can be estimated that there will be an excess prevalence of 8.9% for low birthweight, 9.6% for stunting, 4.8% for underweight, and 11.7% for anemia in Indian children.

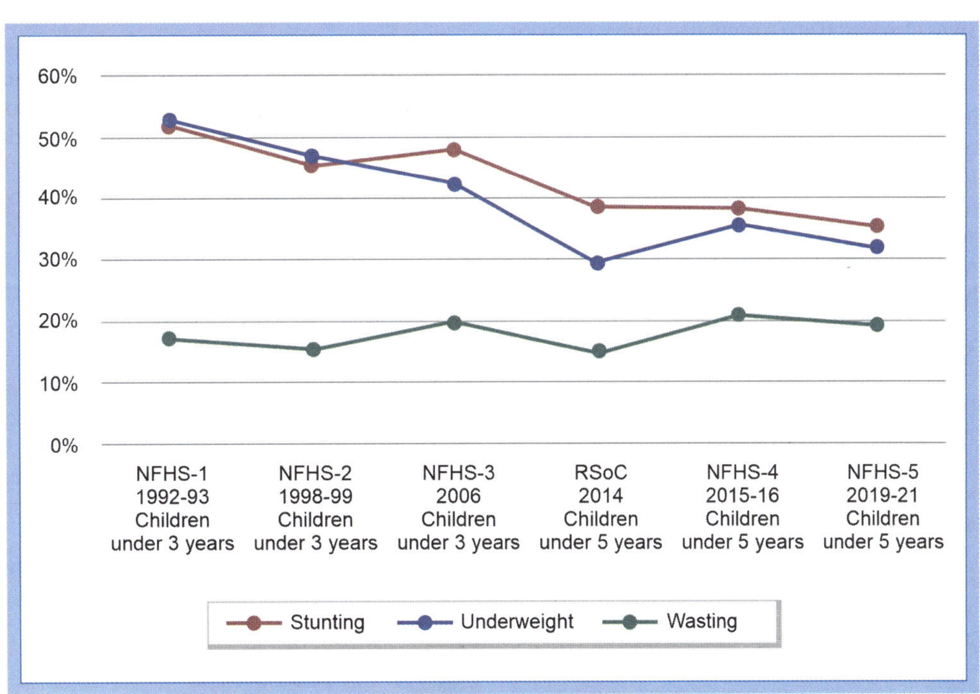

Fig. 9.4: Trends in Nutrition Status in India, 1993–2021

(NFHS: National Family Health Survey)

9.2 Classification of Undernutrition

PE 10.1, PE 10.3

Nutritional deficiency of macronutrients results in undernutrition which may be classified according to the severity, course, and the relative contributions of energy or protein deficit. Severity classifications are based on anthropometric measurements, mainly weight, height, and mid-upper arm circumference (MUAC). For the purpose of these classifications, the term *"expected"* denotes the median (50th centile) value of the reference standard. Growth standards provided by the World Health Organization (WHO) are widely acceptable international growth standards for comparison for under-5 children, while the Indian Academy of Pediatrics (IAP) growth charts are recommended as references for children 5–18 years age.

INDIAN ACADEMY OF PEDIATRICS CLASSIFICATION BASED ON WEIGHT FOR AGE

Once upon a time, this used to be the main classification system to describe the severity of protein-energy malnutrition (PEM) in children. It has lost much relevance in current scenario. Weight of >80% of expected for that age is considered normal. Grades of PEM were categorized as *Grade I* (71–80%), *Grade II* (61–70%), *Grade III* (51–60%) and *Grade IV* (<50%) of expected weight for that age. Alphabet *K* was postfixed in presence of edema. For example, boy weighing 8 kg at 2 years of age with pedal edema (50th percentile for 2 years is 12.3 kg) can be classified as PEM Grade II(k) as per IAP classification.

IAP classification has a major disadvantage that it does not take in account the child's height. Also, the term PEM has gradually fallen out of use.

WELLCOME TRUST CLASSIFICATION

This classification was also based on (a) deficit in bodyweight for age and (b) presence or absence of edema. Children weighing between 60 and 80% of their expected weight for age with edema are classified as *kwashiorkor*. Those weighing between 60 and 80% of expected without edema are known as having *undernutrition*. Those without edema and weighing <60% of their expected weight for age were considered to be having *marasmus*. *Marasmic kwashiorkor* was applied to children with edema and bodyweight <60% of expected. This classification also is now mainly of historical/anecdotal value.

WHO CLASSIFICATION

This classification is based on two anthropometric indicators (stunting and wasting) and one clinical indicator (edema) **(Table 9.1)**.

- ***Wasting*** (measured by deficit in weight-for-height) indicates a deficit in tissue and fat mass and may result either from failure to gain weight or from actual weight loss. It usually signifies *acute onset undernutrition*. A child is considered wasted, if the weight for height/length (WFH/L) is < –2SD (*Z*) score or <80% of the expected. Severe wasting is WFH/L <–3 *Z*-score.
- ***Stunting*** (deficit in height-for-age) signifies accumulated consequences of retarded growth over a prolonged period and generally points toward a *chronic course of undernutrition*. It may also be a residue of past undernutrition or could be due to non-nutritional disorders like genetic short stature or endocrinal disorders. The diagnosis of stunting is based on a height for age (HFA) < –2SD (*Z*) score or <90% of the expected. Severe stunting is HFA < –3SD (*Z*) score.
- Children are classified as having *moderate undernutrition* if they are stunted or wasted.
- Presence of edema along with stunting or wasting indicates *severe undernutrition*.
- A child with *severe wasting* (weight for height/length < –3 *Z*-score or <70% of expected) or *severe stunting* (HFA < –3 *Z*-score or <85% of expected) is considered to have *severe undernutrition*.

Table 9.1 WHO Classification for Undernutrition

	Moderate undernutrition	*Severe undernutrition*
Symmetrical edema *Edematous undernutrition*	No	Yes[a]
Weight for height *(Measure of wasting)*	SD score[b] –2 to –3 (70–79% of expected[c]) *Wasting*	SD score < –3 (<70% of expected) *Severe wasting*
Height for age *(Measure of stunting)*	SD score[b] –2 to –3 (85–89% of expected[c]) *Stunting*	SD score < –3 (<85% of expected) *Severe stunting*

[a]This includes kwashiorkor and marasmic kwashiorkor
[b]SD (*Z*) score = Observed value – Expected value divided by Standard deviation of reference population
[c]Median (50th percentile of WHO standards)

SEVERE ACUTE MALNUTRITION

The term "severe acute malnutrition" was coined by international agencies (WHO and UNICEF) to identify malnourished children at the highest risk of death, and for the purpose of therapeutic feeding in the hospital or community. SAM is defined by (*a*) very low weight for height (below -3 *Z*-scores of the median WHO growth standards), or (*b*) visible severe wasting, or (*c*) presence of nutritional edema, or (*d*) mid-arm circumference below 11.5 cm for children aged between 6 months and 5 years.

Moderate acute malnutrition: A child who has WFH SD between -3 and -2 *Z*-scores of the median WHO growth standards or mid-upper arm circumference between 11.5 and 12.4 cm and has no bilateral pitting edema is classified as having moderate acute malnutrition.

The frequency of undernutrition cannot be easily estimated from the prevalence of commonly recognized clinical syndromes of undernutrition such as marasmus and kwashiorkor because these constitute only the proverbial tip of the iceberg. Cases with mild to moderate undernutrition are likely to remain unrecognized because clinical criteria for their diagnosis are imprecise and difficult to interpret accurately.

IN A NUTSHELL

Undernutrition: Prevalence and Classification

1. Undernutrition can be categorized as macronutrient (protein, fat, and carbohydrates) and micronutrient (vitamins and minerals) deficiency.
2. The spectrum of macronutrient deficiency extends from mild underweight to severe acute malnutrition and includes wasting, stunting, and severe forms such as marasmus and kwashiorkor.
3. Weight-for-age, HFA, and WFH are indicators to assess and grade underweight, stunting, and wasting, respectively.
4. Wasting is an indicator of acute malnutrition while stunting indicates chronic nutritional deficit.
5. Severe acute malnutrition is a life-threatening form of undernutrition and causes maximum mortality.

International Institute for Population Sciences (IIPS) and Ministry of Health and Family Welfare Government of India. (2019-21). National Family Health Survey (NFHS-5), India Report. [online] Available from: https://iipsindia.ac.in/content/national-family-health-survey-nfhs-5-india-report. [Last accessed May, 2025].
International Institute for Population Sciences (IIPS) and ICF. (2017). National Family Health Survey (NFHS-4), 2015-16: India. Mumbai: IIPS. [online] Available from: https://dhsprogram.com/pubs/pdf/FR339/FR339.pdf [Last accessed August, 2025].
UNICEF-WHO-The World Bank Group: Joint child undernutrition estimates: Levels and trends in child undernutrition: 2021. [online] Available at https://www.who.int/publications/i/item/9789240025257. [Last accessed August, 2025].
WHO. WHO child growth standards: length or height-for-age, weight-for- age, weight-for-length, weight-for-height and body mass index-for-age: methods and development. Geneva: World Health Organization; 2006.

9.3 Etiopathogenesis of Undernutrition *PE 10.1*

ETIOLOGY

Undernutrition occurs when the quantity of one or more macronutrients available to body tissues is inadequate to sustain optimal bodily functions, and this is usually accompanied by numerous micronutrient deficiencies. Undernutrition is a broad concept that includes a variety of clinical conditions such as undernutrition; wasting; stunting; kwashiorkor; moderate and severe acute malnutrition; and micronutrient deficiencies. Common causes of undernutrition are discussed below:

Low Birthweight

Undernourished mothers have a high incidence of low birth-weight (LBW) and growth-retarded babies with poor nutritional reserve. These LBW babies are more likely to become under-nourished.

Feeding Habits

Lack of exclusive breastfeeding for first 6 months makes the child prone to early onset of undernutrition. Lack of confidence in the mother coupled with nonavailability of skilled help and social pressures make the mother think that her breastmilk supply is not sufficient to satisfy the nutritional needs of the infant. Artificial feeding is employed in these situations, which is often disastrous for the baby because of the poor quality of the substitute milk, excessive dilution and use of unhygienic feeding bottles and nipples.

Another major cause of undernutrition is delayed introduction of complementary feeding. Introduction of solid or mushy foods is delayed, often beyond 1 year. Most of the times, it is the diluted animal milk or dal water is used to supplement breastfeeds. The amount is also inadequate. According to NFHS-5, only 45.9% of infants aged 6–8 months receive complementary semi-solid foods as recommended.

Parents often withhold food or dilute the milk during episodes of diarrhea. Affluent families may also have irrational beliefs about the nutritional needs of infants and nutritional quality of common foods. Some foods are erroneously believed to be hot or cold in nature. Prevailing dietary practices and cultural taboos on consumption of certain types of foods are the other conditioning factors leading to undernutrition.

Infections and Infestations

Diarrhea, pneumonia, malaria, measles, whooping cough, and tuberculosis precipitate acute undernutrition and aggravate the existing nutritional deficit. Recurrent attacks of diarrhea in preschool children are a major contributory factor. During infections, the child's appetite is impaired; there may be iatrogenic restriction of food by the parents; the patient catabolizes his own tissues to produce the additional heat energy, which is lost during fever. Therefore, such infants lose weight. Metabolic demands for protein during infections are higher. Protein may be lost because of tissue breakdown and in pus and exudates. Also, undernutrition may adversely affect the immune status and make the undernourished individuals more vulnerable to infections. This sets up a vicious cycle of undernutrition-infection-undernutrition.

High Pressure Advertising of Baby Foods

Advertisement of baby foods by baby food manufacturers and social demands on the urban educated working women have encouraged early discontinuation of breastfeeding. Evaporated dry milk powders and packaged foods are expensive. A poor mother tends to conserve on their use and offers diluted milk formula to the infant. Unhygienic feeding practices in the preparation of milk formula result in frequent episodes of diarrhea and diminished absorption of food by the infant.

Social Factors

Repeated pregnancies, inadequate child spacing, food taboos, broken homes, and separation of a child from his parents are the important social factors that may play a part in etiology of undernutrition. Share of women and preschool children is disproportionately less compared with the economically active male adults. Wars and civil unrest exaggerate preexisting under-nutrition in the community. Natural disasters such as floods, earthquakes, and droughts shift the precarious nutritional balance toward the negative side.

Poverty

Poverty is an important determinant of undernutrition. Poor cannot purchase adequate amount of food of the desired quality for meeting their and their family's nutritional requirements. This deprivation adversely affects their capacity for physical work and endurance. They earn less and this starts a vicious cycle of poverty-undernutrition-diminished work capacity. In the new social milieu, non-food expenditure, such as housing, clothing and entertainment has gone up significantly, often at the cost of food.

Large Family Size

Rapid succession of pregnancies adversely affects the nutritional status of the mother—leaving her undernourished and showing poor lactational performance. Per capita availability of food in large families is low and unequally distributed. Share of women and preschool children is disproportionately less.

Predictors of Undernutrition

The proportion of children who are stunted or underweight increases rapidly with the child's age through age 20–23 months. Overall, girls and boys are equally undernourished. Undernutrition is generally lower for first births than for subsequent births and consistently increases with increasing birth order for all measures of nutritional status. Short birth intervals are associated with higher levels of undernutrition. Undernutrition has a strong negative relationship with the mother's education. The percentage of children who are severely underweight is almost five times as high for children whose mothers have no education as for children whose mothers have 12 or more years of education. The nutritional status of children is also strongly related to maternal nutritional status. Undernutrition is much more common for children of mothers whose body mass index is below 18.5 than for children whose mothers are not underweight. Children from households with a low standard of living are twice as likely to be undernourished as children from households with a high standard of living.

PATHOPHYSIOLOGY

Changes in Body Composition and Function

Severe undernutrition causes several changes in structure and function of organ systems. There is a preferential loss of muscle and subcutaneous tissues which in the resting state have a low metabolic activity; while essential organs with high rate of activity, such as brain and heart, are relatively spared. Body fat and total bone mass are reduced.

Fluid and electrolytes: Total body water in undernourished children is increased to 70–80% of body weight as compared to 60% in age matched well-nourished controls. Greater part of this increase is constituted by extracellular fluid. Activity of the sodium pump is reduced. Cell membranes become more permeable leading to increased intracellular sodium levels and reduced total body potassium and magnesium. Fluid and sodium administration, especially in face of clinical dehydration, should be planned with caution in these children. Dehydration should preferably be corrected orally; intravenous fluids are best avoided unless there is shock.

Metabolic alterations: Basal metabolic rate (BMR) is reduced by 30% and energy expenditure due to activity is very low. Heat generation and heat losses are affected so that the child may behave like a poikilotherm. These factors predispose to hypothermia.

Biochemical changes: Synthesis of all proteins is reduced. Capacity of the liver to take up, metabolize, and excrete toxins is severely affected. Gluconeogenesis is impaired leading to increased risk of hypoglycemia. Plasma transferrin concentration is markedly reduced.

Other nutritional deficiencies:

- Anemia occurs because of deficiency of iron, vitamin B_{12}, and folic acid; hookworm infestation may also contribute.
- Vitamin A deficiency may result in keratomalacia.
- Riboflavin deficiency is also common.
- Scurvy may manifest as painful legs and knees, and gum bleeding. Subperiosteal hemorrhages may occur, acutely mimicking osteomyelitis.
- Rickets is also evident in one-third of cases, vitamin D levels are low.

Immunity: Severe undernutrition is a state of relative immunodeficiency. There is impaired *cell-mediated immunity* due to atrophy of thymus and lymphoid tissues. Sensitization to antigens and recognition of earlier sensitization is impaired. Infections requiring cell-mediated immunity (e.g., tuberculosis) tend to be severe. Delayed hypersensitivity reactions (e.g., Mantoux test) are impaired.

- ***Humoral immunity*** is relatively less affected. Circulating antibody levels are normal or elevated because of frequent co-existence of infections. B lymphocyte level and proportion are also preserved. Antibody response to most vaccines (e.g., measles, diphtheria, tetanus, and poliomyelitis) is adequate. However, secretory IgA may be reduced resulting in increased severity, prolonged infectivity, and delayed recovery from infections.
- ***Leukocyte count*** is generally normal in severe undernutrition. Leukopenia may occur because of associated vitamin B_{12} and folic acid deficiency. Chemotaxis is impaired but phagocytosis is usually normal. There is impaired fungicidal and bactericidal capacity of leukocytes.
- ***Physical barriers*** against infection such as skin and mucosal membranes are breached. Skin is thin and ulcerated which is easily penetrated by microbes. Mucosae are atrophic resulting in increased risk of gastrointestinal and respiratory tract infections.

Gastrointestinal system: Salivary glands atrophy. The liver shows fatty infiltration, fat initially appearing in the periportal area, later spreading toward the central hepatic vein. Pancreatic acini are atrophied and zymogen granules are reduced. Intestinal mucosa demonstrates a moderate reduction in the villus height, increase in the width of villi with a tendency to fusion at the base, and change of columnar villus epithelial into cuboidal cells. Total absorptive surface is reduced. Steatorrhea may occur. Lactose malabsorption is common. Abdominal muscles and large intestine are hypotonic resulting in protuberant abdomen. Rectal prolapse is common.

Central nervous system: Growth and development of the brain are adversely affected, especially if undernutrition sets in first 2 years of life which is a period of rapid brain growth. Associated micronutrient deficiencies (e.g., iron, thiamine, vitamin B_{12}, zinc, and iodine) further impair the brain function resulting in lower developmental scores. Lag in development and intelligence (IQ) may persist even after recovery.

Renal impairment: Glomerular filtration rate and renal plasma flow are reduced in severe undernutrition. Capacity of the kidneys to excrete excess acid or water is greatly affected. Urinary phosphate and sodium excretion are reduced.

Endocrine system: Insulin levels are reduced, and the child has glucose intolerance. Cortisol and growth hormone levels are increased.

Cardiovascular system: Cardiac output and stroke volume are reduced. Blood pressure is low and renal perfusion is compromised.

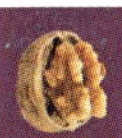

IN A NUTSHELL

Etiopathogenesis of Undernutrition

1. Undernutrition is a common public health problem in under-5 children and multifactorial in origin.
2. Theories of adaptation and free radical injury have been proposed for its pathogenesis.
3. Adrenocortical response to stress of protein and calorie deficiency plays a key role in the development of marasmus and kwashiorkor.
4. Proinflammatory mediators also contribute to impaired growth in undernutrition.
5. Generalized changes in different systems occur in severe undernutrition leading to systemic manifestations.
6. Total body water and serum sodium are increased; whereas potassium is decreased in severe malnutrition.

Bourke CD, Berkley JA, Prendergast AJ. Immune dysfunction as a cause and consequence of malnutrition. Trends Immunol. 2016;37(6):386-98.
Bresnahan KA, Tanumihardjo SA. Undernutrition, the acute phase response to infection, and its effect on micronutrient status indicators. Adv Nutr. 2014;5(6):702-11.
Dipasquale V, Cucinotta U, Romano C. Acute undernutrition in children: pathophysiology, clinical effects, and treatment. Nutrients. 2020; 12(8):2413.
Ghosh-Jerath S, Singh A, Jerath N, Gupta S, Racine EF. Undernutrition and severe acute malnutrition in children. BMJ. 2017;359:j4877.
Guideline: Assessing and Managing Children at Primary Health-Care Facilities to Prevent Overweight and Obesity in the Context of the Double Burden of Malnutrition: Updates for the Integrated Management of Childhood Illness (IMCI). Geneva: World Health Organization; 2017.
International Food Policy Research Institute. Global Nutrition Report 2016: From Promise to Impact: Ending Undernutrition by 2030. Washington, DC: International Food Policy Research Institute; 2016.
Thaxton GE, Melby PC, Manary MJ, Preidis GA. New insights into the pathogenesis and treatment of malnutrition. Gastroenterol Clin North Am. 2018;47(4):813-27.

9.4 Severe Acute Malnutrition

PE 10.1, PE 10.2, PE 10.3, PE 10.4

CLASSIFICATION

Wasting indicates current or acute malnutrition resulting from failure to gain weight or weight loss, represented by low weight-for-height (WFH). Wasting or acute malnutrition is further graded into severe acute malnutrition (SAM) [WFH < –3SD (*Z*) score] and moderate acute malnutrition (MAM) (WFH *Z*-score week –2 to –3) in children based on their WFH *Z*-score or MUAC **(Table 9.2)**.

Table 9.2 Classification of Nutritional Status Based on Mid-upper Arm Circumference (MUAC)

MUAC	*Nutritional status*
12.5 cm or more	Normal
11.5–12.4 cm	Moderate acute malnutrition or wasted
<11.5 cm	Severe acute malnutrition or severely wasted

It has been found that lower the *Z*-score or MUAC, higher is the risk of death. For children in whom WFH *Z*-score is < –3 *Z* and MUAC < 11.5 cm, risk of mortality increases significantly. However, in edematous children with SAM, accumulation of fluid may lead to erroneously higher WFH and MUAC but risk of mortality is more than nonedematous SAM children. Therefore, edema is taken as independent criteria for identifying children with SAM.

DEFINITION

Criteria for identifying children with SAM [*Indian Academy of Pediatrics (IAP) 2013; and WHO 2013*] is given in **Table 9.3**.

MUAC is an age independent criterion particularly used in children 6 months to 5 years. In infants smaller than 6 months of age, the recognition and management of SAM is even more challenging. Hence WHO in 2023, formulated anthropometric criteria to identify children below 6 months

Table 9.3	Criteria for Identifying Children with Severe Acute Malnutrition (SAM)
Age	*Criteria*
6 months to 5 years#	Weight-for-height or length is < –3 SD and/or Mid-upper arm circumference (MUAC) < 11.5 cm and/or Bilateral pitting edema of both feet*
<6 months**	Weight-for-height/length is < –3 SD and/or Bilateral pitting edema of both feet*

#IAP guideline included *severe wasting* as one of the criteria; however, this may be subjective and should be used only when MUAC or weight or height or length measurement is not feasible
*Unilateral edema is not an indicator of SAM and there should not be a known cause of edema such as nephrotic syndrome, congestive heart failure, etc.
**For children with length <45 cm, visible severe wasting is used to identify as SD score charts are not available for infants <45 cm

of age who are at risk of poor growth and development. These include WAZ < –2 SD, WLZ < –3 SD, MUAC <110 mm (for infants between 6 weeks and less than 6 months of age), and failure to gain weight based on two consecutive measurements [*WHO 2023*].

Lower the *Z*-score or MUAC, higher is the risk of death. For children in whom WFH *Z*-score is <–3 *Z* and MUAC <11.5 cm, risk of mortality increases significantly. However, in edematous children with SAM, accumulation of fluid may lead to erroneously higher WFH and MUAC but risk of mortality is more than non-edematous SAM children. Therefore, edema is taken as an independent criteria for identifying children with SAM.

ETIOPATHOGENESIS

Reductive adaptation: The body systems slow down to allow survival on limited calories. When a child's carbohydrate intake is insufficient, fat stores are utilized to provide energy. Later, protein is mobilized from muscles, skin, and gut. Physiological and metabolic changes also take place to conserve energy. These changes take place in an orderly progression, which is called reductive adaptation. A child with SAM conserves energy by reducing physical activity and growth; reducing basal metabolism by slowing protein turnover; reducing the functional reserve of organs; slowing the sodium and potassium pumps in cell membranes and reducing their number; and reducing inflammatory and immune responses.

Consequences of Reductive Adaptation

The functioning of every cell, organ, and system is affected and this puts the child in a very fragile state. Following is a brief description of the effects on different organs:

- The liver is less able to make glucose; so there is increased risk of hypoglycemia and hypothermia. In addition, liver is less able to excrete excess dietary protein and toxins. These changes have implications for feeding. First, long gaps without food must be avoided. This means giving frequent feeds day and night, which is a ready source of glucose. Second, we must limit protein intake to avoid stressing the liver.
- The kidneys are less able to excrete excess fluid and sodium. So, excess fluid and sodium (from feeds or rehydration fluid) can lead to fluid overload.
- The heart is smaller and weaker and has a reduced output. Any excess fluid in the circulation stresses the heart and can lead to death from heart failure. This means that fluid intake must be carefully controlled initially. Also, feeds and rehydration fluid must be low in sodium.
- The gut produces less acid and smaller amounts of enzymes. The intestinal villi are flattened, and motility is reduced. These changes cause bacterial colonization of the small bowel, damage of the mucosa, and deconjugation of bile acids. So, initially, feeds must be small to avoid exceeding the gut's functional capacity, and the composition of feeds should be such that it can easily be absorbed. Feeds should be *enteral, never parenteral*, to reduce the risk of fluid overload. Repair of the gut is also quicker if nutrients are physically present in the lumen.
- During reductive adaptation, sodium leaks into cells due to fewer and slower pumps, leading to excess body sodium. Potassium leaks out of cells and is lost in urine, contributing to electrolyte imbalance, anorexia, fluid retention, and heart failure. So, we need to restrict sodium and provide potassium. We must also provide magnesium to help the potassium get into cells.
- Reduction in muscle mass is accompanied by loss of intracellular nutrients and smaller reserves of muscle glycogen.
- Red cell mass is also reduced, liberating iron. Conversion of harmful free iron to ferritin needs glucose and amino acids, and there may not be enough glucose available to put all the iron into safe storage. Free iron promotes the growth of pathogens and the production of free radicals which damage cell membranes. So, during initial feeding, we need to withhold iron, and provide vitamins and minerals to help mop up free radicals.

CLINICAL FEATURES

SAM without Edema

The most characteristic feature is *visible severe wasting* of muscle and subcutaneous tissues. Child is usually alert, has an emaciated look, and has no edema **(Fig. 9.5)**. Skin is thin, dry, scaly, and wrinkled with loose folds apparent over the gluteal region and thighs. Subcutaneous fat gets depleted as it is used up for providing energy. Buccal pad of fat is the last to disappear because of presence of saturated fats which are utilized after all other sources are depleted. Atrophic muscles make a contour under the thin and wrinkled skin. Bones appear prominent giving a skeleton-like look. Hair are sparse and hypopigmented. Abdomen appears distended because of hypotonia of abdominal wall muscles. Appetite may be normal or reduced depending on whether the child has associated infection.

Other features include sunken eyes due to loss of subcutaneous fat, conjunctival pallor, dryness, Bitot spots, dry eyes and mouth following lacrimal and salivary glands atrophy.

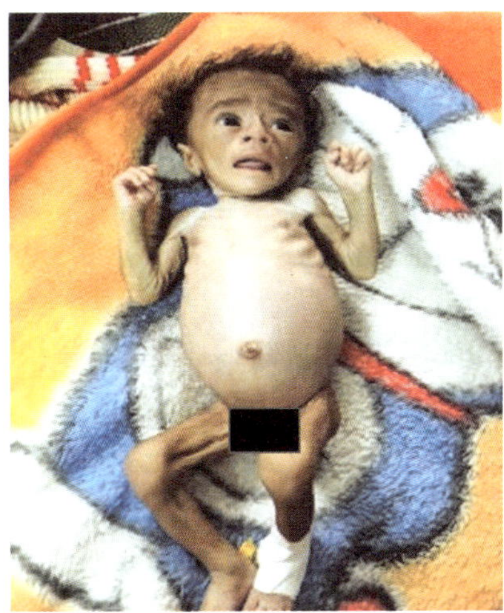

Fig. 9.5: An emaciated grossly wasted child without edema

Courtesy: Prof Praveen Kumar, Lady Hardinge Medical College, New Delhi, India

SAM with Edema

Clinical features resemble the syndrome of kwashiorkor that is described historically as a triad of edema, growth retardation, and psychomotor changes.

Edema: Edema is the clinical manifestation of expansion of extracellular water (ECW) volume caused by prerenal diversion of fluid from the capillary bed to extracellular space. Edema may be caused by (*i*) hypoalbuminemia; (*ii*) retention of fluid and water due to increased capillary permeability because of infection, potassium deficiency being a major contributing factor; and (*iii*) free radical induced damage to cell membranes, induced by infections.

The edema starts in the lower extremities and progresses to involve the upper limbs and the face **(Fig. 9.6)**. The face appears moon-shaped and puffy. The trunk is affected to a lesser extent, and ascites is rare unless there is a coexistent cause such as tuberculosis. In a previously malnourished child, edema is precipitated by debilitating illnesses such as measles or diarrhea. Presence of edema may mask features of severe dehydration secondary to diarrhea in a severely malnourished child.

Psychomotor changes: Children with edematous SAM are lethargic, listless, and apathetic. Play activity and interaction with others is reduced. Child resists attempts to examination. Child loses appetite, and it is difficult to feed orally in the initial phase of dietary management. Child appetite improves once coexistent infection is controlled by antibiotics.

Skin changes: A variety of skin changes have been described in edematous SAM. Dry and scaly skin with cracking is apparent over large areas of trunk and limbs giving mosaic appearance. Most typical skin lesion is *crazy pavement dermatosis* which is characterized by jet black patches over flexures and pressure sites, especially of extremities **(Figs. 9.7A and B)** which later exfoliate to expose raw hypopigmented or reddish skin. Peeling plaques of this dermatosis give appearance of old paint peeling off the surface and is termed *flaky paint dermatosis.* Multiple punctate pinkish areas over the legs are seen in a few cases.

Fig. 9.6: Edematous SAM with skin changes (SAM: severe acute malnutrition)

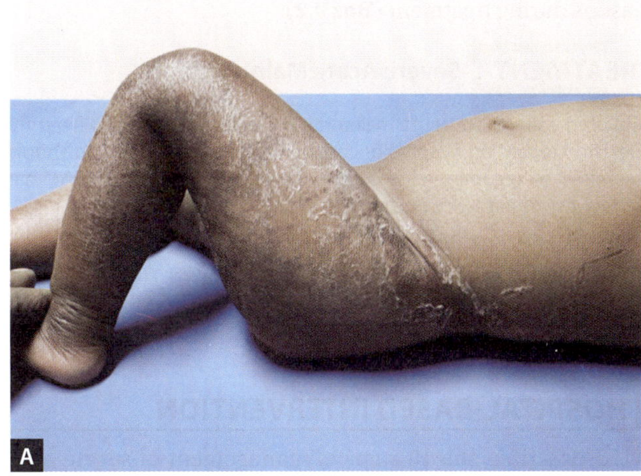

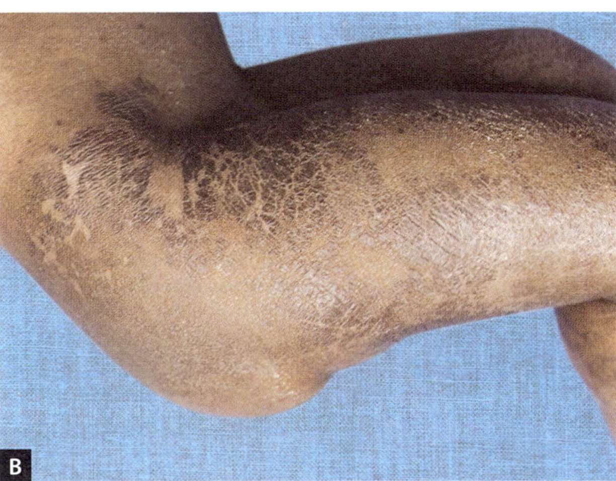

Figs. 9.7A and B: Crazy pavement dermatosis characterized by jet black patches over flexures and pressure sites

Perioral lesions occur frequently which are caused by riboflavin deficiency and zinc deficiency. Deep and indolent ulcerations and fissures in flexures or over pressure points may also occur. Skin changes regress rapidly following successful dietary management of SAM.

Hair changes: Hair become hypopigmented, lustreless, thin, and easily pluckable. The discoloration may be seen only in some segments, often the growing ends. During recovery, segmental discoloration (*flag sign*) is more apparent as the growing part of the hairs gets pigmented. Alternating bands of hypopigmented and normally pigmented hair are sometimes seen when there are multiple periods of nutritional deprivation and nutritional recovery.

Other features include marked wasting, developmental delay, pallor, and features of associated infection and micronutrient deficiencies.

COMPLICATIONS

Complications are listed in **Box 9.1**. These children need to be cared in a nutrition rehabilitation center (NRC) or a health facility. Children with SAM are at risk of death due to various reasons during treatment **(Box 9.2)**.

TREATMENT Severe Acute Malnutrition

Children with severe acute malnutrition need to be treated differently. Decision regarding hospital or community-based intervention should be based on recommended criteria **(Table 9.4)** as child with SAM has higher risk of mortality due to several physiological changes.

Criteria for Hospitalization in Children with SAM

Children with medical complications **(Box 9.1)**, those who fail appetite test **(Box 9.3)** or having 1 or more INMNCI danger signs should be hospitalized and cared in a facility.

HOSPITAL-BASED INTERVENTION

WHO describes the 10 steps of management of severe acute malnutrition. These steps are accomplished in two phases: An initial *stabilization phase* where the acute medical conditions are managed (Steps 1–6); and a longer *rehabilitation phase* (Steps 7–10). Median case fatality rate in children with SAM is very high, i.e., approximately 23.5%, if these management protocols are not kept in mind. The case fatality can be brought down to approximately 7–10% by standard case management protocol. Sequential management of SAM is depicted in **Figure 9.8**.

- The first six steps (Steps 1–6) are related to treatment of complications and can be remembered with the mnemonic SHIELDED.
  S — Sugar deficiency, i.e., hypoglycemia
  H — Hypothermia
  I — Infection and septic shock
  EL — ELectrolyte imbalance
  DE — DEhydration
  D — Deficiencies of iron, vitamins, and other micronutrients.
- Steps 7–10 are related to dietary management which can be remembered by the mnemonic BEST as described below:
  B — Beginning of feeding
  E — Energy dense feeding
  S — Stimulation of emotional and sensorial development
  T — Transfer to home-based diets before discharge or transfer to NRC

Box 9.1 Medical Complications in Severe Acute Malnutrition

1. Edema
2. Persistent vomiting
3. Very weak, apathetic
4. Fever or hypothermia (axillary temperature >38.5°C or <35°C)
5. Children with fast breathing/chest indrawing/cyanosis
6. Extensive skin lesions, eye lesions, post-measles states
7. Diarrhea with dehydration based on history and clinical signs
8. Severe anemia, bleeding, convulsion, or systemic infection
9. Any other general sign that warrants transfer to in-patient facility for assessment or care
10. If caregiver is unable to care for the child at home

Source: Participant Manual for Facility Based Care of Severe Acute Malnutrition. Ministry of Health and Family Welfare, 2013

Box 9.2 Ten Reasons for High Mortality in Severe Acute Malnutrition

1. Inability to distinguish between acute and rehabilitation phases
2. Excessive use of intravenous fluids
3. Fluid overload due to lack of monitoring during rehydration
4. Use of diuretics for edema
5. Use of albumin for edema
6. Not keeping the child warm and euglycemic
7. Low index of suspicion for infection
8. Early use of diets high in protein and sodium
9. Failure to monitor food intake
10. Early treatment of anemia with oral iron

Step 1: Hypoglycemia: Treat and Prevent

Obtain blood sugar. The child may throw seizures or become unconscious due to hypoglycemia (blood sugar <54 mg/dL). If the child is unconscious, lethargic, or convulsing, administer 10% glucose 5 mL/kg intravenously. If the child is conscious, administer 50 mL 10% glucose solution orally or by nasogastric tube. Feeding should be started immediately with F-75 milk-based diet (described in Step 7) and continued every 30 minutes for 2 hours.

If blood sugar continues to be low after 2 hours, give another 50 mL bolus of 10% glucose and continue feeding F-75 every 30 minutes until stable. Thereafter, feeds are given every 2 hourly.

Step 2: Hypothermia: Treat and Prevent

Infants under 1 year of age and those with marasmus, extensive skin loss, or serious infections are prone to get hypothermic (rectal temperature <35.5°C). Cover the hypothermic child with a warmed blanket and place near a heat source (not hot water bottle). Start feeding immediately with F-75. Alternatively, use *kangaroo technique* (placing the child on mother's bare

Table 9.4 Management of Severe Acute Malnutrition

Independent additional criteria	• Poor appetite (failed appetite test) • Acute medical complications • One or more Integrated Management of Childhood Illness (IMCI) danger signs • Severe nutritional edema (+++)		• Appetite good • No medical complications • No criteria needing in-depth assessment or already completed
	↓		↓
Type of therapeutic feeding	**Facility-based**	→	**Community-based**
Intervention	F75 → F100/therapeutic diet And 24-hours medical care		Therapeutic diet basic medical care
Discharge criteria (transition criteria from facility to community-based care)	• Reduced edema and good appetite (with acceptable intake of therapeutic food) • Child eats at least 75% of their calculated therapeutic food for the day • Child does not have any danger signs for at least 24–48 hours prior to transfer time • There is no ongoing weight loss • Nutritional edema is less than +++ • Medical illness for which admission was done has resolved		15–20% weight gain

Infants less than 6 months of age at risk of poor growth and development who have any of the following characteristics should be referred and admitted for inpatient care: (i) one or more Integrated Management of Childhood Illness (IMNCI) danger signs; (ii) acute medical problems or conditions under severe classification as per IMNCI; (iii) edema (nutritional); and (iv) recent weight loss.

Box 9.3 Appetite Test

Procedure: Ask the mother to offer energy dense therapeutic food to the child in a quiet area gently. Child is allowed to drink water while feeding

Interpretation: Passed test, if child eats eagerly. *Failed test*, if refuses therapeutic food even after persistent encouragement

chest or abdomen and covering both of them). Monitor body temperature 2-hourly (half-hourly if heater is used) until it rises to >36.5°.

For prevention of hypothermia in a severely malnourished child, give 2-hourly feeding and cover with a warm blanket, especially during the night. Keep the child dry and let the child sleep with mother at night for warmth.

Step 3: Dehydration: Treat and Prevent

Evaluation of dehydration is difficult in children with severe undernutrition. Skin turgor (elasticity of skin) may be lost either due to loss of the subcutaneous fat or due to loss of extracellular water in dehydration. On the other hand, presence of edema in kwashiorkor may mask the signs of dehydration. As assessment of dehydration is difficult in malnourished children, it is suggested that all children having watery diarrhea should be assumed to have at least *some dehydration*. Presence of weak pulses and oliguria indicate *severe dehydration* or septic shock.

Treatment: Do not use intravenous route to correct dehydration except in presence of shock. Give WHO low osmolarity ORS 5 mL/kg every 30 minutes for 2 hours, orally or by nasogastric tube, then 5–10 mL/kg/h for next 4–10 hours: the exact amount to be given should be determined by how much the child wants, stool loss, and vomiting. Replace the ORS doses at 4, 6, 8, and 10 hours with F-75, if rehydration is continuing at these times. ReSoMal (recommended ORS solution for malnourished children), advocated by WHO is not universally available; and, it can be safely replaced by the standard low osmolarity WHO ORS (glucose and sodium: 75 mMol/L each; potassium: 20 mEq/L; chloride: 65 mEq/L; and citrate: 10 mEq/L).

Return of tears, moist mouth, eyes and fontanel appearing less sunken, and improved skin turgor, may indicate rehydration. However, severely malnourished children may not show these changes even when fully rehydrated. Continuing rapid breathing and pulse during rehydration suggest coexisting infection or overhydration. Signs of excess fluid (overhydration) are increasing respiratory rate and pulse rate, increasing edema, and puffy eyelids. If these signs occur, stop fluids immediately and reassess after 1 hour.

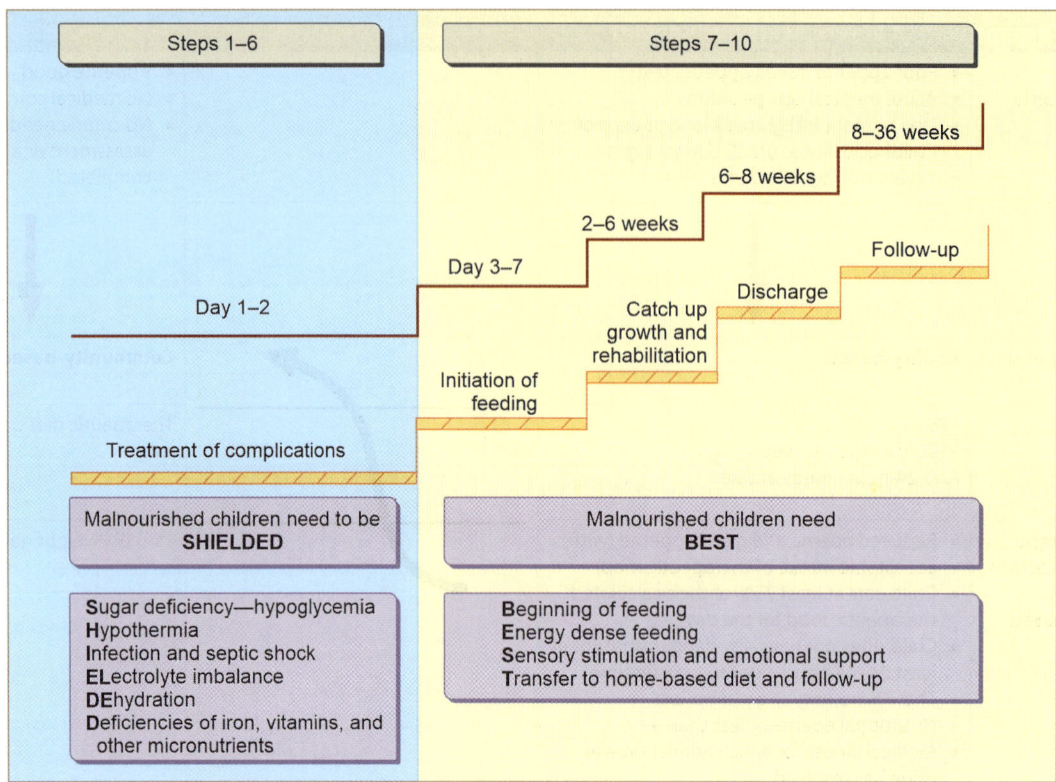

Fig. 9.8: Sequential management of severe acute malnutrition (SAM)

Severe Dehydration

Intravenous therapy should be reserved for children with weak pulse or oliguria to correct severe dehydration. Administer Ringer lactate or N/2 saline in 5% dextrose (15 mL/kg) over 1 hour. If the child fails to improve after the first hour of treatment (15 mL/kg), assume septic shock and manage accordingly (*see* Step 5). If there are signs of improvement (pulse volume improves, and pulse rate decreases), repeat IV fluids at 15 mL/kg over next 1 hour. Then switch to oral or nasogastric rehydration with low osmolarity ORS (100 mL/kg at the rate of 10 mL/kg/h in next 10 hours). Alternate aliquots of ORS can be replaced with starter F-75. If the child cannot be given orally due to paralytic ileus or repeated vomiting, same fluid (100 mL/kg @ 10 mL/kg/h) can be given as N/6 saline in 5% dextrose, intravenously. Maximum attempt should, however, be made to stop IV fluids and shift to feeding F-75 diet, as soon as possible.

To prevent dehydration when a child has continuing watery diarrhea, keep feeding with starter F-75 and replace approximate volume of stool losses with low osmolarity ORS. Give 50–100 mL of ORS after each watery stool. If the child is breastfed, encourage to continue breastfeeding.

Step 4: Electrolyte Imbalance: Treat and Prevent

All severely malnourished children have excess body sodium even though plasma sodium may be low. Therefore, give low sodium fluid (i.e., WHO reduced osmolarity ORS) when rehydrating. Hypertonic saline should not be used even in presence of hyponatremia.

Deficiencies of potassium and magnesium are also present and may take at least 2 weeks to correct. Child should receive extra potassium (3–4 mMol/kg/day) and magnesium (0.4–0.6 mMol/kg/day). Prepare food without salt.

Congestive heart failure: CHF may occur secondary to overhydration, severe anemia, and high sodium intake. Fluid intake must be restricted and frusemide 1 mg/kg IV is given. However, diuretics should never be given to reduce edema in a malnourished child.

Step 5: Infection—Treat and Prevent

The child should be clinically examined for the presence of infections and adequately treated. Most common sites of localized infections are skin, gastrointestinal, respiratory, and urinary tracts. Skin infections are due to *Staphylococcus aureus* or *streptococci*. *Candida* may cause secondary infection over exudative lesions. Skin infections can be prevented by applying barrier cream on raw areas. Perineum should be kept dry. Osteomyelitis is generally caused by *staphylococci*, *H. influenzae*, or *Streptococcus*. Malaria may present with diarrhea and no fever. Always obtain blood culture, chest radiograph, peripheral smear for malarial parasite, and urine culture in a severely malnourished child before starting antimicrobials.

Preferred antibiotics: In severe undernutrition, infections are often hidden. Therefore, antibiotics should be given routinely on admission. If the child appears to have no complications, give oral amoxicillin; and if the child is severely ill (apathetic and lethargic) or has complications (hypoglycemia, hypothermia, broken skin, respiratory tract infection, or urinary tract infection), administer a combination of ampicillin and gentamicin, parenterally. If the child fails to improve clinically within 48 hours, add chloramphenicol. Where specific infections are identified, give specific antibiotics as appropriate.

Continuing diarrhea: Diarrhea should subside during the first week of treatment with cautious feeding. In the rehabilitation phase, loose, poorly formed stools are no cause for concern provided weight gain is satisfactory. Mucosal damage and giardiasis are the two most common causes of continuing diarrhea. Where possible, examine the stools by microscopy. Administer metronidazole (7.5 mg/kg 8-hourly for 7 days), if not already given. Rarely, diarrhea is due to lactose intolerance. Starter F-75 is a low-lactose feed. In exceptional cases, substitute milk feeds with yoghurt or a lactose-free infant formula. Reintroduce milk feeds gradually in the rehabilitation phase.

Tuberculosis: If TB is strongly suspected (contacts with adult TB patient, poor growth despite good intake, chronic cough, chest infection not responding to antibiotics), perform Mantoux test (false negatives are frequent) and chest X-ray. If test is positive or there is a strong suspicion of TB, treat according to national TB guidelines.

Septic shock: Shock from dehydration and sepsis are likely to coexist in severely malnourished children. They are difficult to differentiate on clinical signs alone. Children with dehydration will respond to IV fluids. Those with septic shock will not respond to initial bolus of 15 mL/kg over 1 hour. In this case, give maintenance IV fluids (4 mL/kg/h) while waiting for blood. When blood is available transfuse fresh whole blood at 10 mL/kg *slowly* over 3 hours. Broad-spectrum antibiotics are immediately initiated. Steroids and adrenaline are of no use. If facilities are available, a central venous pressure line should be inserted and the patient should be managed with vasopressors, etc. as for septic shock, in an intensive care unit.

Step 6: Micronutrient Deficiencies

All severely malnourished children should receive vitamins and minerals as follows:

- Vitamin A orally on day 1 (200,000 IU for age >12 months; 100,000 IU for 6–12 months and 50,000 IU for 0–5 months; in case of child >12 months but weighing less than 8 kg, a dose of 1,00,00 IU should be used instead of 2,00,00 IU) unless there is definite evidence that a dose has been given in the last month. In presence of xerophthalmia, the same dose should be repeated on the next day and 2 weeks later. Children receiving F-75, F-100 or RUTF do not require high dose prophylactic vitamin A supplementation; they should receive 5000 IU vitamin A daily (WHO, 2013). If there is corneal clouding or ulceration, give additional eye care in form of antibiotic drops, atropine, and padding.
- Folic acid 5 mg on day 1, followed by 1 mg every day
- Magnesium sulfate 2 mL of 50% solution on day 1
- Vitamin K 2.5 mg IM on day 1
- Give multivitamin supplements, zinc (2 mg/kg/day), copper (0.3 mg/kg/day), and potassium (2 mEq/kg/day) daily for at least 2 weeks.

Anemia: Blood transfusion is required if hemoglobin is <4 g/dL. If there is respiratory distress, transfusion can be given with hemoglobin between 4 and 6 g/dL. Give packed red blood cells 10 mL/kg body weight slowly over 3 hours with furosemide 1 mg/kg IV at the start of the transfusion. It is particularly important that the volume of 10 mL/kg is not exceeded in severely malnourished children. If the severely anemic child has signs of cardiac failure, transfuse packed cells (5–7 mL/kg) rather than whole blood. In mild or moderate anemia, oral iron should be given for 2 months to replenish iron stores but this should not be started until the child has begun to gain weight (usually by the second week), as giving iron in the initial phase can make infections worse.

Step 7: Begin Cautious Feeding (0–7 days)

Start feeding after electrolyte, water imbalance, and infections are brought under control. Do not force food and avoid overloading the system. Vigorous feeding may lead to heart failure and death due to (i) excessive dietary sodium; (ii) rapidly expanding ECF volume; or (iii) activated sodium pump secondary to increased energy supply again leading to increased ECF volume.

The essential features of feeding in the stabilization phase are as follows:

1. Small, frequent feeds of low osmolarity and low lactose
2. Oral or nasogastric (NG) feeds (never parenteral preparations), and
3. ***Calories:*** 100 kcal/kg/day; proteins: 1–1.5 g/kg/day; and fluids: 130 mL/kg/day (100 mL/kg/d if the child has edema).

Route of feeding: Feeds should be initiated as early as possible. If oral feeding is not possible, give nasogastric feeding. Feeding through a nasogastric tube for a few days results in a dramatic change in the behavior of the patient, who then starts accepting oral feeds after a few days. When the child can take fluids by mouth, they should be given frequently and in small amounts. Record the volume taken. If the child is breastfed, encourage to continue breastfeeding.

Type of feed: To start with, milk-based formulas such as starter F-75 containing 75 kcal/100 mL and 0.9 g protein/100 mL (consisting of dried full cream milk powder 35 g or fresh full-cream cow's milk 300 mL, sugar 100 g, vegetable oil 20 g; electrolyte/mineral solution 20 mL; all mixed and volume made up to 1,000 mL) will be satisfactory for most children. Give from a cup or spoon.

The volume of feed is gradually increased and feeding frequency gradually decreased from day 1 to day 7 **(Table 9.5)**.

Use the day 1 weight to calculate how much to give, even if the child loses or gains weight after admission. If the oral intake does not reach 80 kcal/kg/day (105 mL starter formula/kg), give the

Table 9.5 Amount and Frequency of Feed			
Days	*Frequency*	*Vol/kg/feed*	*Vol/kg/day*
1–2	2-hourly	11 mL	130 mL
3–5	3-hourly	16 mL	130 mL
6–7+	4-hourly	22 mL	130 mL

remaining feed by nasogastric tube. Do not exceed 100 kcal/kg/day in this phase. During this phase, diarrhea should gradually diminish and edematous children should lose weight.

Step 8: Energy Dense Feeding

Achieve catch-up growth. Increase in the amount of calories by giving energy dense foods is required once the child is free of complications, shows signs of recovery and the appetite returns after initiation of dietary therapy. This helps the child to restore normal weight for height.

For optimum catch-up growth of severely malnourished children, therapeutic diet should contain energy (150–220 kcal/kg/day) and protein (4–5 g/kg/day). Energy, rather than protein, is the principal determinant of catch up growth rate. The type of foods used during this phase should be energy dense.

The aim should be to achieve a rapid weight gain of >10 g/kg/day.

F-100—the catch-up formula diet: The recommended milk-based F-100 diet contains 100 kcal and 2.9 g protein/100 mL. F-100 consists of dried full cream milk powder 110 g, sugar 50 g, vegetable oil 30 g; electrolyte/mineral solution 20 mL; all mixed and volume made up to 1,000 mL. To change from starter to catch-up formula, replace starter F-75 with the same amount of catch-up formula F-100 for 48 hours then, increase each successive feed by 10 mL. After the transition, give frequent feeds (at least 4-hourly) of unlimited amounts of a catch-up formula to achieve caloric intakes of 150–220 kcal/kg/day and protein intakes of 4–6 g/kg/day. If the child is breastfed, encourage to continue. **Table 9.6** provides a detailed comparison of F-75 and F-100 formula diets.

Ready-to-use therapeutic foods (RUTFs): These are soft or crushable foods used in the domiciliary management of severe undernutrition. These are meant to be consumed without any modification. These are particularly useful in situations where preparation and availability of home-made catch-up food is doubtful. RUTFs have a similar nutrient composition to F-100 but are not water-based and have a longer shelf life. Most RUTFs are made of peanut paste, fats, and added micronutrients and minerals. At least half of the proteins contained in these foods should come from milk products. RUTF has been successfully used in emergency situations globally.

Modified family foods can be used provided they have comparable energy and protein concentrations. These foods can be prepared from mixture of cereal flour (e.g., wheat), pulses (e.g., Bengal gram flour), oil or ghee and jaggery. One example of such energy dense food is *"besan panjiri"* which is prepared by mixing one part each of the above items. It provides 500 calories and 9 g of proteins per 100 g of the preparation. Other such foods can also be prepared based on the local availability and taste. Home available foods can also be used at this stage with added oil and sugar/jaggery to make the food energy dense (e.g., adding oil and curd to *khichdi,* cooking *"parantha"* in place of *"chapati"* and cooking rice with jaggery and oil).

Table 9.6 Milk-based F-75 and F-100 Diets for Severe Acute Malnutrition		
Diets contents (per 100 mL)	*F-75 starter*	*F-100 catch up*
Cow's milk (mL)	30	95
Sugar (g)	9	5
Vegetable oil (g)	2	2
Water (mL)	100	100
Energy (kcal)	75	100
Protein (g)	0.9	2.9
Lactose (g)	1.2	3.8

Step 9: Sensory Stimulation and Emotional Support

Severe undernutrition leads to delayed mental and behavioral development. It is important to provide tender loving care; and a cheerful, stimulating environment. Structured play therapy is essential for at least 15–30 min/day. Encourage physical activity as soon as the child is well enough. Maternal involvement is a must for ensuring complete recovery and also maintaining a good nutritional status in future also.

Step 10: Transfer to Home-based Diet and Prepare for Follow-up

As the child will be ultimately managed at home, it is necessary that the child should be shifted to the adequate quantities of home-based diets. As a general rule, the diet prescribed for the child should be such, which the family can afford to provide for the baby within its limited income, can be easily cooked at home, does not perish easily, is culturally acceptable and easily available in the local market.

Return of appetite, gain in bodyweight with loss of edema, disappearance of hepatomegaly, and rising serum albumin are the early signs of recovery. A child who has achieved 90% weight-for-length can be considered to have completely recovered. This may take 6–8 weeks. The child is still likely to have a low weight-for-age because of stunting.

Good feeding practices and sensory stimulation should be continued at home. Show parent or caregiver how to feed frequently with energy- and nutrient-dense foods. Advise parent/caregiver to bring child back for regular follow-up checks and immunization.

Failure to Respond to Treatment

This is characterized by inadequate weight gain during rehabilitation phase. The rate of weight gain is classified as (i) *Poor:* <5 g/kg/day; (ii) *Moderate:* 5–10 g/kg/day; and (iii) *Good:*

>10 g/kg/day. Possible causes of poor weight gain include (a) inadequate feeding, (b) specific nutrient deficiencies, (c) untreated infection, (d) HIV/AIDS; (e) underlying systemic disorder; and (f) psychological deprivation. A child may have a primary or secondary failure to respond to treatment.

Primary failure to respond may be characterized by the following criteria:

- Failure to regain appetite by day 4;
- Failure to start losing of edema by day 4;
- Failure of disappearance of edema by day 10; or
- Failure to gain weight at least by 5 g/kg of body weight per day by day 10 of therapy.

Secondary failure to respond is said to have occurred, if the child does not gain >5 g/kg/day body weight for 3 consecutive days any time during the rehabilitative phase.

Children who fail to respond to treatment should be screened for persistent diarrhea, giardiasis, shigellosis, amebiasis, otitis media, pneumonia, urinary tract infections, fungal infections, scabies, tuberculosis, helminthiasis, malaria, and HIV/AIDS. If the search proves futile, one should also look for any underlying immunological disease, inborn errors of metabolism and malignancies.

TREATMENT Severe Acute Malnutrition in Less Than 6 Months

Breastmilk is the best source of nutrition in this age group. All possible efforts should be directed toward establishment or re-establishment of effective exclusive breastfeeding by the mother. Supplementary suckling technique (SST) can be utilized to support or re-establish lactation in small or weak infants. In case of failure to re-establish lactation, donor human milk if available should be given. The biggest challenge is in infants where breastfeeding is not possible and nonavailability of a wet nurse or safe donor milk banks.

Supplementary Suckling Technique

Supplementary suckling technique (SST) is a technique used to recommence lactation in mothers who have developed mother's milk insufficiency (MMI) or lactation failure. In SST the F-100 diluted feed 130 mL/kg/day, divided in 6–8 feeds is given through an infant feeding tube of 8-F size. After counseling the mother and taking care of hygiene, one end of the feeding tube is attached to breast with a piece of tape close to the nipple and the other end of the tube put in a cup that contains diluted F-100. The cup is placed 5–10 cm below the level of the nipple so the milk does not flow too quickly and distresses the infant, when he starts suckling at the mother's breast **(Fig. 9.9)**. The sucking stimulates milk production and milk from the bowl through the tube satisfy the need of baby. This keeps the infant at breast for a longer time and stimulates prolactin reflex to produce more milk. Once infant becomes stronger the cup is lowered progressively to about 30 cm below the breast.

Supplementary suckling technique should be done with both breasts alternatively and more than four times per day. At the remaining time, baby should be fed directly from breast or by cup. Gradually, the frequency of SST is decreased. The duration for which SST can be tried ranged from 7 to 14 days. If after few days, the baby does not finish all the supplementary feed, but continues to gain weight, it means that the breast milk is increasing and that the infant is getting enough milk. SST is considered successful if the baby started gaining weight on exclusive breastfeeding.

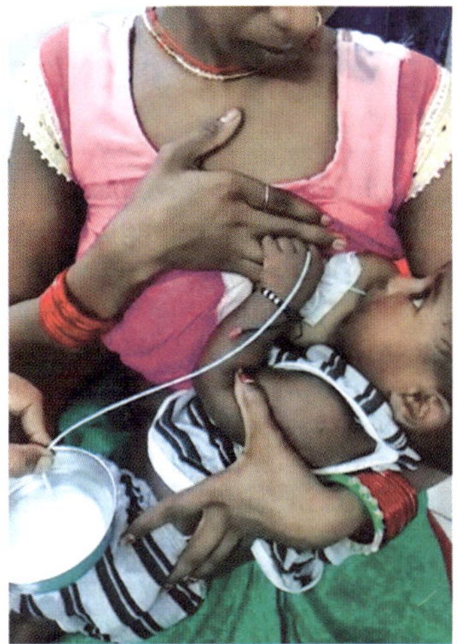

Fig. 9.9: Supplementary suckling technique.

Courtesy: Dr Manisha Maurya, Professor of Pediatrics, MLN Medical College, Prayagraj, Uttar Pradesh

If breastfeeding is insufficient or not possible and there is no edema, commercial generic infant formula or therapeutic diets F-75 or diluted F-100 (diluted by adding 30% water) may be given either alone or as a supplement to the breastfeed. In case the young infant has edema, only F-75 is recommended to supplement the breastmilk. The F-100 diets alone are NEVER used in young infants due to high-renal solute load and the risk of hypernatremic dehydration.

Criteria for Discharge

As per recent WHO recommendations (2023), a child with SAM should be discharged from inpatient to outpatient care if the following criteria are met:

1. Reduced edema and good appetite (with acceptable intake of therapeutic food)
2. Child eats at least 75% of their calculated therapeutic food for the day
3. Child does not have any danger signs for at least 24–48 hours prior to transfer time
4. There is no ongoing weight loss
5. Nutritional edema is less than +++
6. Medical illness for which admission was done has resolved

Ensure that all immunizations have been initiated and mother trained and counseled for care at home. For some children, earlier discharge may be considered, if effective alternative supervision is available.

Early discharge may be considered only if the following criteria are met:

- *The child* is aged >6 months; has completed antibiotic treatment; has good appetite and good weight gain; and has taken potassium/magnesium/mineral/vitamin supplement for 2 weeks (or continuing supplementation at home is possible).
- *The mother/caregiver* is not employed outside the home; is specifically trained to give appropriate feeding; has the financial resources to feed the child; lives within easy reach of the hospital for urgent readmission, if the child becomes ill; can be visited weekly; is trained to give structured play therapy; and is motivated to follow the advice given.
- *Local health workers* are trained to support home care; are specifically trained to examine the child clinically at home, to decide when to refer, to weigh the child, and give appropriate advice; and are motivated.

COMMUNITY-BASED MANAGEMENT OF CHILDREN WITH SEVERE ACUTE MALNUTRITION

This is reserved for children who have passed the appetite test. Community- or home-based management of children with SAM has many advantages as the exposure to hospital-acquired infections is reduced and continuity of care after discharge is ensured. It increases the time available to mothers to spend with family and reduces the risk of possible neglect of siblings. Also, the mothers are able to look after other family responsibilities simultaneously. Treating children with SAM in hospitals is not always desirable or practical in rural settings, and home treatment may be better.

Home-based management (HBM) with energy dense diets or therapeutic foods has better outcomes than standard therapy in hospital. It has been observed that between 60 and 90% of SAM cases, identified through active case finding in community, are without medical complications, and there is adequate evidence that such SAM children can be successfully managed at the home level.

When children are being rehabilitated at home, it is essential to give frequent meals with a high energy and protein content. Aim for achieving at least 150 kcal/kg/day and adequate protein intake (at least 4 g/kg/day). This means feeding the child at least five times per day with foods that contain approximately 100 kcal and 2–3 g protein per 100 g. Home treatment can be food prepared by the caregiver, such as flour porridge, or commercially manufactured food such as ready-to-use therapeutic food (RUTF). Vitamin, iron, and electrolyte/mineral supplements can be continued at home.

Infants and children 6–59 months can be taken off the treatment only if following criteria are met:

1. Weight-for-height/length *Z*-score is equal to or greater than –2 SD of the WHO child growth standards median (WHZ or WLZ ≥ –2 SD).
2. Mid-upper arm circumference (MUAC) is equal to or greater than 125 mm observed for at least 2 consecutive visits/measurements.
3. They have had no nutritional edema for at least 2 consecutive visits/measurements.

Prevention

Undernutrition has twofold adverse impacts. First, due to frequent infections, it causes recurring suffering for children, and second, it puts enormous psychological and financial strain on parents as well as society. Thus, both can be spared if preventive strategies **(Box 9.4)** are adopted.

Box 9.4 Ten Key Interventions to Prevent Undernutrition

1. Timely initiation of breastfeeding within 1 hour of birth
2. Exclusive breastfeeding during the first 6 months of life
3. Timely introduction of complementary foods at 6 months
4. Age-appropriate foods for children 6 months to 2 years
5. Hygienic complementary feeding practices
6. Immunization and biannual vitamin A supplementation with deworming
7. Appropriate feeding for children during and after illness
8. Therapeutic feeding for children with severe acute malnutrition
9. Adequate nutrition and support for adolescent girls to prevent anemia
10. Adequate nutrition and support for pregnant and breastfeeding mothers

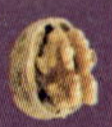

IN A NUTSHELL

Severe Acute Malnutrition

1. Children with weight-for-height/length < –3 *Z*-score of the WHO growth standards or mid-upper arm circumference (MUAC) <11.5 cm or bilateral pedal edema of nutritional origin are classified as SAM.
2. Due to reductive adaptation, children with SAM are at high-risk of hypoglycemia, hypothermia, electrolyte imbalance, infections, and heart failure. Presence of SAM increases risk of mortality in common illnesses such as diarrhea and pneumonia as compared to children without malnutrition.
3. All SAM children with loss of appetite and medical complications should be treated in a health facility while those without complications may be treated in community.
4. World Health Organization has recommended 10 steps of management for children with SAM. Early identification, special therapeutic diet (F-75/F-100), broad-spectrum antibiotic, sodium restriction, and supplementation of potassium and magnesium are integral parts of management.
5. IV fluids should not be used to treat dehydration in children with SAM except in case of shock.
6. During management of infants <6 months with SAM, all possible efforts should be directed toward establishment of exclusive breastfeeding by improving feeding practices and relactation by SST.

Bhatnagar S, Lodha R, Choudhury P, Sachdev HP, Shah N, Narayan S, et al. IAP guidelines 2006 on hospital based management of severely malnourished children. Indian Pediatr. 2007;44:443-61.

Global Nutrition Report. (2022). Executive summary 2022. Global nutrition report. [online] Available from: https://media.globalnutritionreport.org/documents/Executive_summary_2022_Global_Nutrition_Report.pdf [Last accessed August, 2025].

Indian Academy of Pediatrics, Dalwai S, Choudhury P, Bavdekar SB, Dalal R, Kapil U, et al. Consensus Statement of the Indian Academy of Pediatrics on integrated management of severe acute malnutrition. Indian Pediatr. 2013;50(4):399-404.

Ministry of Health and Family Welfare, Government of India. Operational guidelines on facility based management of children with severe acute malnutrition. National Rural Health Mission, New Delhi, India: Ministry of Health and Family Welfare; 2011.
Ministry of Health and Family Welfare Government of India. (2013). Participant Manual for Facility Based Care of Severe Acute Malnutrition. [online] Available from: https://www.medbox.org/document/india-facility-based-care-of-severe-acute-malnutrition-participant-manual#GO [Last accessed August, 2025].
Patwari AK, Kumar S, Beard J. Undernutrition among infants less than 6 months of age: an underestimated public health problem in India. Matern Child Nutr. 2015;11(1):119.
World Health Organization. WHO guideline on the prevention and management of wasting and nutritional oedema (acute malnutrition) in infants and children under 5 years. Geneva: World Health Organization; 2023.
World Health Organization. WHO ETAT Guidelines. Emergency Triage and Treatment. Geneva: World Health Organization; 2016. World Health Organization. WHO Guidelines Approved by the Guidelines Review Committee. Guideline: Updates on the Management of Severe Acute Malnutrition in Infants and Children. Geneva: World Health Organization; 2013.

9.5 Moderate Acute Malnutrition

PE 10.1, PE 10.2, PE 10.3, PE 10.4

DEFINITION

A child who has weight-for-height (WFH) SD score between –3 *Z* and –2 *Z*, or MUAC of 11.5–12.4 cm and has no bilateral pitting edema is classified as having moderate acute malnutrition (MAM).

ETIOPATHOGENESIS

The etiopathogenesis of MAM is generally considered similar to that of the SAM; however, recent studies indicate that MAM could be a result of convergence of multiple factors causing exaggerated dysregulated inflammatory responses and metabolic changes, leading to increases in basal proinflammatory state. Children experience intestinal damage that could be responsible for poor nutrient absorption, reduced intestinal barrier function, increased gut permeability, increased levels of bacterial endotoxin in plasma and a heightened whole blood inflammatory response to bacterial. The elevated levels of serum inflammatory markers observed in MAM suggest that even in the absence of overt infection, there is chronic and low-grade inflammation.

CLINICAL FEATURES

If the dietary intake is deficient for a short period, the body adapts its metabolism to compensate for the deficit to some extent. Energy and protein in the diet are expended more efficiently and nitrogen excretion in the urine and stools is reduced.

If the food deficit persists for a longer period, the malnourished child conserves his energy by curtailing physical activity. Moderately malnourished children appear slow and less energetic. If the nutrition deficit continues longer, the growth of the child is affected; the effect is more visible in weight than in height. With prolonged deprivation, height is also affected. Head circumference is not reduced significantly. As the nutritional deficit exaggerates with the onset of infections, the child may develop severe acute malnutrition.

DIAGNOSIS

Diagnosis of moderate acute malnutrition is based on anthropometric measurements. Weight for height between –3 *Z* and –2 *Z*-score, or mid-upper arm circumference between 11.5 and 12.4 cm without edema classifies a child with MAM.

TREATMENT Moderate Acute Malnutrition

Children with mild and moderate undernutrition are best managed in their home and communities because it is feasible, economical, and effective. Child may receive initial treatment and health education from a nutritional rehabilitation center.

There are two pillars in the management of MAM. One is nutritional education/counseling, that definitely improves the outcome and another is to provide supplementary food through linkages created with services or appropriate supplementary feeding program. All kinds of supplementary foods, e.g., lipid based RUTF, locally produced mixes of various flours, locally processed fortified flour, locally produced corn soy blend (CSB) and milled flour have shown help in recovery.

Daily nutrition supplementation had shown better recovery than weekly supplementation. It is suggested that an energy intake of 25 kcal/kg/d in addition to the standard nutrient requirements of a nonmalnourished child would support a reasonable rate of weight gain without promoting obesity (WHO).

WHO and CMAM (Community Management of Acute Malnutrition) Forum (2014) recommended that children with MAM should receive nutrient-dense supplementary food to provide energy densities between 1.5 and 2.0 kcal g^{-1} (not <0.8 kcal g^{-1}). At least 35 and 45% (not <30%) energy should be derived from fat with minimum 4.5% of the total energy from n-6 polyunsaturated fatty acids (PUFA) and 0.5% from n-3 PUFA. Ratio of linoleic and alpha-linoleic of 5–15, cereal/legume mixtures diet, milk and animal protein sources with protein digestibility corrected amino acid score (PDCAAS) >70% is recommended. Milk powder is suggested to improve amino acid profile, absorption of minerals, e.g., calcium and phosphorus, and as prebiotic. Nutritional recommendations should be complemented with counseling that is feasible, acceptable, and affordable for age-appropriate diet, breastfeeding, and care of child. Demonstration of skill, home visits, and group counseling enhances impact.

All children with moderate acute malnutrition should be assessed for their feeding practices. Counsel parents for adequate amount, frequency, adequate energy density, hygiene, food diversity and active feeding. Parents should learn about the nutritional needs of child and hygienic way of feeding which are important to prevent recurrence of undernutrition. The parents are advised to increase the amount, energy density and diet diversity of the food consumed by the child by all available means. Give a diet chart to the mother which can be modified daily by the mother to provide the variety to the child's food. The diet should provide caloric intake of 150 kcal/kg of the present weight.

All MAM children should be evaluated for any underlying medical conditions, if identified (cleft palate, congenital heart disease, infections, etc.), should be treated or referred for management.

COMPLICATIONS

Main complications of MAM are increased susceptibility to recurrent infections, increased severity of illnesses, progression into SAM, followed by risk of death.

REHABILITATION

To prevent these complications, an effective rehabilitation is of utmost importance. In the post-recovery phase, constant nutritional surveillance is critical to ensure the optimum nutrition and health status, and to provide prompt remedial measure if needed. A regular follow-up should not be limited only to weight gain, but should also take improvement in iron status, height, MUAC, cognitive development along with other micronutrients into account.

PREVENTION

Depending upon the local factors such as functioning markets, household income, and available diet diversity one of three program modalities can be planned for the prevention of MAM.

Blanket supplementary feeding programming in areas with high prevalence of MAM, food insecurity, or high prevalence of chronic undernutrition and micronutrient deficiencies (MNDs).

Cash or voucher programs—where household income is low, this measure increases access and consumption of age-appropriate food for MAM children.

Strong social and behavior change communication (SBCC)/ IYCF-E support—where purchasing power of family is not an issue and local dietary diversity can be utilized.

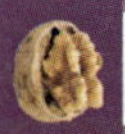

IN A NUTSHELL

Moderate Acute Malnutrition

1. A child who has WFH SD score between −3 Z and −2 Z, or MUAC of 11.5–12.4 cm and has no bilateral pitting edema is classified as having MAM.
2. Complications of MAM are increased susceptibility to recurrent infections, increased severity of illnesses and progression into SAM.
3. Management of MAM includes nutritional education/counseling of parents about age appropriate IYCF practices and care along with supplementary nutrition.

Annan R, Webb P, Brown R. (2014). Management of Moderate Acute Malnutrition (MAM): Current knowledge and practice. UK: CMAM Forum Technical Brief. 2014. pp. 12-5.

Chang CY, Trehan I, Wang RJ, Thakwalakwa C, Maleta K, Deitchler M, et al. Children successfully treated for moderate acute malnutrition remain at risk for malnutrition and death in the subsequent year after recovery. J Nutr. 2013;143(2):215-20.

Global Nutrition Cluster. (2017). Moderate acute malnutrition: a decision tool for emergencies. [online] Available from: https://www.nutritioncluster.net/sites/nutritioncluster.com/files/2021-01/DECISION-TOOL-FOR-MAM_w-exceptional-cicumstances_-May-2017-update-final1.pdf. [Last accessed August, 2025].

Gluning I, Kerac M, Bailey J, Bander A, Opondo C, Trans R. Corrigendum to: The management of moderate acute malnutrition in children aged 6-59 months in low- and middle-income countries: a systematic review and meta-analysis. Soc Trop Med Hyg. 2022;116(3):281.

Lazzerini M, Rubert L, Pani P. Specially formulated foods for treating children with moderate acute malnutrition in low- and middle-income countries. Cochrane database Syst Rev. 2013;6:CD009584.

Lenters L, Wazny K, Webb P, Ahmed T, Bhutta ZA. Treatment of severe and moderate acute malnutrition in low- and middle-income settings: a systematic review, meta-analysis and Delphi process. BMC Public Health. 2013;13:S23.

Patterson GT, Manthi D, Osuna F, Muia A, Olack B, Mbuchi M, et al. Environmental, Metabolic, and Inflammatory Factors Converge in the Pathogenesis of Moderate Acute Malnutrition in Children: An Observational Cohort Study. Am J Trop Med Hyg. 2021;104(5):1877-88.

Stobaugh HC, Bollinger LB, Adams SE, Crocker AH, Grise JB, Kennedy JA, et al. Effect of a package of health and nutrition services on sustained recovery in children after moderate acute malnutrition and factors related to sustaining recovery: a cluster-randomized trial. Am J Clin Nutr. 2017;106(2):657-66.

9.6 Therapeutic Diets

PE 10.5

With the emergence of home-based management approach for SAM children, today there is improved capacity to cost-effectively address the problem of SAM in developing countries, including India. When children are being rehabilitated at home, it is essential to give frequent meals with a high energy and protein content. Aim for achieving at least 150 kcal/kg/day and adequate protein intake (at least 4 g/kg/day). This means feeding the child at least five times per day with foods that contain approximately 100 kcal and 2–3 g protein per 100 g. A practical approach would be using simple modifications of the usual home foods or by use of ready-to-use therapeutic food (RUTF). Home-based management (HBM) with RUTF has been found to be associated with better outcomes than standard therapy in hospital.

READY-TO-USE THERAPEUTIC FOOD

Based on experiences from several countries, WHO and United Nations Children's Fund (UNICEF) have recommended use of ready-to-use therapeutic food (RUTF) for management of children with SAM without complications. These children are managed under an outpatient therapeutic program where they are provided with a high energy *therapeutic food*. RUTF is energy dense ready-to-use paste with at least 50% proteins obtained from milk products. Conventionally, the ingredients used in the production of RUTF are milk powder, vegetable oil, peanuts, sugar, minerals, and vitamins. Paste is homogenized to reduce particle size (<200 μm). RUTF does not need to be mixed with water, thereby avoiding the risk of bacterial proliferation in case of accidental contamination. The product can be safely administered to children with SAM of >6 months of age. It provides sufficient nutrient intake for complete recovery. It can be stored for 3–4 months without refrigeration, even at tropical temperatures. RUTF is consumed with plenty of water every 2–3 hourly in an amount described in **Table 9.7**. While the child is on therapeutic food, breastfeeding should be continued. If the child desires and there is no diarrhea, then even other home-cooked foods may be given.

Characteristics of Ready-to-Use Therapeutic Food

An ideal RUTF should meet the requisite criteria as follows. It should be:

- Caloric dense, high in proteins, vitamins and minerals
- Simple to deliver, to administer, and easy to use
- Fast acting
- Affordable and acceptable cost
- Should not require for trained staff to administer (parents can deliver it to a child)
- Culturally acceptable
- Packed in single-serve packets (each packet may contain fixed amount of calories 400–500 calories)
- Stable with long shelf-life
- Stored in varied climatic conditions and temperature
- Resistant to bacterial contamination.

Table 9.7 Amount of Ready-to-Use Therapeutic Food

Weight (kg)	*Amount of RUTF (g/day)*
3–4.9	105–130
5–6.9	200–260
7–9.9	260–400
10–14.9	400–460

(RUTF: ready-to-use therapeutic food)

Ready-to-Use Therapeutic Food in India

Ready-to-use therapeutic food is not an accepted strategy under RMNCH-A or ICDS program for managing children with SAM. Government of India did not approve the UNICEF activity on the use of RUTF in India. According to the Government of India, for decades good Indian hospitals have successfully treated severe acute malnutrition with local foods. Trials are underway to compare different indigenous nutritional interventions in the community for management of SAM children. A comparison of weight gains with different foods shows that locally made RUTF or even feeding from the modified family pot has similar or sometimes even better weight gains. These findings, however, need further testing and evaluation. The cost of current standard RUTF is the major challenge to large-scale implementation of community-based management of acute undernutrition. Presently in India, there is no commercial RUTF available which can be given to SAM children for community management of SAM.

LOCALLY PREPARED THERAPEUTIC DIETS

Several alternative local food products are now being used for management of children with SAM in community-based programs **(Table 9.8)**. Telangana is using a special formulation "*Balamrutham plus*" in their community-based management

Table 9.8 Sample Home-Based Diet

Foodstuff	*Calories*
• Morning breakfast	
▪ 1 cup (200 mL) milk + 1 tsp sugar	155 (135 + 20)
▪ 1 slice bread (big) + ½ tsp (2.5 g) butter	103 (85 + 18)
▪ 2 biscuits	60
• Lunch	
▪ 1 chapati	80
▪ ½ cup dal	100
▪ ½ cup vegetable (dry)	75
• Evening snack	
▪ 1 banana	90
• Dinner	
▪ 1 cup khichdi	200
▪ 100 mL curd	32
• Night	
▪ 1 cup milk + 1 tsp sugar	155 (135 + 20)
Total = 1,050 kcal	

of acute undernutrition (CMAM) programming. Other states such as Madhya Pradesh (MP), Chhattisgarh, and Odisha have started pilot program using take home ration (THR)-based food intervention in their CMAM program with a target of 150–180 kcal/kg and protein 3.5–5.5/kg through THR based and augmented family foods.

The Cochrane review on the use of alternative diets (home-made RUTF—flour porridge) compared to standard RUTF in improving the clinical outcome of children with SAM in the outpatient setting is inconclusive. The decision regarding the type of diet used in the management can be made based on food accessibility and affordability. An important observation from a recent systematic review is high prevalence of carbohydrate malabsorption (particularly lactose) in infants and children with SAM, which complicates their clinical course and outcome.

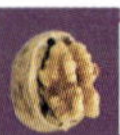

IN A NUTSHELL

Therapeutic Diets

1. The decision regarding the type of diet used in the community management of SAM is based on food accessibility and affordability.
2. WHO and UNICEF have recommended use of ready-to-use therapeutic food (RUTF) for management of children with SAM without complications.
3. RUTF is an energy dense therapeutic food, that contains at least 50% proteins from milk products and could be given to children with SAM of >6 months of age.
4. The cost of current standard RUTF is high. Absence of strict administrative control increases chance of commercial exploitation and misuse of RUTF.
5. Alternative local food products being utilized, range from special formulation as being used in Telangana, to take home ration (THR)-based intervention as seen in Madhya Pradesh (MP), Chhattisgarh, and Odisha with a target of providing 150–180 kcal/kg and protein 3.5–5.5/kg on a daily basis.

Kulkarni B, Mamidi RS. Nutrition rehabilitation of children with severe acute malnutrition: Revisiting studies undertaken by the National Institute of Nutrition. Indian J Med Res. 2019;150(2):139-52.

Kvissberg MA, Dalvi PS, Kerac M, Voskuijl W, Berkley JA, Priebe MG, et al. Carbohydrate malabsorption in acutely malnourished children and infants: a systematic review. Nutr Rev. 2016;74(1):48-58.

Schoonees A, Lombard MJ, Musekiwa A, Nel E, Volmink J. Ready-to-use therapeutic food for home-based treatment of severe acute malnutrition in children from six months to five years of age. Cochrane Database Syst Rev. 2013;2013(6):CD009000.

9.7 Parental Counseling for Undernutrition *PE 10.4*

Parents' counseling plays a pivotal role in the long-term sustained improvement in SAM and MAM as it enables mothers to continue taking proper care at home. Appropriate counseling could prevent the relapse in case of SAM and the deterioration in MAM.

To ensure successful counseling, parents should be communicated succinctly with the help of suitable visual aids such as posters, real foods, etc., especially for the parents who cannot read. In case of hospitalized SAM children, mothers should be encouraged to feed, hold, comfort, and play with their children as much as possible as it would enable them to care better once home. A written card with feeding instructions should be given to parents.

Mothers can be taught to:
- Prepare food
- Feed children
- Bathing and taking care of hygiene
- Play with children, supervise play sessions, and make toys.

Counseling sessions **(Table 9.9)** should start as soon as the child admitted to the facility and continued for whole 14 days with the following schedule including individual and group sessions:

Table 9.9 Counseling Sessions for Parents on Undernutrition

Sr. No.	*Sessions*	*Content*
1.	General hygiene and sanitation (personal and environmental)	• Demonstration—cooking procedure, hand washing, ORS making • Cup, not bottle, should be used for any drink

Contd...

Contd...

Sr. No.	Sessions	Content
2.	Immunization (ANC and children using MCP card)	As instructed in the mother and child protection card/immunization card, bring the child to the health facility for vaccination
3.	Nutritional care for young children	• Provide mixed diets as given to any healthy child • Instead of forcing a child, he should be encouraged to eat by smile or favorable gestures • Feed frequently energy and nutrient dense food
4.	Causes of undernutrition in children	• Do not hold the mother responsible or criticize her for the present nutritional condition of the child as it would demotivate her • Clearly illustrate the gap between what parents have been doing and what needs to be done • Suggest solutions if any specific hurdles in the recovery are noticed
5.	Care of sick children	• Danger sign indicating immediate hospital care: ▪ Not able to drink or breastfeed. Stops feeding ▪ Develops fever ▪ Has fast or difficult breathing. Has a convulsion ▪ Has diarrhea for more than a day, or blood in stool • Basic skills like ORS preparation and identifying danger signs
6.	Appropriate way of cooking food	• Solid foods should include a well-cooked staple cereal • To enrich the energy content, add vegetable oil (5–10 mL for each 100 g serving/half *katori* of approximately 200 mL size) or ghee, or groundnut paste • The cereal should be soft and mashed
7.	How to make nutritious food with available resources at home	• Consider the child's diet routinely consumed • If any specific diet deficit noticed, explain how to prepare a healthy diet with the available ingredients at home
8.	Breastfeeding practices	• Child should continue to be breastfed as often as the he wants • Complementary foods should be given after breastfeeding to avoid replacing breastmilk
9.	Complementary feeding practices	• Explain what to feed, how much to give at each meal, and how many meals and snacks to give • If the child is no longer breastfeeding, animal milk is an important source of energy, protein, minerals and vitamins • Give a variety of well-cooked vegetables, including orange and dark-green leafy ones. If possible, include seasonal fruit, e.g., banana, mango, *cheeku*. Pulses and beans are also good sources of protein. If acceptable, include meat, fish, or eggs in the diet • Give extra food (snacks) between meals in adequate serving size that are energy and nutrients dense, e.g., bread with butter or peanut butter, yoghurt, milk, puddings made with milk, cooked potatoes • Active feeding should be encouraged
10.	Providing sensory stimulation and emotional support through play activities	• Emotional and physical stimulation are crucial for the child's recovery and can reduce the risk of developmental and emotional problems • Give structured play therapy using simple home-made toys at least 15–30 minutes/day individually in addition to the routine play with siblings and peers
11.	Care of mother and family planning	Communicating to mothers the importance of their own health, well-being, and family planning, especially about anemia, personal hygiene, sanitation, diet diversity, and communicable and noncommunicable diseases
12.	Importance of weighing the child and growth monitoring	Highlight the need to record the weight regularly and get it plotted it on the growth chart
13.	Follow-up and care at home after discharge from NRC	• Bring the child to the health facility for health check-up and any prescription. For example, vitamin A supplementation (children aged 9–59 months) for the next dose as advised on discharge and for subsequent 6 monthly doses • Continue advised medication such as vitamins, folic acid (for 2 weeks), and iron (for 2–3 months) at home
14.	Follow-up and recap of all the sessions	Prior to the discharge, review advices and ensure mother's understanding about ingredients to prepare foods at home, number of meals and snacks to feed per day, quantity to feed at each mean or snack, etc.

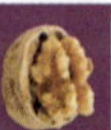

IN A NUTSHELL

Parental Counseling for Undernutrition

1. Counseling of parents is vital for sustained improvement in SAM and MAM children.
2. Counseling sessions should start with first encounter and should continue till the discharge of child from health facility.
3. Mothers should be taught the correct practices to prepare food, make toys, feed, bathe, take care of hygiene, and play with child.

Ashworth A, Ferguson E. Dietary counseling in the management of moderate malnourishment in children. Food Nutr Bull. 2009;30(3 Suppl):S405-33.

Chen Y, Li H. Mother's education and child health: is there a nurturing effect? J Health Econ. 2009;28(2):413-26.

Daniel AI, Bwanali M, Tenthani JC, Gladstone M, Voskuijl W, Potani I, et al. A mixed-methods cluster-randomized controlled trial of a hospital-based psychosocial stimulation and counseling program for caregivers and children with severe acute malnutrition. Curr Develop Nutr. 2021;5(8):nzab100.

Government of Madhya Pradesh. Manual for facility-based management of severe acute malnutrition (SAM) children in Madhya Pradesh 2011. Bhopal, India: Department of Health and Family Welfare; 2011.

9.8 Clinical Approach to a Child with Severe Acute Malnutrition

PE 10.2, PE 10.3

ASSESSMENT OF A CHILD WITH SEVERE ACUTE MALNUTRITION

Initial Workup

Before taking detailed history in a child with SAM, it is important to look for emergency signs. In presence of any of the following emergency signs, immediate treatment should be provided before further evaluation.

- ❖ Not breathing or severe respiratory distress
- ❖ Coma or convulsion
- ❖ Shock/severe dehydration
- ❖ Hypothermia
- ❖ Severe anemia.

If there are no emergency signs, obtain history and examination as described in **Table 9.10** to find out causes (food scarcity and secondary causes), medical complications, and deciding level of treatment. Laboratory tests that should be routinely done on admission include blood glucose, serum electrolytes, hemoglobin, packed cell volume (PCV) in children with severe palmar pallor, and screening for infections. Investigations to identify presence of infections include total and differential leukocyte count; urine routine and microscopic examination; chest X-ray; blood culture and urine culture; Mantoux test; and peripheral smear for malarial parasite. Investigations for secondary causes such as human immunodeficiency virus (HIV), celiac disease, etc., are undertaken as per clinical suspicion.

A representative case study is presented to understand the approach to management of a child with SAM.

Table 9.10 History and Examinations of a Child with Severe or Moderate Acute Malnutrition

History	*Examination*
• Total duration of sickness • Dietary intake of food and fluids • Breastfeeding • Complementary feeds—introduction time, quality, and quantity • Loss of appetite • Any contact with tuberculosis • History of measles in the last 3 months • Known HIV infection • Health of parents • Immunization	• Anthropometric measurements (weight, height or length, and MUAC) • Temperature • Pulse rate or heart rate • Respiratory rate • Capillary refill time • Sensorium • Edema • Lymphadenopathy • Signs of dehydration if history of diarrhea • Palmar pallor • Eye signs for vitamin A deficiency* • Localized signs of infections (ear, throat, skin, and lungs) • Mouth ulcers or oral thrush • Skin changes for dermatosis
Duration and frequency of common complaints: • Diarrhea (watery or bloody) • Vomiting • Fever • Cough	Systemic examination—look for hepatosplenomegaly, any murmur or deformities, hypertonia (cerebral palsy), or sings of meningeal irritation

*One should be very gentle and careful during examination of the eye to prevent the risk of rupture and blindness particularly if the child resists opening of eyes

(HIV: human immunodeficiency virus; MUAC: mid-upper arm circumference)

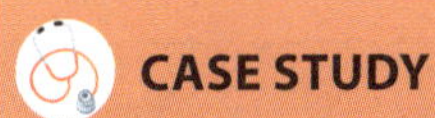

CASE STUDY — Clinical Approach to a Child with Severe Acute Malnutrition

An 18-month-old unimmunized girl is brought to the emergency with frequent loose stools, vomiting, and poor feeding for 7 days. The child is predominantly milk fed (half diluted buffalo's milk with bottle) in addition to some biscuits. Her weight and length are 5 kg and 68 cm, respectively. On examination, she has pallor, weak pulses, cold clammy skin, loss of skin turgor, and sunken eyes.

Assess and classify the nutritional status of this child.

Assessment: The child is obviously malnourished as suggested by her weight and dietary pattern. These children have multiple medical and social problems. The following problems can be identified in this child.

- Acute diarrhea
- Cold clammy skin and weak pulses (severe dehydration and/or septic shock).
- Severe undernutrition and anemia
- Poor feeding (possibility of hypoglycemia and/or infection)
- Faulty feeding (no semi-solids, dilution of milk, bottle feeding)
- Lack of immunization

Classification: Classify severity of undernutrition as per IAP or WHO classification. This child would be classified as *PEM Grade IV* by IAP Classification; and as *severely wasted* and *severely* stunted by WHO classification. Child's weight is 46% of the expected for age (50th percentile at 18 months is 10.8 kg)—*hence PEM IV*. Her length is 84% (<3 SD) of the expected for age (50th percentile at 18 months is 80.9 cm and –3 SD is 71.7 cm)—*hence severely stunted*. The weight for length is 64% (≤3 SD) of the expected (50th percentile for 68 cm is 7.8 kg and –3 SD is 5.5 kg)]—*hence severely wasted*. The child thus has severe acute malnutrition.

Classify state of dehydration: In view of sunken eyes and cold clammy skin, the child is classified as having severe dehydration with shock. Alternatively, the child could be in *septic shock*. Loss of skin turgor may not be a reliable sign in severe acute malnutrition.

Outline the immediate management of this child.

- Admit the child.
- Secure intravenous line and draw samples for blood glucose, blood counts, electrolytes, blood gas, and blood culture.
- Give 25 mL (5 mL/kg) of 10% dextrose IV, if *hypoglycemic*. Give empirically, if blood sugar report is not immediately available.
- Record *temperature* and provide warmth to the child. Keep the child dry, cover with blankets and shift to a warm area.
- *Start fluids for dehydration and shock*. This child has shock which should be initially managed with intravenous fluids. The fluid management in this child would be:
  - *First hour:* 75 mL (15 mL/kg) Ringer lactate or N/2 saline in 5% dextrose intravenously. If there is improvement after 1 hour (pulse rate and respiratory rate decrease and pulse volume improves), repeat 75 mL (15 mL/kg) over next hour. If there is no improvement, consider septic shock and manage in an intensive care setting. In case of improvement, continue fluid administration as below.
    3–12 hours: Put a nasogastric tube and give WHO reduced osmolarity ORS at 50 mL/h (10 mL/kg/h). Replace the ORS doses at 4, 6, 8 and 10 hours with F-75 (50 mL @ 10 mL/kg).
- *Screen and treat for infections:* This child is severely malnourished and has presented with diarrhea, and poor feeding. Start antibiotics immediately and continue even when no organism is identified in urine, stool, or blood culture. The starting antibiotics in this case could be injection ampicillin 100 mg/kg/day (4 divided doses) with gentamicin 7.5 mg/kg/day (three divided doses). Ceftriaxone and vancomycin may be given for severe gram-negative and gram-positive infections, respectively. Obtain a chest X-ray and send urine and stool for culture. Screen for tuberculosis.
- Administer vitamin A 2 Lakh IU orally or 1 Lakh IU intramuscularly.
- Administer vitamin K 2.5 mg IM/IV single dose.
- Administer 2 mL of 50% magnesium sulfate IV and 5 mg of folic acid orally.
- Correct electrolyte disturbances, if any, once serum electrolytes report is available.

Present a detailed plan for dietary management for this child.

Start dietary therapy as soon as possible, if there is no abdominal distention and the bowel sounds are present. Give nasogastric feeds, if the child does not accept orally.

Begin Feeding

Start F-75 diet at 130 mL/kg/day. This child will need 55 mL of F-75 every 2 hourly. This will provide around 100 kcal/kg/day. Continue 2 hourly F-75 for first 2 days. Make the feeds 3 hourly (80 mL @ 16 mL/kg/feed) from day 3 to day 5, and 4 hourly (110 mL @ 22 mL/kg/feed) from day 6. Shift to high energy F-100 diet, if the child's appetite is good (i.e., easily finishes all F-75 feeds orally).

Phase of High-energy Feeding

Readiness to enter this phase is signaled by a return of appetite, usually about one week after admission. When the appetite returns, feed with a cup. Replace starter F-75 with the same amount (110 mL 4 hourly) of catch-up formula F-100 for 48 hours. Increase the amount of F-100 by 10 mL in each successive feed from day 3 onwards till the intake reaches 30 mL/kg/feed (200 mL/kg/day).

Introduce solid foods as early as possible to accustom the child to home-based foods. If the child is able to accept solid home-based foods, she can be shifted to full home-cooked meal providing the desired calories. The high energy therapeutic diets should be continued till the child's weight for height is about 90% of the median.

Preparing the Diet for Home Care

Provide diet chart to the mother which can be modified daily by the mother to provide the variety to the child's food. The diet should provide caloric intake of 150 kcal/kg of the present weight (which should have become 90% of median for that height). Use **Table 9.11** to make a diet chart.

A sample vegetarian North Indian diet for this child has been already depicted in **Table 9.8**. This diet is based on caloric requirement of 1,050 kcal/day (150 kcal/kg) for a 7-kg child. (The weight of this child should have become 90% of median for 68 cm, i.e., 7 kg by this time.) The protein and mineral content is usually adequate, if the diet is wholesome containing foods from all food categories. If the child is unable to consume the suggested amount at one time, divide into frequent small meals. Nonvegetarian foods such as egg, fish, meat, etc., can be included, if culturally acceptable.

Treatment of Micronutrient Deficiencies (Iron, Vitamins, Zinc)

Screen for associated micronutrient deficiency. Pallor of conjunctiva or, palm suggests *anemia. Zinc deficiency* is characterized by perianal rash, redness, and excoriation. Night blindness, Bitot spots, or conjunctival dryness are the pointers of *vitamin A deficiency. Riboflavin deficiency* results in ulceration and excoriation at angle of mouth. Bleeding gums, swelling or pain in lower limbs may suggest scurvy due to *vitamin C deficiency*. Wrist widening, frontal bossing and prominent costochondral junctions are the early features of *rickets*. Clinical deficiency of any micronutrient, if present has to be treated accordingly.

This child is having anemia. Anemia in SAM is multifactorial. Provide iron (3 mg/kg/day), folic acid (0.1 mg/kg/day), vitamin B_{12} (0.1 mg/kg/day), copper (0.3 mg/kg/day) and pyridoxine (70 mg/kg/day).

This child does not have any other symptom or sign of vitamin deficiency but that does not rule out subclinical micronutrient deficiencies. Therefore, administer vitamin D 6 Lakh U orally or intramuscularly (single dose) and zinc (2 mg/kg/day) even when there is no clinical evidence of their deficiency.

Table 9.11 Approximate Calorific Value of Some Cooked Preparations

Preparation	Quantity for one serving	Calories (kcal)
1. Cereal		
Rice	1 cup	170
Phulka	1 no.	80
Paratha	1 no.	150
Puri	1 no.	80
Bread	2 slices	170
Poha	1 cup	270
Upma	1 cup	270
Idli	2 nos.	150
Dosa	1 no.	125
Khichdi	1 cup	200
Wheat porridge	1 cup	220
Semolina porridge	1 cup	220
Cereal flakes with milk (corn/wheat/rice)	1 cup	220
2. Pulse		
Plain *dal*	½ cup	100
Sambar	1 cup	110
3. Vegetable		
With gravy	1 cup	170
Dry	1 cup	150
4. Nonvegetarian		
Boiled egg	1 no.	90
Omelette	1 no.	160
Fried egg	1 no.	160
Mutton curry	¾ cup	260
Chicken curry	¾ cup	240
Fish fried	2 big pieces	190
Fish cutlet	2 nos.	190
Prawn curry	¾ cup	220
Keema kofta curry	¾ cup (6 small koftas)	240
5. Savoury snacks		
Bajji or pakora	8 nos.	280
Besan ka pura	1 no.	220
Chat (dahipakori)	5 pieces	220
Cheese balls	2 nos	250
Dahivada	2 nos	180
Vada	2 nos	140
Masala vada	2 nos.	150
Masala dosa	1 no.	200
Pea-kachori	2 nos.	380
Potato bonda	2 nos.	200
Sago vada	2 nos.	210
Samosa	1 no.	200
Sandwiches (butter 2 tbsp)	2 nos.	200
Vegetable puff	1 no.	200
Pizza (cheese and tomato)	1 slice	200
6. Chutney		
Coconut/groundnut/til	2 tbsp	120
Tomato	1 tbsp	10
Tamarind (with jaggery)	1 tbsp	60
7. Sweets and desserts		
Besan barfi	2 small pieces	400
Chikki	2 pieces	290
Fruit cake	1 piece	270
Rice puttu	½ cup	280
Sandesh	2 nos.	140
Double ka meetha	½ cup	280
Halwa (kesari)	½ cup	320
Jelly/jam	1 tbs	20
Custard (caramel)	½ cup	160
Srikhand	½ cup	380
Milk chocolate	25 g	140
Ice cream	½ cup	200

Contd…

Contd…

1 cup = 200 mL

Source: Dietary Guidelines for Indians, 2nd Ed. National Institute of Nutrition, ICMR; 2011

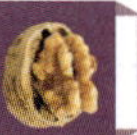

IN A NUTSHELL

Clinical Approach to a Child with Severe Acute Malnutrition

1. After classification of nutritional status all hospitalized SAM children should receive treatment and preventive measures for hypoglycemia, hypothermia, electrolyte imbalance, infections, dehydration and initiation of feeding.
2. Once stabilized feeding should be increased along with focus on sensory stimulation, and preparing mother to provide continue care at home.
3. Management of MAM is done at home/community by providing counseling to mother for IYCF appropriate practices with provision of supplementary food to supply extra 25 kcal/kg/day.

Ministry of Health and Family Welfare, Government of India. Operational guidelines on facility based management of children with severe acute malnutrition. National Rural Health Mission. New Delhi, India: Ministry of Health and Family Welfare; 2011.

World Health Organization. WHO guideline on the prevention and management of wasting and nutritional oedema (acute malnutrition) in infants and children under 5 years. Geneva: World Health Organization; 2023.

World Health Organization, World Food Programme, United Nations System Standing Committee on Nutrition & United Nations Children's Fund (UNICEF). (2007). Community based management of severe acute malnutrition: A joint statement by the World Health Organization, World Food Program, United Nations Standing Committee on Nutrition, United Nations Children's Fund. Geneva: World Health Organization/World Food Program, United Nations Standing Committee on Nutrition/United Nations Children's Fund; 2007. [online] Available from: https://apps.who.int/iris/handle/10665/44295 [Last accessed August, 2025].

9.9 Adolescent Nutrition

PE 10.6

NUTRITIONAL REQUIREMENT

Adolescence is a rapid phase of growth and development as 50% of adult weight and more than 20% of the adult height, and 50% of the skeletal/bone mass is gained during this period. The "growth spurt" results in a 50% increase in calcium and 15% increase in iron requirements. So nutritional requirement increases dramatically and moreover, this period can be the last opportunity for an adolescent to catch up with the growth failure to realize the full growth potential. The recommended dietary allowance (RDA) of Indian adolescents is shown in **Table 9.12**.

Factors Influencing Adolescent Nutrition

- ***Conditioning factors:*** Worm infestations, diarrhea, poor environmental sanitation, and menstruation in girls contribute to malnutrition.
- ***Cultural factors:*** Food habits (eating rice in eastern and southern India and wheat in northern India), custom, beliefs, tradition, attitudes, religion, food fads, cooking practices, and social custom (women taking food at the end) has a bearing on the nutritional intake.
- ***Socioeconomic factors:*** Poverty, ignorance, insufficient education, lack of knowledge regarding nutritive value of foods, large family size may lead to malnutrition and poverty.
- ***Gender issues:*** Girls and young women are discriminated against in both quantity and quality of food. At times they are married early and suffer pregnancy and child birth further compromising their nutrition.
- ***Eating pattern:*** Due to emergence of growing independence adolescent tend to break away from the family eating pattern which is based mainly on availability, convenience, and time rather than nutritive value. They tend to take fast foods, skip meals and breakfast under the influence of peers, mass media, and sociocultural norms of their groups or cliques. Taste preferences are also a major determinant of food choices.

ADOLESCENT UNDERNUTRITION

Malnutrition and Anemia

Adolescent girls are at particularly high risk of anemia and malnutrition. Iron deficiency anemia (IDA) in adolescent girls (up to 66% in some areas) puts a young woman and her future child at risk of premature birth, low birth weight, increased perinatal mortality and maternal mortality. Even boys are found anemic up to 45% in some areas. Iron deficiency anemia also impairs cognitive development and behavior resulting in reduced school performance. It reduces physical performance resulting in reduced work capacity and productivity and thus has economic implications.

Stunting is prevalent in 37.2% boys and 41.0% girls in India. Two-thirds suffer from chronic energy deficiency of the third degree, with body mass index below 16. Almost half of the adolescents of both sexes are not getting even 70% of their daily requirements of energy and a quarter of them are getting <70% of RDA of proteins.

Micronutrient Deficiency

Deficiencies of iodine, iron, and vitamin B_{12} are common among adolescents. The adverse effects of these deficiencies include delayed growth spurt, stunted height, delayed/retarded intellectual development, anemia, and increased risks in childbirth.

Intake of most foods, except cereals, millets, roots and tubers, is below the reference daily intake (RDI) in adolescents. Consumption of green leafy vegetables, fruits, pulses and milk is grossly inadequate. More than 75% of adolescents are consuming <50% of RDA of vitamin A, and 41% of boys and 11% girls are getting <50% of RDA of iron.

Overweight and Obesity

Lifestyle changes related to high-fat diet and low levels of physical activity have resulted in the rising prevalence of overweight

Table 9.12 Recommended Dietary Allowances for Indian Adolescents (ICMR 2020)

Age (years)	Calories	Proteins (g)	Fat (g)	Calcium (mg)	Iron (mg)	Zinc (mg)
Girls						
10–12	2010	33	35	850	28	8.5
13–15	2330	43	40	1000	30	12.8
16–18	2440	46	35	1050	32	14.2
Boys						
10–12	2190	32	35	850	16	8.5
13–15	2750	45	45	1000	22	14.3
16–18	3020	55	50	1050	26	17.6

Source: National Institute of Nutrition, ICMR Guidelines 2020

and obese adolescents (8–12%), particularly in urban areas. Overweight and obesity during childhood and adolescence continue into adulthood, increasing the likelihood of a range of health conditions such as cardiovascular diseases, diabetes, hypertension, stroke, gallbladder disease and some cancers. Obese teenagers are vulnerable to social discrimination. Poor self-esteem and body image are consistently associated with obesity in adolescents.

EATING DISORDERS

Most adolescents are conscious and highly sensitive about the changes in their bodies. They want to conform to the "ideal" body image. As such, they try unhealthy diets and engage in unhealthy eating habits that can lead to eating disorders. Adolescent girls go to extreme measures to remain thin. Most young women want to reduce their weight to be what they believe is more beautiful, attractive, or healthy. Their dieting behavior is supported by their female friends and by commercial advertising. These young women would have iron deficiency anemia, osteoporosis (at present or in later life), amenorrhea, or develop anorexia nervosa or bulimia.

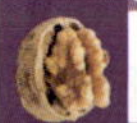

IN A NUTSHELL

Nutrition in Adolescents

1. Some of the important factors influencing nutrition in adolescents include environmental, socioeconomic, cultural, eating patterns and gender issues.
2. Adolescent age group is burdened with triple burden of undernutrition, overweight and obesity and micronutrient deficiencies.
3. Girls are more vulnerable, and the common micronutrients deficiencies are iron, iodine and vitamin.

Bhutta, ZA, Das, JK, Rizvi, A, et al. Nutrition Interventions Review Group, and Maternal and Child Nutrition Study Group. Evidence based interventions for improvement of maternal and child nutrition: what can be done and at what cost? Lancet. 2013;382:452-77.

Black RE, Victora CG, Walker SP, et al. Maternal and Child Nutrition Study Group. Maternal and child undernutrition and overweight in low-income and middle-income countries. Lancet. 2013;382:427-51.

Nutrient Requirements for Indians Recommended Dietary Allowances Estimated Average Requirements—A Report of the Expert Group, 2020 Indian Council of Medical Research India. Updated 2024.

9.10 Obesity

PE 11.1, PE 11.2, PE 11.3, PE 11.4

DEFINITIONS

Obesity is a complex, multifactorial disorder characterized by an excess of adipose tissue to an extent that health may be adversely affected. In simple terms, obesity is a consequence of an energy imbalance where energy intake has exceeded energy expenditure over a considerable period. *Energy intake* is constituted by the food and drink intake, mainly in terms of macronutrients, i.e., carbohydrates, proteins, and fats. *Energy expenditure* occurs through basal metabolism (40–50%), physical activity (30–50%), and dietary thermogenesis (10%).

Positive energy balance occurs when energy intake is greater than energy expenditure. It promotes an increase in energy stores and body weight.

Overweight means a weight more than the average for a given sex, height, and age. Overweight is usually due to obesity but can arise from other causes such as abnormal muscle development or fluid retention.

Obese individuals differ not only according to the degree of excess fat, which they store but also in the regional distribution of that fat within the body. Excess abdominal fat is itself a risk factor for disease as is excess body fat *per se*. It is logical, therefore, in having a method of distinguishing those an increased risk of diseases as a result of abdominal fat distribution, or central obesity, from those with obesity and peripheral fat distribution, in which fat is more evenly and peripherally distributed around the body.

INDICES OF OBESITY

Body Mass Index

Body mass index is a simple index of weight for height that is commonly used to classify overweight and obesity. It is calculated as the weight in kilograms divided by the square of the height in meters (kg/m^2), e.g., the BMI in a 10-year-old girl child who is 50 kg in weight and 132 cm in height will be 28.70 kg/m^2.

$$\text{BMI} = \text{weight (kg)/height (m}^2) = 50 \text{ (kg)} \div 1.32^2 \text{ (m}^2) = 28.7$$

This value of BMI should be plotted on the IAP growth chart (5–18 years) and interpreted as per the cut-offs on the chart **(Figs. 9.10 and 9.11)**. BMI below the 3rd centile signifies undernutrition. BMI above the orange line signifies a BMI that would correspond to an adult-BMI of 23 kg/m^2 suggesting overweight, and a BMI above the red line corresponds to an adult BMI of 27 kg/m^2 indicating obesity. The orange line corresponds to 71th and 75th centile of BMI for boys and girls, respectively. The red line corresponds to 90th and 95th centile of BMI for boys and girls, respectively.

In younger children below 5 years of age, the BMI may be calculated and checked as per the cut-offs on the WHO chart. A BMI *Z*-score [standard deviation score (SDS)] of >+2 or >+3 suggests overweight and obesity, respectively.

Limitations: BMI does not distinguish between weight associated with muscle and weight associated with fat. As a result, the relationship between BMI and body fat content may vary according to body build and proportion. Despite its limitations,

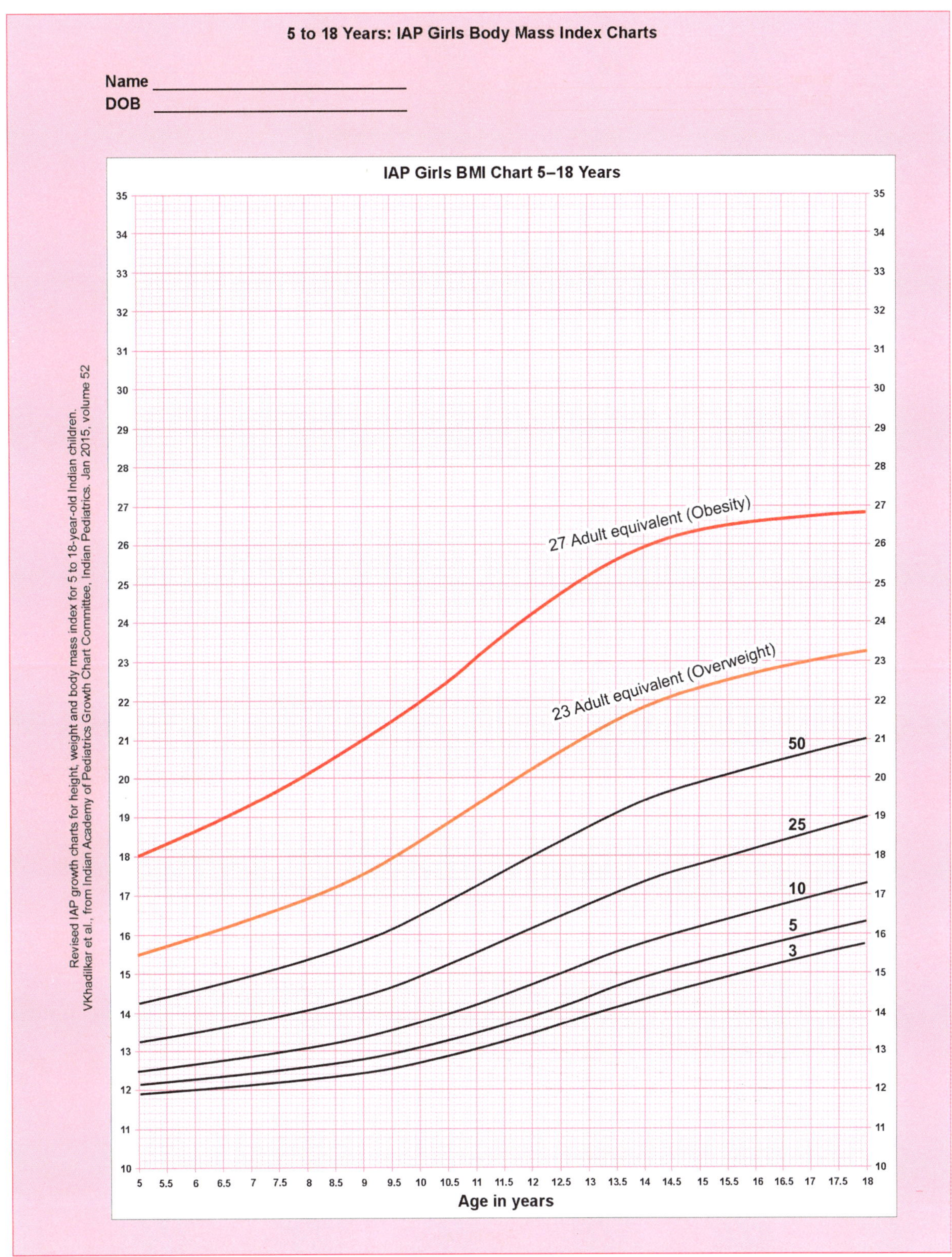

Fig. 9.10: Indian Academy of Pediatrics (IAP) Growth Chart for Body Mass Index (BMI) of girls (5–18 years)

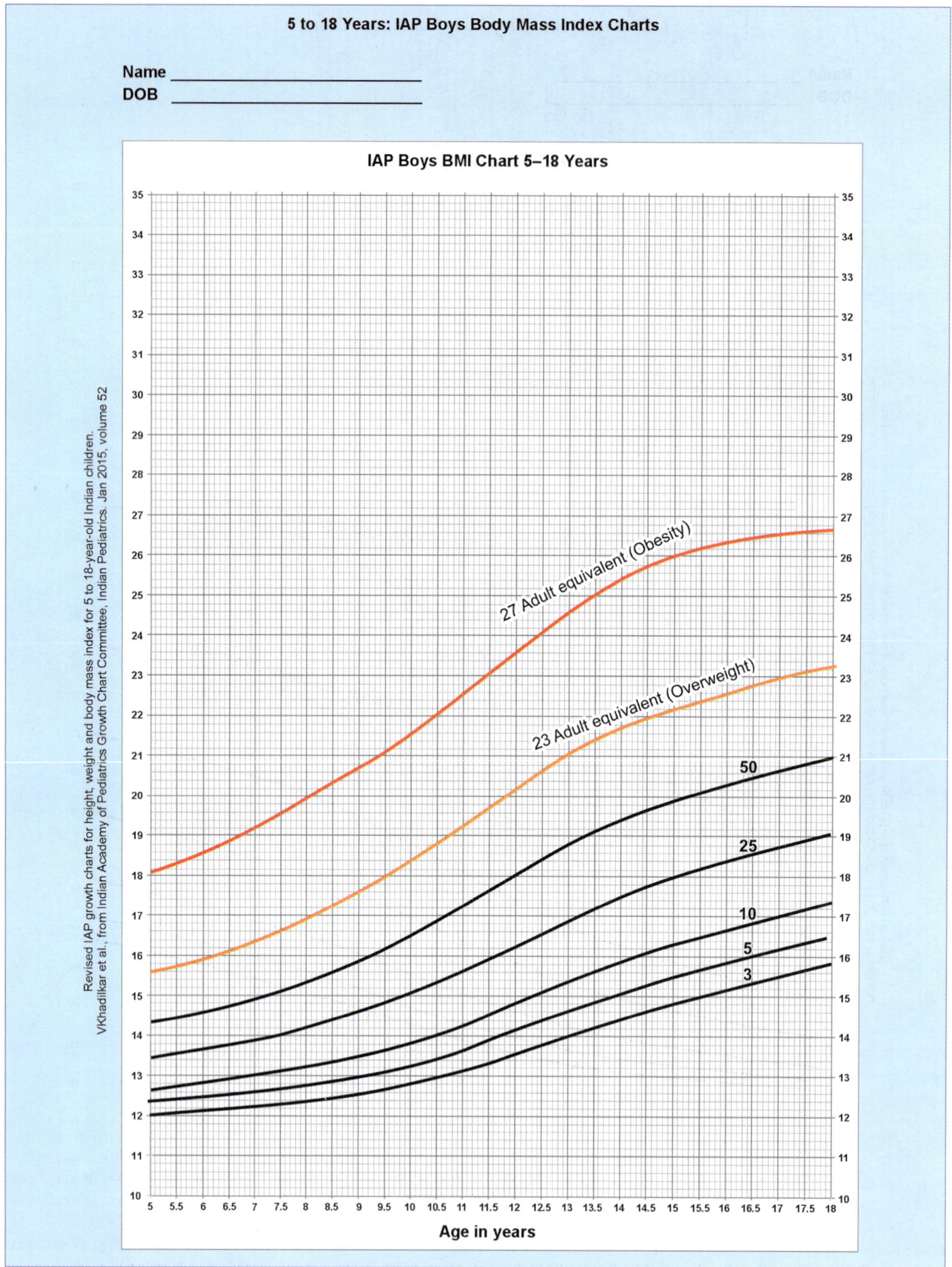

Fig. 9.11: Indian Academy of Pediatrics (IAP) Growth Chart for Body Mass Index (BMI) of boys (5–18 years)

BMI is considered to be the most useful, albeit crude, population level measure of obesity and the risks associated with it.

Waist Circumference and Waist-Hip Ratio: Measures of Abdominal Fat

Abdominal fat mass can vary dramatically within a narrow range of total body fat or BMI. For any accumulation of total body fat, men have on an average twice the amount of abdominal fat than in premenopausal women.

- ***Waist-hip ratio (WHR):*** A high WHR of >1.0 in men and 0.85 in women was accepted for identifying patients with abdominal fat accumulation.
- ***Waist circumference:*** Recent evidence suggests that waist circumference, measured at the midpoint between the lower border of the rib cage and iliac crest, may provide a more practical correlate of abdominal fat distribution and associated ill health.

  The age-wise charts of waist circumference have been collated for use in Indian children.

  - *Advantages:* Waist circumference is a convenient and simple measurement, which is unrelated to height, correlates closely with BMI, and is an approximate index of intra-abdominal fat mass and total body fat. Furthermore, changes in waist circumference reflect changes in risk factors for cardiovascular disease and other forms of chronic disease. This measures the status of central adiposity and increased values are essential for a diagnosis of metabolic syndrome in children.

ETIOLOGY

In most children obesity is caused by a combination of environmental and hereditary factors with an organic cause identified in very few cases (<1%). The causes of childhood obesity are listed here:

- ***Constitutional:*** Environmental factors (95% of all cases)
- ***Pathological:***
  - *Endocrine:* Cushing syndrome, GH deficiency, hypothyroidism, and pseudohypoparathyroidism.
  - *Hypothalamus:* Head injury, infection, brain tumor, and radiation.
  - *Drugs:* Steroids, antiepileptic agents, and estrogen.
  - *Genetic syndromes:* Prader–Willi syndrome, Laurence–Moon syndrome, Bardet–Biedl syndrome, Beckwith–Wiedemann syndrome, and Carpenter syndrome.
  - *Monogenic disorders:* Leptin deficiency/resistance and melanocortin-4 receptor (*MC4R*) gene abnormality.

CONSTITUTIONAL OBESITY

Constitutional obesity results from energy imbalance in association with exogenous or endogenous factors.

Exogenous Factors

Dietary Factors

The fundamental cause of obesity and overweight is an energy imbalance between calories consumed and calories expended. Increased intake of energy-dense foods that are high in fat and carbohydrates is the most important factor.

Carbohydrate and protein balances are usually regulated well by the body. The capacity for storage of fat in humans is unlimited. Therefore, weight gain occurs primarily due to high fat intake leading to anomalous fat balance.

Consumption of sugars also leads to excess energy balance. High protein intake appears to be useful in controlling the body weight, but when consumed in moderation. Frequent consumption of energy dense meals/snacks (grazing) leads to weight gain. The intake of a balanced diet should be encouraged.

Physical Activity Patterns

Physical activity refers to any bodily movement produced by skeletal muscles that result in a substantial increase over the resting energy expenditure.

Physical activity patterns affect total energy expenditure, fat balance, and food intake. A decrease in physical activity levels is a major factor contributing to overweight and obesity. Increased prevalence of obesity has occurred concurrently with a rise in sedentary lifestyles. *Sedentary behavior* is defined as a state when body movement is minimal and energy expenditure approximates resting metabolic rate. As per the WHO and Centers for Disease Control and Prevention (CDC), the guidelines for children and adolescents are mentioned in **Box 9.5**.

Children in low- and middle-income countries are exposed to high-fat, high-sugar, high-salt, energy-dense, micronutrient-poor foods, which tend to be lower in cost but also lower in nutrient quality. These dietary patterns in conjunction with lower levels of physical activity result in sharp increase in childhood obesity.

Environmental Factors

The process of modernization and economic transition has led to industrialization. Motorized transport, mechanized equipment, and labor-saving devices both in home and at work have replaced physically arduous tasks.

Endogenous/Host Factors

Epidemiological, genetic, and molecular studies suggest that there are people who are more susceptible than others to

Box 9.5 Recommendations for Physical Activity

- *Preschool age children:* Physical activity every day throughout the day. Active play through a variety of enjoyable physical activities.
- *Children and adolescents:*
  - At least an average of 60 minutes/day of moderate-to-vigorous intensity, mostly aerobic, physical activity, at least three times a week. Moderate intensity activity would usually be at 5–6 on a scale of 0–10 for an individual. Vigorous intensity activity is usually 7–8 on a scale of 0–10
  - Activities that strengthen muscle and bone should be incorporated at least 3 days a week. These produce an impact or tension on the bones to promote growth, such as running, skipping, and lifting weights
  - Should limit the sedentary time and recreational screen time

becoming overweight and obese. A lifestyle which promotes a positive energy balance would result in obesity more readily in people who have an inherited susceptibility. Apart from diet and lifestyle factors, the following associations are ascribed to multifactorial causation of obesity.

- ***Polygenic obesity:*** Polygenic obesity results from a complex interaction of multiple genetic, social, environmental, and behavioral influences, e.g., single nucleotide polymorphisms of the *PSMA6* and *PSMA3* proteasomal genes affecting gene expression.
- ***Gut microbiota:*** There is emerging association of gut microbiota and obesity as these microorganisms regulate appetite, influence production of short chain fatty acids which are important metabolic regulators and are responsible for epithelial integrity and immunomodulation.
- ***Drugs:*** Certain drugs such as antiepileptics, steroids, and estrogen can result in substantial weight gain. Recent research has implicated the role of various environmental pollutants such as polychlorinated biphenyls (PCBs), dichlorodiphenyldichloroethylene (DDE), and hexachlorobenzene (HCB) in obesity. It is postulated that these chemicals can act as endocrine disruptors even after in utero exposure, to result in permanent physiological changes which can cause obesity in later life. In utero maternal exposure to these chemicals was associated with excess obesity and cardiometabolic risk in children till 4 years of age.

SECONDARY OBESITY

These are uncommon causes of obesity seen in practice.

- ***Monogenic:*** Monogenic obesity is associated with a single gene mutation, insertion or deletion (e.g., a mutation in the leptin/melanocortin pathway, resulting in severe obesity). Loss of function homozygous mutations in leptin (*LEP*) and leptin receptor (*LEPR*) genes are known to result in obesity. Certain genes near which variants have been discovered for children with obesity include fat mass and obesity associated gene (*FTO*), *MC4R* and others such as *ADCY5, ETV5, KCTD15, GNPDA2,* and *TMEM18* loci. Monogenic obesity is identified commonly in consanguineous families.
- ***Syndromic:*** It involves concurrent intellectual disability, dysmorphism, and/or organ-specific developmental abnormalities, e.g., Prader-Willi syndrome, Down syndrome, Albright hereditary osteodystrophy, Bardet-Biedl syndrome, fragile X syndrome, Cohen syndrome, and Carpenter syndrome.
- ***Endocrine:*** These include Cushing syndrome, pseudohypoparathyroidism and hypothyroidism and are discussed in separate chapter.
- ***Hypothalamic:*** This is an extreme form of obesity resulting from functional or anatomical damage to hypothalamus. Ventromedial nucleus (VMN) is involved which is the key regulator of appetite and weight in the human body. Markedly increased and uncontrollable urge to eat is one of the important features of this condition.

EVALUATION OF A CHILD WITH OBESITY

History

The main aim of a detailed history in a child with obesity is to ascertain the cause in terms of energy imbalance and identify any other associated environmental risk factors. The history should also mention the onset and progression of obesity, that will be insidious and slowly progressive in constitutional obesity. In pathological obesity, the onset is sudden and progression is rapid over a period of few weeks to months. These children may also have other systemic features of the underlying systemic disease/disorder.

Dietary history: Record the diet intake by a 24 hours recall. Patterns of frequent snacking, binge eating, and substance abuse (if any), should be noted. The history should also focus on any drugs and supplements that the child is consuming.

History of physical activity and lifestyle: Record it. A detailed family history of obesity and other lifestyle disorders such as type 2 diabetes and cardiovascular disease in adults increases the risk of systemic complications in the child with obesity.

Developmental history: This is essential to identify any developmental delay that can be associated with syndromic or genetic disorders with obesity. Children with constitutional obesity can also have developmental or behavioral issues.

Psychosocial assessment: Many obese adolescent view their bodies in a negative light, believing that others wish to exclude them from social interaction. Body weight appears to be inversely related to both overall self-esteem and body image. Obesity is also associated with depression and anxiety disorders.

Others: The following points should also be elucidated:

- History of maternal gestational diabetes or any other complication of pregnancy such as gestational hypertension and intrauterine growth restriction (IUGR).
- Birthweight, weight gain during infancy, toddler, and adolescent age groups.
- Detailed history of sleep pattern including daytime somnolence.
- History of use of nutritional supplements for weight loss or height gain.
- Menstrual history in girls—age of menarche and menstrual irregularities.

Examination

Apart from routine general and systemic physical examination, following should be recorded in all subjects with overweight and obesity:

- ***Anthropometric measurement***—height, weight, waist and hip circumferences, and BMI.
- ***Signs of insulin resistance***—acanthosis nigricans which are hyperpigmented thick velvety skin patches that can be seen at the posterior and lateral folds of neck, axilla, groin and sometimes at elbows and knees **(Figs. 9.12A and B)**. Skin tags may also be seen.

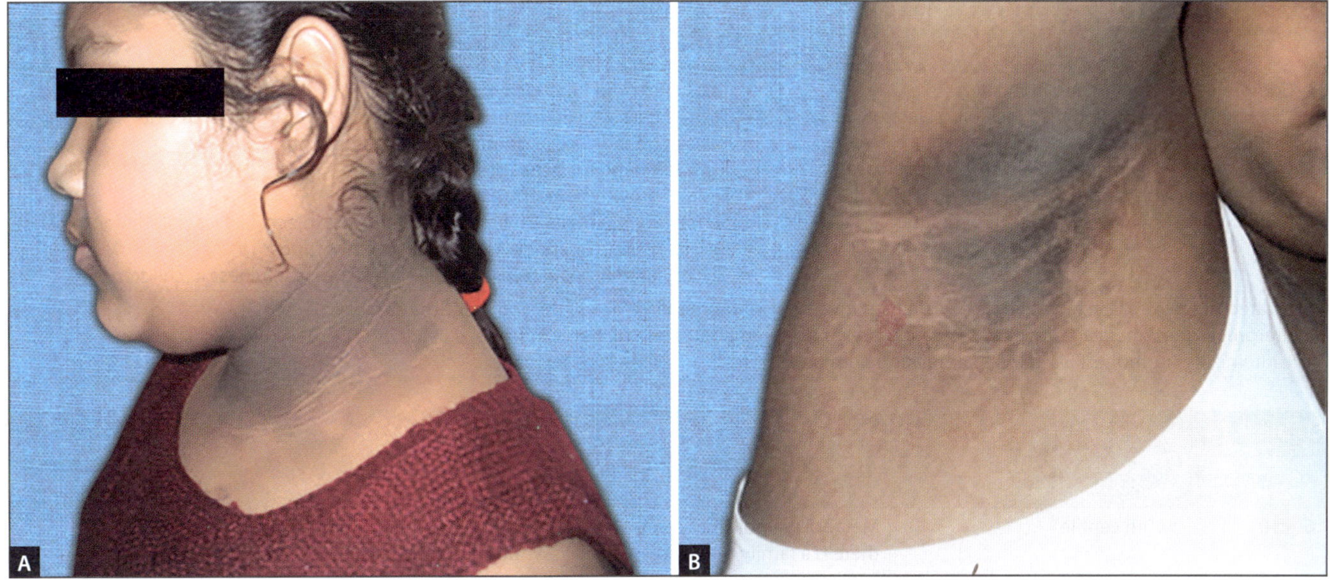

Figs. 9.12A and B: Acanthosis nigricans over (A) Neck; and (B) Axilla

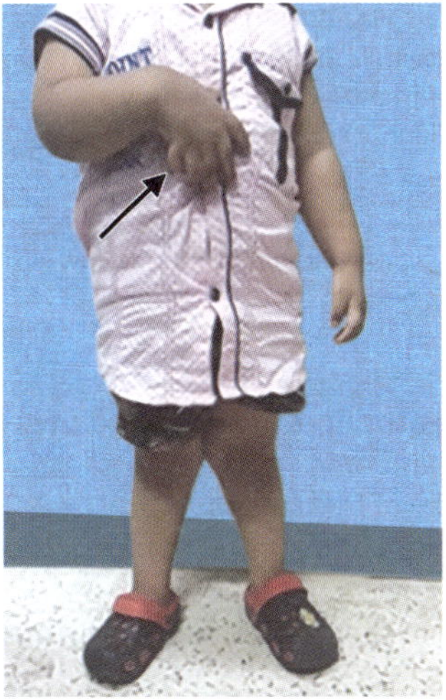

Fig. 9.13: A 3-year-old obese child with Bardet–Biedl syndrome. Note the extra-axial polydactyly. The child had retinal dystrophy and pelvicalyceal dilatation in bilateral kidneys

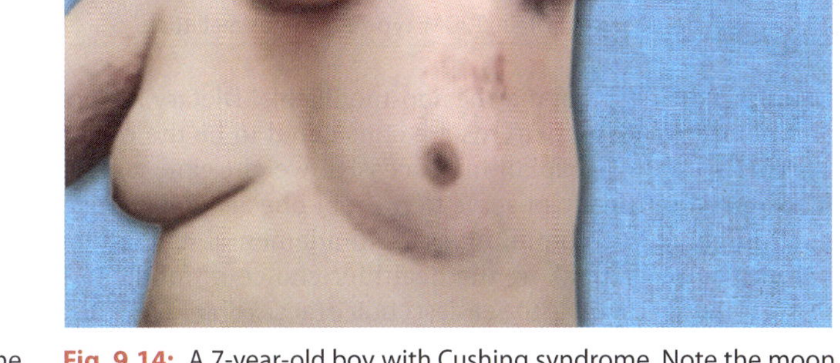

Fig. 9.14: A 7-year-old boy with Cushing syndrome. Note the moon facies, facial plethora, double chin, fullness of supraclavicular fossa, extensive skin striae, and lipomastia

- ***Signs of hyperandrogenism (girls)***—acne, hirsutism, and increased hair fall.
- Any dysmorphic feature/stigmata which may suggest secondary cause of obesity. **Figure 9.13** depicts a 3-year-old child with Bardet–Biedl syndrome showing extra-axial polydactyly in all limbs along with retinal dystrophy. **Figure 9.14** depicts a boy with classical Cushing syndrome, showing striae and gynecomastia.
- ***Pubertal status:*** The pubertal status should be determined. Differentiate lipomastia from true breast enlargement. Increased BMI in girls is associated with early puberty.
- Psychiatric evaluation should be done in all children.

Investigations

Basic and limited laboratory investigations are advisable in obese and overweight children to assess for associated metabolic abnormalities **(Table 9.13)**. When secondary obesity is suspected, a detailed work-up and opinion of concerned specialist may be required. The child also needs to be evaluated for metabolic syndrome **(Table 9.14)**.

PREVENTION OF OBESITY

The susceptibility of individuals to gain weight is affected by genetic and other biological factors, such as sex, age, and

Table 9.13 Blood Investigations Required in Evaluation of Obesity

Investigations routinely required in evaluation of obesity	*Investigations required only if clinical examination is suggestive*
• Complete blood count and blood film • *Liver and renal function tests including electrolytes • Fasting lipid profile • **Oral glucose tolerance test—with 1.75 g glucose/kg body weight with maximum of 75 g (Blood glucose samples at 0 and 120 minutes)	• Tests of thyroid functions • Tests of cortisol axis—overnight dexamethasone suppression test • Tests of gonadal axis—serum LH/FSH/testosterone • X-ray left hand for bone age assessment • Tests of growth hormone axis • Serum vitamin D/parathyroid hormone—in subjects with skeletal symptoms • Serum insulin/C-peptide—only in research settings • Glycosylated hemoglobin (HbA1c)—no proven usefulness in children

*Elevated ALT > 25 U/L in boys and >22 U/L in girls. Investigate if more than twice of this for 3 months or more
**Interpret as per American Diabetic Association cut-offs for prediabetes and diabetes mellitus
(LH: luteinizing hormone; FSH: follicle-stimulating hormone)

Table 9.14 Definition of Metabolic Syndrome in Children as per International Diabetic Federation (IDF)

Age group (years)	*Waist circumference (WC)*	*Serum triglyceride*	*Serum HDL-cholesterol*	*Blood pressure*	*Fasting blood glucose*
6–<10	>90th centile*	Metabolic syndrome¶ cannot be diagnosed, but further measurements should be made if there is a family history of metabolic syndrome, T2DM, dyslipidemia, cardiovascular disease, hypertension and/or obesity			
≥10–<16	>90th centile* or adult cut-off if lower	≥150 mg/dL	<40 mg/dL	Systolic ≥130 mm Hg or diastolic ≥85 mm Hg#	≥100 mg/dL or known T2DM
≥16	WC ≥94 cm for men and ≥80 cm for women plus any two of the next four factors	≥150 mg/dL	<40 mg/dL for men <50 mg/dL for women	Systolic BP ≥130 or diastolic BP ≥85 mm Hg, or treatment of previously diagnosed hypertension	≥100 mg/dL or known T2DM

*WC—depends on ethnicity, age, and gender
#National High Blood Pressure Education Program
¶Metabolic syndrome is defined as presence of central obesity (raised WC) with two or more risk factors (raised triglyceride, low HDL-c, hypertension or dysglycemia)
(HDL: high density lipoprotein; T2DM: type 2 diabetes mellitus)

hormonal activity, that may be non-modifiable. Dietary factors and physical activity patterns are considered to be the major modifiable factors explaining excessive weight gain which, if corrected in time, can serve to prevent obesity. Supportive environments and communities are fundamental in shaping people's choices, making the healthier choice of foods and regular physical activity the easiest choice (accessible, available, and affordable), and therefore preventing obesity.

Universal Prevention

Preventing the development of overweight in normal children is the most cost-effective approach to tackle obesity.

An efficient strategy should primarily address the need for change in the dietary habits and physical activity levels, the two most important issues in obesity prevention.

Diet

For diet, recommendations for populations and individuals should include the following:

- Limit energy intake from total fats and shift fat consumption away from saturated fats to unsaturated fats. Encourage elimination of trans-fatty acids. No fat restriction is required below 2 years. For older children, fats should contribute to 20–30% of total calories.
- Increase consumption of fruits and vegetables, legumes, whole grains, and nuts.
- Limit the intake of free sugars.
- Limit salt (sodium) consumption from all sources and ensure that salt is iodized.
- Fiber content in diet should be approximately equal to age (in years) + 5 g.

Care should be provided to support adequate nutrition during the antenatal period to optimize intrauterine growth pattern, promote exclusive breastfeeding and encourage adequate quantity and quality of complementary feeding. Exclusive breastfeeding has shown to prevent the adulthood risk of obesity, type 2 diabetes, and metabolic syndrome. IAP recommendations to avoid junk food are listed in **Box 9.6**.

Physical Activity

Energy expenditure can be increased by provision of convenient and safe exercise facilities, allocation of time for the activity, parental education, and reduction in screen time. IAP recommends no screen viewing below 2 years of age and <1 hour for older children.

Younger children and toddlers should have daily ½–1 hour of outdoor play. Older children should have moderate to vigorous exercise for 60 minutes daily of which 30 minutes should be during school time. Also, most of daily physical activity should

Box 9.6 Recommendations to Limit Consumption of JUNCS in Childhood

J—Junk food (foods high in fats (saturated and trans-fats, sugars and salts, lacking micronutrients)
U—Ultraprocessed foods
N—Nutritionally inappropriate foods, applicable to homemade food also if cooked in recycled oil, containing high amount of sugar, fat, or salt
C—Caffeinated/colored/carbonated beverages
S—Sweetened sugar beverages

Recommendations:

1. To reduce free sugars to <5% of the total energy intake
2. Fruit juices which contain high content of unprocessed sugars to be avoided in children <2 years of age, not to be offered even as reward or gift
3. Encourage intake of seasonal whole fruits over fruit juices in children and adolescents
4. Fruit juices to be limited to 125 mL per day for children between 2 and 5 years of age and 250 mL per day for >5 years; preferably be given as fresh juices
5. The total sugar content (added plus inherent sugars) to be limited to <30% of total energy for beverages/liquid food and <10% for solid food
6. No caffeinated or carbonated drinks should be consumed by children <5 years of age
7. In school going and adolescents, limit tea/coffee intake to a maximum of half cup/day (100 mL) and in 10–18 years one cup/day, provided no other caffeinated products are being consumed

be aerobic; however, vigorous activities which strengthen muscle and bone should also be included at least three times a week. Activities like dance and sports are other attractive options.

Behavior

Parental motivation, commitment, and simulation of healthy lifestyle are necessary. Older children should be educated and made responsible for their nutrition and exercise pattern. Facilitatory techniques include no stacking of unhealthy foods in house, setting realistic goals for exercise, positive reinforcement on successful diet change or exercise, and timely monitoring.

Targeted Prevention

This is directed at high-risk children who may have a detectable amount of excess weight and at high risk of associated diseases but are not yet obese.

At-risk Approach

"At-risk approach" deals with children who are at particularly high risk of obesity and its consequences. It has four components:

1. Prevention of weight gain
2. Promotion of weight maintenance
3. Management of health risks associated with obesity
4. Promotion of weight loss

An effective "at-risk approach" involves five main stages:

1. Recruitment and referral
2. Comprehensive health assessment
3. Setting appropriate targets
4. Implementing management strategies
5. Monitoring, reward, and evaluation

CRITERIA FOR REFERRAL

The health consequences of obesity range from an increased risk of premature death to several nonfatal but debilitating complaints with impact on immediate quality of life. Obesity is strongly related to major cardiovascular risk factors such as raised blood pressure, glucose intolerance, type 2 diabetes, and dyslipidemia. BMI is thought to account for about 60% of the risk of developing type 2 diabetes, over 20% of that for hypertension and coronary heart disease and between 10 and 30% for various cancers.

- All children with obesity should be referred to institute a multidisciplinary team plan for management. This would require services of a pediatrician to conduct the clinical examination and screen for comorbidities, a dietician to plan the diet plan, and a counselor to advise behavioral modifications for compliance to dietary and physical activity plan. These children also require a regular follow-up to monitor weight reduction and compliance to lifestyle.
- Children with any associated comorbidity (metabolic syndrome, diabetes, hypertension, and secondary obesity) should be referred for further management.

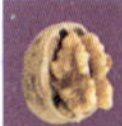

IN A NUTSHELL

Obesity

1. Pediatric obesity is an indolent epidemic with repercussions in adulthood.
2. BMI is the most used parameter to assess obesity.
3. Detailed history and clinical examination are important for eliciting red flag signs.
4. Investigations should be done to detect associated comorbidities like metabolic syndrome.
5. Management approach focuses on preventive measures with conservative treatment options, and limited role of pharmacotherapy or bariatric surgery in children.

Abrego Del Castillo KY, Dennis CL, Wamithi S, et al. Maternal BMI, breastfeeding and perinatal factors that influence early childhood growth trajectories: a scoping review. J Dev Orig Health Dis. 2022;13(5):541-9.
Bull FC, Al-Ansari SS, Biddle S, et al. World Health Organization 2020 guidelines on physical activity and sedentary behaviour. Br J Sports Med. 2020;54(24):1451-62.
Gupta P, Shah D, Kumar P, et al. Indian Academy of Pediatrics Guidelines on the Fast and Junk Foods, Sugar Sweetened Beverages, Fruit Juices, and Energy Drinks. Indian Pediatr. 2019;56(10):849-63.
Kumar S, Kelly AS. Review of Childhood Obesity: From Epidemiology, Etiology, and Comorbidities to Clinical Assessment and Treatment. Mayo Clin Proc. 2017;92(2):251-65.
Thomas-Eapen N. Childhood Obesity. Prim Care. 2021;48(3):505-15.
Weihrauch-Blüher S, Wiegand S. Risk Factors and Implications of Childhood Obesity. Curr Obes Rep. 2018;7(4):254-9.

Piyush Gupta, Nidhi Bedi; and Aashima Dabas (Obesity)

10 CHAPTER Vitamins

AS PER NMC COMPETENCIES

PE12.1	Describe the RDA, dietary sources of vitamin A, its metabolism.	*Ch 10.2*
PE12.2	Describe the causes, clinical features, classification, diagnosis and management of deficiency/excess of vitamin A.	*Ch 10.2*
PE12.3	Describe the causes, clinical features, diagnosis and management of deficiency/excess of vitamin D (rickets and hypervitaminosis D).	*Ch 10.3*
PE12.4	Describe the causes, clinical features, diagnosis and management of deficiency of vitamin E.	*Ch 10.4*
PE12.5	Describe the RDA, dietary sources of vitamin K and their role in health and disease.	*Ch 10.5*
PE12.6	Describe the causes, clinical features, diagnosis, management and prevention of deficiency of vitamin K.	*Ch 10.5*
PE12.7	Describe the causes, clinical features, diagnosis and management of deficiency of B complex vitamins.	*Ch 10.6*
PE12.8	Describe the RDA, dietary sources of vitamin C and its role in health and disease, clinical features of deficiency and management.	*Ch 10.7*

10.1 Introduction

Vitamins are a group of organic nutrients required by the body in minute quantities. They do not contribute to calories but are indispensable for various specific metabolic reactions. Since most vitamins cannot be synthesized in the body in requisite amounts, they need to be supplied in diet.

Vitamins serve diverse functions such as cofactors and coenzymes in enzyme systems (e.g., vitamin B complex), hormones (e.g., vitamin D), and antioxidants (e.g., vitamin E). Their action as cofactors in many enzyme systems makes them essential for various body functions, such as energy production, hematopoiesis, neurological functions, hydroxylation and synthesis of fats, amino acids, nucleic acids, and nucleoproteins. Any aberrations in these critical mechanisms can cause profound changes to the nervous system and to the integrity of skin, mucous membrane, synthesis and repair of connective tissues, and drug metabolism.

The fetus and the infant get adequate vitamins from the mother during pregnancy and lactation. Dietary intake of vitamins may be low or marginal during infancy and early childhood. Vitamin deficiencies may be caused by (1) Deficient intake (ignorance, food fads, and faulty cooking methods); (2) Faulty absorption (malabsorption and chronic diarrhea); (3) Increased losses; (4) Poor utilization (chronic liver disease); or (5) Greater demand. The requirement of vitamins increases in preterm babies, during postoperative stress, infections, and in some genetic metabolic disorders.

Vitamins are classified into (1) *Water-soluble vitamins*: vitamin B complex and vitamin C; and (2) *Fat-soluble vitamins*: vitamin A, vitamin D, vitamin E, and vitamin K.

National Nutrition Monitoring Bureau, NNMB. Technical Report No. 22: Prevalence of Micronutrient Deficiencies. Hyderabad: National Institute of Nutrition, Indian Council of Medical Research; 2003.

The Micronutrient Initiative Global Nutrition Report. https://globalnutritionreport.org/[Last accessed August, 2025].

WHO. Micronutrient. [online] Available from: https://www.who.int/health-topics/micronutrients [Last accessed August, 2025].

WHO. Vitamin and Mineral Requirements in Human Nutrition, 2nd edition. Geneva: WHO; 2005.

Fat-soluble Vitamins

10.2 Vitamin A and Xerophthalmia

PE 12.1, PE 12.2

INTRODUCTION

Vitamin A is a subgroup of retinoids exhibiting the biological activity of retinol. Naturally occurring retinoids include retinol (vitamin A alcohol), retinyl ester (vitamin A ester), retinal (vitamin A aldehyde), and retinoic acid (vitamin A acid). Retinoic acid is the most active form of the vitamin. Vitamin A from the diet is ingested as carotene (from plant sources) and retinal (from animal sources). Out of many different carotene pigments, beta-carotene (provitamin A) yields the highest amount of retinol. The absorption of dietary beta-carotenes varies according to the source, and is generally assumed to be 50%. Absorbed vitamin A is stored in liver as retinyl palmitate. Zinc is required for mobilization of retinyl palmitate to free retinol. Retinol is transported in blood, bound to a retinol binding protein (RBP).

1 μg of retinol = 3.33 international units (IU) of vitamin A

1 IU of vitamin A = 0.6 μg of carotene

60 mg of retinol = 110 mg of retinyl palmitate = 69 mg retinyl acetate = 2 lakh IU of vitamin A

DAILY REQUIREMENTS

The daily requirement values are in terms of retinol equivalents (RE) (ICMR, 2020). If carotenes are the sources, RE is multiplied by 6 assuming a 1:6 conversion efficiency (CE) for all carotenoids except β-cryptoxanthine and α-carotene where a CE of 1:12 is recommended. It is recommended that minimum 50% of retinol equivalents should be derived from animal sources to ensure adequacy in vulnerable groups **(Table 10.1)**.

Table 10.1 Requirements of Vitamin A (Retinol Equivalents) for Different Age Groups

Age group	*RDA (μg/day)*	*EAR (μg/day)*
Men	1,000	460
Women	840	390
Pregnant women	900	406
Lactating women	950	720
Infants		
• 0–6 m	350 (AI)	—
• 6–12 m	350	170
Children		
• 1–3 y	390	180
• 4–6 y	510	240
• 7–9 y	630	290
Boys (10–12 y)	770	360
Girls (10–12 y)	790	370
Boys (13–15 y)	930	430
Girls (13–15 y)	890	420
Boys (16–18 y)	1,000	480
Girls (16–18 y)	860	400

(EAR: estimated average requirement; RDA: recommended dietary allowance; AI: adequate intake; m: months; y: years)
Source: ICMR 2020

DIETARY SOURCES

Breastmilk fulfills the needs of vitamin A entirely for first 6 months of life and continues to be an important source up to 2 years. Preformed vitamin A (retinol) is abundant in fish liver oils, liver, dairy products, and egg yolk. Vegetarian sources of vitamin A are green leafy vegetables, and yellow fruits and vegetables, where it is present as carotenoids **(Fig. 10.1)**.

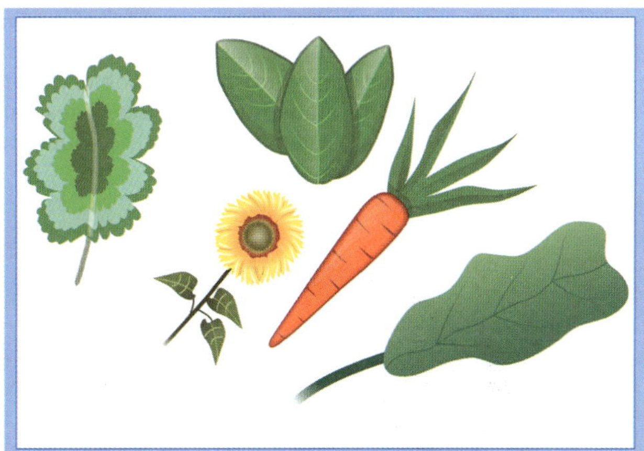

Fig. 10.1: Sources of vitamin A

ROLE IN HEALTH AND DISEASE

Vitamin A is necessary for the integrity of epithelial tissues and functioning of retina and vision. Retinol is necessary for spermatogenesis and integrity of testicular and vaginal epithelium. Patients with vitamin A deficiency have defective dark adaptation. Vitamin A as retinoic acid is involved in growth especially skeletal growth, fertility, and immune response. It is also termed as an anti-infective vitamin. This is attributed to its role in maintaining integrity of epithelial tissue for resisting invasion by pathogens and for functional immune response. Role of vitamin A in reduction of overall child mortality, once hyped, is now being questioned.

VITAMIN A DEFICIENCY

Causes

Insufficient intake of vitamin A (not consuming vitamin A rich fruit, vegetables, etc.) is the most common cause of vitamin A deficiency. Severe malnutrition is another important cause. The requirement of vitamin A is increased in preterm neonates and during infections (e.g., measles and respiratory tract infections) making children prone to its deficiency during these states. Chronic diarrhea, malabsorptive states, and chronic liver disease cause significant vitamin A deficiency.

Clinical Features

Subclinical Deficiency

Respiratory system, urinary tract, intestinal epithelium, and immune system are affected before the deficiency manifests clinically. Subclinical vitamin A deficiency contributes to an increased severity of certain infections and an increased risk of infection related mortality.

Early Features

Defective dark adaptation is the most characteristic early clinical feature, resulting in night blindness.

Xerophthalmia

Prolonged deficiency of vitamin A in the diet results in a syndrome of xerophthalmia, especially prevalent in 6–36 months old. It is often combined with general undernutrition.

- ***Xerosis (dryness) of the conjunctiva*** **(Fig. 10.2)** is usually the first clinical sign. Palpebral conjunctiva loses its sheen and wetness. Wrinkling appears in the conjunctiva which can be appreciated as conjunctival folds when the child moves the eyeball toward the opposite side.
- ***Bitot spots*** are the most characteristic feature of xerophthalmia. These appear **(Fig. 10.3)** as triangular areas on the temporal aspects of junction of cornea with sclera. The spots are made up of heaped up dry masses of conjunctival epithelium. There may be more than one spot measuring from 1-5 mm. The spots are whitish gray, look dry, nonreflective, and may have embedded wrinkles. These are present bilaterally and associated with a muddy conjunctiva.

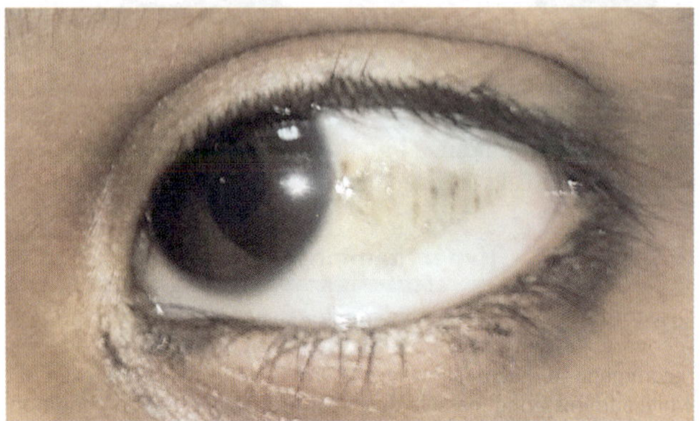

Fig. 10.2: Xerosis of conjunctiva

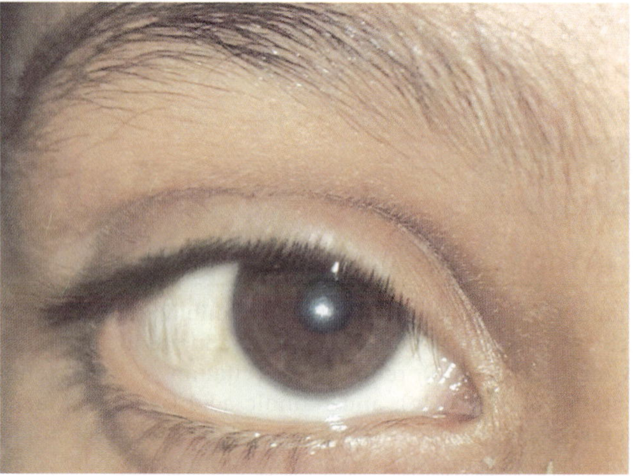

Fig. 10.3: Xerophthalmia: Bitot spot

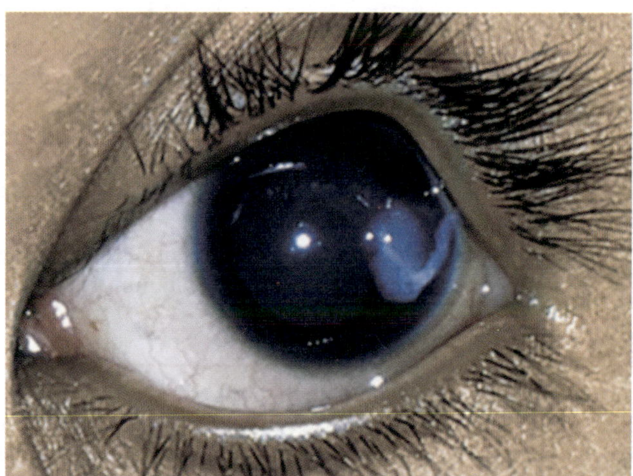

Fig. 10.4: Corneal ulceration—keratomalacia

The spots may be stained black, if the mother has applied *kajal* (*surma*) in the eyes of the infant.

- ***Cornea dries up as the next step:*** A dry cornea is susceptible to exposure injury and can get ulcerated easily. Ulcers are pinpoint initially and later coalesce. The ulceration spreads to involve most of the cornea. This stage is known as *keratomalacia* and is a forerunner to corneal perforation **(Fig. 10.4)**.
- Aqueous humor and iris prolapse out, that ultimately results in corneal blindness. Corneal xerosis is reversible while keratomalacia is irreversible.

The sequence of changes described above remains the same, through the rate of progression may be acute, subacute, or chronic. Serum vitamin A (retinol) level is <20 μg/dL.

On fundoscopy, pale yellow spots can be visualized near the course of retinal vessels and also in the periphery. Vitamin A deficiency is a common cause of preventable blindness in India. **Table 10.2** presents the World Health Organization (WHO) classification for ophthalmic manifestations of vitamin A deficiency.

Table 10.2 World Health Organization Classification of Xerophthalmia

	Primary signs	*Secondary signs*
X1A	Conjunctival xerosis	• XN: Night blindness • XF: Fundal changes • XS: Corneal scarring
X1B	Bitot spots	
X2	Corneal xerosis	
X3A	Corneal ulceration (<1/3 of cornea)	
X3B	Corneal ulceration (>1/3 of cornea)	

Indicators of Vitamin A Deficiency

- Clinically, presence of night blindness is used as the best indicator for vitamin A deficiency (VAD).
- Serum retinol of <0.70 μmol/L is used to identify those at risk for biochemical VAD.

However, the deficiency problem is overestimated if we do not consider coexisting deficiency of iron, zinc, and protein; or take infections into account. Iron deficiency reduces serum retinol levels. Zinc affects metabolism by influencing absorption, transport, and utilization. Protein is needed to mobilize liver reserves into blood. A child with severe acute malnutrition will thus have lower serum retinol level. Serum retinol concentrations can be lowered up to 25% by infections, so C-reactive protein should be estimated while assessing serum retinol levels.

Serum retinol should be measured by high-pressure liquid chromatography (HPLC).

Prevalence cut-offs to define significance of VAD in a population are detailed in **Table 10.3**.

TREATMENT Vitamin A Deficiency

Xerophthalmia can progress from conjunctival xerosis to perforation very rapidly, resulting in blindness. Thus, any evidence of vitamin A deficiency should be treated on priority and emergency basis.

Specific

Immediately on diagnosis, oral vitamin A is administered in a dose of 50,000, 1 lakh, and 2 lakhs IU in children aged <6 months, 6–12 months, and >1 year, respectively. For children >12 months but less than 8 kg, a dose of 1 lakh IU of vitamin A should be used instead of 2 lakh IU. The same dose is repeated next day and 2 weeks later. Parenteral, water-soluble vitamin A administration is recommended (in half the doses suggested earlier) in cases with impaired oral intake, persistent vomiting, and severe malabsorption. Oil-based injections should not be used to treat xerophthalmia.

Local Treatment

Antibiotic drops or ointment should be instilled three times a day to prevent secondary infection in the event of presence of corneal ulcer. Padding the eye prevents dehydration and further corneal exposure. Padding also enhances epithelial healing and reduces pain and photophobia. Mydriatics are necessary; usually atropine drops 1% or ointment is applied once a day.

Table 10.3 Indicators for Recognizing Vitamin A Deficiency in the Community

Vitamin A deficiency in the community	*Prevalence of night blindness in preschool children*	*Serum retinol <0.70 mmol/L in preschool children*
Mild	0–1%	2–10%
Moderate	1–5%	10–20%
Severe	>5%	>20%

Source: World Health Organization, 2009

HYPERVITAMINOSIS A

Causes

Unnecessary intake or high-dose vitamin A supplementation causes hypervitaminosis A. Levels increase either due to enhanced intestinal absorption of vitamin A or diminished chylomicron clearance. Aqueous preparations are 10 times toxic, compared to oil-based retinol preparations. Since, the conversion to the active form of vitamin A is significantly regulated, increased intake of provitamin does not lead to hypervitaminosis.

Clinical Features

Acute Hypervitaminosis A

It causes pseudotumor cerebri manifesting as bulging fontanel, vomiting, and irritability in young infants. Older children may complain of diplopia and headache. Papilledema and cranial nerve palsies are rare. Symptoms and signs improve rapidly on withdrawing vitamin A. Acetazolamide, mannitol, or a therapeutic lumbar tap may be needed in severe cases.

Chronic Hypervitaminosis A

It results in skin desquamation, alopecia, hepatosplenomegaly, bone swellings, and increased intracranial tension. The shaft of long bones may show hyperostosis. Chronic toxicity usually results from intake of medicinal vitamin A over a period of several weeks. Excessive intake of vitamin A is teratogenic during first trimester of pregnancy.

Diagnosis

Diagnosis of toxicity is difficult since serum retinol is not sensitive to toxic level of vitamin A. Even with inconsistent dietary intake of vitamin A, the serum retinol concentrations are maintained within normal range of 1-3 mol/L by homeostatic regulation. Instead, fasting retinyl ester concentrations >10% of total circulating vitamin A could indicate the toxic level. This occurs as a result of overflowing of extra esters into the blood from already saturated hepatic stellate cells and decreased hepatic uptake of vitamin A.

TREATMENT Hypervitaminosis A

Discontinuation of excessive intakes usually results in complete recovery. Prevention is possible by restricting the intake as per recommended dietary allowance (RDA). Caution should be exercised while administering massive doses for prophylaxis and in conditions such as pregnancy and liver disease.

PREVENTION OF VITAMIN A DEFICIENCY

High-risk conditions: Children suffering from measles and severe malnutrition should be administered oral vitamin A (1 and 2 lakh IU each for <1 year and >1 year olds, respectively), on two consecutive days. Those with persistent diarrhea and other prolonged febrile conditions are given one dose in each episode, keeping at least 1 month interval between the two doses.

Diet: Consumption of vitamin A rich food should be encouraged by all pregnant and lactating women and children under 5 years of age, including locally available carotene rich foods, i.e., green leafy vegetables and yellow and orange vegetables and fruits such as pumpkin, carrots, papaya, mango, oranges, along with cereals and pulses. Consumption of milk and milk products, egg, and liver must be promoted. Long-term prevention strategies include nutrition education for dietary diversification, horticultural interventions including home gardening, nutritional supplementation, and selective fortification for risk areas and special groups.

Vitamin A prophylaxis: The program was launched in 1970 with the objective of reducing the disease and preventing blindness due to vitamin A deficiency. The strategy consisted of administration of prophylactic vitamin A as per the following dosage schedule: 100,000 international units (IU) at 9 months with measles immunization, 200,000 IU at 16–18 months, with diphtheria-tetanus-pertussis (DPT) booster, and then 200,000 IU every 6 months, up to the age of 5 years. Other components include health and nutrition education to encourage colostrum feeding, exclusive breast feeding for the first 6 months, introduction of complementary feeding thereafter and adequate intake of vitamin A-rich foods, and early detection and proper treatment of infections.

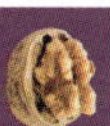

IN A NUTSHELL

Vitamin A and Xerophthalmia

1. Vitamin A and its metabolites play critical role in vision, fetal growth and development, reproduction, gastrointestinal and respiratory function, and immunity. It is part of antioxidant defenses.
2. Sources of vitamin A include fish liver oils, liver, dairy products, egg yolk, green leafy vegetables, yellow fruits, and vegetables such as carrots, papaya, tomatoes, sweet potatoes, mango, broccoli, and spinach.
3. Vitamin A deficiency can lead to xerophthalmia, childhood blindness, anemia, decrease host resistance to infection, and increased risk of mortality in under-5 children.
4. Prevalence of night blindness, Bitot spots, and serum retinol of <0.70 μmol/L are used as the indicators for VAD in a community.
5. Treat all children with clinical signs of VAD as early as possible with massive doses of vitamin A.
6. Vitamin A deficiency in the community can be prevented by improving the availability and consumption of vitamin A by dietary diversification and to strengthen the general nutritional standing of the population; food fortification; and targeted mega-dose vitamin A supplementation to preschool children and during pregnancy.

Awasthi S, Peto R, Read S, et al. Vitamin A supplementation every 6 months with retinol in 1 million pre-school children in north India: DEVTA, a cluster-randomised trial. Lancet. 2013;381(9876):1469-77.

Gupta P. India's Universal Mega-dose Vitamin A Supplement Program: Time to Bid Goodbye! Indian Pediatr. 2021;58(4):311-2.

Imdad A, Mayo-Wilson E, Herzer K, et al. Vitamin A supplementation for preventing morbidity and mortality in children from six months to five years of age. Cochrane Database Syst Rev. 2017;3(3):CD008524.

Mendu VVR, Nair KPM, Athe R. Systematic review and meta-analysis approach on vitamin A fortified foods and its effect on retinol concentration in under 10 year children. Clin Nutr ESPEN. 2019;30:126-30.

Ministry of Health and Family Welfare (MoHFW), Government of India. Comprehensive National Nutrition Survey (CNNS). New Delhi: MoHFW, UNICEF, and Population Council; 2019.

Reddy GB, Pullakhandam R, Ghosh S, et al. Vitamin A deficiency among children younger than 5 y in India: an analysis of national data sets to reflect on the need for vitamin A supplementation. Am J Clin Nutr. 2021;113(4):939-47.

Vijayaraghavan K. National control programme against nutritional blindness due to vitamin A deficiency: Current status & future strategy. Indian J Med Res. 2018;148(5):496-502.

WHO, UNICEF, IVACG Task Force. Vitamin A supplements: a guide to their use in the treatment and prevention of vitamin A deficiency and xerophthalmia, 2nd edition. Geneva: World Health Organization; 1997.

World Health Organization. Serum retinol concentrations for determining the prevalence of vitamin A deficiency in populations. Vitamin and Mineral Nutrition Information System. Geneva: World Health Organization; 2011.

10.3 Vitamin D and Rickets

PE 12.3

METABOLISM

Cholecalciferol (vitamin D_3) and calciferol (vitamin D_2) are biologically equivalent compounds. Vitamin D_3 is synthesized in the skin on exposure of 7-dehydrocholesterol (present under normal skin) to ultraviolet rays in the sunlight. The metabolically active form of vitamin D is $1,25(OH)_2D_3$ which is obtained by conversion of cholecalciferol to 25-hydroxy-cholecalciferol $25(OH)D_3$ in the liver followed by another hydroxylation in the kidney. $1,25(OH)_2D_3$ is a hormone which helps in absorption of calcium and phosphorus in the gut, and promotes bone dissolution, and mineralization, thereby increasing the serum calcium and alkaline phosphatase activity. The feedback control in synthesis is mediated by parathormone which diminishes in response to elevation of serum calcium level inhibiting further synthesis of $1,25(OH)_2D_3$ in the kidney.

DAILY REQUIREMENT

An intake of 400 IU/day is recommended for breastfed infants. As breastmilk is a poor source of vitamin D, this may need to be provided by supplements (400 IU/day from birth to 1 year of age), especially if exposure to sunlight is deficient **(Table 10.4)**.

Table 10.4 Requirements of Vitamin D for Different Age Groups

Age group	RDA (IU/day)	EAR (IU/day)
Men	600	400
Women	600	400
Pregnant women	600	400
Lactating women	600	400
Infants		
• 0–6 m	400 AI	—
• 6–12 m	400 AI	—
Children		
• 1–3 y	600	400
• 4–6 y	600	400
• 7–9 y	600	400
Boys (10–12 y)	600	400
Girls (10–12 y)	600	400
Boys (13–15 y)	600	400
Girls (13–15 y)	600	400
Boys (16–18 y)	600	400
Girls (16–18 y)	600	400

(EAR: estimated average requirement; RDA: recommended dietary allowance; AI: adequate intake; m: months; y: years)

Source: Nutrient Requirements for Indians, ICMR 2024

SOURCES

Fish oils, liver, egg yolk, and fortified foods are main sources of vitamin D besides exposure to sunlight. Milk, including breastmilk, provides very less amounts of vitamin D.

ROLE IN HEALTH AND DISEASE

Vitamin D is a lipid-soluble vitamin that acts as a hormone. Main functions of vitamin D are (1) To enhance intestinal calcium and phosphate absorption; (2) To inhibit parathormone production; and (3) To ensure formation and mineralization of bone.

Apart from these functions 1,25-dihydroxyvitamin D_3, the hormonally active form of vitamin D, generates several extra skeletal biological responses including inhibition of breast, colon, and prostate cancer cell progression; effects on the cardiovascular system; and protection against a number of autoimmune diseases including multiple sclerosis and inflammatory bowel disease. Although there is compelling evidence from the laboratory of extra skeletal beneficial effects of $1,25(OH)_2D_3$, conclusive clinical data for the use of vitamin D and analogs for the treatment or prevention of several disease processes are not yet available. There is no high- or moderate-quality evidence to support the effectiveness of vitamin D supplementation in various diseases such as pneumonia, diarrhea, tuberculosis, human immunodeficiency virus (HIV), asthma, obesity, atopy, and neurodevelopmental conditions.

RICKETS

Vitamin D deficiency (VDD) is common in infants who are dark-skinned and exclusively breastfed beyond 3–6 months of age, particularly in the background of maternal VDD during pregnancy or prematurity. VDD is also common among children who are on vegetarian and unusual diets, use anticonvulsant or antiretroviral medications, or those with malabsorption. Additional risk factors include residence at higher latitudes, winter season, and other causes of low-sun exposure **(Box 10.1)**. Genetic pleomorphism predisposing individuals to VDD rickets has been recently reported.

VITAMIN D DEFICIENCY RICKETS

Vitamin D deficiency in growing children (before closure of epiphyses) leads to *rickets* whereas the manifestations are termed *osteomalacia* in adolescents and adults. The main causes of deficiency are inadequate dietary intake and lack of exposure to sunlight. Poor vitamin D content of milk and vegetarian diets contribute to deficiency of vitamin D.

Clinical Features

Most clinical manifestations of rickets are due to bone changes related to deposition of unmineralized osteoid and softening.

Box 10.1 Etiology of Vitamin D Deficiency

1. Disorders of vitamin D synthesis:
   - Increased skin pigmentation
   - Topical application of sunscreen agents
   - Overclothing preventing sunlight exposure
   - High-rise buildings and urbanization
2. Geographical location:
   - Latitude (>400 North or South)
   - Winter season
   - Air pollution and cloud cover
   - High-altitude
   - Avoidance of sunlight for cosmetic reasons and fear of skin cancer
3. Decreased intake of vitamin D—vegetarianism
4. Decreased maternal vitamin D stores and exclusive breastfeeding
5. Malabsorption:
   - Celiac disease
   - Pancreatic Insufficiency
   - Chronic cholestasis
6. Decreased synthesis or increased degradation of 25(OH)D:
   - Chronic liver disease
   - Drugs (rifampicin, isoniazid, antifungals, and anticonvulsants)
   - Genetic factors

- ***Craniotabes***, the earliest manifestation of rickets, is the ping pong ball feeling of skull in infants on giving pressure over the occipital or parietal bones.
- Frontal and parietal bossing may be evident beyond infancy.
- Anterior fontanel is large and its closure is delayed beyond 18 months.
- There is clinically apparent widening of the wrists **(Fig. 10.5A)**.
- Long bones of legs get deformed when the child starts bearing weight (after 1 year). Anterior bowing of legs, knock knee, and coxa vara are the usual deformities.
- Medial malleolus of tibiae widens giving the appearance of *double malleolus* **(Fig. 10.5B)**.
- Costochondral junctions become prominent to give appearance of a rosary (*rachitic rosary*) **(Fig. 10.6)**. There may be an increase in anteroposterior diameter of chest wall (*pigeon chest*). A horizontal depression (*Harrison's groove*) is seen along the lower border of chest, corresponding to the insertion of diaphragm.
- Scoliosis, kyphosis, or lordosis may occur in severe cases. Deformities of chest and softening of ribs impairs air movement and make the child more prone to respiratory tract infections.
- Abdomen becomes protuberant (*potbelly*) because of marked hypotonia of abdominal wall muscles, visceroptosis, and lumbar lordosis.
- Eruption of primary teeth is delayed.

Diagnosis

The diagnosis of rickets is based on typical skeletal manifestations of wrist widening, rachitic rosary or/and bowlegs in a child at risk of VDD. Radiological changes are confirmatory and the biochemical changes help in finding the etiology of rickets.

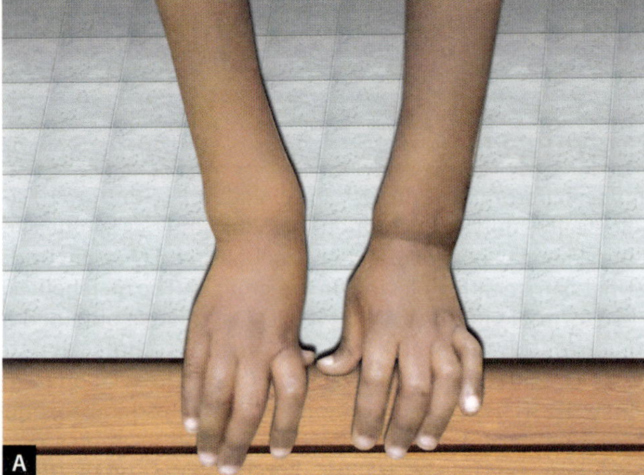

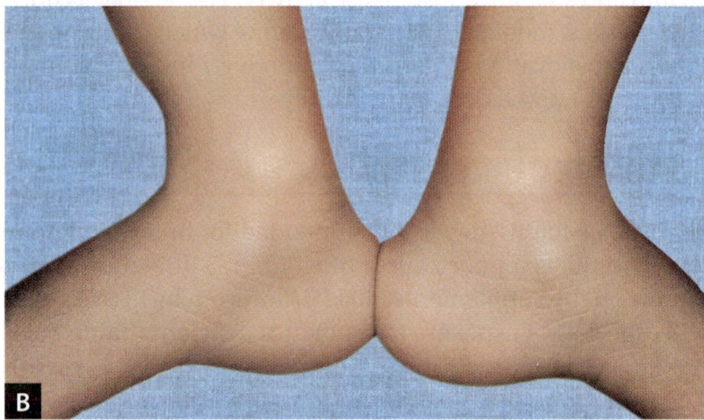

Figs. 10.5A and B: Rickets: (A) Widening of the wrists; (B) Double malleoli

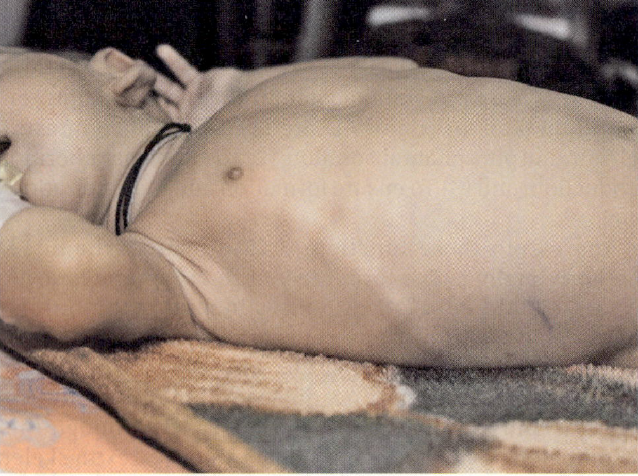

Fig. 10.6: Rachitic rosary: Costochondral junctions become prominent

Skeletal Changes

There is inadequate mineralization of bone matrix at the growth plates due to increased bone resorption secondary to increased parathormone activity, and also because of low calcium and

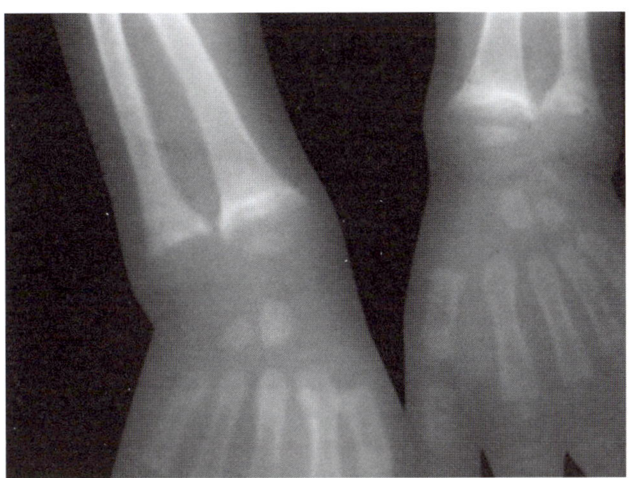

Fig. 10.7: Rickets: Early radiological changes showing cupping and fraying at lower ends of radius and ulna

phosphorus levels in blood. Deposition of unmineralized matrix leads to widening of growth plate and metaphysis causing manifestations such as wrist widening and rachitic rosary. Bone becomes less rigid and is prone to bending, deformities, and fractures. On weight bearing, soft end of bone is compressed leading to flaring of the metaphyses.

Early radiological changes are observed in wrist at lower ends of radius and ulna **(Fig. 10.7)**. In infants, changes are first visible in lower ends of femur and upper end of tibia. The normally convex or flat appearing metaphyses become concave (*cupping*). There is widening of distal end of metaphysis with elongation of both ends (*splaying*). The smooth margin of metaphysis appears irregular (*fraying*). Rachitic rosary may be apparent as beading of costochondral junctions in the chest radiograph. In long-standing cases, the diaphysis is also rarefied due to resorption of cancellous bone.

Biochemical Changes

As a result of decreased absorption of calcium from the gut, there is compensatory increase in parathormone concentration to maintain blood calcium levels (*secondary hyperparathyroidism*). Parathormone acts on osteocytes to release calcium from bones, and also reduces the excretion of calcium by kidneys. There is associated decrease in the renal tubular reabsorption of phosphate. The net result is *normal serum calcium level* and *low serum phosphorus*. An increase in the osteoblastic activity results in *elevation of serum alkaline phosphatase level.*

In later stages, the compensatory increase in parathormone cannot sustain normal calcium level and hypocalcemia occurs.

US Endocrine Society classification based on serum levels of 25(OH)D_3, vitamin D status is classified as: *Severe deficiency*: <5 ng/mL; *Deficient:* <12 ng/mL; *Insufficient* 12-20 ng/mL; *Sufficient:* >20 ng/mL; and *Toxic*: >150 ng/mL.

Flowchart 10.1 depicts the assessment, treatment, and monitoring of children with rickets/VDD as per IAP Guidelines 2021.

TREATMENT Vitamin D Deficiency Rickets

Indications for Treatment

- Children with nutritional rickets, with other symptoms attributable to VDD (e.g., hypocalcemic seizures, tetany, and hypocalcemic dilated cardiomyopathy) and having serum 25(OH)D level <20 ng/mL should be treated for VDD.
- Incidentally detected low serum 25(OH)D level <12 ng/mL in healthy children or <20 ng/mL in those at high-risk should be treated, as per protocol for nutritional rickets.
- Children with clinical pointers toward non-nutritional rickets, should undergo evaluation for etiology of rickets including assessment of serum 25(OH)D levels and parathyroid hormone.

Dose and Duration of Vitamin D Therapy

- *Route:* Oral treatment is the preferred, which more rapidly restores serum 25(OH)D levels than intramuscular treatment. Intramuscular route is to be used only when absorption of oral dose is doubtful, e.g., in malabsorption states. Parenteral administration of mega doses of vitamin D (>300,000 IU) is not recommended.
- *Daily versus Intermittent bolus:* Daily vitamin D therapy is more physiological than bolus doses.
  - *Daily regimes:* Oral cholecalciferol, preferably in a daily dosing schedule, 2,000 IU below 1 year of age and 3,000 IU in older children for minimum of 12 weeks is recommended. Some children may require a longer treatment duration for normalization of alkaline phosphatase and serum 25(OH)D levels. Calcium intake of 50–75 mg/kg/day (not exceeding 500 mg/day) must be ensured either through diet or supplementation in combination with vitamin D.
  - *Intermittent regimes:* If compliance to daily dosing cannot be ensured, intermittent regimens may be prescribed for children above 6 months of age. Oral cholecalciferol five doses of 60,000 IU for cumulative dose not exceeding 300,000 IU with calcium carbonate should be used across different ages. Bolus doses may be administered at interval of 2–4 weeks. Various regimens for treating rickets are summarized in **Table 10.5**.
- Vitamin D_3 is more efficacious than vitamin D_2 to raise serum 25(OH) D level. Most preparations available in the Indian market contain vitamin D_3.

Monitoring During Treatment of Nutritional Rickets

Healing is apparent in 3–4 weeks at the end of long bones in form of a white line of calcification. Thereafter, consumption of 400–600 units of vitamin D_3 per day should be encouraged. Adequate calcium and phosphorus intake should also be ensured.

- Radiographs should be obtained at 4 weeks and 12 weeks after vitamin D therapy in rickets to look for evidence of healing.
- Serum calcium, phosphate, alkaline phosphatase, serum 25(OH)D levels should be performed at 12 weeks after vitamin D therapy to measure response and toxicity.
- If complete radiological healing and normalization of biochemical parameters (serum 25(OH)D >20–50 ng/mL) is not attained in rickets by 12 weeks, therapeutic doses of vitamin D and calcium should be continued. Maintenance dose of vitamin D should be started once complete healing has been achieved.
- *Urine calcium:* Creatinine ratio and renal ultrasonogram should be done when there is hypercalcemia or hypervitaminosis D.

If there is no response after vitamin D supplementation or if there is a family history or if biochemical changes are not typical of VDD, other variants of rickets should be suspected.

- Low phosphate level with aminoaciduria is seen in (1) VDD or malabsorption, (2) hepatic disease or prolonged anticonvulsant therapy, and (3) Fanconi syndrome. Glycosuria indicates Fanconi disease.
- Low phosphate level without aminoaciduria with acidic urinary pH indicates proximal renal tubular acidosis. Urinary pH is normal in familial hypophosphatemia.

Flowchart 10.1: Algorithm for evaluation of rickets

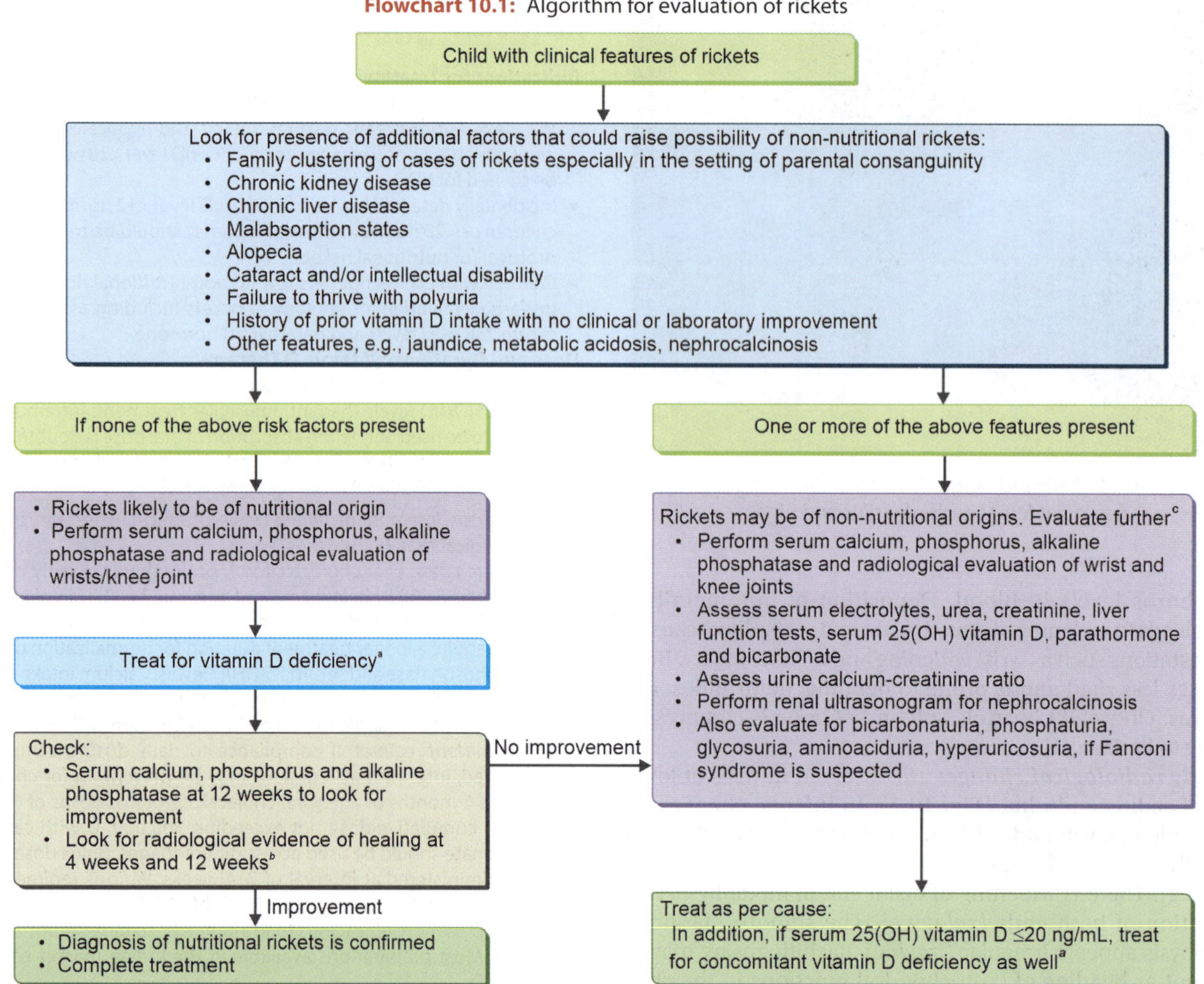

[a]Treatment of vitamin D deficiency includes calcium supplements along with vitamin D

[b]Monitoring of therapy

[c]Other investigations as clinically indicated

Source: Gupta P, Dabas A, Seth A, et al. Indian Academy of Pediatrics Revised (2021) Guidelines on Prevention and Treatment of Vitamin D Deficiency and Rickets. Indian Pediatr. 2022;59(2):142-58

PREVENTION OF NUTRITIONAL RICKETS

Vitamin D Supplementation

Indian Academy of Pediatrics 2021 guidelines recommendation for vitamin D supplementation are as follows:

- For prevention of rickets in infants (0–1 years of age), 400 IU vitamin D/day is recommended. Same dose is safe in preterm babies. Higher doses such as 1,600 IU daily or above can cause toxicity.
- Routine vitamin D supplementation is not recommended during childhood and adolescence, rather sunlight and diet desired to be the main source for providing EAR of vitamin D (400–600 IU/day) in these age-groups, to prevent VDD.
- Routine vitamin D supplementation (minimum 400 IU daily) is recommended in children with underlying high-risk conditions such as children receiving long-term anticonvulsants or glucocorticoids, ketoconazole; chronic kidney disease, chronic liver disease, malabsorption states, hyperparathyroidism, children with nonambulatory states like cerebral palsy, neuromuscular disorders chronic inflammatory diseases, and disorders with extensive cutaneous involvement.
- Routine screening of apparently healthy children for VDD is not recommended. Asymptomatic screened only if they are at risk for VDD.

Maternal Supplementation

Universal vitamin D supplementation is not recommended during pregnancy (WHO) as it does not have any benefit for fetal and neonatal outcomes. Routine calcium supplementation should be ensured during pregnancy and lactation in the dose of 1,200 mg daily or in higher doses of 1.5–2 g for pre-eclampsia.

Table 10.5 Doses for Management of Vitamin D Deficiency or Nutritional Rickets in Children

Age	Daily dose for 12 week[a]	Alternative intermittent does regimen[b]	Maintenance dose (daily)[c]
<6 months	2,000	NA	400
6–12 months	2,000	Equivalent of 2,000 IU/day may be given on a monthly or weekly basis	400
>12 months	3,000	60,000 IU fortnightly (after every 2 weeks) × 5 doses	600

[a]Reassess response after 12 weeks. Ensure daily calcium intake of 50–75 mg/kg/day, not exceeding 500 mg/day

[b]In certain situations, if compliance is not good, intermittent regimens may be prescribed (in children above 6 months of age only)

[c]Ensure daily intake of recommended dose through supplementation or dietary sources. Optimum duration of maintenance vitamin D therapy is not known at present

Sunlight

Sunlight exposure is recommended at least five times a week during noon (11 AM to 3 PM) for children and adolescents across all regions of India to increase serum 25(OH)D levels and prevent VDD. A daily sunlight exposure of 17–30 minutes in infants and 30–45 minutes in older children over 15–40% body surface area is recommended. Sunscreens decrease serum vitamin D levels and should not be routinely used in children. Sunlight exposure is recommended for all ages, the exact duration and body surface area, however, will differ on host and environmental factors.

Diet

Though only vitamin D rich foods may not be enough to meet the requirements, their intake should be encouraged. An adequate intake of calcium, i.e., 500 mg/day in infancy, 600 mg/day in 1–9 years old and 800 mg/day in adolescents should be ensured during childhood to meet the dietary requirements.

HYPERVITAMINOSIS D

Causes

Administration of vitamin D in therapeutic doses for long periods results in toxicity. The upper limit of daily intake of vitamin D is 1,000 IU for infants and 2,000 IU for older children and adults.

Clinical Features

Renal manifestations are secondary to hypercalcemia and hypercalciuria; and include polyuria, nephrocalcinosis, nephrolithiasis, and renal failure. Gastrointestinal manifestations are anorexia, abdominal pain, and constipation. Child may have hypotonia, irritability, disorientation, convulsions, and coma. Death may occur due to cardiac arrhythmias or due to electrolyte abnormalities secondary to dehydration.

Diagnosis

Diagnosis of vitamin D toxicity is confirmed by high serum calcium, hypercalciuria, and high serum vitamin D 25(OH) (>100 ng/mL), hypercalciuria is defined as urinary calcium excretion >4 mg/kg/day or urine calcium-creatinine ratio <0.2 (in age >2 years). Normal upper limit for serum calcium are: birth to 3 months—11.3 mg/dL; 3-6 months—11.2 mg/dL; 6–12 months—11.3 mg/dL; 1–3 years: 11.1 mg/dL; and 4–18 years: 10.7 mg/dL. Serum parathyroid hormone (PTH) is suppressed in vitamin D toxicity.

TREATMENT Hypervitaminosis D

Treatment comprises of elimination of source of excess vitamin D, and management of dehydration and electrolyte abnormalities. Oral prednisolone, calcitonin, and bisphosphonates are effective in decreasing serum calcium.

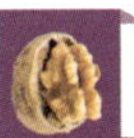

IN A NUTSHELL

Vitamin D and Rickets

1. Vitamin D, the sunshine hormone is required for skeletal health as well as for extra skeletal well-being.
2. Prevention of vitamin D deficiency needs appropriate sunlight exposure, changes in dietary habits, routine supplementation in children below 1 year of age, and food fortification.
3. Vitamin D deficiency in children older than 1 year and adolescents is not very high.
4. Nutritional rickets manifests mostly in infants and toddlers with bony deformities. Vitamin D deficiency in infancy may also present with hypocalcemic seizures.
5. The most common method to determine vitamin D status is serum 25(OH)D. Lower value than 12 ng/mL is considered vitamin D deficiency.
6. Measurement of alkaline phosphatase levels in plasma is a useful screening test for vitamin D deficiency.
7. All prevalent treatment regimens for deficiency with vitamin D_3 are equally effective. Bolus high-dose therapy needs to be avoided.

Cashman KD, Sheehy T, O'Neill CM. Is vitamin D deficiency a public health concern for low middle income countries? A systematic literature review. Eur J Nutr. 2019;58(1):433-53.
Food Safety and Standards Authority of India (FSSAI), Ministry of Health and Family Welfare, Government of India. (2020). Summary of recommended dietary allowances for energy, protein and minerals. [online] Available from: https://www.fssai.gov.in/upload/advisories/2020/01/5e159e0a809bbLetter_RDA_08_01_2020.pdf [Last accessed August, 2025].
Gupta P, Dabas A, Seth A, et al. Indian Academy of Pediatrics Revised (2021) Guidelines on Prevention and Treatment of Vitamin D Deficiency and Rickets. Indian Pediatr. 2022;59(2):142-58.
Gupta P, Dewan P, Shah D, et al. Vitamin D supplementation for treatment and prevention of pneumonia in under-five children: a randomized double-blind placebo controlled trial. Indian Pediatr. 2016;53(11):967-76.
ICMR. Recommended Dietary Allowances and Estimated Average Requirements Nutrient Requirements for Indians–2020. A Report of the Expert Group Indian Council of Medical Research, National Institute of Nutrition. Hyderabad: ICMR; 2020.
Koçyiğit C, Çatlı G, İnce G, et al. Can Stoss therapy be used in children with vitamin D deficiency or insufficiency without rickets? J Clin Res Pediatr Endocrinol. 2017;9(2):150-5.
Meena P, Dabas A, Shah D, et al. Sunlight exposure and vitamin D status in breastfed infants. Indian Pediatr. 2017;54(2):105-11.
Ministry of Health and Family Welfare, Government of India. (2018). Comprehensive National Nutrition Survey (CNNS) 2016-2018. [online] Available from: https://nhm.gov.in/WriteReadData/l892s/1405796031571201348.pdf [Last accessed August, 2025].
Munns CF, Shaw N, Kiely M, et al. Global Consensus Recommendations on Prevention and Management of Nutritional Rickets. J Clin Endocrinol Metab. 2016;101:394-415.
National Institute of Nutrition, Indian Council of Medical Research, Ministry of Health and Family Welfare. (2017). Indian Food composition tables 2017. [online] Available from: https://www.nin.res.in/ebooks/IFCT2017.pdf [Last accessed August, 2025].
Shah D, Gupta P. Vitamin D Deficiency: Is The Pandemic for Real? Indian J Community Med. 2015;40(4):215-7.

10.4 Vitamin E

PE 12.4

ROLE IN HEALTH AND DISEASE

Vitamin E is an antioxidant that protects membrane phospholipids from free radical induced peroxidase damage. It has antineoplastic, anti-inflammatory effect and may raise the concentration of high-density lipoprotein cholesterol. Vitamin E is transported in the body by lipoprotein. Preterm newborns have low tissue stores. As an antioxidant, it is used as a free radical scavenger.

SOURCES

Nuts such as almond and peanut, and polyunsaturated vegetable oils such as canola and olive, are rich sources. Seeds, whole wheat grain, egg yolk, milk fat, butter, green leafy vegetable, liver and fortified cereals, are good sources.

DAILY REQUIREMENT

The suggested requirement of alpha-tocopherol is 0.8 mg/g of dietary essential fatty acids. This is approximately 7.5–10 mg tocopherol per day, depending on the edible oil used. 1 mg of d-alpha-tocopherol provides 1.5 IU activity of vitamin E. Intake of 4–5 mg/day is considered adequate for infants **(Table 10.6)**.

Table 10.6 Requirements of Vitamin E for Different Age Groups

Age group	*RDA (mg/day)*	*EAR (mg/day)*
Men	15	12
Women	15	12
Pregnant women	15	12
Lactating women	19	16
Infants	4–5	—
Children		
1–3 years	6	5
4–8 years	7	6
9–13 years	11	9
Adolescence	15	12

(EAR: estimated average requirement; RDA: recommended dietary allowance; m: months; y: years)

Source: Institute of Medicine (US) Panel on Dietary Antioxidants and Related Compounds. Dietary Reference Intakes for Vitamin C, Vitamin E, Selenium and Carotenoids. Washington (DC): National Academies Press; 2000

VITAMIN E DEFICIENCY

Causes

Vitamin E deficiency might be observed in low-birth-weight infants. Majority of children with vitamin E deficiency have cholestatic disease with coexistent fat malabsorption.

Clinical Features

Clinical manifestations include loss of reflexes, ataxia of trunks and limbs, diminished proprioception, muscle weakness, ptosis, pes cavus, scoliosis, and dysarthria. Low levels of vitamin E in premature infants are associated with hemolytic anemia, hyperbilirubinemia, and intraventricular hemorrhage. In low-birth-weight infants, it may result in anemia, reticulocytosis, thrombocytopenia, and abnormal erythrocyte metabolism. Vitamin E prophylaxis may reduce the incidence of retinopathy of prematurity.

Diagnosis

Alpha-tocopherol level is low with low ratio of serum alpha-tocopherol to serum lipid. In children with abetalipoproteinemia, serum alpha-tocopherol levels are undetectable.

TREATMENT Vitamin E Deficiency

Underlying cause of the deficiency (fat malabsorption and disorders) should be addressed with supplementation of oral vitamin E. Diet should include rich sources of vitamin E such as whole grains, nuts, seeds, vegetable oils, and fortified cereals. A supplement of 15–25 mg/kg once per day or mixed tocopherols 200 IU can be used. If malabsorption is the cause, then intramuscular route can be employed.

VITAMIN E TOXICITY

Vitamin E toxicity occurs due to excessive vitamin supplementation, not due to dietary intake. Vitamin E may inhibit platelet aggregation and also vitamin K-dependent clotting cascade resulting in enhanced risk of bleeding, specifically in patients on anticoagulation or antiplatelet therapy. Life-threatening hemorrhagic stroke, gastrointestinal manifestations, weakness, fatigue, and emotional lability are some of the other complications.

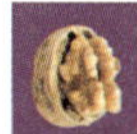

IN A NUTSHELL

Vitamin E

1. Vitamin E is a fat-soluble vitamin with antioxidant properties.
2. It also has antineoplastic and anti-inflammatory properties.
3. Nuts and polyunsaturated vegetable oils are rich sources of vitamin E.
4. Vitamin E deficiency in premature infants is associated with hemolytic anemia.
5. The use of vitamin E with anticoagulants and antiplatelet drugs can increase the risk of bleeding.

Diab L, Krebs NF. Vitamin Excess and Deficiency. Pediatr Rev. 2018;39(4):161-79.

Gomez-Pomar E, Hatfield E, Garlitz K, et al. Vitamin E in the Preterm Infant: A Forgotten Cause of Hemolytic Anemia. Am J Perinatol. 2018;35(3):305-10.

Khadangi F, Azzi A. Vitamin E–The Next 100 Years. IUBMB Life. 2019; 71(4):411-5.

10.5 Vitamin K

PE 12.5, PE 12.6

ROLE IN HEALTH AND DISEASE

Vitamin K is a group of fat-soluble vitamins that includes phylloquinone (vitamin K_1) and menaquinones (vitamin K_2). It is an essential cofactor of the enzyme vitamin K-dependent carboxylase that catalyzes formation of prothrombin. It is also needed for the generation of several proteins involved in hemostasis (blood clotting) and bone metabolism, and other physiological functions. Lately, there has been a significant research interest in the role of vitamin K_2 on osteoporosis, vascular calcification, osteoarthritis, cancer, and cognition.

SOURCES

Phylloquinone is the main dietary form of vitamin K, present primarily in green leafy vegetables (spinach, cabbage, and lettuce). Cheese, egg yolk, and liver contain the vitamin in fair amounts. It has been shown that some amounts (menaquinones) are also formed by the bacterial action of the intestinal flora of human. Therefore, even if required amounts are not supplied by diet, deficiency is not common. Natto (a traditional Japanese food made from fermented soybeans) is a rich source of menaquinones. Vitamin K is stable to heat but unstable to alkalis, acids, and light.

DAILY REQUIREMENT

A normal adult requires about 55 µg of vitamin K per day (ICMR, 2020). Given the data inadequacy to establish an estimated average requirement (EAR) for vitamin K, adequate intakes for all ages based on vitamin K intakes in healthy population groups was established. The adequate intakes for infants are based on the assumption that infants receive prophylactic vitamin K at birth. The current adequate intakes for vitamin K in micrograms (µg) are listed in **Table 10.7**.

VITAMIN K DEFICIENCY

Clinical Features

The risk of developing vitamin K deficiency is higher in newborns not given vitamin K at birth, in people with malabsorption disorders, and in those receiving antibiotics as they destroy vitamin K-producing bacteria in the gut.

Less placental transfer of phylloquinone, low clotting factor levels, and low vitamin K content of breastmilk lead to deficiency in newborns, resulting in hemorrhagic disease of the newborn. Idiopathic vitamin K deficiency of infants or acquired prothrombin complex deficiency is a bleeding disorder of infants between 2 weeks and 2 months old.

Table 10.7 Adequate Daily Intake for Vitamin K

Age	Male	Female
Birth to 6 months	2.0 µg	2.0 µg
7–12 months	2.5 µg	2.5 µg
1–3 years	30 µg	30 µg
4–8 years	55 µg	55 µg
9–13 years	60 µg	60 µg
14–18 years	75 µg	75 µg
19+ years	120 µg	90 µg

Source: Institute of Medicine (US) Panel on Micronutrients. Dietary reference intakes for vitamin A, vitamin K, arsenic, boron, chromium, copper, iodine, iron, manganese, molybdenum, nickel, silicon, vanadium, and zinc. Washington, DC: National Academy Press; 2001

Diagnosis

Serum level of phylloquinone (K_1) <0.15 µg/L are indicative of deficiency and is most commonly used marker. But it does not measure other vitamin K homologues and interference from recent dietary intake. To overcome that issue undercarboxylated prothrombin [protein induced by vitamin K absence/antagonism (PIVKA-II)] is measured (reference range 17.4-50.9 mAU/mL), that acts as an indicator of hepatic vitamin K status. Prothrombin time is elevated. Estimating prothrombin time and PIVKA-II together provides satisfactory results.

TREATMENT Vitamin K Deficiency

Vitamin K deficiency should be prevented by giving 1 mg of intramuscular vitamin K to the newborn at birth. In severe deficiency, 2.5–5 mg of aqueous vitamin K is given parenterally.

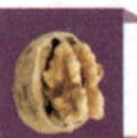

IN A NUTSHELL

Vitamin K

1. Vitamin K is a fat-soluble vitamin that includes phylloquinone (vitamin K_1) and menaquinones (vitamin K_2).
2. Rich source of vitamin K_1 are green leafy vegetables, vegetable oils, while K_2 are present in animal-based and fermented foods cheese.
3. Severe deficiency manifests as bleeding and hemorrhage.
4. Diagnosis is clinically supported by elevated prothrombin time, and PIVKA-II levels.
5. All newborns at birth should receive 1 mg of intramuscular vitamin K to prevent deficiency.

Card DJ, Gorska R, Harrington DJ. Laboratory assessment of vitamin K status. J Clin Pathol. 2020;73(2):70-5.

DiNicolantonio JJ, Bhutani J, O'Keefe JH. The health benefits of vitamin K. Open Heart. 2015;2(1):e000300.

Hand I, Noble L, Abrams SA. Vitamin K and the newborn infant. Pediatrics. 2022;149(3):e2021056036.

Water-soluble Vitamins

10.6 Vitamin B Complex

PE 12.7

INTRODUCTION

Vitamin B complex includes thiamine (B_1), riboflavin (B_2), niacin or pellagra preventing factor (B_3), pyridoxine (B_6), folic acid, cyanocobalamin (B_{12}), pantothenic acid, and biotin.

Being water-soluble, excess amounts are excreted in the urine, rarely posing a threat of toxicity. Since they cannot be stored in the body, they must be supplied in the diet, failing which characteristic deficiency symptoms might arise.

THIAMINE (VITAMIN B_1)

Role in Health and Disease

Thiamine pyrophosphate (TPP) is the coenzyme form of thiamine and is involved in direct oxidative pathway for glucose, synthesis of nucleic acid, and fatty acid synthesis. It maintains good appetite, normal digestion, the muscle tone, and a healthy mental attitude. Its deficiency causes mental and neurological disturbances. It is also required for the synthesis of acetylcholine and gamma-aminobutyric acid (GABA), essential for nerve conduction. In thiamine deficiency, utilization of pyruvic acid is decreased. Therefore, pyruvic acid and lactic acid accumulate in the tissue, and their blood levels are increased.

Sources

Liver, organ meat, egg yolk, fish, dry beans and peas, soybean, peanuts, whole grains, enriched bread, cereals, and dried yeast are rich sources.

Milk and its products, fruits and vegetables are not good sources but add a significant amount to the daily intake, if consumed in sufficient quantities.

Daily Requirement

Normal requirements depend on age, physiological status, level of physical activity, and range between 0.5 and 1.7 mg per day. The dietary allowance according to ICMR (2020) for men is 0.6 mg/1,000 kcal and 0.8 mg/1,000 kcal for women **(Table 10.8)**.

Table 10.8 Requirements of Vitamin B_1 for Different Age Groups

Age group	RDA (mg/day)	EAR (mg/day)
Men		
• Sedentary	1.4	1.2
• Moderate	1.8	1.5
• Heavy	2.3	1.9
Women		
• Sedentary	1.4	1.1
• Moderate	1.7	1.4
• Heavy	2.2	1.8
Pregnant women	2	1.6
Lactating women	2.1	1.7
Infants		
• 0–6 m	0.2 (AI)	—
• 6–12 m	0.4 (AI)	—
Children		
• 1–3 y	0.7	0.6
• 4–6 y	0.9	0.8
• 7–9 y	1.1	1.0
Boys (10–12 y)	1.5	1.3
Girls (10–12 y)	1.4	1.2
Boys (13–15 y)	1.9	1.6
Girls (13–15 y)	1.6	1.3
Boys (16–18 y)	2.2	1.9
Girls (16–18 y)	1.7	1.4

(EAR: estimated average requirement; RDA: recommended dietary allowance; AI: adequate intake; m: months; y: years)
Source: Nutrient Requirements for Indians, ICMR 2024

Deficiency of thiamine is not evident even if deficiency is there, as its requirement is closely related to energy intake.

Thiamine Deficiency

Thiamine is readily lost from rice during the process of milling. Being a water-soluble vitamin, further losses take place during cooking due to leaching of the vitamin into the cooking water, and not due to destruction by heat. Hence, food should be cooked in least amount of water to conserve its thiamine content. Polishing, processing, and cooking destroy the thiamine content of cereals. Thiamine deficiency is characteristically associated with consumption of polished rice as a staple food. Deficiency of vitamin B_1 is also associated with severe malnutrition and chronic alcoholism.

Clinical Features

Thiamine deficiency mainfests as beriberi.

- Initial symptoms are nonspecific such as fatigue, apathy, nausea, and abdominal pain.
- ***Dry beriberi:*** Neuritic form manifests as irritability, ataxia, tenderness of calf muscles, hypotonia, and diminished deep tendon reflexes. A pseudomeningeal form occurs in infants between 8 and 10 months of age. These children present with altered sensorium, signs of raised intracranial pressure, meningeal irritation, and neurologic deficit. This presentation is known as *Wernicke encephalopathy*. Cerebrospinal fluid (CSF) shows pleocytosis and elevated proteins. Infantile form of beriberi is seen in breastfed infants, where the mothers are thiamine deficient. The usual age of onset is between 2 and 3 months.
- ***Wet beriberi:*** This manifests in apparently healthy infants between the ages of 2–4 months with cardiovascular involvement, is characterized by cardiomegaly, edema, and congestive heart failure. Cyanosis and pulmonary edema may also develop and carry a bad prognosis.
- ***Laryngeal variety*** presents with cough and hoarseness of voice, or aphonia.
- Mixed and atypical forms may also occur.

Deficiency of thiamine is not evident even if deficiency is there, as its requirement is closely related to energy intake.

Diagnosis

Decreased levels of red blood cell (RBC) transketolase are seen in thiamine deficiency.

TREATMENT Beriberi

Beriberi is treated with 3–5 mg of thiamine per day, orally, for at least 6 weeks. Parenteral preparations are needed in very sick children, including those having congestive heart failure. Treatment of dependency states requires higher doses.

RIBOFLAVIN (VITAMIN B_2)

Riboflavin enzymes are involved in many oxidative enzyme systems in energy metabolism, synthesis of glycogen and erythropoiesis. Riboflavin is cardinal to cellular growth and tissue respiration. Retina also contains free riboflavin.

Riboflavin-derived coenzymes, flavin mononucleotide (FMN), and *flavin adenine dinucleotide* (*FAD*) are cofactors of numerous enzymes involved in oxidation-reduction reactions. Riboflavin is also involved in antioxidant activity, being a cofactor for the enzymes like glutathione reductase and is required for the metabolism of other vitamins like vitamin B_6, niacin, and vitamin K.

Sources

Eggs, green leafy vegetables, organ meats liver, milk and its products (cheese, whey, curds, and butter milk) are some sources. Wheat, millets, and pulses are fair sources; rice germination increases the riboflavin content of pulses and cereals.

Daily Requirement

The requirement of B_2 is related to energy intake, being 0.9 mg per 1,000 kcal for men and 1.1 mg/1,000 for women per day. It also depends on age, physiological status, and level of physiological activity (**Table 10.9**).

Table 10.9 Requirements of Vitamin B_2 for Different Age Groups

Age group	RDA (mg/day)	EAR (mg/day)
Men		
• Sedentary	2.0	1.6
• Moderate	2.5	2.1
• Heavy	3.2	2.7
Women		
• Sedentary	1.9	1.6
• Moderate	2.4	2.0
• Heavy	3.1	2.6
Pregnant women	2.7	2.3
Lactating women	2.9–3.0	2.4–2.5
Infants		
• 0–6 m	0.4 (AI)	—
• 6–12 m	0.6 (AI)	—
Children		
• 1–3 y	1.1	0.8
• 4–6 y	1.3	1.1
• 7–9 y	1.6	1.3
Boys (10–12 y)	2.1	1.7
Girls (10–12 y)	1.9	1.6
Boys (13–15 y)	2.7	2.2
Girls (13–15 y)	2.2	1.9
Boys (16–18 y)	3.1	2.5
Girls (16–18 y)	2.3	1.9

(EAR: estimated average requirement; RDA: recommended dietary allowance; AI: adequate intake; m: months; y: years)
Source: Nutrient Requirements for Indians, ICMR 2024

Riboflavin Deficiency

Causes

Severe riboflavin deficiency or ariboflavinosis occurs if the diet is deficient in animal protein and leafy vegetables. During cooking, 15–100% of riboflavin is lost depending on the type of food and cooking method (ICMR). Cooking losses can be attributed to leaching of this vitamin into cooking water and also destruction by light.

Clinical Features

Malnutrition, malabsorption, and prolonged diarrhea are the main causes of riboflavin deficiency. For deficiency symptoms to show up, riboflavin intake should be low for several months. Riboflavin deficiency is characterized by lesions in oral cavity, eye, and skin.

- ***Oral lesions:*** Angular cheilosis (fissuring and cracking at the angles of mouth) and glossitis (fissuring, redness, or paleness of tongue; sore, glazed, smooth tongue) are the predominant oral lesions seen in riboflavin deficiency **(Fig. 10.8)**.
- ***Skin lesions:*** The dermatitis may involve the nasolabial folds (nasolabial dysbacea—scaly dermatitis, pruritus, seborrhea, and desquamation). Scrotal dermatitis may be frequently present.

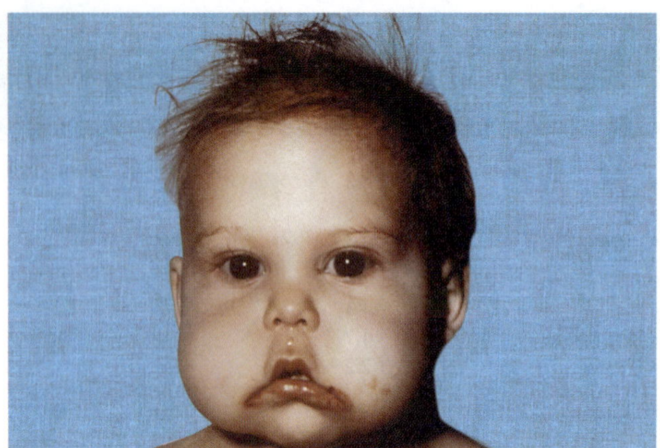

Fig. 10.8: Angular cheilosis

- ***Eye manifestations*** include photophobia, lacrimation, itching, and circumcorneal congestion. Corneal vascularization, keratitis, and opacity may develop in severe cases.

Peripheral neuropathy with hyperesthesia, altered temperature sensation, and pain may be other manifestations.

Diagnosis

Diagnosis is mainly clinical and can be confirmed by a urinary riboflavin excretion of <30 mg in 24 hours.

TREATMENT Riboflavin Deficiency

Treatment consists of 3–10 mg riboflavin PO daily. Parenteral riboflavin may be given in cases resistant to oral therapy.

NIACIN (PELLAGRA PREVENTING FACTOR) (B_3)

Niacin containing cofactors, nicotinamide adenine dinucleotide (NAD) and nicotinamide adenine dinucleotide phosphate (NADP), are important in many biologic reactions such as respiratory chain, deoxyribonucleic acid (DNA) synthesis and repair, fatty acid synthesis, and steroid synthesis. Niacin is essential for functioning of skin, intestinal tract, and nervous system.

It plays an important role in DNA synthesis and repair. Niacinamide is part of coenzymes connected with glycolysis, tissue respiration, and synthesis of macromolecules. In pharmacological doses, it controls blood cholesterol and lipids.

Sources

Cereals, pulses, groundnut, and green leafy vegetables are main sources in vegetarian diet whereas fish, meat and poultry form are for nonvegetarians. Eggs and milk, though contain little niacin, are rich sources of tryptophan which can be converted to niacin.

Daily Requirements

Dietary allowance of niacin is expressed in terms of niacin equivalents. (1 mg niacin equivalent = 1 mg niacin = 60 mg tryptophan). The requirement of B_3 is related to energy intake, based on EAR of 5.6 mg/1,000 kcals for adults **(Table 10.10)**.

Table 10.10 Requirements of Vitamin B_3 for Different Age Groups

Age group	*RDA (mg/day)*	*EAR (mg/day)*
Men		
• Sedentary	14	12
• Moderate	18	15
• Heavy	23	19
Women		
• Sedentary	11	9
• Moderate	14	12
• Heavy	18	15
Pregnant women	13	11
Lactating women	16	13
Infants		
• 0–6 m	2 (AI)	—
• 6–12 m	5 (AI)	—
Children		
• 1–3 y	7	6
• 4–6 y	9	8
• 7–9 y	11	10
Boys (10–12 y)	15	12
Girls (10–12 y)	14	12
Boys (13–15 y)	19	16
Girls (13–15 y)	16	13
Boys (16–18 y)	22	19
Girls (16–18 y)	17	14

(EAR: estimated average requirement; RDA: recommended dietary allowance; AI: adequate intake; m: months; y: years)
Source: Nutrient Requirements for Indians, ICMR 2024

Causes

Niacin deficiency is predominantly seen in populations where maize is the main staple food. Severe malnutrition and anorexia nervosa are other common causes. Maize contains the vitamin in bound form which is poorly bioavailable. High leucine content and low tryptophan content of the maize is one of the major factors contributing to the development of niacin deficiency. Milling leads to loss of niacin. Niacin is stable to the factors encountered during storage and food processing. However, its water solubility destroys it during food preparation, but cooking in sufficient amounts of water reduces its loss. ICMR has estimated an average loss of 25% of this vitamin during cooking.

Pellagra

Pellagra is the classical syndrome resulting from niacin deficiency. *The classical triad of* three D's—*diarrhea, dermatitis, and dementia summarizes the clinical presentation of pellagra.*

Dermatitis of pellagra is characterized by symmetrical hyperpigmented scaly lesions on exposed parts such as hands (*pellagrous glove*), feet (*pellagrous boot*), and neck (*Casal necklace*) **(Figs. 10.9A and B)**. In a severely malnourished child, it is sometimes difficult to differentiate these features from dermatosis of kwashiorkor. The lesions heal promptly following administration of niacin. Neurological features include irritability, apathy, disorientation, and confusion. An acute encephalopathy may develop occasionally. Gastrointestinal disorder symptoms include diarrhea, loss of appetite, nausea, vomiting, and achlorhydria. Neurological manifestations include muscle weakness, mental retardation or dementia, and loss of memory.

Diagnosis

Diagnosis of niacin deficiency is clinical, supported with dietary history.

TREATMENT Pellagra

Supplementation of 50–300 mg/day of niacin with a balanced diet rapidly corrects the deficiency. Severe cases or those with poor-intestinal absorption may require intravenous niacin. Sun exposure should be avoided for skin lesions and emollients can be applied on the affected areas.

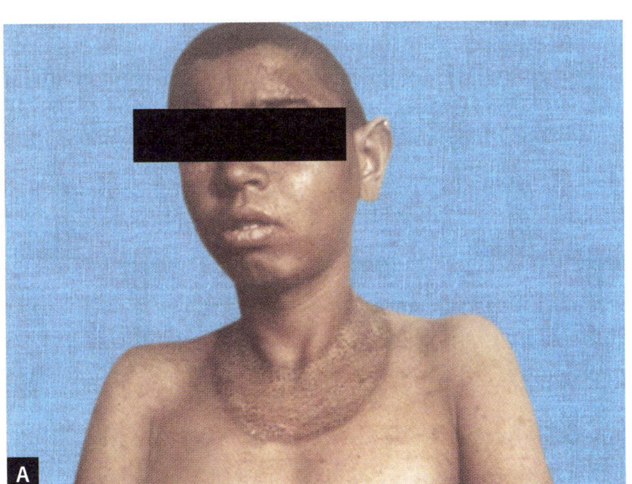

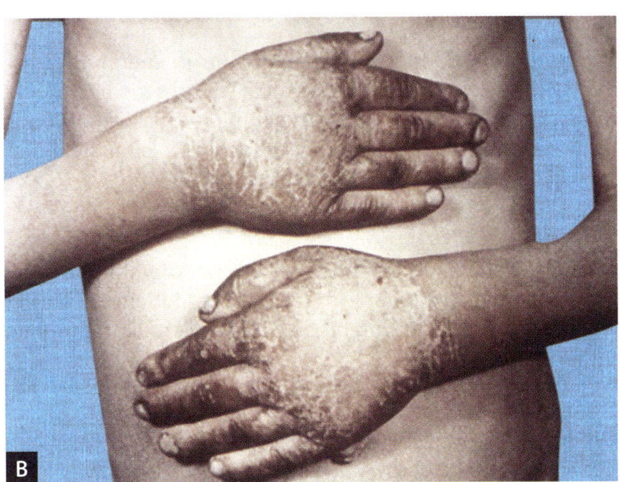

Figs. 10.9A and B: (A) Casal necklace; (B) Pellagrous glove
Source: Public Health Image Library, Centers for Disease Control and Prevention

Niacin Toxicity

Toxicity of niacin is rare with dietary intake but can occur from long-term use of high-dose supplements. Niacin administration can cause vasodilatation, flushing, tingling, and a sensation of warmth, chills, and gastrointestinal upset. Tolerable upper limit (TUL) for niacin is 35 mg/day.

PYRIDOXINE (B_6)

Pyridoxine is essential for normal brain metabolism and growth of infants. Through its active coenzyme form (pyridoxal phosphate), vitamin B_6 is needed for important pathways like gluconeogenesis, synthesis of neurotransmitters such as serotonin, dopamine, taurine, GABA, norepinephrine, and histamine. Along with folic acid, vitamin B_{12} and riboflavin, vitamin B_6 is needed for the metabolism of homocysteine. It is also involved in immune system and nucleic acid metabolism.

Vitamin B_6 has been found to have a beneficial effect in nausea and vomiting of pregnancy and radiation sickness.

Sources

Liver, meat, fish, yeast, cereals, pulses, and peas potatoes, and bananas are rich sources. Milk, eggs, vegetables, and fruits contain only small amount of pyridoxine.

Daily Requirements

Requirement (EAR) of vitamin B_6 for 1,000 kcal is 0.616 mg/day (ICMR, 2020). Vitamin B_6 is stored in the liver during fetal growth and is drawn when required. Requirement of vitamin B_6 for different age groups is depicted in **Table 10.11**.

Table 10.11 Requirements of Vitamin B_6 for Different Age Groups

Age group	*RDA (mg/day)*	*EAR (mg/day)*
Men		
• Sedentary	1.9	1.6
• Moderate	2.4	2.1
• Heavy	3.1	2.6
Women		
• Sedentary	1.9	1.6
• Moderate	1.9	1.6
• Heavy	2.4	2.1
Pregnant women	2.3	1.9
Lactating women	2.07–2.16	1.76–1.82
Infants		
• 0–6 m	0.1 (AI)	—
• 6–12 m	0.6	0.5
Children		
• 1–3 y	0.9	0.8
• 4–6 y	1.2	1.0
• 7–9 y	1.5	1.3
Boys (10–12 y)	2.0	1.7
Girls (10–12 y)	1.9	1.6
Boys (13–15 y)	2.6	2.2
Girls (13–15 y)	2.2	1.8
Boys (16–18 y)	3.0	2.5
Girls (16–18 y)	2.3	1.9

(EAR: estimated average requirement; RDA: recommended dietary allowance; AI: adequate intake; m: months; y: years)
Source: Nutrient Requirements for Indians, ICMR 2024

Pyridoxine Deficiency

Deficiency states are unusual and are either secondary to another disease or to an inborn error of metabolism. Pyridoxine deficiency may be seen after prolonged isoniazid, penicillamine, and hydralazine therapy, and parenteral alimentation.

Clinical Features

Pyridoxine dependency in infancy (due to metabolic disturbances) causes convulsions. Clinical features include failure to thrive, hyperirritability, hyperacusis, microcytic hypochromic anemia, nausea, and vomiting. These include seborrheic dermatitis, peripheral neuritis, and depression.

Diagnosis

Subclinical deficiency can be detected by estimating urinary excretion of pyridoxic acid. In pyridoxine deficiency states, urinary excretion of xanthurenic acid increases after tryptophan loading.

TREATMENT Vitamin E Deficiency

Child should consume a balanced diet. Seizures due to vitamin B_6 deficiency respond to 100 mg of pyridoxine. Further doses are not required with good-dietary intake.

Pyridoxine Dependency

Pyridoxine dependency refers to a condition characterized by increased pyridoxine requirements. Pyridoxine-dependent syndromes include pyridoxine dependent seizures, pyridoxine responsive anemia, and homocystinuria.

Pyridoxine dependency in neonates causes convulsions. Therapeutic trial with intramuscular administration of 100 mg of pyridoxine, in newborn infants not responding to usual seizure management and with a normal metabolic profile is the best method to diagnose pyridoxine-dependent seizures. This should be followed by prolonged administration of pyridoxine 10-100 mg/day orally.

Pyridoxine Toxicity

Taking very high doses of vitamin B_6 supplements may cause neuropathy. TUL for pyridoxine is 100 mg/day.

COBALAMIN (VITAMIN B_{12})

Vitamin B_{12} plays an important role in lipid and carbohydrate metabolism, nucleic acid synthesis, protein synthesis, and affects myelin formation.

Sources

Vitamin B_{12} is present only in foods of animal origin such as liver, meat, eggs, and milk. Fortified cereals and milk are the main sources for vegetarian populations.

Considerable amounts of this vitamin are stored in the liver. Although cobalamin is synthesized by bacteria of intestinal colon, it is not available for absorption.

Daily Requirements

ICMR recommends 2 µg per day EAR for an average Indian adult. Additional allowance of 0.2 µg is sufficient to meet the B_{12} needs of pregnant women. The amount of vitamin B_{12} secreted in breastmilk is in between 0.25 and 0.3 µg, therefore, additional allowance of 0.5 µg per day would suffice during lactation **(Table 10.12)**.

Vitamin B_{12} Deficiency

Causes

Vegans have low serum B_{12} levels which can pose a serious risk of deficiency. Reports indicate that vitamin B_{12} deficiency exists in >30% in adults and in children in India. Vitamin B_{12} malabsorption occurs in blind loop syndrome and tropical sprue, Crohn disease, and intestinal tuberculosis. Vitamin B_{12} deficiency is also seen in methylmalonic aciduria, in breastfed infants of vitamin B_{12} deficient vegetarian mothers, and following administration of drugs such as neomycin, para-amino salicylic acid, and colchicine. Lack of intrinsic factor in the stomach results in failure of absorption of vitamin B_{12} and causes pernicious anemia.

Clinical Features

Anemia: In the bone marrow, erythropoiesis is arrested in the later stages. Bone marrow shows megaloblastic reaction. The immature forms of RBCs, which are larger than the normal cells, enter the circulation. These cells have a short lifespan. The failure of maturation does not prevent hemoglobinization, resulting in *macrocytic normochromic anemia.*

Table 10.12 Requirements of Vitamin B_{12} for Different Age Groups

Age group	*RDA (µg/day)*	*EAR (µg/day)*
Adults	2.5	2
Pregnant women	+ 0.25	+0.20
Lactating women	+ 1.0	+0.8
Infants (0–6 m)	Breast milk	–
Infants and preschool children (6 m to 5 y)		1.0
School children and adolescents (5–17 y)	2.2	2.0

(EAR: estimated average requirement; RDA: recommended dietary allowance; m: months; y: years)
Source: Nutrient Requirements for Indians, ICMR 2024

Deficiency of vitamin B_{12} impairs synthesis of DNA and causes defective myelin formation.

Neuropathy: Demyelination of large nerve fibers of the spinal cord, especially the long tracts and posterior columns occur. Early signs are numbness and tingling sensation in the fingers and toes. Advanced cases result in subacute combined degeneration of the cord.

Newborn: Vitamin B_{12} deficiency occurs in >50% women. Maternal vitamin B_{12} deficiency has been linked to offspring adiposity and insulin resistance. Supplementation of pregnant women with vitamin B_{12} has shown to improve birth weight.

Diagnosis

Diagnosis of vitamin B_{12} require complete blood picture that shows megaloblastic anemia along with low serum level of B_{12} and folic acid.

TREATMENT Cobalamin (Vitamin B_{12}) Deficiency

Serum vitamin B_{12} and folate levels should be estimated prior to therapy. In the presence of strong clinical features of vitamin B_{12} deficiency treatment should be initiated to avoid neurological impairment, while awaiting investigation reports. If coexisting folic acid deficiency is present, vitamin B_{12} should preferably be started 10–14 days before giving oral folic acid. Folic acid should not be prescribed alone as the neurological symptoms due to vitamin B_{12} deficiency may precipitate or worsen.

Pharmacological Therapy

Oral therapy: Oral vitamin B_{12} should be given in empty stomach as food interferes with the absorption. Oral vitamin B_{12} therapy (500 µg in infants and 1,000 µg in older children) may be given every day for a week, every other day for the next week, 2 times a week, once a week, once every 15 days for a month and then once a month to complete at least 3 months duration of therapy. Alternatively, daily oral vitamin B_{12} therapy (500 µg in infants and 1,000 µg in older children) can be given for 3 months.

Parenteral therapy: Parenteral vitamin B_{12} is administered by intramuscular or deep subcutaneous injection. Vitamin B_{12} is rapidly excreted after intravenous administration. Injectable vitamin B_{12} should be used only where a rapid response is needed especially in children with neurological manifestations, severe anemia, pancytopenia or poor compliance with oral medication, underlying malabsorption of vitamin B_{12} or disorders of vitamin B_{12} metabolism. After the initial response with parenteral route, maintenance therapy with oral vitamin B_{12} can be provided. Children with vitamin B_{12} deficiency having mild or moderate anemia may be managed using oral vitamin B_{12} preparations as it is convenient, cheaper, and ensure better compliance.

Start treatment with 25 µg of vitamin B_{12} daily by intramuscular/deep subcutaneous/intravenous route for the initial 2–3 days. This is followed by 100 µg (50 µg in infants) daily for the next 7 days (till 3 weeks in children with neurological features), followed by 100 µg on alternate days for next 7 days, and then 1,000 µg every week over the next 1 month. Further maintenance therapy (1,000 µg monthly) can be given by oral or parenteral route. The intravenous route is used where the patient has thrombocytopenia as giving intramuscular or subcutaneous injections may lead to hematoma formation. Intravenous vitamin B_{12} should be administered as an infusion over 45–60 minutes. There is a need to monitor serum potassium levels in the initial few days of therapy.

Duration of Therapy

Children without neurological manifestations need treatment for at least 3 months, and those with neurological signs and symptoms need at least 6 months of therapy. Children with an irreversible underlying cause of vitamin B_{12} deficiency (e.g., pernicious anemia and inherited disorders of vitamin B_{12} metabolism), underlying malabsorption disorders and those with strict veganism require lifelong vitamin B_{12} therapy.

Dietary Counseling

Age-appropriate, adequate, and diverse complementary foods after 6 months are recommended to optimize the micronutrient intake. Food rich in vitamin B_{12} includes meat, poultry, shellfish, eggs, dairy products, mushrooms, and fermented foods such as curd and yogurt.

Monitoring

The evaluation is done with complete blood counts (CBC) and mean corpuscular volume (MCV) on day 7 in severe anemia, day 14 for moderate anemia, and day 28 for mild anemia. Rise in reticulocyte count is observed within 48–72 hours and peaks at the end of the first week after starting treatment. Hypersegmented neutrophils disappear and MCV begins to fall by day 14. The CBC, including MCV, becomes completely normal by 6–8 weeks. Neurologic improvement begins within the first week and is usually complete in 6–12 weeks. Repeat estimation of serum vitamin B_{12} is not useful as their levels may rise rapidly after administration.

FOLIC ACID (PTEROYLGLUTAMIC ACID)

Folic acid (vitamin B_9) products dihydrofolate and tetrahydrofolate are coenzymes in amino acid and nucleotide metabolism as single-carbon donors. Along with vitamin B_{12}, folic acid has a role in the synthesis of nucleic acids.

Sources

Green leafy vegetables especially spinach and broccoli, asparagus, cereals, beans, nuts, fruits, liver, and yeast, are good sources of folate whereas milk, eggs, and most root vegetables contain folic acid in lesser amounts.

Daily Requirements

During pregnancy, additional intake of 300 µg of folate has been suggested by ICMR to maintain the plasma and red cell folate levels with the normal range **(Table 10.13)**. Folic acid supplementation of 400 µg to the mother is recommended during the periconceptional period to prevent neural tube defects in the offspring. The dose should be hiked to 5 mg per day if there is a history of previous child born with a neural tube defect.

Considering the amount of folate secreted in breastmilk, which is mostly absorbed, an additional allowance of 100 µg is suggested during lactation. Protein deficiency impairs the function of folic acid. Certain conditions such as pregnancy, leukemia, and hemolytic anemia pose extra demands for folic acid requirements.

Table 10.13 Requirements of Vitamin B_9 for Different Age Groups

Age group	*RDA (µg/day)*	*EAR (µg/day)*
Men	300	250
Women	220	180
Pregnant women	570	480
Lactating women	330	280
Infants		
• 0–6 m	25 (AI)	—
• 6–12 m	85	71
Children		
• 1–3 y	120	97
• 4–6 y	135	111
• 7–9 y	170	142
Boys (10–12 y)	220	180
Girls (10–12 y)	225	186
Boys (13–15 y)	285	238
Girls (13–15 y)	245	204
Boys (16–18 y)	340	286
Girls (16–18 y)	270	223

(EAR: estimated average requirement; RDA: recommended dietary allowance; AI: adequate intake; m: months; y: years)
Source: Nutrient Requirements for Indians, ICMR 2024

Folic Acid Deficiency

Risk of folate deficiency is increased during periods of rapid growth as in infancy. It can also result from poor-nutritional intake, malabsorption (celiac disease and inflammatory bowel disease), increased cell turnover (chronic hemolytic anemia), prolonged drug treatment (methotrexate, 6-mercaptopurine, azathioprine, phenytoin, etc.), and some inborn errors of folate metabolism (methylenetetrahydrofolate reductase deficiency).

Clinical Features

Impaired synthesis of DNA in the cells results in abnormal cell division. Tissues with rapidly dividing cells, such as intestinal mucosa and bone marrow are affected in folic acid deficiency. Therefore, megaloblastic anemia and diarrhea are the predominant symptoms.

Other manifestations include glossitis, growth retardation, and impaired immunity. Folic acid deficiency is also associated with increased thrombotic events, which may be related to increased homocysteine levels. Folic acid seems to be protective against development of atherosclerosis and other vascular disease by virtue of its homocysteine lowering effect.

Neural tube defects: Maternal folic acid deficiency during the first trimester (phase of embryogenesis and morphogenesis) is associated with neural tube defects in the fetus. Folic acid is now recommended for preventing both occurrence and recurrence of these congenital disorders. Better folate status in women of reproductive age group may be achieved by increasing the folate-rich food intake, supplementation, or food fortification.

In recent years, both folic acid and vitamin B_{12} deficiency were found to be associated with elevated blood homocysteine level, which in turn was reported to be a major etiological risk factor of cardiovascular disease.

Diagnosis

Peripheral smear showing megaloblastic anemia, along with low serum folate and low RBC folate levels are used as a measure of folate tissue stores.

TREATMENT Folic Acid Deficiency

In case of deficiency states, such as megaloblastic anemia, therapeutic doses of 1–5 mg/day of folate are needed along with vitamin B_{12} for 3–4 weeks. Although small doses of folate can correct the anemia due to B_{12} deficiency, they may aggravate the associated neurologic abnormalities if given alone. Folate deficiency due to antifolate medication requires elimination of the offending drug.

- A daily intake of 400 µg of folic acid in women of reproductive age is recommended to prevent the first occurrence of neural tube defect. It is to be started before conception and continued till the end of 12th week of gestation.
- A daily intake of 4,000 g (4 mg) of folic acid, starting from 1 month before to 3 months after conception, is recommended in pregnant women with previously affected pregnancies, to prevent recurrence.

Folic Acid Toxicity

Toxicity is extremely rare especially from dietary sources. However, tolerable upper intake level is defined as 1,000 µg/day for adults, 300 µg/day for 7–9 years, and 600–800 µg/day for 9–17 years. Higher intake through supplements can mask vitamin B_{12} deficiency.

PANTOTHENIC ACID

It is present in coenzyme A and acyl carrier protein. It acts as H ion donor and receptor in the metabolism of lipids, cholesterol, fatty acids, and sterols.

Sources

Pantothenic acid is widely spread in both plant and animal tissues. Rich sources include yeast, eggs, liver, and cereals. Fair amounts are present in cauliflower, potatoes, and tomatoes.

Daily Requirements

Approximately 10 mg of pantothenic acid is sufficient to satisfy the daily requirement. Dietary intake recommended for infants is 1.5–4.5 mg and 4.5 mg for school children. As not sufficient data is available to derive an EAR for pantothenic acid, instead adequate intake is provided for different age groups **(Table 10.14)**.

TABLE 10.14 Adequate Daily Intake for Pantothenic Acid for Different Age Groups

Age group	*AI (mg/day)*
Men	5
Women	5
Pregnant women	5
Lactating women	7
Infants	
• 0–6 m	2
• 6–12 m	2
Children	
• 1–3 y	2
• 4–6 y	3
• 7–9 y	4
Boys (10–12 y)	5
Girls (10–12 y)	5
Boys (13–15 y)	5
Girls (13–15 y)	5
Boys (16–18 y)	5
Girls (16–18 y)	5

(AI: adequate intake; m: months; y: years)
Source: Nutrient Requirements for Indians, ICMR 2024

Deficiency

Individuals with a mutation in their pantothenate kinase 2 (*PANK2*) gene are likely to have a pantothenic acid inadequacy.

Clinical Features

Specific deficiency results in burning feet syndrome. Other symptoms of deficiency are tiredness, vomiting, depression, disturbed sleep, and muscle weakness.

Diagnosis

Blood concentrations of pantothenic acid below 1 µmol/L (normal 1.6–2.7 µmol/L) and urinary excretion rate <1 mg/day (normal about 2.6 mg/day) are considered low and suggestive of deficiency.

TREATMENT Pantothenic Acid Supplementation

Pantothenic acid is widely distributed in nature and deficiency is uncommon in humans. Provision of at least 5 mg of pantothenic acid per day is sufficient.

BIOTIN

Biotin acts as a cofactor for enzymes needed in gluconeogenesis, fatty acid metabolism, and amino acid metabolism. It also plays key role in insulin receptor transcription and pancreatic β-cell function.

Sources

It is present abundantly in natural foods. Largely, the human requirement is met by synthesis from intestinal bacteria itself. Rich sources include kidney, liver, yeast, egg yolk, legumes, cereals, nuts, vegetables like mushrooms, fruits such as water-melons, bananas, and strawberries. However, meat and cereals are poor sources.

TABLE 10.15 Adequate Daily Intake of Biotin for Different Age Groups

Age group	*AI (μg/day)*
Men	25
Women	25
Pregnant women	25
Lactating women	30
Infants	
• 0–6 m	4
• 6–12 m	5
Children	
• 1–3 y	7
• 4–6 y	9
• 7–9 y	12
Boys (10–12 y)	15
Girls (10–12 y)	16
Boys (13–15 y)	20
Girls (13–15 y)	20
Boys (16–18 y)	25
Girls (16–18 y)	25

(AI: adequate intake; m: months; y: years)
Source: Nutrient Requirements for Indians, ICMR 2024

Daily Requirements

Sufficient data is not available to derive an EAR and RDA for biotin, only adequate intakes could be established **(Table 10.15)**.

Biotin Deficiency

Biotin is widely distributed in food stuffs and deficiency is uncommon. Infants and children receiving total parenteral nutrition without biotin supplementation may develop deficiency. Deficiency may also occur in persons consuming large quantities of raw egg white, which contains avidin, a biotin antagonist.

Clinical Features

Deficiency may result in a periorificial dermatitis, conjunctivitis, anorexia, extreme lassitude, muscle pain, alopecia, and central nervous system abnormalities. Genetic defects with biotin deficiency include Rett syndrome and carboxylase defects.

Diagnosis

Serum biotin levels may not be helpful in the diagnosis as levels do not decrease in the initial phase of deficiency. Increased excretion of 3-hydroxyisovaleric acid in the urine is the most reliable test. Status of propionyl-CoA carboxylase in human lymphocytes is also reliable for determining biotin status.

TREATMENT Biotin Deficiency

Oral administration of 2–5 mg biotin daily for 2–3 weeks corrects the deficiency.

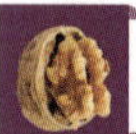

IN A NUTSHELL

Vitamin B Complex

1. Vitamin B complex includes thiamine (B_1), riboflavin (B_2), niacin (B_3), pyridoxine (B_6), cobalamin (B_{12}), biotin, and pantothenic acid, all of which are water-soluble.
2. B-complex vitamins function as coenzymes in several enzymatic reactions.
3. Poor diet can result in deficiency of one or more B-complex vitamins leading to beriberi (thiamine deficiency), pellagra (niacin deficiency), or megaloblastic anemia (B_{12} deficiency).
4. Malabsorption syndromes and drugs can cause secondary deficiency of vitamin B complex.
5. All B-complex vitamins are supplemented together in a deficient person.
6. Folate deficiency in mother is linked to increased incidence of neural tube defects in the offsprings.
7. Folate supplementation is recommended in periconceptional period in women of childbearing age.

Devalia V, Hamilton MS, Molloy AM. Guidelines for the diagnosis and management of cobalamin and folate disorders. Br J Haematol. 2014;166(4):496-513.

ICMR. Recommended Dietary Allowances and Estimated Average Requirements: Nutrient Requirements for Indians–2020. A Report of the Expert Group Indian Council of Medical Research, National Institute of Nutrition. Hyderabad: ICMR; 2020.

Kennedy DO. B vitamins and the brain: Mechanisms, dose and efficacy—A review. Nutrients. 2016;8(2):68.

Lee LW, Yan AC. Skin manifestations of nutritional deficiency disease in children: modern day context. Int J Dermatol. 2012;51(12):1407-18.

Revised Short Summary Report-2024, ICMR-NIN Expert Group on Nutrient Requirement for Indians, Recommended Dietary Allowances (RDA) and Estimated Average Requirements (EAR)-2020.

Shipton MJ, Thachil J. Vitamin B_{12} deficiency—a 21st century perspective. Clin Med (Lond). 2015;15(2):145-50.

Sriram K, Manzanares W, Joseph K. Thiamine in nutrition therapy. Nutr Clin Pract. 2012;27(1):41-50.

Verma D, Chandra J, Kumar P, et al. Efficacy of oral methylcobalamin in treatment of vitamin B_{12} deficiency anemia in children. Pediatr Blood Cancer. 2017;64(12):e26698.

Wan P, Moat S, Anstey A. Pellagra: a review with emphasis on photosensitivity. Br J Dermatol. 2011;164(6):1188-200.

Waddell L. The power of vitamins. J Fam Health Care. 2012;22(1):14,16-20,22-5.

Zempleni J, Hassan YI, Wijeratne SS. Biotin and biotinidase deficiency. Expert Rev Endocrinol Metab. 2008;3(6):715-24.

10.7 Vitamin C and Scurvy

PE 12.8

ROLE IN HEALTH AND DISEASE

Vitamin C (ascorbic acid) is essential for formation of collagen and intercellular matrix in teeth, bones, and capillaries. It is also involved in tyrosine metabolism, adrenal cortical functioning, and electron transport. It is a cofactor in activation of hydroxylating enzymes in oxidation processes. It also helps in transfer of iron from plasma transferrin into tissue ferritin and thus helps in storage of iron in the bone marrow, spleen, and liver.

Being a strong reducing agent, it provides protection to eyes and lungs against oxidizing agents and reduces oxidation of low-density lipoproteins and prevents deposition of atheromatous plaques. It helps in maintenance of vascular integrity through prostacyclin (antiplatelet and vasodilatory effect).

Ascorbic acid is a major antioxidant. It is needed for hydroxylation of collagen, biosynthesis of carnitine and catecholamines, metabolism of the metal ions, and plays a vital role in maintaining vascular integrity through prostacyclin. Ascorbic acid promotes absorption of soluble nonheme iron.

DIETARY SOURCES

Leafy vegetables, citrus fruits, Indian gooseberry (amla), and tomatoes are rich sources of the vitamin. Even roots and tubers such as potatoes, cabbage, leafy greens, and germinating pulses contain considerable amounts of it, as do guavas. Large quantities occur in liver and kidney but not in lean meat. Milk (except human milk), eggs, meat, and poultry are poor in vitamin C. Vitamin C is destroyed in cooking and storage.

DAILY REQUIREMENTS

Requirements are increased during fever, diarrhea, iron deficiency, and hypoproteinemia. Ascorbic acid in a vegetarian meal improves iron absorption, which is important for Indian diet **(Table 10.16)**.

Table 10.16 Requirements of Vitamin C for Different Age Groups

Age group	RDA (mg/day)	EAR (mg/day)
Infants		
• 0–6 m	20	—
• 6–12 m	27	71
Children		
• 1–3 y	27	22
• 4–6 y	32	27
• 7–9 y	43	36
Boys (10–12 y)	54	45
Girls (10–12 y)	52	44
Boys (13–15 y)	72	60
Girls (13–15 y)	66	55
Boys (16–18 y)	82	69
Girls (16–18 y)	68	57

(EAR: estimated average requirement; RDA: recommended dietary allowance; m: months; y: years)
Source: Nutrient Requirements for Indians, ICMR 2024

SCURVY

Severe vitamin C deficiency causes scurvy. The usual age of onset is 6–18 months. Severely malnourished children, and children dependent on boiled animal milk for their nutritional needs are at significant risk of scurvy. Breastfed children are protected as the breastmilk contains enough vitamin C to meet most of the requirements in the first 2 years of life.

Clinical Features

- Irritability, anorexia, low grade fever, fretfulness, and crying on handling are early features of scurvy. This is followed by swelling of limbs with the child assuming a frog-like position (abduction of thighs and slight flexion of knees). Child may be so reluctant to move his limbs that he appears paralyzed (*pseudoparalysis*). After a few days of onset, swelling may show hardening because of calcification of subperiosteal hematoma.
- Hemorrhages occur under the periosteum of long bones, gums, skin, and mucous membranes.
- Gums are swollen and purplish which start bleeding easily during the period of dentition. Petechiae may be seen over the skin. Orbital or conjunctival hemorrhages may also be observed.
- Costochondral junctions become prominent and appear sharp and angular (*scorbutic rosary*) in comparison to the dome-shaped and semicircular prominence of costochondral junction in rachitic rosary. Scorbutic rosary is attributed to separation of epiphyses of ribs and backward displacement of sternum.
- Wound healing is delayed.

Diagnosis

Radiological Features

Diagnosis is based on radiological features, mainly seen at the lower end of femur and upper ends of humerus and tibia.

- Bone assumes a ground glass appearance with a *pencil thin cortex*.
- Metaphyses demonstrate a zone of well-calcified cartilage, referred to as *white line of Frenkel*. White line may also be seen in healing rickets, severe protein energy malnutrition (PEM), plumbism, acute leukemia, and congenital syphilis.
- Epiphyseal centers of ossification are surrounded by a white ring (*Wimberger sign*) **(Fig. 10.10)**. A zone of rarefaction or destruction appears proximal and parallel to the white line. Epiphyseal separation may occur along this line.
- Subperiosteal hemorrhage results in periosteal elevation. Diaphyseal fractures are rare.

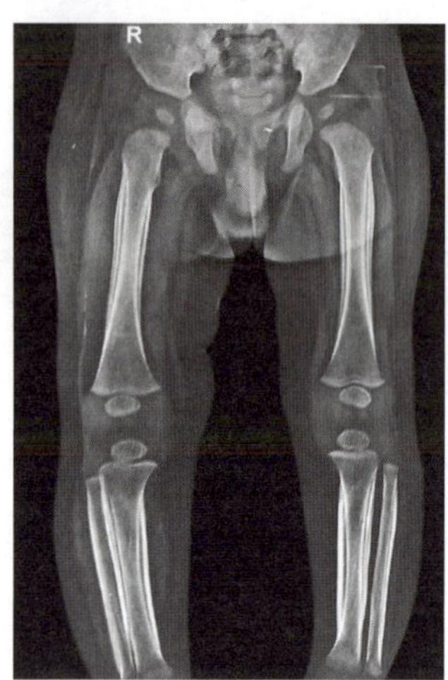

Fig. 10.10: White ring around epiphysis (Wimberger sign), and pencil thin cortex, suggestive of scurvy

Biochemical Diagnosis

Plasma ascorbic acid levels vary widely and cannot be relied upon to detect early vitamin C deficiency. Ascorbic acid content of white blood cell (WBC) offers a sensitive estimate of its status in the body (25–40 mg/100 mg is normal). Fasting vitamin C level >0.6 mg/dL excludes scurvy. Urinary excretion of vitamin C 3–5 hours after a loading dose of 11 mg/kg is >80% in normal subjects.

Differential Diagnosis

Other causes of pseudoparalysis such as septic arthritis, osteomyelitis, and congenital syphilis should be considered.

TREATMENT **Scurvy**

Ascorbic acid 100–200 mg per day provides quick relief. Treatment should continue for 3 months to ensure full recovery. Vitamin C rich foods need to be given.

Toxicity

Vitamin C is well-tolerated and safe, even in high doses. Large amounts of vitamin C intake may be associated with an increased risk of kidney stones and iron overload. The tolerable upper intake level for oral vitamin C for children range from 350 to 2,000 mg/day, at various ages.

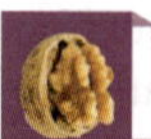

IN A NUTSHELL

Vitamin C and Scurvy

1. Vitamin C is a water-soluble vitamin, lost in cooking as a result of heat and oxidation.
2. Fresh citrus fruits and vegetables (cauliflower, broccoli, and cabbage) are good sources of vitamin C.
3. Deficiency results in scurvy; manifests as petechial hemorrhages, painful and swollen bones, and poor wound healing.
4. Diagnosis is clinically supported by radiological changes.
5. Oral supplementation produces dramatic improvement in symptoms.

Aggarwal A, Shaharyar A, Kumar A, et al. Scurvy in pediatric age group—A disease often forgotten? J Clin Orthop Trauma. 2015;6(2):101-7.

Brickley M, Ives R. Skeletal manifestations of infantile scurvy. Am J Phys Anthropol. 2006;129(2):163-72.

Ceglie G, Macchiarulo G, Marchili MR, et al. Scurvy: still a threat in the well-fed first world? Arch Dis Child. 2019;104(4):381-3.

Fortenberry M, Rucker H, Gaines K. Pediatric Scurvy: How an Old Disease Is Becoming a New Problem. J Pediatr Pharmacol Ther. 2020;25(8):735-41.

Kaur S, Goraya JS. Scurvy in children: Down but not out. Indian J Paediatr Dermatol. 2021;22(2):118-22.

11 CHAPTER Micronutrients, Minerals, and Trace Elements

AS PER NMC COMPETENCIES

PE13.1	Describe the RDA, dietary sources of iron and their role in health and disease, clinical features of iron deficiency, and management.	*Ch 11.2*
PE13.2	Describe the national anemia control program and its recommendations.	*Ch 11.3*
PE13.3	Describe the RDA, dietary sources of iodine and their role in health and disease, deficiency, and goiter control program.	*Ch 11.4*
PE13.4	Describe the RDA, dietary sources of calcium and magnesium and their role in health and disease, clinical features and management of deficiency states.	*Ch 11.6*

Topics available online: ***Free Radicals and Antioxidants; Minerals and Trace Elements; Lead: A Toxic Element; and Food Safety and Adulteration***

11.1 Introduction

Micronutrients are nutrients required in tiny amounts, may be a few micrograms per day, and include various minerals and vitamins. They do not contribute to the energy intake but normal healthy living is not possible without them.

While deficiencies in any of the essential micronutrients can result in health problems, there are a few that are vital to intelligence, immunity, reproduction, and work capacity. They cannot be synthesized endogenously and must be supplied in diet, e.g., vitamin A, iron, iodine, zinc, and folic acid. We have discussed vitamins in the previous chapter. In this chapter, we will focus on minerals and trace elements.

MINERALS

These are small inorganic elements and are indestructible unlike other major nutrients and vitamins. Calcium, phosphorus, potassium, sodium, chloride, magnesium, and sulfur are known as *macrominerals* and are usually required in amounts >100 mg per day, as they are present in relatively higher amounts in body tissues.

TRACE ELEMENTS

The term *trace* is applied to concentrations of element not exceeding 250 μg per g of matrix. The definitive feature of a nutritionally significant trace element is either its essential intervention in physiological processes or its potential toxicity when present at low concentrations in tissues, food, or drinking water. A world health organization (WHO) expert consultation has categorized nutritionally significant trace elements into three groups:

1. ***Essential elements*** such as iron, iodine, zinc, selenium, copper, molybdenum, and chromium.
2. ***Elements which are probably essential***, i.e., manganese, silicon, nickel, boron, and vanadium.
3. ***Potentially toxic element***, some of which may have some essential functions at low levels, i.e., fluorine, lead, cadmium, mercury, arsenic, aluminum, lithium, and tin.

HIDDEN HUNGER

Micronutrients deficiencies are termed as hidden hunger, as they do not give rise to apparent manifestations till the condition becomes severe **(Figs. 11.1A to C)**. Micronutrient malnutrition continues to affect over 2 billion people out of a world population of 7 billion. At least 340 million children younger than 5 years are found to be suffering from micronutrient deficiencies. It is difficult to assess the true burden of micronutrient malnutrition, as it requires laboratory facilities, advanced technology, and other resources.

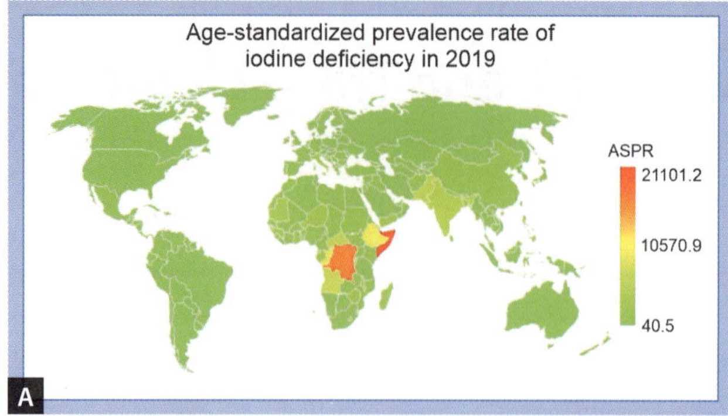

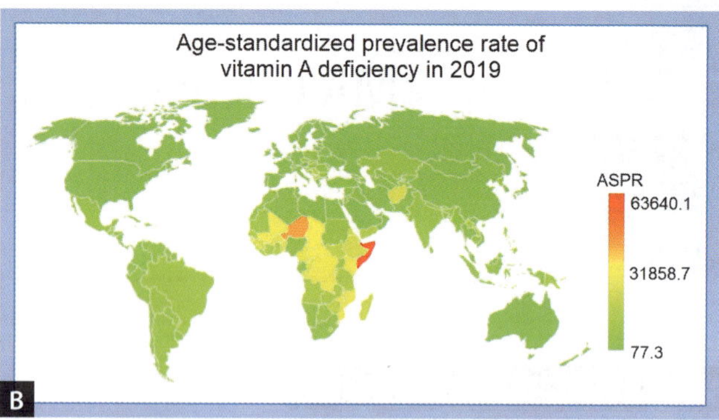

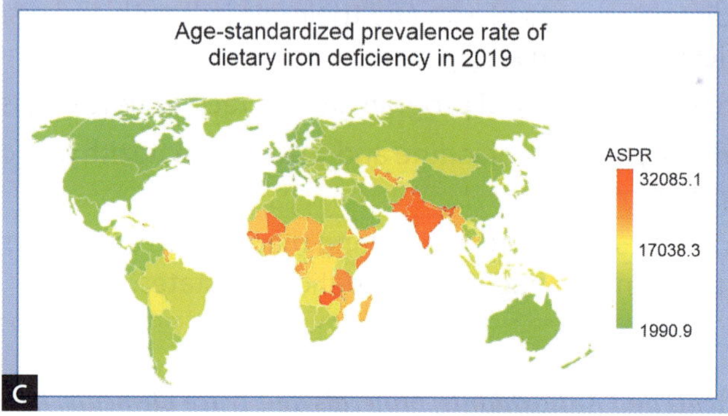

Figs. 11.1A to C: Global age-standardized prevalence rates of (A) Iodine deficiency; (B) Vitamin A deficiency; and (C) Dietary iron deficiency in 2019 (ASPR: age-standardized prevalence rate)

Source: Han X, Ding S, Lu J, et al. Global, regional, and national burdens of common micronutrient deficiencies from 1990 to 2019: A secondary trend analysis based on the Global Burden of Disease 2019 study. EClinicalMedicine. 2022;44:101299

There are several reasons for micronutrient deficiencies. The population may be deficient because they have poor access to micronutrient rich food due to poverty, defective crop growing pattern, deficient soil quality, inappropriate climate, or geographical isolation. Traditional dietary fads may also hinder intake, absorption, or utilization of micronutrient rich foods. Cereal-pulse based Indian diets are qualitatively deficient in iron, calcium, vitamin A, riboflavin, and folic acid, due to low intake of green-leafy vegetables, fruits, and foods of animal origin. The food distribution within the family is also inequitable.

Micronutrient deficiency is clinically evident only in the later stages of the disease, manifesting with impaired work capacity, learning disability, increased susceptibility to infections, and greater risk of death. For the country, it translates into loss of economic productivity and hike in investment on health and education.

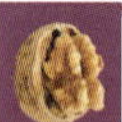

IN A NUTSHELL

Micronutrients, Minerals, and Trace Elements

1. Micronutrients are nutrients required in very small amount, include vitamins, minerals, and trace elements.
2. They are needed for a range of functions as enzymes, hormones, and antioxidants.
3. Their deficiency or excess both can cause detrimental effect on body.
4. Around 20% of total child deaths are attributable to zinc, vitamin A, iron, and iodine deficiency.
5. Many of these deficiencies are preventable through nutrition education and consumption of a healthy diet containing diverse foods, as well as food fortification and supplementation.

Awasthi S, Kumar D, Mahdi AA, et al. Prevalence of specific micronutrient deficiencies in urban school going children and adolescence of India: A multicenter cross-sectional study. PLoS One. 2022;17(5):e0267003.

Berger MM, Shenkin A, Schweinlin A, et al. ESPEN micronutrient guideline. Clin Nutr. 2022;41(6):1357-424. doi: 10.1016/j.clnu.2022.02.015. Epub 2022 Feb 26.

Capone K, Sentongo T. The ABCs of Nutrient Deficiencies and Toxicities. Pediatr Ann. 2019;48(11):e434-e440.

Gombart AF, Pierre A, Maggini S. A Review of Micronutrients and the Immune System-Working in Harmony to Reduce the Risk of Infection. Nutrients. 2020;12(1):236.

Savarino G, Corsello A, Corsello G. Macronutrient balance and micronutrient amounts through growth and development. Ital J Pediatr. 2021;47:109.

Shenkin A, Cuerda C, Berger MM. About micronutrient shortage and definition of deficiency. Nutr Clin Pract. 2022;37(4):966-7.

11.2 Iron

PE 13.1

INTRODUCTION

Iron is an essential micronutrient required for the synthesis of hemoglobin needed for adequate oxygenation of various body tissues and maintain the functioning of RBCs. Besides it has a role in various other functions including enzymatic reactions and immune functions. Iron is present in the body in three forms: Hemoglobin, plasma iron, and tissue iron. Hemoglobin iron constitutes a major part of body iron which gets released into plasma when the RBCs get lysed. The plasma iron is reutilized for synthesis of hemoglobin. The tissue iron is present as ferritin and hemosiderin in liver, spleen, and bone marrow; and myoglobin in muscles and cellular enzymes. Of the available storage forms, ferritin is normally predominant.

DIETARY SOURCES

Good sources of iron include red meat, chicken, fish, beans, spinach and other green leafy vegetables such as amaranth (chaulai sag/dantu), turnip, mint leaves, jaggery and tamarind. Whereas vitamin-rich food increases iron absorption, caffeine containing products like tea and coffee and presence of phytates in diet decreases iron absorption.

DIETARY REQUIREMENT

Nearly 1 mg/day of iron should be absorbed by the body to meet the physiological demands of iron. Since, only 10% of dietary iron is ultimately absorbed, 10–15 mg/day iron is needed.

IRON DEFICIENCY

Iron-deficiency anemia is the most widespread micronutrient deficiency in the world, affecting >1.5 billion people. In 2019, global anemia prevalence was 39.8% (95% UI 36.0%, 43.8%) in children aged 6–59 months, equivalent to 269 million children with anemia (**Fig. 11.2**). Anemia is highly prevalent among the under-5 children, pregnant women, and in every state of India. According to the NFHS-5 data, 67.1% children between 6–59 months are anemic (Hb <11 g/dL). As per CNNS Report 2019, anemia is most prevalent among children under 2 years of age; this may partly be attributed to the initiation of weaning-infection coupled with poor nutritional supplementation. Female adolescents are more likely to suffer from anemia (40%) than male adolescents (18%).

Clinical Features

The most common manifestation of iron deficiency is anemia. The manifestations are insidious in onset. It may present with poor appetite, loss of energy, paleness of body (pallor) and lethargy. There may be a drop in school performance and history of pica. As the pallor progresses, there may be history of dyspnea on exertion. On examination, pallor is the most notable finding. Long standing iron deficiency leads to epithelial tissue changes, koilonychia, platynychia, and loss of tongue papillae. Atrophy of the tongue papillae result in a smooth looking tongue. Tachycardia, systolic murmur and cardiomegaly may ensue if untreated [*Refer* to Chapter 23 (Section 23.4) for details on Iron Deficiency Anemia].

TREATMENT Iron Deficiency

Treatment of IDA includes deworming, oral iron supplementation with 3–6 mg/kg/day of elemental iron and dietary modification. Severe cases may require blood transfusion.

Prevention and Control

To prevent IDA, supplementary foods rich in iron should be initiated as soon as complementary feeding is started, preferably at 6 months of age. Pulses, green leafy vegetables and beans must be included in diet. Vulnerable groups like preterm low birth weight infants need to be supplemented with iron in a dose of 2–4 mg/kg/day starting from 4 to 6 weeks age. Diet of girls attaining menarche should be fortified with iron. Iron supplements are also necessary during adolescence for preventing anemia of puberty. Hookworm infestation should be curbed by regularly deworming children every 6 months and by encouraging them to not walk bare feet.

Weekly Iron and Folic Acid (IFA) Supplementation (WIFS) Program

Government of India has implemented the Weekly Iron and Folic Acid Supplementation (WIFS) program since January 2013, under the National Rural Health Mission (NRHM) in government/aided and municipal schools (nationwide) and Anganwadi centers across all states in India to combat anemia amongst adolescents and preschool children. Weekly prophylactic supplementation of iron is as effective as daily supplementation.

Iron Fortification

The Government of India is implementing fortification of common salt with iron to control IDA in community. The National Institute of Nutrition has successfully fortified the common salt with iron (ferrous sulfate: 3.2 g, sodium acid sulfate: 5 g, and orthophosphoric acid: 3.2 g in 1 kg of common salt).

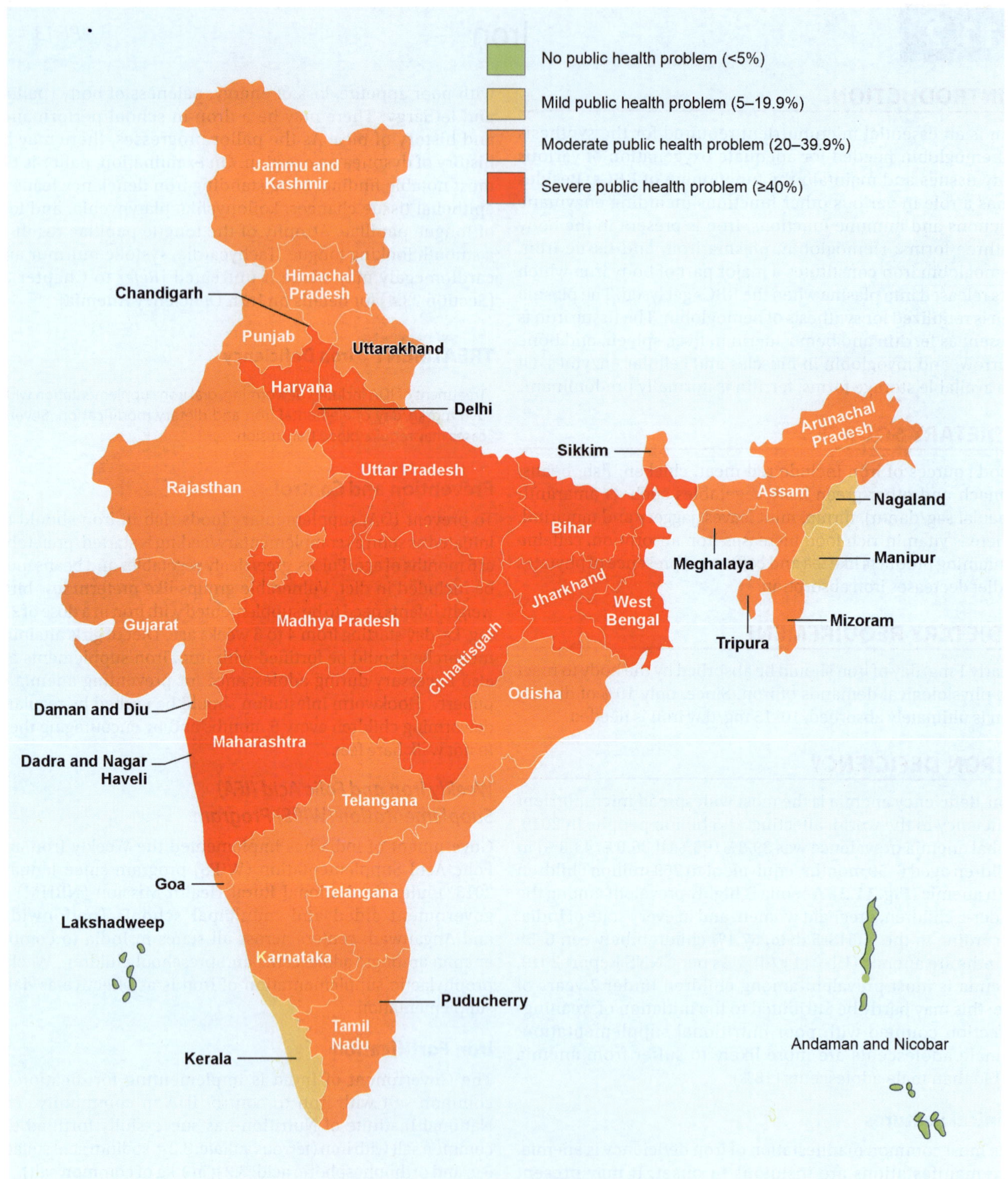

Fig. 11.2: Prevalence of anemia as a public health problem among children aged 1–4 years

Source: Comprehensive National Nutrition Survey (CNNS) National Report. Government of India, UNICEF, and Population Council; 2019

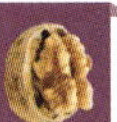

IN A NUTSHELL

Iron

1. Iron is an important component in hemoglobin synthesis.
2. Anemia is the most common presentation of iron deficiency in children.
3. A child with IDA often presents with lethargy, decreased appetite, pallor which may progress to heart failure if untreated.
4. Deworming, iron supplementation and dietary modifications are most important modalities of treatment and prevention.

Chandra J, Dewan P, Kumar P, et al. Diagnosis, Treatment and Prevention of Nutritional Anemia in Children: Recommendations of the Joint Committee of Pediatric Hematology-Oncology Chapter and Pediatric and Adolescent Nutrition Society of the Indian Academy of Pediatrics. Indian Pediatr. 2022;59(10):782-801.
Comprehensive National Nutrition Survey (CNNS) National Report. Government of India, UNICEF, and Population Council; 2019.
Lokeshwar MR, Mehta M, Mehta N, et al. Prevention of iron deficiency anemia (IDA): How far have we reached? Indian J Pediatr. 2011;78(5):593-602.
Thomas DW, Hinchliffe RF, Briggs C, et al. Guideline for the laboratory diagnosis of functional iron deficiency. Br J Haematol. 2013;161(5):639-48.
Zimmerman MB, Hurrell RF. Nutritional iron deficiency. Lancet. 2007;370(9586):511-20.

11.3 National Anemia Control Program

PE 13.2

ANEMIA MUKT BHARAT

History

Anemia is widespread across most age groups across all states in India. The Government of India implemented National Nutritional Anemia Control Program (NNACP) to address this issue and later adopted the National Iron Plus Initiative (NIPI) under Ministry of Health and Family Welfare (MoHFW) in 2013. The other programs were also implemented to address causes of anemia other than iron deficiency such as National Deworming Day for deworming, National Vector Borne Disease Control Program (NVBDCP) for malaria and special efforts for populations affected with hemoglobinopathies and National Program for Prevention and Control of Fluorosis. Considering the slow progress, i.e., <1% per annum reduction in prevalence of anemia from 2005 to 2015, there was a need for intensifying efforts to address all causes of anemia for accelerating decline in its prevalence among all age groups using a multipronged strategy rather than scattered programs.

Objectives

The reduction of anemia prevalence is one of the objectives of the *Prime Minister's Overarching Scheme for Holistic Nourishment (POSHAN) Abhiyaan* launched in March 2018. To mitigate the targets of *POSHAN Abhiyaan* and National Nutrition Strategy set by NITI Aayog, Anemia Mukt Bharat (AMB) strategy has been designed to reduce prevalence of anemia by 3% points per year among children, adolescents and women in the reproductive age group (15–49 years) from 2018 to 2022.

The Strategy

Anemia Mukt Bharat has $6 \times 6 \times 6$ *strategic approach* which includes—six beneficiaries, six interventions, and six institutional mechanisms to implement the program.

- ***Six beneficiaries:*** It aims to reduce the prevalence of anemia in—(1) children 6–59 months age, (2) children 5–9 years age, (3) adolescent girls and boys (10–19 years age), (4) women of reproductive age (20–24 years age), (5) pregnant women, and (6) lactating women (during initial 6 months).
- ***Six interventions:*** AMB program focuses on six interventions—(1) prophylactic iron folic acid supplementation, (2) deworming, (3) intensive year round behavior change communication campaign (Solid body Smart mind campaign) including ensuring delayed cord clamping, (4) testing of anemia using digital methods and point of care treatment, (5) mandatory provision of iron folic acid fortified foods in public health programs, and (6) to address nonnutritional causes of anemia in endemic pockets, with special focus on linkage with malaria, hemoglobinopathies, and fluorosis.
- ***Six institutional mechanisms:*** This program has six institutional mechanisms for implementation and account ability. These include—(1) National Anemia Mukt Bharat unit, (2) intraministerial coordination, (3) strengthening supply chain and logistics, (4) convergence with other ministries, (5) national center of excellence and advanced research on anemia control, and (6) Anemia Mukt Bharat dashboard and digital portal—one stop shop for anemia.

What is New in Anemia Mukt Bharat Program?

- Routine testing and treating for adolescent girls and boys in government and government aided schools (through RBSK) and pregnant women (ANC clinics)
- Delayed cord clamping
- Supplementation of 60 mg elemental iron instead of 100 mg in prophylactic dose of elemental iron for women and adolescents with sugar coated iron folic acid tablets
- Mandating use of fortified food in public health programs

- Special focus on use of iodine and iron double fortified salt
  - Hemoglobin measurement by invasive digital methods and point of care treatment.
  - Using intravenous iron sucrose/ferric carboxymaltose for management of moderately/severely anemic pregnant women.
  - Special focus on newlywed women 20–24 years.
  - Private schools to be covered under program in addition to government/government aided schools
  - Setting up program management units for AMB at national and state levels
  - Quarterly progress reports based on denominator and Health Management Information Systems (HMIS) and award
  - Dedicated AMB dashboard and portal (www.anemiamuktbharat.info)
  - To address nonnutritional causes of anemia by strengthening programs with special focus on linkage with malaria, fluorosis, and hemoglobinopathies
  - Establishment of National Centre of Excellence and Advanced Research on anemia control at All India Institute of Medical Sciences (AIIMS), New Delhi
  - To establish State Institutes of Excellence and Advanced Research on Anemia Control
  - Intensive communication through newly developed communication material and communication activities to create a *Jan Andolan*.

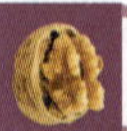

IN A NUTSHELL

National Anemia Control Program

1. Anemia Mukt Bharat focusses on giving prophylactic iron-folic acid (weekly/biweekly) to all children, adolescents, and women of reproductive age, irrespective of anemia.
2. Biannual (on 10th February and 10th August) deworming with oral albendazole is done for all children aged 1–19 years.
3. Delayed cord clamping, behavioral change in children, intensified screening for anemia along with curtailing non-nutritional causes of anemia are other cornerstones for controlling anemia.

Anemia Mukt Bharat. A programme by Ministry of Health and UNICEF. [online] Available from: https://anemiamuktbharat.info/ [Last accessed May 2025].

Joe W, Vishwakarma R, Patel N, et al. Coverage of Iron and Folic Acid Supplementation in India: Progress Under the Anemia Mukt Bharat Strategy 2017-20. Health Policy Plan. 2022;37(5):597-606.

Kapil U, Kapil R, Gupta A. National Iron Plus Initiative: Current status & future strategy. Indian J Med Res. 2019;150(3):239-47.

11.4 Iodine

PE 13.3

INTRODUCTION

Iodine is an essential micronutrient required for the synthesis of thyroid hormones needed for optimal physical growth and development. A healthy human body contains about 20 mg of iodine, 70–80% of which is present in the thyroid gland. Normal functioning of the thyroid gland depends on an adequate supply of iodine in the body.

DIETARY SOURCES

Seafoods and vegetables grown on iodine-rich soil are good sources of iodine. Soil in mountainous regions has low iodine content. In these areas, IDD are common. About 90% of the iodine requirement is met through food, while the rest 10% is obtained through drinking water in an iodine sufficient environment. Daily intake of 10 g of iodized salt having iodine at a minimum level of 15 parts per million (ppm) provides about 150 ppm per day, in addition to iodine present in foods consumed.

DIETARY REQUIREMENT

Dietary requirement for iodine in different age and physiological groups for Indian children is given in **Table 11.1**. The intake should be increased if there is presence of goitrogens in the diet.

"Goitrogens" are chemical substances leading to development of goiter. They interfere with iodine metabolism in the body at various levels. Some of the known goitrogens found in

Table 11.1 Requirements of Iodine for Different Age Groups

Age group	*RDA (µg/day)*	*EAR (µg/day)*
Infants		
0–6 m*	100	—
6–12 m	130	130
Children		
1–3 y	90	65
4–6 y	120	80
7–9 y	120	80
Boys (10–12 y)	150	100
Girls (10–12 y)	150	100
Boys (13–15 y)	150	100
Girls (13–15 y)	150	100
Boys (16–18 y)	17.6	100
Girls (16–18 y)	14.7	100

*AI (Adequate Intake)

(EAR: estimated average requirement; RDA: recommended dietary allowance; m: months; y: years)

Source: ICMR 2020

the environment are thiocyanates, cyanoglycosides, thio-oxazolidone, disulfides, phenols, phthalates, flavonoids, biphenyls, and lithium. Some of these substances are found in abundance in certain tubers and vegetables such as tapioca, cabbage, and cauliflower. Certain varieties of common foodstuffs such as sorghum, finger millet, mustard, and groundnuts are known to contain fair amounts of goitrogens. Cassava, maize, bamboo shoots, sweet potatoes, and millets are other important goitrogens.

IODINE DEFICIENCY

Global status of iodine deficiency is shown in **Figures 11.3A and B**. In India, the entire population is prone to iodine deficiency disorders (IDD) due to deficiency of iodine in the soil. National salt iodization program has substantially reduced the burden of iodine deficiency. Median urinary iodine concentrations (mUIC) <50 μg/L is being considered as suboptimal iodine intake at the population level (WHO).

The Comprehensive National Nutrition Survey (CNNS) 2018 providing national and state level data, reported adequate iodine status (mUIC 100 μg/L and 300 μg/L) in all three age groups—(1) 213 μg/L among preschool children, (2) 175 μg/L among school-age children, and (3) 173 μg/L among adolescents. All states had adequate levels of urinary iodine concentration except Tamil Nadu that showed marginal excess intake with mUIC >300 μg/L (median ~320 μg/L).

Clinical Features

Iodine deficiency leads to a wide spectrum of disorders, which are termed as IDD **(Table 11.2)**. Lack of iodine may

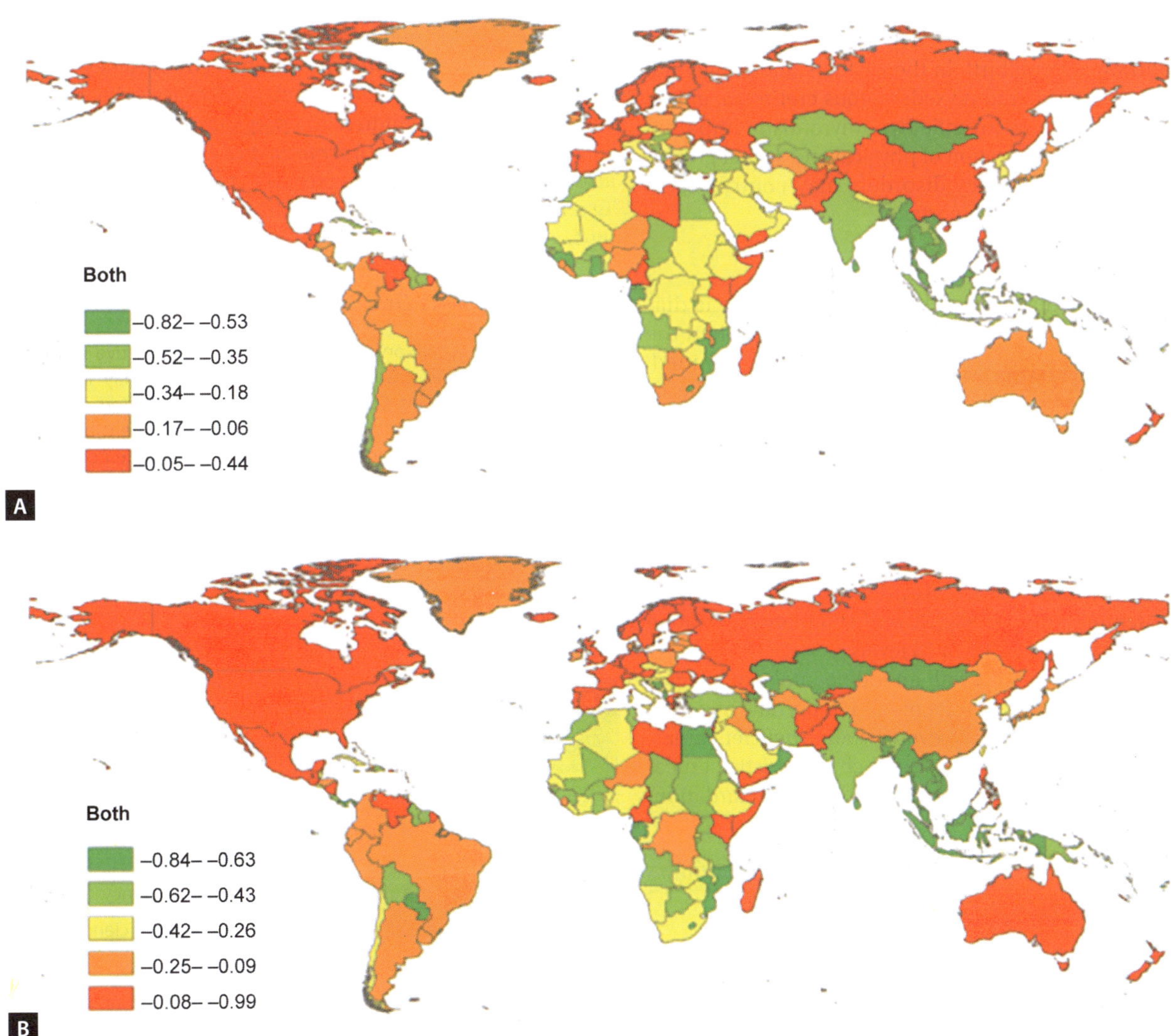

Figs. 11.3A and B: Global EAPC of iodine deficiency age-standardized rates from 1990 to 2019, by country. (A) EAPC of ASI rate; (B) EAPC of age-standardized DALY rate (DALY: disability adjusted life-year)

Source: Zhifei Wu, Yu Liu, Wenjuan Wang. The burden of iodine deficiency. Arch Med Sci. 2024;20(5):1484-94

Table 11.2 Iodine Deficiency Disorders

Physiological groups	*Health consequences of iodine deficiency*
All ages	• Goiter • Hypothyroidism • Increased susceptibility to nuclear radiation
Fetus	• Spontaneous abortion • Stillbirth • Congenital anomalies • Perinatal mortality
Neonate	• *Endemic cretinism* including mental deficiency with a mixture of mutism, spastic diplegia, squint, hypothyroidism, and short stature • Infant mortality
Child and adolescent	• Impaired mental function • Delayed physical development • Iodine-induced hyperthyroidism (IIH)

result in abortion and stillbirth in the mothers and congenital anomalies, neurological and myxedematous cretinism, goiter, and psychomotor defects, juvenile hypothyroidism, impaired mental function, and retardation of physical and sexual growth in children. Iodine deficiency disorders may contribute to increased infant and perinatal mortality.

Goiter

Goiter is an enlargement of the thyroid gland. Goiter is diagnosed when the lateral lobe of the thyroid is larger than the terminal phalanx of the thumb of the child being examined. It may be classified as congenital or acquired, sporadic or endemic. Goiter may be associated with diminished, normal, or increased thyroid function. The size of the goiter is assessed by palpation and stages as given in **Table 11.3**. Ultrasonography provides a more precise and objective method.

Endemic goiter is present when the prevalence in a defined population exceeds 10%. The differential diagnosis is established by epidemiological criteria. Clinical evidence of hypothyroidism is difficult to demonstrate. Usually, thyroid-stimulating hormone (TSH) is elevated with low T4 and T3 levels.

Endemic cretinism occurs with an iodine intake of <25 µg/day in contrast to a normal intake of 80–150 µg/day, affecting up to 10% of population living in severely iodine deficient areas. It is associated with endemic goiter and characteristic clinical features, which include deaf-mutism, squint, mental retardation, characteristic spastic or rigid neuromotor disorder (spastic diplegia), and dwarfism. Two types of endemic cretinism are described:

1. ***Neurological cretinism*** is characterized by deaf-mutism, squint, proximal spasticity, and rigidity more in the lower extremities, disorders of stance and gait with preservation of vegetative functions, occasional signs of cerebellar or oculomotor disturbance, and severe mental deficiency.
2. ***Myxedematous cretinism*** is characterized by retarded psychomotor development, short stature, coarse facial features, and myxedema without deaf mutism. The pathogenesis of endemic cretinism is poorly understood.

Table 11.3 Simplified Classification of Goiter by Palpation

Grade 0	No palpable or visible goiter
Grade 1	A goiter that is palpable but not visible when the neck is in the normal position (i.e., the thyroid is not visibly enlarged). Thyroid nodules in a thyroid which is otherwise not enlarged fall into this category
Grade 2	A swelling in the neck that is clearly visible when the neck is in a normal position and is consistent with an enlarged thyroid when the neck is palpated

Indicators of Iodine Deficiency

Iodine deficiency disorders become a public health problem, when *total goiter rate* (*TGR*) (number with goiters of grades 1 and 2 divided by total examined) is 5% or more in school-children 6–12 years of age. TGR of 5–19.9, 20–29.9, and 30% and more are indicative of mild, moderate, and severe IDD in an area.

Estimate of urinary iodine excretion (UIC) values <100 µg/L in spot urine sample is another method of assessing the iodine status of preschool children and pregnant women **(Table 11.4)**.

Thyroid-stimulating hormone and thyroglobulin (Tg) can also serve as other surveillance indicators for iodine deficiency. Tg reference interval for iodine sufficient school children is 4–40 µg/L.

TREATMENT Iodine Deficiency

Prolonged administration of iodine or thyroxine is effective in reducing the size of the goiter. Goiters while on treatment may shrink with appearance of nodules. Surgical removal of large goiters is useful in airway obstruction and for cosmetic reasons. Treatment of endemic cretinism may eliminate signs of hypothyroidism but neuromotor and intellectual deficiency are irreversible.

Prevention and Control

Iodine deficiency disorders can be prevented by the use of iodinated salt or iodized oil.

Table 11.4 Epidemiological Criteria for Assessing Iodine Nutrition Based on Median Urinary Iodine Concentrations

Median urinary iodine (µg/L)	*Iodine intake*
School-age children	
<20	Insufficient—severe iodine deficiency
20–49	Insufficient—moderate iodine deficiency
50–99	Insufficient—mild iodine deficiency
100–199	Adequate—adequate iodine nutrition
200–299	Above requirements—likely to provide adequate intake for pregnant/lactating women but may pose a slight risk of more than adequate intake in the population

Iodized salt: WHO recommends that iodine concentration in salt should be within 20–40 ppm, to provide 150 µg of iodine per person per day (presuming that 20% iodine is lost during transport, 20% lost during cooking), and average salt consumption is 10 g per person per day. *Mild and moderate IDD* can be eliminated with iodized salt.

Iodized oil: *Severe IDD* areas require administration of iodized oil (1 mL contains 480 mg of iodine), given either orally or parenterally. 1 mL of oil should be dispensed to all females up to 40 years and all males up to 20 years in areas with severe IDD; repeat the dose after 3 years if severe iodine deficiency persists.

NATIONAL IODINE DEFICIENCY DISORDER CONTROL PROGRAM (NIDDCP)

It started in 1962 with the name National Goiter Control Program. The program is directed toward ensuring that only iodized salt is used in India. Based on an assumption that the mean intake of salt is 10 g per day, the recommended level of iodination is 15 ppm of iodine in salt.

Objectives

- Surveys to assess the magnitude of IDD.
- Supply of iodated salt in the place of common salt.
- Resurvey after every 5 years to assess the extent of IDD and the impact of iodated salt.
- Laboratory monitoring of iodated salt and urinary iodine excretion.
- Health education and publicity.

Indicators of Elimination of Iodine Deficiency Disorder

- Proportion of households using adequately iodized salt (>90%).
- Mean urinary iodine level of 100–199 µg/L in general population and 150–249 µg/L in pregnant women.
- Presence of a national program for elimination of IDD, political commitment, legislation on universal salt iodization, education and social mobilization, quality control, and a national database.

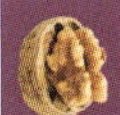

IN A NUTSHELL

Iodine

1. Iodine is essential for normal growth and development.
2. Iodine is required in a small amount, i.e., 150 µg/day. There is no natural food item, which is rich in iodine.
3. Iodine deficiency disorders include fetal loss, stillbirths, cretinism, dwarfism, intellectual disability, spastic diplegia, neonatal or childhood hypothyroidism, and poor school performance. Iodine deficiency is the world's major cause of preventable mental retardation.
4. For assessment of iodine deficiency, indicators used are TGR, urinary iodine excretion, TSH, and thyroglobulin.
5. Iodized salt is the most common mode for prevention of IDD.

Angermayr L, Clar C. Iodine supplementation for preventing iodine deficiency disorders in children. Cochrane Database Syst Rev. 2018;11(11):CD003819.

Eastman CJ, Zimmermann MB, Feingold KR, et al. The Iodine Deficiency Disorders. In: Feingold KR, Anawalt B, Boyce A, et al., (Eds). South Dartmouth (MA): MDText.com, Inc.; 2018.

Menon PSN. Prevention of Iodine Deficiency Disorders in Children in India—the Way Forward. Indian J Pediatr. 2019;86(2):113-5.

Yadav K, Pandav CS. National Iodine Deficiency Disorders Control Programme: Current status & future strategy. Indian J Med Res. 2018;148(5):503-10.

Zhifei Wu, Yu Liu, Wenjuan Wang. The burden of iodine deficiency. Arch Med Sci. 2024;20(5):1484-94.

11.5 Zinc

INTRODUCTION

Zinc is essential for ribonucleic acid (RNA), deoxyribonucleic acid (DNA), and ribosome stabilization and for the functioning of biomembranes. It is a part of the several enzyme systems of the body, e.g., carbonic anhydrase. Zinc also supports normal growth and development during pregnancy, childhood, and adolescence, and is required for sense of taste and smell. Zinc supplementation in under-five children reduces the risk of diarrhea and pneumonia, and results in faster recovery from diarrhea.

SOURCES

Animal foods such as oysters and lean meat are rich sources of zinc and also have high-bioavailability. Zinc contents in animal foods vary with the organs, such as liver, breast, shoulder. Plant foods contain relatively low amounts of zinc and also phytate in plant foods can bind zinc in the intestinal lumen and form an insoluble complex that cannot be digested or absorbed. However, cooking processes, such as soaking, germination, and fermentation of foods can degrade the phytate, thereby improving zinc bioavailability. Furthermore, consumption of animal proteins (e.g., eggs, meat, and cheese) improves the bioavailability of zinc from plant foods.

DIETARY REQUIREMENT

Zinc supplementation (10 mg/day for <6 months, and 20 mg/day for 6 months to 5 years) is now routinely recommended along with oral rehydration solution (ORS) for treatment of all under-five children suffering from diarrhea and is to be continued for 14 days. Overall, the body absorbs 15–21% of dietary zinc from

Table 11.5 Requirements of Zinc for Different Age Groups

Age group	RDA (mg/day)	EAR (mg/day)
Infants		
• 0–6 m	—	—
• 6–12 m	2.5	2.0
Children		
• 1–3 y	3	2.5
• 4–6 y	4.5	3.7
• 7–9 y	5.9	4.9
Boys (10–12 y)	8.5	7.0
Girls (10–12 y)	8.5	7.1
Boys (13–15 y)	14.3	11.9
Girls (13–15y)	12.8	10.7
Boys (16–18 y)	17.6	14.7
Girls (16–18 y)	14.2	11.8

(EAR: estimated average requirement; RDA: recommended dietary allowance; m: months; y: years)

lactovegetarian meals and 40–50% from nonvegetarian diets. Due to poor-zinc bioavailability from plant foods than animal foods, vegetarians may have as much as a 50% higher need for zinc than nonvegetarians. Dietary requirement for zinc are given in **Table 11.5**.

ZINC DEFICIENCY

Zinc deficiency is defined as per **Table 11.6**. In India according to CNNS 19% of 1–4 years old children, 17% of 5–9 years age children, and 32% of 10–19 years old adolescents are zinc deficient. Zinc deficiency is more common in rural areas, poorest households (1–9 years) and in the children not attending school (5–9 years). Male adolescents are more deficient (35%) as compared to female adolescents (28%). State wise in all three age groups zinc deficiency is lowest in Nagaland and highest in Himachal Pradesh (1–9 years) and in Gujarat (10–19 years) **(Fig. 11.4)**.

The main reasons for deficiency are: (1) Low dietary intake of zinc-containing foods and low zinc content of soil, (2) Presence of inhibitors of zinc absorption in cereals and legumes, and (3) High fecal losses of zinc due to recurrent episodes of diarrhea.

CLINICAL FEATURES

Milder form of zinc deficiency, as seen in malnutrition and chronic diarrhea, is characterized by stunting, anorexia, periorificial rash, and excoriation, behavioral changes, and increased susceptibility to infections, especially diarrhea and pneumonia. The typical periorificial (around mouth and anus) distribution of rash is a pointer toward zinc deficiency. A syndrome of growth failure, hypogonadism, anemia, and hepatomegaly due to zinc deficiency was first described in West Asia. Deficiency is also associated with acute and chronic diarrhea, protein-energy malnutrition, immune deficiencies, night blindness, alopecia and lesions of eye and nails **(Table 11.7)**.

Acrodermatitis enteropathica, a severe zinc deficiency state, is an autosomal recessive inborn error of metabolism resulting from a defect in intestinal zinc-specific transporter gene (SCL39A4). The cutaneous manifestations of acrodermatitis enteropathica are dry, scaly, eczematous, or vesicobullous lesions mainly distributed around perioral and perianal regions **(Fig. 11.5)**, limbs may also be involved. Alopecia, severe growth retardation, chronic diarrhea, and immunodeficiency are other common features.

DIAGNOSIS

It is mainly clinical, based on typical rash in a predisposed child. A serum zinc cut-off of 65 µg/dL (9.9 µmol/L) is recommended for identifying zinc deficiency in populations for children aged between 2 and 10 years. The risk of zinc deficiency is of public health concern when the prevalence of low serum zinc concentrations is greater than 20%. Amongst the functional outcomes, height- or length-for-age is the parameter of choice for estimating zinc deficiency in populations.

TREATMENT Zinc Deficiency

Acrodermatitis enteropathica should be treated with 50 mg (infants) or 150 mg (older children) of elemental zinc daily. Clinical deficiency secondary to malnutrition is treated with 2 mg/kg/day of elemental zinc, given for 2 weeks. Zinc supplementation is also required during acute diarrhea, daily dose of 20 mg of elemental zinc for children older than 6 months, and 10 mg for children aged 2–6 months should be started as soon as diarrhea starts and continued for 14 days.

PREVENTION AND CONTROL

The preventive measures include assuring daily intake of foods rich in zinc such as meat and fish whole wheat, nuts, and legumes, as body has no specialized zinc storage. Dietary interactions such as cysteine and histidine enhance zinc absorption while phytates

Table 11.6 Measures of Zinc Deficiency

Time of day and fasting status[a]	Age		
	<10 years	≥10 years	
	Males and females	Nonpregnant females	Male
Morning fasting	<65 µg/dL	<70 µg/dL	<74 µg/dL
Morning nonfasting		<66 µg/dL	<70 µg/dL

[a]Fasting is defined as no food or beverage consumption for at least 8 hours

Source: International Zinc Nutrition Consultative Group, 2012

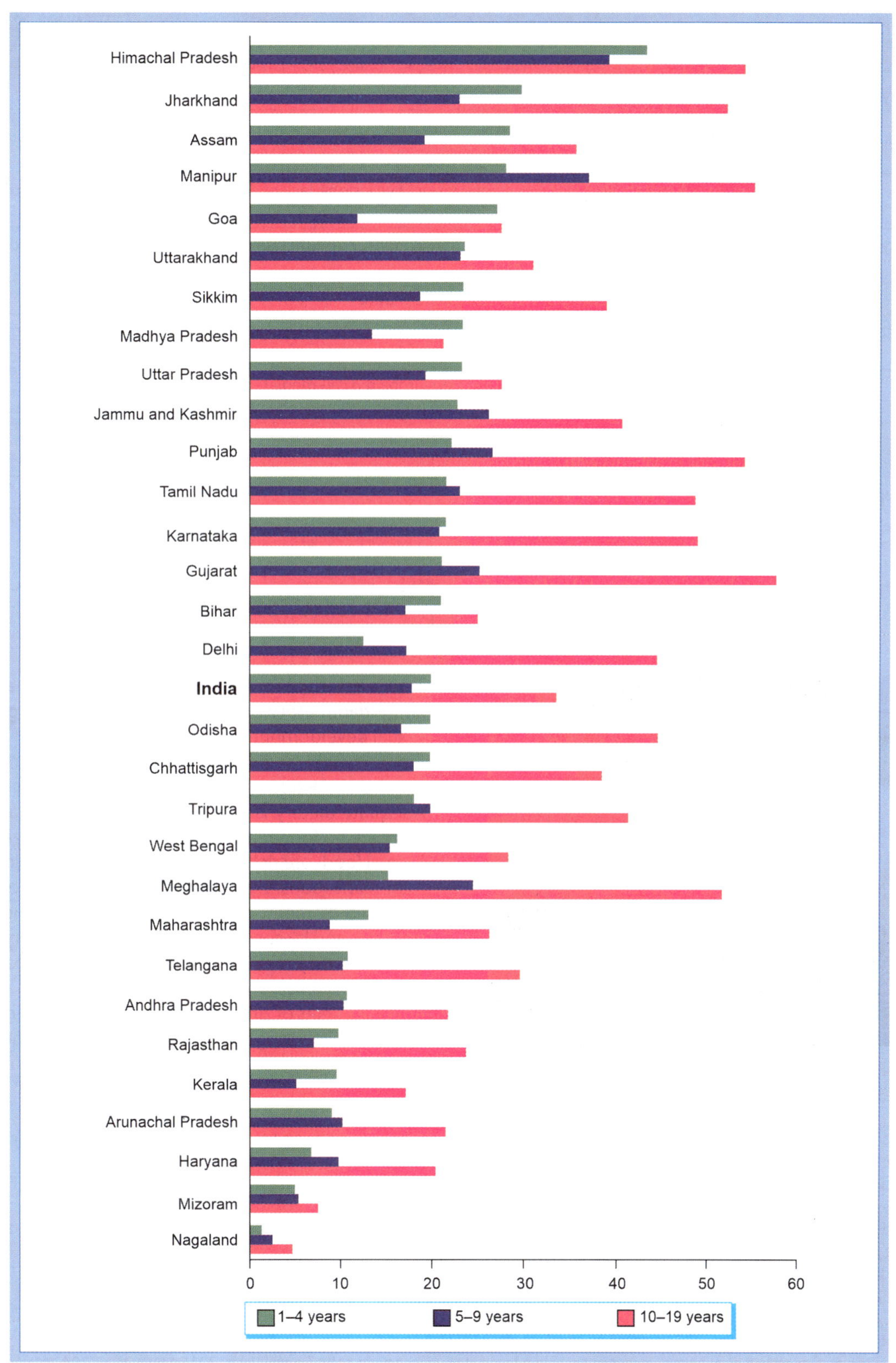

Fig. 11.4: Prevalence of zinc deficiency in Indian states

Source: CNNS Survey, 2019

Table 11.7 Clinical Features of Zinc Deficiency

System	*Signs and symptoms*
Gastrointestinal system	Loss of appetite, diarrhea, anorexia, taste and smell dysfunction, eating disorders, glossitis, and gingivitis
Hair	Early graying of hair, alopecia, and hair loss
Nails	Blackening of nails and nail dystrophy
Eye	Impaired vitamin A metabolism with weakened vision, eye lesions, lack of dark adaptation, photophobia, conjunctivitis, and blepharitis
Central nervous system	Behavioral abnormalities, impaired mental function, cognitive dysfunction, and depressed mood, impaired concentration, and intention tremor, ADHD
Skin	Skin lesions, acne, delayed healing of wounds, and dermatitis
Reproductive system	Problems in the menstrual cycle of women, impaired reproduction, hypogonadism in males, zinc deficiency in the pregnant woman can lead to poor growth in the fetus
Growth and development	Weight loss with increased susceptibility to infections, impaired cell-mediated immunity, thyroid dysfunction, growth failure, delayed sexual maturation, impaired immune function, decreased lean body mass, and bone fractures
General	Hypozincemia during fever may trigger febrile convulsions Reduced RBC zinc in patients with subacute thyroiditis
Manifestations depend on severity of deficiency and other factors	

(ADHD: attention deficit hyperactivity disorder; RBC: red blood cell)

inhibit zinc absorption should be taken in account while planning meal. Other useful strategies are improvement in zinc content of agricultural soil, food fortification, and prevention of diarrhea.

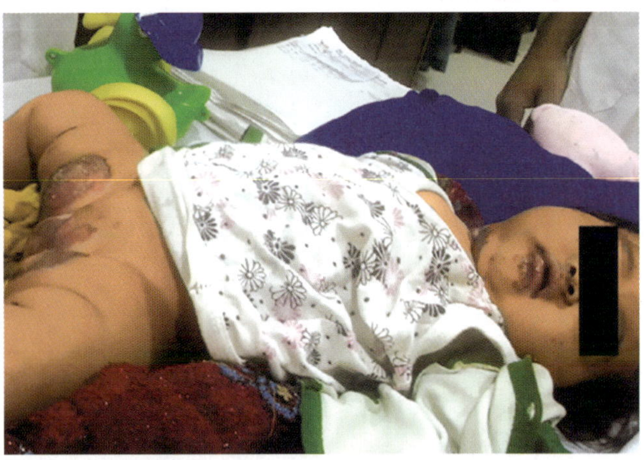

Fig. 11.5: Acrodermatitis enteropathica

Courtesy: Dr Arun Shah, Muzaffarpur, Bihar

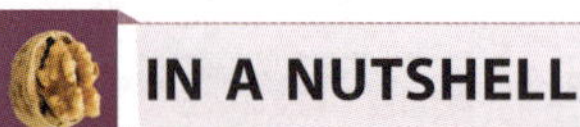

IN A NUTSHELL

Zinc

1. Zinc is essential for immune function and has antioxidant, anti-inflammatory properties, promotes linear growth, and sexual development in children.
2. Zinc is useful as adjunctive therapy in the treatment of common infectious diseases, especially diarrhea.
3. Adequate dietary zinc intake is necessary on daily basis, as there are no functional body stores of available zinc.
4. Animal foods are rich sources of zinc with high bioavailability than plant foods. Zinc bioavailability of plant foods can be increased by methods such as soaking, sprouting and fermentation, and by consuming animal proteins/dairy products.
5. Zinc deficiency may be diagnosed by low plasma zinc levels along with clinical symptoms.
6. Adverse effects of zinc deficiency on cognitive function, taste acuity, and stunting are reversible if detected and treated at an early stage.

Aggarwal R, Sentz J, Miller MA. Role of zinc administration in prevention of childhood diarrhea and respiratory illnesses: a meta-analysis. Pediatrics. 2007;119(6):1120-30.

Chiplonkar SA, Kawade R. Linkages of biomarkers of zinc with cognitive performance and taste acuity in adolescent girls. Int J Food Sci Nutr. 2014;65(4):399-403.

Gopal M, Sunitha K, Arockiasamy J, et al. Micronutrient Deficiency in Pregnancy: Time to Think Beyond Iron and Folic Acid Supplementation. Indian J Community Med. 2022;47(3):425-8.

Gupta S, Brazier AKM, Lowe NM. Zinc deficiency in low- and middle-income countries: prevalence and approaches for mitigation. J Hum Nutr Diet. 2020;33(5):624-43.

ICMR-NIN. (2020). Expert Group on Nutrient Requirement for Indians. [online]Available from: https://www.metabolichealthdigest.com/nutrient-requirements-for-indians-icmr-nin-2020/ [Last accessed August, 2025].

Kloubert V, Rink L. Zinc as a micronutrient and its preventive role of oxidative damage in cells. Food Funct. 2015;6(10):3195-204.

Rerksuppaphol S, Rerksuppaphol L. Zinc supplementation enhances linear growth in school-aged children: A randomized controlled trial. Pediatr Rep. 2018;9(4):7294.

Roy C, Kumar S, Ranjan RD, et al. Genomic approaches for improving grain zinc and iron content in wheat. Front Genet. 2022;13:1045955.

11.6 Calcium and Magnesium

PE 13.4

CALCIUM

Introduction

Calcium is a major element essential for several life processes. An adult man of 60 kg has nearly 1 kg of calcium, most of which is present in the bones. It is required for skeletal and teeth formation as well as their maintenance. It helps in the clotting of blood, neuromuscular excitation, and membrane permeability. The storehouse of calcium is ends of bones, this helps in maintaining the calcium levels in plasma, in case of deficiency.

Dietary Sources

Milk, milk products such as butter milk, skimmed milk, and cheese and millet like *ragi* are rich sources of calcium. A liter of cow's milk provides about 1,200 mg of calcium and human milk about 300 mg. Among vegetable foods, green leafy vegetables especially amaranth, fenugreek, drumstick leaves, tapioca—root vegetables are good sources of calcium.

Daily Requirement

About 20–50% of the calcium in the diet is absorbed, and the absorption is greatly facilitated by vitamin D. Moderate fat content facilitates calcium absorption. Phytic acid (present in cereals), oxalic acid (present in vegetables), and fatty acids make calcium insoluble and, therefore, hinder its absorption. Calcium losses also occur through urine, stools, bile, and sweat. Additional calcium is required during growth period for skeletal development and during lactation for milk secretion. The requirement of calcium as recommended by Indian Council of Medical Research (ICMR) (2020) is given in **Table 11.8**.

Table 11.8 Requirements of Calcium for Different Age Groups

Age group	*RDA (mg/day)*	*EAR (mg/day)*
Infants		
0–6 m	300	—
6–12 m	300	—
1–3 years	500	400
4–6 years	550	450
7–9 years	650	500
Boys (10–12 y)	850	650
Girls (10–12 y)	850	650
Boys (13–15 y)	1,000	800
Girls (13–15 y)	1,000	800
Boys (16–18 y)	1,050	850
Girls (16–18 y)	1,050	850

(EAR: estimated average requirement; RDA: recommended dietary allowance; m: months; y: years)

Source: Nutrient Requirements for Indians, ICMR 2024

HYPOCALCEMIA

Introduction

Hypocalcemia can occur at any age, but much more common in neonates. Causes of hypocalcemia in childhood are given in **Box 11.1**.

Box 11.1 Causes of Hypocalcemia

A. Increased skeletal need or inadequate supply of calcium:
1. Early neonatal hypocalcemia
2. Malabsorption
3. Hungry bone syndrome, e.g., postparathyroidectomy, after rapid healing of severe vitamin D deficiency/dependency rickets

B. Decrease in relative ionized calcium concentration:
1. Chelation, e.g., blood transfusion
2. Respiratory or metabolic alkalosis

C. Phosphate overload:
1. Excessive phosphate intake (cow's milk in the neonate)
2. Acute or chronic renal failure
3. Crush injuries and rhabdomyolysis

D. Hypoparathyroidism and parathyroid hormone (PTH) resistance:
1. Transient (secondary to maternal hypercalcemia)
2. Familial hypocalcemic hypercalciuria (activating mutations of the calcium-sensing receptor)
3. Congenital agenesis and hypoplasia of the parathyroid glands [DiGeorge syndrome, HDR (hypoparathyroidism), deafness, and renal dysplasia syndrome, Kearns–Sayre syndrome, Pearson syndrome, mutations of the GCMB gene]
4. Idiopathic hypoparathyroidism
5. Autoimmune polyendocrinopathy-candidiasis-ectodermal dystrophy (APECED)
6. Post-thyroidectomy or parathyroidectomy
7. Radiation to the neck
8. Iron deposition in parathyroid glands in thalassemia major
9. Pseudohypoparathyroidism (maternally inherited GNAS1 mutations or imprinting defect)

Clinical Features

Neonates can present with jitteriness, irritability, stridor, apnea, tetany, and generalized or focal convulsions.

Older children: Calcium deficiency may lead to tetany (characterized by muscle cramps, numbness, and tingling in limbs), rickets, osteoporosis, joint pains, hypotension, heart failure, arrhythmias, insomnia, and impaired growth.

Diagnosis

Hypocalcemia is diagnosed when total serum calcium is <8 mg/dL (2 mmol/L) or ionized calcium <4.4 mg/dL (1.1 mmol/L) in term infants or weight >1,500 g, <7 mg/dL (1.75 mmol/L) or ionized calcium <4 mg/dL (1 mmol/L) in very low birth weight infants weighing <1,500 g and total serum calcium concentration <2.1 mmol/L (8.5 mg/dL) in children. Ionized calcium is more informative than total or bound form. Serum calcium should always be interpreted in the light of serum albumin.

TREATMENT Hypocalcemia

Intravenous 10% calcium gluconate solution (1–2 mL/kg) should be administered to infants with acute symptomatic hypocalcemia. This is infused over 10 minutes since a rapid injection can cause arrhythmias. Continue oral calcium supplements (50–75 mg/kg/day) after acute symptoms subside.

In infants with hypocalcemia secondary to magnesium deficiency, Intermuscular (IM) 50% magnesium sulfate solution 100 mg/kg or 0.2 mL/kg/dose, usually two doses 12 hours apart are sufficient.

Chronic hypocalcemia associated with parathyroid hormone deficiency/resistance is treated with 15 ng/kg/day (maximum 1.5 µg) calcitriol (1,25-dihydroxy vitamin D) twice daily or with 25 ng/kg (maximum 2.0 µg) alfa-calcidol (1a-hydroxyvitamin D) single dose.

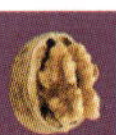

IN A NUTSHELL

Calcium

1. Calcium is an essential mineral required for skeletal and teeth formation, clotting of blood, neuromuscular excitation, and membrane permeability.
2. Milk and milk products such as butter milk, skimmed milk, and cheese and millet like *ragi* are rich sources of calcium.
3. Deficiency of calcium can cause tetany, rickets, osteoporosis, joint pains, hypotension, heart failure, arrhythmias, insomnia, impaired growth, and convulsions in neonates.
4. Serum level of total calcium <8.5 mg/dL is diagnostic for deficiency.

Cooper MS, Gittoes NJ. Diagnosis and management of hypocalcaemia. BMJ. 2008;336(7656):1298-302.

Pepe J, Colangelo L, Biamonte F, et al. Diagnosis and management of hypocalcemia. Endocrine. 2020;69(3):485-95.

Vuralli D. Clinical approach to hypocalcemia in newborn period and infancy: who should be treated? Int J Pediatr. 2019;2019:4318075.

Wosje KS, Specker BL. Role of calcium in bone health during childhood. Nutr Rev. 2000;58(9):253-68.

Zhou P, Markowitz M. Hypocalcemia in infants and children. Pediatr Rev. 2009;30(5):190-2.

MAGNESIUM

Introduction

Magnesium is the most abundant mineral cation in cells, second only to potassium. About 60–70% magnesium is present in bones, 25–30% in muscles, 6–8% in soft tissue, and 1% in extracellular fluid. Magnesium is an essential element, necessary for the synthesis of fatty acids, proteins, and cyclic-adenosine monophosphate (AMP). Magnesium form complexes with phospholipids of cell membranes and nucleic acids. Magnesium ion is extremely important for autonomic control of the heart, for maintaining electrical potential in nerves and muscle membranes. It is an important cofactor of the kinases and is needed for the energy transfer reactions involving adenosine triphosphate (ATP) and creatine phosphate.

Table 11.9 Requirements of Magnesium for Different Age Groups

Age group	RDA (mg/day)	EAR (mg/day)
Infants		
0–6 m	30	—
6–12 m	75	—
Children		
1–3 y	135	111
4–6 y	155	131
7–9 y	215	178
Boys (10–12 y)	270	223
Girls (10–12 y)	255	214
Boys (13–15 y)	355	294
Girls (13–15 y)	325	270
Boys (16–18 y)	405	338
Girls (16–18 y)	335	279

Source: Nutrient Requirements for Indians, ICMR 2024

Sources

Magnesium is present widely in plant foods and meat. Milk is a poor source. Magnesium is the metal ion in chlorophyll. Animal products, legumes, and cereals are good sources of magnesium.

Daily Requirement

Requirement of magnesium is 3–6 mg/kg/day **(Table 11.9)**. About one-third of dietary magnesium is absorbed from the usual Indian diet.

HYPOMAGNESEMIA

Magnesium (Mg) is the third most abundant intracellular cation. Almost all enzymatic processes require magnesium for activation. Approximately 60% of total body magnesium is present in bone, 38% in intracellular compartment, and only <2% in the extracellular fluid. Thus, serum levels of magnesium do not reflect the status of total body stores. Normal serum concentration ranges from 1.2 to 1.9 mEq/L or 1.5–2.3 mg/dL (1 mEq = 12 mg elemental magnesium, conversion factor-divide mEq/L by 0.822 for mg/dL).

Etiology

Prolonged administration of magnesium-free parenteral fluids, prolonged nasogastric suction, infectious diarrhea, steatorrhea, inflammatory bowel disease (IBD), and gastrointestinal neoplasms may cause hypomagnesemia. Several drugs (furosemide, cisplatin, amphotericin, mannitol) can also cause increased urinary loss of magnesium. A congenital defect in tubular reabsorption of magnesium also has been described. Severe hypo-

Box 11.2 Causes of Hypomagnesemia

A. *Gastrointestinal losses:*
1. Acute and chronic diarrhea
2. Malabsorption, syndrome
3. Extensive bowel surgery
4. Acute hemorrhagic pancreatitis

B. *Endocrine:*

5. Hyperparathyroidism
6. Hyperthyroidism
7. Hyperaldosteronism
8. Syndrome of inappropriate antidiuretic hormone secretion (SIADH)

C. *Renal losses:*

9. Prolonged parental fluid therapy
10. Osmotic diuretics (diabetic ketoacidosis)
11. Hypercalcemia
12. Drugs (diuretics, aminoglycosides)
13. Metabolic acidosis
14. Renal disease
15. Chronic pyelonephritis, interstitial nephritis, and glomerulonephritis
16. Diuretic phase of acute tubular necrosis
17. Postobstructive nephropathy
18. Inherited tubular diseases

magnesemia may occur during the recovery phase of diabetic ketoacidosis. Causes of hypomagnesemia are listed in **Box 11.2**.

Clinical Manifestations

Hypomagnesemia results in secondary hypocalcemia. Hence, the prominent manifestations of hypomagnesemia seen are that of hypocalcemia. Hypomagnesemia may manifest clinically as CNS and neuromuscular hyperexcitability. Early manifestations may include painful muscle cramps, nausea, vomiting, and lethargy. At serum magnesium levels <0.7 mg/dL, children may have tremor, hyperactive deep-tendon reflexes, hyper-reactivity to sensory stimuli, muscular fibrillations, positive Chvostek and Trousseau signs, and carpopedal spasms progressing to tetany. Mental status changes may be present and include irritability, disorientation, depression, and psychosis. Reversible respiratory muscle failure may occur in severe hypomagnesemia.

Investigations

Laboratory analysis by atomic absorption spectrophotometry is the most specific technique available to measure total serum magnesium. Hypomagnesemia may be associated with hypokalemia resulting in ECG changes such as ST segment prolongation, and T wave flattening. Severe magnesium deficiency may cause prolonged QT interval and ventricular arrhythmias.

Diagnosis

Serum magnesium <1.2 mEq/L is diagnostic. For magnesium deficiency, a high index of suspicion is needed especially in children with severe acute malnutrition, chronic diarrhea, refractory hypocalcemia, hypokalemia, and ventricular arrhythmias. Urinary excretion of >2 mEq/day or fractional excretion of >2% suggest renal loss of magnesium. Magnesium homeostasis is closely associated with calcium and potassium status and should be evaluated with these two cations.

TREATMENT Hypomagnesemia

Treatment for hypomagnesemia depends on the degree of deficiency and the child's clinical symptoms and signs. Therapy can be oral for children with mild symptoms or IV for children with severe symptoms.
- If hypomagnesemia is mild and the child is asymptomatic, oral replacement is appropriate.
- In children with normal renal function, the therapeutic dose is 0.05–0.1 mL/kg of 50% solution, i.e., 2.5–5 mg/kg of elemental magnesium as slow infusion. With renal impairment, reduce this dose by 50%.
- Magnesium gluconate is preferred oral form given in the doses of 30 mg/day in 3–4 divided doses up to 120 mg/day. Intravenous magnesium is effective for treating torsade de pointes and managing rapid atrial fibrillation. Concomitant deficit of calcium and potassium should also be corrected.
- Continuously monitor electrolytes, deep tendon reflex, renal function, and hemodynamic parameters during replacement.
- In overdose, calcium gluconate, 10–20 mL IV of 10% solution can be given as antidote for clinically significant hypermagnesemia, hypotension, hypocalcemia, and respiratory depression.

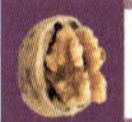

IN A NUTSHELL

Hypomagnesemia
1. Hypomagnesemia (serum magnesium below 1.2 mg/dL) results from diarrhea, steatorrhea, inflammatory bowel disease (IBD), renal disorders, and drugs.
2. Seizures are the most common symptoms. In seizures with hypocalcemia refractory to calcium supplementation, hypomagnesemia should be ruled out.
3. Genetic causes such as Gitelman and Bartter syndrome have hypokalemia and metabolic alkalosis along with hypomagnesemia.
4. Severe hypomagnesemia is treated by slow intravenous (IV) infusion of 50% magnesium sulfate 0.05–0.1 mL/kg, may be repeated 2–3 times q6–8 hourly.

Morooka H, Tanaka A, Kasugai D, et al. Abnormal magnesium levels and their impact on death and acute kidney injury in critically ill children. Pediatr Nephrol. 2022;37(5):1157-65.
Tseng MH, Konrad M, Ding JJ, et al. Clinical and genetic approach to renal hypomagnesemia. Biomed J. 2022;45(1):74-87.

11.7 Prevention of Micronutrient Deficiency

INTRODUCTION

Public health interventions aimed at preventing or correcting micronutrient deficiencies can be expected to reduce both mortality and disability substantially, especially in children. To achieve the maximum benefits, such interventions need to be done on the appropriate scale in deficient populations. Recent estimates indicate that fortification or supplementation with iodine, iron, vitamin A, and zinc are among the most cost-effective interventions available. Most effective strategies are discussed here.

Dietary diversification: New crops to include more micronutrient-rich foods should be planned. Nutrition education should be imparted to improve the cooking and preservation methods to preserve micronutrient. Dietary diversification remains a sustainable long-term solution but is not very useful in communities where micronutrient deficiency is widespread requiring immediate relief.

Supplementation: Micronutrients may be supplemented in a capsule, tablet, or syrup form to the suffering population as a short-term measure to reduce the deficiency quickly.

Food fortification: Micronutrients should be added to an appropriate food that can be enriched—an appropriate food is one that is widely consumed by the target group, is centrally processed, and whose taste and appearance do not change with the addition of the micronutrient. Examples include fortification of common salt with iodine, sugar, and *ghee* with vitamin A, and cereals with iron.

METHODS OF FOOD FORTIFICATION

The appropriate and effective method of fortification will depend on the prevalence of particular micronutrient deficiencies, population affected, dietary intake, available infrastructure, and capacities for food processing. The main fortification vehicles are as follows.

Large-Scale Food Fortification

Large-scale food fortification (LSFF) or industrial fortification is the addition of micronutrients during processing to commonly consumed foods (staple food) such as salt, flours, oil, sugar, and condiments. Universal iodization of salt is the best example of effective mandatory fortification to control IDD.

Wheat and maize flour fortification can be considered when industrially produced flour is regularly consumed by large population groups in a country. Fortification of flour with folic acid, vitamin B_{12}, vitamin A, zinc, and iron has been tried.

Biofortification

Biofortification is the process by which food crops are fortified through plant breeding or agronomically to improve their nutritional value. Biofortification processes include iron biofortification of rice, beans, maize, and sweet potato; zinc biofortification of wheat, rice, beans, sweet potato, and corn; and vitamin A biofortification of sweet potatoes, corn, and cassava. Biofortification also allows simultaneous introduction of multiple micronutrients in a single crop.

Point-of-Use or Home Fortification

Point-of-use fortification is the addition of vitamins and minerals to food that has been cooked and is ready to be eaten. This intervention can be used at schools and refugee camps apart from home; hence, the term "point-of-use" (WHO, 2012) is preferred and for this micronutrient powders (MNPs) are being used. MNPs are single-dose packets containing multiple vitamins and minerals in powder form that can be sprinkled onto food without affecting the taste or color.

MICRONUTRIENT INTERACTIONS

It appears that the effects of iron, vitamin A, and zinc deficiencies are largely independent. However, it is also important to understand the interactions of the essential micronutrients. When provided in supplements, vitamin A may enhance iron status and zinc may increase vitamin A absorption. On the other hand, iron and zinc may interfere with the absorption of each other. It should not be assumed that providing supplements with multiple micronutrients will have the same benefits as supplements with individual micronutrients.

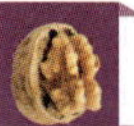

IN A NUTSHELL

Food Fortification

1. Food fortification is the process of enriching the staple food or food that is widely consumed with one or more micronutrients to improve the nutritional quality of the food and provide a public health benefit with minimal risk to health.

Allen L, Benoist B, Dary O, et al. Guidelines on Food Fortification with Micronutrients. Geneva: WHO; 2006.

Athe R, Dwivedi R, Pati S, et al. Meta-analysis approach on iron fortification and its effect on pregnancy and its outcome through randomized, controlled trials. J Family Med Prim Care. 2020;9(2):513-9.

Das JK, Kumar R, Salam RA, Bhutta ZA. Systematic review of zinc fortification trials. Ann Nutr Metab. 2013;62(Suppl 1):44-56.

Hombali AS, Solon JA, Venkatesh BT, et al. Fortification of staple foods with vitamin A for vitamin A deficiency. Cochrane Database Syst Rev. 2019;5(5):CD010068.

Nidhi Bedi and Piyush Gupta

12 CHAPTER Fluid and Electrolyte Balance

AS PER NMC COMPETENCIES

PE15.1	Describe the fluid and electrolyte requirement in health and disease.	*Ch 12.1, Ch 12.2*
PE15.2	Interpret electrolyte report and describe the management of sodium and potassium imbalance.	*Ch 12.3, Ch 12.4* *Ch 12.5, Ch 12.6*
PE15.3	Demonstrate the steps of inserting an IV cannula in a model.	*Ch 12.7*
PE15.4	Demonstrate the steps of inserting an intraosseous line in a mannequin.	*Ch 12.8*

Topics available online: ***Acid-Base Equilibrium, Evaluation of Acid-Base Disorder, and Acid-Base Abnormalities***

12.1 Body Fluids and Electrolytes *PE 15.1*

INTRODUCTION

Total body water (TBW) constitutes approximately 75% of body weight at birth that declines to 60% at 2 years of age and remains at this level until puberty. At the end of puberty TBW in boys remains at 60%, while TBW in girls decreases to 50% of total body weight due to difference in body fat content. Two-thirds of TBW is located within the cells and is termed the *intracellular fluid* (ICF). The remaining one-third of TBW is *extracellular fluid* (ECF) **(Table 12.1)**.

Extracellular fluid includes (*i*) *interstitial fluid* (80%), (*ii*) *plasma* (15–20%), and (iii) *transcellular fluid* (5%). Dehydration occurs because of reduction in interstitial fluid. Transcellular fluids include lymph, cerebrospinal fluid, synovial fluid, humors of the eye, endolymph, perilymph, gastric juices, pleural, pericardial, and peritoneal fluid.

FLUID COMPARTMENTS

Selectively permeable cell membranes separate body fluids into three fluid compartments. The plasma membranes of individual body cells separate intracellular fluid from interstitial fluid and endothelial cells separate interstitial fluid from plasma. The proportion of plasma at all ages is about 6% and that of transcellular water about 2–3%; whereas interstitial fluid declines from maximum at birth to about 18–20% of body weight by 2 years. Plasma along with blood cells constitutes the blood volume.

Table 12.1 Distribution of Body Water

Intracellular fluid (ICF) 67% of total body water (TBW)	*Extracellular fluid (ECF) 33% of TBW*		
Intracellular fluid (ICF)	Interstitial fluid 80% of ECF	Plasma 15–20% of ECF	Transcellular fluid 5% of ECF

Although fluids are in constant motion between the three compartments, the volume of fluid in each compartment at any given time remains fairly constant. Osmosis is the mechanism by which water moves from one compartment to another. As a result, the concentration of the solutes (mainly electrolytes) in the compartments is a major determinant of fluid balance.

Movement across the cell membrane occurs because of osmotic pressure that is related to osmolality. Plasma osmolality is controlled at 285–295 mosm/kg by regulating water intake and excretion. Intravascular volume status is controlled by sodium. Glucose contributes minimally as it is rapidly metabolized in the intravascular compartment except in diabetics. In a crisis, *body prefers to maintain intravascular volume over maintenance of osmolality (refer* **Flowchart 12.1***)*.

ELECTROLYTES

Electrolytes exist as ions, namely positively charged cations (Na^+, K^+, Ca^{2+}, etc.) and negatively charged anions (Cl^-, HCO_3^-). The total number of cations in body is equal to anions. Electrolytes have a greater effect on osmosis (water movement between compartments) than nonelectrolytes because water moves to an area with a greater total number of particles in solution.

In extracellular fluid, the most abundant cation is Na^+. In the intracellular fluid, the most abundant cation is K^+. In extracellular fluid, the most abundant anion is Cl^-, while in intracellular fluid, the most abundant anions are proteins and phosphates (PO_4^{3-}).

Milliequivalent (mEq) is the unit for measurement of electrolytes, calculated as one-thousandth part of the equivalent weight. Equivalent weight of a substance is derived by dividing the atomic weight by valency. For example, equivalent weight of calcium is 20(40/2). Concentration of an electrolyte is expressed in mEq per liter (mEq/L) and can be calculated from mg/L.

Example 1: Calcium level in blood is 10 mg/dL. Converting this into mg/L, we get 100 mg/L. Divide this by equivalent weight of calcium, i.e., 20 and we get 5 mEq/L.

Example 2: The 7.5% solution of sodium bicarbonate contains 7.5 g/dL, i.e., 75,000 mg/L. Molecular weight of sodium bicarbonate ($NaHCO_3$) is 84 (23 + 1 + 12 + 48). The molality of 7.5% $NaHCO_3$ is thus 75,000 ÷ 84 = 892.8 mmol/L, containing 892.8 mEq/L of sodium and 892.8 mEq/L of bicarbonate. One milliliter of 7.5% $NaHCO_3$ thus contains 0.89 mEq of sodium and 0.89 mEq of bicarbonate. Osmolarity of 7.5% sodium bicarbonate is thus 892.8 + 892.8 = 1785 mOsm/L.

FLUID COMPOSITION

The distribution of body fluid is determined by the composition of electrolytes and proteins in different compartments. The composition of plasma and interstitial fluid and major cations and anions in different biological fluids are mentioned in **Tables 12.2 and 12.3**. Despite difference in composition, it is noteworthy that all fluid compartments have similar osmolarity (290 mOsm/L).

REGULATION OF WATER AND SODIUM BALANCE

The main source of body water is from ingested liquids and foods that have been absorbed by the gut. This water is called *preformed water*. The second source of body water is *metabolic water*, the water produced by the various chemical reactions of the body. It amounts to about 200 mL/day. For every 100 calories metabolized, the body loses about 65 mL water in urine, 40 mL by sweating, 15 mL by lungs, and about 5 mL in feces; whereas it gains 15 mL from production as a result of metabolic processes. Thus, 110 mL of water is utilized for every 100 calories metabolized.

The loss of water through sweating depends on the surface area, temperature, and environmental humidity; that from lungs on respiratory rate and humidity of inspired gases; and that in feces on the frequency and fluidity of stools.

Fluid intake is regulated by thirst. When water loss is greater than water gain, the resulting dehydration stimulates thirst. Dehydration causes decreased saliva production with dry mouth and throat. Tactile receptors in the mucosa relay nerve impulses to the thirst center of the hypothalamus, giving rise to a thirst sensation. Dehydration also increases osmotic pressure, stimulating osmoreceptors in the hypothalamus, which in turn stimulate the hypothalamic thirst center. Dehydration decreases blood volume and thus blood pressure, causing the kidneys to activate the *renin-angiotensin system*. Angiotensin II directly stimulates the hypothalamic thirst center. As a result of these mechanisms, the sensation of thirst and the conscious desire to drink are increased. Initially, wetting

Table 12.2 Ionic Composition of Different Fluids

Concentration (mEq/L)	*Plasma*	*Interstitial fluid*	*Intracellular fluid*
Sodium	135–145	144	6
Potassium	3.5–5.5	5	154
Calcium	4.25–5.25	5	—
Magnesium	1.5–2.0	5	40
Bicarbonate	20–26	27	13
Chloride	95–106	118	
Proteins (g/dL)	6–8	—	60
Phosphates	2.6–4.4	5	106
Sulfates	4	4	17

Table 12.3 Major Cations and Anions in Body Fluids

Concentration (mEq/L)	*Gastric juices*	*Ileal fluid*	*Cerebrospinal fluid*	*Diarrheal stool*	*Bile*	*Sweat*
Sodium	20–80	100–140	140	10–90	120–140	10–30
Potassium	5–20	5–15	3	10–80	5–15	3–10
Chloride	100–150	90–130	120	10–110	80–120	10–35

the mouth and throat quenches thirst but, the major inhibition of thirst results from stretch of the stomach and a decrease in the blood osmotic pressure.

Loss of Na^+ (excess sweating, vomiting, diarrhea, coupled with low Na^+ intake or plain water intake) causes the interstitial fluid osmotic pressure to decrease, leading to increased net filtration pressure, net loss of water from the plasma, decreased blood volume, decreased blood pressure, and finally circulatory shock.

Net osmosis into the cell leads to overhydration. As a result, water intoxication occurs, producing neurological symptoms ranging from disorientation to convulsions to coma to death.

Hormones

Aldosterone, antidiuretic hormone, atrial natriuretic peptide, and renin-angiotensin system play a major role in water regulation. Action of all these hormones is ultimately reflected by increased or decreased urine output (as the case may be).

- ***Antidiuretic hormone*** (ADH) synthesized in hypothalamus and secreted from posterior pituitary, increases the permeability of the distal tubules and collecting ducts of the kidney to water, causing increased reabsorption of water.
- ***Aldosterone*** secreted from adrenal cortex in response to production of renin and angiotensin by the kidneys, increases Na^+ reabsorption by the distal convoluted renal tubules, leading to increased obligatory reabsorption of water.
- ***Atrial natriuretic peptide*** produced by right atrial myocyte in response to stretching, cause decrease in Na^+ reabsorption, leading to decreased obligatory reabsorption and increased water loss in the urine (diuresis). Hence, the major site of regulation of water and sodium is the kidney.

The factors regulating water and sodium are depicted in **Flowchart 12.1**.

Flowchart 12.1: Regulation of water and sodium balance

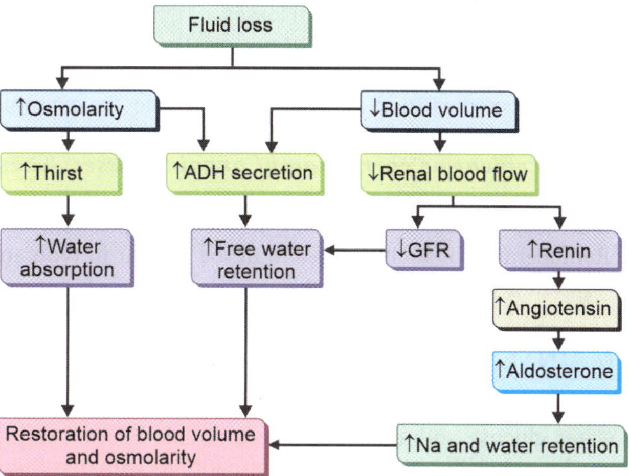

REGULATION OF POTASSIUM BALANCE

Potassium homeostasis is maintained both by renal and extrarenal mechanisms. High serum level of potassium stimulates secretion of aldosterone, which acts upon distal convoluted tubules to reabsorb sodium; and only potassium is excreted. Aldosterone also promotes loss of potassium in colon, sweat, and saliva. Hyperkalemia also stimulates Na^+–K^+ ATPase pump at distal convoluted tubule resulting in sodium absorption and potassium excretion in urine.

The three factors responsible for enhanced movement of potassium into cells are alkalosis, insulin secretion, and catecholamines. Alkalosis causes efflux of H^+ from cells in exchange for K^+. Insulin increases potassium uptake by cells by directly stimulating Na^+–K^+ ATPase activity independent of cyclic-AMP. β-agonists act by stimulating cyclic-AMP via adenylate cyclase enzyme, which in turn activate Na^+–K^+ ATPase pump. All this results in hypokalemia.

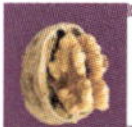

IN A NUTSHELL

Body Fluids and Electrolytes

1. Total body water consists of intracellular fluid (67%) and extracellular fluid (33%).
2. Extracellular fluid (ECF) consists of (i) interstitial fluid (80%); (ii) plasma (15–20%), and (iii) transcellular fluid (5%).
3. Major cations in the body are sodium and potassium. While sodium is mainly in extracellular fluid, most of potassium is intracellular.
4. Major anions include chloride (extracellular), and proteins, phosphates (intracellular).
5. Aldosterone, antidiuretic hormone (ADH), atrial natriuretic peptide (ANP), and renin-angiotensin system hormones are responsible for water regulation.

Kight BP, Waseem M. Pediatric Fluid Management. 2023 Feb 28. In: StatPearls [Internet]. Treasure Island (FL): StatPearls Publishing; 2025.

Young A, Brown LK, Ennis S, et al. Total body water in full-term and preterm newborns: systematic review and meta-analysis. Arch Dis Child Fetal Neonatal Ed. 2021;106(5):542-8.

12.2 Fluid and Electrolyte Requirements *PE 15.1*

FLUID THERAPY

Fluid therapy should follow the *ROSE* (*Resuscitation, Optimization, Stabilization, Evacuation*) concept, more so in critically sick children, so as to provide essential support to the organs and simultaneously avoid fluid overload. It is also important to be aware of four Ds: *drug, dosing, duration, and de-escalation.* Fluid and electrolyte therapy has three major components:

1. ***Provision of maintenance requirements:*** These are required for normal metabolism and include insensible water loss

and urinary losses. Insensible losses include losses through breathing and evaporative skin losses.

2. ***Resuscitation or correction of pre-existing deficits:*** These losses, via renal or extrarenal route, should be estimated and corrected as soon and safely as possible; for example, rehydration therapy for diarrheal dehydration.
3. ***Replacement or correction of ongoing losses:*** These losses mainly occur via the gastrointestinal tract, as in diarrhea, vomiting, etc., or removal (suction, aspiration, etc.). Replacement of such losses should be similar in type and amount to the fluid being lost.

MAINTENANCE FLUID THERAPY

The maintenance fluids are generally composed of a solution of water, glucose, sodium, and potassium. This solution should have a long shelf life, low cost, and compatibility with peripheral intravenous (IV) administration. The goal of maintenance fluid therapy is to deliver basic electrolytes and glucose for metabolic needs and prevent dehydration, electrolyte disorders, ketoacidosis, and protein degradation. Maintenance fluid usually does not provide adequate calories, protein, fat, minerals or vitamins; and children on maintenance fluid lose 0.5–1% of weight each day. Thus, maintenance fluids cannot be substituted for nutrition over long periods of time.

Amount of Maintenance Fluid

Under normal condition, a 10 kg child requires water: 100 mL or 100 kcal/kg/day; sodium 1–3 mEq/100 kcal/day; and potassium 1–2 mEq/100 kcal/day. Holiday and Segar showed that the basal caloric requirements for children are as follows:

Body weight 0–10 kg	:	100 kcal/kg/day
Between 11 and 20 kg	:	1,000 kcal + 50 kcal/kg/day for each kilogram
>20 kg	:	1,500 kcal + 20 kcal/kg/day for each kilogram

For children with normal renal function and under basal metabolic conditions, provision of 50 mL for every 100 kcal consumed per day will replace the normal insensible water losses (IWL), and 66.7 mL/100 kcal consumed per day will replace the average urinary losses. This adds up to 116.7 mL/100 kcal consumed per day as maintenance fluids, if we ignore the minimal losses through stool. But 16.7 mL of water is produced as water of oxidation for every 100 kcal metabolized by the body. So the net requirement comes to 100 mL/100 kcal losses. Using the weight-based calculations for caloric requirements as described above, the total maintenance fluid requirements can thus be calculated as shown in **Table 12.4**.

Composition of Maintenance Fluid

The composition of the maintenance fluid should be such that its osmolality is close to the normal plasma osmolality of 285–295 mOsm/kg. The body also needs 3 mEq/kg of sodium, 2 mEq/kg of potassium and 2 mEq/kg of chloride per day for maintenance of normal homeostasis.

There is increasing evidence that balanced solutions such as PlasmaLyte/PlasmaLyte with 5% dextrose are better for maintenance therapy **(Table 12.5)**. Conventionally or in case of nonavailability, 0.9% saline (NS) and 20 mEq/L of potassium chloride is used, provided the child is passing adequate urine. Hypotonic fluids (such as 0.2% or 1/5 normal saline) should not be used as maintenance fluids because of the risk of hyponatremia.

Neonatal Fluid Requirements

Neonates have a shift of fluid from intracellular to extracellular fluid compartment after birth, which leads to postnatal diuresis and physiologic weight loss in the first week of life (up to 10% of body weight in term neonates and up to 15% in preterm neonates). In addition, neonatal kidneys have limited capacity for solute and water load handling, which leads to the salt and water diuresis in the first 48–72 hours.

Therefore, the fluids for neonates for the first 48 hours are without any electrolytes (10% dextrose only for the initial 48 hours). Total fluids administered are increased on a daily basis by 10–15 mL/kg/day increments, up to a maximum of 150 mL/kg/day by the end of 1 week of life **(Table 12.6)**. Sodium and potassium are added in IV fluids from day 3 of life.

For babies with prematurity, intrauterine growth retardation, and for those who are born to diabetic mothers, it may be necessary to add calcium gluconate (10% solution: 8 mL/kg/day) to initial IV fluids since they are at risk for developing hypocalcemia.

DEFICIT THERAPY

This is best assessed by measuring acute weight loss. Weight loss occurring over a matter of hours or a few days is assumed to be due to fluid deficit, because any significant weight change attributable to nutrition would occur over several days to weeks. The deficit volume should be replenished over 4–6 hours.

Table 12.4 Estimation of Maintenance Fluid Requirements

Body weight	*Fluid*	*Infusion rate*
Up to 10 kg	100 mL/kg/day	4 mL/kg/h
10.1–20 kg	1,000 + 50 mL/kg/day × (wt–10)	40 mL/h + 2 mL/kg/h × (wt–10)
20.1–30 kg	1,000 + 500 + 20 mL/kg/day × (wt–20)	60 mL/h + 1 mL/kg/h × (wt–20)
Maximum	2,400 mL per day	100 mL/h

For obese children, calculate the fluid requirements according to the ideal body weight (wt) and not the actual weight

Table 12.5 Composition of Various IV Fluids

Fluid type	Sodium (mEq/L)	Potassium (mEq/L)	Chloride (mEq/L)	Dextrose (g/L)	Others	Osmolality
Normal saline	154	—	154	—	—	
5% dextrose normal saline	154	—	154	50	—	560
Isolyte P	25	20	22	50	Acetate: 23 Phosphate: 3 Magnesium: 3	
Ringer lactate	130	4	109	—	Lactate: 28 Calcium: 3	278
Half normal saline	77	—	77	—	—	
Hypertonic 3% saline	512	—	512	—	—	
PlasmaLyte	140	5	98	—	Magnesium: 3 Calcium: 3 Acetate: 27 Gluconate: 23	294

Table 12.6 Daily Fluid Requirements in the First Week of Life (mL/kg)

Age (days)	<1,000 g	1,000–1,500 g	>1,500 g
1	80	80	60
2	100	95	75
3	120	110	90
4	130	120	105
5	140	130	120
6	150	140	135
7	160	150	150

If the baseline weight is not known, one has to take recourse to clinical assessment as No, Some, or Severe dehydration. *When body fluids are lost, approximately 60% of that loss originates in the ECF and 40% in the ICF compartments.* The more acute the dehydration, the greater is the proportion of ECF loss; and the more chronic the dehydration, the greater is the proportion of ICF loss. The loss of 1 L of ECF means approximately 140 mEq of sodium and 100 mEq of chloride have got lost. Similarly, the loss of 1 L of ICF implies a concomitant loss of approximately 150 mEq of potassium.

If the child can accept oral fluids, replenishment with standard World Health Organization (WHO) oral rehydration solutions (ORS) over 3–6 hours is the treatment of choice. This is described at length elsewhere. However, if enteral intake is not possible, one would have to administer IV fluids. For a 10% fluid deficit in a 10 kg child, one would need a normal saline preparation. A total of 1,250 mL over 6 hours (1,000 mL deficit + 250 mL maintenance for 6 hours) would take care of deficit and maintenance needs. 2 mL potassium chloride is added per 100 mL fluid if child is passing urine.

REPLACEMENT FLUID THERAPY

Gastrointestinal tract is a potential site of water and electrolyte loss, leading to hypokalemia and dehydration. It is often accompanied with bicarbonate loss in acute diarrhea and may cause metabolic acidosis, which may be accentuated, if volume depletion causes hypoperfusion and a concurrent lactic acidosis. Frequent emesis or massive losses from nasogastric tube in intestinal obstruction may lead to metabolic alkalosis.

The losses are to be replaced every 1–6 hours depending on rate of loss, with very rapid losses being replaced more frequently. Composition of replacement IV fluids is given in **Table 12.5**. Choice and amount of fluid are mentioned below:

- ***Ongoing losses in stool:*** A total of 5% dextrose in 1/4 normal saline + 15 mEq HCO_3^-/L + 25 mEq/L potassium.
- ***Emesis and nasogastric losses:*** Normal saline + 10 mEq/L potassium.
- ***Oliguria or anuria:*** Insensible fluids (400 mL/m^2/24 hours) + replace urine output mL for mL with half-normal saline.
- ***Polyuria (postobstructive diuresis, polyuric phase of renal failure, diabetes mellitus, and diabetes insipidus):*** Insensible fluids: half normal saline (400 mL/m^2/24 hours) + replace urine output mL/mL with a solution based on urinary electrolytes.
- ***Third space losses and chest tube output:*** Isotonic fluid, normal saline, or Ringer lactate mL for mL, every 1–6 hours.
- Surgical drains and chest tubes can produce measurable fluid output and should be replaced when they are significant. Third space losses are due to shift of fluid from intravascular space into interstitial space. The losses cannot be quantified. It can be massive and lead to intravascular volume depletion despite weight gain of children. Thus, replacement of third space is empirical but should be anticipated. Protein losses from chest tubes drainage can be significant and occasionally require 5% albumin as replacement fluid.

Recently, the importance of fluids given as drug diluents and to guarantee catheter patency, i.e., *fluid creep* has been highlighted. These may contribute to a significant volume load, which was not recognized previously.

Fluid Resuscitation in Shock

In most children with *hypotensive* shock, a fluid bolus of 10–20 mL/kg of isotonic crystalloid such as 0.9% saline or Ringer

Flowchart 12.2: Fluid resuscitation in hypotensive shock

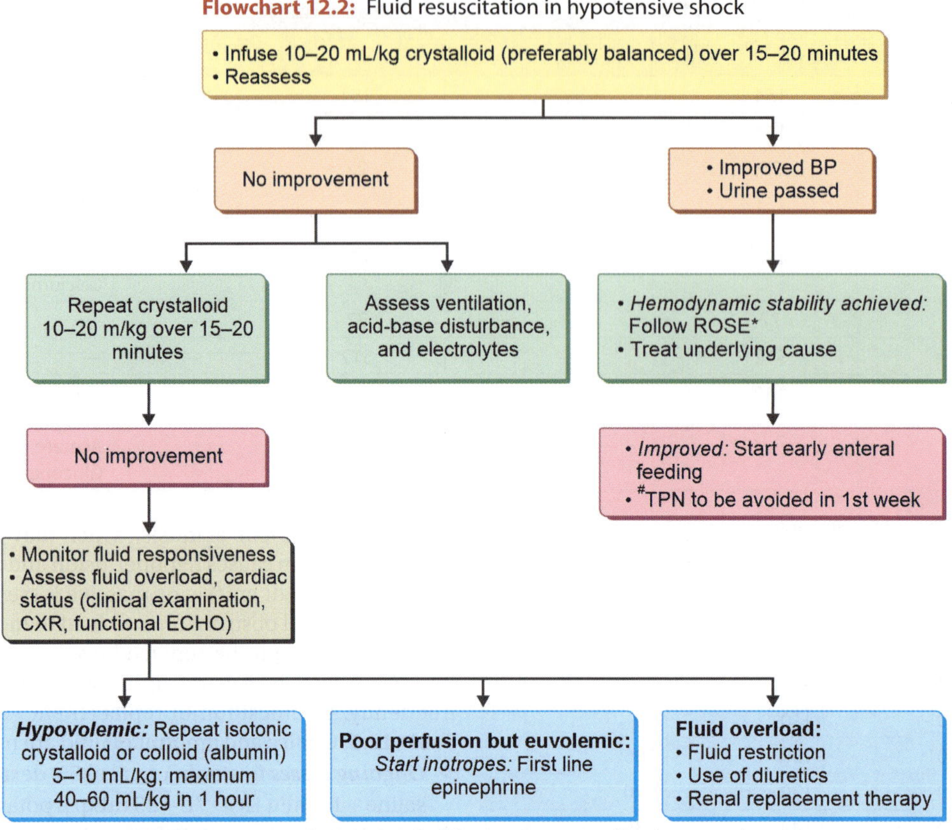

***ROSE:** Resuscitation, Optimization, Stabilization, Evacuation; #Total parenteral nutrition

lactate should be given over 15–20 minutes. Children suffering from septic shock receiving fluid boluses over 5–10 minutes had higher risk of intubation than those receiving over 15–20 minutes, though no difference in mortality was noted. Thus post the Fluid Expansion As Supportive Therapy (FEAST) Trial, it is widely thought that rapid fluid resuscitation may not be the best strategy especially in resource-limited settings. The child is reassessed to determine, if more fluid is required or other form of therapy, i.e., antibiotics, vasopressors should be initiated. Children with hypovolemic shock may require and tolerate fluid boluses of 40–60 mL/kg within first 1 hour of presentation. However, the risk of fluid overload must be monitored. In case of *perfusion abnormality without hypotension*, no fluid bolus is required and maintenance fluids alone suffice. Algorithm of fluid resuscitation is provided in **Flowchart 12.2**.

SPECIAL SITUATIONS

Acute Renal Failure

These children do not pass adequate urine. Thus, the maintenance fluid will consist of only the insensible losses and the volume of fluid lost as urine. Insensible losses (300–400 mL/m^2 of body surface area per day) are replaced volume for volume every 6 hours by 10% dextrose; while urine output is replaced by half NS (N/2 saline).

Correct the hyperkalemia (by administering calcium gluconate, insulin-glucose drip, sodium bicarbonate, or nebulized salbutamol), hyponatremia (fluid restriction, 3% NaCl), hyperphosphatemia (phosphate binders, dietary phosphate restriction) and hypocalcemia (reduce phosphate).

Child presenting with oliguria (urinary output <0.5 mL/kg/h) is initially resuscitated with a fluid challenge of 20 mL/kg of normal saline over 30 minutes. If the child does not pass urine, then think of intrinsic renal or postrenal failure and give a single shot of furosemide 2–4 mg/kg. If there is no response despite both these measures and with rising blood urea levels, restrict the IV fluids and shift to acute renal failure regimen.

> *Example:* **Fluids in acute renal failure**
> Total amount of fluids
> = Amount of insensible fluid losses (300–400 mL/m^2/day) + Urine output + Extrarenal losses
> *Insensible losses are replaced with 10% dextrose and renal losses with N/2 normal saline.*

Congestive Heart Failure

Restrict the maintenance fluid to two-thirds of the normal maintenance with an isotonic crystalloid fluid, such as normal saline or 5% dextrose normal saline (DNS). Maintenance potassium may be added, if needed.

Chemotherapy

Newly diagnosed patients with lymphoreticular malignancies who are being started on induction chemotherapy regimen for the treatment of their malignancy are at risk for tumor lysis syndrome. This results from rapid cell death induced by chemotherapeutic agents. This puts the patients at risk for various metabolic complications, including hyperkalemia, hyperphosphatemia, hyperuricemia, and hypocalcemia.

The fluid of choice in tumor lysis syndrome is crystalloid fluids without potassium. These children are given extra fluids to prevent acute kidney injury, usually 2.5 times the maintenance with a target urine output of 4 mL/kg/h in infants and 100 mL/m^2/h in older children. In addition allopurinol and rasburicase may be required.

Meningitis

Isotonic crystalloid fluids should be used as maintenance fluids in these children. Restriction of fluid because of risk for syndrome of inappropriate antidiuretic hormone (SIADH) secretion is now debatable and not routinely followed. Studies have shown that most of the cases have high ADH because of underlying hypovolemia. Hence, it is important to first ensure that there is euvolemic state. If serum sodium persists to be low even after the underlying volume status is adequate, one should consider fluid restriction. One should avoid overhydration as well.

Syndrome of Inappropriate Antidiuretic Hormone

Fluid restriction to 1,000 mL/m^2/day (500 mL/m^2/day urinary losses + 500 mL/m^2/day nonurinary losses). Details are given under hyponatremia section.

Raised Intracranial Tension

Hypotonic maintenance IV solutions should be avoided in favor of isotonic solutions as they can worsen the cerebral edema. 3% saline and mannitol are also used as antiedema measures.

IN A NUTSHELL

Fluid and Electrolyte Requirements

1. Normally, a child requires 100 mL/kg/day of fluids (0–10 kg body weight). Additional 50 mL/kg/day is required for weight (11–20 kg) and another 20 mL/kg/day for weight >20 kg.
2. Normal plasma osmolality is 285–295 mOsm/kg. Maintenance fluid needs to be iso-osmolar. Balanced isotonic solutions are the first choice.
3. *Deficit therapy in dehydration:* Crystalloids are the preferred solution for intravenous rehydration in diarrheal dehydration.
4. Fluid bolus of 10–20 mL/kg is given over 15–20 minutes in hypovolemic shock. This requirement may go up to 40–60 mL/kg over 1 hour.

Braun CG, Askenazi DJ, Neyra JA, et al. Fluid deresuscitation in critically ill children: comparing perspectives of intensivists and nephrologists. Front Pediatr. 2024;12:1484893.

Malbrain MLNG, Langer T, Annane D, et al. Intravenous fluid therapy in the perioperative and critical care setting: executive summary of the International Fluid Academy (IFA). Ann Intensive Care. 2020;10(1):64.

Weiss SL, Peters MJ, Alhazzani W, et al. Surviving Sepsis Campaign International Guidelines for the management of septic shock and sepsis-associated organ dysfunction in children. Pediatr Crit Care Med. 2020;21(2):e52-e106.

12.3 Hyponatremia

PE 15.2

DEFINITION

Hyponatremia is defined as serum sodium concentration less than 135 mEq/L. It is the most common electrolyte abnormality encountered in pediatric practice with an incidence of 1.5% of all pediatric hospital admissions. Symptoms appear when the serum sodium concentration is less than 125 mEq/L.

ETIOLOGY

Hyponatremia can be produced by three different mechanisms: (i) deficiency in sodium intake, (ii) excessive loss of sodium (renal or extrarenal), and (iii) excessive water retention.

Because the human body protects itself from hyponatremia through an intact thirst mechanism, conditions associated with alteration in thirst mechanism are more prone to hyponatremia. Hyponatremia is also caused by a deficient intake, like in infants fed with hypotonic fluids.

The most common cause of hyponatremia in children is diarrhea. Sodium loss also occurs via the kidneys. Diuretics are the most common culprit followed by salt-losing nephritis, mineralocorticoid deficiency, and cerebral salt-wasting syndrome. Causes are listed below:

- ***Hypervolemic hyponatremia:*** Congestive heart failure, cirrhosis, nephritic syndrome, acute or chronic renal failure.
- ***Hypovolemic hyponatremia*** due to renal loss. Diuretic excess, osmotic diuresis, salt wasting, adrenal insufficiency, proximal renal tubular acidosis, metabolic alkalosis, pseudohypoaldosteronism.
- ***Hypovolemic hyponatremia*** due to extrarenal loss. Vomiting, diarrhea, fistula, excessive sweating, acute pancreatitis, burns, trauma, peritonitis, effusions, ascites.
- ***Normovolemic hyponatremia:*** SIADH, acute leukemia, lymphoma, asthma, empyema, pneumonia, ligation of PDA, cystic fibrosis, meningitis, encephalitis, hypoxic-ischemic encephalopathy (HIE), ventriculoperitoneal shunt, head trauma.

- ***Drugs:*** Chlorpropamide, vincristine, vinblastine, diuretics, clofibrate, carbamazepine, fluphenazine, amitriptyline, morphine, isoproterenol, nicotine, adenine arabinoside, colchicine, barbiturates.
- ***Endocrinal:*** Addison disease, hypothyroidism, congenital adrenal hyperplasia, IV fluid therapy.

Syndrome of Inappropriate Antidiuretic Hormone Secretion (SIADH)

Excessive antidiuretic hormone (ADH) secretion causes water retention and subsequent dilutional hyponatremia despite decreased serum osmolality. It is seen secondary to CNS pathology like infection, trauma, bleed, tumor, etc. Some drugs, e.g., 3,4-methylene dioxymethyl amphetamine or ecstasy; antiepileptics like carbamazepine, valproate, etc., also can cause SIADH. Arterial blood volume may be increased, or normal depending on the underlying clinical condition.

PATHOPHYSIOLOGY

When serum sodium declines, the serum osmolality also decreases. This results in an osmotic gradient across the blood-brain barrier causing water to move into intracellular compartment which has greater osmolality than the ECF. When brain cells swell, enclosed by a rigid skull, the resultant cerebral edema manifests as headache, nausea, vomiting, irritability, and seizures. The brain's adaptation to hyponatremia is accomplished by loss of interstitial fluid into the cerebrospinal fluid, and loss of cellular mainly K^+, Cl^- ions and organic solutes into ECF.

When water moves into the brain, increasing hydrostatic pressure shifts interstitial fluid into cerebrospinal fluid, which subsequently is absorbed through the arachnoid villi. The interstitial fluid is rich in sodium. The brain equilibrates the osmolar gradient by removing this fluid. In addition, intracellular potassium acts similarly with a maximal response occurring in 24 hours. If hyponatremia lasts longer, intracellular amino acids extrude to maintain the osmolar gradient. This shifting of solutes and organic osmolytes plays an important role in protecting the brain from cerebral edema. The resultant hypo-osmolar state makes the brain vulnerable to dehydration secondary to rapid correction of hyponatremia. The optimum speed of correction is not known. However, it should not be more than 0.5 mEq/L/hour. Rapid correction in fully compensated chronic hyponatremia results in a demyelinating lesion in the pons known as central pontine myelinolysis (CPM).

CLINICAL FEATURES

Clinical manifestations are due to decreased serum osmolality and vary from asymptomatic to severe neurologic dysfunctions. The most serious complication is hyponatremic encephalopathy, which if not treated can lead to irreversible brain damage. Neurological symptoms are predominant in hyponatremia, although cardiovascular and musculoskeletal symptoms (including weakness and muscular cramps) are also present. Factors contributing to central nervous system (CNS) symptoms include (*i*) rate of change in serum sodium, (*ii*) level of serum sodium, and (*iii*) duration of the elevated serum sodium level.

Early signs of CNS involvement include anorexia, headache, nausea, and emesis. Advanced signs include impaired response to verbal and painful stimuli, bizarre behavior, hallucinations, obtundation, incontinence, and respiratory insufficiency.

In late stage, children may have decorticate or decerebrate posturing, bradycardia, hypertension or hypotension, altered temperature regulation, dilated pupils, seizure, respiratory arrest, and coma. Renal failure may occur.

LABORATORY WORKUP

Serum sodium, osmolality, urea, creatinine, and urine osmolality should be measured. Urine sodium changes according to the type of hyponatremia.

- First step is to check if hyponatremia is associated with hypo-osmolality (true hyponatremia). If yes, the next step is to determine the volume status and to measure the urine osmolality.
- High urine osmolality suggests hypovolemic hyponatremia. Hyponatremia can also be due to renal insufficiency, adrenal insufficiency, cortisol deficiency, diuretics use, and hypothyroidism.
- Urine sodium is very valuable in differentiating between renal and nonrenal etiology. There is renal retention of sodium in nonrenal causes and urine sodium is characteristically <10 mEq/L (cf. renal causes where urine Na^+ is >20 mEq/L).
- Once the above are ruled out, consider SIADH as it is a diagnosis of exclusion. SIADH is characterized by maintained to normal—high circulatory volume, impaired free water excretion, normal sodium excretion, and hyponatremia, which is refractory to sodium administration in the absence of fluid restriction. Suggestive biochemical parameters are:
  - Urine sodium >30 mEq/L
  - Fractional excretion of sodium (FENa) >0.5%
  - Fractional excretion of urate >11%
- Other laboratory studies include serum aldosterone, cortisol, thyroid function tests, adrenocorticotropic hormone, and ADH.
- Imaging studies, such as radiograph of skull and computed tomography (CT) scan, should be done to delineate intracranial pathology. Ultrasound may reveal an abdominal mass in individuals with bilateral adrenal hyperplasia and adrenal tumor.

CENTRAL PONTINE MYELINOLYSIS

Clinical features include slowly progressive flaccid paralysis, cranial nerve abnormalities (dysphagia or pseudobulbar palsy), alteration of mental status (behavioral changes, depression of sensorium, lethargy), seizures, and coma. The condition is usually fatal in 3–5 weeks. Magnetic resonance imaging (MRI) permits visualization of the brainstem and is sensitive to alterations in white matter. Lesions become apparent 1–2 weeks later.

TREATMENT Hyponatremia

Syndrome of inappropriate antidiuretic hormone usually abates with treatment of underlying etiology. Fluid needs to be restricted to 600 mL/m^2/day. Normal saline alone, may not help to correct hyponatremia. Rather, can aggravate hyponatremia if the urine osmolality is greater than 500 mOsm/kg. Loop diuretics increase urine electrolyte free water clearance and impair urinary concentration, thus helping to correct hyponatremia. Children who do not respond to fluid restriction and have asymptomatic hyponatremia, we increase the oral sodium intake or give oral urea (15–30 g once daily) in order to increase the renal solute load, thereby causing an osmotic diuresis. In children with chronic hyponatremia, correction of sodium should be slow to prevent potential demyelinating lesions. Optimal rate of correction is 0.5 mEq/h, not to exceed serum sodium of 125 mEq/L.

The amount of sodium required to raise serum sodium by a given amount can be calculated by the following formula:

Sodium required (mEq) = Weight in kg × 0.6 ×(125 – observed sodium)

Vaptans (tolvaptan, conivaptan), a nonpeptide vasopressin V2 receptor antagonist, are a new group of drugs used for treatment of hypervolemic hyponatremia, e.g., congestive heart failure and chronic liver failure. In first 2 hours of dosing, vaptans selectively counter the antidiuretic effect of AVP and cause urinary free water diuresis (aquaresis) without loss of electrolyte. They increase sodium levels up to 5–7 mEq/L within 24 hours of administration. Vaptans are associated with serious side effects and hence must be used judiciously as a short-term second line therapy in refractory cases.

Symptomatic Hyponatremia

Hyponatremic encephalopathy is a medical emergency. In symptomatic children, serum sodium should be rapidly raised by IV administration of 3% sodium chloride (3% NaCl, 513 mEq/L) in dose of 2 mL/kg over 10–15 minutes. Bolus may be repeated, maximum 150 mL until symptoms resolve. Aim is an increase in serum sodium 5–6 mEq/L in first 1–2 hours. Serum sodium needs to be monitored every 2 hours.

Seizures resulting from acute water intoxication are not responsive to antiepileptic drugs; however, such seizures respond very well to 3% NaCl.

Each milliliter of 3% NaCl contains approximately 0.5 mEq Na/L. Administering 1 mL/kg of 3% sodium chloride raises the serum sodium by 1.6 mEq. The current evidence suggests that it is safe to raise plasma sodium concentration in chronic hyponatremia by 10–12 mEq/L in first 24 hours and 15–20 mEq/L over the first 48 hours.

IN A NUTSHELL

Hyponatremia

1. Hyponatremia (serum sodium <125 mEq/L) can cause seizures and cerebral edema. It can occur in adrenal insufficiency, syndrome of inappropriate antidiuretic hormone (SIADH), and diarrhea.
2. Symptomatic hyponatremia needs to be treated with 3% NaCl : 2 mL/kg bolus over 10 minutes. Maximum 150 mL.
3. Bolus may be repeated till symptoms improve. Or rise in serum sodium by 5 mEq/L.
4. Monitor serum sodium levels every 2 hours.
5. Hyponatremic encephalopathy is unlikely if no improvement seen after an acute increase in serum sodium of 5–6 mEq/L.
6. Correction in first 48 hours:
   - Not to exceed 15–20 mEq/L.
   - Avoid normonatremia or hypernatremia.

Moritz ML. Syndrome of inappropriate antidiuresis. Pediatr Clin North Am. 2019;66(1):209-26.

Stephanos K, Dubbs SB. Pediatric hematologic and oncologic emergencies. Emerg Med Clin North Am. 2021;39(3):555-71.

12.4 Hypernatremia

PE 15.2

DEFINITION

Hypernatremia is defined as serum sodium concentration of >145 mEq/L. It is characterized by seizures, doughy skin, dehydration; and carries high morbidity and mortality, especially during treatment.

ETIOLOGY

Hypernatremia usually occurs because of pure water depletion (diabetes insipidus), sodium excess (ORS administration), or water depletion exceeding sodium depletion (diarrhea). Important causes are listed here:

- ***Hypovolemic hypernatremia:*** Diarrhea, excessive perspiration, renal dysplasia, obstructive uropathy, osmotic diuresis.
- ***Normovolemic hypernatremia:*** Diabetes insipidus (central and nephrogenic).
- ***Hypervolemic hypernatremia:*** Sodium bicarbonate/NaCl administration, primary hyperaldosteronism, improper infant formula mixing.
- ***Drugs:*** Amphotericin, intravenous immune globulin (IVIG), radiocontrast, mannitol, alcohol intoxication.

PATHOPHYSIOLOGY

As a result of increased extracellular sodium, plasma osmolarity increases, which results in shift of fluid from within the cells, resulting in cell desiccation. Extracellular volume remains normal, but at the expense of intracellular dehydration, which is responsible for the clinical manifestations of hypernatremia.

Hence, urine output and blood pressure may remain preserved in initial stages of hypernatremic dehydration.

The central nervous system has special adaptive capabilities during these episodes with water efflux from neurons during acute phases and increased intracellular concentration of electrolytes. Central nervous system problems occur, if the cellular shrinkage goes beyond a certain limit, causing thrombosis of small arteries and veins. It can also lead to rupture of blood vessels and intracranial bleed.

Chronic hypernatremia (>48 hours)—organic osmolytes start appearing inside the neurons. Some of them move inside the cells, while others are synthesized within the cell. These osmolytes were initially called idiogenic molecules and the primary function is to prevent cellular dehydration. Though the presence of organic osmolytes is protective, it causes significant problems during rehydration. Rapid rehydration results in cerebral edema by relative hypotonic fluids entering the cerebral neurons.

CLINICAL MANIFESTATIONS

Children usually present with irritability, fever, high-pitched cry, lethargy, altered sensorium, seizures, oligoanuria, and increased muscle tone. Skin turgor is reduced and a doughy characteristic feel of the skin is present, when the severity of dehydration results in loss of 10% of body weight. Seizures can occur because of hypernatremia *per se,* however, it is more commonly seen during treatment of hypernatremia because of rapid decline in serum sodium.

LABORATORY EVALUATION

Serum sodium, serum osmolarity, urea, creatinine, and urinary sodium should be estimated in all cases of suspected hypernatremia:

- In euvolemic hypernatremia, urine sodium is variable.
- In hypervolemic hypernatremia, urine sodium is >20 mEq/L and urine osmolarity <800 mOsm/kg.
- In diabetes insipidus, urine osmolarity is usually <300 mOsm/kg (dilute), which increases following desmopressin administration.

Computed tomography and MRI scan of the brain should be done to exclude intracranial tumors, granulomatous diseases (sarcoid, tuberculosis), histiocytosis, and other intracranial pathology. Ultrasound of the kidney is to be done to rule out renal diseases.

Other tests include serum aldosterone, cortisol, ADH, and adrenocorticotropic hormone (ACTH) to exclude associated endocrinal disorders.

TREATMENT Hypernatremia

The management of hypernatremia includes correction of underlying causes and the prevailing hypertonicity.

- ***Correcting hypernatremia:*** While correcting hypernatremia, do not reduce sodium level rapidly. The goal of correction is to decrease plasma sodium by approximately 0.5 mEq/L/h (10–12 mEq/L/24 hours). Rapid reduction of sodium level may cause cerebral edema.
  - The recommended duration of correction is based on serum sodium level (145–157 mEq/L over 24 hours, 158–170 mEq/L over 48 hours, and >170 mEq/L over 72 hours). The rate of correction remains same at 0.5 mEq/L/h.
  - The type of fluid used for correction is 5% half normal saline (N/2) and the amount of fluid is 1.5 times of maintenance requirement. This is best achieved by giving deficit correction and maintenance fluids over 48–72 hours.
  - Once the child starts passing urine, potassium may be added to fluid in a dose of 20 mEq/L to facilitate water absorption into cells.
  - If the serum sodium concentration is >180 mEq/L, peritoneal dialysis should be done using a high glucose and low sodium dialysate.
- ***Replacement fluid:*** The volume of replacement fluid needed to correct the water deficit is determined by the concentration of sodium in the replacement fluid. The replacement volume can be determined as follows:

  Replacement volume = body weight × 0.6 (1–145)/current sodium

  If the child is hypotensive, correct hypotension with crystalloid. Normal saline is preferred over Ringer lactate solution as sodium concentration of the latter may cause a sudden drop of serum sodium. Hyperglycemia may accompany hypernatremia. Insulin treatment is not recommended because sudden drop in hyperglycemia can cause cerebral edema by decreasing plasma osmolality.
- ***Other modalities:***
  - Peritoneal dialysis is indicated for renal failure, obstructive uropathy, or serum sodium level >180 mEq/L.
  - Surgical intervention is recommended for children with renal dysplasia, medullary cystic disease, reflux nephropathy, and polycystic disease.

PROGNOSIS

Mental retardation, intracranial hemorrhage, intracerebral calcification, cerebral infarction, cerebral edema, hypocalcemia, and hyperglycemia may occur in children with hypernatremia. Children, who have recovered from hypernatremia and have recurrent history, will develop neurologic sequelae. The incidence of persistent neurologic abnormality is 11–15% consisting of intellectual deficits, seizure disorders, and spastic plegias. The overall mortality is about 10%.

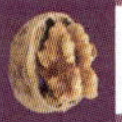

IN A NUTSHELL

Hypernatremia

1. Hypernatremia (serum sodium >145 mEq/L) can occur in diarrhea, diabetes insipidus, and inappropriate oral rehydration solutions (ORS) administration.
2. Hypernatremia presents with lethargy, seizures, coma as blood hypertonicity affects brain cells mainly. In the initial stages, symptoms of dehydration, oliguria, and hypotension may be absent.
3. Hypernatremic dehydration needs correction slowly. Aim is to decrease 0.5 mEq/L/h (10–12 mEq/L/24 hours).
4. Consider renal replacement therapy if serum sodium >180 mEq/L.
5. Consider therapy with desmopressin in central diabetes insipidus (DI) and with thiazides for nephrogenic DI.

Bulfon AF, Alomani HL, Anton N, et al. Intravenous fluid prescription practices in critically ill children: a shift in focus from natremia to chloremia? J Pediatr Intensive Care. 2019;8(4):218-25.
Büyükkaragöz B, Bakkaloğlu SA. Serum osmolality and hyperosmolar states. Pediatr Nephrol. 2023;38(4):1013-25.

12.5 Hypokalemia

PE 15.2

DEFINITION

Hypokalemia is defined as a plasma potassium level <3.5 mEq/L. Clinically, it is characterized by hypotonia, muscle weakness, and cardiac arrhythmia. Most common causes are diarrhea and severe malnutrition. Prognosis is good, if treated on time.

PATHOPHYSIOLOGY

Potassium is essential for transmission of nerve impulses, contraction of cardiac muscle, maintenance of intracellular tonicity, skeletal and smooth muscles, and maintenance of normal renal function. Derangements of potassium regulation often lead to neuromuscular, gastrointestinal, and cardiac conduction abnormalities.

Acute depletion may result from diuretic therapy, primary or secondary hyperaldosteronism, diabetic ketoacidosis, severe diarrhea, vomiting, or inadequate replacement during prolonged parenteral nutrition.

Gradual potassium depletion occurs via renal excretion, through gastrointestinal (GI) loss or because of low intake.

ETIOLOGY

- ***Gastrointestinal and skin losses:*** Vomiting, acute diarrhea, villous adenoma, excessive sweating, severe burns, nasogastric aspiration, laxative use.
- ***Decreased stores:*** Protein-energy malnutrition.
- ***Shift from extracellular to intracellular compartment:*** Insulin, catecholamines therapy, alkalosis, periodic paralysis, refeeding syndrome.
- ***Renal:*** Renal tubular acidosis (RTA), Bartter syndrome, Gitelman syndrome, dialysis, diuretic therapy.
- ***Endocrinal:*** Diabetic ketoacidosis, hyperaldosteronism, Cushing syndrome, steroid therapy.
- ***Drugs:*** Theophylline, verapamil, high-dose penicillin, ampicillin, carbenicillin, aminoglycosides, amphotericin B and cisplatin.
- ***Miscellaneous:*** Hypothermia, cystic fibrosis, hypomagnesemia, acute myelogenous monomyeloblastic or lymphoblastic leukemia.

CLINICAL FEATURES

Muscle weakness is characteristic and initially observed in limbs, followed by trunk and respiratory muscles. In infants, paralytic ileus and gastric dilatation are common. Life-threatening complications include acute respiratory failure from muscle paralysis and cardiac arrhythmias. Occasionally, tachycardia with irregular beats may be heard. Severe hypokalemia may manifest as bradycardia with cardiovascular collapse.

INVESTIGATIONS

The serum level reflects the severity of deficiency.

- Serum potassium <2.5 mEq/L indicates a massive loss of intracellular potassium.
- Urinary potassium <15 mEq/L indicates that extrarenal losses are unlikely.
- Children should also be evaluated for concurrent electrolyte abnormalities and arterial blood gases, which may affect treatment.
- Electrocardiogram (ECG) shows ST segment depression, T wave flattening, prolongation of QT interval, and appearance of U waves **(Fig. 12.1)**. Hyponatremia and alkalosis aggravate ECG abnormalities.
- Although ECG changes may be helpful, if present, their absence should not be taken as normal cardiac conduction. The ECG may be normal or may have only subtle findings prior to clinically significant dysrhythmias.
- Children should also be evaluated for Cushing syndrome, Conn syndrome, or adrenal hyperplasia, if clinical manifestations suggest the diagnosis.
- MRI of brain is indicated in children with suspected pituitary tumor as a cause of hypercortisolism.
- Abdominal ultrasound or CT should be done, if adrenal tumor or hyperplasia is suspected.

TREATMENT Hypokalemia

Medical therapy is aimed at potassium supplementation and correction of underlying causes.

Transient, asymptomatic, or *mild hypokalemia* may resolve spontaneously or may be treated with enteral potassium supplements. Oral dose of potassium is 2–4 mEq/kg/day PO in divided doses to avoid gastric distress.

Symptomatic or *severe hypokalemia* should be corrected with intravenous potassium chloride (1 mL of 10% KCl contains 2 mEq of potassium). The usual dose of IV replacement is 0.5–1 mEq/kg (total dose not to exceed 40 mEq) as infusion over 1 hour. It should be accompanied by continuous ECG monitoring to detect fatal ventricular arrhythmia. If a child is receiving concurrent intravenous fluids, potassium can be infused 40 mEq/L of maintenance fluid.

PROGNOSIS

Mortality is rare except when hypokalemia is severe or occurs in a child with underlying heart disease requiring digoxin therapy, following cardiac surgery or when accompanied by arrhythmia. Short-term morbidity is common including ileus, cardiac dysrhythmia, and muscle weakness or cramping.

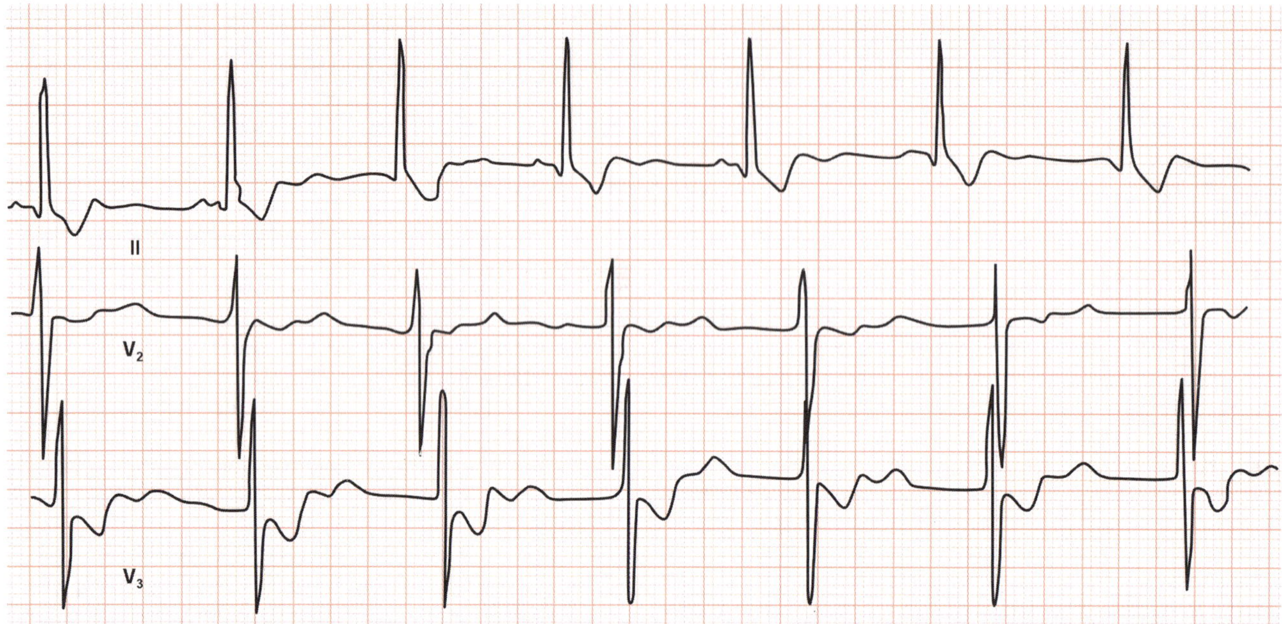

Fig. 12.1: ECG showing prominent U waves suggesting hypokalemia

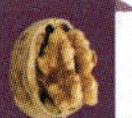

IN A NUTSHELL

Hypokalemia

1. Hypokalemia (serum potassium <3.5 mEq/L) manifests as hypotonia, abdominal distension, and muscle weakness. Hypokalemia is a common finding in children with severe malnutrition.
2. Electrocardiogram (ECG) changes: T wave depression, prolonged QT interval, U wave are helpful in diagnosis and monitoring.
3. Mild hypokalemia is treated by maintenance potassium 2–4 mEq/kg given PO.
4. Severe hypokalemia (serum potassium <2.5 mEq/L) is treated by 0.5–1 mEq/kg infusion over 1 hour under ECG monitoring. Maximum dose not to exceed 40 mEq.
5. Underlying cause must be treated.

Bonilla-Félix M. Potassium regulation in the neonate. Pediatr Nephrol. 2017;32(11):2037-49.

Desloovere A, Renken-Terhaerdt J, Tuokkola J, et al. The dietary management of potassium in children with CKD stages 2-5 and on dialysis-clinical practice recommendations from the Pediatric Renal Nutrition Taskforce. Pediatr Nephrol. 2021;36(6):1331-46.

Kermond R, Mallett A, McCarthy H. A clinical approach to tubulopathies in children and young adults. Pediatr Nephrol. 2023;38(3):651-62.

12.6 Hyperkalemia *PE 15.2*

DEFINITION

Hyperkalemia is defined as a serum potassium level of >5.5 mEq/L and characterized by tachycardia, muscular weakness, and arrhythmia. Most common etiology is impaired excretion of potassium due to renal insufficiency that involves defects in mineralocorticoid, aldosterone, and insulin function. Sudden and rapid onset of hyperkalemia can be fatal.

PATHOPHYSIOLOGY

Potassium is the principal intracellular cation in body and plays a key role in intracellular volume regulation. Total body potassium is approximately 53–55 mEq/kg body weight. Both animal and vegetable foods contain significant amounts of potassium and are consumed every day regardless of the type of diet. Despite the level of consumption, a balance between intake and excretion maintains plasma potassium levels within a narrow range (3.5–4.5 mEq/L). Less than 10% of potassium is excreted through sweat and stool, while kidneys excrete more than 90%. Increased levels of aldosterone stimulate potassium secretion, while low levels inhibit potassium secretion by the cortical collecting duct. In addition, potassium levels are partly responsible for a negative feedback to the adrenal cortex, so that high levels of potassium decrease aldosterone production, while low levels increase the secretion of aldosterone.

ETIOLOGY

- ***Inadequate excretion:***
  - *Renal:* Acute or chronic renal failure, RTA type IV, lupus nephritis.
  - *Adrenal failure*: Hypoaldosteronism, congenital adrenal hyperplasia (salt-losing variant), Addison disease, pseudohypoaldosteronism.
  - *Drugs*: Potassium sparing diuretic, angiotensin-converting enzyme (ACE) inhibitors, nonsteroidal anti-inflammatory drugs (NSAIDs), heparin.
- ***Shift of potassium from tissues to extracellular compartment:***
  - *Metabolic acidosis*
  - *Tissue injury:* Acute rhabdomyolysis, tumor lysis syndrome, burns, surgery, repeated blood transfusions.
  - *Drugs:* Succinylcholine, beta-blockers, digitalis intoxication, malignant hyperthermia (precipitated by inhaled anesthetics).
- ***Increased intake:*** Intravenous or oral, blood transfusions.

CLINICAL MANIFESTATIONS

The history of acute gastroenteritis, decreased urine output, adrenogenital syndrome, chemotherapy, crush injuries, and ingestion of potassium containing preparations should be taken in all children. Clinical findings depend on the degree of hyperkalemia and primarily related to its effects on the heart.

Children with serum potassium levels >8 mEq/L can present with circulatory failure and wide-complex tachycardia or ventricular fibrillation. Other symptoms include weakness of skeletal muscles that progresses to paralysis and respiratory failure. Children may complain of nausea, vomiting, and paresthesias.

Levels exceeding 8.5 mEq/L cause respiratory paralysis and cardiac arrest and are usually fatal. It causes abnormal heart and skeletal muscle function by lowering resting action potential and preventing repolarization and muscle paralysis.

INVESTIGATIONS

Serum urea, creatinine, uric acid, urinalysis, and urine electrolytes including potassium, and ECG should be done in all children. The sequences of changes that occur in ECG in hyperkalemia are mentioned below and shown in **Figures 12.2 and 12.3**:

Serum K^+ > 6.0 mEq/L: T waves tall and tented.

Serum K^+ 7.0–8.0 mEq/L: Prolonged PR interval, P wave flattens, ST segment depression, QRS widens.

Serum K^+ >8.0 mEq/L: The wide QRS merges with the T wave, thus forming a sinusoidal wave. P wave is absent.

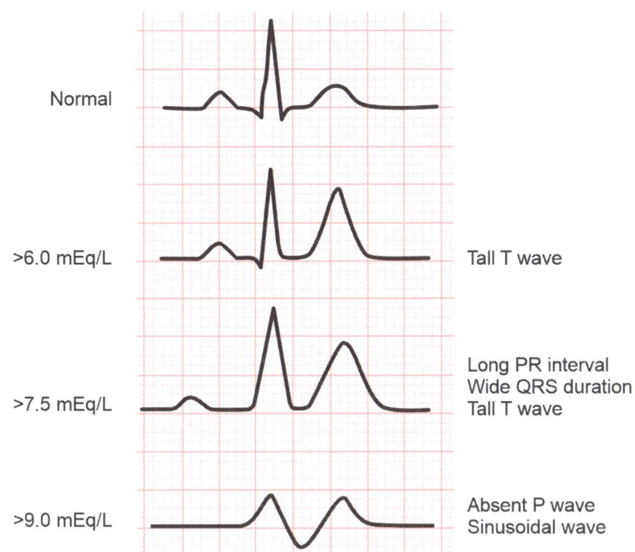

Fig. 12.2: ECG changes at various levels of serum potassium

TREATMENT Hyperkalemia

Firstly, it is important to stop all external sources of potassium. The goals of management include (*i*) counteracting the deleterious electrophysiologic effects of hyperkalemia; (*ii*) shifting potassium intracellularly; (*iii*) removing excess potassium; and (*iv*) identify and, treat the cause. Various approaches to achieve these goals are tabulated in **Table 12.7**.

Mild to Moderate Hyperkalemia

- *Inhaled beta-adrenergic agent* (Salbutamol: 5–10 mg) is effective in lowering serum potassium for 4–6 hours. It induces the intracellular movement of potassium via the stimulation of the Na–K adenosine triphosphate (ATP) pump. However, peak response is unclear; therefore, it is not recommended as the first line of therapy in severe hyperkalemia.
- *Insulin and glucose infusion* (1 mL/kg of 50% dextrose with regular insulin 0.1 units/kg infused over 1 hour) causes a transcellular shift of potassium into muscle cells, thereby temporarily lowering serum levels of potassium. Although the effect is almost immediate, it is temporary and, therefore, should be followed by therapy that actually enhances potassium clearance.
- *Sodium bicarbonate 7.5% IV* (1–2 mEq/kg over 10–30 minutes) is used as a buffer that breaks down to water and carbon dioxide after picking up free hydrogen ions, thus counteracts acidosis by raising blood pH and causes potassium entry into the cell.
- *Sodium polystyrene sulfonate* is an exchange resin that can be used to treat mild-to-moderate hyperkalemia. Each mEq of potassium is exchanged for 1 mEq of sodium. It binds it primarily in the large intestine and decreases total body potassium. The onset of action after oral administration ranges from 2 to 12 hours and is longer when administered rectally.

Severe Hyperkalemia

Calcium gluconate severe hyperkalemia requires immediate therapy consisting of IV 10% calcium gluconate (0.5–1.0 mL/kg over 1–3 minutes under cardiac monitoring) to stabilize the myocardium, rapid decrease of serum levels by alkalinization with sodium bicarbonate and a continuous IV infusion of dextrose and insulin. In a child receiving digitalis, it should be given over half an hour.

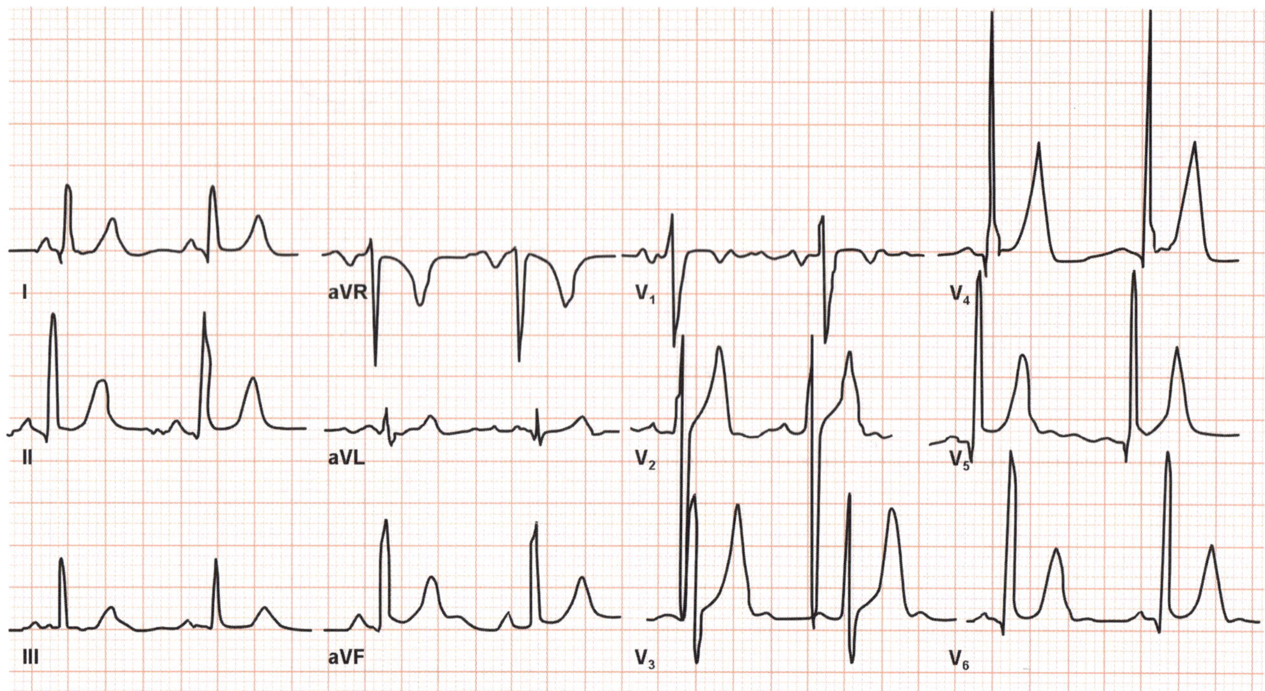

Fig. 12.3: Tall, slender T waves in leads I, II, aVF, and V2–6 in ECG

Table 12.7 Treatment of Hyperkalemia

Goal	*Management modality*
Counteracting the deleterious electrophysiologic effects of hyperkalemia	10% calcium gluconate (1 mg/kg IV)
Shifting potassium intracellularly	• Beta-2 agonist nebulization • Insulin and glucose infusion (1 mL/kg of 50% dextrose with regular insulin 0.1 units/kg infused over 1 hour) • Sodium bicarbonate
Removing excess potassium	Sodium polystyrene sulfonate resin (1 g/kg orally or rectally), peritoneal dialysis and hemodialysis
Identify and treat the cause	Surgical removal of bilateral ureteric stone, fulguration of posterior urethral valve, surgery for pelvic ureteric junction (PUJ) obstruction, etc.

Hemodialysis or peritoneal dialysis (PD) sometimes is necessary to treat severe symptomatic hyperkalemia, which is resistant to drug therapy. Rates of removal with PD are almost equal to the removal rate of Kayexalate. Continuous arteriovenous hemodialysis (CAVHD) or continuous venovenous hemodialysis (CVVHD) hemofiltration with dialysis also has been used to remove potassium. Supportive care may include adequate intravascular volume expansion, if indicated.

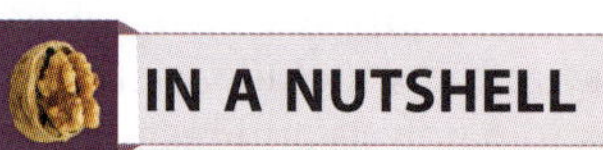

IN A NUTSHELL

Hyperkalemia

1. Hyperkalemia (serum potassium >5.5 mEq/L) is associated with characteristic ECG changes (prolonged PR interval, wide QRS, and tall T waves).
2. Management involves stopping all external sources of potassium, administration of IV calcium gluconate, salbutamol nebulization, glucose-insulin drip, sodium bicarbonate, and Na^+-K^+ exchange resin.
3. Dialysis to be considered in severe hyperkalemia refractory to drugs.

Littmann L, Gibbs MA. Electrocardiographic manifestations of severe hyperkalemia. J Electrocardiol. 2018;51(5):814-7.
Palmer BF, Clegg DJ. Diagnosis and treatment of hyperkalemia. Cleve Clin J Med. 2017;84(12):934-42.

12.7 Intravascular Access

PE 15.3

INTRODUCTION

Intravascular access is essential for administering medications and fluids directly into the intravascular compartment. Intravenous access is the most used method although intra-arterial or catheterization of central veins may be needed in certain situations. Over-the-needle catheters are preferred, their size depending upon the age of the child and caliber of veins. Butterfly/scalp vein needles may be used for cannulating scalp veins but this route is resorted to when other access cannot be obtained.

PERIPHERAL VENOUS ACCESS

Indication: Intravenous access is achieved to provide drugs, fluids, nutrition when administration via gastrointestinal tract is not possible. **Box 12.1 and Figure 12.4** depict the various sites used for IV access.

Box 12.1 Sites of Intravenous Access in the Order of Preference

1. Veins on dorsum of hand
2. Veins of the forearm, median cubital vein in antecubital fossa
3. Veins on dorsum of feet
4. Great saphenous vein at ankle
5. Vein in the center of volar aspect of wrist
6. Scalp veins
7. Proximal great saphenous vein

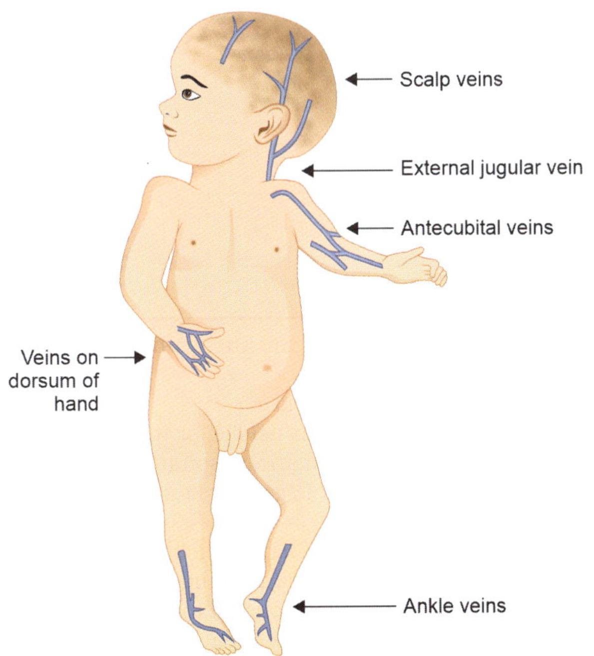

Fig. 12.4: Sites for peripheral venous access

Procedure: Prepare the skin at the point of entry to prevent entry of harmful microorganisms into the bloodstream. Materials required for preparation of skin include gloves, spirit and iodine, and sterile swabs. Once the skin is prepared, over-the-needle cannula (intracath, **Fig. 12.5**) can be inserted at the selected site as detailed in **Table 12.8**.

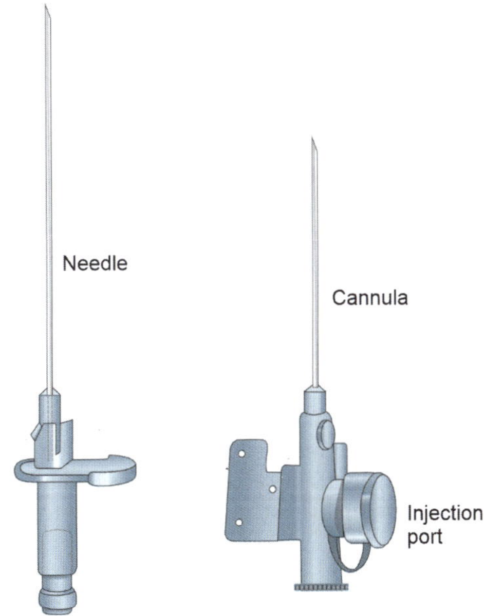

Fig. 12.5: Intravenous cannula

Table 12.8 Insertion of Intravenous Cannula

Action	*Rationale*
Puncture the skin with the bevel of the needle facing upwards and the needle at 30° angle to the skin surface. The point of entry should be 0.5 cm distal to the vein with needle aimed at the course of the vein in its direction of blood flow	To avoid excess trauma to the skin and blockage of the cannula at the time of entry
As soon as the skin is punctured, reduce the angle to almost skin level and advance needle slowly till the needle is felt to have pierced the vessel wall (a slight "pop" may be felt)	A small subcutaneous portion gives better stability to the cannula and reduces cross- puncturing of the vessel wall
Backflow of blood into the set may be seen. If not, gently withdraw the stylet	A good maintained backflow indicates that the cannula is inserted properly inside the vein
As blood appears, advance the cannula into the vein while removing the stylet	This ensures that the cannula remains in vein throughout the insertion

Contd...

Contd...

Action	*Rationale*
If no blood return is seen, draw cannula back and keeping it under the skin, advance again slowly to attempt reinsertion	Repeated removal of the cannula will create multiple puncture sites and increase the risk of contamination
Flush the inserted cannula with some normal saline to confirm patency of the vein and cannula	To ensure that the vein has not been cross-punctured. In case swelling appears just proximal to the site of cannula insertion on flushing, remove the cannula, and do not reattempt cannulation in the same vein

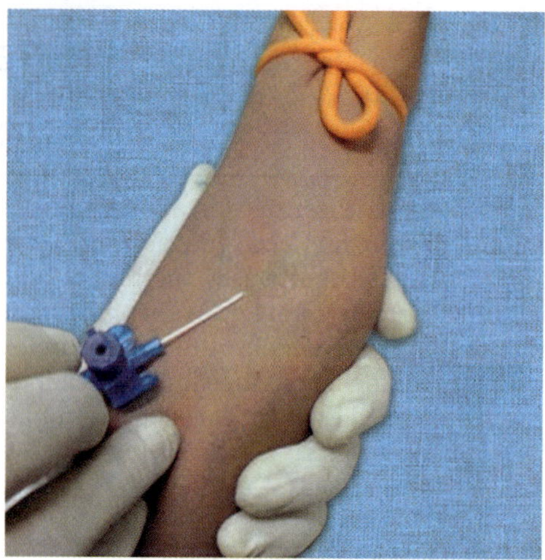

Fig. 12.6: Inserting intravenous cannula

Stretch the overlying skin using one hand to secure the position of vein while inserting the intracath. With another hand, grasp the intracath between the thumb and first finger and insert the cannula along the length of the vein **(Fig. 12.6)**. After obtaining venous access, anchor the intracath with adhesive tapes to the surrounding skin.

Recently use of transillumination and ultrasound-guided intravenous cannulation has shown to increase the chances of successful first attempt in children with difficult venous access.

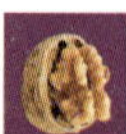

IN A NUTSHELL

Intravascular Access

1. Intravenous access is required to administer fluids, drugs, and nutrition and for monitoring in sick children.
2. Peripheral intravenous (IV) access via transillumination or ultrasound guidance was associated with fewer numbers of attempts and a higher successful first attempt compared to traditional approach in children with difficult access.

Dutt RD, Verma Y, Ranganath B, et al. Comparison of LED-based transillumination device with traditional vein viewing methods for difficult intravenous cannulation in Indian children: a non-randomized controlled trial. Indian J Pediatr. 2023;90(6):548-54.

Kleidon TM, Schults JA, Royle RH, et al. First-Attempt Success in Ultrasound-Guided vs Standard Peripheral Intravenous Catheter Insertion: The EPIC Superiority Randomized Clinical Trial. JAMA Pediatr. 2025:e245581.

Mitchell EO, Jones P, Snelling PJ. Ultrasound for pediatric peripheral intravenous catheter insertion: a systematic review. Pediatrics. 2022; 149(5):e2021055523.

12.8 Intraosseous Cannulation *PE 15.4*

INTRODUCTION

Indications: Intraosseous cannulation is an effective method of vascular access in critically ill or injured child in shock for administration of medications and fluids, if IV access cannot be obtained.

Position: The child is made to lie supine on a firm surface with knees slightly flexed and legs positioned with slight external rotation.

Sites of access: Most common site is the proximal end of tibia 1–3 cm below and medial to the tibial tuberosity. Distal femur and proximal humerus are alternative sites.

PROCEDURE

- Identify the site and clean the area with spirit, povidone iodine, followed by spirit.
- Stabilize the leg on a firm surface.
- Use a standard intraosseous needle for the access. In case of nonavailability, a bone marrow aspiration needle can be used. Alternatively, a thick 18 gauge spinal needle with stylet can be used in emergency.
- Insert the needle perpendicular to the skin. Drill the needle into the bone using a twisting motion. Insert the needle through the cortical bone till there is a sudden loss of resistance once the marrow is entered. Correct spacing

of the needle is indicated by firm placement without any support.

- Remove the stylet and attach a syringe. Aspiration of the bone marrow particles and blood reconfirms the correct placement.
- Remove the syringe and infuse a small amount of saline; and observe for swelling in the insertion site or posteriorly opposite the site.
- Stabilize the needle using tapes and connect the needle to intravenous tubing; and give the desired fluids and medications. All medications, which can be given by IV route, can be given by intraosseous route.
- Check regularly for development of swelling and try to establish an intravenous access as fast as possible as intraosseous access should not ideally be used for >24 hours.

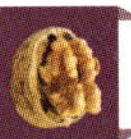

IN A NUTSHELL

Intraosseous Cannulation

1. Intraosseous route is an alternative if peripheral or central access is not attainable.
2. It is especially useful in shock, hypovolemia.
3. The preferred site is anteromedial aspect of tibia, 1–2 cm below the tibial tuberosity.
4. Intraosseous needle, spinal needle, bone marrow biopsy needle are manual devices available for insertion.

Petersen LB, Bogh SB, Hansen PM, et al. An assessment of long-term complications following prehospital intraosseous access: A nationwide study. Resuscitation. 2025;206:110454.

13 CHAPTER

Vaccines and Immunization

AS PER NMC COMPETENCIES

PE18.1	Explain the components of the Universal Immunization Program and the National Immunization Program.	*Ch 13.2*
PE18.2	Explain the epidemiology of vaccine preventable diseases.	*Ch 13.1*
PE18.3	Describe vaccine with regards to classification of vaccines, strain used, dose, route, schedule, risks, benefits and side effects, indications and contraindications.	*Ch 13.3*
PE18.4	Define cold-chain and discuss the methods of safe storage and handling of vaccines.	*Ch 13.4*
PE18.5	Describe immunization in special situations—HIV positive children, immunodeficiency, preterm, organ transplants, those who received blood and blood products, splenectomized children, adolescents, travelers.	*Ch 13.5*
PE18.6	Assess patient for fitness for immunization and prescribe an age-appropriate immunization schedule.	*Ch 13.2*
PE18.7	Educate and counsel a parent for immunization.	*Ch 13.6*
PE18.8	Describe the components of safe vaccine practice—patient education/counselling; adverse events following immunization, safe injection practices, documentation and medicolegal implications.	*Ch 13.6, Ch 13.7, Ch 13.8*
PE18.9	Observe the handling and storing of vaccines.	*Ch 13.4*
PE18.10	Document immunization in an immunization record.	*Ch 13.9*
PE18.11	Observe the administration of UIP vaccines.	*Ch 13.7*
PE18.12	Demonstrate the correct administration of different vaccines in a mannequin.	*Ch 13.7*
PE18.13	Explain the term implied consent in immunization services.	*Ch 13.9*
PE18.14	Enumerate available newer vaccines and their indications including pentavalent pneumococcal, rotavirus, JE, hepatitis A, influenza, COVID, typhoid, IPV and HPV.	*Ch 13.10*

Topics available online: ***The Immune System and Immune Response***

13.1 Basic Concepts of Vaccination

PE 18.2

EPIDEMIOLOGY OF VACCINE PREVENTABLE DISEASES

Epidemiology is a scientific and systematic study of distribution and determinants (causes and risk factors) of health and disease related states and their applications in the prevention, control, and management of health-related problems. It helps to plan and use appropriate strategies such as surveillance, disease specific control, elimination and/or eradication strategies (such as polio eradication and measles elimination). Apart from providing guidelines to healthcare providers, it is an essential resource for policy makers and resource allocation.

In vaccine preventable diseases (VPDs), epidemiology plays a crucial role to assess and monitor the burden of the diseases, surveillance methods, immunization programs, plan out newer strategies and vaccine(s) research. Vaccine epidemiology is defined as the study of the interactions and effects of vaccines and immunization programs on the epidemiology of VPDs. The occurrence of VPDs depends on the susceptibility of the host, virulence of the microorganism, and the suitable environment which facilitates the transmission and this is known as epidemiological triad. Certain terms are used in the basic understanding of the epidemiology of VPDs and these include:

- ***Incidence:*** It is the number of new cases occurring in a defined population during a specified time period or duration.
- ***Prevalence:*** It is the number of total cases (old and new) at a given point of time (point prevalence) or in a specified period of time (period prevalence).
- ***Immunogenicity:*** It is the ability of the antigens to produce the antibodies. It is also defined as the capacity of the vaccine to produce cell-mediated and/or antibody-mediated immunity and/or immunological memory.
- ***Seroconversion:*** It means more than or equal to fourfold increase in the antibody titers from prevaccination to postvaccination level or detectable postvaccination titer in a vaccinee who had no detectable antibody before vaccination.
- ***Seroprotection:*** It implies a state of protection from disease due to the presence of a certain detectable level of antibodies in serum.
- ***Vaccine efficacy:*** It is the ability of the vaccine to protect an individual under experimental conditions. It can be assessed through clinical trials, cohort studies, or case control studies. It is calculated as:

$$\text{Vaccine efficacy} = \frac{\text{Disease incidence in unvaccinated} - \text{Disease incidence in vaccinated}}{\text{Disease incidence in unvaccinated}}$$

- ***Vaccine effectiveness:*** It is the ability of the vaccine to protect the community and is the combination of vaccine efficacy and herd effect.
- ***Herd immunity:*** It is the proportion of immune individuals in a population. Individuals may acquire immunity following a disease or immunization against that disease, e.g., all those who have had chickenpox plus those who have acquired immunity because of varicella immunization shall constitute the immune individuals in a given population.
- ***Herd effect:*** It is the protection offered to unvaccinated members when good proportion (usually >85%) of the population is vaccinated. Herd effect is due to reduced carriage of the causative microorganism by the vaccinated cohort and thus is seen only with vaccines against those diseases where humans are the only source (there is no herd effect for tetanus). An effective vaccine is a prerequisite for good herd effect.
- ***Vaccination:*** The terms vaccine and vaccination are derived from *vacca*, the Latin term for cow. Vaccine was the term used by Edward Jenner to describe material used (i.e., cowpox virus) to produce immunity to smallpox. Vaccination is the process of administering the vaccine which may or may not evoke a protective immune response.
- ***Immunization:*** It is the artificial and purposeful induction of specific immune response by administering specific antigens to stimulate antibody production (active immunization) or by protecting the individual by giving pre-formed antibodies for temporary and short-term immunity (passive immunization). Vaccination and immunization are not synonymous because the administration of an immunobiological cannot be equated automatically with development of adequate immunity.
- ***Immunobiologicals:*** These include antigenic substances or antibody-containing preparations (e.g., globulins and antitoxins) from human or animal donors. These products are used for active or passive immunization or therapy and include vaccines, immunoglobulins, antitoxins, and monoclonal antibodies.

VACCINES

Vaccines are the preparations which contain live (attenuated) or inactivated organisms (such as bacteria or viruses) or fractions (e.g., subunit, polysaccharides, and toxoids) thereof, administered to induce immunity and prevent infectious disease or its sequels. In addition to their antigens, the vaccines also contain few other ingredients such as preservatives, stabilizers and adjuvants. Some vaccines contain highly defined antigens (e.g., the polysaccharide of *H. influenzae* type b or the surface antigen of hepatitis B); others have antigens that are complex or incompletely defined (e.g., *Bordetella pertussis* antigens or live-attenuated viruses). *Toxoid* is a modified bacterial toxin that has been rendered nontoxic, but retains the ability to stimulate the formation of antibodies to the toxin.

Types of Vaccines

Earlier the vaccines had been classified as live attenuated and killed (inactivated) vaccines, but with the advances in vaccine technology and production methods, a newer and relevant

Table 13.1 Types of Vaccines

Types of vaccines	*Vaccines*
Live and attenuated (bacterial and viral)	• *Viral:* Oral polio vaccine (OPV), rotavirus, measles, mumps, and rubella (MMR), varicella, hepatitis A, and yellow fever • *Bacterial:* Bacillus Calmette–Guérin (BCG) and oral typhoid
Inactivated/killed	Injectable polio vaccine (IPV), pertussis component of DTwP, inactivated influenza vaccine (IIV), and hepatitis A
Toxoid	Diphtheria, tetanus vaccines (e.g., DT, TT, Td)
Recombinant (viral subunit)	Hepatitis B, human papilloma virus vaccine
Capsular polysaccharide (unconjugated and conjugated with carrier protein)	*Haemophilus influenzae* type b (Hib), pneumococcal, meningococcal and Vi-typhoid vaccines
Bacterial subunit	Acellular pertussis vaccine in DaPT
Viral vector-based	Coronavirus disease 2019 (COVID-19)

classification is shown in **Table 13.1**. Few of their examples are also included.

Live-attenuated Vaccines

Live-attenuated vaccines are produced by modifying a disease producing (wild) bacteria or virus in a laboratory by repeated culturing. The live-attenuated vaccines have the following characteristics:

- The vaccine virus or bacteria must grow (replicate) in the vaccinated child to produce an immune response.
- The immune response produced is similar to that produced by a natural infection.
- Though live-attenuated virus or bacterium replicates in the host, it usually does not cause the disease unlike the disease caused by wild form. These vaccines are extremely sensitive to heat and light and hence must be handled and stored carefully. These are also sensitive to circulating maternal antibodies.
- Although active infection (with active viral replication) ensues after vaccine administration, usually little or no adverse reaction occurs. Very rarely, live-attenuated vaccine virus could revert to its original virulent form.
- Live vaccines are contraindicated in children with significant immune suppression.

Inactivated/Killed Vaccines

Inactivated vaccines are produced by growing the bacteria or virus in culture media and then inactivating them with either heat and/or chemicals (usually formalin). The vaccines for some viruses and most bacteria are inactivated (killed) or are subunit (purified components) preparations. Some subunits may be conjugated chemically to biologically active proteins (e.g., tetanus toxoid). Inactivated vaccines have the following characteristics:

- Inactivated vaccines cannot cause an infection but they still stimulate a protective immune response.
- These vaccines are less affected by circulating antibodies than the live vaccines.
- As the organisms in the inactivated (killed) vaccines cannot replicate (grow), these vaccines require multiple doses.
- The antibody titers tend to diminish with time and as a result, some inactivated vaccines require periodic supplemental doses to boost the antibody titers.

Other Types of Vaccines

The other types of vaccine such as recombinant vaccines are produced using recombinant deoxyribonucleic acid (DNA) technology or genetic engineering in which the genes for desired antigen of the microorganism are inserted into a vector. Such vaccines provide a very high level of immunity and lifelong protection in healthy individuals (e.g., hepatitis B vaccine). The conjugation of polysaccharide vaccines (e.g., conjugate pneumococcal, *H. influenzae* type b (Hib), and typhoid conjugate vaccine (TCV) with a carrier protein (vehicle) makes them act like T-cell-dependent antigens leading to anamnestic immune response and long-term immune protection. Thus, unlike pure polysaccharide vaccines, conjugated polysaccharide vaccines are used in children <2 years age for prolonged protection.

Immune Globulins

Immune globulins are antibodies usually obtained from human blood in a sterile solution. They are obtained by cold ethanol fractionation of large pools of blood plasma and contain 15–18% protein. Intended for intravenous or subcutaneous administration, immune globulins are primarily indicated for routine maintenance of immunity among certain immunodeficient persons and for passive protection.

Hyperimmune Globulin (Specific)

These are special preparations obtained from blood plasma from donor pools preselected for high antibody content against a specific antigen (e.g., hepatitis B immune globulin, tetanus immunoglobulin (TIG), varicella-zoster immune globulin, and rabies immune globulin.

Others

Antitoxin is a solution of antibodies against a toxin. It can be derived from either human (e.g., tetanus immune globulin) or animal (usually equine) sources (e.g., diphtheria and botulism antitoxin). It is used to confer passive immunity and for treatment. Antibodies of animal origin (animal antisera) are now used less often as they pose risk of reactions to the recipient. The use of such products should be limited strictly to certain indications for which specific Ig preparations of human origin are not available (such as diphtheria and botulism).

Monoclonal antibody (mAbs) is a product with antibodies against a single antigen and is prepared from a single lymphocyte clone in the laboratory. They have been used in the treatment of coronavirus disease 2019 (COVID-19) but are used more often in the treatment of cancers, allergies, and autoimmune disorders. Specific mAbs are now available for use against immediate and passive protection against rabies for the prevention of rabies.

Passive Immunization

Passive immunization is accomplished by administration of preformed antibodies. These antibodies are derived from the pooled plasma of adults by an alcohol fractionation procedure. The antibodies consist primarily of IgG with trace amount of IgA and IgM and are not known to transmit human immunodeficiency virus (HIV), hepatotropic or other infectious disease agents. Large number of donors is used to ensure inclusion of a broad-spectrum of antibodies.

Immunoglobulin and specific hyperimmune Ig are recommended for intramuscular, intravenous or subcutaneous administration. A few of the indications for the use of Ig for passive prophylaxis are as follows:

- Replacement therapy in congenital or acquired immune deficiency disorders.
- Prevention of complications of the disease in a high-risk child, such as those of leukemia, who can develop potentially life-threatening complications when exposed to diseases such as measles or varicella.
- When time does not permit the adequate protection by active immunization alone in postexposure situations such as rabies, hepatitis B, tetanus, and measles.

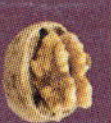

IN A NUTSHELL

Basic Concepts of Vaccination

1. In vaccine preventable diseases (VPDs), epidemiology plays a crucial role to assess and monitor the burden of the diseases, surveillance methods, immunization programs, plan out newer strategies, and vaccine(s) research.
2. Vaccines are a preparation which contain live (attenuated) or inactivated organisms (such as bacteria or viruses) or fractions (e.g., subunit, polysaccharides, and toxoids) thereof, administered to induce active immunity and prevent infectious disease or its sequels.
3. Passive immunization is accomplished by administration of preformed antibodies to provide immediate protection.

Dowdle WR. The principles of disease elimination and eradication. Bull World Health Organ. 1998;76(Suppl 2):23-5.

Lahariya C. Vaccine epidemiology: A review. J Family Med Prim Care. 2016;5(1):7-15.

13.2 National Immunization Program

PE 18.1, PE 18.6

INTRODUCTION

Immunization schedules are the basic framework for the delivery of vaccines and immunization to the individuals and the community. A well-planned immunization schedule should be epidemiologically relevant, immunologically effective, operationally feasible, and socially acceptable.

Various factors that need to be considered for planning the immunization schedule, include (1) Epidemiology of the disease; (2) Age-specific morbidity and mortality; (3) Vaccine effectiveness; (4) Risks of vaccine-related adverse events; (5) Cost-effectiveness; and (6) Healthcare infrastructure.

Vaccines for Universal Immunization are recommended at the youngest age at which a significant risk of disease and its complication exists and at which a protective immunological response can be expected. Logistics and operational feasibility of administering the vaccine at appropriate age without much increase in the cost and number of visits and requirement of the manpower are also important determinants of any immunization schedule.

UNIVERSAL IMMUNIZATION PROGRAM (UIP)

India launched its National Immunization Program as Expanded Program of Immunization (EPI) in 1978. The vaccines and the schedules are revised from time to time based upon disease epidemiology, availability of newer vaccines, regional variations (such as endemicity) and budgetary funding for vaccines and immunization programs. UIP is one of the most cost effective public health interventions responsible for the reduction of vaccine preventable diseases in infants and children. The sustained strengthening of UIP led to eradication of poliomyelitis and India being certified polio free in 2014. The expanding landscape of UIP continues to achieve improving vaccination coverage (Intensified Mission Indradhanush 2017), improving quality (capacity building of human resources), introduction of new vaccines [e.g., pneumococcal conjugate vaccine (PCV) in National Immunization Schedule and roll out of Electronic Vaccine Intelligence Network (eVIN).

NATIONAL IMMUNIZATION PROGRAM (NIP)

The epidemiological patterns of the diseases are often different in different countries and thus the immunization schedule of one country often differs from another. Even within the states, a few disease patterns may vary, e.g., vaccine for Japanese encephalitis is used under NIP in North Eastern states, where this disease is endemic. Besides, childhood immunization is a dynamic and evolving scientific process, thus necessitating the addition of newer vaccines in NIP. The examples of such recent introduction of vaccines under NIP include PCV and rotavirus vaccines, which are known to prevent morbidity and mortality from two leading causes of under <5 mortality namely childhood pneumonia and diarrhea.

Disease patterns and immunization needs may continue to change in future as more information on diseases becomes available and the development of newer vaccines continues to take place. Strategies such as catch-up immunization and

Table 13.2	National Immunization Schedule
Age	*Vaccines*
Birth	BCG, OPV (0), HBV birth dose
6 weeks	Pentavalent-1, bOPV-1, fIPV-1, *rotavirus*-1, and PCV-1
10 weeks	Pentavalent-2, bOPV-2, and *rotavirus*-2
14 weeks	Pentavalent-3, bOPV-3, fIPV-2, *rotavirus*-3, and PCV-2
9–12 months	MR-1, JE-1*, fIPV-3, and PCV-booster
16–24 months	DPT-booster 1, OPV booster, MR-2, JE-2*
5–6 years	DPT-booster 2
10 years	Td
16 years	Td
Pregnancy and mothers	Td-1, Td-2 (4 weeks after Td-1)[#]

*In selected endemic districts.

[#]If mother has received two doses during pregnancy within last 3 years, then only one dose of Td.

(bOPV: bivalent oral polio vaccine; fIPV: fractional dose of injectable polio vaccine; Pentavalent: diphtheria, pertussis, tetanus, Hib and hepatitis B virus (HBV) combination vaccine; PCV: conjugate pneumococcal vaccine; MR: measles and rubella combination vaccine; Td: tetanus and reduced dose diphtheria vaccine; JE: Japanese encephalitis vaccine)

supplementary immunization days (e.g., polio *ravivaar*) are additional tools in NIP. Hence, there is a constant need to revise the recommendations about the vaccines and their scheduling. Besides with the eradication of poliomyelitis from India, the need to address the potential safety issues with oral polio vaccine (OPV) was prioritized, leading to introduction of fractional doses of inactivated polio vaccine (fIPV) under NIP. The currently recommended National Immunization Schedule is shown in **Table 13.2**.

Assess Patient for Fitness for Immunization and Prescribe an Age-appropriate Immunization Schedule

- At every healthcare visit, child's vaccination status must be reviewed to avoid any missed opportunity for vaccination.
- Look out for the general well-being of the child and ask the parents if the child has any complaints and assess accordingly. Ask for any relevant past history of febrile seizures.
- Look out for any contraindications and precautions even if the child has received the vaccine earlier.
- Minor illnesses such as mild fever, cold and/or diarrhea are not contraindications to the use of vaccine and the vaccination should not be delayed to a further date.
- Perform a quick examination and assessment of the child before actual administration of the vaccine(s).
- Write down the following details on the immunization card of the vaccine given as (i) Date, (ii) Vaccine(s) administered, (iii) Batch number and its expiry date or paste the sticker supplied with the vaccine vial, (iv) Prescribe paracetamol to be given only when needed and not prophylactically, (v) Inform parents to report back or consult the health center if they have any concern at home or child has any severe adverse event following immunization (AEFI), and (vi) Schedule a date for further visit and next scheduled dose of vaccination.

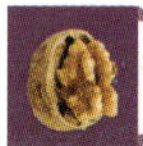

IN A NUTSHELL

National Immunization Program

1. An immunization schedule should be epidemiologically relevant, immunologically effective, operationally feasible, and socially acceptable.
2. Vaccines are recommended at an earliest age when there is a significant risk of disease/complications and at which a protective immunological response is expected.
3. National Immunization Program (NIP) is an evolving and dynamic process which undergoes revision and addition of newer vaccines (e.g., PCV) and local/regional disease patterns (e.g., JE vaccine).
4. Well child visits provide excellent opportunities to assess the immunization status of every child and to avoid any missed opportunities for immunization.
5. Vaccine safety remains an important component of NIP.
6. Minor illnesses such as acute diarrhea and upper respiratory infections should not delay or postpone routine immunization.

Lahariya C. A brief history of vaccines and vaccination in India. Indian J Med Res. 2014;139:491-511.

Ministry of Health and Family Welfare, Government of India. (2024). National Immunization Schedule–Routine Immunnization Manual for Medical Officers. [online] Available from https://mohfw.gov.in/sites/default/files/Routine%20Immunization%20I%20Manual%20For%20Medical%20Officers.pdf [Last accessed August, 2025].

Ministry of Health and Family Welfare. (2022). Focus on Universal Immunization: Dr. Mansukh Mandaviya launches Intensified Mission Indradhanush (IMI) 4.0. [online] Available from https://pib.gov.in/pressreleasepage.aspx?prid=1796099 [Last accessed August, 2025].

Vashishtha VM. Scheduling of vaccines. In: Gupta P, Menon PSN, Ramji S, et al. (Eds). PG Textbook of Pediatrics, 3rd edition. New Delhi: Jaypee Brothers Medical Publishers; 2022. pp. 1112-6.

13.3 Vaccines in National Immunization Schedule under Universal Immunization Program

PE 18.3

BCG (BACILLUS CALMETTE–GUÉRIN) VACCINE

The BCG vaccine is named after a French bacteriologist Albert Calmette and a veterinarian Camille Guérin who are credited with development of BCG strain. BCG is a live-attenuated vaccine and was first used in 1921. The BCG parent strain was obtained from a primary strain of *Mycobacterium bovis*. Danish strain 1331 is used in India to produce BCG vaccine and the vaccine is produced at BCG laboratory, Guindy, Chennai. Other strains prevalent worldwide differ in their morphological and biochemical characteristics as well as immunogenic and reactogenic potential.

CHARACTERISTICS

The BCG vaccine is a live-attenuated vaccine and contains 0.1–0.4 million-colony forming units (CFUs) per dose. It is supplied as lyophilized (freeze-dried) powder in multidose, vacuum-sealed, dark-colored ampoule as the vaccine is light- and heat-sensitive and deteriorates rapidly on exposure to ultraviolet rays. It contains 1% sodium glutamate as preservative. The ampoule needs to be opened carefully by gradually filing at the junction of the neck and the body of the ampoule so the air does not rush in causing the spillage. Normal saline is supplied as the diluent for the vaccine and the reconstituted vaccine must be used within 4–6 hours of its reconstitution. Freeze-dried vaccine can be stored at 2–8°C for up to 1 year.

PROTECTIVE EFFICACY

The BCG vaccine is currently being used in over 100 countries with the objective of preventing disseminated and other life-threatening manifestations of *Mycobacterium tuberculosis* infection in infants and young children. However, it does not prevent infection with *M. tuberculosis*. Various BCG vaccines used throughout the world differ in composition and efficacy. Other factors affecting the vaccine efficacy are endemicity of the disease, heavy bacillary load during primary infection, nutritional status, constant contact with open tuberculosis case, and concomitant HIV disease.

Earlier reports on efficacy of BCG vaccines reported 0–80% protection. However, recent analysis shows that it has relatively high protective efficacy (approximately 80%) against meningeal and miliary tuberculosis in children but no protection against primary infection. Another meta-analysis concluded that BCG vaccine significantly reduced the risk of active tuberculosis cases and deaths. The protective efficacy against pulmonary tuberculosis differs significantly depending on the factors discussed earlier and averages around 50%. Other promising and newer BCG vaccines (such as subunit vaccines) are under development to overcome the limitations of current BCG vaccine.

ADMINISTRATION AND DOSAGE

The vaccine provides cell-mediated immunity which is adequate in newborns. It is given at birth or soon thereafter and till 5 years of age for any unimmunized infant or child. In cases of delayed vaccination, prior tuberculin testing is not required. The vaccine is given intradermally on left deltoid region just above its insertion using tuberculin syringe and a 26G needle. Local antiseptics are not necessary before vaccinating but sterile cotton swabs are advised for local cleaning. Though the standard recommended dose of vaccine is 0.1 mL in NIP, there are recommendations on the usage of lower dose of 0.05 mL in infants <1 month and 0.1 mL thereafter. This vaccination is followed by a development of scar at injection site within 8–12 weeks.

PHENOMENA SEEN AFTER VACCINATION

- ***Day 0:*** Wheal of 5–8 mm develops at the site of injection, which subsides in 20–30 minutes.
- ***2–3 weeks:*** Papule develops.
- ***3–6 weeks:*** Papule increases in size up to 4–8 mm.
- ***6–12 weeks:*** Papule breaks into a shallow ulcer. Healing occurs spontaneously leaving behind a permanent, tiny 4–8 mm, round papery thin scar.

If no local reaction is seen in the local site at the end of 12 weeks, the vaccine should be repeated. Routine tuberculin test is not necessary prior to administration of the second dose.

ADVERSE EFFECTS

The adverse reactions and complications of BCG vaccine are rare. Local ulceration and regional lymphadenitis are major but occasional complications. These events usually resolve spontaneously and medical treatment does not seem to reduce the frequency of suppuration in BCG adenitis. Osteitis and disseminated BCG disease are extremely infrequent in immunocompetent patients. BCG should not be given to a child with severe immunosuppression and symptomatic HIV disease.

OTHER USES

Apart from tuberculosis, BCG vaccine offers some protection against leprosy. BCG has also been used as an immune modulating agent in diseases such as nephrotic syndrome and some cancers especially urinary bladder cancer.

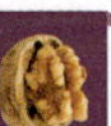

IN A NUTSHELL

BCG Vaccine

1. BCG is a live-attenuated vaccine, which is administered at birth or on first contact after birth. Catch up immunization is given up to 5 years of age.
2. The route is intradermal over the left shoulder in a dose of 0.1 mL.
3. The scar over the site develops by 8–12 weeks but absence of scar does not necessarily indicate absence of immunity.
4. The vaccine protects against the severe and disseminated forms of childhood tuberculosis such as tuberculosis meningitis (up to 80%).
5. After its reconstitution, it must be used within 6 hours and protected from exposure to heat and light.
6. It may rarely cause regional lymphadenitis.
7. Other and newer BCG vaccines such as subunit vaccines and using nonmycobacterial vaccine vectors are under development.

Centers for Disease Control and Prevention. (2025). BCG Vaccine Fact Sheet. [online] Available from https://www.cdc.gov/tb/hcp/vaccines/index.html [Last accessed August, 2025].

Cernuschi T, Malvolti S, Nickels E, et al. Bacillus Calmette-Guérin (BCG) vaccine: A global assessment of demand and supply balance. Vaccine. 2018;36(4):498-506.

Gupta P, Menon PSN, Ramji S, et al. BCG Vaccine. PG Textbook of Pediatrics, 3rd edition. New Delhi: Jaypee Brothers Medical Publishers; 2022. pp. 1129-33.

Mangtani P, Abubakar 1, Ariti C, et al. Protection by BCG vaccine against tuberculosis: A systematic review of randomized controlled trials. Clin Infect Dis. 2014;58(4):470-80.

World Health Organization. BCG Vaccine: WHO position paper, February 2018–Recommendations. Wkly Epidem Rec. 2018;93(8):73-96.

DPT (DIPHTHERIA, PERTUSSIS, AND TETANUS) VACCINES

Diphtheria and tetanus used to cause tremendous childhood mortality in the prevaccination era while pertussis causes prolonged respiratory morbidity in children. Widespread immunization with DPT vaccine has resulted in decline in incidence of these diseases.

Characteristics

The vaccines against diphtheria, pertussis, and tetanus are available in different combinations and formulations. These include:

- Monovalent as tetanus toxoid
- Bivalent as DT (diphtheria and tetanus for pediatric use up to 7 years) and Td (tetanus and diphtheria for older children and adults).
- Trivalent as DTwP containing diphtheria, tetanus and whole cell pertussis; DTaP containing diphtheria, tetanus and acellular pertussis; and Tdap as tetanus, with low dose diphtheria toxoid and acellular pertussis.

Other combinations of DTwP are available with *Haemophilus influenzae type b* (Hib) and HBV vaccine as pentavalent vaccine. DTaP in combination with Hib, HBV, and inactivated polio vaccine (IPV) is available as a hexavalent combination.

Each dose of DTwP vaccine contains diphtheria toxoid 25 Lf, tetanus toxoid as 5–25 Lf and pertussis as >4 IU of formalin inactivated *B. pertussis* cells. DTaP (acellular pertussis) vaccine contains four purified inactivated pertussis antigens (pertussis toxin, filamentous hemagglutinin, fimbrial agglutinogen, and pertactin). DTwP contains aluminum salts as adjuvants which make these vaccines opaque.

Immunity to diphtheria is conferred by antibodies produced against the exotoxin of *Corynebacterium diphtheriae.* Antitoxin levels of 0.1 IU/mL are essential to provide clinical immunity. Diphtheria vaccines contain modified bacterial toxin (toxoid), adsorbed with aluminum hydroxide (adjuvant), which improves the immunogenicity of the vaccine.

Schedule of Administration

The DPT vaccine is indicated for universal and routine immunization of infants. Three primary doses are to be given at 6, 10, 14 weeks of age, separated by a minimum interval of 4 weeks. For a child whose immunization schedule is resumed after deferral or interruption of the recommended schedule, the next dose in the sequence should be given, regardless of the interval since the last dose and the schedule is not reinitiated. The first booster is recommended at 16–24 months and second booster at 5–6 years of age.

The DTwP or DTaP can be used only up to 7 years, and thereafter DT should be used. These vaccines are available in ready to use form and dose is 0.5 mL given intramuscularly in anterolateral thigh. These vaccines are stored at 2–8°C and should never be frozen. If frozen accidentally, the vaccine should be discarded.

The primary doses of DPT are given as pentavalent vaccine (combination of DPT + Hib + HBV) at 6, 10, 14 weeks, under NIP.

Efficacy

The vaccine efficacy after completing three doses of primary immunization is 80%, 70–80%, and 100% for diphtheria, pertussis, and tetanus, respectively. The whole cell vaccine (DTwP) and acellular vaccine (DTaP) have similar efficacy against clinical or culture confirmed pertussis. There are no immunological markers of protection against the pertussis. The protection offered against all the disease components decreases over a period thus requiring booster doses.

Adverse Reactions

The adverse reactions observed after (DTwP) can either be *mild* or *severe.* Mild reactions include redness, edema, induration, tenderness, and sterile abscess at injection site. Most of these effects are attributed to the pertussis component. Drowsiness, fretfulness, vomiting, crying, and slight-to-moderate fever are also seen. These manifestations occur within several hours of the injection and subside spontaneously. Serious adverse effects have been reported but are extremely rare. Local and febrile adverse reactions are less common and less severe with acellular (DTaP) than with whole cell pertussis (DTwP) vaccine.

Contraindications and Precautions

Anaphylaxis or an encephalopathy occurring within 7 days of previous vaccination is an absolute contraindication to pertussis containing vaccine(s). Due to an uncertainty of component causing anaphylaxis in the DPT vaccine, no further immunization with diphtheria, pertussis, and tetanus containing vaccine is recommended. In encephalopathy, pertussis containing vaccines are contraindicated and only diphtheria and tetanus containing vaccines should be used for further doses, if needed.

Conditions such as persistent inconsolable crying >3 hours, hyperpyrexia >40.5°C, and hypotonic-hyporesponsive episodes within 48 hours of vaccination and convulsions with or without fever within 72 hours are not contraindications but are precautions to further doses of DTwP vaccines. An evolving and progressive neurological disease is a relative contraindication to the first dose of DTwP. DTwP can be safely administered to children who have stable neurological disorder. A child who has recovered from diphtheria or tetanus must be actively immunized because amount of toxin responsible for these diseases in humans does not elicit protective immunity.

TETANUS TOXOID

Tetanus toxoid vaccine is prepared by chemically inactivating tetanus toxin called "toxoid", which evokes immune response but does not cause disease. It is given 0.5 mL intramuscularly. It is stored at 2–8°C and should not to be frozen. Adverse reactions associated with this vaccine are pain, swelling at local site, low-grade fever and very rarely, severe allergic reaction. The only contraindication is severe allergy to a vaccine component or prior dose. A child who has recovered from tetanus must be actively immunized because the amount of toxin responsible for disease in humans does not elicit protective immunity. Tetanus antitoxin level of >0.1 IU per mL is considered protective. Tetanus toxoid is recommended for HIV infected children irrespective of presence of symptomatology. In NIP, it is now being replaced with Td vaccine as boosters at 10 and 16 years and as two doses/boosters for pregnant women.

Tdap/Td VACCINES

Although Tdap vaccine is not included in NIP, but this is a vaccine in use for protection of older children against diphtheria, pertussis, and tetanus in private health setups. The immune protection following DTaP vaccines against diphtheria, pertussis, and tetanus is known to wane off over the next 6–12 years, making older children and adolescents vulnerable to diphtheria and pertussis. The standard strength DTwP and DTaP vaccines cannot be used for vaccination of children 7 years and above due to increased reactogenicity. TdaP vaccine is recommended for use in older (>7 years) children and adults for booster doses or catch up vaccination. Adolescents and adults who have never received any dose of Tdap in the past are recommended a single dose of Tdap irrespective of the time interval elapsed after the last vaccine. If TdaP is not available at the facility, it may be substituted with Td vaccine.

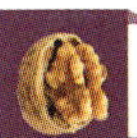

IN A NUTSHELL

DPT (Diphtheria, Pertussis, and Tetanus) Vaccines

1. DPT vaccines are used as combination vaccines in immunization programs as pentavalent vaccines (DPT, Hib, and HBV) in primary immunization schedule in NIP.
2. Immunity against DPT is reported to wane off gradually over a period of 6–12 years and hence regular boosting is recommended for these antigens.
3. DTP (DTwP) is given in three primary doses at 6, 10, and 14 weeks followed by boosters at 16–24 months and 5–6 years. It is then given as Td boosters at 10 and 16 years of age.
4. Most adverse effects of DPT vaccine are attributable to the pertussis component.
5. Anaphylaxis to a previous dose or an encephalopathy within 7 days of vaccination is a contraindication to the further dose of DPT vaccine.
6. Acellular pertussis vaccines (DTaP and TdaP) contain more purified pertussis antigens and are less reactogenic.

Balasubramanian S, Shah A, Pemde HK, et al. IAP Advisory Committee on Vaccines and Immunization Practices 2018-19. Indian Academy of Pediatrics. Recommended immunization schedule and update on immunization for children aged 0 through 18 years. Indian Pediatr. 2018;55:1066-74.

Klein NP, Bartlett J, Fireman B, et al. Waning Tdap effectiveness in adolescents. Pediatrics. 2016;137(3):1-9.

National Rural Health Mission. National Immunization Schedule and Frequently asked Questions. Immunization Hand Book for Health Workers. New Delhi: Ministry of Health and Family Welfare, Government of India; 2006. pp. 17-26.

Sidhu J, Dewan P, Gupta P. Maternal and neonatal tetanus: A journey into Oblivion. Indian Pediatr. 2016;53(12):1057-61.

POLIO VACCINES

Since the year 2014, when WHO declared India polio free, no case of wild polio virus has been reported. Presently, poliomyelitis is endemic in Afghanistan and Pakistan. In the last few years, of the three wild polio viruses (types 1, 2, and 3), two (type 2 and 3) have been declared as eradicated globally in 2015 and 2019 respectively and thus type 1 is responsible for all the reported cases of wild poliovirus infections. Two types of vaccines are available against poliomyelitis, which include live-attenuated OPV and IPV.

ORAL POLIO VACCINE

The OPV which was developed by Sabin is a now a bivalent vaccine containing serotypes 1 and 3 (bOPV). Trivalent OPV (tOPV) with additional type 2 wild virus is no longer in use since 2016. Monovalent type 2 OPV (mOPV), though not in use, has been stockpiled to be used in an event of outbreak. The wild poliovirus is attenuated by repeated passages on nonoptimal tissue culture and then cultured on monkey kidney cells (vero cells) to produce large quantities of the vaccine. OPV is administered orally and to generate an effective response, the vaccine virus must be taken up by the intestinal mucosa.

The immunogenicity and efficacy of OPV is dependent upon mucosal immunity provided by secretory IgA and humoral immunity generated by circulating neutralizing antibodies. After three doses, the seroconversion rate is 73% for type 1, 90% for type 2, and 70% for type 3. It provides a state of local resistance in the gastrointestinal tract, based on mucosal immunity. This gastrointestinal resistance results in a significantly decreased number of successful implantations (challenge), a shorter period of virus excretion upon reinfection challenge, and lower titers of virus excreted. Studies have reported protective effects against paralytic poliomyelitis and interruption of wild poliovirus circulation. The protective efficacy lasts nearly 10 years, even if antibodies are at very low levels or undetectable.

Studies conducted in developing countries, however, report that seroconversion rates even after multiple doses of OPV are lower than those reported from developed countries, particularly against type 1 virus. The reasons proposed for this difference include high prevalence of nonpolio enteroviruses in gut, high incidence of malnutrition including zinc deficiency and diarrhea in children in developing countries, temperature variations in temperate climate, and improper storage. Bivalent OPV is more immunogenic than trivalent OPV due to lesser degree of competition between the virus uptake in the intestinal mucosa.

Administration and Schedule

The OPV is given orally as three primary doses (2 drops) in most immunization schedules, at an interval of 4–8 weeks. The vaccine is given at the same visit as the pentavalent (DPT/Hib/HBV) vaccine for the sake of convenience; hence most countries follow schedule 6, 10, 14 weeks or 2, 4, 6 months although the latter is immunologically preferable. However, in India, due to logistics reasons, primary doses are administered at 6, 10, 14 weeks only. OPV is stored at an outreach facility at 2–8°C. In National Immunization Schedule, hospital-born children are also administered another dose, immediately or within 14 days of birth (zero dose) along with birth dose of BCG and HBV vaccine. This additional early (zero) dose of polio vaccine (OPV) has been noted to enhance seroconversion and protect babies who subsequently receive three conventional doses.

The primary series of OPV is followed by a booster at the age of 15–18 months. In addition, children up to 5 years of age should also receive the pulse-polio doses administered on national immunization days and supplemental NIDs (NIDs and sNIDs), irrespective of previous routine immunization.

Adverse Effects

The OPV is well-tolerated and devoid of any gastrointestinal and systemic side effects. Though a rare occurrence, it can cause a serious adverse event such as vaccine-associated paralytic poliomyelitis (VAPP).

Vaccine-associated Paralytic Poliomyelitis

The most significant adverse effect associated with administration of oral polio vaccine is VAPP. The overall risk is estimated at one case per 2.5 million doses (distribution), or one case per million OPV recipients. In these cases, the live-attenuated poliovirus contained in OPV, while replicating in the intestinal tract of recipient undergoes mutation and regains its neurovirulence. The reverted virus might reach the central nervous system (CNS) and produce disease like the wild poliovirus. The risk of VAPP is higher in patients with B-cell immunodeficiency. VAPP virus is not transmissible to others and there are no outbreaks following it. The clinical features of this illness are identical to those of natural paralytic poliomyelitis due to the wild virus.

Vaccine-derived Poliovirus

Circulating vaccine derived polioviruses (VDPVs) are rare strains of poliovirus that have genetically mutated from the strain in the OPV. The ability to circulate determines whether neurovirulent vaccine-derived viruses may cause outbreaks of VAPP, hence the term "circulating vaccine-derived polioviruses" (cVDPV) has been coined. Clearly cVDPV are deattenuated and wild-like. They have intermediate degrees of virulence and transmissibility, compared to wild and vaccine strains. Polio virus serotype 2 strain has been associated with most of the paralytic polio outbreaks of cVDPVs.

Persistently underimmunized communities are at a risk of cVDPV outbreaks as there are enough susceptible children for the excreted vaccine-derived polioviruses to begin circulating in the community. The lower the population immunity, the longer these viruses survive. The longer they survive, the more they replicate, change, and exchange genetic material with other enteroviruses as they spread through a community. A newer and novel monovalent, type 2 oral polio vaccine with improved genetic stability and lower risk of reversion to neuro virulence (nOPV2) has been developed and is being used in supplementary immunization activities (SIAs) in response to cVDPV2 outbreaks in different countries.

Contraindications

Oral polio vaccine is contraindicated in situations where immunity is unpredictable or definitely compromised, such as immunosuppressed HIV positive children, and those suffering from lymphoreticular malignancies and immune dysfunction. OPV is also contraindicated to household contacts of such persons since there is a risk of acquiring the virus through the secretions of vaccinated contacts. Pregnancy is also a relative contraindication to use of OPV. In all such situations, IPV remains the preferred vaccine. Mild diarrhea is not a contraindication for OPV administration. Repeat dose of OPV should be given, if the child vomits within 10 minutes of administration.

INACTIVATED POLIOVIRUS VACCINE

The IPV was first developed in 1950s by Jonas Salk by the inactivation of polio virus by formaldehyde. The vaccine strain has undergone purification and refinement to become third generation IPV, also known as enhanced IPV (eIPV). With a standardized vaccine potency, eIPV contains 40, 8, and 32 D antigen units of types 1, 2, and 3 viruses, respectively. Another IPV, known as Sabin IPV (sIPV), is in different stages of development to address polio end game strategies and biosafety level issues. IPV is available as a single vaccine and also in combination as DTaP/Hib/HBV, DTaP/IPV (Hexavalent), and DTaP/IPV/Hib (acellular pentavalent), and DTwP/IPV/Hib/HBV, as a whole cell Hexavalent vaccine.

The IPV is a highly immunogenic vaccine and induces neutralizing antibodies against all three poliovirus serotypes in 90–95% children after second dose and in 99% of the vaccinees after the third dose. It produces excellent humoral immunity, as well as local pharyngeal and possible intestinal immunity and thus offers herd protection. The relative benefit of mucosal immunity induced by OPV compared with that of eIPV remains controversial. The secretory antibody response after OPV administration is greater, both in titer and in frequency, than after IPV administration. Consistent with its ability to induce greater secretory antibody response, OPV is also more effective than IPV in preventing and limiting intestinal infection following oral challenge. However, IPV also provides herd immunity, although less than that of OPV, by inhibition of pharyngeal infection by poliovirus and reducing intestinal excretion in vaccinees.

Administration and Schedule

The IPV is available as a single dose vial/prefilled syringe. Routinely, it is given as 0.5 mL intramuscularly. In NIP, the primary series of OPV is combined with a fractional dose (0.1 mL) of IPV (fIPV) given intradermally at ages of 6 and 14 weeks and 9 months on the left side at the insertion of deltoid muscle. The benefits offered by fIPV are to provide protection to a larger number of eligible children, and decreasing the cost of the vaccine with a limited vaccine supply. This is done as a risk mitigation strategy (disease risk reduction) in routine immunization program toward the achievement of global polio eradication. As a strategy for polio eradication in near future, the transition from OPV to IPV all across the world is known as polio endgame strategy.

Safety

The IPV is an extremely safe vaccine with minimal local side effects and rare occurrence of hypersensitivity reactions to vaccine components such as neomycin and polymyxin B. It contains killed poliovirus, and thus never causes VAPP or formation of cVDPV strains.

Indian Academy of Pediatrics (IAP) recommends the use of IPV (0.5 mL, IM) at 6, 10, and 14 weeks followed by booster doses at 16–18 months and 5 years. Based on the epidemiological factors, different schedules of 3 + 1, 2 + 1, and 3 + 0 are used in other countries with a dosing interval of 4–8 weeks in the primary series.

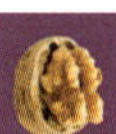

IN A NUTSHELL

Polio Vaccines

1. Two types of vaccines (OPV and IPV) are used against polio viruses.
2. Now we use bivalent OPV (bOPV) with type 1 and type 3 strains. Trivalent OPV, which was used earlier, is no longer available.
3. Protective efficacy lasts nearly 10 years, even if antibodies are nearly undetectable.
4. In NIP, apart from four doses of OPV at birth, 6 weeks, 10 weeks, and 14 weeks, fractional dose IPV (fIPV) is given at a dose of 0.1 mL intradermally at the ages of 6 and 14 weeks and 9 months. IAP recommends full (0.5 mL) doses of IPV given intramuscularly at 6, 10, and 14 weeks followed by two boosters at 16–18 months and 4–6 years, respectively.
5. OPV has rare though serious side effects such as VAPP and VDPV.
6. As a strategy for polio eradication in near future, the transition from OPV to IPV all across the world is known as polio endgame strategy.

American Society for Microbiology. (2022). Polio Vaccines: New Developments on the Road to Eradication. [online] Available from https://asm.org/Articles/2022/July/Oral-Polio-Vaccines-Old-Problems,-New-Solutions [Last accessed August, 2025].

Dunavan CP. Polio's Precarious Future A Review of Polio: The Odyssey of Eradication and an Interview with Dr. T. Jacob John. Am J Trop Med Hyg. 2019;100(3):763-5.

Kasi SG, Shivananda S, Marathe S, et al. Indian Academy of Pediatrics (IAP) Advisory Committee on Vaccines and Immunization Practices (ACVIP): Recommended Immunization Schedule (2020-21) and Update on Immunization for Children Aged 0 Through 18 Years. Indian Pediatr. 2021;58(1):44-53.

National Rural Health Mission. National Immunization Schedule and Frequently Asked Questions. Immunization Hand Book for Health Workers. New Delhi: Ministry of Health and Family Welfare, Government of India; 2006. pp. 17-26.

Peak CM, Lyons H, Voorman A, Gray EJ, Cooper LV, Blake IM, Hawes KM, Bandyopadhyay AS. Monitoring the Risk of Type-2 Circulating Vaccine-Derived Poliovirus Emergence During Roll-Out of Type-2 Novel Oral Polio Vaccine. Vaccines (Basel). 2024 Nov 22;12(12):1308.

World Health Organization. Polio Vaccines: WHO position paper–March 2016. Weekly Epidemiol. 2016;91:145-68.

HAEMOPHILUS INFLUENZAE b VACCINE

Infections due to Hib are common causes of invasive bacterial infections including meningitis, bacteremia, pneumonia, septic arthritis, and epiglottitis in children <5 years of age. Most Hib infections are known to occur before 2 years of age. Besides contributing to high case fatality, Hib infections can leave behind neurologic sequelae such as mental retardation and permanent sensorineural deafness in children. Mass immunization with Hib vaccine has led to virtual elimination of Hib disease from UK and USA and the vaccine has demonstrated excellent efficacy and safety.

CHARACTERISTICS

The Hib vaccine is an inactivated conjugate vaccine consisting of Hib capsular polysaccharide [polyribosyl ribitol phosphate, (PRP)] covalently linked to a carrier protein directly or via an intervening spacer molecule. This process of conjugation changes the polysaccharide antigen from a T-cell independent to T-cell dependent antigen and greatly improves the immunogenicity of the vaccine. It is effective from the age of 6 weeks onward. It also leads to herd effect by reducing the nasopharyngeal carriage of the organism.

The conjugate Hib vaccines differ from one another on the size of PRP molecule, type of carrier protein (e.g., diphtheria toxoid, tetanus toxoid), type of linkage between PRP and carrier proteins and the presence of an adjuvant. All licensed Hib vaccines in India use tetanus toxoid as carrier protein. Hib vaccine is no longer available in a monovalent standalone vaccine but is available as a part of combination vaccines (DTwP/Hib/HBV, DTwP/Hib, and DTaP/Hib/HBV/IPV). The vaccine is stored at 2–8°C.

PROTECTIVE EFFICACY

The Hib conjugate vaccines are very immunogenic and high antibody titers are observed following the completion of primary series. These conjugate vaccines do not interfere with the immunogenicity of other simultaneously administered vaccines. The first, second, and third doses of vaccine give 71%, 89%, and 95–100% vaccine efficacy, respectively. The mean geometric titers of anti-PRP antibodies for long-term protection against the invasive Hib disease are greater than 1.0 μg/mL.

ADMINISTRATION AND SCHEDULE

The Hib vaccine is given by intramuscular route and routine vaccination with Hib vaccine is started at 6 weeks of age and three primary doses of vaccine are given intramuscularly at an interval of 4 weeks. The vaccine is a part of pentavalent vaccine (DTwP/Hib/HBV) in NIP. For an unimmunized child between 6 and 12 months, two primary doses are given at 6–8 weeks interval. For a child between 12 and 15 months, only one primary dose is given. All these children are given a booster dose between the ages of 15 and 18 months. This vaccine is not recommended in healthy children >5 years of age, as Hib is a disease of infants and young children.

ADVERSE EFFECTS

The adverse effects are uncommon and are mild such as local pain, tenderness, and fever. There are no absolute contraindications except for hypersensitivity to the vaccine components.

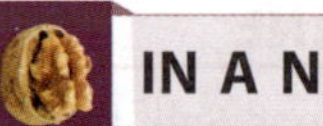

IN A NUTSHELL

***Haemophilus influenzae* Type b Vaccine**

1. *H. influenzae* b can cause invasive diseases such as bacteremia, acute bacterial meningitis, osteomyelitis, septic arthritis, and epiglottitis mostly in first 2 years of life.
2. It is a conjugate vaccine with a carrier protein to make it a T-cell dependent antigen, which improves the immunogenicity of the vaccine.
3. It is used as a pentavalent vaccine (DPT/Hib/HBV) in NIP.
4. It is also available in combination with DTaP and IPV.
5. Catch-up vaccination with one dose is recommended till 5 years of age.

Gavi. (2021). Routine vaccines, extraordinary impact: *Haemophilus influenzae* type b (Hib). [online] Available from https://www.gavi.org/vaccineswork/routine-vaccines/extraordinary-impact-haemophilus-influenzae-type-b-hib [Last accessed August, 2025].

Gupta SK, Sosler S, Lahariya C. Introduction of Hib as Pentavalent (DPT-HepB-Hib) in two states of India. Indian Pediatr. 2012; 49:707-9.

Zarei AE, Almehdar HA, Redwan EM. Hib Vaccines: Past, Present, and Future Perspectives. J Immunol Res. 2016;2016:7203587.

HEPATITIS B VIRUS VACCINES

Hepatitis B infection is a potentially life-threatening disease caused by hepatitis B virus (HBV) and still remains a global health problem. The virus is extremely infectious and even miniscule quantities of serum lead to the accidental transmission of the virus through the parenteral route. With the availability of genetically engineered HBV vaccine in 1986, the prevention of HBV infection has been revolutionized.

CHARACTERISTICS

The HBV vaccine is produced by recombinant DNA technology wherein DNA of HBV is incorporated in the genetic material of the yeast (*Saccharomyces cerevisiae*) which then begins to produce the hepatitis B surface antigen (HBsAg). This method nullifies the risk of transmission of infection from inadvertent contamination and guarantees almost limitless supply of antigen. Recently, a new novel adjuvant vaccine (Heplisav-B) has been approved for use in persons >18 years by Food and Drug Administration (FDA) in two-dose schedule 4 weeks apart.

The HBV vaccine is available as a monovalent (standalone) vaccine which is most widely used in NIP as a birth/1st dose within 24 hours of birth to prevent any vertical transmission of HBV infection from the mother to the newborn baby. If the mother is HBsAg positive, the baby should receive hepatitis B immunoglobulin (HBIG) within 12 hours of birth along with first dose of HBV vaccine using two separate syringes at different injection sites. Following the birth dose, HBV vaccine is administered at 6, 10, and 14 weeks as a combination vaccine along with DPT and Hib vaccines. Different combinations of HBV vaccine with other childhood vaccines are available and are widely used.

PROTECTIVE EFFICACY

Administration of three doses of HBV vaccine in different schedules results in a high degree of seroconversion. Over 95% of vaccinated individuals develop protective level of antibodies (anti-HBs level >10 mIU/mL), 1–3 months after the completion of schedule. This is believed to confer life-long immunity against HBV. Any accidental re-exposure to the virus in future ensures adequate protection due to an anamnestic response. Routine booster doses are not recommended for immunocompetent children and adults.

ADMINISTRATION AND SCHEDULE

The HBV vaccine should be given intramuscularly in anterolateral thigh in infants and deltoid in older children and adults. Injection into gluteal region elicits decreased immune response and must be avoided. The pediatric dose of vaccine is 10 µg/0.5 mL in children up to 12 years. The adult dose is 20 µg/mL. Larger vaccine doses (40 µg) are needed to induce protective antibody in children on hemodialysis and with immunocompromised status.

In an unimmunized child, who has not received the vaccine as per schedule, catch-up immunization should be done by giving three doses in a schedule of 0, 1, and 6 months. Immunologically, 0, 1, and 6 months schedule of HBV immunization is most widely used and proven to be ideal with high antibody titer at the end of immunization series.

ADVERSE EFFECTS

The adverse effects of HBV vaccine are mild and transient which may include fever and soreness at injection site. The only absolute contraindication to HBV vaccine is the occurrence of anaphylaxis to a previous dose or an allergy to vaccine component but is extremely rare.

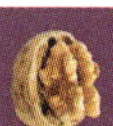

IN A NUTSHELL

Hepatitis B Virus Vaccines

1. HBV vaccine is a recombinant vaccine available as a standalone vaccine and in combination form.
2. The first dose of vaccine (birth dose) is recommended within 24 hours of birth, followed by three doses at 6, 10, and 14 weeks.
3. The vaccine provides long-term protection against HBV infection.
4. No boosters are required in healthy children/adults.
5. Immunocompromised children need double of the recommended dose. Otherwise, an additional vaccine dose can be given at 12 months.
6. The safety profile of the vaccine is well-established.
7. A baby born to an HBsAg positive mother should receive HBIG (within 12 hours of birth) and first dose of HBV vaccine at separate sites to prevent the perinatal transmission of infection to the newborn.

Advisory Committee on Vaccines and Immunization Practices, Indian Academy of Pediatrics. Hepatitis B Vaccine. In: Indra Shekhar Rao M, Kasi SJ (Eds). IAP Guide book on Immunization. New Delhi: Jaypee Brothers Medical publishers; 2022. pp. 140-59.

Bruce MG, Bruden D, Hurlburt D, et al. Antibody Levels and Protection After Hepatitis B Vaccine: Results of a 30-Year Follow-up Study and Response to a Booster Dose. J Infect Dis. 2016;214(1):16-22.

Centres for Disease Control and Prevention (CDC). (2021). Hepatitis B Vaccine Information Statements (VISs). [online] Available from https://www.cdc.gov/vaccines/hcp/current-vis/hepatitis-b.html [Last accessed August, 2025].

Gupta P, Menon PSN, Ramji S, et al. Hepatitis B Vaccine. PG Text book of Pediatrics, 3rd edition. New Delhi: Jaypee Brothers Medical Publishers; 2022. pp. 1144-6.

WHO. (2022). Hepatitis B. [online] Available from https://www.who.int/news-room/fact-sheets/detail/hepatitis-b [Last accessed August, 2025].

ROTAVIRUS VACCINES

Rotavirus infections are the most common cause of acute diarrheal illnesses in children <5 years of age. They are estimated to be responsible for nearly 40% hospital admissions for acute gastroenteritis in children. The vaccine is now used all over the country under routine immunization program since the year 2019.

CHARACTERISTICS

All currently available vaccines against rotavirus are live and attenuated vaccines to be given orally and which aim to mimic the protection given by natural rotavirus infection. Different brands of rotavirus vaccines containing human and bovine human reassortant strains and subgroups are licensed for use in India. The vaccines are available either in monovalent form or in polyvalent form (serotypes G1, G2, G3, G4, and G9). They are effective in the prevention of severe rotavirus gastroenteritis (reduction by 54–60%) and are immunogenic even with their different compositions. The protective effect of rotavirus vaccine lasts through second year of life. Another rotavirus vaccine, Indian Neonatal Rotavirus Live Vaccine, 116E has a strain of Indian origin and is also effective against other serotypes. It has been shown to provide 56% protection in the first year of life. The vaccine is stored between 2 and 8°C.

ADMINISTRATION AND SCHEDULE

Rotavirus vaccines are administered orally as liquid preparations and in variable volumes depending on their constituents. These are recommended either in two or three doses schedule beginning at 6 weeks of age. In NIP, rotavirus vaccine (pentavalent bovine human reassortant vaccine) is administered in a three-dose schedule at 6, 10, and 14 weeks. Specifically prepared multidose vials containing five doses with vaccine vial monitors are provided for government health sectors. Though the vaccine package inserts recommend that rotavirus vaccine should not be given after 32 weeks of age, the maximum upper

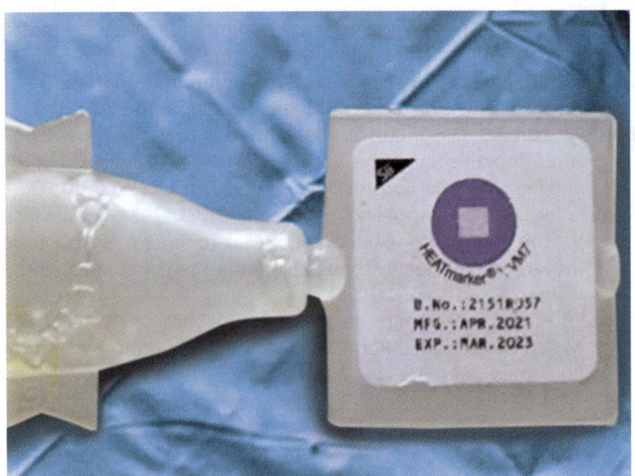

Fig. 13.1: Vaccine vial monitor on rotavirus vaccine.

limit for giving first dose of rotavirus vaccine under NIP is 1 year. In such a situation if any infant who has received first dose, should complete the series by additional two doses at an interval of 4 weeks in the second year. WHO recommends that rotavirus vaccine needs to be given first if it is given in the same session along with other vaccines. Rotavirus vaccine and OPV when administered in same session have no interference and are safe and immunogenic. Multidose rotavirus vaccine vials under NIP come with VVM on their caps/plastic ampoules/vials **(Fig. 13.1)**.

ADVERSE EFFECTS

Side effects are uncommon but fever, vomiting and diarrhea following vaccination can occur and are generally self-limiting. Past history of intussusception and uncorrected gastrointestinal tract malformation are absolute contraindications to the use of vaccine.

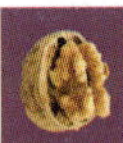

IN A NUTSHELL

Rotavirus Vaccines

1. Rotavirus diarrhea is a leading cause of childhood diarrhea during first 2 years of life.
2. Rotavirus vaccine is an oral and live attenuated vaccine.
3. The schedule for administration is three doses at 6, 10, and 14 weeks. In NIP, a dose of 5 drops is administered.
4. The efficacy is reported to be 50–60% in developing countries such as India.
5. Intussusception is a rare adverse event following vaccine and the benefits of rotavirus vaccination much exceed the risk of rare adverse events.

Bhat N, Vodicka E, Clifford A, et al. The evidence base for rotavirus vaccination in India: Current status, future needs. Vaccine. 2025;44:126551.

Burke RM, Tate JE, Parashar UD. Global Experience with Rotavirus Vaccines. J Infect Dis. 2021;224(12 Suppl 2):S792-800.

Kumar A, Basu S, Vashishtha V, et al. Burden of Rotavirus Diarrhea in Under five Indian Children. Indian Pediatr. 2016;53(7):607-17.

Steele AD, Victor JC, Carey ME, et al. Experiences with rotavirus vaccines: can we improve rotavirus vaccine impact in developing countries? Hum Vaccin Immunother. 2019;15(6):1215-27.

MEASLES CONTAINING VACCINES

Measles is an extremely contagious viral disease with a high burden of childhood morbidity and mortality in developing countries. Till 2017, a monovalent live, attenuated measles vaccine was in use in NIP at the age of 9 months followed by second dose at 15 months. In a two-dose schedule, this monovalent vaccine helped to prevent this highly contagious disease and its serious complications. The Government of India launched a campaign of administering a single dose of measles-rubella (MR) vaccine between the ages of 9 months and 15 years with a goal to further reduce the number of cases occurring annually. MR vaccine is given in a two dose in NIP at 9 months, followed by a second dose between the ages of 16–24 months.

CHARACTERISTICS

Measles-containing vaccines (MCVs) include: (1) MR vaccine and (2) MMR vaccine. Currently, only MR vaccine is an EPI vaccine. MR and MMR vaccines are combination vaccines.

The MCV are live and attenuated viral vaccines. Measles vaccine has its origin from the Edmonston strain, which has been further modified into strains such as Edmonston Zagreb, Schwarz, Moraten, and Edmonston B strains. Mumps vaccines use strains such as Leningrad 3, Urabe, and Jeryl Lynn. The most widely used strain in rubella vaccine is RA 27/3. These vaccines are freeze dried vaccines in single and multiple dose dark-colored vials as these are heat and light sensitive. They are reconstituted with the supplied diluent (sterile water) and stored at 2–8°C even while being used during a session.

PROTECTIVE EFFICACY

The factors that affect the protective efficacy and immunogenicity against measles are the age of the vaccinee as transplacentally derived maternal antibodies may interfere with the vaccine uptake. Efficacy is also affected by intercurrent illnesses and presence of severe malnutrition. Vaccine-induced immunity against measles is life-long after two doses with at least one dose after 1 year of age. Single dose of MMR vaccine has 95% efficacy in preventing mumps and rubella. Duration of vaccine-induced immunity is probably life-long in most vaccine recipients.

ADMINISTRATION AND SCHEDULE

The MCVs are given as subcutaneous injections in a dose of 0.5 mL of reconstituted vaccine on the deltoid region or anterolateral part of thigh. Two dose schedules are followed for MCV. WHO recommends first dose at 12 months followed by second dose at 15–18 months. In India, due to high transmission rates and complications of measles, the first dose of MCV (MR) is scheduled at 9 months (270 completed days) to provide early protection. NIP follows a two-dose schedule of MR vaccine at 9 months of age followed by second dose between 16 and 24 months. The vaccine can be used at ≥6 months of age in case of an outbreak. Catch-up immunization is advised for unimmunized children and adolescents with two doses with a minimum interval of 4 weeks between the two doses.

ADVERSE EFFECTS

The MCVs are safe vaccines. Mild fever and mild measles like maculopapular rash may be seen in 2–5% recipients after 7–12 days. Thrombocytopenia and anaphylaxis are rare. Transient arthralgia may occur following rubella vaccine in adolescents while mumps component can cause high fever and rarely transient parotitis and aseptic meningitis after 2–3 weeks. As there is no preservative in the vaccine, bacterial contamination of the already punctured vials can cause bacterial growth (such as staphylococci) and lead to severe shock (toxic shock syndrome). Thus, all multidose vials should be used within 4–6 hours of opening the vial. All the left over and remaining/partially used multidose vials must be discarded at the conclusion of the session. There is no causal relationship between the MCV and autism, inflammatory bowel disease and Guillain-Barré syndrome.

The MCVs are contraindicated in severe immune deficiency and severe allergic reaction to an earlier dose of the vaccine. Pregnant women should not receive MCV due to the risks to the fetus from the live viral vaccines.

MEASLES AND RUBELLA INITIATIVE

The measles and rubella initiative is an ongoing collaborative partnership between WHO, UNICEF, and countries on a global level for a strategic plan to reduce deaths due to measles and elimination of measles by improving vaccination coverage (>95%) in six WHO regions of the world. This is done by using laboratory-based surveillance, outbreak preparedness, and case management. The need for follow-up MR campaigns is based upon the country specific surveillance data every 3–5 years. The introduction of MR vaccine in national schedule, is a step forward to control of rubella and elimination of congenital rubella syndrome (CRS) in coming years. Separate rubella vaccine is also available to immunize against rubella.

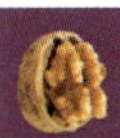

IN A NUTSHELL

Measles Containing Vaccines

1. The MCV are live and attenuated and freeze-dried vaccines available as measles and rubella (MR), and measles, mumps and rubella (MMR).
2. These should be used within 6 hours of reconstitution and any leftover doses should be discarded.
3. All MCVs are immunogenic, effective, and safe to use.
4. Two doses of MR are used at the age of 9 months and between 16 and 24 months in NIP. There is no upper age limit for use.
5. Mumps component is not yet a part of NIP.
6. These are not recommended during pregnancy, in severe immune deficiency, and with a history of anaphylaxis to its previous dose.
7. Measles and rubella campaigns are mass events based on surveillance data to achieve and sustain high levels of population immunity against these VPDs.

Di Pietrantonj C, Rivetti A, Marchione P, et al. Vaccines for measles, mumps, rubella, and varicella in children. Cochrane Database Syst Rev. 2020;4(4):CD004407.

Gupta P, Menon PSN, Ramji S, et al. Measles Vaccine. In: Soni V, Verma S. PG Textbook of Pediatrics, 3rd edition. New Delhi: Jaypee Brothers Medical Publishers Pvt Ltd; 2022. pp. 1149-52.

Kasi SG, Parekh BJ, Wadhwa A, et al. Measles, Mumps and Rubella Vaccines. IAP Q & A on Vaccines and Vaccinology, 1st edition. New Delhi: Jaypee Brothers Medical Publishers; 2021. pp. 204-14.

Vashishtha VM, Yewale VN, Bansal CP, et al. IAP Perspectives on Measles and Rubella Elimination Strategies. Indian Pediatr. 2014;51(9):719-22.

PNEUMOCOCCAL VACCINES

Streptococcus pneumoniae (earlier referred to as *Pneumococcus*) is a major cause of serious bacterial infections in children. Invasive pneumococcal disease (IPD) is an important cause of VPDs in infants and children in the world. With the availability of safe and effective vaccines, immunization with the vaccine is the only available tool to prevent this morbidity and mortality. *S. pneumoniae* can exist as:

- Asymptomatic nasopharyngeal carriage
- Noninvasive pneumococcal diseases such as otitis media and pneumonia
- Invasive pneumococcal diseases (IPDs) such as meningitis, septicemia, osteomyelitis, and endocarditis.

Globally, >90 serotypes of the *S. pneumoniae* are recognized but only 10 serotypes are responsible for most pediatric infections. Out of these, 1, 6, 14, 19, and 23 are the most common. Children <5 years are at a high risk of IPD.

There are two types of pneumococcal vaccines licensed for use in India:

1. Pneumococcal polysaccharide vaccine (PPSV)
2. Pneumococcal conjugate vaccines (PCV)

PNEUMOCOCCAL POLYSACCHARIDE VACCINE

Characteristics

This pneumococcal polysaccharide vaccine (PPSV-23) is composed of purified preparation of pneumococcal capsular polysaccharide and can prevent 88% of invasive disease (pneumonia, meningitis, and bacteremia) caused by *S. pneumoniae*. Each dose of 0.5 mL contains 25 µg of polysaccharide of each of 23 serotypes contained in the vaccine. As this vaccine is an unconjugated polysaccharide vaccine, it is poorly immunogenic in children below 2 years of age. Further, it does not result in immunological memory. The 23-valent PPSV vaccine is licensed for use in older children and adults.

Administration and Schedule

The vaccine is administered either intramuscular or subcutaneously in a single dose of 0.5 mL. Mild local reactions may be seen in 30–50% of vaccine recipients and systemic reactions are uncommon. It can only be given to children above the age of 2 years. It is useful for high-risk children with diabetes, cardiovascular diseases, HIV infection, sickle cell disease, asplenia, and nephrotic syndrome. Revaccination with a single dose is recommended after 5 years. The maximum number of doses for PPSV-23 is restricted to two only due to the lack of boosting effect and even hypo-responsiveness to the vaccine.

PNEUMOCOCCAL CONJUGATE VACCINES

As there is an immunological limitation with the use of PPSV in children below the age of 2 years, PCV have been developed and are being used for several years for prevention of IPD. The capsular polysaccharide is conjugated with an immunological carrier protein to make it a T-cell-dependent antigen. This increases the immunogenicity of the vaccine with an additional advantage of anamnestic response with boosters. It also has the potential to reduce nasopharyngeal carriage.

These vaccines come in different valences with reference to the number of serotypes in them (10, 13 and 14). PCV-10 valent was included in a phased manner in NIP in 2019 and is given as two primary doses at 6 and 14 weeks of age and a booster dose at 9 months. Other PCV with additional strains (PCV 15 and 20) are in use in other countries.

The efficacy and immunogenicity of PCV depends on the serotypes in the vaccine because they induce serotype specific response. There is evidence of extended cross protection for certain serotypes in the same subgroup such as 6A and 6B. All the available PCV have good immunogenicity against IPD.

Administration and Schedule

The PCV are given in a dose of 0.5 mL intramuscularly in a three-dose schedule at 6, 10, and 14 weeks followed by a booster dose between 12 and 15 months. Catch-up immunization has been recommended up to the age of 5 years in a child who has not received it earlier. The common side effects include injection site soreness, malaise, and low-grade fever.

Replacement Disease

While introduction of pneumococcal vaccine on a large scale will reduce the nasal carriage of vaccine serotypes, it is possible that these are replaced by nonvaccine serotypes and finally the overall nasopharyngeal carriage of pneumococci may remain the same. Thus, theoretically, benefit from reducing diseases caused by vaccine serotypes may be partially offset by an increase in the disease caused by nonvaccine serotypes of pneumococci. However, replacement disease is not expected to increase the overall burden of pneumococcal disease.

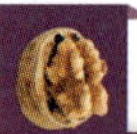

IN A NUTSHELL

Pneumococcal Vaccines

1. Two types of pneumococcal vaccines are licensed for use in India and these include pneumococcal conjugate vaccine (PCV) and polysaccharide 23-valent vaccine (PPSV-23).
2. The PCV (10-valent) is included in NIP in a two-dose schedule at 6 weeks and 10 weeks and a booster dose at 9 months for the prevention of invasive pneumococcal diseases (IPD).
3. The PCV are effective vaccines to prevent IPD caused by the serotypes present in the vaccines.
4. The PPSV-23 is an unconjugated polysaccharide vaccine and is poorly immunogenic in children below 2 years of age. It does not result in immunological memory.
5. The PPSV-23 is mainly used in high-risk children after the use of PCV-10. Minimum gap of 8 weeks is recommended between PCV-10 and PPSV-23.

Daniels CC, Rogers PD, Shelton CM. A Review of Pneumococcal Vaccines: Current Polysaccharide Vaccine Recommendations and Future Protein Antigens. J Pediatr Pharmacol Ther. 2016;21(1):27-35.

Gupta P, Menon PSN, Ramji S, et al. Pneumococcal Vaccines. In: Kumar P, Vashishtha VM (Eds). PG Textbook of Pediatrics, 3rd edition. New Delhi: Jaypee Brothers Medical Publishers Pvt Ltd; 2022. pp. 1167-72.

Kasi SG, Parekh BJ, Wadhwa A, et al. Pneumococcal Conjugate Vaccines. IAP Q & A on Vaccines and Vaccinology, 1st edition. New Delhi: Jaypee Brothers Medical Publishers; 2021. pp. 174-88.

Kobayashi M, Farrar JL, Gierke R, et al. Use of 15-Valent Pneumococcal Conjugate Vaccine Among U.S. Children: Updated Recommendations of the Advisory Committee on Immunization Practices—United States, 2022. MMWR Morb Mortal Wkly Rep. 2022;71:1174-81.

Wiese AD, Huang X, Yu C, et al. Changes in Otitis Media Episodes and Pressure Equalization Tube Insertions Among Young Children Following Introduction of the 13-Valent Pneumococcal Conjugate Vaccine: A Birth Cohort-based Study. Clin Infect Dis. 2019;69(12):2162-9.

World Health Organization. Pneumococcal Conjugate Vaccines: WHO Position Paper. Weekly Epidemiol Rec. 2019;94:85-104.

JAPANESE ENCEPHALITIS VACCINES

Japanese encephalitis mainly affects children of ages <15 years and has significant mortality and neurological morbidity. Japanese encephalitis vaccines are recommended in UIP for children living in districts highly endemic for Japanese encephalitis. The disease is endemic in several states in India especially in North and North Eastern parts of India. Vaccination against the disease is the only effective long-term control measure against Japanese encephalitis.

CHARACTERISTICS

Inactivated mouse brain derived vaccine using Nakayama strain was first to be used. Inactivated vaccine after cultivation in primary hamster kidney cells of the Beijing-3 strain was the second Japanese encephalitis vaccine. Both of these are now no longer in use. Because of rare adverse events such as fatal encephalitis and hypersensitivity with mouse brain vaccine, WHO recommends that only cell culture-derived live vaccines should be used. Cost, efficacy, and safety concerns led to the development of a live-attenuated virus vaccine (SA14-14-2) and more recently, a number of second-generation Japanese encephalitis vaccines are now available.

LIVE-ATTENUATED CELL CULTURE-DERIVED SA 14-14-2 JAPANESE ENCEPHALITIS VACCINE

This vaccine offers long-term protection (single dose followed by a booster 1 year later). This live vaccine contributes to over 50% of global production of Japanese encephalitis vaccine. Initial studies have shown efficacy of 80% and 98% with one and two doses, respectively. The vaccine has been used in endemic areas under public health program by Government of India since 2006. It is not available in private health sector for use.

Other vaccines include JEEV (inactivated vero cell culture derived vaccine from SA 14-14-2 strain) and JENVAC (inactivated vero cell culture derived vaccine from Kolar 821564XY strain). These are inactivated vaccines and are available for use in private sector. JE vaccine is also recommended for travelers to endemic belts for one month or more and/or to frequent travelers to JE endemic regions at least 1 week before travel.

ADMINISTRATION AND SCHEDULE

Live, attenuated cell culture vaccine derived from SA 14-14-2 is given in a dose of 0.5 mL for all ages by subcutaneous route on the upper arm. A two-dose schedule is recommended with first dose given at 9 months and second dose between 16 and 24 months. The vaccine is used in notified endemic districts of India under NIP. The vaccine can also be used for catch-up immunization in susceptible children up to the age of 15 years. The vaccine is safe and may have transient symptoms such as fever, local pain, and rash. It can be safely given concomitantly with other childhood vaccines.

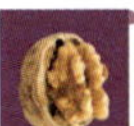

IN A NUTSHELL

Japanese Encephalitis Vaccines

1. Japanese encephalitis mainly affects children of ages <15 years and has significant mortality and neurological morbidity.
2. Inactivated mouse brain derived vaccine is now no longer in use.
3. A live-attenuated vaccine (SA 14-14-2) has been developed and offers long-term protection with a single dose followed by a booster 1 year later.
4. Inactivated vaccines are available for use in private sector.
5. Vaccination against the disease is the only effective long-term control measure against Japanese encephalitis.
6. Japanese encephalitis vaccine is used in notified endemic districts of India under NIP. The vaccine can also be used for catch-up immunization in susceptible children up to the age of 15 years.
7. Japanese encephalitis vaccines can be given simultaneously with other childhood vaccines.

Advisory Committee on Vaccines and Immunization Practices. (2020). Japanese B Encephalitis. [online] Available from https://acvip.org/parents/columns/japanese-encephalitis.php [Last accessed August, 2025].

Ramachandran VG, Smilie C. Japanese Encephalitis Vaccines. In: Gupta P, Menon PSN, Ramji S, et al. (Eds). PG Textbook of Pediatrics, 3rd edition. New Delhi: Jaypee Brothers Medical Publishers; 2022. pp. 1162-4.

Vashishtha VM, Ramachandran VG. Vaccination Policy for Japanese encephalitis in India: Tread with caution. Indian Pediatr. 2015;52:837-9.

OTHER (NON-EPI) VACCINES

The following vaccines are not used under NIP, though these are widely used in private health setup. Besides vaccines under NIP, Indian Academy of Pediatrics (IAP) and its Advisory Committee on Vaccines and Immunization Practices (ACVIP) recommends the use of additional vaccines during childhood and adolescence to offer protection against other VPDs.

TYPHOID VACCINES

The first generation inactivated whole cell typhoid vaccines have been withdrawn because of high reactogenicity. Other vaccines against typhoid include:

- ***Live oral Ty21a*** vaccine is now not available in India, but is used in few other countries as enteric coated capsule. Other live oral typhoid vaccine candidates are under development.
- ***Vi-polysaccharide vaccine:*** It contains 25 μg of Vi capsular polysaccharide antigen in 0.5 mL of phenolic isotonic buffer. It is extracted from *Salmonella typhi* Ty2 and the process of purification and extraction preserves the Vi antigen. As this vaccine is a polysaccharide vaccine, it is not effective in children below 2 years of age and has no immunologic

memory. Serological correlate of protection is anti-Vi antibodies at/above a concentration of 1 μg/mL. The vaccine does not interfere with the interpretation of the Widal test. Efficacy drops over time and the cumulative efficacy at 3 years against culture confirmed typhoid fever is reported as 55–70%. For sustained protection, revaccination should be done once every 3 years. The vaccine needs to be given subcutaneously or intramuscularly in a dose of 0.5 mL to children above 2 years of age. Adverse effects are mild which include fever, local pain, and erythema at injection site. There are no contraindications to its use other than prior severe reaction to vaccine components.

- ***Typhoid conjugate vaccine:*** As the polysaccharide vaccines are not known to induce anamnestic response, the process of conjugation of Vi-polysaccharide of *S. typhi* Ty2 to a protein conjugate such as tetanus toxoid helps to overcome this limitation. Conjugation enhances the immune response and confers T-cell-dependent property to the antigen. Four different brands of typhoid conjugate vaccines (TCV) are licensed for use in India and each single dose of vaccine should contain 25 μg of conjugated Vi antigen suspended in 0.5 mL of isotonic saline. This vaccine is given intramuscularly in a dose of 0.5 mL from the age of 6 months to 45 years. A booster dose is not recommended at present. TCV and MCV can be given simultaneously at the age of 9 months and beyond. The vaccine has to be stored between 2 and 8°C. The vaccine is safe with transient side effects such as mild fever and local reactions at injection site. Other and newer TCVs are currently under different stages of development.

HEPATITIS A VACCINE

Hepatitis A virus (HAV) vaccination is recommended for children who are at increased risk of infection and for those wishing to obtain immunity. Two categories of hepatitis A vaccines, inactivated and live-attenuated vaccines, are currently available in Indian market.

Inactivated Vaccine

Characteristics

Inactivated hepatitis A vaccine is derived from HM 175/GBM strains grown on MRC-5 human diploid cell lines. It is formalin inactivated and aluminum hydroxide is used as adjuvant. The vaccine is stored at 2–8°C. The vaccine does not contain thiomersal.

The HAV vaccine is highly effective and immunogenic in children and adolescents, when administered in the recommended dosages and schedules. There is some evidence that higher doses generate protective antibody levels more rapidly. Although the geometric mean titer (GMT) of antibodies produced after vaccination is lower than those produced by natural infection, they are sufficiently high to provide lifelong immunity following the two doses schedule of HAV vaccine.

Administration and Schedule

The vaccine is administered intramuscularly in children older than 12 months of age in a two dose schedule, given 6 months apart. Seroconversion rates range from 90 to 100% after two doses. Booster is not recommended at present. The standard pediatric dose is 720 EU (0.5 mL) and adult dose (>13 years) 1,440 EU (1.0 mL). The vaccine needs to be stored at 2–8°C. HAV vaccine can be safely given simultaneously with other childhood vaccines.

Adverse Events

The HAV vaccine is a safe vaccine with a few side effects such as fever and pain at injection site that are mild and transient.

Live-attenuated Vaccine

Another HAV vaccine has been prepared from H2 and L-A-1 strain and attenuated after multiple culture passage in human diploid cells. A multicentric study has shown that a single dose schedule was immunogenic and tolerable with minimal reactogenicity. The protective antibodies against HAV are shown to persist for 10–15 years. The vaccine is recommended for use in children >12 months of age and dose is 0.5 mL to be given by subcutaneous route, irrespective of the age.

VARICELLA VACCINE

Characteristics

Varicella vaccine is a live-attenuated viral vaccine derived from the Oka strain of varicella-zoster virus (VZV). The varicella vaccines may vary in their passage numbers in human diploid cells, virus content (between 1,000 and 10,000 PFU), presence of trace antibiotics to ensure sterility and stabilizers. The minimum infectious dose of the vaccine virus should be 1,000 PFU per 0.5 mL dose. The vaccine is not a part of NIP as the disease is not a high priority infectious disease for developing countries including India. A combination vaccine of MMR with varicella (MMRV) had also been in use in India for children between the ages of 1 and 12 years. This vaccine is no longer available.

Varicella vaccine is highly immunogenic and provides >99% efficacy against moderate-to-severe disease in healthy children between the ages of 12 months and 12 years. The immunity induced in vaccine recipients appears to be long lasting, though exact duration of protection is not known.

Although varicella vaccine prevents varicella, breakthrough varicella infections (occurring >42 days after vaccine administration) may occur in 15% of vaccinated children who have seroconverted following vaccination. Most cases of breakthrough infections are milder than infections that occur in unvaccinated children.

Administration

Varicella vaccine is available as a single dose lyophilized product and must be reconstituted with its diluent before its use. It should be used within 30 minutes of reconstitution. The vaccine is administered subcutaneously either in the upper arm or the anterolateral thigh. The vaccine is recommended to be used in a two dose schedule, with the first dose administered at 15 months of age and followed by the second dose after an interval of 3–6 months. Second dose may be given after 4–8 weeks in high-risk children to complete active immunization quickly.

There is some evidence that varicella vaccine may be effective in preventing varicella or modifying the severity of the disease, if given within 3–5 days after exposure to a case of varicella. The vaccine can be used for catch-up immunization in children and adolescents. Vaccination of older children and adolescents will protect at-risk individuals but will not disturb the general epidemiology of the disease. The vaccine can be given safely with all other routine childhood immunizations without any risk of reduced efficacy and lower tolerability.

Adverse Effects

Varicella vaccine is safe and side effects reported are mild and transient. These may include fever, minor injection site reactions, and vaccine-associated rash. Systemic adverse events are uncommon. Varicella vaccine should not be given in moderate and severe illness, immunocompromised children, leukemia, HIV infection, children on corticosteroid therapy and pregnancy. It is recommended that pregnancy should be avoided for 4 weeks following the vaccine.

Passive Prophylaxis

Varicella-zoster immunoglobulin (VZIG) is used for passive prophylaxis in children without evidence of immunity to varicella and who are at high risk for the severe disease and/or its complications. It has to be given intramuscularly in a dose of 125 units for every 10 kg of body weight. The indications include (1) Immunocompromised children, (2) Neonates whose mothers have had varicella 5 days before to 2 days after delivery, and (3) Susceptible pregnant women.

INFLUENZA VACCINES

Characteristics

Vaccines are important tools in the prevention of a highly contagious viral respiratory infection which can be serious in high-risk children and adults. Immunity following infection by one strain may not protect fully against subsequent antigenic variants. As the circulating strains of influenza virus are known to undergo constant antigenic change every year, WHO Global Influenza Surveillance Network (GISN) recommends use of two different set of strains for Northern and Southern hemispheres every year.

The efficacy of influenza vaccine depends on several factors which include the case definition (clinical versus laboratory confirmed), age group, season, and the vaccine strain. The protective efficacy of various influenza vaccines ranges from 31 to 91% and is not uniform for all the subtypes of influenza.

Influenza vaccines are inactivated injectable vaccines (IIV) carrying whole virus, split virus, or a subunit of virus. Vaccine virus is grown in egg or on cell culture. They may either be trivalent or quadrivalent. They contain gelatin as stabilizer and thimerosal as preservative. Another type of influenza vaccine is live-attenuated influenza vaccine (LAIV). It is used as a nasal spray. Even though it is available in other countries, it is not available in India.

Administration and Schedule

The vaccine is not a part of NIP for healthy children. The vaccine is given as 0.5 mL intramuscularly in anterolateral thigh/deltoid muscle to children from 6 months to 8 years in a two-dose schedule at an interval of 4 weeks or more for the first-time recipients. Other children >8 years and adults require one dose. Annual vaccination is recommended for children belonging to high-risk groups including those with chronic systemic diseases, hemoglobinopathy, immunosuppression, and household contacts. A few vaccine recipients may develop short-lasting local and transient systemic reactions such as fever, malaise, and myalgia. The vaccine should be temporarily withheld in moderately sick children till they recover and is contraindicated in those with a history of anaphylaxis to an earlier dose of vaccine or egg.

RABIES VACCINES

Characteristics

Rabies vaccines in India are viral inactivated cell culture vaccines and developed from tissue culture. Vaccines include:

- Human diploid cell vaccine (HDCV)
- Purified chick embryo cell vaccine (PCECV)
- Purified vero cell vaccine (PVCV)
- Purified duck embryo vaccine (PDEV)

All these vaccines are lyophilized products supplied with sterile water as diluent and must be used within 8 hours of reconstitution. The vaccines contain ≥2.4 IU of antigen/intramuscular dose (as per WHO recommendation).

Administration and Schedule

Rabies vaccines are used both for postexposure (PEP) and preexposure (PrEP) prophylaxis from the disease. Since the transmission of rabies virus is almost exclusively through the bite of an infected animal and as the incubation period is relatively long, the use of rabies vaccine as postexposure prophylaxis is possible. The dose of vaccine is 0.5 mL (PCECV) or 1 mL (HDCV) depending upon the product and this must be given intramuscularly regardless of the age or weight of the child. The recommended site of injection is deltoid muscle (>2 years of age) and/or anterolateral part of thigh in infants and young children. The vaccine should never be given in the gluteal region as the subcutaneous fat in this area retards the absorption of the antigen and if it is given inadvertently in this region, that dose is not counted in the schedule and must be repeated. There are no contraindications to the use of these vaccines for postexposure prophylaxis. Fever, local redness, and pain may occur following vaccine administration.

Considered as a gold standard in the rabies prevention, these vaccines satisfy all the criteria of potency, immunogenicity, and safety. The vaccines, whether in use for PrEP or PEP, induce protective antibodies in >99% of vaccine recipients.

The use of *intradermal route* in government sectors helps to reduce the costs resulting in the dose sparing from the vaccine vial when the vaccine can be administered during a session to a larger number of vaccines. National rabies prophylaxis program uses two intradermal doses of 0.1 mL at different sites on day 0, 3, 7, and 28 days. Intradermal schedule is not recommended in private health setup and for immunocompromised persons who should receive standard regimen of total of four doses on day 0, 3, 7, and between 14 and 28 days by *intramuscular route*. There should be no delay in the initiation of PEP regardless of the availability of rabies immunoglobulin.

After the bite, care of the wound and adjoining area is very important. Wound should be immediately washed and flushed with soap or detergent and running water or with water alone for a minimum of 15 minutes to remove the virus. Suturing must be avoided for 1 week as it facilitates the spread of the virus in the deeper tissues and if unavoidable the sutures should be loosely applied after local infiltration of rabies immunoglobulin (RIG). Deeper wounds are to be irrigated with povidone-iodine or ethanol 70%. If indicated, TT should be administered.

Passive prophylaxis is given in all category III bites and category II and III bites in immunocompromised persons **(Table 13.3)**. This is done by the use of RIG or antirabies monoclonal antibodies (MoAb). Antirabies MoAb is highly purified, safe, and effective and should be given along with the rabies vaccine on day 0. It can be given maximally up to 7 days after the exposure and the total amount must be infiltrated in and around the wound. Passive prophylaxis is not required in those who have received PrEP or have received RIG in the past. All wounds irrespective of the categories need thorough wound washing. A bite from any wild animal is considered as category III bite and thus be treated accordingly.

Rabies Vaccine/Passive Prophylaxis for Different Categories

Rabies prophylaxis is based on the category of the exposure/bite **(Table 13.3)**. All wounds irrespective of the categories need thorough wound washing. A bite from any wild animal is considered as category III bite and thus be treated accordingly.

Pre-exposure prophylaxis: This is recommended for persons who are at a high risk of exposure to rabies such as laboratory staff, veterinary doctors, delivery agents, postmen, security personnel, zoo and forest workers, and travelers and residents to endemic regions with extensive outdoor activities. PrEP is not generally practiced in children though it may be discussed with parents who have pets at home. The schedule includes three doses on day 0, 7, and 21–28 days by intramuscular route.

Table 13.3 Postexposure Prophylaxis

Category	*Types of exposure*	*Treatment required*
Category I	• Touching, feeding, or licks of the animal • Licks on the intact skin	No treatment is required as this is not considered an exposure
Category II	• Nibbling of uncovered skin • Minor scratches or abrasions without bleeding • Licks or nibbles on the broken skin	• Use rabies vaccine alone in healthy persons • In immunocompromised, use vaccine and immunoglobulin
Category III	• Single or multiple transdermal bites, abrasions • Licks on broken skin • Contamination of mucous membrane with saliva	Use vaccine and immunoglobulin

MENINGOCOCCAL VACCINES

Routine immunization against meningococcal disease is not recommended in India. A quadrivalent vaccine containing purified bacterial polysaccharide antigen from serogroups A, C, Y, and W135 is available. In India, epidemics are usually caused by type A or C while endemic cases are mainly due to type B. No vaccine is available for protection against group B disease. Group A antigen is immunogenic in children over 3 months of age and group C over 2 years of age.

Types of Vaccines

Vaccines are available as (1) Polysaccharide unconjugated, or (2) Conjugated vaccines. Unconjugated vaccines are not immunogenic in children below 2 years of age and do not induce immunological memory. These are either monovalent (containing serogroup) bivalent (A and C) or quadrivalent (A, C, Y, and W 135).

Polysaccharide-protein conjugate meningococcal vaccines are now available in India. These are effective in infants and younger children and are approved for use from the age of 9 months onward.

Administration

A single intramuscular injection of 0.5 mL is recommended for high-risk children with asplenia and complement deficiencies. During an outbreak, immunization may be recommended to persons at risk. The vaccine is indicated for use (as an adjunct to chemoprophylaxis) in close contacts of patients with the disease, in immune deficiency conditions and travel to high endemicity belt in African Continent. The vaccine is mandatory for Haj pilgrims and residential students in some universities abroad.

Protective Efficacy

Meningococcal vaccines are safe and induce protective antibodies in adults and children over the age of 2 years. However, like other polysaccharide vaccines, it does not produce immunological memory and repeated doses are required for long-term protection. In children over 2 years, a single dose is recommended. Revaccination may be indicated after 2–3 years for children who are first immunized at the age of <4 years and remain at high risk of infection. This interval is increased to 5 years for older children and adults. Side effects are mild and short lasting such as pain and local inflammation.

YELLOW FEVER VACCINE

The vaccine against yellow fever (YF) is a live-attenuated vaccine grown on chick embryo cells. It is available as freeze dried formulation in a single/multiple dose vials with sterile saline as its diluent. The reconstituted vaccine is heat labile and must be used within 1 hour of its preparation. It should be stored between

2 and 8°C. The protective efficacy is between 90 and 100% and according to WHO, a single dose confers lifelong protection.

Yellow fever vaccine is given by subcutaneous or intramuscular route in a dose of 0.5 mL. In endemic countries such as sub-Saharan Africa and Central and South America, the vaccine is administered at 9–12 months of age. In India, it is mandatory for travelers aged 9 months to 60 years who are visiting an endemic country. One dose should be administered at least 10 days before arrival to the endemic country. While pregnancy is considered as a contraindication for the use of vaccine, lactating mothers and persons >60 years can be administered the vaccine by taking adequate precautions.

Yellow fever vaccine has transient adverse effects such as mild fever, headache, and myalgia for 5–10 days. Severe side effects such as anaphylaxis and neurologic reactions are extremely rare.

CHOLERA VACCINES

This vaccine is not recommended for routine use in healthy individuals, its recommended only for the vaccination of persons residing in highly endemic areas and people travelling to such areas and where the risk of outbreak such as during pilgrimages like Kumbh Mela, etc. The whole cell inactivated injectable cholera vaccine has now been withdrawn due to its poor efficacy and high reactogenicity. Subsequently, two types of oral cholera vaccines were developed which are effective and safe to use.

Oral Inactivated Cholera Vaccines

Oral cholera vaccines have been developed which are safe, immunogenic, and effective. Two types of inactivated/killed oral vaccines, including a monovalent (*Vibrio cholerae* O1) and a bivalent (*V. cholerae* O1 and O139) are currently in use globally. A killed whole cell oral cholera vaccine (Shanchol-TM) is currently available for use in India. This bivalent vaccine has been found to be safe and confer significant protection against El Tor cholera in both children and adults and has been in use with reasonably good efficacy and long-term protection. The protective efficacy of two doses is 80–85% by inducing an IgA antibody response and preventing the attachment of *V. cholerae* to the gut receptors. There are three oral cholera vaccines in use in other countries.

The vaccine is available in a ready to use single dose formulation and is given orally as 1.5 mL in a two-dose schedule given 14 days apart. It may cause mild side effects such as abdominal pain and diarrhea in few recipients.

Live-attenuated Vaccine

CVD 103-HgR vaccine is a live-attenuated oral cholera vaccine. It consists of genetically modified *V. cholerae* O1 strain (CVD 103-HgR). This vaccine appears to be safe and immunogenic in children >2 years of age. A single dose confers around 65% protection. Long-term protection is doubtful. This vaccine may be useful in prevention of cholera before or during epidemic. There are a number of live oral vaccines undergoing phase II and phase III trials and the results are promising.

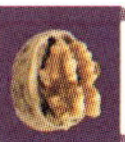

IN A NUTSHELL

Other Vaccines

1. Apart from the vaccines used in NIP, there are a few other vaccines which are widely available and used in private health setups and are recommended for routine use by Indian Academy of Pediatrics (IAP).
2. Amongst different types of typhoid vaccines, typhoid conjugate vaccine (TCV) is preferred due to its improved immunological properties and ability to be used as early as 6 months of age.
3. Hepatitis A vaccines in their scheduled doses provide long-lasting and possibly lifelong protection against the disease in children and adults.
4. Being a live viral vaccine, varicella vaccine should not be given in immunocompromised children, leukemia, HIV infection, and children on corticosteroid therapy.
5. Annual influenza vaccination is recommended for children belonging to high-risk groups such as those with chronic systemic diseases, hemoglobinopathies, immunosuppression, and their household contacts.
6. Following an exposure to potential rabies, there should be no delay in the initiation of recommended rabies postexposure prophylaxis along with the immediate and appropriate wound management and its surrounding area.
7. Meningococcal vaccines are recommended for high-risk situations (e.g., asplenia), and during outbreaks.
8. Meningococcal vaccine is mandatory for Haj pilgrims and residential students in some universities abroad.
9. Yellow fever vaccine is mandatory for all the travelers between the ages of 9 months to 60 years who are visiting endemic regions such as sub-Saharan Africa, Central and South America.
10. Yellow fever vaccine must be administered in a registered or authorized government vaccination center.
11. A killed whole cell oral cholera vaccine is currently available for use in India. It is recommended to be used for those residing in or traveling to endemic regions with a risk of cholera outbreaks.

Advisory Committee on Vaccines and Immunization Practices, Indian Academy of Pediatrics. Meningococcal Vaccines. In: Pemde HK, Vashishtha VM, Yewale VN, et al. (Eds). IAP Guidebook on Immunization 2018-19. New Delhi: Jaypee Brothers Medical Publishers; 2020. pp. 352-66.

Advisory Committee on Vaccines and Immunization Practices, Indian Academy of Pediatrics. Typhoid Vaccines. In: Guduru VK, Kalra A, Vashishtha VM (Eds). IAP Guidebook on Immunization 2018-19. New Delhi: Jaypee Brothers Medical Publishers; 2020. pp. 278-301.

Dutta AK, Swaminathan S, Abitbol V, et al. A Comprehensive Review of Meningococcal Disease Burden in India. Infect Dis Ther. 2020;9(3):537-59.
Kumar R. Varicella Vaccine. In: Gupta P, Menon PSN, Ramji S, et al. (Eds). PG Textbook of Pediatrics, 3rd edition. New Delhi: Jaypee Brothers Medical Publishers; 2022. pp. 1176-8.
Saxena D, Yasobant S, Shah Tushar P. Rabies Vaccine. In: Shah T, Shah A (Eds). Adult Immunization in Office Practice. Jaypee Brothers Medical Publishers; 2023. pp. 116-21.
World Health Organization. Rabies vaccines: WHO position paper–April 2018. Wkly Epidemiol Rec. 2018;93:201-20.
Zhang L. Hepatitis A vaccination. Hum Vaccin Immunother. 2020;16(7):1565-73.

13.4 Vaccine Storage and Cold Chain

PE 18.4, PE 18.9

INTRODUCTION

The term "cold chain" is used to denote a chain of personnel, equipment, and processes which are utilized for maintaining the potency and effectiveness of vaccines by keeping them at recommended temperatures during transportation, distribution, and storage from the site of manufacture to the point of their actual use.

The cold chain plays a crucial role in the immunization process because vaccines are sensitive to heat and light and improper cold chain maintenance can irreversibly affect their potency and efficacy. *This loss of potency can lead to vaccine failure with a negative impact on immunization program.* The vital components of cold chain include the following:

- Proper monitoring, maintenance, handling, and storage of vaccines.
- Transport and storage equipment.
- Trained personnel.

The Government of India has rolled out an Electronic Vaccine Intelligence Network (eVIN) system that digitizes the entire vaccine stock management, their logistics and temperature tracking at all levels of vaccine storage–from national to the sub-district.

HEAT SENSITIVE VACCINES

Vaccines are biological products and, therefore, vulnerable to the extreme temperature variations. All the vaccines are sensitive to heat to some extent but some are more sensitive than others. Repeated exposure to high temperatures has a cumulative damaging effect on vaccine potency. The commonly used vaccines can be ranked according to their sensitivity to heat as shown in **Figure 13.2**. The vaccines sensitive to freezing are shown in **Figure 13.3**.

- Vaccines such as bacillus Calmette-Guérin (BCG), measles, mumps, and rubella (MMR) are both light- and heat-sensitive. These vaccines are supplied in vials made up of dark-brown glass, which protects them against damage from light. Care must be taken to cover and protect them from strong light at all times.
- The diluents must never be frozen and need to be stored between 2 and 8°C.
- Vaccines containing aluminum-based adjuvants [diphtheria, pertussis and tetanus (DPT), DT, TT] are adversely affected by freezing temperatures. If these vaccines are accidentally frozen, they should be discarded.

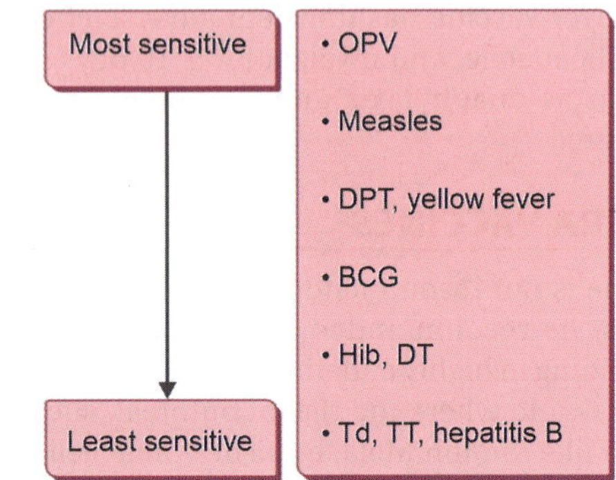

Fig. 13.2: Heat sensitivity of vaccines (BCG: bacillus Calmette–Guérin; DPT: diphtheria, pertussis and tetanus; OPV: oral polio vaccine)

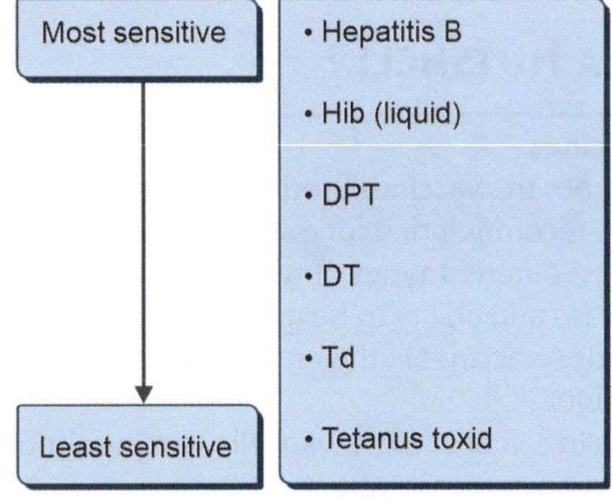

Fig. 13.3: Vaccines sensitivity to cold (DPT: diphtheria, pertussis and tetanus)

STRUCTURE OF COLD CHAIN

The structure of cold chain consists of two aspects, which are complementary to each other.

1. ***Fixed component*** includes walk in coolers, ice-lined refrigerators (ILR), deep freezers and refrigerators, and purpose-built refrigerators **(Fig. 13.4)**. The advantages offered by the purpose-built refrigerators are maintenance of a stable and controlled temperature between +2 and +8°C from top to bottom of the unit, increased storage space and a facility of an alarm to alert the internal temperature fluctuations.
2. The *mobile component* of the chain is represented by isothermal boxes and ice boxes. These make it possible to transport the vaccines to health units and are effective for

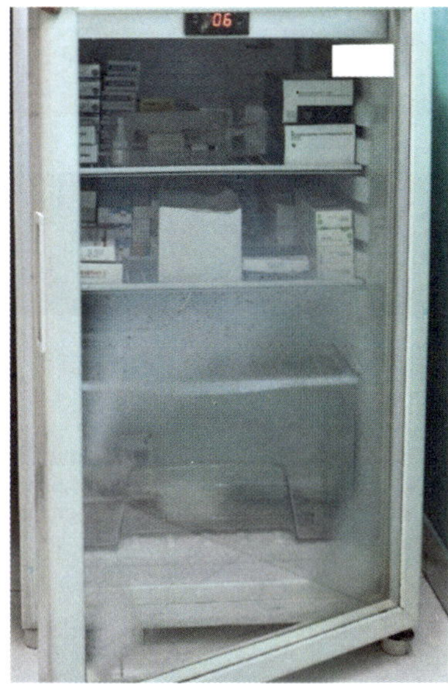

Fig. 13.4: Purpose-built refrigerator

outreach services. Vaccines need to be properly packed with the required number of frozen ice packs. The recommended storage temperature for these components is between +2 and +8°C.

At the higher levels of cold chain, i.e., national and regional, OPV must be kept frozen between -15 and -25°C. Freeze-dried vaccines (BCG, measles, MMR, and yellow fever) may also be kept frozen at -15 to -25°C but it is neither essential nor recommended. All the vaccines at other levels of cold chain should be stored between +2 and +8°C.

Care of Vaccines in Refrigerator

With the use of domestic refrigerators for vaccine storage, the following guidelines must be followed:

- Refrigerator must be at least 10 cm away from the wall to allow proper air circulation. It should be away from direct sunlight.
- Ice packs and water-filled bottles should be kept in freezer compartment and the shelves, respectively.
- Store vaccine boxes or trays with spaces in between to allow air circulation inside the refrigerator.
- No vaccines should be stored in door compartment.
- Voltage control and periodic defrosting (when the ice layer in freezer is >5 mm) are important maintenance issues.
- Vaccines should be used on the "first in and first out" basis.
- Temperature log should be maintained twice daily.

VACCINE VIAL MONITORS

The vaccine vial monitor (VVM) is an indicator applied on each vial of vaccine and helps decide the potency of the vaccine at the time of its use. VVMs were first introduced on the vials of OPV in 1996. The VVM is a small square of heat sensitive material (diacetylene), which on exposure to heat becomes dark in color, thus giving a visual indication about usability of the particular OPV vial. Combined effects of time and temperature lead to gradual and irreversible change in the color of small square from light to dark and the color of outer circle is used as a reference **(Fig. 13.5)**.

Based upon the heat sensitivity of the vaccine(s), there are four types of VVM which include VVM2, VVM7, VVM14, and VVM30. These numbers correspond to the number of days after which VVM reaches its end point when exposed to temperatures at +37°C. VVM2 means that it reaches its endpoint when exposed to temperatures of +37°C for 2 days. Hence, VVM2 is applied to most heat sensitive vaccines.

TO OBSERVE STORAGE AND HANDLING OF VACCINES

To Observe Storage

1. To observe whether the vaccine storage units are appropriately placed at a proper and firm level with good air circulation around the equipment and functioning properly or not.
2. To observe and check proper power supply to the fixed storage device. To ensure that there is a signage of "Do Not Unplug" near the supply point. An uninterruptible power supply (UPS) unit should be used to assure an uninterrupted power supply in case of power failure.
3. To observe and check that the door of the domestic/purpose-built refrigerator is kept closed, opened only when necessary, and the rubber seal fits well.
4. To observe and check if the temperature monitoring device in the storage unit is functional or not. Also check that the temperature reads between 2 and 8°C.
5. To observe the storage of water bottles in the door racks of the domestic refrigerator. They are not needed for certain types of purpose-built units.
6. To observe and check that no food/beverages are stored in the unit with the vaccines and other immunobiologicals.
7. To observe that the vaccines are properly placed in their original package as per recommendations in the unit.
8. There should be no loose vials and exposed prefilled syringes in the unit.
9. Check that no diluents are stored in the freezer unit.
10. Place vaccines and diluents in rows with adequate space for air circulation between them and those with earlier expiry dates in front and others with late expiry in back rows.

To Observe Handling

1. To observe and confirm the vaccine that is to be administered.
2. To observe and check the date of expiry and note the batch number.
3. To observe the VVM for temperature exposure and to confirm the suitability of that specific vial.
4. To observe all the aseptic precautions in the administration of the vaccine.
5. To observe opening of an ampoule or a vial only when the healthcare worker is ready to administer it. Open single use prefilled syringe (PFS) vaccine just before its use.
6. To observe whether the lyophilized vaccines are mixed and reconstituted with their supplied diluents under all aseptic precautions.

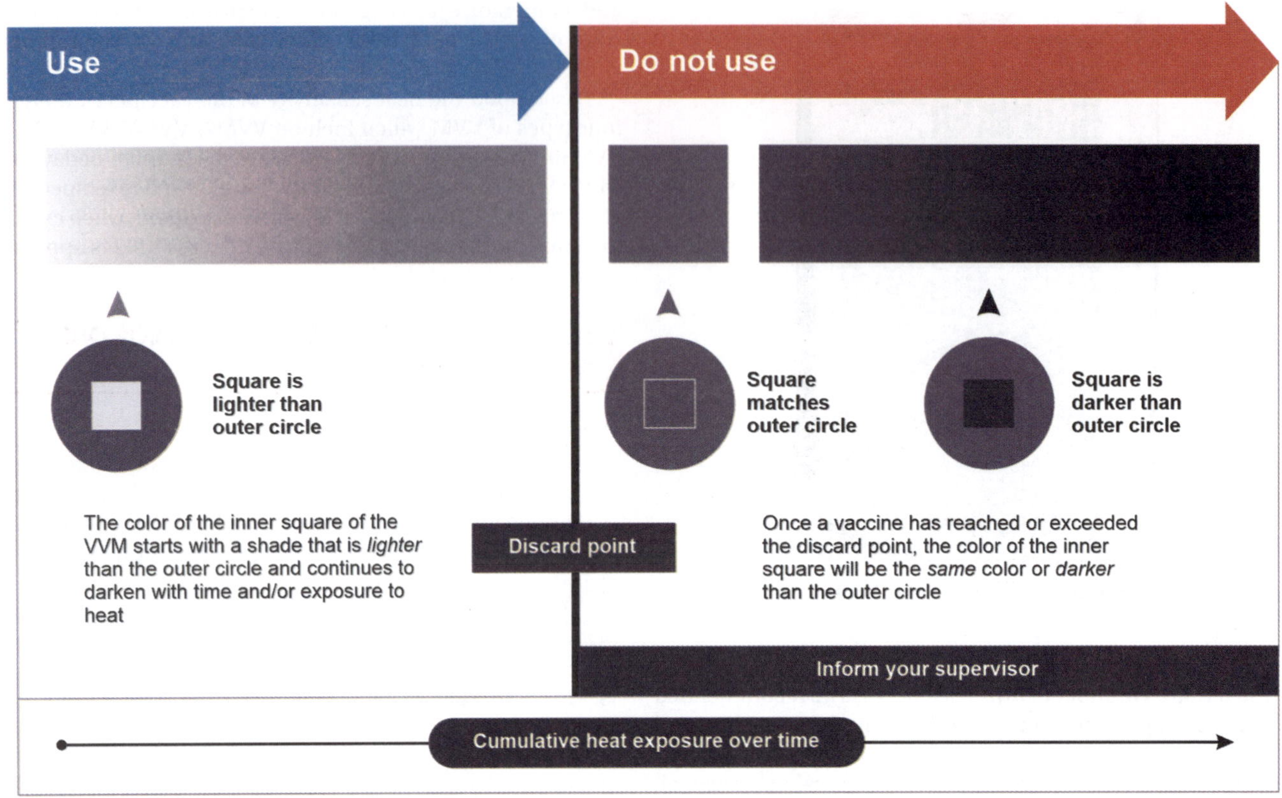

Fig. 13.5: Vaccine vial monitor (VVM) showing cumulative exposure change

Source: WHO. (2021). Vaccine vial monitor. [online] Available from https://www.who.int/publications/m/item/vaccine-vial-monitor [Last accessed November, 2022]

7. To observe that the diluents are brought to near room temperature at the time of administration.
8. To observe that all the vaccines in use (multidose vials) are kept with the ice pack during the session and away from direct sunlight and extremes of temperature.
9. To observe the use of single use auto-disable syringes for the vaccine administration.
10. To observe the proper disposal of the needles and syringes after their use as per the norms of biomedical waste management.

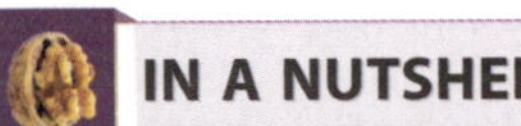

IN A NUTSHELL

Vaccine Storage and Cold Chain

1. Cold chain is an organized structure and function of personnel, equipment, and processes utilized for maintaining the potency and effectiveness of vaccines at recommended temperatures during transportation, distribution, and storage from the site of manufacture to the point of their actual use.
2. Any breech in cold chain can irreversibly affect the vaccine potency contributing to vaccine failure.
3. All the vaccines are sensitive to heat exposure and loss of potency but some of them are more sensitive than others such as OPV, and measles containing vaccines are most heat sensitive.
4. Vaccines such as DPT, DT and TT should never be frozen and if frozen accidentally those should be discarded.
5. Most vaccines and diluents can be stored between 2 and 8°C in the domestic and purpose-built refrigerators.
6. Vaccine vial monitors (VVMs) help the vaccine user to decide the potency of vaccine at the time of its administration.

Gupta A, Gupta R. Study of Cold Chain Practices at Community Health Centres of Damoh District Of Madhya Pradesh. Natl J Community Med. 2015;6(04):528-32.

Gupta P, Menon PSN, Ramji S, et al. Vaccine Storage and Cold Chain. PG Textbook of Pediatrics, 3rd edition. New Delhi: Jaypee Brothers Medical Publishers Pvt Ltd; 2022. pp. 1116-23.

Parekh BJ, Kasi SG, Wadhwa A, et al. Cold Chain Management. In: Parekh BJ, Kasi SG, Wadhwa A, et al. (Eds). IAP Q & A on Vaccines and Vaccinology, 1st edition. New Delhi: Jaypee Brothers Medical Publishers Pvt Ltd; 2021. pp. 54-71.

13.5 Immunization in Specific Situations

PE 18.5

INTRODUCTION

The administration of childhood vaccines is an integral part of an immunization program and is a general recommendation for normal and healthy children. However, there are heterogeneous situations in childhood and adolescence where the benefits of the delivered vaccines may be suboptimal and/or there may be a higher risk of developing AEFI. Such situations where specific needs must be addressed are included under the category of "immunization in specific situations." A few examples of such situations include:

- Preterm and low birth weight (LBW) babies
- Children with immune deficiencies or dysfunction
- Patients with organ transplants
- Recipients of blood and blood products
- Chronic systemic diseases

PRETERM AND LOW BIRTH WEIGHT BABIES

Basic considerations for these situations include:

- In a majority of preterm and LBW babies, with stable clinical conditions immunizations should be carried out at the recommended chronological age and according to the same schedule and precautions as for full-term infants and children.
- The full-recommended doses of the vaccines should be used. Divided or reduced doses are not recommended.
- BCG and birth dose of OPV should be administered as soon as the newborn is in stable condition or just prior to the discharge from the hospital.
- Decreased seroconversion rates might occur among certain preterm and LBW babies who are <2.0 kg at birth, after hepatitis B vaccine. However, if the mother is HBsAg positive or has unknown HBsAg status, the babies should receive HBV vaccine and hepatitis B immunoglobulin (HBIG) prophylaxis within 12 hours of birth for immediate protection. The babies weighing <2.0 kg born to HBsAg negative mothers should receive the first dose of HBV vaccine at 1 month of age or earlier whenever the desired weight is achieved.
- Rotavirus vaccine should be deferred until discharge from the hospital unit to prevent the potential spread of vaccine virus in the nursery. Rotavirus vaccine can be given during follow-up visits after the discharge from the hospital.
- Presence of low muscle mass may require the use of smaller gauge needles (5/8 inch or lesser) for intramuscular route of vaccines.

LAPSED IMMUNIZATIONS

Due to persistence of immunologic memory, longer than routinely recommended intervals between the doses do not impair the immunologic response in case of live and attenuated vaccines which need more than one dose to achieve primary immunity. Similarly, delayed administration of booster doses does not adversely affect the antibody response to vaccines. The interruption of the recommended primary series or an extended and delayed interval for boosters does not need reinitiation of entire vaccination series.

UNKNOWN IMMUNIZATION STATUS

Such children should always be considered as unimmunized and are being susceptible to the disease and age-appropriate recommended immunizations should be administered. There is nothing to suggest that the administration of polio vaccine, hepatitis B vaccine, MMR, Hib, or varicella vaccine to already immune recipients is harmful.

Missed opportunities for immunization are defined as situations when a child visits a health facility and is not immunized. Minor illnesses, such as fever, respiratory infections and diarrhea, and malnutrition, should not be considered as contraindications to immunization and the vaccines should be given as per schedule.

CHILDREN WITH IMMUNE DEFICIENCY OR DYSFUNCTION

These conditions can be primary (such as inherited disorders of T- and B-cell dysfunction, phagocytic function, or complement function) or may be secondary (malignancy, HIV infection, steroids/other immunosuppressive therapy, hematopoietic stem cell transplant and solid organ transplant recipients, and splenectomy/asplenia). The determination of immunocompetence in such children is important.

- All the live vaccines are generally contraindicated in severe immunodeficiency states due to risk of serious disseminated disease because of uncontrolled viral replication. In situations with mild-to-moderate immune deficient states (e.g., anatomical or functional asplenia), these may be given after risk-benefit analysis.
- All the inactivated/killed vaccines can be given but the vaccine immunogenicity and efficacy may be decreased due to their inability to mount adequate immune response. Thus, a higher strength dose or an increased number of doses (e.g., hepatitis B vaccine) may be required.
- Specific serum antibodies should be measured to evaluate immune response. Additional/booster doses need to be given if the antibody titers remain low.
- Transmission of vaccine virus (e.g., OPV) from a household contact to immunocompromised host can occur and hence injectable polio vaccine should be used for children living in the same house. Other immunocompetent persons in the household should be up-to-date with their immunization (e.g., MMR, varicella, and annual influenza vaccine) to minimize the risk of exposure to the immunocompromised child.

CHILDREN ON STEROID THERAPY

Children who are receiving 2 mg/kg/day or 20 mg/day of prednisolone or its equivalent for more than 2 weeks are considered immunosuppressed. Live vaccines should not be given to these children. Killed/inactivated vaccines and toxoids are safe.

Corticosteroid therapy is not a contraindication to administering live vaccines, if:

- The administration is short term (<2 weeks)
- On a low-to-moderate dose (<20 mg prednisolone per day)
- On long-term alternate day therapy
- When steroids are given by topical, inhaled, or intra-articular routes

Children who have received steroid therapy in high doses for >2 weeks should be vaccinated 1 month after stopping the treatment, as it is believed that the immune function would have returned to normal by then.

CHILDREN ON IMMUNOSUPPRESSIVE DRUGS

Whenever feasible, all indicated vaccines should be provided before the initiation of chemotherapy and/or radiotherapy. Children with leukemia, solid tumors, or organ transplants are considered to be immunodeficient. In children with cancer on therapy, live vaccines should not be given during the chemotherapy and for at least 6 months after stopping such immunosuppressive treatment. The need for additional and booster doses of vaccines is also determined by the earlier immunization status of the child, degree of immunosuppression caused by the disease, and the immunosuppressive therapy. Inactivated vaccines given during chemotherapy might need to be repeated after immune competence is regained. Patients receiving other drugs and biological agents (e.g., ILs, GM-CSF) are also immunosuppressed and should not be given live viral vaccines at least for 3 months after stopping the therapy.

Children who have received a highly suppressive chemotherapy and hematopoietic stem cell transplant (HSCT) should be revaccinated with all age-appropriate vaccines as they are virtually unimmunized and unprotected *due to the loss of memory responses after marrow ablation.*

HIV INFECTION

Children infected by HIV are vulnerable to severe, recurrent, or unusual infections by vaccine preventable pathogens. The efficacy and safety of vaccines depends on the degree of immunodeficiency. In general, in early life, most vaccines are safe and efficacious as the immune system is relatively well-preserved. The duration of protection may be compromised as there is impairment of memory response with immune attrition. HIV infected children with CD4+ counts <200/mm^3 mount a suboptimal or a negligible immune response. Efficacy and safety are significantly lower in advanced disease. Consideration should be given to readministering childhood immunizations to such children when their immune status has improved following antiretroviral therapy. Vaccination of a baby born to an HIV positive mother but with an indeterminate HIV status should be as per the normal schedule.

CHILDREN WITH SPLENECTOMY/ASPLENIA

Children with anatomic or functional asplenia (such as sickle cell disease, splenectomy, and following radiotherapy) are at an increased risk of infections with encapsulated organisms especially with *S. pneumoniae, N. meningitidis,* and *H. influenzae* b. Vaccines against these organisms should be considered at least 2 weeks before elective splenectomy. If these vaccines are not administered before emergency surgery, they should be given 2 weeks after the surgery.

RECIPIENTS OF BLOOD/BLOOD PRODUCTS

Administration of blood products (packed red blood cells, whole blood, plasma, and platelets) and antibodies containing products (e.g., IVIG, specific immunoglobulins for rabies, or HBV) can interfere with the immune responses to the live vaccines depending on the amount of antigen specific antibodies present in the blood/blood products. Some basic principles to follow are:

- Live parenteral vaccines (e.g., MMR and varicella) should not be given simultaneously or at an interval shorter than the recommended duration with the blood products. Based upon the blood product, this interval varies from 3 to 11 months.
- Inactivated, subunit (polysaccharide, recombinant vaccines, and toxoids) and oral live vaccines (rotavirus and OPV) can be given before, after, or concurrently with these products.
- Subcutaneous administration of yellow fever vaccine (live vaccine) can be given, if necessary.
- Different sites and separate injections must be used for both the vaccines and the blood product, if concurrent use is needed.
- Washed RBC transfusion greatly decreases the proportion of antibodies in the product and hence no minimum interval is required between the vaccines.

In exceptional situations such as a high-risk child, live parenteral vaccine may be given before the minimum prescribed interval between the two but the dose must not be counted.

SOLID ORGAN TRANSPLANTS

Children due for solid organ transplant (SOT) must complete their age-appropriate immunizations before the scheduled transplant as the ongoing disease process, immunosuppressive treatment, and organ failure can contribute to decreased vaccine responses. Inactivated and live vaccines need to be completed at least 2 and 4 weeks prior to transplant procedure, respectively. This should be followed by documentation of antibody responses and seroconversion before the transplant. MMR and varicella vaccines may be administered between 6 and 11 months, if the transplant is scheduled before the age of 1 year.

Following transplant, inactivated vaccines can be given after 6 months and there may be a need for booster doses (e.g., HBV vaccine). Inactivated influenza vaccine can be given within 1–2 months and then annually while all the live vaccines are contraindicated post-transplant. All the household persons and healthcare workers in contact with SOT patient should receive influenza, varicella, and MMR vaccines to reduce the risk of these VPDs in the transplanted child.

CHILDREN WITH COCHLEAR IMPLANTS

Children with cochlear implants are more prone to acute bacterial meningitis than normal children. Such children should be up to date in their routine immunization. In addition they should be immunized with pneumococcal conjugate vaccine (PCV) and influenza vaccine. In children >24 months, the dose of PCV should be followed by PPSV (23), 8 weeks later. The immunization is best completed at least 2 weeks before the scheduled implant.

CHILDREN WITH CHRONIC SYSTEMIC DISEASES

Children with systemic and chronic diseases (e.g., nephrotic syndrome and chronic liver diseases) have an increased risk of infectious diseases and their complications. These children should be offered vaccines for which they are eligible on an individual basis depending upon their previous immunization status. Children with chronic liver diseases must be protected against hepatitis B and hepatitis A infections. Children with chronic cardiac and pulmonary diseases need protection with pneumococcal vaccine and annual dose of influenza vaccine. Unless there is an associated immunodeficiency along with systemic disease, live vaccines can be administered.

IMMUNIZATION OF ADOLESCENTS

Adolescents represent an important additional target group for immunization. The need for adolescent immunization is based on the following considerations:

- Adolescents may or may not have received full courses (including timely boosters) and other vaccines either due to earlier unavailability or lack of access.
- They present unique challenges for immunization due to their lifestyle and potential risk-taking behaviors and other social issues.
- Immunity provided by childhood vaccines (such as diphtheria, pertussis, and tetanus) starts waning off and needs boosting.
- Epidemiological shift of diseases (e.g., hepatitis A, varicella, and pertussis) due to increasing coverage of childhood immunization makes adolescents vulnerable to these VPDs.
- Timely administration of vaccines such as HPV in adolescent girls can prevent cervical cancer in adulthood.
- Visits for immunization provide opportunities for counseling services to follow a healthy lifestyle.
- National immunization schedule has at present diphtheria and tetanus booster (Td), JE vaccine in endemic regions and MR vaccine in campaign programs. If any adolescent has not received or completed the course of recommended vaccines, he/she should be offered catch-up immunization on an individualized basis. These include MMR, hepatitis B, hepatitis A, TCV, and varicella vaccines. Any eligible/missed immunization needs to be completed as catch up immunization.

VACCINES FOR TRAVELERS

With the COVID-19 pandemic, the need for vaccines for domestic and international travel has been strengthened during the past 2 years. WHO has recommended that all the travelers to international destinations should be up-to-date with the routine vaccinations for the prevention and transmission of VPDs. This depends upon the earlier vaccination history, age of the traveler, pre-existing comorbidities and regions to be visited and the times of travel such as mass gatherings/religious events (e.g., Haj and Kumbh Melas). The purpose of vaccines for travelers is for own protection, possible transmission, and not to bring back the disease-causing microorganisms to his/her country. Few general recommendations are as follows:

- All the travelers must be familiar with the travel advisories on the official websites of home nation, countries in transit, and the destination country.
- All the vaccines/doses must be completed 2–4 weeks before the travel.
- All the vaccine records must be easily accessible and kept handy.
- Yellow fever vaccine is mandatory for travelers to and from endemic countries as Africa and South America.
- Meningococcal vaccine is mandatory for Haj pilgrimage, and study in UK, USA, and certain other countries.
- Bivalent OPV is required (one dose) within past 12 months and at least 4 weeks before travel to countries such as Afghanistan, Nigeria, and few other Asian and African counties. IPV is alternatively acceptable in few countries.
- Travelers to regions/countries where cholera and/or Japanese encephalitis are endemic should be given specified vaccines.

COMBINATION VACCINES

A combination vaccine consists of two or more separate immunogens that have been physically combined in a single preparation. Certain combination vaccines, such as DTwP/Hib/HBV, DTaP/Hib/IPV, DTaP/Hib/HBV/IPV, MR, MMR vaccines are available and are in use for many years. The presence of symbol (/) indicates that the vaccines are supplied in a premixed form and are given as a single injection. Vaccines such as DPT, OPV, and IPV are also considered as combination of different antigens. The prerequisites for combining two or more different antigens into a single vaccine are:

- The combination should not decrease purity, potency, efficacy, and safety of any of the individual components.
- Combination vaccine should not be inferior with respect to any of its individual components.

Advantages

The benefits of combination vaccines include:

- Reduced number of injections.
- Reduced pain and anxiety to the child and parents.

- Reduced number of visits and better compliance.
- Successful implementation of immunization programs (such as MR vaccine campaigns).
- Improved logistics and reduced burden on storage and handling.

Limitations

- Combination of different antigens into one vaccine may lead to chemical incompatibility or immunologic interference that may be difficult to overcome.
- The process of production of combination vaccines is different from that of mixing two vaccines in a single vaccine vial.
- Different vaccine schedules may cause certain degree of uncertainty and confusion.
- Combination product must fit into immunization schedule without much compromise in the recommended age and interval of individual vaccines.
- Rarely the occurrence of an adverse event following combination vaccine can cause uncertainty over the specific cause of antigenic reaction.

Considering these factors, only licensed combination vaccines should be used. Additionally, separate vaccines should not be combined at the time of administration unless approved by regulatory authority.

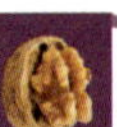

IN A NUTSHELL

Immunization in Specific Situations

1. Live vaccines are generally contraindicated in patients with significant immunosuppression such as patients with congenital or acquired immunodeficiency, patients on cancer chemotherapy, immunosuppressive therapy, and transplant recipients.
2. Children who have received steroid therapy in high doses for more than 2 weeks should be vaccinated 1 month after stopping the treatment.
3. Live vaccines should not be given during the chemotherapy and for at least 6 months after stopping such immunosuppressive treatment.
4. All inactivated or killed vaccines can be given to immunosuppressed individuals however, the immune response may be suboptimal. Immunosuppressed patients are most vulnerable to catch infections, so all efforts should be made to provide the maximum number of safe vaccinations which are permissible.
5. Vaccines should be spaced appropriately with the antibody containing blood products. In case of lapsed, unknown, incomplete or catch-up immunization, there is no need to restart the immunization series.
6. In a majority of preterm and LBW babies, immunizations should be carried out at the recommended chronological age and according to the same schedule and precautions as for full-term infants and children. The full recommended doses of the vaccines should be used.
7. In case of lapsed, incomplete, or catch-up immunization, there is no need to restart the immunization series.
8. Any child who has an unknown vaccination status should be considered as an unimmunized child and should receive the recommended age-appropriate vaccines.

American Academy of Pediatrics. Immunization in special clinical circumstances. In: Pickering LK, Baker CJ, Kimberlin DW, et al. (Eds). Red Book: 2018 Report of the Committee on Infectious Diseases, 28th edition. Elk Grove Village, IL: American Academy of Pediatrics; 2009.

Casswall TH, Fischler B. Vaccination of the immunocompromised child. Expert Rev Vaccines. 2005;4(5):725-38.

Centers for Disease Control and Prevention (CDC). General Recommendations on Immunization. Recommendations of the Advisory Committee on Immunization Practices (ACIP). MMWR. 2019;60:1-61.

L'Hullier AG, Kumar D. Immunizations in solid organ and hematopoeitic stem cell transplant patients: A comprehensive review. Hum Vaccin Immunother. 2015;11(12):2852-63.

Naqvi A, Fadoo Z, Alvi S. Vaccination guidelines for children with cancer and hematopoietic stem cell transplantation living in resource-poor countries. Pediatr Blood Cancer. 2010;54(1):3-7.

Rubin GI, Levin MJ, Ljungman P, et al. 2013 IDSA clinical practice guidelines for vaccination of the immunocompromised host. Clin Infect Dis. 2014;58(3):309-18.

13.6 Parental Education, Counseling, and Ethical Issues

PE 18.7, PE 18.8

- Introduce yourself, be patient and calm, and inform the need and protection the child needs from timely immunization.
- Accept the concerns and doubts, if any, the parents have and avoid any judgment and discuss their issues in a scientific and empathetic way.

- Inform parents that the child's well-being and safety from VPDs by immunization is a shared interest between the parents and the healthcare professionals.
- Give them the relevant information about the vaccine(s) to be administered.
- Inform and discuss with them about the information available on internet, though useful, cannot always be relied upon as it may not be always based on science and the reliability of the source of information. Dispel the myths spread by antivaccine lobbies.
- Tell them that the benefits of vaccines far outweigh the risks of contacting the disease and its complications. Give them an example such as that of smallpox eradication and polio eradication.
- Avoid missed opportunities by explaining and counseling for multiple vaccines in one visit and continuing with scheduled vaccination even with mild disease.
- Tell them that the side effects are generally mild, can be managed easily, and serious events are extremely rare.
- Maintain a positive body language and a soft tone throughout the communication and the counseling.
- Avoid technical jargons as much as much possible (e.g., seizures and hyperpyrexia).
- Be honest and transparent, give options of free vaccines available at government centers (public health) versus options of paid vaccine in private setup.
- Explain the reason for the precautionary need to wait for 20 minutes after the vaccination in the vaccination center premises.

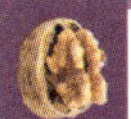

IN A NUTSHELL

Parental Education, Counseling, and Ethical Issues

1. Providing relevant information and addressing parents' concern about vaccines to be given is an essential step in childhood immunization.
2. Being transparent and patient during communication helps to allay parents' anxiety and hesitancy, if they have any.
3. Inform them that prevention of VPDs is a shared responsibility between the healthcare providers, families, and the community for the control of infectious diseases.

American Academy of Pediatrics. Talking with vaccine hesitant parents. [online] Available from https://www.aap.org/en/patient-care/immunizations/communicating-with-families-and-promoting-vaccine-confidence/talking-with-vaccine-hesitant-parents/ [Last accessed September, 2025].

Marotta S, McNally VV. Increasing Vaccine Confidence Through Parent Education and Empowerment Using Clear and Comprehensible Communication. Acad Pediatr. 2021;21(4):S30-1.

Murhekar, Manoj V, et al. Evaluating the effect of measles and rubella mass vaccination campaigns on seroprevalence in India: a before-and-after cross-sectional household serosurvey in four districts, 2018–2020. The Lancet Global Health. 2022;10(11):e1655-4.

Otsuka-Ono H, Hori N, Ohta H, et al. A childhood immunization education program for parents delivered during late pregnancy and one-month postpartum: a randomized controlled trial. BMC Health Serv Res. 2019;19:798.

Sankaranarayanan S, Jayaraman A, Gopichandran V. Assessment of Vaccine Hesitancy among Parents of Children between 1 and 5 Years of Age at a Tertiary Care Hospital in Chennai. Indian J Community Med. 2019;44(4):394-6.

13.7 Administration of Vaccines (Safe Vaccine Practices)

PE 18.8, PE 18.11, PE 18.12

INTRODUCTION

Improper administration of vaccine may pose a risk of adverse events including transmission of infection to recipient as well as to the healthcare provider. Safe and proper administration practices include appropriate counseling and communication with parents, safe injection practices and administration, infection control and documentation, and taking care of possible adverse events following immunization.

ROUTE AND SITE OF ADMINISTRATION

The vaccines should always be administered by their recommended route and at appropriate site. Deviation from the recommended route might reduce vaccine efficacy and/or increase local side effects. The routes of administration for childhood vaccines are intradermal (BCG, fIPV, and rabies can also be given), subcutaneous (measles, MMR, varicella), intramuscular (DPT, TT, hepatitis B, IPV, typhoid, PCV, influenza, rabies), oral (OPV, rotavirus vaccine), and intranasal (influenza).

The method of administration is partly determined by the presence of adjuvants in some vaccines and such vaccines should be given intramuscularly to avoid local irritation, inflammation, and granuloma formation. Adjuvants are the agents (mostly aluminum salts), which are distinct from the antigen and enhance the immunogenicity of the vaccines. The common vaccines that contain adjuvant include DPT, DT, TT, Hib, and hepatitis B virus (HBV) vaccines.

- Intradermal administration is mainly recommended for BCG vaccination. It is also recommended for fIPV in government hospitals/centers and for mass scale immunization for rabies vaccine. BCG is given intradermal at the site of deltoid insertion. A 3/8–3/4 inch, 26 gauge needle is used. The needle is inserted into epidermis at angle parallel to the long axis of the upper arm.
- The subcutaneous injections are administered at a 45° angle usually in the thigh in infants and in the upper outer triceps area for children older than 12 months, using a 5/8 inch 23–25 gauge needle.

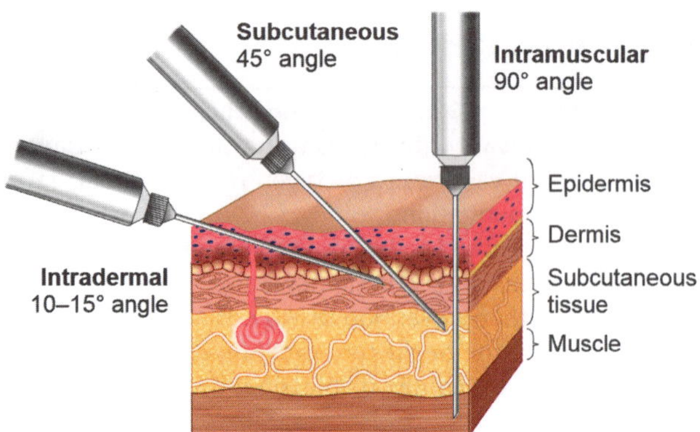

Fig. 13.6: Parenteral routes of vaccine administration
Source: WHO

- The intramuscular injections are given at a 90° angle preferably into the anterolateral aspect of the thigh (infants <12 months) as it provides a large muscle mass. A 23–25 gauge needle with a length of 5/8–1 inch is appropriate for intramuscular vaccines in infants and children. The gluteal region should not be used for vaccine administration due to the potential risk of injury to sciatic nerve and a decreased immunogenic response to the vaccine. The deltoid muscle should be used for intramuscular injection, if the muscle mass is adequate in children older than 12 months.
- Oral vaccines should be administered slowly over inside of the cheek to prevent gag reflex.
- Separate sites should be used, if multiple vaccines are to be given during the same visit. If two vaccines are to be given in the same limb, these should be separated from each other by at least one inch, so that any local reaction can be differentiated.

  Figure 13.6 shows parenteral routes of administration of vaccines.

  1. Patient anxiety during the procedure must be addressed. Assurance should be given and pain and fever management should be taken care of after the procedure.
  2. Safe injection practices and waste disposal are mandatory components of any vaccine(s) administration.
  3. The procedure should be followed by complete documentation and record keeping for future visits and further references.

NON-STANDARD PRACTICES

The recommendation for the dosage, site, and route of administration of immunobiologicals must be followed as any deviations from these recommendations can result in inadequate protection of the vaccine recipient. A few examples of such practices include the gluteal/intradermal administration of HBV vaccine, which results in substantially lower immunogenicity of the vaccine. Similarly, the doses of rabies vaccine given in gluteal region should not be counted as valid doses and should be repeated. Use of reduced dosages given at multiple immunization visits that equal a full dose is also not recommended.

INFECTION CONTROL AND STERILE TECHNIQUES

The administration of vaccines should observe appropriate steps and precautions to minimize infection.

- The hands should be cleansed either with an alcohol-based waterless antiseptic hand rub or washed with soap and water between each patient contact.
- The needle and syringes used for injection must be sterile and disposable to minimize the risk of contamination and a separate needle and syringe should be used for each injection.
- The changing of needle between drawing the vaccine from the vial and injecting it into the recipient is not necessary.
- The vaccines should never be mixed in the same syringe unless specifically licensed for such use.

Injection Safety

WHO estimates that at least 50% of world's 12 billion injections administered each year are unsafe and pose serious health risks to recipients, healthcare workers, and the public. Unsafe injection practices can cause local infections such as abscess and nerve injury and result in transmission of number of infections such as HBV, HCV, and HIV. Improving the safety of injection is an important component of universal precautions. WHO has defined safe injection as the one which (1) does not harm the patient, (2) does not expose the health worker to an avoidable risk, and (3) does not result in waste that puts other people at risk. The essential steps for a safe injection include:

- Preparation with clean hands in a clean area.
- Medication to be drawn in from a sterile vial.
- Use of sterile equipment at an appropriate site.
- Immediate discarding of needles and syringes to prevent needle stick injuries, in labeled puncture-proof containers located in the same room where the vaccines are administered. Needles should not be recapped before being placed in the container for appropriate disposal.
- Use of auto-disable (AD) syringes is being promoted in the NIP. AD syringes are single use, self-locking syringes designed in such a way that these are rendered unusable after single use.
- Syringes and needles should be disposed of as per the standard guidelines of the biomedical waste disposal and must not be reused.

TIMING AND SPACING ISSUES

While immunizing children, it is important to follow certain guidelines to derive the maximum benefit from the vaccines and to minimize the cost and the risk associated with vaccination. Optimal response to a vaccine depends upon multiple factors including the nature of the vaccine and the age and immune status of the recipient.

Spacing of Multiple Doses

The vaccines should be given as closely as possible to the recommended immunization schedule. Inactivated vaccines do not interfere with the immune response to other inactivated or live vaccines. An inactivated vaccine can be administered either simultaneously or any time before or after a different inactivated or live vaccine.

There should be at least 4 weeks interval between the live injected vaccines (measles, MMR, and varicella), if they are not administered on the same day. This is important to eliminate or reduce the interference from the vaccine given first on the vaccine given later. The dose of vaccine given too close to each other could reduce the efficacy of the vaccine. The recommended minimum interval for DPT and bOPV vaccines in primary immunization is 4 weeks.

Simultaneous Administration

Most of the childhood vaccines can be safely and effectively given simultaneously (during the same visit but not combined in the same syringe). Simultaneous administration of vaccines can improve the vaccine compliance and result in significant improvement of immunization rates in children. Simultaneous administration of most live and inactivated vaccines does not result in decreased antibody response or an increased rate of adverse reactions. The rates of adverse reactions seen after the use of combination vaccines are similar to those seen after the most reactogenic component, if given separately.

Spacing with Immunoglobulins

The presence of circulating antibody, e.g., immunoglobulins may reduce immune response to a vaccine antigen. Inactivated vaccines are not affected by immunoglobulins and thus can be given before, after, or at the same time as the immunoglobulins. Blood (whole blood, packed cells, and plasma) and other antibody containing blood products can inhibit the immune response to measles and rubella vaccines for a period ranging from 3 to 11 months depending upon product and dose. The effect of blood and immune globulin preparations on response to mumps and varicella vaccines is unknown.

The length of time that interferes with injectable live virus vaccine (other than yellow fever) can persist after the antibody-containing product is a function of the amount of antigen-specific antibody contained in the product. Thus, after an antibody-containing product is received, live vaccines (other than yellow fever, and rotavirus) should be delayed until the passive antibody has degraded. The recommended interval for administration of measles vaccine after administration of tetanus immunoglobulin, rabies immunoglobulin, packed red blood cell (RBC)/whole blood transfusion, and intravenous immunoglobulins is 3 months, 4 months, 6 months, and 8–11 months, respectively. Response to OPV, and yellow fever vaccine is not affected by antibody containing products and thus these vaccines can be given simultaneously or separated by any interval after blood products.

DOCUMENTATION AND RECORDKEEPING

Recordkeeping is an important aspect of good immunization practices. The availability of vaccines with different brand names, different combinations, and vaccination at different places often results in confusion. Improper records may result in missing or duplication of doses and improper schedules.

The ideal vaccination record should have date of vaccination, product administered, brand name, lot or batch number, expiry date, site and route of administration, and details of healthcare provider. The record should be clearly legible.

PREPAREDNESS FOR LIFE-THREATENING ADVERSE EVENTS FOLLOWING IMMUNIZATION

There should be functional resuscitation in place. It should be equipped with resuscitation facilities and medications (adrenalin, hydrocortisone, and normal saline) to treat anaphylaxis or any allergic reactions. The vaccinee should be observed for 15–20 minutes following vaccination.

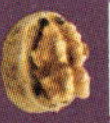

IN A NUTSHELL

Administration of Vaccines (Safe Vaccine Practices)

1. Do not deviate from the recommended route, site, and technique of administration.
2. Infection control and safe vaccination practices need utmost attention.
3. Proper documentation of vaccine administered is essential.
4. Vaccination setup should be well-prepared to manage life-threatening events like anaphylaxis.
5. Proper communication with parents regarding need, safety, efficacy, and cost of vaccine is a must.

Agrawal M. Immunization Agents. Immunization in Practice: Facts & FAQs, 1st edition. Mumbai: Bhalani Publishers; 2022. pp. 13-24.

CDC. (2020). Vaccine Safety Information for Health Care Providers. [online] Available from https://www.cdc.gov/vaccine-safety/hcp/clinical-safety/index.html#:~:text=Administering%20vaccines&text=While%20severe%2C%20life%2Dthreatening%20reactions,Reporting%20System%20(VAERS). [Last accessed August, 2025].

Centre for public impact. (2017). The Universal Immunization Program in India. [online] Available from https://centreforpublicimpact.org/public-impact-fundamentals/the-universal-immunisation-programme-in-india/[Last accessed August, 2025].

Gupta P, Menon PS, Ramji S, et al. Vaccine Administration Practices. PG Text Book of Pediatrics, 3rd edition. New Delhi: Jaypee Brothers Medical Publishers; 2022. pp. 1107-11.

Purple Book. IAP Guidebook on Immunization. Indian Academy of Pediatrics Advisory Committee on Vaccines and Immunization Practices (ACVIP). In: Rao IS, Kasi SG (Eds). New Delhi: Jaypee Brothers Medical Publishers; 2022. pp. 37-48.

13.8 Adverse Events Following Immunization (AEFI) *PE 18.8*

INTRODUCTION

All the vaccines are proven to be extremely safe but like any other drug, they carry with them a potential and rare risk of adverse reactions in the vaccinee. According to WHO, AEFI is defined as "any untoward medical occurrence which follows immunization though does not necessarily have a causal relationship with the usage of the vaccines." AEFI may include one or more of unintended or unfavorable sign, symptoms, disease, or laboratory finding.

CLASSIFICATION OF ADVERSE EVENTS FOLLOWING IMMUNIZATION (AEFI)

The AEFI are classified based on their severity as follows:

- ***Minor AEFI:*** These events are generally due to the host's immune response to the vaccine ingredients including the adjuvants, stabilizers, and antigens. These present commonly as local reactions such as pain, redness, and swelling at the injection sites and systemic symptoms such as fever, irritability, and malaise.
- ***Severe AEFI:*** These are similar to minor AEFI but with an increased severity and/or intensity such as high-grade fever or an increased injection site swelling extending beyond nearest joint subsequent to pentavalent vaccine. Severe refers to the intensity of the specific event, but the event itself may be of relatively minor medical significance. Such patients do not need hospitalization and do not have any sequelae.
- ***Serious AEFI:*** This event is considered serious if it:
  - Results in death, hospitalization, or persistent disability.
  - Occurs in clusters.
  - Causes parental or community concern.
  - Results in birth defect in the unborn fetus.

As AEFI surveillance forms an integral part of immunization program, AEFI are also classified into cause-specific categories:

- ***Vaccine product-related reaction:*** This is caused or precipitated due to one or more of inherent properties of vaccine product or its ingredients such as excessive injection site swelling due to DPT vaccine.
- ***Vaccine quality defect-related reaction:*** This is due to a quality defect in the vaccine or its delivery device provided by the manufacturer. This is extremely rare as good manufacturing practices (WHO-GMP) are being followed by vaccine manufacturers.
- ***Immunization error-related reaction:*** Inappropriate handling, ignoring contraindications, or inappropriate administration of the vaccine are programmatic errors which can contribute to these reactions. Thus, by its nature, such AEFI are preventable.
- ***Immunization-related anxiety reaction:*** This is often due to anxiety or fear of injections particularly in mass immunization campaigns in older children. A syncope in an adolescent is a common example of this reaction.
- *Coincidental event:* This reaction is due to causes other than those mentioned earlier and have a likelihood of a chance association with vaccine administration.

TREATMENT Adverse Events Following Immunization

Most minor AEFI are of short duration and subside within 48–72 hours. These can be treated symptomatically by antipyretics and analgesics for a short duration.

Serious AEFI such as severe allergy or anaphylaxis (1 per 1,000,000 vaccine doses), hypotensive-hyporesponsive episodes (HHE), convulsions, and toxic shock syndrome need close monitoring and must be managed on an emergency basis. A child with anaphylaxis should be made to lie flat and given oxygen. Adrenaline is given at a dose of 0.01 mL/kg (maximum 0.5 mL). The dose can be repeated after 5 minutes, if needed. The child should be admitted for 24 hours even if the recovery is immediate.

PREVENTION

Appropriate storage and handling of vaccines, proper vaccine administration technique, and observing valid precautions and contraindications are important steps in the prevention of AEFI. Communication with the parents/caregivers about the vaccine and possible adverse effects should be done. Availability of the resuscitation equipment and its functioning should be confirmed along with access to adrenaline, oxygen, hydrocortisone, and intravenous fluids (Ringer lactate) for emergency use. Since allergic reactions can be of variable severity and anaphylaxis is an unpredictable event, all the vaccine recipients must be observed in the health setup for 15–30 minutes following vaccine administration.

REPORTING OF ADVERSE EVENTS FOLLOWING IMMUNIZATION

Effective and spontaneous reporting of AEFI is the first step to ensure that the vaccine products are safe and are being safely administered. AEFI reporting should be done as quickly as possible. It helps to formulate an immediate decision for further action and necessary investigations. The health workers and medical personnel should report all serious AEFI to Medical Officer (MO) of nearest primary health center or the District Immunization Officer within 24 hours. The district administration forwards these reports to state and central health authorities. AEFI should be reported following the use of any vaccine in a government hospital or in a private hospital/clinic.

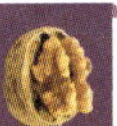

IN A NUTSHELL

Adverse Events Following Immunization

1. All the vaccines are extremely safe but have a rare risk of AEFI in the vaccinee.
2. AEFI may manifest as an unfavorable sign, symptom, disease, or a laboratory finding.
3. AEFI are classified based upon their severity as minor, serious, or severe variety.
4. Most minor AEFIs are self-limiting and can be easily managed by symptomatic treatment and counseling.
5. Serious AEFI must be treated and managed on an emergency basis.
6. Prevention and timely reporting of AEFI are essential steps for vaccine safety.

Ministry of Health and Family Welfare, Government of India. Adverse events following immunization. Immunization Handbook for Health workers. New Delhi: Ministry of Health and Family Welfare, Government of India; 2018. pp. 107-26.

Pandey D, Mehta G, Sachdeva M, Tripathi R. Adverse Event Following Immunization (AEFI) in Children: An Analysis of Reporting in VigiAccess. Drug Res (Stuttg). 2022;72(8):435-40.

Pemde H. Adverse events following immunization. IAP Guidebook on Immunization 2018-2019, 3rd edition. New Delhi: Jaypee Brothers Medical Publishers; 2020. pp. 69-83.

Vashishtha VM, Prajapati BS. Adverse events following immunization against vaccination. FAQs on Vaccines and Immunization Practices, 2nd edition. New Delhi: Jaypee Brothers Medical Publishers; 2015. pp. 63-75.

WHO. (2021). Reporting form for AEFI. [online] Available from https://www.who.int/publications/m/item/reporting-form-for-aefi [Last accessed January 2025].

13.9 Participation in Immunization

PE 18.10, PE 18.13

DEMONSTRATE WILLINGNESS TO PARTICIPATE IN THE NATIONAL AND SUBNATIONAL IMMUNIZATION DAYS (NIDs AND SNIDs)

Mass immunization campaigns, known as NIDs or supplementary immunization activities (SIAs), are strategic programs for the eradication of the diseases such as poliomyelitis. This supplementary immunization is intended to complement and not replace routine immunization schedules. Pulse polio immunization (PPI) program was started in 1990s and included vaccination of all children under the age of 5 years against the polio virus on NIDs and sNIDs. Such mass immunization activities are also termed as Supplementary Immunization Activities (SIAs) and have been carried out using measles and rubella (MR) containing vaccines for children between 9 months to 15 years of age to accelerate efforts towards measles elimination.

As PPI is one of the largest public health interventions as a part of National Health Mission, it requires massive logistics and an organized infrastructure with large number of healthcare workers and nongovernmental agencies to vaccinate millions of children within in a limited time duration.

Willingness to participate in such NIDs gives an opportunity to learn about national health programs, provides practical hands-on experience in the administration of vaccines, and observe and study the logistics and related issues during the day long sessions.

IMPLIED CONSENT IN IMMUNIZATION SERVICES

Parents must be informed and made aware of the vaccine(s) the child is eligible and fit to receive and would be receiving during their visit. Though a written consent is not mandatory, an informed consent is taken as implied consent for the immunization and the parents need to agree verbally as per their free choice and free from duress of the family or health professional. The legal age of consent is 18 years and hence child or adolescent in the age group 6–17 years cannot provide consent to vaccination and so consent is normally required from their parent or legal guardian. As a legal safeguard, the healthcare professional must practice and follow basic and appropriate standards of care during the immunization procedures and must possess adequate facility to manage AEFI.

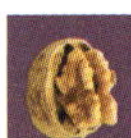

IN A NUTSHELL

Participation in Immunization

1. Supplementary immunization activities such as NIDs are meant to complement and not replace the national and routine childhood immunization.
2. Participation in mass immunization programs provides an active opportunity to have hands on experience and be aware of the logistic issues in the administration of the vaccines.
3. A written consent is not mandatory for childhood immunization and informed consent is taken as an implied consent.
4. Appropriate and basic standards of care must be adhered to during and after vaccine administration.

Das MK, Arora NK, Mathew T, Vyas B, Sindhu M, Yadav A. Documentation of vaccine handling and service delivery at outreach immunization sessions across 27 districts of India. Heliyon. 2018;4(12):e01059.

Ministry of Health and Family Welfare, Government of India. Managing an Immunization Session. Immunization Handbook for Health Workers. New Delhi: Ministry of Health and Family Welfare, Government of India; 2018. pp. 87-105.

13.10 Newer Vaccines

PE 18.14

INTRODUCTION

These "newer vaccines" have been approved in recent years as alternative to existing vaccines or as vaccines against diseases for which no active prophylaxis is available presently or are under trial phase. Some such as dengue and malaria vaccines are available for limited clinical use in other countries.

Various vaccines including those for COVID-19, dengue fever, malaria, HIV, chikungunya, hepatitis C, hepatitis E, Epstein–Barr virus, enterovirus, respiratory syncytial virus, and parainfluenza virus are under various phases of clinical trials. Therapeutic vaccines are being investigated against cancers, rheumatoid arthritis, multiple sclerosis, Alzheimer disease, and type I diabetes.

COVID VACCINES

The vaccines against the new virus, SARS-CoV-2, have been developed in a record time of a few months following the onset of pandemic, as compared to an average time of 10–12 years taken for development of any other vaccine. Several vaccine development technologies were utilized in the process and few of these were recombinant viral vector vaccines (Covishield), inactivates virus (Covaxin) mRNA (Moderna).

Characteristics

There are several target antigens for COVID-19 vaccines and vaccines targeting the spike (S) protein elicit potent humoral and cellular immune response against the virus. The receptor binding domain (RBD) on the S1 subunit of the S protein is especially important since this protein binds specifically to the ACE-2 receptor on the human cell which is the crucial step in infection with SARS-CoV-2. The "N" protein is more conserved and induces long-lived memory T cells in humans. The "N" protein can provide a potentially viable addition to "S" protein to accord cross-protective and long-lasting T-cell immunity against SARS-CoV-2. The results of initial studies for Covaxin and Covishield have shown efficacy of >77% and >70% against all severity COVID-19 infections, respectively.

Administration and Schedule

As many as 13 vaccines had been rolled out under emergency use authorization (EUA) or with full authorization in different countries. Since July 2022 onwards, India approved the use of COVID-19 vaccines (Covishield and Covaxin).

Most COVID-19 vaccines have a two-dose schedule with an interval of 21–28 days between them.

HUMAN PAPILLOMAVIRUS VACCINES

Human papillomavirus (HPV) is responsible for various clinical conditions in both genders including premalignant conditions which can progress to cancer. Of about 13 oncogenic genotypes, HPV-16 and HPV-18 infections lead to cervical cancer. HPV can also cause vulvar cancer, vaginal cancer, oropharyngeal cancer, penile cancer, and anogenital warts. The interval between the acquisition of HPV infection and progression to invasive carcinoma is 10–20 years or longer.

Characteristics

The current HPV vaccines are based on noninfectious virus like particles (VLP) produced by recombinant technology and are highly immunogenic. Three HPV vaccines are currently available and marketed in many countries worldwide. All of these vaccines are to be administered if possible before the onset of sexual activity, i.e., before first exposure to HPV infection.

1. ***Bivalent HPV vaccine:*** It contains purified viral L1 protein for HPV types 16 and 18. It is available in one-dose or two-dose vials or prefilled syringes for intramuscular use.
2. ***Quadrivalent HPV vaccine:*** It contains purified viral L1 protein for HPV types 6, 11, 16, and 18. It is available in 1-dose vials or prefilled syringes for intramuscular use.
3. ***Nanovalent HPV vaccine:*** A newer vaccine with 9 HPV serotypes has recently been licensed for clinical use.

Protective Efficacy

About 70–80% of women develop antibodies to HPV after natural infection and the degree of protection is low. HPV vaccination elicits much stronger and robust antibody production. As the vaccine was introduced in 2006, the exact duration of protection is not known. The mechanism of protection involves both the cellular immune responses and neutralizing IgG antibodies. Long-term efficacy has been demonstrated against cervical cancer and precancerous lesions. As of now, there is no need of boosters.

Administration and Schedule

For all HPV vaccines, the vaccination schedule depends on the brand of vaccine, valence of vaccine, and age of the vaccine recipient.

Bivalent HPV vaccine (Cervarix-GSK): It was approved for use in girls in India. For age 9–14 years, a two-dose schedule (0.5 mL given intramuscularly at 0 and 6 months) is recommended. For age ≥15 years, 3 doses (0.5 mL at 0, 1, and 6 months) are recommended.

Quadrivalent HPV vaccine (Gardasil 4-MSD): This vaccine is approved for use in girls above the age of 9 years and in women till the age of 45 years. For girls aged 9–13 years, this vaccine can be administered according to a two-dose schedule (0.5 mL at 0 and 6 months). For girls 14 years of age and older, the vaccine should be administered according to a 3-dose schedule (0.5 mL at 0, 2, and 6 months).

Nanovalent HPV vaccine (Gardasil 9-MSD): This vaccine is approved for use both in males (9–15 years) and females (9–26 years) as three-dose schedule in India (0.5 mL at 0, 2, and 6 months).

Adverse Effects

The HPV vaccines are safe to administer and can be associated with mild fever and local reactions. Postvaccination syncope (fainting) has been reported among adolescents, hence it is recommended to give vaccines in lying down position and observe the child for 15–30 minutes after vaccination.

Gender neutral vaccination is the universal vaccination with HPV vaccines irrespective of the sex of the vaccine recipient. Traditionally, HPV vaccination was promoted in India as, "only female vaccine" for prevention of carcinoma of cervix, vulva, anogenital, and oropharyngeal region. It is also helpful in males for prevention of penile, anogenital, oropharyngeal cancer, and anal warts. Vaccinating both males and females help to reduce HPV disease and transmission and increase herd immunity.

DENGUE VACCINE

There are various challenges in the development of vaccines against dengue fever such as prevalence of four different serotypes (types 1, 2, 3, and 4), lack of animal model, and poor growth of dengue virus in cell culture. Various vaccine technologies have been tried for development of dengue vaccines including live-attenuated vaccine, inactivated virus vaccine, recombinant subunit vaccines or from VLPs, plasmids, or viral vectors.

Dengvaxia (CYD-TDV), by Sanofi Pasteur is the first licensed dengue vaccine to receive authorization for use in endemic countries of Asia and Latin America. This is a live recombinant tetravalent vaccine that has been evaluated as a three-dose series at 0, 6, and 12 months in phase III clinical studies. Mixed safety and efficacy data in phase III trials have led to concerns and controversy. Data suggested increased risk of severe dengue in primary seronegative individuals, so it can be considered for individuals who have laboratory confirmed evidence of prior dengue infection. It has been registered for use in individuals between the ages of 9 and 45 years who are living in endemic areas with high transmission. However, due to complexities such as increased risk of severe dengue in seronegative persons, WHO recommends that it should be only given to children and adults who have had confirmed prior dengue infection. It has not been implemented in regular immunization schedule. It is not available in India.

There is felt need for safe and effective vaccines which can be administered to young children and which can be given to individuals irrespective of immune status. There are several other vaccine candidates under evaluation in clinical trials, including live-attenuated vaccines, as well as subunit, DNA and purified inactivated vaccines. Additional technological approaches, such as virus-vectored and VLP-based vaccines, are under evaluation in preclinical studies.

MALARIA VACCINE

Despite years of research, an effective malaria vaccine still eludes the scientific community. It is difficult to formulate an effective vaccine against malaria due to complex life cycle of parasite, different stages of the parasite, and involvement of two host organisms. The vaccines can be broadly grouped into pre-erythrocyte vaccines, blood stage vaccines, and transmission blocking vaccines. Most of the research is for vaccine against *Plasmodium falciparum*. A malaria vaccine RTS, S/AS01 (Mosquirix) is approved for use by WHO in high endemic countries of sub-Saharan Africa. The research continues for the development of recombinant protein and attenuated whole organism vaccine against malaria.

HIV VACCINE

The main obstacle in development of vaccine is the peculiarity of the virus which dampens the immune system. HIV isolates are highly variable with a vast genetic divergence so vaccine needs to be broad enough to map all the variability. Various vaccines such as whole inactivated vaccines, live-attenuated vaccines, VLPs, recombinant vaccines, subunit vaccines, and DNA vaccines are under evaluation. None of them is approved for clinical use.

FUTURE TECHNOLOGIES

Vaccines research and development are a constantly evolving process with the commitment of prevention and the improvement of public health all across the world. Not only infectious diseases, the potential vaccines have a broad perspective to address the issues of allergies, cancers, and other progressive diseases such as neurological diseases. As the vaccine development and production have expanded, a paradigm shift has recently taken place to use vaccines for disease treatment in addition to the disease prevention. Alternative methods of vaccine delivery and the field of genomics are likely to further the scope of vaccines in human health and diseases in the coming decades. Virus linked particles (VLPs) from other infectious agents hold a platform and promise for future developments in vaccinology.

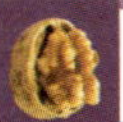

IN A NUTSHELL

Newer Vaccines

1. There are many COVID vaccines at the various stages of development and are based on different vaccine technologies. Few of them have been rolled out under emergency use or wit full authorization. In general mRNA vaccines have shown the highest efficacy, but requirement of ultracold temperature of cold chain and high cost are big challenges. Viral vector based vaccines are most popular globally. Subunit vaccines might race ahead, going forward with their high safety and efficacy.
2. Bivalent, quadrivalent and nanovalent HPV vaccines are available. All these HPV vaccines are highly immunogenic and highly efficacious in preventing HPV infection.
3. *Dengvaxia (CYD-TDV)*, by Sanofi Pasteur is the first licensed dengue vaccine to receive authorization. Due to its mixed safety and efficacy data, it is not available in India.
4. Despite years of research, an effective malaria vaccine still eludes the scientific community.

Bhatta M, Nandi S, Dutta S, et al. Coronavirus (SARS-CoV-2) a systematic review for potential vaccines. Hum Vaccin Immunother. 2022; 18(1):1-18.

Centers for Disease Control and Prevention. Human Papillomavirus (HPV) Vaccine safety. [online] Available from https://www.cdc.gov/vaccine-safety/vaccines/hpv.html. [Last accessed August, 2025].

Chung YH, Beiss V, Fiering SN, et al. COVID-19 vaccine frontrunners and their nanotechnology design. ACS Nano. 2020;14(10):12522-37.

Dong Y, Dai T, Wei Y, et al. A systematic review of SARS-CoV-2 vaccine candidates. Signal Transduct Target Ther. 2020;5(1):237.

Food and Drug Administration. Highlights of prescribing information. Gardasil 9 (human papillomavirus 9-valent vaccine, recombinant). Silver Spring, MD: US Department of Health and Human Services, Food and Drug Administration; 2014.

Giuliano AR, Palefsky IM, Goldstone S, et al. Efficacy of quadrivalent HPV vaccine against HPV infection and disease in males. N Engl J Med. 2011;364(5):401-11.

Kaur SP, Gupta V. COVID-19 vaccine: A comprehensive status report. Virus Res. 2020;288:198114.

Kheirvari M, Liu H, Tumban E. Virus-like Particle Vaccines and Platforms for Vaccine Development. Viruses. 2023;15(5):1109.

Nossal G. Vaccines of the future. Vaccine. 2011;29:D111-5.

Pormohammad A, Zarei M. Ghorbani S, et al. Efficacy and safety of COVID-19 vaccines: A systematic review and meta-analysis of randomized clinical trials. Vaccines (Basel). 2021;9(5):467.

WHO. (2018). Dengue Vaccine: WHO Position Paper, September 2018. [online] Available from https://www.who.int/publications/i/item/dengue-vaccines-who-position-paper-september-2018 [Last accessed August, 2025].

WHO. Human papillomavirus vaccines: WHO position paper. Wkly Epidemiol Rec. 2017;92(19):241-68.

WHO. Malaria Vaccine: WHO Position Paper, January 2016. Vaccine. 2018;36(25):3576-7.

CHAPTER 14

Infections and Infestations

AS PER NMC COMPETENCIES

PE31.1	Describe the epidemiology, clinical features, clinical types, complications of tuberculosis in children and adolescents.	*Ch 14.3*
PE31.2	Describe the various diagnostic tools for childhood tuberculosis.	*Ch 14.3*
PE31.3	Describe the various regimens for management of tuberculosis as per national guidelines.	*Ch 14.3*
PE31.4	Describe the preventive strategies adopted and the objectives and outcome of the national tuberculosis control program.	*Ch 14.3*
PE31.5	Elicit, document and present history of contact with tuberculosis in every patient encounter, identify BCG scar and interpret a Mantoux test.	*Ch 14.3*
PE31.6	Interpret blood tests in the context of laboratory evidence for tuberculosis.	*Ch 14.3*
PE31.7	Describe the various samples for demonstrating the organism, e.g., gastric aspirate, sputum, CSF, FNAC.	*Ch 14.3*
PE31.8	Enumerate the indications, discuss the limitations of methods of culturing *M. tuberculosis* and the newer diagnostic tools for tuberculosis including BACTEC CBNAAT and their indications.	*Ch 14.3*
PE31.9	Enumerate the common causes of fever and describe the etiopathogenesis, clinical features, complications and management of fever in children.	*Ch 14.1, Ch 14.2*
PE31.10	Enumerate the common causes of fever and describe the etiopathogenesis, clinical features, complications and management of child with exanthematous illnesses like measles, mumps, rubella and chickenpox.	*Ch 14.4, Ch 14.5 Ch 14.6, Ch 14.7*
PE31.11	Enumerate the common causes of fever and discuss the etiopathogenesis, clinical features, complications and management of child with diphtheria, pertussis, tetanus.	*Ch 14.8, Ch 14.9 Ch 14.10*
PE31.12	Enumerate the common causes of fever and discuss the etiopathogenesis, clinical features, complications and management of child with typhoid.	*Ch 14.11*
PE31.13	Enumerate the common causes of fever and discuss the etiopathogenesis, clinical features, complications and management of child with dengue, chikungunya and other vector-borne diseases.	*Ch 14.12, Ch 14.13*
PE31.14	Enumerate the common causes of fever and discuss the etiopathogenesis, clinical features, complications and management of children with common parasitic infections, malaria, leishmaniasis, filariasis, helminthic infestations, amebiasis, giardiasis.	*Ch 14.14, Ch 14.15 Ch 14.16, Ch 14.17 Ch 14.18, Ch 14.19 Ch 14.20, Ch 14.21 Ch 14.22, Ch 14.23 Ch 14.24*

Topics available online: ***Influenza, Coronavirus Disease 2019 and MIS-C, HIV in Children, and Rickettsial Diseases***

14.1 Fever *PE 31.9*

INTRODUCTION

Fever is a condition in which the body's temperature is elevated as a result of the body's thermostat (i.e., hypothalamus) being reset to a higher than usual temperature. Fever occurs in response to a variety of insults, infection being the most common. Fever is induced by pyrogens. Bacteria, fungi, viruses, malignancies, connective tissue disorders, certain drugs, and trauma may endogenously stimulate production of pyrogens.

- Common ***endogenous pyrogens*** include interleukin-1 (IL-1), tumor necrosis factor (TNF), and interferon. Other endogenous pyrogens include IL-6, IL-11, leukemia inhibitory factor (LIF), ciliary neurotropic factor (CNTF), and oncostatin-M.
- ***Exogenous pyrogens*** include the bacterial cell wall component lipopolysaccharide (LPS), enterotoxins, and exotoxins. Exogenous pyrogens can induce production of endogenous pyrogens via activation of Toll signaling, and both endogenous and exogenous pyrogens stimulate the synthesis of prostaglandins (PG). Prostaglandin E2 (PGE2) is the ultimate endogenous pyrogen. It resets the temperature of the hypothalamus. Aspirin acts as an antipyretic by inhibiting cyclooxygenase (COX) 1 and 2, the rate limiting enzyme in PGE2 synthesis. Ibuprofen is also a COX-inhibitor.

DEFINITION

Body (rectal) temperature normally fluctuates between 36.6°C in the morning and 37.9°C in the evening. Because of the normal variation in body temperature, there is no single value that can be used as cut-off to define fever. However, a clinically significant fever is generally defined as a rectal temperature of 100.4°F (38°C) or higher. This is equivalent to an oral temperature of 99.5°F (37.5°C), and axillary (armpit) temperature of 99°F (37.2°C).

Fever above 41.5°C (107°F) is called *hyperpyrexia* and warrants aggressive antipyretic therapy because of risk of irreversible organ damage. Usual underlying etiology of hyperpyrexia includes meningitis, pneumonia, bacteremia, and heatstroke in tropical climates. Acetaminophen (paracetamol), nonsteroidal anti-inflammatory drugs (NSAIDs) and steroids are effective antipyretics.

Fever may be beneficial in the sense that it increases host defense mechanisms, augments immunological functions, and suppresses growth of some microbes. However, there is no overwhelming evidence against use of antipyretic therapy for fever in children. Fever in children increases the risk of febrile seizure and should, therefore, be cautiously handled.

INITIAL ASSESSMENT

Before proceeding to identifying the etiology of fever, it is essential to clinically assess the child for vital signs and severity of illness. This includes assessing the general look and behavior of the patient, measurement of temperature, heart rate, respiratory rate, capillary refill time, blood pressure, and pulse oximetry. Watch the patient for any evidence of cyanosis or dehydration (in form of dry mucosa, decreased skin turgor, and bulging or depressed fontanel). The criteria to define tachycardia, tachypnea, and hypotension are shown in **Table 14.1**.

- All children with cardiopulmonary compromise should be provided with immediate life-saving resuscitative procedures to ensure earliest restoration of airway, breathing, and circulation.
- SpO_2 <94% is considered hypoxia. It should be aggressively managed with oxygen and respiratory support, if needed.
- Capillary refill time of >3 seconds suggests poor perfusion and demands immediate intervention in form of isotonic fluids and inotropes.

High body temperature, on its own, does not identify those with serious illness. One should not also use the duration of fever to predict the likelihood of serious illness.

ETIOLOGY OF FEVER

The most common cause of fever in children is a viral infection. In viral infection, fever is usually short-lived and signs are usually more generalized than those with bacterial infection. Common viral and bacterial illnesses such as cold, gastroenteritis, ear infections, croup, and bronchiolitis are the most likely illnesses known to cause short fevers. The classical signs of an upper respiratory tract infection are coryza, inflamed tympanic membranes, fever, or tonsillitis. Bacterial tonsillitis and otitis media are difficult to differentiate from viral causes, but a bacterial otitis media is more likely to be unilateral. Viral infections usually resolve within a week of onset. Persistence of fever for a longer period demands thorough investigation. The term "fever of unknown origin" has been used to denote fever persisting for >21 days.

EVALUATION OF A FEBRILE CHILD

A good history and thorough examination are essential for the early diagnosis of fever in childhood. The history should include questions regarding characteristics of fever (onset,

Table 14.1 Cut-off Values for Heart Rate, Respiratory Rate, and Blood Pressure

Tachycardia	*Tachypnea*	*Hypotension (1–10 years)*
<12 months: >160 beats/min	*<2 months:* >60 breaths/min	*<1 year:* SBP <70 mm Hg
12–24 months: >150 beats/min	*2–12 months:* >50 breaths/min	*1–10 years:* SBP <(70 + age × 2)
2–5 years: >140 beats/min	*1–5 years:* >40 breaths/min	*>10 years:* SBP <90 mm Hg

intensity, duration, and type of fever—continuous, remittent, or intermittent); localizing symptoms of fever; vaccination; past history of any significant illnesses such as congenital heart disease or tuberculosis; and family history of members with fever; and recent history of contact with infectious disease.

Ask about any other symptom that the child is having. This will give an important clue in localizing the disease to a particular system. Examination should take note of the following:

- *General condition*—whether alert, active, playful, irritable, lethargic, or comatose?
- *Rash*—if present, appeared on which day of fever? Describe the rash—macular, papular, maculopapular, vesicular, or pustular.
- Examination for pallor, icterus, clubbing, edema.
- Examination of eyes for conjunctivitis and ears for suppurative otitis media.
- *Throat examination* for tonsillar enlargement (tonsillitis), pharyngeal membrane (for diphtheria).
- Examination of *neck*, axillae, and inguinal region for lymphadenopathy.
- Palpation of *abdomen* for hepatosplenomegaly or other abdominal masses or tenderness.
- Examination of genitalia for any swelling, pain, or redness.
- Examination of *chest* for any abnormal chest signs.
- Examination of *bones and joints* for swelling or tenderness.
- *Cardiovascular system* examination for murmurs.
- Rule out *neck rigidity* and other *meningeal signs*.

Once an appropriate history has been taken and examination performed, the next steps are to (*i*) localize the fever to a particular organ system by presenting complaints; and to (*ii*) identify the probable etiology of fever, depending upon its duration, and clinical examination.

Localizing the Focus of Fever

Every effort should be made to delineate the system involved, based on following localizing symptoms:

Exanthematous fevers: Rash, mucosal erythema, nodules, pustules, maculopapular rash.

Upper respiratory tract: Cough, cold, coryza, throat pain, difficulty in swallowing, earache, hoarse voice, stridor, regional lymphadenopathy.

Lower respiratory tract: Cough, difficult and fast breathing, wheezing, chest pain, sputum production.

Urinary tract: *Upper*—vomiting, abdominal pain, diarrhea; *Lower*—burning micturition, frequency, urgency, hematuria.

Gastrointestinal and hematological systems: Pallor, rash, bleeding from any site, petechiae, ecchymosis, lymph node enlargement, joint or bone pains, lump in abdomen.

Central nervous system (CNS) involvement: Vomiting, nausea, headache, altered sensorium, seizures, abnormal movements, abnormality of tone, opisthotonus, neck rigidity, irritability, and photophobia.

Hepatobiliary system: Jaundice, abdominal distension, diarrhea, and vomiting.

Table 14.2 Etiology of Fever based on Presenting Features

Symptom	Possible etiologies
Cough and coryza	Viral fever
Rash	Exanthematous illnesses such as measles, rubella, chickenpox, erythema infectiosum, roseola infantum, herpes simplex; or other illnesses such as meningococcemia, dengue, Henoch–Schönlein purpura, leukemia, and Kawasaki disease
Ear pain	Acute suppurative otitis media (ASOM)
Skin boils	Abscess, pustules, cellulitis, impetigo
Fast breathing and cough	Pneumonia, bronchiolitis, pleural effusion, tuberculosis
Joint swelling	Septic arthritis, rheumatic fever, tubercular arthritis, connective tissue diseases
Vomiting	Gastritis, gastroenteritis, viral hepatitis, meningitis, enteric fever
Diarrhea	Gastroenteritis, enteric fever, dysentery
Urinary frequency, burning micturition, or crying during micturition	Urinary tract infection
Chills or pallor or jaundice	Malaria, hepatobiliary involvement
Altered sensorium	Meningoencephalitis (bacterial, viral, tubercular), cerebral malaria, enteric encephalopathy, brain abscess
Abdominal pain	Gastroenteritis, appendicitis, liver abscess, hepatitis, cholecystitis

Cardiovascular system: Dyspnea, palpitation, chest pain, pedal edema, prominent neck veins, and cough.

Musculoskeletal system: Joint swelling, pain, or limited movements in a muscle group or joint.

Identify the Etiology of Fever

Short Duration Fevers

Fever of <2-week duration is usually infectious in origin, and due to viruses, bacteria, or protozoa. Many of these patients recover completely, even before a precise diagnosis is made or treatment is given. These children may present with or without localizing manifestations. Localizing symptoms can give a clue as to the etiology of fever, as detailed in **Table 14.2**.

Prolonged Fever

Fever lasting for >2 weeks requires a different approach. Infections remain the most important cause of prolonged fever; however, noninfectious causes are also responsible. Common causes of prolonged fever are listed below:

- ***Infections:*** Tuberculosis, urinary tract infections, human immunodeficiency virus (HIV), chronic fungal infections, etc.
- ***Inflammatory disorders:*** Rheumatoid arthritis, systemic lupus erythematosus, Kawasaki disease, and other connective tissue disorders including polyarteritis nodosa, Behçet's disease, Wegener's granulomatosis.

Box 14.1 Etiology of Fever with Rash, Lymphadenopathy, and Hepatosplenomegaly

A. Fever with hepatosplenomegaly
- *Infectious causes:* Malaria, enteric fever, kala-azar, tuberculosis, infectious mononucleosis, brucellosis, echinococcosis, TORCH infection, dengue, septicemia, and infective endocarditis
- *Malignancies:* Leukemias, lymphomas, histiocytosis, infantile hemangioendothelioma, hepatoblastoma, and metastasis
- *Connective tissue diseases:* Systemic lupus erythematosus (SLE); systemic juvenile idiopathic arthritis (JIA), sarcoidosis, scleroderma, and rheumatic fever
- *Chronic hepatitis/chronic liver disease:* Autoimmune hepatitis, chronic hepatitis B/C, and Wilson's disease

B. Fever with rash
- *Infectious causes:* Meningococcemia, dengue, measles, rubella, varicella, roseola infantum, erythema infectiosum, herpes simplex, and lupus vulgaris.
- *Malignancies:* Leukemia and histiocytosis
- *Vasculitis:* Henoch–Schönlein purpura, Kawasaki disease, rheumatic fever, systemic JIA, and SLE

C. Fever with lymphadenopathy and/or hepatosplenomegaly
- Suppurative lymphadenitis (bacterial, often accompanying pharyngitis, tonsillitis, dental infections, scalp infections)
- Tuberculosis
- Lymphoma (Hodgkin and non-Hodgkin lymphomas)
- Histiocytosis
- Acute lymphoblastic leukemia (ALL)
- HIV infection
- Connective tissue disorders such as systemic JIA or sarcoidosis
- Kawasaki disease

(TORCH: toxoplasmosis, rubella cytomegalovirus, herpes simplex)

- ***Malignancies:*** Lymphoma (including Hodgkin disease), leukemia, hepatoblastoma, Wilms' tumor, neuroblastoma, brain tumors, etc.
- ***Endocrine causes:*** Thyrotoxicosis, diabetes insipidus.
- ***Hematological and immune deficiency disorders:*** Spherocytosis, agranulocytosis, hemolytic anemia, disorders of T or B cells, disorders of phagocytosis.
- ***Neurologic disorders:*** Familial dysautonomia, hypothalamic and third ventricle lesions, anhidrotic ectodermal dysplasia.
- ***Miscellaneous causes:*** Drug fever, periodic fever, factitious fever.

Box 14.1 provides a detailed list of common causes of fever associated with hepatosplenomegaly, rash, or lymphadenopathy. When fever has been persistent for a week, and no cause has been found, serious consideration should be given to hospital admission to confirm pyrexia and initiate investigations.

TREATMENT Fever

The primary objective of treating a child with fever is to improve the comfort of the child. The primary focus should not be on normalization of body temperature; though this is acceptable as a secondary outcome, following measures taken to make the child (and parents) comfortable. A summary of guidelines on management of fever are highlighted in **Boxes 14.2 to 14.4**. There are two major methods of antipyresis:

1. *Nonpharmacological:* Environmental measures, fluids, and hydrotherapy; and
2. *Pharmacological:* Antipyretics.

Nonpharmacological Antipyresis

Nonpharmacological methods include environmental modifications, increased fluid intake, and sponging or hydrotherapy.

Box 14.2 NICE (National Institute for Care and Health Excellence) Guidelines, 2013

1. For infants <4 weeks, body temperature should be measured in axilla with an electronic thermometer. For children 4 weeks–5 years, electronic thermometer in axilla or infrared tympanic thermometer should be used
2. Forehead chemical thermometers are not recommended due to poor reliability
3. Antipyretic agents do not prevent febrile convulsions and hence not to be used specifically for this purpose
4. Use antipyretics only till child appears distressed
5. Tepid sponging is not recommended for treatment of fever
6. Children with fever should not be underdressed or overwrapped

Source: Fever in under 5s: Assessment and initial management. National Institute for Care and Health Excellence Guidelines, 2013

Box 14.3 Italian Pediatric Society Guidelines, 2017

1. For infants <4 weeks, body temperature should be measured in axilla with an electronic thermometer. For children 4 weeks to 5 years, electronic thermometer in axilla or infrared tympanic thermometer should be used
2. Use of paracetamol/ibuprofen is not recommended prophylactically to reduce the incidence of fever and local reactions in children undergoing vaccination
3. Combined or alternating use of paracetamol/ibuprofen is not recommended
4. Ibuprofen is not recommended in chickenpox/Kawasaki disease
5. Preventive use of ibuprofen is not recommended in prevention of febrile seizure
6. Paracetamol/ibuprofen is contraindicated in known case of NSAID induced asthma but not in other febrile children with asthma

(NSAID: nonsteroidal anti-inflammatory drug)

Source: Chiappini E, Veturini E, Principi N, et al. 2016 Update of the Italian Pediatric Society Guidelines for Management of Fever in Children. J Pediatr. 2017;180:177-83.e1

Box 14.4 Consensus Guidelines on Febrile Child Presenting to the Emergency Department in India 2017

1. Rectal temperature is the preferred method of temperature determination in very young children
2. Temporal artery and tympanic membrane thermometer can be used for quick access of temperature
3. Evaluation and management of well looking child is based on defined age groups: neonate (<28 days), young infant (29–90 days), old infant and young child (91 days to 2 years) and children >2 years
4. In patients with fever without localization, chest X-ray is mandatory for neonates whereas in young infants, chest X-ray is indicated, if temperature >102.2°F, leukocyte count >20,000/mm^3 or respiratory distress is present

Source: Mahajan P, Batra P, Thakur N, et al. Consensus Guidelines on Evaluation and Management of the Febrile Child Presenting to the Emergency Department in India. Indian Pediatr. 2017;54:652-60

Environmental Measures

Environmental measures include placing the child in cool and airy environment (21–22°C), which enhances heat loss by convection. Minimal clothing, i.e., dressing the child in only one layer of clothing is advocated as this further enhances heat loss. Some theories even support a gentle body massage to dilate the cutaneous blood vessels, which further increases heat dissipation.

Hydration

As fever increases, the metabolic loss of the body also needs to be compensated. For each 1°C rise of temperature above 37.2°C, there is an increase in insensible water loss of 7 mL/kg body weight/day. Hence, extra fluid intake is advised in febrile patients. For each 1°C of increase in temperature, a 12% increase in fluid intake is recommended.

Sponging or Hydrotherapy

It is considered the mainstay of nonpharmacological antipyresis. External cooling lowers the temperature of febrile patients by evaporation, conduction, and convection. Evaporation is rated as the most effective physical mean of promoting heat loss in febrile children because it has the least capacity to induce shivering. External cooling acts by impairing the overwhelming effect or mechanisms that have been evoked by elevated thermoregulatory set point, rather than by lowering the elevated set point. The capacity of external cooling to lower core temperature is limited because it induces both cutaneous vasoconstriction and shivering. Therefore, unless concomitant antipyretic therapy or other pharmacological methods are used to abolish shivering, external cooling is vigorously opposed in febrile patients by thermoregulatory mechanisms endeavoring to maintain elevated temperature.

Sponging should be done by continuous wiping of the body with tepid water (28–30°C) from head to toe for 15–20 minutes. Sponging action ensures that water film is constantly moving thus maximizing heat conduction. Tepid sponging acts by conduction of heat from skin to the cooler water.

Studies indicate that use of hydrotherapy alone is clearly inferior for reduction of fever for periods >30 minutes after initiation of treatment. However, external cooling could still be of value, if it potentiates activity of antipyretics.

Results of randomized trials comparing the combination of antipyretics and physical methods with antipyretics alone have provided mixed results. In four out of seven such studies, the combination treatment was superior to use of antipyretics alone for reduction of temperature during first 30 minutes of initiation of therapy and overall. In three other studies, both modes of treatment were equally effective in lowering temperature. It is recommended to administer antipyretic drugs at least 30 minutes before sponging.

However, main disadvantage of hydrotherapy as compared to use of drugs is patient discomfort and shivering. Shivering not only impedes cooling during fever but also imposes considerable metabolic burden. Studies in volunteers have shown that shivering increases the oxygen consumption, respiratory minute volume, respiratory quotient, increase in percentage of carbon dioxide in exhaled air during exposure to cold and increase in mean arterial pressure. Perhaps in febrile patients with cardiovascular disease, external cooling can cause coronary artery vasoconstriction by cold press or response and thus decreases coronary perfusion. Sponging, though rapid in reduction of temperature, has an ill sustained effect. Indications for immediate sponging with lukewarm water include the following: (i) febrile delirium; (ii) febrile seizure; or (iii) fever >41.1°C. Paracetamol should be given 30 minutes prior to sponging. Heatstroke requires cold water sponging. An absorbent towel should be soaked, rinsed, and placed on the legs, trunk, and forehead in order to reduce the body temperature. Hydrotherapy should be continued till the body temperature comes down to 38°C.

Pharmacological Antipyresis

Commonly available antipyretics are aspirin, paracetamol, indomethacin, mefenamic acid, and ibuprofen. Aspirin was the first antipyretic used in children. However, after reports of its association with causation of Reye's syndrome, aspirin is not recommended in children.

Mechanism of Action

Paracetamol, aspirin, and other NSAIDs all seem to block conversion of arachidonic acid to PGE2 by inhibiting COX, the enzyme that catalyzes rate limiting step from arachidonic acid of prostacyclin H2 the precursor of all PG isomers. Paracetamol and NSAIDs differ with respect to their relative potencies as inhibitors of peripheral and CNS COX. Paracetamol is nearly as effective as aspirin and 10% as effective as indomethacin in inhibiting central COX but only 5% as effective as aspirin and 0.02% as effective as indomethacin in inhibiting peripheral COX. Brain COX is more sensitive to inhibition by paracetamol than spleen COX and thus the relatively weak action of paracetamol against peripheral COX accounts for its poor anti-inflammatory response.

Available Drugs

Paracetamol: It is clearly established as the most commonly used standard antipyretic and analgesic. The recommended dose is 15 mg/kg at 4–6 hourly intervals not exceeding 60 mg/kg/day. Compared to 10 mg/kg, the dose of 15 mg/kg maintains lower temperature for longer time and is more effective in decreasing the mean temperature from baseline. Paracetamol reduces the temperature by 2–3°F after 2 hours of intake. The rate of fall of temperature is directly related to the initial temperature. Greater the initial temperature, greater is the fall after drug intake and vice versa. Hence, drug administration in low grade temperature may not lead to any significant fall. On the other hand, antipyretic treatment in high grade fevers (>104°F) would result in reduction of temperature by 2°F, thus failing to touch the baseline.

Ibuprofen: It belongs to propionic acid group of NSAIDs. Efficacy of paracetamol and ibuprofen has been compared in several studies, with variable results. Some studies have shown greater antipyretic effect with 10 mg/kg of ibuprofen as compared to 15 mg/kg of paracetamol. Ibuprofen has the advantage of longer duration of antipyresis (8 hours) as compared to paracetamol (4 hours).

Ibuprofen can also be used as a first-line antipyretic. Recent evidence indicates that there is no difference in the safety and effectiveness of paracetamol and ibuprofen in the care of a healthy child with fever. There is evidence that combining these two drugs is more effective than using them alone. However, this should not be followed as a routine because of associated risk of inappropriate dosages. The practice of alternating ibuprofen and paracetamol has limited value.

Choice of Antipyretic

With extensive commercial claims and counterclaims about the antipyretic drugs, the decision regarding the use of antipyretic should be based on personal experience, scientific data regarding efficacy, safety, duration of effect, and cost. Aspirin and paracetamol are equally effective at similar doses. Ibuprofen is also efficacious and has longer duration of action. In therapeutic dosages, aspirin is more toxic and causes considerable gastritis, gastrointestinal bleeding, impaired platelet function, diminished urinary excretion of sodium, Reye's syndrome, and blunted immune response. These side effects are known to occur less frequently with ibuprofen and none with paracetamol. Paracetamol can be used in children with asthma, with sensitivity to aspirin or ibuprofen, coagulation disorders, peptic ulcer, or reflux esophagitis. No association has been seen with the use of acetaminophen and development of Reye's syndrome in children or adolescents who have influenza or chickenpox. Thus, paracetamol is considered to be the safest antipyretic in children at therapeutic dosages.

PARENTAL EDUCATION

As fever is so common and causes considerable parental anxiety and concern, parents should be counselled adequately. Most parents suffer from so-called fever phobia and hence parental education will be an important step toward decreasing this. Fever issues such as what is fever, what is high grade fever, are all fever harmful and should be treated, which fever should be treated and how, when should a doctor be consulted need to be addressed. Parents should be told that fever is a protective response of body and helps to fight the disease.

The facts that *(i) fever per se is just a symptom of underlying illness and not a disease itself;* and *(ii) underlying disease and not thermometer should be treated* needs to be highlighted. Low fevers in absence of associated risks are harmless and should be left untreated. Medicines should be used only when indicated. Aspirin use for control of fever should be discouraged in children. Febrile children should be advised to drink plenty of water and wear as little as possible. The fact that febrile seizures occur in minority of children and are benign and do not cause any permanent brain damage or epilepsy should be told to the parents to prevent unnecessary panic. In children who have a history of such seizure, close monitoring is required. Parents should be told about the danger signs of fever and when to consult a doctor. This will prevent unnecessary phone calls and outpatient attendance.

HEAT HYPERPYREXIA

Heat hyperpyrexia is not an unusual cause of fever in tropical countries where ambient temperature may go as high as 45°C. Heat hyperpyrexia may occur even without exposure of the child to the direct sunlight. The predisposing factors include high temperature and humidity in the environment, unsuitable clothing, dehydration and debilitating illness, such as malaria, pneumonia, measles, and renal disorders.

Invariably, heat hyperpyrexia is associated with cessation of sweating. Children with ectodermal dysplasia and absence of sweat glands are more prone to develop episodes of heat hyperpyrexia.

The onset of high fever may be quite sudden. The rectal temperature may exceed 42–43°C. The skin appears hot and dry (without sweating). Tachycardia and tachypnea are present. The loss of consciousness occurs early. The patient may develop peripheral circulatory failure and hemorrhages.

Headache, faintness, abdominal discomfort, and delirium are usually of the complaining symptoms. The liver and kidney failure may complicate heat hyperpyrexia.

TREATMENT Heat Hyperpyrexia

When the temperature exceeds 41°C, body of the child below the neck should be immersed in the cold water without further delay to prevent irreversible brain damage. The parents should be reassured that this seemingly drastic measures will not induce shock. Ice cold bath does not cause significant vasoconstriction. The rectal temperature should be recorded continuously, and the hydrotherapy should be discontinued as the temperature falls <38°C.

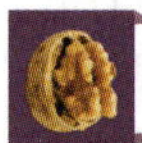

IN A NUTSHELL

Fever

1. Fever is defined as rectal temperature of 100.4°F or higher.
2. The height and duration of fever should not be considered as a criterion to judge the severity of the illness.
3. Paracetamol 15 mg/kg/dose is the optimal symptomatic treatment for fever.
4. Combined or alternating use of paracetamol and ibuprofen should be avoided.

Chiappini E, Venturini E, Remaschi G, et al. 2016 Update of the Italian Pediatric Society Guidelines for management of fever in children. J Pediatr. 2017;180:177-83.e1.

Green C, Krafft H, Guyatt G, et al. Symptomatic fever management in children: a systematic review of national and international guidelines. PLoS One. 2021;16(6):e0245815.

Gupta H, Shah D, Gupta P, et al. Role of paracetamol in treatment of childhood Fever: a double-blind randomized placebo-controlled trial. Indian Pediatr. 2007;44(12):903-11.

Hamilton JL, Evans SG, Bakshi M. Management of fever in infants and young children. American family physician. 2020;101(12):721-9.

Mahajan P, Batra P, Thakur N, et al. Consensus guidelines on evaluation and management of the febrile child presenting to the emergency department in India. Indian Pediatr. 2017;54:652-60.

McIntyre J. Management of fever in children. Arch Dis Child. 2011;96(12):1173-4.

NICE–National Institute for Care and Health Excellence. (2019). Fever in under 5s: assessment and initial management. [online] Available from https://www.nice.org.uk/guidance/ng143 [Last accessed August, 2025].

Sarkar R, Mishra K, Garg VK. Fever with rash in a child in India. Indian J Dermatol Venereol Leprol. 2012;78(3):251-62.

Section on Clinical Pharmacology and Therapeutics; Committee on Drugs, Sullivan JE, Farrar HC. Fever and antipyretic use in children. Pediatrics. 2011;127(3):580-7.

Sherman JM, Sood SK. Current challenges in the diagnosis and management of fever. Curr Opin Pediatr. 2012;24(3):400-6.

Walsh A. Available evidence does not support routine administration of antipyretics to reduce duration of fever or illness. Evid Based Nurs. 2011;14(2):58-9.

Young PJ, Saxena MK, Beasley RW. Fever and antipyresis in infection. Med J Aust. 2011;195(8):458-9.

14.2 Fever without Focus

PE 31.9

INTRODUCTION

Fever without focus refers to fever, not presenting with any other symptom-complex. It is further categorized as "fever without localizing sign" and "fever of unknown origin".

Fever without localizing signs or fever without a source is defined as fever for less than a week without adequate explanation after a thorough history and physical examination. This should be differentiated from *fever of unknown origin (FUO)* defined as fever (rectal temperature >38.3°C) of >3-week duration documented by a healthcare provider, for which the specific diagnosis could not be established even after 1 week of admission and investigation in a hospital setting. The recent literature has shown the duration of FUO to vary from 1 to 3 weeks in different settings.

FEVER WITHOUT LOCALIZING SIGNS

These children are represented by short duration fever (<7 days), having no symptoms or signs that could indicate involvement of a particular system or a probable etiology.

These children represent an important group because of higher risk of occult bacteremia and serious bacterial infections (range 5–20%). Therefore, it may sometimes become essential to start specific and empirical treatment without establishing an etiological diagnosis.

Approach to a child with fever without localizing signs will primarily depend upon his/her age; as the risk of occult bacteremia, risk of severe bacterial infection, and common etiological diagnosis are different for newborn, young infants (1–3 months), and children (3 months to 3 years).

Neonates and Fever without Localizing Signs

Newborns having a fever without any localizing signs are the most tricky to evaluate. Evaluation should start with consideration of possibility of dehydration, fever, especially in tropical climate. Such infants would usually respond to increased fluid intake and control of environmental temperature.

Serious bacterial infection (SBI) should be considered a possibility even in an apparently otherwise healthy neonate with fever, if there is no response to these measures. SBI includes meningitis, pneumonia, urinary tract infection, osteomyelitis, septic arthritis, and occult bacteremia. In India, *Haemophilus influenzae* (*H. influenzae*) B and *Streptococcus* are still considered as important causes of SBI, besides *Klebsiella*, *Staphylococcus aureus*, and *Escherichia coli (E. coli)*. In recent times, the incidence of SBI caused by *H. influenzae* and *Streptococcus* has come down due to vaccination against these infections. Malaria, scrub typhus, dengue, and chikungunya should also be considered as strong possibilities in endemic areas.

All febrile neonates without focus should be hospitalized. Initial management should consist of environmental cooling subjected to sepsis screen (blood counts, urine microscopy, blood culture, urine culture, chest X-ray, and peripheral smear for malarial parasite, peripheral blood smear for band forms, toxic granules, vacuolization, and immature/total neutrophil ratio, rickettsial, dengue, and chikungunya serology in endemic cases). Cerebrospinal fluid examination should also be done in children who appear lethargic or fail to breastfeed.

Empirical antibiotics should be started. Cefotaxime 150–200 mg/kg/day or ceftriaxone 100 mg/kg/day are the initial agents of choice. Ampicillin (100 mg/kg/day IM or IV q 12 hours) should be added in infants <4 weeks of age, to cover *Listeria* and enterococci.

Fever in Young Infants between 1 and 3 Months of Age

Febrile infants <3 months with diminished spontaneous activity, lethargy, respiratory compromise (tachypnea, chest retraction, and grunting), diminished muscle tone, mottled cool extremities, irritability, and weak sucking are at high risk. They must be evaluated for sepsis by complete blood count, lumbar puncture, blood culture, urine analysis, urine culture, and chest radiograph. *H. influenzae, E. coli, Pneumococcus, Enterococcus,* and *Neisseria meningitidis* infections are a major cause of bacterial infections at this age.

Infants 1–3 months of age with fever who appear well and had been previously healthy, and have a normal physical examination, can be categorized as at "low-risk" or "high-risk" for serious bacterial infections by certain investigations. Several criteria are available to classify them into one of these two categories.

As per *Rochester criteria,* well-looking infants are at low risk if they have a white blood cell count 5,000–15,000/mm^3, a band count of <1,500 cells/mm^3, and a normal urine (<10 white blood cells per high power field), and normal stool (<5 pus cells per high power field) microscopy. Such infants can be watched safely without starting antibiotics, till the reports of blood and urine culture are available.

Fever without Focus in 3 Months to 3-year-old

Viral infections are responsible for majority of children having nonlocalizing fever in this age group. However, serious bacterial infection can also occur due to *Streptococcus pneumoniae, Neisseria,* and *H. influenzae.* Risk factors for occult bacteremia in these children include rectal temperature >39°C, white blood cells (WBC) count >15,000/mm^3, raised erythrocyte sedimentation rate (ESR), and raised C-reactive protein. Rectal temperature >40°C and WBC count >25,000/mm^3 indicate a higher probability of serious bacterial infection. Management options are detailed in **Flowchart 14.1**.

Infants with moderate to high-risk factors should be treated with ceftriaxone [50–80 mg/kg/day in one or two divided doses intravenous (IV) or intramuscular (IM)]. Infants who do

Flowchart 14.1: Management of fever without focus in young children

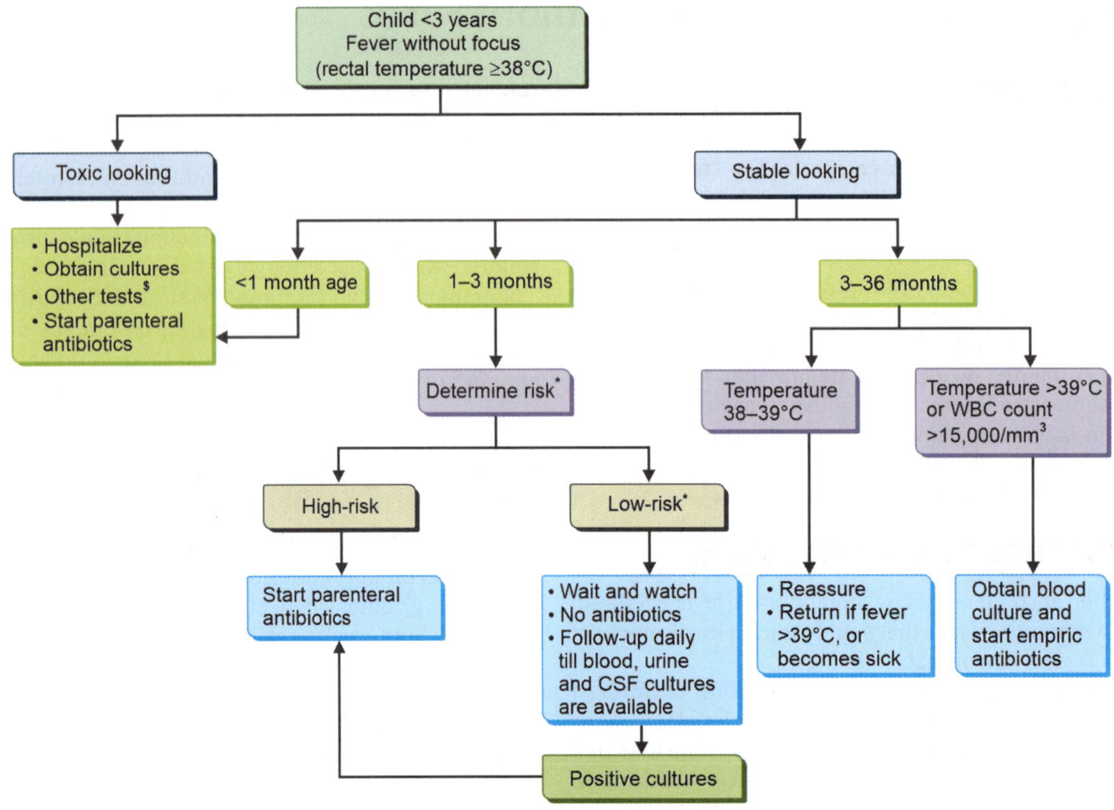

*Determine risk based on history, examination, and laboratory studies; *Low risk*: Normal history and physical examination; WBC 5,000–15,000/mm^3; band cell <1,500/mm^3; urine pus cells <10/hpf; stool pus cells <5/hpf; normal chest radiograph; and CSF <8 lymphocytes/mm^3

$Other tests include WBC count; urine and stool microscopy; chest X-ray; CSF Gram stain. Cultures include that of blood, urine, and CSF

not satisfy the above criteria for low-risk should be started on injection ceftriaxone.

FEVER OF UNKNOWN ORIGIN

Definition

Fever of unknown origin is defined as fever (rectal temperature >38°C) of >3 weeks duration documented by a healthcare provider, for which the specific diagnosis could not be established even after 1 week of admission and investigation in a hospital setting.

Nosocomial or healthcare-associated FUO refers to hospitalized children receiving acute care in whom infections or fever were absent on admission but in whom a fever of 38.0°C or more occurs on several occasions, for at least a week.

Neutropenic FUO is defined as multiple readings of >38°C in a child with absolute neutrophil count <500/mm^3, after at least 3 days of investigations including at least 48 hours of incubation of cultures.

Human immunodeficiency virus-associated FUO: This is defined as temperature more than or equal to 38.3°C or (≥101°F) on several occasions over a period of 4 weeks for outpatients or >3 days for hospitalized patients with HIV infection when appropriate investigations for 3 days, including 2 days incubation of cultures, reveal no source.

Etiology

Fever of unknown origin in children is usually due to infection, connective tissue, or autoimmune diseases. Malignancies should also be considered in the differential diagnosis. Drug fever is another differential diagnosis in a child receiving certain drug for a long time.

In a 2011 systematic review of 18 studies of FUO including 1,338 children (<18 years of age), the most common causes of FUO were as follows:

- *Infection*—51% of cases; 59% of infections were bacterial; the most common bacterial infections were tuberculosis and typhoid fever in resource-poor countries.
- No diagnosis or resolution before diagnosis—23% of cases.
- *Rheumatologic disease*—9% of cases, most commonly juvenile idiopathic arthritis and SLE.
- *Neoplastic disorder*—6% of cases, most commonly leukemia and lymphoma.

Other causes included Kawasaki disease, inflammatory bowel disease, factitious fever, hemophagocytic lymphohistiocytosis, immunodeficiency, familial Mediterranean fever, non-specified autoimmune diseases, and drugs.

Infections: Epidemiologically relevant infections must be considered first in differential diagnosis. Pulmonary or extrapulmonary tuberculosis, typhoid and paratyphoid fevers, malaria and kala-azar, amebic hepatitis and amebic liver abscess, and subacute bacterial endocarditis should always be excluded by appropriate clinical, laboratory, and radiological evaluation.

Other common infectious causes of FUO include hidden abscesses, especially in liver, urinary tract, pelvic viscera, ovaries, retroperitoneum, lungs, pleural cavity, mediastinum, subdiaphragmatic region, bones, and brain. Urinary tract infections, infections of bone and joints, spirochetal and chlamydial infections, infectious mononucleosis, cytomegalovirus (CMV) infection or hepatitis, and fungal diseases such as candidiasis, histoplasmosis, coccidioidomycosis, and cryptococcosis also result in prolonged undiagnosed fever.

Rickettsial infections (e.g., typhus, Q fever), brucellosis, leptospirosis, and relapsing fever are rare but should be considered in differential diagnosis, if epidemiologically relevant. Nosocomial infections with unusual organisms, e.g., *anaerobic bacilli*, should be considered in differential diagnosis of patient who had received various antibiotics, especially aminoglycosides, for several days in the hospital.

Malignancies: Hodgkin disease, non-Hodgkin lymphoma, leukemia, aleukemia, preleukemia, neuroblastoma, and CNS tumors may also result in FUO.

Autoimmune diseases: Systemic onset juvenile idiopathic arthritis (JIA), systemic lupus erythematosus, Still's disease, polyarteritis nodosa, mixed connective tissue disorders, rheumatic fever, vasculitis, and drug fever should also be considered in the differential diagnosis of FUO.

Granulomatous disorders: Sarcoidosis, inflammatory bowel disease, and hypertriglyceridemia can also present as FUO.

Other causes: These include various neurological, hematological, genetic, and miscellaneous disorders as already detailed under causes of prolonged fever. Several metabolic abnormalities, such as diabetes insipidus or mellitus and hyperthyroidism, may also not be diagnosed early. Factitious fever should be a possibility if fever persists for >6 months without diagnosis.

EVALUATION OF FEVER

Before starting to investigate, it is essential to document fever and observe the type of fever. The onset, type, and character of fever and the course of illness should be evaluated clinically to arrive at the possible diagnosis. Hodgkin disease has a typical *Pel–Ebstein* type of fever (3–10 days cycles of febrile and afebrile periods). Fever with chills and rigors suggests malaria, urinary tract infection, abscesses, or nosocomial infections.

Clinical Examination

Detailed history-taking and a frequently repeated physical examination remain the most important clinical tools for diagnosis. History of any skin rash, nature of medications, travel to an endemic area, exposure to certain animals, and heavy metals are especially important. While examining the child, particular attention should be paid to evaluation of skin, fundus, throat, lymph nodes, genitalia, and sinuses.

Detailed eye inspection including that of cornea, conjunctiva, orbit, uveal tract, and retina may point toward many infectious, collagen vascular, malignant or metabolic disorders.

Laboratory Tests

Appropriate laboratory investigations such as total leukocyte count, differential leukocyte count, peripheral blood smear examination for malaria, and filaria (night blood) are routinely performed. Similarly, simple serological tests for typhoid, brucellosis, leishmaniasis, rickettsiosis, toxoplasmosis and amebiasis, and bacteriological culture of blood for *Salmonella* and *Brucella* should be undertaken.

Repeated microscopic examination and cultures of blood, urine, throat, sputum, stool for bacterial and fungal infections should be carried out at periodic intervals. If specifically indicated, cultures of bone marrow, cerebrospinal fluid, gastric aspirate, lymph node aspirate, and liver aspirate for aerobic and anaerobic bacteria, mycobacteria and fungi may prove to be invaluable. Serology should also be repeated to look for any rising antibody titer. Modern molecular diagnostic techniques, e.g., polymerase chain reaction (PCR), are now available for diagnosis of several infectious agents. A variety of immunological tests for detection of various autoantibodies are now available to rule out various autoimmune disorders.

Procedures

Radiograph of the chest, barium studies of gastrointestinal tract, ultrasonography, whole body computed tomography (CT) scan, radionuclide scans, and magnetic resonance imaging (MRI) are the important noninvasive diagnostic procedures that may be required for diagnosis. Imaging studies, particularly of CNS, abdomen, pelvis, and heart, may supply substantial clues. Lymphangiography can be resorted to, for demonstrating retroperitoneal, iliac, and periaortic lymph nodes.

Endoscopic evaluation of respiratory, genitourinary, and gastrointestinal tracts may help. Skin tests are not much useful except the purified protein derivative (PPD) test for *Mycobacterium*. Biopsies of lymph node, liver, and bone marrow are routinely carried out in prolonged undiagnosed fevers. If indicated, skin, pleura, muscle, kidneys, etc., can also be biopsied.

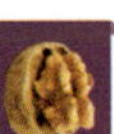

IN A NUTSHELL

Fever without Focus

1. Fever without localizing signs or fever without a source is defined as fever for ≤1 week without adequate explanation after a thorough history and physical examination.
2. Fever of unknown origin (FUO) is defined as fever (rectal temperature >38.3°C) of >3 weeks duration documented by a healthcare provider, for which the specific diagnosis could not be established even after 1 week of admission and investigation in a hospital setting.
3. The most common causes of FUO in developing countries are typhoid and tuberculosis.

Chow A, Robinson JL. Fever of unknown origin: a systematic review. World J Pediatr. 2011;7(1):5-10.
Chusid MJ. Fever of unknown origin in childhood. Pediatr Clin North Am. 2017;64(1):205-30.
Harris JA. Managing fever without a source in young children: the debate continues. Am Fam Physician. 2007;75(12):1774, 1776.
Machado BM, Cardoso DM, de Paulis M, et al. Fever without source: evaluation of a guideline. J Pediatr. 2009;85(5):426-32.
Sur DK, Bukont EL. Evaluating fever of unidentifiable source in young children. Am Fam Physician. 2007;75(12):1805-11.
Trapani S, Fiordelisi A, Stinco M, Resti M. Update on fever of unknown origin in children: focus on etiologies and clinical approach. Children (Basel). 2023;11(1):20.
Varghese GM, Trowbridge P, Doherty T. Investigating and managing pyrexia of unknown origin in adults. BMJ. 2010;341:C5470.

14.3 Tuberculosis

PE 31.1, PE 31.2, PE 31.3, PE 31.4, PE 31.5, PE 31.6, PE 31.7, PE 31.8

INTRODUCTION

Tuberculosis (TB) is a chronic infectious disease caused by *Mycobacterium tuberculosis (MTB)*. The disease is widely prevalent throughout the world. Due to improved standard of living and better sanitation, the incidence of TB has steadily declined in the affluent and developed countries. However, it is still a major public health problem in the economically underprivileged countries of Asia, Africa, and South America.

BURDEN OF TUBERCULOSIS

In 2020, 86% of new TB cases occurred in the 30 high TB burden countries. Eight countries accounted for two-thirds of the new TB cases: India, China, Indonesia, Philippines, Pakistan, Nigeria, Bangladesh, and South Africa. India has the highest TB burden in the world accounting for about one-fourth of the estimated incident cases globally in 2013. As per Global TB report 2018, an estimated 2.2 lakh children become ill with TB each year in India (22% of global TB burden) with a slightly higher burden among males. Pulmonary TB (PTB) is the most common form in children, but the extra-PTB forms a larger proportion of TB cases when compared to adults.

EPIDEMIOLOGY

Agent: Tuberculosis in humans is caused mostly by *M. tuberculosis*. These are nonspore forming, nonmotile, obligate aerobe, and acid fast bacilli.

Transmission: The infection is spread by an open adult TB patient, who discharges tubercle bacilli in the sputum or nasopharyngeal secretions during bouts of coughing or sneezing. Young children rarely spread TB because the small amounts of tubercle bacilli in the endobronchial secretions and poor coughing force, are not sufficient to suspend infectious particles of adequate size in the air. The infected sputum spitted carelessly by open cases of TB dries up and the tubercle bacilli are suspended in the dust and air. The usual mode of infection is through inhalation of droplets of infected secretions.

Host Factors

- ***Environment:*** Children living in overcrowded apartments with inadequate ventilation and little sunlight are at high risk. Damp and unhygienic living conditions are important predisposing factors.
- ***Malnutrition:*** Undernourished children are more susceptible to develop TB due to decreased immunity. TB may precipitate severe acute malnutrition.
- ***Infections:*** A quiescent tuberculous infection may flare up after an attack of measles or whooping cough.
- ***Immunodeficiency:*** Children with primary or secondary immunodeficiency are more prone to develop disease after tuberculosis infection and to develop disseminated TB.

PATHOGENESIS

The most common portal of entry of *M. tuberculosis* is lungs. The tubercle bacilli multiply in alveoli and produce local infection. Most are killed while some survive in macrophages and are carried to the draining regional lymph nodes. The parenchymal lesion together with enlarged regional lymph nodes is known as primary complex (Ghon focus). These tubercle bacilli are carried to other organs via blood and lymphatic vessels. Disseminated disease develops when large number of bacilli enter these organs or when host is immunocompromised.

CLINICAL FEATURES

Systemic Manifestations

Persistent fever of >2 weeks without a known cause, weight loss of >5%, or no weight gain in past 3 months despite adequate nutrition or failure of nutritional rehabilitation in children with severe acute malnutrition should arouse suspicion of tuberculosis.

Pulmonary Tuberculosis

Primary Pulmonary Tuberculosis

The inflamed area at the point of entry of tubercle bacilli is called the "primary focus". Its size varies from a few millimeter to 1 or 2 cm. Some tubercle bacilli travel to the regional lymph nodes via the draining lymphatic vessels and cause an inflammatory reaction there. The primary focus, the draining lymphatics, and the inflamed regional lymph nodes are collectively called the *"primary complex"*.

Primary complex occurs most commonly in the subpleural region and all the lobar segments are at equal risk. Primary TB has larger regional lymphadenitis as compared to pulmonary focus. Lymph node may cause bronchial obstruction leading to collapse-consolidation. It may erode the bronchus to cause endobronchial TB, which causes intraluminal obstruction of bronchus. The focus may erode into blood stream to cause miliary TB, which is characterized by small nodules homogeneously distributed in the lungs. Primary TB has lesser symptoms and signs as compared to chest X-ray findings. Mild breathlessness and nonproductive cough are the most common symptoms. Systemic symptoms such as fever, weight loss, anorexia, and night sweats are uncommon.

Progressive Pulmonary Tuberculosis

Further development of the primary complex depends on the host defenses. If the resistance of the host is good, the primary complex heals by itself. When the host defenses are poor, primary complex progresses further resulting in progressive primary TB. Primary focus continues to enlarge, and the center shows liquefactive necrosis and cavity formation. Significant signs and symptoms are present in the form of dyspnea, productive cough, high fever, weight loss, and reduced appetite.

Reactivation TB occurs due to reactivation of a previous focus. It is more common in adults and rare in children.

Tuberculous Lymphadenitis (Scrofula)

It is characterized by progressive enlargement of lymph nodes for >2 weeks. It is usually unilateral, firm, non-tender, fixed to underlying, and overlying tissues. Lymph nodes may get matted, fluctuate, and may rupture to form sinuses and fistulae.

Pleural Effusion

Effusion develops when subpleural pulmonary focus or caseated lymph node discharges acid-fast bacilli into the pleural space. It presents with high fever, cough, discomfort, and pain on the affected side of the chest. The pain becomes worse with deep breathing and coughing. The affected side of the chest is less mobile, the intercostal spaces appear full, the trachea is shifted to the opposite side, vocal fremitus is decreased, percussion note is stony dull, and the breath sounds are distant.

Pericardial Tuberculosis

Tuberculous pericarditis is the most common cardiac manifestation of TB. It occurs due to direct invasion or due to lymphatic drainage from subcarinal lymph nodes. It presents with low nonspecific features (fever, weight loss), breathlessness, pericardial friction rub, distant heart sounds, and pulsus paradoxus. If diagnosed late, constrictive pericarditis may develop.

Abdominal Tuberculosis

Tuberculosis of abdomen may present with colicky abdominal pain, vomiting, and constipation. The abdomen feels characteristically doughy. The rolled-up omentum and enlarged lymph nodes may appear as irregular nodular masses. There may be frank ascites, intestinal obstruction, or hepatosplenomegaly.

Central Nervous System Tuberculosis

Tuberculous Meningitis

Tuberculous meningitis (TBM) is the most serious complication of TB in children. It occurs due to lymphohematogenous dissemination of bacilli leading to formation of caseous lesions in cerebral cortex and meninges. Initially, the child becomes dull and has low-grade fever (*Stage 1*). This is followed by onset of meningeal signs (neck rigidity) and signs of raised intracranial tension (alteration of consciousness, convulsions). There may be paralysis of one side of the body along with deviation of face, eye movements due to involvement of the cranial nerves (*Stage 2*). In the *Stage 3*, the child passes into deep coma and develops abnormal central type of respiration.

Tuberculoma

These are tumor-like lesions formed due to conglomeration of tubercles, which contain caseous material or calcifications. Children present with fever, headache, seizures, and focal neurological deficits. Its close differential diagnosis is neurocysticercosis.

Osteoarticular Tuberculosis

Bone TB most commonly involves vertebrae. Tubercular spondylitis leads to Gibbus deformity and kyphosis, known as Pott's spine.

Genitourinary Tuberculosis

It is rare in children occurring mostly due to lymphohematogenous spread of infection. Renal tuberculosis is usually unilateral presenting with sterile pyuria, hematuria, dysuria, and flank pain. Genital TB affects adolescent girls and boys. It affects most commonly the fallopian tubes followed by endometrium, ovaries, and cervix in girls and manifests with abdominal pain and menstrual abnormalities. In boys, epididymis and testes are affected and manifests as painless nodular swelling of scrotum.

Disseminated Tuberculosis

In all cases of tuberculosis, lymphohematogenous spread of tubercle bacilli to distant organs such as liver, spleen, meninges, skin, bone marrow, eyes, lung apices, bones and joints occurs, which is mostly asymptomatic. Clinical features develop only when bacilli load is heavy and immune response of the host is suppressed. The patients present with hepatosplenomegaly, lymphadenopathy, meningitis, skin tuberculids, bone, and joint tuberculosis.

Miliary Tuberculosis

It is a form of disseminated TB with two or more organ involvement occurring due to massive dissemination of bacilli into the blood stream. Infants, malnourished, and immunocompromised children are at higher risk. The onset of the illness is sudden presenting with fever, dyspnea, delirium, and convulsions. Chest X-ray reveals characteristic miliary mottling (uniform-sized nodules of <2–3 mm in diameter homogeneously distributed in both the lung fields).

Congenital Tuberculosis

It occurs due to transmission of infection from mother to the baby through placenta and sometimes by aspiration of amniotic fluid. It presents at birth or by 2nd–3rd week of life as fever, failure to thrive, refusal to feed, respiratory distress, hepatosplenomegaly, lymphadenopathy, abdominal distension, and skin lesions.

Tuberculosis in Human Immunodeficiency Virus Patients

Tuberculosis infection, TB disease, recurrent and relapse of TB occur at higher rate in untreated HIV patients as compared to non-HIV patients. Also, TB is severe, progressive, and difficult to diagnose in such patients. *Four-symptom screening* for TB should be done during every visit to the antiretroviral therapy (ART) center. Children should be assessed for current cough, fever, poor weight gain, and contact history of TB. Any child found positive on history should undergo detailed investigations and examination to rule out TB. Also, all children with TB should be screened for HIV infection.

CASE DEFINITIONS OF TUBERCULOSIS

- ***Presumptive tuberculosis:*** Person who presents with symptoms or signs suggestive of TB.
- ***Microbiologically confirmed TB case:*** A microbiologically confirmed TB case refers to a presumptive TB case from whom a biological specimen is positive for acid fast bacilli, or positive for *MTB* on culture, or positive for TB through rapid diagnostic molecular test.
- ***Pulmonary tuberculosis (PTB):*** Any bacteriologically confirmed or clinically diagnosed case of TB involving the lung parenchyma or the tracheobronchial tree, including tuberculous intrathoracic lymphadenopathy (mediastinal and/or hilar), without radiographic abnormalities in the lungs.
- ***Miliary TB*** is classified as PTB because there are lesions in the lungs. A person with both PTB and miliary TB should be classified as having PTB.
- ***Extrapulmonary tuberculosis (EPTB):*** Any bacteriologically confirmed or clinically diagnosed case of TB involving organs other than the lungs (e.g., pleura, peripheral lymph nodes, abdomen, genitourinary tract, skin, joints and bones, meninges).
- ***Contact:*** Any person exposed to a person with TB.
- ***New TB patient:*** A TB patient who has never had treatment for TB or has taken anti-TB drugs for <1 month is considered as a new TB patient.
- ***Previously treated TB:*** A patient who has received 1 month or more of anti-TB drugs from any source in the past.
- ***Recurrent TB patient:*** A TB patient previously declared as successfully treated (cured/treatment completed) and is subsequently found to be microbiologically confirmed TB is a recurrent TB patient.
- ***Treatment after failure:*** These are the patients who have previously been treated for TB and whose treatment failed at the end of their most recent course of treatment.
- ***Treatment after lost to follow-up:*** A TB patient previously treated for TB for 1 month or more and was declared lost to follow-up (LFU) in his/her most recent course of treatment and subsequently found to be microbiologically confirmed.
- ***Monoresistance (MR):*** A TB patient, whose biological specimen is resistant to one first-line anti-TB drug only.
- ***Polydrug resistance (PDR):*** A TB patient, whose biological specimen is resistant to more than one first-line anti-TB drug, other than both isoniazid (INH) and rifampicin (R).
- ***Multidrug resistance (MDR):*** A TB patient, whose biological specimen is resistant to both first-line drugs, based on the INH and R, with or without resistance to other drugs.
- ***Rifampicin resistance:*** Resistance to R detected using phenotypic or genotypic methods, with or without resistance to other anti-TB drugs excluding INH. Patients, who have any R resistance, should also be managed as if they are an MDR-TB case.
- ***Extensively drug-resistant (XDR):*** An MDR TB case whose biological specimen is additionally resistant to a fluoroquinolone (ofloxacin, moxifloxacin, or levofloxacin) and a second-line injectable anti-TB drug (kanamycin, amikacin, or capreomycin) from a quality assured laboratory.

NATIONAL TUBERCULOSIS PROGRAM

- The *National Tuberculosis Control Program (NTCP)* was launched by the Government of India in 1962. It focused primarily on bacillus Calmette–Guérin (BCG) vaccination as preventive strategy for tuberculosis.

- *Revised National Tuberculosis Control Program (RNTCP)* was launched in 1997, which adopted *Directly Observed Treatment Short Course (DOTS) strategy*.
- In 2020, RNTCP was renamed as *National Tuberculosis Elimination Program (NTEP)* to achieve the goals of *Revised National Strategic Plan (NSP) for Tuberculosis Elimination 2017–2025*.
- The *end TB strategy* announced by WHO targets to reduce TB deaths by 90% and 95%, and incidence by 80% and 90%, by 2030 and 2035, respectively. The government of India aims to eliminate TB from our country by 2025, ahead of the global target.
- The vision of NSP is tuberculosis free India with zero deaths, disease, and poverty due to tuberculosis. Its goal is to achieve a rapid decline in burden of tuberculosis, morbidity, and mortality to achieve elimination of TB in India by 2025. Its four basic pillars are: *"detect-treat-prevent-build" (DTPB)*.
- *NIKSHAY* is a web-based surveillance system for TB to facilitate notification of TB cases from both government and private health sectors. *Nikshay Poshak Yojana* is a scheme under national health mission to provide financial support for nutritional rehabilitation of notified TB cases.

DIAGNOSIS

The diagnosis of TB is based on clinical features, history of contact with an open infective case, demonstration of hypersensitivity to tuberculin (*Mantoux test*), evidence of radiological lesions suggestive of TB (X-ray of chest, ultrasound abdomen, or CT brain), and laboratory investigations (elevated ESR, demonstration of tubercle bacilli in the sputum, gastric lavage or bronchial aspirate), or histopathology of affected lymph nodes. There is a paradigm shift in diagnostic strategy from conventional smear microscopy to molecular methods of diagnosis due to their higher sensitivity. *NTEP approved rapid Nucleic Acid Amplification Tests (NAAT)* such as Xpert Rif/Truenat have made it possible to detect MTB with much higher sensitivity and rapidity as compared to smear and culture respectively. *Cartridge-based nucleic acid amplification test (CB-NAAT)* is the new diagnostic modality that can detect the deoxyribonucleic acid (DNA) of *Mycobacterium* in body fluids and tissues. These tests also detect R resistance, a surrogate for MDR-TB.

In addition, NTEP also recommends *line probe assays (LPA)*, which are multiplex NAAT—to test for resistance to R, INH, and other second line drugs (fluoroquinolones and second-line injectables). Under the strategy called *Universal Drug Sensitivity Testing (U-DST)*, each likely patient of tuberculosis should be tested for presence of MTB as well as R resistance. Current algorithm for evaluation of pulmonary TB in children is shown in **Flowchart 14.2**.

Tests for Tuberculosis Infection

Mantoux Test (Tuberculin Test)

It involves administration of PPD RT 23 with Tween 80 equivalent. One, two, and five tuberculin units PPD are available in India. PPD should be stored at a temperature of 2–8°C. It should be discarded if >30 days have passed after opening the vial or expiry date is passed. Antigen should not be drawn into the syringe >1 hour before use. The standard tuberculin test recommended is Mantoux test.

Procedure: Injection is given intradermally on volar aspect of the left forearm. Patient's forearm is exposed with the palm side up with the elbow slightly flexed. A total of 0.1 mL of a suitable dilution of tuberculin (PPD RT23 equivalent) is taken in a 1 mL tuberculin syringe. The injection is given 2–4 inches below the elbow. The site is cleaned using spirit swab. The skin is stretched taut, and the tuberculin syringe is inserted at 5–15° angle keeping the bevel of the needle up. A weal of 5 mm should be raised. The needle should be removed without rubbing or massaging the area. The patient is asked to keep the area clean and dry and to avoid scratching.

Reading the test: The reaction is read after 48–72 hours. As the induration may not always be visible, ballpoint, or palpatory methods are used to read the induration. The edges of the induration are located using the fingertips. Alternatively, the induration may be detected by the ballpoint method. A ballpoint pen is used to draw a line starting 1–2 cm away from the skin reaction and moving toward its center. An increased resistance is felt when the pen reaches the margin of the induration. The distance between the ends of the opposing lines at the margins of the induration is measured. Using a millimeter ruler, the widest diameter of the induration perpendicular to the long axis of the forearm is measured.

Interpretation: Width of induration of >10 mm in the horizontal plane is considered positive and indicates exposure to tubercle bacilli. Ten millimeter cut-off is recommended using 1 TU PPD RT23. This cut-off may be used for strengths of PPD up to 5 TU. A negative tuberculin reaction does not rule out TB, especially in children with malnutrition, severe disseminated tubercular disease or those receiving steroids.

The skin test reaction is depressed in malnutrition; very young age; immunosuppression by corticosteroids, live-virus vaccines, viral infections (measles, mumps, varicella, influenza), and overwhelming tuberculosis. False-positive reactions may be caused by infection with nontuberculous mycobacteria and prior BCG vaccination.

Interferon Gamma Release Assays

These assays detect interferon gamma generation by peripheral mononuclear cells in response to specific *M. tuberculosis* antigens [early secretion antigen target (ESAT 6) and culture filtrate protein 10 (CFP 10)]. Two commercially available interferon gamma release assays (IGRAs) are: T-SPOT.TB and QuantiFERON-TB. These tests can be used to detect latent TB in low prevalence settings in place of tuberculin skin test.

Diagnostic Tests for Pulmonary Tuberculosis

Chest X-ray

Chest X-ray should be performed in all cases with suspected tuberculosis. Highly suggestive lesions are—miliary shadows,

Flowchart 14.2: Evaluation of pulmonary TB among children with no risk factors for drug resistance

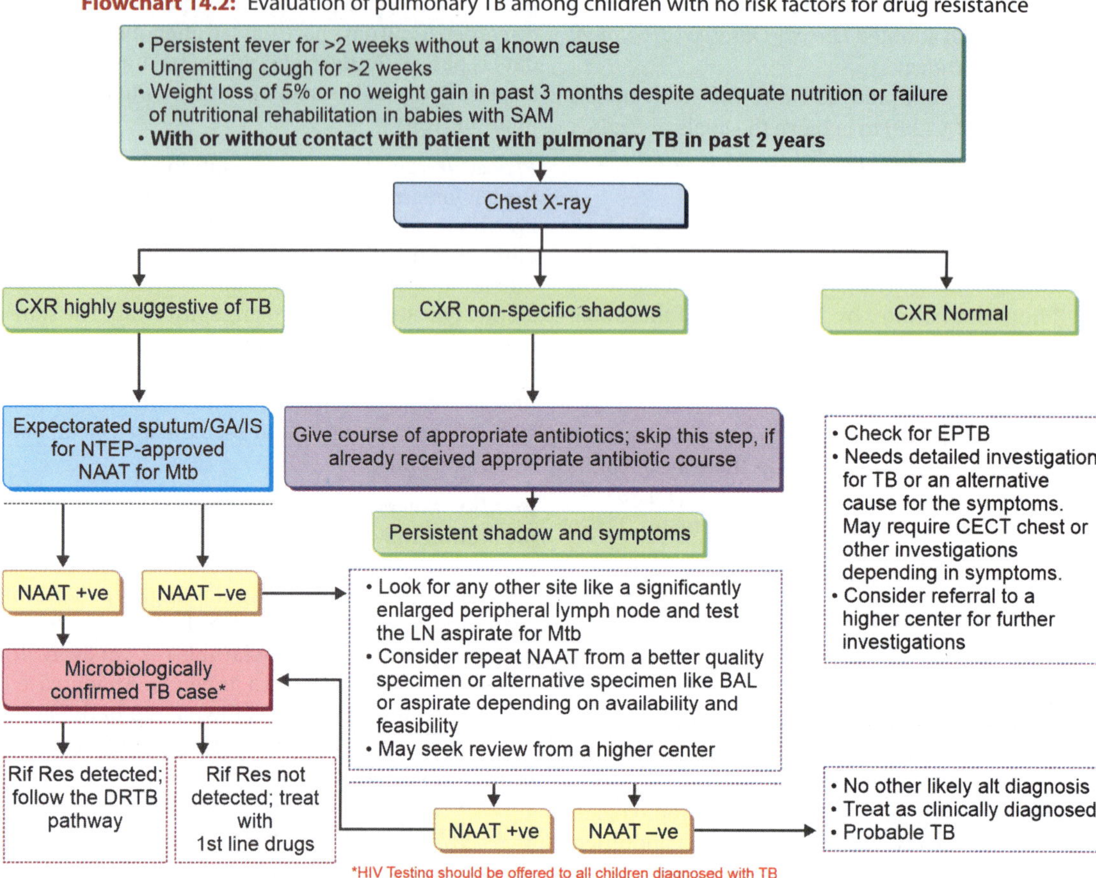

(DRTB: drug-resistant TB; GA: gastric aspirate; NAAT: rapid nucleic acid amplification test)
Source: National Tuberculosis Elimination Program Pediatric TB management guideline 2022

hilar and mediastinal lymphadenopathy, and chronic fibro-cavitary parenchymal lesions. Nonspecific chest X-ray patterns refer to those other than highly suggestive ones such as consolidations, nonhomogeneous shadows, etc. Persistence of nonspecific shadows after antibiotic course in a symptomatic child should raise suspicion of tuberculosis. But these shadows may be due to other conditions such as interstitial lung disease or bronchiectasis. Persistent nonspecific shadows in an asymptomatic child may be due to healed parenchymal lesions, and pleural thickening.

Computed Tomography (CT Scan)

CT scans are crucial for evaluating children with persistent pneumonia or unexplained fever, despite being costly and involving significant radiation. Specific CT patterns can suggest tuberculosis (TB), including: Necrotic mediastinal lymphadenopathy, centrilobular nodules with tree-in-bud pattern, and cavities with surrounding consolidations. Chest CT scans also enable guided biopsies for tissue diagnosis.

Ultrasonography (USG)

USG helps assess pleural fluid collection, differentiate thymus and lymph nodes, and identify optimal sites for aspiration or biopsy in peripheral lesions.

Bacteriology

The gold standard for diagnosis of tuberculosis is demonstration of acid-fast bacilli (AFB) in body fluids and tissues. Various samples for demonstration of AFB are sputum, gastric aspirate, cerebrospinal fluid (CSF), and fine-needle aspiration cytology (FNAC).

Samples:

- ***Gastric aspirate:*** Since most children are unable to expectorate the sputum, early morning gastric aspirate is a preferred sample for AFB demonstration. After overnight fasting of at least 6 hours, an appropriate sized gastric tube is passed in the stomach before the child rises and content is aspirated. Thereafter, stomach is washed with 15–30 mL of normal saline and the content is aspirated again. Sample is sent immediately to the laboratory.
- ***Induced sputum:*** After overnight fast children are nebulized with salbutamol followed by hypertonic (3%) normal saline. Chest physiotherapy is done. Older children may expectorate at the end of the procedure while in young children nasopharyngeal aspirate can be collected.
- ***Bronchoalveolar lavage:*** Bronchoscopy followed by bronchoalveolar lavage is used to collect the respiratory secretions especially in cases of persistent pneumonia.

Methods

1. ***Ziehl–Neelsen (ZN) staining:*** ZN staining of the samples such as sputum, gastric aspirate, CSF remained the primary strategy for bacteriological confirmation of tuberculosis for long. ZN stain can reveal AFB only if sample contains >10,000 bacilli/mL. The paucibacillary nature of pulmonary TB in children, inability to expectorate sputum and lack of skills or facilities for collection, and processing of nonsputum specimens at the diagnostic centers further decreased the use of this diagnostic modality.
2. ***Cartridge-based nucleic acid amplification tests (CBNAATs):*** CBNAAT is a fully automated real-time PCR-based test, which can detect both TB and resistance to rifampicin in <2 hours. RNTCP approved CBNAAT (Xpert-Rif/Truenat) has proved to be a rapid method for microbiologic confirmation of TB. The test is more sensitive than conventional microscopy as it requires just above a hundred DNA copies (organisms) per milliliter of the specimen as compared to tens of thousands for a smear. This has led to a paradigm shift in diagnostic strategy from conventional smear microscopy to molecular methods of diagnosis.
   Cartridge-based nucleic acid amplification tests can be used on various respiratory (sputum, gastric aspirate, and bronchoalveolar lavage fluid) and nonrespiratory (CSF, pus, lymph node aspirates, and other tissues) specimens. Pleural fluid and ascitic fluid are suboptimal samples for CBNAAT. Also, it should not be used for blood. It has a high specificity (around 100%) but sensitivity is 92% for bronchial washing and around 60% for pleural fluid.
   Negative CBNAAT does not rule out TB. It can detect tubercular DNA even after starting treatment for up to 1 month. Its advantages are simplicity to use, rapidity of result, and high specificity. Disadvantages are that it is far more expensive as compared to smear examination and requires electrical supplies and temperature control facilities.
3. ***Line probe assays (LPA):*** These are molecular tests used to detect *Mycobacterium tuberculosis* and test for resistance antitubercular drugs. LPA has relatively lower sensitivity so it can be used directly only in smear positive specimens or after isolating MTB on culture. First line LPA (FL-LPA) detects rifampicin and isoniazid resistance. Second line LPA (SL-LPA) detects resistance to fluoroquinolones and second line injectables.
   In children with signs and symptoms of pulmonary TB, CBNAAT should be used as the initial diagnostic test for TB and detection of R resistance on sputum, gastric aspirate, nasopharyngeal aspirate, or stool, rather than conventional smear microscopy/culture and phenotypic drug susceptibility testing (DST).
4. ***Culture:*** Lowenstein-Jensen (LJ) medium is the conventional medium used for culture of *M. tuberculosis.* It contains glycerol as carbon source and ammonium as nitrogen source. Although the method is simple, it requires around 3–6 weeks for isolation of organisms and another 2–4 weeks for drug susceptibility testing. To reduce the time required for isolation, selective liquid culture media such as BACTEC (Becton Dickinson and Company) radiometric assay and mycobacterial growth indicator tube (MGIT) system are preferred. These methods have reduced the time of isolation to 1–3 weeks and time for drug susceptibility to 3–5 days.

Serodiagnostic tests: Antibodies to various antigens of MTB can be detected by enzyme-linked immunoassay (ELISA). Sensitivity and specificity of these tests depend upon the antigens against which antibodies are measured. These tests have no role in diagnosis of TB at present.

Diagnostic Tests for Extrapulmonary Tuberculosis

- ***Fine-needle aspiration cytology (FNAC) and biopsy:*** In tubercular lymphadenitis, FNAC should be done for AFB stain/CBNAAT, culture, and histology. Demonstration of AFB in the specimen may be positive in 20–70% of patients. Histology shows necrosis and epithelioid granuloma formation. If results are inconclusive, histopathology and AFB demonstration can be done in biopsy specimens.
- ***Pleurocentesis and pleural fluid examination:*** If chest X-ray is suggestive of pleural effusion, pleural fluid examination for cytology, biochemistry, and smear examination for AFB is done. Tubercular pleural effusion is characterized by elevated protein, leukocytosis with lymphocytic predominance, and elevated adenosine deaminase (ADA) levels.
- ***Paracentesis and ascitic fluid examination:*** In suspected tubercular peritonitis, ascitic fluid examination should be done, which shows exudate with lymphocytic pleocytosis and elevated protein.
- ***Lumbar puncture and CSF examination:*** In suspected tubercular meningitis, CSF examination is done. Typically, CSF is clear with lymphocytic leukocytosis, elevated protein, mildly low sugar, and elevated ADA levels.
- ***Neuroimaging:*** CECT head may show tuberculoma, dilated ventricles, periventricular ooze, infarcts, and basal meningeal enhancement suggestive of CNS tuberculosis.
- ***Ultrasonography (USG) abdomen:*** USG abdomen should be done in suspected abdominal tuberculosis. Findings suggestive of TB are: Mesenteric lymphadenopathy (>15 mm), thickened mesentery, dilated bowel loops, and ascites.

TREATMENT Tuberculosis

Principles of Treatment

The principles of treatment are listed below:

- The diagnosis should be made early.
- The treatment should be prompt, adequate, vigorous, and prolonged depending on the severity of the illness.
- More than one antitubercular drug should be used simultaneously for prevention of development of drug-resistant tubercle bacilli.
- Nutrition of the child should be improved by nutritionally balanced diet with adequate calories and protein. The diet should be supplemented by vitamins and minerals to improve the host resistance.
- Intercurrent infections should be prevented or treated vigorously.
- Every effort should be made to trace the reservoir of infection or the open infective case in the family or extra familial contacts and he or she should be treated.
- The living condition should be improved by better hygienic measures and improved sanitation.

Table 14.3 Anti-TB-drug Dosages for Children as per NTEP Guidelines 2022

		Range (mg/kg/day)	Average (mg/kg/day)	Maximum dose (mg)
Rifampicin	R	10–20	15	600
Isoniazid	H	7–15	10	300
Pyrazinamide	Z	30–40	35	2,000
Ethambutol	E	15–25	20	1,500
Streptomycin	S	15–20	20	1,000

(NTEP: National Tuberculosis Elimination Program)

- The child should be exposed to adequate sunlight and living apartment should be well ventilated.

Drugs

Antitubercular drugs are divided into two major categories:

1. ***First-line drugs:*** Majority of patients can be successfully treated with these drugs. These drugs are effective with minimal toxicity. These include INH, R, ethambutol, and pyrazinamide. Streptomycin is no longer a first line drug and is used only in case of non-availabilty or resistance to amikacin.
2. ***Second-line drugs:*** These are used in drug resistant cases or in situations where first-line drugs cannot be used due to either toxicity or some other constraints. These include ethionamide, amikacin, kanamycin, capreomycin, cycloserine, ofloxacin, etc. The following dosages of anti-TB medicines are recommended for the treatment of TB in children **(Table 14.3)**.

National Tuberculosis Elimination Program (NTEP) 2022 tuberculosis treatment guidelines are shown in **Tables 14.4 to 14.6**. The algorithm for evaluation of children with suspected drug resistance is shown in **Flowchart 14.3**. The standard regime consists of two phases: (1) intensive phase, and (2) continuation phase.

Table 14.4 Drug Regimen for Rifampicin-sensitive Tuberculosis as per NTEP Guidelines, 2022

*Type of patent**	*Regimens*
New microbiologically confirmed pulmonary TB	2HRZE+ 4HRE#
New clinically diagnosed pulmonary TB	
New microbiologically confirmed extrapulmonary TB	
New clinically diagnosed extrapulmonary TB	
Previously treated TB^ (recurrence, treatment after loss to follow-up, treatment after failure)	

*Molecular testing for rifampicin resistance shall be done in all new cases in children with suspected TB at diagnosis.

#In case of neurological, bone, joints and spinal TB the continuation phase is extended to 10 months. In disseminated forms, the continuation phase might be extended to 7 months.

^All retreatment cases are to be evaluated as per DR-TB algorithm. They were earlier treated with CAT II or retreatment regimen, which is now withdrawn. Their treatment should be based on drug sensitivity, particularly for R and H. In case they are found to be drug sensitive, they shall be started on the above regimen as for a new case.

(E: ethambutol, H: isoniazid; NTEP: National Tuberculosis Elimination Program; R: rifampicin; Z: pyrazinamide)

Table 14.5 Drug Regimen for Pediatric Drug-resistant Tuberculosis as per NTEP Guidelines, 2022

Type of tuberculosis	*Treatment regimes*	*Special considerations*
RR/MDR-TB Shorter oral Bedaquiline containing regime	*Intensive phase* (4–6) Mfx^h Km Eto Cfz ZH^h E (6) Bdq *Continuation phase* (5) Mfx^h Cfz Z E	• Recommended for pulmonary cases or nonsevere forms of EPTB like isolated lymph node disease or pleural effusion, etc. • Not exposed to reserve drugs • Send tests for SLI and FQ class resistance, continue this regimen only if sensitive to these two drug classes
MDR-TB/MDR-TB + FQ resistance/XDR–TB[#,$,+] Longer oral regime	*(18–20) Lfx (Mfxh) Lzd (1) Cfz Cs* *(6–9) Dlm (Bdq)*	• Not for severe EPTB such as intracranial TB or disseminated TB • Not for children <6 years • Bdq to be replaced by Dlm in 6–17 years of age • Lfx to be replaced by Mfx^h if FQ class resistance • No separate intensive or continuation phase
MDR-TB (EP)/ Or MDR-TB + FQ resistance/XDR–TB Longer oral regime	*Intensive phase* (6–9) Amika Mfx^h Lzd Cfz Eto Cs *Continuation phase* (18) Mfx^h Lzd (1) Cfz Cs	Disseminated or severe extrapulmonary disease
Resistance to INH (with or without any non-rifampicin first-line drug resistance)^	Uniphasic regime (6) Lfx R E Z	Can be extended to 9–12 months in extensive pulmonary disease and extrapulmonary disease like bone or intracranial

*Shorter MDR-TB regimen is of 9–11 months with 4–6 months of IP containing injectables and 5 months of CP. If the IP is prolonged, the injectable is only given three times a week in the extended intensive phase.

#All oral longer MDR-TB regimens are of 18–20 months.

$New drugs such as Bdq and Dlm would be given for 6 months duration while the dose of Lzd will be tapered to 10 mg/kg/day (maximum 300 mg) after the initial 6–8 months of treatment.

+This regimen will also be used for treatment of XDR-TB patients with 20 months duration.

^All oral H monopoly DR-TB regimen is of 6 months with no separate IP/CP.

(Bdq: bedaquiline; Cs: cycloserine; Cfz: clofazimine; Dlm; delamanid; E: ethambutol; EPTB: extrapulmonary TB; Fq: fluoroquinolones; Eto: ethionamide; H^h: high dose isoniazid; Km: kanamycin; Lfx: levofloxacin; Lzd: linezolid; MDR: multidrug resistant; Mfx^h: high dose moxifloxacin; NTEP: National Tuberculosis Elimination Program; RR: rifampicin resistant; SLI: second-line injectables; XDR: extensively drug resistant; Z: pyrazinamide)

Table 14.6 Tuberculosis Drug Formulations and Dosages for Children as per NTEP Guidelines, 2022

Weight band (kg)	*Dose (0–18 years)*
4–7	1 P + 1 E
8–11	2 P + 2 E
12–15	3 P + 3 E
16–24	4 P + 4 E
25–29	3 P + 3 E + 1 A
30–39	2 P + 2 E + 2 A

(H: isoniazid, R: rifampicin, Z: pyrazinamide, E: ethambutol; Number preceding the letter denotes number of pediatric or adult formulations; NTEP: National Tuberculosis Elimination Program; Pediatric formulation (P) H50, R 75, Z 150 + E 100 (E separate tab); adult formulation (A) H 75, R 150, Z 400, E 275)

1. ***Intensive phase:*** The goal of this phase is to eliminate the bacterial load and prevent the emergence of drug-resistant strains. Four drugs, including at least three bactericidal drugs are used during this phase to initiate the therapy. This phase usually lasts for 2 months.
2. ***Continuation phase:*** During this phase, at least three drugs are used to continue and complete the therapy. The phase lasts from 4–6 months. The total duration of therapy may range from 6 months to 1 year, depending on the extent of disease. Steroids (prednisolone) are indicated in cases of tuberculous meningitis, pericarditis, peritonitis, or terminally ill children with miliary TB.

National Tuberculosis Elimination Program has introduced daily therapy with dispersible tablets in fixed dose combinations (FDC) for children. Younger children get 3-drug FDCs (HRZ) along with 100 mg ethambutol tablets. Older children can also get, in addition, 4-drug FDCs (RHZE) to meet their drug dosages. Isoniazid and rifampicin are in a ratio of 2:3 and the average dose of isoniazid is around 10 mg/kg/day. These drugs are given free of cost in public sector. **Tables 14.3 and 14.6** show TB drug formulations and dosages as per NTEP guidelines, 2022. Addition of pyridoxine (10 mg/day) with isoniazid containing regimens is recommended because of the risk of peripheral neuropathy due to higher dosages.

PREVENTION

Tracing the Source of Infection

Effort should be made to trace the source of infection in the family and extra-familial contacts of every child with TB. The extrafamilial contacts should include school teachers, food vendors, domestic servants, and frequent visitors to the household. The open infective case should be treated vigorously to make him/her noninfective.

Health Education

The community should be educated about the mode of infection of TB, early symptoms, methods of prevention, and treatment. Hygienic living with good environmental sanitation should be propagated. The living apartments should be well ventilated with good sanitation. Dampness should be avoided. Milk should always be boiled before use. Adults should be advised not to spit indiscriminately.

BCG Vaccination

Bacillus Calmette-Guérin vaccination is an extremely useful measure to reduce the incidence of TB and its serious complications. BCG vaccine should be given at birth. Catch-up vaccination can be done till 1 year of age as per universal immunization program of India and up to 5 years as per IAP. It is given intradermal in left upper arm at a dose of 0.05 mL until

Flowchart 14.3: Algorithm for evaluation of children with suspected drug-resistant tuberculosis

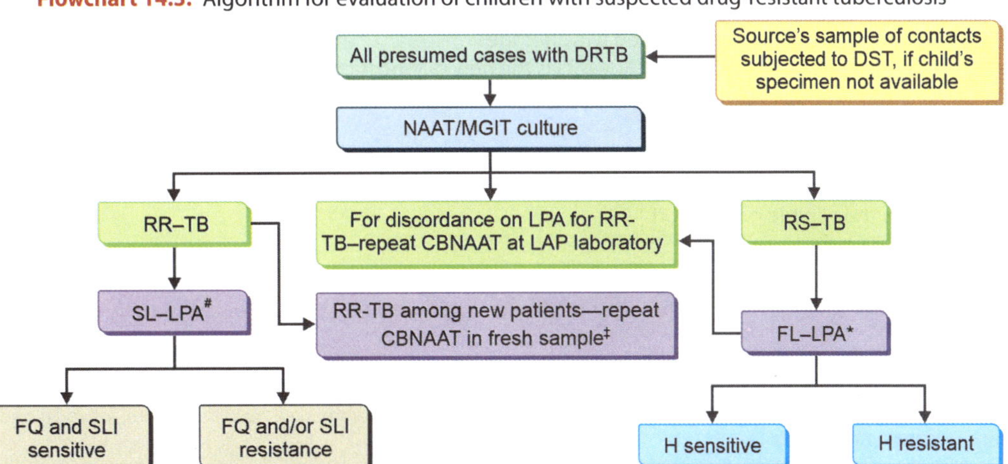

**First-line* LPA (FL-LPA) may be done directly if smear positive; else, send for MGIT followed by FL-LPA to evaluate for R and H resistance
#*Second-line* LPA (SL-LPA) may be done directly (if smear positive; else send for MGIT followed by SL-LPA or liquid culture DST (Mfx 2.0, km, Cm Lzd)
‡If Rifampicin resistant on repeat test, DRTB regimen is initiated; if repeat test shows Rifampicin resistance not detected or if result is unavailable, DSTB regimen is initiated

(DRTB: drug-resistant TB; GA: gastric aspirate; NAAT: rapid nucleic acid amplification test; NTEP: National Tuberculosis Elimination Program)
Source: National Tuberculosis Elimination Program—Indian Academy of Pediatrics guideline for management of childhood tuberculosis 2020

1 month and 0.1 mL beyond age 1 month. There is no visible change at the vaccination site for 1–2 weeks after injection. A papule develops after 2–3 weeks, which increases to a size of 4–8 mm by the end of 5–6 weeks. This papule often heals with ulceration and results in a scar after 6–12 weeks. BCG revaccination is not indicated even if no BCG scar is formed by 12 weeks postvaccination.

Tuberculosis Preventive Treatment/ TB Preventive Therapy

Household contact is a person who shared the same enclosed living space as the index case for one or more nights or for frequent or extended daytime periods during the 3 months before the start of current treatment. Latent tuberculosis infection (LTBI) is a state where the person has TB infection without evidence of active TB disease. Mantoux test and IGRA detect LTBI. Tuberculosis preventive treatment (TPT) decreases the risk of active disease by almost 90% in patients with LTB infection. TPT is recommended in the following situations:

- Children under 5 years of age who are household contacts of microbiologically confirmed pulmonary TB cases should be provided with TPT after ruling out active TB.
- In children and adolescents (5–15 years) who are household contacts of microbiologically confirmed pulmonary TB cases, TPT should be started if they are found to have LTBI.
- Infants born to a mother with tuberculosis during pregnancy should be offered TPT after ruling out congenital TB.
- Children and adolescents (1–15 years) living with HIV should be given TPT after ruling out TB irrespective of contact status.
- Infants (<12 months) living with HIV should also be given TPT if they are contacts of pulmonary TB, after ruling out active TB.
- Tuberculosis preventive treatment is also recommended for tuberculin skin test positive children who are receiving immunosuppressive therapy (children with nephrotic syndrome, acute leukemia, etc.).

Isoniazid is recommended for TPT at a dose of 10 mg/kg/day for 6 months. In contacts of MDR-TB cases TPT is not recommended currently. A close follow-up for 2 years after exposure is recommended for early identification of the disease.

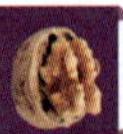

IN A NUTSHELL

Tuberculosis

1. Tuberculosis (TB) is caused by a bacterium *Mycobacterium tuberculosis.*
2. Although TB affects lungs more commonly, it can affect any organ of the body.
3. About one-quarter of the world's population has a TB infection.
4. Tuberculosis is spread from person-to-person through the air. When people with lung TB cough, sneeze, or spit, TB bacilli are suspended in the air. Inhalation of this air causes TB infection in the person.
5. Two TB-related conditions are: Latent TB infection (no symptoms) and TB disease where clinical manifestations of disease are present.
6. Tuberculosis can present with fever, cough, weight loss, loss of appetite, and other organ specific manifestations.
7. Diagnosis of TB is based on clinical features, history of contact with an open infective case, positive Mantoux test, evidence of radiological lesions suggestive of TB [X-ray of chest, ultrasound abdomen, or computed tomography (CT) brain], and laboratory investigations (elevated erythrocyte sedimentation rate (ESR), demonstration of tubercle bacilli in the sputum, gastric lavage, or bronchial aspirate), or histopathology of affected lymph nodes.
8. *Cartridge-based nucleic acid amplification test (CB-NAAT)* is the new diagnostic modality that can detect the deoxyribonucleic acid (DNA) of *Mycobacterium* in body fluids and tissues. These tests also detect rifampicin (R) resistance, a surrogate for multidrug resistance (MDR) TB.
9. Tuberculosis is curable with a combination of antitubercular drugs for a proper duration.
10. Disease can be prevented by bacillus Calmette–Guérin (BCG) vaccination, contact tracing, good hygiene, and tubercular preventive therapy to the eligible population.

Pediatric TB management guideline 2022. National Tuberculosis Elimination Program. Central TB Division, Ministry of Health and Family Welfare, New Delhi.

Piskur ZI, Mykolyshyn LI. Comorbidities at the tuberculosis among children. Wiad Lek. 2021;74(10 pt 1):2433-38.

Singh V, Parakh A. What is new in the management of childhood tuberculosis in 2020? Indian Pediatr. 2020;57(12):1172-6.

Sudbury EL, Clifford V, Messina NL, et al. *Mycobacterium tuberculosis*-specific cytokine biomarkers to differentiate active TB and LTBI: a systematic review. J Infect. 2020;81(6):873-81.

Tahan TT, Gabardo BMA, Rossoni AMO. Tuberculosis in childhood and adolescence: a view from different perspectives. J Pediatr (Rio J). 2020;96(Suppl 1):99-110.

Vlad RM, Smădeanu ER, Becheanu GB, et al. The diagnostic challenges in a child with intestinal tuberculosis. Rom J Morphol Embryol. 2021;62(4):1057-61.

WHO consolidated guidelines on tuberculosis: module 5: management of tuberculosis in children and adolescents. Geneva: World Health Organization; 2022.

14.4 Measles *PE 31.10*

INTRODUCTION

Measles is a highly contagious disease caused by a virus belonging to the Paramyxoviridae family. The illness is characterized by fever, upper respiratory symptoms, a pathognomonic enanthem (i.e., Koplik spots), followed by an erythematous maculopapular rash starting between 3 and 7 days after onset of fever. The rash heals leaving a browny pigmentation. The entire course of uncomplicated measles lasts for about 7–10 days. Serious and fatal complications include pneumonia, diarrhea, and encephalitis. Infection confers lifelong immunity.

EPIDEMIOLOGY

Measles has the greatest incidence in children <2 years of age, especially in developing nations. However, no age is exempt. More than 80% of cases occur in under-fives. Both sexes are equally affected; however, complication rates are higher in males.

Before the vaccine became available in 1960s, measles used to kill between 7 and 8 million children per year and caused 135 million episodes per year worldwide. It still accounts for 25 million cases and more than half a million deaths each year, majority of these occurring in the developing world. These deaths represent 50–60% of deaths due to all vaccine-preventable diseases.

The disease burden has been high in India, despite availability of an effective vaccine. This is because of inadequate coverage under routine immunization [83%, (United Nations International Children's Emergency Fund) UNICEF data], and nonavailability of a second opportunity for measles vaccination. With introduction of second dose of measles-containing vaccine in the National Immunization Program, and increasing coverage, there is a hope to control measles morbidity and mortality in near future.

Transmission

Spread of infection: Measles spreads from the infected person to a normal individual by the respiratory route or conjunctivae. Transmission mainly occurs through large droplet or small droplet aerosols. Sometimes large droplets or direct person-to-person contact may also spread the disease. As measles virus is highly contagious, a 5% susceptible population is sufficient to sustain periodic outbreaks in otherwise highly vaccinated populations.

Period of communicability: Infection is spread from the secretions of nose and throat usually 4 days before and 5 days after the appearance of rash.

ETIOLOGY

Measles is caused by a ribonucleic acid (RNA) virus classified as morbillivirus. The virus is composed of an outer envelope and internal helical nucleocapsid. Envelope contains proteins F, H, and M, and has spikes on its surface. The virus is rapidly inactivated by heat and ultraviolet rays. Man is the only natural host and source of measles virus. Carrier state does not exist.

PATHOGENESIS

Measles virus is spread by aerosol and enters the susceptible host by the respiratory route. Initial infection and viral replication occur locally in tracheal and bronchial epithelial cells. This leads to primary viremia (day 2–3) that infects local lymphatic tissues, perhaps carried by pulmonary macrophages. Following the amplification of measles virus in regional lymph nodes, a predominantly cell-associated viremia disseminates the virus to various organs prior to the appearance of rash.

This secondary viremia (day 5–7) is responsible for systemic symptoms. Two types of giant cells are seen in measles: Warthin–Finkeldey cells of reticuloendothelial system and epithelial giant cells of respiratory and other epithelia. In individuals with deficiencies in cellular immunity, the virus causes a progressive and often fatal giant cell pneumonia. Measles causes an immunosuppression marked by decrease in delayed-type hypersensitivity, interleukin-12 production, and antigen-specific lymphoproliferative responses that persist for weeks to months after the acute infection. Immunosuppression may predispose individuals to severe bacterial infection, particularly bronchopneumonia, a major cause of measles-related mortality among younger children.

Immunity

An attack of measles makes the individual immune for whole life against subsequent infections. Serum antibodies to viral hemagglutinin, hemolysin, and complement are observed following an infection. Hemagglutinin inhibiting and neutralizing antibodies appear after 2 weeks, peak at 4–6 weeks, and decrease over a year, but persist lifelong. Children with defective cell-mediated responses are more prone to die from progressive measles infection. Acute measles results in a temporary defect in neutrophil motility. T lymphocytes, B, and null lymphocytes are reduced. Interferon response appears after 10 days and coincides with recovery from acute infection.

Transplacental immunity: Measles antibodies are transferred from mother to fetus, which protect the infant for first 6–9 months of life. These antibodies may interfere with live-attenuated measles vaccination.

CLINICAL FEATURES

Incubation period: The incubation period from exposure to onset of symptoms ranges from 8 to 12 days.

Prodromal phase: Measles is marked by an acute onset of moderate grade fever. It is associated with cough, coryza, rhinitis, conjunctivitis, malaise, and anorexia. Fever is almost continuous, exceeds 101°F and persists for at least 1 week.

Enanthematous phase: On the second or third day of fever, Koplik spots appear on the buccal mucosa. These appear as bluish-gray specks or "grains of sand" on a red base at the level of premolars. They may also occur on lips, palate, conjunctivae, gums, and vagina. These spots begin 1–2 days before the onset of rash and start fading or sloughing as the exanthematous rash appears.

Exanthematous phase: The rash appears on 4th day. It begins on the face and neck, near the hairline; it then proceeds to the trunk, extremities, palms, and soles and lasts for about 5 days. Patients appear most ill during the first or second day of the rash. The rash is erythematous and maculopapular. It blanches on pressure during the initial 2–3 days. In later stage, the rash does not blanch and starts darkening.

Rash may be absent in patients with underlying deficiencies in cellular immunity. Children with partial immunity develop a "*modified measles*" that is a milder illness with less severe symptoms and shorter duration of fever and rash. *Hemorrhagic measles* is a severe form characterized by generalized bleeding, altered sensorium, convulsions, coma, and a high fatality rate.

Generalized lymphadenopathy, mild hepatomegaly, and appendicitis may occur because of generalized involvement of lymphoid tissue.

Recovery phase: The rash starts disappearing after 5 days in the sequence in which it had appeared, leaving behind desquamated areas, that spares the palms and soles. Fever subsides 5–7 days after appearance of rash.

COMPLICATIONS

Mortality

Mortality from measles is often the result of complications that follow the derangement in immune system and respiratory mucosa. Malnutrition, underlying malignancy, or immunodeficiency, and low serum retinol (vitamin A) levels predispose to a more severe and complicated disease course. The most common cause of death from measles is pneumonia. Case fatality rate is highest in under-five children.

Morbidity

Pneumonia: It is the most common complication in Indian context, whereas otitis media is most common in western countries. Laryngotracheobronchitis, bronchiolitis, sinusitis, mastoiditis, retropharyngeal abscess, and tracheitis are other respiratory complications of measles. Primary tuberculosis may flare up following measles.

Pneumonia may be caused either by the measles virus itself (measles pneumonia) or because of superimposed bacterial infection by *Staphylococcus aureus, Streptococcus pneumoniae, H. influenzae,* or gram-negative bacilli including *Klebsiella, Escherichia coli,* and *Pseudomonas.*

Encephalitis: Approximately 1 in every 1,000 patients with measles develops encephalitis. As thought earlier, it is not due to the measles virus *per se*. Encephalitis following measles is now considered to be a postinfection and immune-mediated disorder. Usual symptoms include altered sensorium and seizures. The onset occurs in the first week of illness. Approximately one-third develop long-term sequelae. Case fatality rate of measles encephalitis ranges from 10 to 20%.

Subacute sclerosing panencephalitis (SSPE): This is a degenerative CNS disease that can result from a persistent measles infection. The mean incubation period for SSPE is approximately 10.8 years (range 7–13 years). SSPE is characterized by behavioral and intellectual deterioration, followed by myoclonic epilepsy. The disease is progressive in nature finally leading to extrapyramidal symptoms in form of dystonia and rigidity. Dementia, coma, and death follow. There is no definitive cure.

Diarrhea and dysentery: Gastrointestinal epitheliums are characterized by giant cell formation, manifesting as diarrhea and vomiting. This may get prolonged as persistent diarrhea, especially in malnourished children. Appendicitis may occur due to lymphoid tissue blocking its lumens. Rare complications include hepatitis and ileocolitis.

Others: Myocarditis, Stevens-Johnson syndrome, bacteremia, cellulitis, acute glomerulonephritis, and consumption coagulopathy are other complications of measles. Measles can precipitate edematous malnutrition.

DIFFERENTIAL DIAGNOSIS

Measles needs to be differentiated from other causes of fever with maculopapular rash, including rubella, infectious mononucleosis, roseola, fifth disease, group A streptococcal infection, meningococcemia, dengue fever, rickettsial infections, mycoplasma infections, and Kawasaki disease. Koplik spots, if present, are pathognomonic of measles. However, they are present in 50–70% children only and rest may still pose a diagnostic challenge.

Rubella is a milder disease with a characteristic postoccipital lymphadenopathy. Infectious mononucleosis should be suspected, if there is generalized lymphadenopathy and hepatosplenomegaly. Children with dengue fever have a rash that is confluent and also involves palms and soles. Meningococcal and streptococcal rashes are characterized by petechiae, purpura, associated with a generalized toxic look. Rash of roseola infantum (caused by herpesvirus-6) typically starts from trunk and is associated with periorbital edema. Fifth disease caused by human parvovirus B19 (HPV19) is characterized by an erythematous rash on the cheeks, giving these children a typical "*slapped cheek*" appearance.

DIAGNOSIS

The diagnosis of measles is primarily clinical and routine laboratory investigations are not essential. According to World Health Organization (WHO), *measles is clinically diagnosed in a person presenting with fever and maculopapular rash (non-vesicular) and cough, coryza, or conjunctivitis.* White cell count is usually low with relative lymphocytosis. ESR and CRP are not elevated. Serologic confirmation requires demonstration of immunoglobulin M (IgM) antibodies in serum. These last for almost a month after an acute infection. A fourfold rise in immunoglobulin G (IgG) titer between exanthematous and convalescent samples collected 2–4 weeks later is also diagnostic. The virus can be isolated from respiratory secretions, blood, and urine during the prodromal, enanthematous, and exanthematous phases.

TREATMENT Measles

Treatment is by and large supportive and symptomatic.

World Health Organization and UNICEF recommend *administration of two doses of vitamin A* supplements given 24 hours apart, to all children diagnosed with measles, in communities where measles related mortality is >1%. There is evidence that administration of vitamin A reduces severity of disease and mortality due to measles by 50%. Giving vitamin A at the time of diagnosis can help prevent eye damage and blindness.

Fever is controlled by paracetamol and hydrotherapy. Moderate degree of cough need not be suppressed. Cough helps in clearing of mucus from the lungs. Very irritating cough may be relieved by saline nebulization.

The child is given adequate fluids orally. If there is vomiting, fluids are given intravenously. Nutrition should be maintained by a good high protein diet. Appropriate antibiotics should only be reserved for secondary bacterial pneumonia. Body and oral hygiene are important. Child should be given a bath daily.

PREVENTION

The Vaccine

Live-attenuated measles virus is used as the vaccine. The most popular strains of vaccine-viruses, namely *Schwartz, Moraten,* and *Edmonston-Zagreb* were derived by further attenuation from the *Edmonston B* strain, which itself was attenuated from the *Edmonston A* strain. Many vaccines are available, either as monovalent vaccine or in combination with measles, mumps, rubella, or varicella (MMR or MMRV). The protective response to each component of these antigens, in a combination vaccine, remains unaltered.

The vaccine is given subcutaneously. Its shelf-life is at least 1 year at 4–8°C. The minimum recommended potency is 1,000 median cell culture infectious doses of virus. Diluents must not be frozen. After reconstitution, its potency drops rapidly and loses all potency after 1 hour at 37°C. Moreover, several cases of staphylococcal toxic shock syndrome with high mortality have occurred in India after giving reconstituted measles vaccine stored for one or more days. For these two reasons, reconstituted vaccine should be used within 4–6 hours. Leftover doses must be discarded.

Age at Vaccination

Residual maternal antibody in the infant's serum neutralizes the immunogenic property of the vaccine, and it should be offered at an age when most infants would have lost these antibodies. Therefore, in developing countries, the recommended minimum age is 9 months. A total of 85–95% of those vaccinated at the age of 9 months, develop antibodies in adequate titer. Second dose is to be given between 16 and 24 months.

Under UIP, 2 doses of measles-containing vaccines are administered. First dose is given at 9–12 months of age as measles-rubella (MR) vaccine and second dose as MR/MMR (measles mumps rubella) vaccine at 16–24 months of age. IAP recommends 3 doses of MMR vaccine at 9 months, 15 months and 4–6 years of age, respectively. Catch up vaccination may be done with doses of MR vaccine at an interval of 4–8 weeks till 5 years of age under UIP. IAP recommends catch up till 18 years of age.

Adverse Events

Depending upon the strain of vaccine-virus, 10–20% of vaccines may develop mild to moderate fever about 6–8 days after receiving measles vaccine. It lasts for 1–3 days and is not associated with malaise. A total of 1–5% of children may develop a few red spots on the trunk during this period. Treatment for primary tuberculosis is not a contraindication. Since measles vaccine does not seem to aggravate primary tuberculosis, screening is not necessary before immunization.

Measles Vaccine as Aerosol

The *Edmonston-Zagreb* strain of vaccine-virus grown in human diploid cells has been successfully administered as an aerosol to immunize infants against measles. By utilizing the respiratory route, it is hoped to avoid neutralization by any maternal IgG antibodies that may be present. Hence, it is possible to successfully immunize children as young as 4–6 months. In a recent trial conducted in India, it was observed that the aerosolized vaccine was safe and resulted in 85% seroconversion between 9 and 12 months of age, but it was slightly inferior to the subcutaneous vaccine.

Contraindications

These include pregnancy, history of anaphylactic reactions to egg protein, history of anaphylaxis to neomycin, significantly immunocompromised states such as leukemia, administration of antimetabolites, radiations, or corticosteroids, and recent administration of immunoglobulin within last 3 months. Symptomatic and asymptomatic HIV infection is *not* a contraindication for measles vaccination because of risk of severe life-threatening measles in children with HIV infection. Interestingly, immunization with live measles vaccine within 72 hours of exposure to a case of measles may modify the illness and provide protection in certain cases. Therefore, measles exposure is not a contraindication for active immunization. Rather in school-based outbreaks, it should be the measure of choice.

Passive Immunization

Exposure to measles may necessitate administration of immunoglobulin (IG) in a susceptible person. Immunoglobulin must be given within 6 days of exposure in a dose of 0.25 mL/kg body weight, intramuscularly. Immunoglobulin administration is justified for children who are <1 year old, immunocompromised, and for pregnant women.

Measles Control and Elimination

In April 2012, the partners [WHO, UNICEF, Centers for Disease Control and Prevention (CDC), United Nations (UN)] of the *Measles Initiative* introduced a global plan to tackle measles and rubella jointly by using a combined measles-rubella vaccine. This Global Measles and Rubella Strategic Plan 2012–2020 (MRSP 2012–2020) was aimed at control of measles, rubella and congenital rubella syndrome. The aim was to reduce measles deaths worldwide by 95% by 2015; and to eliminate measles and rubella in at least five of six WHO regions by 2020. MRSP 2021–2030 now aims at elimination of measles and rubella which are defined as "the absence of endemic measles and rubella transmission in a defined geographical area (e.g., region or country) for ≥12 months in the presence of a well-performing surveillance system".

India joined other countries in the WHO South-East Asia Region in 2019 to aim for measles and rubella elimination by 2023. This goal was a revised version of the previous objective to eliminate measles and control rubella and congenital rubella syndrome by 2020. To achieve this goal, India developed a national strategic plan aimed at achieving and sustaining measles and rubella elimination by year 2023 by four key strategies:

1. Achieving >95% coverage with measles and rubella containing vaccine
2. Sensitive case based MR surveillance
3. Rapid response to measles outbreaks
4. Setting up accredited MR laboratory network.

Measles can be eradicated because man is the only reservoir of the virus, the disease occurs due to only one serotype, and an effective vaccine is available.

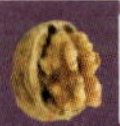

IN A NUTSHELL

Measles

1. Measles is a highly contagious acute viral illness lasting for 7–10 days that confers lifelong immunity against further episodes. It is the leading cause of death amongst all the vaccine-preventable diseases.
2. The virus spreads by the respiratory route or conjunctivae. Period of infectivity is usually 4 days before and 5 days after the onset of rash.
3. Measles is characterized by a generalized maculopapular rash lasting ≥3 days; temperature of ≥38.3°C (101°F) and presence of cough, coryza, or conjunctivitis. Koplik spots, if present, are pathognomonic of measles.
4. Common complications include pneumonia, diarrhea, and encephalitis.
5. Uncomplicated measles generally resolves on its own within 7–10 days. Treatment is mainly symptomatic. Vitamin A should be given to all children diagnosed with measles.
6. WHO and UNICEF recommend administration of two doses of measles containing vaccine to ensure adequate protection against the disease.

Murugan R, Van der Ende K, Dhawan V, et al. Progress Toward Measles and Rubella Elimination—India, 2005–2021. MMWR Morb Mortal Wkly Rep. 2022;71(50):1569-75.

Measles and rubella strategic framework 2021–2030. Geneva: World Health Organization; 2020. Weekly Report. 2022;71(50):1569-75. Available from https://iris.who.int/bitstream/handle/10665/339801/9789240015616-eng.pdf. [Last accessed August, 2025].

14.5 Mumps

PE 31.10

INTRODUCTION

Mumps is a self-limiting, vaccine-preventable, acute viral infection of the parotid and other salivary glands. It is characterized by fever, and bilateral tender swelling of salivary glands. Aseptic meningitis is the most common sequel.

The annual global incidence of mumps is 100–1,000 per 100,000 population with epidemic peaks every 2–5 years. Natural infection with mumps virus confers lifelong protection.

EPIDEMIOLOGY

Transmission: Man is the only known host. Virus is transmitted through saliva or by respiratory droplets. The virus may also be found in urine and cerebrospinal fluid. Subclinical infections are very common. These may transmit the infection to susceptible persons. The disease is most likely to transmit from 2 days before to 5 days after appearance of parotitis. Carrier state does not exist.

Host factors: Mumps is commonly a disease of children with peak incidence in 5–15 years. Infantile period is protected because of the presence of transplacental antibodies. Mumps occurring in adults produces more severe disease. Mumps infection during early pregnancy increases the risk of abortion.

ETIOLOGY

Mumps is caused by the virus belonging to paramyxovirus group. It is an RNA virus and contains hemolysin, neuraminidase, and hemagglutinin. The virus can be obtained from the saliva swab of the infected patients 7 days before and 7 days after the onset of salivary gland swelling. There is only one serotype of the virus.

PATHOGENESIS

The virus enters human body through the inhalational route and seeds the epithelium of upper respiratory tract, where it replicates. Absorption of virus in host cell is facilitated by HN (hemagglutinin-neuraminidase) surface glycoprotein, while F (fusion) glycoprotein mediates viral penetration into the cell. This is followed by regional lymphoid invasion and viremia. Mumps virus selectively targets the salivary glands, CNS, pancreas, testes, heart, liver, kidneys, thyroid, and joints. The virus evokes a lymphocytic response in infected tissue, with ultimate necrosis of the salivary epithelium. Mumps virus enters the CNS via the choroid plexus. Cerebrospinal fluid is also characterized by a lymphocytic response. Focal ischemic infarcts are observed in the testis.

CLINICAL FEATURES

Incubation period: The incubation period varies from 12 to 25 days with a median 16–18 days.

Prodromal symptoms: Initial symptoms consist of fever, malaise, headache, vomiting, and nausea. Fever is mild to moderate. Appetite is impaired.

Presenting features: The disease can vary from a mild upper respiratory illness to viremia with widespread systemic involvement. The most common presentation is a parotitis that occurs in 30–40% of affected children. Other reported sites of infection are the testes, pancreas, eyes, ovaries, CNS, joints, and kidneys. Infection with mumps virus is asymptomatic in 20–30% of cases.

Parotitis: Classic mumps is characterized by enlargement of the parotid and other salivary glands; parotitis is bilateral in three-quarters of cases; and other salivary glands are involved in 10% of cases. Swelling of parotid is preceded by pain near the ear lobe, difficulty in swallowing and chewing. Swelling initially appears on one side of the cheek. Within 72 hours, it becomes bilateral. Swelling results in obliteration of the angle of the jaw and lifting of the ipsilateral ear lobe, upward and outward. The swelling increases in size for 3–4 days. Disease may remain unilateral in 30% cases. Lymphatic obstruction in facial and neck planes may result in local edema, extending up to sternum.

Recovery: Fever subsides within 3–5 days. Parotid swelling starts receding after 5 days. It may take 10–14 days for the swelling to subside completely.

COMPLICATIONS

Aseptic meningitis: Aseptic meningitis is the most common complication of mumps. It occurs in up to 10% of all children with mumps, more often in males. Asymptomatic pleocytosis in CSF occurs in 50% of all children with mumps. Symptomatic meningitis occurs in 15% cases, characterized by severe headache aggravated by movement, photophobia, and neck stiffness due to spasm of the spinal muscles.

Mumps meningitis is a benign condition that appears within a few days of parotid swelling, although some meningitis patients do not have any parotid swelling. Patients recover within 7 days without complications but require hospitalization during the course of the illness. Death due to mumps is exceedingly rare and is mostly caused by mumps encephalitis.

Meningoencephalitis: Encephalitis, though less common than meningitis, can occur before, with, or after appearance of parotid swelling. *Early onset encephalitis* occurs within 1–2 weeks of onset of swelling and is due to mumps infection of the brain. *Late onset encephalitis* is an immune-mediated demyelinating condition.

Other neurological manifestations of mumps include cerebellar ataxia, acute disseminated encephalomyelitis (ADEM), cranial nerve involvement (facial and auditory), transverse myelitis, and Guillain–Barré syndrome. Although most patients recover without prolonged sequelae, the mortality rate is reported to be up to 1.4%.

Orchitis, epididymitis, and oophoritis: Epididymo-orchitis occurs in about 25% of postpubertal adolescents who contact mumps. Testicular atrophy occurs in about one-third of them, but sterility is rare. In postpubertal adolescent girls, mastitis and oophoritis can occur.

Pancreatitis: It is seen in about 4% of patients with mumps. There is evidence suggesting that mumps virus can infect human pancreatic β cells and may trigger the onset of insulin-dependent diabetes mellitus in some individuals. Additional rare complications include nephritis, arthritis, thrombocytopenic purpura, mastitis, thyroiditis, and keratouveitis.

DIFFERENTIAL DIAGNOSIS

A parotid swelling needs to be differentiated from an enlarged cervical lymph node. For this, draw an imaginary line bisecting the long axis of the ear to the angle of jaw. A cervical lymph node usually lies posterior to this imaginary line, while a parotid swelling overlies this line.

Differential diagnoses of a parotid swelling include suppurative parotitis caused by *Staphylococcus aureus*, which is usually unilateral and is extremely painful. There may be a pus discharge from Stensen's duct. Parotitis can also be caused by other viruses including parainfluenza, influenza, HIV, Epstein-Barr virus, and cytomegaloviruses.

Noninfective parotitis is caused by collagen vascular disorders (SLE, Sjögren syndrome), malignancies (leukemia, lymphoma), and obstruction of Stensen's duct due to calculus.

DIAGNOSIS

Diagnosis is primarily clinical. According to WHO, *clinical diagnosis of mumps is made in presence of acute onset of unilateral/bilateral, tender, self-limited swelling of the parotid or other salivary gland, lasting 2 or more days and without any other apparent cause.* Laboratory investigations are usually not required. Mumps virus can be isolated from nasopharyngeal swabs, urine, blood, and fluid from buccal cavity typically from 7 days before up until 9 days after the onset of parotitis. Mumps infection can be confirmed by demonstrating significant (4-fold) rise in mumps-specific IgG antibody between acute and convalescent titers or a positive mumps IgM. IgG titer can be detected by complement fixation, hemagglutination inhibition, or enzyme immunoassay. Polymerase chain reaction (PCR) can be used to detect viral antigen. Lymphocytosis or leukopenia may be present. Serum amylase level may be elevated. CNS infections usually exhibit a lymphocytic pleocytosis in cerebrospinal fluid, with hypoglycorrhachia.

TREATMENT Mumps

No specific treatment is available for mumps. Supportive care and outpatient follow-up are indicated for uncomplicated infections. Fever should be treated with paracetamol. Adequate hydration should be maintained. Warm salt water gargles, soft foods, and extra fluids may also help relieve symptoms. Children are advised to suck on lozenges that stimulate the salivary secretions and reduces the swelling earlier.

Complications due to mumps should be treated based on presentation. Management of complicated mumps infection should include testicular ultrasonography for orchitis, ice-packs applied to scrotal area for swelling, scrotal support and anti-inflammatory agents, intravenous hydration for severe pancreatitis, and symptomatic management for meningitis or encephalitis. Classic mumps with no major complications can be managed on an outpatient basis with supportive care and good follow-up.

PREVENTION AND CONTROL

Care of Contacts

Children should not be allowed to go to school for 10 days after the onset of parotid swelling. Mumps immunoglobulin has no role. As with measles, mumps vaccine can be given after exposure to provide protection against future exposures. If the disease develops in such contacts, who have been given mumps vaccine following exposure, no additional risk or reactions are conferred on the individuals.

Active Immunization

A live-attenuated preparation of mumps vaccine is available as a part of combined MMR vaccine. A single dose confers lifelong immunity and 98% seroconversion. In developing countries, the priority for mumps prophylaxis is low. Most commonly, the vaccine consists of the Jeryl Lynn strain. Other strains in use are Leningrad-3 (erstwhile Soviet states); Urabe (Japan, France, Italy), L-Zagreb (Croatia, India, Slovenia), and Rubini (Switzerland). All vaccines offer >90% seroconversion. The ideal age for vaccinating children is 15–18 months. The vaccine is administered in a dose of 0.5 mL subcutaneously (as MMR). MMR can be given to individuals who are already immune to one or more component viruses of the vaccine. The mumps component is still not a part of national schedule in India. A few states are giving it as part of MMR vaccine at 15–18 months. IAP recommends 3 doses of MMR vaccine (9 months, 16–24 months, and 4–6 years).

Adverse events: Adverse events to mumps vaccine are rare. Aseptic meningitis is reported in 0.1–100 per 100,000 vaccines.

Contraindications: These include pregnancy, history of anaphylactic reaction to egg, persons with immunodeficiency disorders or those receiving immunosuppressives and persons who have received immunoglobulins or blood transfusion recently in the past 3 months. For such patients, who cannot be vaccinated, it is advisable to vaccinate their close susceptible contacts. Vaccine-virus is not transmitted by immunized persons.

Global Efforts

By 2015, a total of 121 countries or regions had included vaccination against mumps in their national immunization programs, mostly as MMR vaccine. Most countries in Africa and South-East Asia region have not adopted this strategy and the incidence of mumps remains high in these areas.

Mumps Control

Mumps can be controlled through high (>90%) routine coverage with an effective mumps-containing vaccine administered at 12–18 months of age. Lower immunization coverage (<80%) fails to interrupt circulation of the mumps virus in the community and results in an epidemiological shift with increase in the number of cases in adults. The strategies for elimination are outlined below:

1. Achieving high (>90%) coverage with a first dose of mumps-containing vaccine at the age of 12–18 months.
2. Ensuring a second opportunity for immunization, if coverage with the first dose is <80%.
3. Conducting catch-up immunization of susceptible cohorts; the target age group should be that in which susceptibility to mumps is highest.

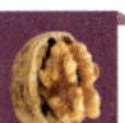

IN A NUTSHELL

Mumps

1. Mumps is a self-limiting, acute viral illness causing inflammation of parotid and other salivary glands. Natural infection confers lifelong protection.
2. Meningoencephalitis is the most important complication of mumps infection.
3. The differential diagnosis includes cervical lymphadenopathy, suppurative (bacterial) parotitis, viral parotitis, and non-infective parotitis caused by collagen vascular disorders, malignancies, and salivary gland calculus.
4. The management is mainly supportive. Spontaneous recovery occurs in 2 weeks.
5. The disease can be prevented by administration of the mumps vaccine, available as a component of MMR vaccine.

Almansour I. Mumps Vaccines: Current Challenges and Future Prospects. Front Microbiol. 2020;11:1999.

Di Pietrantonj C, Rivetti A, Marchione P, et al. Vaccines for measles, mumps, rubella, and varicella in children. Cochrane Database Syst Rev. 2020;4(4):CD004407.

Su SB, Chang HL, Chen AK. Current status of mumps virus infection: epidemiology, pathogenesis, and vaccine. Int J Environ Res Public Health. 2020;17(5):1686.

Vaidya SR, Hamde VS. Is it right time to introduce mumps vaccine in India's universal immunization program? Indian Pediatr. 2016;53(6):469-73.

Zerbo O, Modaressi S, Glanternik JR, et al. Identification and description of mumps cases in a non-outbreak setting and evaluation of the effectiveness of mumps-containing vaccines over time. Hum Vaccin Immunother. 2020;16(12):3098-02.

14.6 Rubella

PE 31.10

INTRODUCTION

Rubella in children is a mild disease characterized by mild fever, rash, and lymphadenopathy. Most of the times, the infection may pass off unnoticed. The primary infection *per se* does not result in significant mortality or morbidity. However, if a pregnant woman is infected with rubella virus, serious consequences can occur in her fetus. The infant may be born with *congenital rubella syndrome* with multisystem involvement (brain, heart, eyes, and ears). Congenital rubella is the most important cause of preventable deafness in children. It is estimated that >46,000 cases occur in South-East Asian countries alone every year.

The risk of fetal infection is 50% or higher, if the mother acquires infection during first 4 weeks of gestation. It declines to about 25% between 23 and 26 weeks and then rises again to 70% for rubella infections acquired during the latter part of pregnancy.

Maternal rubella infection during the phase of embryogenesis, i.e., the first trimester, results in congenital defects in up to 90% of the offspring. The risk is reduced to 25% at 15–16 weeks. Fetal rubella infection beyond 16 weeks of intrauterine gestation does not result in congenital defects.

EPIDEMIOLOGY

Rubella virus is a ribonucleic acid (RNA) virus and can be isolated from the nasopharynx, throat, urine, and cerebrospinal fluid, during the acute illness. Man is the only source of infection.

Rubella is mainly a disease of children, though it affects all age groups. Transmission occurs by droplet spread and the virus enters the host by respiratory route. Postnatal rubella is infective from 7 days before to 14 days (median 5 days) after the appearance of rash. Natural infection confers lifelong immunity. Subclinical infections are common.

Transplacental protection remains for 6–9 months. Transplacental spread of virus results in congenital rubella. Affected infants may continue to shed virus in nasopharyngeal secretions and urine for a year or more following birth.

PATHOLOGY

Rubella virus enters the human host by respiratory route, lodges in local epithelium, replicates, and spreads to regional lymph nodes. This is followed by a viremic phase lasting for 2 weeks.

Fetal infection occurs by transplacental spread. The virus replicates extensively in the fetus and persists in the neonate and even in infant, resulting in widespread tissue damage, primarily in brain, heart, and auditory nerve. The exact mechanism of cellular injury is not clear, but ischemia, chromosomal breaks, and mitotic arrests could be one of the possible reasons.

CLINICAL FEATURES

Postnatal Infection

Incubation period of rubella is 14–21 days. Half of the infections are subclinical and asymptomatic. It is difficult to differentiate this illness from other viral fevers of the childhood. Sore throat and fever herald the onset of disease. Suboccipital, posterior auricular, and anterior cervical lymph nodes enlarge by 7th day. A macular rash appears within 24 hours after the onset of fever. It first appears on face and neck and spreads centrifugally to involve the whole body.

On the first day of appearance of exanthema, small pink-colored ring lesions and petechiae also appear on the soft palate. These are known as *Forchheimer spots* and are pathognomonic of rubella infection. The rash lasts for 3 days and then fades away without any residual pigmentation or desquamation.

Postnatal rubella needs to be differentiated from other exanthematous fevers including measles, roseola, erythema infectiosum, and infectious mononucleosis, based on their typical clinical features.

Complications occur rarely, and include encephalitis, thrombocytopenia, arthritis, and a progressive rubella panencephalitis (similar to SSPE associated with measles), myocarditis, and infective polyneuritis.

Congenital Rubella Syndrome

Fetal infection with rubella during the first trimester may lead to abortion in 10% and stillbirth in 4% of pregnancies.

The rest of the infected fetuses are born with congenital rubella syndrome: Most common manifestations in the affected newborn include: (*i*) microcephaly, (*ii*) deafness, (*iii*) cardiac anomalies (patent ductus arteriosus, pulmonary stenosis, or septal defects), (*iv*) mental retardation, (*v*) congenital cataract, (*vi*) hepatosplenomegaly; and (*vii*) thrombocytopenia. Infants are born small for gestational age. Uncommon manifestations include extramedullary hematopoiesis, dermal erythropoiesis, and meningoencephalitis.

Late onset disease: The infected infant may be asymptomatic in the neonatal period and develop evidence of congenital rubella syndrome subsequently. Late onset manifestations include: (*i*) diabetes mellitus, (*ii*) thyroid dysfunction, (*iii*) psychomotor defects, and (*iv*) ocular abnormalities.

The newborn infant can shed virus up to the age of 18 months and serve as an important source of infection to other pregnant mothers. There is no treatment and prognosis is generally poor.

DIAGNOSIS

Presence of rubella IgM or a fourfold rise in rubella IgG titer from paired acute and convalescent sera provides evidence of ongoing or recent rubella infection. Viral isolation is not routinely used for diagnosis.

PREVENTION

Active Immunization

Childhood rubella is too benign a disease to warrant routine prophylaxis. Immunization is intended solely to prevent congenital rubella syndrome. Two possible approaches are: (a) either to selectively immunize adolescent girls and/or women of childbearing age; or (b) to achieve universal immunization of infants and young children of both sexes.

1. The *first approach of adolescent immunization* will result in a decrease in the incidence of congenital rubella syndrome (CRS). However, elimination of CRS cannot be achieved with this strategy, because it would require every susceptible woman to be effectively immunized. Unvaccinated girls who refuse vaccination will still be exposed to circulating rubella virus in male population and children.
2. The *second approach of childhood immunization* will reduce the circulation of virus. However, pregnant women will continue to be exposed to rubella in adults.

It is now realized that combining in universal immunization of infants and children with vaccination of adolescent girls and adult women is the most effective approach to eliminate rubella and congenital rubella syndrome.

The Vaccine

Most of the currently-licensed vaccines are based on the live-attenuated RA27/3 strain of rubella virus, propagated in human diploid cells. The RA27/3 vaccine can be stored at 4°C for at least 5 years. Each dose of this vaccine, which is given by the subcutaneous route, contains a defined number of active virus particles (>1,000 TCID 50). Other attenuated rubella vaccine strains, such as the Matsuba, DCRB 19, Takahashi, Matsuura, and TO-336 strains are used primarily in Japan; the BRD-2 strain is used in China. Efficacy ranges from 95 to 100%.

As the vaccine consists of live-attenuated virus, it should be given only after maternal antibodies have disappeared; the recommended minimum age is 9 months. Vaccine-induced immunity is generally lifelong. The vaccine is often combined with measles and mumps vaccine. Adverse reactions to rubella vaccine include lymphadenopathy, arthralgia, and transient skin rash, all of which are self-limiting. As per IAP, it is given as 3 doses of MMR vaccine at 9 months, 15–24 months and 5 years of age. Under NIS, it as given as 2 doses of MR vaccines at 9–12 months and 16–24 months of age.

Contraindications: Pregnancy is an absolute contraindication for rubella vaccination. Like measles and mumps, rubella vaccine cannot be administered, if there is a history of immunoglobulin administration or blood transfusion in last 3 months. Immunocompromised states (except HIV infection) are also contraindications for rubella vaccination. After puberty, immunization should be advised only after estimation of hemagglutination inhibition antibody titer and if pregnancy can be effectively avoided for at least 8 weeks.

Postexposure Prophylaxis

If a pregnant mother is suspected of having been exposed to possible rubella during early pregnancy, hemagglutination inhibition (HI) antibody titer in the blood should be obtained immediately and after 3–6 weeks interval, irrespective of the occurrence of any rash. A fourfold or greater increase in HI antibody titer indicates rubella infection. If the infection is confirmed, medical termination of pregnancy should be advised.

Surveillance

Methods for surveillance of congenital rubella syndrome include hospital record review, deaf/blind surveys, clinician reporting, and active search for cases with congenital rubella syndrome after outbreaks of acquired rubella. Serological surveillance among antenatal women can be used to monitor the impact of the immunization program.

Indian Initiative

As per WHO recommendations, the National Technical Advisory Group on Immunization (NTAGI) in India recommended the inclusion of rubella vaccination in Universal Immunization Program (UIP), in February 2014.

In accordance with the NTAGI recommendations, Government of India (GOI) decided to introduce a *Rubella Initiative* as a part of the nationwide measles-rubella (MR) campaign in two stages—the first stage targeted to cover a wide age range of children and adolescents aged 9 months to 15 years with the MR vaccine. This was followed by the second stage that entailed inclusion of measles-rubella (MR) vaccine in the routine immunization programs in a two-dose schedule at 9–12 months and at 16–24 months of age. These campaigns, by vaccinating all young people between 9 months and 15 years, rapidly interrupted the spread of rubella virus. As part of this initiative, mass vaccination campaigns for children and adolescents aged 9 months–15 years, with MR vaccine were planned in the country in four phases from July 2015 to March 2017. MR vaccine was chosen over MMR, given the comparatively lower cost of the vaccine and a less significant mumps disease burden in the country.

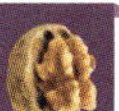

IN A NUTSHELL

Rubella

1. Rubella is a mild viral illness characterized by mild fever, rash, arthralgia, and lymphadenopathy.
2. Fetal rubella infection occurs due to transplacental spreads from infected mothers.
3. Congenital rubella syndrome is characterized by a triad of sensorineural deafness, ophthalmologic, and cardiac abnormalities.
4. Rubella can be eliminated by active immunization.

Dewan P, Gupta P. Burden of congenital rubella syndrome in India: a systematic review. Indian Pediatr. 2012;49(5):377-99.

Di Pietrantonj C, Rivetti A, Marchione P, et al. Vaccines for measles, mumps, rubella, and varicella in children. Cochrane Database Syst Rev. 2020;4(4):CD004407.

Plotkin SA. Rubella eradication: not yet accomplished, but entirely feasible. J Infect Dis. 2021;224(12 Suppl 2):S360-66.

World Health Organization. Progress in control and elimination of rubella and congenital rubella syndrome worldwide, 2012–2020. Wkly Epidemiol Rec. 2022;97(6):33-44.

14.7 Varicella (Chickenpox) *PE 31.10*

INTRODUCTION

Chickenpox is a highly infectious disease caused by primary infection of varicella-zoster virus. The illness is characterized by an exanthematous vesicular rash with a centripetal distribution. The rash typically begins as maculopapular lesion on first day of fever. The course is usually benign and lasts for about 7 days. Chickenpox infections give lifelong immunity. However, varicella-zoster virus can remain latent and can recur years later as herpes zoster (shingles). Primary disease is vaccine preventable.

EPIDEMIOLOGY

Varicella-zoster virus is an enveloped deoxyribonucleic acid (DNA) virus that is transmitted from person-to-person by direct contact, droplet, airborne spread, or fomites. Only 1 serotype is known. Man is the only reservoir. Infectivity is maximum during prodromal period and completely wanes when eruptions become crusted. Crusts from chickenpox lesions do not contain live virus. Period of infectivity ranges from 48 hours prior to appearance of rash, up to 3–7 days after the rash appears. Varicella virus is transmitted to 65–86% of susceptible household contacts. This secondary attack rate is lower in a school setting. Subclinical varicella is almost non-existent.

PATHOGENESIS

Airborne virus enters the oropharynx through inhalation by droplet infection. Primary seeding occurs in tonsillar tissue and mucosa of the upper respiratory tract. Virus replication for initial 10 days is followed by primary viremia that spreads the virus to reticuloendothelial system. No clinical symptoms occur. Skin lesions appear only during the secondary viremic phase that lasts for 3–7 days. Infectious virus is carried to vesicular fluid and back to respiratory mucosa, from where it is shed, transmitting infection to susceptible contacts. The virus may be transported to the dorsal root of spinal cord, where a latent infection is established. Reactivation of this focus at a later stage results in herpes zoster.

CLINICAL FEATURES

Chickenpox occurs at all ages (including neonates) with peak incidence between 2–8 years. The median incubation period is 14–16 days (range 10–21 days). The disease ushers in with fever and malaise. Prodromal symptoms also include headache, sore throat, and backache. The rash appears within 24 hours of the onset of prodrome. At times, prodromal symptoms may be absent, and the illness may straightaway begin with a rash.

Fever is usually moderate, usually between 102 and 103°F, but may rise to 106°F. Fever usually resolves after 3–4 days of appearance of rash.

Evolution of the Rash

The rash begins as crops of macules, which evolve into papules and then vesicles. The vesicles are initially filled with clear fluid that soon becomes cloudy. The vesicles persist for 3–4 days, become pustular and then form crust. The vesicles may be round, oval, elliptical, or irregular, often surrounded by red areola. The lesions first appear over face, scalp, or trunk; and then spread to whole body. Palms and soles are spared. The lesions measure 5–10 mm in diameter. New lesions may keep occurring for 1 week. Most children have >250 lesions. Lesions of different stages, i.e., macules, papules, vesicles, and scabs can be seen simultaneously. Lesions tend to be more abundant on covered than exposed parts of the body. By the time of vesicle formation, there is excessive itching. Vesicles may also be observed over conjunctiva, palate, tongue, and buccal mucous membranes.

Vesicles dry up within 1–2 days, starting from the center, forming crusts and scabs. Scabs fall off in 10–20 days. Underlying skin becomes hypo- or hyperpigmented that stays for days to weeks. Permanent scarring is unusual.

COMPLICATIONS

Bacterial Infections

Secondary skin infection due to group A *Streptococcus* and *Staphylococcus aureus* results in cellulitis, erysipelas, and skin abscesses. Bacteremic spread may lead to pneumonia, osteomyelitis, and septic arthritis.

Neurological Complications

Neurological complications occur toward the end of first week of illness as the rash reaches maturity. The most common manifestation is a pure cerebellar ataxia, which has an excellent prognosis.

Meningoencephalitis is a dreaded complication with 5–25% mortality. Acute disseminated encephalomyelitis (ADEM) is a rare form of postvaricella encephalitis with cerebral demyelination. It presents with cranial nerve involvement, long tract signs, and convulsions. Transverse myelitis, acute infantile hemiplegia, and Guillain-Barré syndrome are the other neurological complications. Chronic neurological sequelae are rare.

Pneumonitis

Varicella pneumonia appears 3–5 days after the onset of rash. These children present with acute respiratory distress and hemoptysis and diffuse nodular infiltration in chest radiograph.

Others

Myocarditis, pericarditis, endocarditis, hepatitis, glomerulonephritis, appendicitis, keratoconjunctivitis, arthritis, thrombocytopenia, and purpura fulminans are the other notable complications. Immunocompromised children, adolescents, and pregnant women are at increased risk of severe disease. Children with AIDS can develop chronic chickenpox lasting for months.

CONGENITAL VARICELLA

If the mother contacts chickenpox in the first trimester, there is 2% risk of the baby developing congenital varicella embryopathy. The child may be born with multiple malformations, including cicatricial scarring of the limbs, cortical atrophy, limb hypoplasia, digital defects, retinitis, and cataract.

VARICELLA NEONATORUM

If the maternal rash appears <5 days before delivery or up to 2 days after delivery, there is 17–30% risk that the baby will receive a large inoculum without maternal antibody. Such babies are at a very high risk of disseminated disease with death (fatality rate can be as high as 30%, if not treated in time) from pneumonitis, and should be protected at birth by giving varicella-zoster immunoglobulin (VZIG). Neonatal varicella may still occur in 50% of these, despite VZIG administration, however, the disease is mild. If symptoms develop, the baby should receive intravenous acyclovir (10 mg/kg every 8 hours).

DIAGNOSIS

The diagnosis of varicella is essentially clinical and routine laboratory investigations are not essential. Rapid laboratory diagnosis can be made by electron microscopy or by immunofluorescence. Varicella-zoster virus (VZV) can be identified quickly by direct fluorescence assay of cells from cutaneous lesions or by polymerase chain reaction amplification testing. Although multinucleated giant cells (Tzanck smear) can be detected with nonspecific strains, they do not help to differentiate between varicella virus and herpes simplex virus infections and have poor sensitivity. IgG antibodies to VZV can be detected by several methods and a 4-fold rise in antibody titer is also confirmatory of acute infection. Leukopenia is typical during the first 72 hours; followed by lymphocytosis. Liver enzymes are also mildly elevated.

TREATMENT Varicella (Chickenpox)

Supportive Therapy

No treatment is usually required and bed rest is unnecessary except in ill children. Paracetamol will control prodromal symptoms and fever. Aspirin should not be given because of the risk of Reye's syndrome. Calamine lotion will normally soothe pruritus; if not, an antihistaminic should be tried. If the enanthem is severe, careful oral toilet is needed. Lesions on the conjunctiva should be protected from secondary infection.

Specific Therapy

Acyclovir therapy is not recommended routinely for treatment of uncomplicated chickenpox in the otherwise healthy child because of marginal benefit, cost of the drug, and low risk of complications of the disease. Oral acyclovir to healthy children within 24 hours of onset of rash decreases the duration of rash by 1 day and number of new lesions by only 25%.

Indications for acyclovir in varicella infection are as follows:

- Chronic cutaneous or pulmonary disorders
- Those receiving short term, intermittent or aerosolized corticosteroids
- Those receiving long-term salicylate therapy
- Immunocompromised patients including those with HIV infection and malignancies
- Disseminated varicella infection including pneumonia, encephalitis, severe hepatitis, or thrombocytopenia.

Intravenous acyclovir therapy is indicated for severe disease and for varicella in immunocompromised patients. Intravenous acyclovir (10 mg/kg q 8 hours IV) initiated within 72 hours of development of initial symptoms decreases the progression of the disease in high-risk patients. The treatment is continued for 7–10 days. Oral acyclovir (20 mg/kg/dose) given as 4 doses/day for 5 days should be used for the other indications mentioned above. Treatment should be initiated as early as possible, within 24 hours of rash. Foscarnet is the only available drug for acyclovir resistant varicella.

Cloxacillin can be used to treat skin infections. More severe sepsis will require appropriate antibacterial chemotherapy, which should be guided by swabbing of the affected lesions and by cultures of the blood and of any pus.

BREAKTHROUGH VARICELLA

Varicella vaccine administered as a 1-dose regimen to healthy children offers 85% protection (range 44–100%). Vaccinated children can thus suffer from varicella. Breakthrough varicella is defined as varicella occurring in a child who was vaccinated at least 42 days prior to eruption of the rash with one dose of varicella vaccine and caused by wild type varicella virus. Rash occurring between 14 and 42 days after vaccination can also be due to vaccine strains.

Breakthrough varicella is usually a mild disease. It is predominated by a maculopapular rash; vesicles are less frequent. Number of lesions is <50. These children are less likely to transmit the disease to others, i.e., the secondary attack rate of breakthrough varicella is lower than classical varicella. Recipients of two-dose varicella vaccine are less likely to have breakthrough varicella as compared to those having received one dose only.

PREVENTION

Active Immunization

Two doses of live virus vaccine are recommended by the IAP to prevent varicella in healthy children. Protective efficacy of two-dose regimen is 98–100%. First dose is administered at 15 months of age and second dose is given 3 months later. For those >13 years of age 2 doses should be given at an interval of at least 4 weeks. Varicella vaccine should not be given within 4 weeks of MMR vaccination; however, both can be given simultaneously.

Postexposure Prophylaxis

Varicella vaccine, if given within 3–5 days of exposure, can prevent or modify the disease in household contacts. Chemoprophylaxis with acyclovir is not an established mode of prevention.

Varicella-zoster immunoglobulin is recommended for newborns whose mothers have varicella 5 days before to 2 days after delivery. Other susceptible high-risk contacts (pregnant women, immunocompromised children, and hospitalized, premature infants born <28 weeks or <1,000 g birth weight) should also be given VZIG.

Varicella-zoster immunoglobulin is given as 125 IU/10 kg with a maximum dose of 625 IU. Minimum dose is 62.5 IU for less than or equal to 2 kg and 125 IU for 2–10 kg. Varicella vaccination should be given almost 5 months after VZIG administration.

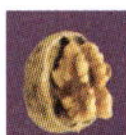

IN A NUTSHELL

Varicella (Chickenpox)

1. The rash typically begins as maculopapular lesion on first day of fever, as crops of macules, which evolve into papules and then vesicles.
2. If the maternal rash appears <5 days before delivery or up to 2 days after delivery, the baby should be protected by giving VZIG.
3. For all postexposure prophylaxis, administration of VZIG should be as soon as possible, ideally within 4 days for maximum efficacy, but maximum within next 10 days.
4. The most common complication of varicella is a pure cerebellar ataxia, which has an excellent prognosis.
5. First dose of varicella vaccine should be given between 15 and 18 months and second dose between 4 and 6 years.

Committee on Infectious Diseases. Policy statement—prevention of varicella: update of recommendations for use of quadrivalent and monovalent varicella vaccines in children. Pediatrics. 2011;128(3):630-2.

Gershon AA, Gershon MD, Shapiro ED. Live attenuated varicella vaccine: prevention of varicella and of zoster. J Infect Dis. 2021;224(12 Suppl 2):S387-97.

Javed S, Javed SA, Tyring SK. Varicella vaccines. Curr Opin Infect Dis. 2012;25:135-40.

Lachiewicz AM, Srinivas ML. Varicella-zoster virus post-exposure management and prophylaxis: a review [published correction appears in Prev Med Rep. 2020 Dec 13;20:101283]. Prev Med Rep. 2019;16:101016.

Partridge DG, McKendrick MW. The treatment of varicella-zoster virus infection and its complications. Expert Opin Pharmacother. 2009;10(5):797-812.

Smith CK, Arvin AM. Varicella in the fetus and newborn. Semin Fetal Neonatal Med. 2009;14(4):209-17.

Zhang Z, Suo L, Pan J, et al. Two-dose varicella vaccine effectiveness in China: a meta-analysis and evidence quality assessment. BMC Infect Dis. 2021;21(1):543.

14.8 Diphtheria *PE 31.11*

INTRODUCTION

Diphtheria is an acute infectious disease caused by a toxin produced by the gram-positive bacillus *Corynebacterium diphtheriae* (*C. diphtheriae*). Infection may result in an asymptomatic carrier state, or clinical disease. The illness is characterized by moderate fever and sore throat; adherent membrane of the tonsils, pharynx, or nose; and severe toxemia.

THE PROBLEM STATEMENT

Diphtheria used to be a leading cause of death in children until the introduction of a vaccine 50 years back. WHO estimates that there are about 100,000 cases and up to 8,000 deaths every year worldwide. In the last decade, epidemics were reported in Russia, Ukraine, and other countries of the former USSR. The epidemics began in 1990 and since then have spread to 15 countries. The death rate was as high as 50% among children under 2 years in Turkmenistan. These epidemics are largely due to decreasing immunization coverage among infants and children, waning immunity to diphtheria in adults, and an irregular supply of vaccines.

Diphtheria is endemic in India. Exact figures on prevalence are not available, but of late, the incidence has shown a decline mainly due to widespread vaccination coverage of under-fives.

EPIDEMIOLOGY

Eighty percent of cases occur in individuals <15 years of age. Both sexes are equally affected. Diphtheria occurs more often in the autumn and winter months. Transplacental immunity acquired from the mother protects the offspring during first 8–10 weeks of life. Infection can occur in immunized, partially immunized, or unimmunized individuals.

Mode of Spread

Diphtheria is acquired by contact with a carrier or a person with the disease. Bacteria are transmitted by airborne droplet liberated during coughing, sneezing, or talking. Fomites and dust may at times serve as mode of transmission of infection. Bacteria may enter the host through respiratory tract, abraded skin, eyes, genitalia, middle ear, or umbilicus in the neonate. Once infected, the patient remains infective to others till the virulent bacilli are present in the lesions, usually for a period of 2–4 weeks.

Carriers: For every case of clinical diphtheria, there exist 20 asymptomatic carriers in the community. The organism is carried in nose or throat. The carrier state may be temporary or chronic.

ETIOLOGY

The infection is caused by *C. diphtheriae*, also known as Klebs-Loeffler bacilli.

Corynebacterium diphtheriae secretes a potent exotoxin. This exotoxin is the major determinant of pathogenicity of the organism. The toxin causes reversible early cardiac damage and late neurological lesions. Diphtheria toxin is lethal to man in a dose of 130 μg/kg body weight.

Both toxigenic and nontoxigenic strains of *C. diphtheriae* can cause disease; however, cardiac and neurological sequels are observed following infection with toxigenic strains only.

PATHOGENESIS

Diphtheria is a rapidly developing, acute, febrile infection, which involves both local and systemic pathology. The primary local lesion develops in the upper respiratory tract and involves necrotic injury to epithelial cells. As a result of this injury, blood plasma leaks into the area and a fibrin network forms which is interlaced with rapidly growing *C. diphtheriae* cells. This membranous network covers the site of the local lesion and is referred to as the pseudomembrane. The membrane is adherent to underlying tissues.

The diphtheria bacilli do not tend to invade tissues below or away from the surface epithelial cells at the site of the local lesion. At this site, they produce the toxin that is absorbed and disseminated through lymph channels and blood to the susceptible tissues of the body. Degenerative changes in these tissues, which include heart, muscle, peripheral nerves, adrenals, kidneys, liver, and spleen, result in the systemic pathology of the disease.

The pathogenicity of *C. diphtheriae* thus includes two distinct phenomena:

1. ***Invasion of the local tissues of the throat***, which requires colonization and subsequent bacterial proliferation. Not much is known about the adherence mechanisms of *C. diphtheriae*; and
2. ***Toxigenesis (bacterial production of the toxin):*** The diphtheria toxin causes the death of eukaryotic cells and tissues by inhibiting protein synthesis in the cells.

Although the toxin is responsible for the lethal symptoms of the disease, the virulence of *C. diphtheriae* cannot be attributed to toxigenicity alone, since a distinct invasive phase apparently precedes toxigenesis. Diphtheria toxin may also play an essential role in the colonization process.

CLINICAL FEATURES

Incubation period is 2–5 days (range 1–10 days). Onset of symptoms is acute with moderate fever (39°C) and nonspecific symptoms, often resembling viral upper respiratory infection. Fever is associated with chills, malaise, weakness, prostration, sore throat, and headache. Further symptoms depend on the site of involvement:

- ***Nasal diphtheria*** is characterized by a serosanguineous or seropurulent nasal discharge.

- ***Tonsillar diphtheria*** manifests with dysphagia, sore throat, and cervical lymph node enlargement.
- ***Laryngeal diphtheria*** should be suspected, if the child presents with cough, hoarse voice, inspiratory stridor, and dyspnea.

Examination reveals general toxic and ill-looking anxious child, who has difficulty in breathing. Typical hallmark of the disease is presence of a thick, gray, and leathery membrane covering the affected area; i.e., tonsils, soft palate, oropharynx, nasopharynx, uvula, or laryngeal walls and folds. Attempt at scraping the pseudomembrane causes bleeding of the underlying mucosa.

Pharynx shows marked congestion and edema. Regional lymph nodes of the neck are involved. Extensive anterior and submandibular cervical lymphadenopathy imparts a *bull's neck* appearance. The child may hold the head in extension. It can be associated with dysphonia.

Presence of the membrane over larynx results in respiratory obstruction that may manifest itself as stridor, wheezing, cyanosis, accessory muscle use, and retractions. Untreated, it may progress to respiratory failure.

COMPLICATIONS

Exotoxin of diphtheria typically affects the heart, nerves, and kidneys. Cardiac toxicity typically occurs after 1–2 weeks of illness following improvement in the pharyngeal phase of the disease, and manifests as myocarditis or arrhythmia. Neurological toxicity involves both cranial and peripheral nerves and symptoms may appear as early as in the beginning of 2nd week of illness. A latent period of up to 3 months is also described. Renal complications consist of tubular necrosis and proteinuria.

Cardiac complications: Myocarditis is seen in as many as 60% of patients (especially if previously unimmunized). It can present acutely with congestive heart failure, circulatory collapse, or in a more subtle way with progressive dyspnea, diminished heart sounds, cardiac dilatation, and weakness. Atrioventricular blocks, ST-T wave changes, and various dysrhythmias may be seen.

Neurologic toxicity: It is proportional to the severity of the pharyngeal infection. Most patients with severe disease develop neuropathy. Deficits include regurgitation of swallowed fluids due to paralysis of the soft palate and posterior pharyngeal wall; oculomotor and ciliary paralysis accounting for cranial neuropathies; and dysfunction of facial, pharyngeal, or laryngeal nerves.

Peripheral neuritis develops anywhere from 10 days to 3 months after the onset of pharyngeal disease. It manifests itself initially as a motor defect of the proximal muscle groups in the extremities. The weakness is usually symmetrical and simulates Guillain-Barré syndrome. Various degrees of dysfunction exist, ranging from diminished deep tendon reflexes to complete motor paralysis. Occasionally, a glove-and-stocking neuropathy pattern can be observed. All nerve damage due to diphtheria eventually resolves.

CUTANEOUS DIPHTHERIA

Cutaneous diphtheria begins as a painful lesion resembling an erythematous pustule, which breaks down to form an ulcer covered with a gray membrane. The lesion usually develops at a site of previous trauma or a primary dermatologic disease. It follows an indolent course, typically lasting weeks to months. Occasionally, it may cause respiratory diphtheria.

TREATMENT Diphtheria

If diphtheria is strongly suspected, specific treatment with *antitoxin* and *antibiotics* should be initiated immediately while bacteriological investigations are still pending. Antitoxin therapy is the mainstay of treatment. Antibiotic therapy is required to eradicate the organism and prevent spread. Mechanical airway obstruction and myocarditis are the main causes of death in toxigenic disease and careful supportive management is required.

Diphtheria Antitoxin

Diphtheria antitoxin is hyperimmune serum produced in horses. Antitoxin will only neutralize circulating toxin that is not yet bound to tissue; thus prompt administration is critical. Delayed administration increases the risk of late effects such as myocarditis and neuritis. Before antitoxin is administered, the patient should be tested for sensitivity to horse serum and if necessary, desensitized. The dose of antitoxin to be administered depends upon the site and extent of the diphtheritic membrane, the degree of toxicity, and the duration of illness. **Table 14.7** indicates the suggested dose range for various clinical situations.

If acute anaphylaxis develops, intravenous epinephrine (0.2–0.5 mL of 1:1,000 solution) be administered immediately by intravenous injection. Antitoxin is probably of no value for cutaneous disease, although some centers advocate 20,000–40,000 units of antitoxin because toxic sequels have been reported. Vigorous cleaning of the wound with soap and water and administration of antibiotics is recommended.

Antibiotics

Antibiotic treatment is necessary to eliminate the organism and prevent spread; it is not a substitute for antitoxin treatment. The antibiotics of choice are erythromycin or penicillin. The recommended dose regimens are as follows:

Penicillin, preferably crystalline penicillin (100,000–150,000 units/kg/day q 6 hours) IV or intramuscular procaine penicillin G (2,5000–50,000 units/kg/day) in two divided doses or parenteral erythromycin (40–50 mg/kg/day, maximum 2 g) are the initial therapeutic options. One can shift to oral administration of erythromycin (40–50 mg/kg/day in four divided doses) or oral penicillin V (125–250 mg four times daily) when the patients is able to swallow. Antibiotic treatment should be continued for 14 days.

Table 14.7 Dosage of Antitoxin for Diphtheria

Type of diphtheria	*Dosage (units)*	*Route*
Nasal	10,000–20,000	IM/IV
Tonsillar	15,000–25,000	IM/IV
Pharyngeal or laryngeal	20,000–40,000	IM/IV
Combined types or delayed diagnosis	40,000–60,000	IV
Severe diphtheria with respiratory obstruction or bull-neck	40,000–10,0000	IV or part IV and part IM

(IM: intramuscular; IV: intravenous)

Treatment of Carriers

Carriers should be treated with erythromycin 40 mg/kg/day for 7–10 days or a single intramuscular dose of benzathine penicillin (0.6 megaunits for <30 kg weight and 1.2 megaunits for >30 kg). Cultures should be obtained after 2 weeks. If positive, give an additional course of erythromycin for 10 days. Antitoxin is not recommended for asymptomatic carriers.

Unimmunized carriers should receive a full schedule of active immunization. Previously immunized carriers should receive a booster dose if the previous dose was received more than a year ago.

PREVENTION

Better control of diphtheria depends on high immunization coverage, prompt recognition and management of diphtheria cases, and rapid identification and effective management of close contacts to prevent further spread of outbreaks.

Isolation of the Patient

Communicability in untreated persons usually lasts for 2 weeks. If treated adequately communicability lasts for <4 days. The patient should be isolated until this period is over or two cultures from nose and throat are negative.

Care of the Contacts

The management of close contacts depends on whether the contact can be kept under surveillance for minimum 7 days or not. The management is given in **Flowchart 14.4**. There is no role of prophylactic diphtheria antitoxin in unimmunized close contacts. *Schick test*, previously recommended to assess the presence of circulating antibody to exotoxin and immune status of the individual with respect to diphtheria, is no longer in current use.

Flowchart 14.4: Care of contacts of a patient with diphtheria

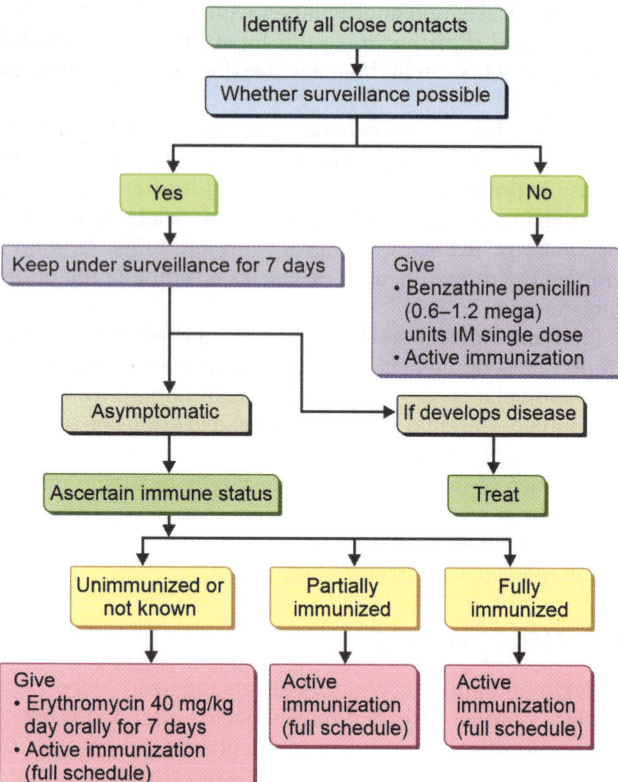

Active Immunization

The aim is to immunize the infant before the effect of transplacental acquired immunity against diphtheria is over. The vaccine currently in use is a toxoid, and available as diphtheria-pertussis-tetanus (DPT) vaccine. Immunization does not eliminate *C. diphtheriae* in skin or nasopharynx.

Primary immunization consists of three doses of DTP (as combination like pentavac vaccine) at an interval of 4-6 weeks, starting from 6th weeks after birth. First booster is given at 18 months and a second booster at 5 years. In view of increased cases of diphtheria in adolescents and adults and increased severity of the disease in this population, IAP recommends tetanus-reduced dose diphtheria-reduced dose acellular pertussis (Tdap) vaccine at 10 years, Td at 16–18 years and revaccination with Td vaccine every 10 years thereafter. Also, National Immunization Schedule by Government of India has recommended continued revaccination at 10 and 16 years with Td vaccine and subsequent revaccination with Td vaccination every 10 years. Catch up immunization under 7 years is done by DTP vaccine in 0,1 and 6 month schedule while that in children above 7 years is done by Tdap/Td vaccine in 0, 1, 6 month schedule. (Td)/Tdap vaccine contains not >2 limit of flocculation (Lf) unit of diphtheria toxoid per dose as compared to 25 Lf in DPT preparation.

All patients suffering from diphtheria should undergo active immunization because the attack of disease, by itself, may not confer immunity against subsequent infections. The immunization coverage with three doses of DPT vaccine in infants is still far from satisfactory in India as compared to rest of the world.

Replacement of TT with Td

In the light of recent diphtheria outbreaks affecting older children and younger adults in developing countries and the resurgence of the disease in industrialized countries, it has become clear that periodic administration of booster doses of diphtheria toxoid is needed to ensure long-lasting protection of all individuals against diphtheria. It has, therefore, been recommended to replace TT with Td in a phased manner. As a priority, TT should be replaced by Td in all countries that have had DTP-3 coverage of 70% or more for 5–7 years. Where boosters of DT are given at school age, replacing the first dose of DT with Td simplifies delivery programmatically. In India, TT has been replaced by Td at 10 and 16 years of age as well as during pregnancy in national immunization schedule.

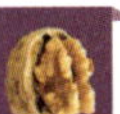

IN A NUTSHELL

Diphtheria

1. Diphtheria is caused by gram-positive bacteria *Corynebacterium diphtheriae (C. diphtheria)*, which produce a toxin.
2. Diphtheria spreads from person-to-person, usually through respiratory droplets from coughing or sneezing.
3. Invasion of local tissue of nose, throat, and larynx produces fever, malaise, nasal discharge, sore throat, dysphagia, stridor, dyspnea, and cervical lymphadenopathy.
4. Absorption of toxins into the circulation produces myocarditis and polyneuropathy.
5. Demonstration of *C. diphtheriae* in throat swab smear examination and culture isolates is diagnostic of diphtheria.
6. Treatment includes antitoxins and antibiotics.
7. Primary prophylaxis against diphtheria includes routine vaccination with diphtheria containing vaccines.
8. Secondary prophylaxis includes immunization of close contacts with diphtheria containing vaccines and/administration of antibiotics.

Dash N, Verma S, Jayashree M, et al. Clinico-epidemiological profile and predictors of outcome in children with diphtheria: a study from Northern India. Trop Doct. 2019;49(2):96-101.

Efstratiou A, Engler KH, Mazurova IK, et al. Current approaches to the laboratory diagnosis of diphtheria. J Infect Dis. 2000;181(Suppl 1):S138-45.

Truelove SA, Keegan LT, Moss WJ, et al. Clinical and epidemiological aspects of diphtheria: a systematic review and pooled analysis. Clin Infect Dis. 2020;71(1):89-97.

WHO laboratory manual for the diagnosis of diphtheria and other related infections. Geneva: World Health Organization; 2021.

14.9 Pertussis (Whooping Cough)

PE 31.11

INTRODUCTION

Whooping cough is a highly communicable illness caused by a coccobacillus *Bordetella pertussis* (*B. pertussis*). The illness affects all ages, but the effects and course are more pronounced in infants and young children. The disease is characterized by paroxysmal bouts of cough lasting for almost a month.

EPIDEMIOLOGY

Age: Pertussis is typically a disease of young children. A significant epidemiological shift has been observed in many industrialized countries, indicating a higher incidence of pertussis among previously vaccinated schoolchildren, adolescents, and adults. Even neonates can be affected as immunity to pertussis is not transmitted transplacentally.

Sex: There is a female predilection for pertussis.

Nutritional status: Incidence of pertussis as well as mortality due to pertussis is more in children whose body weight is <60% of the expected weight.

Environment: Whooping cough is more common in winter and spring. Overcrowding, poor socioeconomic status, and low level of parental education are related with higher mortality.

Mode of Spread

Man is the only known host of *B. pertussis*. Transmission occurs directly *via* respiratory secretions. Bacteria are spread by droplets discharged from the nose or throat of an infected person, usually in close contact. Pertussis is highly contagious during the first week of illness with a secondary attack rate of almost 100% in susceptible contacts. Communicability then decreases rapidly, but may persist up to 21 days. Fomites do not constitute a major route of transmission.

Adults with overt or subclinical infection are important sources of infection for young children. People with asymptomatic infection are less likely to transmit the disease than individuals with symptomatic infection. Asymptomatic chronic carriers of *B. pertussis* are uncommon.

ETIOPATHOGENESIS

Bordetella pertussis is a gram-negative coccobacillus, which colonizes ciliated epithelium. The pathogenic effects are mediated through various antigens, or their products produced by the organism. *B. pertussis* has two major antigens, i.e., FHA or filamentous hemagglutinin antigen and LPF or lymphocytosis producing factor. *B. pertussis* also produces several toxins, of which pertussis toxin (PT) is the most important virulence factor. It also acts as a mediator for attachment to respiratory cells. Filamentous hemagglutinin also mediates attachment of *B. pertussis* to respiratory epithelium. Both PT and hemagglutinin produce protective antibodies that prevent clinical disease. Therefore, any vaccine aiming to prevent pertussis should contain both these antigens.

Bordetella pertussis also produces tracheal toxin (TCT), adenylate cyclase toxin (ACT), dermonecrotic toxin (DNT), and several agglutinogens. TCT disturbs mucociliary clearance and damages the epithelium. Adenylate cyclase toxin and PT inhibit phagocytic functions. TCT, DNT, and ACT contribute to local damage while PT is primarily responsible for systemic manifestations. Pertussis is not a single toxin disease such as diphtheria and tetanus.

CLINICAL FEATURES

The incubation period ranges from 7 to 14 days. Natural history is classically described in three phases; i.e., (*a*) Catarrhal phase; (*b*) Paroxysmal phase; and (*c*) Convalescent phase.

During the *catarrhal phase*, the disease is usually indistinguishable from cough and cold, sometimes with mild fever. After about 10 days, the cough worsens, and the disease progresses into *paroxysmal phase* with bouts of coughing; the child's face becomes congested passing from red to blue during bouts. The classical whoop occurs due to a rescue inspiration at the end of coughing. Post-tussive vomiting may occur. This phase may continue for about 2 weeks without improvement. If there are no complications, the disease progresses to *convalescent phase,* which may last for up to 3 months. In clinical practice, the paroxysmal and convalescent phases may be considered as one. Relapses back to paroxysmal coughing are common. The disease is also known as "cough of 100 days". The cough is exhaustive and scaring for the child and family.

The disease may have an atypical presentation in infants <3 months of age. The whoop may be absent in babies who may lack strength to mount paroxysms. These children are at high risk and the disease can present as serious respiratory infection or a cough proceeding to apneic attacks. Also, young infants are especially vulnerable since protective antibodies present in childhood decline in adults and hence, there is little passive protection of the newborn by maternal antibodies.

COMPLICATIONS

Complications are related to pressure effects resulting from paroxysms or occur because of respiratory or neurological involvement.

- ***Pressure effects*** lead to venous congestion causing subconjunctival hemorrhages, skin petechiae, nose bleeds, and hemoptysis. Intracranial hemorrhage is rare. Raised intracranial pressure due to incessant cough may also enlarge several hernias. Persistent coughing may result in increased intrathoracic pressure. Resultant barotrauma can cause air leak, i.e., pneumothorax.
- ***Secondary infection*** in lungs may occur and should be suspected in any child with high temperature. Atelectasis, interstitial pneumonia, and bronchiectasis are other reported respiratory complications. Pertussis can flare up a pre-existing focus of tuberculosis in lungs, especially in malnourished children.
- ***Neurological sequelae*** are the most serious complication. They may be toxin-mediated or the sequelae of hypoxia. CNS manifestations include loss of consciousness, convulsions, or encephalopathy, which may lead to brain damage, morbidity, or death. Neurological complications occur in 3–5% and can also manifest as motor deficits, visual and auditory loss, and aphasia.

DIAGNOSIS

Case Definition

Whooping cough should be *suspected* whenever there is a history of severe cough lasting for 2 weeks or more. This definition has 84–92% sensitivity and 3–90% specificity, during outbreaks.

Whooping cough is *probably suspected*, if any of the following exists in a case:

- Prolonged coughing followed by a period of apnea and cyanosis, or in older children paroxysms of coughing followed by vomiting, or a typical breath intake and "whoop", or subconjunctival hemorrhages
- Exposure to a suspect case in the previous 3 weeks
- Epidemic of whooping cough in the area or
- Lymphocytosis of 15,000/mm^3 or more.
- A probable case is *confirmed,* if there is laboratory evidence of *B. pertussis* from the culture or immunofluorescence of nasopharyngeal secretions. The nasopharyngeal diagnosis is provided by a perinasal sample, which requires a special cotton swab on a long flexible wand. The swab needs to be placed in a culture medium such as Stuarts, and, though storage overnight in a refrigerator is permissible, rapid transport to the laboratory for planting improves the chance of positive result.

DIFFERENTIAL DIAGNOSIS

Other causes of protracted cough include those caused by adenovirus, respiratory syncytial virus (RSV), enterovirus, influenza virus, parainfluenza virus and *Mycoplasma.*

INVESTIGATIONS

Recovery of the organism is easier at early stages of illness. A positive culture on Bordet–Gengou medium is the gold standard of diagnosis. Peripheral smear shows absolute lymphocytosis. Direct immunofluorescent assay (DFA) of nasopharyngeal aspirate has variable sensitivity and specificity. It should be emphasized that no single serologic test is highly specific and sensitive. Newer serological methods include PCR and ELISA techniques for detection of pertussis toxin and filamentous hemagglutinin.

TREATMENT Pertussis (Whooping Cough)

Antibiotics

Once in the paroxysmal phase, drug therapy makes little impact on the course of the illness. An antibiotic (erythromycin is highly effective) should always be given to render the sufferer noninfectious and prevent the spread of disease. This is normally achieved after 5 days of erythromycin; however, treatment is best continued for 2 weeks as a few individuals remain culture positive even after 1 week of antibiotics. Azithromycin is the drug of choice for neonatal pertussis.

- Erythromycin is given in a dose of 40 mg/kg/day orally, in four divided doses for 2 weeks. The newer macrolides (e.g., azithromycin, clarithromycin), are potential alternatives for patients who cannot tolerate erythromycin.
- Azithromycin is typically administered in doses of 10–12 mg/kg/day PO once a day for 5 days.
- Clarithromycin is administered at 15–20 mg/kg/day PO in 2 divided doses, not to exceed 1 g/day for 5–7 days.
- Trimethoprim-sulfamethoxazole (trimethoprim 8 mg/kg/day and sulfamethoxazole 40 mg/kg/day) in two divided doses is another antibiotic option.

Supportive Treatment

Adjunct therapy should center on five principles of care:

1. Avoid provoking paroxysms of coughing
2. Comforting during paroxysms
3. Clearing away mucus and vomit during paroxysms to prevent inhalation
4. Early recognition and treatment of complications
5. Maintaining good hydration and reasonable nutrition.

Humidification of the air diminishes the viscosity of mucus and the affected child can bring it out more easily. Mild sedation should be done to allay anxiety. Salbutamol has no role in preventing incidence or reducing the severity of paroxysms.

Care of Contacts

The Committee on Infectious Diseases of the American Academy of Pediatrics currently recommends promptly treating all household and other close contacts (e.g., children and staff at daycare centers) with erythromycin to limit secondary transmission. This is regardless of the age or immunization status of contacts. A 14-day course of oral erythromycin (40–50 mg/kg/day in four divided doses) is recommended for close contacts. Some experts prefer the estolate preparation in young infants because of more effective absorption, which may lead to decreased dosing and less frequent dosing intervals.

PREVENTION

Natural disease does not provide lifelong immunity. Similarly, pertussis vaccination protects the individual for a maximum period of 10–20 years. However, universal immunization of children with pertussis vaccine is essential for control of pertussis. Since protective antibodies against this disease do not cross the placenta, early immunization is desired. The National Immunization Schedule of India advocates pertussis vaccination as DPT at 6, 10, and 14 weeks of age. This is to be followed by two boosters at 18–24 months and at 5 years of age.

Pertussis vaccine has limited impact on the circulation of *B. pertussis* even in countries with high vaccination coverage. Nonimmunized children and adults may serve as reservoirs for the infection and occasionally transmit *B. pertussis* to unimmunized young infants.

Acellular Pertussis Vaccine

Studies have indicated that DPT with a whole cell pertussis (wP) component is responsible for frequent reactions. These reactions are both unpleasant and at times dangerous. This led to the development of acellular pertussis vaccine in the year 1981 in Japan. The acellular vaccine predominantly contains PT as the essential component, and different amounts of filamentous hemagglutinin (FHA), pertactin (PRN), and fimbrial hemagglutinins 1, 2, and 3 (FIM 1, 2, 3). Recent studies have demonstrated a better efficacy of whole cell vaccine for primary immunization, as compared to acellular vaccine.

The Indian Academy of Pediatrics (IAP) recommends use of whole cell pertussis vaccine for primary immunization. Academy also recommends use of tetanus-diphtheria-acellular pertussis (Tdap) vaccine during each pregnancy to protect very young infants. Recently, Government of India has replaced TT vaccine by Td vaccine during pregnancy. WHO also recommends continuation of the whole cell pertussis vaccine in countries with limited resources.

Future research will be concentrated on the development of a genetically engineered product, which carries the additional advantage of reduction in the number of required dosages for primary immunization.

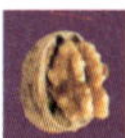

IN A NUTSHELL

Pertussis (Whooping Cough)

1. Pertussis, caused by *Bordetella pertussis (B. pertussis)*, is a toxin-mediated disease, presenting as a typical whooping cough. The illness usually lasts for 3 months.
2. Diagnosis is established by isolation of organism on Bordet–Gengou medium.
3. Management is mostly supportive, targeted toward comforting the patient and monitoring for complications.
4. Azithromycin is effective, if given in the first week of illness.
5. Immunization with three doses and two boosters of DPT vaccine prevents pertussis with 70–90% efficacy.

Cherry JD, Grimprel E, Guiso N, et al. Defining pertussis epidemiology: clinical, microbiologic and serologic perspectives. Pediatr Infect Dis J. 2005;24:S25-34.

Decker MD, Edwards KM. Pertussis (whooping cough). J Infect Dis. 2021;224(12 Suppl 2):S310-20.

Mathew JL. Acellular pertussis vaccines pertinent issues. Indian Pediatr. 2008;45(9):727-9.

Polinori I, Esposito S. Clinical findings and management of pertussis. Adv Exp Med Biol. 2019;1183:151-60.

Yeh SH. Pertussis: persistent pathogen, imperfect vaccines. Expert Rev Vaccines. 2003;2:113-27.

Zasztowt-Sternicka M, Jagielska AM, Nitsch-Osuch AS. Pertussis vaccination in pregnancy—current data on safety and effectiveness. Ginekol Pol. 2021;92(8):591-4.

14.10 Tetanus

PE 31.11

INTRODUCTION

Tetanus is caused by an anaerobic bacterium, *Clostridium tetani* (*C. tetani*), which produces a neurotoxin called tetanospasmin. The disease is characterized by generalized muscle rigidity and spasms, lockjaw, and opisthotonus and carries a significant morbidity and mortality. Majority of cases are reported from developing countries; with 50% of these occurring in neonates. Mortality is 30–50% even with optimal treatment.

India has been declared free from neonatal and maternal tetanus on May 15, 2015. *Elimination of neonatal tetanus is defined as less than one case in 1,000 live births in every district across the country.* Maternal tetanus is considered eliminated once neonatal tetanus elimination has been achieved. Nagaland was the last state in India to achieve neonatal and maternal tetanus elimination.

ETIOLOGY

Clostridium tetani is a gram-positive, anaerobic, motile, rod-shaped bacterium. The organism bears spores at its terminal end giving it a typical drumstick appearance. While the bacillus is an obligate anaerobe, its spores remain viable at ambient oxygen concentrations. The spores are highly resistant to extremes in temperature and humidity and can survive indefinitely. Spores are ubiquitous in soil and in the feces of many animals and of humans.

MODE OF SPREAD

Tetanus organism or spores may enter the body through a puncture wound, or laceration, following an acute injury. Recent surgery also accounts for several cases. Nonacute etiologies include chronic wounds, IV drug use, and complications of diabetes. Other etiologies include otitis media (*otogenic tetanus*), intranasal foreign bodies, corneal abrasions/ulcers/foreign bodies, dental procedures, injections, abortion, childbirth, and burns. Neonatal tetanus follows infection of the umbilical stump of a newborn delivered to an unimmunized mother. Lack of immunization is the greatest risk factor for contracting tetanus. Tetanus is not transmitted from man-to-man by direct spread.

PATHOGENESIS

Spores of *Clostridium* are carried into the wounds along with soil, dirt, or dust. The spores may not germinate immediately due to unfavorable tissue conditions. They may activate well after the wound has healed, which may account for the cases of tetanus that have no identifiable source. When conditions such as gross contamination or tissue injury favor anaerobic proliferation, the spores germinate into mature bacilli, which then form the toxins *tetanolysin* and *tetanospasmin*.

Tetanolysin has an uncertain role in clinical tetanus; it may contribute to an anaerobic environment by damaging viable tissue. *Tetanospasmin* is primarily responsible for the clinical manifestations of tetanus. Tetanospasmin is highly lethal with 1 mg of toxin being enough to kill 6,40,000 mice. It enters peripheral nerves and travels via the axonal retrograde transport system to the CNS. Tetanospasmin then enters presynaptic neurons and disables neurotransmitter release, most importantly, the inhibitory neurotransmitters gamma-aminobutyric acid (GABA) and glycine. This results in a disinhibition of end-organ neurons, such as motor neurons and those of the autonomic nervous system. This accounts for the muscle spasms characteristic of tetanus and for the autonomic instability seen with severe tetanus.

Recovery involves synthesis of new presynaptic components and their transport to the distal axon. This takes about 2–3 weeks before clinical improvement begins.

CLINICAL FEATURES

The median incubation period is 7 days; 73% of patients develop their first symptom between 4 and 14 days after an injury. The rapidity of incubation and onset correlates with the severity of disease. There are four clinical forms of tetanus representing the extent and location of neurons involved: Generalized, local, cephalic, and neonatal.

Generalized Tetanus

The initial symptom is trismus (*lockjaw*) secondary to masseter muscle spasm in 50–75% of cases. *Risus sardonicus*, the "ironical smile of tetanus", can occur due to facial muscle contraction. Nuchal rigidity and dysphagia may also be initial complaints. As the disease spreads, generalized muscle spasms occur, either spontaneously or to minor stimuli such as touch or noise. Opisthotonus, a tonic contraction very similar to decorticate posturing, is classically described with tetanus. Severe spasms can result in vertebral fractures, long bone fractures, and detachment of tendons from their insertions. Unfortunately for the patient, mental status is not affected and spasms are felt with severe pain. In the acute phase, death may result from acute respiratory failure due to diaphragmatic paralysis and/or laryngeal spasms. With intensive medical intervention, including paralysis and mechanical ventilation, such deaths can be averted.

In patients surviving beyond the acute phase, autonomic instability is the major cause of death, with a fatality rate of 11–28%. Autonomic instability occurs several days after the onset of generalized spasms and manifests as labile hypertension, tachycardia, and pyrexia. Arrhythmias and myocardial infarction are the most common fatal events. The exact mechanism of this syndrome is unclear but likely involves disinhibition of the sympathetic nervous system.

Local Tetanus

Only a particular muscle group, which is close to the site of injury, is involved. The rigidity may linger for weeks to months and often self-resolves without sequelae. What appears to be localized tetanus may instead be the first symptom of generalized tetanus. Case-fatality rate is 1%.

Cephalic Tetanus

Injury to face, eyes, ears, neck, following tonsillectomy, or dental extraction may result in isolated involvement of cranial nerves, known as cephalic tetanus. Cephalic tetanus uniquely results in cranial nerve palsies and muscle spasms. The seventh cranial nerve is most often involved, followed by the 6th, 3rd, 4th, and 12th in decreasing order of frequency. Cephalic tetanus also presents with trismus, but in 42% of cases, cranial nerve deficits precede the onset of trismus. In such cases, cephalic tetanus is easily misdiagnosed. With its predilection for the 7th cranial nerve, it commonly mimics Bell's palsy. Head trauma and otitis media are commonly cited etiologies. About two-thirds of the patients progress to generalized tetanus and the overall mortality is 15–30%.

Neonatal Tetanus

This is a generalized tetanus that occurs in the newborn around the first week of life. It occurs characteristically in a newborn of an unimmunized mother, where the umbilical cord was cut by unsterile and unconventional means. Symptoms begin with nonspecific irritability and poor feeding, and rapidly progress to generalized spasms. The portal of entry of spores is the freshly cut umbilical cord.

The risk of contracting neonatal tetanus is directly related to the cleanliness of delivery conditions and to maternal immunization, since passive transfer of maternal immunoglobulins is protective. Mortality is very high (50–100%) due to the high load of toxin per kilogram body weight in neonates.

DIAGNOSIS

The diagnosis of tetanus is clinical. There are no laboratory tests, which can diagnose or rule out tetanus. Fortunately, the presentation of tetanus is so characteristic that a presumptive diagnosis can be made in most cases. The differential diagnoses are discussed below:

- Trismus can be caused by *peritonsillar or odontogenic abscesses* and *dystonic reactions*. These can be ruled out by history and examination.
- ***Strychnine poisoning*** can closely resemble generalized tetanus; strychnine disables glycine release such tetanospasmin but does not affect GABA release. A strychnine level should be sent for all suspected cases of tetanus.
- ***Hypocalcemia*** causing tetany is another mimic, which can easily be ruled out.
- Other entities that cause diffuse muscle spasms, such as seizures, *toxidromes*, and encephalopathy are accompanied by changes in mental status.
- Processes that affect muscles locally, such as *myopathies* or *neuropathies*, tend to cause weakness rather than spasm and rigidity. In addition, neuropathies are associated with sensory deficits, which is not a feature of tetanus.
- Cephalic tetanus without trismus can be easily mistaken for *Bell's palsy, CNS tumor*, or *stroke*; with the inevitable appearance of trismus and muscle spasm, the diagnosis becomes clear.
- Neonatal tetanus initially presents much such as a host of other disorders, including infectious, toxic, and *metabolic etiology*. However, once generalized spasms begin, the diagnosis is obvious.

As an aid in clinical diagnosis, a bedside "spatula test" for tetanus has been described. A spatula is inserted into the pharynx. If the patient gags and tries to expel the spatula, the test is negative for tetanus; if the patient bites the spatula due to reflex masseter spasm, the test is positive for tetanus.

TREATMENT Tetanus

Treatment strategies involve three management principles:

1. Organisms present in the body should be destroyed to prevent further toxin release.
2. Toxin present in the body, outside the CNS should be neutralized.
3. The effects of toxin already in the CNS should be minimized.

Neutralization of unbound toxin: Human tetanus immune globulin 3,000–6,000 units is given intramuscularly.

Removal of the source of infection: Where present, obvious wounds should be surgically debrided. Antibiotics are administered to eradicate clostridia.

- *Penicillin* has been widely used for many years but is a GABA antagonist and associated with convulsions.
- *Metronidazole* is probably the antibiotic of choice. It is safe and comparative studies with penicillin suggest equally good results.

Control of Rigidity and Spasms

It is best achieved by a combination of avoidance of unnecessary stimulation and sedation with a benzodiazepine. Benzodiazepines augment GABA agonism by inhibiting an endogenous inhibitor at the GABA receptor. Diazepam may be given by various routes, is cheap and widely used, and doses as high as 100 mg/h have been used. Midazolam has been used with less apparent accumulation.

Additional sedation may be provided by anticonvulsants, particularly phenobarbitone (which further enhances GABAergic activity) and phenothiazines, usually chlorpromazine. Propofol has been used for sedation with rapid recovery on stopping the infusion.

When sedation alone is inadequate, neuromuscular blocking agents and intermittent positive pressure ventilation may be required for a prolonged period. Pancuronium (long-acting), vecuronium (short-acting), and intrathecal baclofen have been used.

Control of Autonomic Dysfunction

Sudden cardiac death can occur due to autonomic dysfunction in severe tetanus. The cause remains unclear but plausible explanations include sudden loss of sympathetic drive, catecholamine-induced cardiac damage, and increased parasympathetic tone or "storms".

Benzodiazepines, anticonvulsants, and morphine are beneficial for controlling the autonomic dysfunction. Morphine is particularly useful as cardiovascular stability may occur without cardiac compromise. Proposed mechanisms of action include replacement of endogenous opioids, reduction in reflex sympathetic activity, and release of histamine. Phenothiazines, particularly chlorpromazine, are another useful sedative; anticholinergic and alpha-adrenergic antagonism may contribute to cardiovascular stability.

Other drugs that have been used to control autonomic dysfunction include a combination of *alpha- and beta-adrenergic receptor blocking agents*. The alpha-adrenergic agonist clonidine has been used orally or parenterally, with variable success. Acting centrally, it reduces sympathetic outflow, thus, reducing arterial pressure, heart rate, and catecholamine release from the adrenal medulla. Peripherally, it inhibits the release of norepinephrine from prejunctional nerve endings. Other useful effects include marked sedation and anxiolysis.

Magnesium sulfate has been used both in artificially ventilated patients to reduce autonomic disturbance and in nonventilated patients to control spasms. Magnesium is a presynaptic neuromuscular blocker, blocks catecholamine release from nerves and adrenal medulla, reduces receptor responsiveness to released catecholamines, is an anticonvulsant and a vasodilator. Hypotension and bradyarrhythmia may occur. It is, therefore, mandatory to maintain levels in the therapeutic range.

Supportive Intensive Care Treatment

Nutrition should be established as early as possible. Enteral nutrition is associated with a lower incidence of complications and is cheaper than parenteral nutrition. Percutaneous gastrostomy may avoid the complications associated with nasogastric tube feeding and is easily performed in the intensive care unit under sedation.

PREVENTION

Primary Immunization

Tetanus immunization should be started at the age of 6 weeks along with diphtheria and pertussis immunization. Three doses of DPT are recommended, 4–6 weeks apart. First booster is given at 18 months and the second between 5 and 6 years of age. Thereafter, a booster of tetanus and adult diphtheria vaccine (Td) is advocated at 10 and 16 years of age as per national immunization schedule, India.

IAP recommends Tdap vaccine at 10 years followed by Td vaccine at 16 years and every 10 years thereafter.

Catch up vaccination in less than 7 years age includes DTwP/DTaP at 0, 1, 6 months. In those older than 7 years, first dose should be Tdap/Td followed by Td at 1 and 6 months.

Prevention of Neonatal Tetanus

Aseptic delivery: The delivery should be conducted by a trained birth attendant, umbilical cord should be cut with a sterile blade, and application of extraneous and indigenous substances on the umbilical stump should be actively discouraged.

Maternal active immunization: Tetanus toxoid should be administered to all pregnant women. According to the National Schedule on Immunization, two doses of tetanus toxoid are recommended between 20 and 36 weeks of pregnancy, given a month apart. In previously immunized women, a single dose given at around 32–34 weeks is considered sufficient.

Prevention of Tetanus following Injury

Care of the wound: Any wound, abrasion, etc., should be thoroughly cleaned with water immediately, if nothing else is available. Foreign bodies and debris in the wound should be removed. Soil, dirt, necrotic tissue should not be allowed to remain at the injury site.

Immunization: The need for immunization is determined by the state, extent, cleanliness of the wound, and previous immune status **(Table 14.8)**. In case of minor clean wounds, passive immunization is not required. Active immunization is offered only in previously unimmunized or partially immunized individuals, or if the last dose of booster was given <10 years. Severe or contaminated wounds in previously immunized individuals do not require either active or passive immunization provided the individual has received a booster of tetanus toxoid in the last 5 years.

In previously immunized (where the last dose was given >10 years ago) and unimmunized individuals, one dose of toxoid is given shortly after the injury, followed by completion according to primary immunization schedule.

Passive immunization: It is provided with tetanus immune globulin (TIG), given intramuscularly within 3 days of injury. A single intramuscular dose of 5,000 units is sufficient to neutralize systemic toxin, but total dose of 3,000–6,000 units is also recommended. TIG does not cross the blood–CSF barrier. If TIG is not available, equine-derived or bovine-derived tetanus antitoxin (TAT) is used. The usual dose of TAT is 50,000–1,00,000 units with half given intramuscularly and rest intravenously, is sufficient for toxin neutralization. Active immunization can be given alongside passive immunization. However, the injection of globulin and toxoid should be given in separate syringes at two different sites.

Table 14.8 Tetanus Prophylaxis in Wound Management

	Doses of TT	*Clean and minor wounds*	*All other wounds*[#]	*Given in past*
	Td/Tdap	TIG*	Td/Tdap	TIG*
Unknown, <3 doses, and immunodeficient	Yes	Yes	Yes	Yes
≥3 doses	No[†]	No	No[‡]	No

[#]Including, but not limited to, wounds contaminated with dirt, feces, soil, and saliva; puncture wounds; avulsions; and wounds resulting from missiles, crushing, burns, and frostbite.
*TIG: tetanus immunoglobulin (250–500 IU IM).
[†]Yes, if >10 years since last dose.
[‡]Yes, if >5 years since last dose.
(Tdap: tetanus toxoid and reduced quantity diphtheria and acellular pertussis; TT: tetanus toxoid)

ELIMINATION OF MATERNAL AND NEONATAL TETANUS

World Health Organization added tetanus toxoid vaccine in its Expanded Program on Immunization (EPI) in the year 1974. Almost 15 years later, by 1989, only a quarter (27%) of pregnant females was receiving the standard doses of tetanus toxoid. Year 1990 was initially set as target by WHO to achieve the goal of neonatal tetanus elimination, defined as <1 case/1,000 live births per year in all districts of a country; it was later extended to 1995. By the end of 1999, there were 57 countries that had yet not achieved this goal.

In the year 2000, WHO, UNICEF, and United Nations Population Fund (UNFPA) partnered to relaunch their efforts to achieve the goal of neonatal tetanus elimination. As neonatal tetanus depends mainly on tetanus immunization of the mother during pregnancy, the goal of elimination of maternal tetanus was also added to this initiative, which was rechristened "Maternal and Neonatal Tetanus Elimination Program" (MNTE), and year 2005 was set as the cut-off year to achieve this goal. However, 19 countries are yet to achieve this goal. India was one of the last from a few countries to be declared free of maternal and neonatal tetanus on 15th May, 2015.

The strategies recommended to achieve and maintain the goal of MNT elimination include strengthening of routine immunization, surveillance, implementation of supplementary immunization activities (SIAs), targeting women of child-bearing age with three doses of properly spaced injections with tetanus toxoid in selected high-risk areas, and the promotion of clean deliveries.

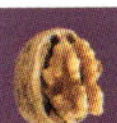

IN A NUTSHELL

Tetanus

1. Tetanus is caused by an anaerobic bacteria, *Clostridium tetani,* which produces a neurotoxin called tetanospasmin.
2. The disease is characterized by generalized muscle rigidity and spasms, lockjaw, and opisthotonus and carries a significant morbidity, and mortality. Difficulty in swallowing, restlessness, irritability, and headache are early manifestations.
3. Laryngeal and respiratory muscle spasms can lead to airway obstruction and asphyxia.
4. Neonatal tetanus manifests within 3–12 days of birth.
5. Diagnosis is mainly clinical.
6. Human tetanus immunoglobulin (TIG) is recommended to be given immediately. Penicillin is the antibiotic of choice.
7. The average mortality is 45–55%. For neonatal tetanus, the mortality is 60–70%.
8. Active immunization is the best method to prevent tetanus.

Nguyen KH, Srivastav A, Lindley MC, et al. Parental vaccine hesitancy and association with childhood diphtheria, tetanus toxoid, and acellular pertussis; measles, mumps, and rubella; rotavirus; and combined 7-series vaccination. Am J Prev Med. 2022;62(3):367-76.

Njuguna HN, Yusuf N, Raza AA, et al. Progress toward maternal and neonatal tetanus elimination—worldwide, 2000-2018. MMWR Morb Mortal Wkly Rep. 2020;69(17):515-20.

Rao MI, Kasi SG, editors. Indian Academy of Pediatrics. *IAP Guidebook on Immunization*. 2022–2023 ed. New Delhi: Indian Academy of Pediatrics; 2023.

Rhinesmith E, Fu L. Tetanus disease, treatment, management. Pediatr Rev. 2018;39(8):430-32.

World Health Organization. (2018). Saving mothers, saving children: Elimination of maternal and neonatal tetanus in India. [online] Available from https://www.who.int/india/news/feature-stories/detail/saving-mothers-saving-children-elimination-of-maternal-and-neonatal-tetanus-in-india [Last accessed August, 2025].

Yusuf N, Raza AA, Chang-Blanc D, et al. Progress and barriers towards maternal and neonatal tetanus elimination in the remaining 12 countries: a systematic review [published correction appears in Lancet Glob Health. 2022;10(2):e185]. Lancet Glob Health. 2021;9(11):e1610-17.

Yusuf N, Steinglass R, Gasse F, et al. Sustaining maternal and neonatal tetanus elimination (MNTE) in countries that have been validated for elimination—progress and challenges. BMC Public Health. 2022;22(1):691.

14.11 Enteric Fever (Typhoid)

PE 31.12

INTRODUCTION

Typhoid fever is a severe multisystemic infection caused by *Salmonella typhi (S. typhi).* Similar illness can be caused by related but less virulent *Salmonella paratyphi (S. paratyphi)* (paratyphoid fever). Enteric fever is a collective term and refers to all illnesses caused by these organisms. The disease is characterized in endemic areas by the classic prolonged high-grade fever, sustained toxemia, gastrointestinal symptoms, and splenomegaly. Enteric fever is potentially fatal, if untreated.

EPIDEMIOLOGY

Salmonella typhi and *S. paratyphi* infections occur worldwide but primarily in developing nations where sanitary conditions are poor. Typhoid and paratyphoid fevers are endemic in Asia (especially the Indian subcontinent), Africa, Latin America, the Caribbean, and Oceania. Typhoid fever affects 13–17 million people yearly and kills an estimated 600,000. In endemic areas, children aged 5–19 years are at the highest risk of infection. However, children between 1 and 5 years are also susceptible. This age group is at highest risk of morbidity and mortality because of waning passively acquired maternal antibody and lack of acquired immunity.

In young children, the clinical syndrome is often a nonspecific febrile illness that is not recognized as typhoid fever. Early antibiotic therapy has transformed a previously life-threatening illness of several weeks duration with an overall mortality rate approaching 20% into a short-term febrile illness with negligible mortality.

Mode of Spread

S. typhi is excreted in the feces of infected persons. A person with active typhoid fever may also spread the organism through urine, respiratory secretions, or vomitus. The food can be contaminated by flies, which carry the bacilli from feces of an infected or carrier individual. Contaminated water or unpasteurized milk are the other sources of infection.

Reservoir: Man is the only true reservoir of *S. typhi.* Carrier state can occur in convalescent patients (temporary carriers excrete the bacilli for 6–8 weeks). *Chronic carrier* is defined as an individual who continues to excrete the organism in feces for 3 months or longer. This state develops in 3–5% of individuals having suffered from *S. typhi* infection. Chronic carrier state is less frequent in children and more often observed in females. In certain cases, carrier state persists lifelong. The bacilli are carried to the gallbladder of a carrier. These carriers serve as a major source of infection to the community.

Environmental factors: Transmission of *S. typhi* is dependent on a multitude of *environmental, social, and cultural factors.* Cases occur more frequently during summer and rainy season, peaking with the onset of monsoons. Proper and adequate supply of potable water, proper excreta disposal system, hygienic personal and food habits, practicing of strict hand washing, pasteurization of milk, and health awareness are instrumental in preventing its transmission. Low socioeconomic groups who may not have access to the above-mentioned facilities are more prone to suffer from typhoid fever.

ETIOLOGY

Salmonella typhi is a gram negative, motile bacillus. It has three antigens, namely (*a*) somatic cell wall O antigen, a lipopolysaccharide, (*b*) flagellar H antigen, and (*c*) Vi (virulence) antigen, a polysaccharide capsular antigen, which is T-cell independent. Vi antigen also interferes with phagocytosis by preventing binding of C3 to the surface of the bacterium. Systemic immunity to typhoid can be achieved through induction of antibodies to either O and H antigen or Vi polysaccharide antigen. *S. typhi* can survive at extremely low freezing temperature and drying, and, therefore, can be transmitted through ice, frozen foods, and dust.

PATHOGENESIS

Children are typically infected with *S. typhi* and *S. paratyphi* through contaminated food and beverages. Infective dose is 10^5–10^8 organisms. After ingestion by the host, the bacteria invade through the gut and multiply within the mononuclear phagocytic cells in the liver, spleen, lymph nodes, and Peyer's patches of the ileum. The infected macrophage provides *Salmonella* a vehicle safe from other elements of the immune system and in which it can multiply and travel. It passes through the mesenteric lymph nodes into the thoracic duct and the lymphatics beyond to seed the reticuloendothelial tissues—liver, spleen, bone marrow, and lymph nodes. In these, it multiplies until some critical density is reached.

From blood or from the liver via bile ducts, it infects the gallbladder and re-enters the gastrointestinal tract in the bile, spreading to other hosts via stool. In addition, it occasionally invades the urinary tract and spreads via urine. After primary intestinal infection, further seeding of the Peyer's patches occurs through infected bile. They may become hyperplastic and necrotic with infiltration of mononuclear cells and neutrophils, forming ulcers that may bleed through eroded blood vessels or perforate the bowel wall, causing peritonitis. The host induces cytokines such as interferon alpha, interleukin (IL)-12, and tumor necrosis factor-alpha, which recruit macrophages and leads to high fever of the disease. Probability of clinically evident disease is more with a higher number of infecting particles, reduced gastric acidity, and possession of Vi antigen by the bacteria.

CLINICAL FEATURES

Salmonella typhi infection can be asymptomatic, subclinical, or present with the classical illness, as described below.

Incubation Period

The incubation period of typhoid fever varies with the size of the infecting dose and averages 7–14 (range, 3–60) days. In paratyphoid infection, the incubation period ranges from 1 to 10 days. During the incubation period, 10–20% of patients have transient diarrhea (enterocolitis) that usually resolves before the onset of the full-fledged disease. As bacteremia develops, the incubation period ends. Patients often experience chills, diaphoresis, anorexia, dry cough, a dull frontal headache, and myalgia before the onset of a high fever. About 20–40% of patients present with abdominal pain.

Classical Typhoid Fever

The classic manifestations of enteric fever include fever, toxemia, delirium, abdominal pain, constipation, and hepatosplenomegaly.

First week: Fever occurs in 75–85% of patients in the first week and is often initially remittent but becomes steady. The individual's temperature often rises to as high as 103–104°F (39–40°C) by the beginning of second week. Constipation often develops early and is likely due to obstruction at the ileocecal valve by swollen Peyer's patches. It may last for the entire duration of illness. At approximately the end of the first week of illness, some patients develop bacterial emboli to the skin known as *rose spots*. Rose spots constitute a subtle, extremely sparse (often ≤5 spots), salmon-colored, blanching, truncal, maculopapular rash with 1- to 4-cm lesions that generally resolve within 2–5 days. They are uncommon in dark-skinned individuals. Relative bradycardia and a dicrotic pulse are also common during this stage of illness.

Second week: During the *second week* of illness, the child may look toxic—appearing, anorexic and apathetic with sustained fever and significant weight loss. The abdomen is slightly distended, often with a tympanic note. Spleen becomes palpable by 7th day of illness. The patient may have a thready pulse, tachypnea, conjunctivitis, and crackles over the lung bases and may enter into a *typhoid state* of apathy, confusion, and even psychosis.

Some individuals may produce liquid, foul, green-yellow diarrhea (pea soup diarrhea). Rare complications of enteric fever include pancreatitis, meningitis, orchitis, and osteomyelitis.

Untreated, the patient may die or recover in 3–4 weeks. Mortality is 10% in untreated cases, and <1% in those treated. Death ensues from overwhelming toxemia, myocarditis, intestinal hemorrhage, or perforation due to necrotic Peyer's patches.

COMPLICATIONS

Intestinal perforation and hemorrhage may occur in <1% subjects during the 2nd week of illness. The presentation can be in the form of frank blood in stools, abdominal distension, acute abdominal emergency, peritonitis, abdominal guarding, rigidity, and shock. Other common complications are hepatitis, cholecystitis, cholangitis, bronchitis, and encephalopathy. Uncommon complications include myocarditis, transverse myelitis, Guillain-Barré syndrome, cerebellar ataxia, osteomyelitis, arthritis, pancreatitis, nephritic syndrome, parotitis, orchitis, etc.

DIFFERENTIAL DIAGNOSIS

During the initial 1 week, typhoid fever needs to be differentiated from common febrile illness that present without localizing signs such as viral fever, malaria, and dengue fever. Once spleen appears, other differential diagnoses that need consideration include malaria, hepatitis, infectious mononucleosis, rickettsial disease, leptospirosis, and brucellosis. Undiagnosed enteric fever beyond 2 weeks will need to be differentiated from tuberculosis, leukemia, and collagen vascular diseases.

DIAGNOSIS

Laboratory Diagnosis

Hematology: Blood counts usually show a normal or low normal leukocyte count. There is always a moderate neutropenia leading to relative lymphocytosis. Thrombocytopenia and proteinuria may be observed.

Blood culture remains the gold standard for diagnosis of typhoid fever. It is positive in >75% patients during the first week of illness. Bone marrow cultures are highly sensitive (90%) for diagnosis of typhoid fever. In some children with negative bone marrow cultures, duodenal string cultures have been positive. Stool and urine cultures may also reveal *Salmonella* after 2 weeks of the illness.

Serology: The Widal agglutination test measures antibodies against the somatic (O) antigen, and the flagellar (H) antigens of salmonellae. These antibodies are usually detectable only by the end of first week of illness, and rise progressively during the course of illness. Widal test is said to be positive, if antibody titer to "O" antigen is >1:160 after 7 days of onset of illness; or it demonstrates a 4-fold rise between the paired sera, collected in the first week, and then at least 2 weeks later. Widal test is of no diagnostic utility on a single sample, if obtained in first week of illness or in areas of endemicity. The somatic antigen O is common for both typhi and paratyphi, while H antigen is specific for *S. typhi, paratyphi A,* and *paratyphi B.*

TREATMENT Enteric Fever (Typhoid)

General Supportive Therapy

General supportive measures such as use of antipyretics, maintenance of hydration, appropriate nutrition and prompt recognition and treatment of complications are extremely important for a favorable outcome. The child should continue to have normal diet and no food should be restricted. In areas of endemic disease, 90% or more of typhoid cases can be managed at home with proper oral antibiotics and good nursing care. Close follow-up is necessary to look for development of complications or failure to respond to therapy.

Patients with persistent vomiting, inability to take oral feed, severe diarrhea, and abdominal distension usually require parenteral antibiotic therapy preferably in a hospital.

Antimicrobial Therapy

Chloramphenicol (50–75 mg/kg/day in 4 divided doses given for 14–21 days) has been the standard treatment for enteric fever in children. Ampicillin (100–200 mg/kg/day in 4 divided doses), amoxicillin (100 mg/kg/day in 4 divided doses), cotrimoxazole (6–8 mg/kg of trimethoprim/day), and furazolidone (10 mg/kg/day), each given for 14 days have also been used with equivocal results. This therapy can still be used for uncomplicated typhoid fever sensitive to these drugs.

Since 1990, use of chloramphenicol has been associated with drug resistance, high relapse rate, high rate of continued and chronic carriage, bone marrow toxicity, and high mortality. This has resulted in the decreasing trends of its usage. At the same time, number of culture positive cases of typhoid fever resistant to multiple conventional anti-typhoid drugs is being reported with increasing frequency from all over the world.

Multidrug resistant *S. typhi* (MDRST) refers to strains, resistant to all the three drugs in first-line treatment, i.e., chloramphenicol, ampicillin, and cotrimoxazole. Fluoroquinolones (ciprofloxacin, ofloxacin, gatifloxacin) emerged as effective drug for enteric fever caused by MDRST. The dosage is 20 mg/kg in two divided doses at 12 hours interval orally or 10 mg/kg/day q 12 hours IV. The temperature comes down in 4–5 (range of 3–10) days. Treatment should be continued for 7–10 days. Fluoroquinolones, such as ciprofloxacin, are effective but their frequent use in children is not yet cleared officially except when the benefits far exceed the possible risk to the growing cartilage.

However, many children with MDRST typhoid fever also fail to respond to quinolones, taking a very long time to attain defervescence, and continued constitutional discomfort. These cases show *in vitro* resistance to nalidixic acid. Nalidixic acid is also a quinolone. Though not used in treatment of enteric fever, resistance to nalidixic acid by *S. typhi* is considered a surrogate marker of resistance to other quinolones that are used for treating enteric fever; e.g., ciprofloxacin and ofloxacin. These strains are now known as nalidixic acid resistant *S. typhi* (NARST). In children with quinolone and resistant *S. typhi* infection, 3rd generation cephalosporins are the initial drug of choice. Of the oral third generation cephalosporins, cefixime, and cefpodoxime proxetil are used. Of parenteral preparations—ceftriaxone, cefotaxime, and cefoperazone are used—ceftriaxone being the most convenient.

Current Guidelines

Uncomplicated typhoid fever: Oral third generation cephalosporin; e.g., cefixime (20 mg/kg/day × 10–14 days) should be the drug of choice as empiric therapy. If by 5 days, there is no clinical improvement and the culture report is inconclusive, add a second-line drug; e.g., azithromycin (8–10 mg/kg/day × 7 days).

Severe typhoid fever: The drug of choice is parenteral third generation cephalosporin; e.g., ceftriaxone 60–75 mg/kg/day for 10–14 days. Azithromycin 20 mg/kg/day for 7 days should be added if there is no response in 5–7 days.

Steroids: Corticosteroid therapy is indicated in children with altered mental state or shock. Dexamethasone in a dose of 3 mg/kg is administered stat followed by another 8 doses of 1 mg/kg at six hourly intervals. Prolonged therapy with steroids increases the relapse rate.

PREVENTION

Active Immunization

Current typhoid fever vaccines include oral live-attenuated Ty21a vaccine, parenteral Vi polysaccharide and Vi-polysaccharide (Vi-PS) capsular conjugate vaccines. Oral live attenuated Ty21a vaccine is not available in India. Vi-PS is not immunogenic in children below 2 years of age and has no immune memory so it is recommended in children above 2 years of age. It is part of immunization schedule of few selected districts including Delhi. Its revaccination is advised every 3 years. Typhoid conjugate vaccine is recommended by IAP at 6-9 months of age in single dose as it is immunogenic even in children under 2 years of age and confers long lasting immunity.

Sanitation Measures

Typhoid fever cannot be controlled by immunization alone. The prime importance should be given to proper sanitation methods for food handling and preparation, safe water supply, proper sewage disposal, strict hand washing, and adequate maintenance of personal and food hygiene. It is important to make the community aware of the potential hazards of using contaminated food or water. Health education regarding importance of good hygiene should be imparted.

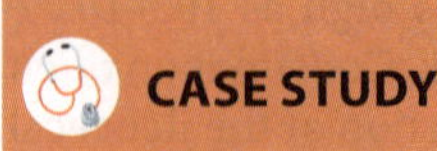

CASE STUDY — Typhoid Fever: Continuous Fever of 1–2 Weeks with Abdominal Symptoms and Splenomegaly

A 7-year-old boy was brought to the emergency room with continuous, high grade fever for 10 days. Mother also complained of lethargy and anorexia for last 5 days. This was associated with nonbilious and non-projectile vomiting for last 2 days. There was no history of dark yellow urine, rash, urinary complaints, abdominal distension, or any other localizing symptoms.

Outline the specific clues you will look for in the physical examination.

Our patient is a 7-year-old boy with complaints of prolonged fever, lethargy, and vomiting, so we will first look for vitals (HR, RR, BP, CFT) degree of fever, consciousness level, any signs of dehydration, icterus, edema, lymphadenopathy, rash, and signs of raised intracranial pressure (ICP). We also need to examine the abdomen for any distension, hepatosplenomegaly or other intra-abdominal lump/mass, shifting dullness, and bowel sounds.

Examination revealed a normal built, toxic looking child, with temperature 104°F, RR—28/min, HR—98/min, BP—98/64 mm Hg. The pulse volume was normal, and CFT was <3 seconds. There was no dehydration, icterus, edema, rash, lymphadenopathy, or signs of raised ICP. Abdomen was slightly distended. Liver was palpable 3 cm below right costal margin and spleen was palpable 2 cm below left costal margin. Both liver and spleen were soft and nontender. Liver span was 9 cm. Bowel sounds were sluggish.

Summarize the case and discuss the differential diagnosis.

A 7-year-old boy presented with high grade fever for 10 days with vomiting, toxic appearance, lethargy, mild hepatosplenomegaly, and without any other systemic or neurological signs.

Differential diagnosis will include enteric fever, malaria, dengue fever, UTI, and viral hepatitis (anicteric).

- Fever of >1 week with vomiting, toxic look, lethargy, and mild hepatosplenomegaly is in favor of *enteric fever*.
- Prolonged fever, vomiting, toxic look, lethargy, mild hepatosplenomegaly can all be seen in *malaria*. However, continuous nature of fever is not that common in malaria.
- Absence of rash, edema, shock, and bleeding rules out *dengue fever* to some extent. In second week of illness, dengue fever either recovers or has led to some complication.
- *Anicteric viral hepatitis* can present with fever, and lethargy. However, fever usually subsides in 1 week and spleen is generally not palpable. A nontender liver does not favor viral hepatitis. Absence of urinary symptoms keeps possibility of urinary tract infection (UTI) little lower but you should keep in mind that upper UTI can present with high grade fever and vomiting without any urinary symptoms. Hepatosplenomegaly in this child does not favor the diagnosis of UTI.

Other less common but important differential diagnoses are infectious mononucleosis, sepsis, leptospirosis, brucellosis, rickettsial diseases, and kala-azar (in endemic areas).

Outline the investigations needed to make a final diagnosis, in order of importance.

Initially we will order blood culture, Widal test, peripheral smear for malarial parasite (PS-MP), rapid malarial antigen (RMA), complete blood counts, kidney and liver function tests, urine microscopy and culture, and abdominal ultrasonography.

Investigations revealed total leukocyte count of 4,800/mm³, N32 L60 E2 M6, platelet count of 1.4 lakhs/mm³, negative RMA and PS MP, Widal agglutination test TH 1:320–1:320. Urine albumin was 1+ and microscopy was WNL. Liver enzymes were not elevated. Blood culture results were not available in 48 hours. Ultrasonography (USG) abdomen revealed a few mesenteric lymph nodes with largest measuring 7 mm (which can be normal). Liver and spleen echotexture was normal. A relative neutropenia and positive Widal test suggest the diagnosis of enteric fever.

Outline the specific antibiotic therapy for this patient.

We can start with oral antibiotics if the vomiting can be controlled with antiemetic. However, the child will need to be given intravenous antibiotics if vomiting persists. Cefixime (15–20 mg/kg/day × 10 days) is the drug of choice for oral therapy. Ceftriaxone (75–100 mg/kg/day divided in two equal doses for 10 days) is preferred for parenteral therapy.

After 4 days of treatment with IV ceftriaxone, patient was still febrile. Toxic look had disappeared, vitals were stable, and vomiting had subsided. What will you do now?

In enteric fever, the fever usually takes 4–5 days to resolve. Our patient is showing signs of improvement (nontoxic look, no vomiting, vitals stable, return of appetite), thus we will continue same treatment. The second drug (azithromycin 20 mg/kg/day) will need to be added, only if the fever does not subside after completing 7 days of IV ceftriaxone. Also, by this time, blood culture and sensitivity report should be available that can guide further therapy.

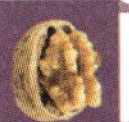

IN A NUTSHELL

Enteric Fever (Typhoid)

1. Typhoid fever is a severe multisystemic infection caused by *Salmonella typhi*. Similar illness can be caused by related but less virulent *Salmonella paratyphi* (paratyphoid fever).
2. Enteric fever is characterized in endemic areas by the classic prolonged high-grade fever, sustained toxemia, gastrointestinal symptoms, and splenomegaly.
3. Complications of typhoid are seen in 10–15% with intestinal perforation and bleeding being the most serious.
4. Blood culture is the gold standard for diagnosis. Widal test is positive from 2nd week onward.
5. Third generation cephalosporins are the first-line treatment. Azithromycin can be added for nonresponders (after a week).

Cao Y, Karthikeyan AS, Ramanujam K, et al. Geographic pattern of typhoid fever in India: a model-based estimate of cohort and surveillance data. J Infect Dis. 2021;224(224 Supple 5):S475-83.

Carey ME, MacWright WR, Im J, et al. The Surveillance for Enteric Fever in Asia Project (SEAP), Severe Typhoid Fever Surveillance in Africa (SETA), Surveillance of Enteric Fever in India (SEFI), and Strategic Typhoid Alliance Across Africa and Asia (STRATAA) Population-based Enteric Fever Studies: A Review of Methodological Similarities and Differences. Clin Infect Dis. 2020;71(Suppl 2):S102-S110.

Crump JA. Progress in Typhoid Fever Epidemiology. Clin Infect Dis. 2019;68(Suppl 1):S4-S9.

Marchello CS, Birkhold M, Crump JA. Complications and mortality of typhoid fever: a global systematic review and meta-analysis. J Infect. 2020;81(6):902-10.

Mukhopadhyay B, Sur D, Gupta SS, et al. Typhoid fever: Control & challenges in India. Indian J Med Res. 2019;150(5):437-47.

Neupane DP, Dulal HP, Song J. Enteric fever diagnosis: current challenges and future directions. Pathogens. 2021;10(4):410.

Sinha B, Chandola TR, Goyal N, et al. Incidence of enteric fever in a pediatric cohort in North India: comparison with estimates from 20 years earlier. J Infect Dise. 2021;224(5):S558-67.

Syed KA, Saluja T, Cho H, et al. Review on the recent advances on typhoid vaccine development and challenges ahead. Clin Infect Dis. 2020;71(Suppl 2):S141-50.

14.12 Dengue

PE 31.13

INTRODUCTION

Dengue infections are characterized by an acute febrile illness, usually seen in the tropics and Africa, and caused by four closely related virus serotypes of the genus *Flavivirus*, family *Flaviviridae*. Dengue virus is transmitted to humans by *Aedes aegypti* (*A. aegypti*) mosquito. The disease is characterized by a biphasic fever and may be associated with hemorrhagic manifestations. In 10–20% cases, the patient develops shock because of plasma leakage into the third space.

Dengue is recognized as the most important mosquito-transmitted viral disease in terms of morbidity and mortality. Worldwide, children <15 years comprise 90% of patients with dengue fever.

CLINICAL SPECTRUM

Dengue virus infection may be asymptomatic, lead to a benign illness, or may present as a serious illness with severe manifestations.

Traditionally, symptomatic dengue virus infections in children were categorized into three groups: (*i*) undifferentiated dengue fever; (*ii*) dengue fever; and (*iii*) dengue hemorrhagic fever (DHF), further subclassified as without or with shock; i.e., dengue shock syndrome (DSS). Case definitions were available for each of the diagnosis.

However, it was being realized that this classification was at times difficult to apply in clinical settings, was not able to categorize all patients with dengue, and was missing out cases with severe dengue.

The WHO classification in 2009 categorized children with dengue fever into two broad groups; i.e., (*i*) dengue fever, and (*ii*) severe dengue. The first group; i.e., dengue fever is further categorized as being with or without presence of *warning signs*. **Figure 14.1** depicts the suggested dengue case classification and levels of severity according to the new guidelines. It is important to note that even patients without warning signs can develop severe dengue!

- ***Nonsevere manifestations*** consist of a biphasic fever, generalized body ache, rash, and a positive *tourniquet test*. These may or may not be associated with warning signs.
- ***Warning signs*** should be detected by close observation of the patient, so as to institute early and aggressive therapy. These include (*i*) abdominal pain or tenderness; (*ii*) persistent vomiting; (*iii*) clinical fluid accumulation (edema, pleural effusion, ascites); (*iv*) mucosal bleeds; (*v*) hepatomegaly by >2 cm; and (*vi*) hemoconcentration as evidenced by increasing hematocrit with concomitant and rapid fall in platelet count.
- ***Severe manifestations*** include (*i*) severe hemorrhage; (*ii*) profound shock; and (*iii*) multisystem involvement. Presence of any one of these three criteria is sufficient for making a diagnosis of severe dengue infection.

Expanded dengue syndrome is a term introduced in 2011, which refers to unusual and severe involvement of liver, kidney, brain, or heart in association with dengue.

National Vector Borne Disease Control Program Nomenclature

Recently, the National Vector Borne Disease Control Program (NVBDCP) has accepted the revised WHO classification for dengue as shown in **Figure 14.1**. There may be asymptomatic subjects who may be tested positive for dengue. Among symptomatic patients, they can be classified into three categories—mild, moderate, and severe dengue **(Flowchart 14.5)**.

ETIOLOGY

Dengue fever is caused by a virus, which has at least four serotypes (1, 2, 3, and 4). These are antigenically very similar but do not offer a complete cross-protection after infection by any one of them. Infections in human by a serotype will produce lifelong immunity against reinfection by the same serotype. Subsequent infection (secondary infection) by another serotype results in severe dengue.

EPIDEMIOLOGY

Vector

The most common vector is a mosquito, *A. aegypti*. Female mosquito bites the man during daytime. After feeding on a person with viremia, the female mosquito can transmit dengue immediately or after a period of 10–14 days (extrinsic incubation period). The extrinsic incubation period is a critical factor in successful transmission of the disease. A lower environmental temperature increases the extrinsic incubation period, which in turn, decreases the transmission. Once the mosquito becomes infective, it remains so till it dies. The flight range of an adult *A. aegypti* mosquito is not >25–50 m in an urban environment.

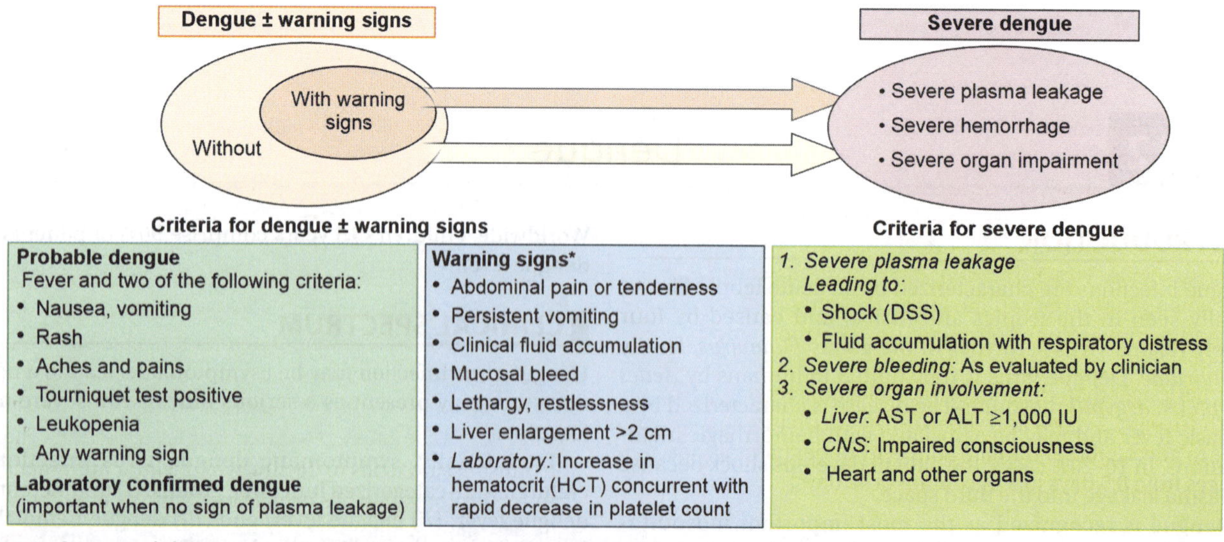

Fig. 14.1: Suggested dengue case classification and levels of severity (ALT: alanine aminotransferase; AST: aspartate aminotransferase; CNS: central nervous system; DSS: dengue shock syndrome)

*Require strict observation and medical intervention

Source: Reproduced with permission from: Handbook for Clinical Management of Dengue. WHO; 2012. Available from http://whqlibdoc.who.int/publications/2009/9789241547871_eng.pdf

Flowchart 14.5: Clinical case classification of dengue infection

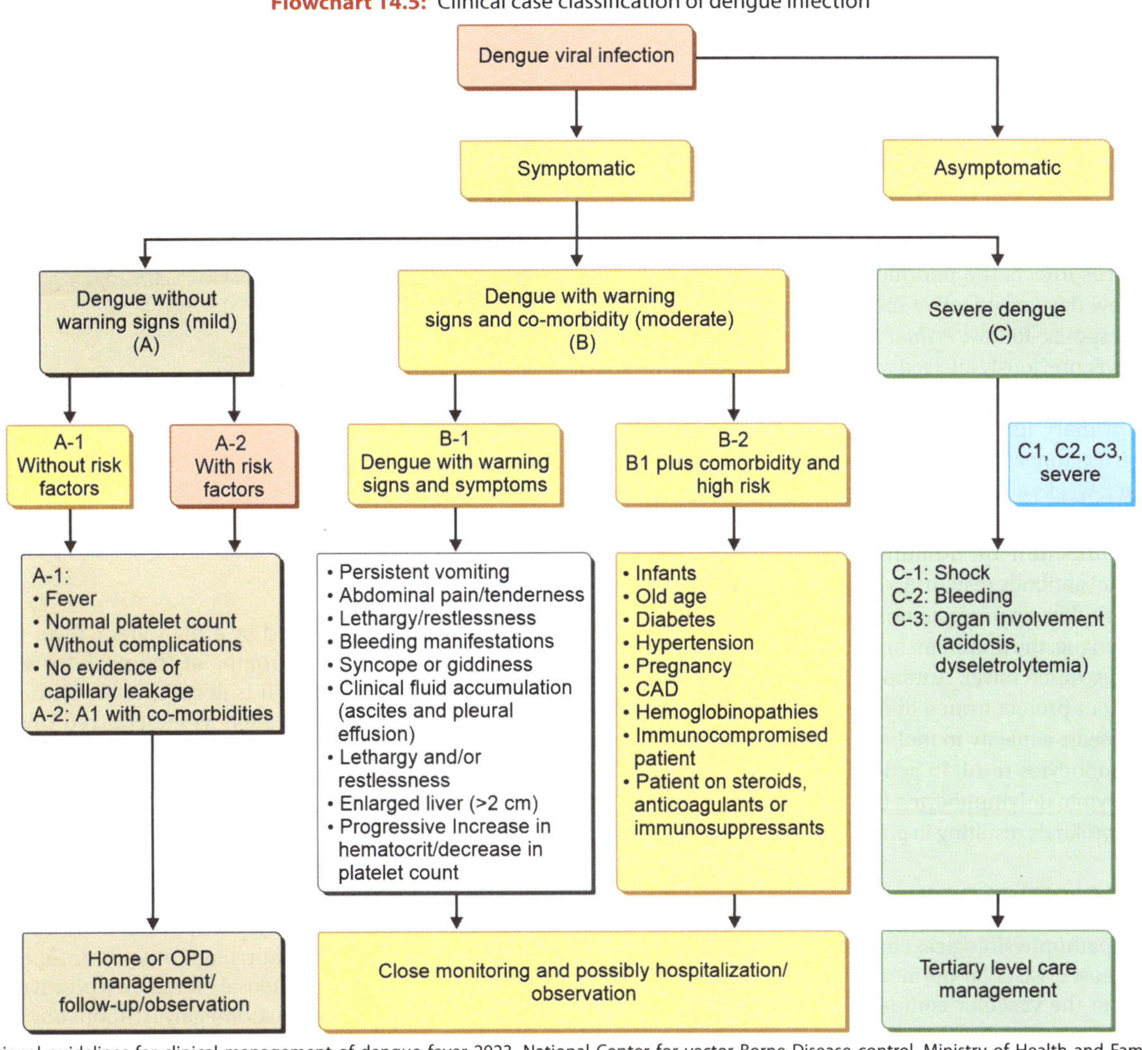

Source: National guidelines for clinical management of dengue fever 2023. National Center for vector Borne Disease control. Ministry of Health and Family Welfare. Government of India. Available from https://ncvbdc.mohfw.gov.in/Doc/National%20Guidelines%20for%20Clinical%20Management%20of%20Dengue%20Fever%202023.pdf. [Last accessed February, 2025]

However, the vector can be transported by water, land, and air travel contributing to the transmission. For dengue transmission, the number of infected female mosquitoes per house is important. Usually this number is small, and in an Indian epidemic it was observed to be just one per household. The minimum vector density, below which the dengue transmission ceases, is still unknown. The *A. aegypti* mosquito breeding is not necessarily related to the ambient temperature. The mosquito has been found at altitudes as high as 2,200 m above sea level. Vectors must survive longer than the sum of the initial nonfeeding period after birth (usually 2 days) and the extrinsic incubation period to be able to infect another human. Longevity under natural conditions ranges from 8.5 days to a maximum of 42 days.

Host

People at all ages are susceptible to dengue. Severe dengue occurs at high frequency in (*a*) infants; and (*b*) children having experienced a previous dengue infection. The first attack gives only temporary and partial protection against the other three virus types and subsequent infections with other serotypes are possible. Nonsevere dengue occurs in children and adults at equal frequency. Bronchial asthma and AIDS are significantly associated with severe dengue.

Environmental Factors

In many tropical countries, a positive association between rainfall or larval density and dengue incidence has been documented. However, dengue epidemics have also been recorded in those areas where rainfall is unusually low. The transmission occurs, only if the ambient temperature is above 16°C. Therefore, the transmission tends to decline when winter approaches. This is due to prolongation of extrinsic incubation period beyond the longevity of mosquito.

Transmission Risk Factors

When a member of a household is infected with dengue, other family members are at risk. Dengue spread is facilitated in any vector-infested place where people congregate, such as schools, temples, cinema halls, offices, hospitals, factories, etc.

In utero transmission: Dengue infection of pregnant women may result in passive transfer of antidengue IgG to the fetus or a congenital infection. These infants with maternal antibody are at a higher risk of developing severe dengue.

PATHOGENESIS

Dengue virus infects the peripheral blood mononuclear cells within a few days of infective mosquito bite. Two patterns of immune response follow: *Primary* and *secondary* (*anamnestic*). Persons never previously infected with a *flavivirus*, nor immunized with a *flavivirus* vaccine (e.g., yellow fever, Japanese encephalitis), mount a primary IgM antibody response when infected with dengue virus, appearing within 2–3 days of defervescence and peaking at 2 weeks after the onset of symptoms. Antidengue IgG appears afterwards. Individuals with immunity due to previous *flavivirus* infection or immunization mount a secondary (anamnestic) antibody response when infected with dengue virus. In secondary *flavivirus* infections, which account for most cases of severe dengue, the dominant immunoglobulin is IgG; the levels of IgM being much lower. Antibody against a strain of dengue virus does not protect from a different strain of virus. Rather, it may increase its capacity to multiply in human monocytes. The infected monocytes result in activation of cross-reactive CD4+ and CD8+ cytotoxic lymphocytes. Cytotoxic lymphocytes mediate release of cytokines resulting in plasma leakage and hemorrhage.

PATHOPHYSIOLOGY

Two main pathophysiological changes occur in dengue. These are (*i*) increased vascular permeability that gives rise to loss of plasma from the vascular compartment leading to hemoconcentration, low pulse pressure, and other signs of shock; and (*ii*) disorder in the hemostasis involving thrombocytopenia, vascular changes, and coagulopathy.

Secondary dengue infection results in formation of immune complexes and activation of complement system. Tumor necrosis factor alpha (TNF-α), interferon, and interleukin-2 are elevated, and C1q, C3–C8, are depressed. As a result, vasoactive amines are released from the platelets. These cause massive release of water, electrolytes, and plasma proteins from the blood vessels and lead to hypovolemic shock. Increased vascular permeability is mediated through the nitric oxide pathway. Platelet defects are both quantitative and qualitative. Thus, a patient with a normal platelet count may still have a prolonged bleeding time. Maculopapular and petechial rashes are present. In these lesions, dengue antigen, IgM, and complement (C3) have been observed.

CLINICAL FEATURES

Dengue infections have a wide clinical presentation. Following an incubation period of 3–7 days, the illness is characterized by three distinct phases, in that chronological order: (*i*) febrile phase, (*ii*) critical phase, and (*iii*) phase of recovery.

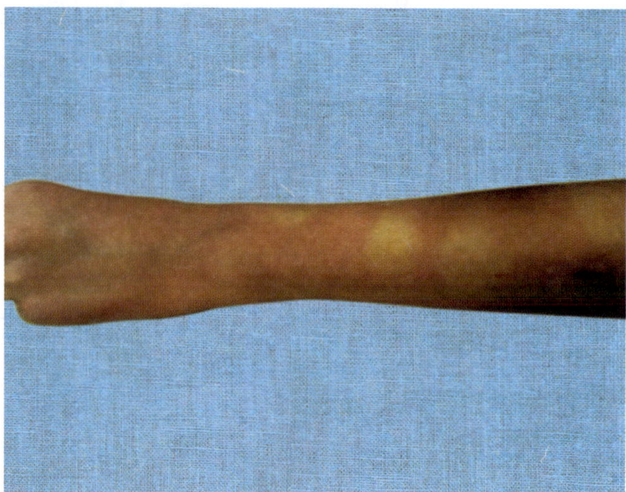

Fig. 14.2: Cutaneous flushing of forearm with blanching on applying pressure

Febrile Phase

This phase is characterized by a high-grade fever up to 104°F, abrupt in onset. Fever remains at the peak for 48–72 hours before it starts declining. It is accompanied with nonspecific constitutional symptoms such as generalized myalgia, body ache, anorexia, nausea, vomiting, and headache. Parents may notice an erythematous rash, especially over the extremities. There may be flushing of skin with compromised cutaneous circulation **(Fig. 14.2)**. Some children may have associated sore throat, or arthralgia. These features, by themselves, are, however, not sufficient to arrive at a diagnosis of dengue fever.

Dengue should be strongly suspected, if above features are associated with mild hemorrhagic manifestations including petechial hemorrhages, mucosal bleeds, or a positive tourniquet test. Presence of tender hepatomegaly (without obvious icterus) strongly favors possibility of dengue infection.

The febrile phase lasts for 2–3 days.

Complications: High fever in this phase can cause dehydration, febrile delirium, and febrile seizures in children <5 years of age.

Critical Phase

Onset of the critical phase is closely linked to the time of defervescence that occurs by 3rd day of illness. Not all children with dengue infection enter this phase. Many children improve progressively after defervescence (nonsevere dengue).

All children in defervescence phase need to be closely monitored for the *warning signs* as described earlier. Those manifesting with one or more of these signs are likely to enter the critical phase.

Critical phase is characterized by an increase in capillary permeability, initially presenting as rising hematocrit. This is preceded by a fall in the platelet count. Increased capillary permeability results in leakage of plasma into the third space. Clinically, this manifests as polyserositis, i.e., with fluid accumulation in body spaces–pleural effusion and ascites. Plasma leakage from the intravascular compartment into the third space results in hemoconcentration in the vascular bed, reflected by a rising hematocrit. Increase in hematocrit is directly proportional to the volume of plasma lost from the vascular compartment.

Epigastric discomfort, tenderness at right costal margin, and generalized abdominal pain are common. Liver becomes palpable. Petechiae may be present over extremities, axillae, face, and palate.

Leakage of a significant volume of plasma leads to hypovolemia, hypoperfusion, and shock. Hypoperfusion may result in multiple end-organ impairment, metabolic acidosis, and disseminated intravascular coagulation. Consumption coagulopathy results in hemorrhage that may cause a fall in hematocrit. End organ impairment manifests with hepatitis, myocarditis, or encephalitis. Children developing profound shock, severe hemorrhage, or multisystem involvement are at higher risk of mortality and thus are said to having *severe dengue infection*. These children need aggressive management.

This phase lasts for 48 hours.

Recovery Phase (Plasma Reabsorption Phase)

Plasma starts coming back to the intravascular compartment, provided the patient survives the critical phase of plasma leakage and shock. Onset of this phase is characterized by an improvement in general well-being and appetite. Urine output improves, and abdominal pain subsides. Though this is the phase of improvement, child should be monitored carefully for hypervolemia. Reabsorption of leaked plasma plus administration of excess intravenous fluid may result in fluid overload, pulmonary edema, and congestive heart failure, manifesting as dyspnea, tachycardia, and raised jugular venous pressure. Cardiovascular manifestations (bradycardia, arrhythmias) are also reported during this phase.

Hematocrit value either normalizes or may show a decline below normal. Platelet count starts improving.

This phase lasts for 48–72 hours. Thus, most patients with dengue fever run a typical course of disease lasting from 7 to 10 days **(Fig. 14.3)**.

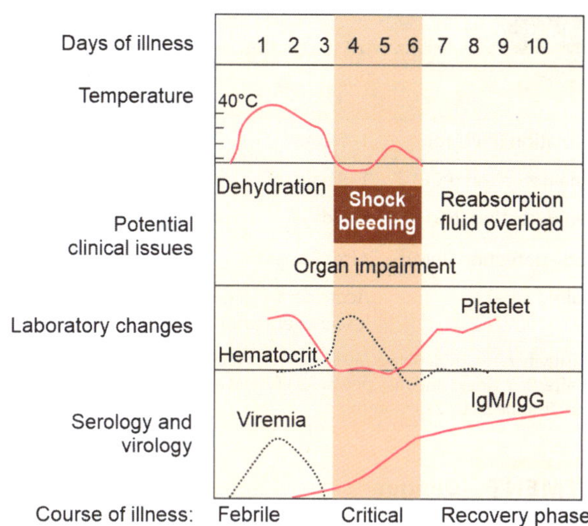

Fig. 14.3: The course of dengue illness

Source: Reproduced with permission from: Handbook for Clinical Management of Dengue. WHO, 2012

SEVERE DENGUE

Children and adolescents with severe dengue have a more protracted course and recovery may take 10–14 days. Dengue shock is characterized by a narrow pulse pressure <20 mm Hg, cold extremities, delayed capillary refill time, weak pulse, and tachycardia. Skin becomes cool, blotchy, and congested. Major bleeding can occur from gastrointestinal tract or brain. Organ impairment manifests as hepatic failure, renal failure, myocarditis, or encephalopathy.

LABORATORY STUDIES

Hematological Tests

The clinical diagnosis is corroborated by raised hematocrit and thrombocytopenia.

- A hematocrit level rise of >20% is a sign of hemoconcentration and precedes shock. The hematocrit level should be monitored at least every 24 hours to facilitate early recognition of warning signs and every 3–4 hours in severe dengue.
- Thrombocytopenia has been demonstrated in up to 50% of children with dengue. Platelet count of <100,000 cells/mL indicates onset of critical phase and typically occurs before defervescence and the onset of shock. The platelet count should also be monitored at least every 24 hours initially. Leukopenia, often with lymphopenia, is observed near the end of the febrile phase of illness. Lymphocytosis, with atypical lymphocytes, commonly develops before defervescence or shock.

Biochemical Profile

Prothrombin time is prolonged. Activated partial thromboplastin time is prolonged. Low fibrinogen and elevated fibrin degradation product levels are signs of disseminated intravascular coagulation. Hyponatremia is the most common electrolyte abnormality in critical phase. Metabolic acidosis and elevated blood urea are observed in those with shock. Serum glutamic pyruvic transaminase (SGPT) levels are elevated. Low serum albumin levels are a sign of hemoconcentration.

Serodiagnosis

Serum specimens should be sent to the laboratory for serodiagnosis, PCR, and viral isolation. Because the signs and symptoms of dengue fever are nonspecific, attempting laboratory confirmation of dengue infection is important. Serodiagnosis is based on (*i*) detection of viral nonstructural protein (NS1) during initial illness; (*ii*) detection of IgM antibodies to dengue; or (*iii*) 4-fold rise in dengue IgG in paired samples. **Table 14.9** outlines the desired timing of these tests for confirming the diagnosis.

Table 14.9 Diagnostic Tests for Dengue Fever

Diagnostic method	*Timing of test (after disease onset)*	*Validity*
Virus isolation (culture)	1–5 days	++++
Genome detection (PCR)	1–5 days	++++
Antigen detection (NS1)	1–5 days	+++
Antibody detection (IgM)*	After 5 days	++
IgG (paired sera)	Acute sera 1–5 days; convalescent sera after 15 days	+

*IgM positivity rates: by 3–5 days (50%), 5–7 days (80%), 10 days (90%). IgG appear after 1–2 weeks and may persist for life. IgM appears between 3 and 10 days and disappears by 2–3 months

TREATMENT Dengue

The mainstay of treatment is supportive therapy. Increased oral fluid intake is recommended to prevent dehydration. Supplementation with intravenous fluids may be necessary to prevent dehydration and significant hemoconcentration. Fever is managed with paracetamol. Aspirin and nonsteroidal anti-inflammatory drugs should be avoided as these drugs may worsen the bleeding tendency associated with some of these infections. Shock is managed with isotonic fluids. Packed cell transfusion is indicated in refractory shock or if there is significant bleeding.

Patients with known or suspected dengue fever should have their platelet count and hematocrit measured daily from the 3rd day of illness until 1–2 days after defervescence. Patients with a rising hematocrit level or falling platelet count should be monitored more frequently.

Management of dengue illness can be discussed in three steps:

Step 1: Overall assessment

Step 2: Diagnosis and severity assessment

Step 3: Categorizing into mild, moderate, or severe dengue and treating accordingly.

Overall Assessment

History and examination: Emphasis in history should be on assessment of warning signs. Physical examination should concentrate on hemodynamic assessment, to determine the presence and extent of shock, confirming or detecting the warning signs; and checking for bleeding manifestations, abdominal tenderness, mental state, and hydration. Tourniquet test is a must.

Investigations: Initial investigations should include a hematocrit, WBC count, platelet count, and tests to confirm the diagnosis, as described in the section on laboratory diagnosis. In critical phase, additional tests need to be done and include liver function test, renal function test, chest X-ray, serum electrolytes, and ultrasound abdomen.

Deciding on Need of Hospitalization

Determine the phase of disease (febrile, critical, recovery) and severity (nonsevere, severe) of dengue, as per criteria outlined earlier. The child will require admission if any of the following criteria is fulfilled:

- Presence of any of warning signs
- Signs and symptoms of hypotension
- Bleeding from any site
- Renal, hepatic, or CNS involvement
- Pleural effusion or ascites
- Rising hematocrit, and
- Platelet count <50,000/mm^3.

Categorize Patients in Mild, Moderate, or Severe Dengue (Table 14.10)

This step is aimed to place the patient in an appropriate group (A, B, or C) to decide on future course of action, as follows:

- *Mild:* Patients, who may be sent home.
- *Moderate:* Patients need close monitoring or hospitalization.
- *Severe:* Patients requiring tertiary level care.

Mild Dengue: Home Management

All children who are tolerating oral fluids, passing urine at least once in 6 hours, and not having any of the warning sign can be sent home. Following management needs to be advised:

- Encourage fluid intake; can give ORS, fruit juice, etc.
- Paracetamol (15 mg/kg/dose) if the child is uncomfortable because of fever. Avoid aspirin, ibuprofen, mefenamic acid, and nimesulide.
- Monitor at home for fluid intake, urine output, fever, obvious bleeding, and altered sensorium.
- Bring back if any of the above is present or the child develops any of the warning signs.

Moderate Dengue: Hospital Management

Presence of warning sign should place the patient in Group B. Other indications for hospitalization have been outlined above. Management plan is as follows:

- Obtain baseline hematocrit.
- Start isotonic IV fluids (normal saline or ringer lactate) @ 5–7 mL/kg/h for 1–2 hours.

Table 14.10 Treatment of Dengue

Category	*Patient characteristics*	*Treatment*
Mild	Accepting orally, passing urine adequately and no warning signs*	Home therapy • Increased oral fluids, paracetamol
Moderate	• Warning signs* present • High-risk infants, old age, pregnancy, comorbid conditions**	Hospitalize • Monitor hematocrit, platelets, vitals • Intravenous fluids—titrated as per hematocrit • If worsens, manage as severe dengue
Severe	• Severe bleeding • Severe shock • Severe organ dysfunction—hepatic, CNS, heart, kidney • Severe metabolic disorder	Intensive care • Monitor hematocrit, platelets, vitals • Treatment of shock—normal saline bolus • Blood transfusion for severe bleeding or clinical worsening. Judicious use of platelets • Supportive treatment for organ failure • Watch for signs of fluid overload, and treat, if detected (oxygen, frusemide)

**Warning signs:* Abdominal pain, persistent vomiting, mucosal bleed, hepatomegaly, clinical fluid accumulation, lethargy, hemoconcentration, thrombocytopenia.

**Comorbid conditions include hypertension, diabetes, thyroid illness, renal disease, hemoglobinopathy, hepatitis, heart disease.

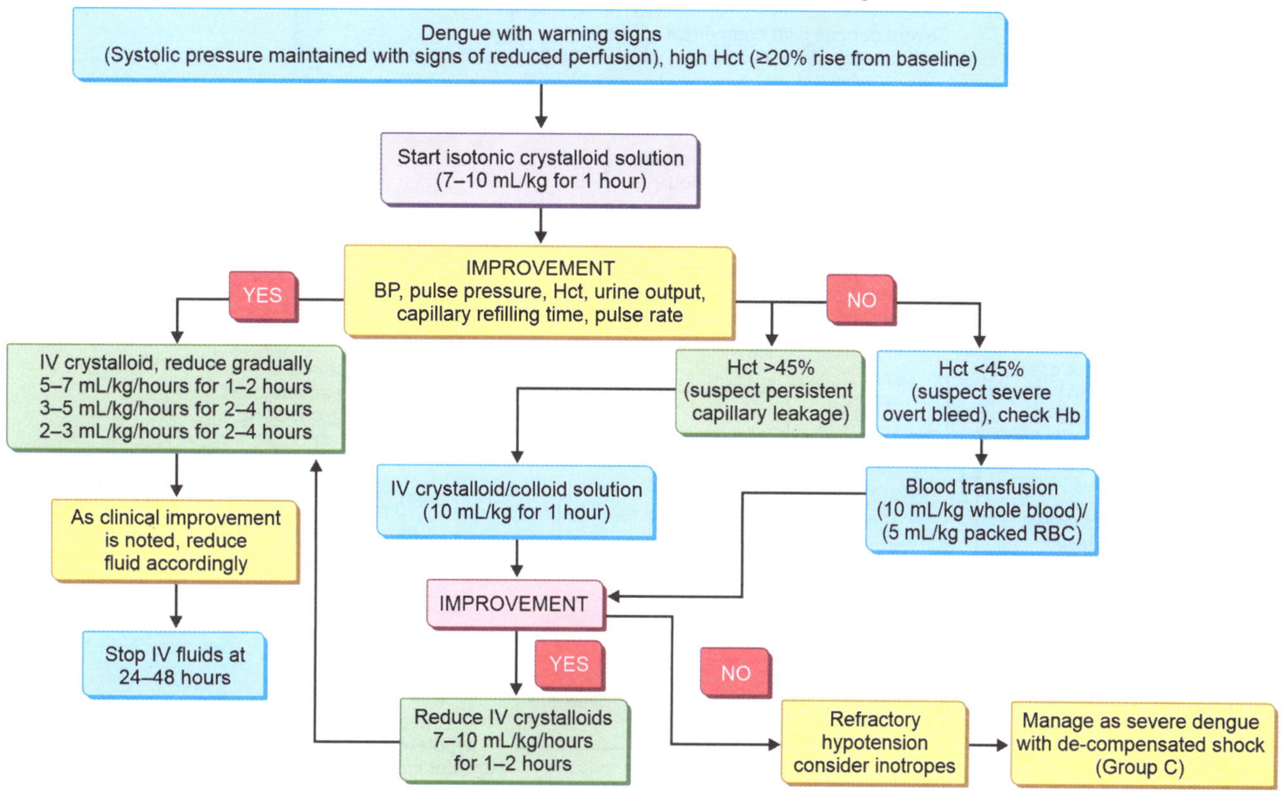

Flowchart 14.6: Management of moderate dengue

(Hct: hematocrit; IV: intravenous)

Source: National guidelines for clinical management of dengue fever 2023. National Center for vector Borne Disease control. Ministry of Health and Family Welfare. Government of India. Available from https://ncvbdc.mohfw.gov.in/Doc/National%20Guidelines%20for%20Clinical%20Management%20of%20Dengue%20Fever%20 2023.pdf. [Last accessed February, 2025]

- Reassess hematocrit and clinical status.
  - If improving, decrease to 3 mL/kg/h for another 2-4 hours and then continue within 1.5 mL/kg/h for 2-4 hours.
  - If clinical status worsens or hematocrit rises, increase rate of fluids to 10 mL/kg/h for 1-2 hours.
- Reassess clinical status, repeat HCT, and review fluid infusion rates, till the child is better.
  - If the child improves, maintain minimum IV fluids @ 0.5 mL/kg/h for 24-28 hours. Stop fluids when child demands and accepts adequate oral fluids, and food.
  - Those who worsen or develop profound shock, bleeding or multisystem involvement, manage as in **Flowchart 14.6**.

Severe Dengue: Emergency Treatment

Emergency treatment is required in children with severe dengue or those in critical phase, as follows:

- Obtain hematocrit, blood count, and other organ function tests, as indicated.
- *Compensated shock:* This stage is characterized by low systolic blood pressure (SBP), narrow pulse pressure (<20 mm Hg), and rise in hematocrit (>20%). In these children, fluid resuscitation is started at 10–20 mL/kg/h over 1 hour, and further directed as per **Flowchart 14.7**.
- *Hypotensive shock:* Administer isotonic fluid bolus 20 mL/kg in 15 minutes. For further management, follow the algorithm depicted in **Flowchart 14.8**. Colloids may be needed in refractory shock.
- *Hemorrhagic complications:* Suspect severe bleeding, if there is an unexplained fall in hematocrit, refractory shock not responding to 40–60 mL/kg of fluid, and persistent or worsening metabolic acidosis. Packed cell transfusion 10 mL/kg over 2–3 hours can be life-saving in these children.
- *Monitoring:* This essentially remains the basic prerequisite for treating children with severe dengue, in an emergency setting.
  - Monitor vital signs and peripheral perfusion 1–4 hourly unless patient is out of critical phase. Monitor hematocrit before and after fluid replacement, then 6–12 hourly.
  - Monitor blood glucose and other organ dysfunction both clinically and biochemically.
  - A typical monitoring chart for dengue fever should record the following: Body temperature, heart rate, blood pressure, pulse volume, capillary refill time, abdominal pain, appetite, vomiting, and bleeding.

Role of Platelets

There is not much evidence for platelet transfusion or fresh frozen plasma for severe bleeding. Platelet transfusions should not be used prophylactically. Its use has neither shown to prevent progression to severe bleeding nor does it shorten the bleeding time and may instead be associated with severe side effects. Platelet transfusion should be restricted to cases with severe bleeding or when platelet counts are below 10,000/mm^3. Platelets obtained by single donor apheresis are preferred as they raise the platelet count by 30,000–50,000 as compared to random donor platelets, which result in rise by 5,000–10,000/unit.

Flowchart 14.7: Algorithm for management of severe dengue with compensated shock

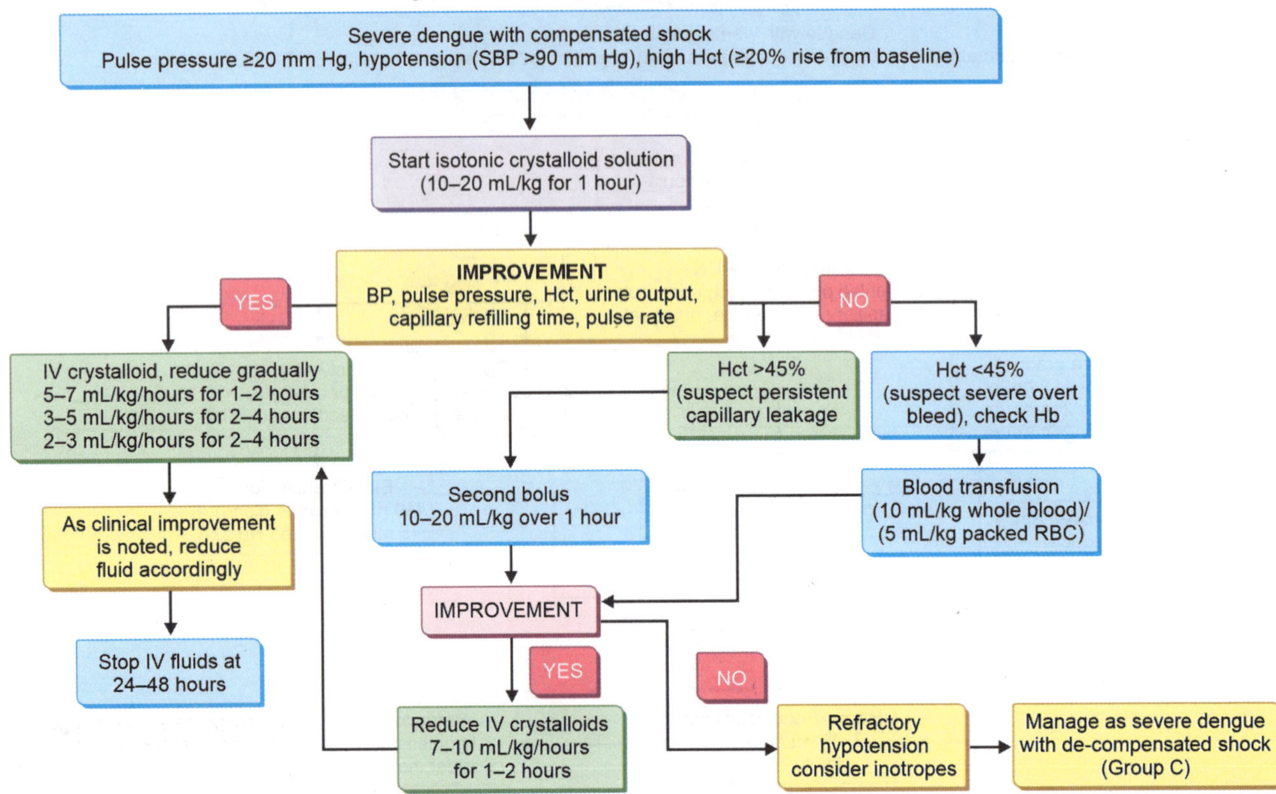

(Hct: hematocrit; IV: intravenous)

Source: National guidelines for clinical management of dengue fever 2023. National Center for vector Borne Disease control. Ministry of Health and Family Welfare. Government of India. Available from https://ncvbdc.mohfw.gov.in/Doc/National%20Guidelines%20for%20Clinical%20Management%20of%20Dengue%20Fever%202023.pdf. [Last accessed February, 2025]

Treatment of Fluid Overload

A patient with dengue can have fluid overload due to excessive or rapidly transfused IV fluids, use of hypotonic fluids, and inappropriate use of fresh frozen plasma or platelets. Another important reason is continuation of IV fluids even during the phase of plasma reabsorption and recovery.

These children may present with features of pulmonary edema or congestive heart failure. Following management is suggested:

- Oxygen therapy
- Discontinuation/reduction of IV fluids.
- Frusemide 0.1–0.5 mg/kg/dose once or twice daily, maintaining serum potassium.
- Look for occult hemorrhage and transfuse packed cells.

Criteria for Discharge

Patient should be discharged only if he/she has been afebrile for at least 24 hours, passing urine normally, having improved appetite, has no respiratory distress, has a stable hematocrit and platelet count is >50,000/mm^3.

CASE STUDY **Dengue Fever—Fever with Rash with Shock**

A 10-year-old boy arrived in emergency room with complaints of high-grade continuous fever accompanied with chills and rigors, myalgia, and loss of appetite for 4 days. The child had also developed nonitchy erythematous macular rashes on whole body involving the palms and soles, since morning. He also complained of abdominal pain and vomiting. The mother noticed that from past 1 hour, the child's limbs were cold to touch.

What are the other points you would like to ask in history?

In a child presenting with fever, rash, abdominal symptoms, and cold extremities indicating impaired perfusion, think of dengue fever, typhoid fever, and meningococcemia. Ask for history of bleeding from any site, altered sensorium, abnormal body movements, neck pain, any preceding history of sore throat or pain, presence of similar symptoms in other family members/neighborhood.

There was no complaint of bleeding from any site. Neurological status was normal. There was history of similar illness in the locality, being diagnosed as dengue fever. Examination revealed temperature of 104.5°F, RR—34/min, HR—112/min, BP—86/52 mm Hg, and erythematous blanchable macular rashes all over body mainly distributed over extremities. Abdomen was distended. Tenderness was noted in right hypochondrium over a palpable liver 2 cm below right subcostal margin. Rest of systemic examination was well within normal range.

Discuss the differential diagnosis for this patient?

A febrile patient with rashes all over body on 4th day of fever with cold extremities alarms us toward possibility of dengue fever with shock. Other similar cases in the neighborhood support the diagnosis. Other possible differential for this patient can be meningococcemia, enteric fever, rickettsial fever, severe sepsis with shock, or algid malaria.

Flowchart 14.8: Algorithm for management of severe dengue with hypotensive decompensated shock

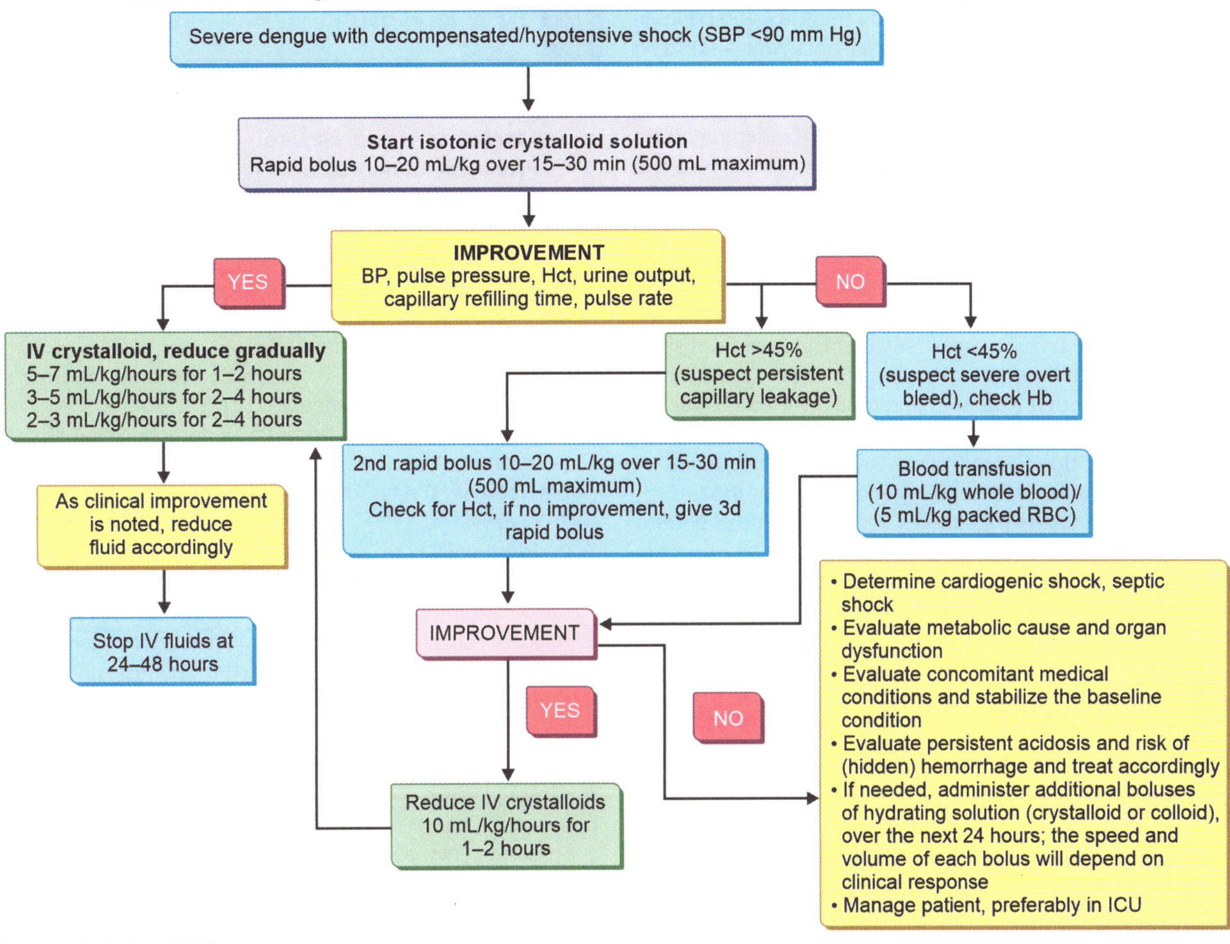

(Hct: hematocrit; IV: intravenous)

Source: National guidelines for clinical management of dengue fever 2023. National Center for vector Borne Disease control. Ministry of Health and Family Welfare. Government of India. Available from https://ncvbdc.mohfw.gov.in/Doc/National%20Guidelines%20for%20Clinical%20Management%20of%20Dengue%20Fever%202023.pdf. [Last accessed February, 2025]

How will you confirm the diagnosis?

The most useful diagnostic test for dengue fever on day 4 of fever, will be documentation of NS1 antigen. This antigen can be demonstrated in serum from day 2 onwards. IgM antibodies against virus appear only on 4–5 days of fever, and may be negative in this child.

How will you manage this child?

This child is having cold extremities and hypotension, which indicate shock. The illness will be classified as *severe dengue*. The child needs to be hospitalized and immediately started on intravenous (IV) fluids to expand the intravascular volume. Initial fluid should consist of normal saline bolus @10–20 mL/kg over 1 hour. Further management will depend on response to initial therapy.

Laboratory criteria for definitive diagnosis include one or more of the following:

- Isolation of the dengue virus from serum, plasma, leukocytes, or autopsy samples.
  - Demonstration of NS1, a glycoprotein induced by the virus between 1 and 4 days of illness, has a high sensitivity and specificity.
  - Demonstration of a 4-fold or greater change in reciprocal immunoglobulin G (IgG); or presence of immunoglobulin M (IgM) antibody titers to one or more dengue virus antigens in paired serum samples.
  - Demonstration of dengue virus antigen in autopsy tissue via immunohistochemistry or immunofluorescence or in serum samples via enzyme immunoassay.
  - Detection of viral genomic sequences in autopsy tissue, serum, or cerebral spinal fluid (CSF) samples via polymerase chain reaction (PCR).

PREVENTION AND CONTROL

Aedes aegypti should be the main target of surveillance and control.

Surveillance

Mainly two indices are used for measuring the vector density. There are (*a*) *House index;* and (*b*) *Breteau index.* House index is defined as the percentage of houses positive for the larvae; and Breteau index as the number of containers positive for the larvae per 100 houses. These indices measure larval infestation rather than adult mosquito density.

Long-term Vector Control

Adequate water supply is a must. Sprays of larvicides are recommended in high-risk localities. All objects that may collect water (old tyres, broken jars, empty tins, and bottles) should be disposed off. Water should be changed routinely in water coolers, flower vases, and overhead tanks. Coolers, if not in use, should be drained and mopped dry. Large tanks with taps should be kept covered. Management of roof tops, porticos, and sunshades to be encouraged. Health education should be provided regularly in schools and through mass media. Sensitize and involve the community for detection of *Aedes* breeding places and their elimination.

Biological and Chemical Control

Use of larvivorous fishes in ornamental tanks, fountains, or biocides can kill the larval stages. Use chemical larvicides such as "Abate" in big breeding containers. Aerosol space spray during daytime may be another option in high density areas. In recent years, interest in mosquito-killing (entomopathogenic) fungi is reviving, mainly due to continuous and increasing levels of insecticide resistance and increasing global risk of mosquito-borne diseases. Focus is on species belonging to the genera *Lagenidium, Coelomomyces, Entomophthora, Culicinomyces, Beauveria,* and *Metarhizium.*

Vaccine Development

Development of a multivalent vaccine against all four serotypes seems necessary. Progress in vaccine development is slow because these viruses grow poorly in cell culture and there is no acceptable animal model for dengue illness.

Few available dengue vaccines which have completed phase III trial are: Dengvaxia, Qdenga and Tetravax DV.

Dengvaxia, also known as chimeric yellow fever-tetravalent dengue vaccine (CYD-TDV) is a live recombinant tetravalent dengue vaccine administered in a three-dose schedule (0, 6, 12 months) in 9–45 years age group. It uses yellow fever virus as backbone. Its use led to severe dengue manifestations in dengue-naive children due to antibody dependent enhancement. In these children, vaccine acted as first dengue infection and on subsequent natural dengue infection, severe manifestations happened. So, this vaccine is recommended only in persons with evidence of a past dengue infection.

Qdenga, also known as Takeda vaccine (TAK-003) is also a tetravalent vaccine in which genes of Dengue viruses 1,3 and 4 are inserted into the genome of attenuated dengue virus 2 backbone. It is recommended in individuals aged 4–60 years in a two-dose schedule regardless of previous dengue infection. Dengvaxia and Qdenga are not available in India.

Tetravax DV, also known as butantan DV is a combination of four monovalent attenuated dengue viruses 1-4. It is under trial in India too.

An ideal dengue vaccine should cover all age groups, 4 serotypes, may be administered irrespective of previous immune status and prevent not only severe dengue including death and hospitalizations due to dengue but milder cases too. There is no ideal dengue vaccines till now.

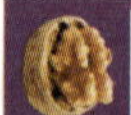

IN A NUTSHELL

Dengue

1. Dengue is an acute viral illness caused by four viruses 1–4; and spread by *Aedes* mosquito.
2. Clinical presentation consists of a biphasic fever, myalgia, arthralgia, and hemorrhagic manifestations, lasting over 3–7 days. The most vulnerable stage is soon after defervescence (critical phase) characterized by increased capillary permeability.
3. Increased capillary permeability and coagulopathy are major pathogenic abnormalities.
4. Thrombocytopenia occurs both due to bone marrow suppression and immune-mediated destruction.
5. Serological diagnosis is possible by detecting non-structural (NS) antigen 1 between 2–5 days, detection of IgM antibodies between 5–10 days, or fourfold rise in IgG antibodies after 7–10 days.
6. Children with warning signs should be hospitalized. Those with severe shock, severe bleeding, and organ involvement need management in intensive care unit (ICU) setting.
7. Fluid therapy is the mainstay of treatment. Crystalloid is the fluid of choice during resuscitation. Best guide to fluid therapy is hematocrit.

Chakravarti A, Arora R, Luxemburger C. Fifty years of dengue in India. Trans R Soc Trop Med Hyg. 2012;106(5):273-82.

Dash N, Aby R, Kumar M, et al. Infant dengue a 10-year experience from a tertiary center in South India. Am J Trop Med Hyg. 2021;105(2):435-9.

Ghosh A, Dar L. Dengue vaccines: challenges, development, current status and prospects. Indian J Med Microbiol. 2015;33(1):3-15.

National guidelines for clinical management of dengue fever 2023. National Center for vector Borne Disease control. Ministry of Health and Family Welfare. Government of India. Available from https://ncvbdc.mohfw.gov.in/Doc/National%20Guidelines%20for%20Clinical%20Management%20of%20Dengue%20Fever%202023.pdf. [Last accessed February, 2025].

Rajesh NT, Alagarasu K, Patil JA, et al. Serotype-specific differences in the laboratory parameters among hospitalized children with dengue and genetic diversity of dengue viruses circulating in Tamil Nadu, India during 2017. J Med Virol. 2020;92(8):1013-22.

Santhosh Kumar M, Kamaraj P, Khan SA, et al. Seroprevalence of dengue infection using IgG Capture ELISA in India, 2017-2018. Am J Trop Med Hyg. 2021;105(5):1277-80.

Sinha B, Goyal N, Kumar M, et al. Incidence of lab-confirmed dengue fever in a pediatric cohort in Delhi, India. PLoS Negl Trop Dis. 2022;16(4):e0010333.

Sreenivasan P, Geetha S, Kumar AS. WHO 2009 warning signs as predictors of time taken for progression to severe dengue in children. Indian Pediatr. 2020;57(10):899-903.

World Health Organization. (1997). Dengue haemorrhagic fever. Diagnosis, treatment, prevention and control. [online] Available from http:// apps.who.int/iris/bitstream/10665/41988/1/9241545003_eng.pdf [Last accessed November, 2022].

World Health Organization. (2021). Dengue and severe dengue. Factsheet. [online] Available from https://www.who.int/news-room/fact-sheets/detail/dengue-and-severe-dengue [Last accessed August, 2025].

14.13 Chikungunya

PE 31.13

INTRODUCTION

Chikungunya is a debilitating nonfatal dengue-like mosquito-borne arboviral disease. The term "chikungunya" comes from African Makonde language, meaning "to become contorted", and describes the bent over appearance of affected people with joint pain.

EPIDEMIOLOGY

Burden of Disease

Chikungunya was first described in an outbreak in Tanzania in 1952 and is now prevalent in over 60 countries of Africa, Asia, Europe, and America. It is reported mainly from Africa, South-East Asia including India and Pakistan. It occurs principally during the rainy season. It has re-emerged in the country after a gap of 3 decades. In 2019, 12,205 laboratory confirmed chikungunya cases were reported in 21 Indian states and three union territories. Majority of the cases were reported from Karnataka followed by Maharashtra and Telangana. Currently, disease is endemic in 24 Indian states and six union territories.

Agent

Chikungunya virus (CHIKV) is an RNA virus that belongs to the *Alphavirus* genus of the family *Togaviridae*. Humans are considered to be the major source or reservoir of Chikungunya virus.

Vector

Mosquitoes are the vector for CHIKV. Both *A. aegypti* and *Aedes albopictus* (*A. albopictus*) have caused large outbreaks of chikungunya. *Aedes aegypti* is confined to the tropics and subtropics whereas *A. albopictus* occurs in temperate regions also. Both the species are found outdoors while *A. aegypti* is also found indoors. These mosquitoes bite during daytime.

Transmission

Chikungunya virus is transmitted to humans via mosquitoes. When an uninfected virus feeds on an infected person, the virus enters the gut of the mosquito and replicates there from where virus disseminates to the salivary glands of the mosquito. When this mosquito feeds on an infected person, the virus is transmitted to that person.

CLINICAL FEATURES

The incubation period ranges from 2 to 6 days. The disease has two stages–acute and chronic. Acute stage is febrile phase lasting for up to 15 days and is characterized by abrupt onset high grade fever and severe polyarthralgia. Arthralgia is usually bilateral, mainly involving small joints of ankles, wrists and hands. Other manifestations include myalgia, headache, nausea, vomiting, and rashes. Rash may appear at the outset or several days into the illness; its development often coincides with defervescence, which takes place around day 2 or day 3 of the disease. The rash is maculopapular and most intense on trunk and limbs and may desquamate. The disease is self-limiting and resolves in 2 weeks. However, few patients develop chronic stage, which is characterized by polyarthralgia and polyarthritis of small joints, which can last up to several years. Complications such as retinitis, uveitis, cranial nerve palsies, Guillain–Barré syndrome, myocarditis, and nephritis have been observed in few cases. A full-blown disease is most common among adults, in whom the clinical picture may be dramatic. Severe cases of chikungunya can occur in the elderly, in the very young (newborns) and in those who are immunocompromised. Dengue and Zika have many clinical features common to chikungunya. Hemorrhagic manifestations are rare and shock is not seen in chikungunya, unlike dengue.

DIAGNOSIS

Chikungunya should be suspected when epidemic disease occurs with the characteristic triad of fever, rash, and rheumatic manifestations. The virus may be detected in the blood during the first few days of infection (up to 5 days) using virological methods particularly reverse transcriptase-polymerase chain reaction (RT–PCR). Serological test such as ELISA to detect CHIKV IgM antibody is the method of choice in the later stages of CHIKV infection (>5 days postinfection). CHIKV-specific IgG antibody ELISA in paired serum samples from the acute and convalescent phase of CHIKV infection can also be used for serodiagnosis. A rise of four-fold or more is suggestive of recent CHIKV infection.

TREATMENT Chikungunya

No specific antivirals are approved for CHIKV. Management is supportive and includes antipyretics for fever, analgesics for arthralgia, plenty of fluids and rest. Paracetamol and acetaminophen are recommended to reduce fever and pain. Aspirin and nonsteroidal anti-inflammatory drugs should be avoided until dengue is ruled out as there is risk of bleeding.

PREVENTION

Person infected with CHIKV can spread disease to others during the first week of illness by mosquito bites. So, all efforts should be made to avoid further mosquito bites. Measures should be taken to avoid breeding of mosquitoes and to avoid mosquito bites such as use of mosquito repellents, full sleeve clothes, etc.

One live-attenuated Chikungunya vaccine known as IXCHIQ is available in US. Centers for Disease Control and Prevention (CDC) recommends the vaccine for: travelers to areas with high risk of Chikungunya transmission, laboratory workers who handle the virus and adults 18 years and older who are at high risk of exposure to the virus.

PROGNOSIS

In most patients, full recovery occurs from the infection, but in some cases joint pain may persist for several months, or even years. Unlike dengue, serious complications are not common in chikungunya. Once an individual is recovered, he/she is likely to be immune from future infections.

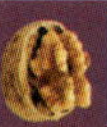

IN A NUTSHELL

Chikungunya

1. Chikungunya is a mosquito-borne arboviral disease transmitted to humans by infected *Aedes* mosquitoes caused by the chikungunya virus (CHIKV).
2. Predominant clinical features include high fever and severe polyarthralgia. Other symptoms include muscle pain, headache, joint swelling, nausea, and rash.
3. The disease mostly occurs in Africa, Asia, and the Indian subcontinent.
4. Dengue and Zika are the close differentials of the disease.
5. No antiviral is approved for CHIKV. Treatment is mainly supportive and includes antipyretics for fever, analgesics for pain, plenty of fluids to prevent dehydration and rest.
6. Currently no vaccine is approved for CHIKV.
7. Prevention includes measures to reduce breeding of mosquitoes and protection from mosquito bites.

Barr KL, Vaidhyanathan V. Chikungunya in infants and children: is pathogenesis increasing? Viruses 2019;11(3):294.
CDC. Chikungunya vaccine [online]. Available from https://www.cdc.gov/chikungunya/prevention/chikungunya-vaccine.html#cdc_generic_section_1-chikungunya-vaccine. Last accessed February 2025.
The Translational Research Consortia (TRC) for Chikungunya Virus in India. Current Status of Chikungunya in India. Front Microbiol. 2021;12:695173.
Ward CE, Chapman JI. Chikungunya in children: a clinical review. Pediatr Emerg Care. 2018;34(7):510-15.
World Health Organization. (2020). Factsheet-Chikungunya. [online] Available from https://www.who.int/news-room/fact-sheets/detail/chikungunya [Last accessed Augsut, 2025].

14.14 Malaria *PE 31.14*

INTRODUCTION

Malaria (*mal*-foul; *aria*-air) is one of the most important parasitic diseases of humans. It is associated with high morbidity and mortality, accounting for nearly 1.5–2.5 million deaths all over the world every year. More than half of these deaths occur in children under 5 years of age. In recent years, there has been a resurgence of malaria due to increasing drug resistance, environmental changes, population migration, and inconsistent national malaria control programs.

EPIDEMIOLOGY

Transmission: Malaria is spread to humans during the bite of an infected female anopheline mosquito. Female mosquitoes require blood meal to produce eggs. Male mosquitoes do not suck blood but feed on plant juices. Rarely, malaria may be transmitted by blood transfusion, transplacentally (congenital malaria), or through contaminated needles.

Vector: Malaria is spread from person-to-person by mosquitoes belonging to genus *Anopheles*. *Anopheles culicifacies* and *Anophele stephensi* are important vectors in India. The former is more active in rural areas, and later in urban areas. *Anopheles minimus* is an efficient vector in North-East India. Transmission of malaria is directly proportional to the density of the vector.

Environment: The transmission of malaria is profoundly influenced by climate. Malaria is common during rainy season because stagnant water and high humidity favor mosquito breeding and survival. Edges of streams, water-tanks, pits, cisterns, and overhead tanks are favored breeding sites of the mosquito. Irrigation schemes, dams, deforestation, urbanization, floods, and agricultural practices can influence mosquito populations and alter patterns of malaria transmission. Malaria is uncommon at altitudes 2,000 m above sea-level.

ETIOLOGY

Malaria is caused by *Plasmodium,* an obligate intracellular protozoon. Five species of *Plasmodium* are responsible for disease in humans:

1. *Plasmodium falciparum (P. falciparum)*—malignant tertian malaria
2. *Plasmodium vivax (P. vivax)*—benign tertian malaria
3. *Plasmodium ovale (P. ovale)*—ovale malaria
4. *Plasmodium malariae (P. malariae)*—quartan malaria, and

5. *Plasmodium knowlesi (P. knowlesi)*—fifth human malaria parasite

Plasmodium falciparum accounts for nearly all deaths and severe disease due to malaria. In India, most cases of malaria are caused by *P. vivax* (60–65%) and *P. falciparum* (35–40%). *P. malariae* accounts for only 1% of cases, mainly from a few districts of Karnataka (Hasan and Tumkur). *P. ovale* is very occasionally reported. *P. knowlesi*, a causative agent of simian malaria, has been reported from forested areas of Southeast Asia. No case is yet reported from India.

Life Cycle of Malarial Parasite (Fig. 14.4)

Infection with malaria begins when *sporozoites*, the infective stage of the parasite, are inoculated into subcutaneous capillaries as female mosquito takes a blood meal. Sporozoites are carried rapidly via the bloodstream to the liver where they begin a period of asexual reproduction. Salient characteristics of malaria parasites are given in **Table 14.11**.

Pre-erythrocytic (exoerythrocytic) schizogony (hepatic or tissue phase): In liver cells, *sporozoites* multiply asexually over a

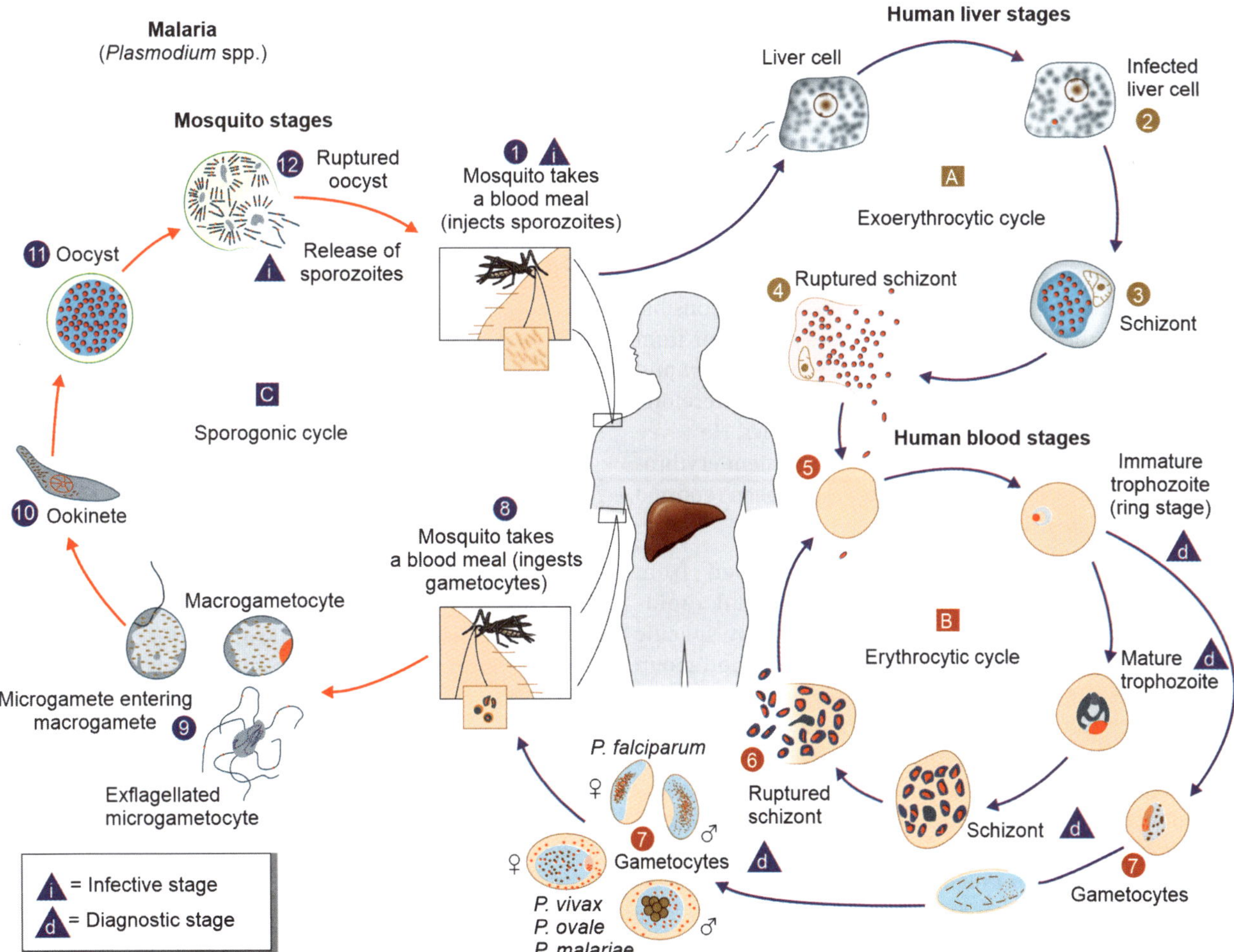

Fig. 14.4: Life cycle of malaria. The malaria parasite life cycle involves two hosts. During a blood meal, a malaria infected female *Anopheles* mosquito inoculates sporozoites into the human host (1). Sporozoites infect liver cells (2) and mature into schizonts (3), which rupture and release merozoites (4). [Of note, in *P. vivax and P. ovale,* a dormant stage (hypnozoites) can persist in the liver and cause relapses by invading the bloodstream weeks, or even years later.] After this initial replication in the liver [exoerythrocytic schizogony (A)], the parasites undergo asexual multiplication in the erythrocytes [erythrocytic schizogony (B)]. Merozoites infect red blood cells (5). The ring stage trophozoites mature into schizonts, which rupture releasing merozoites (6). Some parasites differentiate into sexual erythrocytic stages (gametocytes) (7). Blood stage parasites are responsible for the clinical manifestations of the disease. The gametocytes, male (microgametocytes) and female (macrogametocytes), are ingested by an *Anopheles* mosquito during a blood meal (8). The parasites' multiplication in the mosquito is known as the sporogonic cycle (C). While in the mosquito's stomach, the microgametes penetrate the macrogametes generating zygotes (9). The zygotes in turn become motile and elongated (ookinetes) (10) which invade the midgut wall of the mosquito where they develop into oocysts (11). The oocysts grow, rupture, and release sporozoites (i), which make their way to the mosquito's salivary glands. Inoculation of the sporozoites (12) into a new human host perpetuates the malaria life cycle

Source: Public Image Health Library. CDC-DPDx/Alexander J. da Silva, PhD, Melanie Moser

Table 14.11 Salient Characteristics of Malaria Parasites

Characteristics	*P. falciparum*	*P. vivax*	*P. ovale*	*P. malariae*
Exoerythrocytic cycle (days)	5.5	8	9	15
Erythrocytic cycle (hours)	48	48	48	72
No. of merozoites per hepatic schizont	40,000	10,000	15,000	2,000
Persistent exoerythrocytic cycle	No	Yes	Yes	No
Relapses	No	Yes	Yes	No
Recrudescence	Yes	Yes	Yes	Yes
Red cells parasitized	All	Reticulocytes	Reticulocytes	Old

period of 6–15 days to form thousands of merozoites in a *hepatic* or *tissue schizont*. The swollen hepatocyte finally ruptures, releasing *merozoites* into bloodstream. These merozoites invade erythrocytes but cannot reinfect hepatocytes or start a fresh cycle of pre-erythrocytic schizogony. This phase is asymptomatic.

In *P. vivax* and *P. ovale* infections, intrahepatic sporozoites do not develop immediately but remain dormant in liver for a period ranging from weeks to years before reproduction begins. These "sleeping" forms, or *hypnozoites*, are responsible for *relapses* with these two species. Relapses can occur from *P. vivax* till 2–4 years. On the other hand, *P. falciparum* and *P. malariae* do not form hypnozoites in liver, and, therefore, relapses do not occur in infections with these species. However, *recrudescence* of infection can occur due to persistent erythrocytic forms. Recrudescence from *P. malariae* has been reported up to 5 years after the primary infection.

Erythrocytic schizogony: Merozoites, released from ruptured hepatocyte, enter the bloodstream and rapidly invade erythrocytes. Attachment is mediated by specific erythrocyte surface receptors, for example, Duffy blood group antigen for *P. vivax* and glycophorins for *P. falciparum*. *P. vivax* and *P. ovale* primarily invade immature erythrocytes. *P. malariae* invades mature erythrocytes only, limiting parasitemia (number of infected erythrocytes) to <2%. In contrast, *P. falciparum* invades both mature and immature erythrocytes and parasitemia can be as high as 60%. Inside the red blood cells, malarial parasites are known as *trophozoites*. During early phase of development (<12 hours), the young trophozoites appear as *"ring forms"*. Approximately 36 hours after merozoite invasion, repeated nuclear division occurs (*merogony*) and erythrocyte bursts to release 6–32 daughter merozoites. These invade uninfected erythrocytes and cycle is repeated until it is contained by the host's immunity, antimalarial drugs, or a combination of both.

After a period of erythrocytic schizogony, some parasites differentiate into sexual forms known as *microgametocytes* (male) and *macrogametocytes* (female). These usually appear within 3–15 days of the onset of symptoms and are not associated with any illness. Further development of the parasite takes place in the mosquito.

Sexual development: When a female mosquito takes a blood meal on an infected person, gametocytes are ingested, which undergo further development in the stomach (midgut) of the mosquito (sporogony). The development of malarial parasite in mosquito culminates in the formation of sporozoites, the infected form which migrate to the salivary gland of the mosquito. The female mosquito is now infective and ready to transmit infection to humans at the next bite.

PATHOPHYSIOLOGY

The pathophysiology of malaria is complex and results from interaction between malarial parasite and human host. Only blood-stage parasites are involved in the pathogenesis and clinical manifestations of malaria; exoerythrocytic stages, gametocytes and sporozoites do not induce pathophysiological changes.

Cytokines: In response to rupture of infected erythrocytes, pro-inflammatory cytokines such as tumor necrosis factor (TNF) and interleukins (IL-1, IL-6, IL-8) are produced by the cells of macrophage-monocyte system. Cytokines are responsible for many clinical manifestations of malaria, particularly fever and malaise.

Cytoadherence, sequestration, and rosetting: These phenomena are essential to the pathogenesis of falciparum malaria.

- After 24–36 hours of merozoite invasion, infected erythrocytes become sticky and adhere to venular and capillary endothelium. This is known as *cytoadherence*. The stickiness of erythrocytes is due to the appearance of knob-like projections consisting of histidine-rich protein (HRP).
- *Sequestration* refers to the disappearance of infected erythrocytes containing mature forms of *P. falciparum* from circulation. This is the reason why the mature forms of *P. falciparum* are rarely found in the peripheral blood and the degree of parasitemia may be greatly underestimated.
- Erythrocytes containing mature forms of *P. falciparum* also adhere to uninfected erythrocytes, a process known as *rosetting*. This is particularly prominent in cerebral malaria. Rosetting may promote cytoadherence by reducing blood flow.

The net effect of these events is impaired microcirculation and dysfunction of various organ systems.

Immune Response to Malaria Parasite

Immune response in malaria is complex and not completely understood. Immunity against malaria develops gradually, is incomplete at best, and is not lifelong. Malarial parasite can elude host immune system by its ability to express antigens on the erythrocyte surface that change during the infection (*antigenic diversity*). This has also hampered the efforts to develop effective vaccine against malaria.

In endemic regions, newborns and young infants are protected against malaria by antibodies acquired transplacentally and through breastmilk, and high levels of fetal hemoglobin (HbF), which retards the development of the parasite.

Clinical Correlates

Clinical manifestations of malaria are related to the red cell destruction and the host's response to this phenomenon. The periodicity of malarial paroxysm depends on the duration of erythrocytic cycle of the parasite. Paroxysms occur every 48 hours (*tertian*) in *P. vivax*, *P. ovale*, and *P. falciparum* infections and every 72 hours (*quartan*) in *P. malariae* infection. Generally, it requires 5–7 days before enough schizonts rupture at the same time and infection becomes synchronized. Therefore, malarial paroxysms are absent in the beginning of the disease. Often, in patients with asynchronous infections where >1 brood of parasites is developing in the blood at different times, periodicity is not found, and fever may occur daily (quotidian). This is particularly true for *P. falciparum* infections where fever may never regularize to a tertian or subtertian (every 36 hours) pattern.

CLINICAL FEATURES

The incubation period (time from sporozoite inoculation to the onset of fever) ranges from 9 to 40 days (shortest for *P. falciparum*, longest for *P. malariae*). It can be prolonged by partial immunity and chemoprophylaxis. The clinical features of malaria range from an asymptomatic infection to life-threatening illness. Manifestations are determined by the immune status of the host which, in turn, is determined by previous exposure to malaria.

- ***In stable high transmission settings*** where people are continuously exposed to a constant rate of malarial inoculations and where inoculation rates are high, partial immunity to the clinical disease is acquired early in childhood. This situation prevails in much of sub-Saharan Africa and parts of Oceania. In such circumstances, severe malaria is confined to young children and becomes infrequent with increasing age.
- ***With unstable malaria transmission pattern,*** which prevails in much of Asia and Latin America, the inoculation rates (number of bites by mosquitoes carrying infected sporozoites) fluctuate widely over seasons and years. This prevents development of immunity. In such situations, severe malaria can affect both children and adults.

Uncomplicated Malaria

It is defined as symptomatic infection without signs of severity and/or evidence of organ dysfunction (described under severe malaria). The clinical picture of uncomplicated malaria is common to all four species. It must be understood that there are no distinctive features of malaria in children. Fever may not follow any definite pattern and may be irregular, continuous, remittent, or intermittent in nature. Typical malarial paroxysms consisting of fever spikes, chills, and rigors occurring at regular intervals are uncommon, particularly in children <5 years of age. The initial symptoms of malaria are nonspecific and similar to the symptoms of a viral illness. They include anorexia, malaise, irritability, headache, myalgia, and slight fever. As infection continues, the child may develop high fever, headache, vomiting, diarrhea, pallor with or without jaundice.

The classical malarial paroxysm, though uncommon in children, occurs more commonly with *P. vivax* and *P. ovale* infections than with other species, and consists of three successive stages, namely, the *cold stage*, the *hot stage* and the *sweating stage*. Cold stage is characterized by sudden rise of temperature; feeling of intense cold (*chills*) prompting the need for warmth or cover, and shivering with or without teeth chattering (*rigors*). There is peripheral vasoconstriction and gooseflesh. The rigors usually last 10–30 minutes but may last up to 90 minutes. The hot stage follows—the patient feels hot and fever becomes high grade. There is severe headache, myalgia, vomiting, tachypnea, palpitation, delirium, and prostration. The hot stage lasts 2–6 hours. It is followed by the sweating stage, which is characterized by drenching sweats and rapid fall in temperature. Defervescence usually takes 2–3 hours. The entire paroxysm may last 8–12 hours. In between paroxysms, the patient appears well.

There are a few findings in uncomplicated malaria. Spleen becomes palpable toward the end of first week of illness; it is soft and occasionally tender. The liver may be enlarged, soft, and sometimes tender. There may be anemia and slight jaundice. Absence of lymphadenopathy and skin rash is useful negative findings in malaria. Without effective treatment for *P. falciparum,* severe malaria may develop rapidly.

Severe Malaria

It is defined as acute malaria with signs of severity and/or evidence of vital organ dysfunction. Almost all severe morbidity and mortality in malaria are caused by *P. falciparum.* The high virulence of *P. falciparum* is attributed to its tendency to produce high parasitemia, cytoadherence, sequestration, and rosetting capacity, and antimalarial drug resistance.

Severe malaria is defined as occurrence of one or more of the following in the presence of *P. falciparum* asexual parasitemia. The features include (*i*) impaired consciousness, (*ii*) prostration; (*iii*) severe anemia (hemoglobin <5 g/dL or hematocrit <15%), (*iv*) acute renal failure, (*v*) jaundice, (*vi*) hypoglycemia (blood glucose <40 mg/dL), (*vii*) shock, (*viii*) disseminated intravascular coagulation, (*ix*) repeated convulsions (>2 episodes a day), (*x*) acidemia, (*xi*) pulmonary edema, and (*xii*) hyperparasitemia (>10%). Untreated severe malaria is almost always fatal. Even with treatment, the mortality remains unacceptably high (15–20%).

Although *P. vivax* is known to be a benign malaria, rarely it can cause severe disease with life-threatening end-organ involvement, similar to *P. falciparum* malaria.

Cerebral Malaria

This is the most dreaded complication of *P. falciparum* infection. Very rarely, *P. vivax* infection can also cause cerebral malaria.

Clinical manifestations: The onset is generally sudden but may be gradual. The child has high fever for a few days followed by coma and seizures. There may be pallor, jaundice, or splenomegaly. However, their absence does not exclude cerebral malaria.

Cerebral malaria is a diffuse, symmetric encephalopathy. Focal signs are rare. Neurological signs are variable and include deep coma (Glasgow Coma Scale <11), variable muscle tone and tendon reflexes, absent abdominal reflexes, upgoing plantar in half the patients, opisthotonus, and decerebrate or decorticate posturing. Meningeal signs and cranial nerve abnormalities are absent. Papilledema is rare but retinal hemorrhages are found in 15% of cases. Disconjugate gaze is common.

Pathology: Cerebral malaria is characterized by blockage of capillaries and venules with erythrocytes containing *P. falciparum*. Cerebral edema does not occur in cerebral malaria and anti-edema agents such as mannitol and steroids are not useful in this condition. The exact cause of coma is not clear. It may be related to cytokine-induced production of nitric oxide, which is a potent inhibitor of neurotransmission. Cerebrospinal fluid is generally normal. Some patients may have slight pleocytosis and moderate elevation of protein while glucose remains normal.

Prognosis: Untreated cerebral malaria is fatal. With appropriate therapy, the mortality rate is 15% in children, 20% in adults and up to 50% in pregnant women. Recovery is fast and generally complete. Most children regain consciousness within 24–48 hours. Neurological sequels in the form of hemiparesis, ataxia, cortical blindness, mental retardation, and aphasia are seen more in children (10%) than in adults (3%).

Anemia

Life-threatening anemia can develop rapidly in malaria. It may lead to high output cardiac failure and sudden death. Anemia in malaria is more severe than expected from the destruction of parasitized erythrocytes. Other contributing mechanisms include destruction of unparasitized erythrocytes by immune mechanisms, dyserythropoiesis, increased splenic clearance of parasitized as well as unparasitized erythrocytes, and hemolysis associated with blackwater fever. At times, malarial anemia is superimposed on pre-existing nutritional anemia. Anemia is normocytic, normochromic, and reticulocyte count is low or normal.

Blackwater Fever

This is characterized by sudden and massive, intravascular hemolysis and the passage of "Coca-Cola" colored urine due to hemoglobinuria. In severe cases, renal failure may develop. Blackwater urine can occur in three situations: (*i*) when G-6-PD deficient patients are given oxidant drugs regardless of whether they have malaria or not; (*ii*) when patients of G-6-PD deficiency develop malaria and receive quinine; and (*iii*) when patients with normal G-6-PD levels receive quinine. The mechanism of quinine-induced hemolysis is not known as it is not an oxidant drug. Probably hypersensitivity to quinine is responsible for hemolysis.

Hypoglycemia

It is the most common biochemical abnormality in severe malaria, observed in 30% of children with cerebral malaria. Factors responsible for hypoglycemia include cytokine-induced suppression of gluconeogenesis and increased glucose consumption caused by fever, anaerobic glycolysis, infection, and malarial parasites. This is further aggravated by quinine-stimulated pancreatic insulin secretion. Pregnant women appear to be especially susceptible to quinine-induced hypoglycemia. It is not possible to detect hypoglycemia clinically as the manifestations are indistinguishable from severe malaria. Therefore, frequent blood glucose monitoring is recommended in sick children. Quinine-stimulated hypoglycemia can be prevented by giving quinine infusion slowly over 4 hours in 5% or 10% dextrose solutions.

Algid Malaria

Majority of patients with severe malaria remain well perfused and warm, but some develop shock with cold extremities. This is known as algid malaria (*algid*—cold). This may result from secondary gram-negative bacteremia and hypovolemia (dehydration and, rarely hemorrhage). Patients with severe malaria are vulnerable to bacterial infections due to transient immunosuppression.

Other Features

Renal failure, pulmonary edema, jaundice, disseminated intravascular coagulation (DIC), and metabolic acidosis are other important manifestations of severe malaria. Renal failure is caused by acute tubular necrosis following obstruction of renal microvasculature by sequestrated erythrocytes. Glomerulonephritis is very rare. Pulmonary edema occurs due to increased pulmonary capillary permeability, a finding not observed in others vascular beds. It is sometimes precipitated by excessive parenteral fluid therapy. Jaundice occurs due to hemolysis, hepatic dysfunction, and cholestasis. Frank hepatic failure suggests concomitant viral hepatitis or another diagnosis. DIC is caused by the activation of coagulation cascade by the parasitized erythrocytes and cytokines. Metabolic acidosis is attributed to anaerobic glycolysis, failure of liver and kidney to clear lactate, and lactate production by the parasite.

Congenital Malaria

Congenital malaria can be caused by the first four species of malaria parasite. It usually occurs in a nonimmune mother. Symptomatic congenital malaria is rare in areas with stable malaria transmission pattern, probably due to transplacental transfer of protective maternal IgG antibodies. In endemic areas, it is an important cause of abortion, stillbirths, premature births, and intrauterine growth restriction. Placenta may be black in color due to malaria pigment and parasites may be seen in tissue sections, although the maternal blood smear may be negative. Maternal treatment is inadequate to cure the fetus. The incubation period ranges from 2 to 8 weeks. Clinical manifestations include fever, irritability, failure to thrive, pallor, jaundice, and hepatosplenomegaly. Because there are no exoerythrocytic stages in congenital *P. vivax* and *P. ovale* infections, radical cure with primaquine is not required.

Chronic Complications of Malaria

Repeated malarial infections can cause chronic complications such as tropical splenomegaly syndrome, nephrotic syndrome (*P. malariae*), endemic Burkitt's lymphoma, and endomyocardial fibrosis.

Tropical splenomegaly syndrome: It is also known as hyperreactive malarial splenomegaly. It is considered to be an aberrant immunological response to repeated malarial infection. All the four species of *Plasmodium* can be associated with this condition. Constant stimulation of the reticuloendothelial system by circulating antigen-antibody complexes result in the enlargement of liver and spleen.

The essential features are residence in a malaria endemic area, massive splenomegaly, mild to moderate hepatomegaly, elevated serum IgG and IgM malarial antibody levels, and hepatic sinusoidal lymphocytosis with Kupffer cell hyperplasia. There may be anemia, leukopenia, and thrombocytopenia. Low grade fever may be present. Most children have growth retardation. Parasites are absent in the peripheral blood. Therapy consists of prolonged antimalarial chemoprophylaxis (chloroquine and/or proguanil) for at least 1 year. Chemoprophylaxis acts by removing the antigenic stimulus from repeated malarial infections, thus permitting the patient's immune system to return to normal. Response is generally seen within 3 months. There is no role of splenectomy.

Relapse and Recrudescence

Relapse results from persistence of parasites (hypnozoites) in the liver and their subsequent release into circulation. Only *P. vivax* and *P. ovale* produce hypnozoites and thus are capable of relapsing. Relapse occurs in approximately half of those infected in Southeast Asia; the frequency is lower in Indian subcontinent (15–20%) and may occur as long as 5 years after initial infection.

Relapses are not seen in *P. falciparum* and *P. malariae* infections as there is no persistent exoerythrocytic stage (hypnozoites) in these infections. However, they may give rise to repeated episodes of parasitemia called recrudescence; either by long-term persistence of erythrocytic stages (e.g., within a sequestration site) or the continuation of erythrocytic schizogony at low levels for a prolonged period. Recrudescence can also occur following *P. vivax* and *P. ovale* infections. The main importance of differentiating relapse from recrudescence is that, whereas recrudescence is amenable to standard chemotherapy, relapse requires a specific treatment with primaquine (*radical cure*) to eradicate the infection.

LABORATORY DIAGNOSIS

The diagnosis of malaria is based on clinical criteria (clinical diagnosis) supplemented by the detection of parasites in the blood (parasitological or confirmatory diagnosis). Clinical diagnosis alone has very low specificity and in many areas parasitological diagnosis is not currently available. The decision to provide antimalarial treatment in these settings must be based on the prior probability of the illness being malaria. One needs to weigh the risk of withholding antimalarial treatment from a patient with malaria against the risk associated with antimalarial treatment when given to a patient who does not have malaria.

Parasitological Diagnosis

Peripheral Blood Smear

This is the gold standard for making the diagnosis of malaria. Both thick and thin smears should be prepared. Thick smear is used for the parasite detection while thin smear is used for species identification. Thick film is 20–40 times more sensitive than thin film as it contains more blood. Thick film can detect as little as 0.001% parasitemia (~50 parasites/µL) and is the only way to quantitate parasitemia. The timing of blood smears with fever spikes is less important than repeating it 2–3 times a day for making a diagnosis. It should be kept in mind that a single negative smear does not exclude malaria and repeated smears should be obtained in a strongly suspected case. The main problem with microscopic diagnosis is that it is time consuming and requires a skilled person.

Plasmodium falciparum can be recognized in peripheral smear by ring forms and crescent-shaped gametocytes, intense parasitemia (S2%), and multiple infection in a single erythrocyte. Other species of parasite have all stages in peripheral blood. Even in the absence of parasitemia the diagnosis of acute malaria can be suspected by, the presence of malaria pigment (*hemozoin*) in monocytes or neutrophils.

Alternate diagnostic methods are used, if the laboratory does not have sufficient expertise in detecting malarial parasite in the peripheral blood smear.

Rapid Diagnostic Tests

These are immunochromatographic tests that detect parasite-specific antigens in a blood sample. Rapid diagnostic tests (RDTs) are available in different formats such as dipsticks, cassettes or cards in which a colored line shows that plasmodial antigens have been detected. RDTs are simple to perform and interpret, and do not require electricity, special equipment or skilled personnel. Current tests are based on the detection of histidine-rich protein 2 (HRP2), which is specific for *P. falciparum*, pan-specific or species-specific parasite lactate- dehydrogenase (pLDH) (e.g., OptiMal), or other pan-specific antigens such as aldolase. With the different tests that are currently available, the procedure may involve 2–6 steps and take 5–30 minutes. National vector-borne Disease Control Program supplies RDT kits for detection of *P. falciparum* in areas where microscopy is not feasible within 24 hours of sample collection.

High temperature and humidity in the field settings may affect test performance leading to unpredictable sensitivity. Sensitivity for *P. falciparum* ranges from comparable to good microscopy (>90% at 100–500 parasites/µL of blood) to very poor (40–50%). Sensitivity is generally lower for other species particularly at parasite densities <500/μL. Therefore, negative RDT should not preclude treatment in a strongly suspected case, especially in severe clinical disease. One drawback of this method is that HRP2 antigen levels remain elevated for weeks after parasite clearance, thus giving false-positive results. Further, RDTs do not quantitate *P. falciparum* parasitemia.

Other Methods

Quantitative buffy coat (QBC) method: Unlike mature erythrocytes, malarial parasites contain DNA that can be stained with acridine orange and easily visualized by fluorescence microscopy. This method is faster and more sensitive than routine microscopy but species identification is less accurate.

Polymerase chain reaction: Although the test is sensitive and specific, it has limited utility due to nonavailability in most places. It has the potential to identify genes which confer drug resistance.

Serology: Antimalarial antibodies are of little diagnostic help in endemic areas since their levels remain elevated for months to years after an attack.

Histidine-rich protein 2 of P. falciparum (PfHRP2): It is a water-soluble protein that is produced by the asexual stages and gametocytes of *P. falciparum,* expressed on the red cell membrane surface, and shown to remain in the blood for at least 28 days after the initiation of antimalarial therapy. Several RDTs targeting PfHRP2 have been developed.

Plasmodium aldolase: It is an enzyme of the parasite glycolytic pathway expressed by the blood stages of *P. falciparum* as well as the nonfalciparum malaria parasites. Monoclonal antibodies against *Plasmodium* aldolase are pan-specific in their reaction and have been used in a combined "P.f/P.v" immunochromatographic test that targets the pan-malarial antigen (PMA) along with PfHRP2.

Parasite lactate dehydrogenase (pLDH): It is a soluble glycolytic enzyme produced by the asexual and sexual stages of the live parasites and it is present in and released from the parasite-infected erythrocytes. It has been found in all four human malaria species, and different isomers of pLDH for each of the four species exist. With pLDH as the target, a quantitative immunocapture assay, a qualitative immunochromatographic dipstick assay using monoclonal antibodies, an immunodot assay, and a dipstick assay using polyclonal antibodies have been developed.

The Choice between RDT and Microscopy

The choice between RDTs and microscopy depends on local circumstances, including the skills available, the usefulness of microscopy for other diseases found in the area, and the case-load. Where the case-load of fever patients is high, microscopy is likely to be less expensive than RDTs. Microscopy has further advantages in that it can be used for speciation and quantification of parasites, and identification of other causes of fever. However, in places where most malaria patients are treated outside the health services, for example, in the home or by private providers; microscopy is generally not feasible in such circumstances, but RDTs may be. The following conclusions and recommendations are based on evidence summarized by recent WHO consultations:

- In *areas of low to moderate transmission*, prompt parasitological confirmation of the diagnosis is recommended before treatment is started. This should be achieved through microscopy or, where not available, RDTs.
- In *areas of high stable malaria transmission*, the prior probability of fever in a child being caused by malaria is high. Children <5 years of age should, therefore, be treated based on a clinical diagnosis of malaria. In older children and adults including in pregnant women, a parasitological diagnosis is recommended before treatment is started.
- In *all suspected cases of severe malaria*, a parasitological confirmation of the diagnosis of malaria is recommended. In the absence of or a delay in obtaining parasitological diagnosis, patients should be treated for severe malaria, on clinical grounds.

TREATMENT Malaria

Early diagnosis and treatment of cases of malaria aims at:
- Complete cure
- Prevention of progression of uncomplicated malaria to severe disease
- Prevention of deaths
- Interruption of transmission and
- Minimizing risk of selection and spread of drug-resistant parasites.

Antimalarial Drugs

There are two broad categories of antimalarials:
- *Schizonticidal drugs* are used for clinical and parasitological cure. These are chloroquine, amodiaquin, quinine, quinidine, pyremethamine, proguanil, sulfadoxine and pyremethamine, mefloquine, halofantrine, and artemisinin.
- *Gametocidal drugs* act on hypnozoites and gametocytes, and prevent relapses. These include primaquine and 8-amodiaquins.

In the past, chloroquine was effective in nearly all cases of malaria. Emergence of chloroquine-resistant species has now necessitated the use of alternate drugs.

Artemisinin Derivatives

Artemisinin or *quinghaosu* (pronounced as "ching-how-soo") is extracted from the leaves of the Chinese herb *Artemisia annua*. The drug acts on late stage ring parasites and trophozoites. Artesunate, artemether, and artemotil (arteether) are the available derivatives. They clear parasitemia more rapidly than any other antimalarial drug, and are remarkably well tolerated. The only significant adverse effect is type I hypersensitivity reactions manifesting as urticaria. These drugs also reduce the gametocytes carriage and thus the transmissibility of malaria. However, their use may be associated with a high recrudescence rate (10%) after monotherapy, so they are usually combined with other antimalarials for clinical treatment. Also monotherapy is discouraged to protect them from resistance. Artesunate has better pharmacokinetic properties than other artemisinin derivatives as it is water soluble and can be given by IV or IM route. Studies in children demonstrate equal efficacy of quinine, artesunate, and artemether. Artemether is administered IM as it is formulated in oil, and may have erratic absorption in severely ill patients. Unlike quinine, artemisinin derivatives do not need dosage adjustment in renal or hepatic impairment or produce hypoglycemia. Artesunate solution should be prepared freshly for each administration and should not be stored. Dose-dependent neurotoxicity affecting brainstem nuclei in animals have not been observed in humans.

Mefloquine

It is used for the treatment of uncomplicated chloroquine-resistant malaria. Mefloquine should not be used as a monotherapy for the treatment of severe malaria. For the treatment of falciparum infection, mefloquine in combination with artemisinin derivatives is used in a dose of 25 mg/kg. For *P. vivax* malaria, the dose is 15 mg/kg stat. The elimination half-life is 14–28 days. It destroys early trophozoites. Only oral formulation is available. Gastrointestinal side effects-like nausea and vomiting occur in 10–15% of patients. The dose should be repeated, if the patient vomits within 1 hour. Less frequent side effects include nightmares, ataxia, suicidal tendencies, anxiety neurosis, hallucinations, psychosis, seizures, and altered sensorium. Splitting the 25 mg/kg dose into two parts (15 mg and 10 mg/kg) and giving at an interval of 6–24 hours increases absorption and improves tolerability. The drug is not recommended for persons involved with activity requiring fine coordination and special performance (*e.g.,* airplane crews, operators of dangerous equipment).

Treating Uncomplicated Malaria

Children with uncomplicated malaria are treated with oral drugs (**Box 14.5**). Parasitological confirmation of diagnosis, either by light microscopy or rapid diagnostic tests, is required before starting treatment in uncomplicated malaria. Chloroquine remains the drug of choice in sensitive regions. WHO recommends combinations of antimalarials for the treatment of uncomplicated falciparum malaria acquired in chloroquine-resistant regions. In India, resistance to chloroquine has been reported from all regions.

Artemisinin Combination Therapy

Antimalarial combination therapy (ACT) refers to the simultaneous use of two or more blood schizonticidal drugs with independent modes of action. The purpose of combination therapy is to improve therapeutic efficacy and to delay the emergence of resistance to single antimalarial drugs. When one of the partner drugs is the artemisinin derivative it is known as *artemisinin combination therapy*.

Artemisinin derivatives are effective against all antimalarial parasites. In mixed malarial infections, ACTs are also the treatment of choice. The duration of artemisinin therapy is variable depending on whether the partner drug is rapidly or slowly eliminated. When used in combination with rapidly eliminated drugs (tetracycline, doxycycline, clindamycin) artemisinin compounds are given for 7 days but when given in combination with slowly eliminated drugs (lumefantrine, mefloquine, amodiaquine, sulfadoxine-pyrimethamine), a 3-day course suffices. Artemether-lumefantrine (AL) is available as co-formulated tablets and suspension. It should be emphasized that AL should be taken with milk or fatty meal to increase absorption from gut. Inadequate fat intake may cause low blood levels, with resultant treatment failure.

In 3-day course, the dose of artesunate is 4 mg/kg once a day. In 7-day course, the dose is 2 mg/kg once a day. The dosing schedules of artemether-lumefantrine and artesunate-mefloquine are given in **Tables 14.12 and 14.13**, respectively.

Box 14.5 Antimalarial Chemotherapy for Uncomplicated Malaria

- *Chloroquine-sensitive malaria**
  Chloroquine 10 mg/kg on first and second day and 5 mg/kg on third day. Repeat the dose if child vomits within 30 minutes.
- *Chloroquine-resistant malaria** (mostly *P. falciparum*, rarely *P. vivax*)
  - *First-line antimalarial combinations* (3-day regimen)
    Artemisinin combination therapy (ACT)
    - Artemether-lumefantrine (most preferred)
      OR
    - Artesunate + mefloquine
      OR
    - Artesunate + amodiaquine
      OR
    - Artesunate + sulfadoxine-pyrimethamine (not preferred due to increasing resistance to S-P)
  - *Second-line antimalarial combinations* (to be used when first-line antimalarial combinations fail) (7-day regimen)
    - Artesunate + clindamycin or doxycycline or tetracycline
      OR
    - Quinine + clindamycin or doxycycline or tetracycline
  - *Single drug treatment* (unsuitable for *P. falciparum*; may consider for *P. vivax*)
    - Mefloquine 15 mg base/kg as a single dose
      OR
    - Quinine 10 mg salt/kg three times a day for 7 days
      OR
    - Sulfadoxine-pyrimethamine as a single dose (no longer recommended)

*To achieve radical cure in *P. vivax* malaria, primaquine should be given 0.25 mg base/kg, once a day for 14 days in low malaria-transmission regions after excluding G6PD deficiency. For falciparum malaria, a single dose of primaquine (0.25 mg/kg) is given for gametocidal action

Treatment of Severe Malaria

Severe malaria is a medical emergency and is treated with parenteral drugs **(Box 14.6)**. Delay in treatment raises mortality significantly. Therefore, when faced with a critically sick child having an illness compatible with severe malaria and no alternative diagnosis, antimalarial treatment must be started even before the diagnosis is confirmed. It is important to remember that a single negative smear or a negative RDT does not exclude malaria.

Artemisinin derivatives and quinine are the mainstay of treatment because of their activity against chloroquine-resistant *P. falciparum*. Recently, artemisinin derivatives are being used increasingly due to reported resistance to quinine. Artemisinin derivatives are easier to administer and are marginally superior to quinine in reducing mortality in severe malaria only in areas where there is quinine resistance as seen

Table 14.12 Dosing Schedule for Artemether-Lumefantrine

		Dose of artemether (mg) and timing					
Weight (kg)	*Age (years)*	*0 hour*	*8 hours*	*24 hours*	*36 hours*	*48 hours*	*60 hours*
5–14	<3	20	20	20	20	20	20
15–24	3–8	40	40	40	40	40	40
25–34	9–14	60	60	60	60	60	60
>34	>14	80	80	80	80	80	80

Table 14.13 Dosing Schedule for Artesunate + Mefloquine

Age	Dose in mg (no. of tablets)					
	Artesunate (50 mg)			Mefloquine (250 mg)		
	Day 1	Day 2	Day 3	Day 1	Day 2	Day 3
5–11 months	25 (1/2)	25	25	–	125 (1/2)	
1–6 years	50 (1)	50	50	–	250 (1)	
7–13 years	100 (2)	100	100	–	500 (2)	250 (1)
>13 years	200 (4)	200	200	–	1,000 (4)	500 (2)

Box 14.6 Antimalarial Chemotherapy for Severe Malaria

- Artesunate* weight >20 kg: 2.4 mg/kg IV or IM on admission (0 hour), then at 12 hours, 24 hours, and then once daily for 6 days (total 7 days)
  Weight <20 kg: 3.0 mg/kg
  OR
- Artemether* 3.2 mg/kg IM on admission followed by 1.6 mg/kg IM daily for 6 days (total 7 days)
  OR
- Quinine 20 mg salt/kg (loading dose)** diluted in 10 mL/kg of 5–10% dextrose IV over 4 hours, followed 8 hours after starting the loading dose with 10 mg salt/kg (maintenance dose)*** over 4–8 hourly, until the child can swallow oral quinine*** 10 mg/kg three times daily to complete 7 days of treatment

*Following initial improvement when patient starts taking orally, add doxycycline 3.5 mg/kg once a day for 7 days except for children <8 years where add clindamycin 10 mg/kg 2 times a day for 7 days.

**Loading dose should be omitted if the patient has received quinine or mefloquine in last 24 hours.

***If parenteral therapy is needed for >48 hours-reduce the maintenance dose of quinine by one-half to one-third (5–7 mg salt/kg/dose) to avoid accumulation.

in various clinical trials. Death from severe malaria often occurs within hours of admission to hospital, and so it is essential that therapeutic concentrations of antimalarials are achieved as soon as possible. With loading dose of quinine, effective blood levels are attained by the end of 4-hour infusion. Without loading dose, therapeutic levels may not be reached in the first 12 hours of therapy, an unacceptable delay in the treatment of severe malaria. Quinine may be given intramuscularly (IM), if intravenous infusion is not possible. For IM administration, quinine should be diluted with normal saline to concentrations of 60–100 mg/mL, and first dose should be split 10 mg/kg to each thigh. Therapeutic drug levels are similar for both routes of administration. However, IV route is preferred as quinine IM may be erratically absorbed in severe malaria particularly in patients with shock. Quinine should be given slowly by infusion and never by IV bolus injection as lethal hypotension may occur. Following initial parenteral treatment, once the patient starts accepting orally, the same drug (quinine or artesunate or artemether) is continued orally to complete a full 7-day course of treatment. In addition, the patient is also given doxycycline or clindamycin for 7 days. Recently, artemisinin combination therapy (ACT), artesunate plus amodiaquine or artemether plus lumefantrine, has also been proposed following parenteral treatment.

Supportive Therapy

Fluid and electrolyte requirements should be individualized. Dehydration and shock should be corrected. Septicemia may complicate severe malaria in children. Therefore, cover these children with broad-spectrum antibiotic, such as ceftriaxone after taking blood culture. Avoid overhydration as it may precipitate pulmonary edema. In cerebral malaria, the fluids should be restricted to two-thirds of usual maintenance requirements. Packed red cells are transfused for severe anemia. Fever is controlled by paracetamol and tepid sponging. Acid-base disturbances should be corrected. Blood sugar should be checked three or four times a day to detect hypoglycemia. Exchange transfusion may be beneficial, if parasitemia exceeds 5%. Renal failure is managed appropriately. Seizures are controlled with diazepam and phenobarbitone or phenytoin. Prophylactic anticonvulsants are not recommended. There is no role of steroids, heparin, low-molecular-weight dextrans, prostacycline, deferoxamine, pentoxifylline, and anti-TNF-α monoclonal antibodies in the treatment of cerebral malaria. The role of mannitol in cerebral malaria is uncertain. Some authorities advocate mannitol, only if there is definite evidence of raised intracranial pressure such as strongly positive Macewen sign, unequal pupils, papilledema, and deepening coma. With appropriate therapy, patients show signs of clinical and laboratory improvement within 48–72 hours.

Treatment of Relapse and Recrudescence

Relapsing malaria (*P. vivax* and *P. ovale*) is treated with a standard course of chloroquine or ACT (outlined under uncomplicated malaria) followed by primaquine 0.25 mg/kg orally per day for 14 days (radical cure). Primaquine should be taken with food to minimize abdominal discomfort. G-6-PD screening test should be performed before starting this drug. In severe G-6-PD deficiency, primaquine should not be given as it can lead to severe hemolysis. In mild to moderate G-6-PD deficiency, primaquine 0.75 mg/kg once a week for 8 weeks can be given with a minimal risk of hemolysis. *P. vivax* and *P. ovale* infections acquired congenitally or through blood transfusion do not produce relapses as they lack exoerythrocytic (hepatic) cycle. In high transmission settings, radical cure is generally considered unnecessary as the risk of reinfection is high.

Treatment Failure

It is defined as failure of fever and parasitemia to resolve or recur during a follow-up period of S28 days. Failure to respond within 3 days is referred to as *early treatment failure* and that between 4 and 28 days as *late treatment failure*. The treatment failure could be clinical or based on nonresolution of parasitemia. Absence of parasitemia on day 28 is labeled as *adequate clinical and parasitological response* (ACPR).

It is important to know that although drug resistance may lead to treatment failure, not all treatment failures are caused by drug resistance.

Treatment failure can also occur due to incorrect dosing, poor compliance, poor drug quality, incorrect drug administration in the home and reduced drug absorption due to individual variation in bioavailability. In a clinically suspected case, it should be confirmed by blood smear examination.

- HRP2-based tests should not be used to document treatment failure as they remain positive for weeks even after effective therapy.
- In falciparum malaria, treatment failure within 2 weeks of receiving a therapy is due to recrudescence and should be treated with a second-line antimalarials. Failure after 2 weeks could be due to recrudescence or new infection and can be retreated with the first-line ACT. However, mefloquine should not be reused within 28 days of first treatment due to higher risk of neuropsychiatric disturbances (seizures, encephalopathy, psychosis).
- In *P. vivax* malaria, treatment failure within 16 days of starting treatment of the primary infection suggests recrudescence due to chloroquine-resistant parasites. Treatment failure between days 17–28 may be either a recrudescence or a relapse. Beyond 28 days, any recurrence suggests a relapse.
- Chloroquine-resistant *P. vivax* infection is treated with quinine for 7 days, or mefloquine (15 mg/kg) as a single dose, or amodiaquine 10 mg/kg once a day for 3 days, or with ACTs as outlined in **Box 14.5**.
- Avoid the use of sulfadoxine-pyrimethamine as parasite has developed resistance to this combination in many areas.

MALARIA VACCINES

The World Health Organization (WHO) recommends the RTS,S/AS01(Mosquirix) and R21/Matrix-M vaccines to prevent malaria in children **living in malaria endemic areas** like Ghana, Kenya, and Malawi, **prioritizing areas of moderate and high transmission**. The vaccines are given in a series of four doses, starting around five months of age.

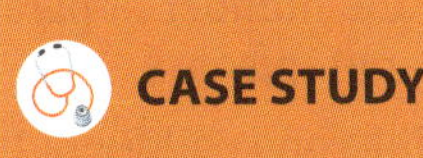

Malaria—Intermittent Fever of Short Duration (<1 week) with Splenomegaly

A 7-year-old girl presented with intermittent high grade fever accompanied with chills and rigors for 5 days. Fever used to get relieved with excessive perspiration. The child was relatively better in between fever episodes. Examination revealed temperature of 104°F, RR—34/min, HR—112/min, BP—108/64 mm Hg. There was mild pallor, no icterus, no rash, no edema, no lymphadenopathy. Examination of the abdomen revealed a soft, nontender liver 2 cm palpable below the right costal margin (liver span 7.0 cm) and palpable spleen 2 cm (soft, nontender) below left costal margin. There was no evidence of free fluid in abdomen. Other systemic examination was normal.

What are the differential diagnoses in this child?

Common differential diagnoses for short duration fever (of <7 days) with mild hepatosplenomegaly without any other localizing signs or symptoms are (a) uncomplicated malaria, (b) infectious mononucleosis, (c) viral hepatitis, and (d) dengue fever. Enteric fever is another possibility, but splenomegaly in enteric fever usually appears in the second week of illness. Here it was present on 5th day of fever.

- *Malaria:* Points in favor include intermittent fever with characteristic hot and cold cycle (relief of fever with excessive perspiration), relative well-being of child in between fever episodes, and presence of hepatosplenomegaly. Tertian and quotidian fever, i.e., fever every third day as in *P. vivax* and fever every day (as in *P. falciparum*) are not characteristic of malaria in children.
- *Infectious mononucleosis:* Intermittent fever with hepatosplenomegaly is in favor. Absence of sore throat, lymphadenopathy, rash, and toxic appearance are against the diagnosis.
- *Viral hepatitis:* Fever is usually low grade and icterus is usually present. This may be early phase of illness and icterus may be late finding or this may be a case of anicteric hepatitis. A child with hepatitis also remains anorexic, and is not well in between fever episodes (points against).
- *Dengue fever:* Fever in dengue is usually biphasic and not continuous. Absence of myalgia, bone pains, rash, edema, bleeding manifestations, and shock are also against the diagnosis.
- *Urinary tract infection (UTI):* Absence of urinary complaints such as frequency, urgency, dysuria are against UTI. However, fever may be the sole presentation of upper UTI.

Outline the investigations to confirm your diagnosis?

Peripheral blood smear examination for detection of malarial parasite is the gold standard test for diagnosis of malaria. Rapid diagnostic tests (RDTs) for malarial antigen are indicated, if peripheral blood smear is negative but suspicion of malaria is high. Investigations to rule out other possibilities include complete blood counts, peripheral smear for atypical lymphocytes, blood culture, liver enzymes, and urine microscopy and culture.

Peripheral smear revealed large-sized RBCs containing ring form and trophozoites of malarial parasite. Large chromatin dots, ameboid cytoplasm with Schüffner dots suggested P. vivax infection. Hb was 8.2 g/dL, leukocyte count 6,100/mm³, and platelet count was 54,000/mm³. Liver function and urine examination were normal.

What is your final diagnosis? Name the drug of choice for treatment.

This is a case of *uncomplicated malaria* (absence of neurological manifestations, anemia, coagulopathy, hematuria, metabolic and electrolyte abnormalities, shock, respiratory problems, jaundice classifies above patient as uncomplicated malaria caused by *P. vivax*).

Drug of choice will be oral chloroquine (25 mg/kg to be given over a period of 3 days).

As relapse is common in vivax malaria (due to presence of hypnozoites/sleeping forms), the child will also need to be treated with primaquine 0.25 mg/kg/day for 14 days (after ruling out G6PD deficiency), since primaquine can trigger hemolytic anemia in G6PD deficient individual.

The fever did not respond even after 3 days of chloroquine?

Ensure that the compliance was good and the child was receiving the correct dose. Consider chloroquine-resistant *vivax malaria* or mixed infection of more than one species of *Plasmodium*. Treat the child with ACT combination therapy (artemether + lumefantrine is most preferred combination).

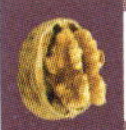

IN A NUTSHELL

Malaria

1. In India, most cases of malaria are caused by *P. vivax* (60–65%) and *P. falciparum* (35–40%).
2. Malaria is spread to humans during the bite of an infected female anopheline mosquito.
3. Typical malarial paroxysms consisting of fever spikes, chills, and rigors occurring at regular intervals are uncommon in children <5 years of age.
4. Microscopy is the gold standard of diagnosis; rapid diagnostic tests (RDTs) are reserved for areas without skilled microscopist.
5. For uncomplicated *P. vivax* malaria, chloroquine is the drug of choice.
6. All cases of falciparum and complicated malaria should be treated with artemisinine combination therapy (ACT).
7. Mosquito control is the most effective way to prevent malaria.

Basu S, Sahi PK. Malaria: an update. Indian J Pediatr. 2017;84(7):521-8.
Chan XHS, Win YN, Haeusler IL, et al. Factors affecting the electrocardiographic QT interval in malaria: A systematic review and meta-analysis of individual patient data. PLoS Med. 2020;17(3):e1003040.
Greenwood B, Zongo I, Dicko A, et al. Resurgent and delayed malaria. Malar J. 2022;21(1):77.
Infectious Diseases Chapter, Indian Academy of Pediatrics, Kundu R, Ganguly N, et al. Management of malaria in children: update 2008. Indian Pediatr. 2008;45(9):731-5.
Mathew JL. Artemisinin derivatives versus quinine for severe malaria in children: a systematic review and meta-analysis. Indian Pediatr. 2010;47:423-8.
Mousa A, Al-Taiar A, Anstey NM, et al. The impact of delayed treatment of uncomplicated *P. falciparum* malaria on progression to severe malaria: a systematic review and a pooled multicentre individual-patient meta-analysis. PLoS Med. 2020;17(10):e1003359.
Thwing J, Eisele TP, Steketee RW. Protective efficacy of malaria case management for preventing malaria mortality in children: a systematic review for the Lives Saved Tool. BMC Public Health. 2011;11(Suppl 3):S14.
WHO guidelines for malaria, 30 November 2024. Geneva: World Health Organization; 2024. Available from https://doi.org/10.2471/B09146. [Last accessed February, 2025].
World Health Organization. (2021). Global technical strategy for malaria 2016–2030, 2021 update. [online] Available from https://www.who.int/publications/i/item/9789240031357 [Last accessed August, 2025].
World Health Organization. (2025). WHO Guidelines for malaria. [online] Available from https://www.who.int/publications/i/item/guidelines-for-malaria [Last accessed August, 2025].

14.15 Visceral Leishmaniasis

PE 31.14

INTRODUCTION

Leishmaniasis is caused by parasites of the genus *Leishmania,* which are transmitted to humans by female sandflies of the genus *Phlebotomus.* There are three major clinical forms of leishmaniasis—visceral leishmaniasis, cutaneous leishmaniasis, and mucocutaneous leishmaniasis. In India, only visceral and cutaneous forms of leishmaniasis occur. The term kala-azar (*Kala*—black; *Azar*—sickness) for this disease denotes hyperpigmentation seen in patients with visceral leishmaniasis. Infection may be asymptomatic.

The disease is world-wide in distribution and occurs on all continents except Australia and Antarctica. In India, kala-azar is most often reported from Bihar, West Bengal, Jharkhand, and Eastern UP. Of the 1-3 lakh cases reported annually in India, 90% occur in Bihar alone.

ETIOLOGY

There are at least 30 species of *Leishmania.* Visceral leishmaniasis in the Indian subcontinent is most often caused by *L. donovani.*

Parasites are present in the human host as *amastigotes,* which are nonflagellated, round or oval (*Leishman-Donovan bodies*), and as flagellated *promastigotes* in the sandfly and in the culture medium. Amastigotes live and multiply in the cells of the mononuclear phagocyte system, which includes blood monocytes, macrophages, histiocytes, Kupffer cells, and reticuloendothelial cells in spleen and lymphoid tissue.

EPIDEMIOLOGY

Vector Phlebotomus argentipes (sandfly) is the only vector responsible for Indian kala-azar. It breeds in cattle sheds, and eggs are laid above the water-line during seasonal floods. Sandflies are small insects, about one-fourth of a mosquito. Life cycle lasts for more than a month; however, duration depends on temperature and other ecological conditions. They prefer high relative humidity, warm temperature, high subsoil water, and abundance of vegetation. These are ecologically sensitive insects, fragile and cannot withstand desiccation. The sandfly is a light-avoiding mosquito.

Parasite load is measured by an index known as average parasite density (APD). APD depends on the number of parasites per high power field in a stained smear of spleen.

Host: Indian kala-azar primarily affects adults and children <10 years of age, sparing infants. Mostly poor socioeconomic groups of population primarily living in rural areas are affected.

Environment: The conditions that permit outbreaks of kala-azar include a heavy rainfall, increased relative humidity, high ambient environmental temperature, plenty of vegetation, and subsoil water. Rural areas lying within 600 feet above sea level are more susceptible. Primitive housing and low standards of hygiene increase the risk of transmission. Infection rate is usually highest among the people living at the edge of foci (forest or desert) close to zoonotic cycle.

Mode of Spread

Transmission: Female sandflies feeding on infected persons ingest parasitized cells. Amastigotes transform into promastigotes, which develop and multiply in the insect's gut and migrate to the proboscis (salivary glands). The female sandfly becomes infective to man after an external incubation period of 6-9 days, ready to transmit infection to the human. Infection occurs when an infected female sandfly bites a person and injects parasites into the human host. Male sandflies feed on fruit juices and do not suck blood. Rarely, visceral leishmaniasis can be transmitted by blood transfusion, sexual intercourse, accidental needle prick, or congenitally.

Reservoir: Man appears to be the only reservoir of infection for visceral leishmaniasis in India. However, in other geographical areas, dogs, cats, jackals, and rodents, also act as reservoirs.

PATHOGENESIS

Following the bite of an infected sandfly, promastigotes enter reticuloendothelial cells, transform into amastigotes and multiply. Parasites spread hematogenously within macrophages to the liver, spleen, bone marrow, and lymphoid tissue. The protective immune response in visceral leishmaniasis is primarily cell mediated (CMI), which results in subclinical infection and spontaneous cure in many cases. Failure of CMI to develop leads to the clinical syndrome of visceral leishmaniasis. Anti-leishmanial antibodies are not protective in nature. Defective CMI correlates with increased suppressor cell activity and decreased production of interferon-gamma, interleukin-1, and interleukin-2 by mononuclear cells. The *leishmanin skin test* (*Montenegro test*) detects delayed-type hypersensitivity to leishmanial antigens. The test is negative during active disease and becomes positive 3–6 months after recovery. For every case of visceral leishmaniasis, there are about 30 subclinical infections. Malnutrition and HIV predispose to clinical disease.

CLINICAL FEATURES

The *incubation period* is generally 2–8 months, although it may be as long as 2 years.

The onset is insidious in most cases. The typical manifestations of kala-azar consisting of prolonged fever (>2 weeks), weight loss, abdominal discomfort, emaciation, pallor, marked splenomegaly, and moderate hepatomegaly generally appear a few months after the onset of illness. However, a more rapid clinical course over 1–2 months has been observed in some patients. Fever may not follow any definite pattern. It may be high or low grade, remittent, intermittent, or continuous. The *"double-rise"* of temperature in a day (*double quotidian*), although characteristic, is an uncommon finding. The patient does not appear "toxic".

Splenic enlargement is seen in nearly all cases. It is huge, firm, smooth, and nontender unless there has been a recent infarct. Moderate hepatomegaly is seen in over 80% of cases. Unlike African visceral leishmaniasis, lymphadenopathy is infrequent in kala-azar. Hyperpigmentation of skin is characteristic and occurs in late stages of disease, affecting the face, hands, and upper trunk.

Pancytopenia is common. Anemia is attributed to autoimmune hemolysis, hypersplenism, ineffective erythropoiesis, co-existing nutritional deficiencies, and gastrointestinal blood loss. Progressive emaciation occurs in all cases. Cough and diarrhea are common. Appetite is generally well maintained. There may be petechial hemorrhages, epistaxis, and gum bleeding. Pedal edema may occur due to hypoalbuminemia. Jaundice is uncommon. DIC and cirrhosis of liver are rare complications of visceral leishmaniasis. Diminished cell-mediated immunity may account for the high incidence of secondary infections, mainly pneumonia, septicemia, measles, tuberculosis, dysentery, otitis media, and cancrum oris. Without treatment, death occurs within 2 years in 80–90% of patients, usually from secondary infection or gastrointestinal hemorrhage.

Recently, visceral leishmaniasis has been recognized as an opportunistic infection in HIV infected persons. It may also result from reactivation of subclinical infection in HIV infected individuals. The presentation may be atypical with prominent gastrointestinal tract involvement and absence of hepatosplenomegaly.

Post-kala-azar dermal leishmaniasis (PKDL): This is sequel to infection with *L. donovani*. Up to 20% of patients of Indian kala-azar may develop PKDL, 1–10 years after successful treatment of visceral leishmaniasis. Hypopigmented macules and papules appear over chin, lips, neck, extensor surfaces of the arms, trunk, and legs, sparing the scalp, palms, soles, axillae, and perineum. There may be nodular skin lesions. Clinically, PKDL may be confused with lepromatous leprosy, but peripheral nerves are spared. Skin lesions may persist for up to 20 years, and such patients may act as chronic reservoir of infection.

DIFFERENTIAL DIAGNOSIS

The differential diagnosis for visceral leishmaniasis includes all conditions, which present with prolonged fever and hepatosplenomegaly such as, malaria, tropical splenomegaly syndrome, lymphoma, and leukemia, tuberculosis, schistosomiasis, portal hypertension, brucellosis, etc.

DIAGNOSIS

Laboratory Diagnosis

Demonstration of Parasites

Identification of parasites in tissue specimens [Leishman-Donovan (LD) bodies] or by culture on *Novy-McNeal-Nicolle* (NNN) medium provides a definitive diagnosis of VL. The positivity rate is highest for splenic aspirate (>95%), followed by bone marrow or liver (85%), buffy coat (70%), and African lymph node (65%). Splenic aspiration is safe in experienced hands but is contraindicated if the prothrombin time exceeds control value by 5 seconds or more, or platelet count is below 40,000/mm^3. Under these circumstances, bone marrow aspiration can be performed safely, although the yield rate is slightly low. Recently, PCR has been successfully employed to detect parasites in tissue specimens.

Serological Tests

Antibodies are readily detectable by several methods. These include enzyme immunoassay, indirect immunofluorescence, and direct agglutination tests. In general, serological tests have sensitivity >90% but with lower specificity.

A dipstick ELISA using recombinant K39 (rK39) antigen has shown a sensitivity and specificity close to 100%. The test is rapid, easy to perform, and much less invasive compared to splenic or bone marrow aspiration. Since, it remains positive for long periods, it is of no use in cases of relapse or reinfection. In micro-ELISA format, titers to rK39 decrease following successful therapy and tend to rise in cases of relapse, thus making it useful to recognize treatment failures.

Another kala-azar latex agglutination-based antigen detection test in urine has been developed (KaTex), which is highly specific, unfortunately its sensitivity is low, but it turns negative at the end of successful therapy.

Napier's aldehyde *test* was used in past for the diagnosis of kala-azar. The test has very low sensitivity and specificity and is no longer in use.

TREATMENT Visceral Leishmaniasis

Antimonials: Until now the pentavalent antimonials were the drug of choice for the therapy of visceral leishmaniasis. However, increasing resistance to these compounds in India, particularly in Bihar, has led to frequent treatment failures. Therefore, antimonials are not used as first-line agent in Bihar. However, it is still effective against visceral leishmaniasis in other parts of India, although resistant cases have been reported from these areas. The main reason for employing this agent is easy availability and low cost. Sodium antimony gluconate (sodium stibogluconate) containing 100 mg antimony (stibium) per mL or meglumine containing 85 mg antimony per mL are equal in efficacy and toxicity when used in equivalent doses. IM injections are painful and better avoided. IV injections should be diluted 1:10 with 5% dextrose and infused slowly over 20 minutes. Adverse effects include vomiting, fatigue, arthralgia, myalgia, abdominal pain, elevated serum transaminases, lipase and amylase levels, bone marrow depression, and ECG abnormalities, including nonspecific ST and T-wave changes and T-wave flattening or inversion. Weekly ECG monitoring is recommended during therapy. Rarely, there may be prolongation of QTc interval.

Pentamidine: It has been used in cases unresponsive to antimony compounds. However, resistance to this agent is now common and its use is associated with serious side effects such as hypotension, hypoglycemia, renal damage, injection abscess, and diabetes. Because of these drawbacks, it is no longer preferred at present.

Amphotericin B desoxycholate: It is 400 times more potent than antimony compounds against *Leishmania*. The main side effects include fever, chills, thrombophlebitis, hypokalemia, and renal failure. Liposomal amphotericin B is very safe and effective drug. It is the drug of choice for antimony-resistant kala-azar. Compared to conventional amphotericin, its concentration in reticuloendothelial cells is 10 times more, and toxicity 10 times less. The drug is costly. The cure rate is less in patients co-infected with HIV.

Paromomycin: It is an aminoglycoside with good activity against *Leishmania*, in doses of 15 mg of paromomycin sulfate (11 mg/kg base) intramuscularly for 21 days.

Miltefosine: It originally developed as an antineoplastic drug, has demonstrated a cure rate of >90% in visceral leishmaniasis. It was the first oral drug active against *Leishmania*. Gastrointestinal side effects are frequent but mild in nature. Miltefosine is contraindicated in pregnancy and in women of child-bearing age, unless women use appropriate contraception.

Sitamaquine: It is another oral drug undergoing phase 3 trials.

Aminosidine: It is an aminoglycoside similar to paromomycin, has also been found to be effective.

Current Treatment Guidelines

Currently liposomal amphotericin B is the drug of choice for the treatment of visceral leishmaniasis in regions with widespread resistance to antimony compounds. Even a single dose infusion of liposomal amphotericin B has shown cure rates equivalent to conventional amphotericin B infusions (15 alternate-day infusions). There is ever growing threat of development of resistance in parasites, and thus combination therapy is being tested now. A combination of drugs, including liposomal amphotericin B (single dose), miltefosine (7 days), and paromomycin (10 days) have been used successfully. Research is also being carried out on newer delivery systems of amphotericin B, such as nanoparticles and cochleates to improve drug efficacy.

In addition to specific therapy, patients may require broad-spectrum antibiotics for intercurrent infection, packed RBCs, and nutritional care. The treatment options for visceral leishmaniasis are summarized in **Table 14.14**.

Response to Treatment

Fever, spleen size, hemoglobin, blood cell counts, serum albumin, and body weight are useful indicators of progress. In most patients, the fever subsides within 7 days, blood counts and hemoglobin levels rise, the patient feels better, and spleen becomes smaller within 2 weeks. Parasitological cure should be documented at the end of therapy by splenic or bone marrow aspiration. As relapses are common in this disease, patient should be followed for at least 6 months before a long-term definite cure is pronounced. The spleen may take 6 months to 1 year to regress completely. Relapse is suggested by an increase of spleen size, a fall in hemoglobin levels and should be confirmed by the demonstration of parasites.

PREVENTION AND CONTROL

Early diagnosis, complete treatment, and vector control are the main components of the control program. Spread of the disease is prevented by controlling the source of infection and eradicating the vector. All infected patients should be identified and treated intensively. Patients with post-kala-azar dermal leishmaniasis are a rich reservoir of infection and pose a special public health problem.

Table 14.14 Treatment of Visceral Leishmaniasis

Drug	*Dose and duration*
Liposomal amphotericin B. Drug of first choice in antimony-resistant cases	3 mg/kg IV on days 1–5, and again on day 10
Amphotericin B deoxycholate	0.5–1.0 mg/kg IV on alternate days for 4 weeks
Miltefosine	2.5 mg/kg/day orally in 1–2 doses orally for 4–6 weeks
Paromomycin sulfate	15 mg/kg (11 mg/kg base) IM for 28 days
Pentamidine	4 mg/kg IV or IM three times a week for 8 weeks
Sodium antimony gluconate (sodium stibogluconate) or meglumine antimoniate. Drug resistance is common	20 mg/kg once a day IV or IM for 30 days

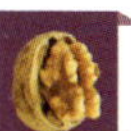

IN A NUTSHELL

Kala-azar

1. Kala-azar is caused by parasites of the genus *Leishmania,* which are transmitted to humans by female sandflies of the genus *Phlebotomus*.
2. The typical manifestations consist of high fever often with rigors, abdominal discomfort, emaciation, pallor, marked splenomegaly, and moderate hepatomegaly. There is no lymphadenopathy.
3. Diagnosis is based on demonstration of amastigotes in bone marrow or splenic aspirates. K39 antigen-based rapid diagnostic tests are increasingly being used for the diagnosis of kala-azar.
4. Liposomal amphotericin B or multidrug therapy is preferred treatment.

Bhattacharya SK, Choudhury TK. Visceral leishmaniasis in children. Ann Pediatr Child Health. 2020;8(4):1183.

Goyal V, Das VNR, Singh SN, et al. Long-term incidence of relapse and post-kala-azar dermal leishmaniasis after three different visceral leishmaniasis treatment regimens in Bihar, India. PLoS Negl Trop Dis. 2020;14(7):e0008429.

Prestes-Carneiro LE, Spir PRN, Fontanesi M, et al. Unusual manifestations of visceral leishmaniasis in children: a case series and its spatial dispersion in the western region of São Paulo state, Brazil. BMC Infect Dis. 2019;19:70.

Safavi M, Eshaghi H, Hajihassani Z. Visceral leishmaniasis: kala-azar. Diagn Cytopathol. 2021;49(3):446-8.

World Health Organization. (2023). Leishmaniasis. [online] Available from "https://www.who.int/news-room/fact-sheets/detail/leishmaniasis" https://www.who.int/news-room/fact-sheets/detail/leishmaniasis [Last accessed February, 2025].

14.16 Filariasis

PE 31.14

INTRODUCTION

Filarial worms are nematodes that reside in the lymphatics and subcutaneous tissues. Eight filarial species are known to infect humans, the most important being *Wuchereria bancrofti (W. bancrofti), Brugia malayi (B. malayi), Onchocerca volvulus,* and *Loa loa*. Their chief characteristics, geographical distribution, vectors responsible for transmission, and site of localization in the human body are depicted in **Table 14.15**.

Infections are transmitted by both larvae (carried by insects) and adult worms (carried in lymphatics or subcutaneous tissues of man). Adults give birth to microfilariae, which circulate in the blood or skin. Microfilariae are ingested again by the insect vector, where they develop into new infective larvae. Adult worms live for many years; microfilariae from 3 months to 2 years.

Lymphatic Filariasis

Lymphatic filariasis is caused by *W. bancrofti, B. malayi,* or *Brugia timori* (*B. timori*). These thread-like parasites reside in the lymphatic system of the host. Lymphatic filariasis remains a public health problem of considerable magnitude in many tropical countries of the world especially in Southern and South-East Asia, Pacific and Eastern Africa.

MAGNITUDE OF THE PROBLEM

Global

As of 2018, 51 million people were infected with lymphatic filariasis. In 2020, around 863 million people in 50 countries were living in endemic requiring preventive chemotherapy

Table 14.15 Characteristics of Filariae

Organism	*Distribution*	*Vector*	*Location*
Wuchereria bancrofti	India, China, Indonesia	Culex, Anopheles, Aedes	Lymphatics
Brugia malayi	India, China, Indonesia	Aedes, Mansonia, Coquillettidia	Lymphatics
Brugia timori	Indonesia	Anopheles	Lymphatics
Onchocerca volvulus	South and Central America, Africa	Blackfly (*Simulium*)	Skin, eye
Loa loa	West and Central Africa	Deerfly (*Chrysops*)	Subcutaneous
Mansonella ozzardi	South and Central America, Caribbean	Midges (*Culicoides*)	Undetermined
Mansonella perstans	Africa, South and Central America	Midges (*Culicoides*)	Body cavities
Mansonella streptocerca	West and Central Africa	Midges (*Culicoides*)	Subcutaneous

to stop the spread of infection. A decline of 74% has occurred in disease prevalence since the start of WHO's Global Programme to Eliminate Lymphatic Filariasis in 2000. Since 2000, >925 million people have received mass drug administration (MDA). In 2020, 863.2 million population required MDA, and 358.8 million people (41.6%) in 28 countries have been treated. MDA was implemented in a population of 451.3 million people living in the 1,164 implementation units (IUs). MDA was not implemented in 17 countries. A total of 86.3% of these IUs achieved effective coverage. **Figure 14.5** depicts a map of countries where lymphatic filariasis is endemic and status of mass drug administration in 2016.

India

India contributes to 40% of the global filariasis burden and 50% of the global population at risk of infection. Largest proportion of people receiving preventive therapy lives in India and it is one of the countries to achieve 100% coverage of MDA along with Maldives and Thailand in the Southeast Asia region. National Filaria Control Programme (NFCP) was launched in the country in 1955. MDA started as mass campaign from 2004. Initially single dose of diethylcarbamazine (DEC) only was given. In the year of 2007, dual therapy with DEC and albendazole started, which was replaced in 2018 by triple drug therapy (IDA), i.e., DEC + Albendazole + Ivermectin in selected districts. In India, 99.4% of the cases are caused by *Wuchereria bancrofti (W. bancrofti)*, whereas *B. malayi* is responsible for 0.6% of the problem, mostly in Kerala.

EPIDEMIOLOGY

Agent

Life cycle in mosquito: The mosquito ingests the microfilariae from man by biting and taking a blood meal. Mosquito serves as an intermediate host inside which the microfilariae develop into the larval stage. The larva undergoes transformation into various stages; namely, L1, L2, and L3. Only L3 larvae are infective. The duration of larval development is 10–14 days in case of *W. bancrofti* and 7–10 days in case of *B. malayi*, and *B. timori*. Again, when the mosquito takes a blood meal from another man, some of the infective larvae will escape and actively enter the human host. The microfilariae of *W. bancrofti* are 290 μm long.

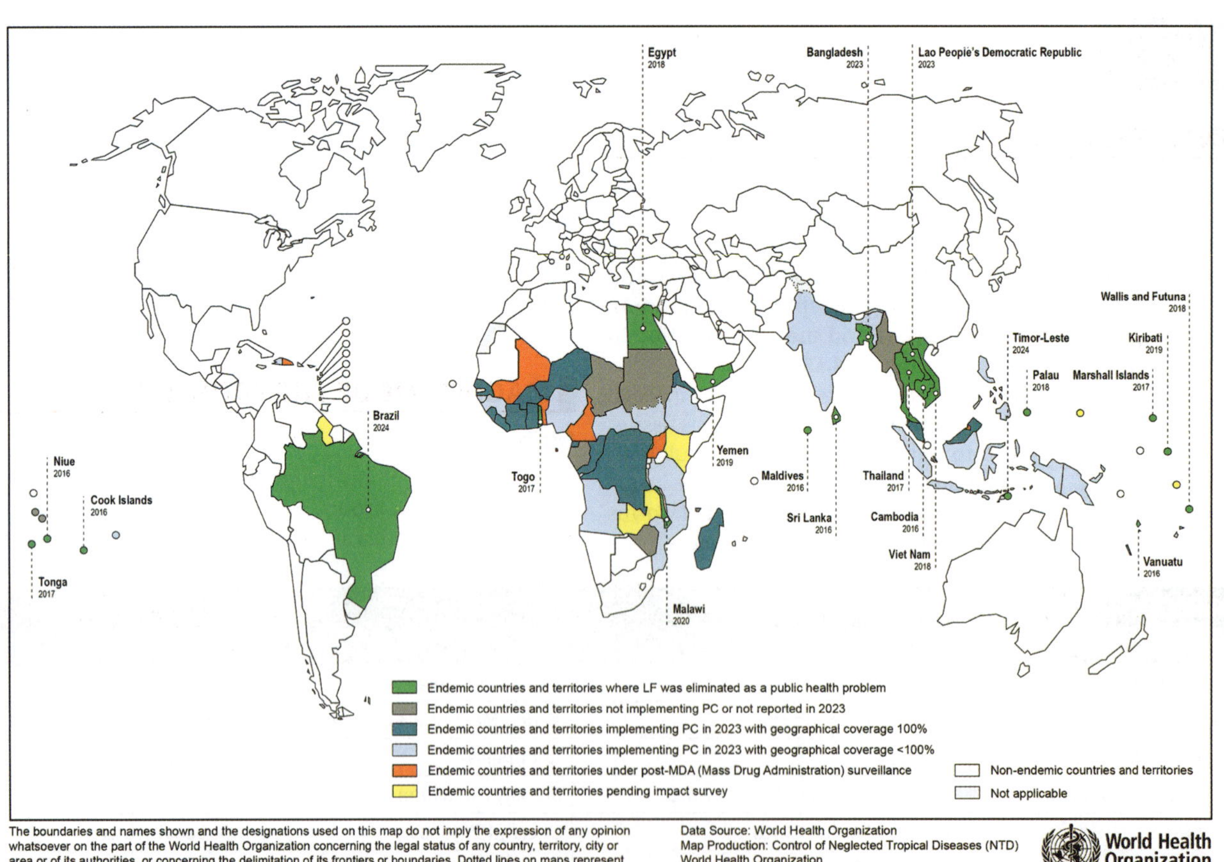

Fig. 14.5: Distribution of lymphatic filariasis and status of preventive chemotherapy in endemic countries, 2024

Source: WHO preventive chemotherapy joint reporting form. Annual country report 2024. https://www.who.int/images/default-source/maps/lf_2024.png?sfvrsn=73a1fd43_2

In humans L3 larva develops into L4 stage in the lymphatics and then to adult male or female worm. Female adult produces microfilariae which migrate to the bloodstream from the lymphatics. The time period from the entrance of L3 to the appearance of microfilariae in the peripheral blood is known as "pre-patent" period, and is estimated to be 3 months for *B. malayi* and 9 months for *Wuchereria*. An adult worm may live for 5–10 years in the lymphatic channels of man.

Periodicity

The microfilariae show a characteristic periodicity in the course of 24-hour cycle, i.e., they can be detected in the peripheral blood only during certain hours. *Wuchereria bancrofti* and *B. malayi* can be nocturnal, periodic or subperiodic. *B. timori* is by and large nocturnal periodic.

- ***Nocturnal periodic:*** The microfilarial density is markedly increased in the peripheral blood during night hours. This is the most common variant in India and mainly observed in urban slums and rural areas.
- ***Nocturnal subperiodic:*** Microfilariae can be found in peripheral blood at all hours with a slight increase in density during the night hours. This strain of *W. bancrofti* is found in Thailand and Vietnam.
- ***Diurnal subperiodic:*** Microfilariae are demonstrable at all times with a slight increase in density during the day-time. This is a rural strain occurring in the Eastern Pacific islands.

It is important to determine microfilarial periodicity in a given area to know the best time for blood samplings to detect microfilaremia.

Vectors

Wuchereria bancrofti is mainly transmitted in India through *C. quinquefasciatus*, and *B. malayi* through *Mansonia annulifera* and *Mansonia uniformis* mosquitoes. It is important that the local vectors and their biting behavior are established. Ideal measurement of the intensity of transmission of filarial infections is not available.

Reservoir

Wuchereria bancrofti in India has no animal reservoir. However, for *B. malayi,* reservoirs have been observed in cats, dogs, and monkeys. Prevalence and intensity of microfilaremia in human population are measured by microfilaria rate and microfilarial density.

- ***Microfilaria (MF) rate:*** It is expressed as the percentage of microfilaria positive people among the total number of people examined and indicates the prevalence status of a given area.
  - *Area of low endemicity:* MF rate <5%
  - *Area of medium endemicity:* MF rate 5–10%
  - *Area of high endemicity:* MF rate >10%
  - The average microfilariae rate in India has come down from 1.24 (2004) to 0.53 (2013) in recent years.
- ***Microfilarial density in the blood:*** It is the number of microfilariae per unit volume (20 mm^3) of blood sample. Microfilarial density has a better association with disease rate than microfilaria rate. Individuals with high microfilarial densities are most likely to be sources of reinfection for the treated community. Following mass therapy, a high number of such persons in the community indicates inadequate coverage of the area or drug refusal.

Mode of Spread

The infected mosquito bites man and deposits the larvae in the skin. These may remain in the skin or cross this barrier to enter the lymphatics. Congenital transmission of *W. bancrofti* from mother to child has also been reported.

Host Factors

Persons of all age groups are susceptible to an infection with filariae. However, the maximum incidence is observed in young adults. The youngest infant reported to be microfilaremic with *B. malayi* was 3.5-month-old.

Environmental Factors

Lymphatic filariasis, such as cholera and leprosy, is a disease associated with poverty, illiteracy, and insanitary living conditions. Environmental factors such as ineffective drainage and sewage systems help in collection of unwanted water, and promote mosquito breeding. The maximum life span of the mosquito is observed during the hot and humid climates resulting in high transmission rate.

CLINICAL FEATURES

Incubation period: Following the inoculation of infective larvae into man, a time lag of 8–16 months may elapse before the clinical symptoms appear.

Asymptomatic Amicrofilaremia

In most of the endemic areas, there will be a group among the population, who have been exposed to the infective larvae but do not show either microfilariae in the blood or clinical symptoms suggestive of filariasis. This group of population is referred to as asymptomatic amicrofilaremic.

Until and unless a reliable immunodiagnostic test is developed to determine whether these people have any evidence of exposure, it is impossible to find out whether this population is (*i*) free from infection; (*ii*) having subclinical infection; or (*iii*) having sub-threshold microfilaremia.

Asymptomatic Microfilaremia

Microfilariae appear in the peripheral blood following the "pre-patent" period. In several patients, these may persist in the blood without giving rise to any clinical symptoms for years together. These cases are also commonly observed in endemic areas and are referred to as having asymptomatic microfilaremia.

Symptomatic Microfilaremia (Acute Stage)

Acute clinical manifestations are characterized by recurrent attacks of fever, associated with inflammation of the lymph nodes (lymphadenitis) and lymph vessels (lymphangitis). Episodes can recur as frequently as 10 times a year, and they usually subside spontaneously over a period of 7–10 days. Lymph nodes are enlarged. Both upper and lower limbs are involved in bancroftian and brugian infections. Genital lymphatic involvement occurs exclusively in bancroftian infections.

Chronic Stage

Lymphadenitis may progress to lymphatic obstruction resulting in changes associated with elephantiasis. The chronic signs usually do not develop before the age of 25 years. In bancroftian filariasis, major chronic signs consist of hydrocele, chyluria, lymphedema and elephantiasis. In brugian filariasis, leg below the knee and arm below the elbow are characteristically involved. Lymphedema can be classified as follows:

- ***Grade I:*** Pitting edema, reversible on elevation.
- ***Grade II:*** Nonpitting edema, not reversible.
- ***Grade III:*** Elephantiasis, gross increase in volume with dermatosclerosis and papillomatous lesions. During stage III, microfilariae disappear from blood.

Occult Form (Tissue Phase)

Microfilariae are not found in the blood but may be found in the tissues. Tropical pulmonary eosinophilia is a classical example. Classical clinical manifestations are not present. Remnants of microfilaria surrounded by clumps of eosinophils are sometimes found in lungs. The syndrome is characterized by nocturnal paroxysmal cough, hypereosinophilia, increased bronchovascular markings, increased titers of filarial IgE antibodies, and a good therapeutic response to DEC.

Extrapulmonary symptoms may occur in 15% patients and consist of hepatosplenomegaly and lymphadenopathy. Untreated cases may result in restrictive lung disease, interstitial fibrosis, and respiratory failure.

DIAGNOSIS

Detection of Microfilariae

- Microfilariae can be detected in blood, urine (in chyluria), hydrocele fluid, or tissues. Examination of a *thick night blood film* is still the best method for fieldwork.
- ***DEC provocative test:*** It provokes the microfilariae in the lung capillaries to be released into peripheral circulation. It is used when night blood collection is impossible. One hundred milligram of DEC (2 mg/kg in children) is given by mouth during daytime, and peripheral blood is examined 35–40 minutes later. The test is much less sensitive as compared to night film method.
- ***Concentration techniques:*** Membrane filter concentration method is a very sensitive test for detecting low density microfilaremia. Venous samples of 1–10 mL are required. These are filtered using nucleopore membrane filters of 3–5 μm porosity. The filters are then dried, stained, and examined under the microscope.
- Microfilariae in urine or hydrocele fluid can be detected by centrifuging the sample and examining the sediment microscopically.

Detection of Adult Worm

It may be possible in biopsies of lymph nodes.

Lymphatic Imaging

Contrast lymphangiography carries the risk of lymphatic damage. Lymphoscintigraphy is another safe technique, which can demonstrate lymphatic abnormalities even in asymptomatic patients.

Immunodiagnosis

There is no universal diagnostic test that can provide most specific and sensitive information needed both for individual cases and population-based studies. Secondly, no clear-cut criteria exist to define the appropriate negative controls and significance of a positive test in an amicrofilaremic, asymptomatic resident of an endemic area. Lastly, ample information is not available on various antibody responses to the defined filarial antigens during the natural course of infection and effect of treatment on such responses. The research is progressing on both antigen and antibody detection assays. Some success has been achieved with monoclonal antibody-based assays to detect and quantify filarial antigens in serum, urine, and other body fluids in persons with lymphatic filariasis.

Serological tests, that would enable to (*a*) identify microfilaremic individuals; (*b*) detect all individuals with current active infections; or (*c*) quantify the adult worm burden prior to and following chemotherapy, will greatly facilitate filaria surveys and constitute invaluable tools to monitor the impact of control programs.

Recently, a rapid day blood immunochromatographic card test (ICT) for detection of infection has been found to be highly specific and more sensitive in India as compared to the night blood smear examination. Though costlier, it has the advantage of an on-the-spot day blood detection of parasite carriers in large numbers. The other newer diagnostics include Og4C3 antigen assay in human whole blood and sera and DNA probes for infection detection in man/vector.

Xenodiagnosis

After feeding on the suspected patients, the vector mosquitoes are dissected after 2 weeks and microfilaremia can be demonstrated. This may be useful in diagnosis of cases with low density microfilaremia.

TREATMENT Filariasis

Drugs

Diethylcarbamazine (DEC), ivermectin, and albendazole are the three main drugs for treatment of filariasis:

- *Diethylcarbamazine:* DEC has been the drug of choice for lymphatic filariasis for 5 decades, both at individual and community levels. DEC is active against adult worms, microfilariae, and stage L3, L4 larvae *in vivo*. Microfilariae of *W. bancrofti* in hydrocele fluid are not affected by DEC. DEC reduces the prevalence and incidence of adenolymphangitis, reduces frequency of attacks, and reduces the likelihood of developing chronic obstructive lesions. However, patients with large hydrocele or elephantiasis with deformities do not show any response to DEC. DEC is also the drug of choice for tropical pulmonary eosinophilia. Relapses are not uncommon following DEC therapy.

- *Ivermectin:* It is a macrolide antibiotic with a wide spectrum of activity against many nematodes. A single oral dose (200–400 µg/kg of body weight) has been found to be effective, but is associated with high recurrence rates (5–40%) after 6 months of treatment in bancroftian infections. For *B. malayi*, the effect is slow but sustained.

  Ivermectin and DEC regimens induce similar clearance of microfilaremia in bancroftian filariasis. However, the parasite clearance is much more sustained with DEC (for >6 months) in heavily infested individuals.
- *Albendazole* has also been shown to be having good filaricidal activity.

Treatment of Individual Cases

The goal is to destroy and eliminate the parasite, and reduce or prevent morbidity. Both albendazole and DEC have been shown to be effective in killing the adult-stage filarial parasites (necessary for complete cure of infection). The dose is 6 mg/kg body weight per day for 6 days a week for 2 weeks of 12 to a total doses of DEC. Repeated courses may be required for complete parasitic cure especially endemic areas. This should be accompanied with rigorous hygiene of the affected limbs, and measures to minimize super-infection and promote lymph flow.

Treatment of Community

The objectives are to (*a*) reduce morbidity by treating clinical cases of filariasis; (*b*) reduce transmission by treating people with microfilaremia; and (*c*) interrupt transmission and eliminate the parasite. The treatment is offered on mass or selective basis. Recent studies have shown that single doses of diethylcarbamazine (DEC) have the same long-term (1-year) effect in decreasing microfilaremia as the formerly-recommended 12-day regimens of DEC and, even more importantly, that the use of single doses of 2 drugs administered concurrently (optimally albendazole with DEC or ivermectin) are 99% effective in removing microfilariae from the blood for a full year after treatment. This therapeutic modality has facilitated the new efforts to eliminate lymphatic filariasis.

- *Mass treatment:* The treatment is given to all community members irrespective of whether they have microfilaremia or not except pregnant women, children <2 years and seriously ill patients. Single dose mass therapy has been found to be as effective as 12-day therapy as a public health intervention. However, very high (>85%) coverage is required to achieve interruption of transmission.
- *Selective treatment:* Only microfilaria positive persons or persons with clinical manifestations are treated after being selected by large scale clinical and blood film screening. Selective treatment is more suitable for low endemicity areas.
- *DEC medicated salt:* Common salt medicated with DEC (1–4 g of DEC/kg of salt) was used in Lakshadweep islands. It eliminated 90% of circulating microfilaria in 80% of initial carriers and reduced the disease rate by 20%. Trials in Puducherry, Kerala, and Andhra Pradesh have also been successful. It has led to a belief that administration of DEC medicated salt is a simple, rapid, safe, inexpensive, efficient prophylactic, and practical tool for the filariasis control. Concurrent medication of salt with DEC and iodine has no adverse effects.

PREVENTION AND CONTROL

The control programs for lymphatic filariasis are aimed at (*a*) decreasing morbidity; (*b*) reducing transmission; and (*c*) interrupting the transmission cycle.

Reduction of Morbidity

The morbidity can be reduced by recognizing clinical cases of filariasis and treating them. This will require a team whose members are well versed with clinical manifestation of this disease. DEC has to be made available through the primary healthcare system.

Reducing Transmission

Methods to reduce transmission may aim at the parasite or at the vector. Parasite control can be achieved with mass or selective DEC treatment, medication of salt with DEC, or annual single dose DEC treatment with or without albendazole/ivermectin. Vector control may be achieved by physical, chemical or biological means, and is aimed at either the adult mosquito or its larvae. Determine the breeding site, feeding habits, biting densities, resting habits and infection and infectivity rates pertaining to the concerned mosquito.

- ***Antilarval measures:*** These consists of insecticide sprays (chlorpyrifos or methoprene for *Culex quinquefasciatus*), breeding of larvivorous fish (*Gambusia* and *Poecilia*), and use of microbial agents (*Bacillus sphaericus* 1593; which produces a potent insecticidal exotoxin, effective against larvae of *Culex*). Environmental modification may include proper drainage, conversion of swamp lands to fields, filling of land depressions, removal of aquatic plants, and use of buoyant polystyrene balls in pit latrines to prevent access of Culex to the water for oviposition.
- ***Antiadult measures:*** House spraying of insecticides is not that effective for control of filariasis, because many important vectors do not rest indoors. Vector control by insecticide spraying requires long efforts and is less cost-beneficial against filariasis as compared to malaria. Moreover, adult *Culex quinquefasciatus* is widely resistant to organochlorine compounds.
- ***Decreasing contact between vector and human population:*** The frequency of contact can be reduced by providing better housing, use of mosquito nets and screens, repellent coils, and proper clothing and covering of breeding sites. Mosquito nets with impregnated insecticide (permethrin or deltamethrin) can be used.

Interrupting Transmission

This should be the ultimate and ideal goal. This may not become feasible due to longevity of the adult worms and limited resources of manpower and finance in most endemic countries. Once accomplished, the need for continuing maintenance of control program can be avoided.

Community Involvement

Community must be motivated to take part in control of filariasis. This includes imparting of adequate education on the nature of the disease and the effectiveness of DEC in reducing transmission and morbidity. The individuals should be taught to self-protect from mosquito bites; and at the same time strive for better environmental sanitation to reduce mosquito breeding sites.

PROGRAM TO ELIMINATE LYMPHATIC FILARIASIS

The Global Program to Eliminate Lymphatic Filariasis (GPELF) was launched by WHO in 2000 with the goal of eliminating lymphatic filariasis as a public health problem by the year 2020. The twofold strategy is—interrupting transmission using combinations of two medicines delivered to entire populations at risk, a strategy known as mass drug administration (MDA) and alleviating suffering and disability by introducing basic measures, such as improved hygiene and skin care, to people with lymphedema and by providing surgery for men with hydrocele. GPELF is now part of a comprehensive program of Neglected Tropical Diseases (NTD) control efforts, in which preventive chemotherapy, vector control, and morbidity management are increasingly integrated and delivered as multi-intervention packages at the global, national, and local levels.

In most countries, the program is based on once-yearly administration of single doses of two drugs given together: albendazole (400 mg) plus either diethylcarbamazine (6 mg/kg) or ivermectin (200 μg/kg), the latter in areas where either onchocerciasis or loiasis is also endemic. This yearly, single-dose treatment has to be carried out for at least 5 years. The number of rounds required to reduce the prevalence of microfilaremia to <1% appears to depend on three key factors: baseline prevalence of microfilaremia, the population's compliance with MDA, and the efficiency of the vector (as well as the presence of vector-control measures). In areas with intense transmission and less compliance, a longer duration of MDA may be required.

An alternative community-wide regimen with equal effectiveness is the use of common table/cooking salt fortified with DEC in the endemic region for a period of 1 year. This should be associated with appropriate community education programs to increase awareness.

Strategy in India

The National Health Policy 2002 aimed at elimination of lymphatic filariasis by 2015. The strategy for achieving the goal of elimination was by annual mass drug administration of DEC (single dose) for 5 years or more to the population excluding children <2 years, pregnant women, and seriously ill persons in affected areas to interrupt transmission of disease. Annual mass drug administration with single dose of DEC was launched as National Filaria Day on 5th June, 2004. In India, the at-risk population is 600 million. In 2009, MDA with DEC and albendazole was delivered in all endemic districts of India. In 2018 triple drug therapy (IDA), i.e., DEC + Albendazole + Ivermectin is launched initially in five selected districts.

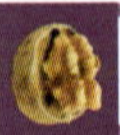

IN A NUTSHELL

Filariasis

1. Lymphatic filariasis is a parasitic infection caused by filarial worms.
2. Filarial worms are the nematodes that reside inside the lymphatic system of the body.
3. The disease spreads from person-to-person by mosquito bites.
4. The infection may remain asymptomatic or present with recurrent attacks of fever, lymphadenitis, and lymphangitis. Chronic stage is characterized by lymphedema and hydrocele. Tropical eosinophilia may occur due to involvement of lungs.
5. Diagnosis is made by detection of microfilariae in peripheral blood smear.
6. Diethylcarbamazine (DEC) is the drug of choice for filariasis.
7. Preventive measures include prevention of mosquito bite and mass drug administration of DEC, albendazole and/ivermectin.

Local Burden of Disease 2019 Neglected Tropical Diseases Collaborators. The global distribution of lymphatic filariasis, 2000-18: a geospatial analysis [published correction appears in Lancet Glob Health. 2021;9(10):e1371]. Lancet Glob Health. 2020;8(9):e1186-94.

Modi A, Vaishnav KG, Kothiya K, et al. Lymphatic filariasis elimination endgame in an urban Indian setting: the roles of surveillance and residual microfilaremia after mass drug administration. Infect Dis Poverty. 2021;10(1):73.

Paramanik M, Sarkar N, Chandra G. Awareness and impact of Lymphatic Filariasis among school children in rural endemic areas of West Bengal, India. J Vector Borne Dis. 2020;57(4):295-300.

Sawers L, Stillwaggon E. Economic costs and benefits of community-based lymphedema-management programs for lymphatic filariasis in India. Am J Trop Med Hyg. 2020;103(1):295-302.

World Health Organization. (2023). Lymphatic Filariasis Factsheet. [online] Available from https://www.who.int/news-room/fact-sheets/detail/lymphatic-filariasis [Last accessed February, 2025].

14.17 Amebiasis *PE 31.14*

INTRODUCTION

Amebiasis is caused by the protozoa *Entamoeba histolytica (E. histolytica)*, and usually presents with dysentery or diarrhea. The ameba may spread to various organs, the most common being the liver where it manifests as amebic liver abscess. *E. histolytica* can be differentiated antigenically and by molecular methods from *E. dispar*, which is nonpathogenic and responsible only for asymptomatic infection.

EPIDEMIOLOGY

Entamoeba histolytica has a worldwide distribution and is endemic in developing countries due to low socioeconomic conditions. It is the third leading cause of parasitic death in the world after malaria and schistosomiasis. It is estimated that approximately 10% of the world's population; i.e., 600 million people are infected, with an annual mortality of 40,000–110,000.

Prevalence rates vary widely with the population studied, from around 1% in the industrialized nations to 50–80% in the tropics. The exact number of persons infected by pathogenic strains is still not clear but from the data available from a few such reports, the asymptomatic carriage seems to predominate with a prevalence of 10% and only 1% for pathogenic strains. In India, the prevalence rates vary from 5 to 50% depending upon the population and geographical region.

Mode of Spread

The infection is transmitted by ingestion of food or water contaminated with fecal material containing cysts of *Entamoeba*. The source of contamination may be the food handlers or flies. Cysts can remain viable and infective in water and feces for several days. Sexual transmission is also reported.

Young, immunocompromised, and malnourished children, and those receiving steroids are at a higher risk of severe *E. histolytica* infection. Other factors contributing to increased transmission include low socioeconomic status, overcrowding, lack of safe water supply, and poor sanitation.

ETIOLOGY

Entamoeba histolytica exists in nature in two forms: Cyst or a trophozoite **(Figs. 14.6A and B)**. Cysts (10–18 μm) are oval or round, asymmetrical with four nuclei. They are easily destroyed by most disinfectants and by heating to 55°C but may survive chlorination of water and in water at low temperature. Cyst is the infective stage of the parasite. Asymptomatic human cyst carriers are the principal reservoir of infection. There is no animal reservoir.

PATHOGENESIS

Following ingestion, cyst hatches in the small intestine to produce eight trophozoites. Trophozoites colonize and invade the colonic mucosa where they multiply and spread laterally underneath the intestinal epithelium producing characteristic "flask-shaped or teardrop ulcers". These lesions are commonly found in cecum, transverse colon, and sigmoid colon. There is little local inflammatory response. Some ameba trophozoites become cyst and are passed in the stool to survive for weeks in a moist environment. On the other hand, some trophozoites invade the intestinal mucosa and spread *via* bloodstream to the liver, lung, and brain.

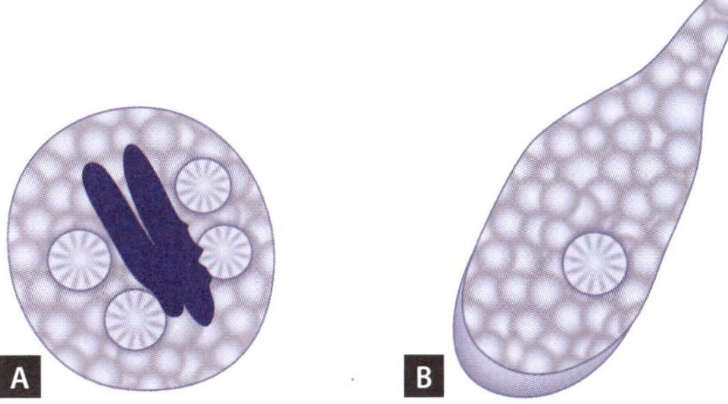

Figs. 14.6A and B: *Entamoeba histolytica:* (A) Cyst; (B) Trophozoite

Extraintestinal Complications

They arise from spread of infection through portal circulation. Amebic liver abscess develops because of toxin release and hepatocyte damage. It is seen more frequently in the right lobe of the liver (posterosuperior part); 5–20% have abscess in the left lobe. Single liver abscess is found in 95% of instances. Its contents are chocolate-colored and viscid (described as anchovy-sauce appearance), usually sterile, and contain no neutrophils. Amebae are located at the periphery of abscess. The abscess may regress, rupture, or disseminate. Transdiaphragmatic rupture of liver abscess into the pleural space may result in amebic empyema and pulmonary amebiasis. The abscess may also rupture into the peritoneum (2–5%), or pericardial cavity (<1%).

CLINICAL FEATURES

Entamoeba histolytica infection is asymptomatic in 90% of patients. About 4–10% of persons infected with *E. histolytica* develop amebic colitis; while <1% develop disseminated disease, including amebic liver abscess.

Intestinal Disease (Amebic Colitis)

Incubation period for symptomatic disease varies from 2 weeks to months. Acute intestinal amebiasis presents with colicky abdominal pain, tenesmus, and frequent loose stools containing mucus and blood. The stool may be positive for occult blood. Fever is seen in only one-third of patients and constitutional symptoms are rare. Examination may reveal diffuse tenderness in the cecal or rectosigmoid junction areas. The course of illness may be protracted lasting for weeks or even months. Rarely, a reactive collection of edematous granulation and fibrous tissue called an ameboma can grow into the lumen, causing pain, obstruction and, possibly, intussusception. Chronic amebiasis presents with intermittent diarrhea, which is often followed by constipation due to spasm of the large intestines, fatigue, and weight loss. Toxic megacolon, pneumatosis coli (intramural air), and peritonitis can also occur. Acute amebic dysentery should be differentiated from that caused by *Shigella, Salmonella, Campylobacter, E. coli* and *Yersinia*.

Amebic liver abscess develops in <1% of infected persons, often months to years after exposure. A past history of amebic dysentery is forthcoming in only 20% of patients and only 10% have concomitant intestinal symptoms. The child presents with high fever with chills and rigors, abdominal pain, distension and tender hepatomegaly, and appears toxic. Pain in the upper abdomen is intense and radiates to the shoulder. Jaundice is uncommon and observed in only 10–15% cases.

Abscess may rupture into pleural space, peritoneum, and pericardium, requiring emergency drainage. Mortality in children in ruptured abscess can be up to 25%.

INVESTIGATIONS

The amebic liver abscess needs to be differentiated from pyogenic liver abscess, hepatoma, and hydatid cyst of the liver.

Parasite detection: Microscopic examination of formed stool for cysts; or diarrheal stool for trophozoites is necessary for the diagnosis of intestinal infection with *E. histolytica*. Diarrheal stools must be examined within 1 hour of collection to look for motility of trophozoites. Stool microscopy cannot distinguish *E. histolytica* from *E. dispar* infection, unless phagocytosed erythrocytes are seen in trophozoites (seen in *E. histolytica*). Stool antigen testing may also distinguish the two species.

A complete examination of stool for cysts includes wet-mount in saline, an iodine-stained wet mount, and a fixed trichrome-stained preparation. These preparations not only delineate cyst morphology but also distinguish bacillary from amebic dysentery. At least three stool specimens taken on consecutive days should be examined to exclude amebic infection of the intestines, since excretion of cysts may be intermittent. However, detection of amebic cysts, even with associated gastrointestinal symptoms does not necessarily indicate acute infection.

Stool contains plenty of erythrocytes but a few leukocytes in patients with amebic colitis unlike bacillary dysentery where the inflammatory cells especially polymorphonuclear cells are replete.

Sigmoidoscopy followed by aspiration of mucosal lesions or biopsy is valuable in symptomatic sick patients, where other tests fail to provide conclusive evidence. It is difficult to demonstrate the amebae in the liver aspirate.

Liver aspirate: The aspirate is usually sterile on culture. Trophozoites may be present in the aspirate and can be demonstrated only from the wall of the abscess.

Serology: In extraintestinal amebiasis and *invasive* amebiasis, antibody detection by ELISA is the most sensitive test. Indirect hemagglutination (IHA) test may be done for invasive intestinal disease or liver abscess. IHA is usually negative in asymptomatic carriers. Serological response as detected by CIE or ELISA becomes negative 6–12 months after infection. IHA, on the other hand, may stay positive for as long as 10 years following complete recovery.

Radiology: Chest radiograph in case of a liver abscess shows elevated diaphragm and pleural reaction on the *right* side in a child with liver abscess. Ultrasound, CT, MRI, or isotope scan can localize the exact site of abscess.

Others: Leukocytosis, anemia, high ESR, and elevated alkaline *phosphatase* are common in amebic liver abscess. There is no eosinophilia in invasive disease.

TREATMENT Amebiasis

Due to the possibility of its invasive nature and severe extraintestinal manifestations, all children with *E. histolytica* infection, whether symptomatic or not, should be treated.

- *Luminal amebicides*, such as diloxanide furoate and iodoquinol act on only those organisms that are present in the intestinal lumen.
- *Tissue amebicides*, such as metronidazole, tinidazole, chloroquine, and dehydroemetine are effective in the treatment of invasive amebiasis but are less effective for luminal clearance.

A combination of a luminal and a tissue amebicide is thus advocated for complete parasite clearance in invasive disease. Metronidazole is the most popular drug for management of both intestinal and extraintestinal forms of amebiasis and till date, there is no evidence of resistance against this agent.

Invasive Amebiasis

Both intestinal and extraintestinal amebiasis should be treated initially with a tissue amebicide such as (*a*) oral metronidazole 35–50 mg/kg/day in three divided doses for 7–10 days; or (*b*) tinidazole 50 mg/kg/day once daily for 3–5 days. Tinidazole is as efficacious as metronidazole but the treatment duration is shorter with fewer adverse effects. Following this, all children should be given a course of luminal amebicide:

(*a*) Diloxanide furoate 20 mg/kg/day in three divided doses for 7 days; or (*b*) paromomycin 25–35 mg/kg/day in three divided doses for 7 days; or (*c*) iodoquinol 30–40 mg/kg/day in three divided doses for 20 days. Either of paromomycin, diloxanide furoate, or iodoquinol may be used to treat asymptomatic carriers, given in the regimen same as for invasive disease. Reinfection is quite common, even after complete cure.

- For cases of *Fulminant amebic colitis*, therapy with dehydroemetine, 1 mg/kg/day subcutaneously or IM, may be instituted. Broad-spectrum antibiotics may also be needed.
- Intestinal perforation or ruptured amebic liver abscess or toxic megacolon may warrant surgical intervention.

Amebic Liver Abscess

It should also be treated with the same regime as advocated for invasive amebiasis, above. Image-guided aspiration is indicated in (*i*) large abscess; (*ii*) left lobe abscess; (*iii*) impending rupture of abscess; or (*iv*) failure to improve after 4–6 days of treatment with amebicidal drugs. Percutaneous drainage of abscess under USG guidance is preferred over open surgical drainage. Chloroquine may be a useful additive drug as it concentrates in liver. Abscess cavity resolves slowly over a period of several months.

PREVENTION

Prevention involves avoiding fecal contamination of food and water and adopting good handwashing technique. Boiling and purification of drinking water by filtration are important preventive measures. The use of night soil (human feces) for fertilization of crops should be avoided. No prophylactic drug or vaccine is available.

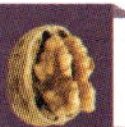

IN A NUTSHELL

Amebiasis

1. Amebiasis [caused by *Entamoeba histolytica (E. histolytica)]* is spread by fecal-oral route.
2. Clinical spectrum may vary from asymptomatic cyst carriers, explosive diarrhea, dysentery, subacute protracted course with GI symptoms, to persistent diarrhea.
3. Diagnosis is by stool microscopy of at least three samples.
4. Treatment of choice for amebiasis is metronidazole.
5. *E. histolytica* may spread hematogenously to result in liver abscess.

Centers for Disease Control and Prevention (CDC). CDC Yellow Book 2024: Health Information for International Travel. New York: Oxford University Press, 2023. available from https://wwwnc.cdc.gov/travel/yellowbook/2024/infections-diseases/amebiasis. [Last accessed, February 2025].

Gonzales MLM, Dans LF, Sio-Aguilar J. Antiamoebic drugs for treating amoebic colitis. Cochrane Database Syst Rev. 2019;1(1):CD006085.

Gupta S, Smith L, Diakiw A. Amebiasis and amebic liver abscess in children. Pediatr Clin North Am. 2022;69(1):79-97.

Lal SB, Venkatesh V, Kumar A, et al. Liver Abscess in children-experience from a single tertiary care center of North India: etiology, clinical profile and predictors of complications. Pediatr Infect Dis J. 2021;40(5):e179-84.

Li J, Cui Z, Li X, et al. Review of zoonotic amebiasis: epidemiology, clinical signs, diagnosis, treatment, prevention and control. Res Vet Sci. 2021;136:174-81.

14.18 Giardiasis *PE 31.14*

INTRODUCTION

Giardia lamblia (also known as *G. intestinalis* or *G. duodenalis)* is an important flagellated protozoan enteropathogen of humans. It affects 2.5 million people annually, and is the most common parasite infection of humans worldwide. The clinical manifestations range from asymptomatic carrier state to acute and persistent diarrhea, and malabsorption syndrome. Children appear to be more severely affected than adults. Humoral immunodeficiency (such as X-linked agammaglobulinemia and common variable immune deficiency) is associated with chronic *Giardia* infection. Malnourished and children with cystic fibrosis are particularly predisposed to giardiasis. Breast milk contains glycoconjugates and secretory IgA that provide protection against giardiasis.

EPIDEMIOLOGY

Giardiasis is spread by fecal-oral contamination, the prevalence being higher in populations with poor sanitation, close contact, and oral-anal sexual practices. The disease is commonly water-borne because *Giardia* is resistant to the chlorine levels in normal tap water. Boiling may inactivate the cyst. Food-borne transmission is rare but can occur with ingestion of raw or undercooked foods.

Reservoir: Man and contaminated water supply remain the major reservoirs of *Giardia*.

ETIOLOGY

The parasite exists in the form of trophozoites (10–20 mm × 5–15 mm) or cysts (8–10 mm) **(Figs. 14.7A and B)**. Trophozoites colonize the proximal small intestine. Cysts are excreted in the feces; these are the infective stage of the parasite.

The life cycle of *Giardia* consists of two stages—the feco-orally transmitted cyst and the disease-causing trophozoite. Cysts are passed in a host's feces, remaining viable in a moist

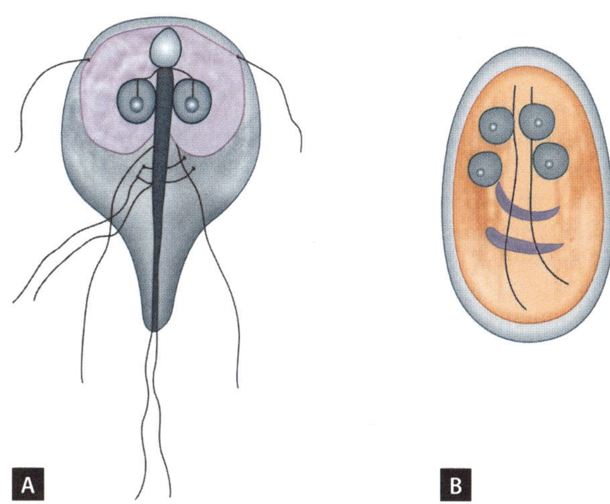

Figs. 14.7A and B: *Giardia lamblia:* (A) Trophozoite; (B) Cyst

environment for months. Ingestion of at least 10–25 cysts can cause infection in humans. When a new host consumes a cyst, the host's acidic stomach environment stimulates excystation. Each cyst produces two trophozoites. These trophozoites migrate to the duodenum and proximal jejunum, where they attach to the mucosal wall by means of a ventral adhesive disk and replicate by binary fission.

PATHOGENESIS

Growth of trophozoites is promoted by bile, glucose, and relative hypoxia. The trophozoites colonize the duodenum and proximal jejunum of the host. Each trophozoite has four pairs of flagella and two nuclei. The trophozoites carry a ventral disk on its concave surface, which enables their attachment to the intestinal wall. The powerful sucking disk of the trophozoite causes mechanical irritation and damage to the microvilli of the small bowel mucosa resulting in deficiency of brush border enzyme activities. As the detached trophozoites pass through the intestine, they undergo encystations to form oval cysts containing four nuclei. Cysts pass in stools of infected persons and can remain viable for up to 2 months in soil. Unlike amebiasis, there are no invasive or locally destructive lesions.

Parenchymal involvement of the pancreas has been incriminated for the reported steatorrhea and decreased trypsin activity. In other cases, fat malabsorption observed in giardiasis is attributed to bacterial overgrowth in the duodenum and upper jejunum and bile salt deconjugation liberating free bile acids. Immunological studies have shown decreased levels of secretory IgA in duodenal aspirates and depressed T-cell function.

CLINICAL FEATURES

Asymptomatic carriage is the most common form of infection.

In symptomatic cases, incubation period after ingestion of cysts is 1–2 weeks.

In acute infections, there may be a sudden onset of explosive watery (nonbloody) foul smelling diarrhea along with abdominal distension, flatulence, nausea, anorexia, and epigastric cramps. There is no blood or mucus in stools. The illness may last 3 or 4 days and is usually self-limiting in normal immunocompetent children.

Some infections may have a *subacute onset* with a protracted course, with persistent or recurrent mild to moderate symptoms such as brief episodes of loose foul smelling stools accompanied by flatus and abdominal distension. Between exacerbations, the stools are mushy or there may be constipation. Abnormal stool pattern may alternate with normal bowel movements. Symptoms last for 2–4 weeks.

Thirty to fifty percent children develop *persistent diarrhea*. Children with chronic giardiasis show lactose malabsorption, steatorrhea, iron deficiency anemia, and failure to thrive. Unlike *E. histolytica* infection, there is no extraintestinal spread of infection. Chronic giardiasis can cause growth failure and stunting. Repeated *Giardia* infections can lead to cognitive impairment.

Rarely, patients with giardiasis also present with reactive arthritis or asymmetric synovitis, usually of the lower extremities. Rashes and urticaria may be present as part of a hypersensitivity reaction.

INVESTIGATIONS

Diagnosis is made by examining diarrheal stools for trophozoites or cysts. At least three specimens of stools collected on alternate days (detection rate 90%) are examined microscopically, because the multiplication and passage of the giardial cysts is often intermittent. Sensitivity of a single stool examination is only 50%. Stool does not contain blood or leukocytes. Trophozoites are usually seen only in watery diarrhea but can also be detected by endoscopic brush cytology or intestinal biopsy. A duodenal aspirate or biopsy may yield high concentration of *Giardia*. Biopsy of the duodenum is not routinely recommended but may be done in patients with clinically suspected giardiasis, negative stool tests, negative duodenal fluid aspirate, absent secretory IgA level, hypogammaglobulinemia or chlorhydria. Another test may be recommended, if the microscopic examination of stool is negative, *viz.*, the "String test". A weighted piece of string is swallowed till it reaches the duodenum. The trophozoites adhere to the string and may be visualized microscopically after withdrawal of the string.

Stool enzyme immunoassay or direct immunofluorescence tests for *Giardia* are the preferred tests for diagnosis. Blood cell counts are normal. There is no eosinophilia as there is no tissue invasion.

TREATMENT Giardiasis

All symptomatic cases—acute and persistent diarrhea, failure to thrive, and malabsorption syndrome—require drug treatment. Asymptomatic cyst carriers require no therapy except for control of outbreaks. The drug of choice may be tinidazole or nitazoxanide. Tinidazole has very high efficacy (>90%) and need for only a single-dose therapy, while nitazoxanide has fewer side effects. A cheaper alternative may be metronidazole. Second-line alternatives include furazolidone, albendazole, and quinacrine. The treatment of giardiasis is given in **Box 14.7**.

Box 14.7 Treatment of Giardiasis

A. *First-line therapy*
   1. *Tinidazole:* >3 years, 50 mg/kg, single dose, oral
   2. *Nitazoxanide:*
      - *1–3 years:* 100 mg BD for 3 days, oral
      - *4–11 years:* 200 mg BD for 3 days, oral
      - *>12 years:* 500 mg BD for 3 days, oral
   3. *Metronidazole:* 15 mg/kg/day in 3 divided doses for 5–7 days

B. *Second-line therapy*
   1. *Albendazole:* >6 years—400 mg once a day for 5 days
   2. *Furazolidone:* 6 mg/kg/day in four divided doses for 10 days
   3. *Quinacrine:* 6 mg/kg/day in 3 divided doses for 5 days

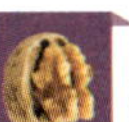

IN A NUTSHELL

Giardiasis

1. Giardiasis is caused by a protozoan *Giardia lamblia.*
2. The clinical manifestations range from asymptomatic carrier state to acute and persistent diarrhea, and malabsorption syndrome.
3. Giardiasis is spread by feco-oral contamination, the prevalence being higher in populations with poor sanitation, close contact, and oral-anal sexual practices.
4. Diagnosis is made by examining diarrheal stools for trophozoites or cysts.
5. The drug of choice is tinidazole or nitazoxanide.

Benedict K, Roellig D. Giardiasis. CDC Yellow Book 2024: Travel-Associated Infections & Diseases [online]. Available from https://wwwnc.cdc.gov/travel/yellowbook/2024/infections-diseases/giardiasis. [Last accessed, February 2025].
Leung AKC, Leung AAM, Wong AHC, et al. Giardiasis: an overview. Recent Pat Inflamm Allergy Drug Discov. 2019;13(2):134-43.
Mmbaga BT, Houpt ER. Cryptosporidium and giardia infections in children: a review. Pediatr Clin North Am. 2017;64(4):837-50.
Tejman-Yarden N, Eckmann L. New approaches to the treatment of giardiasis. Curr Opin Infect Dis. 2011;24(11):451-6.

14.19 Cryptosporidiosis

PE 31.14

INTRODUCTION

Cryptosporidium parvum causes cryptosporidiosis, primarily presenting as watery diarrhea. Children <2 years and immunocompromised children, especially AIDS and HIV-infected children are prone to this infection. The parasite is resistant to chlorination.

The infection is acquired by feco-oral route through ingestion of oocysts. The oocysts excyst in the small intestine where the sporozoites are released. Each oocyst releases four sporozoites. Sporozoites invade the jejunum.

CLINICAL FEATURES

The infection presents with nonbloody watery diarrhea following an incubation period of 2–12 days. Vomiting may be seen in >80% of infected children. Fever occurs in about 50% of infected children. In immunocompetent persons, the disease is self-limiting, though oocysts may be shed for months. In immunocompromised patients, severe constitutional symptoms and affection of the biliary tract and pancreas may occur.

DIAGNOSIS

Infection is detected by microscopic examination of stool using modified acid-fast staining wherein the oocysts appear as small, spherical bodies (2–6 mm). At least three stool samples should be examined as shedding of oocysts is intermittent. However, ELISA is the investigation of choice. Biopsy of the intestine may reveal *Cryptosporidium* organisms in the microvillus border especially in the jejunum. Histopathology of the intestine reveals villus atrophy, epithelial flattening, and inflammation of the lamina propria.

TREATMENT Cryptosporidiosis

Treatment includes adequate rehydration along with nitazoxanide given for 3 days duration. The dose is as follows: 1–3 years: 100 mg BD, PO; 4–11 years: 200 mg BD, PO; and ≥12 years: 500 mg BD, PO.

Carter BL, Stiff RE, Elwin K, et al. Health sequelae of human cryptosporidiosis: a 12-month prospective follow-up study. Eur J Clin Microbiol Infect Dis. 2019;38(9):1709-17.
Chalmers RM, Alexander C. Defining the diagnosis of cryptosporidiosis. Lancet Infect Dis. 2021;21(5):589-90.
Hlavsa M, Roellig D. Cryptosporidiosis. CDC Yellow Book 2024. Travel-Associated Infections & Diseases [online]. Available from https://wwwnc.cdc.gov/travel/yellowbook/2024/infections-diseases/cryptosporidiosis. [Last accessed, February 2025].
Wang B, Castellanos-Gonzalez A, White AC Jr. Novel drug targets for treatment of cryptosporidiosis. Expert Opin Ther Targets. 2020;24(9):915-22.

14.20 Helminthic Infestations and Ascariasis

PE 31.14

INTRODUCTION

Intestinal parasites are of two main types, *viz.*, single-cell protozoa and multicellular metazoan called helminths (worms). These are usually transmitted by feco-oral route. Rarely, they may enter the human body by penetrating through skin or sexual route. In their adult form, the helminths cannot multiply in the human body, while protozoa can multiply inside the human body.

Box 14.8	Common Intestinal Parasitic Infections and Infestations

Protozoa
- *Entamoeba histolytica*, E. dispar*, Giardia lamblia, Cryptosporidium parvum, Isospora belli,* and *Cyclospora*

Helminths
- *Nematodes (soil transmitted helminths)*
  - *Type 1:* Direct transmission by infective ova: *Enterobius vermicularis*, Trichuris trichiura**
  - *Type 2:* Ova infective after development in soil: *Ascaris Lumbricoides*
  - *Type 3:* Penetration of skin: *Ancylostoma duodenale, Necator Americanus,* and *Strongyloides stercoralis*
- *Trematodes: Fasciolopsis buski, Echinostoma* spp., and *Heterophyses heterophyes*
- *Cestodes: Taenia saginata* (beef tapeworm), and *Taenia solium* (pork tapeworm)

*Except these parasites (which inhabit the large intestine), and all others inhabit small intestine

- Common intestinal protozoa include *Giardia, Entamoeba, Cryptosporidium, Isospora,* and *Cyclospora.*
- Helminths may be classified as *nematodes* (roundworms), *trematodes* (flatworms), and *cestodes* (tapeworms). Common intestinal helminths are listed in **Box 14.8**.

Parasites can live within the intestines for years without causing any symptoms or manifest with abdominal pain, diarrhea, dysentery, weight loss, malabsorption, rash or perianal itching, nausea, vomiting, bloating, belching, vaginitis, or passage of worms in stool. Uncommon symptoms may include joint pain, chest pain, cough, memory loss or mental symptoms, and organ infiltration.

ASCARIASIS (ROUNDWORM)

Ascariasis is the most common human helminthic infection, infecting about 1.3 billion and causing 60,000 deaths annually. Infection is most prevalent in tropical and subtropical climates due to lack of sanitary facilities or the use of human feces as fertilizer. Preschool children are most vulnerable to infection due to their hand to mouth behavior. Infection may also be acquired through ingestion of contaminated fruits and vegetables. Most infected individuals are asymptomatic due to low worm load. Clinical manifestations occur due to pulmonary hypersensitivity and intestinal complications.

PATHOGENESIS

Ascaris lumbricoides causes the disease. Infection is acquired through ingestion of embryonated eggs. Larvae hatch in the small intestine, invade the intestinal mucosa, migrate to the lungs *via* the venous circulation, break into the alveoli, ascend through bronchi and trachea, and return via swallowing to the small intestine, where they develop into adult worms. After an interval of 2–3 months, female worms start producing eggs. A gravid female can produce up to 200,000 eggs a day, which pass with the feces. Under favorable environmental conditions, eggs embryonate and become infective after 5–10 days. Ascaris eggs are remarkably resistant to environmental stresses and can remain infective for several years.

The lifespan of adult worms is 1–2 years. Man is the only reservoir of infection.

CLINICAL FEATURES

Symptoms may be produced by migration of larvae through lungs (*pulmonary ascariasis*) or the presence of adult worms in the intestine (*intestinal ascariasis*).

Pulmonary ascariasis presents as Loeffler's syndrome; characterized by fever, cough, dyspnea, wheeze, urticaria, eosinophilia, and lung infiltrates. Pulmonary ascariasis should be differentiated from other causes of Loeffler's syndrome, namely, visceral larva migrans caused by *Toxocara canis* or hookworm, schistosomiasis, pulmonary aspergillosis, and tropical pulmonary eosinophilia.

Intestinal manifestations of ascariasis result because of adult worms; and include abdominal distension, vomiting, vague abdominal discomfort, and irritability. The child may pass adult worms in the vomitus or feces. In heavy worm infestation, small bowel obstruction can occur due to a mass of entangled worms. Occasionally worms migrate to aberrant sites such as biliary and pancreatic ducts, where they can cause cholecystitis, cholangitis, pancreatitis, and rarely intrahepatic abscess.

COMPLICATIONS

Worms can also pass across the intestinal wall and cause peritonitis. As parasites compete with host for nutrients, heavy worm infestation may be associated with poor growth and nutritional deficiencies in young children.

DIAGNOSIS

The diagnosis is established by identification of characteristic eggs in stool samples by microscopy. The eggs are round or oval (45–70 mm × 35–50 mm), brownish, with a thick mamillated covering. Occasionally, adult worm in feces or vomitus can be recognized by its large size and smooth cream colored surface. Blood eosinophilia, prominent during early migratory phase (pulmonary ascariasis), decreases to minimal levels in established infection. Ultrasound can identify worms in pancreaticobiliary ducts. Occasionally, worms can be incidentally diagnosed on contrast studies of the gastrointestinal tract, appearing as *string shadows* due to barium in the alimentary canal of the worms, or as linear filling defects outlined by contrast media.

TREATMENT Ascariasis

Adult worms in the gastrointestinal tract can be killed by single dose albendazole (400 mg, PO, for all ages), or mebendazole (100 mg BD for 3 days or 500 mg PO, single dose for all ages). Single dose of pyrantel pamoate (11 mg/kg) or ivermectin (150–200 mg/kg) is also effective. Nitazoxanide given for 3 days may be as effective as single dose albendazole. Piperazine citrate (75 mg/kg/day, 2 days) is recommended in heavy infestations at risk of intestinal obstruction, and biliary infestation. Severe obstruction may require surgery.

Re-infections can occur in endemic areas in >80% of the population.

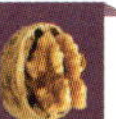

IN A NUTSHELL

Ascariasis

1. Ascariasis is the most common human helminthic infection caused by *Ascaris lumbricoides*.
2. Intestinal manifestations of ascariasis because of adult worms; and include abdominal distension, vomiting, vague abdominal discomfort and irritability.
3. Pulmonary ascariasis presents as Loeffler's syndrome; characterized by fever, cough, dyspnea, wheeze, urticaria, eosinophilia, and lung infiltrates.
4. Ascariasis is diagnosed by microscopic examination of stool specimen for eggs.
5. Treatment of choice is albendazole or mebendazole.

Leung AKC, Leung AAM, Wong AHC, et al. Human ascariasis: an updated review. Recent Pat Inflamm Allergy Drug Discov. 2020;14(2):133-45.
Mohd-Shaharuddin N, Lim YAL, Ngui R, et al. Expression of Ascaris lumbricoides putative virulence-associated genes when infecting a human host. Parasit Vectors. 2021;14(1):176.
Siviero I, de Almeida UVB, Penna CRR, et al. Abdominal complications of ascariasis in childhood. J Pediatr (Rio J). 2024;100(5):460-7.

14.21 Ankylostomiasis (Hookworm) (*Ancylostoma Duodenale, Necator Americanus*)

PE 31.14

INTRODUCTION

Hookworm infestation is one of the most prevalent helminthic diseases, affecting >500 million humans and causing iron deficiency anemia. Infection is more common in rural areas of tropical and subtropical regions. Most infected persons are asymptomatic. Hookworm disease develops when worm load is high. Two species of hookworm, *Ancylostoma duodenale (A. duodenale)* and *Necator americanus (N. americanus)* are found exclusively in humans while less common zoonotic species *Ancylostoma caninum*, *Ancylostoma braziliense,* and *Ancylostoma ceylanicum* may affect humans.

PATHOGENESIS

Filariform larva is the infective stage of the parasite. Infection occurs when larvae in soil penetrate the skin (*N. americanus* and *A. duodenale*) or when they are ingested through contaminated food and water (*A. duodenale*). Following skin penetration, larvae reach lungs *via* systemic circulation, break into the alveoli, ascend through bronchi and trachea, and are swallowed to reach the small intestine, where they develop into mature worms. Orally ingested infective larvae may either undergo extraintestinal migration or remain in the intestine to develop into mature worms. Adult worms inhabit jejunum, measure 1 cm in length, and use buccal teeth (*A. duodenale*) or cutting plates (*N. americanus*) to attach to the bowel mucosa and suck blood. *A. duodenale* sucks blood at the rate of 0.15 mL/worm/day. Additional 0.05 mL blood is lost as hemorrhage from the abandoned feeding site. Blood loss is less for *N. americanus.*

Adult hookworms produce thousands of eggs daily, which pass into soil where rhabditiform larvae are released which mature into the filariform larvae. Ova fail to develop into larva, if it gets dried, or the surrounding temperature drops below 13°C. The lifespan of adult worm ranges from 1 to 5 years. Man is the only reservoir.

CLINICAL FEATURES

Symptoms due to larvae appear 1–2 weeks after infections and those due to ova appear after 42–45 days of infection.

Infective larvae may produce a pruritic maculopapular eruption known as *ground itch* at the site of skin penetration. Larvae migrating through lungs may also cause transient lung infiltration, but this is less common than with *Ascaris.* Nonspecific complaints such as abdominal pain, anorexia, and diarrhea have also been attributed to the hookworm infection.

Chronic blood loss due to hookworm infection causes iron deficiency anemia and occasionally, hypoproteinemia. Only heavily infected children become symptomatic. Children with light infections have minimal blood loss and, thus, may have hookworm infection but not hookworm disease. Sometimes children may develop a yellow-green pallor known as "chlorosis". *A. duodenale* infection during infancy may be associated with diarrhea, failure to thrive, and severe anemia.

DIAGNOSIS

The diagnosis is established by identifying the characteristic oval hookworm eggs in the feces. Eggs of the two species are indistinguishable. Blood examination reveals microcytic hypochromic anemia, occasionally with eosinophilia. Hypoalbuminemia may be seen in heavy infections.

TREATMENT **Hookworm Infestations**

Eradication of worms is achieved with albendazole (400 mg, PO, single dose, for all ages), or mebendazole (100 mg, PO, twice a day for 3 days). Pyrantel pamoate orally (11 mg/kg once daily for 3 days) is also effective. Anemia is treated with oral iron therapy. Severe anemia may require a packed cell transfusion.

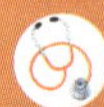

CASE STUDY **Hookworm Infestation**

Mother of an 8-year-old boy presented with chief complaint that her child appears to be pale than before. This was associated with history of pain in the abdomen and loose stools over the last 4–5 months. There was no history of fever, red-colored urine, yellowish discoloration of eyes, abdominal distension, rash, petechiae, bleeding from any site, or black-colored foul smelling stools. There was no history of blood transfusion in the child or any other family member. Dietary history was appropriate for age.

On examination, there was moderate pallor over conjunctiva, palms, and soles. There was no icterus, edema, or significant lymphadenopathy. Abdominal examination revealed no hepatosplenomegaly. Rest of the systemic examination was normal.

Summarize your impression of this child.

This child presented with moderate pallor of insidious onset without any evidence of bleeding, fever, jaundice, and/or hepatosplenomegaly. This ruled out involvement of reticuloendothelial or hepatobiliary system. Abdominal pain and abnormal bowel habits point toward an abdominal cause of anemia. It is possible that the child was having occult bleeding from the gastrointestinal (GI) tract. Nutritional deficiency of iron leading to anemia was unlikely since dietary intake was reported to be normal.

How will you investigate this child?

Firstly, I would like to examine the peripheral smear to identify the morphology of RBCs and look for any abnormal cells. I will also get the hemoglobin level and blood counts. Secondly, to look for blood loss from GIT, I will order a stool occult blood test.

Blood examination revealed following: Hb 7.0 g/dL, microcytic hypochromic RBC and no features of hemolysis. WBC and platelet counts were normal. Stool for occult blood was positive.

On further questioning, you realize that child belongs to a rural area and spends quite some time walking barefoot in the fields. Does that change/modify your diagnosis? How will you confirm it?

A strong possibility exists for hookworm infestation, which typically presents with anemia (without fever or RES involvement) in a physically active child. A stool microscopic examination should be done for at least 3 days, consecutively, for ova/cyst of *Ancylostoma duodenale* or *Necator americanus*. Stool examination for ova/cyst by Lugol Iodine preparation showed eggs of *Ancylostoma duodenale*. Clinical presentation (age of the child, rural residence, anemia, abdominal complaints); peripheral smear findings (microcytic hypochromic anemia, normal WBC, and platelets counts); and presence of occult blood in stool support the diagnosis of hookworm infestation.

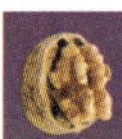

IN A NUTSHELL

Ankylostomiasis (Hookworm)

1. Hookworm infestation in humans is caused by two species *Ancylostoma duodenale* and *Necator americanus*.
2. Clinical features include anorexia, abdominal pain, diarrhea, iron deficiency anemia due to blood loss and hypoproteinemia (occasionally).
3. Diagnosis is made by demonstration of ova in stools.
4. Treatment includes administration of albendazole, mebendazole, and pyrantel pamoate.

Ajjampur SSR, Kaliappan SP, Halliday KE, et al. Epidemiology of soil transmitted helminths and risk analysis of hookworm infections in the community: results from the DeWorm3 Trial in Southern India. PLoS Negl Trop Dis. 2021;15(4):e0009338.

Umbrello G, Pinzani R, Bandera A, et al. Hookworm infection in infants: a case report and review of literature. Ital J Pediatr. 2021;47(1):26.

14.22 Enterobiasis (Pinworm) *PE 31.14*

INTRODUCTION

Enterobius vermicularis (Pinworm or Threadworm) is a small (1 cm long), white, thread-like nematode that lives in the cecum, appendix, ileum, and ascending colon. Eggs are not usually liberated in the gut. Rather, gravid females migrate at night into the perianal region and release up to 15,000 eggs there. The egg becomes infective within 6 hours. Perianal scratching causes transfer of eggs to fingernails. Infection occurs when eggs are ingested. Eggs take 35–60 days to develop into adult worms. The larvae hatch and mature within the intestine. The adult worm lives for about 2 months.

PATHOGENESIS

Man is the only reservoir. Larvae enter the human body by oral route. Transmission occurs by any of the following methods:

1. Most commonly from perianal region to the mouth.
2. By ingestion of viable eggs present in soiled bed linen and other contaminated objects.
3. Via mouth or nose from contaminated eggs in dust.
4. ***Retroinfection:*** Eggs hatch near anus and larvae migrate up the bowel.

Pinworm can infect all age groups, but prevalence is highest in 5–14-year-old children. Worm burden tends to be higher in younger age group. There appears to be no sex predilection. Pinworm usually affects all members of the family as it is easily transmitted from one child or person to a new host. The infection is common in lower socioeconomic regions where personal hygiene is poor. Ova usually contaminate the area beneath the fingernails. The lack of proper hygiene favors the transmission.

CLINICAL FEATURES

Perianal itching, especially in night is the most common complaint. The exact cause of itching is not known but is believed to be due to migration of worm in the perianal region. Pruritus ani may be associated with anorexia, weight loss, irritability, and enuresis.

Itching also leads to restless sleep, irritability, and enuresis. Complications include ectopic lesions such as vulvitis. Rarely, the worm may migrate to ear, nose, liver, kidney, and lungs.

DIAGNOSIS

Direct visualization of the adult worm or microscopic detection of eggs confirms the diagnosis, but only 5% of infected persons have eggs in their stool. The "*cellophane tape test*" can serve as a quick way to clinch the diagnosis. This test consists of touching tape to the perianal area several times, removing it, and examining the tape under direct microscopy for eggs. The test should be conducted right after awakening on at least three consecutive days. This technique can increase the test's sensitivity to roughly 90%.

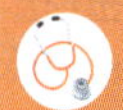

CASE STUDY Enterobius Infestation

A 3-year-old girl was brought to pediatric outpatient department with chief complaint of excessive itching in the periurethral area. There was no history of fever, burning micturition or increase in itching during or after micturition. There was no history of foul smelling vaginal discharge, constipation, or history of similar illness in the family. The itching typically increased during night time. On examination, child had poor personal hygiene. Vitals and systemic examination were normal. Local examination revealed erythema in perianal and periurethral area with scratch marks. There was no rash or vaginal discharge.

Enumerate causes of periurethral itching. What is the likely possibility in this case and how will you confirm the diagnosis? It may be difficult for a small child to localize the symptoms to periurethral or perianal area. Therefore, causes for localized itching in periurethral area could be: (1) Urinary tract infection (UTI), (2) vaginitis, (3) anal fissure, and (4) pinworm infestation. Absence of fever, burning micturition, and normal urine culture, and microscopy examination will rule out UTI. Absence of foul smelling vaginal discharge rules out vaginitis. No history of constipation or hard stools with excessive straining rules out anal fissure. Scabies is also less likely, since there is no rash and no family history of itching.

Pinworm infestation appears to be most probable diagnosis, with a history of poor personal hygiene and excessive itching during night. Cellophane test is the investigation of choice.

Cellophane test was done for three consecutive days. On 2 days, it revealed eggs of *Enterobius vermicularis*. Child was given albendazole and mother was counseled to maintain personal hygiene.

TREATMENT Enterobiasis (Pinworm)

Infected persons and their family members should be treated with a single oral dose of mebendazole (100 mg PO for all ages) or albendazole (400 mg, PO) and repeated after 2 weeks again to achieve a cure rate of 90–100%. Single dose of pyrantel pamoate (11 mg/kg), or ivermectin (150–200 mg/kg) are also highly effective.

Pinworm infection may be difficult to eradicate due to repeated autoinfection. Maintenance of personal hygiene remains the key to prevent autoinfections. Morning bath and frequent change of underclothing are important.

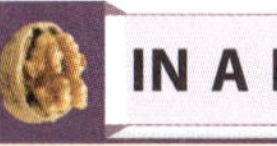

IN A NUTSHELL

Enterobiasis (Pinworm)

1. Clinical features include perianal itching, anorexia, weight loss, and enuresis.
2. Diagnosed by demonstration of adult worms or ova in stool specimen.
3. Difficult to eradicate due to repeated autoinfection.
4. Treatment includes drug therapy with albendazole or mebendazole and maintenance of personal hygiene.

Gunaratna GP, Dempsey S, Ho C, et al. Diagnosis of enterobius vermicularis infestations. J Paediatr Child Health. 2020;56(12):1994.

Özdil K, Karataş N, Zincir H. Low socioeconomic level and enterobius vermicularis: a interventional study to children and their mothers in home. Zoonoses Public Health. 2020;67(8):882-91.

Wendt S, Trawinski H, Schubert S, et al. The diagnosis and treatment of pinworm infection. Dtsch Arztebl Int. 2019;116(13):213-9.

14.23 Trichuriasis (Whipworm) *PE 31.14*

The normal habitat of *Trichuris trichiura* is the cecum, ascending colon, and appendix. Adult worms measures 3–5 cm in length. The anterior three-fourths portion of the worm is threaded into superficial mucosa and the short posterior part is free in the lumen of the gut. Infection is transmitted directly by ingestion of embryonated eggs in contaminated food, water, and hands or indirectly through flies and other insects. Larva escapes from the eggs in small intestine moving down to lodge in cecum. The average lifespan of the adult worm is up to 1 year. Infection is most common in the 5–15 years of age.

Incubation period is usually 60 days. Infection is asymptomatic in most cases due to low worm load. Adult worms suck approximately 0.005 mL blood per worm per day that is not sufficient to cause significant anemia. Heavy worm loads are associated with dysentery, anemia, rectal prolapse, epigastric pain, abdominal distension, hypoproteinemia, and growth retardation. Trichuriasis frequently co-exists with amebiasis, roundworm or hookworm infestation.

Diagnosis is made by identification of characteristic "barrel-shaped eggs" in the feces. Blood eosinophilia is minimal. Mebendazole (100 mg twice a day for 3 days or 500 mg single dose, PO, for all ages) is recommended and associated with a cure rate of 70–90%. A single dose of albendazole (400 mg) or ivermectin (150–200 mg/kg) is an effective alternative.

Badri M, Olfatifar M, Wandra T, et al. The prevalence of human trichuriasis in Asia: a systematic review and meta-analysis. Parasitol Res. 2022;121(1):1-10.

Schachter J, Alvarinho de Oliveira D, da Silva CM, et al. Whipworm infection promotes bacterial invasion, intestinal microbiota imbalance, and cellular immunomodulation. Infect Immun. 2020;88(3):e00642-19.

14.24 Taeniasis (Tapeworm) *PE 31.14*

INTRODUCTION

These worms are also known as the pork tapeworm [*Taenia solium (T. solium)*] and beef tapeworm (*T. saginata*), reflecting the principal intermediate hosts for each of them. Man is the only definitive host for both the parasites. *T. solium* consists of a scolex with suckers and hooks, by which it attaches to the intestinal wall. Hooks are absent in *T. saginata*. Usually only one adult worm is found in the intestine, which may live for up to 25 years.

Intermediate stage of *T. solium* is known as cysticercus. Cysticercus, on its own can also infect humans. The resultant disease—cysticercosis—can practically involve almost any part of the body.

PATHOGENESIS

Infection with adult tapeworm (taeniasis) is acquired by ingestion of undercooked pork and beef, containing infectious cysticerci. Human cysticercosis, on the other hand, is acquired by consumption of food and water contaminated with eggs of *T. solium*. Therefore, cysticercosis may occur in persons who do not eat pork. Infection can also arise by autoinfection, if eggs reflux from intestine into the stomach from reverse peristalsis. Persons infected with an adult *T. solium* may also infect themselves with the eggs by the feco-oral route.

CLINICAL FEATURES

Most infections with adult worms are asymptomatic. Some children may develop nonspecific complaints such as nausea, pain in abdomen, and diarrhea. Carriers have an increased risk of developing cysticercosis by repeated autoinfection. Rarely, adult worms can cause intestinal obstruction, cholangitis, appendicitis, and pancreatitis.

Cysticercosis

Infection with the intermediate stage (larvae) of *T. solium* results in cysticercosis. The intermediate stage of beef tapeworm is non-infectious to humans. Neurocysticercosis is the most common parasitic infection of the CNS and may account for as high as 20–50% cases of unprovoked seizures. Following ingestion, eggs develop into larvae in the small intestine. Larvae migrate across the intestinal wall and are carried to the target organs by bloodstream. The common target organs for cysticerci are brain, muscle, and subcutaneous tissue. The larvae mature into cysticerci in about 2 months. The size of cysticerci varies from 2 mm to 2 cm. Clinical manifestations depend on the location, number and size of cysts in the brain and host inflammatory response. Viable cysts generally do not elicit a strong response. On the other hand, degenerating cysts provoke a vigorous host response. Most cysts remain viable for 5–10 years. Neurocysticercosis may manifest as partial or generalized seizure, raised intracranial tension, focal neurological deficits, or disturbances in consciousness or behavior.

DIAGNOSIS

The diagnosis of taeniasis is established by the demonstration of eggs or proglottids in the stools. Patients may pass motile segments of worms through anus. Diagnosis of neurocysticercosis is made by MRI of brain. Details of diagnosis and management of neurocysticercosis are discussed in chapter on Neurological Disorders.

TREATMENT Taeniasis (Tapeworm)

Treatment of taeniasis is similar for both infestations. A single dose of niclosamide (50 mg/kg) or praziquantel (25 mg/kg) is effective. Purgation is not essential.

Cysticercosis needs to be treated with albendazole (15 mg/kg twice daily) for 15–30 days or praziquantel 50–100 mg^3 times a day for 30 days.

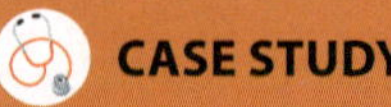

CASE STUDY Neurocysticercosis

An 8-year-old boy was brought to pediatric emergency with right sided focal seizures lasting for >5 minutes. This episode was aborted with intravenous lorazepam after checking for airway, breathing, and circulation. This episode was not preceded or associated with fever, altered sensorium, behavioral abnormalities, headache, vomiting, rash, blurring of vision, or neck stiffness. There was no past history of seizures. On examination, vitals, and blood pressure were normal. Child was oriented to time, place, and person. General physical examination was normal. Neurological examination was normal. Systemic examination was also normal.

What is the likely diagnosis?

Seizures lasting for >5 minutes are labeled as status epilepticus. The most common cause of a focal seizure, in an otherwise normal child (without any neurodevelopmental or systemic manifestations), in our setting is an irritative lesion in the brain—most likely neurocysticercosis or tuberculoma. Absence of fever, altered sensorium, and meningeal signs rules out meningitis or encephalitis. Also, there was no focal neurological deficit, blood pressure was normal, and bilateral pupils were reacting to light equally; so, possibility of stroke involving thrombus or hemorrhage is also less likely. At present, this episode cannot be labeled as epilepsy, since that is defined as >1 episode of seizures, at least 24 hours apart.

How will you confirm your diagnosis?

I would like to get a neuroimaging done, preferably magnetic resonance imaging (MRI) of brain. MRI T2 and fluid-attenuated inversion recovery (FLAIR) images reveal a ring enhancing lesion with surrounding edema. This was associated with an eccentrically placed scolex of cysticercosis within the lesion. These findings are consistent with neurocysticercosis. Tuberculosis was ruled out by doing a chest X-ray and Mantoux test.

How will you treat this child?

I would like to start the child on an antiepileptic agent, preferably carbamazepine (to be continued for at least 2 years, from the date of last seizure activity) along with oral steroids (prednisolone 2 mg/kg/day orally × initial 3 days) to reduce the pericystic edema. After 3 days of administering steroids, I would prescribe albendazole (10 mg/kg/day PO) for 28 days.

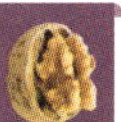

IN A NUTSHELL

Taeniasis (Tapeworm)

1. Caused by *Taenia solium* and *Taenia saginata*.
2. Manifestation includes nausea, abdominal pain, and diarrhea. Rarely, intestinal obstruction, cholangitis, pancreatitis may develop.
3. Central nervous system (CNS) involvement presents with seizures and is known as neurocysticercosis.
4. Treatment includes niclosamide or praziquantel.

Lateef M, Nazir M, Zargar SA, et al. Epidemiology of *Taenia saginata* taeniasis with emphasis on its prevalence and transmission in a Kashmiri population in India: a prospective study. Int J Infect Dis. 2020;98:401-5.

Sankhyan N, Kadwa RA, Kamate M, et al. Management of neurocysticercosis in children: Association of Child Neurology Consensus Guidelines. Indian Pediatr. 2021;58(9):871-80.

Silva CV, Costa-Cruz JM. A glance at *Taenia saginata* infection, diagnosis, vaccine, biological control and treatment. Infect Disord Drug Targets. 2010;10(5):313-21.

Singanamalla B, Singh B, Saini L, et al. Disseminated cysticercosis-a tropical curse. J Pediatr. 2020;217:213.

WHO guidelines on management of *Taenia solium* neurocysticercosis [Internet]. Geneva: World Health Organization; 2021. EXECUTIVE SUMMARY. Available from: https://www.ncbi.nlm.nih.gov/books/NBK573846/. [Last accessed February, 2025].

14.25 Rational Use of Antibiotics

PE 31.14

INTRODUCTION

Antimicrobials are boon to the humanity in the management of infectious diseases. But use of antimicrobials inappropriately has led to the emergence of resistance to antibiotics. Rational use of antibiotics is need of the hour to curb antimicrobial resistance.

ANTIMICROBIAL RESISTANCE

Antimicrobial resistance (AMR) develops when bacteria, viruses, fungi, and parasites change over time and become resistant to various antimicrobials. AMR is a natural process occurring over time due to genetic changes in the organisms. Factors which accelerate the AMR are: misuse and overuse of antimicrobials; poor access to clean water, poor sanitation and hygiene; poor infection prevention and control practices; poor access to diagnostic and therapeutic facilities; lack of awareness and lack of legislative enforcement. These resistant organisms spread faster from one person to the other. Over the last few decades AMR has become a major health hazard and has made infections difficult to treat.

Indian Network for Surveillance of Antimicrobial Resistance (INSAR) group has reported prevalence of 41% methicillin-resistant *Staphylococcus aureus* (MRSA) in India. Multidrug resistant enterobacteriaceae due to the production of extended spectrum β-lactamases (ESBL) has also emerged in India. AMR is also prevalent against tuberculosis, malaria and HIV infections.

RATIONAL USE OF ANTIMICROBIALS

Antibiotics should be used only when required. A precise clinical diagnosis should be made based on clinical features and investigations. All possible efforts should be made to document the site of infection and causative microorganisms. Possible cultures should be sent. An appropriate antibiotic should be chosen based on efficacy, safety, suitability, and cost. One should have knowledge of local sensitivity pattern by ongoing research. Right dose, route and duration should be decided. Clinical response should be followed, and de-escalation should be considered when appropriate. Audit on antibiotic prescription should take place regularly.

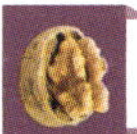

IN A NUTSHELL

Rational Use of Antibiotics

1. Antimicrobial resistance is a growing concern.
2. All possible efforts should be made to prevent misuse and overuse of antibiotics.

Antimicrobial stewardship programmes in health-care facilities in low- and middle-income countries. A practical toolkit. Geneva: World Health Organization; 2019.
Optimizing the Use of Antibiotic Agents in the Pediatric Intensive Care Unit: A Narrative Review. Pediatric Drugs. 2021;23:39-53.

14.26 Antimicrobial Stewardship (AMS) *PE 31.14*

INTRODUCTION

Stewardship is defined as "the careful and responsible management of something entrusted to one's care". Antimicrobial stewardship (AMS) is defined as "a cluster of interventions targeted toward the improvement and monitoring of appropriate antimicrobial use by selecting the most optimal drug regimen including the type of drug used, the dose, the duration of therapy, and the route of administration". **Table 14.16** lists some common areas for improving antibiotic prescribing. AMS is one of the three "pillars" of health system strengthening approach, the other being infection prevention and control (IPC) and medicine and patient safety. Antimicrobial stewardship program is an organizational or system-wide healthcare strategy to promote appropriate use of antimicrobials through the implementation of evidence-based interventions. The goals of antimicrobial stewardship programs are optimization of the use of antimicrobials, improvement of patient outcomes, reduction of antimicrobial resistance, and healthcare-associated infections, and reduction of healthcare costs.

BASIC AMS INTERVENTIONS

1. Educating the health personnel about AMS.
2. Development and updation of patients' medical record to provide complete information of antibiotics used.
3. Patients receiving antibiotic treatment should have written indications.
4. Antibiotic treatment for patients who are prescribed three or more broad-spectrum antibiotics should be reviewed.
5. The dose of antibiotics prescribed should be reviewed.
6. Surgical antibiotic prophylaxis where it is prescribed for >24 hours and where a single dose is appropriate should be reviewed.
7. Local guidelines for treatment of common clinical conditions such as community-acquired pneumonia, urinary tract infections, skin and soft tissue infection should be developed.
8. Basic microbiology laboratory facilities and regular surveillance activities should be established.

Many countries have developed their own AMS programs. In India too, programs have been started but the situation is not very promising and much more need to be done.

National Action Plan on Antimicrobial Resistance (NAP-AMR)

In India, Core Working Group on AMR has drafted the NAP-AMR. India's National Action Plan on Antimicrobial Resistance (NAP-AMR) focuses on six key areas:

1. Raising awareness about AMR through communication, education, and training.

Table 14.16 Nine Common Areas for Improving Antibiotic Prescribing

Prescriptions	*What to improve*
Overprescribing	Antibiotics are prescribed when not needed, e.g., fever without evidence of infection, asymptomatic urinary tract colonization, viral infections, malaria, inflammatory conditions
Overly broad spectrum	More broad-spectrum antibiotics (WATCH and RESERVE antibiotics) are prescribed than are necessary (e.g., surgical prophylaxis)
Unnecessary combination therapy, including certain fixed dose combinations	Multiple antibiotics are used, particularly with overlapping spectra and in combinations that have not been shown to improve clinical outcomes
Wrong antibiotic choice	Wrong antibiotic(s) are prescribed for particular indications/infections
Wrong dose	Antibiotics are prescribed with the wrong dose (over- or underdosing)
Wrong dose interval	Antibiotics are prescribed with the wrong dose interval (too much time between doses)
Wrong route	Antibiotics are prescribed by the wrong route (e.g., IV instead of oral)
Wrong duration	Duration of antibiotic treatment should be optimized (e.g., antibiotics prescribed for too long a period, prolonged surgical prophylaxis)
Delayed administration	Administration of the antibiotic(s) is delayed from the time of prescription. Repeat doses are not administered in a timely way, which is critical in the case of septic shock and other serious infections

Source: Antimicrobial stewardship programmes in health-care facilities in low- and middle-income countries. A WHO practical toolkit. World Health Organization 2019

2. Enhancing surveillance to improve understanding and tracking of AMR.
3. Preventing infections through effective infection control measures.
4. Promoting responsible use of antimicrobials in humans, animals, and food.
5. Encouraging research, innovation, and investment to combat AMR.
6. Strengthening India's global leadership on AMR efforts.

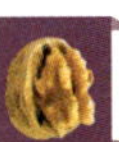

IN A NUTSHELL

Antimicrobial Stewardship (AMS)

1. Antimicrobial resistance is a natural process, which is accelerated due to misuse and overuse of antibiotics.
2. Antimicrobial stewardship involves a cluster of interventions targeted toward the improvement and monitoring of appropriate antimicrobial use.
3. Antibiotic prescribing can be improved by avoiding over prescription, broad spectrum, wrong antibiotic, wrong dose, wrong duration, and wrong route of antibiotics.
4. AMS program has been adopted by many countries, but it is still in nascent stage.

Antimicrobial stewardship programmes in health-care facilities in low- and middle-income countries. A practical toolkit. Geneva: World Health Organization; 2019.

Bedi N, Gupta P. Antimicrobial stewardship in pediatrics: An Indian perspective. Indian Pediatr. 2016;53(4):293-8.

Fay MJ, Bryant PA. Antimicrobial stewardship in children: where to from here? J Paediatr Child Health. 2020;56(10):1504-7.

Mzumara GW, Mambiya M, Iroh Tam PY. Antimicrobial stewardship interventions in least developed and low-income countries: a systematic review protocol. BMJ Open. 2021;11(8):e047312.

Nair M, et al. India's National Action Plan on Antimicrobial Resistance: a critical perspective. Journal of Global Antimicrobial Resistance. 2021;27:236-8.

Subramaniam G, Girish M. Antibiotic resistance—a cause for reemergence of infections. Indian J Pediatr. 2020;87(11):937-44.

World Health Organization. (2019). Antimicrobial stewardship programmes in health-care facilities in low- and middle-income countries. A practical toolkit. [online] Available from https://iris.who.int/handle/10665/329404 [Last accessed August, 2025].

Piyush Gupta, and Aaradhana; with Pooja Dewan (HIV; online only) and Atul Kulkarni (Rickettsial Diseases; online only)

15 CHAPTER

Care of the Normal Newborn

AS PER NMC COMPETENCIES

PE19.1	Define the common neonatal nomenclatures including the classification newborn and describe the characteristics of a normal term neonate and high-risk neonates, explain the care of a normal neonate.	*Ch 15.1, Ch 15.3* *Ch 15.6, Ch 15.7*
PE19.2	Perform neonatal resuscitation on a manikin.	*Ch 15.2, Ch 15.6*
PE19.3	Assessment of normal neonate. Explain the follow up care for neonates including breastfeeding, temperature maintenance, immunization, importance of growth monitoring and red flags.	*Ch 15.3, Ch 15.4* *Ch 15.5, Ch 15.6* *Ch 15.7, Ch 15.9* *Ch 15.10, Ch 15.11*
PE19.9	Describe the temperature regulation in neonates, clinical features and management of neonatal hypothermia.	*Ch 15.8*

15.1 Neonatal Nomenclature *PE 19.1*

Neonate/newborn: The infant from birth up to 4 weeks (28 days) is called a neonate or a newborn.

Early neonatal period: First week (7 days) of life is called early neonatal period.

Late neonatal period: This extends from 7th completed day to 28th day of life.

In utero transport: Transfer of a pregnant mother to a better equipped center before delivery (in utero), with the aim to salvage the high-risk fetus.

Live born: A live born neonate is the product of conception irrespective of weight or gestational age that, after separation from mother, shows any evidence of life such as breathing, heartbeat, pulsation of umbilical cord, or definitive movement of voluntary muscle.

Stillbirth: A fetal death (a product of conception that, after separation from mother does not show any evidence of life) at a gestation age of 20 weeks or more or weighing more than 500 g is defined as a stillborn or stillbirth.

Term: A newborn delivered between 37 and 41 weeks of gestation irrespective of birth weight.

Preterm: A newborn delivered before 37 completed weeks of gestation.

Post-term: A baby delivered at or after completed 42 weeks of gestation.

Low birth weight (LBW): A newborn baby weighing <2,500 g at birth.

Very low birth weight (VLBW): A newborn baby weighing <1,500 g at birth.

Extremely low birth weight (ELBW): A newborn baby weighing <1,000 g at birth.

Small for gestational age (SGA): Neonates with birth weight <10th percentile for that gestational age, also known as small for date (SFD).

Appropriate for gestational age (AGA): Neonates with birth weight between 10th and 90th percentile for that gestational age.

Large for gestational age (LGA): Neonates with birth weight >90th percentile for gestational age, also known as large for date (LFD).

Thermoneutral range of temperature: The ideal environmental temperature for a newborn, at which the basal metabolic rate (BMR) of the baby is at minimum, oxygen utilization is least, and baby maintains a core temperature between 36.5 and 37.5°C.

Warm chain: A chain of 10 steps to maintain a warm body temperature of a newborn during transport and stay in the hospital or home.

Normal neonate: A normal neonate is one that is born single, at term, weighs 2,500–4,000 g at birth, is able to establish normal respiration immediately after birth and does not have any obvious significant congenital anomaly or any other problem which can pose a threat to it.

15.2 Neonatal Resuscitation *PE 19.2*

NORMAL TRANSITION

With the birth of a baby, there is a sudden transition from intrauterine to extrauterine existence. At birth, the most significant event is breathing of the baby followed by transition from fetal to neonatal circulation. In the fetus the role of lungs, i.e., exchange of gases is taken care of by the placenta and the lungs are nonfunctional and filled with fluid. At birth, the baby is delivered, and the umbilical cord is cut. The placenta can no longer take care of the exchange of gases. The baby breathes immediately so that the lungs get filled with air, pushing the fluid out **(Fig. 15.1)** and exchange of gases can take place. Simultaneously, the blood flow to the lungs increases facilitating exchange of gases. This also leads to gradual closure of the ductus arteriosus as the blood hitherto flowing through it is shunted to the lungs.

If the baby does not initiate respiration or cannot maintain effective breathing, the lungs do not get inflated and remain filled with fluid. As the alveoli do not get filled with air, there is no exchange of gases. Respiratory failure and hypoxia ensues and may even lead to death of the baby.

Most newborns make a smooth transition and no intervention is needed. Majority (85%) of the babies begin breathing soon after birth. Few babies (≈10%) start breathing after initial steps and only 5% babies will need active intervention in the form of positive pressure ventilation (PPV). Very few babies (≈0.2%) will need advanced resuscitation, i.e., chest compressions and medications **(Fig. 15.2)**.

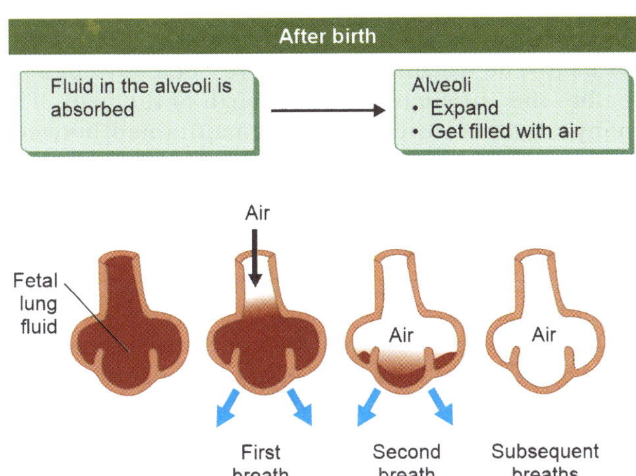

Fig. 15.1: Air replaces fluid in the alveoli when baby takes the first breath

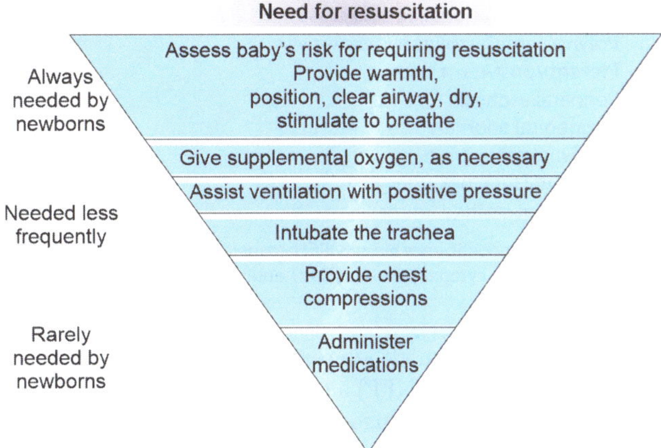

Fig. 15.2: Inverted triangle of need for resuscitation at birth

WHO NEEDS RESUSCITATION

High-risk babies **(Box 15.1)** are more likely to need some resuscitation measures, but a baby who has no risk factors may also need to be resuscitated. The need for intervention cannot be predicted prior to the birth of the baby, and every birth is to be considered a potential emergency where immediate resuscitation may be needed. Preparedness, training of healthcare workers and a protocolized approach while taking care of babies at birth can save many newborn lives.

Unlike adults, the primary focus of neonatal resuscitation (NNR) is to establish effective and quick ventilation. The newborns requiring resuscitation have an essentially normal heart and it is the primary failure of respiration which leads to compromised exchange of gases.

RESUSCITATION GUIDELINES

American Heart Association (AHA) and American Academy of Pediatrics (AAP) have formulated guidelines for resuscitation

Box 15.1 High-risk Newborns

A. High-risk maternal factors:
- *Maternal age:* <16 years, >40 years
- Poor socioeconomic status
- Drug addiction/alcoholism/smoking
- *Diabetes:* Pregestational, gestational
- *Hypertension:* Pregestational, pregnancy induced
- *Chronic medical disease:* Renal, cardiovascular, and anemia
- Bad obstetric history
- Premature rupture of membranes
- *Intrauterine infections:* TORCH, HIV, and hepatitis B

B. Fetal factors:
- Multiple gestation
- Intrauterine growth retardation
- Large for gestational age/macrosomia
- Polyhydramnios/oligohydramnios
- Preterm/post-term baby
- Perinatal asphyxia
- Congenital anomaly
- Fetal distress
- Abnormal fetal position
- Meconium-stained liquor

(HIV: human immunodeficiency virus; TORCH: toxoplasmosis, other (e.g., syphilis, HIV), rubella, cytomegalovirus (CMV), and herpes simplex virus)

of newborn at birth which are revised periodically. Neonatal resuscitation program (NRP) algorithm suggested by them is followed world over. The algorithm is a stepwise flowchart in which the *hexagons denote assessment* and *rectangles denote actions needed* **(Fig. 15.3)**.

COMPONENTS OF NEONATAL RESUSCITATION

The key components of NNR are:

- ***Preparedness before birth:*** All preparations need to be done before the birth of the baby. Precious time is lost if complete prior preparation has not been done.
- ***Anticipation:*** Need for resuscitation must be anticipated before each birth.
- ***Training*** of healthcare workers is extremely important for the success of resuscitation. Anyone involved in newborn care must be trained in basic steps of resuscitation, i.e., till PPV. Each birth must be attended by at least one person who is trained in basic steps of NNR.
- ***Availability*** of appropriate and sterilized equipment and consumables **(Box 15.2)**.
- ***Effective communication*** amongst the members of the team responsible for resuscitation of the baby. There should be a team leader and all members should know about their roles and responsibilities.

  Important questions that should be asked before the birth of the baby which will help in planning for resuscitation are:
  - What is the expected gestational age of the baby?
  - Is the amniotic fluid clear?
  - Are there any additional risk factors?
  - What is the plan of umbilical cord management?

INITIAL STEPS OF RESUSCITATION

As soon as the baby is born, a quick assessment should be done and following should be noted:

- Is the baby term gestation?
- Does the baby have good muscle tone? Healthy term babies have flexed extremities indicating good muscle tone.
- Is the baby breathing or crying?

If the answers to all the questions are *yes*, then the baby can be kept in skin-to-skin contact with the mother and initial steps can be performed and routine care can be given over the mother's abdomen or chest **(Fig. 15.4)**. The mother and the baby are then covered with a sheet or towel to keep them warm. In all vigorous term and preterm babies, the cord clamping should be delayed for at least 30–60 seconds to allow additional blood to flow from the placenta to the baby. This has been found to be beneficial for the newborn baby. If the answer to *any* of the above questions is *no*, the baby should be brought to the radiant warmer for the initial steps.

The initial steps should be completed within 30 seconds of the baby's birth. Some of the steps can be performed simultaneously. The initial steps of resuscitation over the mother abdomen or chest are:

1. ***Warmth:*** Warmth is maintained by immediately keeping the baby in skin-to-skin contact with the mother. The baby is then covered with a warm and dry towel/sheet.
2. ***Drying:*** The baby is also dried immediately by a warm, dry towel/sheet.
3. ***Position:*** The baby should be positioned over the mother's abdomen to ensure that the airway is open.
4. ***Secretions:*** The secretions should be cleared, if necessary, by wiping the mouth and the nose by a soft cloth. Gentle suction may be required in a few babies who have difficulty in clearing their secretions.

After the initial steps are over, the baby should be continuously monitored for breathing, color, and temperature. If the baby is brought to a radiant warmer, the initial steps should be done as follows:

1. ***Warmth:*** The baby is placed under the radiant warmer, so that it can be observed carefully and there is no loss of heat. The warmer should have been switched on before the anticipated time of birth of the baby. The baby's temperature should be maintained between 36.5 and 37.5°C.
2. ***Dry:*** The baby is immediately dried with a warm and dry towel. The first towel which gets wet should be removed and another warm and dry towel should be used.
3. ***Stimulate:*** If the baby is breathing well or crying vigorously, no further stimulation is needed. But, if the newborn fails to have adequate respiration, then brief tactile stimulation should be given to the baby in the form of a gentle rub over the back, trunk or extremities **(Fig. 15.5)**. Vigorous stimulation or shaking the baby should never be done.
4. ***Positioning:*** The baby should be positioned supine with the neck in the "sniffing position" or slight extension **(Fig. 15.6)**. This will open the airway and help the baby breathe easily. The neck should not be hyperextended or

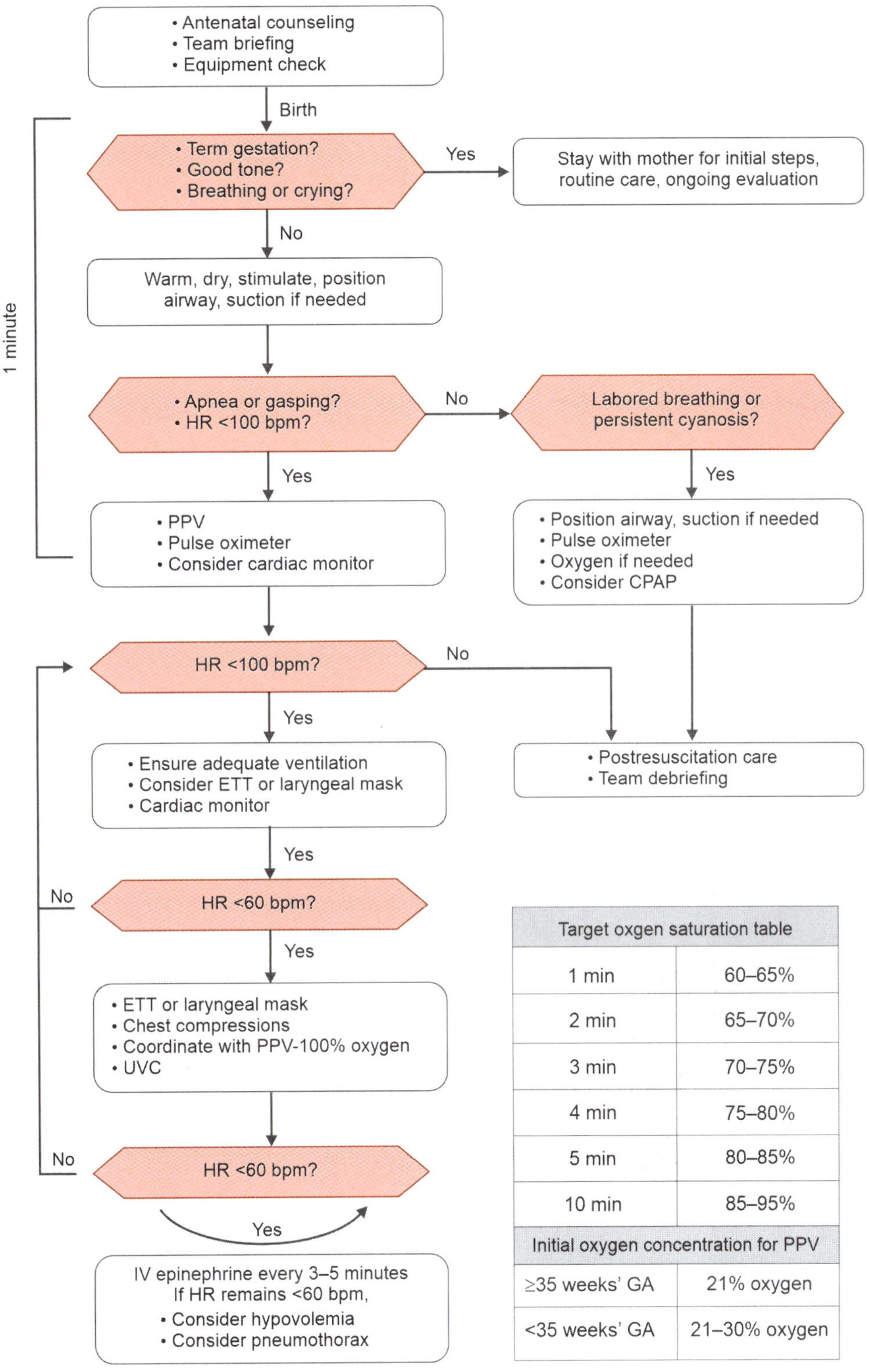

Target oxgen saturation table	
1 min	60–65%
2 min	65–70%
3 min	70–75%
4 min	75–80%
5 min	80–85%
10 min	85–95%
Initial oxygen concentration for PPV	
≥35 weeks' GA	21% oxygen
<35 weeks' GA	21–30% oxygen

Fig. 15.3: Neonatal resuscitation program algorithm

Box 15.2 List of Equipment for Neonatal Resuscitation

- *Warm:*
  - Preheated warmer
  - Warm towels
  - Cap
  - Plastic wrap and thermal mattress for babies <32 weeks
- *Clear airway:*
  - 10F or 12F suction catheter
  - Suction machine/central suction
  - Mucus extractor
- *Auscultate:*
  - Stethoscope
- *Ventilate:*
  - Flow meter set to 10 L/min
  - Oxygen blender
  - Self-inflating bag
  - Term and preterm masks
  - 8F orogastric tube
  - Cardiac monitor (optional)
- *Oxygenate:*
  - Device to deliver free-flow oxygen
  - Pulse oximeter
- *Intubate:*
  - Laryngoscope with blade no. 0 and 1
  - Endotracheal tubes
  - Waterproof tape
  - Scissors
- *Medicate:*
  - Epinephrine (0.1 mg/mL)
  - Normal saline
  - Supplies for placing umbilical venous catheter and administering medications

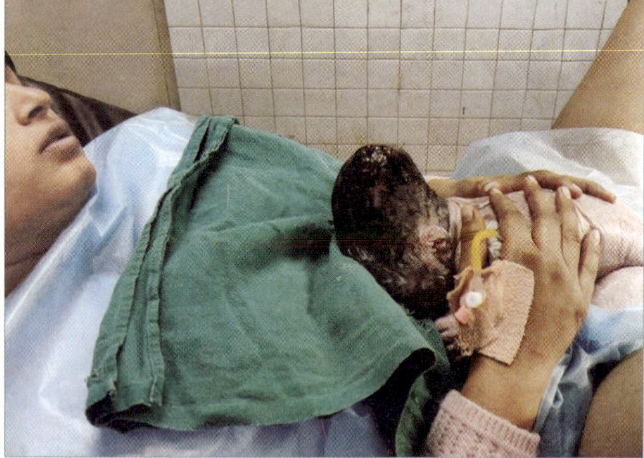

Fig. 15.4: Baby delivered over the mother's abdomen

Courtesy: Dr Sweta Kumari, UCMS, Delhi

flexed. To maintain proper position of the baby a small shoulder roll should be placed under the shoulders of the baby.

5. ***Suction:*** Routine suctioning of the airway is not recommended for all the babies. Secretions may be cleared if the baby is not breathing or does not have good respiratory efforts, or if the secretions are obstructing the airway and interfering in the baby's breathing. Suction should be brief and gentle. It should not be vigorous or deep. This may lead to vagal stimulation,

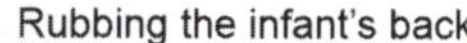

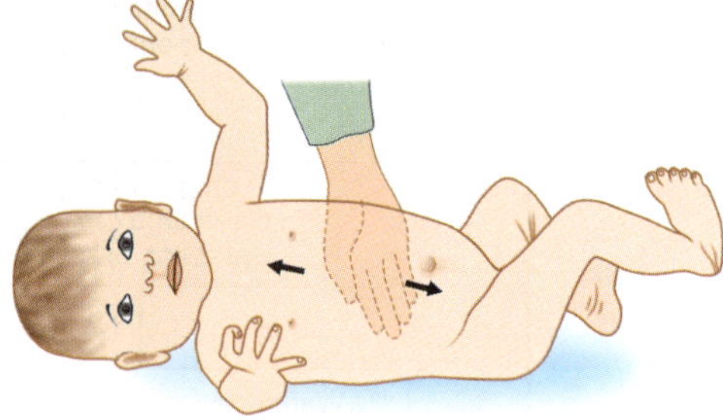

Fig. 15.5: Tactile stimulation

bradycardia, or apnea. The mouth should always be suctioned before the nose.

After performing these steps, the baby should be assessed for respiration and heart rate. If the baby is breathing effectively, then heart rate should be assessed by keeping the stethoscope over the left side of the chest of the baby. Heart rate can be estimated by counting for 6 seconds and multiplying by 10 to get the heart rate in beats per minute (bpm), e.g., if 8 heart beats are counted in 6 seconds, this is multiplied by 10 and we get the heart rate as 80 bpm. The baby's heart rate should be 100 bpm or more. If the heart rate ≥100 bpm, the baby is breathing well and does not have central cyanosis, the baby can be given to the mother for skin-to-skin contact and kept under ongoing evaluation.

Free-flow Oxygen

If the heart rate ≥100 bpm, the baby is breathing well but appear to have persistent central cyanosis, a pulse oximeter must be placed on the right hand/wrist to assess baby's saturation. Peripheral cyanosis, i.e., cyanosis only on hands and feet is normal in babies soon after birth and does not need any

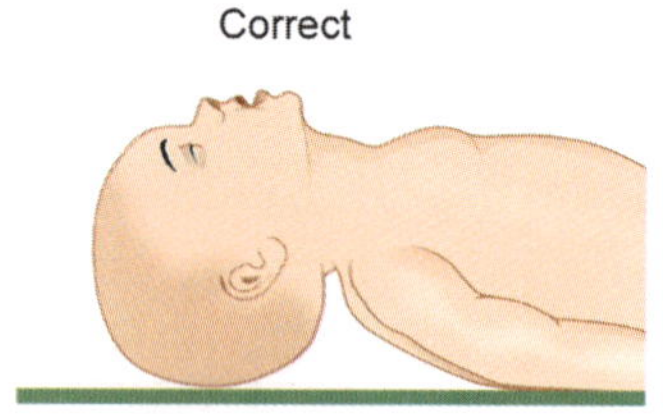

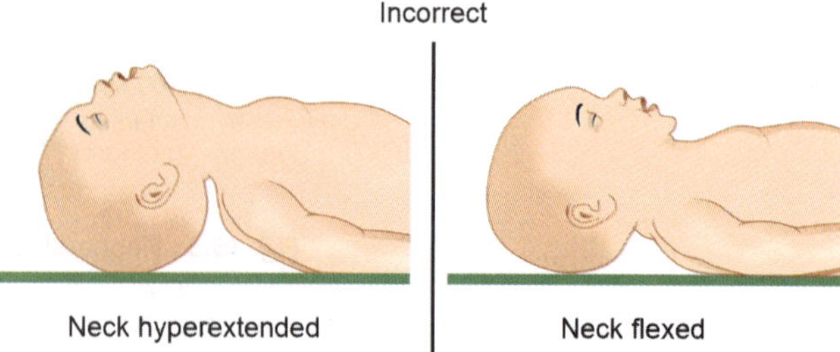

Fig. 15.6: Positioning of the baby

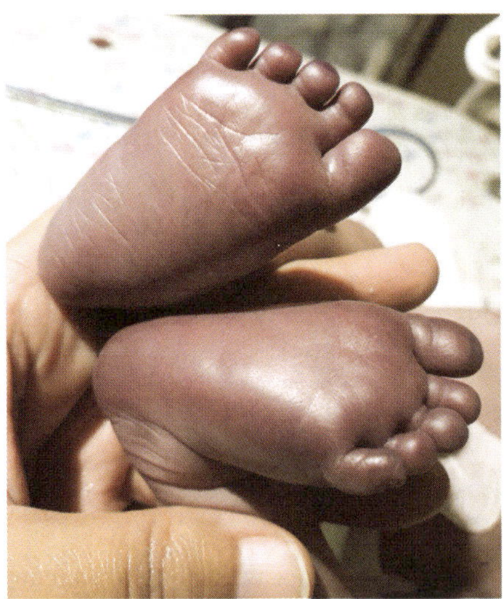

Fig. 15.7: Acrocyanosis

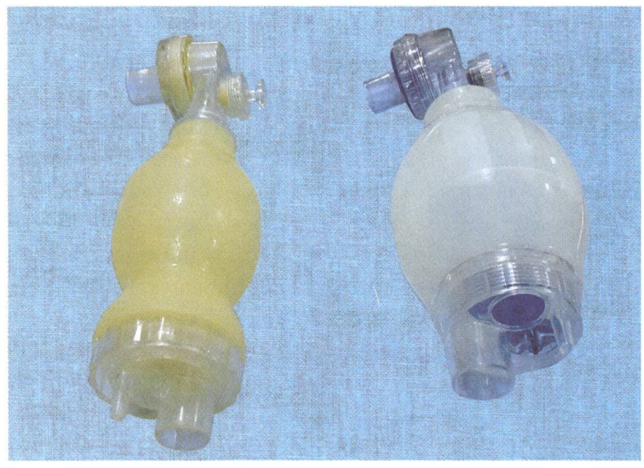

Fig. 15.8: Self-inflating bag of different sizes

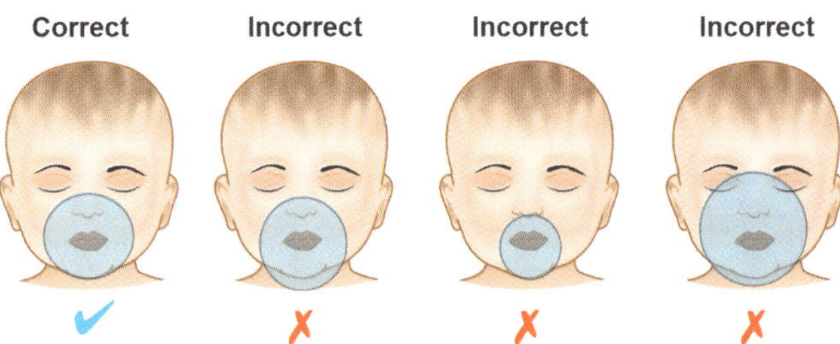

Fig. 15.9: Choosing an appropriate size face mask

intervention **(Fig. 15.7)**. The saturation monitored in the right hand should be compared to the target saturation for the baby in the first 10 minutes after birth **(Table 15.1)**. If the monitored saturation is less than the target range for the baby's age, supplemental oxygen should be started by holding an oxygen tubing close to the baby's mouth and nose. The concentration of the delivered oxygen (FiO_2) can be adjusted as per the monitored saturation of the baby. Ideally, a blender should be used to deliver the exact FiO_2 needed. If the baby has labored breathing or persistently low saturations despite delivering 100% oxygen, continuous positive airway pressure (CPAP) or PPV can be tried.

POSITIVE PRESSURE VENTILATION

Indications of starting PPV after initial steps of resuscitation are:
- The baby is still apneic and not breathing, *or*
- Has gasping respiration, *or*
- Has a heart rate of <100 bpm.

If PPV is indicated, it should be started without any further delay. If a baby needs PPV, one should be able to initiate within first minute of birth which is the golden minute of resuscitation. Quick assessment of the baby, initial steps of resuscitation, identification of need for PPV, and initiation of PPV should be done within this 1 minute. It should always be remembered that ventilation of the newborn lungs is the single most important and effective step in NNR. Timely identification of need for PPV and its initiation can prevent a lot of neonatal deaths and disease. PPV is delivered to the baby with the help of a self-inflating bag/flow inflating bag/T piece resuscitator and mask. Following must be considered while giving PPV to the newborn:
- Appropriate size self-inflating bag should be used (250 mL/500 mL) **(Fig. 15.8)**.
- Appropriate size face mask must be selected. The mask must rest on the chin and cover the mouth and the nose but not the eyes **(Fig. 15.9)**. A tight seal between the mask and the mouth and nose is very crucial for effective ventilation. Proper seal can be ensured only if the mask is of appropriate size and method of application of the mask to the baby's mouth and nose is correct.
- One can hold the mask over the baby's mouth and nose by one hand and start ventilating with the other hand by squeezing the self-inflating bag.
- All babies needing PPV must have their saturation monitored by connecting a pulse oximeter to their right hand/wrist.
- Babies with gestational age ≥35 weeks should be started PPV with FiO_2 of 21%, i.e., room air (no oxygen source should be connected to the self-inflating bag).
- Babies with gestational age <35 weeks should be started PPV with FiO_2 21–30%.
- After initiation of PPV, the FiO_2 is then adjusted based on the measured saturation by the pulse oximeter and the target saturation for the baby.

Table 15.1	Target Oxygen Saturation for Newborn in the Delivery Room
1 minute	60–65%
2 minutes	65–70%
3 minutes	70–75%
4 minutes	75–80%
5 minutes	80–85%
10 minutes	85–95%

Technique of Giving Positive Pressure Ventilation

The baby is ventilated at the rate of 40–60 breaths per minute. This rate is achieved by counting out loud "*breathe*, two, three, *breathe*, two, three, *breathe*, two, three" The self-inflating bag is squeezed every time one says "breathe" and the bag is released at "two, three" to allow the baby to breathe out/exhale. As one starts ventilating the baby, a gentle rise and fall of the chest should be visible with each breath. Increase in heart rate is the most important indicator of effective PPV. If there is no increase in heart rate within first 15 seconds of PPV and the chest movements are not observed while breaths are being delivered, this indicates ineffective PPV. In that case, to deliver effective ventilation, ventilation corrective steps should be taken. The ventilation corrective steps are denoted by an acronym "MRSOPA". This acronym denotes the following *M*ask adjustment, *R*epositioning of the head and neck of the baby, *S*uction of the mouth and nose to clear any secretions, *O*pening the mouth of the baby, increasing *P*ressure while ventilating the baby, and use of *A*lternate airway such as intubation or use of laryngeal mask airway. If chest movements are seen with each breath delivered, then PPV should be continued for 30 seconds.

After 30 seconds of effective PPV that moves the chest, baby's heart rate is checked again.

- ***If the heart rate is ≥100 bpm:*** Ventilation should be continued at the same rate of 40–60 breaths per minute and the baby should be monitored for chest movement, heart rate, and respiratory efforts. As the baby starts breathing on its own, the rate of PPV is gradually reduced and slowly stopped as baby's breathing becomes regular. PPV can be stopped when the baby's respiratory efforts are good, and the heart rate is ≥100 bpm.
- ***If the heart rate is at least 60 but <100:*** PPV should be continued till the baby shows improvement. Simultaneously, one must monitor the rate of ventilation, chest movement, and adjust FiO_2 to meet target saturation. If prolonged PPV is needed the baby should preferably be intubated, if not done till now. Cardiac monitor should also be attached, if available, by this time. Additional help must also be called by this time to assist in resuscitation. If PPV needs to be given for longer than several seconds, placement of orogastric tube should be considered as gas may enter the esophagus and stomach by prolonged PPV. Putting an orogastric tube will give vent for the gas in the stomach.
- ***If the heart rate is <60 bpm:*** Additional measures such as cardiac compression and medication may be needed. This will be discussed subsequently.

Good to Know

- A CO_2 detector device can be put between the PPV self-inflating bag and mask. This can help us identify that the delivered PPV is effective, and ventilation is inflating and aerating the lung.
- Laryngeal mask airway may be used in situation when one has not been able to deliver effective PPV by self-inflating bag and face mask and intubation is not possible.
- Initial ventilation pressure should be 20–25 cmH_2O.

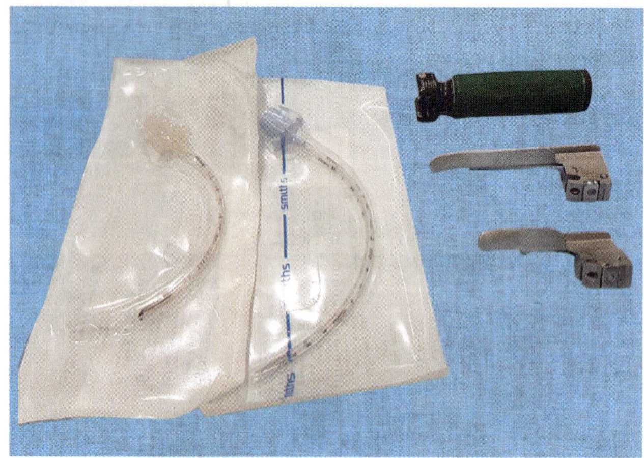

Fig. 15.10: Laryngoscope with term and preterm blade

ENDOTRACHEAL INTUBATION

Indications of endotracheal intubation are:

- If the baby's heart rate remains <100 bpm and is not increasing after effective PPV with bag and mask ventilation.
- Before starting chest compressions.
- For PPV in a patient with suspected congenital diaphragmatic hernia.
- If PPV is needed for prolonged time, intubation can be considered for improved efficacy and ease.
- If surfactant is to be administered.

A person skilled in intubation should be available if the need for intubation arises. Intubation should ideally be completed within 30 seconds. Laryngoscope with right size of blade should be used **(Fig. 15.10)**. Also, appropriate size endotracheal tube should be used for intubation **(Table 15.2)**. The endotracheal tube insertion length can be estimated by the gestational age of the baby or by measuring the nasal-tragus length of the baby and adding 1 cm to it. Once inserted the endotracheal tube should be fixed securely. The endotracheal tube should be positioned so the tip lies 1–2 cm below the vocal cords. The correct placement of the endotracheal tube can be confirmed by:

- Bilateral chest movement on giving PPV.
- Presence of equal breath sounds on both the sides of the chest.
- Condensation inside the endotracheal tube.
- Exhaled CO_2 detection.

Table 15.2 Endotracheal Tube Size for Babies According to Birth Weight and Gestational Age

Weight	*Gestational age*	*Endotracheal tube size (internal diameter)*
<1,000 g	<28 weeks	2.5 mm
1,000–2,000 g	28–34 weeks	3.0 mm
>2,000 g	>34 weeks	3.5 mm

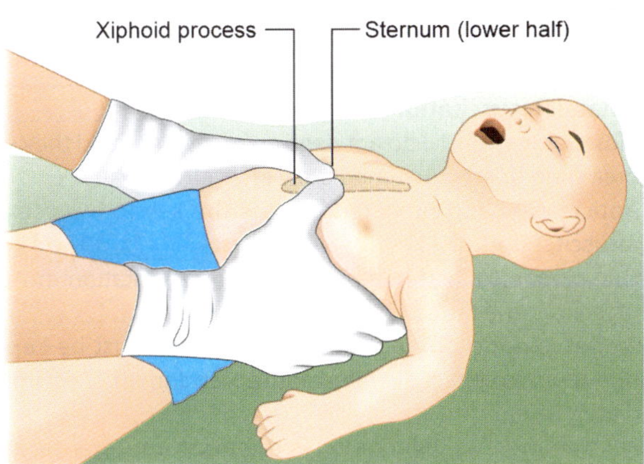

Fig. 15.11: Two-thumb technique for chest compression

CHEST COMPRESSIONS

If after 30 seconds of PPV that ventilates the lungs, the baby's heart rate <60 bpm, chest compressions should be started immediately. In all babies in whom chest compression is needed:

- The baby should be intubated if not done till now.
- Delivered FiO_2 should be increased to 100%.
- At least two people trained in neonatal resuscitation must be available.

Technique of Giving Chest Compressions

Two thumb technique is used for cardiac compressions in neonates. Both the thumbs are placed on the sternum in the center just below the imaginary line joining the baby's nipples. The torso of the baby is encircled with both hands and the back of the baby is supported by the fingers **(Fig. 15.11)**. Both the thumbs are pressed downward with sufficient pressure together to depress the sternum by approximately one-third of the total anteroposterior diameter of the chest. The compression rate should be around 90 compressions per minute. The compressions have to be coordinated with PPV, which is now given at a rate of 30 breaths per minute. To achieve these 90 compressions and coordinated 30 breaths, rhythm used is *"one-and-two-and-three-and breathe-and"*. Cardiac compressions are given at *"one, two, three"* and chest is released at each *"and"* while a breath is delivered at *"breathe"*. Compressions should be paused when a breath is delivered. The ratio of compression to ventilation is maintained at 3:1. The cycle of compressions and PPV should continue for 60 seconds before the heart rate is checked again. If the heart rate is ≥60 bpm, cardiac compressions are stopped and PPV is continued at the rate of 40–60 breaths per minute. If the heart rate remains <60 bpm after 60 seconds of cardiac compressions and PPV, then emergency vascular access is needed for epinephrine administration.

MEDICATIONS

Medications are rarely needed in NNR. The route of choice for drug administration is intravenous and cannulation of the umbilical vein is recommended. Intraosseous route can be used as an alternative route if umbilical venous access is not possible. Insertion of peripheral intravenous catheter is not recommended for emergency medication administration as it may be more time consuming or unsuccessful.

Epinephrine: It is indicated when heart rate remains <60 bpm after 60 seconds of coordinated cardiac compressions and ventilation with 100% FiO_2 **(Table 15.3)**.

Volume expanders: They are indicated when the baby is not responding to the steps of resuscitation and there are signs of shock or a history of acute blood loss. The fluid of choice is normal saline (0.9%), ringer lactate may also be used. Packed red blood cells may be used if severe fetal anemia is suspected.

Decision to stop resuscitation: Newly born babies who do not have a detectable heart rate after 10–20 minutes of resuscitation, stopping resuscitation may be considered.

Good to Know

Preterm babies need special precautions while resuscitation. Some points to take care are:

- They are more likely to need resuscitation.
- They are also at increased risk of developing complications.
- Additional resources may be needed such as, trained personnel, CPAP device, and need for surfactant administration.
- If the baby <32 weeks of gestational age, a plastic bag or plastic wrap should be used to cover the baby to prevent evaporative heat loss **(Fig. 15.12)**.

Table 15.3 Drug Dose for Neonatal Resuscitation in Delivery Room

Drug	Route	Dose	Remarks
Epinephrine 0.1 mg/mL Or 1 mg/10 mL (1:10,000)	Intravenous/ intraosseous	0.02 mg/kg (0.2 mL/kg) *Range:* 0.01–0.03 mg/kg (0.1–0.3 mL/kg)	• Give it as quickly as possible • Flush with 3 mL normal saline • Can be repeated every 3–5 minutes
	Endotracheal	0.1 mg/kg (1 mL/kg) *Range:* 0.05–0.1 mL/kg (0.5–1 mL/kg)	• May be given while venous access is being established • No flush needed • Give several breaths to distribute the drug into the lungs
Normal saline (0.9%) O Rh negative blood if severe fetal anemia suspected	Intravenous/ intraosseous	10 mL/kg	Administer over 5–10 minutes

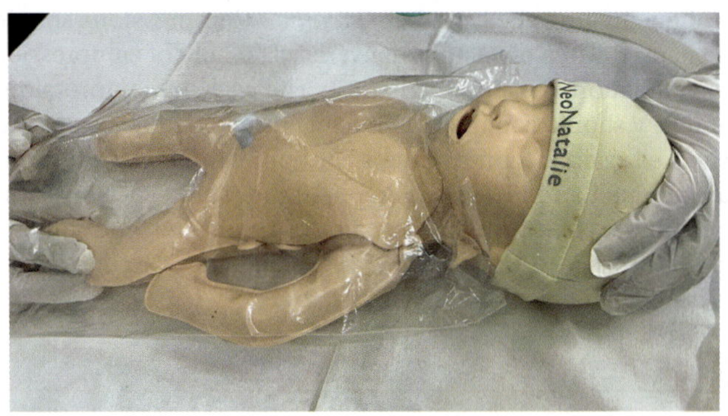

Fig. 15.12: Preterm baby in a plastic wrap

Courtesy: Dr Satvik Bansal, Gwalior

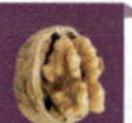

IN A NUTSHELL

Neonatal Resuscitation

1. Most babies (~85%) do not need any assistance and they start breathing or crying immediately after birth.
2. Anticipation and preparedness are the key to a successful resuscitation.
3. One person trained in basic neonatal resuscitation must be present at the time of birth of a baby.
4. All babies who do not need resuscitation must be kept in skin-to-skin contact over the mother's abdomen/chest immediately after birth.
5. Positive pressure ventilation is the most important step in neonatal resuscitation.

American Heart Association and American Academy of Pediatrics. Textbook of Neonatal Resuscitation, 8th edition. New Delhi: CBS Publishers; 2021.
National Health Mission, Ministry of Health and Family Welfare, Government of India. (2020). Navjaat Shishu Suraksha Kaaryakram. [online] Available from https://nhm.gov.in/images/pdf/programmes/child-health/guidelines/NSSK/NSSK-Resource-Manual.pdf [Last accessed May, 2025].

15.3 Care of the Newborn at Birth *PE 19.1, PE 19.3*

INTRODUCTION

The birth of a baby is a significant medical event and all births irrespective of presence or absence of high-risk factors should be considered as a potential medical emergency. Therefore, it is very important that we should be prepared to take care of a baby before its birth. There should be a smooth transition of the baby from in utero to the external environment at birth. We should facilitate this smooth transition to avoid any problems, detect them early, and manage them accordingly. Things that should be taken care of at the time of birth are given here.

TEMPERATURE MAINTENANCE

The temperature of the delivery room should be kept at 26–28°C. The radiant warmer should be switched on before the birth of the baby **(Fig. 15.13)**. Prewarmed, dry, and sterile towels must be ready for the baby. The baby should be dried immediately after birth and the wet towel should be removed. The baby is kept on the mother's abdomen for skin-to-skin contact and then covered with a warm and clean cloth/towel.

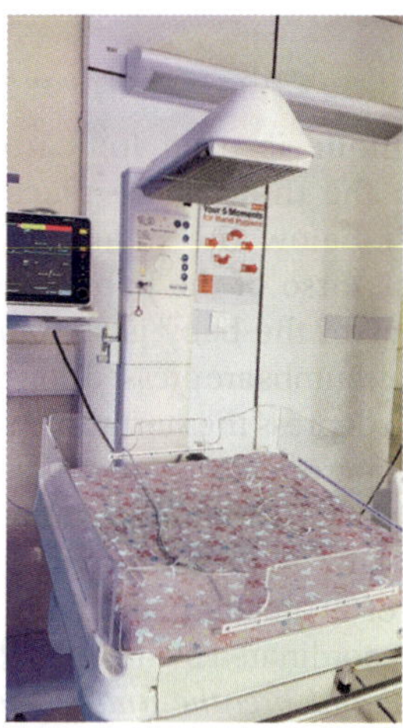

Fig. 15.13: Radiant warmer ready before the birth of the baby

HANDLING THE BABY

Follow universal precautions while handling a baby. Handwashing by personnel to prevent infection of the baby should be done before touching a newborn baby. Wipe off all the blood but the vernix should not be forcefully removed as it prevents hypothermia in the baby. It is important to observe how the baby responds to being handled. There is no need to routinely suction the mouth and nose of the baby at birth. Routine stomach wash by passing a nasogastric tube is also not needed. It is also important that the baby should be handled gently.

PREVENTION OF INFECTION

As the mother and the baby both are at risk of infection during the process of delivery, therefore, it is of utmost importance to follow the steps of cleanliness also known as the "clean chain." Preparedness even before the delivery plays a key role in maintenance of asepsis. The components of the clean chain are:

During Delivery

Five Cs of a clean delivery are:

1. ***Clean hands:*** All healthcare workers must do hand hygiene.
2. ***Clean delivery surface***
3. ***Clean cord:*** Nothing should be applied to the umbilical cord and it should be kept clean. Sterile blade or scissors must be used to cut the cord.
4. ***Clean tie:*** The cord should be tied with a sterile clamp or a clean thread.
5. ***Clean cloth*** for the baby and mother.

After Delivery

1. The baby should be handled only after thorough hand washing.
2. The baby should be given exclusive breastfeeds.
3. The cord should be kept clean and dry.
4. Clean cloth should be used for tying as a diaper.

The caregiver should wash hands well after changing diapers of the baby and the perineum of the baby must be cleaned properly after the diapers have been soiled.

Care of the Umbilical Cord

The umbilical cord is a good medium for bacterial growth. Therefore, it is extremely important to ensure that it is kept clean and dry. Umbilical cord of the baby should be clamped 1–3 minutes after birth of the baby. This allows some extra blood to flow from the mother to the baby and prevents anemia later in infancy. A disposable and sterile cord clamp should be used to clamp the cord. The cord can also be clamped using a clean rubber band or strong thread. The cord should be cut with a sterile blade. The length of the cord left should be only 3–4 cm **(Fig. 15.14)**. The clamp/tie should be around 2 cm from the base of the cord and another 1–2 cm of the cord should be left beyond the clamp before cutting. A long cord that hangs around on the abdomen may get soiled in the genital area and is prone to infections.

Care of the Eyes

The eyes should be cleaned using a soft, clean, and wet cloth from the inner canthus (corner) of the eye to the outer canthus. Separate pieces of cloth should be used for each eye and discarded after cleaning.

PHYSICAL EXAMINATION

After stabilization, the baby should be examined. Care must be taken that the ambient temperature is appropriate for the baby to prevent hypothermia. The baby should ideally be examined under a radiant warmer. After quick assessment, the baby is covered well again. The baby must be assessed for color and any breathing difficulty. The skull should be examined for any abnormal swelling or shape and for any cuts or injury during delivery. The movements of all four limbs must be observed. There may be decreased movement of any limb due to fracture or neurological injury **(Fig. 15.15)**.

Congenital Anomalies

A detailed but quick assessment must be done for any congenital malformation that may need urgent attention like meningomyelocele **(Fig. 15.16)** or omphalocele **(Fig. 15.17)** (herniation of the abdominal contents through the umbilical cord), or ambiguous genitalia. The anal opening must also be checked and spine should be examined. Sometimes, there may be no anal orifice but just a dimple at the site **(Fig. 15.18)**. Deformities such as deformed feet [congenital talipoequinovarus deformity (CTEV)] **(Fig. 15.19)**, cleft palate and lip **(Fig. 15.20)**, and polydactyly **(Fig. 15.21)**, do not need immediate management but should be identified at birth.

Sex Determination

The sex of the baby must be assigned soon after birth and the family and the mother should be informed. Controversy may sometimes arise because of the sex of the baby. Rarely, the baby may have ambiguous genitalia **(Fig. 15.22)**, i.e., the sexual

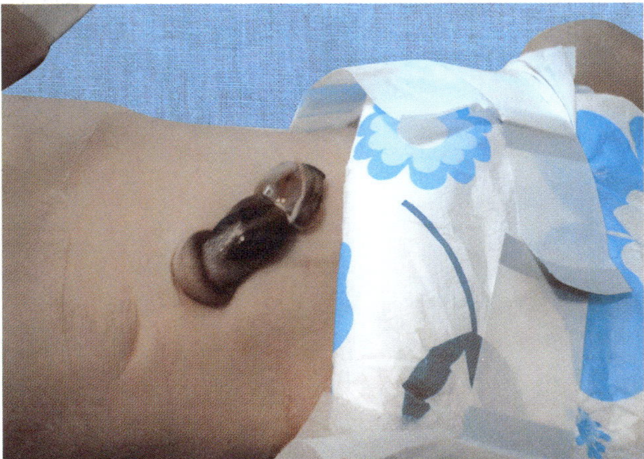

Fig. 15.14: Appropriate length of umbilical cord left after cutting

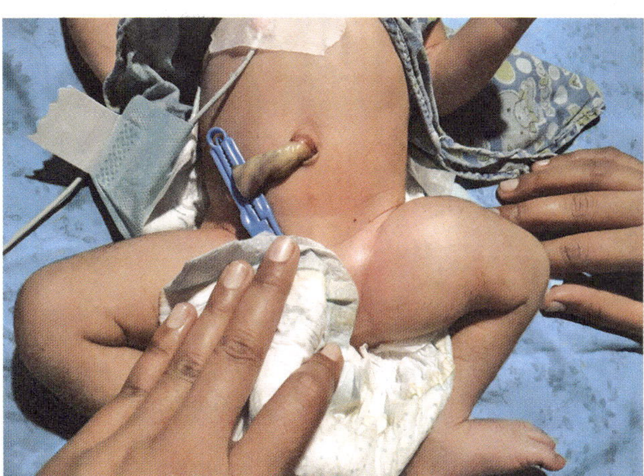

Fig. 15.15: Baby with fracture left femur appearing as swelling

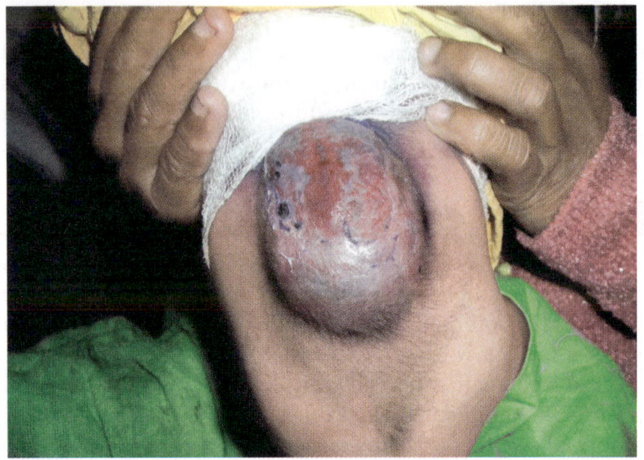

Fig. 15.16: Lumbar meningomyelocele

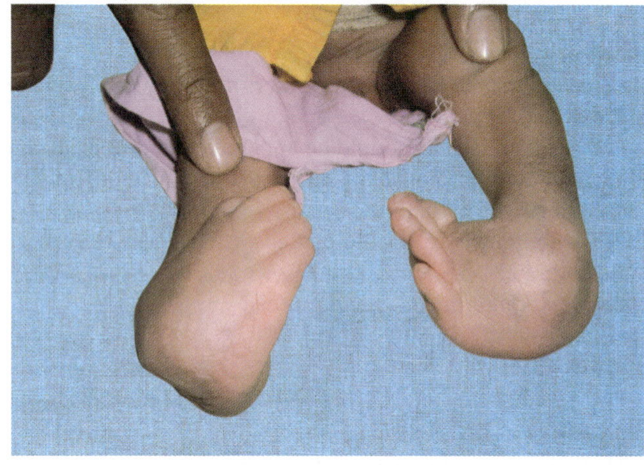

Fig. 15.19: Bilateral congenital talipes equinovarus deformity

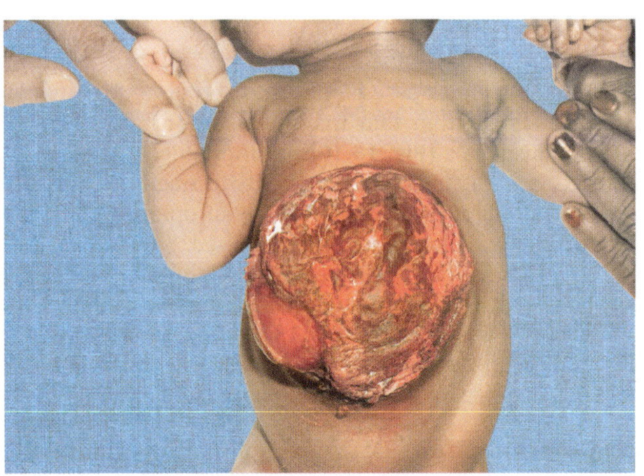

Fig. 15.17: Omphalocele

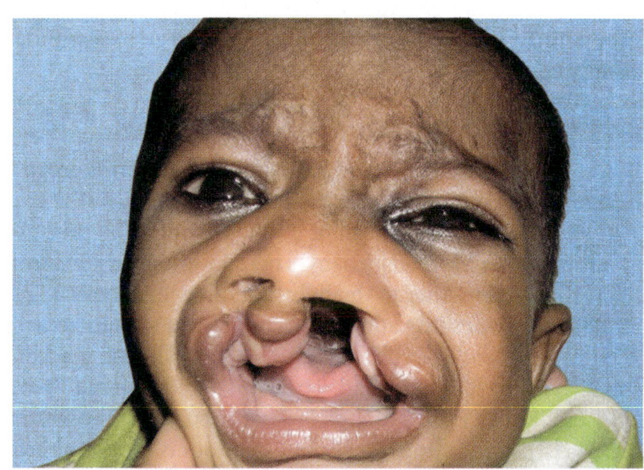

Fig. 15.20: Cleft lip and palate

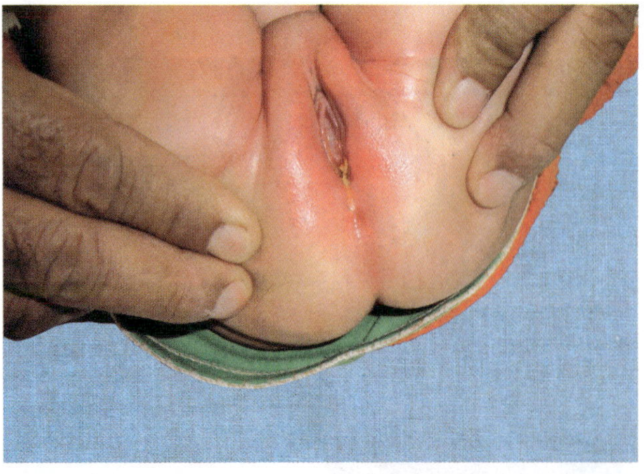

Fig. 15.18: Absent anal opening

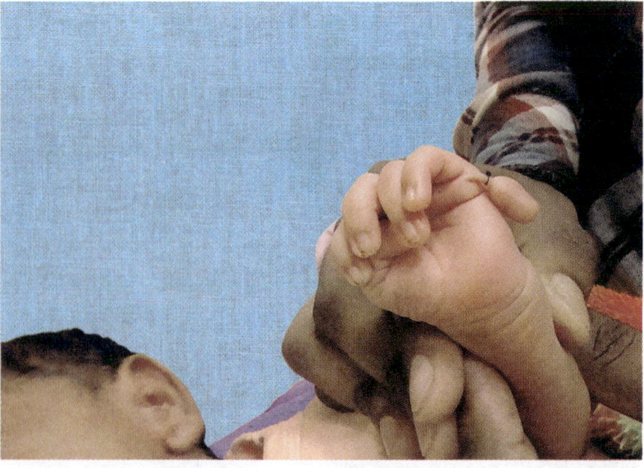

Fig. 15.21: Polydactyly

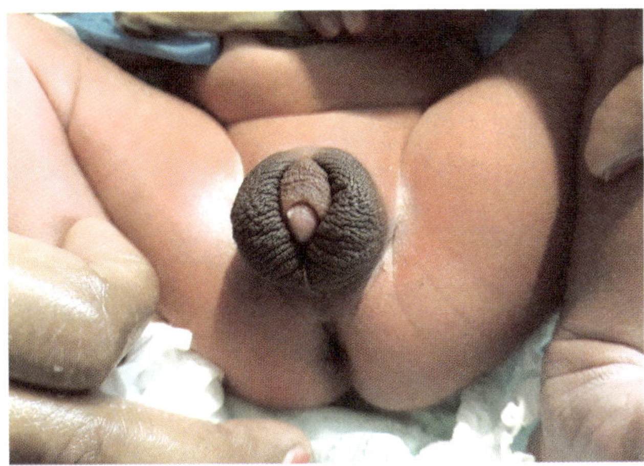

Fig. 15.22: Ambiguous genitalia

characters of the baby do not consort to either of the sex. In case of ambiguous genitalia the family should be told and counseled accordingly.

Weight

After the baby has stabilized, it should be weighed using a digital weighing machine (discussed later).

Injection Vitamin K

Injection vitamin K1 should be given to all newborns at birth. Intramuscular 1 mg of vitamin K1 is given to newborns with birth weight ≥1,000 g and 0.5 mg for babies who weigh <1,000 g on the anterolateral aspect of thigh. Newborns are prone to vitamin K deficiency as it is not transferred to the baby from the mother and it takes time before the baby can produce vitamin K in its own body. Moreover, the mother's milk is also deficient in vitamin K. Deficiency of vitamin K presents as bleeding from any site (skin, mouth, gastrointestinal, urine, and intracranial) and needs urgent management.

Record Keeping

A proper record should be kept for each baby which should include gender of the baby, name of the mother and father, time and date of birth, birth weight, details of resuscitation done, treatment given if any (including vitamin K), or any other relevant information like the human immunodeficiency virus (HIV) or hepatitis B status of the mother.

Baby Identification

An identification band displaying the details of the baby should be tied on the baby's wrist or arm and footprint must be taken.

IMMUNIZATION

All babies should be immunized at birth with bacillus Calmette-Guérin (BCG), oral polio vaccine (OPV) (zero dose), and hepatitis B (birth dose). OPV can be given up to 14 days of age. Hepatitis B vaccine should be given on the first day of life.

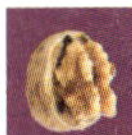

IN A NUTSHELL

Care of the Newborn at Birth

1. Temperature maintenance is the most important aspect that must be take care of while handling a baby.
2. Umbilical cord of the baby who does not need resuscitation should be clamped 1–3 minutes after birth of the baby.
3. Infection control measures and asepsis should be followed while taking care of a baby.
4. Nothing should be applied on the umbilical cord and it should be kept clean and dry.
5. A quick and thorough examination of the baby is done at birth to rule out any obvious congenital anomalies.
6. Injection vitamin K1 is given to all babies at birth to prevent its deficiency.

National Health Mission, Ministry of Health and Family Welfare, Government of India. Operational guidelines on Injection Vitamin K Prophylaxis at Birth (in facilities). [online] Available from http://nhm.gov.in/images/pdf/programmes/child-health/guidelines/Vitamin_K_Operational_Guidelines.pdf [Last accessed May, 2025].

National Health Mission. Ministry of Health and Family Welfare, Government of India. Navjaat Shishu Suraksha Karyakram. [online] Available at https://nhm.gov.in/images/pdf/programmes/child-health/guidelines/NSSK/NSSK-Resource-Manual.pdf [Last accessed May, 2025].

World Health Organization. Early essential newborn care. [online] Available from https://apps.who.int/iris/rest/bitstreams/1246772/retrieve [Last accessed May, 2025].

15.4 Initial Assessment and Care

PE 19.3

INTRODUCTION

All babies need to be assessed periodically in the first 48 hours of birth and at least twice a day until discharge.

- The purpose of first examination of the baby after stabilization is to ensure that the baby has had a smooth transition from intrauterine life to extrauterine life. Immediate assessment should be done for the pattern of respiration, color, posture, alertness, activity, and breastfeeding.
- Ongoing monitoring helps in early identification of babies with danger signs and complications. Vital monitoring every half an hour for first 2 hours then every 12 hourly or as and when indicated should be done.

PREREQUISITES FOR EXAMINING

Hands must be washed, dried, and warm. The baby must be exposed adequately before examining. Examining a baby immediately after a feed should be avoided as this may lead to regurgitation.

Monitor Temperature

Constant monitoring of temperature is important for newborn babies. Newborns are prone to becoming hypothermic. There is no urgency in bathing a baby after birth. Bathing can be postponed till the cord falls especially in LBW babies and in winter months. A term healthy baby can be bathed on second or third day of life.

Prevention of Infection

The mother and the other family members should be educated about the importance of hygiene in a newborn. The baby should be sponged daily with a soft, clean absorbent cloth from head to toe with lukewarm water, and then dried immediately. The baby should be dressed in clean, soft front open clothes which should be changed daily or as and when they get soiled.

The healthcare workers also need to be sensitized about the need of handwashing (with soap and water) before touching a baby and in between two babies to prevent transmission of infection from one baby to another.

Initiate Breastfeeding

Breastfeeding should be initiated within 1 hour of birth irrespective of mode of delivery. Breastfeeding within an hour of birth could prevent 20% of newborn deaths. It should be ensured that the mother is frequently breastfeeding her baby. Mothers, especially primigravida, need a lot of support and counseling to establish breastfeeding in the first few days. The baby should receive frequent breastfeeds all throughout the day and especially at night. This not only gives nutrition to the baby but also keeps the baby warm.

CARE OF THE EYES

Routine use of antibiotic eye drops is not recommended. The eyes should be cleaned daily using a soft, clean, and wet cloth from the inner canthus (corner) of the eye to the outer canthus. Sometimes due to blockage of the nasolacrimal duct in newborns, there is excessive lacrimation (watering) from eyes. This makes the eyes sticky. This condition resolves in most babies by 3–6 months of age. A simple massage in which firm and sustained pressure is applied on the nasal bone just besides the inner corner of the eye should be done 4–5 times in a day. Antibiotic eye drops are needed in case of pus discharge from the eyes.

CARE OF THE SKIN

The baby's skin is very soft and sensitive. Application of lotions and powder should be avoided. Nonmedicated soap (with a neutral pH) can be used for bath. Massage should be done once a day with any oil as it improves the circulation. Massage of the baby many times in day should be avoided. Sometimes, a baby may be allergic to a specific oil and may develop a rash. In such a case, the oil used should be changed.

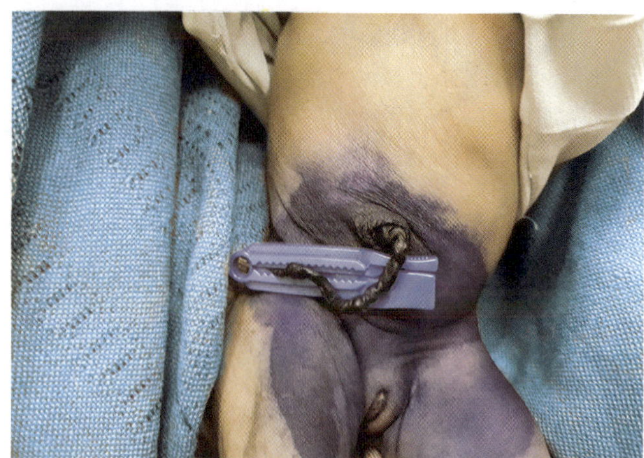

Fig. 15.23: Gentian violet paint applied to the umbilical cord: this is a wrong practice

CORD CARE

After the cord is cut, it slowly starts drying and finally separates from the body and falls off by 7–10 days. It should be cleaned while giving bath or sponging the baby. Nothing should be applied on the cord like antibiotic ointment/powder/bandage or cotton soaked in betadine or gentian violet paint **(Fig. 15.23)**. A moist or a wet cord facilitates the growth of bacteria further. Risk of infection to the cord is maximum in the first 3 days of life. The cord should be examined daily to look for any redness around it or any pus discharge **(Fig. 15.24)**. This should be treated with antibiotics.

DANGER SIGNS

A neonate who (1) is active, (2) cries vigorously, (3) has good reflexes, (4) feeds well on the breast, and (5) has warm and pink palms and soles is essentially a healthy baby.

If any of the danger signs **(Box 15.3)** is present, the baby needs immediate attention.

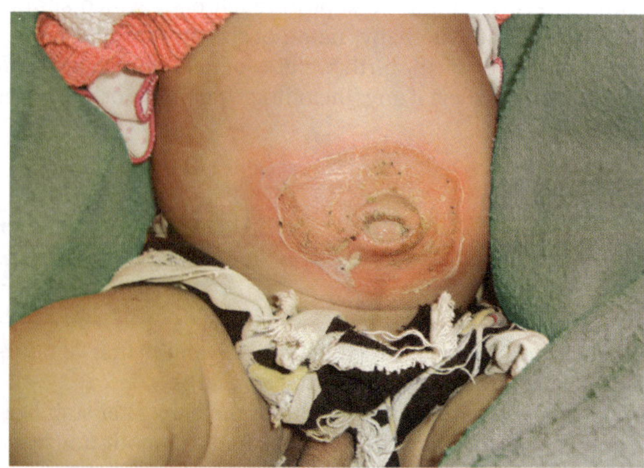

Fig. 15.24: Umbilical sepsis

Box 15.3	Danger Signs in a Newborn

1. Hypothermia/fever
2. Lethargy
3. Excessive crying
4. Bleeding from any site
5. Cyanosis
6. Yellow palms and soles
7. Inability to accept breastfeeds
8. Difficulty in breathing
9. Abdominal distention
10. Bilious vomiting
11. Persistent vomiting
12. Convulsions

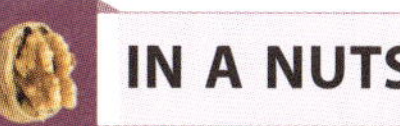

IN A NUTSHELL

Initial Assessment and Care

1. All newborns must have ongoing evaluation for the first 48–72 hours.
2. Breastfeeding must be initiated within 1 hour of birth irrespective of the mode of delivery.
3. Care of the eyes, cord, and skin of the baby is important.
4. Maintenance of temperature and infection control are extremely important for newborn babies.

National Health Mission, Ministry of Health and Family Welfare. Facility based newborn care. [online] Available from http://nhm.gov.in/images/pdf/programmes/child-health/guidelines/operational_guidelines_for_fimnci.pdf [Last accessed May, 2025].

National Health Mission, Ministry of Health and Family Welfare. Integrated Management of Neonatal and childhood illnesses. [online] Available from https://nhm.gov.in/images/pdf/programmes/child-health/guidelines/imnci_chart_booklet.pdf [Last accessed May, 2025].

World Health Organization. (2017). WHO recommendations on newborn health: guidelines approved by the WHO Guidelines Review Committee. [online] Available from https://apps.who.int/iris/handle/10665/259269 [Last accessed May, 2025].

15.5 Assessment of Weight and Gestation *PE 19.3*

ANTHROPOMETRIC EXAMINATION

Weight

The baby is weighed after initial stabilization at birth, using preferably a digital weighing machine **(Fig. 15.25)**. All precautions must be taken to prevent hypothermia and infection during the process.

- The sheet over the pan of the weighing machine should be sterile, dry, and warm.
- A fresh sheet should be used for each baby.
- The weighing machine should have a broad base and should be kept on a stable, hard surface to prevent the baby from falling.

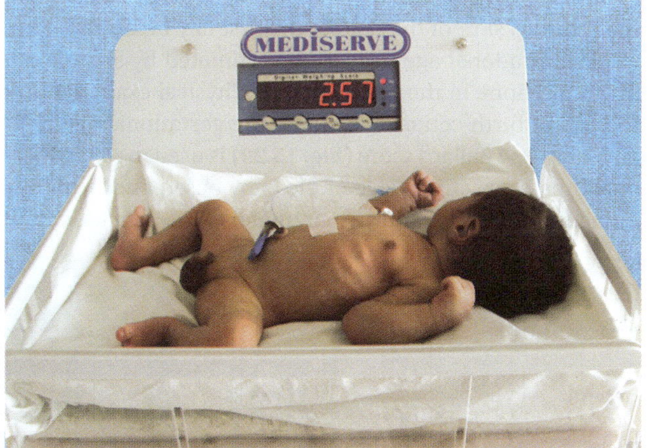

Fig. 15.25: Weighing a baby after birth

Classification of Newborn According to Weight

Weight is the single most important prognostic factor for morbidity and mortality. Newborns are classified based on birth weight as given in **Table 15.4**.

The birth weight charts according to the gestational age are available, according to which the baby is categorized appropriately **(Fig. 15.26)**.

- ***Small for date or small for gestational age (SGA):*** These babies have a birth weight <10th percentile for their gestational age. These babies have much higher morbidity and mortality. These babies have a malnourished look with less subcutaneous fat and wrinkled skin **(Figs. 15.27A and B)**.
- ***Appropriate for gestational age:*** The birth weight of these babies lies between 10th and 90th percentile for their gestational age.
- ***Large for gestational age:*** The birth weight of these babies is >90th percentile for their gestational age.

Length

The length of the baby is measured using an infantometer **(Fig. 15.28)**. The head end is fixed and the foot end can be

Table 15.4 Classification of Newborn According to the Birth Weight

Classification	*Birth weight (grams)*
Low birth weight	<2,500
Very low birth weight	<1,500
Extremely low birth weight	<1,000

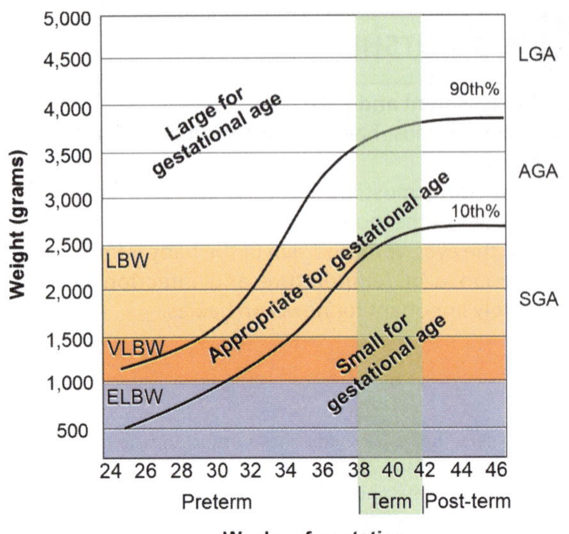

Fig. 15.26: Classification of a baby according to birth weight and gestational age

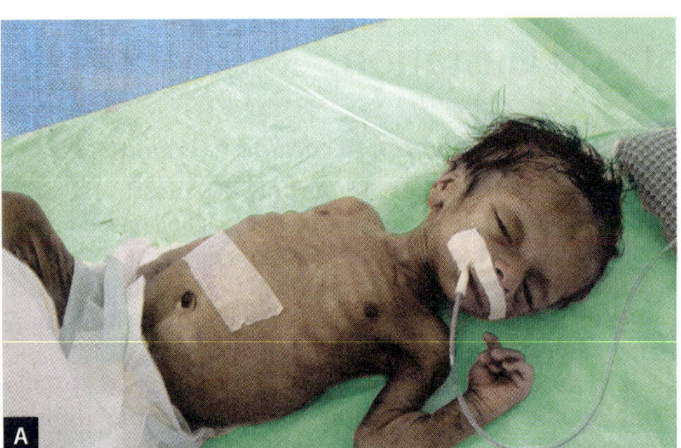

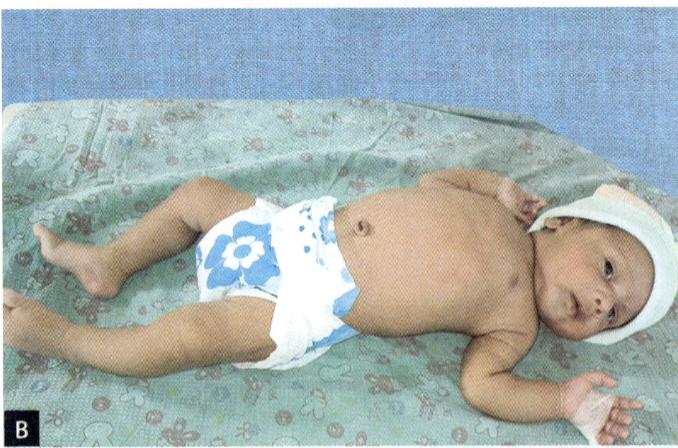

Figs. 15.27A and B: (A) Small for gestational age baby; (B) Appropriate for gestational age baby

adjusted so that it touches the soles of the feet. The baby is made to lie on the infantometer. The head of the baby is stabilized at the head end and the body is straightened and the knees are pressed down, the feet are held at 90° to the base such that the toes point upward. The length is then noted in cm. The length of a term baby is around 50 cm.

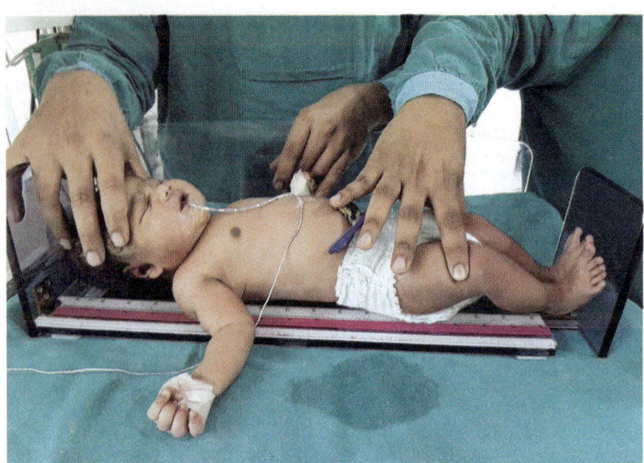

Fig. 15.28: Measuring length of a baby using an infantometer

Head Circumference

The head circumference should be taken after 24 hours of birth. The baby may have a caput succedaneum at birth due to which the head circumference will be falsely increased. In vaginal delivery, there is molding of the skull to facilitate the passage of the skull through a narrow birth canal which may give a falsely low head circumference at birth. The normal head circumference of a term baby is 33–35 cm. An abnormally small or large head may be due to some central nervous system disorder and must be evaluated thoroughly.

GESTATIONAL AGE ESTIMATION

The gestational age calculation is done with respect to the 1st day of the last menstrual period of the mother. The classification of a newborn according to the gestational age at birth is given in **Table 15.5**. An accurate gestational age can be calculated, if the mother is sure of the date of the first day of last menstrual period. Gestational age can also be estimated by an antenatal ultrasound done in the first trimester. Physical examination of the baby at birth can also estimate the gestational age of the baby. The New Ballard score **(Fig. 15.29)** is used to calculate the approximate gestational age of the baby based on the physical and neuromuscular maturity parameters. An estimation of the

Table 15.5 Classification of Newborn According to the Gestational Age

Classification	*Gestational age*
Preterm	<37 weeks
Term	37–41 weeks
Post-term	>41 weeks

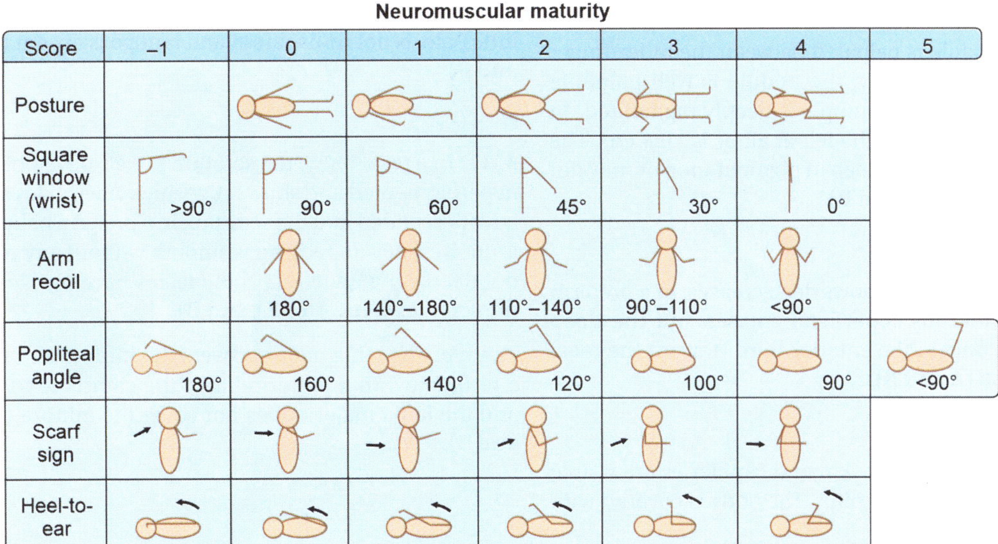

Neuromuscular maturity

Score	−1	0	1	2	3	4	5
Posture							
Square window (wrist)	>90°	90°	60°	45°	30°	0°	
Arm recoil		180°	140°–180°	110°–140°	90°–110°	<90°	
Popliteal angle	180°	160°	140°	120°	100°	90°	<90°
Scarf sign							
Heel-to-ear							

Physical maturity

Skin	Sticky, friable, transparent	Gelatinous, red, translucent	Smooth, pink, visible veins	Superficial peeling and/or rash, few veins	Cracking pale areas, rare veins	Parchment deep cracking, no vessels	Leathery, cracked, wrinkled
Lanugo	None	Sparse	Abundant	Thinning	Bald areas	Mostly bald	
Plantar surface	Heel-toe 40–50 mm: −1 <40 mm: −2	> 50 mm, no crease	Faint red marks	Anterior transverse crease only	Creases anterior ⅔	Creases over entire sole	
Breast	Imperceptible	Barely perceptible	Flat areola, no bud	Stippled areola, 1–2 mm bud	Raised areola, 3–4 mm bud	Full areola, 5–10 mm bud	
Eye/Ear	Lids fused Loosely: −1 Tightly: −2	Lids open, pinna flat, stays folded	Slightly curved pinna, soft, slow recoil	Well-curved pinna, soft, but ready recoil	Formed and firm, instant recoil	Thick cartilage, ear stiff	
Genitals male	Scrotum flat, smooth	Scrotum empty, faint rugae	Testes in upper canal, rare rugae	Testes descending, few rugae	Testes down, good rugae	Testes pendulous, deep rugae	
Genitals female	Clitoris prominent, labia flat	Prominent clitoris small labia minora	Prominent clitoris enlarging minora	Majora and minora equally prominent	Majora large, minora small	Majora cover clitoris and minora	

Maturity rating

Score	Weeks
−10	20
−5	22
0	24
5	26
10	28
15	30
20	32
25	34
30	36
35	38
40	40
45	42
50	44

Fig. 15.29: New Ballard score

gestational age assessment is necessary to identify whether the baby needs special attention or needs to be referred for admission to a neonatal intensive care unit (NICU). Any baby who is born preterm or post-term may need special care.

Certain physical parameters can help in differentiating a term baby from a preterm one. The following parameters are useful in estimating the gestational age.

Elastic Recoil

The external ear is made up of cartilage, which has a property to recoil when folded. If the ear of a term baby is folded and then released, it recoils back immediately to its original shape and position. The ear also feels firm in a term baby. In a preterm baby, the ear recoils back slowly and does not feel firm.

Breast Nodule

The breast bud or nodule is palpated between the index finger and the thumb. In a term baby, the nodule is well palpable and measures >0.5 cm and the nipple is deeply pigmented. In a preterm, the nodule may not be felt at all or is <0.5 cm. The nipple in a preterm baby is not deep in pigmentation or may not be perceivable **(Figs. 15.30A and B)**.

Plantar Creases

In a term baby, the entire sole shows deep creases. In a preterm baby, there are numerous superficial creases, but the deep creases are present only in the anterior third (toward the toes) of the feet **(Figs. 15.31A and B)**.

Lanugo and Skin

A preterm baby has transparent skin and capillaries are visible under it. The baby appears very pink. The body is covered with excessive hair called lanugo. In a term baby, the skin appears a little pale, is not transparent and lanugo is absent **(Figs. 15.32A and B)**.

Genitalia

Male: In a term baby, the scrotum is well-developed, the skin is hyperpigmented and shows rugosities or wrinkles and the testes have descended into the scrotum. In a preterm baby, the scrotum is not well-developed and is smooth without any rugosities. It is not deeply pigmented and the testes have not descended into the scrotum **(Figs. 15.33A and B)**.

Female: The labia majora covers the minora and the clitoris in a term baby. In a preterm baby, the clitoris is very prominent and the labia majora does not cover the minora **(Figs. 15.34A and B)**.

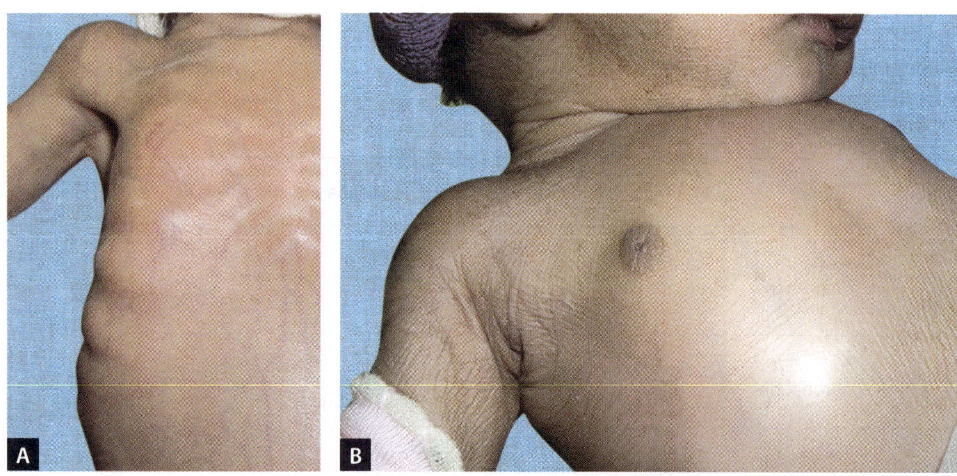

Figs. 15.30A and B: Breast nodule: (A) Preterm baby; (B) Term baby

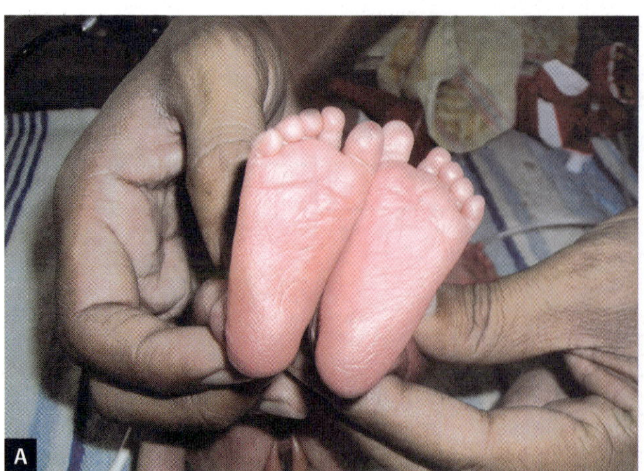

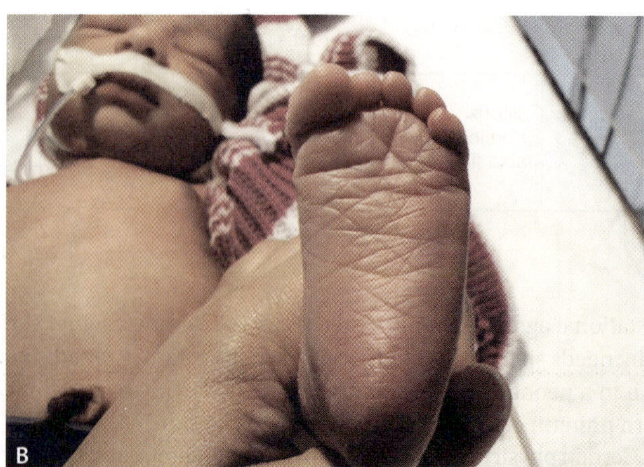

Figs. 15.31A and B: Plantar creases: (A) Preterm baby; (B) Term baby

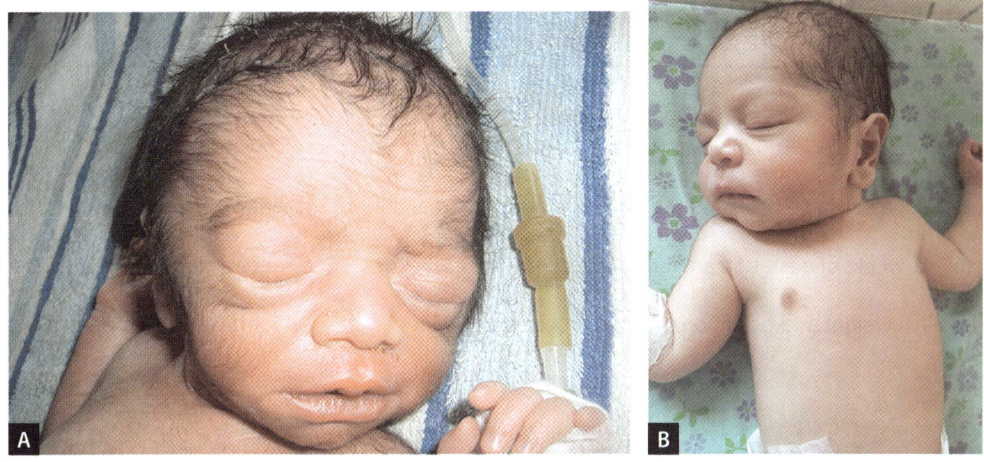

Figs. 15.32A and B: Lanugo and skin: (A) Preterm baby; (B) Term baby

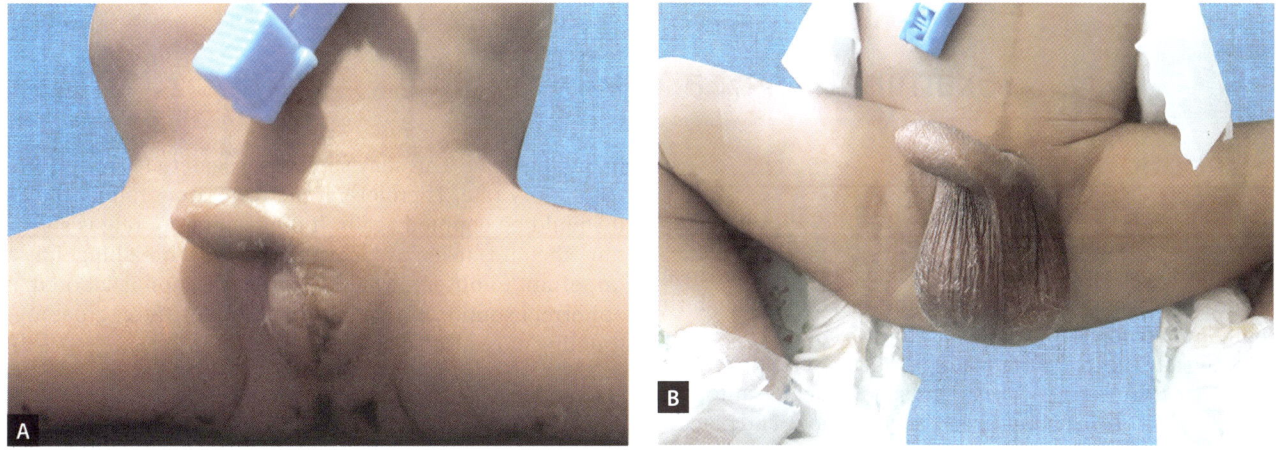

Figs. 15.33A and B: Male genitalia: (A) Preterm baby; (B) Term baby

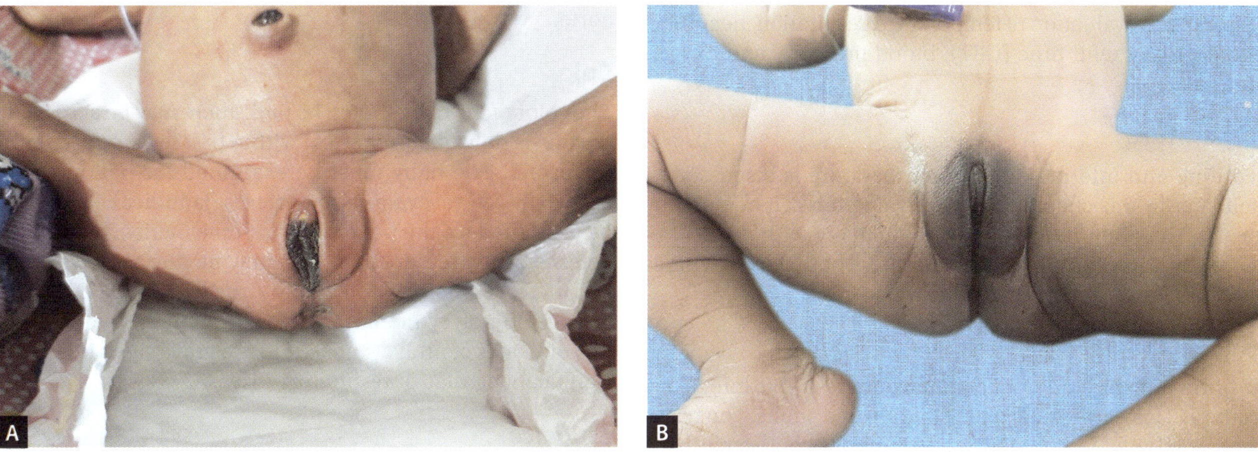

Figs. 15.34A and B: Female genitalia: (A) Preterm baby; (B) Term baby

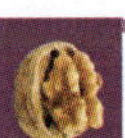

IN A NUTSHELL

Assessment of Weight and Gestation

1. A term baby should weigh between 2,500–4,000 g at birth.
2. A baby with a birth weight of <2,500 g is classified into low birth weight (LBW), very low birth weight (VLBW), and extremely low birth weight (ELBW).
3. The gestational age of a baby can be estimated from the last menstrual period, antenatal ultrasound in the first trimester or New Ballard score.
4. Babies born at 37–41 weeks of gestation are term babies, born <37 weeks are preterm babies, and born >41 weeks are post-term babies.
5. According to the birth weight and gestation of a baby it can be classified into, small for gestation, appropriate for gestation, and large for gestation.

Ballard JL, Khoury JC, Wedig K, et al. New Ballard Score, expanded to include extremely premature infants. J Pediatr. 1991;119(3):417-23.
Ballard score. (2019). The Ballard Score Maturational Assessment of Gestational Age in Newly Born Infants. [online] Available from https://ballardscore.com [Last accessed May, 2025].
World Health Organization. (2004). ICD-10: International statistical classification of diseases and related health problems, tenth revision, 2nd edition. [online] Available from https://apps.who.int/iris/handle/10665/42980 [Last accessed May, 2025].

15.6 Examination of a Newborn

PE 19.1, PE 19.2, PE 19.3

INTRODUCTION

Three thorough examinations must be done in a newborn before the baby is discharged (1) at birth, (2) at 24 hours, and (3) at the time of discharge. But periodic evaluation is needed in all newborns, frequency depends upon the gestational age, birth weight, and any complications that they develop. For a baby presenting after birth from another healthcare setting or home, a detailed history must be taken. This should include antenatal history, a detail history about events at birth, mode and place of delivery, resuscitation required, and treatment given. A detailed and thorough examination should follow.

VITAL SIGNS

These include evaluation of temperature, respiration, heart rate, color, capillary refill time (CRT), blood pressure, and oxygen saturation.

Temperature

Recording and interpretation of temperature is discussed in detail later in this chapter. A quick evaluation can be done by touching the abdomen and sole of the baby with dorsum of hand. Baby is having normal temperature, if both the extremities and the abdomen are warm to touch.

Respiratory Rate

The normal respiratory rate of a newborn is 40–60/min. They breathe at a faster rate than older children and adults. The respiratory rate should be counted for 1 minute. Newborns may have irregular respiration known as periodic breathing, they have brief periods of rapid breathing followed by slow breathing or no breathing at all. This may sometimes lead to falsely increased respiratory rate. Therefore, if the respiratory rate is ≥60/min, it should be counted again. If the respiratory rate is still ≥60/min, then it is taken as tachypnea, i.e., fast breathing. It is also important to observe whether the respiration is labored. Any abnormal sounds of respiration such as stridor, groaning, or grunting must also be noted.

Heart Rate

The heart rate of a newborn is also more than that of older children and adults, i.e., 120–160/min. Pulse rate may not correlate with the heart rate and if the baby is hypothermic, it may be difficult to feel the pulse. All peripheral pulses should be palpated, they are weak in case of hypothermia, shock, or coarctation of aorta.

Color

The color of the baby should be pink, there may be acrocyanosis (cyanosis only of peripheries) within first few hours after birth is normal. The baby must be examined for pallor, cyanosis especially central cyanosis and icterus (jaundice). Pallor should be examined on the palm or face. Some babies may appear to be excessively red in color. This may be due to polycythemia, i.e., increased hemoglobin. Newborns who are SFD are prone to develop polycythemia. Cyanosis present on the tongue and lips indicates central cyanosis and is a grave sign and is seen in significant cardiac or respiratory disease.

Jaundice

We do not look for jaundice in the conjunctiva of a newborn as we do in older people. The newborn keeps the eye closed most

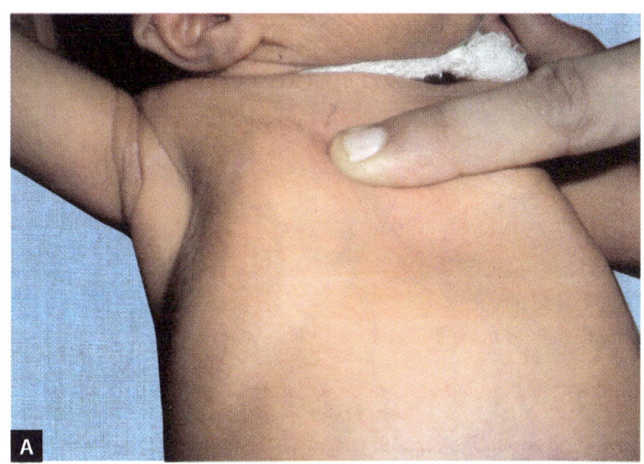

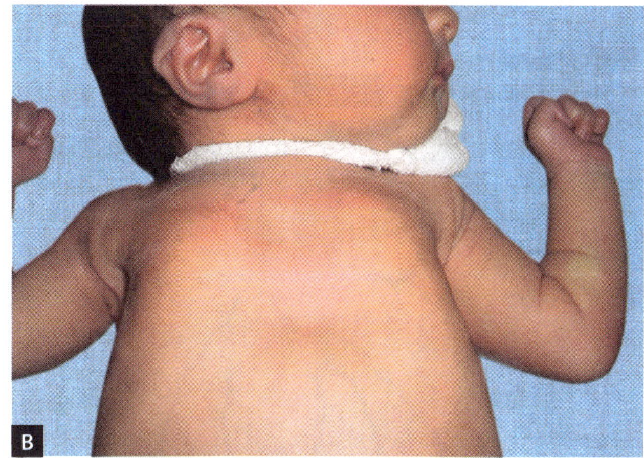

Figs. 15.35A and B: Method of examination of jaundice in a newborn

of the times and it is difficult to visualize the conjunctiva. It is easily seen on the skin **(Fig. 15.35A)**, by pressing on the skin with the index finger at a bony prominence for around 3-5 seconds and then the finger is lifted **(Fig. 15.35B)**. The finger is pressed to blanch the skin so the yellowish discoloration can then easily be seen. Jaundice first appears on the face and then progresses downward to the abdomen and extremities.

Capillary Refill Time

Capillary refill time is seen to assess the circulation of the baby. As the name suggests it is the time taken for the capillaries to refill after they have been emptied. CRT in newborns is always assessed over the sternum. The skin over the sternum is pressed with the index finger for around 5 seconds to blanch the skin and empty the capillaries and then released. The time for the capillaries to refill, i.e., for the skin color to return to normal over the blanched area is noted. The time can be noted by counting "one thousand one, one thousand two, one thousand three,......" If the color returns over the blanched area completely, before the count of "one thousand and three," this indicates that the CRT is <3 seconds, which is the normal value. If it takes longer for the color to return to normal, i.e., ≥3 seconds, the CRT is prolonged, which may be a sign of shock.

Blood Pressure

Blood pressure is not routinely measured in healthy newborns. If indicated, it should be measured using an appropriate-sized neonatal cuff (disposable neonatal cuffs are available in five sizes).

SpO_2 Monitoring

Monitoring of percent saturated hemoglobin is a good screening tool to evaluate the respiratory and cardiac status of the baby. It is also used to screen for critical congenital heart diseases. This is done with the help of a pulse oximeter. The probe is attached to the wrist or feet and connected to the pulse oximeter and the reading is displayed on the monitor **(Fig. 15.36)**. The saturation of newborns should be 90–95%.

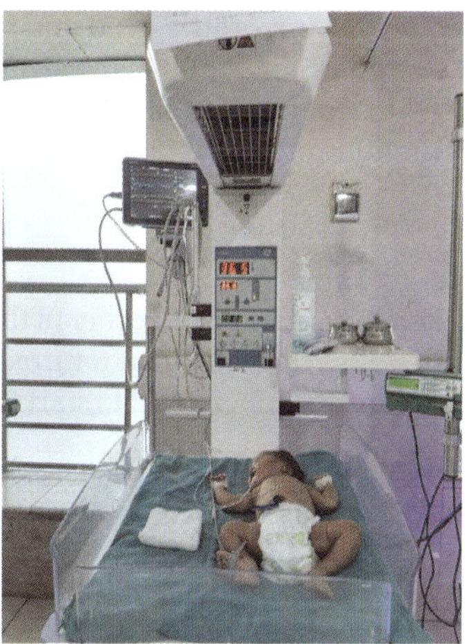

Fig. 15.36: Measurement of oxygen saturation

GENERAL EXAMINATION

Cry and Activity

The cry of a baby tells a lot about the condition of the baby. A healthy cry is loud and consolable, accompanied by active movements of the limbs. A central nervous system insult may lead to a shrill, high-pitched cry which is inconsolable. A baby with hypothyroidism may have a hoarse cry. Newborn with asphyxia or septicemia may have a feeble cry or may not cry at all, even on giving stimulus. A healthy baby should be active and have good body movements with active extension and flexion of all the limbs. A dull or a lethargic baby is difficult to arouse and lies with both the upper and lower limbs extended due to poor tone.

Neonatal Reflexes

Neonatal reflexes tell us about the neurological status of a baby.

Moro Reflex

The baby's head and trunk are lifted from the examination couch and then gently allowed to fall on the couch. The hand should

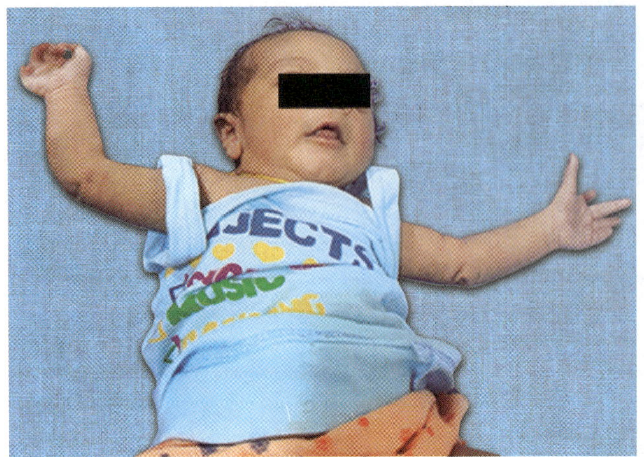

Fig. 15.37: Moro reflex

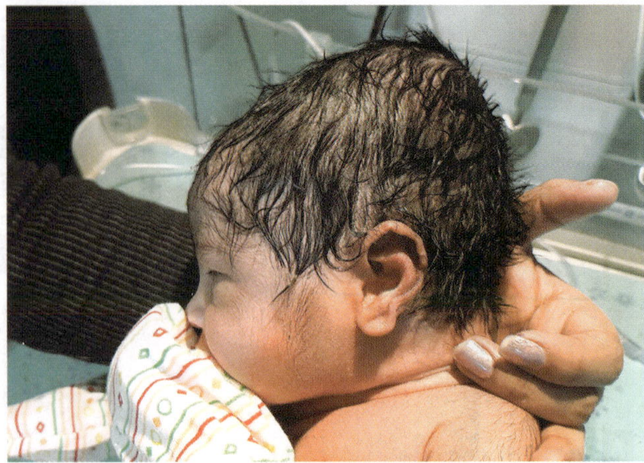

Fig. 15.38: Caput succedaneum

be kept on the couch to support the head and body when they fall back. There is sudden abduction of the arms and extension of the forearms with opening up of the hands. This is then followed by adduction and flexion of the arm and forearm **(Fig. 15.37)**.

Rooting Reflex

This reflex is elicited by touching the corner of the baby's mouth or the cheek gently with a finger. The baby turns its head toward the stimulus and opens the mouth as if to start feeding.

Sucking Reflex

If one touches the upper and lower lips and gently introduces the finger into the baby's mouth, the baby starts sucking on it.

Grasp Reflex

A touch or stroke on the palm of the baby with a finger will elicit this reflex in which the baby grasps the finger tightly.

HEAD-TO-TOE EXAMINATION

Head

Head should be examined for any swelling or abnormal shape.

- Caput succedaneum is a swelling over the scalp which is present at birth or just after birth **(Fig. 15.38)**. It is normally seen after a vaginal delivery due to venous collection of blood. It subsides in next 24–48 hours and needs no treatment.
- Cephalohematoma is also a swelling on the scalp which appears after second day of life and may increase in size for next 2–3 days. This is due to bleeding under the periosteum. It is usually present on the parietal bones **(Fig. 15.39)**. Cephalohematoma does not need any treatment but takes 2–3 months to resolve. This may contribute to jaundice in a newborn.
- Encephalocele and occipital meningocele are other swellings that may be present on the scalp **(Fig. 15.40)**.
- Anterior fontanel must also be examined in a newborn. It is a soft area between the skull bones **(Figs. 15.41A and B)**. It should be soft and at or below the level of the skull bones. A tense or a bulging anterior fontanel is a grave sign and indicative of asphyxia, meningitis, or hydrocephalus.

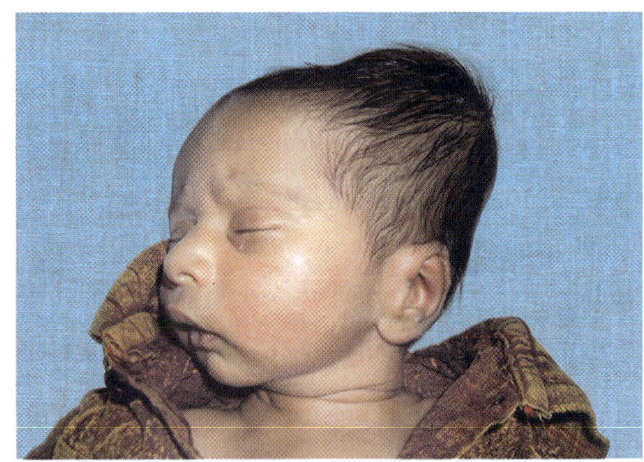

Fig. 15.39: Cephalohematoma

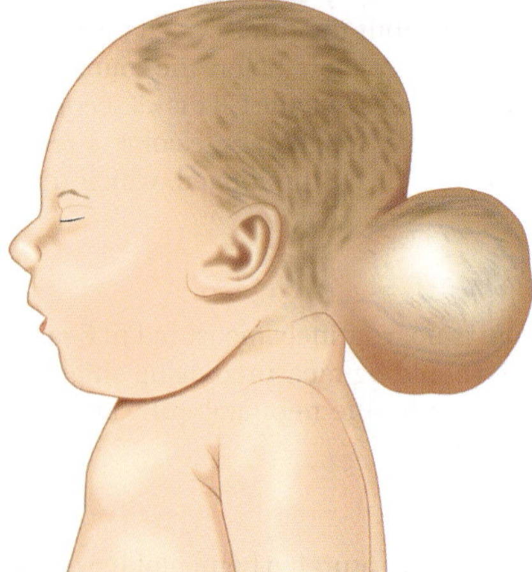

Fig. 15.40: Encephalocele

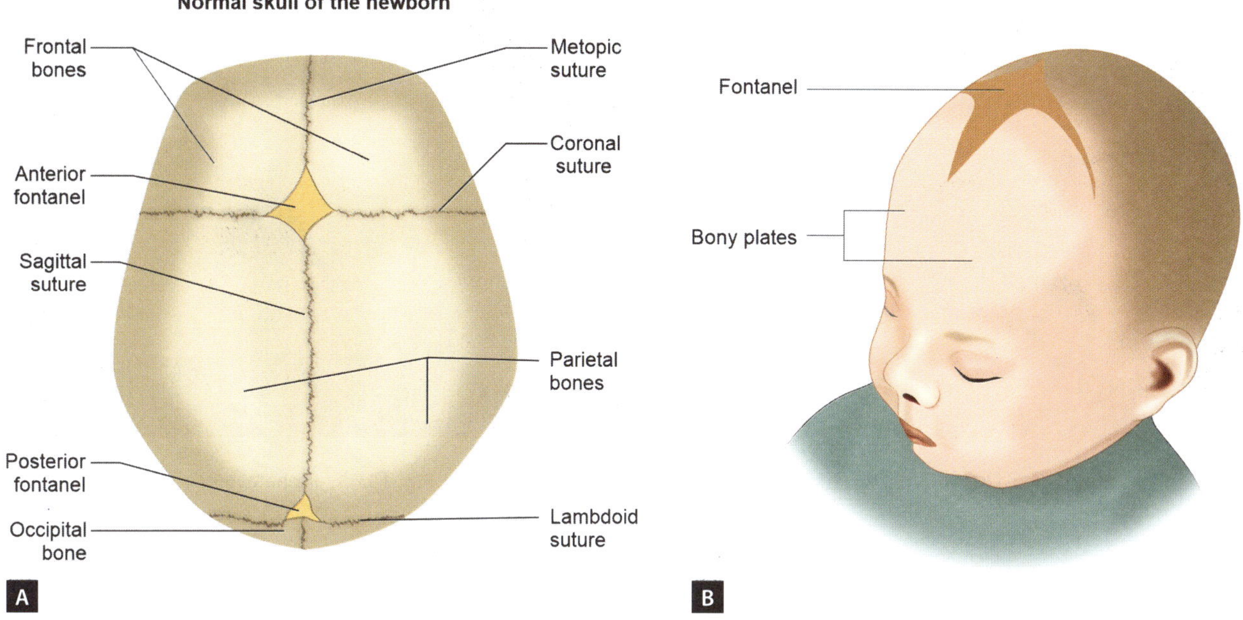

Figs. 15.41A and B: Anterior fontanel

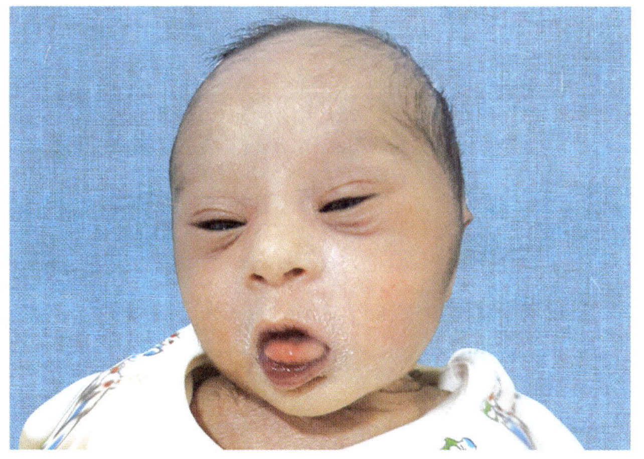

Fig. 15.42: Down syndrome

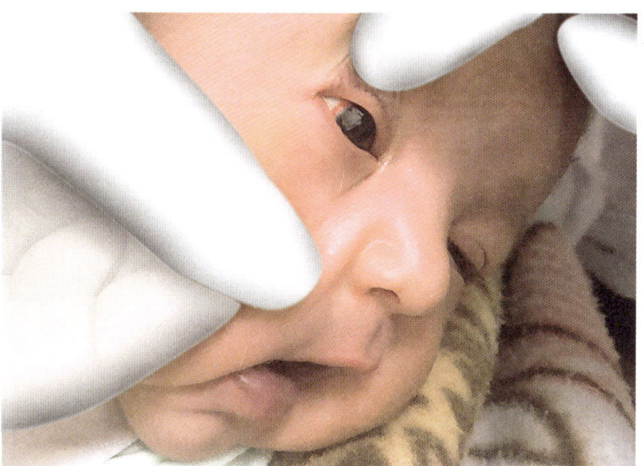

Fig. 15.43: Subconjunctival hemorrhage

Face, Eyes, Mouth, Ears

Face

Facial symmetry should be seen. An abnormal looking face or facial dysmorphism can be due to some chromosomal abnormality like Down syndrome **(Fig. 15.42)**.

Eyes

The eyes may show subconjunctival hemorrhage or bleed **(Fig. 15.43)**, which is a normal finding especially in babies born vaginally. The bleed resolves in a week. The eyes may show redness and purulent discharge. There may be watering from one or both eyes.

Mouth

The mouth must be examined for cleft lip and cleft palate. There may be oral candidiasis (oral thrush) **(Fig. 15.44)**, which is a white curdy material sticking to the tongue and oral mucosa. This is a painful condition for the baby and it may stop feeding well. This needs treatment with local antifungal agent. Prenatal teeth may rarely be present **(Fig. 15.45)**. Sometimes, a tongue is attached to the floor of the mouth by a tag known as tongue tie. This usually causes a lot of apprehension in the parents. This generally needs no treatment and the parents need to be reassured.

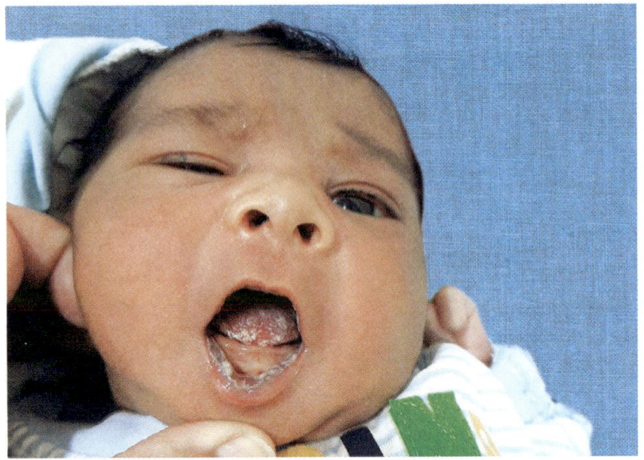

Fig. 15.44: Oral candidiasis

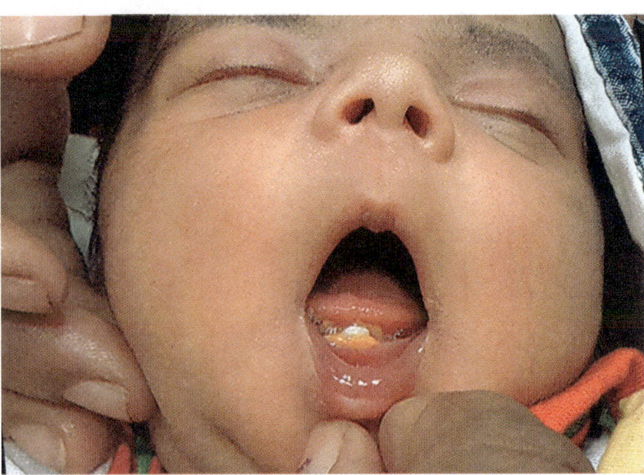

Fig. 15.45: Prenatal teeth

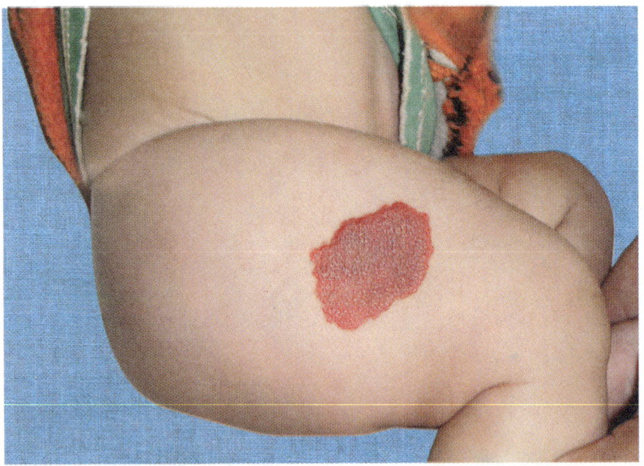

Fig. 15.46: Strawberry hemangioma

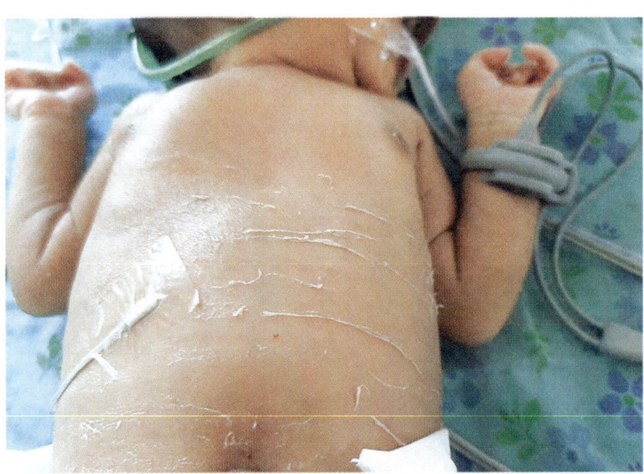

Fig. 15.47: Peeling of skin in post-term baby

Ears

The ears may be of abnormal shape or preauricular tags may be present. There may be discharge from the ears, which will need to be treated promptly with antibiotics.

Skin

Skin should be examined for any abnormal pigmentation like hemangioma **(Fig. 15.46)**, skin tags, dimple, and tuft of hair on the lower back. Preauricular tags (just in front of the ear) may be associated with renal anomalies. Post-term babies have dry skin which peels off at many places **(Fig. 15.47)**. An SFD baby has wrinkled skin. Staphylococcal scalded skin syndrome is an extensive infection of skin in newborns **(Fig. 15.48)**.

Chest

It should be examined for nipples, shape and symmetry, and any deformity. There may also be signs of respiratory distress such as intercostal or subcostal retraction and chest indrawing.

Abdomen

The abdomen of a newborn is slightly distended. It may also appear distended immediately after a feed, especially in a preterm baby. A significantly distended abdomen can be seen in intestinal obstruction, anal atresia, and necrotizing enterocolitis **(Fig. 15.49)**. Liver and spleen may be normally palpable in a newborn, but they are soft in consistency. There may be umbilical or inguinal hernia **(Fig. 15.50)**, in which there is a swelling which increases each time the baby cries.

Genitalia

Both testes should be descended in the scrotum in the term male baby. If they are not felt in the scrotum, the testes may just be present above the scrotum in the inguinal region. If testes are not felt in a term baby **(Fig. 15.51)**, he must be evaluated further. In a preterm male baby, the testes may not have descended into the scrotum.

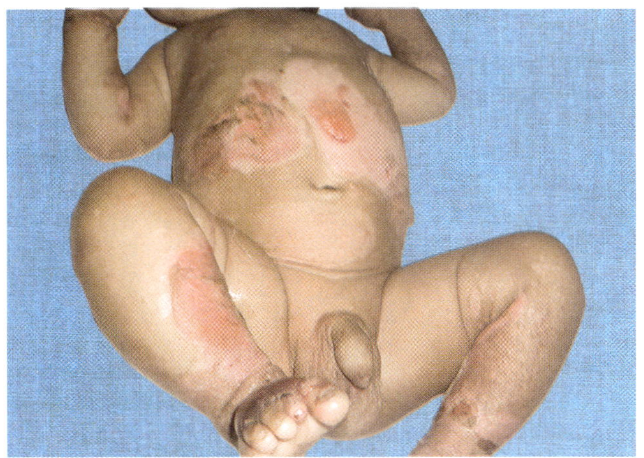

Fig. 15.48: Staphylococcal scalded skin syndrome

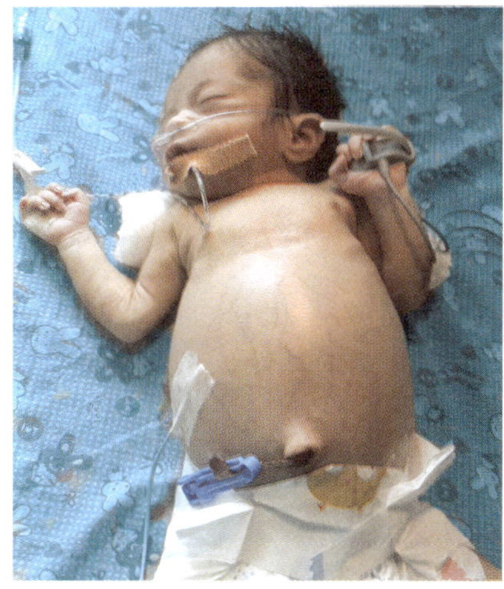

Fig. 15.49: Abdominal distention due to necrotizing enterocolitis

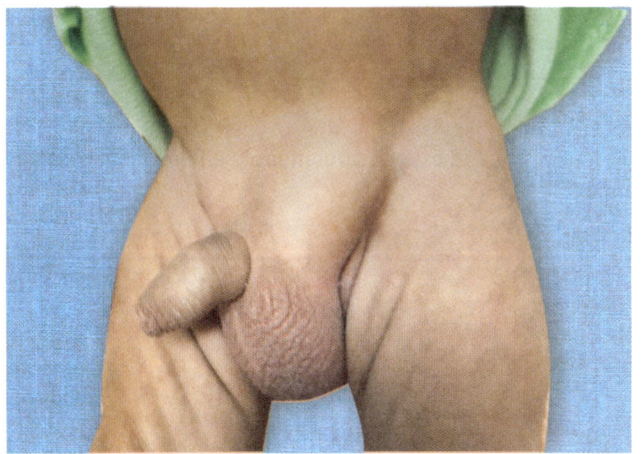

Fig. 15.50: Left inguinal hernia

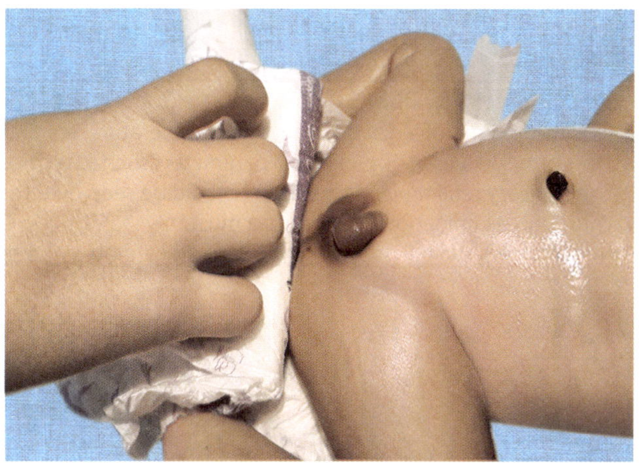

Fig. 15.51: Bilateral undescended testis

- ***Hydrocele*** is a swelling of the scrotum due to accumulation of fluid. This usually requires no intervention and resolves with time.
- It is also normal for newborns to have *phimosis*, i.e., the prepuce or the foreskin on the penis cannot be retracted. This causes a lot of anxiety in the parents. They should be advised not to forcefully retract the foreskin. It just needs reassurance as the phimosis will correct itself with time.

Spine and Limbs

Any swelling over the spine could be meningocele. A dimple or tuft of hair over the lower back may indicate a hidden spinal deformity **(Fig. 15.52)**. Curvature of the spine must also be checked for any abnormality. All four limbs should be examined for movement of all joints. Decreased movement of the upper limbs can be due to fracture of the humerus during delivery **(Fig. 15.53)**. Abnormal position of the upper limb can be due to nerve injury during delivery **(Fig. 15.54)**.

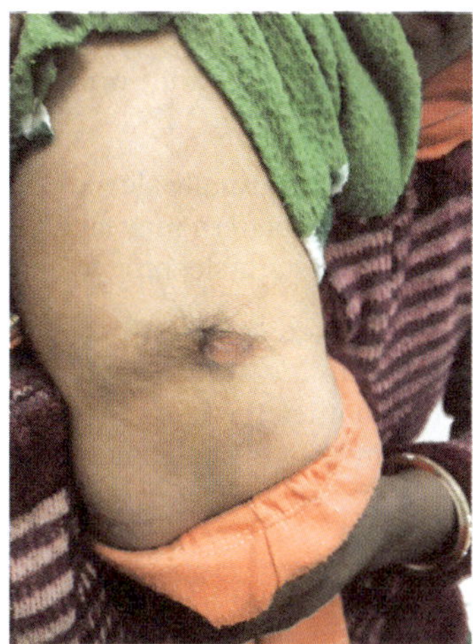

Fig. 15.52: Tuft of hair on the back

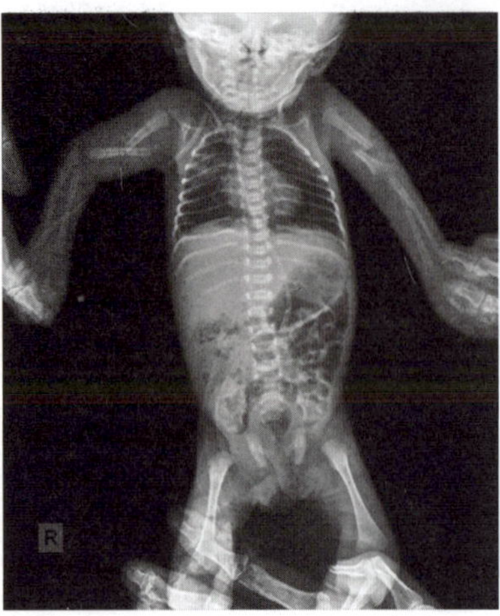

Fig. 15.53: X-ray showing bilateral fracture of humerus

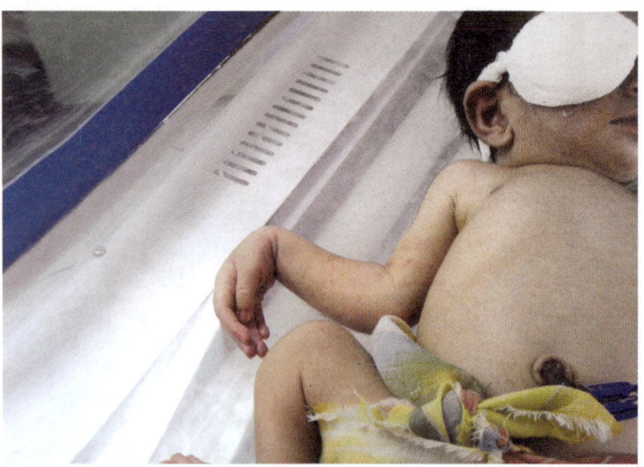

Fig. 15.54: Brachial plexus injury: Erb's palsy

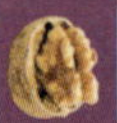

IN A NUTSHELL

Examination of a Newborn

1. Vital monitoring of a newborn includes temperature, respiratory rate, heart rate, capillary refill time, oxygen saturation.
2. The normal values of physiological parameters such as respiratory rate, heart rate, and oxygen saturation are different in newborns.
3. The capillary refill time of a newborn should be seen over the sternum.
4. Thorough examination of a baby is a must.
5. Neonatal reflexes tell us about the neurological status of the baby.

Gupta P. Clinical methods in Pediatrics, 5th edition. New Delhi: CBS publishers; 2020.
Hasen. Cloherty and Stark's manual of neonatal care (South Asian edition). Gurugram, Haryana: Wolters Kluwer; 2020.

15.7 Common Neonatal Problems *PE 19.1, PE 19.3*

NORMAL VARIATIONS

Hiccups, yawning, and sneezing are normal and usually not associated with any illness.

Sleeping pattern: Newborns usually sleep during the day and are awake in the night. This pattern may take some time before it normalizes and the baby starts sleeping in the night.

Feeding pattern: A newborn demands breastfeeds every 1.5–2 hours, as the mother's milk is easy to digest and the stomach gets empty very fast. The mother, therefore, develops a false belief that the baby is constantly crying and her milk output is less.

REGURGITATION

The tone of the lower esophageal sphincter is poor in newborns, therefore, they tend to regurgitate after feeds. The baby spits out the swallowed milk in the process. While feeding, the baby also swallows some air along with the milk. When the baby burps, this swallowed air is taken out by the baby. Along with air, some amount of milk is also taken out. This is a normal physiological phenomenon. This decreases as the baby grows older and the tone of the sphincter increases. A baby with physiological regurgitation grows well, is alert, healthy looking and gains good weight.

VOMITING

Vomiting can also be because of pathological causes. Some congenital anomalies of the stomach and intestines may present with vomiting such as ileal or duodenal atresia and pyloric atresia/stenosis. Vomiting can also be due to many other nonabdominal causes such as sepsis, raised intracranial tension, renal anomalies, and inborn errors of metabolism. Therefore, one must be careful before labeling vomiting as physiological.

Vomiting is pathological, if it is bile-stained, associated with abdominal distention or constipation, poor weight gain, or weight loss. Such newborns should be thoroughly evaluated for cause of vomiting.

BOWEL AND BLADDER

Meconium

A normal breastfed baby has a variation in frequency of stools. In the first 2–3 days of life, the newborn passes dark green sticky stools known as meconium **(Fig. 15.55)**. Normally, a term newborn should pass meconium once within first 24 hours of birth. If a healthy, term baby does not pass meconium on the first day of life, this could be due to hypothyroidism, imperforate anus or Hirschsprung disease. The stools after 3–4 days then become thin, watery, and yellowish to greenish yellow.

Stools

A normal breastfed baby may pass stools which may vary in frequency from one to as many as 12–15 per day. The gastrocolic reflex in newborns leads to passage of stools every time the baby feeds. This is falsely taken as "loose motions" or diarrhea by many mothers and they start top feeds thinking that their milk is not "suiting" the baby. This does not require any medication and mother just needs reassurance.

On the other extreme, a breastfed baby may pass stool once in 4–5 days. This is not constipation, the stool is soft and the baby has no discomfort in passing stools. There is no associated abdominal distention or vomiting. This needs to be differentiated from the constipation which some babies develop when given animal milk.

A constipated baby passes hard stools which may be associated with blood and the baby has difficulty in passing stools. Also, there may be associated abdominal distention and vomiting. Constipation may be due to feeding with animal milk or deficiency of thyroid hormone or a surgical condition like congenital megacolon Hirschsprung disease. This needs to be properly evaluated.

Urine

A newborn baby must pass urine within 48 hours of birth. A normal, healthy baby should pass urine at least 5–6 times in 24 hours. It is normal for newborns to cry just before and after passing urine or stool. It should not be mistaken for difficulty in passage of urine or stool.

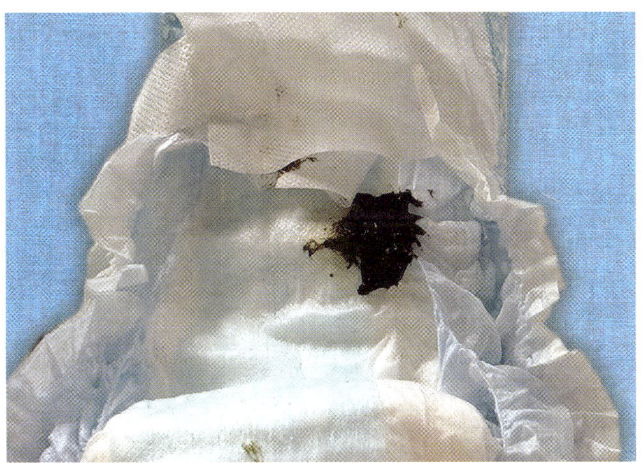

Fig. 15.55: Meconium

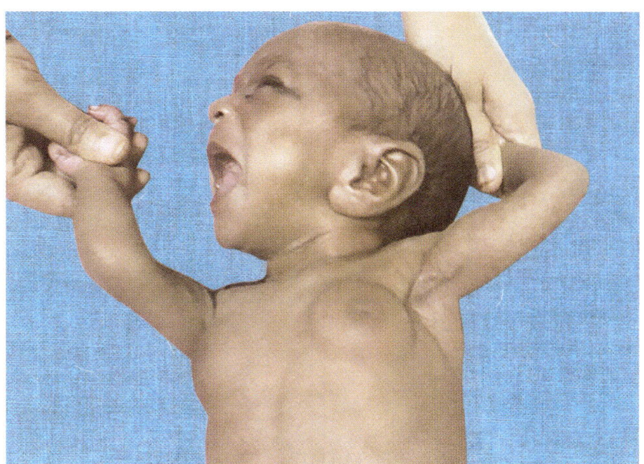

Fig. 15.56: Mastitis neonatorum

MASTITIS NEONATORUM

Engorgement of both breasts is a normal physiologic phenomenon in babies of both sexes due to maternal progesterone and estrogen transferred from the mother. There is swelling of the breast **(Fig. 15.56)** and there may be milk discharge especially on squeezing. This needs no treatment and subsides within a week or two on its own. It is a common practice to press the enlarged breasts and express milk out of it. This can be harmful as it may lead to infection and formation of breast abscess.

VAGINAL BLEEDING AND DISCHARGE

Female newborns may have vaginal bleeding by the end of the first week of life. This is a normal hormonal withdrawal response and the bleeding stops in 4–5 days without any treatment. Whitish thick vaginal discharge may occur in female babies from day 2–3 of life and subsides in a week.

WEIGHT PATTERN

All newborns lose weight in the first 4–5 days of life. Newborns have excessive body water at the time of birth, which is shed after birth leading to weight loss **(Fig. 15.57)**. A term baby may lose 7–10% of the birth weight and preterm babies may lose as much as 15–20%. After initial loss in weight, the baby starts gaining weight. A term baby regains its birth weight by 10 days and preterm babies by 14 days. After this, the baby starts gaining weight by 20–30 g/day.

PHYSIOLOGICAL JAUNDICE

Majority of newborns develop jaundice by day 3 of life. The serum bilirubin increases for next 3–4 days and then decreases such

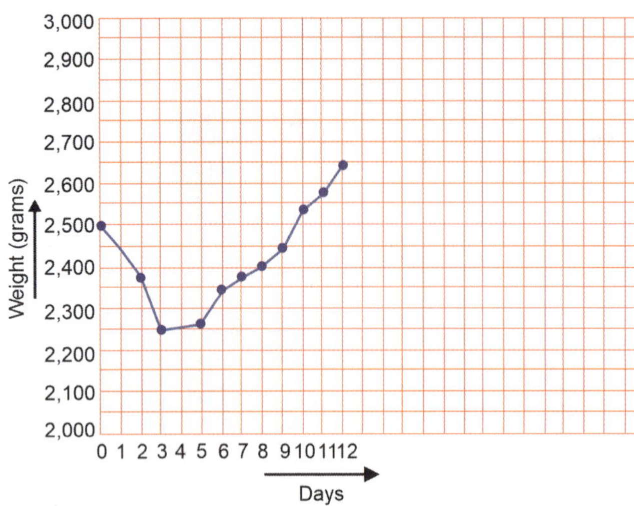

Fig. 15.57: Normal weight pattern of a term healthy baby

that jaundice is not visible by day 10 in most babies. In preterm babies, the jaundice may persist longer.

The jaundice is pathological, if:

- It appears within 24 hours of birth
- Persists beyond 14 days
- Palms and soles are also stained at any time
- Passage of clay-colored stools
- Passage of high-colored urine

Pathological jaundice must be evaluated and may need treatment.

SKIN

Erythema toxicum: Newborns develop a confluent reddish rash all over the body by 2–3 days of life **(Fig. 15.58)**. This fades away in next 3–4 days.

Mongolian spot: This bluish discoloration on the back, buttocks, or legs is seen in many babies **(Fig. 15.59)**. It is a large irregular and well-defined lesion usually seen on the lower back (lumbosacral region). This fades away with time by 1 year of age.

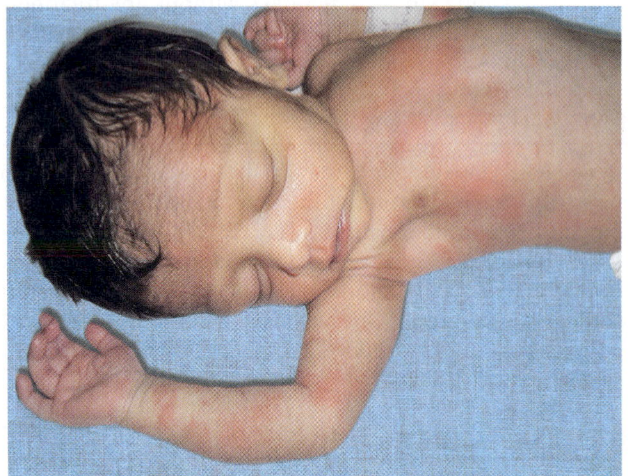

Fig. 15.58: Erythema toxicum neonatorum

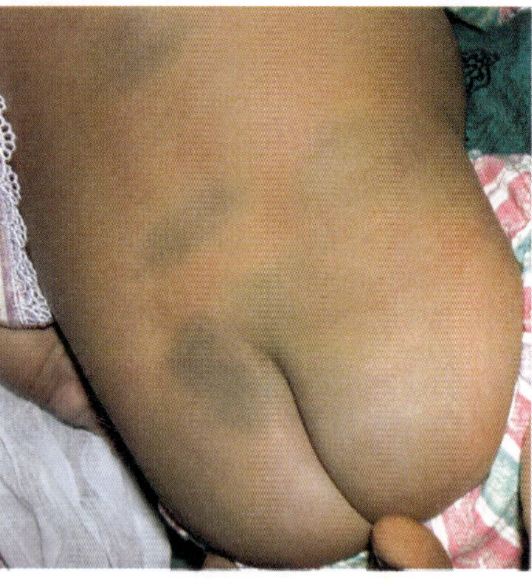

Fig. 15.59: Mongolian spot

Epstein pearl: This is a small, white, and glistening pearl-like inclusion cyst present on the hard palate or tip of penis and is of no significance **(Fig. 15.60)**.

Salmon patch: These are capillary malformations seen on the face typically on the forehead and upper eyelid. They resolve by 1 year of life.

Milia: These are small pinpoint-sized whitish lesions present on the face and nose, which disappear in weeks to months.

NATAL TEETH

Rarely newborns may have the lower central incisors at birth. They may be extracted, if interfering with breastfeeding.

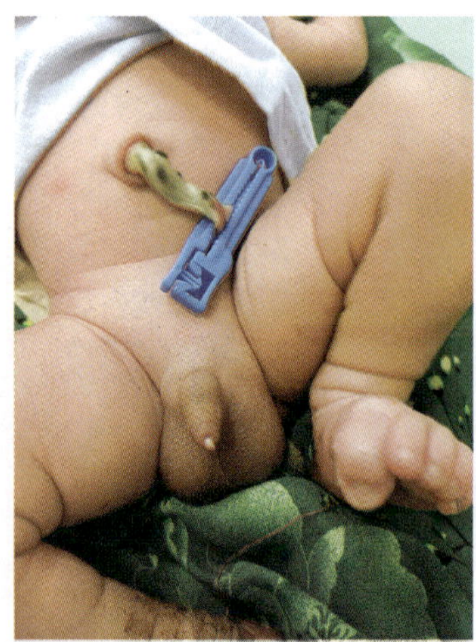

Fig. 15.60: Penile Epstein pearl

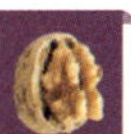

IN A NUTSHELL

Common Neonatal Problems

1. It is essential to understand the normal physiological patterns of a baby as they are different from older children.
2. A healthy term baby should pass meconium within first 24 hours and urine within first 48 hours of birth.
3. Most babies develop physiological jaundice by day 3 of life which subsides by day 10 of life.
4. It is important to differentiate between physiological and pathological jaundice.
5. Vaginal bleeding by day 4–5 of life is a normal physiological phenomenon in female babies, it subsides in 3–4 days.

Eichenwald EC, Hansen AR, Martin CR, et al. Cloherty and Stark's manual of neonatal care (South Asian edition), 8th edition. Gurugram, Haryana: Wolters Kluwer; 2021.
Parthasarathy A. Care of a normal newborn. In: Menon PSN, Nair MKC (Eds). IAP textbook of Pediatrics, 7th edition. New Delhi: Jaypee Brothers Medical Publishers; 2019. pp. 46-49.
World Health Organization. (2017). WHO recommendations on newborn health. [online] Available from https://apps.who.int/iris/handle/10665/259269 [Last accessed May, 2025].

15.8 Maintenance of Temperature

PE 19.9

INTRODUCTION

Temperature maintenance is one of the most important aspects of neonatal care. All newborns are prone to hypothermia, this risk increases when the baby is preterm, LBW, or sick. Therefore, temperature of newborns should be maintained whether they are healthy or sick. The newborns are prone to hypothermia because of the following factors:

- The response to cold is not well-developed in the newborns, especially those who are preterm and sick.
- A newborn at birth has a sudden transition from 37°C in the mother's uterus to the room temperature which is generally lower than this. This leads to rapid fall in temperature of the baby. At birth, the baby is wet with the amniotic fluid, which contributes to the evaporative heat loss.
- A baby cannot shiver to produce heat and, therefore, lacks an important protective mechanism.
- The body surface area of the newborn is more in relation to its weight and so loses more heat.

All the above factors are aggravated in preterm and LBW babies.

BROWN FAT

Brown fat and subcutaneous fat is present around the adrenal glands, kidneys, and interscapular region in term newborns. It protects them from hypothermia. The brown fat generates heat and causes nonshivering thermogenesis. On catecholamine stimulation, burning of this brown fat releases heat, which is carried to the rest of the body through blood. Brown fat is deposited late in the gestation and therefore, deficient in preterm and LBW babies. Shivering thermogenesis is not developed in newborns.

THERMONEUTRAL ENVIRONMENT

This is the narrow range of environmental temperature in which the baby maintains a normal body temperature with minimum basal metabolic rate (BMR) and oxygen consumption and also thrives well. All babies should be nursed in a thermoneutral environment. This thermoneutral range of temperature varies with the gestational age and postnatal day of life of the baby. The temperature range is higher for lesser gestational age and postnatal age.

Ways of Heat Loss

The normal newborn loses heat mainly by four mechanisms **(Fig. 15.61)**:

1. ***Conduction:*** The baby loses heat to the objects and surfaces in direct contact with it, like the tray on which the baby is received or the sheet in which the baby is wrapped. Therefore, all the surfaces with which the baby comes in contact with should be warm.

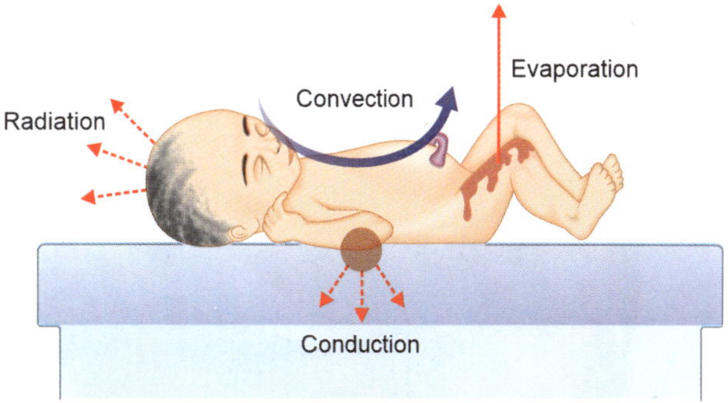

Fig. 15.61: Mechanism of weight loss in a newborn

2. ***Evaporation:*** The baby also loses heat through its wet body by the process of evaporation. As the water evaporates from the body surface, the baby becomes hypothermic. At birth, the baby is wet with amniotic fluid and should be dried immediately and wrapped in a warm, dry towel.
3. ***Convection:*** This is the process through which the baby loses heat due to the current of air around it. Newborn babies should be kept in a room where there is no draught of air, but should be well-ventilated. There should not be much activity or movement around the baby as it causes air currents. The baby's bed should be away from the doors and windows.
4. ***Radiation:*** The baby also loses heat to other surfaces and objects in the vicinity, which are not in direct contact with the baby, such as the furniture, equipment, and walls. The ambient temperature of the NICU or the room where the baby is kept should be maintained between 26 and 28°C, so that other objects in the room also become warm. The warmer or the bed of the baby should not be kept too close to the walls.

ASSESSMENT OF TEMPERATURE

Temperature must be recorded in all healthy newborns every 3–4 hourly in the first 24 hours of life and then 6–8 hourly subsequently in the postnatal ward. Newborns that are sick must be cared for under a servo-controlled radiant warmer under constant temperature monitoring.

The temperature of a newborn is routinely measured in the axilla, but it can also be measured in the rectum or on the skin. A digital thermometer is used to measure temperature.

Axillary Temperature

The thermometer is placed in the axillary pit against the roof and the baby's arm is then held close to its body **(Fig. 15.62)**. The temperature should be read when the thermometer gives a beep. The axillary temperature is as good as the rectal temperature and is the preferred most of the times, it is also easy to take and safe.

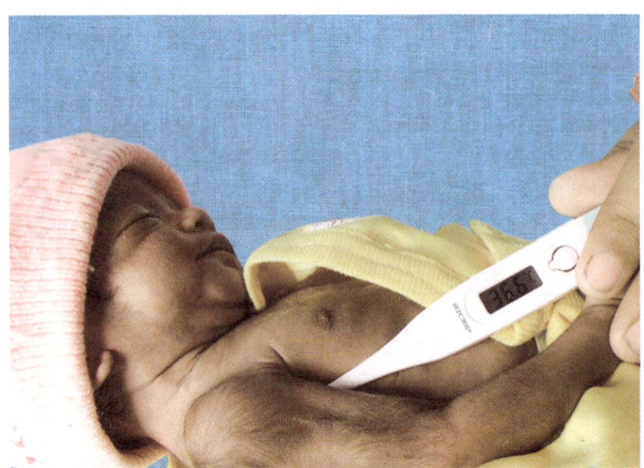

Fig. 15.62: Measurement of axillary temperature

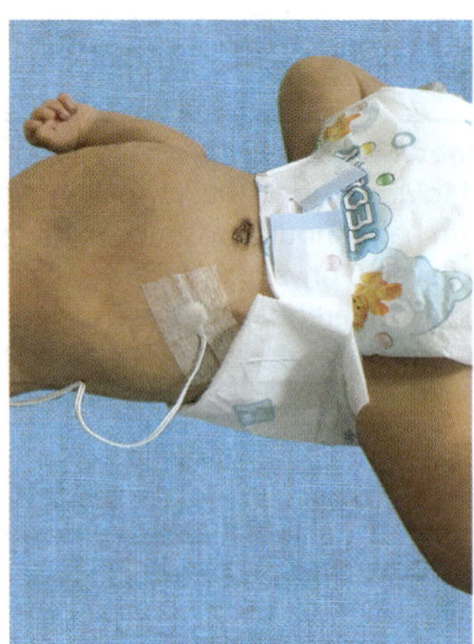

Fig. 15.63: Skin probe to measure temperature in a newborn

Rectal Temperature

Measurement of rectal temperature is indicated only in very sick, hypothermic babies and requires a special low reading thermometer. It carries a risk of rectal perforation, if done by an untrained person.

- For measuring rectal temperature, the lower limbs of the baby are lifted and the bulb of the thermometer is greased and inserted into the rectum backward and upward around 3 cm in term babies and 2 cm in preterm babies.

Skin Temperature

The skin temperature of the baby is measured using a thermistor probe which is attached to the skin of baby over the upper abdomen **(Fig. 15.63)**. Care must be taken that the metallic surface of the probe is in contact with the skin of the baby. The temperature measured by the probe is displayed on the display board. If the probe gets displaced, the baby can get hypo- or hyperthermic. The desired skin temperature should be set at 36.5–37°C.

Interpretation of Temperature

The normal temperature of a newborn is 36.5–37.5°C. Temperature below 36.5°C is known as hypothermia. Temperature >37.5°C is known as hyperthermia **(Table 15.6)**. A rough assessment of temperature can also be done by touching the baby by

Table 15.6 Grading of Axillary Temperature in a Newborn

Classification	Axillary temperature (°C)
Normal temperature	36.5–37.5
Cold stress/mild hypothermia	36.0–36.4
Moderate hypothermia	32.0–35.9
Severe hypothermia	<32.0
Hyperthermia	>37.5

Table 15.7 Classification of Hypothermia by Touch

Classification	Peripheries/feet	Abdomen
Normal	Warm	Warm
Cold stress	Cold	Warm
Hypothermia	Cold	Cold

the dorsum of hand. Grading of the temperature can be done by touching the abdomen and feet of the baby **(Table 15.7)**. This is a very good method of assessment of temperature at home by the mother especially by those who cannot read a thermometer.

PREVENTION OF HYPOTHERMIA

A warm chain should be maintained throughout in the delivery room, NICU, or the postnatal ward.

Warm Chain

Baby must be kept warm at the place of birth, during transportation from hospital to home or within the hospital. Try to minimize all sources of heat loss and promote heat gain. The "warm chain" is a set of 10 steps carried out at birth and later, to reduce the occurrence of hypothermia in all newborn babies **(Box 15.4)**.

1. ***Warm delivery room:*** The delivery room should be kept warm, and temperature of the room should be kept at 25–28°C. The temperature of the NICU where sick newborns are kept should be maintained at 28°C ± 2°C. A radiant warmer should be available in every delivery area, which should be switched on before the delivery so the ambient temperature under the warmer is maintained by the time baby is delivered. Babies with lesser gestational age and birth weight need higher ambient temperature to maintain their temperature.
2. ***Warm resuscitation:*** In the entire process of resuscitation, temperature needs to be maintained. The towels used for drying and wrapping, oxygen if needed, the baby tray, pan of the weighing machine, etc., should all be warm.
3. ***Immediate drying:*** The baby should be immediately dried after birth using a sterile, warm, and dry towel. This towel which becomes wet should be removed after drying and the baby should be wrapped in another warm and dry towel.
4. ***Skin-to-skin contact:*** Skin-to-skin contact should be started immediately after birth, if the baby does not require any resuscitation and is breathing normally. The baby should be kept on the mother's abdomen even before the cord is cut in case of a vaginal delivery or over the chest of the mother in case of cesarean section for at least an hour.
5. ***Postpone bathing:*** The vernix which keeps the baby warm should not be removed. The baby should not be given bath soon after birth. Bathing can be postponed till the baby is a weekold in LBW babies. A baby should not be given a bath if the ambient environment is cold or the weight of the baby <2,000 g. A healthy baby can be given a bath on second day of life.
6. ***Breastfeeding:*** The baby should be started on breastfeeds within 1 hour of birth and then onward given frequent breastfeeds.
7. ***Rooming in:*** The mother and the baby should be kept together in the same room and close to each other on the same bed. The postnatal ward should also be kept warm (25–28°C).
8. ***Cover the baby well:*** The baby should be covered well and made to wear appropriate clothes according to the season and temperature **(Fig. 15.64)**. Special emphasis should be laid on covering the head and the hands and feet.
9. ***Warm transport:*** If there is need to refer the baby to another health facility, utmost care should be taken for temperature maintenance during transport. Special electrical blankets which keep the baby warm on the way can be used. The baby should be well-covered and transported in a closed vehicle. Skin-to-skin contact is a useful method of maintaining temperature during transport.

Box 15.4 10 Steps of Warm Chain in Newborn

1. Warm delivery room
2. Warm resuscitation
3. Immediate drying after birth
4. Skin-to-skin contact
5. Breastfeeding
6. Postpone bathing
7. Appropriate clothing and bedding
8. Rooming in
9. Warm transport
10. Training and awareness of healthcare workers

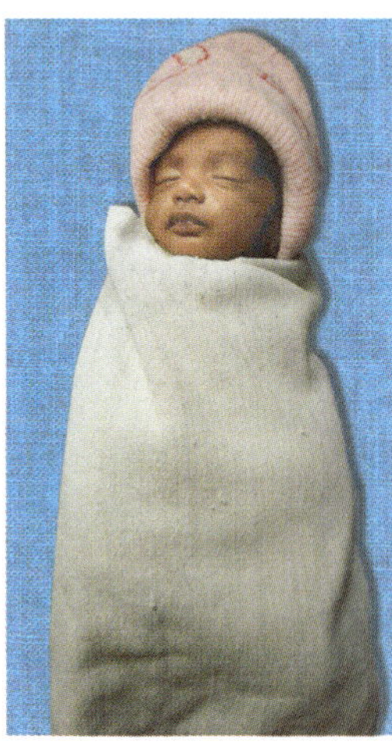

Fig. 15.64: Appropriately covered baby

10. ***Awareness:*** It is essential to build awareness among healthcare workers and the family members of the baby regarding prevention, identification, and management of hypothermia. The mother and the family should be counseled at discharge regarding the steps for prevention of hypothermia.

KANGAROO MOTHER CARE

This is an indigenous technique used to prevent and manage hypothermia, which is very simple and easy and does not require any expertise or expensive equipment.

The newborn is kept in skin-to-skin contact with the mother or any other family member. The baby is placed on the bare chest of the mother between both the breasts in an upright posture **(Fig. 15.65)**. The baby should not wear any clothes except for the cap, socks, and the mittens. The baby should also wear a diaper. The head of the baby should be turned to one side so that the baby can breathe comfortably. The baby should be held close to the mother's body in close contact with the mother's skin. The baby is held snugly in this position with the help of a shawl or a special gown so that both the mother and the baby are comfortable and there is no risk of the baby slipping **(Fig. 15.66)**. The mother can sit or lie down as per her convenience. The mother can wear a front open gown to facilitate kangaroo mother care (KMC). The baby is allowed to breastfeed in between.

The KMC can also be given by the father or any other family member, if the mother is not available or sick. KMC should be given for as long as possible in a day but a minimum of 3 sittings lasting for an hour each must be done. This technique is especially useful for maintaining the temperature of LBW and preterm babies in the hospital as well as at home after discharge. All babies except those who are critically ill can be given KMC, even if they are receiving oxygen or intravenous fluids.

Advantages of Kangaroo Mother Care

- Maintains temperature of the baby.
- Keeps the vitals of the baby such as heart rate and respiratory rate stable.
- Babies receiving KMC show better weight gain.

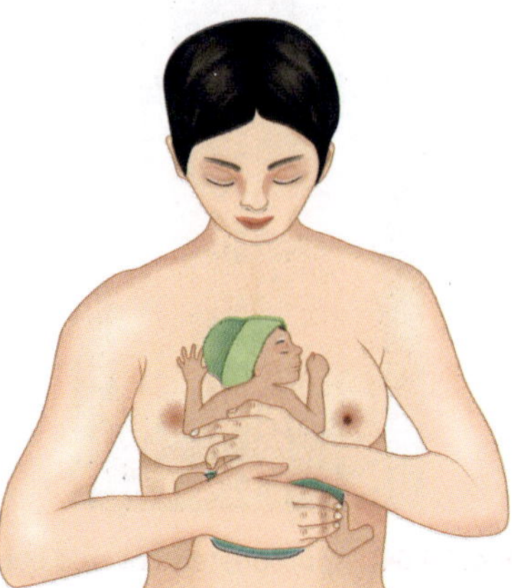

Fig. 15.65: Kangaroo mother care position of the baby

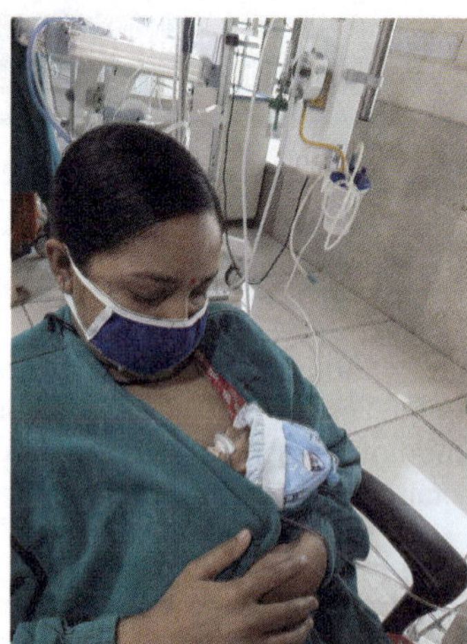

Fig. 15.66: Mother doing Kangaroo mother care

- This also reduces incidence of infection in the baby.
- KMC improves the emotional bonding between the mother and the baby.
- It helps in initiation and continuing exclusive breastfeeding and maintains milk output in the mother.
- It reduces the duration of hospital stay of the baby.

HYPOTHERMIA

Clinical Features

Clinical features of hypothermia are very varied and nonspecific. Apart from being cold to touch, the baby may become dull, lethargic, and stop feeding well. There may be convulsions, bleeding from any site, respiratory distress, or abdominal distention in case of severe hypothermia. It can lead to hypoglycemia, shock, and even death.

TREATMENT Hypothermia

- ***Cold stress or mild hypothermia:*** One must look for the cause of hypothermia and remove it, like low ambient room temperature, open doors and windows leading to current of air, inappropriate clothing, wet clothes, or diaper. Sometimes, malfunction of the radiant warmer may lead to hypothermia. The baby must be clothed well and covered with a blanket. KMC can be started to maintain the temperature of the baby. The mother should be encouraged to breastfeed the baby frequently.
- ***Moderate hypothermia:*** In case the baby is sick, then external heat must be provided. If possible, the baby must be kept under a radiant warmer as it provides regulated heat and there is no risk of overheating. If, radiant warmer is not available, any other source of heat can be used to bring up the ambient room temperature but the heat should never be directed toward the baby. As these sources of heat deliver unregulated heat, there is a danger of overheating the baby and may even cause death. Hot water bags are strictly contraindicated as it can cause burns, if the temperature of water inside the bag is very high. KMC can also be helpful in managing these babies.
- ***Severe hypothermia:*** Babies with severe hypothermia must be managed aggressively. They need to be started on intravenous fluids, oxygen, and antibiotics. Vitals, such as heart rate, respiratory rate, and CRT, must be monitored regularly.

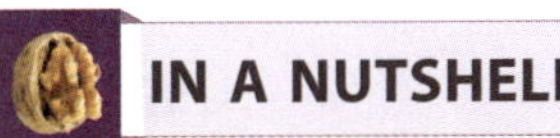

IN A NUTSHELL

Maintenance of Temperature

1. Temperature maintenance is most important aspect of neonatal care.
2. Axillary temperature of the baby should be 36.5–37.5°C.
3. Newborns, especially preterm and low birth weight babies are extremely prone to lose heat and become hypothermic because of various factors.
4. Hypothermia is the single most common factor adversely affecting neonatal outcomes.
5. Kangaroo mother care (KMC) is a simple tool to prevent hypothermia and promote weight gain in preterm and low birth weight babies.

Maternal health and safe motherhood programme division of family health world health organization. Thermal Control of the Newborn: a practical guide. [online] Available from https://apps.who.int/iris/bitstream/handle/10665/60042/WHO_FHE_MSM_93.2.pdf [Last accessed May, 2025].

Ministry of Health and Family Welfare, Government of India, National Health Mission. Facility Based Integrated Management of Neonatal and Childhood Illness (F-IMNCI). [online] Available from https://nhm.gov.in/images/pdf/programmes/childhealth/guidelines/facility_based_care [Last accessed May, 2025].

Royal Children's Hospital, Melbourne. Clinical guidelines: Assisted thermoregulation. [online] Available from https://www.rch.org.au/rchcpg/hospital_clinical_guideline_index/Thermoregulation_in_the_Preterm_Infant/ [Last accessed May, 2025].

15.9 Follow-up Care

PE 19.3

DISCHARGING A NEWBORN

Following must be ensured before discharging a baby:

- Breastfeeding has been established and the mother is confident in breastfeeding.
- The vitals of the baby such as heart rate, respiration, and color are normal and the baby is active and sucking well.
- The baby has been immunized with BCG, OPV_0, and Hepatitis B (birth dose).
- The mother and the family members have been counseled about the care of the baby at home.

Following points must be seen when the baby comes for follow-up visits:

- ***Growth monitoring:*** Weight, length, and head circumference should be noted and plotted on the WHO chart to identify any growth faltering.
- ***Development assessment*** should be done for early identification and intervention in case of any developmental problems.
- ***Details of feeding*** must be asked especially if there is growth faltering, or the mother is not exclusively breastfeeding her baby. The mother must be praised if she is exclusively breastfeeding her baby. If the mother is not exclusively breastfeeding her baby, she should be counseled to do so.
- ***Vaccinations*** status of the baby should be enquired.
- Any other ***medical issues*** of the baby must also be looked into.
- ***Mother's queries*** about her baby must be answered.
- ***Health issues of the mother*** should also be addressed.

RED FLAG SIGNS IN A FOLLOW-UP VISIT

- A baby who is not being exclusively breastfed, i.e., a baby who is being given water, *ghutti*, honey, any animal milk like cow, buffalo, goat, etc., or anything else apart from the breast milk
- ***Baby who is not growing well:*** This can be identified if the baby's weight, length, or head circumference is below the normal for the baby's age and gender.
- Baby who is not developing as per its age. If the baby has not achieved the milestones proper for its age according to the development charts.
- Baby who shows signs of a medical illness.

World Health Organization. Early essential newborn care. [online] Available from https://apps.who.int/iris/rest/bitstreams/1246772/retrieve [Last accessed May, 2025].

15.10 Parental Counseling *PE 19.3*

Once the baby is ready to be discharged, the family members and the mother must be counseled and educated about different aspects of care of the baby at home.

- ❖ The family members must be educated about importance of exclusive breastfeeding till 6 completed months, its benefits to the baby, harms of giving animal milk. Exclusive breastfeeding is giving only mother's milk to the baby till 6 completed months of age. Nothing else like water, animal milk, water, or *ghutti* should be given.
- ❖ The mother and other family members should also be counseled regarding healthy and hygienic rearing practices such as care of the cord, no kajal application in eyes, personal hygiene of the baby and others in the family, and hand hygiene.
- ❖ The family members must be told how to keep the baby warm, about identification of hypothermia at home and its immediate management.
- ❖ The mother must be explained about the danger signs in a newborn. She must consult a healthcare worker in case any danger signs are identified by her. The danger signs are:
  - The baby appears dull/cries excessively
  - The baby does not accept feeds well
  - Difficulty in breathing
  - Baby is cold to touch
  - Bleeding from any site
  - Baby has yellow palms and soles/appears blue or pale
  - Convulsions
  - Excessive vomiting/abdominal distention
  - Any other feature which the mother's thinks is abnormal
- ❖ The mother should be explained about the next follow-up visit and next vaccination.
- ❖ The mother should be advised regarding her diet and contraception.

Moyer VA. Effective guidelines for counseling parents before discharging a newborn. Am Fam Physician. 2006;73(5):771.
Parthasarathy A, Menon PSN, Nair MKC. Parent counselling, Care of newborn. IAP textbook of Pediatrics, 7th edition. New Delhi: Jaypee Brothers Medical Publishers; 2019. pp. 56-9.

15.11 Infection Control *PE 19.3*

INTRODUCTION

Newborns have immature immune system to fight against infection. The fetus is generally not posed with any infection in utero as the environment is sterile. The response to infection is, therefore, neither prompt nor adequate. Infection in newborns is still one of the most common causes of mortality. We can prevent a lot of deaths of newborn babies by simple methods which prevent infection.

ASEPSIS IN DELIVERY ROOM

The infection control in a newborn should start right from the delivery room. Proper asepsis should be maintained while conducting a delivery. Follow the five Cs, i.e., clean hands, clean delivery surface, clean cord and clean blade, clean tie, and clean cloth.

ASEPSIS DURING RESUSCITATION

All the equipment used for NNR should be clean and sterile. Disposables should be freely available in the delivery room and baby area. Reusable items such as the sheets, self-inflating bags and masks, and laryngoscopes, should be autoclaved after each use. Stethoscope, thermometers, measuring tapes and probes, should be disinfected with isopropyl alcohol.

HANDWASHING

Handwashing is the single most important intervention which can prevent infection. This is cheap, easy to perform, and does not require any expertise. All health personnel handling the baby should do proper handwashing for 40–60 seconds before entering the baby care area and should do hand hygiene with soap and water or alcohol-based hand rub for 20–30 seconds before and after touching a baby, before doing an aseptic procedure, after body fluid exposure risk, and after touching baby's surroundings. Any soap can be used to wash hands. Hands once washed should be dried in air or using sterile single use wipes.

ASEPSIS DURING FEEDING

Exclusive breastfeeding brings down the risk of infection in the newborns by almost ten times. Bottle feeding carries a very high risk of infection, as they are difficult to clean. Colostrum must be given to all the babies.

In a rare case scenario where a baby must be fed expressed breastmilk or top feeds, it should be given by *katori* and spoon or *paladai*. The utensils used should be thoroughly washed and autoclaved or boiled in a pressure cooker for 15–20 minutes.

GENERAL CARE

The baby should be sponged daily with a soft, clean cloth, if not given a bath. It should be dressed in clean and soft clothes. Diapers should be changed regularly and perineal area cleaned thoroughly after passage of stool/urine. Nothing should be applied on the cord.

The mother and the caregiver should take care of his/her personal hygiene. He/she should wash hands properly after changing diapers and before feeding a baby, if the baby is on spoon or *paladai* feeds.

ASEPSIS IN NEONATAL INTENSIVE CARE UNIT

It is most important to maintain strict asepsis in the NICU. Written housekeeping protocols must be available in the unit and all the staff should be trained regarding the procedures involved. A check must be kept from to time to see whether the protocols are being followed or not.

Availability of disinfectants for the floor, surfaces, and equipment should always be ensured in the unit. Proper pictorial charts such as those for handwashing and biomedical waste disposal, must be displayed at appropriate places. A clearly designated area for keeping clean and dirty utility items must be there.

Thorough handwashing must be done by anyone entering the NICU. All jewelry, watch, and threads should be removed. Nails should be clean and short. The sleeves are folded up to above the elbow before handwashing.

Universal precautions must be followed before every procedure. The prerequisites for maintaining asepsis in the NICU are:

- 24 × 7 running water supply and soap
- Easy availability of disinfecting agents
- Free availability of disposables
- Elbow operated taps
- Strict adherence to the asepsis protocols.

DISINFECTION PROTOCOLS IN NEONATAL INTENSIVE CARE UNIT

The following disinfection and sterilization protocols should be followed:

- ***Radiant warmers:*** The walls and the mattress should be cleaned daily by a light detergent solution and dried. A thorough cleaning must be done after dismantling every week and when a new baby is being shifted. The mattress must be changed as soon as the surface covering is torn. If the warmer is not occupied by a baby, then it should be cleaned with surface disinfectant.
- ***Oxygen hoods:*** They should be cleaned with a mild detergent daily and in between babies.
- ***Resuscitation bags and mask:*** They should be sterilized weekly by soaking in 2% glutaraldehyde for 4–6 hours and after each use. After removing from glutaraldehyde, the bag and the mask should be rinsed with distilled water and dried and then wrapped in sterile linen. Care must be taken that the bag is dismantled before disinfection and sterilization. Most of the self-inflating bags and masks are autoclavable, so they can be alternatively sent for autoclaving instead of using gluteraldehyde.
- ***Laryngoscope:*** If visibly soiled, the blade of the laryngoscope should be washed with detergent and water and then cleaned with 70% isopropyl alcohol or soaked in 2% glutaraldehyde for 15–20 minutes. Wash thoroughly after removing from glutaraldehyde solution.
- ***Weighing machine:*** It should be wiped with surface disinfectant.
- ***Feeding utensils:*** They should be cleaned with soap and water and boiled in water for 20 minutes after each use.
- ***Thermometers, measuring tapes, blood pressure cuffs, and stethoscopes:*** They should be disinfected with 70% isopropyl alcohol daily and before each use.
- ***Floors and walls:*** They must be cleaned with 3% phenol or 5% lysol. Sweeping of the floor or dry dusting should not be done. Instead wet mopping of the floor should be done at least 3 times a day.
- ***Linen and blanket covers:*** Autoclaved linen should be used each time.

Visitor Policy in Neonatal Intensive Care Unit

A defined policy for visitors should be formulated for each unit in the hospital. The policy for an NICU should be formulated keeping in mind the baby's health, safety, and confidentiality.

- The parents should be encouraged to visit their babies uninterrupted. This improves outcomes of the babies and helps in establishing breastfeeding and enhances milk output in mothers.
- No visitors may be allowed during rounds or during procedures.
- Anyone showing signs and symptoms of an infection or illness should not be allowed to enter the NICU.
- To keep a check on the noise levels in the NICU, the mobile phones should be kept switched off or on silent mode.
- All the visitors including the mother should perform complete and proper hand scrub before entering. The visitor's/mother's personal hygiene should also be observed and they should be advised accordingly.

Visitor Policy in the Postnatal Ward

Too many people and relatives should not crowd around the baby and touch the baby. Entry to the room where the mother and her newborn are kept should be restricted especially if the baby is an LBW or a preterm baby. LBW and preterm babies are more prone to infections than the term babies. Therefore, all the precautions should be very strictly followed while handling them.

- The mother and family members should be counseled about all infection control measures that should be taken at home.
- Health workers or family members suffering from a contagious or infectious disease should not handle the baby.

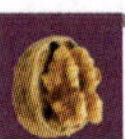

IN A NUTSHELL

Infection Control

1. Newborns are very susceptible to infections and sepsis is the leading cause of neonatal mortality.
2. Hand hygiene is the most important step toward asepsis.
3. Infection control measures must be strictly followed in delivery room, postnatal ward, and especially in neonatal intensive care unit (NICU).
4. There should be written protocols for disinfection and sterilization of all items in equipment in NICU.
5. Simple procedures such as feeding and handling a baby can also transmit infection to a newborn.

National Health Mission, Ministry of Health and Family Welfare. Facility based newborn care. [online] Available from http://nhm.gov.in/images/pdf/programmes/child-health/guidelines/operational_guidelines_for_fimnci.pdf [Last accessed May, 2025].

16 CHAPTER

Care of the High-risk Newborn

AS PER NMC COMPETENCIES

PE19.4	Describe the etiology, clinical features and management of birth asphyxia.	*Ch 16.3*
PE19.5	Describe the etiology, clinical features and management of respiratory distress in newborn including meconium aspiration and transient tachypnea of newborn.	*Ch 16.5*
PE19.6	Explain the etiology, clinical features and management of birth injuries.	*Ch 16.4*
PE19.7	Explain the etiology, clinical features and management of hemorrhagic disease of newborn.	*Ch 16.12*
PE19.8	Describe the clinical characteristics, complications and management of low birth weight (preterm and small for gestation).	*Ch 16.2*
PE19.10	Describe the temperature regulation in neonates, clinical features and management of neonatal hypoglycemia.	*Ch 16.8* *Ch 16.9*
PE19.11	Explain the etiology, clinical features and management of neonatal hypocalcemia.	*Ch 16.10*
PE19.12	Describe the etiology, clinical features and management of neonatal seizures.	*Ch 16.7*
PE19.13	Explain the etiology, clinical features and management of neonatal sepsis.	*Ch 16.11*
PE19.14	Describe the etiology, clinical features and management of perinatal infections.	*Ch 16.14*
PE19.15	Describe the etiology, clinical features and management of neonatal hyperbilirubinemia.	*Ch 16.13*
PE19.16	Identify clinical presentations of common surgical conditions in the newborn including TEF, esophageal atresia, anal atresia, cleft lip and palate, congenital diaphragmatic hernia and causes of acute abdomen.	*Ch 16.16*
PE19.17	Describe the risk factors, clinical features, diagnosis and management of oxygen toxicity.	*Ch 16.15*

16.1 Newborn Survival

INTRODUCTION

Neonatal deaths contribute to highest proportion of deaths among children below 5 years of age. Neonatal mortality rate (NMR), defined as number of neonates (≤28 days) dying per 1,000 live births, has declined globally, however, at a slower rate compared to infant and under-five mortality resulting in increasing contribution of neonatal mortality to under-five deaths. Neonatal deaths per 1,000 live births occurring before first 7 days of life constitute the early neonatal mortality rate (ENMR) and those occurring between 7 and 28 days of life constitute late NMR.

GLOBAL SCENARIO

Approximately 2.3 million newborns die annually worldwide (2022 estimates). Neonatal deaths have decreased from 2.8 million in 2015 to 2.3 million in 2022, a 17% reduction. This is lower than the decline in post-neonatal under-5 deaths, which fell from 3.3 million to 2.6 million, a 21% decrease. The global

NMR is currently 17 per 1,000 live births, ranging from 3 per 1000 in Europe and Northern America to 27 per 1,000 in Sub-Saharan Africa.

INDIAN SCENARIO

India's current neonatal mortality rate (NMR) in 2020 is 20 per 1,000 live births, higher than the global average of 17. Infant mortality and under-five mortality rates are 28 and 32 per 1,000 live births, respectively, with 71% of infant deaths and 62% of under-five deaths occurring during the neonatal period. NMR varies from 4 per 1,000 in Kerala to 31 per 1,000 in Madhya Pradesh. Early neonatal mortality rate (ENMR) is 15 per 1,000, while late NMR is 5 per 1,000. The first week of life accounts for 47% of total under-five deaths, with the decline in early NMR being slower than that of late NMR.

CAUSES OF NEONATAL MORTALITY

About 46% of under-five deaths occur in the neonatal period and contributory causes are enlisted here:
- Preterm birth complications (16.6%)
- Intrapartum-related events (11.0%)
- Infections (lower respiratory tract infection, sepsis and meningitis, and diarrhea) (8.1%)
- Congenital abnormalities (4.5%)
- Injury (0.3%)
- Tetanus (0.1%)
- Other (5.3%)

In India, there is marked discrepancy in the NMR of the different states and various districts in a state. NMR of rural areas is twice compared to urban areas. NMR is also higher among female neonates due to gender-based differences in care seeking attitude of the parents. Maternal malnutrition is the predominant risk factor, to which 83.0% of neonatal deaths in India could be attributed. Teenage pregnancy increases the risk of neonatal mortality and low birth weight (LBW) by almost 50%. NMR is also higher in states with lower per capita gross domestic product (GDP) and among tribal communities.

Perinatal Mortality and Stillbirth Rate

According to World Health Organization (WHO), a baby born with no signs of life with a birth weight over 1,000 g, gestational age ≥28 weeks, and/or, length >35 cm constitutes per 1,000 total birth is stillbirth rate. A baby may be either antepartum or intrapartum stillborn and intrapartum stillbirths are largely preventable by providing access to high-quality care during delivery, including ongoing intrapartum monitoring and timely intervention in case of complications. Global stillbirth rate was reported to be 13.9 per 1,000 total births with worst affected regions being sub-Saharan Africa and South Asia. UNICEF estimated the stillbirth rate to be 13.9 per 1,000 total births in 2019 in India. There is vast inequality in the distribution of stillbirths across the regions of the world and proportion of antepartum and intrapartum stillbirths also vary across the nations. Preventable intrapartum stillbirth constitutes almost 50% of all stillbirths in South Asian and African regions compared to just 6% in Western Europe and Northern America. Timeliness and quality of intrapartum care is indicated by intrapartum stillbirths. Perinatal mortality rate consists of stillbirths and early neonatal deaths per 1,000 total births. Both stillbirth rates and perinatal mortality rates are underestimated as stillbirths are extremely difficult to capture and may be misclassified.

PREVENTION OF NEWBORN DEATHS

The global Every Newborn Action Plan (ENAP) launched in 2014, provides evidence-based interventions to prevent newborn deaths and stillbirths all over the globe. India adopted ENAP strategies and put forth the vision and strategies to prevent newborn deaths and stillbirths in India in the form of India Newborn Action Plan (INAP). The revised aim is to bring down the NMR to a single digit (<10 per 1,000 per year) by 2030.

The packages of care with greatest impact on ending preventable neonatal deaths and stillbirths include:
- ***Care during labor:*** It consists of skilled care at birth, basic and comprehensive obstetric care and care of preterm birth with use of antenatal corticosteroids.
- ***Care around birth and the first week of life:*** It includes essential newborn care with hygienic care, thermal control, support for breastfeeding, and if required, newborn resuscitation.
- ***Care for the small and sick newborn:*** It comprises interventions to deal with infections (antibiotics for sepsis, meningitis, pneumonia, and diarrhea), provision of extra-thermal care (kangaroo mother care), and support for feeding for small or preterm babies (including cup and nasogastric tube feeding and intravenous fluids), infection prevention, safe oxygen therapy, case management of jaundice and possibly surfactant, and respiratory support.

Recognition of High-risk Newborn

High-risk newborns are those who need special attention and close observation because of presence of certain adverse factors. Healthcare personnel and parents should be aware of these situations and be prepared for the associated difficulties. Factors associated with high-risk neonates are listed in **Table 16.1**.

Danger Signs

Danger signs are the clinical features which may suggest that the neonate is sick and needs early referral to an appropriate healthcare facility. Parents and health workers should be aware of these signs so that there is no undue delay in seeking care. WHO recognizes nine signs as danger signs to identify sick neonates **(Table 16.2)**.

TREATMENT High-risk Neonates

- Anticipate the need of resuscitation, a skilled team should be present for delivery.
- The cord blood and placenta should be saved after delivery.
- Observation for at least 72 hours after delivery for development of complications.
- Admission to the neonatal unit at earliest suspicion and provision of appropriate management.
- Transfer to higher facility, if necessary.
- At discharge, parents should be made aware of the possible danger signs.

Table 16.1 Factors Associated with High-risk Newborn

Maternal conditions	*Associated risk for fetus or neonate*
	Age at delivery
Over 35 years	Chromosomal abnormalities, macrosomia, intrauterine growth restriction (IUGR), blood loss (abruption and placenta previa)
Teenage pregnancy	IUGR, prematurity, child abuse/neglect (mother herself may be abused)
	Personal factors
Poverty	Prematurity, infection, IUGR
Lack of antenatal care	Prematurity, IUGR
Smoking	IUGR, increased perinatal mortality
Drug, alcohol abuse	IUGR, fetal alcohol syndrome, withdrawal syndrome, sudden infant death syndrome (SIDS), child abuse/neglect
Poor nutritional status	LBW/IUGR
Trauma (acute, chronic)	Fetal demise, prematurity
	Medical history
Diabetes mellitus macrosomia/birth injury	Congenital anomalies, stillbirth, respiratory distress syndrome (RDS), hypoglycemia
Thyroid disease	Goiter, hypothyroidism, hyperthyroidism, IUGR, stillbirth, prematurity
Renal disease	IUGR, stillbirth, prematurity
Urinary tract infection	Prematurity, sepsis
Heart, lung disease	IUGR, stillbirth, prematurity
Hypertension (chronic or pre-eclampsia)	IUGR, stillbirth, asphyxia, prematurity
Anemia	IUGR, stillbirth, asphyxia, prematurity, hydrops
Isoimmunization (Rh, ABO, minor blood groups)	Stillbirth, anemia, jaundice, hydrops
	Obstetric history
Past history of infant with prematurity, jaundice, RDS, or anomalies	Same with current pregnancy

Contd...

Contd...

Maternal conditions	*Associated risk for fetus or neonate*
Maternal medications	IUGR, congenital anomalies
Bleeding in early pregnancy	Stillbirth, prematurity
Hyperthermia	Fetal demise, fetal anomalies
Bleeding in third trimester	Stillbirth infection/sepsis
Premature rupture of membranes, fever, infection	Infection, prematurity
	Fetal conditions
Multiple gestation	Twin-twin transfusion syndrome, IUGR, asphyxia, birth trauma
Intrauterine growth restriction (IUGR)	Fetal demise, congenital anomalies, asphyxia, hypoglycemia, polycythemia
Macrosomia	Congenital anomalies, birth trauma, hypoglycemia
Abnormal fetal position	Congenital anomalies, birth trauma, hemorrhage hydrops, asphyxia
Abnormality of fetal heart rate or rhythm	Congestive heart failure, heart block
Decreased activity	Fetal demise, asphyxia
Polyhydramnios	Anencephaly, other central nervous system (CNS) disorders, neuromuscular disorders, problems with swallowing (e.g., esophageal atresia), diaphragmatic hernia, omphalocele, gastroschisis, trisomy, tumors, hydrops, isoimmunization, anemia, cardiac failure, intrauterine infection, maternal diabetes
Oligohydramnios	IUGR, placental insufficiency, postmaturity, fetal demise, intrapartum distress, renal agenesis, pulmonary hypoplasia
	Conditions of labor and delivery
Premature labor	Respiratory distress syndrome (RDS)
Labor occurring 2 weeks or more after term	Stillbirth, asphyxia, meconium aspiration
Maternal fever	Infection/sepsis
Maternal hypotension	Stillbirth, asphyxia
Rapid labor	Birth trauma, intracranial hemorrhage
Long labor	Stillbirth, asphyxia, birth trauma
Abnormal presentation	Birth trauma, asphyxia
Uterine tetany	Asphyxia
Meconium-stained amniotic fluid	Stillbirth, asphyxia, meconium aspiration syndrome, persistent pulmonary hypertension
Prolapsed cord	Asphyxia, intracranial hemorrhage
Cesarean section	RDS, retained fetal lung fluid/transient tachypnea, blood loss

Contd...

Contd...

Maternal conditions	*Associated risk for fetus or neonate*
Obstetric analgesia and anesthesia	Respiratory depression, hypotension, hypothermia
Placental anomalies: • Small placenta • Large placenta • Torn placenta • Vasa previa	 • IUGR • Hydrops, maternal diabetes • Blood loss • Blood loss
Immediate neonatal conditions	
Prematurity Low birth weight/IUGR	RDS, other consequences of prematurity
Foul smell of amniotic fluid or membranes	Infection
Low 5-minute Apgar score	Prolonged transition (especially respiratory)
Birth weight >4 kg	Perinatal asphyxia, trauma, hypoglycemia, RDS
Absent/delayed cry	Perinatal asphyxia
Congenital malformations	Risk depends on organ-system involved

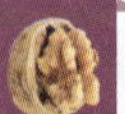

IN A NUTSHELL

Newborn Survival

1. Neonatal mortality rate (NMR) for India was reported to be 20 per 1,000 live birth for the year 2020 contributing to more than one-fourth of global neonatal deaths.
2. Approximately 70% of the total infant deaths occur in the neonatal period.
3. More than one-third of deaths occurring in entire neonatal period occur in first 24 hours of life.
4. Prematurity, low birth weight (LBW), asphyxia, and sepsis are the major causes of newborn deaths.
5. Revised India Newborn Action Plan (INAP) is aimed to bring down the NMR to a single digit by 2030, by timely recognition and prompt quality management of high-risk newborns.

Chawla D, Darlow BA. Development of Quality Measures in Perinatal Care–Priority for Developing Countries. Indian Pediatr. 2018;55(9):797-802.

Datta V, Ghosh S, Aquino LD. Progressing towards SDG 2030 goals with system changes: the India Newborn Action Plan. BMJ Open Qual. 2022;11(Suppl1):e001971.

Table 16.2 The 9 Danger Signs in Newborns

1. Very low temperature (<35.4°C)
2. High temperature (<37.5°C)
3. Not able to feed well
4. Fast breathing (respiratory rate ≥60/min)
5. Abnormal movements/convulsions/staring or blinking of eyes/lip smacking
6. Lethargy/no movements/movements only when stimulated

7. Chest indrawing

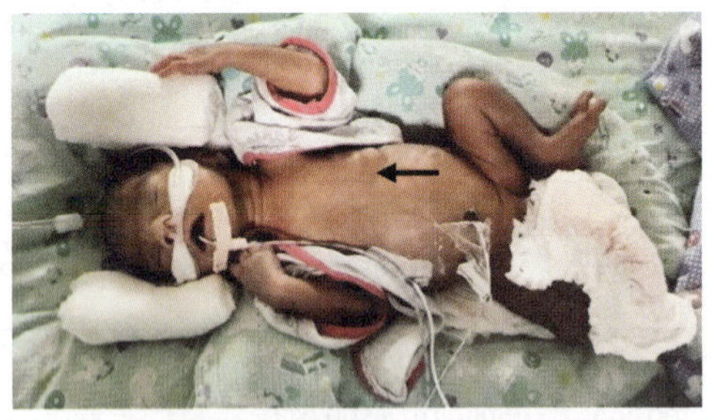

8. Yellow soles

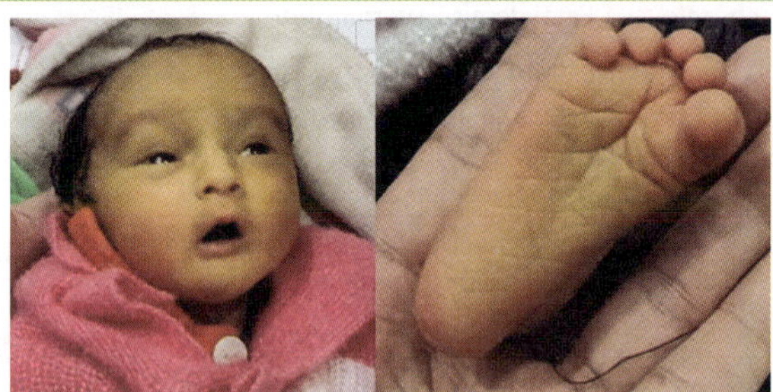

9. Signs of local infection: Umbilicus red or draining pus, skin boils, etc.

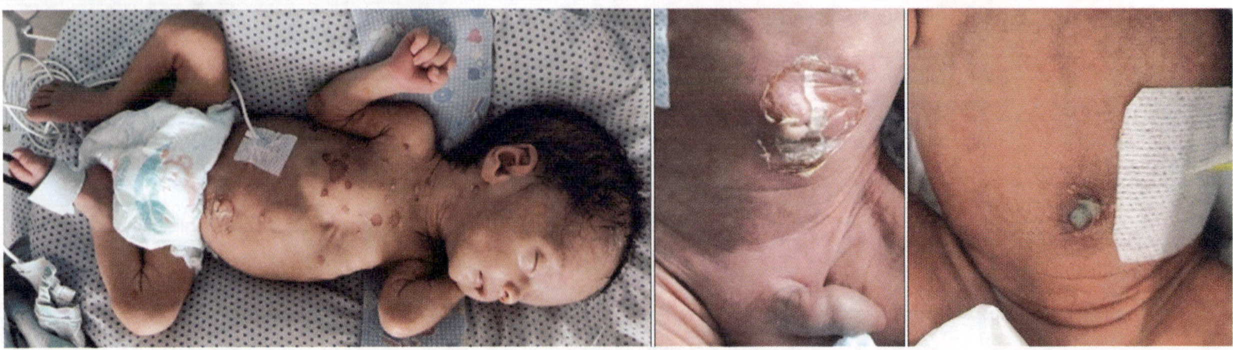

Kumar H, Sarin E, Alwadhi V, et al. A Novel Approach to Promote Evidence-Based Development of District Maternal and Newborn Health Plans in Two States in India. Indian J Community Med. 2022;47(1):66-71.
Ministry of Health and Family Welfare, Government of India. (2014). India Newborn Action Plan. [online] Available from https://nhm.gov.in/images/pdf/programmes/inap-final.pdf [Last accessed August, 2025].
Registrar General of India. Sample Registration System (SRS) Statistical Report 2020. New Delhi: 2022.
Singh S, Nayak MK, Routray PK, et al. Quality Assessment of Stillbirth Review: A Pilot Study in Ten High-Priority Districts in Odisha. Indian J Community Med. 2021;46(3):430-3.
Sitrin D, Perin J, Vaz LM, et al. Evidence from household surveys for measuring coverage of newborn care practices. J Glob Health. 2017;7(2):020503.
UNICEF, WHO, The World Bank, and United Nations. Levels & Trends in Child Mortality. Report 2023—Estimates Developed by the UN Inter-agency Group for Child Mortality Estimation. New York: 2023.

16.2 Low Birth Weight

PE 19.8

INTRODUCTION

Birth weight <2,500 g irrespective of gestational age is defined as (LBW). Global LBW prevalence was estimated to be 14.6% in 2015 with 90% of LBW births occurring in low- and middle-income countries, mainly southern Asia (48%) and sub-Saharan Africa (24%). According to National Family Health Survey-5 (2019–2021), the prevalence of LBW in India is 18%. These babies require additional care and resources as approximately 80% of neonatal deaths and 50% of infant deaths occur in LBW infants.

The LBW babies are prone to malnutrition, recurrent infections, and neurodevelopment handicaps. There is evidence to suggest that LBW infants are more likely to develop diabetes mellitus, obesity, hypertension, and coronary artery disease in later life. LBW, therefore, is a key risk factor of adverse outcome throughout life.

TYPES OF LOW BIRTH WEIGHT

A newborn baby may be LBW due to birth before 37 weeks of gestation (preterm LBW) or more commonly, born at term gestation but LBW due to intrauterine growth restriction (IUGR) (term LBW). Two-thirds of LBW neonates in our country are term babies. At times, an LBW neonate may be both preterm and having IUGR.

SYMMETRIC AND ASYMMETRIC INTRAUTERINE GROWTH RESTRICTION

The IUGR babies are further categorized as *symmetric* or *asymmetric* IUGR based on type and timing of prenatal insult, anthropometric parameters involved and outcome. The difference between the two is summarized in **Table 16.3**.

Ponderal index (PI) is used to differentiate between the symmetrical and asymmetrical babies with IUGR. It is calculated as follows:

$$[(\text{Weight in gram/length in cm}^3) \times 100]$$

The index is <2 in asymmetric IUGR and >2 in symmetric IUGR (>2.5 in term appropriate for gestational age newborn).

ETIOLOGY OF LOW BIRTH WEIGHT

The LBW is multifactorial in etiology. Several responsible factors are listed:

Table 16.3 Difference Between Symmetrical and Asymmetrical Intrauterine Growth Restriction

Features	*Symmetrical*	*Asymmetrical*
Prevalence	Less common [20–30% of all intrauterine growth restriction (IUGR)]	More common (70–80% of all IUGR)
Time of prenatal insult	First and second trimester	Usually third trimester
Causes	Chromosomal, genetic, teratogenic, and infectious etiologies	Poor maternal nutritional status, placental insufficiency, and hypertensive disorders of pregnancy
Antenatal ultrasound	Proportionately decreased head circumference (HC), abdominal circumference (AC), biparietal diameter, and femur length	Only abdominal circumference decreased, HC, and length are spared
Cell number	Decreased	Normal
Cell size	Normal	Decreased
Postnatal anthropometry	All parameters (HC, length, and weight) reduced	Reduced weight, HC normal, and length low to normal
Ponderal index	>2	<2
Features malnutrition	Less common	More marked (loose skin folds, scaphoid abdomen, prominent ribs, and triangular facies)

1. Poor nutritional status of the mother (prepregnancy weight <40 kg, height less than 145 cm, body mass index (BMI) <18.5.
2. Poor weight gain during pregnancy.
3. Maternal anemia and trace element deficiency.
4. Maternal infections including toxoplasmosis, others (Syphilis, hepatitis B), rubella, *Cytomegalovirus* (CMV), and herpes simplex (TORCH) and other intrauterine infections.
5. Chronic maternal diseases of heart, kidneys, lungs, or liver.
6. Multiple pregnancy, frequent pregnancies, short inter-pregnancy interval, and teenage pregnancy.
7. Maternal hypertension, pregnancy-induced hypertension (PIH).
8. Heavy physical work particularly in third trimester.
9. Lack of antenatal care, postmaturity.
10. Tobacco use, alcohol, or drug addiction in mother.

Most of the above factors can cause preterm delivery as well as growth restriction. Additional causes of preterm birth include cervical incompetence, previous preterm delivery, premature rupture of membranes, maternal genital tract colonization, chorioamnionitis, and uterine anomalies such as bicornuate uterus.

Preterm Low Birth Weight versus Term Intrauterine Growth Restriction Low Birth Weight

There are differences in the physical characteristics of term LBW and preterm LBW newborns **(Figs. 16.1A and B)**. They are summarized in **Table 16.4**. Preterm baby is diagnosed based on period of gestation calculated from the first day of last menstrual period of the mother. If it is <37 weeks, the baby is preterm.

Ultrasonography is very useful in estimating gestational age during antenatal period. In first trimester, crown-rump length accurately predicts gestational age while in second and third trimesters, measurement of biparietal diameter (BPD) and fetal femur length best predict gestational age.

Table 16.4 Differences Between Preterm and Term Intrauterine Growth Restriction (IUGR) Newborns

Characteristic	*Preterm*	*Term IUGR*
Appearance	Small baby with extended limbs and less activity and alertness	Small body size, emaciated or marasmic look with loose folds of skin, extremities well flexed, active and alert
Behavior	Sleepy most of the time	Alert/hyperalert appearance
Skin	Red, gelatinous, translucent	Pink, pale, opaque, rough, dry, wrinkled, peeling
Lanugo	Abundant	Mostly absent
Ear Pinna Cartilage Curvature recoil	Poorly developed Poorly formed Poorly developed Poor	Well-developed Well-formed Well-developed Good
Sole creases	Absent or only in anterior third	Present all over the sole
Areola with breast nodule	Areola poorly formed and depigmented, nodule barely palpable	Well-formed pigmented areola and palpable firm nodule
Genitalia—male • Scrotum • Rugae • Median raphe • Color • Testes	 • Small sized, smooth surface • Absent • Absent • Pink • Undescended	 • Pendulous, bigger in size • Present • Present • Darkly pigmented • Descended
Genitalia—female • Labia • Clitoris	 • Labia minora not covered with majora • Enlarged	 • Labia minora well-covered with majora • Small
Muscle tone	Less	Good
Abdomen	Normal in appearance	May be scaphoid

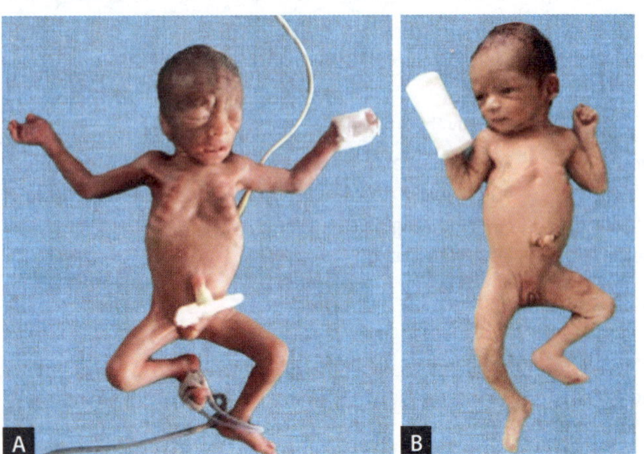

Figs. 16.1A and B: (A) Preterm low birth weight; (B) Term low birth weight

Problems of Term Intrauterine Growth Restriction Low Birth Weight Neonates

- Perinatal asphyxia
- Hypothermia, hypoglycemia, hypocalcemia
- Meconium aspiration syndrome
- Persistent pulmonary hypertension of newborn
- Pulmonary hemorrhage
- Polycythemia/hyperviscosity
- Poor postnatal growth
- Infection
- Higher incidence of degenerative diseases, such as diabetes mellitus, hypertension, and atherosclerosis later in life.

Problems of Preterm Low Birth Weight Neonates

- Perinatal asphyxia
- ***Respiratory:*** Respiratory distress syndrome (RDS), apneic spells, congenital pneumonia, and bronchopulmonary dysplasia (late complication)
- ***Cardiovascular:*** Patent ductus arteriosus and hypotension
- ***Central nervous system:*** Periventricular/intraventricular hemorrhage, periventricular leukomalacia and neurodevelopmental handicaps
- ***Gastrointestinal and hepatobiliary:*** Feeding intolerance, gastroesophageal reflux, necrotizing enterocolitis, indirect hyperbilirubinemia and cholestatic jaundice
- ***Thermoregulation:*** Hypo-/hyperthermia
- ***Immunologic:*** Repeated infections
- ***Nutrition:*** Poor growth
- ***Metabolic:*** Hypo-/hyperglycemia, hypocalcemia and metabolic bone disease of prematurity
- ***Renal:*** Late metabolic acidosis and electrolyte imbalance
- ***Hematological:*** Anemia, disseminated intravascular coagulation, vitamin K deficiency bleeding
- ***Skin:*** High transepidermal water loss and skin abrasions
- ***Eye:*** Retinopathy of prematurity, myopia and strabismus
- ***Ear:*** Hearing impairment

TREATMENT Low Birth Weight

Care at Delivery

- The baby may require resuscitation and admission to the neonatal intensive care unit (NICU). Therefore, delivery should take place in a hospital with facilities for neonatal care. In utero transport is far safer than transport of a sick baby after birth.
- Delivery should be attended by health professionals skilled in neonatal resuscitation.
- Not all babies require hospital care. An otherwise healthy LBW newborn with a birth weight of 1,800 g or above or gestation of 34 weeks or more can be managed at home with assistance from a health worker.
- Indications for admission:
  - Birth weight <1,800 g
  - Gestation <34 weeks
  - Not able to take feeds from the breast or by cup (irrespective of birth weight and gestation) or
  - Sick neonate (irrespective of the birth weight or gestation).

Maintenance of Temperature

The LBW babies are prone to hypothermia due to large surface area, poor insulation due to decreased subcutaneous fat, large evaporative heat loss due to thin skin, and less heat production due to poor stores of brown adipose tissue. A hypothermic baby has increased oxygen demand and may develop hypoglycemia, apnea, acidosis, hypoxemia, bleeding diathesis, respiratory failure, shock, and eventually death.

- *Rooming-in:* The temperature can be maintained at home or hospital by keeping mother and baby together in the same bed under a single blanket.
- *Kangaroo mother care (KMC):* This is a low tech readily available alternative to radiant heat warmers and incubators to keep babies warm. There are other benefits of KMC such as enhanced breastfeeding, better bonding between mother and baby, better weight gain, and reduced risk of sepsis. For all these reasons, KMC needs to be widely popularized and practiced in resource-limited settings **(Fig. 16.2)**.

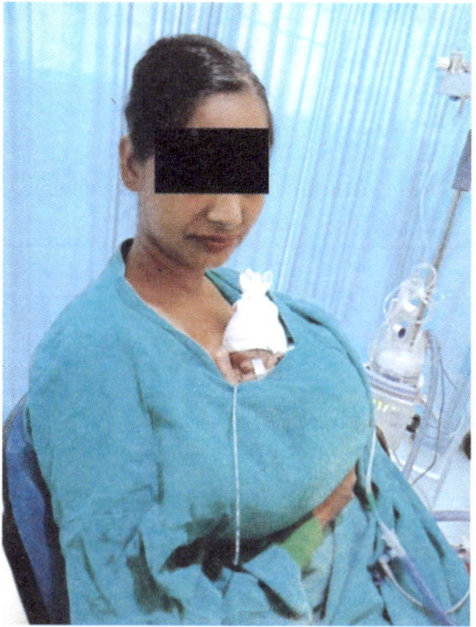

Fig. 16.2: Kangaroo mother care

- *The baby should be clothed well*: At least two or three layers of clothes are generally required. If the room is not warm enough, woolen sweater should also be put on. Feet should be covered with socks, hands with mittens, and head with a cap. Further, the room where an LBW baby is kept should be warmed using electrical heater, especially in winter months. The baby should not be kept directly in front of electrical heater. This may produce thermal injury.
- *Monitor temperature*: If the baby is maintaining normal body temperature, both trunk and soles/palms should be warm to touch and pink in color. In early stages of hypothermia, the trunk is warm but the soles and palms are cold to touch and bluish in appearance. The mother should be educated and trained in the touch technique to detect hypothermia in the early stages. This condition, known as cold stress, can be managed by providing KMC and keeping the room warm.
- *In the hospital*, apart from the above methods, overhead radiant warmer or incubator may be used to keep the baby warm. Regular monitoring of axillary temperature should be carried out in all sick babies.

Intravenous Fluids

Sick LBW babies who cannot be given oral or gavage (tube) feeding should be given intravenous fluids. Fluid requirement of LBW babies are summarized in **Table 16.5**. Key points to remember are:

- On day 1, the fluid requirements range from 60 to 80 mL/kg.
- The daily increment in fluid volume is around 15 mL/kg till day 7 by which time a baby should be getting around 150 mL/kg/day.
- Initiate fluid therapy with plain 10% dextrose. For newborns weighing below 1 kg, 5% dextrose is preferred to avoid hyperglycemia.
- Sodium (3 mEq/kg/day) and potassium (2 mEq/kg/day) are added after 48 hours by which time most babies will pass urine. Isolyte-P is a readymade electrolyte containing solution which can be used after 48 hours of age.
- For administering intravenous fluids to the neonate, a small volume infusion set/syringe pump should be used. Fluid therapy should be carefully monitored. Too rapid infusion may result in pulmonary edema or even death in a small baby.

Nutrition

Nutrition is an essential part of the care of LBW newborns. Their little reserves of fat and carbohydrate are rapidly depleted unless provided sufficient nutrients. Inability to take oral feeds and limited feeding tolerance of these infants make feeding a challenging task. Type of milk initiation and progression of feeds is described here.

Table 16.5 Fluid Requirements (Intravenous or Oral) of Neonates (mL/kg Body Weight/Day)

Day of life	*Birth weight*	
	>1,500 g	*≤1,500 g*
1	60	80
2	75	95
3	90	110
4	105	125
5	120	140
6	135	155
7 onward	150	170

Choice of milk: First choice for feeding LBW remains mother's own milk in the absence of which pasteurized donor human milk is the next best option. The least preferred milk is formula milk. Human milk feeding is the preferred choice as it is associated with lesser risk of infection, better cognitive development but accompanied by slower growth compared to formula fed babies. LBW neonates fed exclusively with human milk may develop iron deficiency, osteopenia, zinc, vitamin Aand vitamin D deficiency therefore nutrient supplementation is required as described later.

Mode, initiation, and progression of feeding: The method of feeding depends on the gestation, postnatal age, and presence or absence of sickness and vigor (feeding effort) of the baby. The options include breastfeeding, cup/*paladai* feeding, or tube feeding (nasogastric/orogastric). **Table 16.6** describes the gestational age and feeding skill-based mode of feed initiation and progression in LBW neonates.

Volume of feeding: Stable LBW neonates weighing 1,000–2,499 g may be started with full feeds on day 1 without intravenous fluids while those weighing <1,000 g are started on intravenous fluids (consisting of total parenteral nutrition in the form of glucose, amino acids, and intralipids) and tube feeds which is increased gradually. Volume of feeds at the time of initiation and daily increments are described in **Table 16.7**. However, severely growth restricted neonates with abnormal Doppler flows in umbilical artery should be kept nil orally along with total parenteral nutrition on day 1. From day 2 onward, feeds can be introduced and increased as described for neonates <1,000 g with careful monitoring for feed intolerance.

Prefeed Aspiration

For tube-fed babies, prefeed aspiration of stomach contents need not be done routinely before each feed for diagnosis of feeding intolerance. It is better to measure baseline abdominal girth. If prefeed abdominal girth increases by 2 cm or more from baseline, gastric contents should be aspirated and its volume and color noted.

- If the aspirate is milky and volume is <25% of previous feed and baby is otherwise stable, continue feeding.
- If the aspirate is milky and volume is 25–50% of previous feed and baby is otherwise stable, miss that feed and again check for the next feed.
- If the aspirate is bilious/hemorrhagic or the baby is looking sick, stop feeding and consider the possibilities of paralytic ileus, infection, hypokalemia, or early necrotizing enterocolitis.

Trophic Feeding

Trophic feedings are defined as giving very small volumes of feeds (up to 24 mL/kg/day) every 4–6 hours for the purpose of gut maturation rather than nutrient delivery. Trophic feeds are indicated when clinical condition of the newborn precludes normal volume enteral feeding.

In the past, these newborns would have remained nil per orally for a few days. Keeping a newborn baby nil orally for a few days can produce intestinal changes including involution of gut villi, mucosal thinning, and loss of intestinal enzymes. Trophic feeding prevents these changes.

Trophic feeds can be started on the first day in newborns who are hemodynamically stable. Benefits of trophic feedings (gut priming) include less feeding intolerance, earlier progression to full enteral feedings, and improved weight gain. It is best to start trophic feedings with breastmilk.

Table 16.6 Gestational Age, Maturation of Feeding Skills, and Guide for Feed Initiation

Gestation	*Feeding skill*	*Clinical implication*	*Remark*	*Progression of feeds*
<28 weeks	No sucking, immature gut motility	Start on intravenous (IV) fluids	Initiate minimal enteral feeds (trophic feeds) (10–20 mL/kg)	If baby tolerates minimal enteral feeds, increase tube feed volume taper and stop IV fluid
28–31 weeks	Sucking bursts develop, however, there is no coordination between sucking, swallowing, and breathing	Start with orogastric tube feeding	Monitor for feed intolerance (increase in abdominal girth, bilious vomiting), if present start IV fluids and stop feeding	Try *katori* spoon feeding once baby is 32–33 weeks postmenstrual age and gives cues (waking, fussing, sucking on hands, stable tone, and vital signs) for oral feeding readiness, also put the baby on mother's empty breast (after milk expression) for non-nutritive sucking (NNS); once baby starts accepting cup feeds well, increase cup feed frequency and taper and stop tube feeds
32–34 weeks	Mature sucking pattern seen and coordination between breathing swallowing begins	Start with *katori* spoon/cup/ *paladai* feeding	Closely watch for spillage of milk and whether the baby takes adequate amount, if intake is poor shift to tube feeding	Put on mother's breast before each feed for NNS; taper and stop cup feed if mother is confident
>34 weeks	Mature sucking pattern, coordinated breathing-swallowing reflex	Start with breastfeeding	Monitor for latching and effective sucking in the absence of which *katori* spoon feeding should be tried	

Table 16.7 Volume of Feeds at the Time of Initiation and Progression in Low Birth Weight Neonates			
Birth weight	*Volume of feed at the time of initiation*	*Daily increments*	*Maximum volume*
<1,000 g	10–20 mL/kg/day with total parenteral nutrition	30–40 mL/kg/day	180 mL/kg/day
1,000–1,500 g	80 mL/kg/day	20 mL/kg/day	180 mL/kg/day
≥1,500 g	60 mL/kg/day	20 mL/kg/day	180 mL/kg/day

Assessing Adequacy of Feeding

Adequacy of nutrition can be judged by assessing growth of a LBW baby. Weight should be recorded daily and head and length measurements should be taken weekly.

All newborns lose weight in the first week of age. Term newborns may lose 5–10% of their birth weight while preterm newborns may lose up to 10–15% of their birth weight. All newborns should regain birth weight by 10–14 days of age and should gain weight at a rate of about 15–20 g/kg/day. IUGR infants may not lose much weight and may start gaining weight early. A baby should gain at least 125 g each week. Poor weight gain may indicate inadequate intake, cold stress, infection, anemia, or other systemic disorders.

Adequately breastfed baby will pass light colored urine at least 6–8 times a day. If a baby is passing urine <6 times a day and the urine is concentrated, i.e., dark yellow in color, it indicates that the baby is not getting enough breastmilk.

Supplements

All LBW babies should receive intramuscular vitamin K 0.5 mg at birth to prevent vitamin K deficiency bleeding. Fortification of human milk with multicomponent human milk fortifier (HMF) should be done for all neonates with birth weight <1,800 g being fed with mother's own milk or donor human milk. HMF enriches human milk with extra calories, proteins vitamins, minerals, and iron. Fortification is started when feed volume exceeds 100 mL/kg/day. Depending on the birth weight and type of feeding additional supplements are required as described in **Table 16.8**.

Prevention of Infection

The LBW babies are prone to develop infections and mortality due to high sepsis. Following measures are helpful in preventing infections:

- Ensure exclusive breastfeeding and avoid prelacteal feeds.
- Handwashing by the health professionals, mother, and family members before touching the baby.
- For cup-feeding, mother should wash her hands before expressing the milk into a clean cup. Cup should be cleaned by washing with soap and water and then putting it in boiling water for 5 minutes. Alternatively, cup can be cleaned by pouring boiling water into the cup and leaving it there for a few minutes.
- Keep the umbilical stump dry. Do not apply anything over it.
- Avoiding unnecessary handling of the baby by multiple persons.

Immunization

The LBW infants should be immunized at the same chronological age as term appropriately grown infants and according to the national immunization schedule. LBW does not increase the incidence of vaccine-related adverse events, and the dose should not be reduced for any vaccine.

OUTCOME OF LOW BIRTH WEIGHT BABIES

Outcome of LBW newborn is determined by birth weight, gestational age, underlying etiology, extent, and timing of IUGR, immediate postnatal complications, and catch up growth.

- For similar birth weight, preterm newborn perform worse than IUGR newborns in the immediate postnatal period, due to greater immaturity of their organ systems.
- Compared to appropriately grown newborn, IUGR babies experience higher morbidity and mortality.
- Asymmetric IUGR infants have more favorable outcome thansymmetric IUGR infants due to better potential for growth.
- Overall, former IUGR infants remain shorter (less height) and lighter (less weight) compared to their normal siblings.
- Recent studies suggest that certain diseases such as diabetes mellitus, insulin resistance, obesity, and cardiovascular

Table 16.8 Supplements to be Started for Low Birth Weight Neonates				
	Birth weight <1,500 g			
	Till 40 weeks PMA			
Supplements	*Unfortified breastmilk*	*HMF fortified breastmilk*	*After 40 weeks PMA*	*Birth weight 1,500–2,499 g*
Calcium	140–160 mg/kg/day once 100 mL/kg/day feeds are reached	Not needed	–	–
Phosphorus	70–80 mg/kg/day once 100 mL/kg/day feeds are reached	Not needed	–	–
Iron	2 mg/kg/ day at 2 weeks	Not needed	2 mg/kg/day till 2 years of age	2 mg/kg/day from 4 weeks till 2 years
Multi-vitamins	1 mL once 100 mL/kg/day feeds are reached	1 mL once 100 mL/kg/ day feeds are reached	–	–
Vitamin D	800–1,000 IU/day	Not needed	800–1,000 IU/day till 2 years of age	400 IU/day from 2 weeks till 2 years of age

(HMF: human milk fortifier)

disease are more common in adults who were IUGR/ LBW at birth. These pathologies may be a consequence of "programming" in which an insult occurring at a critical stage of human development may result in a long-lasting effect on the structure and function of the organism (*Barker's hypothesis*). Mechanisms underlying these morbidities are poorly understood.

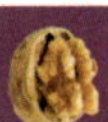

IN A NUTSHELL

Low Birth Weight

1. In India, 5 million LBW infants (<2,500 g) are born every year and account for 30% of the total of 20 million LBW babies born globally.
2. Newborn infant can be LBW because of intrauterine growth restriction (IUGR) or prematurity.
3. Poor maternal nutrition is the principal risk factor for LBW.
4. The major immediate complications encountered in LBW are difficult resuscitation, respiratory distress syndrome, apnea, hypotension, hypothermia, hypoglycemia, necrotizing enterocolitis, intracranial hemorrhage, feeding difficulties, and vulnerability to infections, and iatrogenic complications.
5. Breastmilk remains the choice of feeding in LBW along with mineral and vitamin supplements.
6. Nearly three-fourths of neonatal deaths and half of infant deaths occur amongst LBW infants.

Boel L, Hixson T, Brown L, et al. Noninvasive respiratory support in preterm infants. Paediatr Respir Rev. 2022;43:53-9.

Gebeyehu NA, Gelaw KA, Azeze GA, et al. Knowledge, attitude, and practice towards kangaroo mother care among postnatal women in Ethiopia: Systematic review and meta-analysis. PLoS One. 2022;17(5):e0265411.

Kaempf JW, Guillen U, Litt JS, et al. Change in neurodevelopmental outcomes for extremely premature infants over time: a systematic review and meta-analysis. Arch Dis Child Fetal Neonatal Ed. 2022:fetalneonatal-2022-324457.

Karlsson V, Blomqvist YT, Ågren J. Nursing care of infants born extremely preterm. Semin Fetal Neonatal Med. 2022;27(3):101369.

Kim YJ, Shin SH, Park HW, et al. Risk factors of early pulmonary hypertension and its clinical outcomes in preterm infants: a systematic review and meta-analysis. Sci Rep. 2022;12(1):14186.

Mabrouk A, Abubakar A, Too EK, et al. A Scoping Review of Preterm Births in Sub-Saharan Africa: Burden, Risk Factors and Outcomes. Int J Environ Res Public Health. 2022;19(17):10537.

Ramaswamy VV, Abiramalatha T, Bandyopadhyay T, et al. ELBW and ELGAN outcomes in developing nations-Systematic review and meta-analysis. PLoS One. 2021;16(8):e0255352.

Samouilidis A, Beltsios ET, Mavrovounis G, et al. The use of antenatal dexamethasone in late preterm and term pregnancies to improve neonatal morbidity and mortality: A Systematic Review and Meta-Analysis. Cureus. 2022;14(8):e27865.

Thanigainathan S, Abiramalatha T. Early fortification of human milk versus late fortification to promote growth in preterm infants. Cochrane Database Syst Rev. 2020;7(7):CD013392.

Venkataramani M, Ogunwole SM, Caulfield LE, et al. Maternal, infant, and child health outcomes associated with the special supplemental nutrition program for women, infants, and children: A Systematic Review. Ann Intern Med. 2022;175(10):1411-22.

Walsh V, Brown JVE, Copperthwaite BR, et al. Early full enteral feeding for preterm or low birth weight infants. Cochrane Database Syst Rev. 2020;12(12):CD013542.

WHO ACTION Trials Collaborators. The World Health Organization ACTION-I (Antenatal CorTicosteroids for Improving Outcomes in preterm Newborns) Trial: a multi-country, multi-centre, two-arm, parallel, double-blind, placebo-controlled, individually randomized trial of antenatal corticosteroids for women at risk of imminent birth in the early preterm period in hospitals in low-resource countries. Trials. 2019;20(1):507.

Yadav A, Siddiqui N, Debata PK. Two-hourly versus Three-hourly Feeding in Very Low Birthweight Neonates: A Randomized Controlled Trial. Indian Pediatr. 2021;58(4):320-4.

Yadav DK, Shukla GS, Gupta N, et al. Maternal and Obstetric Factors Associated with Low Birth Weight. J Nepal Health Res Counc. 2020;17(4): 443-50.

Zaveri A, Paul P, Saha J, et al. Maternal determinants of low birth weight among Indian children: Evidence from the National Family Health Survey-4, 2015-16. PLoS One. 2020;15(12):e0244562.

16.3 Perinatal Asphyxia and Hypoxic-Ischemic Encephalopathy

PE 19.4

INTRODUCTION

Perinatal asphyxia is the second most common cause of neonatal death after prematurity-related complications and is the leading cause of neurodevelopmental disability in children. The term perinatal asphyxia is preferred to birth asphyxia as asphyxial injury may occur before, during, or after birth.

Hypoxic-ischemic encephalopathy (HIE) refers to the characteristic neurological manifestations in term and near-term newborns which develop soon after birth following perinatal asphyxia. HIE occurs at a rate of approximately 3–5 cases per 1,000 full-term live births, half of which progress to moderate to severe HIE.

DEFINITION

Perinatal asphyxia may be defined as hypoxic insult to the fetus severe enough to cause metabolic acidosis, neonatal encephalopathy, and multiorgan system dysfunction. The National Neonatology Forum of India has defined asphyxia as "gasping or ineffective breathing or lack of breathing at 1 minute of life." The essential criteria for diagnosing perinatal asphyxia as outlined by the American Academy of Pediatrics (AAP) are as follows:

- Umbilical artery metabolic or mixed acidemia with pH <7.0 or base deficit ≥12 mmol/L, or both
- Apgar score of <5 at 5 minutes and 10 minutes
- Magnetic resonance imaging (MRI) or MR spectroscopy brain showing injury consistent with acute hypoxia-ischemia
- Evidence of multiorgan system dysfunction

ETIOLOGY

Perinatal asphyxia is multifactorial in origin. In most cases (>90%), the asphyxia insult occurs during the antepartum or intrapartum period. Postpartum insult is responsible for the remaining cases of perinatal asphyxia.

Prepartum Insult

Placental insufficiency during the antepartum or intrapartum periods results in an inability to provide oxygen and remove carbon dioxide and hydrogen ion from the fetus leading to perinatal asphyxia. Causes of placental insufficiency include:

- ***Impaired maternal*** oxygenation as in maternal hypoxia due to anemia, pulmonary, cardiac, or neurologic disease in the mother.
- ***Decreased blood flow from the mother to the placenta*** as in maternal infection, shock, dehydration, and hypotension.
- ***Decreased blood flow from the placenta to the fetus*** as in placental abruption, cord prolapse, cord entanglement, true knot, cord compression, and abnormality of the umbilical vessels.
- ***Impaired gas exchange across placenta or fetal tissues*** as in maternal hypertension, vascular disease, diabetes, drug abuse, postmaturity, placental calcification, infarct, or fibrosis, etc.
- ***Increased fetal oxygen requirement*** as in fetal anemia, fetal infection, or IUGR.

Postpartum Causes

Postpartum insults occur secondary to pulmonary, cardiovascular, or neurologic insufficiency during immediate postpartum period.

PATHOPHYSIOLOGY

Perinatal asphyxia results in lack of oxygen (hypoxia) and lack of perfusion (ischemia) to various organs. The most vulnerable organ to be affected by hypoxic-ischemic injury is brain, as neonatal brain has very high requirements for oxygen and baseline blood flow. Hypoxic insult to the fetus initiates *diving seal reflex*, causing shunting of blood to brain, heart, and adrenals and away from lungs, gut, kidneys, liver, spleen, and skin, in an attempt to maintain perfusion to more vital organs.

Biochemically, hypoxia impairs cerebral oxidative metabolism, resulting in increase in lactate, fall in pH (acidosis), and decrease in adenosine triphosphate (ATP) levels. Acidosis causes myocardial depression and reduced cardiac output. During prolonged hypoxia, hypotension develops and cerebral blood flow is compromised, and a combined hypoxic and ischemic insult leads to further failure of oxidative phosphorylation. Brain injury in HIE occurs in two phases, primary and secondary energy failure:

1. ***Primary energy failure*** during initial insult impairs ion pumps, leading to accumulation of Na^+, Cl^-, H_2O, and Ca^{++} intracellularly; and K^+ and neurotoxic excitatory amino acids—glutamate and aspartate, extracellularly. After reperfusion of previously ischemic tissues, there is a brief period of normal cerebral metabolism, followed by development of secondary energy failure.
2. ***Secondary energy failure*** is characterized by generation of oxygen free radicals which along with inflammation, altered growth factors, and protein synthesis further produce neuronal damage by brain cell apoptosis and necrosis over the next several days to week.

The therapeutic window occurring between primary and secondary energy failure is approximately 6 hours as determined by animal studies. Pathologically, brain damage occurs mainly in cerebral cortex and basal ganglia in term newborns. In preterm newborns, the insult predominantly involves periventricular white matter. The pathophysiology is summarized in **Flowchart 16.1**.

CLINICAL FEATURES

Clinical manifestations and course vary depending on the severity of hypoxic-ischemic insult. The clinical picture is described as mild, moderate, and severe as given in **Table 16.9**.

Mild Hypoxic-ischemic Encephalopathy

Transient abnormalities are observed, such as poor feeding, irritability, or excessive crying or sleepiness. Muscle tone may be slightly increased and deep tendon reflexes may be brisk.

Moderate Hypoxic-ischemic Encephalopathy

The infant is lethargic, with significant hypotonia, and diminished deep tendon reflexes. The grasp, Moro, and sucking reflexes may be sluggish or absent and the baby may develop occasional periods of apnea. Seizures may occur within the first 24 hours of life, most commonly within first 12 hours.

Flowchart 16.1: Pathophysiology of neuronal injury in hypoxia ischemia

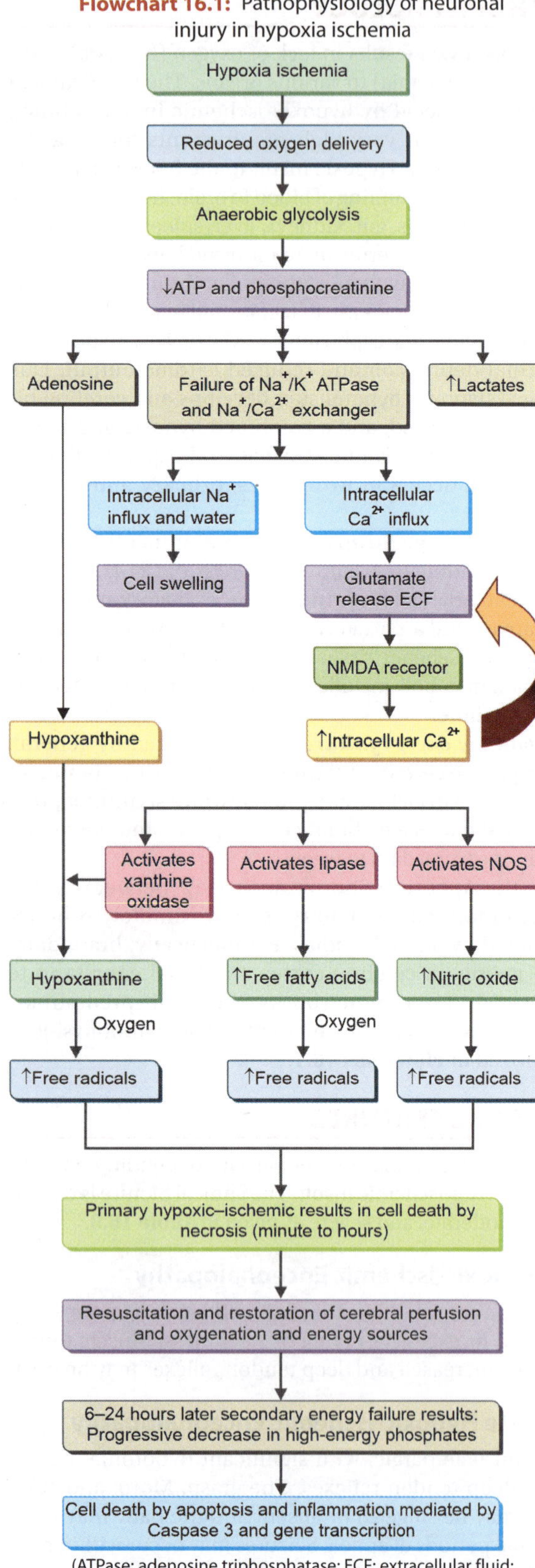

(ATPase: adenosine triphosphatase; ECF: extracellular fluid; NMDA: N-methyl D-aspartate; NOS: nitric oxide synthase)

Table 16.9 Grading of Neonatal Hypoxic-ischemic Encephalopathy

	Grade I (mild)	*Grade II (moderate)*	*Grade III (severe)*
Conscious level	Irritable/ hyperalert	**Lethargic**	**Comatose**
Tone	**Either**[a] mildly abnormal (hypo/hyper)	**Moderately abnormal** (hypotonic or dissociated)	**Severely abnormal** (hypotonia)
Suck	**Or**[b] abnormal	Poor	**Absent**
Primitive reflexes	Exaggerated	**Depressed**	**Absent**
Seizures	**Absent**	Present	Present
Brainstem reflexes	**Normal**	**Normal**	Impaired
Respiration	Tachypneic	Occasional apnea	**Severe apnea**

The features in **bold** must be described to meet the minimum requirements for each grade. Features not in bold may be present but are not required to make the syndrome assignment

[a/b]: Either abnormal tone or abnormal suck should accompany altered conscious level to assign grade I

Source: Adapted from Fenichel

Severe Hypoxic-Ischemic Encephalopathy

The baby becomes comatosed and may not respond to any physical stimulus. Breathing becomes irregular, and baby may require ventilatory support. Tone is decreased and deep tendon reflexes are depressed. Neonatal reflexes (e.g., sucking, swallowing, grasp, and Moro) are absent. Disturbances of ocular motion, such as a skewed deviation of the eyes, nystagmus, bobbing, and loss of "doll's eye" (i.e., conjugate) movements may be revealed by cranial nerve examination. Pupils may be dilated, fixed, or poorly reactive to light.

Seizures occur in up to 50% newborns with HIE and may be subtle, tonic, or clonic. Anterior fontanel may be full or bulging due to cerebral edema. Irregularities of heart rate and blood pressure (BP) are common during the period of reperfusion injury, as is death from cardiorespiratory failure. These neonates would eventually die or have permanent neurologic sequelae.

Organ System Involvement

In addition to brain, perinatal asphyxia may affect kidneys, heart, lungs, intestine, and liver. Organ systems involved following a hypoxic-ischemic events include the following:

- ***Renal:*** After brain, kidney is the next most affected organ in perinatal asphyxia. Hypoxic-ischemic insults lead to acute tubular necrosis with oliguria.
- ***Heart:*** Reduced myocardial contractility, severe hypotension, passive cardiac dilatation, and tricuspid regurgitation.
- ***Lungs:*** Respiratory distress due to pulmonary edema, hemorrhage, and pulmonary hypertension.

- ***Liver:*** Deranged liver function, hyperammonemia, and coagulopathy.
- ***Gastrointestinal system:*** Poor peristalsis, delayed gastric emptying, and necrotizing enterocolitis.
- ***Hematologic:*** Increased nucleated red blood cells (RBCs), neutropenia or neutrophilia, thrombocytopenia, and coagulopathy.

INVESTIGATIONS

There are no confirmatory laboratory tests to diagnose perinatal asphyxia. Tests are helpful to assess the severity of brain injury and to monitor the functional status of systemic organs.

- ***Blood glucose:*** It should be monitored frequently. Both hypoglycemia (blood glucose <45 mg/dL) and hyperglycemia (blood glucose >125 mg/dL) are to be avoided.
- ***Serum electrolytes:*** Daily assessment of serum electrolytes, especially calcium, is valuable until the infant's status improves. Markedly low serum sodium, potassium, and chloride levels in the presence of reduced urine flow and excessive weight gain may indicate acute tubular damage particularly during the initial 2–3 days of life.
- ***Renal function tests:*** Blood urea and serum creatinine.
- ***Liver function tests:*** To assess the degree of hypoxic–ischemic injury.
- ***Coagulation*** prothrombin time and partial thromboplastin time.
- ***Blood gas monitoring:*** To assess acid-base status, and to avoid hyperoxia, hypoxia as well as hypercapnia and hypocapnia.
- ***Neuroimaging:*** Neuroimaging is helpful in demonstrating diffuse or focal brain injury and predicting long-term outcome. Cranial ultrasound has better predictive ability in preterm infants while cranial computed tomography (CT) is more useful in term infants. MRI is the imaging modality of choice for the diagnosis and follow-up of infants with moderate-to-severe HIE. MRI can reveal specific patterns of brain injury in both preterm and term neonates which may not be demonstrated by other imaging modalities.
- ***Electroencephalogram (EEG):*** It is a valuable tool in predicting outcome. Burst suppression, low voltage, or electrocerebral inactivity are associated with poor outcome.

TREATMENT Perinatal Asphyxia and Hypoxic-Ischemic Encephalopathy

The management of perinatal asphyxia is essentially supportive. Initial resuscitation and stabilization are important for prevention of perinatal asphyxia and HIE. A normal metabolic state including glucose, calcium, and acid-base balance should be maintained.

Supportive Therapy

1. *Intravenous fluids:* An intravenous line should be started with 10% dextrose at 60 mL/kg/day.
2. *Perfusion and blood pressure:* Hypotension is common in infants with HIE and is due to myocardial dysfunction, capillary leak syndrome, and hypovolemia. It should be promptly treated. A systemic mean arterial BP of at least 45–50 mm Hg is desirable for term infants, 35–40 mm Hg for infants weighing 1,000–2,000 g and 30–35 mm for infants <1,000 g to maintain cerebral perfusion. Vasopressor agents like dobutamine or dopamine should be used if BP is low.
3. *Maintenance of temperature:* Temperature should be closely monitored and maintained in the normal range of 36.5–37.5°C. Recent studies suggest that term and late preterm infants with moderate to severe encephalopathy with evidence of intrapartum asphyxia undergoing *therapeutic hypothermia* have better outcomes in terms of mortality or major neurodevelopmental disability. Modest hypothermia (33–34°C) may be beneficial by virtue of preventing energy depletion, inhibiting glutamate release, and inhibiting apoptosis. Hyperthermia is also detrimental as it increases the metabolic and energy expenditure and induces neuronal injury.

   Temperature must be monitored closely from the start in the delivery room. The radiant warmer should not be turned off until after resuscitation and determination of eligibility for therapeutic hypothermia.
4. *Glucose:* Blood glucose level should be kept at 75–100 mg/dLto provide adequate substrate for the brain. If the baby is hypoglycemic, a bolus of 2 mL/kg of 10% dextrose should be administered followed by a continuous glucose infusion at a rate of 6 mg/kg/min.
5. *Calcium:* Calcium level should be kept in the normal range (9–11 mg/dL). Hypocalcemia is a common metabolic alteration in the HIE. A subnormal serum Ca^{++} level may compromise cardiac contractility and may cause seizures. Hypercalcemia should be avoided as it can enhance neuronal injury.
6. *Pulmonary dysfunction:* Delayed fluid clearance and pulmonary hypertension may manifest with respiratory distress so ventilator support should be provided and carefully monitoring of paO_2, $paCO_2$ should be done to avoid acidosis, hypoxia, hyperoxia, and hypocarbia.
7. *Nutrition:* Trophic feeds may be started with breastmilk and increased only after rewarming has started and sedation depth has decreased.
8. *Coagulation profile:* Coagulation profile should be monitored for neonates with perinatal asphyxia undergoing therapeutic hypothermia as liver injury in HIE and cooling both increase bleeding tendency.

Seizure Management

The HIE is the most common cause of seizures in the neonatal period occurring most commonly in first 12–24 hours of life. Seizures may be focal or multifocal, brief or may be recurrent especially in first 24 hours. Phenobarbitone is the first-line anticonvulsant in neonates with efficacy of controlling seizures in 50% of the infants only. Second-line drugs include phenytoin and benzodiazepines with levetiracetam emerging as an important anticonvulsant due to its attractive characteristics such as CYPP450 independence, intravenous formulation available, 100% oral bioavailability, no drug interactions, and no protein binding but its efficacy and safety is yet to be established. Anticonvulsants are usually only required in the first week because seizures are "acute symptomatic" and burn out with time. Occasionally, longer-term therapy is required in severely affected infants. Cochrane review does not support prophylactic anticonvulsants in HIE.

Cerebroprotective Interventions

Brain-sparing or cerebroprotective interventions are being studied for improving the outcome of perinatal asphyxia. These include therapeutic hypothermia, free radical scavengers, antagonists of excitotoxic amino acids, calcium channel blockers, etc.

The only recommended cerebroprotective agent till date is therapeutic hypothermia. It is standard of care for neonates with moderate-severe HIE and should be initiated within 6 hours after birth, the therapeutic window between primary and secondary energy failure phases.

Standard clinical tools in the form of modified Sarnat exam should be used to evaluate for encephalopathy within the first hour of birth. If baby is delivered at a center not equipped with therapeutic hypothermia machines should make an early communication (within 1 hour of birth) with a therapeutic hypothermia center to facilitate patient selection and expedite initiation of treatment and transfer. Once a patient meets all criteria for therapeutic hypothermia, start passive or active cooling with a goal temperature of 33.5°C ± 0.5°C as soon as possible, with close attention to core temperature. Cooling is continued for 72 hours followed by slow rewarming. At the end of 72 hours of therapeutic hypothermia, the newborn is rewarmed at a rate of 0.5°C every 2 hours until patient reaches 36.5°C which should take approximately 10–12 hours. Both total body and head cooling have been shown to be safe and effective. Infant undergoing therapeutic hypothermia should be sedated to provide comfort and prevent shivering which can increase metabolism.

Significant adverse effects noted with cooling are sinus bradycardia and thrombocytopenia seen in 5% and 31% of the patients, respectively.

Cerebral edema is an uncommon complication of HIE. Drugs such as mannitol, steroids, and furosemide used in past are no longer recommended.

Monitoring

Early detection of complication by clinical and biochemical monitoring and prompt management is essential to prevent extension of cerebral injury.

Regular clinical assessment should be made by recording respiratory rate, heart rate, capillary filling time, blood pressure, temperature, and oxygen saturation. Urine output should be monitored. Biochemical monitoring consists of estimation of blood sugar by dextrostix, hematocrit, serum electrolytes (Na, K), serum calcium, blood urea nitrogen (BUN), creatinine, blood gases, and pH.

Oxygenation should be kept in the normal range by monitoring transcutaneous or arterial PaO_2 or percent oxygen saturation (SpO_2) by pulse oximetry. PaO_2 should be maintained between 60 and 80 mm Hg and SpO_2 should be maintained between 90 and 94%. Hypoxia should be treated with O_2 and, if required, ventilation. Hyperoxia should always be avoided. CO_2 levels should be kept in the normal range by maintaining $PaCO_2$ between 35 and 45 mm Hg.

PROGNOSIS

The mortality is 20% and 30% of survivors have neurodevelopmental sequelae. Long-term handicaps include developmental delay, cerebral palsy, microcephaly, seizures, blindness, deafness, and problems with cognition, memory, fine motor skills, and behavior.

Predictors of poor outcome: The presence of one or more of the following features is associated with poor outcome: Failure to establish respiration by 5 minutes of life; Apgar score of 3 or less at 5 minutes; onset of seizures within 12 hours; refractory seizures; stage III HIE; persistent oliguria (<1 mL/kg/h) for the first 36 hours of life; inability to establish oral feeds by 1 week; abnormal EEG and failure to normalize by day 7; and abnormal CT, MRI in postasphyxial period.

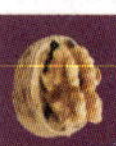

IN A NUTSHELL

Perinatal Asphyxia and Hypoxic-Ischemic Encephalopathy

1. Perinatal asphyxia is the second most common cause of neonatal death after infections.
2. Hypoxic-ischemic encephalopathy (HIE) refers to the characteristic neurological manifestations which develop following perinatal asphyxia.
3. Brain damage occurs mainly in cerebral cortex and basal ganglia in term newborns. In preterm newborns, the insult predominantly involves periventricular white matter.
4. Seizures occur in up to 50% newborns with HIE and are mostly subtle.
5. Sarnat staging is used for grading the severity of HIE.
6. Therapeutic hypothermia is the most promising neuroprotective intervention to date for infants with moderate to severe HIE.
7. The mortality is 20%; and 30% of survivors have neurodevelopmental sequelae including cerebral palsy and intellectual disability.

Agut T, Alarcon A, Cabañas F, et al; eurUS.brain group. Preterm white matter injury: ultrasound diagnosis and classification. Pediatr Res. 2020;87(Suppl 1):37-49.

Aker K, Støen R, Eikenes L, et al. Therapeutic hypothermia for neonatal hypoxic-ischaemic encephalopathy in India (THIN study): a randomised controlled trial. Arch Dis Child Fetal Neonatal Ed. 2020; 105(4):405-11.

Dorner RA, Burton VJ, Allen MC, et al. Preterm neuroimaging and neurodevelopmental outcome: a focus on intraventricular hemorrhage, post-hemorrhagic hydrocephalus, and associated brain injury. J Perinatol. 2018;38(11):1431-43.

Gilles FH, Leviton A. Neonatal white matter damage and the fetal inflammatory response. Semin Fetal Neonatal Med. 2020;25(4):101111.

Iribarren I, Hilario E, Álvarez A, et al. Neonatal multiple organ failure after perinatal asphyxia. An Pediatr (Engl Ed). 2022;97(4):280.

Krishnan V, Kumar V, Variane GFT, et al; Newborn Brain Society Guidelines and Publications Committee. Need for more evidence in the prevention and management of perinatal asphyxia and neonatal encephalopathy in low and middle-income countries: A call for action. Semin Fetal Neonatal Med. 2021;26(5):101271.

Mathew JL, Kaur N, Dsouza JM. Therapeutic hypothermia in neonatal hypoxic encephalopathy: A systematic review and meta-analysis. J Glob Health. 2022;12:04030.

Thayyil S, Pant S, Montaldo P, et al; HELIX consortium. Hypothermia for moderate or severe neonatal encephalopathy in low-income and middle-income countries (HELIX): a randomised controlled trial in India, Sri Lanka, and Bangladesh. Lancet Glob Health. 2021;9(9): e1273-85.

Wassink G, Harrison S, Dhillon S, et al. Prognostic Neurobiomarkers in Neonatal Encephalopathy. Dev Neurosci. 2022;44(4-5):331-43.

16.4 Birth Injuries

PE 19.6

INTRODUCTION

Injuries to the infant that result from mechanical forces (i.e., compression and traction) during the birth process are categorized as birth trauma. Significant birth injury occurs in 6–8 newborns per 1,000 live births. In general, larger infants are more susceptible to birth trauma.

FACTORS PREDISPOSING TO INJURY

Primigravida, cephalopelvic disproportion, small maternal stature, maternal pelvic anomalies, fetal macrosomia (large-for-date infants, especially infants weighing more than 4,500 g), prolonged or precipitate labor, deep transverse arrest of descent of presenting part of the fetus, oligohydramnios, abnormal presentation (breech), use of midcavity forceps or vacuum extraction, versions and extractions, very low birth weight infant or extreme prematurity, multiple gestation, large fetal head, and fetal anomalies.

TYPES OF INJURIES

The following injuries can be encountered during birth trauma:

- ***Soft tissue injuries:*** Abrasions, ecchymosis, lacerations, and subcutaneous fat necrosis
- ***Skull:*** Caput succedaneum, cephalhematoma, and linear fractures
- ***Face:*** Subconjunctival hemorrhage and retinal hemorrhage
- ***Nerve injuries:*** Brachial plexus injury, cranial nerve and spinal cord injuries
- ***Musculoskeletal injuries:*** Clavicular fractures, fractures of long bones, and sternocleidomastoid injury
- ***Intra-abdominal injuries:*** Liver hematoma, splenic hematoma, adrenal hemorrhage, and renal hemorrhage

Soft Tissue Injuries

Abrasions and lacerations occur because of scalpel cuts during cesarean section or instrumental delivery (i.e., vacuum and forceps). Infection remains a risk, but most of them healuneventfully. Management consists of careful cleaning, application of antibiotic ointment, and surgical suturing, if necessary. Other common injuries, such as caput succedaneum and cephalhematoma, have been discussed in the previous chapter.

Nerve Injuries

Brachial plexus injury occurs most commonly in large babies, frequently with shoulder dystocia or breech delivery. Incidence for brachial plexus injury is 0.5–2.0 per 1,000 live births. Most cases are of Erb palsy. Entire brachial plexus involvement occurs in 10% of cases.

- ***Duchenne-Erb palsy*** (lesion in C5–C6) is the most common type of brachial plexus injury and is associated with lack of shoulder motion. The involved extremity lies adducted, prone, and internally rotated with flexion of the wrist and fingers in the characteristic waiter's tip posture. Moro, biceps, and radial reflexes are absent on the affected side. Grasp reflex is usually present.
- ***Klumpke paralysis*** (C7–8, T1) is rare and results in weakness of the intrinsic muscles of the hand; grasp reflex is absent. If cervical sympathetic fibers of the first thoracic spinal nerve are involved, this will lead to ipsilateral Horner syndrome.

TREATMENT Erb/Klumpke Paralysis

X-ray of shoulder and upper arm should be done to rule out bony injuries. Diaphragmatic palsy should be excluded. Management is expectant. "Statue of liberty" splinting should be avoided due to the risk of contractures in the shoulder girdle. Physiotherapy with passive movements should be started within 7–10 days, when the postinjury neuritis has resolved. Prognosis depends on the extent of injury, whether nerve roots are intact (excellent outcome) or avulsed (guarded outcome). Significant clinical improvement within 2 weeks means normal or near-normal function will be eventually restored. Most babies recover fully by 3 months. Surgery is recommended in those with poor biceps function at 3 months after electromyography and nerve conduction studies.

Cranial nerve and spinal cord injuries result from hyperextension, traction, and overstretching with simultaneous rotation; they may range from localized neuropraxia to complete nerve or cord transection.

Clavicular Fracture

Clavicle is the most frequently fractured bone in the neonate during birth. It is an unpredictable unavoidable complication of normal birth. Some correlation with birth weight, midforceps delivery, and shoulder dystocia exists. The infant may present with pseudoparalysis. Examination may reveal crepitus, palpable bony irregularity, and sternocleidomastoid muscle spasm. Radiographic studies confirm the fracture. Healing usually occurs in 7–10 days. In order to decrease pain, arm motion may be limited by pinning the infant's sleeve to the shirt. Assess other associated injury to the spine, brachial plexus, or humerus.

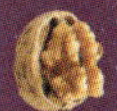

IN A NUTSHELL

Birth Injuries

1. Injuries during birth may be inflicted to soft tissues, skull, face, nerves, muscles, bones, or the viscera.
2. *Duchenne-Erb palsy* (lesion in C5–C6) is the most common type of brachial plexus injury and is associated with lack of shoulder motion.
3. *Klumpke paralysis* (C7–8, T1) is rare and results in weakness of the intrinsic muscles of the hand.
4. Cranial nerve and spinal cord injuries result from hyperextension, traction, and overstretching with simultaneous rotation; they may range from localized neuropraxia to complete nerve or cord transection.

Berényi M, Szeredai M, Cseh Á. Neonatal brachial plexus palsy—early diagnosis and treatment. Ideggyogy Sz. 2022;75(7-08):247-52.
Huang H, Yang M, Zhou H, et al. Method of shoulder delivery and neonatal outcomes: A meta-analysis of prospective controlled studies. Natl Med J India. 2018;31(6):324-8.
Romero S, Pettersson K, Yousaf K, et al. Perinatal outcome after vacuum assisted delivery with digital feedback on traction force; a randomised controlled study. BMC Pregnancy Childbirth. 2021;21(1):165.
Uhing MR. Management of birth injuries. Pediatr Clin North Am. 2004;51:1169-86.

16.5 Respiratory Distress in Newborn

PE 19.5

INTRODUCTION

Respiratory distress in the neonate is defined as presence of any one of the following features: (1) Respiratory rate >60/min; (2) subcostal or intercostal retractions; and (3) expiratory grunt. Cyanosis may or may not be present.

ETIOLOGY

The etiology of respiratory distress in newborn depends on the age of onset of symptoms, gestational age, maternal factors, and feeding and infant care practices. The causes of respiratory distress in neonates are summarized in **Table 16.10**. Salient features of common neonatal disorders presenting with respiratory distress are described in **Table 16.11**.

RESPIRATORY DISTRESS SYNDROME

Respiratory distress syndrome is characterized by onset of respiratory distress in a preterm newborn soon after birth. The incidence is inversely related to the gestational age. Approximately 50% of newborn infants delivered at 26–28 weeks of gestation develop RDS, whereas the disease becomes infrequent after 34 weeks, affecting <5%.

Pathophysiology

Respiratory distress syndrome is caused by deficiency of the surfactant in the lungs. Pulmonary surfactant is synthesized and secreted by type II epithelial cells in alveolus. The major constituents of surfactant are (1) Dipalmitoyl phosphatidylcholine (lecithin) and phosphatidylglycerol, (2) Apoproteins (surfactant proteins A, B, C, D), and (3) Cholesterol.

Surfactant synthesis begins at 20–24 weeks of gestation. Mature levels of surfactant are usually present after 34 weeks. Surfactant diminishes the surface tension of the water film that lines alveoli, thereby decreasing the tendency of alveoli to collapse at the end of expiration. With surfactant deficiency, the lungs become diffusely atelectatic (collapsed), triggering inflammation, and pulmonary edema. Because blood passing through the atelectatic portions of lung is not oxygenated (due to right to left intrapulmonary shunt), the infant becomes hypoxemic. Lung compliance is decreased, thereby increasing the work of breathing. In severe cases, the diaphragm and intercostal muscles fatigue, and CO_2 retention and respiratory acidosis develop. Pathogenesis of RDS is summarized in **Flowchart 16.2**.

Risk Factors

Besides prematurity, other risk factors include multifetal pregnancies, maternal diabetes, cesarean section, asphyxia, and hypothermia. Risk decreases with fetal growth restriction, preeclampsia or eclampsia, maternal hypertension, prolonged rupture of membranes, maternal opiate addiction, and antenatal corticosteroid use.

Histopathology

Lungs appear deep purplish red and are liver-like in consistency. Microscopically, there is diffuse atelectasis, pulmonary edema, pulmonary vascular congestion, hemorrhage, and

Table 16.10 Causes of Respiratory Distress in Neonates

Category	*Cause*
Respiratory	Respiratory distress syndrome, transient tachypnea of the newborn, meconium aspiration syndrome, pneumonia, sepsis, pneumothorax and other air-leak syndromes, pulmonary hemorrhage, pulmonary hypoplasia, persistent pulmonary hypertension of the newborn, congenital deficiency of surfactant proteins B or C
Cardiac	Congestive heart failure from any cause, e.g., patent ductus arteriosus (PDA) in a preterm baby or transposition of great arteries (TGA), etc.
Neurologic	Perinatal asphyxia, intracranial hemorrhage and birth trauma
Hematologic	Polycythemia and severe anemia
GIT	Necrotizing enterocolitis, abdominal distension from any cause
Surgical causes	Tracheoesophageal fistula, diaphragmatic hernia, bilateral choanal atresia, congenital lobar emphysema, cystic adenomatoid malformation of the lung
Miscellaneous	Septicemia, hypothermia, hypoglycemia, hemorrhage, metabolic acidosis and shock

Table 16.11 Salient Findings in Common Causes of Respiratory Distress in Newborns			
Clinical condition	*Pathogenesis*	*Clinical features*	*Diagnosis*
Respiratory distress syndrome	• Results from surfactant deficiency in preterm • Most common respiratory disorder among infants born at <32 weeks gestation • Lower gestational age and birth weight, lack of exposure to antenatal corticosteroids, perinatal asphyxia, and maternal diabetes are important risk factors	Presents at or soon after birth with tachypnea, grunting, chest retractions, nasal flaring, and hypoxia	• ***Chest X-ray (CXR):*** Low lung volume with a fine granular or "ground-glass" appearance with air bronchograms • In mild RDS, a diffuse, linear granular pattern is most common
Transient tachypnea of newborn	Delayed clearance of fetal lung fluid History of maternal diabetes and delivery by cesarean section is present	Mild-to-moderate respiratory distress begins soon after birth and gradually improves during the first 48–72 hours of life	***CXR:*** Normal to mildly overexpanded lungs with a diffuse hazy appearance and increased interstitial streaky shadowing extending to the periphery. Small pleural effusions, typically seen as prominence of the interlobar fissures
Meconium aspiration syndrome	• Partial and/or complete airway obstruction by the meconium • Inflammation • Pulmonary hypertension • Surfactant inactivation	• Respiratory distress in an infant born through MSAF with radiographic findings which do not suggest a different etiology is usually diagnosed as MAS • Clinical picture ranges from mild respiratory distress, with minimal or no oxygen requirement and without CO_2 retention, to severe respiratory distress requiring mechanical ventilation, inhaled nitric oxide (iNO), and extracorporeal membrane oxygenation (ECMO) • Severity of the disease is related to the degree of associated PPHN	***CXR:*** Shows lung hyperexpansion with or without heterogeneous patchy infiltrates to complete opacification of the thorax. Some infants born with MSAF demonstrate radiographic findings of significant parenchymal disease even when they have only minimal or no clinical signs of respiratory distress. Others with minor X-ray changes may develop severe MAS
Pneumonia	• Neonatal pneumonia is classified as early or late onset • Most early-onset pneumonias are acquired congenitally from transplacental inoculation or perinatally from the maternal vaginal tract • Late-onset pneumonia is often a nosocomial complication of mechanical ventilation	• Early-onset pneumonia presents within the first week of life with respiratory distress and systemic signs of sepsis including poor perfusion, lethargy, and jaundice • Late-onset presents after the first week of life with respiratory distress	CXR in late-onset pneumonia is diffusely hazy, similar to RDS, but in contrast to early-onset pneumonia, the lungs often exhibit normal or hyperexpansion with heterogeneously distributed densities
Pneumothorax	Occurs spontaneously or because of infection, meconium aspiration, lung malformation or ventilator barotraumas	The clinical presentation of pneumothorax varies from an incidental finding on CXR to severe respiratory distress and cardiovascular collapse	• ***CXR:*** Air in the pleural space with compression of the affected lung, flattening of the diaphragm, and shift of the mediastinum to the contralateral side • A lateral decubitus X-ray with the affected side up is often helpful in cases of small air leaks
Pulmonary hemorrhage	Common risk factors include prematurity, asphyxia, patent ductus arteriosus, coagulopathy, infection, and severe respiratory distress	It is an acute, often severe form of pulmonary edema that ranges in clinical presentation from a small amount of fresh, frothy blood from the airway to catastrophic bleeding and cardiopulmonary collapse	CXR range from patchy infiltrates to complete opacification of one or more lung fields

Contd...

Contd...

Clinical condition	*Pathogenesis*	*Clinical features*	*Diagnosis*
Persistent pulmonary hypertension (PPHN)	• Maladaptation of the pulmonary vasculature, where the vasculature is structurally normal but constricted, and is associated with lung parenchymal diseases such as MAS, RDS, pneumonia, and sepsis • Remodeled pulmonary vasculature with normal lung parenchyma (idiopathic PPHN; 10%) • Hypoplastic pulmonary vasculature as occurs in patients with lung hypoplasia secondary to congenital diaphragmatic hernia (CDH) or oligohydramnios	Newborns with PPHN present with labile and/or profound hypoxemia and differential cyanosis (higher preductal SpO_2 and PaO_2 compared to postductal measurements	• The chest X-ray may show normal sized heart or cardiomegaly • If there is no associated pulmonary pathology, vascularity may be normal or decreased • Echocardiography is essential in distinguishing PPHN from congenital heart disease • Echo may show flattened or septum bowed to the left suggestive of pulmonary hypertension. Color Doppler may reveal evidence of tricuspid regurgitation
Congenital diaphragmatic hernia	• Results from failure of the pleural peritoneal fold to close early in gestation • Greater lung hypoplasia and presence of the liver in the thorax are associated with decreased survival rates • Pulmonary vasculature is also abnormal and hypermuscular resulting in persistent pulmonary hypertension of the newborn (PPHN)	• Postnatally cyanosis, retraction tachypnea and grunting are commonly seen • On examination, abdomen is scaphoid, anteroposterior diameter of the chest is increased, mediastinum is shifted, and bowel sounds may be heard in the chest • Presentation may be delayed in the less severely affected babies	***CXR:*** Shows air-filled loops of bowel within the hemithorax, compression of the lung on the affected size, and contralateral displacement of the mediastinum
Esophageal atresia with or without tracheoeso-phageal fistula	It is the most common surgical condition leading to respiratory distress	• Neonates present soon after birth with frothing from the mouth or choking with attempted feeds or with manifestations of aspiration pneumonitis • An obstruction to the passage of an orogastric tube at about 10 cm from mouth is usually diagnostic	***CXR:*** Coiling of an orogastric tube in upper pouch is diagnostic

Flowchart 16.2: Pathogenesis of respiratory distress syndrome

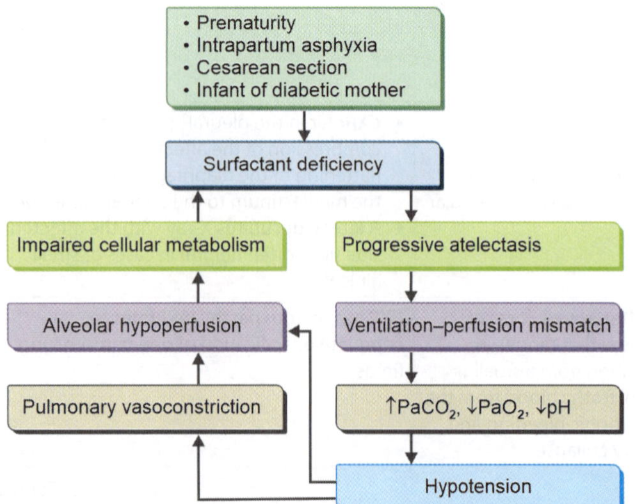

evidence of injury to respiratory epithelium. *Hyaline membranes*, a characteristic feature of RDS, consist of acidophilic, homogeneous, or granular membranes, lining the alveoli, alveolar ducts, and respiratory bronchioles. Hyaline membranes may not be seen, if a baby dies within 6–8 hours of birth. Although, hyaline membranes are characteristic of RDS but they are not pathognomonic and may be seen in other conditions such as pneumonia.

Clinical Manifestations

Tachypnea (respiratory rate >60/min) appears immediately or within 6 hours after delivery. This is often associated with chest retractions and flaring of alae nasi. Another characteristic feature of RDS is the *expiratory grunt*. This sound is produced due to exhalation against a partially closed glottis, due to an attempt by the baby to maintain some alveolar volume. Expiratory grunt may also be heard in severe pneumonia. Cyanosis appears, as hypoxia ensues. Atelectasis and respiratory failure are characterized by lethargy, irregular breathing, and apnea.

Table 16.12 Respiratory Distress Score (Downe Score)			
Score	0	1	2
Respiratory rate	40–60/min	60–80/min	>80/min
Oxygen requirement	None	≤50%	>50%
Retractions	None	Mild-to-moderate	Severe
Grunting	None	With stimulation	At rest
Breath sounds	Normal	Decreased	Barely heard

Assessment of the Severity of Respiratory Distress

The severity of RD can be judged clinically by the respiratory score (Downe score) **(Table 16.12)**. The score is used in babies who are breathing spontaneously, including those receiving continuous positive airway pressure (CPAP). A score of <5 indicates mild RD, a score of 5–8 moderate RD, and a score of >8 severe RD.

Another important commonly used score to quantify respiratory distress is Silverman and Andersen score **(Table 16.13)**. It is very useful for resource limited settings as it includes purely clinical examination related points and there is no need of equipment in the form of pulse oximeter. It is an easy, quick, and objective method to grade the severity of respiratory distress in sick neonates without physically disturbing them. A total score of 0–3, 4–6, and >6 signify mild, moderate, and impending respiratory failure, respectively.

Diagnosis

Diagnosis of RDS is made, if a preterm baby develops respiratory distress within 6 hours of age, with characteristic radiological findings with or without hypoxia and hypercarbia in arterial blood gas (ABG) analysis. Radiological features include fine reticulogranular pattern in both the lung fields, reduced lung volume, air bronchograms, blurring of heart borders and margins of diaphragm, and complete white-out of lungs (ground-glass appearance) in late stages **(Fig. 16.3)**.

Assessment of Fetal Lung Maturity

Respiratory distress syndrome can be anticipated prenatally using tests of fetal lung maturity, which measure surfactant levels in the amniotic fluid. The amniotic fluid can be obtained by amniocentesis or collected from the vagina (if membranes have ruptured). Risk of RDS is low when lecithin/sphingomyelin (L/S) ratio in the amniotic fluid is >2. Exceptions include infants of diabetic mothers, perinatal asphyxia, and Rh hemolytic disease where despite L/S ratio above 2, the baby may still develop RDS.

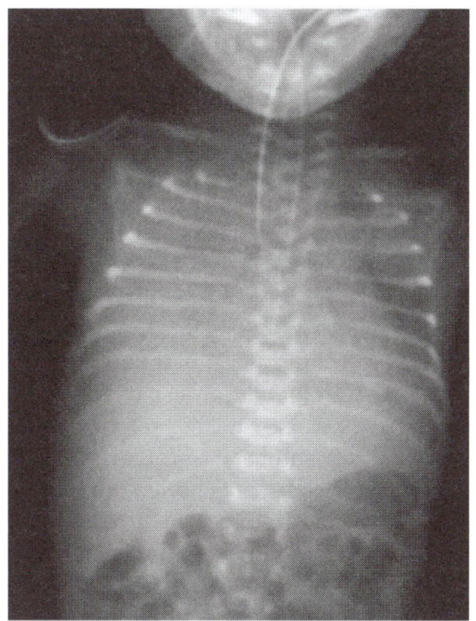

Fig. 16.3: X-ray of respiratory distress syndrome showing diffuse haziness, air bronchogram, and blurring of heart borders and diaphragm. This diffuse haziness gives a ground-glass appearance, also known as white-out lungs

Postnatally, lung maturity can be assessed by the *Shake test* on gastric aspirate. 1 mL of amniotic fluid or gastric aspirate of the baby is mixed with 1 mL of absolute alcohol in a test tube. The test tube is shaken for 15 seconds and allowed to stand for 15 minutes. The amount of air bubbles at the meniscus is noted and graded as follows:

- \+ : One-third of meniscus has bubbles
- ++ : Two-thirds of meniscus has bubbles
- +++ : One row along the circumference of meniscus has bubbles
- ++++ : More than one row of bubbles

The risk of hyaline membrane disease is minimal if the test is more than ++.

Differential diagnosis includes early onset sepsis, transient tachypnea of the newborn, persistent pulmonary hypertension, meconium aspiration syndrome, pulmonary edema, and congenital cardiopulmonary anomalies.

Table 16.13 Silverman-Anderson Retraction Score					
Score	Upper chest retraction	Lower chest retraction	Xiphoid retraction	Nasal flaring	Grunt
0	Synchronous	None	None	None	None
1	Lag on inspiration	Just visible	Just visible	Minimal	Stethoscope only
2	See saw	Marked	Marked	Marked	Naked ear
A score of >6 is indicative of impending respiratory failure					

TREATMENT Respiratory Distress Syndrome (RDS)

Treatment for neonatal respiratory distress can be general supportive measures and disease-specific.

1. *Antenatal corticosteroids:* Respiratory distress syndrome can be prevented by using antenatal corticosteroids to pregnant women between 24 and 34 weeks of gestation with threatened preterm labor. A complete course consists of two doses of betamethasone (12 mg intramuscular) at 24 hourly interval or four doses of dexamethasone (6 mg intramuscular) at 12 hourly interval. Tocolytics can be used to allow time for steroids to take effect or for safe transfer where appropriate. Antenatal steroids can also be considered for cesarean not in labor up to 39 weeks. In late preterm pregnancy at risk of early birth, a course of antenatal steroids may also be considered provided there is no evidence of chorioamnionitis. A single repeat course of steroids may be given in threatened preterm birth before 32 weeks of gestation if the first course was administered at least 1–2 weeks earlier, however, multiple courses of steroids are not recommended due to fear of brain damage to the fetus.
2. *Delivery room stabilization:* Cord clamping at birth should be delayed by at least 1 minute. To prevent heat loss, baby should be stabilized in a plastic bag under a radiant warmer. In a spontaneously breathing preterm baby, breathing is gently supported using CPAP. ECG and pulse oximetry should be used to guide heart rate response to stabilization. Resuscitation is initiated with about 21–30% oxygen and titrated up or down as needed to maintained saturations in the ranges provided by neonatal resuscitation algorithm. Intubation at birth is considered only for those not responding to the above, although early intubation and surfactant may be required for babies who demonstrate early signs of severe RDS such as chest retractions and high oxygen requirements.
3. *Continuous positive airway pressure:* The CPAP is simple, safe, effective, cheap, and noninvasive alternative to mechanical ventilation to provide initial respiratory support in RDS. In CPAP, a continuous distending pressure of 6–8 cmH_2O is given through nasal prongs. It works by preventing alveolar atelectasis, thereby reducing work of breathing. CPAP is utilized in spontaneously breathing babies. Intractable apnea is a contraindication for CPAP. Regular monitoring of ABG is essential. A PaO_2 <50 mm Hg and/or a $PaCO_2$ >60 mm Hg indicate CPAP failure and need for mechanical ventilation.
4. *Maintenance of temperature:* The baby should be kept under servo-controlled radiant warmer with a set temperature of 36.5°C. Excessive handling should be avoided.
5. *Intravenous fluids and nutrition:* Parenteral nutrition should be started immediately with amino acids and lipids. Total fluid rate should be limited to 60–80 mL/kg/day. Enteral feeding with mothers' milk should also be initiated on day 1 if the baby is stable. Monitoring of urine output, body weight, and serum electrolytes should be done and fluids are adjusted accordingly. Excessive fluid intake is harmful and may lead to patent ductus arteriosus (PDA) and bronchopulmonary dysplasia (BPD).
6. *Surfactant administration:* Surfactant reduces the mortality and complication rates of RDS, and shortens the duration of mechanical ventilation. Natural, animal derived surfactants, bovine or porcine, are better than synthetic preparations. The dose is 100–200 mg/kg. Conventionally, surfactant is instilled directly into the lungs through endotracheal tube on mechanical ventilation. After surfactant administration, baby should be extubated to CPAP, a method called as intubation, surfactant, and extubation to CPAP (INSURE) instead of continued mechanical ventilation to prevent lung injury.

   To prevent intubation and lung injury resulting from positive pressure ventilation specialized catheters are available which can be used to instill surfactant while the baby is breathing spontaneously on CPAP. This method is termed as less invasive surfactant administration (LISA) helping to avoid intubation and improve respiratory outcomes.

   Regarding timing of surfactant administration, in symptomatic babies, early rescue therapy (within 2 hours) is better than delayed therapy (<2 hours). Surfactant administration in the delivery room before onset of significant respiratory distress is indicated for newborns requiring intubation in delivery room for stabilization. Neonates on CPAP showing worsening in the form of increasing Silverman-Andersen score even at FiO_2 >0.30 and CPAP pressure of at least 6 cm H_2O, should be treated with surfactant. Dose may be repeated 6–12 hours later if significant respiratory distress persists. Babies should be extubated to CPAP or noninvasive positive pressure ventilation (NIPPV) immediately following surfactant, and judgment needs to be made if an individual baby will tolerate this. For those who require mechanical ventilation, aim is to ventilate for as short a time as possible, avoiding hyperoxia, hypocarbia, and volutrauma.
7. *Mechanical ventilation:* It is a life-saving but invasive therapy which has greatly improved the outcome of respiratory distress. Mechanical ventilation should be considered when baby has moderate-to-severe respiratory distress, CPAP fails to maintain blood gases within normal range, or there is intractable apnea. Many types of ventilators are available to provide respiratory support. In newborn, time-cycled, pressure-limited, continuous flow ventilators are most frequently used conventional ventilators. Synchronized intermittent mandatory ventilation (SIMV), which synchronizes with the newborn's own respiratory effort, is the most used mode of ventilation. The main complication of mechanical ventilation is ventilator-induced lung injury (VILI) including air leaks and BPD. VILI can be reduced by using lowest inspiratory pressures while using pressure-controlled ventilation, use of volume targeted ventilation to limit the volumes delivered during each respiratory cycle and oxygen concentrations to maintain adequate gas exchange (PaO_2 >50 mm Hg; $PaCO_2$ <55 mm Hg). High-frequency oscillatory ventilation (breath rate >150/min) may be useful when conventional ventilation fails.

   Caffeine therapy should be used routinely to minimize the need for ventilation. Babies should be maintained on noninvasive respiratory support in preference to mechanical ventilation if possible. In preterm babies receiving oxygen, the saturation target should be between 90 and 94%.
8. *Hemodynamic support:* Hypotension is common in preterm newborn with RDS. On day one, the acceptable lower limit of mean arterial pressure (MAP) approximates gestational age in weeks. After day 3, most babies under 26 weeks' gestation have MAP >30 mm Hg. In the absence of blood pressure measurement, capillary refill time (CRT) may be used to assess circulatory status. Prolonged CRT (>3 seconds) is treated by infusing normal saline bolus 10 mL/kg slowly over 20–30 minutes followed by dopamine infusion @ 5–10 µg/kg/min, if needed.
9. *Antibiotics:* Antibiotics should be used judiciously and stopped early when sepsis is ruled out.
10. *Pain management:* Protocols should be in place for monitoring pain and discomfort and consideration given for nonpharmacological methods of minimizing procedural pain and judicious use of opiates for more invasive procedures.

Prognosis

Acute complications include air leaks (pneumothorax, pneumomediastinum, and pulmonary interstitial emphysema), PDA, intracranial hemorrhage, and infection. Long-term complications are retinopathy of prematurity, BPD, neurodevelopmental impairments, and other complications of prematurity. Antenatal steroids, surfactant replacement therapy, CPAP, mechanical ventilation, and good supportive care have reduced mortality of RDS to <10%.

PNEUMONIA

Pneumonia is an important cause of respiratory distress and mortality in the newborn. It may present soon after birth as a part of early onset sepsis (congenital or intrauterine pneumonia), or later in the neonatal period as a more localized disease. Since pneumonia shares the same risk factors, causative organisms, and clinical manifestations with neonatal sepsis, its diagnosis and management are discussed under sepsis. Radiological features of pneumonia are shown in **Figure 16.4**.

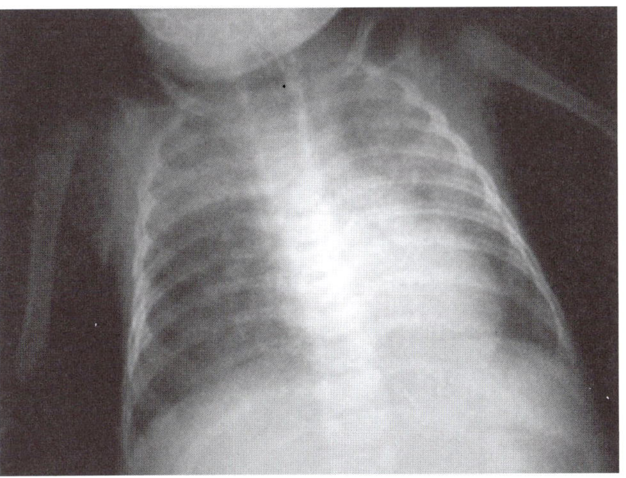

Fig. 16.4: X-ray showing bilateral diffuse haziness suggestive of pneumonia, more so in upper zones

MECONIUM ASPIRATION SYNDROME

Meconium aspiration syndrome (MAS) is characterized by respiratory distress soon after birth in a term or post-term newborn delivered through *meconium-stained amniotic fluid (MSAF), whose symptoms cannot be explained otherwise.* MSAF occurs in 10–15% of total live births. Meconium aspiration syndrome develops in 5–10% of newborns delivered through MSAF.

Etiopathogenesis

Fetal distress (e.g., from hypoxia caused by umbilical cord compression or placental insufficiency or from infection) may cause the fetus to pass meconium into the amniotic fluid before delivery. In the presence of fetal distress, gasping by the fetus can lead to the aspiration of meconium before, during, or immediately after delivery. Aspirated meconium blocks airways and causes release of cytokines and other vasoactive substances, resulting in pulmonary hypertension. The net effect is ventilation-perfusion mismatch and arterial hypoxemia. The pathogenesis of MAS is summarized in **Flowchart 16.3**.

Clinical Manifestations

These include tachypnea (respiratory rate >60/min) appearing soon after delivery, nasal flaring, chest retractions, cyanosis or desaturation, bilateral crepitations, barrel-shaped chest due to air trapping; and greenish yellow staining of the umbilical cord, nail beds, or skin.

Chest X-ray findings include patchy infiltrates, coarse streaking of lung fields, areas of hyperinflation and atelectasis, flattening of diaphragm, and air leaks **(Fig. 16.5)**.

Flowchart 16.3: Pathogenesis of meconium aspiration syndrome

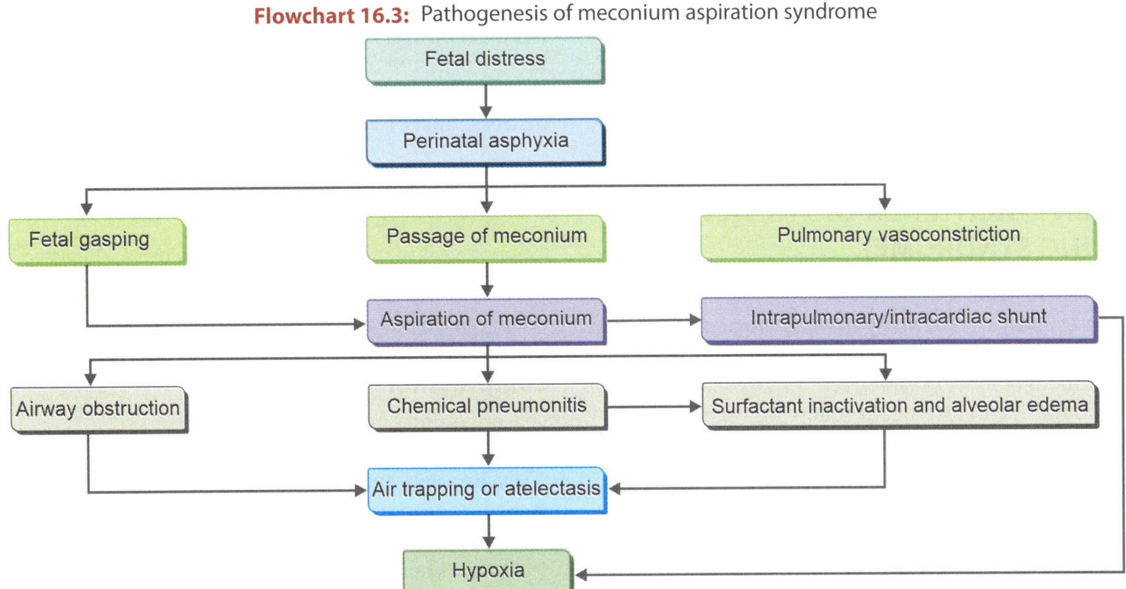

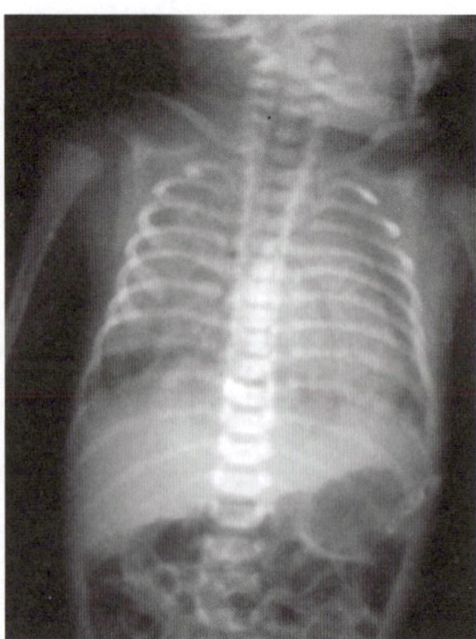

Fig. 16.5: Chest X-ray showing bilateral patchy infiltrates in meconium aspiration syndrome

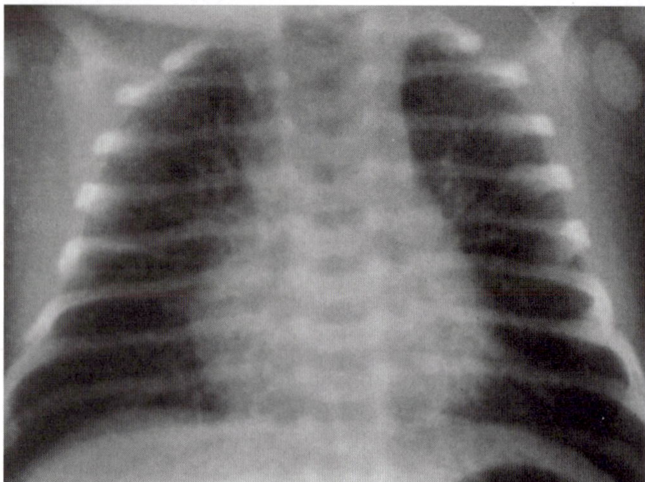

Fig. 16.6: Chest X-ray showing streaky perihilar markings with fluids in the interlobar fissures suggesting transient tachypnea of newborn

TREATMENT Meconium Aspiration Syndrome

1. *Management in delivery room*: Prenatal hypopharyngeal suctioning and postnatal endotracheal intubation and suctioning of vigorous infants are not effective. As per Neonatal Resuscitation Program (NRP) 2020 guidelines, intubation and suctioning of nonbreathing infants (nonvigorous) is not required and positive pressure ventilation should be started if baby remains apneic and heart remains <100/min after initial steps.
2. *Supportive management* such as maintenance of temperature, intravenous fluids, oxygen inhalation, oral or parenteral nutrition, and inotropic support for shock.
3. *Antibiotics* (usually ampicillin and an aminoglycoside), if risk factors for sepsis are present.
4. *Regular monitoring* of pulse oximetry and ABG analysis.
5. *Mechanical ventilation*: It is required if there is severe hypoxemia (PaO_2 <50 mm Hg) and/or hypercarbia ($PaCO_2$ >60 mm Hg).
6. *Other therapies*: Since surfactant may be inhibited by meconium, surfactant replacement therapy may be considered, if baby's condition does not improve. Sildenafil, magnesium sulfate, or inhaled nitric oxide (iNO) therapy may be considered for persistent pulmonary hypertension of the newborn (PPHN).
7. Extracorporeal membrane oxygenation (ECMO) is indicated in intractable respiratory failure.

TRANSIENT TACHYPNEA OF THE NEWBORN (WET LUNG SYNDROME)

Transient tachypnea of the newborn (TTN), also known as wet lung syndrome, is respiratory distress caused by delayed resorption of fetal lung fluid. TTN usually affects term and late preterm infants (34–36 weeks) delivered by cesarean section without labor. But it can also occur following vaginal delivery. Maternal diabetes and asthma are also risk factors for TTN.

Pathophysiology

Alveolar epithelium secretes fetal lung fluid which is required for normal lung growth and development in utero. At the time of birth, under the influence of hormones and other chemicals, alveolar epithelium changes from secretory mode to absorptive mode, leading to absorption of lung fluid from alveoli to the interstitium and then to pulmonary capillaries and lung lymphatics. Delay in clearance of fetal lung fluid results in transient pulmonary edema that characterizes TTN.

Diagnosis

Rapid respirations, grunting, and retractions begin soon after delivery, and cyanosis may occasionally develop. Chest X-ray shows normal or hyperinflated lungs with streaky perihilar markings with fluids in the interlobar fissures **(Fig. 16.6)**. Rapid recovery within 2–3 days helps differentiate it from other causes of respiratory distress in newborn. In severe cases, baby may need respiratory support in the form of continuous positive airway pressure and occasionally even mechanical ventilation. TTN is a diagnosis of exclusion and other causes of respiratory distress must be ruled out.

TREATMENT Transient Tachypnea of the Newborn

Supportive management should be provided as discussed in RDS. TTN is a self-limited disease and the outcome is good.

Common Conditions Causing Pulmonary Compression

- Congenital diaphragmatic hernia
- Pneumothorax, congenital lobar emphysema, and congenital cystic adenomatoid malformation (CCAM)
- Eventration of diaphragm and pleural effusions (especially chylothorax)
- Congenital lung cysts

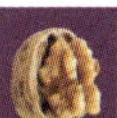

IN A NUTSHELL

Respiratory Distress in Newborn

1. Respiratory distress in newborn can be because of respiratory, metabolic, cardiac, central nervous system (CNS), or surgical causes.
2. It is important to assess severity of respiratory distress by using a respiratory distress score.
3. Common causes include RDS in preterm neonates and MAS and pneumonia in term neonates.
4. Surgical causes must be ruled out as these are correctible by surgical intervention.
5. Hyaline membrane disease (HMD) is the most important cause of respiratory distress in preterm neonates. The clinical features are related to surfactant deficiency and manifest as tachypnea, intercostal retractions, and grunt.
6. Surfactant should be used as early rescue in infants who need intubation and those who continue to need >30–35% oxygen despite adequate CPAP support.
7. Early CPAP support is the mainstay of treatment for HMD.
8. Antenatal steroids are highly cost-effective in decreasing the incidence of HMD and its complications. They must be given to all women with threatened preterm delivery from 24 to 34 weeks of gestation.
9. Amnioinfusion and tracheal suction after birth are no longer recommended as strategies for prevention of meconium aspiration syndrome.
10. ECMO must be considered in select cases of refractory hypoxic respiratory failure.

Chen IL, Chen HL. New developments in neonatal respiratory management. Pediatr Neonatol. 2022;63(4):341-7.

Condò V, Cipriani S, Colnaghi M, et al. Neonatal respiratory distress syndrome: are risk factors the same in preterm and term infants? J Matern Fetal Neonatal Med. 2017;30(11):1267-72.

Daniyan O, Ezeanosike O, Obu D, et al. Use of off-label compounded oral sildenafil in the management of persistent pulmonary hypertension of the newborn: a case report. J Cardiovasc Thorac Res. 2022;14(2): 141-3.

Gupta BK, Saha AK, Mukherjee S, et al. Minimally invasive surfactant therapy versus InSurE in preterm neonates of 28 to 34 weeks with respiratory distress syndrome on non-invasive positive pressure ventilation: a randomized controlled trial. Eur J Pediatr. 2020;179(8):1287-93.

Gupta N, Bruschettini M, Chawla D. Fluid restriction in the management of transient tachypnea of the newborn. Cochrane Database Syst Rev. 2021;2(2):CD011466.

Jena SR, Bains HS, Pandita A, et al, On Behalf Of Sure Group. Surfactant therapy in premature babies: SurE or InSurE. Pediatr Pulmonol. 2019;54(11):1747-52.

Permall DL, Pasha AB, Chen XQ. Current insights in non-invasive ventilation for the treatment of neonatal respiratory disease. Ital J Pediatr. 2019;45(1):105.

Raimondi F, Migliaro F, Corsini I, et al. Lung Ultrasound Score Progress in Neonatal Respiratory Distress Syndrome. Pediatrics. 2021;147(4):e2020030528.

Sheikh M, Nanda V, Kumar R, et al. Neonatal outcomes since the implementation of no routine endotracheal suctioning of meconium-stained non-vigorous neonates. Am J Perinatol; 2022.

Strand ML, Perlman JM. Contemporary management of infants born through meconium stained amniotic fluid. Semin Perinatol. 2022;46(6):151625.

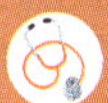

CASE STUDY Newborn with Respiratory Distress

A 34-week male baby delivered by cesarean section developed fast breathing soon after birth and was brought to the neonatal unit. There is a history of premature rupture of membrane 24 hours before delivery. The birth weight of the baby is 1,500 g. On examination, the axillary temperature is 37.2°C, respiratory rate is 82/min with moderate retractions and intermittent grunting. Bilateral air entry in the chest is poor and there is no cyanosis. Heart rate is 148/min. Capillary refill time (CRT) is 2 seconds. Blood sugar is 55 mg/dL.

What is the likely diagnosis? What is minimal diagnostic workup?

Early-onset sepsis with intrauterine pneumonia is the most likely diagnosis due to presence of maternal risk factor for infection. Other differential diagnoses include respiratory distress syndrome (RDS) and transient tachypnea of newborn (TTN).

We will like to obtain a chest X-ray and do a septic screen including total blood counts, C-reactive protein, and blood culture. If facilities are available, arterial blood gas should also be done. A shake test can be done on the gastric aspirate to see for lung maturity. This could help in ruling out RDS.

How will you manage this baby?

National Neonatology Forum (NNF) of India has popularized the abbreviation TABC-FM-FM-CF to deal with all aspects of care in a sick newborn admitted to a healthcare facility. This approach simplifies care of a sick baby and ensures comprehensive management, including stabilization, medications, monitoring, communication, and follow-up advice. Let us manage this baby step by step by following this approach:

- T—*Temperature:* Nurse the baby prone under radiant warmer
- A—*Airway:* Ensure open airway
- B—*Breathing:* Provide oxygen by hood (2–4 L/min) or nasal cannula. Monitor oxygen saturation by attaching to a pulse oximeter. Consider CPAP/ventilation, if the child fails to maintain SpO_2 between 90 and 94%.
- C—*Circulation:* No need of fluid bolus as CRT is normal (<3 seconds).
- F—*Fluids:* Baby should be given intravenous fluids as feeding is not possible due to illness. Fluid requirement on day 1 in a preterm child = 80 mL/kgof 10% dextrose = 80 × 1.5 = 120 mL that can be given as 40 mL 8 hourly intravenous.
- M—*Medications:* Injection vitamin K 1 mg intramuscular, if not received before. Start first-line antibiotics after taking sample for blood culture [ampicillin (50 mg/kg/dose 8 hourly) and gentamicin (2.5 mg/kg/dose 12 hourly)].
- F—*Feeding* should not be started initially as the baby is sick.

- M—*Monitor:* Respiratory rate (RR), heart rate (HR), CRT, temperature, SpO_2, and urine output.
- C—*Communication*: Inform parents what is wrong with the baby and what you are doing. Update them frequently on the progress of the baby.
- F—*Follow-up:* This point will be covered at the time of discharge.

After 24 hours, baby is stable, C-reactive protein (CRP) is positive and total white blood cell (WBC) count is 4,800/mm³. Chest X-ray showed bilateral diffuse infiltrates suggestive of intrauterine pneumonia. SpO_2 is 92% with oxygen 2 L/min. Sepsis workup suggests infection. Final confirmation awaits blood culture report.

How will you proceed further?

Investigations have confirmed the presence of pneumonia, so the antibiotics will be continued for 10 days. Initiate breastfeeding as soon as respiratory distress settles down (RR <60/min, no retractions or grunting). Advise regarding temperature maintenance, exclusive breastfeeding.

F—*Follow-up:* Advise first follow-up after 1 week and then fortnightly for two more visits. Subsequently, follow-up visits should coincide with immunization schedule. Assess growth and development and treat medical problems as they arise pressures to avoid rupture of contralateral lung. Ionotropic support may be needed to maintain blood pressure and peripheral circulation. Pulmonary hypertension of the newborn (PPHN) may require sildenafil or inhaled nitric oxide (iNO) therapy. Some babies may require high frequency oscillatory ventilation and extracorporeal membrane oxygenation (ECMO) to maintain life.

16.6 Apnea in Newborn

INTRODUCTION

Apnea in the newborn is defined as cessation of breathing for longer than 20 seconds, or of shorter duration, if accompanied by bradycardia, or oxygen desaturation.

PATHOGENESIS

Apneic spells are common in preterm newborns. More immature the baby, higher is the risk of apnea. Up to one-fourth of preterm infants below 34 weeks of gestation have at least one episode of apnea.

Apnea of prematurity arises due to physiologic immaturity of respiratory control mechanisms. Possible mechanisms include developmental immaturity of brainstem respiratory center, altered chemoreceptor response to hypoxia and hypercarbia, and intrinsic instability of upper airway muscles leading to airway obstruction.

Apnea of prematurity generally begins 24 hours after birth and no later than day 7 of life. Apnea that develops after 1 week of age signifies an underlying illness other than apnea of prematurity, such as infection, hypothermia, hypoglycemia, PDA, and intraventricular hemorrhage.

CLASSIFICATION

Apnea of prematurity is classified as: (1) Central, (2) obstructive, or (3) mixed.

- ***Central apnea*** is defined as the cessation of both airflow and inspiratory efforts. It is caused by immaturity of medullary respiratory control centers, insufficient neural impulses from the respiratory centers in the medulla reach the respiratory muscles, and the infant stops breathing.
- ***Obstructive apnea*** is the cessation of airflow in the presence of continued inspiratory efforts. It is caused by obstructed airflow or neck flexion causing opposition of hypopharyngeal soft tissues, nasal occlusion, or reflex laryngospasm.
- ***Mixed apnea*** contains elements of both central and obstructive apnea. Most apneic spells are mixed in origin.

Periodic Breathing

Apneic spells should be differentiated from periodic breathing which is a normal developmental characteristic of neonatal breathing.

Periodic breathing is characterized by alternation between regular breathing for 10–15 seconds and apneic pauses of 3–10 seconds. It is common in preterm babies but is also seen in term neonates and young infants. In most cases, periodic breathing accounts for 2–6% of the breathing time in healthy term neonates and as much as 25% of the breathing time in preterm neonates. There is no associated change in heart rate or color. Periodic breathing diminishes over 6–8 weeks of age. It is attributed to immaturity of respiratory control mechanism in newborns. It requires no treatment and has no prognostic significance.

ETIOLOGY OF APNEA

Important secondary causes of neonatal apnea are mentioned here:

- ***Infection:*** Septicemia, meningitis, and pneumonia
- ***Central nervous system:*** Intracranial bleed, perinatal asphyxia, and seizures
- ***Respiratory:*** Respiratory distress syndrome and obstructive airway disorders
- ***Metabolic:*** Hypoglycemia and hypocalcemia
- ***Gastrointestinal tract (GIT):*** Necrotizing enterocolitis and gastroesophageal reflux
- ***Cardiovascular (CVS):*** Patent ductus arteriosus and congestive heart failure
- ***Developmental:*** Apnea of prematurity

❖ ***Others:*** Hypothermia, hyperthermia, anemia, drug-induced depression, and polycythemia

EVALUATION

Evaluation should include a thorough history and physical examination to rule out the causes outlined earlier, determination of blood glucose and calcium, arterial blood gases, sepsis workup and other investigations based on probable etiology. Pulse oximetry may be helpful for measuring the severity and duration of oxygen desaturation.

TREATMENT Neonatal Apnea

1. Gentle tactile stimulation by flicking the soles of feet or rubbing the trunk with hand may abort apneic spell.
2. Nurse the baby in prone position. This stabilizes the chest wall and may reduce apnea.
3. Skin-to-skin care during kangaroo mother care combines optimal body positioning with tactile and kinesthetic stimulation resulting in decrease in risk of apnea compared to neonates undergoing conventional care.
4. Nasal patency should be maintained, however, avoid vigorous pharyngeal suction to prevent vagal stimulation and use heated humidified gases to prevent drying up of nasal secretions, and use appropriately sized nasal cannulas.
5. Maintain temperature.
6. Ensure normoglycemia (blood sugar >45 mg/dL and normocalcemia (serum calcium >7 mg/dL).
7. Supplemental oxygen, if there is hypoxia. Maintain oxygen saturation between 88 and 94%.
8. *Pharmacotherapy:* Drugs are indicated, if apneic episodes occur >2–3 times or bag and mask ventilation is required.
   - *Methylxanthines* (caffeine and aminophylline) are the mainstay of therapy for apnea of prematurity. They act by stimulating respiratory center, antagonism of adenosine that can produce respiratory depression, and improving diaphragmatic contractility.
     - *Caffeine citrate:* The loading dose of caffeine is 20 mg/kg of caffeine citrate (10 mg/kg of caffeine base) orally or intravenously over 30 minutes, followed by maintenance dose of 5–8 mg/kg (2.5–5 mg/kg of caffeine base) once a day, beginning 24 hours after the loading dose. In addition to reducing apnea-related symptoms, methylxanthines facilitate extubation and reduce the need for mechanical ventilation. Monitor the neonate for side effects of caffeine in the form of tachycardia, cardiac dysrhythmias, seizures, feeding intolerance, and increased metabolic demand, leading to diminished growth in preterm infants.
     - *Aminophylline:* The dose of aminophylline is 5–6 mg/kg intravenous infusion over 20 minutes as loading dose followed by 1.5–2 mg/kg intravenous every 8 hours as maintenance therapy, beginning 12 hours after loading dose.
     - Caffeine is preferred over aminophylline as it has lesser side effects and can be administered as once daily dose.
     - Methylxanthines are discontinued at 32–34 weeks of gestation, if no apneic spells have occurred for 5–7 days.
   - *Doxapram* is central and peripheral stimulant. It is used when methylxanthines fail. Side effects, such as "gasping syndrome," preclude its routine use.
9. Investigate and treat the underlying cause, if identified.
10. Ventilate, if above measures fail.

- Correct anemia and packed red cell transfusion is planned according to postnatal age and need for respiratory support.
- If baby does not respond to tactile stimulation, use bag and mask ventilation to resuscitate the baby.
- *Continuous positive airway pressure:* CPAP is useful in obstructive or mixed apnea. It splints the airway and thereby prevents obstruction. CPAP is indicated when drug therapy fails. Other noninvasive respiratory supports used for apnea of prematurity include non-invasive intermittent positive pressure ventilation and heated humidified high-flow nasal cannula.
- *Mechanical ventilation*: Intractable apnea not responding to above measures should be managed with mechanical ventilation.
- *Discharge:* Otherwise healthy preterm neonates should be apnea-free at least for 7 days before discharge.

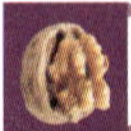

IN A NUTSHELL

Apnea in Newborn

1. Apnea in the newborn is defined as cessation of breathing for longer than 20 seconds, or of shorter duration, if accompanied by bradycardia, or oxygen desaturation.
2. Apnea of prematurity generally begins 24 hours after birth and no later than day 7 of life.
3. Apnea of prematurity is classified as: (1) Central, (2) obstructive, or (3) mixed.
4. *Methylxanthines* (caffeine and aminophylline) are the mainstay of therapy for apnea of prematurity.

Miao Y, Zhou Y, Zhao S, et al. Comparative efficacy and safety of caffeine citrate and aminophylline in treating apnea of prematurity: A systematic review and meta-analysis. PLoS One. 2022;17(9):e0274882.

Samouilidis A, Beltsios ET, Mavrovounis G, et al. The use of antenatal dexamethasone in late preterm and term pregnancies to improve neonatal morbidity and mortality: a systematic review and meta-analysis. Cureus. 2022;14(8):e27865.

Zhao J, Gonzalez F, Mu D. Apnea of prematurity: from cause to treatment. Eur J Pediatr. 2011;170:1097-105.

16.7 Neonatal Seizures

PE 19.12

INTRODUCTION

Seizures are the most common neurological emergency in newborns with an incidence ranging from 1 to 5 per 1,000 live births. Neonatal age is the period of highest incidence of seizures in life. Newborn babies are more prone to seizures due to immaturity of brain. Seizures are more common in preterm newborns than in term babies and inversely related to gestational age of the baby. Most cases of neonatal seizures are either due to underlying cerebral insult or secondary to a systemic disorder. Idiopathic seizures are rare in neonates.

PATHOPHYSIOLOGY

Seizures occur when a large group of neurons undergo excessive, synchronized depolarization. Depolarization can result from excessive excitatory amino acid release (e.g., glutamate) or deficient inhibitory neurotransmitter, e.g., gamma-amino-butyric acid (GABA). Moreover, GABA may temporarily act as an excitatory neurotransmitter via an alteration in chloride gradient and transportation in the immature brain. Another potential mechanism is disruption of ATP-dependent resting membrane potentials, which causes a flow of sodium into the neuron and potassium out of the neuron.

Seizures in the neonatal period are characterized by prominence of focal ictal characteristics and rarity of generalized seizures due to reduced connectivity within the brain. It is also responsible for frequent recurrent seizures in neonates and poor response to antiepileptic drugs (AEDs).

ETIOLOGY

- ***Hypoxic-ischemic encephalopathy:*** This is the most common cause of neonatal seizures, constituting 50–65% of all cases. Most seizures (50–65%) due to HIE start within 12 hours, remaining have an onset within 24–48 hours, and are subtle in nature. Such seizures may be severe and difficult to treat, but they tend to subside after about 5–7 days even without treatment.
- ***Ischemic stroke:*** This is more likely in neonates with polycythemia or with thrombophilia due to a genetic disorder but may also occur without any risk factors. Stroke typically occurs in the middle cerebral artery distribution or watershed zones. Seizures resulting from stroke tend to be focal.
- ***Infections*** such as meningitis and sepsis may cause seizures.
- ***Hypoglycemia*** (blood glucose <45 mg/dL) should be suspected in neonates whose mothers have diabetes, who are small for gestational age, or who have hypoxia-ischemia or other stresses. Prolonged or recurrent hypoglycemia may cause permanent brain damage.
- ***Hypocalcemia*** [serum total calcium (Ca) level <7.0 mg/dLor ionic Ca level <4 mg/dL] is an important cause of seizures in newborns. It may be early onset (first 3 days of life) or late onset (after 3 days of age, usually 1 week). *Early onset hypocalcemia* is associated with prematurity and complications of birth. *Late onset hypocalcemia* is seen in neonates fed with high-phosphate milk, such as cow's milk or in very low birth weight neonates with associated metabolic bone disease of prematurity.
- ***Intracranial hemorrhage***, including subarachnoid, intracerebral, and intraventricular hemorrhage, may cause seizures. Intraventricular hemorrhage, which occurs in premature infants, results from bleeding in the germinal matrix.
- ***Hypernatremia or hyponatremia*** [serum sodium (Na) >150 mEq/L or <125 mEq/L] may cause seizures.
- ***Hypomagnesemia*** is a rare cause of seizures, which may occur when the serum magnesium level is <1.4 mEq/L. Hypomagnesemia often occurs with hypocalcemia and should be considered in neonates with hypocalcemia, if seizures continue after adequate calcium therapy.
- ***Inborn errors of metabolism*** (e.g., amino or organic aciduria) can cause neonatal seizures. Rarely, pyridoxine deficiency or dependency causes seizures.
- ***Other causes*** include CNS malformations, maternal substance abuse (e.g., cocaine, heroin, and diazepam), familial, kernicterus, etc.

CLASSIFICATION OF NEONATAL SEIZURES

The clinical manifestations of seizures in neonates differ from those seen in older children. Due to immaturity of brain, generalized seizures rarely occur in neonates. Relatively advanced development of limbic system may account for predominance of subtle seizures in neonates. During the neonatal period, any unusual repetitive or stereotypic movement may represent a seizure. Alterations in autonomic functions such as blood pressure or heart rate may also represent seizure activity. Apnea may also be a manifestation of seizure in neonates. Classification of neonatal seizures is summarized as follows:

- ***Subtle seizure:*** Most common seizure type. *Eye signs*—staring, deviation, blinking, etc. *Buccal-oral-lingual*: chewing, sucking, and lip smacking; *Limbs*—cycling, swimming, and rowing; *Systemic*—apnea. Heart rate may help to decide whether apnea represents a seizure phenomenon or not. In epileptic apnea, there is tachycardia, as opposed to bradycardia seen in nonepileptic apnea. It may be difficult to differentiate subtle seizures from extremes of normal behavior. Many subtle seizures are thought to arise from the basal ganglia because of diminished cortical inhibition. Further, depression of the cortex with anticonvulsants may not alter these seizures.
- ***Clonic seizure:*** These consist of rhythmic movements of muscle groups in a focal distribution, which consist of a rapid flexion phase followed by a slower extensor movement.

Clonic seizures may be focal or multifocal. These usually involve one limb or one side of the body jerking rhythmically at 1–4 times per second. Most common etiology is a metabolic abnormality—hypoglycemia or hypocalcemia; may be a clue to an underlying focal neuropathology, e.g., hemorrhage or cerebral infarction. Prognosis is good.

- ***Tonic seizure:*** Sustained flexion or extension of axial or appendicular muscle groups involving limbs or trunk or deviation of the head. It may mimic decerebrate or decorticate posturing. May be focal or generalized. Background EEG patterns tend to have multifocal or generalized voltage depression. These are indicative of severe neocortical dysfunction or damage and are often difficult to treat with anticonvulsants.
- ***Myoclonic seizure:*** These consist of rapid, isolated jerks which can be generalized, multifocal or focal in an axial or appendicular distribution lacking the slow return phase of the clonic movement complex. EEG background activity tends to be low-voltage, slow-wave activity, or a burst suppression pattern with focal sharp waves. Myoclonic seizures reflect injury at multiple levels of the neuraxis from the spinal cord, brainstem to cortical regions. These can also occur in a very severe form of encephalopathy and are associated with poor long-term outcome. Another cause is drug withdrawal (especially opiates). If it occurs during sleep, then it is probably "benign neonatal sleep myoclonus."

It is important to distinguish seizures from jitteriness. *Jitteriness or tremulousness* consists of symmetrical rapid movements of the hands and feet, is stimulus sensitive, and may be initiated by sudden movement or noise. It can be abolished by holding the extremity or repositioning the baby, a feature which helps differentiate it from seizures. There are no associated eye movements and EEG is normal. An approach to neonate presenting with abnormal movements is shown in **Flowchart 16.4**.

INVESTIGATIONS

Evaluation begins with a detailed history and a physical examination.

- ***Biochemical evaluation:*** Investigations include measurement of plasma glucose, Na, K, Cl, HCO_3, Ca, and Mg; and

Flowchart 16.4: An approach to neonate presenting with abnormal movements

Approach to neonatal seizures
↓
Neonate with abnormal movements
↓

Seizures
Features:
- Do not end with tactile or motor suppression
- Cannot be induced by a stimulus
- Often involve eye deviation and autonomic changes

Jitteriness
Features:
- Rapid motor activities as tremor or shake
- High frequency, low amplitude, and oscillatory (not jerking movement)
- Can be ended by flexion or holding the limb
- Induced by a stimulus
- No autonomic changes
- Causes include maternal substance abuse, metabolic disorder, hypoglycemia, perinatal insult

Benign neonatal sleep myoclonus
Features:
- Seen in term, healthy, and thriving neonate
- *Age:* From birth to 3 months
- *Character of movements:* Multifocal jerks seen in transition to and during sleep
- *Timing:* Only present during sleep
- Upon wakening, the jerking ceases
- Most common entity misdiagnosed as seizure

Causes (of seizures)

Day 1–4
- HIE
- Drug withdrawal (maternal drug use of narcotic or barbiturates)
- *Drug toxicity:* Lidocaine, Penicillin
- IVH
- *Acute metabolic disorders:* Hypocalcemia, sepsis, hypoglycemia, hypomagnesemia, hyponatremia or hypernatremia
- *Inborn errors of metabolism:* Galactosemia, hyperglycinemia, urea cycle disorders, pyridoxine deficiency and pyridoxal-5-phosphate deficiency (must be considered at any age)

Day 4–14
- *Infection:* Meningitis encephalitis
- *Metabolic disorders:* Hypocalcemia, Cow's milk, persistent hypoglycemia
- *IEM:* Galactosemia, fructosemia, leucine sensitivity
- Drug withdrawal, maternal drug use of narcotics or barbiturates
- Benign neonatal convulsions, familial and nonfamilial
- Kernicterus
- Developmental delay, epilepsy, neonatal diabetes syndrome

Age 2–8 weeks
- *Infection:* HSV, Enterovirus, bacterial
- *Head injury:* Subdural hematoma, child abuse
- *IEM:* Aminoacidurias, urea cycle defects, organic acidurias, neonatal adrenoleukodystrophy
- *Malformations of cortical development:* Lissencephaly, focal cortical dysplasia, tuberous sclerosis, Sturge-Weber syndrome

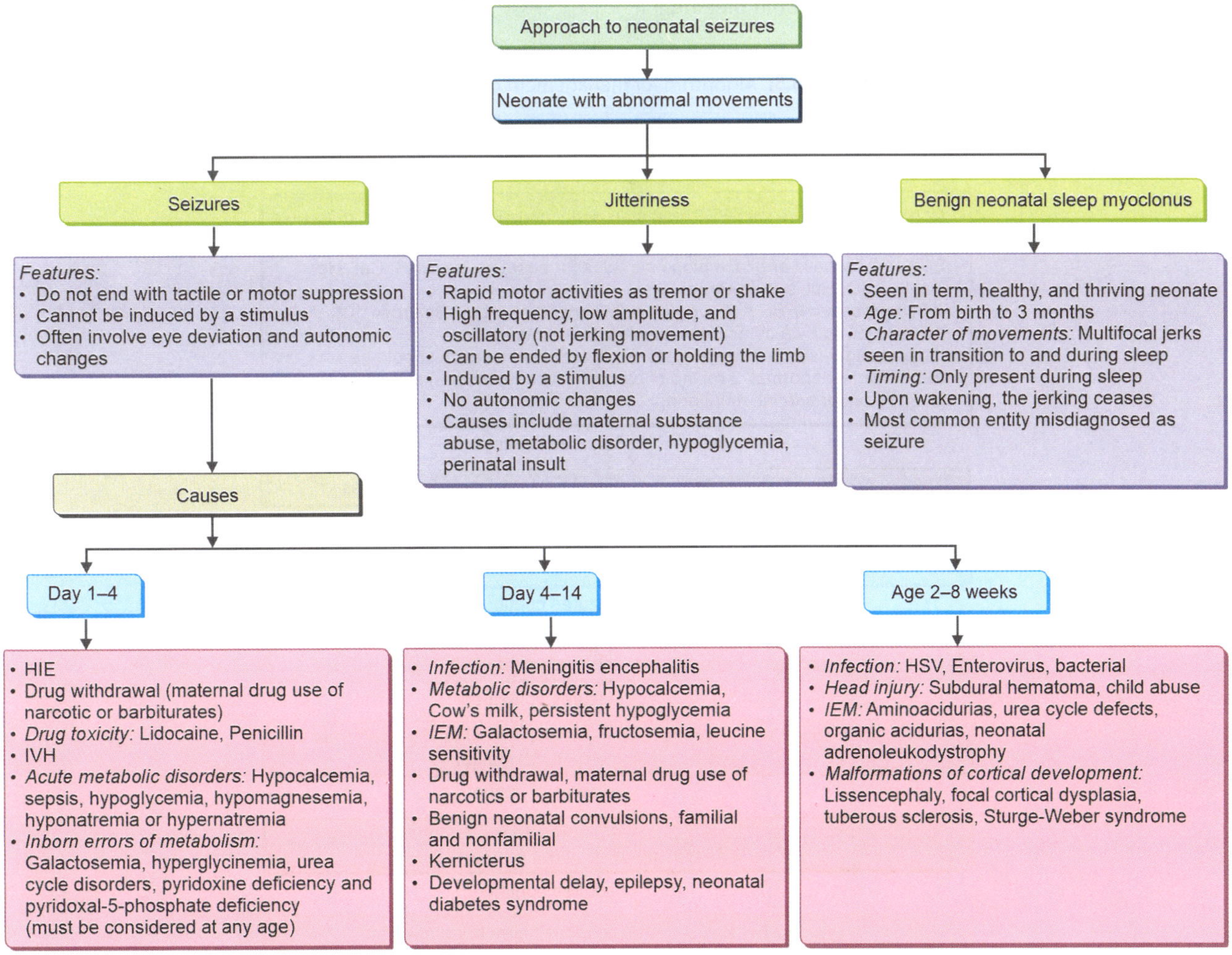

(IEM: inborn errors of metabolism; IVH: intraventricular hemorrhage; HIE: hypoxic-ischemic encephalopathy; HSV: herpes simplex virus)

lumbar puncture for cerebrospinal fluid (CSF) analysis (cell count and differential, glucose, and protein) and culture. The need for other metabolic tests (e.g., arterial pH, blood gases, serum bilirubin, urine amino, or organic acids) or tests for commonly abused drugs depends on clinical suspicion.

- ***Electroencephalogram:*** EEG is considered the gold standard for the diagnosis of seizures in newborns and paroxysmal events not associated with corresponding change in EEG activity are not classified as seizures. Seizures with EEG correlate are referred as electroclinical seizures which can be further classified as motor events (automatisms, focal clonic, focal tonic, myoclonic, and epileptic spasms) or nonmotor events (autonomic and behavioral arrest). EEG seizures without corresponding clinical correlate are called as electrographic seizures. EEG (waking and sleep) is essential, especially when it is difficult to determine whether the neonate is having seizures; EEG is also helpful for monitoring response to treatment.
- ***Neuroimaging:*** Most infants should have a cranial CT because it can detect intracranial bleeding and some brain malformations. Cranial ultrasonography may detect intraventricular bleeding but not subarachnoid bleeding; it may be preferred as a bedside test for very sick infants who cannot be moved to radiology. Diffusion-weighted MRI may detect ischemic tissue within a few hours but is usually done after the 2nd day to look for parenchymal damage.

TREATMENT Neonatal Seizures

Important aspects of management of neonatal seizures is mentioned here and outlined in **Flowchart 16.5**.

Initial Management

The first step in treatment is to identify the potentially treatable cause. The steps of management are outlined here:

- Stabilize and monitor temperature, airway, breathing, circulation, and oxygenation.
- Take a brief history and clinical examination comprising of:
  - *Birth history:* Enquire about gestational age, history of maternal diabetes, IUGR, maternal drug use, traumatic delivery, prolonged labor, and history suggestive of perinatal asphyxia.
  - *Family history of seizures:* With similar presentation and transient nature in siblings or parent suggests benign familial neonatal convulsions (ask grandparents as parents often do not know), history of neurocutaneous stigmata should be asked.
  - *Age at onset:* Right from birth, few hours later, or after days.

Flowchart 16.5: Algorithm for management of neonatal seizures

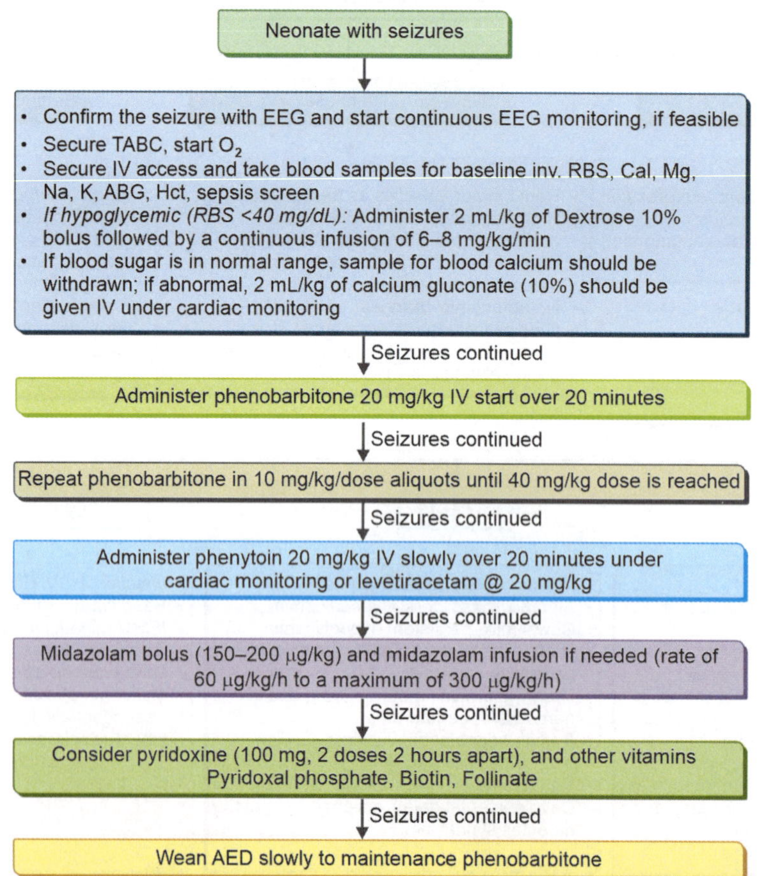

(EEG: electroencephalogram; IV: intravenous; TAB: temperature, airway, breathing, circulation; RBS: random blood sugar; AED: antiepileptic drugs)

- Identify and treat metabolic disorders. Send samples for blood sugar, calcium, and ABG immediately and proceed accordingly. If laboratory facility is not available, give a trial of dextrose and calcium empirically before starting anticonvulsants:
  - *Hypoglycemia (blood glucose <45 mg/dL):* 10% dextrose 2 mL/kg, followed by continuous infusion at the rate of 6 mg/kg/min.
  - *Hypocalcemia (serum calcium <7 mg/dL):* 10% calcium gluconate 2 mL/kg under cardiac monitoring. Add calcium gluconate in intravenous fluid (5–8 mL/kg/day) in documented hypocalcemia.
  - *Hypomagnesemia:* If seizures persist despite correction of hypocalcemia, 0.25 mL/kg of 50% magnesium sulfate should be administered intramuscularly.
- If at least one EEG-confirmed seizure occurs and no immediately correctable cause is there then start AED, phenobarbitone 20 mg/kg slow intravenously. Phenobarbitone can be repeated in aliquots of 5–10 mg/kg/dose every 30 minutes up to a total loading dose of 40 mg/kg, if seizures are not controlled. Maintenance dose is 5 mg/kg/day in two divided doses, beginning 24 hours later. There is a danger of respiratory depression beyond 20 mg/kg loading dose.
- If seizures persist, administer phenytoin 20 mg/kg slow intravenous loading dose followed by 5 mg/kg as maintenance dose, beginning 24 hours later. Other option at this stage is levetiracetam intravenous 20 mg/kg.
- Persistence of seizures after loading dose of phenobarbitone and phenytoin or levetiracetam is an indication to start midazolam drip (Bolus—150–200 µg/kg followed by infusion at the rate of 60 µg/kg/hto a maximum of 300 µg/kg/h).

If seizures persist, a trial of pyridoxine 50–100 mg slowly may be given intravenously. In pyridoxine dependency/deficiency, there is a dramatic response to pyridoxine.

Duration of Antiepileptic Therapy

Unlike older children and adults, anticonvulsants are not used for a long period in neonates. Most experts suggest early termination of seizure medications, to minimize side effects and because neonatal seizures typically abate within days, independent of the therapeutic intervention, and have a low risk of early recurrence.

Monotherapy is the most appropriate strategy to control seizures. Attempts should be made to stop all antiepileptic drugs and discharge the baby to only oral phenobarbitone at 3–5 mg/kg/day. The natural history of seizures due to various etiologies may be used to guide duration of therapy.

For seizures due to moderate hypoxic-ischemic brain injury, subarachnoid hemorrhage, or treatable and reversible metabolic disorders, medical therapy can be discontinued early, preferably within 7 days of seizure treatment or prior to discharge.

If neurological examination is persistently abnormal at discharge, AED is continued and the baby is reassessed at 1 month. If the baby is normal on examination and seizure free at 1 month, AED is discontinued over 2 weeks. If neurological assessment is not normal, or infant has a history of status epilepticus, an EEG is obtained. If EEG is not overtly paroxysmal, AED is tapered and stopped. If EEG is overtly abnormal, the infant is reassessed in the same manner at 3 months and then 3 monthly till 1 year of age.

PROGNOSIS

The outcome depends on the underlying etiology of seizures. In late onset hypocalcemia, prognosis is excellent with normal outcome in 100% of the babies. Subarachnoid hemorrhage also carries favorable prognosis (90% normal). About 50% of neonates with seizures due to perinatal asphyxia, meningitis, hypoglycemia, and early hypocalcemia develop normally. Neonatal seizures due to cerebral dysgenesis carry uniformly bad prognosis.

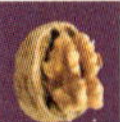

IN A NUTSHELL

Neonatal Seizures

1. Common causes of neonatal seizures include HIE, ischemia,hypoglycemia, hypocalcemia, CNS infections, dyselectrolytemia, and metabolic errors.
2. Neonatal seizures are classified as subtle, clonic, tonic, or myoclonic. They may be unifocal or multifocal.
3. Phenobarbitone is the first drug of choice in treatment of neonatal seizures.
4. Early stopping (48–72 hours) of antiepileptic drug is now advised as to prevent long-term side effects.
5. Long-term prognosis of babies with neonatal seizures stronglydepends on gestation age, etiology, and interictal EEG pattern.
6. Parental counseling and regular neurodevelopmental screening has to be done in babies with neonatal seizures till the age of 2 years to prevent long-term abnormal neurological outcome.

Hahn J, Olson DM. Etiology of neonatal seizures. NeoReviews. 2004;5(8):e327-35.

Mehta N, Shellhaas RA, McCulloch CE, et al. Seizure Burden, EEG, and Outcome in Neonates With Acute Intracranial Infections: A Prospective Multicenter Cohort Study. Pediatr Neurol. 2022;137:54-61.

Mizrahi EM, Pressler RM. The International League Against Epilepsy New Classification of Neonatal Seizures. Pediatrics. 2022;150(5):e2022058114.

Molloy EJ, El-Dib M, Juul SE, et al; Newborn Brain Society Guidelines and Publications Committee. Neuroprotective therapies in the NICU in term infants: present and future. Pediatr Res; 2022.

Mussavi M, Khanzadeh S, Valaei F, et al. Brain CT Scan, Sonography and EEG Findings in Neonates with Seizure. Iran J Child Neurol. 2022;16(3):183-91.

Volpe JJ. Neonatal seizures. Neurology of the Newborn, 4th edition. Philadelphia: Saunders; 2001. pp. 178-214.

16.8 Neonatal Hypoglycemia

PE 19.10

INTRODUCTION

Hypoglycemia is the most common metabolic disorder of newborn infants. Even asymptomatic hypoglycemia can cause brain damage. Anticipation, prevention, and early treatment are essential to reduce morbidity and mortality, and long-term neurodevelopmental sequelae.

DEFINITION

Hypoglycemia is defined as a blood glucose level of <45 mg/dL (2.2 mmol/L) in all newborns irrespective of birth weight or gestational age.

NEONATES AT RISK

- Preterm and LBW neonates especially those weighing <2.0 kg
- Post-term infants
- Infants of diabetic mother
- Any sick neonate requiring intensive care such as perinatal asphyxia, hypothermia, poor and/or delayed feeding, sepsis, shock, RDS, MAS, and polycythemia. Hypoglycemia can occur any time during illness.
- Infants whose mothers received treatment with beta-adrenergic drugs or oral hypoglycemic agents
- Congenital syndrome such as Beckwith-Wiedemann syndrome
- Inborn errors of metabolism

DIAGNOSIS

Infants with low blood glucose concentrations may remain *asymptomatic*. In these at-risk infants, hypoglycemia is usually detected by routine screening of blood glucose.

In *symptomatic* infants, signs of hypoglycemia are non-specific and reflect responses of the nervous system to glucose deprivation. The common symptoms include the following jitteriness or irritability, lethargy, limpness, weak- or high-pitched cry, poor feeding, vomiting; hypothermia, poor respiratory effort or apnea, tachypnea, dusky color or cyanosis, seizures, and coma.

Screening for Hypoglycemia

Capillary blood glucose can be estimated at bedside by a glucometer as a point of care screening. However, it should be remembered that glucometers are not sensitive to detect very low glucose concentrations. In cases of very low glucose concentrations, laboratory confirmation is necessary. Newborns at risk of hypoglycemia should be screened at 2, 6, 12, 24, 36, and 48 hours, and if indicated at 72 hours of age.

TREATMENT Neonatal Hypoglycemia

Asymptomatic hypoglycemia and blood glucose concentration between 25 and 45 mg/dL.

Give a breastfeed and repeat blood glucose after 1 hour.

Symptomatic neonate or blood glucose is <25 mg/dL.

Establish an intravenous line and give a bolus of 2 mL/kg body weight of 10% glucose intravenous slowly over 1 minute.

- Start infusion of dextrose-containing fluid at the daily maintenance volume according to the neonate's age to provide a glucose infusion rate (GIR) of 6 mg/kg/min.
- Check blood glucose 30 minutes after starting the infusion of glucose or any change in GIR.
- If the blood glucose remains below 45 mg/dL, GIR is increased in steps of 2 mg/kg/min to a maximum of 12 mg/kg/min.
- If hypoglycemia continues even after reaching a GIR of 12 mg/kg/min, start hydrocortisone 5 mg/kg/day intravenous in two divided doses for 24–48 hours.
- Once the blood glucose levels remain above 45 mg/dL for over 24 hours, begin tapering GIR in steps of 2 mg/kg/min every 6 hours ensuring blood glucose levels above 45 mg/dL before changing GIR. If blood sugar drops below 45 mg/dL any time, go back to the previous GIR.
- Begin breastfeeding. If the baby cannot be breastfed, give expressed breastmilk using *katori* spoon and/or *paladai*.
- As the baby's ability to feed improves, slowly decrease (over 2–3 days) the volume of intravenous fluids while increasing the volume of oral feeds. Do not discontinue the glucose infusion abruptly to prevent rebound hypoglycemia.

Refractory Hypoglycemia

It is defined as failure to maintain normal blood sugar levels despite a glucose infusion of 12 mg/kg/min or when stabilization is not achieved by 7 days of therapy. Important causes are as follows:

- *Endocrine disorders*: Congenital hypopituitarism, adrenal insufficiency, hypothyroidism, hypothalamic deficiency, glucagon deficiency, and epinephrine deficiency.
- *Hyperinsulinemic states*: They are islet cell hyperplasia, hyperfunction, focal/diffuse hyperinsulinism, Beckwith–Wiedemann syndrome, and insulin-producing tumors.
- *Inborn errors of metabolism:*
  - Defects in carbohydrate metabolism, e.g., fructose intolerance, galactosemia, and glycogen storage disorders.
  - Defects in amino acid metabolism, e.g., maple syrup urine disease.
  - Mitochondrial disorders.
  - Fatty acid oxidation defect.

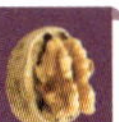

IN A NUTSHELL

Neonatal Hypoglycemia

1. Hypoglycemia in newborns is defined as blood glucose <45 mg/dL.
2. Preterm, IUGR, LBW babies, infants of diabetic mother; and neonates with sepsis, asphyxia, hypothermia, RDS are predisposed to hypoglycemia.
3. Asymptomatic hypoglycemic infants can be given a breastfeed and reassessed after 1 hour.
4. Symptomatic infants or those with blood glucose <25 mg/dL should be administered glucose infusion @ 6 mg/kg/min, which can be gradually increased to 12 mg/kg/min. If still no response, steroids may be tried.
5. Prolonged neonatal hypoglycemia can lead to permanent brain damage.

Abramowski A, Ward R, Hamdan AH. Neonatal Hypoglycemia. In: StatPearls [Internet]. Treasure Island (FL): StatPearls Publishing; 2022.
Dani C, Corsini I. Guidelines for Management of Neonatal Hypoglycemia: Are They Actually Applicable? JAMA Pediatr. 2020;174(7):638-9.
Thornton PS, Stanley CA, De Leon DD, et al; Pediatric Endocrine Society. Recommendations from the Pediatric Endocrine Society for Evaluation and Management of Persistent Hypoglycemia in Neonates, Infants, and Children. J Pediatr. 2015;167(2):238-45.
Wight NE, Academy of Breastfeeding Medicine. ABM Clinical Protocol #1: Guidelines for Glucose Monitoring and Treatment of Hypoglycemia in Term and Late Preterm Neonates, Revised 2021. Breastfeed Med. 2021;16(5):353-65.

16.9 Infant of Diabetic Mother

PE 19.10

INTRODUCTION

Diabetes has long been associated with maternal and perinatal morbidity and mortality. Approximately 6% of pregnancies are complicated by maternal diabetes mellitus (80% of which are gestational).

FETAL EFFECTS OF MATERNAL HYPERGLYCEMIA

Glucose and amino acids can traverse the placental membrane. On the other hand, insulin is unable to cross from maternal to fetal circulation. The fetus is subjected to high levels of glucose during times of maternal hyperglycemia. The fetus responds to hyperglycemia with pancreatic beta-cell hyperplasia and increased insulin levels. The combination of hyperglycemia and insulin, in the presence of increased fetal amino acids, increases fat and glycogen stores, resulting in increased body weight associated with hepatosplenomegaly and cardiomegaly, without an increase in head circumference (macrosomia) **(Fig. 16.7)**.

Elevated insulin levels may inhibit the maturational effect of cortisol on the lung, including the production of surfactant from type 2 pneumocytes. This puts the fetus at risk for developing RDS after birth.

Moreover, poor glycemic control during embryogenesis can result in a 4–8 fold increase in congenital malformations, such as cardiac defects, CNS defects (including anencephaly and spina bifida), genitourinary, and limb defects.

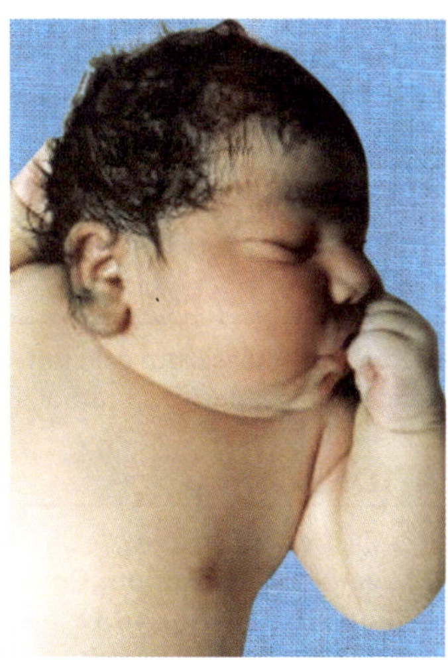

Fig. 16.7: Infant of diabetic mother. Note chubby facies and hairy pinna

NEONATAL COMPLICATIONS

- ***Macrosomia:*** Premature birth, difficult delivery, perinatal asphyxia, and birth trauma.
- ***Intrauterine growth retardation:*** It occurs if maternal diabetes is complicated by microvascular disease.
- ***Metabolic:*** Hypoglycemia, hypocalcemia, and hypomagnesemia.
- ***Pulmonary:*** RDS and TTN.
- ***Hematologic:*** Polycythemia, hyperbilirubinemia, thrombocytopenia, and arterial/venous thrombosis.
- ***Cardiac:*** Asymmetric septal hypertrophy; cardiomyopathy.
- ***CNS:*** Spina bifida, anencephaly, and caudal regression syndrome.
- ***GIT:*** Small left colon syndrome, duodenal, or anorectal atresia.

TREATMENT **Infant of Diabetic Mother**

Management at Delivery

Macrosomia leads to increased risks of shoulder dystocia, clavicular fracture, brachial plexus injury, facial nerve injury, cephalohematoma, perinatal asphyxia, and neonatal mortality at delivery. Tight glucose control during pregnancy will prevent these complications.

Management of Hypoglycemia

Hypoglycemia is a major problem in infant of diabetic mothers (IDM). *In clinically stable newborn with normal blood glucose values (>45 mg/dL),*start breastfeeding within 1/2 hour of birth and continue feeding every 2–3 hours. Screening for and treatment of hypoglycemia should be instituted early. Blood glucose levels are checked at 1, 3, 6, 12, 24, 36, and 48 hours. Hypoglycemia (blood glucose <45 mg/dL) may be symptomatic or asymptomatic. Depending on blood glucose levels and clinical condition of the newborn, the baby is managed as discussed in the previous section on hypoglycemia:

All babies born to diabetic mothers should be closely observed for other problems and managed accordingly.

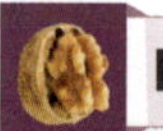

IN A NUTSHELL

Infant of Diabetic Mother (IDM)

1. Poor glycemic control in pregnancy is associated with increased risk of adverse fetal and neonatal outcomes.
2. Fetal macrosomia is associated with increased risk of perinatal asphyxia, birth trauma, neonatal hypoglycemia, polycythemia, and asymmetrical septal hypertrophy.
3. All IDMs must be carefully examined for malformations and monitored for respiratory distress, hypoglycemia, hypocalcemia, and polycythemia.
4. All IDMs with respiratory distress must undergo a chest skiagram and echocardiography (to exclude cardiac malformation and asymmetric septal hypertrophy).
5. Only symptomatic IDMs need to manage in NICU, the others can be managed in a well-baby area with adequate monitoring.

Grev JE, Munger KM, Scott SM. Infant of a Diabetic Mother. SD Med. 2020;73(7):323-7.

Khandare J, Ds M, Ananthan A, et al. Is Routine Monitoring for Hypoglycemia Required in Intramural Asymptomatic Infant of Diabetic Mother? An Audit in a Tertiary Care Hospital. J Trop Pediatr. 2020;66(2):194-200.

Kokhanov A. Congenital Abnormalities in the Infant of a Diabetic Mother. Neoreviews. 2022;23(5):e319-27.

Korkut S, Oğuz Y, Bozkaya D, et al. Evaluation of the Effects of Delayed Cord Clamping in Infants of Diabetic Mothers. Am J Perinatol. 2021;38(3):242-7.

Moss CR. Neonatal Hypocalcemia in the Infant of a Diabetic Mother. Neonatal Netw. 2020;39(4):200-4.

16.10 Neonatal Hypocalcemia *PE 19.11*

INTRODUCTION

Hypocalcemia is defined as total serum calcium <7 mg/dL (1.75 mmol/L) or ionized fraction <4 mg/dL (1 mmol/L).

CLASSIFICATION

Neonatal hypocalcemia is classified as *early-onset* and *late-onset* depending on the age of manifestation. Common causes of hypocalcemia are summarized in **Box 16.1**.

Box 16.1 Causes of Hypocalcemia in Neonates

Early hypocalcemia:

- Preterm and intrauterine growth restriction (IUGR)
- Infants of diabetic mother (IDM)
- Perinatal asphyxia
- Hypoparathyroidism
- Maternal hyperparathyroidism
- CATCH-22 and DiGeorge syndrome
- Hypomagnesemia

Late hypocalcemia:

- Excess phosphate intake by feeding with cow's milk or cow's milk-based formula
- Bicarbonate or lipid infusion
- Phototherapy
- Acute kidney injury
- Maternal vitamin D deficiency

(CATCH 22: cardiac defects, abnormal facies, thymic hypoplasia, cleft palate, and hypocalcemia resulting from 22q11 deletions)

- Early-onset hypocalcemia is defined as hypocalcemia occurring *within first 3 days* after birth.
- Late-onset hypocalcemia develops *after third day of life*, usually manifested at the end of the first week.

CLINICAL FEATURES

Most infants with early-onset hypocalcemia are asymptomatic and are identified by routine screening. Infants with late-onset hypocalcemia usually present with signs of hypocalcemia including severe neuromuscular irritability, jitteriness, or seizures. Seizures may be multifocal or focal clonic in nature. These neonates can rarely present with laryngospasm, bronchospasm, or pylorospasm.

TREATMENT **Neonatal Hypocalcemia**

Asymptomatic Hypocalcemia

Most infants with early-onset hypocalcemia recover with nutritional support alone. Adequate calcium intake should be ensured by initiating early feedings. For neonates on parenteral nutrition, calcium is supplemented as 50 mg/kg/day of elemental calcium (10% calcium gluconate solution) given as a continuous infusion.

Symptomatic Hypocalcemia

Most infants with late-onset hypocalcemia are symptomatic and require treatment with 10% calcium gluconate 1–2 mL/kg intravenously. The solution is diluted with equal amount of 5% dextrose and infused slowly over 5–10 minutes strictly under heart rate monitoring. Infusion should be stopped at earliest sign of bradycardia. The dose can be repeated in 10 minutes, if no response occurs. After acute therapy, maintenance calcium should be started. Infusion sites are monitored regularly for any extravasation which may result in necrosis and subcutaneous calcifications. After initial management, treatment should be directed against the underlying disease causing hypocalcemia.

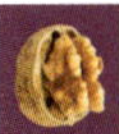

IN A NUTSHELL

Neonatal Hypocalcemia

1. Neonatal hypocalcemia is defined as total serum calcium <7 mg/dL or ionized fraction <4 mg/dL (1 mmol/L).
2. Hypocalcemia is early-onset (0–3 day of life) or late-onset (after 3 days).
3. Most children are asymptomatic. Multifocal clonic seizure is the most important clinical manifestation.
4. Hypocalcemia should be treated with parenteral calcium gluconate infusion.

Cho WI, Yu HW, Chung HR, et al. Clinical and laboratory characteristics of neonatal hypocalcemia. Ann Pediatr Endocrinol Metab. 2015;20:86-91.
Jain A, Agarwal R, Sankar MJ, et al. Hypocalcemia in the newborn. Indian J Pediatr. 2010;77:1123-8.
Levy-Shraga Y, Dallalzadeh K, Stern K, et al. The many etiologies of neonatal hypocalcemic seizures. Pediatr Emerg Care. 2015;31:197-201.
Thomas TC, Smith JM, White PC, et al. Transient neonatal hypocalcemia: presentation and outcomes. Pediatrics. 2012;129:e1461-7.

16.11 Neonatal Sepsis

PE 19.13

INTRODUCTION

Neonatal sepsis is a clinical syndrome characterized by systemic signs of infection in association with a positive blood culture in the first month (28 days) of life. It encompasses various infections of the newborn such as pneumonia, septicemia, meningitis, arthritis, osteomyelitis, and urinary tract infections (UTIs). Newborn babies are highly vulnerable to infection due to immaturity of their immune defense mechanisms.

INCIDENCE

World Health Organization estimates that 1 million deaths per year are due to neonatal sepsis and 42% of these deaths occur in first week of life. The incidence of neonatal sepsis in India is estimated to be 38/1,000 live births in tertiary care hospitals as compared to 1–5/1,000 in West. Sepsis is also the most common cause of neonatal mortality in India, accounting for 30–50% of neonatal deaths in the community. The higher incidence of infection may be due to increased prevalence of maternal genital tract infections, unhygienic delivery practices, high proportion of LBW babies, and poor infant feeding and rearing practices.

CLASSIFICATION

Depending on the age of onset, two patterns of the disease have been recognized:

Early-onset Sepsis

The signs and symptoms of sepsis appear within first 72 hours of birth. The source of pathogens is the maternal genital tract or the delivery area. Respiratory distress due to congenital (intrauterine) pneumonia is the predominant manifestation of early onset sepsis. Risk factors for development of early-onset sepsis (EOS) include:

Obstetric Risk Factors

- Prolonged (>18 hours) rupture of membranes.
- Clinical chorioamnionitis defined as intrapartum maternal fever (>37.8°C) with two or more features: fetal tachycardia (>160/min), uterine tenderness, malodorous vaginal discharge or maternal leukocytosis (>15,000 leukocytes/dL).
- Multiple (≥3) per vaginum examinations in 24 hours.
- Maternal group B *Streptococcus* (GBS) colonization.

Neonatal Risk Factors

- ***Very low birth weight (<1,500 g) and prematurity (<35 weeks of gestation):*** The incidence of septicemia is 10–20 times more in very low birth weight babies than in average birth weight babies. This is primarily due to poor host defense mechanisms in these infants.
- ***Male sex:*** Male babies are at higher risk of developing infection, suggesting the possibility of sex-linked factor in host susceptibility.

Late-onset Sepsis

The signs and symptoms of sepsis appear after 72 hours of age. The pathogens are acquired from community or hospital (nosocomial). Late-onset sepsis commonly presents as septicemia, pneumonia, or meningitis. Risk factors of late-onset sepsis (LOS) include:

- Very low birth weight
- Lack of breastfeeding

- Indiscriminate use of antibiotics—it encourages development of resistant organisms
- Frequent handling
- Presence of central venous catheters
- Delayed enteral feeding
- Prolonged hyperalimentation
- Mechanical ventilation
- Improper hand washing techniques; and
- Unhygienic infant feeding and rearing practices.

ETIOLOGY

Predominant causes of neonatal sepsis in India are gram-negative organisms such as *Klebsiella pneumoniae, Escherichia coli, Acinetobacter baumannii, Pseudomonas,* and *Citrobactor*. Gram-positive organisms, e.g., *Staphylococcus aureus, Staphylococcus albus,* and *Enterobacter* spp. are less frequent. In contrast to Western countries where GBS is a predominant pathogen responsible for neonatal sepsis, it is isolated in a very few cases in India. *Candida* sp. (*C. albicans, C. tropicalis,* etc.), can also cause LOS in very low birth weight neonates exposed to broad-spectrum antibiotics.

CLINICAL MANIFESTATIONS

The clinical picture of neonatal sepsis is highly variable. The signs and symptoms may be minimal, subtle, or nonspecific. This may cause delay in diagnosis with serious consequences. The early features of septicemia are lethargy, sluggishness, poor feeding, poor cry, irritability, hypothermia, and loss of or inadequate weight gain.

There should be high index of suspicion of sepsis. Otherwise diagnosis can be easily missed. Sometimes the baby does not "look well", appears off color, and is less alert/active. This may be an important clue to diagnosis. Parents are very perceptive and concerned about the subtle changes in the behavior and activity of their infants and their concerns should not be easily dismissed. A baby requires careful observation and meticulous examination for the following systemic manifestations:

- ***Respiratory:*** Tachypnea, apnea, retractions, grunting, and cyanosis
- ***Cardiac:*** Tachycardia, and shock in late stages
- ***GIT:*** Vomiting, diarrhea and abdominal distention, and hepatosplenomegaly
- ***Renal:*** Oliguria due to renal failure
- ***CNS:*** Excessive irritability, full fontanel, seizures, staring look, hypotonia/hypertonia, and apneic spells. It is uncommon to find neck rigidity in neonatal meningitis
- ***Hematologic:*** Pallor, disseminated intravascular coagulation, icterus, and bleeding spots
- ***Skin:*** Impetigo, cellulitis, sclerema, bleeds, and petechial spots
- ***Miscellaneous:*** Metabolic acidosis and hypoglycemia.

INVESTIGATIONS

Direct Evidence of Infection

Blood Culture

The diagnosis of septicemia can be made reliably only by recovery of the organism from blood culture or other normally sterile body fluids. It is the gold standard test for confirming neonatal septicemia. Blood culture should always be obtained before starting antibiotics. 1–2 mL of blood is sufficient for culture as neonates have high degree of bacteremia. The ratio of blood to culture medium should be 1:10. All blood cultures should be observed for at least 48 hours before declaring them negative. It is now possible to detect bacterial growth within 12–24 hours by using newer bacteriological techniques such as BACTEC and BACT ALERT.

Lumbar Puncture

Meningitis may coexist without any clinical signs. Therefore, lumbar puncture should be performed on all cases of suspected sepsis. The interpretation of CSF findings is problematic in neonates because of higher cell count (up to 32 cells/mm^3 with 60% of these cells being polymorphs) and increased protein levels (120–150 mg/dL) as normal values.

The CSF samples should be cultured immediately to avoid loss of viability of organisms. Gram stain should also be done. Apart from culture and Gram stain, other parameters to be evaluated are—total white blood cell (WBC) count, neutrophil count, glucose, and protein. Traditionally, the following cut-offs have been used—>30 cells, >60% of polymorphs, glucose <50% of blood glucose, protein >150 mg/dL in term babies, and 180 mg/dL in preterm babies.

It is important to remember that CSF, WBC, and glucose rapidly fall with time, giving spurious results. If the lumbar puncture is traumatic, the CSF should be sent for Gram stain and culture. If the neonate is too sick, lumbar puncture should be deferred, until stabilization is achieved.

Indirect Evidence of Infection

Sepsis Screen

Sepsis screen refers to a combination of several tests in an attempt to improve the diagnosis of neonatal sepsis early in the course of illness. In general, sepsis screen has shown little increase in positive predictive value (if a test is abnormal, disease is present), although negative predictive value (if a test is normal, disease is absent) has improved remarkably. The main value of this screen lies in excluding infection rather than confirming the diagnosis of infection. If repeat screen is still negative 12–24 hours later, then infection can be excluded confidently. A sepsis screen consists of:

- Total leukocyte count <5,000/mm^3
- Absolute neutrophil count <1,800/mm^3
- Immature (band cells + myelocytes + metamyelocytes) to total neutrophils ratio >0.2
- Raised erythrocyte sedimentation rate (μESR) (>15 mm/h)
- Raised CRP (>10 mg/L).

If two or more tests are positive in a neonate with maternal risk factors then it is reasonable to initiate antibiotic therapy after taking blood culture.

Complete blood count: Leukopenia (<5,000/mm^3) is more common than leukocytosis (>25,000/mm^3) in neonatal sepsis. Neutropenia (<1,800/mm^3) is a better predictor of septicemia. However, certain conditions such as birth asphyxia and toxemia of pregnancy may be associated with neutropenia in the neonate.

Apart from these, thrombocytopenia (platelet count <100,000/mm^3) and presence of Döhle bodies (aggregates, of rough endoplasmic reticulum), toxic granulation (eosinophilic granules in the cytoplasm), and vacuolization in neutrophils can also be taken as additional parameters to diagnose sepsis.

Acute phase reactants: In the presence of inflammation due to infection, hepatocytes under the influence of interleukin (IL)-1, rapidly synthesize certain proteins. These are known as acute phase reactants. These include CRP, fibrinogen, haptoglobin, etc.

The levels of certain proteins such as prealbumin, fibronectin, and transferrin, decrease in response to infection. These are known as negative reactants. CRP has a sensitivity of 87% and specificity of 83% in predicting infection. Serial changes in CRP levels are more useful in diagnosing infection and in assessing response to therapy.

Cytokines and Other Markers

Cytokines are being studied for their potential usefulness in diagnosing neonatal septicemia. Two such cytokines are tumor necrosis factor (TNF) and IL-6. The levels increase early in the course of illness. Other potential markers of infection include serum fibronectin, soluble CD14, and procalcitonin. Recently, polymerase chain reaction (PCR) has been successfully employed in the diagnosis of neonatal septicemia.

Other Investigations

Chest X-ray, blood glucose, urea, creatinine, electrolytes, ABGs,and coagulation studies provide useful information for determining supportive management.

Problems in Diagnosis

No laboratory test can rapidly confirm or exclude neonatal sepsis. Therefore, one must use one's clinical judgment taking into account maternal/neonatal risk factors and infant's condition. Since, neonatal sepsis can progress rapidly in a matter of a few hours, it is justified to start antibiotics in symptomatic babies before diagnostic results are available. For asymptomatic babies with maternal or obstetric risk factors for infection, antibiotics are started, if two or more tests in sepsis screen are positive. The subsequent duration of antibiotic therapy is based on the clinical course and the results of laboratory tests.

TREATMENT Neonatal Sepsis

Specific Therapy

Antibiotics are the mainstay of therapy. These should be started after the diagnostic studies are complete. It is not always essential to wait for the results of laboratory tests before starting antibiotics.

Choice of Antibiotics

This is based on the knowledge of the prevalent organisms responsible for septicemia and their antibiotic sensitivity. A combination of ampicillin and an aminoglycoside (gentamicin or amikacin) is a good choice for early-onset septicemia and late-onset community-acquired infections. If there is associated meningitis, the preferred combination is ampicillin and cefotaxime. For community-acquired septicemia of staphylococcal origin, cloxacillin and an aminoglycoside are preferred. If there is concern regarding methicillin-resistant *S. aureus* (MRSA), use vancomycin instead of cloxacillin. **Table 16.14** describes the choice of antibiotics in various settings of neonatal sepsis and **Table 16.15** details the dosages of antibiotic in neonates.

Aminoglycosides: The choice is based on sensitivity pattern, cost, safety profile, and efficacy record. Where resistant organisms are unlikely, gentamicin is preferred choice because of its low cost. For resistant organisms, amikacin is selected. Netilmicin has got highest antistaphylococcal activity but has the disadvantage of high cost. Tobramycin has very good activity against *Pseudomonas.*

Third generation cephalosporins: Cefotaxime, ceftriaxone, and ceftazidime have good activity against gram-negative bacilli. Compared to aminoglycosides, they are safer, do not require monitoring of serum concentrations, and have better penetration through meninges. For these reasons, they are preferred, especially if there is associated meningitis. Only ceftazidime has antipseudomonal activity. Although third generation cephalosporins have only modest activity against *S. aureus,* cefotaxime has better antistaphylococcal coverage than other third generation cephalosporins. Ceftriaxone has the potential to displace bilirubin from albumin. For this reason, ceftriaxone is not used in newborn babies for treating septicemia.

The duration of antibiotic therapy is 10–14 days for septicemia, 14–21 days for meningitis, and at least 28 days for osteomyelitis/arthritis. Intrathecal or intraventricular instillation of antibiotics for neonatal meningitis is not beneficial, and may, in fact, be harmful due to release of bacterial products due to very rapid bacterial killing, resulting in exuberant host inflammatory response with further tissue damage.

Supportive Therapy

- Temperature maintenance—set temperature at 36.5°C.
- *Circulation:* If perfusion is poor as evidenced by capillary refill time (CRT) of >3 seconds—infuse normal saline 10 mL/kg over 20–30 minutes. Repeat the same dose 1–2 times, if perfusion continues to be poor. Start dopamine at the dose of 5–10 µg/kg/min, if CRT is still prolonged.
- *Respiration:* Maintain an oxygen saturation of 88–94%.
- Correction of hypoglycemia, hypocalcemia, and metabolic acidosis.
- Management of renal failure.
- Control of seizures with phenobarbitone.
- Fresh frozen plasma or platelets or packed RBCs for disseminated intravascular coagulation (DIC).
- Vitamin K, if not received before or having active bleeding.
- Assisted ventilation for respiratory failure.
- Phototherapy and exchange transfusion, if required, for severe hyperbilirubinemia.
- *Nutrition:* If baby is hemodynamically unstable, start total parenteral nutrition. As soon as stability is achieved, start orogastric feeding and gradually shift to breastfeeding. Mother must be advised to express her breastmilk frequently during the period the baby is kept nil orally.

Adjunctive Therapy

Exchange transfusion: Exchange transfusion may be beneficial in septic neonates presenting with DIC, sclerema, and significant hyperbilirubinemia. It helps by removing bacteria and bacterial toxins, providing immune factors like immunoglobulins, neutrophils, and macrophages and by improving tissue perfusion. However, this modality has procedure-related morbidity and mortality, especially in very sick infants and, therefore, has limited scope in management of neonatal septicemia.

Intravenous immunoglobulin (IVIG): A recent clinical trial has confirmed that IVIG is not beneficial in neonatal septicemia. Other therapies such as granulocyte colony-stimulating factor (G-CSF), granulocyte macrophage colony-stimulating factor (GM-CSF), activated protein C,and pentoxifylline are still under evaluation for the treatment of neonatal sepsis.

<table>
<tr><th>Table 16.14</th><th colspan="4">Choice of Antibiotics and Duration of Therapy for Neonatal Sepsis</th></tr>
<tr><th>Type of sepsis</th><th>Empirical choice of antibiotics</th><th>Rationale</th><th>Comments</th><th>Duration</th></tr>
<tr><td>Early-onset sepsis</td><td>Ampicillin + Gentamicin</td><td>GBS is sensitive to ampicillin and gentamicin is effective against E. coli</td><td>Gram-negative pathogens, mostly resistant to this combination, are predominant agents causing EOS in developing countries; empirical therapy should be individualized for each hospital</td><td rowspan="2">Since 96% of bacteremic cultures obtained before initiating antibiotic therapy become positive by 48 hours and 98% are positive by 72 hours, so empirical antibiotics should be stopped after 48–72 hours once cultures are documented to be negative</td></tr>
<tr><td>Late-onset sepsis</td><td>Stable neonates:
Cloxacillin+ Gentamicin
Neonates with cardiorespiratory compromise:
Vancomycin + Cefotaxime</td><td>Coagulase negative Staphylococcus aureus (CoNS) is the main pathogen for LOS</td><td>Gram-negative bacteria, Klebsiella spp., E. coli, Acinetobacter spp. are the predominant pathogens causing LOS in developing countries and almost two-thirds of them in hospital setup and one-third in community settings are resistant to 3rd generation cephalosporins; Staphylococcus aureus is also an important pathogen for LOS and almost half of them are methicillin resistant; again empirical therapy for LOS should be individualized for each hospital; consider empiric antifungal coverage for invasive candidiasis for severe sepsis unresponsive to antibiotics, infants on chronic parenteral nutrition, or those with unexplained cytopenias</td></tr>
<tr><th colspan="5">Treatment of infections by organ systems</th></tr>
<tr><th>Organ system affected</th><th>Pathogen</th><th>Choice of antibiotics</th><th colspan="2">Duration of therapy</th></tr>
<tr><td>Bacteremia without a focus</td><td>All the microbes</td><td>–</td><td colspan="2">10–14 days</td></tr>
<tr><td rowspan="4">Bacterial meningitis</td><td>GBS meningitis</td><td>Ampicillin + aminoglycoside</td><td colspan="2">At least 14 days after CSF sterilization</td></tr>
<tr><td>Gram-negative meningitis</td><td>Third generation cephalosporin (cefotaxime)</td><td colspan="2">At least 21 days or for 14 days after the first negative CSF culture</td></tr>
<tr><td>Listeria monocytogenes and Enterococcus</td><td>Ampicillin + aminoglycoside</td><td colspan="2">At least 14 days after CSF sterilization</td></tr>
<tr><td>Staphylococcus aureus</td><td>Vancomycin + third generation cephalosporin</td><td colspan="2">14–21 days</td></tr>
<tr><td rowspan="2">Pneumonia</td><td>Early-onset</td><td>Ampicillin + aminoglycoside</td><td colspan="2">7–10 days</td></tr>
<tr><td>Late-onset</td><td>Vancomycin + third-generation cephalosporin</td><td colspan="2">7–10 days</td></tr>
<tr><td rowspan="2">UTI</td><td>Early-onset</td><td>Ampicillin + aminoglycoside</td><td colspan="2" rowspan="2">7–14 days for uncomplicated UTI; urine culture may be repeated after 2–3 days of starting antibiotics if anatomical abnormality is suspected; renal USG should be performed after clinical stabilization; voiding cystourethrogram is usually done 3–6 weeks after completion of antibiotic treatment to detect vesicoureteral reflux</td></tr>
<tr><td>Late-onset</td><td>Vancomycin + aminoglycoside</td></tr>
<tr><td>Osteomyelitis and septic arthritis</td><td>–</td><td>Vancomycin + aminoglycoside/ third-generation cephalosporin</td><td colspan="2">Joint infections require surgical drainage; duration of therapy is 4–6 weeks for uncomplicated cases; MRSA osteomyelitis is treated for 8 weeks for osteomyelitis; IV antibiotics are continued until clinical improvement and normalization of inflammatory markers</td></tr>
<tr><td>Omphalitis</td><td></td><td>Cloxacillin + gentamicin or Vancomycin + aminoglycoside if MRSA is prevalent in community settings
Consider adding clindamycin or metronidazole if anaerobic infection is suspected from fowl smelling umbilical discharge or history of maternal chorioamnionitis</td><td colspan="2">10 days; switch to oral therapy once clinical improvement is documented</td></tr>
</table>

(CSF: cerebrospinal fluid; EOS: early-onset sepsis; GBS: Group B *Streptococcus*; IV: intravenous; LOS: late-onset sepsis; MRSA: methicillin-resistant *S. aureus*; UTI: urinary tract infection; USG: ultrasonography)

Table 16.15 Dose of Antibiotics for Neonatal Sepsis

Antibiotic	Dose	Frequency		Route
		<7 days age	>7 days age	
Ampicillin	50–100* mg/kg/dose	12 hourly	8 hourly	IV
Cloxacillin	50 mg/kg/dose	12 hourly	8 hourly	IV
Gentamicin	5 mg/kg/dose	24 hourly	24 hourly	IV
Amikacin	15 mg/kg/dose	24 hourly	24 hourly	IV
Cefotaxime	50 mg/kg/dose	12 hourly	8 hourly	IV

*Higher dose is given in meningitis
(IV: intravenous)

OUTCOME AND PROGNOSIS

Mortality due to neonatal septicemia ranges from 15 to 40%. Early onset septicemia, LBW, DIC, meningitis, shock, sclerema, and multiorgan failure carry poor prognosis.

PREVENTION

The only preventive intervention for EOS is intrapartum antibiotic prophylaxis (IAP) with penicillin (preferred agent), ampicillin, or cefazolin given for ≥4 hours before delivery. It is useful against GBS EOS only. The indications for IAP include positive antenatal rectovaginal swab cultures for GBS, unknown maternal colonization status with gestation <37 weeks, ROM >18 hours, or temperature >100.4°F (>38°C), GBS bacteriuria during the current pregnancy and previous infant affected with invasive GBS disease.

Interventions to prevent LOS are summarized in **Box 16.2**.

SUPERFICIAL INFECTIONS

Pyoderma

- It is characterized by pustules, are most commonly found in axillae, groin, neck, and periumbilical area.
- *S. aureus* is the causative bacteria.
- Diagnosis can be confirmed by Gram staining of the pus aspirated from the pustules, which reveals neutrophils and gram-positive cocci.
- A few small lesions in a healthy term infant can be treated with topical mupirocin alone. Multiple big lesions in a healthy neonate necessitate oral antibiotics like cefadroxil or amoxicillin-clavulanate combination (for 5–7 days). Big lesions should be pricked with a sterile needle, and cleaned with betadine solution.
- In more extensive lesions, septicemia or lesions in a preterm infant, detailed sepsis screen including blood culture should be sent and the baby should be treated with intravenous cloxacillin and aminoglycosides (or antibiotics as per sensitivity pattern) for 7–10 days.

Omphalitis

- Omphalitis is characterized by erythema or induration of the periumbilical area along with purulent discharge from the umbilical stump. Causative organisms include both gram-positive and gram-negative species.
- Omphalitis may spread to cause abdominal wall cellulitis or septicemia. Management consists of a full sepsis screen including blood culture and oral/parenteral cloxacillin and aminoglycosides (or antibiotics as per sensitivity pattern) for 7–10 days.

Conjunctivitis (Ophthalmia Neonatorum)

Conjunctivitis is characterized by inflammation of the conjunctiva within the first month of life. Inflammation can be caused by a local irritant (chemical conjunctivitis) or by bacteria (*Neisseria gonorrhoeae*, *Chlamydia trachomatis*, staphylococci, streptococci, and gram-negative spp.) and herpes simplex virus (HSV).

- ***Chemical conjunctivitis:*** It is most commonly seen with silver nitrate prophylaxis, requires no specific treatment, and usually resolves within 48 hours.

Box 16.2 Strategies to Prevent Late-onset Neonatal Sepsis

1. *Hand hygiene:* Soap or hand gel before and after patient contact; no artificial nails, complex rings, or nail polish; audit of hand hygiene practice with feedback
2. *Environmental control:* Proper bed space cleaning, environmental cleaning, and minimizing crowding
3. Early feeding with human milk
4. *Central line care:* Bundling the care of central lines
5. Fluconazole prophylaxis for extremely low birth weight neonates
6. *Ventilator-associated pneumonia (VAP):* Prevention of VAP includes daily assessment of readiness to extubate, elevating the head of the bed for infants, oral care with colostrum, and hand hygiene
7. *Clean delivery services* and hygienic cord care; chlorhexidine application may be beneficial for infants in resource-poor settings for prevention of omphalitis
8. *Antibiotic stewardship:* Limiting empiric therapy to the narrowest-spectrum agents that cover likely pathogens circulating in unit, avoiding prolonged or unnecessary antibiotic therapy for suspected or proven infections, prospective surveillance of antibiotic use, with feedback and interventions

Immunoglobulin therapy, lactoferrin, probiotics, recombinant granulocyte colony-stimulating factor (G-CSF), granulocyte-macrophage colony-stimulating factor (GM-CSF), pentoxiphylline, exchange blood transfusion are of questionable benefit.

- ***Gonococcal conjunctivitis:*** It is present with chemosis, lid edema, and purulent exudate beginning 1–4 days after birth. There may be clouding of cornea or panophthalmitis with loss of vision. The disease is generally bilateral. In suspected cases, the infant should receive single dose of ceftriaxone 25–50 mg/kg intravenous or intramuscular (not to exceed 125 mg) at birth.
- ***Chlamydial conjunctivitis:*** It presents with variable degrees of inflammation, eye discharge, and eyelid swelling 5–14 days after birth. It is treated with erythromycin (50 mg/kg/day in four divided doses) for 14 days. Only topical treatment alone is not adequate, and is unnecessary when systemic therapy is given.
- Other bacterial infections can be treated with local ophthalmic ointments, such as erythromycin or gentamicin.

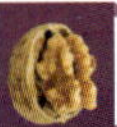

IN A NUTSHELL

Neonatal Sepsis

1. Sepsis is among the top three causes of neonatal deaths.
2. Major pathogens causing infections in neonates in developing countries are *Klebsiella pneumoniae*, *Staphylococcus aureus*, *E. coli*, and *Pseudomonas*.
3. Neonatal sepsis presents with nonspecific and subtle features, which often overlap with common noninfectious conditions.
4. Blood cultures should be obtained in every suspected case prior to start of antibiotics.
5. A combination of ampicillin and an aminoglycoside (gentamicin or amikacin) is a good choice for early-onset septicemia and late-onset community-acquired infections.
6. If there is associated meningitis, the preferred combination is ampicillin and cefotaxime.
7. Hand hygiene is the single most important preventive measure for sepsis.

Alnemri A, Darwish ARA, Baqawi B, et al. Quality assessment of clinical practice guidelines for neonatal sepsis using the Appraisal of Guidelines for Research and Evaluation (AGREE) II Instrument: A systematic review of neonatal guidelines. Front Pediatr. 2022;10:891572.

Gurudas G, Arjun R, Jain N, et al. Prevalence of Group B *Streptococcus* in pregnant women in Kerala and relation to neonatal outcomes: a prospective cross-sectional study. J Trop Pediatr. 2022;68(6):fmac092.

Mathias S, Balachander B, Bosco A, et al. The effect of exchange transfusion on mortality in neonatal sepsis: a meta-analysis. Eur J Pediatr. 2022;181(1):369-81.

Morowitz MJ, Katheria AC, Polin RA, et al. The NICU Antibiotics and Outcomes (NANO) trial: a randomized multicenter clinical trial assessing empiric antibiotics and clinical outcomes in newborn preterm infants. Trials. 2022;23(1):428.

Nair NS, Lewis LE, Dhyani VS, et al. Factors Associated With Neonatal Pneumonia and its Mortality in India: A Systematic Review and Meta-Analysis. Indian Pediatr. 2021;58(11):1059-61.

Poulsen A, Bech CM, Lund S, et al. Risk factors for neonatal sepsis in Sub-Saharan Africa: a systematic review with meta-analysis. BMJ Open. 2022;12(9):e054491.

Razak A, Alhaidari OI, Ahmed J. Interventions for reducing late-onset sepsis in neonates: an umbrella review. J Perinat Med; 2022.

Ting JY, Dunn MS, Chodhury J. Summary of Antimicrobial Therapy for Commonly Encountered Conditions in the Neonatal Intensive Care Unit: A Canadian Perspective. Front Pediatr. 2022;10:894005.

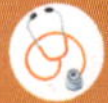

CASE STUDY Newborn with Sepsis and Meningitis

A 5-day-old male baby (weight 1,550 g) is brought to the neonatal unit with complaints of multiple pustules on the back, umbilical discharge, and excessive irritability. The baby was born at 34 weeks and the birth weight was 1,700 g. The axillary temperature is 37.2°C, extremities are warm, RR is 52/min without retractions and grunting. Bilateral air entry in the chest is equal and there is no cyanosis. Heart rate is 148/min. Color is pink, CRT is 5 seconds. Blood sugar is 65 mg/dL. There are no signs of bleeding from any site. Anterior fontanel is tense and bulging.

What is your diagnosis? Justify.

Diagnosis: Preterm LBW with late-onset sepsis, pyoderma, umbilical sepsis, meningitis, and shock. Presentation of disease after 72 hours of age suggests a late-onset disease. Prolonged CRT beyond 3 seconds is suggestive of shock. Excessive irritability and bulging anterior fontanel point to a CNS problem: Could be meningitis or intracranial bleed. However, other evidence of infection (pustules and umbilical discharge) favors an infective cause such as meningitis. This child needs to have a complete septic workup including blood counts, blood culture, chest X-ray, and a lumbar puncture. Neuroimaging (ultrasound/CT of cranium) should also be obtained.

How will you manage this baby?

- Child is having a normal temperature which needs to be maintained.
- Management of shock should be the priority. Infuse normal saline bolus 10 mL/kg over 20 minutes, and reassess for the need of second bolus.
- Start maintenance intravenous fluids. On day 5 of life, the normal requirement is 120 mL/kg of Isolyte P per day, i.e., 204 mL given as 68 mL 8 hourly intravenous.

- Medications to be given on priority will include (1) injection vitamin K 1 mg intramuscular, if not received before; and (2) intravenous antibiotics. The antibiotics should be chosen so as to cover staphylococcal infections (*S. aureus* is the most common cause of umbilical sepsis and pustules), and gram-negative infections (*Klebsiella, E. coli, Proteus* are the usual cause of neonatal meningitis). First-line drugs will consist of a combination of cloxacillin (50 mg/kg/dose 8 hourly) and cefotaxime (50 mg/kg/dose 8 hourly). It there is no response in 48 hours, change antibiotics according to the culture reports.
- Feeding will depend on clinical improvement and feeding readiness of the baby. Tube feeding or cup feeding can be offered to the child once he stabilizes.
- Monitor the temperature, respiration, color, and CRT.
- Communicate with caregivers. Inform parents about the baby's condition and stay in touch.

Lumbar puncture revealed a turbid CSF, with 480 cells/mm^3, 90% polymorphs, protein 180 mg/dL and CSF glucose 24 mg/dL with corresponding blood glucose 75 mg/dL. CRP is positive. After 4 hours of your treatment, the child developed repeated episodes of multifocal clonic seizures.

Outline further management of this child.

Since the blood glucose is normal, hypoglycemia is unlikely to be the cause of seizures. Obtain serum calcium. Control the seizures by administration of phenobarbitone 20 mg/kg IV over 20 minutes. Continue maintenance phenobarbitone 3–5 mg/kg/day in two divided doses, after 24 hours. Since meningitis is established, continue intravenous antibiotics for 2–3 weeks. Repeat vitamin K 1 mg intramuscular every week for the duration of antibiotics. Stop phenobarbitone 5–7 days after the last episode of seizure. Monitor head circumference weekly for hydrocephalus. Discuss with parents the progress of the baby. Plan the first follow-up after 1 week of discharge and next two visits every fortnight, and then coincide subsequent visits with immunization schedule. Advise regarding exclusive breastfeeding, prevention of infection, temperature maintenance, immunization, danger sign evaluation, and early care seeking. Assess growth and development in each follow-up visit.

16.12 Bleeding Newborn

PE 19.7

HEMOSTASIS IN THE NEWBORN

- ***Clotting factors:*** The concentrations of most of the clotting factors, especially vitamin K-dependent factors (II, VII, IX, and X) and contact factors (XI, XII, prekallikrein, and high molecular weight kininogen) are reduced in term newborns compared to older children and adults. The levels are even lower in the premature infants. Only factors V, VIIIc, and XIII are present in concentrations approaching those of adult levels. Coagulation proteins do not cross the placental barrier. Fetus starts synthesizing coagulation factors by 10 weeks of intrauterine life.
- ***Platelets:*** Platelet numbers are similar in premature, term infants, and adults, though their function may be somewhat impaired. Megakaryocytes are seen in yolk sac by 5 weeks of gestation and in liver and spleen by 10 weeks. Platelets first appear in circulation by 5 weeks.
- *Antithrombin* III, plasminogen, and protein C levels are also low in the neonates, especially in the premature infants.

CAUSES OF NEONATAL BLEEDING

Bleeding could result from disorders of platelets, coagulation proteins, and disruption of vascular integrity.

- ***Coagulation disorders:***
  - *Congenital deficiencies:*
    - *X-linked recessive:* Hemophilia A (factor VIII) and hemophilia B (factor IX)
    - *Autosomal recessive (rare):* Factors V, VII, X, XI, XII, XIII, afibrinogenemia
  - *Acquired deficiencies:*
    - Vitamin K deficiency bleeding (also known as hemorrhagic disease of newborn)
    - DIC
    - Liver disorders
- ***Platelet disorders:***
  - *Thrombocytopenia (platelet count <150 × 10^9/L):*
    - *Decreased platelet production*: Congenital infections (e.g., CMV, rubella), certain syndromes (e.g., thrombocytopenia absent radius, Fanconi syndrome), Wiskott-Aldrich syndrome.
    - Increased platelet consumption, e.g., sepsis and disseminated intravascular coagulation, maternal autoimmune disease [e.g., immune thrombocytopenia (ITP), systemic lupus erythematosus (SLE)], neonatal alloimmune thrombocytopenia, maternal thiazide intake, IUGR with toxemia of pregnancy, necrotizing enterocolitis, and heparin-induced thrombocytopenia.
  - *Impaired platelet function* is rare in the newborn except for decreased platelet adhesiveness associated with indomethacin therapy; and von Willebrand disease.
- ***Combined platelet and coagulation factor disorders:***
  - DIC
  - Hepatic dysfunction due to shock, infection, and neonatal hepatitis
- ***Disorders of vascular integrity:*** Hemangioma or vascular malformations, which may rupture and directly bleed, or sequester platelets, and secondarily cause bleeding.

CLINICAL MANIFESTATIONS

Signs and symptoms vary with the cause of bleeding, magnitude of blood loss, and the underlying disease. Signs of abnormal bleeding tendency include petechiae, excessive bruising, prolonged bleeding from puncture sites, umbilical oozing, gastrointestinal bleeding, hematuria, pulmonary hemorrhage, subgaleal hemorrhage, and intracranial hemorrhage. When blood loss is large, the infant may present with signs of hypovolemia (pallor, weak pulses, tachycardia, hypotension, and metabolic acidosis).

EVALUATION OF BLEEDING NEONATE

History

Family history of bleeding diathesis, maternal medications (aspirin, phenytoin, thiazides, and hydralazine), information about pregnancy and delivery, and any illness, medication, anomalies, or procedures done to the infant.

Physical Examination

The clinical appearance of a bleeding neonate as "sick looking" or "well looking" is helpful in differential diagnosis.

- ***Sick neonate:*** Consider infection, DIC, asphyxia, NEC, liver disease, and renal vein thrombosis.
- ***Well neonate:*** Consider vitamin K deficiency bleeding, immune thrombocytopenia, and inherited clotting factor deficiencies.
- Petechiae, small ecchymosis, or mucosal bleeding suggest a platelet disorder.
- Large bruises or hematomas or prolonged bleeding from venipuncture sites indicate DIC, vitamin K deficiency bleeding, liver disease, or inherited clotting factor defects.
- Hepatosplenomegaly, growth restriction, microcephaly, retinal findings suggest intrauterine infection.
- Deformity and shortening of forearms suggest absence of radii—thrombocytopenia-absent radius (TAR) syndrome.
- Hemangiomas point to Kasabach-Merritt syndrome.

Laboratory Tests

- ***Peripheral blood smear:*** To find out number and size of platelets and the presence of fragmented RBCs as seen in DIC. The presence of large platelets (megathrombocytes) points to immune destruction of platelets.
- ***Platelet count:*** Significant bleeding from thrombocytopenia is associated with platelet counts below 20,000–30,000/mm³. Depending on platelet count, thrombocytopenia is defined as mild (100,000–150,000/mm³), moderate (50,000–100,000 mm³), and severe (<50,000 mm³). Depending on the age of onset, thrombocytopenia is defined as early onset (within the first 72 hours of life) or late onset (after 72 hours of age). Approach to thrombocytopenia is depicted in **Flowchart 16.6 and Table 16.16**.
- Prothrombin time (PT)
- Partial thromboplastin time (PTT)
- ***Fibrin degradation products (FDP):*** Elevated levels suggest DIC.
- ***D-dimer test:*** D-dimers are produced from the action of plasma on fibrin clot. Normal values are <0.5 g/μL. Elevated levels are observed in DIC and deep vein thrombosis.
- ***APT test:*** Differentiates fetal blood from maternal blood. The test should be performed when a possibility of swallowed maternal blood is kept in an otherwise healthy baby with hematemesis or melena soon after birth.

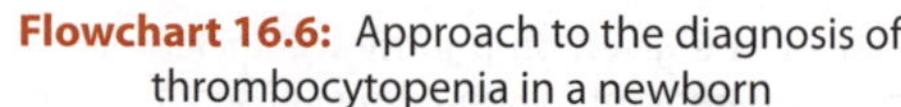

Flowchart 16.6: Approach to the diagnosis of thrombocytopenia in a newborn

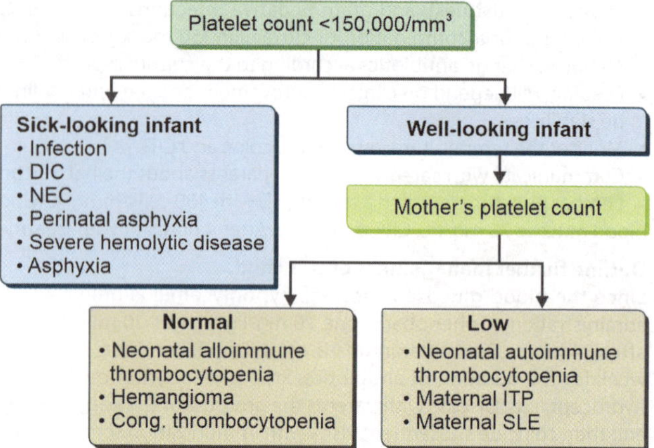

Table 16.16 Approach to the Diagnosis of Bleeding Neonate with Normal Platelet Count

Condition	Appearance	PT	PTT
Vitamin K deficiency bleeding	Well	↑	↑
Hemophilia	Well	N	↑
von Willebrand disorder	Well	N	N or ↑
Platelet function disorder	Well	N	N
Hepatic disease	Sick	↑	↑

(PT: prothrombin time; PTT: partial thromboplastin time)

- ***Maternal platelet count:*** Low in neonatal autoimmune thrombocytopenia while it is normal in neonatal alloimmune thrombocytopenia.

VITAMIN K DEFICIENCY BLEEDING

Etiology

Vitamin K deficiency bleeding is also known as *hemorrhagic disease of the newborn*. Incidence is 1 in 200–400 neonates not given vitamin K prophylaxis. Vitamin K is required for the activity of clotting factors II, VII, IX, and X. It acts by creating calcium-binding sites in these proteins by carboxylating glutamic acid residues. Other vitamin K-dependent proteins are proteins C, S, Z, and osteocalcin.

Neonates are vulnerable to vitamin K deficiency bleeding due to poor transplacental passage of vitamin K from mother to fetus and inadequate hepatic vitamin K stores. This is further aggravated by low vitamin K content of breastmilk and absence of bacterial flora in intestine responsible for vitamin K synthesis.

Clinical Features

Clinically, vitamin K deficiency bleeding presents as prolonged bleeding from multiple sites in an otherwise well baby. Three patterns are described:

1. ***Early hemorrhagic disease:*** It presents within first 24 hours of life. Clinical features include cephalohematoma,

intracranial, intrathoracic, and intra-abdominal hemorrhages. It is associated with maternal drug use, e.g., warfarin, anticonvulsants, salicylates, and antituberculous drugs. These drugs interfere with vitamin K stores or function.

2. ***Classical hemorrhagic disease:*** This is the most common type of vitamin K deficiency bleeding. It presents between 1 and 7 days of age, most commonly on day second and third day of life. Clinically, it manifests as bleeding from umbilicus and puncture sites and gastrointestinal hemorrhage (hematemesis or hematochezia/melena). Intracranial hemorrhage may also occur but is rare.
3. ***Late or delayed hemorrhagic disease:*** Manifests after 1 week of age, usually between 2 and 16 weeks of life. This is rare in infants who have received parenteral vitamin K at birth. Intracranial hemorrhage is the most dreaded complication. Predisposing factors include chronic diarrhea, cholestatic liver disease, malabsorption syndromes, cystic fibrosis, etc.

Diagnosis

Vitamin K deficiency bleeding should be suspected in a bleeding neonate who is otherwise well looking and not sick. There is prolonged bleeding from multiple sites and absence of petechial and purpuric spots in the skin.

Laboratory tests reveal a normal platelet count and prolongation of PT and PTT. Thrombin time (TT), fibrinogen and FDP levels are normal. Serum vitamin K levels are difficult to measure. However, in vitamin K deficiency, the levels of precursor proteins—proteins induced in vitamin K absence (PIVKA)—are elevated. This can be used as a sensitive indicator of vitamin K deficiency.

TREATMENT Hemorrhagic Disease of Newborn

Vitamin K_1 1–5 mg slow intravenously stops bleeding in a few hours. If there is active bleeding, the baby should also be given 10 mL/kg of fresh frozen plasma.

Prevention

Administer 0.5 mg or 1 mg of vitamin K_1 intramuscularly to neonates weighing less than or more than 1 kg, respectively at birth to all infants. This practice has virtually eliminated the problem of hemorrhagic disease of the newborn. Intramuscular route is both safe and effective way to prevent this disorder. There is no evidence that intramuscular vitamin K at birth is associated with increased risk of childhood malignancies, as was reported earlier. Oral vitamin K is not effective in preventing late disease.

Infants on broad-spectrum antibiotics for >2 weeks should receive weekly vitamin K (0.5 mg). Mothers receiving phenytoin or phenobarbitone should be given vitamin K_1 10 mg intramuscular 24 hours prior to delivery to prevent early hemorrhagic disease.

IN A NUTSHELL

Bleeding Newborn

1. Bleeding could result from disorders of platelets, coagulation proteins, and disruption of vascular integrity.
2. The clinical appearance of a bleeding neonate as "sick looking" or "well looking" is helpful in differential diagnosis.
3. Vitamin K deficiency bleeding (hemorrhagic disease of the newborn) presents as prolonged bleeding from multiple sites in an otherwise well baby.
4. Levels of precursor proteins—proteins induced in vitamin K absence (PIVKA)—are elevated in vitamin K deficiency.
5. Administer 0.5 mg or 1 mg of vitamin K_1 intramuscularly to neonates weighing less than or more than 1 kg, respectively at birth to all infants.

Eden RE, Coviello JM. Vitamin K Deficiency. In: StatPearls [Internet]. Treasure Island (FL): StatPearls Publishing; 2022.

Kher P, Verma RP. Hemorrhagic Disease of Newborn. In: StatPearls [Internet]. Treasure Island (FL): StatPearls Publishing; 2022.

Matusiak K, Patriquin CJ, Deniz S, et al. Clinical and laboratory predictors of fetal and neonatal alloimmune thrombocytopenia. Transfusion. 2022;62(11):2213-22.

National Library of Medicine. Drugs and Lactation Database. Bethesda (MD): National Library of Medicine; 2006.

Prasath A, Grafius A, Bonanno M, et al. Alloimmune Neutropenia in a Neonate: Case Report and Review of Literature. Antibodies (Basel). 2022;11(4):63.

Sellers A, Lew A, Tudyk M, et al. Hemorrhagic Disease of the Newborn: A Case Series Illustrating Preventable Harm. J Pediatr Health Care. 2022:S0891-5245(22)00237-1.

16.13 Neonatal Hyperbilirubinemia

PE 19.15

INTRODUCTION

Physiological jaundice occurs in nearly two-thirds of newborns, with excellent outcome. However, in 3-5% of newborns, serum bilirubin levels can exceed physiological limits, raising concerns of brain damage.

BILIRUBIN METABOLISM

Bilirubin is derived from the breakdown of heme proteins in the reticuloendothelial system. Three-fourths of the bilirubin come from destruction of senescent erythrocytes. The remaining 25%, known as early labeled bilirubin, is derived from hemoglobin released by ineffective erythropoiesis in bone marrow, and other heme-containing proteins in tissues such as myoglobin, cytochromes, catalase, peroxidase, and from free heme. 1 g of hemoglobin gives rise to 34 mg of bilirubin. The normal term newborn produces about 6-10 mg/kg/day of bilirubin, in comparison to 3-4 mg/kg/day in the adult. Bilirubin metabolism is summarized as follows (also see **Fig. 16.8**).

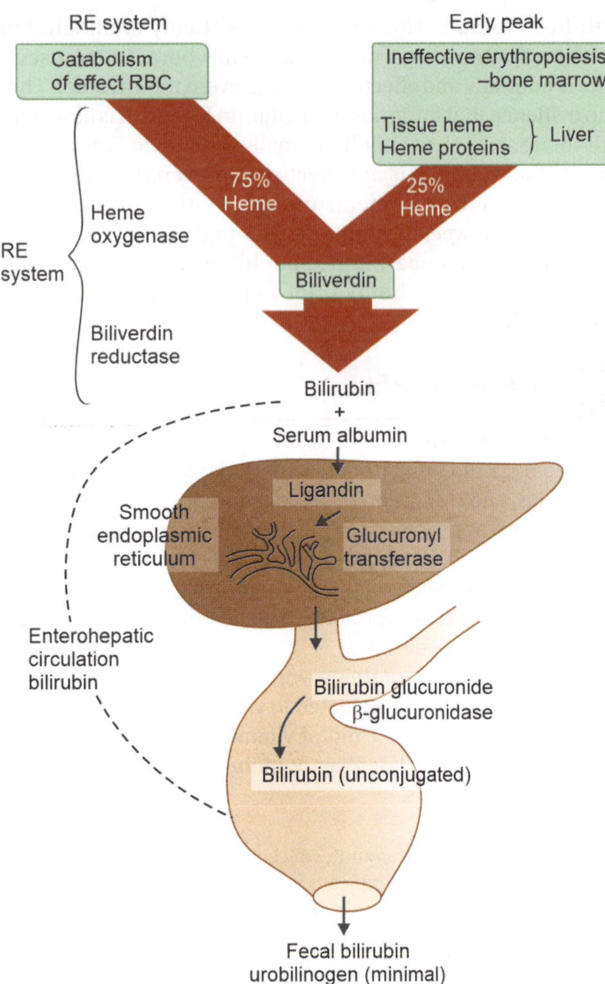

Fig. 16.8: Metabolism of bilirubin

- Bilirubin is bound to albumin for transport in the blood. This bound bilirubin does not enter the CNS and is nontoxic.
- Upon reaching the liver, bilirubin enters the liver cell and gets bound to ligandin which helps to transport it to smooth endoplasmic reticulum, the site of conjugation in hepatocyte.
- Uridine diphosphate glucuronyl transferase 1 A1 (UGT1A1) enzyme causes conjugation with glucuronic acid to produce mono- and di-glucuronides which are water-soluble and are excreted in bile.
- The conjugated bilirubin is transported with the bile to the gut. The sterile newborn gut contains beta-glucuronidase, an enzyme which converts bilirubin glucuronide into unconjugated bilirubin. Unconjugated bilirubin gets reabsorbed into the circulation; this is called enterohepatic circulation.
- With frequent feeding, early colonization of gut occurs. These bacteria reduce bilirubin glucuronide into stercobilinogen which is excreted in stool, thus preventing the enterohepatic circulation.

PHYSIOLOGICAL MECHANISMS OF NEONATAL JAUNDICE

Neonatal jaundice occurs due to the following mechanisms:

- *Increased bilirubin production*
  - Higher erythrocyte mass
  - Shorter RBC lifespan (90 days versus 120 days)
  - Increased ineffective erythropoiesis
  - Increased turnover of nonhemoglobin heme proteins
- *Reduced hepatic metabolism:*
  - Defective uptake
  - Defective conjugation
- *Increased enterohepatic circulation* due to high levels of intestinal-glucuronidase, paucity of intestinal bacteria, and decreased gut motility.

ASSESSMENT OF JAUNDICE

In newborns, the jaundice is detected by blanching the skin with finger, revealing the yellow staining of skin and subcutaneous tissues. The baby should be examined preferably in daylight for better appreciation of jaundice.

Jaundice is seen first in the face at serum bilirubin levels of 5–6 mg/dL and then progresses in a cephalocaudal manner to the trunk and extremities. In adults, sclera appears icteric when serum bilirubin exceeds 2 mg/dL. It is difficult to detect jaundice in eyes of a newborn as unlike adults, neonates keep their eyes shut because of physiological photophobia.

Kramer described the approximate serum bilirubin level with the level of skin discoloration which can be used as a rough guide to the level of jaundice **(Fig. 16.9)**. Once palms and soles are distinctly yellow stained, serum bilirubin exceeds 15 mg/dL. After phototherapy is started, skin gets bleached and it becomes difficult to assess jaundice clinically.

Transcutaneous Bilirubinometry

This is a noninvasive method to assess serum bilirubin levels. The device measures the intensity of yellow staining of skin and subcutaneous tissues and the value is displayed as either transcutaneous bilirubin index or a bilirubin value which correlate reasonably well with serum bilirubin levels. There is no trauma to the baby and repeated measurements can be done. It is a good screening method.

PHYSIOLOGICAL JAUNDICE

This is defined as jaundice in healthy babies during the first few days of life due to physiological reasons. It appears on second or third day of life, rises at a rate <5 mg/dL/day; peaks at 4–5 days of age; and spontaneously disappears by 10–14 days of life. It is always indirect reacting hyperbilirubinemia and serum bilirubin levels do not exceed 15 mg/dL. Apart from jaundice, these neonates have no other problem. Term infants with physiological jaundice do not require any treatment and outcome is excellent.

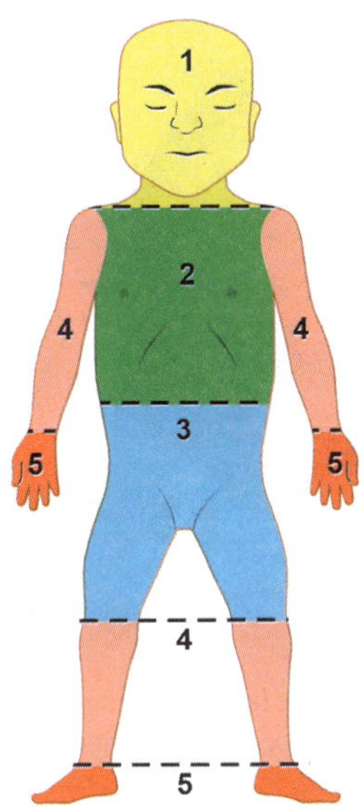

Area of body	Level	Range of bilirubin (mg/dL)
Face	1	5–6
Chest	2	6–10
Abdomen and thigh	3	10–12
Legs	4	12–15
Palms/soles	5	>15

Fig. 16.9: Cephalocaudal progression of jaundice (Kramer's rule)

PATHOLOGICAL JAUNDICE

Neonatal jaundice is considered pathological, if it appears on day 1 of age; persists beyond 2 weeks; total serum bilirubin levels exceed 15 mg/dL or conjugated serum bilirubin is >2 mg/dL or >20% of total bilirubin; rise in serum bilirubin level is >0.5 mg/dL/h; or associated with signs of illness.

Causes of Jaundice

- Jaundice appearing within 24 hours of age
  - *Hemolytic disease of newborn:* Rh, ABO, and minor group incompatibility
  - Intrauterine infections
  - Glucose-6-phosphate dehydrogenase (G6PD) deficiency
  - Hereditary spherocytosis
  - Crigler-Najjar syndrome
  - Alpha-thalassemia
- Jaundice appearing between 24 and 72 hours of life
  - Physiological
  - Septicemia
  - Polycythemia
  - *Concealed hemorrhages:* Cephalohematoma, subarachnoid bleed, and intraventricular hemorrhage
- Jaundice appearing after 72 hours
  - Septicemia
  - Idiopathic jaundice
  - Hypothyroidism
  - Metabolic disorders

Common causes of pathological jaundice in India include blood group incompatibilities, infections, idiopathic jaundice (breastmilk jaundice), G6PD deficiency, bruising, and cephalohematoma.

BREASTMILK JAUNDICE

Breastmilk jaundice is a misnomer since no factor in breastmilk has consistently been shown to be causative of jaundice in neonates and this terminology should be better avoided. It is more appropriate to term this condition as idiopathic jaundice. Labeling the condition as breastmilk jaundice may undermine the efforts to promote breastfeeding.

Diagnosis

Breastmilk jaundice is suspected in an otherwise healthy exclusively breastfed neonate whose physiological (unconjugated) jaundice fails to decline after first week of birth, and persists beyond 2 weeks of birth. The exact cause is not known. Male gender, East Asian ancestry, and genetic mutations are likely to play a role.

TREATMENT **Breastmilk Jaundice**

Phototherapy is indicated, if serum bilirubin exceeds 20 mg/dL, and exchange transfusion, if serum bilirubin reaches 25–30 mg/dL. Some people advocate stopping breastfeeding for 48 hours if serum bilirubin levels are approaching 25 mg/dL. Temporary interruption of breastfeeding may be followed by fall in serum bilirubin values. With reintroduction of breastmilk, there may be some rise in serum bilirubin levels but does not reach the previous high levels. However, in majority of cases the jaundice can be managed without need of stopping breastfeeding.

BILIRUBIN-INDUCED NEUROLOGIC DYSFUNCTION (BIND)

Unconjugated bilirubin is neurotoxic. Conjugated bilirubin does not cause brain damage. Severe unconjugated hyperbilirubinemia can result in neuronal damage. *Bilirubin-induced neurologic dysfunction (BIND)* refers to clinical manifestations of bilirubin toxicity in the neonatal period. The term *kernicterus* is reserved for the chronic and permanent sequelae of bilirubin toxicity. This condition is characterized by yellow staining of the basal ganglia and brainstem nuclei and involves diffuse neuronal damage. The entire spectrum is now known as *kernicterus spectrum disorders* (KSDs).

Predisposing Factors

The risk of BIND depends on serum bilirubin levels, gestational age, underlying cause of jaundice, and other comorbid conditions. Factors predisposing to bilirubin toxicity include acidosis, birth asphyxia, hypercarbia, hypoglycemia, pyogenic meningitis, intracranial hemorrhage, and drugs displacing bilirubin from albumin (e.g., ceftriaxone and diazepam).

Factors other than serum bilirubin levels such as asphyxia, hypercarbia, and sepsis may be involved in producing brain injury in jaundiced preterm newborns. Thus, bilirubin toxicity in preterm newborns may be a function of their overall clinical status rather than serum bilirubin levels *per se*.

Neurotoxic Risk Factors

The neurotoxicity risk factors described in AAP guidelines are mentioned here:

- Gestational age <38 weeks and this risk increases with the degree of prematurity
- Albumin <3.0 g/dL
- Isoimmune hemolytic disease (i.e., positive direct antiglobulin test), G6PD deficiency, or other hemolytic conditions
- Sepsis
- Significant clinical instability in the previous 24 hours

What is the Highest Bilirubin Value that is Safe?

There is no single value of serum bilirubin which is considered safe for all neonates. In term neonates with hemolytic disease, kernicterus rarely occurs with bilirubin levels <20 mg/dL. In case of nonhemolytic jaundice, serum bilirubin levels up to 25 mg/dL are generally considered safe in otherwise healthy term newborns. However, in premature babies, brain damage may occur at lower bilirubin levels, so called "low bilirubin kernicterus."

Clinical Features

- ***Early phase (first 1–2 days):*** Poor sucking, hypotonia, lethargy, high-pitched cry, and loss of Moro reflex.
- ***Intermediate phase (3–7 days):*** Hypertonia, opisthotonus, retrocollis, fever, seizures, bulging of anterior fontanel. Many babies die in this phase. Most survivors develop chronic sequelae **(Fig. 16.10)**.
- ***Advanced phase (>1 week):*** Pronounced opisthotonus (hypotonia may replace hypertonia after 1 week of age), apnea, seizures, coma, and death.

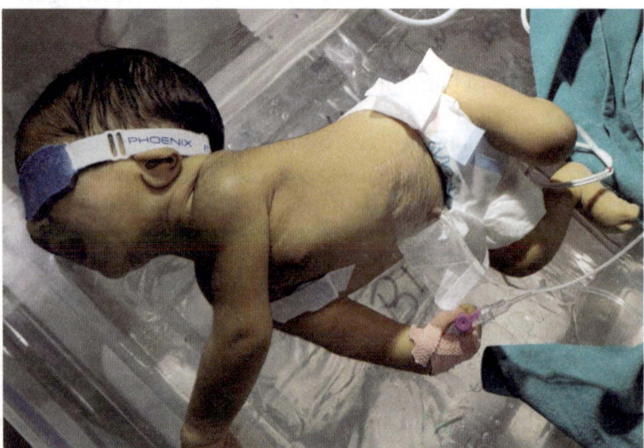

Fig. 16.10: Neonate with acute bilirubin encephalopathy with shrill cry and opisthotonic posturing

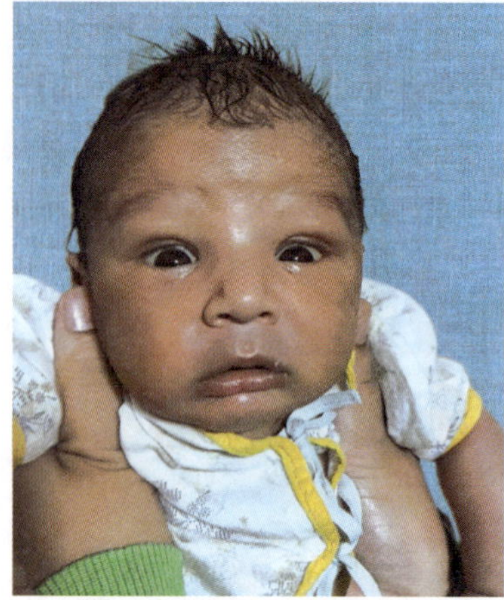
Fig. 16.11: Kernicteric facies with sun setting sign, eyelid retraction, and stunned look

- ***Chronic phase (first year):*** Hypotonia, brisk tendon reflexes, and delayed development.
- ***After first year:*** Choreoathetosis, tremors, upward gaze palsy, sensorineural hearing loss, dental dysplasia, and mental retardation.

Kernicteric facies **(Fig. 16.11)** in acute bilirubin encephalopathy includes setting-sun sign (i.e., paresis of upward gaze) with eyelid retraction, which together comprise the *Collier sign*, and facial dystonia. The infant with kernicteric facies appear stunned, scared, or anxious and it may persist for at least 2–3 weeks after acute bilirubin encephalopathy.

WORKUP FOR PATHOLOGICAL JAUNDICE

- ***Review maternal and perinatal history:*** Age of onset of jaundice, any other sign of illness, color of urine and feces, previous sibling with jaundice for blood group incompatibility, maternal illness during pregnancy, traumatic delivery, delayed cord clamping, oxytocin use, birth asphyxia, delayed feeding, delay in meconium passage, feeding status of the baby, and difficulty in breastfeeding.
- ***Physical examination:*** Excessive weight loss (>10% of body weight), signs of dehydration, bruising, cephalohematoma, prematurity, small for gestation, polycythemia, pallor—hemolysis; petechiae—sepsis, TORCH infections, hepatosplenomegaly—features of acute bilirubin encephalopathy.
- ***Laboratory tests:*** Total serum bilirubin, direct and indirect, blood group and Rh of mother, and baby, direct Coombs test, hematocrit, reticulocyte count, peripheral smear for RBC morphology, evidence of hemolysis, sepsis screen, thyroid profile, G6PD assay, TORCH titers, if indicated.

PREDICTION OF SEVERE HYPERBILIRUBINEMIA

Predischarge serum bilirubin or transcutaneous bilirubin plotted on an hour-specific bilirubin nomogram is useful in identifying newborns at high risk for developing significant hyperbilirubinemia.

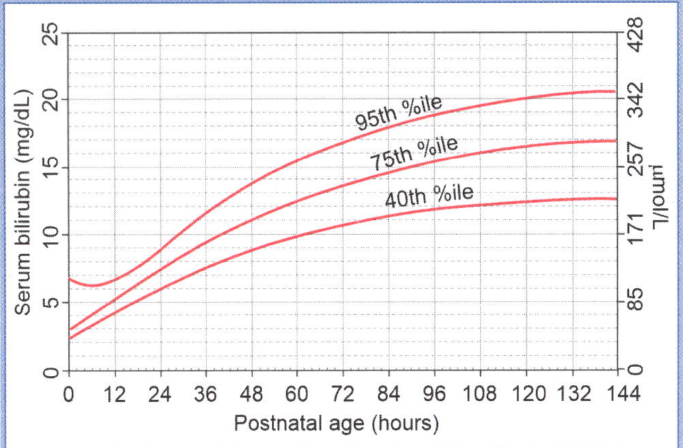

Fig. 16.12: Neonatal bilirubin nomogram

Recently new hour specific nomogram has been published **(Fig. 16.12)** that clarifies that newborns with predischarge total serum bilirubin (TSB) >75th percentile are at higher risk for subsequently exceeding the 95th percentile. Therefore, follow-up within 24 hours is desired. Risk factors for development of severe hyperbilirubinemia in infants of 35 or more weeks of gestation are listed below:

- Lower gestational age (i.e., risk increases with each additional week <40 weeks).
- Jaundice in the first 24 hours after birth.
- Predischarge transcutaneous bilirubin (TcB) or TSB concentration close to the phototherapy threshold.
- Hemolysis from any cause, if known or suspected based on a rapid rate of increase in the TSB or TcB of >0.3 mg/dL per hour in the first 24 hours or >0.2 mg/dL per hour thereafter.
- Phototherapy before discharge
- Parent or sibling requiring phototherapy or exchange transfusion
- Family history or genetic ancestry suggestive of inherited RBC disorders, including G6PD deficiency.
- Exclusive breastfeeding with suboptimal intake.
- Scalp hematoma or significant bruising.
- Down syndrome.
- Macrosomic infant of a diabetic mother.

TREATMENT Hyperbilirubinemia

The aim of therapy is to maintain serum bilirubin levels within safe range and thus prevent brain damage. This is achieved by phototherapy and/or exchange transfusion. In addition, any comorbid condition or a treatable etiology needs to be specifically addressed.

Phototherapy

Mechanism of Action

Phototherapy converts toxic water insoluble unconjugated bilirubin to nontoxic water-soluble photoisomers which can be excreted in bile and urine without the need for hepatic conjugation. There are two types of reactions (1) configurational isomerization, and (2) structural isomerization.

- *In configurational isomerization,* native isomers of bilirubin, 4Z, 15Z is converted to 4Z, 15E isomer which can be excreted by the liver without the need for conjugation. This is a reversible reaction.
- In *structural isomerization*, the native bilirubin molecule is converted to lumirubin which can be readily excreted in bile and urine. This is an irreversible reaction. Structural isomerization mainly accounts for phototherapy-induced reduction in serum bilirubin levels.

In addition to photoisomerization reactions, photooxidation can also occur during phototherapy but it has minor contribution to the effects of phototherapy. The most effective light spectrum for phototherapy is 420–480 nm. There is no role of prophylactic phototherapy.

Technique of Giving Phototherapy

Various phototherapy devices used include fluorescent tubes (CFL), light-emitting diodes (LED), halogen lamps, and fiberoptic systems (biliblanket). Fluorescent tubes are most used. These could be cool-white or special blue tube lights.

- Baby is placed under phototherapy naked except for eye patches to shield eyes from intense light. There is no need to cover the genitalia in male infants.
- The distance between the baby and phototherapy lights should be around 30 cm. Shorter distance can lead to overheating.
- Turn the baby sideways every 2–3 hours for maximal skin exposure.
- Monitor skin temperature as baby can develop hypo- or hyperthermia.
- Phototherapy is given continuously except breaks for breastfeeding.
- Offer breastfeeding frequently. Generally, there is no need to give extra fluids in breastfed babies as increasing the frequency of breastfeeding will meet the requirement.

Side Effects

- Increased insensible water loss can cause dehydration. Increasing the frequency of breastfeeding will take care of this problem.
- *Loose green stools:* No treatment is needed.
- *Skin rashes:* Harmless, no need to discontinue phototherapy.
- *Bronze baby syndrome*: Occurs if baby has conjugated hyperbilirubinemia.
- *Hypo- or hyperthermia:* Monitor temperature frequently.

Intensive phototherapy should be initiated if total serum bilirubin thresholds are reached as shown in **Figures 16.13 and 16.14** based on gestational age, hyperbilirubinemia neurotoxicity risk factors, and age of the infant in hours.

Exchange Transfusion

It is the most effective method to reduce serum bilirubin levels. However, the procedure has inherent risks to the baby. Complications include infection, metabolic disturbances, hypoglycemia, hypocalcemia, bleeding, necrotizing enterocolitis, volume overload, and thrombosis/embolic phenomenon.

Choice of Blood

- *For ABO incompatibility:* O Rh compatible blood cross-matched against mother and infant. One may use type O packed red cells resuspended in AB plasma to ensure that no anti-A or anti-B antibodies are present.
- *For Rh isoimmunization:* O negative blood cross-matched against mother and infant.

Indications

- *At birth:*
  - Hydrops fetalis due to Rh hemolytic disease
  - Cord blood bilirubin >4.5 mg/dL
  - Cord blood hemoglobin <11 g/dL
- *After birth:*
  - Rise in bilirubin values >1 mg/dL/h despite phototherapy
  - Serum bilirubin levels >20 mg/dL in hemolytic jaundice
  - Serum bilirubin levels >25–30 mg/dL in nonhemolytic jaundice
  - Clinical suspicion of acute bilirubin encephalopathy

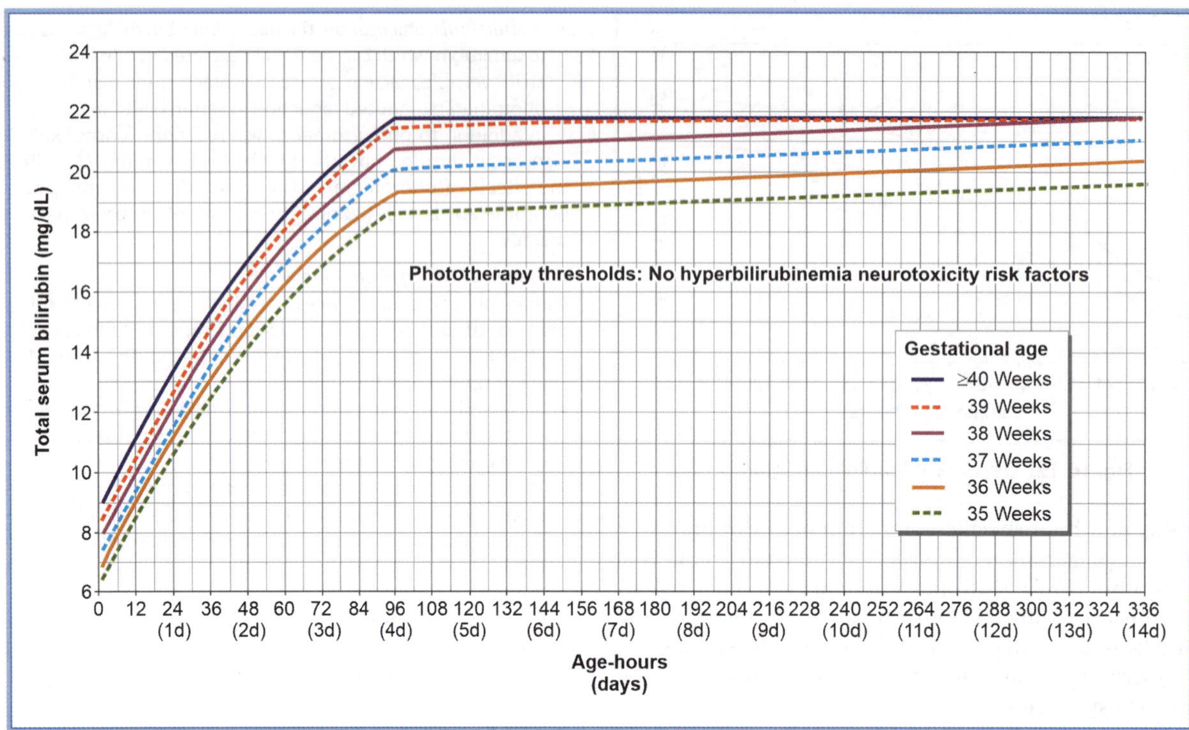

Fig. 16.13: Guidelines for phototherapy in hospitalized infants of 35 or more weeks of gestation without neurotoxicity risk factors (described earlier in this chapter)

Source: Practice Guideline, American Academy of Pediatrics, 2022

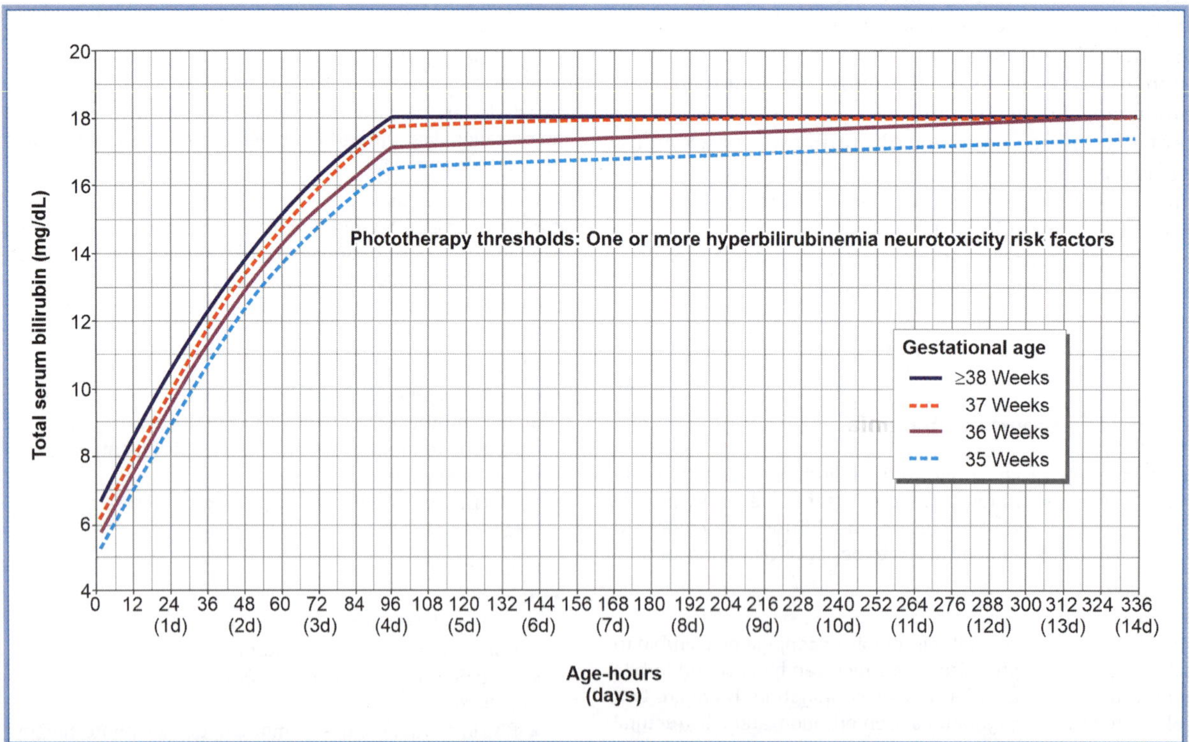

Fig. 16.14: Guidelines for phototherapy in hospitalized infants of 35 or more weeks of gestation with one or more neurotoxicity risk factors (described earlier in this chapter)

Source: Practice Guideline, American Academy of Pediatrics, 2022

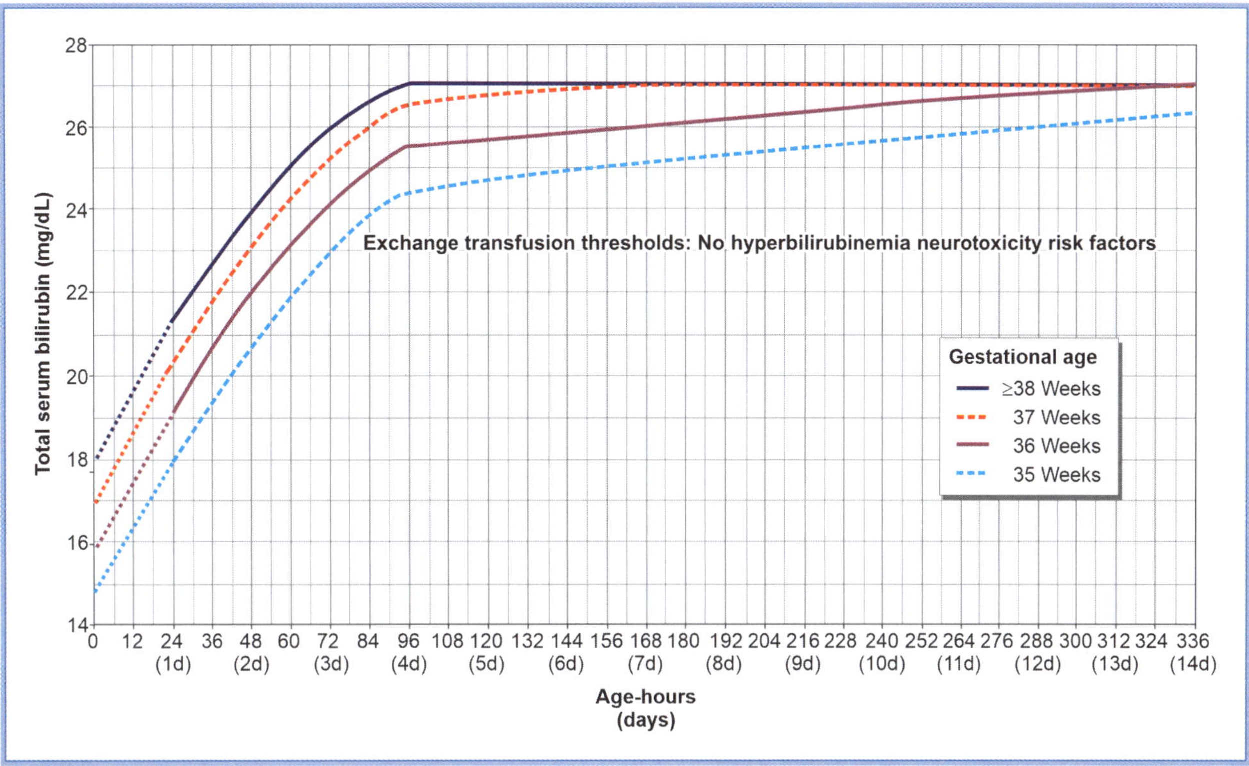

Fig. 16.15: Guidelines for exchange transfusion in infants of 35 or more weeks of gestation without neurotoxicity risk factors (described earlier in this chapter)

Source: Practice Guideline, American Academy of Pediatrics, 2022

Mechanism

Exchange transfusion removes bilirubin, antibodies, sensitized RBCs, and corrects anemia. Normally, double volume exchange transfusion is carried out (normal blood volume 80 mL/kg). This replaces 87% of infant's blood volume and serum bilirubin levels decline by 50%. The guidelines for exchange transfusion in neonates >35 weeks are detailed in **Figures 16.15 and 16.16**.

Management of hyperbilirubinemia in LBW babies is described in **Table 16.17**.

Pharmacological Therapy for Unconjugated Hyperbilirubinemia

- *Intravenous immunoglobulin:* It is effective in preventing immune-mediated hemolysis due to Rh and ABO hemolytic disease. The dose is 0.5–1.0 g/kg intravenously over 2–4 hours. It inhibits hemolysis by blocking Fc receptors on reticuloendothelial cells, thereby preventing them from taking up and lysing antibody-coated RBCs. It has no role in nonimmune-mediated hemolysis or nonhemolytic jaundice.
- *Metalloprotoporphyrins* such as tin and zinc protoporphyrins can reduce bilirubin levels by inhibiting heme oxygenase, enzyme necessary for the conversion of heme to biliverdin. These agents are still experimental, and more data is needed on efficacy and safety.
- *Inhibitors of enterohepatic circulation:* These agents include charcoal, agar, and cholestyramine. The efficacy is doubtful.
- *Phenobarbitone:* It is an inducer of hepatic microsomal enzymes and increases bilirubin conjugation and excretion. However, it is not used due to its side effects and late-onset of action.

Is there any Beneficial Role of Bilirubin?

It has been recognized that bilirubin has antioxidant properties. Newborn babies have inadequately developed antioxidant defenses. Bilirubin may serve as a transient antioxidant in the first a few days of life before antioxidant defense mechanisms mature. This may explain near universal elevation of bilirubin levels in neonate.

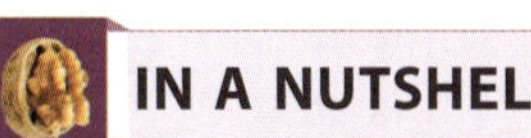

IN A NUTSHELL

Neonatal Hyperbilirubinemia

1. Bilirubin is derived from the breakdown of heme from destruction of RBCs.
2. Jaundice appears first on the face at serum bilirubin levels of 5–6 mg/dL and then progresses in a cephalocaudal manner to the trunk and extremities. Staining of palms and soles indicates serum bilirubin >15 mg/dL and considered a danger sign.
3. Neonatal jaundice is considered pathological, if it appears on day 1 of age; persists beyond 2 weeks; total serum bilirubin levels exceed 15 mg/dL or conjugated serum bilirubin is >2 mg/dL or >20% of total bilirubin; rise in serum bilirubin level is >0.5 mg/dL/h; or associated with signs of illness.
4. Unconjugated bilirubin is neurotoxic. Severe unconjugated hyperbilirubinemia can result in neuronal damage (kernicterus/bilirubin encephalopathy). Conjugated bilirubin does not cause brain damage.
5. Phototherapy forms the backbone of effective management of unconjugated hyperbilirubinemia.

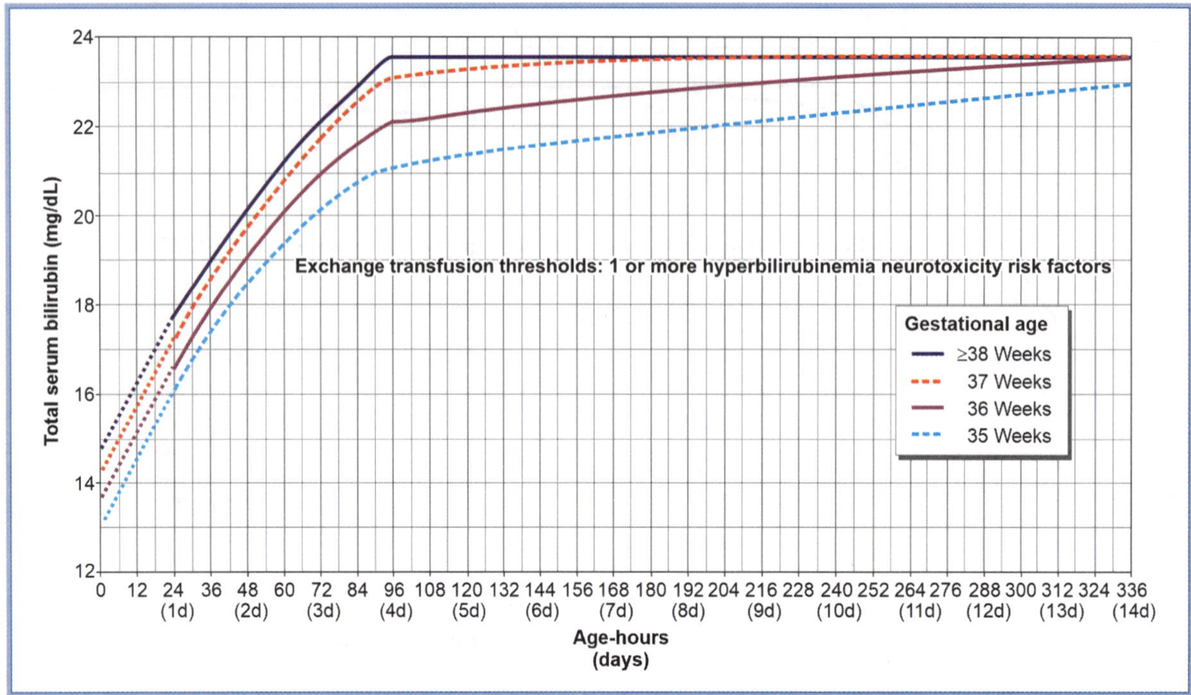

Fig. 16.16: Guidelines for exchange transfusion in hospitalized infants of 35 or more weeks of gestation with one or more neurotoxicity risk factors (described earlier in this chapter)

Source: Practice Guideline, American Academy of Pediatrics, 2022

Table 16.17 Guidelines for Management of Hyperbilirubinemia in Low Birth Weight Neonates

	Total serum bilirubin (mg/dL)	
Birth weight (g)	*Phototherapy*	*Exchange transfusion*
≤1,500	5–8	13–16
1,500–1,999	8–12	16–18
2,000–2,499	11–14	18–20

Fawke J, Wyllie J, Udaeta E, et al. International Liaison Committee On Resuscitation Neonatal Life Support Task Force. Suctioning of clear amniotic fluid at birth: A systematic review. Resusc Plus. 2022;12:100298.

Gazzin S, Jayanti S, Tiribelli C. Models of bilirubin neurological damage: lessons learned and new challenges. Pediatr Res; 2022.

Kemper AR, Newman TB, Slaughter JL, et al. Clinical Practice Guideline Revision: Management of Hyperbilirubinemia in the Newborn Infant 35 or More Weeks of Gestation. Pediatrics. 2022;150(3):e2022058859.

Kuzniewicz MW, Li SX, McCulloch CE, et al. Predicting the Need for phototherapy After Discharge: Update for 2022 Phototherapy Guidelines. Pediatrics. 2022;150(3):e2022058020.

Lazarus G, Francie J, Roeslani RD, et al. Role of ursodeoxycholic acid in neonatal indirect hyperbilirubinemia: a systematic review and meta-analysis of randomized controlled trials. Ital J Pediatr. 2022;48(1):179.

Olusanya BO, Emokpae AA. Use of Transcutaneous Bilirubin to Determine the Need for Phototherapy in Resource-Limited Settings. Neonatology. 2017;111(4):324-30.

Sampurna MTA, Ratnasari KA, Irawan ZS, et al. Evaluation of a mobile application tool (BiliNorm) to improve care for newborns with hyperbilirubinemia in Indonesia. PLoS One. 2022;17(6): e0269286.

Sherbiny HS, Youssef DM, Sherbini AS, et al. High-intensity light-emitting diode vs fluorescent tubes for intensive phototherapy in neonates. Paediatr Int Child Health. 2016;36(2):127-33.

So V, Khurshid F. Treatment practices and implementation of guidelines for hyperbilirubinemia and rebound hyperbilirubinemia. J Neonatal Perinatal Med. 2022;15(2):335-43.

Zhang M, Tang J, He Y, et al. Systematic review of global clinical practice guidelines for neonatal hyperbilirubinemia. BMJ Open. 2021;11(1):e040182.

16.14 Intrauterine and Perinatal Infections

PE 19.14

INTRODUCTION

The maternal infections that are transmissible in utero at several stages of the pregnancy can be caused by many organisms, of which the members of the TORCH complex, namely *Toxoplasma gondii*, Rubella virus, CMV, and the HSV. These infections are associated with inadvertent outcomes including abortion, LBW, intrauterine fetal death, stillbirth, and congenital malformations especially when they are acquired during the first trimester of the pregnancy. Other well-described causes of in utero infection include syphilis, *Enteroviruses*, Varicella-Zoster virus and *Parvovirus* B19. *Zika* virus is the latest addition to the group of intrauterine infections.

Transmission: The intrauterine infection is more likely to be transmitted to the fetus if the maternal infection is primary and occurs later in the pregnancy. The severity of fetal disease is more if infection is acquired in the first trimester.

CLINICAL FEATURES

Intrauterine infections may be suspected either on the basis of laboratory results obtained during pregnancy or clinical manifestation in the newborn which include features such as hydrops fetalis, microcephaly, seizures, cataract, hearing loss, congenital heart diseases, hepatosplenomegaly, jaundice, rash, and thrombocytopenia. Though the clinical symptoms are overlapping, there are some features more common in one infection than the other as summarized in **Table 16.18**. Clinical spectrum and features of each infection are described here:

Congenital Toxoplasmosis

Most (70–90%) infants infected with *T. gondii* are asymptomatic at birth. More severe manifestations usually indicate infection earlier in gestation, whereas fetal infections occurring in the third trimester are usually subclinical at birth. The classic diagnostic triad of symptoms (chorioretinitis, hydrocephalus, and intracranial calcifications) is rare. More common manifestations include anemia, seizures, jaundice, splenomegaly, hepatomegaly, and thrombocytopenia. Newborns showing mild or no signs and symptoms are still at high risk for development of late manifestations and sequelae of the disease which include chorioretinitis and motor and cerebellar dysfunction. Approximately 20% of infants are noted to have retinal lesions at birth, but up to 90% of untreated congenitally infected infants develop chorioretinitis, into and including early adulthood.

Congenital Syphilis

Most affected infants will be asymptomatic at birth, but clinical signs usually develop within the first 3 months of life. The most common signs of early congenital syphilis (<2 years old) include hepatosplenomegaly, rash, condylomata lata, watery nasal discharge (snuffles), jaundice, anemia or edema, and skeletal abnormalities (osteochondritis, periostitis, and pseudoparalysis). Late congenital syphilis in an untreated older child (>2 years old) may have stigmata with bony changes (frontal bossing, short maxilla, high palatal arch, Hutchinson teeth, and saddle nose), interstitial keratitis, and sensorineural deafness, among others. The Centers for Disease Control and Prevention (CDC) 2015 case definition for congenital syphilis includes the following:

Laboratory Criteria for Diagnosis

Demonstration of *Treponema pallidum* by darkfield microscopy, PCR, or immunohistochemical (IHC) test, or special stains of specimens from lesions, placenta, umbilical cord, or autopsy material.

Table 16.18 Clinical Findings Associated with Selected TORCH Infections

Infection	*Hepato-splenomegaly*	*Cardiac lesion*	*Skin lesions*	*Hydro-cephalus*	*Micro-cephaly*	*Intracranial calcifications*	*Ocular disease*	*Hearing deficits*
Toxoplasmosis	+	(–)	Petechiae, purpura, maculopapular rash	++	+	Diffuse intracranial calcifications	Chorioretinitis	(–)
Treponema pallidum	+	(–)	Petechiae, purpura, maculopapular rash	(–)	(–)	(–)	Chorioretinitis, glaucoma	(–)
Rubella	+	PDA, PS, myocarditis	Petechiae, purpura	+	(–)	(–)	Chorioretinitis, cataracts, microphthalmia	++
CMV	+	+	Petechiae, purpura	(–)	++	Periventricular calcifications	Chorioretinitis	++
HSV	+	Myocarditis	Petechiae, purpura, vesicles	+	+	(–)	Chorioretinitis, cataracts	+

(CMV: Cytomegalovirus; HSV: herpes simplex virus; PDA: patent ductus arteriosus)

Case Classification

- ***Probable:*** Infant whose mother had untreated or inadequately treated syphilis at delivery, regardless of signs in the infant, or an infant or child who has a reactive nontreponemal test for syphilis [venereal disease research laboratory (VDRL), rapid plasma reagin (RPR) or equivalent] and any one of the following:
  - Any evidence of congenital syphilis on physical examination
  - Any evidence of congenital syphilis on radiographs of long bones
  - A reactive CSF VDRL test
  - An elevated CSF cell count or protein (without other cause)
- ***Confirmed:*** Case that is laboratory confirmed.

Congenital Rubella

The classic picture of congenital rubella syndrome (CRS) is a small for age infant with a constellation of anomalies which include sensorineural deafness (66%), cataracts (78%), cardiac defects (58%), and ocular abnormalities. Cardiac manifestations include PDA, pulmonary artery stenosis and coarctation of aorta. Eye findings are microphthalmia, corneal opacity and glaucoma. Features common to other perinatal infections such as the blueberry muffin rash, hepatosplenomegaly, and thrombocytopenia may also be present. Delayed manifestations include a higher incidence of diabetes mellitus, hypertension, panencephalitis, and behavioral disorders.

Congenital Cytomegalovirus Infection

The CMV infection is the most common congenital infection and a leading cause of birth defects and childhood disabilities. Primary CMV infection in mother can be transmitted in up to 30–40% of pregnancies. Only 1% of fetuses are infected, if the mother is having recurrent/secondary CMV infection. Most infected children (90%) are asymptomatic, 10% of these develop hearing loss, global developmental delay, microcephaly in first year of life. Symptomatic infection (10%) can be fulminant (liver failure, chorioretinitis, and bleeding neonate), or present with low birth weight, microcephaly, or UGR.

DIAGNOSIS

Viral culture, PCR, and disease-specific serology are the usual investigations for diagnosis of congenital infections. Of these, serological diagnosis (especially on a single sample) is highly unreliable. Preferred diagnostic tests for common intrauterine infections are listed in **Table 16.19**.

A stepwise approach to a child with suspected TORCH infection is given here:

- ***Step 1:*** *Estimate cord blood total IgM antibody*
  - *<18–20% mg:* Infection less likely, but still possible.
  - *>20% mg:* High likelihood of infection, proceed to steps 2–5. If negative, pursue expanded TORCH for *Parvovirus*, Epstein–Barr virus (EBV), hepatitis B virus (HBV), etc.
- ***Step 2:*** *Perform CMV urine culture*
  - If positive, confirms congenital CMV
  - If negative, excludes CMV, go to step 3
  - If no facility for culture—estimate IgM
    - If positive, indicates infection (high chances)
    - If negative, estimate IgG and repeat after 4 weeks. Run both samples together. Four-fold rise indicates infection.
- ***Step 3:*** *Estimate toxoplasma IgG*
  - If negative, rules out congenital toxoplasmosis, go to step 4
  - If positive, get IgM done
    - IgM positive indicates disease
    - IgM negative does not rule out disease, repeat IgG after 3–4 weeks for four-fold rise.
- ***Step 4:*** *Perform rubella serology*
  - Rubella IgG
    - If negative, rules out infection, immunize mother
    - If positive, not diagnostic, do IgM
  - Rubella IgM antibody
    - If positive, confirms congenital rubella
    - If negative, does not rule out rubella, repeat after 4 weeks or demonstrate low avidity antibodies
  - Rubella viral cultures
- ***Step 5:*** *Investigate for HSV infection*
  - HSV culture (most definite)
    - If positive, perinatal herpes present
    - If negative, does not rule out herpes
  - IgM antibodies to HSV
    - If negative, does not rule out herpes
    - If positive, not diagnostic, estimate IgG
      - If positive, perinatal infection
      - If negative, does not rule out herpes
  - CSF PCR in HSV encephalitis

Table 16.19 Diagnostic Tools for Common Intrauterine Infections

Congenital infection	*Best diagnostic test*
CMV	Viral isolation/PCR of urine, saliva in first 2 weeks
Herpes	Viral isolation: skin, CSF, stool, urine, eye; PCR: CSF
Rubella	Rubella IgM, low avidity IgG; viral isolation: urine, CSF, oral cavity
Toxoplasmosis	Toxo IgM (80% sensitivity), CSF PCR, IgA and IgE in references labs
Syphilis	IgM FTA-ABS, dark field microscopy, and serial VDRL

(CMV: cytomegalovirus; CSF: cerebrospinal fluid; FTA-ABS: fluorescent treponemal antibody absorption; Ig: immunoglobulin; PCR: polymerase chain reaction; VDRL: venereal disease research laboratory)

TREATMENT Intrauterine and Perinatal Infections

There is no specific treatment for congenital rubella infection. For CMV, available drugs include ganciclovir, foscarnet, and cidofovir. These are helpful only in severe symptomatic cases. Acyclovir is the drug of choice for congenital HSV infection, to be given for 2–3 weeks. Congenital toxoplasmosis is treated with a combination of sulfadiazine, pyrimethamine, and folinic acid for 1 year. Spiramycin may be used in last 6 months. Steroids are given for chorioretinitis and disseminated disease.

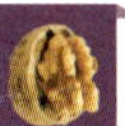

IN A NUTSHELL

Intrauterine and Perinatal Infections

1. The acronym *TORCH-S [Toxoplasma gondii*, rubella virus, *Cytomegalovirus* (CMV), herpes simplex virus (HSV), and syphilis] captures the main list of organisms that cause congenital infections in the newborn.
2. These infections are associated with inadvertent outcomes including abortion, low birth weight, intrauterine fetal death, stillbirth, and congenital malformations especially when they are acquired during the first trimester of the pregnancy.
3. Other well-described causes of in utero infection include syphilis, *Enteroviruses*, Varicella–Zoster virus and *Parvovirus* B19. *Zika* virus is the latest addition to the group of intrauterine infections.
4. *Cytomegalovirus*, rubella, and toxoplasmosis are the most common causes of chronic intrauterine infections in the fetus and newborn.
5. Herpes simplex infection is characterized by the triad of cutaneous, ophthalmic, and neurologic involvement.
6. Congenital tuberculosis should be suspected in newborns who have nonresolving pneumonia, persistent fever, and hepatosplenomegaly, in the absence of any bacterial pathogen isolated on culture.
7. Congenital Zika virus infection results in microcephaly.

American Academy of Pediatrics. Rubella. In: Pickering LK, Baker CJ, Kimberlin DW (Eds). Red book: 2012 report of the Committee on Infectious Diseases, 29th edition. Elk Grove Village (IL): American Academy of Pediatrics; 2012. p. 629.

American Academy of Pediatrics. Syphilis. In: Kimberlin DW, Brady MT, Jackson MA, et al. (Eds). Red Book: 2015 Report of the Committee on Infectious Diseases, 30th edition. Elk Grove Village, IL: American Academy of Pediatrics; 2015. pp. 755-68.

Bialas KM, Swamy GK, Permar SR. Perinatal cytomegalovirus and varicella zoster virus infections: epidemiology, prevention, and treatment. Clin Perinatol. 2015;42(1):61-75.

Jamali Moghadam SR, Bayrami S, Jamali Moghadam S, et al. Zika virus: a review of literature. Asian Pac J Trop Biomed. 2016; 6(12):989-94.

James SH, Kimberlin DW. Neonatal herpes simplex virus infection: epidemiology and treatment. Clin Perinatol. 2015;42(1):47-59.

Kimberlin DW, Baley J; Committee on Infectious Diseases, Committee on Fetus and Newborn. Guidance on management of asymptomatic neonates born to women with active genital herpes lesions. Pediatrics. 2013;131(2):383-6.

Kimberlin DW, Jester PM, Sánchez PJ, et al. Valganciclovir for symptomatic congenital cytomegalovirus disease. N Engl J Med. 2015;372(10):933-43.

Neu N, Duchon J, Zachariah P. TORCH infections. Clin Perinatol. 2015;42(1): 77-103.

16.15 Oxygen Toxicity in Newborns

PE 19.17

INCIDENCE

Oxygen toxicity in newborns, particularly in preterm infants, is a significant concern due to their dependency on supplemental oxygen for respiratory distress syndrome (RDS). The incidence is notably high among neonates requiring prolonged oxygen therapy, with complications such as bronchopulmonary dysplasia (BPD) and retinopathy of prematurity (ROP) affecting nearly 40% of extremely preterm infants (<28 weeks of gestation). The risk escalates with higher oxygen concentrations and extended exposure periods.

ETIOLOGY

The core issue behind oxygen toxicity lies in excessive oxygen exposure, resulting in the production of harmful reactive oxygen species (ROS). Several factors influence susceptibility:

- ***Prematurity:*** Immature antioxidant systems in preterm infants make them highly vulnerable.
- ***Prolonged oxygen exposure:*** High oxygen concentrations (>50% FiO_2) elevate risk.
- ***Oxidative stress:*** Hyperoxia-induced ROS cause cellular damage.
- ***Genetic variations:*** Some infants may have diminished antioxidant enzyme activity, increasing susceptibility.

PATHOGENESIS

Oxygen toxicity arises from oxidative stress induced by hyperoxia. Hyperoxia leads to the overproduction of reactive oxygen species (ROS), including superoxide anions, hydroxyl radicals, and hydrogen peroxide. Neonates, particularly preterm infants, lack sufficient protective enzymes such as superoxide dismutase and catalase, which impairs their antioxidant defense. Consequently, oxidative damage disrupts cell membranes through lipid peroxidation, leading to apoptosis and tissue inflammation. The inflammatory response is exacerbated by cytokines like TNF-α and IL-6, which further contribute to lung tissue injury. Hyperoxia also disrupts retinal vessel formation, resulting in retinopathy of prematurity (ROP) and potential blindness.

CLINICAL MANIFESTATIONS

Pulmonary effects: **Bronchopulmonary dysplasia (BPD)**—characterized by alveolar simplification, fibrosis, and prolonged respiratory support dependency; and **acute lung injury**—leads to surfactant dysfunction, atelectasis, and oxygen dependence.

Ophthalmologic effects: **Retinopathy of prematurity (ROP)**—excess oxygen prevents normal retinal vascularization, resulting in neovascularization and potential retinal detachment.

Neurological effects: **White matter injury**—oxidative stress damages brain tissue, increasing the risk of periventricular leukomalacia and subsequent **neurodevelopmental delay**.

Cardiovascular effects: **Pulmonary hypertension** leading to long-term hypertension risks.

DIAGNOSIS

Oxygen toxicity is primarily diagnosed through clinical evaluation, imaging, and laboratory tests. Pulse oximetry and blood gas analysis are essential for monitoring oxygen saturation and PaO_2. Chest radiography helps identify lung changes indicative of BPD. Retinal examination is used to detect early signs of ROP. MRI scan can reveal white matter abnormalities linked to oxidative stress.

TREATMENT Oxygen Toxicity

Management focuses on reducing oxygen exposure and mitigating oxidative damage:

- *Optimizing oxygen therapy*: Maintaining SpO_2 within safe limits (90–95% in preterm infants).
- *Use of antioxidants*: Vitamin A, E, and glutathione precursors help counteract oxidative damage.
- *Steroids*: Dexamethasone may reduce inflammation in BPD but is used cautiously due to adverse effects.
- *Supportive care*: Mechanical ventilation strategies such as volume-targeted ventilation to minimize lung injury.
- *Retinal interventions*: Anti-VEGF therapy or laser photocoagulation for advanced ROP.

PREVENTION

Preventing oxygen toxicity requires careful oxygen management strategies. Targeted oxygen therapy involves avoiding hyperoxia by using guidelines for oxygen saturation limits. Oxygen weaning protocols emphasize the gradual reduction of oxygen to minimize exposure. Early antioxidant support is crucial, encouraging maternal nutrition rich in antioxidants during pregnancy. Noninvasive ventilation methods such as CPAP and nasal cannula help reduce exposure to high oxygen concentrations. Surfactant therapy is also employed to reduce the need for prolonged mechanical ventilation in preterm infants.

Behnke J, Dippel CM, Choi Y, et al. Oxygen toxicity to the immature lung—Part II: The unmet clinical need for causal therapy. Int J Mol Sci. 2021;22(19):10694.

Cherian S, Morris I, Evans J, Kotecha S. Oxygen therapy in preterm infants. Paediatr Respir Rev. 2014;15(2):135-41.

Darlow BA, Morley CJ. Oxygen saturation targeting and bronchopulmonary dysplasia. Clin Perinatol. 2015;42(4):807-23.

Kapadia V, Wyckoff MH. Oxygen therapy in the delivery room: What Is the right dose? Clin Perinatol. 2018;45(2):293-306.

Kayton A, Timoney P, Vargo L, Perez JA. A review of oxygen physiology and appropriate management of oxygen levels in premature neonates. Adv Neonatal Care. 2018;18(2):98-104.

Nguyen TC, Madappa R, Siefkes HM, et al. Oxygen saturation targets in neonatal care: A narrative review. Early Hum Dev. 2024;199:106134.

16.16 Common Surgical Conditions *PE 19.16*

TRACHEOESOPHAGEAL FISTULA

Tracheoesophageal fistula (TEF) is a congenital communication between the trachea and esophagus. Approximately 17–70% of children with TEFs have associated developmental anomalies such as Down syndrome, duodenal atresia, and cardiovascular defects. As per gross classification, there are five types of TEF with type C, blind upper esophageal pouch, and lower esophageal pouch communicating with the trachea, being the most common type **(Fig. 16.17)**.

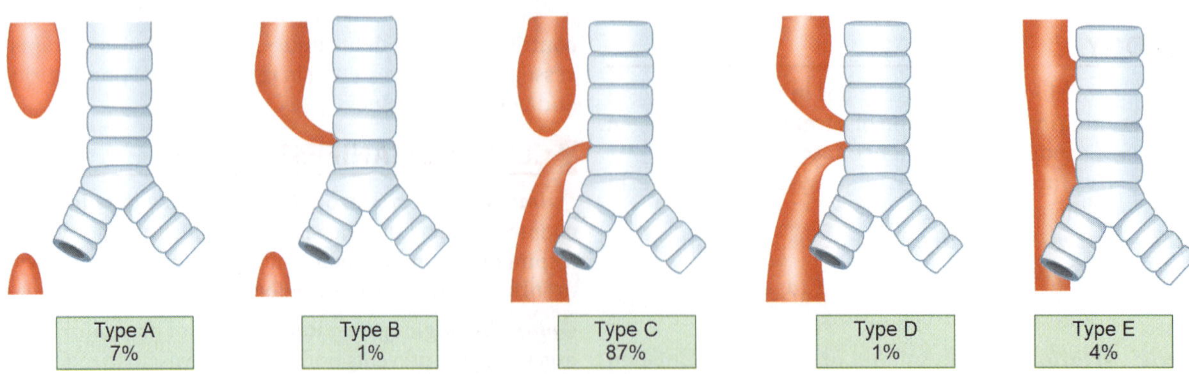

Fig. 16.17: Types of tracheoesophageal fistula with incidence

Clinical Features

Neonates with TEF usually develop copious, fine white frothy bubbles of mucus in the mouth and nose. Secretions recur despite suctioning. Infants may develop rattling respiration and episodes of coughing and choking in association with cyanosis. Symptoms worsen during feeding in the presence of a TEF.

Diagnosis

Fetal diagnosis: Esophageal atresia in the fetus should be suspected in presence of maternal polyhydramnios. Absence of stomach gas on prenatal ultrasound is another indication of esophageal atresia.

Diagnosis in the neonate is confirmed when an orogastric tube cannot be passed beyond 10 cm. Plain chest radiographs may reveal tracheal compression and deviation. Absence of a gastric bubble indicates esophageal atresia without a TEF or esophageal atresia with a proximal TEF. X-ray is usually done after putting an orogastric tube and pushing around 10 mL of air; coiling of the tube within dilated blind pouch of esophagus can be seen.

TREATMENT Tracheoesophageal Fistula

The baby should be kept nil orally and given intravenous fluids. The baby is nursed supine or in semi-upright position with frequent suctioning of esophageal pouch to avoid aspiration of secretions. Surgical repair is undertaken at the earliest.

CONGENITAL DIAPHRAGMATIC HERNIA

The incidence is 1 in 4,000 live births. Herniation of abdominal visceral contents through the posterolateral foramen of Bochdalek (more common) or the anterior foramen of Morgagni (rare) leads to diaphragmatic hernia. Maldevelopment of the posthepatic mesenchymal plate and closure of pleuroperitoneal canal, which is crucial for normal diaphragmatic development, result in congenital diaphragmatic hernia (CDH). Presence of abdominal viscera in the chest during fetal life also prevents normal development of the lungs. Defect is more common on the left side.

Clinical Features

Cyanosis, tachypnea, grunting, and retraction are commonly seen soon after birth. On physical examination, the abdomen is scaphoid, the anteroposterior diameter of the chest is increased, mediastinal shift may be noted, breath sounds are absent on the affected side, and bowel sounds may be heard in chest.

Diagnosis

Prenatal diagnosis can be made on ultrasonography. There may be maternal polyhydramnios. The advantage of prenatal diagnosis is that baby can be delivered in a center where surgery can be done. Postnatal diagnosis is made from the chest radiograph which shows air-filled bowel loops in the chest cavity with nonvisualization of diaphragmatic margin, mediastinal shift, and a relative paucity of abdominal gas **(Fig. 16.18)**. Findings can be confirmed on ultrasonography.

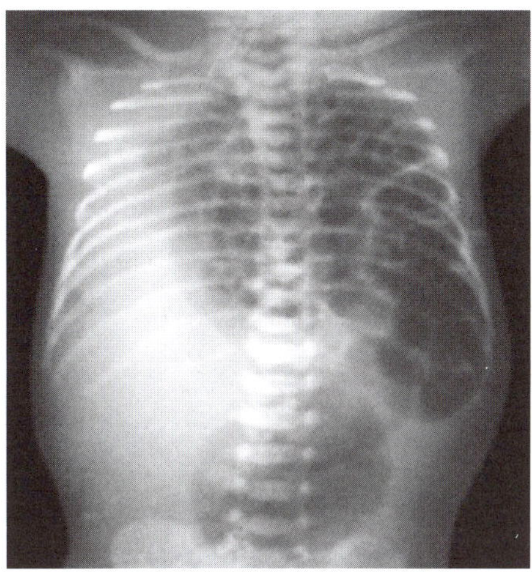

Fig. 16.18: Chest X-ray showing air-filled bowel loops in the left chest cavity with nonvisualization of left dome of diaphragm and mediastinal shift to the right; suggestive of left-sided diaphragmatic hernia

After initial stabilization, definitive treatment is surgical repair. Severe cases diagnosed antenatally have been successfully managed with ex utero intrapartum treatment (EXIT) procedure. EXIT involves maternal laparotomy, partial delivery of fetus through the uterine opening, fetal intubation followed by either complete delivery or immediate institution of ECMO.

TREATMENT Congenital Diaphragmatic Hernia

Bag and mask ventilation is contraindicated in babies with known or suspected diaphragmatic hernia as it causes bowel distention and increases the mediastinal shift further which affects the contralateral lung and also compromises cardiac function. If needed, use bag and endotracheal tube to provide ventilation in these babies.

After admission in NICU, baby is given supportive care. Mechanical ventilation should be done with low inspiratory.

EVENTRATION OF THE DIAPHRAGM

It results from maldevelopment of the diaphragm muscle which is replaced by a thin membranous structure. It usually presents in older children but in newborns it may be difficult to differentiate from CDH. The treatment consists of diaphragmatic plication which can be carried out either by thoracotomy or laparotomy.

CLEFT LIP AND CLEFT PALATE

Cleft lip and palate **(Fig. 16.19)** are common congenital malformations with incidence of cleft lip with or without cleft palate being 1:1000 whereas incidence of isolated cleft palate is 1:2500. Isolated cleft palate occurs uniformly across different ethnicities, whereas incidence of cleft lip with or without cleft palate varies with race with incidence being higher among Asians followed by

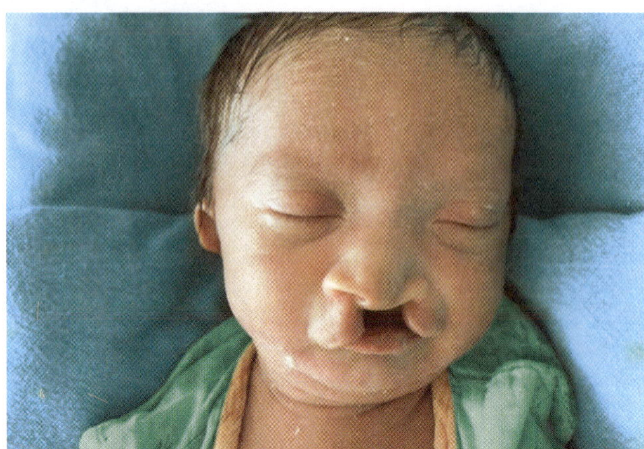

Fig. 16.19: Neonate with cleft lip and palate

Caucasians and Africans. Gender prediction also varies in both the entities:

- ***For isolated cleft palate:*** Male:female—0.5:1
- ***For cleft lip and palate:*** Male:female—2:1

Etiology

Approximately 40% of the cases of cleft lip and palate and isolated cleft palate have following additional congenital anomalies and syndromes in the form of congenital heart defects, hydrocephalus, and urinary tract defects (9.7%), CHARGE syndrome (CHD7), velocardiofacial syndrome (TBX1, COMT), and Apert syndrome (FGFR2). Neonates with isolated cleft palate are twice more likely have associated anomalies compared to cases with both cleft lip/palate. Various exposures associated with cleft lip and palate are smoking, pregestational and gestational diabetes, alcohol abuse, anticonvulsants and deficiency of folate, and vitamins B_6 and B_{12}.

Diagnosis

Prenatal diagnosis: Detection rate of cleft lip and palate varies from 0 to 70% by 2D ultrasound performed between 18 and 20 weeks of gestation. Isolated cleft palate is less likely to be detected prenatally. 3D ultrasound has better detection rate for orofacial clefts.

Postnatal diagnosis: Diagnosis is made clinically and ultrasound of abdomen and head and echocardiography are important to diagnose the associated anomalies.

TREATMENT Cleft Lip and Cleft Palate

Multidisciplinary team is needed for managing orofacial clefts.

- All the neonates with orofacial clefts should be evaluated for feeding difficulties as lack of seal may result in breastfeeding failure especially in babies with cleft palate. Cleft specific bottles with a long teat are available to bottle feed the babies but hygienic practices should be well explained to the parents before advising bottles.
- To decrease cleft width, improve nasal symmetry, and improve psychological outcomes for caregivers, lip taping (tape applied across the cleft lip), and nasoalveolar molding (NAM) are suggested in the neonatal period.
- Definitive lip repair is performed at age 3 months (10 weeks) when baby weighs at least 4.5 kg and hemoglobin level is 10 g/dL. The three prerequisites for surgery is also referred as rule of 10 seconds and first described by Wilhelmsen and Musgrave. Operative technique for repair of unilateral and bilateral cleft lip is called as Millard or Fisher technique and Millard technique, respectively. Palatoplasty is typically done between 9 and 12 months of age which improves speech outcomes especially if soft palate is repaired before 12 months.

Complications of Cleft Lip and Palate Repair

Complications of unilateral cleft lip repair include deficient vermilion or a whistle deformity, muscular dehiscence, and nasal asymmetry. Complications of cleft palate repair include palatal fistula, obstructive sleep apnea, and velopharyngeal dysfunction. Neonates with cleft palate are at higher risk of sensorineural, conductive, and mixed hearing loss.

ACUTE ABDOMEN IN NEONATES

Clinical entities comprising acute abdomen in neonates and their causes are enlisted here.

Acute Peritonitis

Necrotizing enterocolitis (NEC): NEC is an inflammatory disease of the bowel wall with or without necrosis, in the absence of mechanical obstruction, affecting 5–10% of preterm infants weighing <1,000 g. Clinical presentation consists of vomiting, abdominal distention, shock, intestinal hemorrhage, and perforation **(Fig. 16.20)**.

Spontaneous intestinal perforation (SIP): SIP is focal small bowel perforation affecting approximately 2% of extremely LBW neonates. It presents as a gasless abdomen or as an asymptomatic pneumoperitoneum **(Fig. 16.21)** at an earlier postnatal age than NEC. SIP is characterized by significantly lower morbidity and mortality compared to NEC.

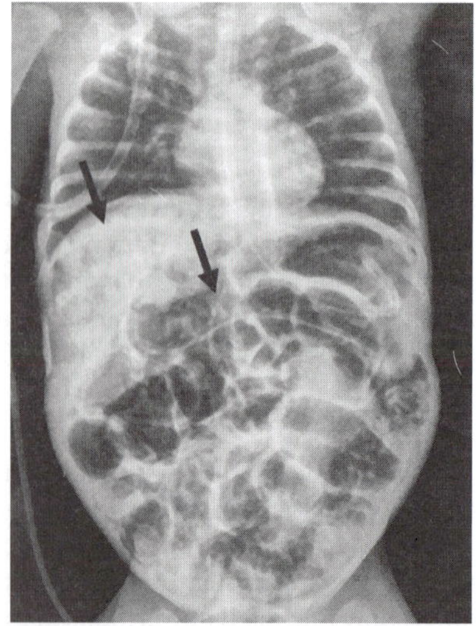

Fig. 16.20: Necrotizing enterocolitis—portal venous gas and presence of gas within the wall of the intestine

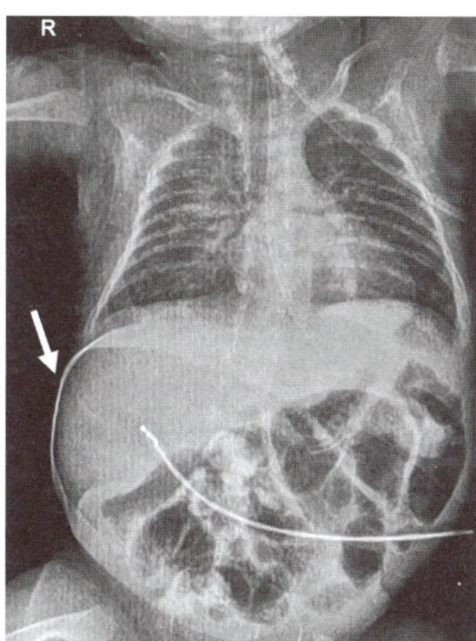

Fig. 16.21: Bowel perforation—free air over the liver shadow, pneumoperitoneum

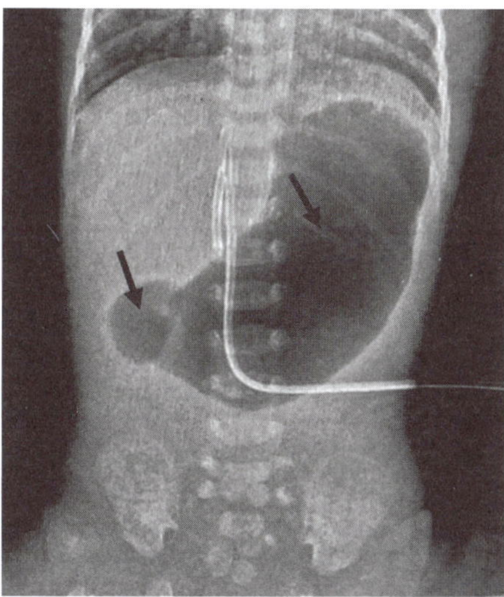

Fig. 16.22: Double bubble (dilated stomach and duodenal cap)—suggestive of duodenal atresia, Ladd bands, and annular pancreas

Intestinal Obstruction

Neonatal intestinal obstruction affects 1 in 2,000 live births and can be mechanical or functional. Various causes of intestinal obstruction include duodenal atresia, malrotation and midgut volvulus, jejunoileal atresia **(Fig. 16.22)**, intestinal duplications, Meckel diverticulum, meconium ileus **(Fig. 16.23)**, Hirschsprung disease, and anorectal malformations. Congenital duodenal atresia or stenosis is the most common of the intestinal atresia. Malrotation refers to all abnormalities of intestinal position and attachment.

Features of intestinal obstruction include maternal polyhydramnios in the antenatal period, bilious emesis, failure to pass meconium in the first day of life, and abdominal distention (more common in lower obstructions). The presence of bile-stained vomiting in the newborn is a life-threatening emergency, with at least 20% of such infants requiring emergency surgical intervention after evaluation. Bilious in a neonate is malrotation until proven otherwise.

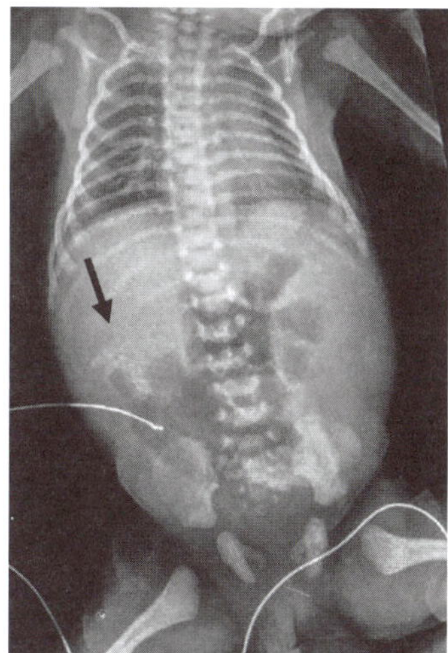

Fig. 16.23: Abdominal calcifications in meconium ileus

Ascites

Neonatal ascites may result from heart failure, chylous ascites, biliary leak, and urinary ascites.

Abdominal Mass

Most common abdominal mass is multicystic dysplastic kidney in neonates. Other common causes include unilateral hydronephrosis, hemorrhagic neuroblastoma, and intraperitoneal cysts. Ultrasonography is important to evaluate the cause of abdominal mass.

Abdominal Bleeding

Bleeding in the intestinal tract is more often part of systemic illness leading to DIC. Peptic ulceration in areas of ectopic gastric mucosa in Meckel's diverticulum and intestinal duplications may also manifest with bleeding.

Abdominal Wall Abnormalities

Gastroschisis and exomphalos are most common abdominal wall defects. The intestines prolapse alongside and usually to the right of the umbilical cord, through a small defect, and lie free in the amniotic cavity in gastroschisis. It is associated with midgut atresia in 10% of the cases.

Exomphalos is a defect in which the bowel is enclosed within a membrane formed by the base of the umbilical cord. It is often associated with other abnormalities, including trisomy, congenital heart disease, and the Beckwith-Wiedemann syndrome.

TREATMENT Acute Abdomen in Neonates

Antenatal ultrasound may provide clue to various gastrointestinal anomalies as summarized in **Table 16.20**. Neonates suspected to have gastrointestinal anomalies should be transported in utero to centers providing neonatal surgeries and postoperative care. Neonates with abdominal wall defects are prone for fluid and heat loss through the defect requiring utmost care of temperature and fluid and electrolyte balance.

Table 16.20 Antenatal Ultrasound Clues to Gastrointestinal Anomalies

Findings	*Differentials*	*Comments*
Persistent small volume stomach and polyhydramnios	Esophageal atresia	Proximal pouch distention is intermittent so unreliable, magnetic resonance imaging (MRI) may help
Polyhydramnios and distended stomach (Single bubble)	Gastric outlet obstruction (pyloric atresia)	–
Double bubble of dilated stomach and duodenal bulb, polyhydramnios	Duodenal atresia, Ladd bands, and annular pancreas	Malrotation of gut occurs in 29% of cases
Triple bubble and polyhydramnios	Very proximal jejunal atresia	–
Multiple dilated, fluid-filled loops, and polyhydramnios	Distal jejunal and ileal atresia	Small intestine is considered dilated if diameter is >7 mm
Hyperechoic debris filling distended loops	Meconium ileus	On MRI, meconium is hyperintense on T1-weighted images and intermediate on T2
Defects of the abdominal wall, intra-abdominal cysts, fetal ascites, and solid organ	–	–

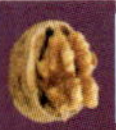

IN A NUTSHELL

Common Surgical Conditions

1. Neonates with tracheoesophageal fistula usually develop copious, fine white frothy bubbles of mucus in the mouth and nose at birth. Diagnosis in the neonate is confirmed when an orogastric tube cannot be passed.
2. Presence of air-filled bowel loops in the chest cavity with nonvisualization of diaphragmatic margin, mediastinal shift, and a relative paucity of abdominal gas, in chest X-ray suggests congenital diaphragmatic hernia.
3. Cleft lip repair is performed at age 3 months (10 weeks) when baby weighs at least 4.5 kg and hemoglobin level is 10 g/dL.
4. Features of intestinal obstruction include maternal polyhydramnios in the antenatal period, bilious emesis, failure to pass meconium in the first day of life, and abdominal distention.
5. Most common abdominal mass is multicystic dysplastic kidney in neonates.
6. Double bubble (dilated stomach and duodenal cap) in abdominal X-ray is suggestive of duodenal atresia.

de la Hunt MN. The acute abdomen in the newborn. Semin Fetal Neonatal Med. 2006;11(3):191-7.
Do WS, Lillehei CW. Malrotation: Management of Disorders of Gut Rotation for the General Surgeon. Surg Clin North Am. 2022;102(5):837-45.
Lohsiriwat V. Anorectal emergencies. World J Gastroenterol. 2016;22(26):5867-78.
Marques AT, Estevão-Costa J, Soares H, et al. Short and Medium-term Outcomes of Omphalocele and Gastroschisis: A Survey from a Tertiary Center. Rev Bras Ginecol Obstet. 2022;44(1):10-8.
Rich BS, Bornstein E, Dolgin SE. Intestinal Atresias. Pediatr Rev. 2022;43(5):266-74.
Worley ML, Patel KG, Kilpatrick LA. Cleft Lip and Palate. Clin Perinatol. 2018;45(4):661-78.

16.17 Transport and Referral of a Sick Newborn

INTRODUCTION

Transporting a sick neonate to a healthcare facility is a difficult task in India due to limitations such as lack of well-organized transport services, long geographical distances, and virtual lack of linkage between peripheral and tertiary level hospitals. The problem is further compounded by poor infrastructure and poverty and ignorance of parents.

During transport, a baby struggles not only with illness and physiological immaturity but also with other factors such as noise, vibrations, sudden jerks, and temperature variation which can further compromise the already sick baby. Therefore, large numbers of newborns die en route while being transported to the healthcare facility.

If the birth of a high-risk neonate is anticipated, it is far better to safely transport the baby in utero rather than shift a sick baby to a hospital after birth under hostile conditions. Nevertheless, if transport of a sick baby becomes necessary, it is important to understand the principles of neonatal transport and practical issues involved to optimize the outcome.

Neonatal transport encompasses not only transfer from community to the healthcare facility, but also transfer between two hospitals, or transport even within the different sectors of the same hospital such as radiology and pediatric surgery services. Transport also includes transfer of a baby back to community hospital or home from higher healthcare facility. The rules and requirements of transport remain the same regardless of the level of transport.

PRINCIPLES OF SAFE AND STABLE TRANSPORT

Prepare Well Before Transport

- ***Assess:*** Carefully assess the condition of the baby before transport. Transport only if there is a definite indication. Referring a newborn for a minor problem unnecessarily stresses the baby and the parents and brings bad name to the doctor.
- ***Communicate:*** Explain to parents the condition of the baby and the reasons for referral well before taking the decision to transport. Give them enough time to organize and arrange for the journey. It should not come as a surprise to parents to immediately shift the sick baby to a hospital. Tell them where to go and whom to contact in the hospital. If possible, the institution/facility where the referral is being made should also be informed telephonically beforehand, so that they are also well-prepared to receive the baby.
- ***Correct hypothermia before transport:*** Other than the illness itself, hypothermia is a major killer of babies during transport. Therefore, correction and prevention of hypothermia is crucial for the wellbeing of the baby. If the baby is hypothermic (temperature <36.5°C), normalize the temperature before transport. Take measures to keep baby warm during transport as mentioned here.
- ***Stabilize the baby before transport:***
  - Clear the airway of secretions
  - Resuscitate and oxygenate, if required
  - Give a feed if the baby is able to suckle
  - Put an intravenous line and start 10% dextrose or maintenance intravenous fluid with Isolyte P, if indicated. Secure intravenous cannula properly.
  - Give medications including antibiotics, if indicated
  - Administer injection vitamin K, if not given before
  - Make sure that neck is not flexed during transport
- ***Documentation:*** A proper referral note should be written which includes relevant history including maternal and birth details, present condition of the baby, need for referral and treatment given along with dosage, and reports of investigations, X-rays, etc. If the baby is having severe jaundice, or jaundice appeared on day 1 of life, send 2–3 mL of maternal blood in double oxalate vial for further workup and management.
- ***Encourage mother to accompany the baby:*** As far as possible, mother should accompany the baby for breastfeeding, providing kangaroo mother care and other supportive care to the baby on the way. If it is not possible for mother to accompany the baby, father or some other close relative should go with the baby.
- ***Arrange for trained healthcare provider to accompany on the way:*** A doctor/nurse/trained dai/health worker should accompany the baby to provide care to the baby during transport.
- ***Provide bag and mask, mucus extractor, and portable O_2 cylinder.***

Care During Transport

The accompanying person should be explained to ensure the following:

- ***Ensure warm feet and warm transport:*** During transport, baby is likely to become hypothermic due to cold environment and air turbulence. Maintaining thermal stability is crucial for baby's survival. Baby's hands and feet should remain warm to touch during transport. If the baby passes urine or stool, wipe her promptly and remove the wet linen. During transportation, warmth can be ensured by following:
  - *Skin-to-skin care (kangaroo mother care):* This is the most effective, safe, and convenient method to maintain temperature during transport.
  - *Covering the baby:* Cover the baby fully with clothes (or cotton) including the head and the limbs. Nurse the baby next to the mother or another adult during transport.
  - *Improvised containers:* Different workers have used thermocol box, basket, padded pouch, plastic covering, etc., for ensuring temperature stability during transport. The ideal mode of transport is transport incubator but this is rarely available. The use of rubber hot water bottle is fraught with considerable danger due to accidental burns to the baby, if the bottle is not wrapped properly or remains in contact with baby's body. It is, therefore, best avoided. But if no other means of providing warmth is available, this method may be employed, making sure that the hot water bottle is wrapped in four-layered clothing.
- ***Ensure an open airway:***
  - Keep the neck of the baby in slight extension
  - Do not cover the baby's mouth and nose
  - Gently wipe the secretions from the nose and the mouth with a cotton or cloth covered finger.
  - Attendants can be trained to use mucus extractor to remove secretions from mouth.
- ***Check breathing:*** Watch baby's breathing. If the baby stops breathing, provide tactile stimulation by rubbing the back or flicking the soles. Accompanying health worker can use bag and mask ventilation in the event of apnea not responding to tactile stimulation.
- ***Provide feeds:*** If baby is able to suckle on the breast, she should be offered breastfeeds. If she can take cup-feeding, expressed breastmilk can be provided carefully. If the distance is long, a nasogastric catheter may be inserted and gavage feeding given. In that case, the amount and interval of feed should be specified. If the baby is on intravenous fluids, the measured volume set should contain no more fluid than is needed for the duration of journey.

In recent years, although neonatal care has improved in many government and private hospitals, neonatal transport has not kept pace with it. There is an urgent need to improve the neonatal transport facilities in the country to optimize the outcome of these newborns.

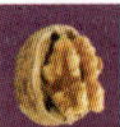

IN A NUTSHELL

Transport and Referral of a Sick Newborn

1. Infants requiring advance medical and/or nursing care exceeding what is available in their current settings will need transfer to a higher health facility.
2. Prior stabilization and adequate care during transport is essential to avoid hypoglycemia, acidosis, and mortality.
3. Neonatal transport programs require appropriate referral systems, management structures, and trained transport personnel.
4. The key components of neonatal transport are human resources, vehicles and equipment, communication, family support, and documentation.

Abdul Wahab MG, Thomas S, Murthy P, et al. Factors Affecting Stabilization Times in Neonatal Transport. Air Med J. 2019;38(5):334-7.
Bellini C, De Angelis LC, Secchi S, et al. Helicopter Neonatal Transport: First Golden Hour at Birth Is Useful Tool Guiding Activation of Appropriate Resources. Air Med J. 2020;39(6):454-7.
Bellini C. Neonatal transport. A red snapshot. Acad Emerg Med. 2022;29(3):391.
Kozuki N, Guenther T, Vaz L, et al. A systematic review of community-to-facility neonatal referral completion rates in Africa and Asia. BMC Public Health. 2015;15:989.
Ramji S. Newborn Care at First Referral Health Facilities. Indian J Pediatr. 2016;83(6):491-2.
Sacks E, Brizuela V, Perrotta C. It's the Destination and the Journey—A Mapping of the Challenges in Transport and Referral for Maternal and Newborn Health in Pandemics and Beyond. Front Public Health. 2021;9:612409.

16.18 Follow-up of High-risk Neonates

INTRODUCTION

With the improvement in the quality of neonatal care in India, more and more sick neonates including extremely low birth weight (ELBW) ones are surviving today. Unfortunately, the incidence of long-term morbidities and adverse outcome such as blindness, deafness, cognitive and learning disabilities, and behavioral problems continue to be high in the survivors. Timely and appropriate interventions are, therefore, of utmost importance to prevent or modify most of these disabilities. All neonatal healthcare facilities should have a structured follow-up program involving a multidisciplinary team.

OBJECTIVES

The objective of follow-up is to provide a continuum of specialized care to high-risk neonates **(Box 16.3)** and to identify early deviation of growth, development, or behavior from normal and provide support and interventions as indicated. Prior to discharge, a detailed medical and neurological assessment, neurosonogram, and screening for retinopathy of prematurity (ROP) and hearing loss should be initiated. A psychosocial assessment of the family should also be done. The neonate "at risk" of neurodevelopmental disability must be identified before discharge from birth admission.

FOLLOW-UP TEAM

Regular follow-up program requires a multidisciplinary team approach involving a team consisting of primary care neonatologist/pediatrician, pediatric neurologist, developmental therapist, radiologist, ophthalmologist, audiologist, physiotherapist, cardiologist, orthopedician, social worker, and dietician.

Box 16.3 High-risk Neonates Who Need Regular Follow-up

1. Very low birth weight (<1,500 g)
2. Gestational age at birth <32 weeks
3. Small for date (<3rd centile) or large for date (>97th centile)
4. Major morbidities in postnatal period:
    - Perinatal asphyxia with hypoxic-ischemic encephalopathy
    - Neonatal sepsis/meningitis
    - Respiratory distress syndrome
    - Meconium aspiration syndrome
    - Shock requiring inotropic/vasopressor support
    - Acute kidney injury
    - Seizures
    - Intraventricular hemorrhage
    - Periventricular leukomalacia
    - Chronic lung disease
    - Congenital cardiac conditions
5. Persistent hypoglycemia or hypocalcemia
6. Mechanical ventilation for >24 hours
7. Bilirubin encephalopathy
8. Necrotizing enterocolitis
9. Surgical conditions such as diaphragmatic hernia, tracheoesophageal fistula, and intestinal obstruction
10. Major malformations
11. Infants born to HIV-positive mothers
12. Inborn errors of metabolism/other genetic disorders

TREATMENT Follow-up of High-risk Neonates

- Early intervention program (early stimulation) must be started in the NICU once the neonate is medically stable.
- Timely specific intervention must be ensured after detection of deviation of neurodevelopment from normal.

NEONATAL GROWTH CHARTS FOR FOLLOW-UP

Common growth charts used in different Indian setups to assess fetal and postnatal growth include Fenton and Olsen charts. None of these charts meet the Indian standards of fetal and neonatal growth, as data of both charts are derived from the neonates of developed countries. To complement the WHO Multicenter Growth Reference Study (MGRS), the International Fetal and Newborn Growth Consortium for the 21st century (INTERGROWTH-21st) developed similar standards for fetuses, newborn infants, and the postnatal growth of preterm infants. Primary data were collected from a population-based sample of healthy pregnant women and their babies in eight countries including India. INTERGROWTH-21st included newborn standards for birth weight, length, and head circumference. It is the first international standards for fetal growth and newborn size at birth as per gestational age and sex. In absence of any exclusive Indian data, we can use these charts in Indian NICUs. Separate charts are available for boys and girls for newborn size at birth (33–43 weeks). Postnatal growth charts for preterm neonates from 27 to 64 weeks are also available (*See* **Annexures**).

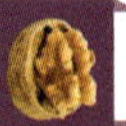

IN A NUTSHELL

Follow-up of High-risk Neonates

1. High-risk newborns should be followed to identify early deviation of growth, development, or behavior from normal and provide support and interventions, if needed.
2. Prior to discharge, a detailed medical and neurological assessment, neurosonogram, and screening for retinopathy of prematurity (ROP) and hearing loss should be initiated.
3. International Fetal and Newborn Growth Consortium for the 21st century (INTERGROWTH-21st) has developed standards for fetus, newborn infants, and the postnatal growth of preterm infants.

Chisholm P, Arasu A, Huertas-Ceballos A. Thames Regional Perinatal Group Outcomes Group. Neurodevelopmental follow-up for high-risk neonates: current practice in Great Britain. Arch Dis Child Fetal Neonatal Ed. 2017;102(6):F558-9.

Doyle LW, Anderson PJ, Battin M, et al. Long term follow up of high risk children: WHO, why and how? BMC Pediatr. 2014;14:279.

Novak I, Morgan C. High-risk follow-up: Early intervention and rehabilitation. Handb Clin Neurol. 2019;162:483-510.

Nwabuobi C, Odibo L, Camisasca-Lopina H, et al. Comparing INTERGROWTH-21st Century and Hadlock growth standards to predict small for gestational age and short-term neonatal utcomes. J Matern Fetal Neonatal Med. 2020;33(11):1906-12.

Villar J, Cheikh Ismail L, Victora CG, et al. International standards for newborn weight, length, and head circumference by gestational age and sex: the Newborn Cross-Sectional Study of the INTERGROWTH-21st Project. Lancet. 2014;384:857-68.

Villar J, Giuliani F, Fenton TR, et al. INTERGROWTH-21st Consortium. INTERGROWTH-21st very preterm size at birth reference charts. Lancet. 2016;387:844-5.

Vipulaguna D, Jahan I, Girish M, et al. Early Interventions for Infants at Risk for Developmental Impairment: The South Asian Perspective. Indian J Pediatr. 2022;89(3):254-61.

Voller SMB. Follow-up care for high-risk preterm infants. Pediatr Ann. 2018;47(4):e142-6.

Yitayew M, Chahin N, Rustom S, et al. Fenton vs. Intergrowth-21st: Postnatal Growth Assessment and Prediction of Neurodevelopment in Preterm Infants. Nutrients. 2021;13(8):2841.

Sriparna Basu and Poonam Singh

17 CHAPTER

Disorders of Kidneys and Urinary Tract

AS PER NMC COMPETENCIES

PE20.1	Enumerate the etiopathogenesis, clinical features, complications and management of urinary tract infection in children.	*Ch 17.2*
PE20.2	Enumerate the etiopathogenesis, clinical features, complications and management of acute post-streptococcal glomerulonephritis in children.	Ch 17.5
PE20.3	Describe the approach and referral criteria to a child with proteinuria.	*Ch 17.6, Ch 17.7*
PE20.4	Describe the approach and referral criteria to a child with hematuria.	*Ch 17.4, Ch 17.5*
PE20.5	Enumerate the etiopathogenesis, clinical features, complications and management of acute renal failure in children.	*Ch 17.8, Ch 17.9*
PE26.4	Explain the etiopathogenesis, clinical features and management of hemolytic uremic syndrome.	*Ch 17.9*
PE20.6	Enumerate the etiopathogenesis, clinical features, complications and management of chronic renal failure in children.	*Ch 17.10*
PE20.7	Enumerate the etiopathogenesis, clinical features, complications and management of Wilms tumor.	*Ch 17.11*
PE20.8	Perform and interpret the common analytes in a urine examination.	*Ch 17.1*
PE20.9	Interpret report of plain X-ray of KUB.	*Ch 17.1*

Topics available online: ***Anatomy and Physiology of Kidney; Cystic Kidney Diseases; and Genitourinary Malformations***

17.1 Evaluation of Genitourinary System *PE 20.8, PE 20.9*

HISTORY-TAKING

The genitourinary system is composed of kidneys, ureters, bladder, urethra, and genital organs, and the spectrum of genitourinary diseases ranges from congenital abnormalities, infections, inflammation, injuries, to tumors. Disorders of the urinary tract can have varied presentations such as obstructive symptoms, infections related symptoms, symptoms of bladder dysfunction, to complex congenital malformations. Few important symptoms related to genitourinary system are defined in **Table 17.1**.

Symptoms of kidney disorders include hematuria, oliguria, hypertension, and edema. The congenital abnormalities of kidney and urinary tract (CAKUT) may present with refractory rickets, oliguria, anemia, short stature, metabolic acidosis, or hypertension.

Disorders of ureter usually present with compromise of the urethral lumen due to intrinsic or extrinsic factors. The children present typically with either symptoms of ureteral obstruction like flank pain, pain abdomen, or back pain; or with symptoms of urinary tract infections (UTIs) such as fever, hematuria, nausea, and vomiting. The symptoms of UTI differ according to the age of the child **(Table 17.2)**. While fever is the most common presenting symptom of infants and young children, symptoms such as abdominal pain, dysuria, frequency, loin pain increase

Table 17.1 Definitions Related to Genitourinary System Symptoms

Terminology	*Definition*
Hesitancy	Difficulty in initiating micturition
Straining	A voluntary increase in abdominal pressure for initiating or maintaining voiding
Weak stream	Poor urinary stream of urine
Intermittency	Multiple stops and start spurts during voiding
Frequency	• Normal—three to eight times in a day • *Decreased frequency*—three or fewer voids • *Increased frequency*—eight or more voids per day
Urgency	An immediate and urgent compelling need to void
Dysuria	Burning micturition or discomfort during micturition. Initial dysuria suggests a urethral origin while terminal dysuria suggests a bladder origin
Incontinence	• Uncontrollable leakage of urine • *Continuous incontinence*—applicable to children of all ages, where leakage is continuous and almost exclusively seen in anatomical anomalies • *Intermittent incontinence*—leakage of urine in discrete amounts either during the day or night • *Daytime incontinence*—while awake • *Enuresis*—incontinence during sleep or night time
Primary enuresis	Intermittent incontinence of urine exclusively during night (enuresis) in a child who was previously dry for <6 months
Secondary enuresis	Intermittent incontinence of urine exclusively during night (enuresis) in a child who was previously dry for >6 months

the likelihood of diagnosis in older children. Features such as recurrent UTI, constipation, holding maneuvers, poor urinary stream, less frequency of voiding may suggest an underlying bowel-bladder dysfunction.

Hematuria is another important and ominous sign of urological disorders.

Voiding History

An accurate voiding history is most important for diagnosing bladder disorders or voiding disorders. The patient's age and expectations of urinary control may dictate the concerns about voiding habits. However, even in infants, the pattern of wetting of the diapers may provide clue to the diagnosis. Parents need to be specifically questioned about the lower urinary tract (LUT) symptoms. Normal voiding frequency is three to eight times during daytime. Anything below is called as decreased frequency and above is increased frequency. The symptoms range from *storage phase related symptoms* such as frequency, urgency, incontinence, nocturia to *voiding* symptoms such as hesitancy, straining, poor urinary stream, and dysuria. A precise voiding frequency/volume diary along with mention of associated bladder symptoms is advised to be maintained by the parents. Episodes of enuresis along with urine volume are recommended to be recorded for 7 nights and a 48-hour diary for

Table 17.2 Age-wise Clinical Presentation of Urinary Tract Infection

Infants <3 months	*Toddlers*	*Children and adolescents*
1. Nonspecific symptoms 2. Fever 3. Vomiting 4. Irritability 5. Poor feeding 6. Lethargy 7. Failure to thrive 8. Hematuria 9. Jaundice 10. Urosepsis	1. Fever 2. Abdominal pain 3. Vomiting 4. Loin tenderness 5. Poor feeding 6. Lethargy 7. Irritability 8. Hematuria	1. Dysuria 2. Frequency 3. Dysfunctional voiding 4. Abdominal pain 5. Loin tenderness 6. Fever, malaise 7. Vomiting 8. Hematuria

daytime incontinence or frequency. A 7-day bowel diary is also recommended in childhood voiding disorders.

In diagnosing a bladder pathology, it is exceedingly important to take a thorough bowel elimination history. Bowel symptoms have been found in up to half of patients with voiding dysfunction. The symptoms related to bowel-bladder dysfunction include history of recurrent UTIs, holding maneuvers like Vincent's curtsy, wetting of undergarments, constipation, presence of thickened bladder wall, and postresidual volume >20 mL.

An extensive history of recurrent UTI and antenatal history with results of ultrasound scans aids in making a diagnosis. Additionally, it is important to elicit history of known malformations of kidney and urinary tract or spinal cord, any associated behavioral, psychological problems, and finally a note of drinking habits including the quantity, type, and timing of fluid intake. A comprehensive approach to voiding disorders is described in **Table 17.3 and Flowchart 17.1**.

Neurogenic bladder: Abnormal innervation of bladder results in either a continuous or intermittent incontinence. They present as either storage related symptoms (frequency, incontinence, urgency, nocturia), voiding symptoms (hesitancy, straining, poor urinary stream), holding maneuvers, genital or LUT pain, dribbling of urine, urinary retention, or feeling of incomplete voiding.

Enuresis: Incontinence can also occur in apparently normal children in the absence of anatomical and neurogenic lesions. The diagnosis is made only after 5 years with symptoms lasting for a minimum duration of 3 months with a minimum of 1 episode per month.

Urolithiasis: Urolithiasis refers to the presence of stones along the urinary tract. The two most characteristic presenting symptoms of stones are pain and hematuria. The pain is often acute and colicky in nature, occurring anywhere from flank till groin depending on the location of the stone. UTI and acute kidney injury (AKI) may be other rare manifestations of stones.

Disorders of the Lower Urinary Tract

Abnormal anatomy of LUT: This includes congenital anatomical malformations and almost exclusively present as continuous

Table 17.3 Evaluation of Voiding Disorders

Incontinence specific history	• Age at onset, duration, severity of symptoms • Symptoms of LUT/bladder dysfunction—storage related symptoms (frequency, incontinence, urgency, nocturia), voiding symptoms (hesitancy, straining, poor urinary stream), genital or LUT pain, dribbling of urine, urinary retention or feeling of incomplete voiding • Continuous or intermittent incontinence • Voiding diary—frequency and volume of voids chart • History of bowel habits, stools diary • Fluid intake diary—frequency/volume/timing • Enuresis alone or presence of daytime symptoms and other LUT dysfunction symptoms • Holding maneuvers • Treatment, family, and psychosocial history • Past history of recurrent UTI
Physical examination	• Examination of back—look for spinal/sacral anomalies like sacral dimple, tuft of hair, lipoma suggesting underlying spinal dysraphism • Abdominal examination—palpable kidneys, bladder • Lower limbs—assess for tone, power sensations • Perineum—anal sphincter tone, perineal sensation, trauma, anorectal malformations • Genital examination—look for hypospadias, labial adhesions, ambiguous genitalia
Urinalysis	Look for urinary tract infection, diabetes mellitus
Imaging studies	• Ultrasound kidney, ureter, and bladder (KUB) • Ultrasound of bladder—pre- and post-void residue, bladder thickness • Micturating cystourethrography • MRI spine
Urodynamic studies	Uroflowmetry

(LUT: lower urinary tract; UTI: urinary tract infection)

Flowchart 17.1: Approach to voiding disorders

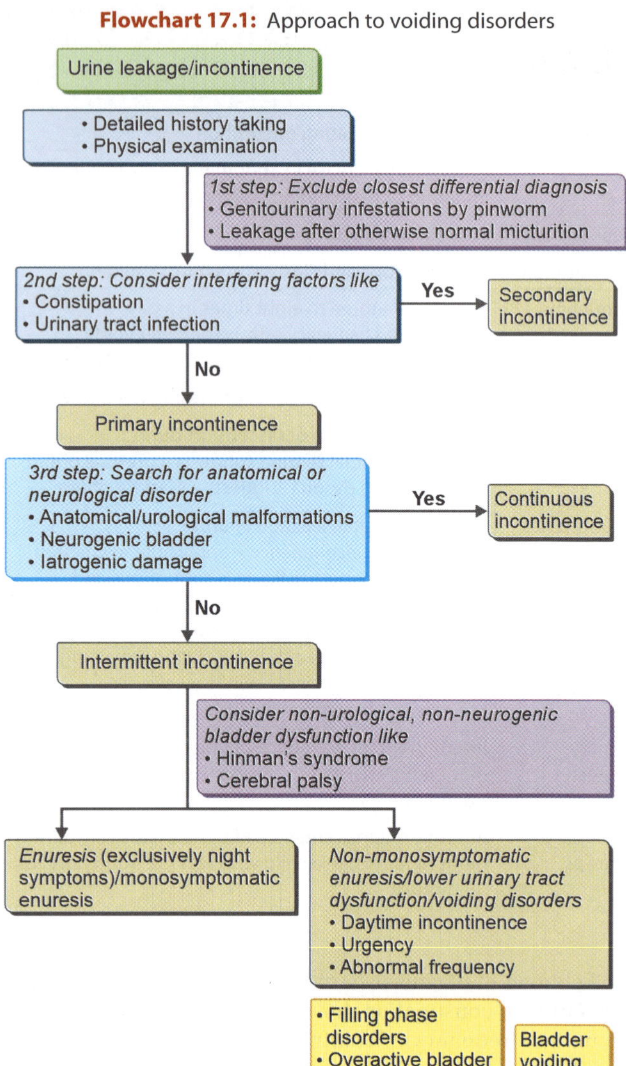

incontinence. Incontinence refers to the uncontrolled leakage of urine. Examples include bladder exstrophy, prune belly syndrome, ureterocele, urogenital sinus, etc. The abnormalities of LUT are usually associated with spinal cord anomalies which develop at the same time as LUT.

PHYSICAL EXAMINATION

A significant proportion of genitourinary tract conditions are evident on a careful physical examination (more often the anatomical or neurological defects). Always look for features of underlying structural or neurological abnormality in a case of UTI like distended bladder (suspected neurogenic bladder), palpable, enlarged kidneys (hydronephrosis), tight phimosis, vulval synechiae, palpable fecal mass in the colon, patulous anus, neurological deficit in lower limbs, urinary incontinence, anorectal malformation, or meningomyelocele. Spine examination is essential to look for any hairy patch, lipoma, cutaneous/dermal malformation, postanal dimple which might indicate an underlying spinal dysraphism. A careful genital examination is also warranted for recognizing conditions such as epispadias, cryptorchidism, ambiguous genitalia, and vulval synechiae.

INVESTIGATIONS

Urinalysis

A freshly collected urine sample preferably within 1 hour, is used for urinalysis. The samples may be collected as clean catch midstream sample in toilet trained older children, or by catheterization and rarely by suprapubic aspiration. The urine samples may be grossly examined for appearance and odor, followed by a microscopic examination of the centrifuged sample to look for the presence of cells, casts, and crystals.

- ***Color:*** The color of the urine is usually clear. Red colored urine can be caused by discoloration due to blood (hematuria), hemoglobin (hemoglobinuria) and myoglobin (myoglobinuria). Foods such as beetroot and berries and medications such as riboflavin and methylene blue can change the urine color.
- ***Urine dipsticks:*** This serve as a useful point-of-care investigation in children with suspected hematuria, proteinuria, or UTI. Proteinuria is an important indicator of renal disease rather than a urological disease and can be quantified by urine dipstick or 24 hours urine collection or urine protein: urine creatinine ratio. Blood in urine is detected by the presence of red blood cells (RBCs) on microscopic examination. Though dipstick can also show positive test with RBCs in urine, false positive test is encountered with hemoglobin or myoglobin. A combined positive leukocyte esterase and nitrite test on urine dipsticks provide a good sensitivity and specificity profile in diagnosing UTI.
- ***Microscopic analysis*** of a freshly collected sample of urine is used for confirming the presence of RBCs, bacteria, cellular casts, and crystals. The urine sample is centrifuged for 5 minutes before analyzing the sample. The normal upper limit of RBCs in a centrifuged sample is 2–4 RBCs per high power field (hpf). Urological origin hematuria is expected to have eumorphic or normal RBCs in contrast to dysmorphic RBCs in glomerular origin hematuria. In heathy children, upper limit of leukocytes is 4 per hpf. A neutrophilic dominant leukocyturia suggests UTI.

Plain X-ray Kidney, Ureter, and Bladder

The plain X-ray kidney, ureter, and bladder (KUB) has limited utility and is not routinely ordered though it is a useful tool for identifying conditions like renal calculi **(Fig. 17.1)**. However, uric acid and cystine stones are radiolucent. X-ray is also useful identifying any ureteric stents or any evident vertebral anomalies overlying the spinal dysraphism.

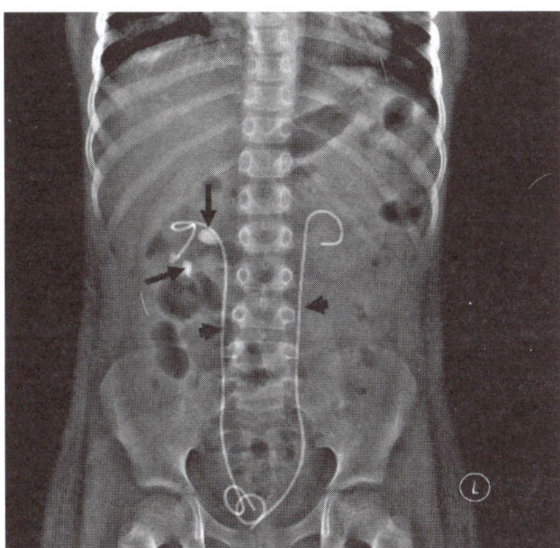

Fig. 17.1: X-ray kidney, ureter, and bladder (KUB) showing right-sided renal calculi (arrows) and bilateral double J stents in situ in the both ureters (arrow heads)

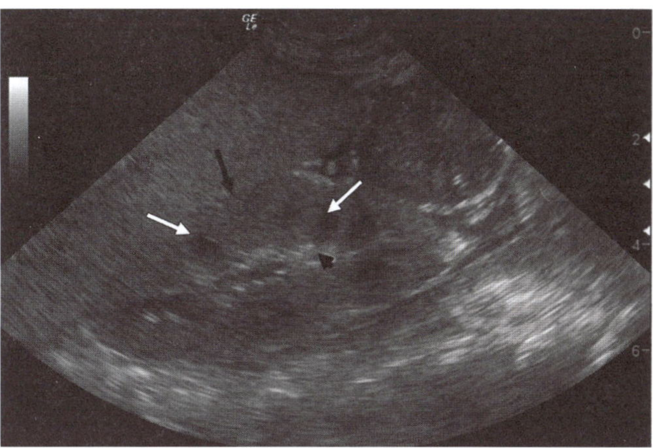

Fig. 17.2: Ultrasound kidney, ureter, and bladder (KUB) of a 4-year-old child showing normal cortex (black arrow), medullary pyramids (white arrow), and renal pelvis (black arrowhead) with normal corticomedullary differentiation and echogenicity

Ultrasonography

Ultrasound is a noninvasive, easily available modality useful in the evaluation of KUB **(Fig. 17.2)**. Ultrasonography can evaluate renal size, position, anatomy, urinary bladder masses, anomalies, and prevoid and postvoid bladder volume. Bladder is usually evaluated when full, though kidneys and ureters are evaluated after micturition.

Indications

- Measurement of renal size and echogenicity
- Diagnosis of hydronephrosis
- Bladder wall thickness as a part of evaluation of voiding disorders
- Structures around the urinary tract that may obstruct the kidney and bladder
- Renal masses
- Nephrocalcinosis
- Cystic renal disease

Micturating Cystourethrography

Micturating cystourethrography helps in diagnosing and grading the vesicoureteral reflux (VUR). It is also a critical investigation in identifying obstructive uropathies like posterior urethral valves (PUV).

DISORDERS OF THE URETHRA AND EXTERNAL GENITALIA

Posterior Urethral Valves

Posterior urethral valves are characterized by presence of sail-like membrane folds in posterior urethra causing severe bladder outlet obstruction in male infants. It is the most common cause of LUT obstruction in male infants and important cause of end stage kidney disease in them. The condition is diagnosed prenatally by typical ultrasound findings of bilateral hydronephrosis, dilated posterior urethra, and thickened bladder. Postnatally they may present with poor urinary stream, recurrent UTIs, renal failure, or presence of bilateral hydroureteronephrosis on ultrasound which can then be confirmed by micturating cystourethrogram (MCU).

Hypospadias

Hypospadias refers to a congenital condition where there is abnormal opening of the urethra on the underside of penis instead of at the tip. These patients have associated renal abnormalities such as ureteral duplications, mild hydronephrosis, and malrotations in 20% of cases. In infants and children, hydronephrosis is identified during evaluation of the UTI, urinary incontinence, flank pain, or in presence of a large thickened bladder wall.

Cryptorchidism

Cryptorchidism or undescended testis is common developmental abnormality, with higher prevalence in premature infants **(Fig. 17.3A)**. It is classified by its location in either abdomen, inguinal canal, superficial inguinal pouch, or upper scrotum. It is rarely located in ectopic sites. Long-term morbidities of the condition include testicular malignancy, infertility, and psychological impact of empty scrotum.

Micropenis

A micropenis is an otherwise well-formed penis which measures 2–2.5 standard deviations below the mean stretched penile length for the age. A stretched length of <2 cm is considered abnormal in newborns. In girls, look for vulval synechiae **(Fig. 17.3B)**.

Anorectal Malformations

The prevalence of urinary tract anomalies increases in the presence of anorectal malformations such as rectoperineal fistula, imperforate anus, and cloacal exstrophy **(Fig. 17.3C)**. The most common structural anomalies of urinary tract in these patients include hydronephrosis, megaureter, and VUR. The

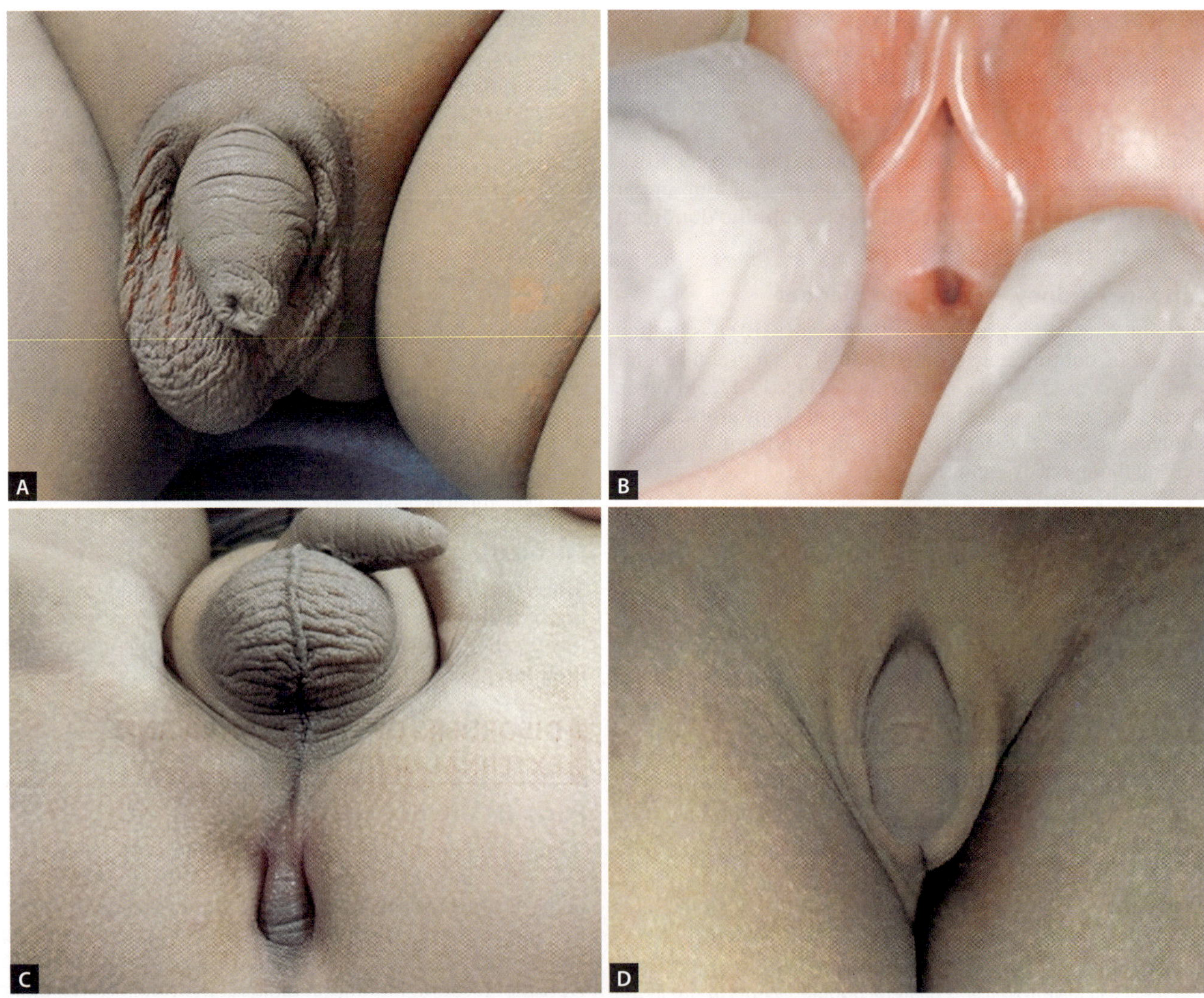

Figs. 17.3A to D: (A) Left undescended testis; (B) Vulval synechiae; (C) Anorectal malformation; (D) Ambiguous genitalia showing an undervirilized male

complex variants especially those with tethered cord tend to deteriorate early and progress to end-stage renal disease (ESRD).

Ambiguous Genitalia

Ambiguous genitalia can manifest as either the female external genitalia appearing virilized (e.g., enlarged clitoris, posterior labial fusion, and inguinal or labial mass), or male external genitalia that may appear undervirilized (bilateral nonpalpable testicles, micropenis, association of hypospadias, and undescended testicles). This overt genital ambiguity **(Fig. 17.3D)** should prompt an evaluation for disorders of sex development (DSD).

CASE STUDIES

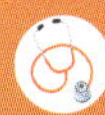

CASE STUDY 1 Asymptomatic Bacteriuria

The parents of a 4-year-old girl are worried about a urine culture report growing Escherichia coli 10,000 CFU/mL. She is asymptomatic. There is no history of fever, dysuria, flank pain, urgency, or constipation. On examination child has no dehydration and is active.

How will you manage the child?

In the absence of symptoms the child is most likely to have asymptomatic bacteriuria. Asymptomatic bacteriuria is estimated to be seen in 3% of school going children and 1% of adolescents. UTI is diagnosed only in the presence of symptoms and a positive urine culture.

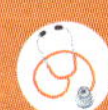

CASE STUDY 2 Urinary Tract Infection

An 8-month-old male infant presented with history of dribbling of urine and poor urinary stream since birth. Parents of the infant revealed past history of recurrent UTI. He was referred for further evaluation.

How will you evaluate this infant?

Children with non-*E. coli* UTI below 2 years of age, and those with recurrent UTI in any age group must undergo renal ultrasound, MCU, and DMSA scan to identify the underlying etiology. As the child has recurrent UTI, the child underwent all three investigations. Ultrasound revealed bilateral gross hydronephrosis with thickened bladder wall (3 mm). The MCU revealed the presence of PUV with bilateral grade V secondary VUR. Dimercaptosuccinic acid (DMSA) radionuclide scan revealed the presence of renal scars. Any child presenting with poor urinary stream should be suspected to have an obstructive uropathy.

IN A NUTSHELL

Evaluation of Genitourinary System

1. The major symptoms of genitourinary system include hematuria, genitourinary pain, incontinence, bladder storage, or voiding phase related symptoms, obstructive symptoms, and urinary tract infection related symptoms.
2. The symptoms of UTI in young children may be nonspecific and need high degree of suspicion.
3. Always evaluate for underlying structural abnormality contributing to ascending infection.
4. Comprehensive history and physical examination are an import adjunct in making diagnosis of voiding disorders.
5. Look for external markers of disorders of genitourinary system on physical examination, including pallor, short stature, edema, palpable kidneys, palpable bladder, sacral dimple, hairy patch, lower limb neurological deficits, and patulous anus.
6. Perform a careful genital examination at birth to identify disorders such as hypospadias and cryptorchidism.
7. Specific investigations like urinalysis, imaging tests such as X-ray kidney, ureter, and bladder, ultrasonography (USG) KUB, micturating cystourethrography, computed tomography (CT), and radionuclide studies as indicated aid in confirming the diagnosis of urinary tract disorders.

Daley SF, Gomez Rincon M, Leslie SW. Enuresis. 2024 Dec 11. In: StatPearls [Internet]. Treasure Island (FL): StatPearls Publishing; 2025.

Docimo SG, Austin P, Canning D, et al. The Kelalis-King-Belman Textbook of Clinical Pediatric Urology. London: CRC Press; 2019.

Hari P, Meena J, Kumar M, et al; Indian Society of Pediatric Nephrology. Evidence-based clinical practice guideline for management of urinary tract infection and primary vesicoureteric reflux. Pediatr Nephrol. 2024;39(5):1639-68.

Vande Walle J, Rittig S, Bauer S, et al; American Academy of Pediatrics; European Society for Paediatric Urology; European Society for Paediatric Nephrology; International Children's Continence Society. Practical consensus guidelines for the management of enuresis. Eur J Pediatr. 2012;171(6):971-83.

17.2 Urinary Tract Infections *PE 20.1*

INTRODUCTION

Urinary tract infections (UTI) are common bacterial infections in children. They may indicate underlying unsuspected anomalies of the urinary tract. Rapid treatment of UTI and appropriate intervention for any associated anomalies are crucial to prevent future complications. Up to 15% of children have risk of residual permanent renal injury after a first febrile UTI, which may result in impaired renal growth, recurrent pyelonephritis, hypertension, or end stage renal disease (ESRD).

DEFINITION

Urinary tract infection is an infection affecting any part of the kidneys or urinary tract, diagnosed by the growth of a significant number of colonies of a single bacterial species in the urine specimen of a symptomatic child.

PREVALENCE

Urinary tract infections constitute nearly 6% of all acutely ill children below 5 years, affecting around 1.7% of boys and 8.4% of girls in the first 10 years of life. During the first year of life boys and girls are almost equally affected, but later, UTI is more common in girls. The rate of UTI for uncircumcised boys is 4–20 times higher than that for circumcised boys.

CLASSIFICATION

Classification According to Site

- ***Cystitis (infection of the lower urinary tract):*** Cystitis refer to infection of the urinary bladder or urethra, usually associated with localizing symptoms such as dysuria, stranguria, frequency, urgency, incontinence, hematuria, or suprapubic pain.
- ***Pyelonephritis (infection of the upper urinary tract):*** This is a diffuse infection of the renal pelvis and parenchyma. The child usually presents with symptoms including fever ≥39°C, loin pain, and systemic toxicity. Infants and young children may have nonspecific signs such as poor appetite, lethargy, irritability, vomiting, or diarrhea.

Though prognosis is different for UTI affecting lower versus upper tract, differentiating between the two may not always be possible clinically. For practical purposes, if UTI is associated fever, it is called acute febrile UTI, which is to be considered as acute pyelonephritis.

Classification According to Episode

- ***First episode of UTI***
- ***Recurrent UTI:*** Second and all subsequent episodes of UTI

ETIOLOGY

The most common cause of UTI in all age groups is *E. coli* (85–90%). Other agents include *Klebsiella pneumoniae, Proteus mirabilis,* other *Enterobacteriaceae, Enterococcus* species, *Pseudomonas aeruginosa*, and *Staphylococcus saprophyticus. Saprophyticus* may be the cause of UTI in sexually active, female, adolescents. Infection with *Candida* may be seen in immunocompromised children, neonates, especially preterm neonates in intensive care settings or children receiving prolonged antibiotic therapy.

PATHOGENESIS

Urine formed in the body is normally sterile. Infection of the urinary tract occurs either as an ascending infection, or by hematogenous spread, with the former being the most common route of spread. The microbes belonging to the fecal flora or from perineal colonization may travel through the urethra to infect the urine. In males who are uncircumcised, bacteria below the prepuce is a significant source. The infected urine may reach the kidneys causing inflammation in the kidneys leading to pyelonephritis.

Uropathogenic *E. coli* adhere to the uroepithelium with the help of adhesive type 1 pili, following which they internalize and proliferate to form large, intracellular communities. Host factors which prevent infection include regular bladder emptying, uni-directional flow of urine and production of antimicrobial peptides. Inflammatory process is initiated when the bacteria overcome the innate host immune defenses, resulting in release of inflammatory mediators and subsequent tissue damage. Acute pyelonephritis may ultimately lead to tubulo-interstitial fibrosis and renal parenchymal scarring. Hematogenous spread, which is seen less commonly, may occur in the setting of infective endocarditis or sepsis in neonates.

PREDISPOSING FACTORS

- ***Sex:*** While UTI occurs in both genders almost equally in children below 1 year of age, girls tend to have a higher incidence of UTI after infancy. Girls have a shorter urethra that puts them at higher risk of retrograde infection. Uncircumcised boys also carry a higher risk of UTI if the prepuce is not retracted and cleaned regularly.
- ***Urethral instrumentation:*** Catheterization of urethra, if done in a nonsterile technique or if kept for prolonged periods (as in intensive care settings) predisposes to UTI. However, in those children who require prolonged catheterization, it is recommended not to routinely change catheters, unless there is obstruction or any other significant reason. Routine change of urinary catheters results in microtraumas which predispose them to UTI.
- ***Obstructive uropathy:*** Congenital anomalies leading to obstruction to outflow of urine cause urinary stasis within the urinary tract that serves as a good medium for bacterial multiplication and subsequent UTI.
- ***Vesicoureteral reflux (VUR):*** This refers to the retrograde flow of urine from the bladder into ureters, during detrusor contraction. VUR promotes the ascent of bacteria into the renal pelvis, and hence is an important risk factor for recurrent pyelonephritis.
- ***Bladder bowel dysfunction (BBD):*** There is a strong association of BBD with VUR and UTI. Improper voiding technique is the main cause of BBD, in which bladder contractions are suppressed by inappropriate contraction of pelvic floor muscles and external sphincter, without any neuronal or congenital anatomical abnormalities. This results in increased voiding pressures, incomplete voiding, and defecation. Constipation causes rectal distension which compresses the adjacent bladder neck and trigonal region, resulting in detrusor overactivity and voiding dysfunction. Incomplete voiding and stasis of urine promotes recurrent UTI by uropathogenic bacteria of gut. In addition, BBD can aggravate retrograde flow of urine in children with VUR, and cause delayed spontaneous resolution of VUR.

CLINICAL FEATURES

Neonates and infants: Neonates and infants with pyelonephritis or urosepsis usually present with nonspecific symptoms such as fever or hypothermia, irritability, lethargy, neonatal jaundice, vomiting, poor feeding, failure to thrive.

Pre-school children: Children younger than 2–3 years of age may not complain of localizing symptoms, rather may present with high fever without a focus (38.5°C or higher) or fever with excessive cry, diarrhea, cloudy urine, or vomiting.

Older children: In case of cystitis, they may present with localizing dysuria, stranguria, frequency, urgency, incontinence, or suprapubic pain. Fever, systemic toxicity, flank pain, or renal angle tenderness suggest an upper urinary tract involvement. Recent onset of enuresis or foul-smelling/turbid urine should also alert to the possibility of UTI.

PHYSICAL EXAMINATION

A complete physical examination is required to exclude any other source of fever. When UTI is suspected, one should search for signs of constipation, palpable kidneys, palpable bladder, stigmata of spina bifida, or sacral agenesis. The genitalia should be examined for phimosis, labial adhesion, postcircumcision meatal stenosis, abnormal urogenital confluence, cloacal malformations, vulvitis, or epididymoorchitis.

DIAGNOSIS

Collection of Urine Specimen

Urine sample must be collected before any antimicrobial agent is given. It is essential to use a method for collection of urine which is appropriate for the age and toilet-trained status of the child, as this affects the rate of contamination and influences interpretation of the results.

- ***Methods of collection of urine specimen:***
  - ***Suprapubic aspiration:*** It is the best method for obtaining an uncontaminated urine sample, but is an invasive procedure. Ultrasound guidance may be used to demonstrate the presence of urine in the bladder.
  - ***Transurethral catheter specimen:*** It may be an alternative to suprapubic aspiration, although the rates of contamination are higher than suprapubic method.
  - ***Clean-voided, mid-stream urine:*** It is a convenient, noninvasive method for obtaining a urine specimen with acceptable contamination rates.
    Perineal adhesive bags attached to the genitalia has high contamination rate and is strongly discouraged.
    In toilet-trained children, a *clean-voided midstream urine sample* is most preferred. The genitalia should be cleaned beforehand to reduce the contamination rate.
    In non-toilet trained, clinically stable children, neonates and infants: Clean-catch collection of urine is to be attempted. Bladder stimulation by suprapubic rubbing with gauze soaked in cold saline, or suprapubic tapping along with lumbar paravertebral massage, may be tried in such infants, to obtain a midstream, clean-voided specimen. If unsuccessful, urine sample may be collected by catheterization or suprapubic aspiration. For sick infants, catheterization and suprapubic aspiration are preferred at the outset, to avoid delay in initiating treatment.

Urinalysis

Urine Microscopy

The specimen must be examined fresh (within 1 hour after voiding, maintained at room temperature or <4 hours after voiding with refrigeration) to ensure validity of the findings.

- ***Significant pyuria:*** It is defined as >10 leukocytes per mm^3 in a fresh uncentrifuged sample, or >5 leukocytes per high-power field in a centrifuged sample.
  However, pyuria may also occur in conditions such as fever, glomerulonephritis, renal stones, or presence of foreign body in the urinary tract. *Pyuria in the absence of significant bacterial growth in urine culture is not sufficient to diagnose UTI.*
- ***Bacteriuria:*** Bacteria detected in urine microscopy has good sensitivity and excellent specificity for diagnosing UTI.

Rapid Dipstick-based Tests

Urine dipstick (having chemical pads for detecting both leukocyte esterase and nitrite) is a convenient bedside screening test for detecting UTI and may be used as a first-line screening test for UTI. Presence of leukocyte esterase (surrogate marker for pyuria) or urinary nitrite (which is converted from dietary nitrates in the presence of most gram-negative enteric bacteria in the urine) are indicators of urinary infection.

Urine nitrite test: The conversion of dietary nitrates to nitrites by bacteria requires approximately 4 hours in the bladder. Hence, this test is not a sensitive marker for infants and young children, who empty their bladders frequently. Negative nitrite test results do not rule out UTI. Moreover, not all urinary pathogens reduce nitrate to nitrite. Meta-analyses of many studies have reported pooled sensitivity and specificity of urine nitrite test as around 49% and 98%, respectively, for diagnosing UTI.

Leukocyte esterase test: The sensitivity of this test pooled from a combination of studies is around 79% while its specificity is around 87% for diagnosing UTI. False-positive results are seen in conditions other than UTI where pyuria may occur, such as fever resulting from any condition, after vigorous exercise, glomerulonephritis, and renal stones.

Pooled analysis has shown that combination (presence of either a positive leukocyte esterase or nitrite) has optimal sensitivity (84%) and specificity (88%).

Urine Culture

The diagnosis of UTI is confirmed on the basis of quantitative urine culture results in a symptomatic child.

Urine specimens should be processed promptly for culture. If this is not possible, then it should be refrigerated at 4°C for

Table 17.4 Colony Count Criteria for the Diagnosis of UTI

Method of collection of urine	*Colony count*
Suprapubic aspiration	$>10^3$ CFU/mL
Urethral catheterization	$>10^4$ CFU/mL
Mid-stream, clean catch	$>10^{4,5}$ CFU/mL

(CFU: colony-forming unit; UTI: urinary tract infection)

Source: Guidelines of the Indian Society of Pediatric Nephrology

up to 12–24 hours, to prevent the growth of organisms that can occur if urine is kept at room temperature.

Urine culture results are considered significant based on defined cut-offs for colony forming units (CFUs) of bacteria of a single species, which differ for different methods of collection of urine **(Table 17.4)**. As the same organism which colonizes the distal urethra and periurethral region may cause UTI, thus a low colony count may be present in a specimen obtained through voiding or catheterization even when bacteria are not present in bladder urine.

Asymptomatic bacteriuria: Urine culture showing significant colony counts of single uropathogenic bacteria **(Table 17.4)** in the absence of symptoms, is considered asymptomatic bacteriuria. It indicates colonization of the bladder by nonvirulent bacteria that are incapable of activating a symptomatic response. Asymptomatic bacteriuria is a benign condition, which does not cause renal injury and should not be treated. Eradication of these organisms is often followed by symptomatic infection with more virulent strains.

TREATMENT Urinary Tract Infection

Treatment of Urinary Tract Infection

Treatment involves administration of antibiotics along with adequate hydration and antipyretics. Treatment should be started promptly, after collecting urine sample for investigations. Oral antibiotics are preferred over intravenous antibiotic therapy for treatment of acute febrile UTI in all children except: (i) infants less than 2 months of age, (ii) severely ill patients, and (iii) patients who are unable to ingest oral antibiotics.

Antimicrobials for Treatment of Urinary Tract Infection

The choice of empirical antibiotic should be guided by local antimicrobial sensitivity patterns. For acute febrile UTI, a third-generation cephalosporin or co-amoxiclav is preferred as initial empirical antibiotic, while for cystitis, a first-generation cephalosporin (cephalexin, cefadroxil) or co-amoxiclav is preferred. If there is satisfactory clinical response, the initial empirical therapy need not be changed later based on the patient's urine culture/sensitivity report. A list of antibiotics along with their dosages and schedule is provided in **Table 17.5**.

Duration of Treatment

The duration of therapy is 7–10 days for acute febrile UTI and 3–7 days for cystitis and uncomplicated UTI. In those receiving parenteral therapy, once the child shows clinical improvement with resolution of fever and toxicity (usually within 24–48 hours), the route of administration of antimicrobials can be changed to oral to complete the course of therapy.

Table 17.5 Antibiotics for Treatment of Urinary Tract Infection in Children

Antibiotic	*Dose (mg/kg/day)*
Parenteral	
Ceftriaxone	75–100 (two divided doses)
Cefotaxime	100–150 (two to three divided doses)
Amikacin	10–15 (single daily dose)
Gentamicin	5–6 (single daily dose)
Ampicillin	100 (in three divided doses)
Oral medications	
Cefixime	8–10 (in two divided doses)
Co-amoxiclav	Amoxicillin 30–40 (in three divided doses)
Ciprofloxacin	15–20 (in two divided doses)
Ofloxacin	15–20 (in two divided doses)
Cephalexin	50–70 (in two to three divided doses)
Cotrimoxazole	6–10 (of trimethoprim) (two divided doses)

Indications of Repeat Urine Culture

A repeat urine culture is not necessary unless there is persistence of fever and toxicity despite 72 hours of adequate antibiotic therapy. In patients with prolonged fever and lack of clinical improvement, infection with resistant uropathogens or the presence of congenital uropathy or urinary tract obstruction should be considered. In such cases, immediate ultrasound examination is necessary. Otherwise, routine urine cultures should not be performed in asymptomatic children.

Supportive Therapy

- Encouraging a liberal fluid intake
- Antipyretics
- Alkalinization of urine is not necessary.

Evaluation after the First Urinary Tract Infection

Radiological evaluations are recommended after the first episode of UTI in children. They include ultrasonography (USG), micturating cystourethrography, MCU, and renal scintigraphy with dimercaptosuccinic acid (DMSA). These help to identify anatomical abnormalities of the genitourinary tract, vesicoureteral reflux (VUR), obstructed urine flow, renal damage, or scarring.

Most guidelines lately agree to the practical and less intense approach of radiological imaging after the first episode of UTI. A screening ultrasound should be performed in every child after the first episode of febrile UTI. An MCU is indicated only if (i) USG findings are abnormal, or (ii) UTI is caused by non-*E. coli* uropathogens in children below 2 years of age, or (iii) recurrent UTI. A DMSA scan to detect permanent scanning, is to be done 4–6 months after UTI, in children with (i) high grade VUR (III-V) or (ii) recurrent UTI.

Urinary Tract Ultrasonography

An ultrasonogram provides information on kidney size, number, location, presence of hydronephrosis, dilatation of ureters, urinary bladder anomalies, and postvoid residual urine. Ultrasonography should be done soon after the diagnosis of UTI.

Renal Scintigraphy

The DMSA scintigraphy is a sensitive technique for detecting renal parenchymal infection and permanent cortical scarring. However, DMSA during acute UTI does not provide any additional information for alteration of management. Thus it is recommended to be carried out 4–6 months after the diagnosis of UTI. Patients having hydronephrosis without any evidence of VUR should be evaluated by diuretic renography using 99m Tc-labeled diethylenetriaminepentaacetic acid (DTPA) or mercaptoacetylglycine (MAG3). These two latter techniques assess the renal function and give an idea about obstructive/non-obstructive drainage.

Micturating Cystourethrogram

The MCU detects VUR and provides anatomical details regarding the bladder and the urethra. An MCU may be performed any time after completion of antibiotic therapy for UTI. It should be done with aseptic precautions, under cover of prophylactic antibiotics, in order to prevent infection following catheterization. Oral amoxicillin in a dose of 50 mg/kg, one hour before the procedure, and 25 mg/kg 6 hours later, or, intramuscular gentamicin (2–3 mg/kg) given 30 minutes before MCU by intramuscular route, are preferrred.

Direct Radionuclide Cystography (DRCG)

It is an alternative to MCU for detection of VUR. It involves less radiation than MCU, but anatomical details are not well-delineated.

Prevention of Recurrent Urinary Tract Infection

About 10–30% children may experience recurrence of UTI, underlying high-grade VUR and BBD being important risk factors for recurrence.

General advice: Parents should encourage their children to have adequate fluid intake and regular voiding with complete emptying of bladder each time. Constipation should be avoided. Parents should be instructed to seek prompt medical evaluation (ideally within 48 hours) in case of future febrile illnesses, to ensure that recurrent infections can be detected and treated promptly.

Bowel bladder dysfunction (BBD): This is characterized by abnormal patterns of micturition, without any neuronal or congenital anatomical abnormalities. Such children have increased voiding pressures with incomplete voiding and defecation and are prone to recurrent UTI. All toilet-trained children with UTI should be evaluated for BBD by a thorough history, clinical examination and voiding diary. Children found to have BBD are to be managed with urotherapy along with treatment of constipation.

Table 17.6 Antimicrobials for Prophylaxis of Urinary Tract Infection

Drug	*Dosage (mg/kg/day)*	*Remarks*
Cotrimoxazole	2 (trimethoprim) + 10 (sulfamethoxazole) bedtime dose	Avoid in infants <3 months of age and G6PD as single deficiency
Nitrofurantoin	1–2 as single daily dose	• Gastrointestinal upset • Avoid in infants <3 months of age • G6PD deficiency and renal insufficiency
Cephalexin	10 as single daily dose	Drug of choice in first 3–6 months of life

(G6PD: glucose-6-phosphate dehydrogenase)

Prophylaxis for Urinary Tract Infection

Long-term antibiotic prophylaxis is recommended to prevent recurrent febrile UTI episodes in following situations:

- Children with high-grade (Grade III-V) VUR.
- Children with recurrent febrile UTI with BBD, irrespective of VUR.

The commonly used drugs for prophylaxis include cotrimoxazole, nitrofurantoin, and cefalexin, usually as a single bedtime dose, which is one-fourth of regular dose **(Table 17.6)**. Mere presence of urinary tract obstruction [e.g., posterior urethral valves (PUV)], urolithiasis, neurogenic bladder, antenatally detected hydronephrosis awaiting evaluation, or clean intermittent catheterization, does not merit long-term antibiotic prophylaxis. In case of breakthrough UTI, change of the medication being used for prophylaxis is usually not necessary. Also, there is no role for antibiotic cycling for prophylaxis.

Antibiotic prophylaxis is to be continued till the age of 2 years, provided they satisfy all three criteria: (i) toilet training, (ii) absence of BBD, and (iii) no febrile UTI in the preceding 1 year.

Vesicoureteric Reflux

Vesicoureteral reflux refers to the retrograde flow of urine from the bladder into ureters, during detrusor contraction. It can be primary (idiopathic) or secondary due to anatomical obstruction or neurogenic bladder. If urine is infected, it facilitates the movement of bacteria from the bladder to upper urinary tract and causes renal parenchymal infection. VUR is found in 30–50% children and 40–50% infants presenting with UTI. Its severity is graded using the International Study Classification from Grade I–V.

Conventional therapy for VUR has been antibiotic prophylaxis and surgical intervention. Systematic reviews have concluded that the outcome after 5-years following surgical ureter re-implantation and antibiotics versus antibiotic prophylaxis alone, was similar in terms of development of new renal scars, though number of breakthrough UTIs were lower in the surgery plus antibiotic group.

As renal scarring is the most critical outcome determining future ESRD, antibiotic prophylaxis being non-invasive, have been preferred for long-term prophylaxis of VUR. However, mere presence of VUR does not merit antibiotic prophylaxis, the latter being indicated only in children with high-grade (Grade III-V) VUR. In case of parental preference, or with recurrent breakthrough febrile UTI on antibiotic prophylaxis, surgical treatment of VUR may be advised: Ureter re-implantation being preferred over endoscopic correction, due to higher success rates of the former with regard to VUR resolution.

Follow-up

Children with VUR should be kept under long-term follow-up in order to detect recurrent UTI and any complications of VUR like renal scarring, hypertension, or proteinuria. Lower grades of VUR resolve faster than higher grades, with median time to resolution being around 38, 98, and 156 months for grade I/II, III, and IV/V, respectively. While ultrasound should be performed periodically to monitor the kidney growth, there is no need to repeat cystography for documenting resolution of VUR. However, an MCU is to repeated if surgery for VUR is planned. Though DRCG has lower radiation compared to MCU, it is inferior in terms of delineation of urethral anatomy. Routine DMSA scans to detect new scars are not required, unless the child has breakthrough UTI. Routine urine microscopy and culture is not required, unless child is symptomatic.

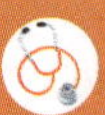

CASE STUDY Urinary Tract Infection

A 20-month-old boy was brought with fever for 4 days, associated with vomiting and poor feeding. The child was sick looking with temperature of 39°C. No other abnormal findings were observed.

In such a child without any focus for fever, if you suspect urinary tract infection, what additional points will you ask in history?

If we suspect UTI, we should enquire about the infant's urinary stream—whether he has a poor stream, whether urine stream is interrupted, whether he appears to have difficulty and seems to apply undue pressure while micturition, whether urine flows in drops, instead of a good projectile stream. These features would be suggestive of bladder outlet obstruction like PUV (the most common congenital cause of obstructive uropathy in boys), which is known to cause urinary retention, secondary VUR , and pyelonephritis.

Further, we should enquire about constipation. We should also enquire about any weakness in lower limbs since birth, any history of lumbosacral spine surgery which would suggest neurogenic bladder. Additionally, any document of antenatal ultrasound should be asked for, to look for any congenital urogenital anomaly.

How will you collect urine sample from this child? What investigations will you ask for and how will you send the samples? How will you confirm the diagnosis of UTI?

As the child is 20-month-old, he is not expected to be toilet-trained. The most suitable method for collection here would be by transurethral catheterization.

Two samples of urine should be collected one for microscopy and the other for culture. The urine samples should be plated for culture within 2 hours. If delay is inevitable, the samples should be refrigerated and can be kept up to 12–24 hours.

Urinary tract infection will be confirmed if urine culture shows growth of a single organism with >10,000 colony forming units (CFU)/mL. Urine microscopy showing leukocytes >5/hpf in a centrifuged sample, would support the diagnosis.

What further investigations should be done in this child after confirmation of UTI? When should these investigations be done?

After confirmation of UTI, this child needs to be evaluated by ultrasonography of kidneys and urinary tract. The ultrasonography should be done soon after the UTI. If the USG is abnormal, or culture shows non-*E. coli* uropathogens, he needs to undergo MCU. Further DMSA is to be done after 4–6 months if high-grade (Grade III-V) VUR is detected in MCU.

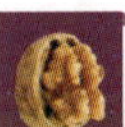

IN A NUTSHELL

Urinary Tract Infections

1. The diagnosis of urinary tract infection (UTI) is made based on the growth of a single species of bacteria with a significant colony count in an appropriately collected urine specimen, in a child with symptoms suggestive of UTI.
2. In toilet-trained children, urine is to be collected as a midstream clean-catch specimen. In children who are not toilet-trained, either a catheterized sample or a sample by suprapubic aspiration or stimulated clean-voided sample may be taken. Urine collected from urobags is strongly discouraged.
3. For management purposes, UTI associated with fever and systemic toxicity or acute febrile UTI is considered to be acute pyelonephritis, while UTI with symptoms restricted to lower urinary tract, without fever is taken as cystitis. Accordingly, empirical antibiotics and duration of treatment are decided.
4. Ultrasound of the kidneys and urinary tract is to be done in all children after first UTI. Micturating cystourethrogram and DMSA nuclear scans are to be done only in selected indications.
5. Long-term antibiotic prophylaxis for prevention of recurrences of UTI is required in (1) presence of high grade (Grade III-V) vesicoureteral reflux, or (2) recurrent febrile UTI irrespective of VUR.

Hari P, Meena J, Kumar M, et al; Indian Society of Pediatric Nephrology. Evidence-based clinical practice guideline for management of urinary tract infection and primary vesicoureteric reflux. Pediatr Nephrol. 2024;39(5):1639-68.

Hoberman A, Chesney RW, RIVUR Trial Investigators, et al. Antimicrobial prophylaxis for children with vesicoureteral reflux. N Engl J Med. 2014;370:2367-76.

Meena J, Hari P. Vesicoureteral reflux and recurrent urinary tract infections. AJPN. 2019;2(2):61-70.

Mori R, Lakhanpaul M, Verrier-Jones K. Diagnosis and management of urinary tract infection in children: summary of NICE guidance. BMJ. 2007;335:395-7.

Stein R, Dogan HS, Hoebeke P, et al. European Association of Urology; European Society for Pediatric Urology. Urinary tract infections in children: EAU/ESPU guidelines. Eur Urol. 2015;67(3):546-58.

Subcommittee on Urinary Tract Infection, Steering Committee on Quality Improvement and Management, Roberts KB. Urinary tract infection: clinical practice guideline for the diagnosis and management of initial UTI in febrile infants and children 2 to 24 months. Pediatrics. 2011;128(3):595-610.

Tullus K, Shaikh N. Urinary tract infections in children. Lancet. 2020; 395(10237):1659-68.

Williams G, Hodson EM, Craig JC. Interventions for primary vesicoureteric reflux. Cochrane Database Syst Rev. 2019;2(2):CD001532.

17.3 Edema

INTRODUCTION

Edema is characterized by an increase in interstitial fluid volume and tissue swelling that can either be localized or generalized. Severe generalized edema is known as anasarca. More localized interstitial fluid collections include ascites (peritoneal cavity) and pleural effusions (pleural cavities).

PATHOGENESIS

The extracellular fluid consists of plasma (in capillaries) and interstitial volume (in interstitial space). The movement of fluid between these spaces is determined by the balance of hydrostatic and oncotic pressures in these compartments, and the permeability of the capillary wall that separates them. This is summarized in the following equation:

Net filtration = K_f (change in hydrostatic pressure) – σ (change in oncotic pressure) $J_v = K_f(P_c - P_i) - \sigma(\pi_c - \pi_i)$

K_f = the ultrafiltration coefficient accounting for capillary wall permeability and surface area

σ = reflection co-efficient

P_c = capillary hydrostatic pressure

P_i = interstitial hydrostatic pressure

π_c = capillary oncotic pressure

π_i = interstitial oncotic pressure

For edema to be detected, the interstitial volume is usually expanded by several liters. The physical forces that govern the exchange of fluid between the interstitial and plasma spaces are known as Starling forces.

At equilibrium, fluid is filtered into the interstitial space at the arterial portion of capillaries due to relatively elevated capillary hydrostatic pressure. At the venous portion, fluid tends to go back into the capillary from the interstitial space because of the increased oncotic pressure. Remaining fluid in the interstitial space is usually taken up by lymphatics. Edema formation results from a derangement of one or more of Starling forces across a capillary bed that promotes net fluid movement from the plasma to the interstitial space. This can involve one or more of the following mechanisms:

- Increase in capillary hydrostatic pressure (congestive heart failure)
- Decrease in capillary oncotic pressure (hypoalbuminia state)
- Increase in the permeability of the capillary (drug, viral or bacterial infection, and allergic angioedema)
- Obstruction of lymphatic flow (malignancy with obstruction).

Role of Kidneys

Edema in congestive heart failure is due to stimulation of sodium retention by the kidneys. Fall in cardiac output is associated with a decrease in effective arterial blood volume. Therefore, the kidneys attempt to correct this deficit in arterial blood volume by activating sympathetic nervous system and renin-angiotensin system. Renin acts on angiotensin to release angiotensin I, which is broken down to angiotensin II. Angiotensin II has generalized vasoconstrictor properties and causes constriction of efferent renal arterioles. This increases sodium reabsorption from proximal tubule independently. It also stimulates production of aldosterone by zona glomerulosa, which in turn enhances sodium reabsorption by collecting tubule. In heart failure, not only aldosterone secretion is elevated but the biologic half-life of it also prolonged.

In acute glomerulonephritis, kidney failure, and nephrotic syndrome, the arterial blood volume as well as the interstitial volume is increased. The secretion of arginine vasopressin (AVP) and endothelin is also elevated that contributes to renal vasoconstriction, sodium retention, and edema. Arterial distension and/or sodium load also stimulate release into circulation of ANP, which causes arteriolar and venous dilatation, excretion of sodium and water by augmenting GFR, inhibiting sodium reabsorption in proximal tubule and inhibiting release of renin and aldosterone.

Regardless of whether sodium retention is the primary or secondary event, the kidneys play an important role in generalized edema.

EDEMA IN DISEASE STATES

Physiology is described in **Table 17.7**.

Edema of Cardiac Diseases

In addition to activation of renin-angiotensin system as described earlier, the defective systolic emptying of chambers of heart and impairment of ventricular relaxation promotes an accumulation of blood in heart and venous circulation. The increase in venous blood volume causes increase in capillary and lymphatic hydrostatic pressure and leads to edema formation.

In impairment of right ventricular function, pressures in systemic veins and capillaries rise, thereby augmenting the transudation of fluid into interstitial space and enhancing peripheral edema. The elevated systemic venous pressure is also transmitted to thoracic duct with consequent reduction of lymph drainage with further increase in accumulation of fluid.

In *left sided dysfunction*, there is increase in pulmonary venous and capillary pressure leading to pulmonary edema.

Nephrotic Syndrome and Other Hypoalbuminia States

There is decreased plasma oncotic pressure due to massive protein losses into urine. This facilitates shift of water into interstitial compartment and leads to hypovolemia and activation of renin-angiotensin system.

Cirrhosis Edema

This is characterized by obstruction to hepatic venous outflow, expansion of splanchnic blood volume, and increased hepatic lymph formation. Intrahepatic hypertension also acts a potent stimulus for renal sodium retention and systemic vasodilation and reduction of effective arterial blood volume as well. The

Table 17.7 Physiological Mechanisms and Diagnosis of Diseases Causing Edema

Clinical condition	*Mechanism of edema*	*Clinical findings*	*Investigations*
Nephrotic syndrome	• Cytokine • Aldosterone • Oncotic pressure	Anasarca, frothy urine, dependent edema	Spot urine protein/creatinine >2 mg/mg, or 24-hour urinary protein >40 mg/m²/h, serum or >1 g/m² day, and serum albumin <3 g/dL
Acute kidney injury	Intravascular volume	Oliguria, hypertension, orthopnea, dependent edema, seizures, encephalopathy	Serum urea, creatinine, serum electrolytes, urinalysis, ABG analysis, chest X-ray, ultrasound for kidney, ureter and bladder
Congestive heart failure	• Cardiac output • Renin • Angiotensin • Aldosterone	Orthopnea, paroxysmal nocturnal dyspnea, dependent edema, raised JVP, bilateral basal crepts, tender hepatomegaly	Chest X-ray, ECG, echocardiogram
Cirrhosis	• Portal hypertension • Aldosterone • Prostaglandin • Oncotic pressure	Hematemesis, malena, esophageal varices, caput medusae, ascites, dependent edema, palmar erythema, spider angiomata	Ultrasound scan of the liver, liver biopsy, serum albumin, prothrombin time and INR upper gastrointestinal tract endoscopy
Edematous malnutrition	Oncotic pressure	Weight between 60th and 80th percentile, dependent edema, psychomotor changes, dermatoses, hypopigmented hairs	Serum albumin
Idiopathic edema	• Renin • Angiotensin or • Aldosterone	Dependent edema	Serum albumin
Inflammation	Cytokine mediated	Redness, heat, swelling, pain	Acute phase reactants, blood culture
Deep venous thrombosis	Venous obstruction, lymphatic obstruction	Phlegmasia cerulea dolens, Homan sign, lymphadenopathy	Doppler flow study of superficial and deep veins, lymphogram

Urine for proteinuria should be tested in the morning first voided sample. Normal <0.5 mg/mg in 6 months to 2 years and <0.2 mg/mg in children aged >2 years of age. Dipstick test detects urine albumin, which reacts with tetrabromophenol blue and produces different shades of green color according to concentration of albumin in urine, and graded as: Negative (<10 mg/dL), Trace (10–29 mg/dL), + (30–100 mg/dL), ++ (100–300 mg/dL), +++ (300–1,000 mg/dL) and +++ (>1,000 mg/dL). It is useful for home monitoring of degree of proteinuria.

secondary hypoalbuminemia due to reduced hepatic synthesis also reduces plasma oncotic pressure and blood volume, which in turn activate renin-angiotensin system, renal sympathetic nerves, and sodium retention.

Serum aldosterone is elevated by liver failure due to defective metabolism of this hormone. Initially, fluid accumulates in peritoneal cavity but later peripheral edema and generalized edema may appear.

TREATMENT Edema

Treatment should always focus on correcting the underlying cause of the edema.

- *Localized edema*: Local edema caused by infection, hypothyroidism, or an autoimmune reaction, should be treated with antibiotics, thyroid replacement, and steroids, respectively.
- *Generalized edema:* Restrict salt (sodium intake 1–2 mEq/kg/d or 15–35 mg/kg salt) and water intake. Diuretics are usually recommended for generalized edema of unknown etiology.

If the edema is the result of decreased cardiac function, inotropic agents such as digoxin or dobutamine may be useful in addition with afterload reduction with ACE inhibitors or ARB. In nephrotic syndrome, furosemide and/or spironolactone, prednisolone or other immunosuppressives are the therapeutic modality. Similarly, if edema seems to be caused by glomerulosclerosis or hyperfiltration, ACE inhibitor may be beneficial. In cases of AKI, dialysis may be required for excess fluid removal. Nutritional support is required for patients of kwashiorkor.

Diuretics should not be used for prolonged period. Since it also stimulates the production of aldosterone, it may aggravate cyclical edema of adolescents. In fact, the metabolic alkalosis that arises from the inhibition of chloride reabsorption may result in a worsening of the edema because of a decrease in oncotic pressure. This may be a contributing factor in the production of the idiopathic edema associated with the use of diuretics.

Albumin infusions (20% salt poor albumin, 0.5–1 g/kg over 3–4 hour, and furosemide 1–2 mg/kg, IV, at the end of infusion) are helpful in transient management of patients. Ascites reinfusion, in which ascitic fluid is transferred back into the vascular space either by removal and subsequent reinfusion through a peripheral vein or by continuous reinfusion with a peritoneal-atrial, or LeVeen shunt can be useful in treatment of children with cirrhosis.

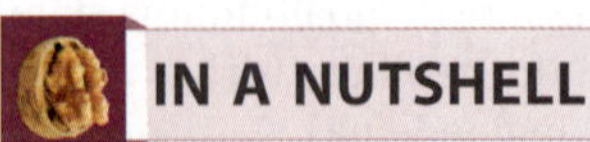

IN A NUTSHELL

Edema

1. Edema in renal diseases starts from periorbital region. Degree of edema is more in nephrotic syndrome than acute glomerulonephritis.
2. Main etiology of edema in nephrotic syndrome is decreased plasma oncotic pressure due to hypoalbuminemia and aggravated by activation of renin-angiotensin system.
3. Measures to reduce edema include salt restriction, diuretic therapy (furosemide and/or spironolactone), and infusion of salt poor albumin (20%) in presence of features of hypovolemia.

Clark AL, Cleland JG. Causes and treatment of oedema in patients with heart failure. Nat Rev Cardiol. 2013;10(3):156-70.
Elwell RJ, Spencer AP, Eisele G. Combined furosemide and human albumin treatment for diuretic-resistant edema. Ann Pharmacother. 2003;37:695-700.
Hwang SJ, Tsai JH, Lai YH, et al. Plasma atrial natriuretic peptide and natriuretic responses to water immersion in patients with nephrotic syndrome. Nephron. 1991;58:330-8.
Sinha A, Bagga A, Banerjee S, et al; Expert Group of Indian Society of Pediatric Nephrology. Steroid sensitive nephrotic syndrome: Revised Guidelines. Indian Pediatr. 2021;58(5):461-81.
O'Brien JG, Chennubhotla SA, Chennubhotla RV. Treatment of edema. Am Fam Physician. 2005;71(11):2111-7.
Teoh CW, Robinson LA, Noone D. Perspectives on edema in childhood nephrotic syndrome. Am J Physiol Renal Physiol. 2015;309(7):F575-82.

17.4 Hematuria

PE 20.4

DEFINITION AND ETIOLOGY

Hematuria refers to the presence of >5 RBCs per mm^3 in fresh uncentrifuged urine specimen or >5 per hpf in centrifuged specimen. Hematuria may be *gross* (visible to the naked eye) or *microscopic* (detected only on urine microscopy).

The incidence of gross hematuria has been reported as 0.13% and the majority has an easily recognizable and an apparent cause. Asymptomatic isolated microscopic hematuria occurs in 0.41–4% of school-aged children.

The causes of hematuria in children and newborn are given in **Box 17.1 and Table 17.8**, and vary from benign (e.g., UTI) to a serious one (malignancy).

PATHOPHYSIOLOGY

The RBCs can originate from any point along the urinary tract, but the most common site of bleeding is from the glomeruli. Thus, hematuria is usually classified as *glomerular* and *nonglomerular.*

Glomerular hematuria: In glomerular disorders, RBCs cross the endothelial-epithelial barrier of the glomeruli and enter the capillary lumen through the discontinuities in the capillary wall, which leads to dysmorphism of the RBCs.

During this passage, the morphology of RBC is modified (*dysmorphic RBCs*) by its intrinsic deformability, intraglomerular capillary pressure, size of the gaps, thickness of the glomerular basement membrane, variation in urine pH, and osmotic pressure, and effects of the renal tubular enzymes.

Glomerular bleeding is usually smoky brown or coca cola colored due to hematin formation from hemoglobin in an acidic environment **(Fig. 17.4)**. RBC cast develop when RBCs are entangled in the glomerular protein matrix.

Nonglomerular hematuria: It is caused by direct injury to the tubulointerstitium by infections, stones, or ischemic necrosis of the papilla. Nonglomerular bleeding is usually bright red or pink in color **(Fig. 17.5)**. The shape of RBCs remain normal (isomorphic RBC). RBC casts are absent.

Distinguishing features of glomerular versus nonglomerular hematuria are listed in **Table 17.9.**

Box 17.1 Causes of Hematuria in Newborn

1. Renal artery/vein thrombosis
2. Autosomal recessive polycystic kidney disease
3. Urinary tract infection
4. Obstructive uropathy
5. Trauma
6. Bladder catheterization

EVALUATION OF A CHILD WITH HEMATURIA

Step 1

History and Physical Examination

Eliciting a good history helps us to narrow down the various etiologies of hematuria. The history should include the color of urine (smoky brown color or bright red color), onset, duration, frequency (*Recurrent:* IgA nephropathy, Alport syndrome, thin glomerular basement membrane disease), with or without pain, timing of hematuria (hematuria at the onset of micturition suggests urethral bleeding, continuous hematuria throughout micturition suggests bleeding from ureter/kidneys), and terminal hematuria (at the end of urination) suggests bleeding from bladder. Familial hematuria is seen in Alport's syndrome, thin glomerular basement membrane disease and renal stone disease. History should also differentiate true hematuria from other causes of red urine. Some of the causes of pseudohematuria are listed in **Box 17.2.**

Also elicit history of any recent trauma, strenuous exercise, headache, visual disturbances, seizures, and features of heart failure.

- History of sore throat or impetigo 2–4 weeks prior to the onset of hematuria favors poststreptococcal glomerulonephritis.
- History of fever, dysuria, flank pain that may radiate down to the groin favors UTI or nephrolithiasis.

The physical examination should include measurement of blood pressure, assessment for edema, and recent weight gain, abdomen examination for tenderness/masses, skin examination for rash/purpura/eczema **(Fig. 17.6)**, and examination of genitalia.

Step 2

Urine Analysis

Urine dipstick: A positive test indicates presence of RBCs, hemoglobin, or myoglobin in urine. The reagent strip utilizes the pseudoperoxidase activity of hemoglobin or myoglobin to catalyze the reaction between hydrogen peroxide and the chromogen tetramethylbenzidine to produce an oxidized chromogen which has a *green-blue color.* It is important to briefly dip the strip in the urine, tap off excess urine, and read the strip

Table 17.8 Causes of Hematuria in Children

Glomerular causes	*Nonglomerular causes*
Primary: • Poststreptococcal glomerulonephritis (most common) • IgA nephropathy • Benign familial hematuria • Rapidly progressive glomerulonephritis • Membranoproliferative glomerulonephritis • Focal segmental glomerulosclerosis • Alport syndrome • Acute interstitial nephritis • Nail Patella syndrome *Systemic:* • Hemolytic uremic syndrome (HUS) • Henoch–Schönlein purpura (HSP) • Goodpasture syndrome • Systemic lupus erythematosus (SLE) • Polyarteritis nodosa • Thrombotic thrombocytopenic purpura • Systemic infections (malaria, leptospirosis, infective endocarditis, snake bite envenomation, and DIC)	• Urinary tract infection (most common) • Nephrolithiasis (most common) • Viral hemorrhagic cystitis • Hypercalciuria • Trauma • Tumors (Wilms tumor and rhabdoid tumors) • Tuberculosis • Strenuous exercise • *Vascular:* Renal artery/vein thrombosis, AV malformations • *Anatomic abnormalities:* Ureteropelvic junction obstruction, posterior urethral valves, urethral diverticula/prolapse, autosomal dominant polycystic kidney disease, multicystic dysplastic kidney • Coagulopathies • *Hemoglobinopathies:* Sickle cell disease • *Drugs:* NSAID, cyclophosphamide, and anticoagulants • Menstruation

(AV: arteriovenous; DIC: disseminated intravascular coagulation; IgA: immunoglobulin A; NSAID: nonsteroidal anti-inflammatory drug)

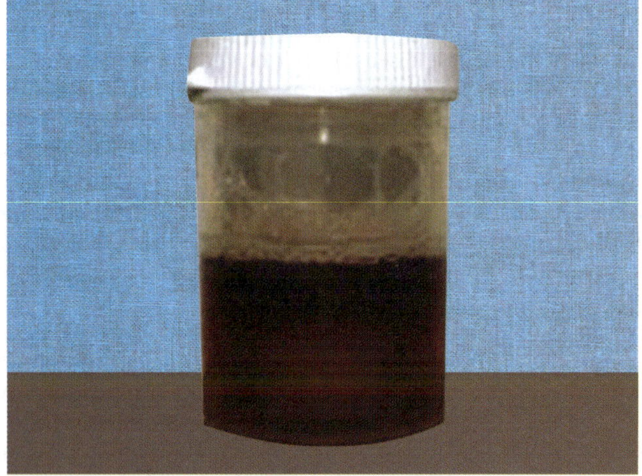

Fig. 17.4: Cola-colored urine in poststreptococcal glomerulonephritis

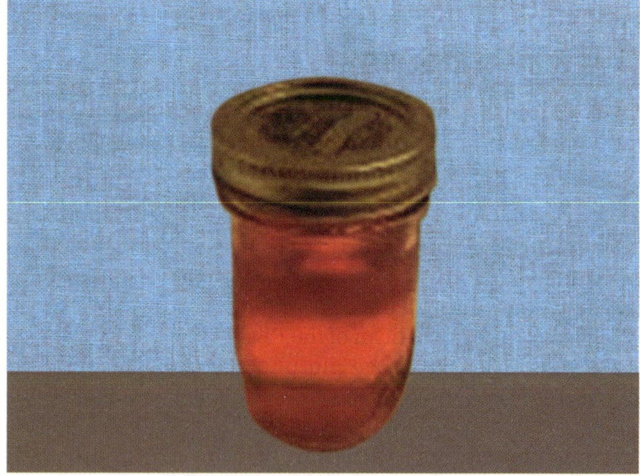

Fig. 17.5: Hematuria in a boy with vesical calculus

Table 17.9 Distinguishing Features of Glomerular from Nonglomerular Hematuria

Features	*Glomerular hematuria*	*Nonglomerular hematuria*
Color	Smoky brown or coca cola color	Bright red/pink color
Proteinuria	2+ or more	<2+
Dysmorphic RBCs	>20%	<15%
RBC cast	Present	Absent
Blood clots	Absent	May be present

at the recommended time interval (usually 1 minute). The test can detect as small as 150 μg/L of hemoglobin in urine. Urine dipsticks have a sensitivity of 100% and specificity of 99%.

Box 17.2 Causes of Pseudohematuria [Red Urine not due to Red Blood Cells (RBCs) in Urine]

1. *Drugs:* Chloroquine, phenazopyridine, rifampicin, deferoxamine, nitrofurantoin, iron-sorbitol, phenolphthalein
2. *Food:* Beetroot, black berries, food coloring
3. *Metabolites:* Porphyrins, methemoglobinuria, bile pigments, homogentisic acid, urates, tyrosine, melanin
4. *Others:* Hemoglobinuria, myoglobinuria

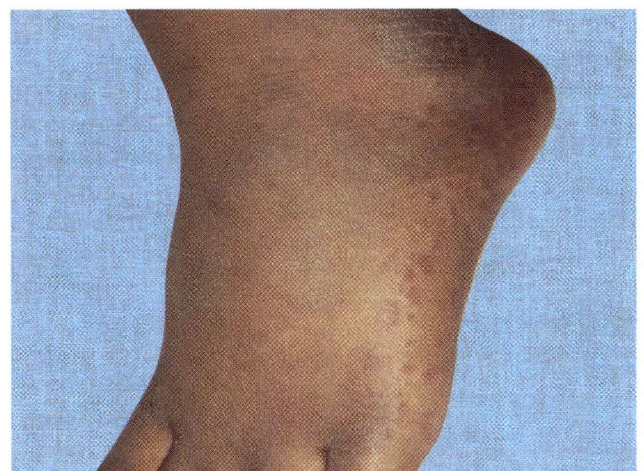

Fig. 17.6: Purpuric lesions in a child with Henoch–Schönlein purpura

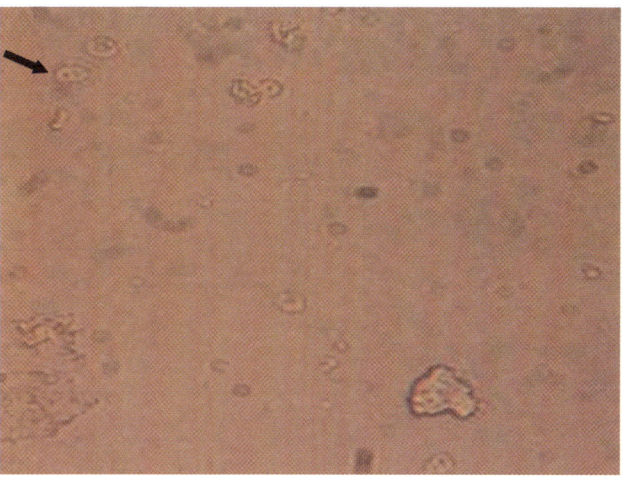

Fig. 17.7: Dysmorphic red blood cells (RBCs) seen in urine microscopy

Dipstick is positive both in hemoglobinuria and myoglobinuria. To differentiate both, add ammonium sulphate to the urine sample and centrifuge it. Ammonium sulphate precipitates hemoglobin but not myoglobin. If the supernatant is clear, the pigment is hemoglobin. If the supernatant is red, the pigment is myoglobin.

Microscopy: A 10 mL of freshly voided urine, preferably passed in the morning, collected by midstream clean-catch method should be subjected for microscopic examination as RBCs are better preserved in fresh concentrated and acidic urine. This urine is centrifuged at 3,600 revolutions per minute for 5 minutes and the presence of >5 RBCs per high-power field (under 40X suggests microscopic hematuria). Identification of dysmorphic RBCs require light microscopy that can be confirmed by staining with Wright's stain or phase contrast microscopy. RBC morphology should be examined at least in 10 hpfs and the presence of >20% dysmorphic RBC is suggestive of glomerular hematuria **(Fig. 17.7)**.

Step 3

Additional Investigations

Further evaluation is guided by the history, physical examination, and initial urine analysis findings. Some of the investigations ordered are urine culture (UTI), Urine calcium-creatinine ratio (hypercalciuria), urine spot protein/creatinine ratio or 24 hour urine protein excretion (glomerular hematuria), blood urea/serum creatinine (renal failure), serum C3 (poststreptococcal glomerulonephritis), antistreptolysin O (ASO) titer (poststreptococcal glomerulonephritis), antinuclear antibodies (ANA) (systemic lupus erythematosus), USG abdomen and pelvis with Doppler (UTI, urolithiasis, tumors, anatomic abnormalities), CT abdomen (renal masses or vascular malformations), complete hemogram with peripheral smear (sickle cell disease, hemolytic uremic syndrome (HUS), Henoch-Schönlein purpura (HSP), coagulation profile [prothrombin (PT), activated partial thromboplastin time (aPTT)] for coagulopathies, and renal biopsy.

Box 17.3 Indications for Renal Biopsy in Children with Hematuria

1. Significant proteinuria
2. Abnormal renal function tests
3. Recurrent persistent hematuria
4. Serologic abnormalities (abnormal complement, ANA, or dsDNA levels)
5. Recurrent gross hematuria
6. A family history of end-stage renal disease

(ANA: antinuclear antibody; dsDNA: double-stranded deoxyribonucleic acid)

The indications of renal biopsy in children with hematuria are listed in **Box 17.3**. An algorithmic approach to evaluation of hematuria is given in **Flowchart 17.2**.

TREATMENT Hematuria

Treatment of hematuria depends on the underlying etiology. The indications for referral to a pediatric nephrologist/urologist includes microscopic hematuria associated with macroscopic hematuria and or nephrotic range proteinuria, hypertension, family history of hematuria, ultrasound showing mass/stones/nephrocalcinosis/cysts, etc., and urine calcium creatinine ratio >0.2 on >2 occasions. Supportive treatment includes restriction of physical activity, plenty of fluid intake, alkalinization of urine (to prevent acute tubular, necrosis), and blood transfusion (in presence of severe anemia).

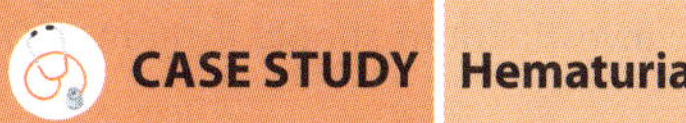

CASE STUDY Hematuria

A 10-year-old boy is brought to the outpatient department for passing red-colored urine. His mom says that it is scary and the family is very anxious.

Flowchart 17.2: Algorithmic approach to a child with red urine/hematuria

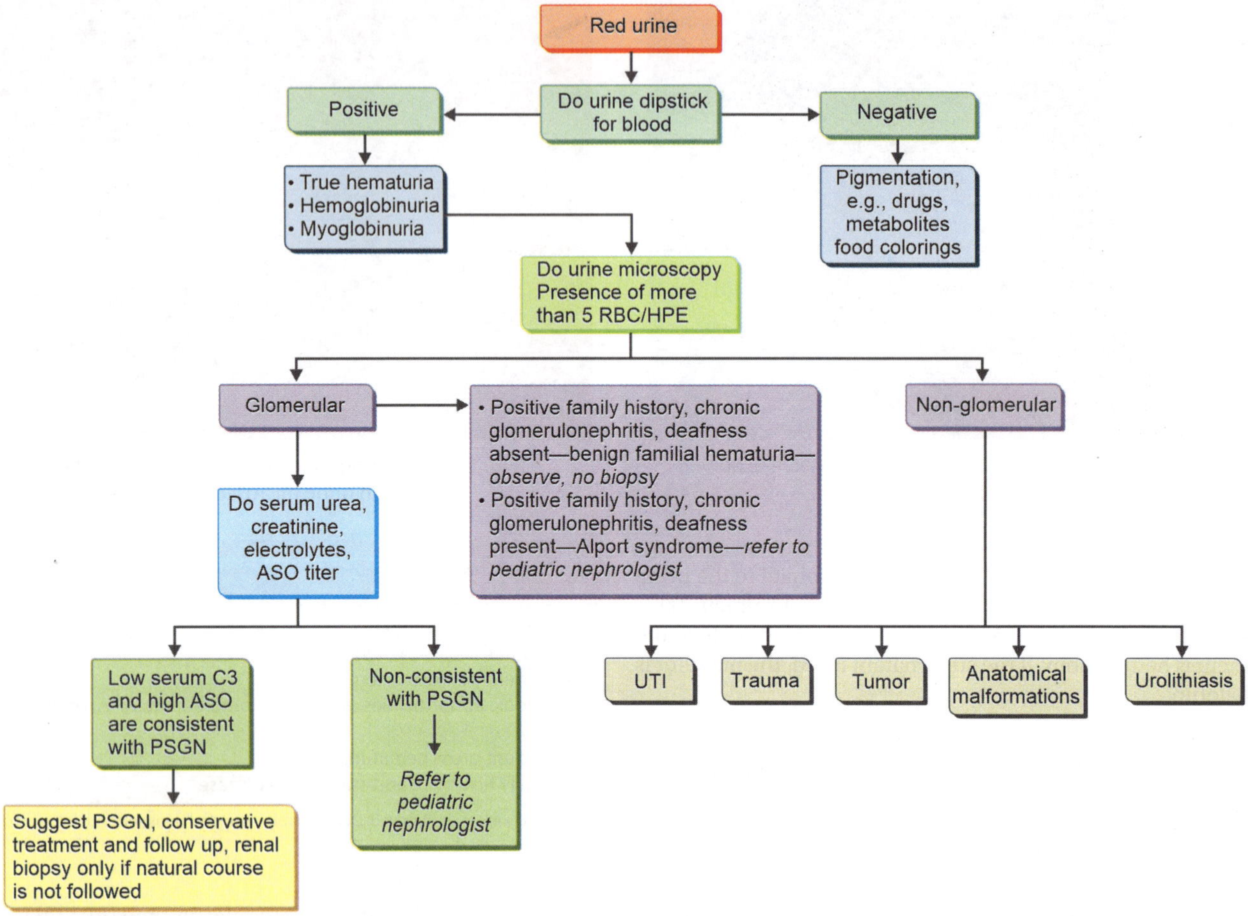

Red urine

Do urine dipstick for blood

Positive

- True hematuria
- Hemoglobinuria
- Myoglobinuria

Negative

Pigmentation, e.g., drugs, metabolites food colorings

Do urine microscopy Presence of more than 5 RBC/HPE

Glomerular

- Positive family history, chronic glomerulonephritis, deafness absent—benign familial hematuria—*observe, no biopsy*
- Positive family history, chronic glomerulonephritis, deafness present—Alport syndrome—*refer to pediatric nephrologist*

Do serum urea, creatinine, electrolytes, ASO titer

Low serum C3 and high ASO are consistent with PSGN

Suggest PSGN, conservative treatment and follow up, renal biopsy only if natural course is not followed

Non-consistent with PSGN

Refer to pediatric nephrologist

Non-glomerular

UTI | Trauma | Tumor | Anatomical malformations | Urolithiasis

(ASO: antistreptolysin O; RBC: red blood cell; HPF: high power field; PSGN: poststreptococcal glomerulonephritis; UTI: urinary tract infection)

What should be the first step?

Confirm presence of hematuria by urine microscopic examination.

Urine analysis reveals cola-colored urine and microscopy shows plenty of RBCs with 30% dysmorphic of RBCs.

What is your impression?

The findings are suggestive of glomerular hematuria.

How will you further proceed with this case?

The age of presentation and urine microscopy favors the possibility of poststreptococcal glomerulonephritis (PSGN). History of sore throat or skin lesions 2–4 weeks preceding the onset of this illness adds to the diagnosis of PSGN. Also one should enquire about history of reduced urine output/headache/visual disturbances/seizures/breathlessness to rule out complications of PSGN if any. Clinical examination should include assessment for pedal edema, measurement of blood pressure and performing a thorough systemic examination. Further investigations should include ASO titer and serum C3 levels.

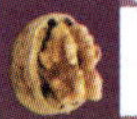

IN A NUTSHELL

Hematuria

1. Hematuria is defined as presence of >5 RBC/hpf in a centrifuged urine sample. It needs to be differentiated from other common causes of red urine such as hemoglobinuria, myoglobinuria, and drug intake (e.g., rifampicin).
2. The most common screening test for hematuria is urine dipstick which is confirmed by urine microscopy.
3. Glomerular causes should be differentiated from nonglomerular causes of hematuria on the basis of dysmorphic RBCs and RBCs casts.
4. Glomerulonephritis, urinary tract infection, and renal stones are the most common causes.
5. Management of hematuria depends upon the underlying etiology.

Avellino GJ, Bose S, Wang DS. Diagnosis and management of hematuria. Surg Clin North Am. 2016;96(3):503-15.
Bignall ONR 2nd, Dixon BP. Management of hematuria in children. Curr Treat Options Pediatr. 2018;4(3):333-49.
Bolenz C, Schröppel B, Eisenhardt A, et al. The investigation of hematuria. Dtsch Arztebl Int. 2018;115(48):801-7.
Kallash M, Rheault MN. Approach to persistent microscopic hematuria in children. Kidney360. 2020;1(9):1014-20.
Pade KH, Liu DR. An evidence-based approach to the management of hematuria in children in the emergency department. Pediatr Emerg Med Pract. 2014;11(19):1-13.
Pan CG, Avner ED. Clinical evaluation of the child with hematuria. In: Kliegman RM, Stanton BF, St.Geme JW, (Eds). Nelson Textbook of Pediatrics, 20th edition. Philadelphia: Elsevier; 2016. pp. 2494-6.
Phadke KD, Vijayakumar M, Sharma J, et al. Indian Pediatric nephrology group. Consensus statement on evaluation of hematuria. Indian Pediatr. 2006;43:965-73.
Vedula R, Iyengar AA. Approach to diagnosis and management of hematuria. Indian J Pediatr. 2020;87(8):618-24.
Vijayakumar M, Nammalwar BR. Diagnostic approach to a child with hematuria. Indian Pediatr. 1998;35:525-32.
Viteri B, Reid-Adam J. Hematuria and proteinuria in children. Pediatr Rev. 2018;39(12):573-87.

17.5 Glomerulonephritis

PE 20.2, PE 20.4

INTRODUCTION

Glomerulonephritis refers to a group of diseases characterized by inflammation and proliferation of cells within the glomerulus. The inflammatory changes may be triggered by immunological mechanism following insult with an infectious agent or sometimes by nonimmune mediated injury.

Glomerulonephritis may manifest clinically as (1) *acute nephritic syndrome* (most common), (2) asymptomatic hematuria and/or proteinuria, (3) nephrotic syndrome, or (4) rapidly progressive glomerulonephritis (RPGN).

- ***Acute nephritic syndrome*** is defined as acute onset of hematuria (gross or microscopic) and proteinuria in the presence of edema, hypertension, and oliguria.
- ***Nephrotic syndrome*** is characterized by heavy proteinuria leading to hypoalbuminemia, edema, and hyperlipidemia.

Table 17.10 compares salient features differentiating acute nephritic and nephrotic syndrome.

Table 17.10 Differences Between Nephritic and Nephrotic Syndrome

	Nephritic syndrome	*Nephrotic syndrome*
Onset	Acute	Insidious
Edema	Minimal, turgid, usually periorbital, sometimes generalized	Severe, pitting, generalized often involves scrotal region
Hypertension	Present in more than two-thirds patients	Uncommon
Urine output	Decreased	Normal/decreased
Circulatory volume	Hypervolemia	Hypovolemia
Hematuria	50–70% gross, microscopic in all cases	20% have microscopic hematuria
Proteinuria	1+ or 2+ on dipstick spot Up/Uc 0.2 to 2	>2+ on dipstick spot Up/Uc >2
Serum cholesterol	Normal	Increased
Serum albumin	Normal/minimal decrease	Low
Glomerular filtration rate	Decreased	Normal

Spot Up/Uc—spot urinary protein-creatinine ratio

ETIOLOGY

The most common cause of acute nephritic syndrome is postinfectious glomerulonephritis (PIGN) that occurs following a group A beta-hemolytic *Streptococcus* (GABHS) infection. Besides GABHS, acute PIGN may result from various other infective agents **(Box 17.4)**. Some of the authors propose a new term infection related glomerulonephritis (IRGN) for glomerulonephritis arising during an ongoing process of bacterial infection. The clinical features of PIGN consist of period of infection, resolution of infection, latency period and then an acute GN. Although many other micro-organisms can cause glomerular damage, IRGN typically refers to bacterial infections. Chronic glomerulonephritis caused by systemic lupus erythematosus nephritis and membranoproliferative glomerulonephritis (MPGN) may present as acute nephritic syndrome. Other conditions presenting with acute nephritic syndrome are listed in **Box 17.5**.

ACUTE POSTSTREPTOCOCCAL GLOMERULONEPHRITIS

Acute PSGN continues to be the most common cause of acute nephritis in children globally. It accounts for over 90% of the cases hence the term "acute poststreptococcal glomerulonephritis" is often used synonymously with AGN. It primarily occurs in developing countries. The annual incidence ranges from 9.5 to 28.5 per 100,000 individuals in underdeveloped nations. Though PSGN remains the most common cause of AGN in children epidemiology among adults has shifted and staphylococcal related

Box 17.4 Infectious Agents Associated with Acute Postinfectious Glomerulonephritis

1. *Bacterial: Streptococcus* group A, C, G, *Streptococcus viridans, Staphylococcus (aureus and albus), Pneumococcus, Neisseria meningitidis, Mycobacteria, Salmonella typhi, Klebsiella pneumoniae, and Escherichia coli*
2. *Viral*: Coxsackievirus, echovirus, cytomegalovirus, Epstein–Barr virus, hepatitis B, C, HIV, rubella, measles, varicella, influenza, adenovirus, COVID-19 and mumps
3. *Fungal: Coccidioides immitis*
4. *Protozoal: Plasmodium malariae, Plasmodium falciparum, Schistosoma mansoni, Toxoplasma gondii, and filariasis*

Box 17.5 Conditions Presenting as Acute Nephritic Syndrome

1. Acute postinfectious glomerulonephritis
2. Membranoproliferative glomerulonephritis
3. IgA nephropathy
4. Henoch–Schönlein purpura nephritis
5. Systemic lupus erythematosus nephritis
6. Vasculitis
7. Goodpasture syndrome (anti-GBM disease)
8. Hemolytic uremic syndrome

(GBM: glomerular basement membrane; IgA: immunoglobulin A)

glomerulonephritis now is more prevalent than post-streptococcal in developed countries. Poststreptococcal glomerulonephritis is an immune-mediated glomerular injury that occurs 1–4 weeks after GABHS, *Streptococcus pyogenes* infection. Longer latent period of 2–4 weeks is seen after skin infections as compared to 1–2 weeks seen after throat infection.

Acute glomerulonephritis may also evolve after infection at other sites such as pneumonia, meningitis, sepsis or deep-seated abscess, and chronic bacterial infections (ventriculoperitoneal shunts, subacute bacterial endocarditis).

Epidemiology

The PSGN is still the most common glomerulopathy in developing countries. It occurs after throat or skin infection by certain nephritogenic strains.

- M serotypes 2, 47, 49, 55, 57, and 60 are associated with nephritis following skin infections and types 1, 2, 3, 4, 12, 25, and 45 following upper respiratory infection.
- In tropical countries like India with hot and humid climate it is seen after pyoderma in summer while in temperate climate it occurs in winter, months after streptococcal pharyngitis.

Pathogenesis

Deposition of immune complexes (antigen-antibody complexes) in glomerular tufts is the key pathogenic event. Several mechanisms have been proposed for the event:

- Formation of immune complexes in circulation and deposition in glomeruli.
- Implantation of nephritogenic antigen in glomeruli and formation of immune complexes in situ.
- Molecular mimicry plays role as antibodies form against streptococcal antigens and bind to normal glomerular antigens due to cross reactivity among them.
- Activation of complement pathway directly by implanted antigen in glomeruli.

Due to certain M serotypes being non-nephritogenic, recent studies have refuted M proteins as "the nephritogenic antigen" in pathogenesis of PSGN. Investigators have proposed nephritis-associated plasmin receptor (NaPlr), streptococcal pyrogenic exotoxin B (SPEB), and its zymogen precursor as nephritogenic. Formation of immune complexes by above mechanisms induces cascade of events, i.e., complement pathway activation, production of cytokines, infiltration of leukocytes, and cellular proliferation in glomerular mesangium and endocapillary.

The inflammatory reaction in glomerular tufts decreases the GFR. The reduction in GFR causes decreased reabsorption of solutes and water in the proximal tubules hence causing sodium and water retention. This results in expansion of extracellular volume, edema, and hypertension. The serum albumin levels are normal or slightly reduced hence do not play role in hemodynamics. The increased extracellular fluid (ECF) volume appropriately suppresses renin-angiotensin-aldosterone axis. The C3 levels are low due to alternate complement pathway activation. C4 levels when low denote classic complement pathway activation also.

Clinical Features

The clinical presentation of PSGN varies from asymptomatic, microscopic hematuria to the full-blown acute nephritic syndrome. PSGN most frequently affects children from 3 to 12 years of age but may affect any age group. Males are twice more commonlyaffected than females. The onset of disease is usually 1–2 weeks after an antecedent pharyngitis and 3–4 weeks after pyoderma.

The clinical manifestations depend on severity of kidney involvement. Mild cases may present with microscopic hematuria with some proteinuria with or without hypertension. A typical patient of PSGN presents with sudden onset of gross hematuria, edema, oliguria, hypertension, and mild azotemia. Active or healed skin lesions **(Fig. 17.8)** might be seen over the extremities. Prodromal symptoms such as malaise, low-grade fever, lethargy, anorexia, and headache may be present.

Gross hematuria is present in 30–70% of patients while microscopic hematuria is a universal finding. Urine is smoky or cola-colored. Gross hematuria may be present for a few hours in a day and usually subsides in 1–2 weeks. Microscopic hematuria may last for an year. A few patients may have relapses of gross hematuria after vigorous exercise or viral illness later.

Edema is present in majority of patients and often noticed in morning as mild periorbital puffiness **(Fig. 17.9)**. It results due to retention of salt and water. Unrestricted fluid and salt intake may cause edema in peripheries, sometimes causing pleural effusion, and ascites.

Oliguria is often present. Anuria is infrequent and when persistent, requires close monitoring for rapidly progressive glomerulonephritis.

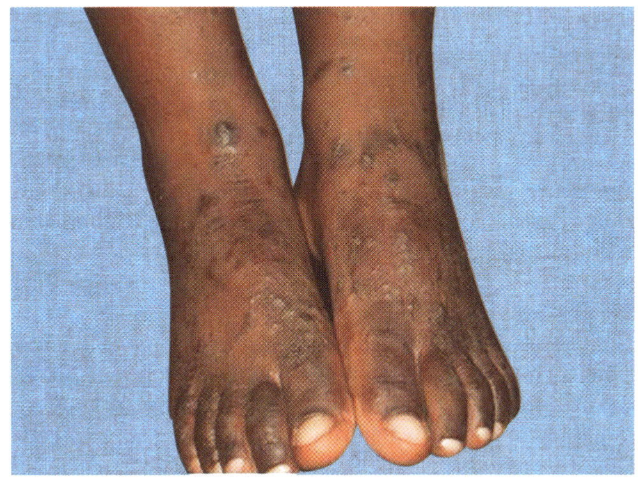

Fig. 17.8: Post-pyoderma scars

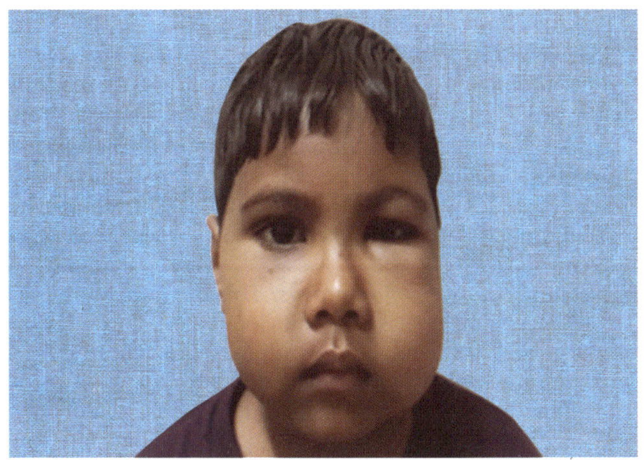

Fig. 17.9: Facial edema in a child with acute poststreptococcal glomerulonephritis (PSGN)

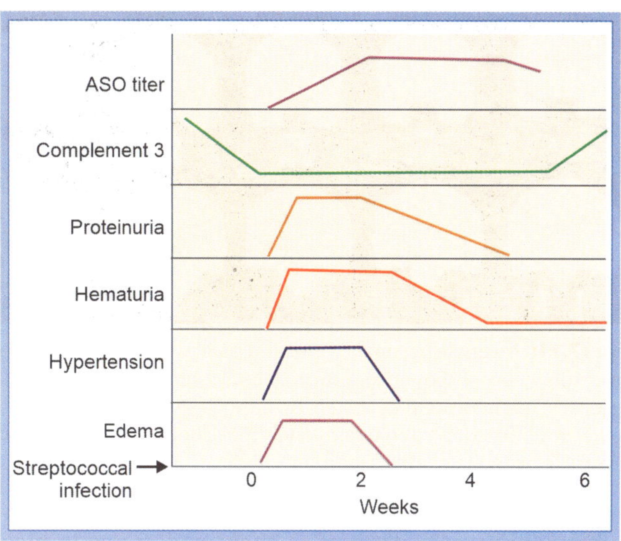

Fig. 17.10 Clinical course of poststreptococcal glomerulonephritis (ASO: antistreptolysin O)

Hypertension is mild and present in 70% of patients. It manifests as headache, blurred vision, seizures, and sometimes altered sensorium. It is transient and resolves after onset of diuresis and recovery of renal function. Severe hypertension requiring multiple antihypertensives and persisting beyond 4 weeks suggests RPGN or chronic glomerulopathy.

Course of Disease and Complications

The acute phase usually lasts for 4–6 weeks **(Fig. 17.10)**. Gross hematuria resolves in 1–2 weeks. Azotemia, edema, and hypertension resolve once diuresis ensues. However, microscopic hematuria may persist for 1–2 years.

Patients may present with one or more complications of acute glomerulonephritis.

- ***Acute pulmonary edema:*** Salt and water retention causes expansion of extracellular fluid volume resulting in circulatory congestion which is the most common complication. Severe hypertension and hypervolemia may lead to pulmonary edema.
- ***Hypertensive encephalopathy:*** 10% of cases of PSGN may present with altered sensorium due to sudden increase in blood pressure which impairs cerebral autoregulation resulting in cerebral edema. Infrequently, children with acute PSGN may present with features of posterior reversible encephalopathy syndrome (PRES). PRES is a rare clinico-radiologic syndrome manifesting with headache, seizures, altered sensorium, visual disturbances, and characteristic lesions on neuroimaging predominantly affecting the posterior regions of the brain.
- ***Acute kidney injury:*** Most cases would have modest derangement of renal functions. However, 1% patients of PSGN may develop oligoanuria, severe hypertension, anemia, rapidly increasing blood urea nitrogen (BUN), and creatinine. Hyperkalemia, hyperphosphatemia, metabolic acidosis, and uremia refractory to medical treatment would require dialysis.
- ***Nephrotic syndrome:*** 2% of cases may present with edema, gross hematuria, hypertension, and massive proteinuria.
- ***Rapid progressive glomerulonephritis:*** A course of rapidly progressive ("crescentic") glomerulonephritis occurs in <1% of cases. RPGN is characterized by acute nephritic syndrome with rapid deterioration in renal function (>50% decrease in GFR) within days to weeks and histopathological evidence of crescents affecting >50% of glomeruli.

Diagnosis

Examination of *urine specimen* reveals 1+/2+ proteinuria, dysmorphic RBCs, and RBC casts in most cases. Nephrotic range proteinuria, white blood cells (WBCs), and WBC casts may be found infrequently.

Hemogram may reveal mild anemia which is dilutional due to expansion of ECF volume. Thrombocytopenia is rare, and when present suggests other etiology such as systemic lupus erythematosus and HUS.

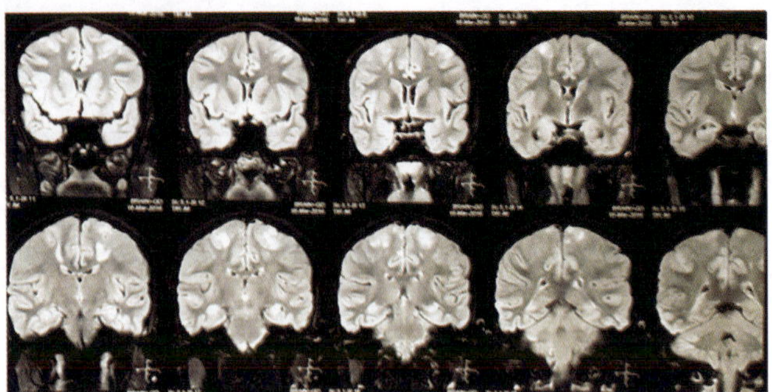

Fig. 17.11: Magnetic resonance imaging brain with fluid-attenuated inversion recovery sequence shows bilateral symmetric hyperintense lesions in parieto-occipital parenchyma in a 9-year-old child with acute poststreptococcal glomerulonephritis suggestive of posterior reversible encephalopathy syndrome (PRES)

Tests for *renal function* often show modest rise in blood urea, creatinine, and potassium. Worsening of renal functions suggested by rapid increase in blood urea and creatinine suggest RPGN and requires prompt evaluation and management.

Tests for *complement studies* show low CH 50 (total complement activity) and low C3 levels (alternate complement pathway activation). C4 levels may decrease in few cases which denotes classic complement pathway activation. 15% of PSGN patients may demonstrate normal complement levels.

Chest X-ray is indicated when the patient has respiratory distress.

Neuroimaging in children with hypertensive encephalopathy, CT scan of brain may reveal nonenhancing hypodensities of cerebral white matter in bilateral parietooccipital lobes. The lesions are best visualized with MRI with fluid attenuated inversion recovery (FLAIR) sequence. T2-weighted MRI images **(Fig. 17.11)**, at the height of symptoms, characteristically show diffuse hyperintensity selectively involving the parietooccipital white matter.

Tests for Evidence of Streptococcal Infection

- ***Culture from throat and skin*** depending upon site of infection
- ***ASO (normal levels <200 U/L)*** levels increase in nephritis associated with pharyngitis. Titers done early may be normal hence serial titers are more relevant. Mean time of significant titers is 3 weeks and continues to rise till 4 weeks. The sensitivity of ASO titers is 60–97% and specificity is 80% as reported in various studies.
- ***Antideoxyribonuclease-B and antihyaluronidase antibodies:*** They increase in nephritis associated with pyoderma. When two antibodies are tested, sensitivity increases from 60 to 80%.
- ***Streptozyme test:*** A slide hemagglutination test that detects antibodies to deoxyribonuclease-B, nicotinamide adenine dinuclease (NADase), streptolysin-O, hyaluronidase, and streptokinase.

Renal Biopsy

Renal biopsy is not required for diagnosis of PSGN but is done when indicated to rule out other conditions. Indications of renal biopsy are (1) rapidly progressive disease; (2) gross hematuria, hypertension and/or deranged renal functions persisting for >2 weeks; (3) normal complement levels; (4) evidence of systemic disease; and (5) persistent low C3 for >12 weeks.

Light microscopy shows diffuse hypercellularity of endothelial and mesangial cells and infiltration of the glomerular tuft with polymorphonuclear cells. Immunofluorescence microscopy shows granular deposits of IgG and C3 in capillary loop and mesangium.

Differential Diagnosis

A child presenting with acute nephritic syndrome with low C3 and evidence of recent streptococcal infection is most likely a case of PSGN. However, some other conditions can present with similar picture of acute nephritic syndrome.

- ***IgA nephropathy:*** Children present with gross hematuria within 24–48 hours of upper respiratory tract infection. It is also called "*synpharyngitic hematuria.*" Recurrent episodes are common. Urinalysis is often found normal at presentation since it is transient. Complement levels are normal.
- ***Membranoproliferative glomerulonephritis:*** Mean age of presentation is 10 years. It is a chronic glomerulonephritis. Sometimes may present as acute exacerbation of chronic glomerulonephritis after an episode of upper respiratory tract infection. Proteinuria is often massive. Renal functions may be deranged at presentation. It is sometimes diagnosed when renal biopsy is done for persistent low C3 levels in a child diagnosed as PIGN.
- ***Systemic lupus erythematosus:*** This is more common in adolescent females. It is a chronic glomerulonephritis but may present with acute nephritic syndrome with nephrotic range proteinuria. Other systemic features [fever, rash, arthritis, anemia, thrombocytopenia, central nervous system (CNS) involvement] may be present. C3 and C4 levels are low. ANA, double-stranded deoxyribonucleic acid (DNA) antibodies are present. Renal biopsy establishes the diagnosis.
- ***Henoch-Schönlein purpura:*** It presents after a viral prodrome with fever, palpable purpuric rash (lower limbs), abdominal pain, joint pain, and swelling. Involvement of gastrointestinal system and joints may be several days to weeks after rash. Renal involvement is found in 50% of the cases, usually presents as hematuria, gross or microscopic. Proteinuria, hypertension, acute renal failure, and nephrotic syndrome may be present. Complement levels are normal. It is a clinical diagnosis as laboratory findings are nonspecific.

Approach to diagnosis of a child with acute nephritic syndrome is depicted in **Flowchart 17.3**.

TREATMENT Poststreptococcal Glomerulonephritis

Treatment of patient with acute PSGN is supportive until the resolution of symptoms occurs. Eradication of triggering agent by administration of antibiotics after onset of symptoms does not ameliorate the severity of nephritis.

- Bedrest and limitation of activity is advised.
- *Fluid and sodium restriction:* Low salt diet and restriction of fluids remains the mainstay of management in mild cases.

Flowchart 17.3: Approach to a case of acute nephritic syndrome

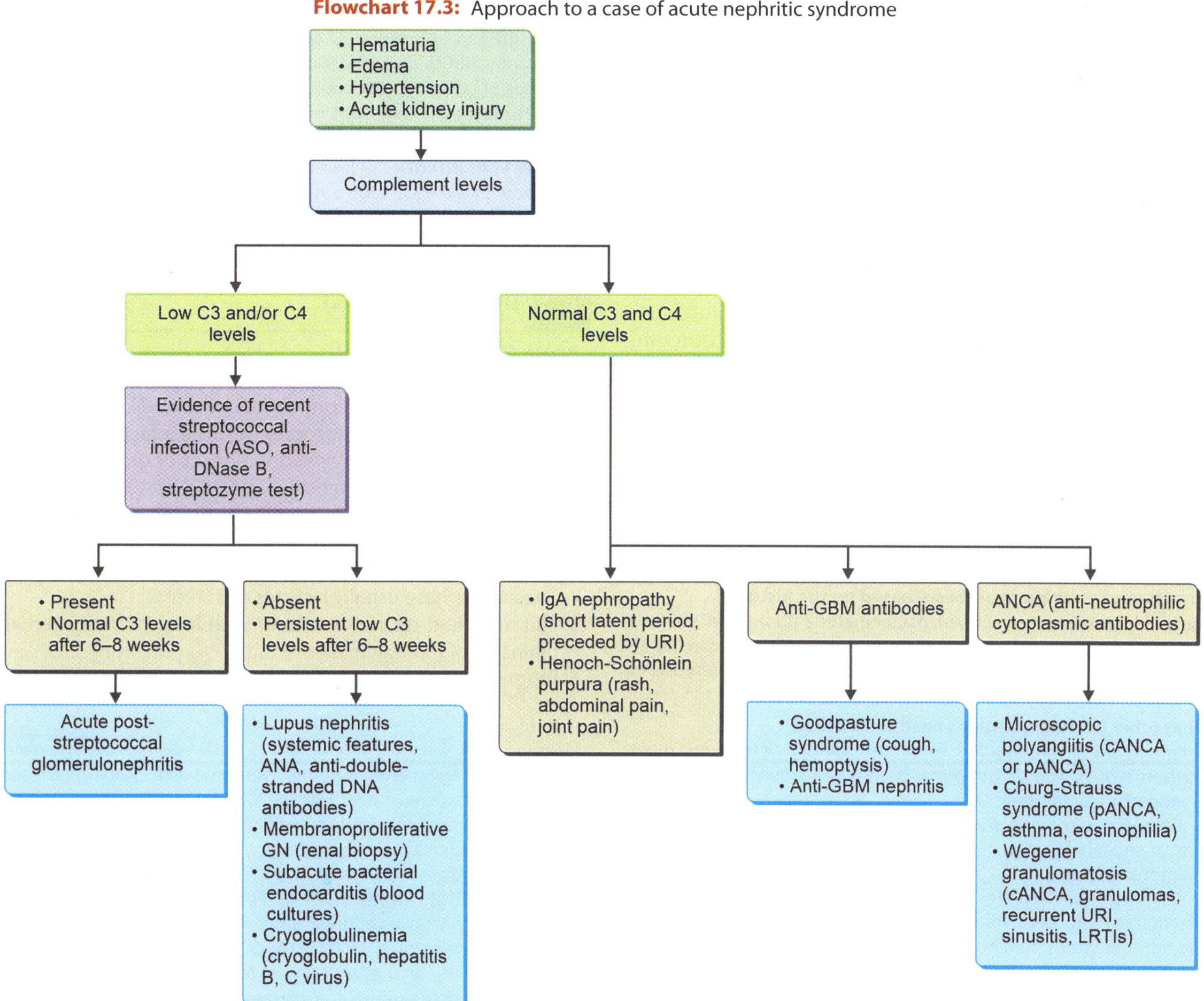

(ANA: antinuclear antibody; ASO: antistreptolysin O; DNA: deoxyribonucleic acid; DNase B: deoxyribonuclease B; GBM: glomerular basement membrane; GN: glomerulonephritis; IgA: immunoglobulin A; LRTIs: lower respiratory tract infections; URI: upper respiratory infection)

- *Diet:* Potassium restricted diet if hyperkalemia is present. Protein restriction is required if azotemia is present.
- *Edema:* Fluid and sodium restriction along with loop diuretics decrease edema.
- *Hypertension:* Furosemide (1–2 mg/kg/day in 2–3 divided doses) is the drug of choice for control of hypertension in acute glomerulonephritis and it also decreases hyperkalemia. Higher doses may be given for pulmonary edema. Oral nifedipine 0.25–0.5 mg/kg every 4–6 hours is given if BP is not controlled with diuretics. In patients with hypertensive emergency intravenous labetalol or nitroprusside infusion is given for 24–48 hours.
- *Hyperkalemia:* Potassium is restricted in diet. Sodium polystyrene sulfonate resin in dose of 0.5–1 g/kg/per dose every 4–6 hourly can be given orally. If still uncontrolled other measures as glucose insulin infusion and nebulization with salbutamol, may help.
- *Dialysis:* This is done in patients with refractory hyperkalemia, acidosis, uremia, hypertension, and fluid overload.
- *Antibiotics:* These are indicated in children with active streptococcal pharyngitis or pyoderma or when throat culture is positive. Single dose of benzathine penicillin 0.6 million units or oral penicillin V 125 mg, every 6 hours for 7–10 days, are adequate treatment. Erythromycin or azithromycin is the treatment of choice in children allergic to penicillin. The antibiotic therapy limits the spread of nephritogenic streptococci to susceptible contacts but does not alter the course of acute glomerulonephritis.
- *Steroids:* There is no role of steroids in treatment of acute PSGN. Patients with >30% crescents on renal biopsy are often treated with methylprednisolone pulses, although there is no evidence that aggressive immunosuppressive therapy has a beneficial effect in patients with rapidly progressive crescentic disease.

Prevention

Adequate treatment of streptococcal infection with a 10 day course of antibiotic therapy prevents the transmission of nephritogenic strains during epidemics and also protects against glomerulonephritis. Hence, it is important to diagnose streptococcal pharyngitis which is suggested by temperature >38°C, tonsillar exudate, soft palate petechiae, and anterior cervical lymphadenopathy.

Prognosis

Majority of children of PSGN recover completely without any sequelae. Recurrences are extremely rare. 1% of cases may develop rapid progressive course which has guarded prognosis. Management of complications adequately decreases mortality. There is scant long-term data of AGN due to other infections (nonstreptococcal) but in general have favorable outcome. Progression to chronic glomerulonephritis occurs in <2% of cases which may slowly progress to ESRD.

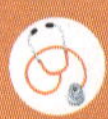

CASE STUDY Acute Nephritic Syndrome

A 7-year-old boy presented with puffiness around eyes more in early morning and headache for 4 days. He was passing cola-colored urine. The day before he passed urine only twice and that too in small volumes.

What is your working hypothesis, based on the history?

The child has presented with edema, hematuria (to be confirmed by urine examination), oliguria, and hypertension (to be confirmed by BP measurement). The symptoms point toward a possible diagnosis of acute glomerulonephritis.

What other leading questions need to be asked?

Symptoms of systemic disorders: Fever, rash, joint pains (systemic lupus erythematosus, HSP), abdominal pain (HSP), cough, hemoptysis (Goodpasture syndrome)

Complications of the disease: Seizures, altered sensorium (hypertensive encephalopathy), rapid breathing, and difficulty in breathing (pulmonary edema).

Past history: History of antecedent sore throat or cutaneous infection (streptococcal infection). Latent period between sore throat and onset of symptoms since shorter period of 2–4 days is suggestive of IgA nephropathy.

The child had chickenpox 1 month back; later, a few lesions developed purulent discharge. He was prescribed oral antibiotics for a week by his pediatrician but they discontinued after 3 days. On examination, he was tachypneic with respiratory rate of 32/min, PR 98/min, BP 164/100 mm Hg, and jugular venous pressure (JVP) was raised. He had periorbital puffiness and pedal edema. He had hyperpigmented spots all over body. Chest examination revealed bilateral basal crepitations. Liver was palpable 4 cm below right subcostal margin. Heart sounds and neurological examination were normal.

What is the probable diagnosis now? Outline the investigation to be done to confirm the diagnosis?

The child presented with gross hematuria, edema, oliguria, and hypertension (acute nephritic syndrome) 1 month after superadded bacterial infection of varicella, the probable diagnosis is acute poststreptococcal glomerulonephritis.

The relevant investigations are urine routine microscopy, blood urea, serum creatinine, serum electrolytes, serum albumin, cholesterol, chest X-ray, electrocardiogram (ECG), C3 level, ASO titer, and anti-DNase B.

Urine examination revealed urine protein 2+, full field RBCs, 30% dysmorphic, a few WBCs. Other investigations revealed blood urea 65 mg/dL, serum creatinine 1.2 mg/dL, sodium 138 mEq/L, potassium 5 mEq/L, serum albumin 3.4 mg/dL, cholesterol 180 mg/dL, C3 34 mg/dL, ASO titer 300 U/L, anti-DNase B 2,000 U/mL. Chest X-ray revealed bilateral fluffy infiltrates and ECG was normal.

Interpret above findings in view of clinical diagnosis.

The child has hematuria of glomerular origin (RBCs, RBC casts, dysmorphic RBCs), azotemia (raised urea and creatinine), low C3, and evidence of past streptococcal infection (elevated ASO and DNase B). All these favor the diagnosis of PSGN. Chest X-ray findings suggest associated pulmonary edema.

Outline your priorities in immediate management of this child.

We need to take care of pulmonary edema and hypertension. Intravenous furosemide 1–2 mg/kg needs to be urgently administered.

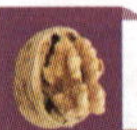

IN A NUTSHELL

Acute Glomerulonephritis

1. Most common cause of acute nephritic syndrome is post-infectious glomerulonephritis that occurs following a group A beta-hemolytic *Streptococcus* (GABHS) infection.
2. PSGN is characterized by sudden onset of gross hematuria, edema, oliguria, hypertension, and mild azotemia.
3. Clinical presentation of acute nephritic syndrome along with low complements and evidence of recent streptococcal infection establishes the diagnosis.
4. The acute phase usually lasts for 4–6 weeks.
5. Salt and fluid restriction along with loop diuretics remain mainstay of management.
6. Prognosis is good and recurrences are extremely rare.

Alhamoud MA, Salloot IZ, Mohiuddin SS, et al. A Comprehensive review study on glomerulonephritis associated with post-streptococcal infection. Cureus. 2021;13(12):e20212.

Chen TH. Childhood posterior reversible encephalopathy syndrome: clinicoradiological characteristics, managements, and outcome. Front Pediatr. 2020;8:585.

Eison TM, Ault BH, Jones DP, et al. Poststreptococcal acute glomerulonephritis in children: clinical features and pathogenesis. Pediatr Nephrol. 2011;26(2):165-80.

Gunasekaran K, Krishnamurthy S, Mahadevan S, et al. Clinical characteristics and outcome of post-infectious glomerulonephritis in children in Southern India: A prospective study. Indian J Pediatr. 2015;82(10):896-903.

Iyengar A, Kamath N, Radhakrishnan J, Estebanez BT. Infection-related glomerulonephritis in children and adults. Semin Nephrol. 2023;43(5):151469.

Kambham N. Postinfectious glomerulonephritis. Adv Anat Pathol. 2012;19(5):338-47.

Orlando C, Milani GP, Simonetti, G.D, et al. Posterior reversible leukoencephalopathy syndrome associated with acute postinfectious glomerulonephritis: systematic review. Pediatr Nephrol. 2022;37:833-41.

Stratta P, Musetti C, Barreca A, et al. New trends of an old disease: the acute post-infectious glomerulonephritis at the beginning of the new millennium. J Nephrol. 2014;27:229-39.

RAPIDLY PROGRESSIVE GLOMERULONEPHRITIS

Rapidly progressive glomerulonephritis is characterized by acute nephritic syndrome with rapid deterioration in renal function (>50% decrease in GFR) within days to weeks and histopathological evidence of crescents affecting >50% of glomeruli. Rapidly progressive glomerulonephritis and crescentic glomerulonephritis term is often used synonymously. RPGN is caused by varied renal disorders. Certain conditions may have similar presentation of RPGN but are without crescents as in HUS.

Pathogenesis

Crescents are formed by infiltration of inflammatory cells and proliferation of parietal and visceral epithelial cells in Bowman space. Severe glomerular injury is caused by immune complexes (systemic infections) and antibodies to glomerular and cellular antigenic components [antineutrophil cytoplasmic antibodies (ANCA), antiglomerular basement membrane (anti-GBM), ANA, double-stranded DNA antibodies).

Classification

Crescentic glomerulonephritis is categorized as:

- ***Immune complex mediated glomerulonephritis:*** It is most common cause of RPGN in children accounting for 50–75% of causes in most series. This group includes diseases that result in granular deposits of immunoglobulins and/or complements along capillary wall and mesangium in immunofluorescence microscopy. Primary glomerulonephritis as IgA nephropathy, postinfectious glomerulonephritis and systemic diseases like systemic lupus erythematosus are diseases which lead to immune complex mediated glomerulonephritis.
- ***Pauci-immune glomerulonephritis:*** 15–40% cases are caused by pauci-immune glomerulonephritis. Small vessel vasculitis as in microscopic polyangiitis, Wegener's granulomatosis and renal limited vasculitis cause extensive crescent formation and necrotizing glomerulonephritis without or minimal deposition of immune complexes. 80% of cases have ANCA in blood.
- ***Antiglomerular basement antibody-mediated glomerulonephritis:*** It causes RPGN in 12–15% of cases. It is most severe form of RPGN. Immunofluorescence shows linear deposits of immunoglobulin G with or without C3 along capillary walls.

Clinical Features

Most common presentation is of acute nephritic syndrome with rapid derangement of renal functions often complicated by hypertensive emergency and acute pulmonary edema. Investigations and clinical features of different categories of RPGN are listed in **Table 17.11**.

TREATMENT Rapidly Progressive Glomerulonephritis

Management of a child with RPGN includes supportive management of fluids, electrolytes, hypertension, nutrition, and specific therapy. High dose steroids and cytotoxic therapy constitute the mainstay of specific management. Intravenous pulse methylprednisolone is given in a dose of 15–20 mg/kg for 3–6 days followed by oral prednisolone 1.5–2 mg/kg/day for 4 weeks. Steroids are then tapered over 3 months and then continued on alternate days for 6 months to 1 year. Alternatively, intravenous pulse cyclophosphamide in a dose of 500–750 mg/m² every 3–4 weeks for 6 pulses is given along with steroids or oral cyclophosphamide in a dose of 2–2.5 mg/kg/day for 12 weeks.

Maintenance immunosuppression is with azathioprine, alternate day prednisolone, or mycophenolate.

Plasmapheresis may be required in patients who do not respond to pulse steroid therapy, in anti-GBM nephritis, and in ANCA associated RPGN with severe renal involvement and/or pulmonary hemorrhage.

Table 17.11 Causes, Clinical Features, and Diagnosis of Rapidly Progressive Glomerulonephritis

	Causes	*Other clinical features*	*Specific investigations*
• Immune complex mediated • Low serum complement C3	Postinfectious glomerulonephritis	History of antecedent streptococcal infection, evidence of septic foci	↑ ASO, ↑ anti-DNase B, renal biopsy—diffuse proliferative GN with IgG and C3 deposits in mesangium and along capillary walls
	Membranoproliferative glomerulonephritis	Acute nephritic syndrome postviral prodrome, anemia	Low C3 ± low C4, renal biopsy—mesangial proliferation and thickening of the peripheral GBM with C3 and IgG deposits
	Systemic lupus erythematosus	Fever, malaise, joint pain, anemia, seizures	Low C3, low C4, ANA, anti-dsDNA, renal biopsy—diffuse proliferation with subendothelial deposits and full house (deposits of all Ig class) in IF
Normal complement	• IgA nephropathy • Henoch–Schönlein purpura	• History of recurrent episodes of gross hematuria after URI • Fever, joint pain, abdominal pain, palpable purpura	• ↑ serum IgA, renal biopsy—mesangial hypercellularity with mesangial IgA deposits • Essential clinical diagnosis • Renal biopsy s/o mesangial hypercellularity with mesangial IgA deposits
• Pauci-immune systemic vasculitis • No systemic vasculitis	• Microscopic polyangiitis • Wegener granulomatosis • Churg–Strauss syndrome • Renal limited vasculitis	• Vasculitic rash over lower limbs • Cough, sinusitis, subglottic stenosis, nasal deformity • Recurrent wheezing episodes, no extrarenal features	• pANCA +, extrarenal non-granulomatous lesions, renal biopsy—necrotizing crescentic glomerulonephritis • cANCA (70–90%) extrarenal granulomatous lesions, renal biopsy—focal necrotizing crescentic glomerulonephritis • Eosinophilia, renal biopsy—necrotizing crescentic glomerulonephritis • Renal biopsy—necrotizing crescentic glomerulonephritis
Antiglomerular basement antibody mediated	Goodpasture syndrome anti-GBM nephritis	Hemoptysis, pulmonary hemorrhage	Presence of anti-GBM antibodies, renal biopsy—crescentic glomerulonephritis with linear IgG deposition along the glomerular capillaries in IF

(ASO: antistreptolysin O; DNase B: deoxyribonuclease B; IF: immunofluorescence; IgA: immunoglobulin A; IgG: immunoglobulin G; GBM: glomerular basement membrane; GN: glomerulonephritis; pANCA: perinuclear antineutrophil cytoplasmic antibody; URI: upper respiratory infection)

Prognosis

Outcome of RPGN has improved in last few years. 60–70% of patients have recovery of renal function. Resolution of renal parameters depends on underlying disease, histopathology, proportion of crescents, extent of tubulointerstitial scarring and fibrosis. Poststreptococcal crescentic glomerulonephritis has better prognosis than lupus, MPGN, pauci-immune or anti-GBM associated RPGN.

Risk factors for kidney failure included oliguria, dialysis requirement at onset, estimated GFR, proportion of fibrous crescents, and pauci-immune glomerulonephritis as the underlying etiology. Almost one in every four patients with crescentic glomerulonephritis progress to kidney failure.

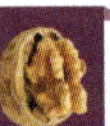

IN A NUTSHELL

Rapidly Progressive Glomerulonephritis

1. RPGN is loss of kidney function over a short period (days to weeks).
2. Clinical manifestations are those of severe acute nephritic syndrome with heavy proteinuria.
3. Evolving GN with progressively deteriorating renal functions need urgent renal biopsy.
4. Renal histology is characterized by presence of crescents in >50% of glomeruli.
5. Intensive immunosuppressive therapy with IV steroids and cyclophosphamide is initiated. Patients with pauci-immune and anti-GBM disease need plasmapheresis during induction phase.
6. Renal outcome depends on severity of disease at presentation, underlying cause, and promptness of therapy.

Appel GB, Kaplan AA. Overview of the classification and treatment of rapidly progressive (crescentic) glomerulonephritis. In UpToDate. Post, Glassock R J, Fervenza FC (Ed) Waltham, MA. [Last accessed August, 2025].

Hoschek JC, Dreyer P, Dahal S, et al. Rapidly progressive renal failure in childhood. Am J Kidney Dis. 2002;40(6):1342-7.

Kher KK. Acute glomerular diseases in children. Open Urol Nephrol J. 2015;26:8.

Meena J, Nangla P, Ojha S, et al. Etiology, clinical profile, and outcomes of crescentic glomerulonephritis in children: a systematic review. Pediatr Nephrol. 2025;40(3):675-684. doi: 10.1007/s00467-024-06521-3.

Rutgers A, Sanders JS, Stegeman CA, et al. Pauci-immune necrotizing glomerulonephritis. Rheum Dis Clin North Am. 2010;36:559-72.

17.6 Proteinuria

PE 20.3

INTRODUCTION

Proteinuria is commonly seen in kidney diseases and is an important prognostic marker. Proteinuria can be *transient* or *persistent*. While the former is usually benign, the latter indicates the presence of an underlying kidney disease and is a well-recognized risk factor for cardiovascular disease and mortality. Hence, monitoring for proteinuria is essential in all patients in whom the kidneys are affected.

DEFINITIONS

- On a 24 hour urine sample, a value >100 mg/m^2/day (or >4 mg/m^2/h) is considered *proteinuria*. Proteinuria of >1,000 mg/m^2/day (or >40 mg/m^2/h) is known as *nephrotic range proteinuria.*
- On a spot urine sample, proteinuria is defined as urinary protein/creatinine ratio (Up/Uc) of ≥0.2 mg protein/mg creatinine. Nephrotic range proteinuria is defined as Up/Uc >2.
- On dipstick analysis of the first morning urine sample, a value ≥1+ on multiple occasions is abnormal and needs to be investigated. Nephrotic range proteinuria is manifested by 3+ or 4+ proteinuria on dipstick testing.
- While the spot and 24-hour samples estimate total proteinuria (including albumin and other tubular proteins like beta-2 microglobulin), the dipstick usually estimates albuminuria only. Albuminuria is defined as urine albumin/creatinine ratio >30 mg/g; a value 30–300 mg/g is considered *microalbuminuria*. The dipstick protein usually remains negative unless albuminuria is >300 mg/g creatinine.

EPIDEMIOLOGY

Transient proteinuria is relatively common and is seen in 5–15% of school-going children on a single random urine sample. Exercise, fever, and trivial infections may lead to transient proteinuria and is usually self-limiting. Only 0.1–0.5% of these children have persistent proteinuria on repeat testing. Nephrotic syndrome has an incidence of 1.2–16.9 per 100,000 children per year, varying by ethnicity and region.

ETIOLOGY

Based on etiology, proteinuria can be classified as *transient, orthostatic, overflow,* or *persistent.*

Transient or Functional Proteinuria

At least 30–50% of children with proteinuria may have transient, nonrecurring proteinuria. Transient proteinuria is known to occur with fever, strenuous exercise, emotional stress, exposure to extreme cold, epinephrine administration, abdominal surgery or congestive heart failure and after seizures.

It resolves spontaneously after the cessation of the precipitating factor, and detailed evaluation is usually not recommended.

Orthostatic (Postural) Proteinuria

Orthostatic proteinuria accounts for up to 60% of all cases of asymptomatic proteinuria reported in children, with an even higher incidence in adolescents. Variations in the quantity of daily protein excretion have been observed. If all laboratory tests (such as blood urea, serum creatinine, serum albumin, serum cholesterol) and clinical findings (such as blood pressure, growth) are normal except for persistently elevated protein excretion, the possibility of orthostatic proteinuria should be investigated, particularly if the child is older than 6 years of age. This is best done by using the *orthostatic test*.

The child is instructed to urinate just before going to bed at night and to discard the urine. He or she must remain supine all night and urinate the next morning immediately after arising. This urine sample is kept separate and labeled "supine" or "recumbent." Additional urine samples are then collected and pooled during the next 12–16 hours, while the patient maintains normal daily activity. The final sample should preferably be collected in the evening, just before the patient goes to bed; this pooled sample should be labeled "active" urine. The duration of collection time for the latter sample can be shortened to 12 hours or less. In patients with orthostatic proteinuria, the supine sample will be free of protein, but the evening sample will contain protein. Children with orthostatic proteinuria usually have Up/Uc <1. Yearly follow-up is recommended for children diagnosed with this condition.

Overflow Proteinuria

Overflow proteinuria occurs when the plasma concentration of certain small proteins exceeds the capacity of the tubules to reabsorb the filtered protein. Examples include the presence of immunoglobulin light chains in the urine in multiple myeloma, hemoglobinuria in intravascular hemolysis, myoglobinuria in rhabdomyolysis, and amylasuria in acute pancreatitis.

Persistent Proteinuria

The finding of at least two positive urine tests showing proteinuria, out of three specimens would suggest persistent proteinuria and warrants a thorough workup. Persistent proteinuria can be secondary to glomerular or tubular etiologies.

Glomerular Proteinuria

Nephrotic syndrome and acute poststreptococcal glomerulonephritis are the main causes of glomerular proteinuria in children.

- ❖ In nephrotic syndrome patients have heavy or "nephrotic range" proteinuria.
- ❖ Proteinuria in acute postinfectious glomerulonephritis (most commonly poststreptococcal) is usually 1+ or 2+; accompanied by hematuria, and generally has a good outcome without long-term sequelae.
- ❖ Other important causes of proteinuria include focal segmental glomerulosclerosis (FSGS), membranous nephropathy (MN), HSP nephritis, lupus nephritis, and MPGN. Human immunodeficiency virus (HIV) infection has emerged as an important cause of proteinuria and nephrotic syndrome in both adults and children.

Other congenital and acquired urinary tract anomalies such as hydronephrosis, polycystic kidney disease, reflux nephropathy, and renal dysplasia may also manifest with proteinuria. In the absence of nephrotic syndrome, glomerular proteinuria may be the only sign of renal damage in many patients with early chronic kidney disease (CKD).

Tubular Proteinuria

Proteinuria, with or without hematuria, occurs in patients with tubulointerstitial diseases of diverse etiologies. When the GFR is normal, the proteinuria is usually of tubular origin. As the GFR decreases as a result of significant nephron loss, hemodynamic mechanisms contribute to glomerular proteinuria.

In general, the proteinuria of tubulointerstitial disease is mild (<1 g per 24 hours). Characteristically, tubular proteinuria is predominantly composed of low molecular weight (LMW) proteins. Some tubular diseases that can manifest as isolated LMW proteinuria during childhood include Dent disease, Lowe syndrome, and Fabry disease.

MECHANISMS OF PROTEIN HANDLING BY THE KIDNEYS

The glomerular filtration apparatus, a complex membrane with selective permeability, is composed of three main cellular barriers: (1) glomerular basement membrane, (2) Fenestrated endothelium, and (3) Podocytes along with their specialized junctions called "split diaphragm." This assembly prevents the passage of large molecules such as albumin (molecular weight 65 kDa). In addition to the size barrier, the glomerular capillary wall contains negative charge which helps in repelling other negatively charged molecules like albumin. These specialized structures thus prevent leaking of plasma proteins into the urine. Recently, there is heightened recognition of the role of podocytes in proteinuria as evidenced by the discovery of numerous single gene defects (e.g., *NPHS1, NPHS2, WT1, PLCE1*, etc.), involving the podocytes and leading to nephrotic syndrome. Proteinuria thus indicates a defect in the integrity of the glomerular filtration barrier (GFB). While the macromolecules like albumin do not cross the GFB, LMW proteins like beta-2 microglobulin are freely filtered across the GFB but are completely reabsorbed in the proximal tubule. Interference in proximal tubular reabsorption, due to a variety of hereditary (e.g., Fanconi syndrome, Dent disease) or acquired (e.g., reflux nephropathy, interstitial nephritis) causes, leads to tubular proteinuria.

Healthy children usually excrete minute amounts of protein, i.e., <100 mg/m^2/day or 4 mg/m^2/h. Out of these, Tamm–Horsfall protein, a glycoprotein secreted by the ascending limb of loop of Henle, contributes to 50% of the total protein excreted in the urine while albumin comprises <30%. The remaining is contributed by plasma proteins such as immunoglobulins, transferrin, and beta-2 microglobulin. This modest amount of physiological proteinuria is not usually detected on routine dipstick testing. Also, the dipstick examination generally does not pick up tubular proteinuria.

How does Persistent Proteinuria Cause Renal Injury?

Several mechanisms have been identified by which proteinuria may induce kidney damage:

- Release of lysosomal enzymes into the cytoplasm of protein-reabsorbing tubules may induce inflammation.
- Filtration of cytokines or chemokines may provoke cell proliferation, inflammatory cell infiltration, and activation of infiltrating cells.
- Filtration of novel antigens may function as antigen-presenting cells and initiate cellular immune response.
- Filtration of lipoproteins and absorption by proximal tubules may activate inflammatory pathways causing cell injury.
- The alternative complement cascade gets activated in this inflammatory milieu and accentuates cell damage.
- Ischemic tubular injury may follow the release of vasoconstricting molecules.
- Release of fibrosis-promoting factors from the injured cells leads to interstitial fibrosis.
- Iron that is filtered into the tubular fluid may be directly cytotoxic or may have indirect effects as a consequence of iron-catalyzed synthesis of reactive oxygen metabolites.
- The tubules may be obstructed by proteinaceous casts.

ESTIMATION OF PROTEINURIA

Dipstick Method

A frequently used screening method for detection of proteinuria is urinary dipstick, which primarily detects albumin, leaving LMW proteins undetected. A color reaction between urinary albumin and tetrabromophenol blue produces various green hues based on the concentration of albumin in the sample, which is graded as follows:

Trace (15 mg/dL);
1+ (30 mg/dL);
2+ (100 mg/dL);
3+ (300 mg/dL); and
4+ (2,000 mg/dL)

Because it is the concentration of urine protein that is measured, false-negative results may occur with very dilute urine. Conversely, false-positive results may occur with very alkaline or concentrated urine specimens in the presence of contaminating antiseptics, such as chlorhexidine and benzalkonium chloride, or after the administration of radiographic contrast, e.g., after intravenous pyelogram (IVP). **Box 17.6** summarizes the causes of false-positive or false-negative dipstick results.

An alternative method is to measure urinary protein in patients with suspected proteinuria by using protein precipitation with sulfosalicylic acid. This technique provides a quantitative estimate of all the urinary proteins including LMW proteins hence is not specific for albuminuria.

Heat Coagulation Test

In a test tube, take 2 mL of urine sample. The test tube is then inclined and the surface is heated on a flame. The formation of a coagulum indicates the presence of albumin.

Box 17.6 Causes of False-positive or False-negative Dipstick Results

- *False-positive results:*
  - Concentrated urine
  - Alkaline urine
  - Contamination by antiseptics (e.g., chlorhexidine, benzalkonium) and antibiotics (e.g., penicillins)
  - Administration of radiographic contrast
  - Gross hematuria
  - Contamination by vaginal secretions
- *False-negative results:*
  - Diluted urine
  - Acidic urine
  - Microalbuminuria/low molecular weight proteinuria

Urinary Protein/Creatinine Ratio

In contrast to adults, since an accurately timed or 24-hour urine collection may not be feasible in children, the Up/Uc of a spot urine specimen (preferably the first morning sample) is commonly used for estimation of protein excretion in children. This Up/Uc ratio has been shown to correlate with the 24-hour urine protein excretion, especially since an early morning spot testing rules out confounding factors such as postural proteinuria. A value of >0.2 is abnormal in children older than 2 years; with values >2 suggesting nephrotic-range proteinuria.

APPROACH TO EVALUATION OF PROTEINURIA

The initial evaluation of proteinuria should comprise of a complete history, including family history of renal disease/stones, recent upper respiratory infections, gross hematuria, changes in weight, and changes in urine output. The physical examination should include measurements of height, weight, and blood pressure, identification of edema, ascites and pallor, and palpation of the kidneys in newborn infants. A urinalysis should be performed, and blood obtained for determination of electrolytes, BUN, creatinine, and serum albumin levels, as well as a complete blood count and complement C3 levels. A quantitative assessment of urinary protein excretion should be made, using a spot urine sample for the Up/Uc ratio.

TREATMENT Proteinuria

Management depends on the underlying etiology of proteinuria. Nephrotic syndrome in children should be managed with corticosteroids as per the Indian Society of Pediatric Nephrology guidelines. Postinfectious glomerulonephritis is usually self-limiting, and a renal biopsy is not indicated in most cases, except in atypical circumstances such as rapidly rising creatinine levels, absence of hypocomplementemia at diagnosis, or persistent hypertension/nephrotic range proteinuria. Other etiologies such as polycystic kidneys may be easily identified from an ultrasound of the kidneys and urinary bladder. Orthostatic proteinuria usually has a benign course, and extensive work up is not required apart from annual follow-up.

Restriction on the child's lifestyle and physical activity is not necessary. While avoiding excessive salt intake is desirable, protein restriction is not recommended and routine protein intake in the diet should be allowed. In patients with glomerular proteinuria, therapy with an ACE inhibitor or angiotensin receptor blockers (ARB) can bring about a significant reduction in proteinuria. ACE inhibitors and ARB have an established antiproteinuric effect which is, to some extent, independent of hypertension control. The mechanism of their antiproteinuric effect is by selective vasodilatation of the efferent arteriole which lowers the filtration pressure and, hence, the amount of albumin in the ultrafiltrate.

PROGNOSIS

Long-term follow-up studies have documented the benign nature of orthostatic proteinuria, although rare cases of glomerulosclerosis have been identified later in life in patients who were initially found to have proteinuria with an orthostatic component. Transient proteinuria, which is most often associated with fever, stress, dehydration, or exercise, is not considered to be indicative of underlying renal disease.

Persistent Proteinuria as an Indicator of Renal Disease and its Progression

On the basis of population-based studies in adults with CKD, persistent proteinuria is considered both a maker of kidney disease, as well as, its progression. It reflects the severity of underlying kidney damage. In children, proteinuria has been significantly correlated with a decline in GFR, both in glomerular and tubular disorders. Current strategies to prevent CKD progression, a concept known as *renoprotection*, aim at controlling blood pressure and reducing urinary protein excretion.

Persistent Proteinuria as a Risk Factor for Cardiovascular Disease

Obesity is considered an independent risk factor for CKD, hypertension, and cardiovascular disease in children and adults. Obesity-related glomerulopathy, presenting as proteinuria and progressive renal dysfunction, is increasing even in children. Severe persistent proteinuria may be a long-term risk factor for atherosclerosis in children. As the severity of proteinuria increases, it is associated with a variety of metabolic disturbances that contribute to cardiovascular disease, e.g., hypercholesterolemia, hypertriglyceridemia, and hypercoagulability. In some patients, other factors such as hypertension, renal insufficiency, and steroid therapy may also contribute to the risk for cardiovascular disease.

Flowchart 17.4 depicts the algorithm for diagnostic evaluation of children with proteinuria.

Flowchart 17.4: Algorithm for diagnostic evaluation of children with proteinuria

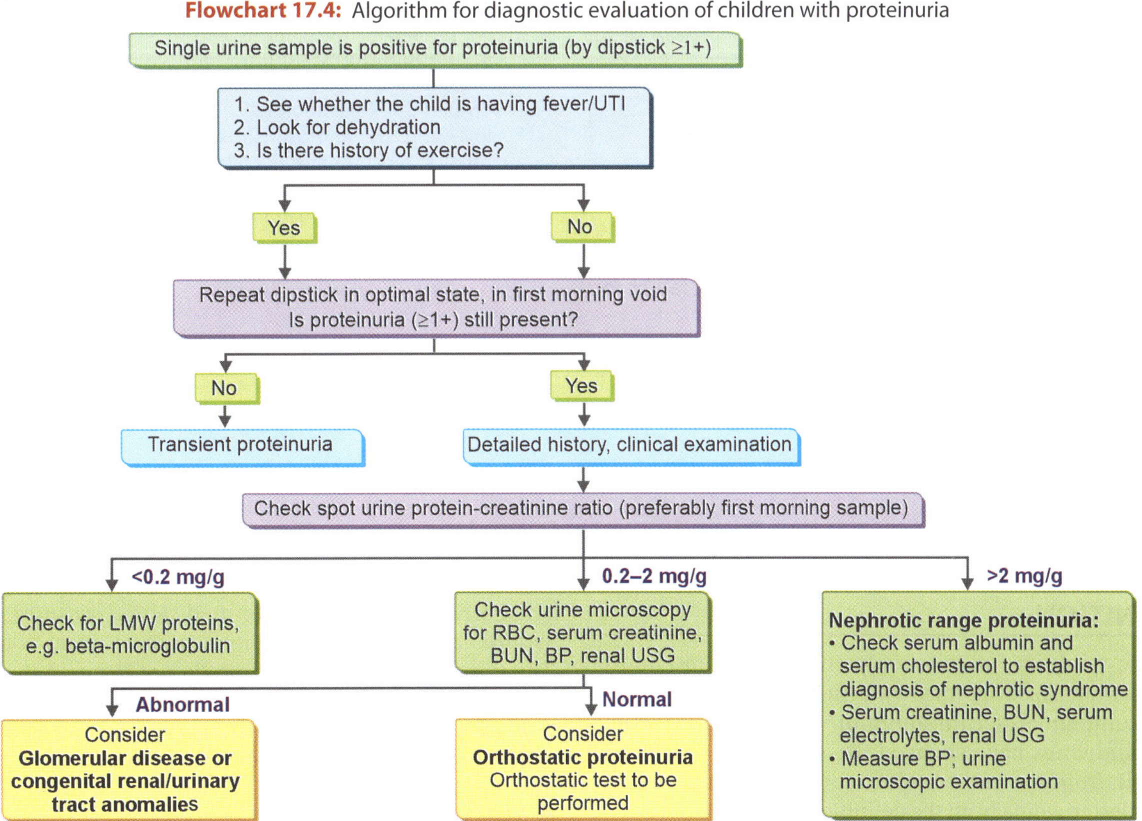

(BP: blood pressure; BUN: blood urea nitrogen; UTI: urinary tract infection; LMW: low molecular weight; RBC: red blood cell; USG: ultrasonography)

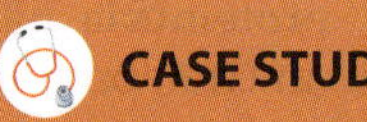

CASE STUDY **Proteinuria in Poststreptococcal Glomerulonephritis**

A 7-year-old girl is brought to the pediatric outpatient department with complaints of puffiness of the face, and oliguria for the past 3 days. There is no history of cola-colored urine. However, there is history of pyoderma over the legs 3 weeks ago, which are now healed. On examination, child has periorbital puffiness and pedal edema. Blood pressure is recorded to be 134/88 mm Hg (>95th centile for age, sex, and height). Rest of the examination is unremarkable. On bedside dipstick testing, the child was found to have 2+ proteinuria with few RBCs.

What is the most likely cause of proteinuria in this child?
Post-streptococcal glomerulonephritis is the most likely diagnosis, since there is a history of pyoderma 3 weeks ago, following which subnephrotic range proteinuria, oliguria, and hypertension have been documented.

What other investigations are needed to confirm the diagnosis?
Microscopic hematuria is required to confirm the diagnosis. Hence, a urinalysis is required to be done. Blood urea, serum creatinine, ASO and C3 levels should be performed in all cases of suspected PSGN.

Urinalysis demonstrated RBC casts with 20 RBC per hpf. Blood urea was 30 mg/dL and serum creatinine was 0.4 mg/dL. Serum C3 levels were very low. ASO was 400 units/L.

What is the role of immunosuppressive therapy as an antiproteinuric measure in this case?
The investigations confirm PSGN. Most cases of PSGN are benign and self-limiting. Proper fluid management along with strict input-output monitoring, blood pressure control, and judicious use of diuretics is vital. Immunosuppressive medications like methylprednisolone pulse therapy is generally not required in most patients, except when complicated by rapidly progressive glomerulonephritis.

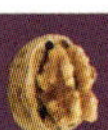

IN A NUTSHELL

Proteinuria

1. Persistent proteinuria indicates the presence of an underlying kidney disorder and is recognized as a marker and mediator of progressive renal insufficiency, as well as a risk factor for cardiovascular disease.
2. Glomerular proteinuria is more severe than tubular proteinuria.
3. Therapeutic measures to control persistent proteinuria are considered an integral part of renoprotective strategies.

Daehn IS, Duffield JS. The glomerular filtration barrier: a structural target for novel kidney therapies. Nat Rev Drug Discov. 2021;20:770-88.

Huang Y, Yang X, Zhang Y, et al. Correlation of urine protein/creatinine ratios to 24-h urinary protein for quantitating proteinuria in children. Pediatr Nephrol. 2020;35:463-8.

Fogo AB, Harris RC. Crosstalk between glomeruli and tubules. Nat Rev Nephrol. 2024.

Hawkins A, Scobell RR. Evaluation and management of proteinuria in children. Curr Treat Options Peds. 2024;10:228-36.

Imam AA, Saadeh SA. Evaluation of proteinuria and hematuria in ambulatory setting. Pediatr Clin North Am. 2022;69:1037-49.

Jang KM, Cho MH. Clinical approach to children with proteinuria. Child Kidney Dis. 2017;21:53-60.

Kamath N, Iyengar A, George N, et al. Risk factors and rate of progression of CKD in children. Kidney Int Rep. 2019;4:1472-7.

Kidney Disease: Improving Global Outcomes (KDIGO) CKD Work Group KDIGO 2024 Clinical Practice Guideline for the Evaluation and Management of Chronic Kidney Disease. Kidney Int. 2024;105:S117–S314.

Mann N, Sun H, Majmundar AJ. Mechanisms of podocyte injury in genetic kidney disease. Pediatr Nephrol. 2024.

Meliambro K, He JC, Campbell KN. Podocyte-targeted therapies—progress and future directions. Nat Rev Nephrol. 2024;20:643-58.

Sinha A, Bagga A, Banerjee S, et al. Steroid sensitive nephrotic syndrome: Revised Guidelines. Indian Pediatr. 2021;58:461-81.

van Biljon G, Meintjes CJ, Becker PJ, Karusseit VOL. Risk factors for progression of chronic kidney disease: An investigation in prepubertal children. Nephrology (Carlton). 2023;28:276-82.

van den Belt SM, Heerspink HJL, Gracchi V, et al. Early proteinuria lowering by angiotensin-converting enzyme inhibition predicts renal survival in children with CKD. J Am Soc Nephrol. 2018;29:2225-33.

Viteri B, Reid-Adam J. Hematuria and proteinuria in children. Pediatr Rev. 2018;39:573-87.

17.7 Nephrotic Syndrome

PE 20.3

DEFINITION

Nephrotic syndrome is commonly encountered in children and is characterized by massive proteinuria (>1 g/m²/day), hypoalbuminemia (serum albumin <3 g/dL), and edema. Recent guidelines have changed the serum albumin cut-off to <3 g/dL from the earlier value of <2.5 g/dL and removed hypercholesterolemia from the definition.

Nephrotic syndrome is commonly known to have a relapsing-remitting course. In most (85–90%) children with idiopathic nephrotic syndrome, the disease is sensitive to therapy with oral corticosteroids, and is termed *steroid sensitive nephrotic syndrome (SSNS)*. The prognosis in these cases is favorable. The remaining 10–15% children do not respond to a 6 weeks course of daily corticosteroids and are labeled *steroid resistant nephrotic syndrome (SRNS)*. Patients with SRNS overall have an unfavorable prognosis when compared to SSNS.

EPIDEMIOLOGY

Nephrotic syndrome has an annual incidence ranging from 1.2 to 16.9 per 100,000 children, with the highest incidence in those of south Asian ancestry. In India, the incidence is about 9–10/lac population.

ETIOLOGY

Nephrotic syndrome occurs due to disturbances in the glomerular filtration barrier, leading to loss of large amounts of albumin in the urine. It is *primary (idiopathic)* in 90–95% cases. *Secondary causes* can be identified in approximately 5–10% cases.

Primary Nephrotic Syndrome

Primary (idiopathic) nephrotic syndrome is histologically dominated by *minimal change disease (MCD)*, seen in approximately 80% of cases. An overwhelming majority of these cases are typically steroid sensitive in whom a kidney biopsy is not performed. Therefore, the true incidence of MCD may be even higher.

The next most common histological variant is *FSGS*. This variant is more commonly seen in SRNS and is considered a risk factor for progression to CKD. Other histopathological variants encountered in primary (idiopathic) nephrotic syndrome include *mesangioproliferative glomerulonephritis (MesPGN), MGN* and MPGN. While MesPGN usually has a favorable prognosis, the other histological variants often manifest with SRNS or atypical clinical features such as gross hematuria, hypertension, or kidney dysfunction; necessitating a kidney biopsy.

Secondary Nephrotic Syndrome

Secondary nephrotic syndrome occurs due to systemic diseases such as systemic lupus erythematosus, HSP, sickle cell disease, Hodgkin lymphoma, and amyloidosis or with infections such as HIV, parvovirus B19, hepatitis B, and hepatitis C. Intrauterine infections with syphilis, malaria, and cytomegalovirus are well known to cause secondary nephrotic syndrome. It can also follow administration of nonsteroidal anti-inflammatory drugs (NSAIDs), penicillamine, gold, toxins, or allergens. Detailed evaluation including a kidney biopsy may be required to establish the diagnosis in such cases.

PATHOGENESIS

The precise pathogenesis of childhood nephrotic syndrome still remains an enigma. Infections such as viral upper respiratory infections trigger a Th2 cytokine bias, increasing the levels of interleukin (IL)-4, IL-10, and IL-13. It is postulated that these interleukins may bind to receptors located on podocytes, causing effacement of their foot processes. This leads to disruption of the glomerular filtration barrier resulting in massive albuminuria, thereby leading to hypoalbuminemia. Hypoalbuminemia reduces the plasma oncotic pressure, leading to fluid shift from the intravascular to the interstitial compartment. Fluid shift manifests in the form of periorbital puffiness, pleural effusion, ascites, pedal edema, or anasarca. The liver synthesizes lipoproteins to compensate for the loss of low-density lipoprotein (LDL) receptors (LDL-r, which are proteins) in the urine, resulting in hypercholesterolemia.

Evidence for an immunological basis for the disease was historically noted by the observation of the disease going into remission after exposure to measles (which suppresses the cell-mediated immunity), and relapsing following a bee or wasp sting. This led to the introduction of steroids, which now have an established place in the management of the disease.

Evidence for a genetic basis for childhood nephrotic syndrome also exists in the form of familial clustering of the disease (even in steroid sensitive patients), in a few cases. Genetic mutations in genes such as *NPHS1, NPHS2, WT1, PLCE1,* and *LAMB2* are reported in congenital nephrotic syndrome (age of onset <3 months) as well as infantile nephrotic syndrome. Genetic studies in pediatric nephrotic syndrome are currently recommended for familial SRNS, congenital nephrotic syndrome, initial steroid resistance (first episode of nephrotic syndrome being steroid resistant), and children with dysmorphic features resembling a genetic disorder on clinical examination.

CLINICAL FEATURES

Age of Onset

The median age of onset of nephrotic syndrome is 4 years (range 2–6 years). Onset before 1 year of age or >15 years of age is a predictor of non-MCD and may require a renal biopsy to establish the histological variant.

Presenting Features

The classical presenting feature is that of a viral upper respiratory tract infection in association with periorbital puffiness followed by progression of edema to involve the whole body (anasarca). Some children may develop localized fluid collections such as neck edema, pleural effusion, ascites, scrotal/penile/vulval, or pedal edema. Edema can also occur over the sacrum (dependent area) in children who are bed-ridden. The edema is pitting in nature, and may be accompanied by oliguria.

Children with initial episode of nephrotic syndrome tend to present with more edema than those with relapses. This is because the parents recognize proteinuria early at home (often even before the onset of significant edema) in cases of relapse, which leads to early presentation to the hospital.

Although mild transient hypertension is quite common (due to activation of the renin-angiotensin-aldosterone axis, consequent upon fluid shift from the intravascular to the interstitial compartment), it is important to note that persistent or severe hypertension is an atypical finding and points toward a non-MCD. Similarly, even though transient microscopic hematuria is common, gross (macroscopic) hematuria is extremely unusual.

Complications as Presenting Features

Other presenting clinical features in children with nephrotic syndrome that could be related to the development of complications include the following:

- ***Serious infections*** such as spontaneous bacterial peritonitis (fever, abdominal pain, guarding or rigidity over the abdomen, mucoid diarrhea, sick looking child), pneumonia (fever, dyspnea, cough, lung crepitations), cellulitis (fever with inflamed limb), or rarely UTI. Spontaneous bacterial peritonitis is the most common severe infection, caused by *Streptococcus pneumoniae.*

- ***Thromboembolic complications*** arising from cerebral venous thrombosis, deep vein thrombosis, or renal vein thrombosis (because of hypercoagulable state due to loss of antithrombin III in urine, protein C and S deficiency, compounded by volume depletion, sepsis, and diuretic use).
- ***Hypovolemic shock*** due to massive redistribution of intravascular fluid to the interstitial compartment leading to hypotension.

Clues to Secondary Etiology

Although primary (idiopathic) nephrotic syndrome is the most common entity, one should always look out for features suggestive of secondary etiology of nephrotic syndrome such as malar rash (lupus), palpable purpura (HSP), hepatosplenomegaly or arthritis (lupus), gross hematuria or cola-colored urine (IgA nephropathy, lupus, and MPGN).

Features of Steroid Toxicity

Children with long-standing disease and/or those on prolonged steroid therapy may develop features of steroid toxicity such as short stature, obesity, posterior subcapsular cataract, glaucoma, abdominal striae, moon face, hypertension, gastritis, and fractures due to osteoporosis.

INVESTIGATIONS

It is essential to demonstrate the presence of massive proteinuria and hypoalbuminemia (serum albumin <3 g/dL) to make a diagnosis of nephrotic syndrome. Serum cholesterol >200 mg/dL is no longer an essential criterion for defining nephrotic syndrome but may be used as a corroborative evidence for diagnosis.

Proteinuria

Massive proteinuria is defined as an urine albumin of 3+ or 4+ in an early morning urine specimen, by urinary dipstick, 20% sulfosalicylic acid test, or heat coagulation test. Another useful test is the spot Up/Uc performed on an early morning urine specimen (a value >2 indicates nephrotic range proteinuria). Other methods of demonstrating nephrotic range proteinuria include estimating urine protein in 24-hour urine sample (>1 g/m^2/day or >40 mg/m^2/h). However, collection of 24-hour urine samples in children is often cumbersome and difficult. Hence, a spot Up/Uc on an early morning sample is often used.

Plasma Proteins

Total serum protein is reduced and albumin level is <3 g/dL. Serum IgG and IgA are reduced and IgM levels can be elevated. Complement C3 level is normal.

Hyperlipidemia

There are increased serum levels of cholesterol, triglycerides, LDL and very low-density lipoproteins (VLDL). Levels of high-density lipoprotein (HDL) may be low, normal, or elevated. The hyperlipidemia is due to increased synthesis of lipoproteins in response to hypoalbuminemia and decreased lipoprotein lipase activity. Although hyperlipidemia was an essential component of the definition of nephrotic syndrome, the recent recommendations no longer mandate this testing for making a diagnosis of nephrotic syndrome.

Other Investigations during the Initial Episode

- ***Blood urea, serum creatinine:*** These are usually normal in idiopathic nephrotic syndrome.
- ***Serum sodium, potassium:*** Hyponatremia may be noticed due to hemodilution. Hypokalemia may develop during resolution of edema with spontaneous or induced diuresis.
- ***C3:*** Indicated in children with gross hematuria only.
- Mantoux test and chest radiographs if clinically indicated to rule out tuberculosis (TB).
- HBsAg and ANA if clinical examination suggests features of hepatitis or lupus, respectively.

Routinely performing blood and urine cultures in the absence of clinical indications is not advised. Similarly, abdominal paracentesis for ascites in children with nephrotic syndrome should not be done as a routine. This procedure should be reserved for clinical suspicion of peritonitis (*diagnostic tap*) or therapeutic management of severe ascites leading to breathing difficulty (*therapeutic tap*).

RENAL BIOPSY

Most children with nephrotic syndrome do not require a kidney biopsy. Indications for kidney biopsy are listed in **Box 17.7**.

DIFFERENTIAL DIAGNOSIS

Differential diagnoses include other renal causes of anasarca such as acute nephritic syndrome and AKI. Acute nephritic syndrome (most commonly due to PSGN) presents with gross or microscopic hematuria (often with cola-colored urine) in association with subnephrotic range proteinuria (Up/Uc 0.2–2); often accompanied by hypertension, oliguria, or edema (lesser edema than nephrotic syndrome).

Other causes of anasarca such as acute liver failure, constrictive pericarditis, protein losing enteropathy, and congestive heart failure should be ruled out by appropriate history, examination, and investigations.

Box 17.7 Indications of Renal Biopsy in Nephrotic Syndrome

- *At onset of nephrotic syndrome:*
  - Gross hematuria, persistent microscopic hematuria, low C3 levels
  - Sustained hypertension
  - Renal failure not attributable to hypovolemia
  - Suspected secondary cause, e.g., lupus, immunoglobulin A (IgA) nephropathy, etc.
  - Age of onset >15 years
- *After initial treatment:*
  - Proteinuria persisting despite 6 weeks of daily prednisolone at 2 mg/kg/day
  - Before starting treatment with cyclosporine A or tacrolimus

TREATMENT Nephrotic Syndrome

Dietary Modifications

Children with nephrotic syndrome should be advised to reduce salt intake during relapses to prevent edema from increasing. Salt should not be added to salads and fruits, and high salt foods such as pickles and salted snack items should be avoided during edema. Not >30% of diet should be derived from fat; and saturated fat should be restricted in the diet in view of hypercholesterolemia. A balanced diet, adequate in proteins (1.5–2 g/kg/day) is recommended. In children with persistent proteinuria, 2–2.5 g/kg/day protein is recommended.

Diuretics

Diuretics are not routinely advised in children with nephrotic syndrome to decrease edema. Their use can be accompanied by hazards such as reduction in intravascular volume (that is already often low in nephrotic syndrome) as well as thrombotic complications. Diuretics are advised only in cases with significant ascites leading to respiratory distress; or persistent weight gain to the extent of >7%. In these situations alone, oral furosemide (1–4 mg/kg daily), spironolactone (2–4 mg/kg/day), hydrochlorothiazide (1–2 mg/kg/day) or metolazone (0.2–0.4 mg/kg/day) can be administered.

In edema refractory to diuretics and steroids, 20% intravenous human albumin infusion (0.5–1 g/kg) is recommended; and this can be accompanied by a careful aseptic abdominal paracentesis for massive ascites. Albumin infusions are also administered for management of severe hypoalbuminemia with hemoconcentration and hypovolemic shock. It is important to consider albumin infusion only after establishing normal kidney function, as patients may develop pulmonary edema if given in AKI.

Control of Hypertension and Dyslipidemia

Hypertension, if present, can be treated with furosemide (1–2 mg/kg/day), enalapril (0.2–0.5 mg/kg/day), or amlodipine (0.1–0.6 mg/kg/day).

Statins are not recommended for management of SSNS. In SRNS, they may be administered in the presence of persistent dyslipidemia for >3–6 months (despite dietary control/exercise/medications to control nephrotic syndrome).

Identify and Treat Infections

Children with nephrotic syndrome are more prone to develop infections due to low serum IgG levels, defective cell-mediated immunity and defective opsonization of capsulated antigens due to loss of complements in urine. Spontaneous bacterial peritonitis is the most common severe infection, and is often caused by *S. pneumoniae* and occasionally by gram-negative organisms like *E. coli*. These children present with tender ascites. Aspiration of the ascitic fluid might reveal >100 cells with at least 50% being polymorphs. Spontaneous bacterial peritonitis should be treated with parenteral third generation cephalosporins (cefotaxime or ceftriaxone) for 7–10 days.

Specific Therapy

Prednisolone is the mainstay of management in nephrotic syndrome. The duration of administration of prednisolone for the initial episode and subsequent relapses is different. Serious infections (if any) should be managed with appropriate course of antibiotics before starting steroids.

Terms used in Childhood Nephrotic Syndrome

For the management of children with nephrotic syndrome; it is essential to know some terminologies **(Table 17.12)**.

Management of initial episode: The first episode of SSNS is treated with oral prednisolone at a dose of 2 mg/kg/day (maximum 60 mg) in single or divided doses for 6 weeks, followed by 1.5 mg/kg (maximum 40 mg) as a single morning dose on alternate days for the next 6 weeks (total duration 12 weeks). Prednisolone is abruptly discontinued thereafter.

Table 17.12 Terminologies Used in the Management of Childhood Nephrotic Syndrome

Remission	Urine albumin nil or trace for 3 consecutive days
Relapse	Urine albumin 3+ or 4+ for 3 consecutive days (Up/Uc >2), having been in remission previously
Infrequently relapsing nephrotic syndrome	<2 relapses in 6 months of initial therapy, or <4 relapses in any 12 months
Frequently relapsing nephrotic syndrome	2 or more relapses within the first 6 months of initial therapy, ≥3 relapses in any 6 months; or ≥4 relapses in 1 year
Steroid dependent nephrotic syndrome	2 consecutive relapses when on alternate day steroids or within 14 days of discontinuation of steroids
Steroid resistant nephrotic syndrome	Lack of complete remission despite therapy with daily prednisolone at a dose of 2 mg/kg (or 60 mg/m^2) daily for 6 weeks

Pneumococcal vaccine (to prevent spontaneous bacterial peritonitis and pneumonia) and varicella vaccine are advised 4–6 weeks after stopping steroids. Live vaccines should not be administered while on steroids and younger siblings should not receive oral polio vaccine while the patient is on steroids or other immunosuppressive medications.

Remission is usually achieved in majority of children with MCD after 10–14 days of starting prednisolone. *Those who do not go into remission despite treatment with prednisolone at a dose of 2 mg/kg (60 mg/m^2/day) for 6 weeks are categorized as SRNS,* and require renal biopsy.

Management of relapse: The disease recurs in most patients (>75%); and almost half of them develop frequent relapses or steroid dependence.

Infrequently relapsing nephrotic syndrome: Each relapse should be treated with prednisolone 2 mg/kg/day daily (maximum 60 mg) in single or divided doses till remission, as defined by nil/trace urine albumin for 3 consecutive days (usually takes 1–2 weeks), followed by 1.5 mg/kg on alternate days (maximum 40 mg) as a single dose in the morning for 4 weeks. Hence, the usual duration of treatment of a relapse is 5–6 weeks. Prednisolone is abruptly discontinued thereafter. Parents should be taught to perform and grade urine albumin with dipstick and maintain a diary at home. In an event of 3+ or 4+ albumin for 3 consecutive days, they should be asked to contact the hospital for initiation of treatment of a relapse. It is important to detect relapses before the appearance of significant edema to prevent complications.

Frequently relapsing and steroid dependent nephrotic syndrome: Frequent relapses are more common in children (1) who are <3 years of age at onset of disease, (2) who take >2 weeks to achieve remission; and those (3) who relapse within 6 months of initial treatment.

If the definition of frequently relapsing or steroid dependent nephrotic syndrome is satisfied (as in **Table 17.12**), then, after treatment of the relapse (for 5–6 weeks, as mentioned in the preceding section), the prednisolone is not discontinued, but tapered by 0.25 mg/kg every 4 weeks and brought down to <0.5–0.7 mg/kg on alternate days, so that remission is maintained. This minimum dosage of prednisolone on every alternate day is administered to maintain remission for a period of 9–18 months, along with calcium and vitamin D supplements to prevent osteoporosis.

If, on the contrary, the prednisolone threshold, to maintain remission, is higher than 0.5–0.7 mg/kg or if features of corticosteroid toxicity are seen (cataract, glaucoma, short stature, obesity, etc.), additional use of the following immunomodulators is suggested, that would act as steroid-sparing agents:

1. *Levamisole* 2–2.5 mg/kg on alternate days orally for a period of 2–3 years. The main side effects of levamisole include leukopenia, flu-like symptoms, hepatotoxicity, and vasculitis. The leukocyte count should be monitored every 3–4 monthly.
2. *Cyclophosphamide* 2–2.5 mg/kg daily for 12 weeks orally (cumulative dosage should not exceed 168 mg/kg). During therapy with cyclophosphamide, high dose steroids (1.5 mg/kg alternate day) are continued and thereafter rapidly tapered once the course of cyclophosphamide is completed. Leukopenia and gonadal toxicity are the chief adverse effects. The leukocyte count should be monitored 2 weekly during this 12-week period of administration of the drug and further doses are withheld if total leukocyte count is <4,000 per mm^3.
3. *Mycophenolate mofetil* 800–1,200 mg/m^2/day daily for 2–3 years given orally. Steroids are gradually tapered and stopped by 3–6 months while mycophenolate is continued for 1–2 years. The principal side effects include gastrointestinal discomfort such as abdominal pain, vomiting, and diarrhea, and other rare side effects such as leukopenia and transaminitis. The leukocyte count should be monitored every 3–4 monthly.
4. *Cyclosporine* 4–6 mg/kg/day in two divided doses daily for 2–3 years along with alternate day tapering doses of prednisolone.

   Adverse effects include acne, gum hypertrophy, hirsutism, hypercholesterolemia, hypertension, and nephrotoxicity. Estimation of serum creatinine is required every 3 months along with an annual lipid profile.
5. *Tacrolimus* is administered at a dose of 0.1–0.2 mg/kg in two divided doses daily for 2–3 years. Adverse effects include hyperglycemia, diarrhea, and neurotoxicity (which may manifest as headache, seizures). Estimation of serum creatinine and blood glucose is required every 3 months.

STEROID RESISTANT NEPHROTIC SYNDROME

Children with SRNS are best managed by a pediatric nephrologist. Renal biopsy is essential in all such patients prior to initiation of therapy. If the renal biopsy shows MCD, FSGS, or MesPGN, treatment with calcineurin inhibitors (CNI) (cyclosporine or tacrolimus) is initiated and continued for 1–2 years. ACE inhibitors (enalapril), alternate day tapering doses of prednisolone and calcium/vitamin D supplements are administered additionally. Patients have to be monitored regularly for blood pressure, renal functions, and side effects of the drugs and doses adjusted accordingly. Patients not responding to CNI or developing side effects to such therapy should be promptly referred to a pediatric nephrologist for further care.

MONITORING ADVERSE EFFECTS OF STEROIDS

A close monitoring of weight, growth velocity (height gain/year), and blood pressure, and evaluation for features of steroid toxicity is essential. These include cushingoid features and ophthalmological complications (posterior subcapsular cataract and glaucoma). Annual ophthalmological screening of children receiving long-term steroids for these complications is recommended. Calcium and vitamin D supplements should be prescribed for children receiving long-term steroids to prevent osteoporosis.

Steroids should never be prescribed on an empty stomach, to prevent peptic ulcers. Proton pump inhibitors or H_2 blockers are not routinely required in all patients receiving steroids but may be considered in those who develop signs/symptoms of gastritis. Patients on steroid sparing agents should be regularly monitored for side effects as elucidated earlier.

LONG-TERM OUTCOME

The long-term outcome of SSNS is excellent, with studies reporting that majority of the children (60–80%) outgrow the disease by puberty. There is a tendency to fewer relapses per year after the first decade of life in most patients. Response to steroids is the most important prognostic factor in children with nephrotic syndrome, irrespective of the histological variant identified on biopsy (if done).

On the contrary, long-term prognosis of SRNS is unfavorable, with 50% of patients progressing to advanced stages of CKD within 10 years of diagnosis of SRNS especially if unresponsive to treatment.

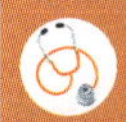

CASE STUDY Nephrotic Syndrome

A 4-year-old girl presents with periorbital puffiness and pedal edema for 15 days accompanied by abdominal distension and decreased urine output. There is no past history of similar episodes. There is no history of fever, cough, respiratory distress, jaundice, dyspnea, palpitations, joint pain, abdominal pain, or red colored urine.

List the probable diagnoses in this patient based on the above history.

In view of history of generalized edema and oliguria, possibilities of nephrotic syndrome, PSGN, and AKI should be considered.

On examination, the child has anasarca with stable vitals. The blood pressure is 98/62 mm Hg. There is no palpable purpura, malar rash, cola-colored urine, jaundice, arthritis, or hepatosplenomegaly. First morning urine sample revealed an *albumin* of 4+ on dipstick examination with a spot Up/Uc of 3.4. *There are no RBCs on urinalysis. Serum albumin is 1.8 mg/dL, blood urea 24 mg/dL, and serum creatinine 0.5 mg/dL.*

Mention the most likely diagnosis and justify the same.

The investigations point toward a diagnosis of nephrotic syndrome as the patient fulfils the criteria for massive proteinuria and hypoalbuminemia which define nephrotic syndrome.

Will you perform a renal biopsy to confirm the diagnosis?

Renal biopsy should not be performed since there are no atypical features in this patient. Blood urea and serum creatinine are usually normal in most patients with nephrotic syndrome.

How will you manage this patient?

As this is the first episode of nephrotic syndrome, patient should be started on oral prednisolone at 2 mg/kg and given daily for 6 weeks followed by 1.5 mg/kg on alternate days for another 6 weeks after which steroids are abruptly stopped. Patient is advised dipstick monitoring at home and regular follow-up.

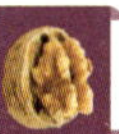

IN A NUTSHELL

Nephrotic Syndrome

1. Nephrotic syndrome is commonly encountered in children and is known to have a frequent relapsing-remitting course.
2. It is characterized by massive proteinuria (>1 g/m²/day) and hypoalbuminemia (serum albumin <3 g/dL).
3. Renal biopsy is not required in majority of the patients with nephrotic syndrome.
4. Most patients respond very well to steroids and have an excellent long-term prognosis. Patients with frequent relapses or steroid dependence require additional steroid-sparing agents.

Chan EY, Boyer O. Childhood idiopathic nephrotic syndrome: recent advancements shaping future guidelines. Pediatr Nephrol. 2024.

Kidney Disease: Improving Global Outcomes (KDIGO) Glomerular Diseases Work Group. KDIGO 2021 Clinical Practice Guideline for the Management of Glomerular Diseases. Kidney Int. 2021;100:S1-S276.

Sinha A, Bagga A, Banerjee S, et al. Steroid Sensitive Nephrotic Syndrome: Revised Guidelines. Indian Pediatr. 2021;58:461-81.

Trautmann A, Boyer O, Hodson E, et al. IPNA clinical practice recommendations for the diagnosis and management of children with steroid-sensitive nephrotic syndrome. Pediatr Nephrol. 2023;38:877-919.

Vivarelli M, Gibson K, Sinha A, Boyer O. Childhood nephrotic syndrome. Lancet. 2023;402:809-24.

Vasudevan A, Thergaonkar R, Mantan M, et al. Consensus Guidelines on Management of Steroid-Resistant Nephrotic Syndrome. Indian Pediatr. 2021;58:650-66.

17.8 Acute Kidney Injury

PE 20.5

INTRODUCTION

Acute kidney injury (AKI) is a clinical condition characterized by rapid decline in GFR leading to oliguria/anuria, retention of nitrogenous waste products (urea, creatinine), and electrolyte and acid-base disturbances. AKI accounts for 3–5% of children admitted in hospitals. In neonates, the incidence of AKI was reported as 30%, varying with gestational age; 47.9% in gestation of ≥22 to <29 weeks, 18.3% between ≥29 and <36 weeks and 36.7% in ≥36 weeks as observed in Assessment of World wide Acute Kidney Epidemiology in Neonates (AWAKEN) study. Overall incidence of AKI in children and young adults was reported to be 27% and severe AKI in 11.6% of cases in intensive care settings, as reported by Assessment of Worldwide Acute Kidney Injury Renal Angina, and Epidemiology (AWARE) study.

Kidney Disease Improving Global Outcomes (KDIGO) defined AKI as presence of any of the following criteria: Increase in serum creatinine by ≥0.3 mg/dL within 48 hours, or by ≥1.5 times from baseline which is known or presumed to occur within previous 7 days, or urine output <0.5 mL/kg/h for 6 hours.

Oliguria is defined as urine output <0.5 mL/kg/h in neonates, <1 mL/kg/h in infants; and <500 mL/m²/day in older children. Although the kidneys perform multiple roles (e.g., metabolic, endocrine, fluid, and electrolyte balance), but the estimated glomerular filtration rate (eGFR) is accepted as the index of functioning renal mass, which is calculated by the following formula:

$$\text{GFR (mL/min/1.73 m}^2) = K \times \frac{\text{Height (cm)}}{\text{Cr (mg/dL)}}$$

K = 0.33 for preterm infants, 0.45 for term infants, 0.55 for children and adolescent females, and 0.70 for adolescent males.

CLASSIFICATION

Previously AKI was classified using the criteria of *R*isk, *I*njury, *F*ailure, *L*oss, and *E*nd-stage kidney failure (*RIFLE*). The adult RIFLE criteria was based on changes in serum creatinine from baseline, an abrupt decrease in urine output, and the length of kidney replacement required at later stages. A modified pediatric RIFLE (pRIFLE) criteria has been used based on decrease in estimated creatinine clearance (eCCl) and reduction in urine output for children patients in the intensive care unit setting **(Table 17.13)**. Later on KDIGO proposed classification and staged AKI for severity to be used in infants and children and also modified for use in neonates, and currently the recommended classification for staging of AKI **(Table 17.14)**.

ETIOLOGY

In Neonates

(*i*) Septicemia; (*ii*) birth asphyxia; (*iii*) obstructive uropathy; (*iv*) renal vein thrombosis; (*v*) multicystic dysplastic kidney (MCDK).

In Older Children

The AKI may be classified into *prerenal azotemia* caused by acute renal hypoperfusion with intact renal parenchyma; *renal*

Table 17.13 Pediatric-modified RIFLE (pRIFLE) Criteria

	Estimated CCl	*Urine output*
Risk	eCCl decrease by 25%	<0.5 mL/kg/h for 8 hours
Injury	eCCl decrease by 50%	<0.5 mL/kg/h for 16 hours
Failure	eCCl decrease by 75% or eCCl <35 mL/min/1.73 m²	<0.3 mL/kg/h for 24 hours or Anuric for 12 hours
Loss	Persistent failure >4 weeks	
End stage	End-stage renal disease (persistent failure >3 months)	

(eCCl: estimated creatinine clearance, calculated using the Schwartz formula)

Table 17.14 KDIGO Classification for Staging of AKI

KDIGO staging of AKI (Adapted from KDIGO Clinical Practice Guidelines for AKI, 2012)

- *Stage 1:* Increase in serum creatinine 1.5–1.9 times baseline, or increase ≥0.3 mg/dL or urine output <0.5 mL/kg/h for a duration of 6–12 hours
- *Stage 2:* Elevation in serum creatinine 2.0–2.9 times baseline, or urine output <0.5 mL/kg/h for ≥12 hours
- *Stage 3:* Increase in serum creatinine ≥3.0 times baseline, or increase in serum creatinine to ≥4 mg/dL or initiation of kidney replacement therapy or decrease in eGFR <35 mL/min/1.73 m^2 in patients below 18 years of age
- Urine output <0.3 mL/kg/h for ≥24 hours, or anuria for 12 hours

Modified KDIGO for Neonates (Adapted from Jetton and Askenazi, 2014)

- *Stage 1*:* Creatinine based criteria are same or urine output ≤1 mL/kg/h but >0.5 mL/kg/h
- *Stage 2*:* Creatinine based criteria are same or urine output ≤0.5mL/kg/h for 24 hours
- *Stage 3*:* Creatinine based criteria are same or serum creatinine is ≥2.5 mg/dL
- Urine output ≤0.3 mL/kg/h for 24 hours or initiation of kidney replacement therapy

*Reference (baseline) creatinine is the lowest previous value

azotemia caused by acute diseases of renal parenchyma of tubular damage due to ischemic insult or toxins; and *postrenal azotemia* because of obstructive uropathy. The different causes of AKI are presented in **Table 17.15**.

PATHOPHYSIOLOGY

Regardless of the cause of AKI, reduction in renal blood flow represents a common pathologic pathway for decrease in GFR. The decreased renal blood flow eventually leads to ischemia and cell death. This initial ischemic insult triggers production of oxygen free radicals and enzymes that continue to cause cell injury even after restoration of blood flow. The tubular cell damage results in disruption of tight junctions between cells, allowing back leak of glomerular filtrate and further decrease in GFR. In addition, dying cells slough off into tubules forming obstructing casts, which further decrease GFR and lead to oliguria.

CLINICAL FEATURES

A child with AKI presents with oliguria or anuria associated with facial puffiness, pedal edema, and acidotic breathing. There may be associated hematuria, hypertension, convulsions, and encephalopathy. There may be a history of preceding events such as gastroenteritis, viral exanthems, boils and drugs intake such as penicillin, sulfonamides, vancomycin, amphotericin B, or aminoglycosides.

LABORATORY INVESTIGATIONS

Kidney Functions

Urea and electrolytes: Blood urea and serum creatinine are increased. Serum sodium is either normal or decreased, and potassium is increased or low (HUS). Serum calcium level is normal or reduced and phosphate is increased. Arterial blood gas analysis shows features of metabolic acidosis (decreased pH and low bicarbonate).

Relation of serum creatinine with GFR:
- ❖ Creatinine 1.0 mg/dL—normal GFR
- ❖ Creatinine 2.0 mg/dL—50% reduction in GFR
- ❖ Creatinine 4.0 mg/dL—70–80% reduction in GFR
- ❖ Creatinine 8.0 mg/dL—90–95% reduction in GFR

Table 17.15 Etiology of Acute Kidney Injury

Prerenal	*Renal*	*Postrenal*
• Hypovolemia ▪ Hemorrhage ▪ Gastrointestinal losses ▪ Hypoproteinemia ▪ Burns ▪ Renal or adrenal diseases with salt wasting • Hypotension ▪ Septicemia ▪ DIC ▪ Hypothermia ▪ Hemorrhage ▪ Heart failure • Hypoxia ▪ Pneumonia ▪ Respiratory distress syndrome	• Glomerulonephritis ▪ Postinfectious ▪ SLE ▪ MPGN ▪ RPGN ▪ Anaphylactoid purpura • Acute tubular necrosis ▪ Heavy metals/drugs ▪ Chemicals ▪ Hemoglobin/myoglobin ▪ Shock ▪ Ischemia • Hemolytic uremic syndrome • Renal vein thrombosis • Acute interstitial nephritis (drugs/infection) • Developmental ▪ Cystic disease ▪ Hypoplasia/dysplasia • Hereditary nephritis	• Obstructive uropathy ▪ Ureteropelvic junction obstruction ▪ Ureterocele ▪ Posterior urethral valve ▪ Tumor • Vesicoureteral reflux • Acquired ▪ Stones ▪ Blood clots

(DIC: disseminated intravascular coagulation; MPGN: membranoproliferative glomerulonephritis; RSGN: rapidly progressive glomerulonephritis; SLE: systemic lupus erythematosus)

Table 17.16 Renal Failure Indices

Index	Functional oliguria	Intrinsic renal failure
Urinary sodium (mEq/L)	<20 (<30)	>40 (>60)
Urinary osmolality (mOsm/kg)	>500 (>400)	<300 (<350)
Blood urea creatinine ratio	>20:1	<20:1
Urine plasma osmolality ratio	>1.5 (>2)	<0.8–1.2 (<1.1)
FENa (%)*	<1 (<3)	>1 (>10)
Fractional excretion of urea**	<35%	>35%

**This is more sensitive and specific than FENa in differentiating between prerenal and renal cause of AKI especially when diuretics have been administered.

$$\text{Fractional excretion of Na (FENa)} = \frac{\text{Urine Na}^+ \times \text{Serum creatinine}}{\text{Urine creatinine} \times \text{Serum sodium}} \times 100$$

*Exceptions
- Intrinsic renal failure with FENa <1% (urinary tract obstruction, acute glomerulonephritis, hepatorenal syndrome, and radiologic contrast induced acute tubular necrosis).
- Pre-renal AKI with FENa >1% are patients on diuretics, pre-existing chronic kidney disease and patient with bicarbonaturia

Renal failure indices: These help in differentiating functional oliguria from intrinsic kidney failure. Common indices are urinary sodium, osmolality, functional excretion of urea, and sodium, and ratios of blood urea creatinine, and urine versus plasma osmolality. Expected values are listed in **Table 17.16**. However, utility of these indices is not reliable if the patient has received sodium containing fluids and/or furosemide before estimation.

Urine examination: It should be done for proteinuria, hematuria, pus cells, eosinophils, red cell casts, or granular casts. Urine culture should also be done to rule out associated UTI.

Furosemide stress test: It is used to assess the function of renal tubular integrity and need of dialysis. In this test, patient of AKI with euvolemia, furosemide (intravenous administration 1 mg/kg in naive or 1.5 mg/kg, if previously exposed to furosemide) is given and urine output is monitored and output of >2 mL/kg within 2 hours is taken as responsive. Non-responsive cases are at risk of development of stage 3 AKI and need of dialysis in critically ill children.

Other Investigations

Hematological parameters: Hemoglobin may be low due to severe hemolysis, dilutional anemia, and precipitation of pre-existing nutritional anemia. Total leukocyte counts are either normal or increased as in sepsis induced AKI or HUS (mostly neutrophils), or allergic interstitial nephritis (eosinophilia). Peripheral blood smear may show features of hemolysis in HUS, malaria and G6PD deficiency. Absolute platelet count is decreased in AKI secondary to HUS, lupus nephritis, malaria and disseminated intravascular coagulation.

Imaging: Chest X-ray is done to rule out cardiomegaly and pulmonary edema.

ECG: It is done to detect hyperkalemia. Look for tall tented T wave, widening of QRS complex, ST segment depression, prolongation of PR interval, absent P wave, and complete heart block.

USG abdomen: Ultrasonography of KUB is required to rule out hydronephrosis, hydroureter, loss of corticomedullary differentiation, stones, clots, and tumors.

Color Doppler flow: This is indicated for suspected renal vein thrombosis and renal arterial stenosis/thrombosis.

Kidney biopsy: Indicated for children in whom prerenal and postrenal AKI has been excluded and cause of intrinsic AKI is unclear, e.g., vasculitis, glomerulonephritis, and interstitial nephritis.

Renal Angina Index

Renal angina index (RAI) was developed for prediction of occurrence of severe AKI in intensive care unit (ICU) setting. It is based on presence of two variables as *risk factors* and *kidney injury*. Total score ranges between 1 and 40 and is obtained from multiplication of risk and injury scores. *Risk* (ICU admission–1 score, solid organ/bone marrow transplant–3 score, ventilation and inotrope use–5 score) and kidney *injury* [no change in estimated creatinine clearance (eCCl) or fluid overload (FO) <5%–1 score, decreased eCCl 0–24% or FO ≥5%–2 score, decreased eCCl 25–49% or FO ≥10%–4 score, decreased eCCl ≥50% or FO ≥15%–score 8] scores were considered. A RAI score of ≥8 within first 12 hour of ICU admission had an increased risk for prediction of severe AKI (KDIGO stages II and III) on day 3 of admission (Odds ratio 3.21; 95% confidence interval 2.20–4.67).

BIOMARKERS OF ACUTE KIDNEY INJURY

The rise in serum creatinine in AKI is a late phenomenon and it occurs when 50% of the kidney function is already lost. Certain urinary biomarkers such as neutrophil associated gelatinase lipocalin A (NGAL), kidney injury molecule-1, N-acetyl-beta-D-glucosaminidase activity, IL 18, and plasma cystatin C have been found to be helpful to detect early AKI. Of these, NGAL is considered better and has modest sensitivity and specificity for early diagnosis of AKI following cardiac surgery, sepsis, and contrast induced nephropathy. Newer biomarkers such as tissue inhibitor of metalloproteinases-2 (TIMP-2) and insulin like growth factor-binding protein 7 (IGFBP7) have shown utility in early detection of AKI. The combination of detection of TIMP2-IGFBP7 (*Nephrocheck*) in urine has been approved by FDA for early detection of AKI in severely ill children. In addition, combination of urinary NGAL and RAI has shown better specificity for detection of severe AKI.

TREATMENT Acute Kidney Injury

Recovery from AKI is mainly dependent upon restoration of kidney blood flow. In prerenal involvement, correction of dehydration and restoration of kidney blood flow is usually sufficient. With intrinsic renal conditions, removal of toxins and initiation of therapy for glomerular disease results in normalization of kidney function. Relief of urinary obstruction in postrenal cause results in prompt normalization of blood flow to renal tissue.

Prerenal Acute Kidney Injury

Immediate correction of dehydration is achieved by intravenous administration of 20 mL/kg of normal saline over 20 minutes. Repeat the same dose if dehydration persists. After volume resuscitation, hypovolemic patients usually void within 2 hours.

Consider diuretic therapy (furosemide 2–4 mg/kg intravenous), if the child does not pass urine, as a single dose. Failure to pass urine following diuretic treatment requires evaluation for intrinsic or postrenal causes of AKI.

Treatment of Intrinsic (Renal) Acute Kidney Injury

Patients with normal intravascular volume should be given 5% dextrose, 400 mL/m^2/24 hours (insensible loss) plus amount of fluid lost in urine/stool/blood (mililitre for mililiter) by N/2 saline. Children with marked hypervolemia may require further restriction of fluid. Further, composition of fluid can be changed according to serum electrolyte report. Fluid intake, urine/stool output, weight, blood pressure, and serum biochemistry need to be monitored on daily basis. In a suspected case of PUV, catheterization of bladder is to be done to drain the urine and later voiding cystourethrogram to confirm the diagnosis. **Table 17.17** summarizes a problem based management approach in a child with AKI.

Kidney Support Therapy

Various modalities of kidney support therapy are there to treat AKI depending upon the facilities and technical expertise available. Peritoneal dialysis (PD) in younger children and intermittent hemodialysis (IHD) or sustained low-efficiency dialysis (SLED) or continuous kidney replacement therapy (CKRT) in older age group can be undertaken.

Clinical indications: Deteriorating neurological status, intractable seizures, congestive heart failure, pulmonary edema, hypertension, features of volume overload, bleeding diathesis due to uremic platelet dysfunction, and anuria >24 hours.

Biochemical indications: Blood urea >200 mg/dL, rate of rise of blood urea >20 mg/dL/day, hyperkalemia >6 mEq/L, refractory hyperphosphatemia, and persistent metabolic acidosis.

Peritoneal Dialysis

It does not require vascular access and sophisticated equipment, so is the preferred dialytic procedure in younger children. In resource-limited settings, it is the preferred mode of dialysis and one session can last up to 72 hours. Repeat session can be done after a gap of 12–24 hours. It provides good clearance and corrects metabolic alterations such as hyperkalemia and acidosis efficiently.

Table 17.17 Management of Complications of Acute Kidney Injury

Problem	*Treatment*	*Remarks*
Fluid overload	*Fluid restriction:* 400 mL/m^2/day of 5% dextrose for insensible losses; N/2 saline for urine output (replace mL by mL), single dose of furosemide in oliguric patients	Monitor other losses and replace as appropriate
Pulmonary edema	• Oxygen • Dopamine 5–10 µg/kg per minute • Furosemide (one dose only) 2–4 mg/kg IV	Monitor by CVP line; peritoneal dialysis with hypertonic glucose initial few cycles/hemodialysis
Hypertension	*Symptomatic:* • Labetolol infusion 0.25–3 mg/kg/h, preferred over sodium nitroprisside • Sodium nitroprusside 0.5–8 µg/kg per minute infusion or labetalol infusion 0.25–3 mg/kg/h • Furosemide (one dose only) 2 mg/kg IV • Nifedipine 0.25 mg/kg orally • *Asymptomatic:* Salt restriction, furosemide treatment	Watch for fluid overload and hypernatremia; consider dialysis
Hyperkalemia	• *Acute emergency:* Calcium gluconate (10%), 0.5–1 mL/kg over 5–10 minutes • *Less urgent:* Salbutamol 5–10 mg nebulization • Sodium bicarbonate (7.5%), 1–2 mEq/kg over 15–20 minutes • Glucose (50%) 0.5–1 g/kg with 0.1–02 units/kg insulin • Calcium resonium 1g/kg/day	• Stabilizes cell membranes; prevents arrhythmia • Shifts potassium into cells • Shifts potassium into cells • Shifts potassium into cells • Given orally or rectally
Hyponatremia	• Fluid restriction is mainstay of therapy (1/2 to 2/3 rd of maintenance) • If sensorial alteration or seizures, 3% saline 3 mL/kg over 20 minutes • mEq of Na required = 0.6 × weight (kg) × 125–observed Na • Tolvaptan (Vasopressin-2 receptor antagonist) oral therapy can be effective in refractory hyponatremia	• Hyponatremia mostly due to fluid excess • 12 mL/kg of 3% saline raises sodium by 10 mEq/L (correction not more than 10 mEq/L in first 24 hours)
Anemia	• Packed red blood cells 3–5 mL/kg; when hemoglobin <5 g/dL • Consider exchange transfusion	Monitor blood pressure
High serum phosphate	• Phosphate binders (calcium carbonate, acetate) • Dietary phosphate restriction	Avoid aluminum-containing agents
Metabolic acidosis	$NaHCO_3$ (7.5%) mEq = 0.3 × weight (kg) × 12 – observed HCO_3	If intractable, consider dialysis

Hemodialysis

Technically, it involves placement of catheter in the vessel, hemodialysis machine, dialyzer and patient should be hemodynamically stable. Two processes (diffusion and convention) are involved. The patient's blood is passed through a semipermeable membrane (dialyzer) and dialytic fluid in a counter current mechanism. In diffusion, solutes move from higher (patients' blood) to lower (dialysate) until equilibrium is attained. In convection, ultrafiltration leads to excessive fluid clearance from the body from a positive (blood) or to negative (dialysate) pressure gradient through dialyzer.

Continuous Kidney Replacement Therapy (CKRT)

The CKRT causes slower fluid removal and solute clearance over longer treatment durations (24 hours per day). It is useful in hemodynamically unstable patients with AKI. However, it is expensive, and requires skilled personnel to perform the procedure. The different modalities of CKRT are continuous venovenous hemofiltration (CVVH), continuous venovenous hemodialysis (CVVHD), and continuous venovenous hemodiafiltration (CVVHDF). The hemodialysis aggravates hemodynamic instability with a high rate of fluid and solute removal, whereas CKRT causes slow and constant removal of water and solutes from the plasma and is preferred option for managing unstable patients with AKI.

Sustained Low-efficiency Dialysis

The blood flow rate is slower than intermittent hemodialysis and can be undertaken in hemodynamically unstable patients. It provides adequate small solute clearances in such patients and procedure lasts for about 8–12 hours.

Supportive Care

Nutritional support: Requirements are as follows: energy 20–30 kcal/kg/day; carbohydrate 3–5 g/kg/day; fat 0.8–1 g/kg/day; protein intake of 0.8–1.0 g/kg/day in noncatabolic AKI patients without need for dialysis; 1.0–1.5 g/kg/day in patients with AKI on kidney support therapy; and 1.7 g/kg/day in patients on CKRT and hypercatabolic patients. Protein should be of high biological value. Vitamin and micronutrients should be supplemented.

Treat anemia with fresh packed RBCs transfusion (if Hb <7 g/dL), as old blood contains increased amount of potassium. Use antibiotics to treat the infection. Doses of the antibiotics are modified as per **Table 17.18**.

Antimicrobials needing dose reduction in AKI: Principle of 4 Ds (drug, duration, dosing and de-escalation) should be followed. Antibiotics which do not require dose modifications at all are azithromycin, cefaclor, cloxacillin, and linezolid. Antibiotics which can be given at normal dose safely up to a fall of GFR of 40 mL/min/1.73 m^2 include ceftriaxone, cefotaxime, cefixime, ciprofloxacin, cefuroxime proaxetil, ampicillin, amoxicillin, trimethoprim, clarithromycin, erythromycin, clindamycin, and metronidazole.

Prevention of AKI

Avoidance of hypovolemia, prompt fluid resuscitation in children who are in need of fluid therapy and avoidance of nephrotoxic medications are some of the important measures to reduce occurrence of AKI in sick children. The actions such as NINJA (**N**ephrotoxic **I**njury **N**egated by **J**ust in time **A**ction) using electronic alerts incorporated into the patient's treatment records is useful to prevent drug-induced AKI. It is a quality initiative program which was applied in non-critically sick hospitalized patients, who were on more than three nephrotoxic medications on the same day or an intravenous aminoglycoside over three consecutive days, and then monitoring of daily serum creatinine level during exposure period and 2 days after exposure ending; it yielded decreased AKI rates obtained by statistical modelling. Administration of single dose of theophylline within first hour of neonates with severe birth asphyxia provided evidence in prevention of AKI.

Table 17.18 Dose Modification of Antibiotics According to Glomerular Filtration Rate (GFR mL/min/1.73 m^2)

Drug	*GFR: 40*	*GFR: 10*	*Anuric*
Paracetamol	Normal dose	50%, ↑ interval	50%, ↑ interval
Amikacin	40% od	20% od	10% od
Gentamicin	60% bid	10% od	5% od
Ceftriaxone	Normal dose	80% od	50% od
Ceftazidime	50% bid	15% od	10% od
Vancomycin	30% od	5% od	15 mg/kg, followed by 1.9 mg/kg/day
Ciprofloxacillin	Normal dose	50% od	33% od
Amoxicillin	Normal dose	30% bid	15% od
Amoxicillin + Clavulanic acid	Normal dose	25% bid	15% od
Phenobarbitone	80%	30%	25%
Phenytoin	Normal dose	Normal dose	Normal dose
Ranitidine	Normal dose	50% bid	50% bid
Steroids	Normal dose	Normal dose	Normal dose

Outcome

Acute kidney injury consists of three phases: (1) oliguric phase, (2) diuretic phase, and (3) postdiuretic recovery phase. *Oliguric phase* lasts for about 5–10 days, followed by *diuretic phase* leading to increase in urine output (2–3 L/day) and it is due to inability of damaged tubules to concentrate urine which results in loss of excess fluid. In *recovery phase*, general condition improves and there is normalization of renal function. Recovery of AKI due to prerenal causes such as acute tubular necrosis and interstitial nephritis is good.

Outcome of the AKI depends upon the nature of underlying disease process and stage of AKI. It carries a mortality of 20–50%. The risk of mortality is 2.5 times higher in risk, 5.4 times in injury, and 10.1 times in failure stage of AKI. Contributors for mortality include anuria >72 hours, cortical necrosis, severe AKI (KDIGO stages II and III), multiorgan failure, need for ventilation, sepsis, shock, and fluid overload. Medical management may be necessary for prolonged period to treat sequel of AKI including CKD, hypertension, renal tubular acidosis, etc. Patients recovering from AKI need long-term follow-up as there may be development of proteinuria, hypertension, and low eGFR (<90 mL/min/1.73 m^2) in some proportion of cases.

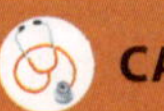

CASE STUDY Acute Kidney Injury

A 4-year-old boy presented with history of high grade fever, frequent loose stools, and vomiting for 2 days, followed by decreased urine output, mild periorbital puffiness, and fast breathing. There is no history of dysentery, sore throat, skin lesions, headache, red urine, and seizures.

On physical examination, child was well-nourished and had puffiness of face with pedal edema. There was no evidence of skin or mucosal bleeding. His pulse rate was 92/min, regular, fair volume, respiratory rate 22/min, blood pressure 160/90 mm Hg, and JVP was not raised. He had acidotic breathing. Microscopic examination of urine showed only hyaline casts.

Mention the most likely diagnosis. Justify.

Presence of edema and oliguria, preceded by infective diarrhea, points toward a possibility of AKI. Since there is no dehydration, AKI is unlikely to be prerenal in origin. Probable etiology is acute tubular necrosis.

Enumerate relevant investigations to confirm your diagnosis in order of priority.

The relevant investigations in order of priority are: (1) peripheral blood smear to look for evidence of hemolysis (schistocytes) and thrombocytopenia (to rule out HUS); (2) serum urea and creatinine to classify AKI as per KDIGO criteria, (3) ABG analysis for evidence of metabolic acidosis, anion gap, and hyperkalemia; (4) C3 and C4 levels to reveal type of glomerulonephritis (low C3 in PIGN, and MPGN and both C3 and C4 low in systemic lupus erythematosus nephritis); and (5) serum electrolytes for evidence of hyperkalemia and treatment as per severity of hyperkalemia.

Monitoring and treatment

Child needs regular recording of weight, blood pressure, urine output, fluid overload, and replacement of losses. Manage complications such as hyperkalemia, hypertension, seizures, pulmonary edema, and metabolic acidosis. Kidney replacement therapy should be instituted early for better recovery and for shorter duration of hospital stay.

List important complications in this child.

Expect hyperkalemia, cardiac arrhythmias, metabolic acidosis, hypertensive encephalopathy, and left ventricular failure.

Basu RK, Kaddourah A, Goldstein SL, AWARE Study Investigators. Assessment of a RAI for prediction of severe acute kidney injury in critically ill children: a multicentre, multinational, prospective observational study. Lancet Child Adolesc Health. 2018;2(2):112-20.

Filho LT, Grande AJ, Colonetti T, et al. Accuracy of neutrophil gelatinase-associated lipocalin for acute kidney injury diagnosis in children: systematic review and meta-analysis. Pediatr Nephrol. 2017;32(10):1979-88.

Greenberg JH, Coca S, Parikh CR. Long-term risk of chronic kidney disease and mortality in children after acute kidney injury: a systematic review. BMC Nephrol. 2014;15:184.

Goldstein SL, Dahale D, Kirkendall ES, et al. A prospective multi-center quality improvement initiative (NINJA) indicates a reduction in nephrotoxic acute kidney injury in hospitalized children. Kidney Int. 2020;97(3):580-8.

Jetton JG, Askenazi DJ. Acute kidney injury in the neonate. Clin Perinatol. 2014;41:487-502.

Jetton JG, Boohaker LJ, Sethi SK, et al. Incidence and outcomes of neonatal acute kidney injury (AWAKEN): A multicentre, multinational, observational cohort study. Lancet Child Adolesc Health. 2017;1(3):184-94.

Kaddourah A, Basu RK, Bagshaw SM, et al; AWARE investigators. Epidemiology of acute kidney injury in critically ill children and young adults. N Engl J Med. 2017;376:11-20.

KDIGO Clinical Practice Guideline for Acute Kidney Injury. [2012] Kidney International Supplements. [online] Available from https://kdigo.org/wp-content/uploads/2016/10/KDIGO-2012-AKI-Guideline-English.pdf [Last accessed December, 2022].

Krishnasamy S, Sinha A, Bagga A. Management of acute kidney injury in critically ill children. Indian J Pediatr. 2023;90:481-91.

Krishnasamy S, Sinha A, Lodha R, et al. Furosemide stress test to predict acute kidney injury progression in critically ill children. Pediatr Nephrol. 2025;40(1):243-51.

Meena J, Kumar J, Thomas CC, et al. Diagnostic accuracy of renal angina index alone or in combination with biomarkers for predicting acute kidney injury in children. Pediatr Nephrol. 2022;37(6):1263-75.

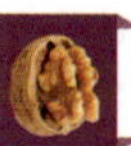

IN A NUTSHELL

Acute Kidney Injury

1. AKI is classified using the KDIGO criteria.
2. The common causes of AKI in newborns are sepsis and birth asphyxia, while acute tubular necrosis following severe dehydration due to acute gastroenteritis is the leading cause in children.
3. The use of biomarkers TIMP2-IGFBP7 (Nephrocheck) is an useful kit for early detection of AKI.
4. Hyperkalemia in AKI is a serious biochemical abnormality and can be treated with salbutamol nebulization, intravenous calcium gluconate administration, glucose-insulin infusion, and dialysis.
5. Recovery of kidney function is good in acute tubular necrosis, while it is poor in cortical necrosis.
6. The patients of AKI need long-term follow-up for development proteinuria, hypertension, and reduction in eGFR.

17.9 Hemolytic Uremic Syndrome

PE 20.5, PE 26.4

INTRODUCTION

Hemolytic uremic syndrome is one of the important causes of AKI in children below 3 years of age. The diagnostic criteria include (1) microangiopathic hemolytic anemia (hemoglobin <10 g/dL), evidence of hemolysis in peripheral blood smear as ≥2% schistocytes) and either raised lactic dehydrogenase of >450 IU/Lor markedly decreased haptoglobin) (2) thrombocytopenia (platelets count <1.5 lac/mm^3), and (3) AKI (>50% rise in serum creatinine from the baseline). Exclusion of disseminated intravascular coagulation and thrombotic thrombocytopenic purpura is required before consideration of diagnosis of HUS.

CLASSIFICATION

(Adapted from Indian Society of Pediatric Nephrology Consensus Guidelines, 2019)

- ***Shiga toxin associated HUS:*** This is caused by Shiga toxin producing *E. coli* (STEC), *Shigella dysenteriae* type 1 and *Campylobacter*.
- ***Pneumococcal HUS:*** This is caused by invasive infection caused by neuraminidase producing *Pneumococcus pneumoniae*.
- ***Infection associated HUS:*** This is caused by infections such as influenza (H1N1), HIV, coxsackie virus, parvovirus B19, varicella, malaria, dengue, *Rickettsia*, corona virus disease of 2019 (COVID 19), leptospira, and hepatitis A, B, C.
- ***Secondary HUS*** may follow bone marrow or solid organ transplantation, or associated with cancer chemotherapy, autoimmune disorders (systemic lupus erythematosus, antiphospholipid syndrome, scleroderma), malignant hypertension, and drug-induced (cyclosporine A, tacrolimus, sirolimus, and clopidogrel).
- ***Defect in cobalamin metabolism*** due to homozygous or compound heterozygous mutation in methylmalonic aciduria and homocystinuria type C.
- ***Atypical HUS (aHUS):*** It can occur in hereditary conditions (mutations in complement factor H (CFH), complement factor I (CFI), CFB, CD 46, C3, and thrombomodulin), autoimmune (anti-CFH antibodies, dysregulation of alternate complement pathway), cobalamin C defects, and diacylglycerol kinase E mutation and homozygous or compound heterozygous mutations in *ADAMTS13*. Anti-CFH antibodies could be detected in 6–10% of aHUS.

ETIOPATHOGENESIS

About 80% cases of diarrhea associated HUS are caused by STEC. Most important serotype is O157 with or without flagella type H7. However, in Indian subcontinent or Africa, *S. dysenteriae* type 1 is the major cause.

The pathology of HUS is broadly described as *thrombotic microangiopathy* (TMA) in which mixed platelet-fibrin thrombi occur in capillaries, arterioles, and sometimes arteries in the absence of vascular inflammation, and fibrin deposition. Toxin-induced endothelial injury, cell retraction, or detachment expose procoagulant material in the subendothelial matrix and cause local thrombosis. Red cells and platelets get injured while traversing these damaged vessels. Though microvascular injury occurs mainly in kidneys, other organs specially brain may also be affected.

CLINICAL MANIFESTATIONS

Shiga Toxin-associated Hemolytic Uremic Syndrome

A prodromal phase of acute dysentery with abdominal pain and vomiting precedes by 1–14 days. The onset of illness is sudden causing AKI; about 50% of patients are anuric. If urine output is there, hematuria and proteinuria are associated features. Hypertension and hypervolemia are also present at the time of presentation.

Systemic manifestations include severe hemorrhagic colitis (10–20%), central nervous system involvement (20%), hepatitis (40%), and acute pancreatitis (20%). The nervous system involvement leads to focal or generalized seizure, stupor, coma, hemiparesis, cortical blindness, and brain stem involvement. Myocarditis, cardiogenic shock, and pulmonary edema are the other manifestations.

Atypical Hemolytic Uremic Syndrome

It is suspected when infections, cobalamin associated, and secondary causes of HUS are excluded. These cases represent about 10% of HUS in children. Kidney failure has a remitting and relapsing course. There may be positive family history. Decline in kidney function leads to end-stage kidney disease in patients over a period of months to years. Neurological symptoms can also occur.

INVESTIGATIONS

In addition to hemogram, peripheral smear reveals evidence of red cell fragmentation as schistocytes, burr cells, and helmet cells. Direct Coombs test is negative and there is reticulocytosis and thrombocytopenia. Coagulation tests are normal. Plasma urea, creatinine, and lactic dehydrogenase levels are increased. Urine microscopy may reveal microscopic hematuria and proteinuria. Stool/rectal swab culture is done for detection of STEC and polymerase chain reaction for *STX1, STX2* and *EAE* genes. Assays for C3, C4 anti-CFH antibodies, and cell flow cytometry for CD46 expression on neutrophils are done. Screening for mutations in CFH, CFI, CFB, and C3, thrombomodulin, DGKE and CD46 by direct sequencing or next generation sequencing can also be performed in evaluation of atypical HUS. In addition, multiplex ligation-dependent probe amplification for detection of copy number variations for CFHR1-5 and CFH can also be undertaken. High plasma levels of total homocysteine (>50–100 μmol/L) with normal levels of vitamin B_{12} and folate can be detected in cobalamin C defect associated HUS. Blood samples can be collected in 3.2% sodium citrate and stored at -20 to -70 °C in suspected HUS for *ADAMTS13* activity assay.

TREATMENT Hemolytic Uremic Syndrome

The basic management of HUS includes removal of antibodies by plasma exchange (PEX), stoppage of antibody production by immunosuppression, blockade of complement cascade activation, and supportive therapy for AKI (treatment of anemia, hypertension, correction of fluid, and electrolyte disturbances and dialytic support).

Therapy of Specific Conditions

Shiga Toxin-associated HUS

Therapy mainly includes adequate hydration with normal saline, use of appropriate antibiotics in dysentery and management of AKI. Plasma exchange is not recommended unless the patients have severe neurological or cardiac involvement.

Anti-factor H Antibody-associated Atypical Hemolytic Uremic Syndrome

Plasma exchange and immunosuppression are main stay of therapy. Plasma exchange (daily for 5–7 days, then gradual taper) is preferred over plasma infusions for removal of antibodies. Immunosuppression should be started once there are raised levels of anti-FH antibodies. Prednisolone (1 mg/kg/day) is given for 4 weeks, then alternate days and gradual taper over 12 months. In addition, pulse therapy with intravenous cyclophosphamide (500 mg/m^2) every 4 weeks, 3–5 doses) or rituximab infusion 375 mg/m^2, two doses at 7 days interval can also be given. Maintenance therapy with mycophenolate mofetil (500–750 mg/m^2, two divided doses) or azathioprine (1–2 mg/kg/day) and low dose prednisolone (0.2–0.3 mg/kg, alternate days) are needed for 18–24 months to reduce the relapses.

As per Indian Society of Pediatric Nephrology guidelines, therapy with Eculizumab (a humanized monoclonal anti-C5 antibody) can be undertaken in specific situation such as there is no remission despite 7–10 cycles of PEX, presence of seizures, cardiac dysfunction, complications because of PEX or problem of vascular access and genetic defects in complement regulation.

Defective Cobalamin Metabolism

Treatment of cobalamin deficiency includes parenteral hydroxycolbalamin (1 mg daily injections till homocysteine levels fall between 40-60 μmol/L), oral betaine (250 mg/kg/day in three divided doses) and folate supplementation (5–30 mg in 2–3 divided doses per week) are provided.

Atypical Hemolytic Uremic Syndrome

Eculizumab, which prevents cleavage of C5 in to C5a and C5b and further formation of C5b-9 complex. It is given for complement dysregulated HUS in developed countries. But this drug is expensive and is now available in India and can be used depending upon affordability, as per guidelines recommendation. Newer FDA approved molecule *Ravulizumab*, having longer half-life as C5 inhibitor, and other agents *Crovalimab* (inhibits C5b6 deposition on endothelial surface) or *Iptacopan* (inhibits factor B) are currently under clinical trial and may be available as therapeutic option, if found efficacious.

Therefore, presently plasma exchange is the treatment option available in our country. It is provided daily initially until hematological remission (platelets >100,000/μL, schistocytes <2%, LDH less than upper limit of normal for 2 consecutive days) with exchange fluid as fresh frozen plasma. Exchanges are done at 60–75 mL/kg/day and tapering over next 4–6 weeks. Maintenance therapy with plasma infusions is continued every 2 weeks for patients with pathogenic variations in complement genes such as CFH and CFI. There is no role of plasma exchange in infection associated HUS, confirmed STEC HUS with no cardiac and neurological involvement and pathogenic variants in CD46 and DGKE.

Outcome

These patients need long-term follow up for at least 5 years for detection of relapses of HUS, hypertension, proteinuria, and development of chronic kidney disease. There are lesser chances of progression to end-stage kidney disease or mortality in patients, who are treated with eculizumab as compared to those who received plasma therapy. Recurrence of disease can occur in follow-up or even in transplanted kidney also.

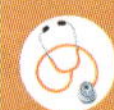

CASE STUDY Hemolytic Uremic Syndrome

A 2-year-old girl presented in emergency with passage of decreased urine output for 24 hours. There was a history of frequent passage of stool mixed with blood 10 days back, and now developed decreased urine output and swelling over the body.

What physical findings you will look for in this patient?

I will look for puffiness of face, pedal edema, acidotic breathing, and evidence of skin and mucous membrane bleeding, and will record blood pressure for evidence of hypertension.

What is most likely diagnosis?

The most likely diagnosis in this patient is HUS as she had history of dysentery followed by oliguria, edema, and bleeding but other causes of AKI should be excluded.

Mention relevant investigations to confirm diagnosis.

Hemoglobin for degree of anemia, complete blood count, peripheral blood smear examination for thrombocytopenia, and features of hemolysis such as fragmented RBCs, schistocytes, burr cells, and reticulocytosis. Kidney function tests (serum urea, creatinine, sodium, potassium) must be done to assess the severity of AKI. Stool culture for Shiga toxin producing organisms and detection of virulence genes on fecal extracts or cultures [*STX1, STX2,* and *eae* by polymerase chain reaction (PCR)]. The levels of C3, C4, and assay of anti-CFH antibody and CD 46 flow cytometry are performed.

Outline management of this patient.

The child should be given restricted fluid intake (400 mL/m^2/day) and institution of early peritoneal or hemodialysis. Hypertension should be treated with calcium channel blocker and/or beta blocker. Meticulous recording of urine output, kidney function tests, and blood pressure should be done during hospitalization and in the follow-up also. Etiology based specific therapy should also be instituted.

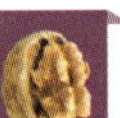

IN A NUTSHELL

Hemolytic Uremic Syndrome

1. Hemolytic uremic syndrome (HUS) consists of a triad of microangiopathic hemolytic anemia, thrombocytopenia, and acute kidney injury.
2. HUS is broadly classified into Shiga toxin associated HUS, infection associated HUS, cobalamin C deficiency HUS, secondary HUS, and atypical HUS.
3. Blood samples for specific investigations like anti-factor H antibodies, C3 level, total homocysteine, and CD46. Flow cytometry should be undertaken before performing plasma exchange.
4. In patients with anti-FH antibodies positive, plasma exchange (4–6 weeks) and immunosuppression are instituted.
5. In patients with anti-FH antibodies negative, genetic testing should be performed. Plasma exchange initially for 4–6 weeks, followed by plasma infusions are recommended. Eculizumab is the drug for complement blockade. Newer agents *Ravulizumab* or Crovalimab or *Iptacopan* may find a place as therapeutic option in future.
6. Treatment is mainly supportive. Dialysis is required in 50–60% cases of HUS.

Abou-Ismail MY, Kapoor S, Citla Sridhar D, Nayak L, Ahuja S. Thrombotic microangiopathies: An illustrated review. Res Pract Thromb Haemost. 2022;6(3):e12708.

Bagga A, Khandelwal P, Mishra K, et al. Indian Society of Pediatric Nephrology. Hemolytic uremic syndrome in a developing country: Consensus guidelines. Pediatr Nephrol. 2019;34:1465-82.

Jokiranta TS. HUS and atypical HUS. Blood. 2017;129(21):2847-56.

Loirat C, Fakhouri F, Ariceta G, et al. An international consensus approach to the management of atypical haemolytic uremic syndrome in children. Pediatr Nephrol. 2016;31:15-39.

Vivarelli M, Barratt J, Beck LH Jr, Fakhouri F, Gale DP, Goicoechea de Jorge E, et al. The role of complement in kidney disease: conclusions from a kidney disease: Improving Global Outcomes (KDIGO) Controversies Conference. Kidney Int. 2024;106(3):369-91.

17.10 Chronic Kidney Disease (CKD) *PE 20.6*

INTRODUCTION

Chronic kidney disease (CKD): It is defined as abnormalities of kidney structure or function, present for >3 months, with or without decreased GFR; or any patient who has GFR <60 mL/min/1.73 m^2 lasting for at least 3 months with or without kidney damage (structure or function).

End-stage kidney disease (ESKD): This is characterized by decline of kidney function to a degree when life cannot be sustained without replacement of kidney function either in form of dialysis or transplantation.

ETIOLOGY

The prevalence of pediatric CKD ranges between 15 and 74.7 cases per million children. Various renal registries across the world reported that congenital anomalies of kidneys and urinary tract (CAKUT) is the most common cause of CKD (48–59%) and grade 5D (34–43%), followed by glomerulonephritis (5–14% and 15–29%, respectively) in children below 20 years of age.

The CAKUT is the most common cause of CKD in children below 5 years. Glomerulonephritis is responsible for most cases of CKD in older children.

- ***Congenital anomalies of kidney and urinary tract (60% cases):*** Hypoplasia, dysplasia ± reflux nephropathy, and obstructive nephropathy.
- Focal segmental glomerulosclerosis (5–10%)
- ***Glomerulonephritis*** (5–10%) lupus nephritis, Henoch-Schönlein purpura, IgA nephropathy, and MPGN.
- ***Hereditary:*** Familial juvenile nephronophthisis, Alport syndrome, ARPKD, and familial nephrotic syndrome.
- ***Metabolic:*** Cystinosis and oxalosis.
- ***Vascular:*** Renal vein thrombosis.
- ***Renal cortical necrosis:*** HUS (atypical).
- ***Other:*** Prune-Belly syndrome and bilateral Wilms tumor.

STAGES OF CHRONIC KIDNEY DISEASE (TABLE 17.19)

Systemic hypertension, acidosis, and proteinuria are the most important independent risk factors for progression of CKD. Other factors are underlying kidney disease, polymorphic genetic variation, hyperphosphatemia, dyslipidemia, and insulin resistance.

CLINICAL PRESENTATION

The onset is usually insidious. The clinical manifestations are usually nonspecific and include fatigue, anorexia, headache,

Table 17.19 Kidney Disease Improving Global Outcomes (KDIGO) Grading of Chronic Kidney Disease

Grading	GFR (mL/min/1.73 m²)	Terms
G1	≥90	Normal or high
G2	60–89	Mildly decreased
G3a	45--59	Mildly to moderately decreased
G3b	30–44	Moderately to severely decreased
G4	15–29	Severely decreased
G5 G5D	<15	• Kidney failure • Kidney failure treated by dialysis

Source: Adapted from Clinical Practice Guidelines on CKD, 2012

lethargy, vomiting, polyuria, polydipsia, and growth failure. On physical examination, majority of patients are anemic and have high blood pressure. In children with congenital kidney abnormalities, growth retardation, and osteodystrophy are present. In any child having severe unexplained anemia, growth retardation, hypertension, and acidotic breathing, CKD is most the likely diagnosis. Other clinical manifestations are mentioned in **Table 17.20**.

Anemia in CKD

Anemia is common in children with CKD and manifests in stages III and IV or when GFR falls to 25–35 mL/min/1.73 m². The causes of anemia include erythropoietin deficiency, iron deficiency, blood loss (phlebotomy, hemodialysis, gastrointestinal), hemolysis, malnutrition, B12 or folate deficiency, bone marrow suppression, chronic or acute inflammation, carnitine deficiency, and associated systemic diseases such as systemic lupus erythematosus or malignancy. The etiology of iron deficiency in CKD includes blood losses, poor dietary intake, poor absorption, and depletion of iron store during recombinant human erythropoietin therapy (rHuEPO). Clinical manifestations include fatigue, depression, decreased quality of life, decreased exercise tolerance, impaired cognitive function, and loss of appetite.

Table 17.20 Clinical Manifestations of Chronic Kidney Disease

Kidney	Edema, hematuria, proteinuria, hypertension, oliguria/polyuria
Metabolic	Hypocalcemia, metabolic acidosis, hyperkalemia/hypokalemia, hyperphosphatemia, hyperglycemia, and hyperlipidemia
Hematological	Anemia, bleeding tendency
Cardiovascular	Congestive heart failure, hypertension, pericarditis
Gastrointestinal	Anorexia, vomiting, gastroesophageal reflux disease (GERD), gastroduodenal ulcer
Neurological	Fatigue, poor concentration, headache, drowsiness, loss of memory, slurred speech, muscle weakness and cramps, psychosis, ataxia, tremors, asterixis, seizures, coma, mental retardation, peripheral neuropathy (motor, sensory or autonomic), and encephalopathy
Dermatological	Pruritus, dermatitis
Reproductive	Delayed sexual development
Musculoskeletal	Muscle weakness, growth retardation, renal osteodystrophy
Miscellaneous	Failure to thrive, polyuria, dehydration

Renal Osteodystrophy

Renal osteodystrophy occurs usually late in children with CKD and is characterized by osteopenia, osteoporosis/rickets, osteosclerosis, and osteitis fibrosa cystica. *Osteitis fibrosa cystica* is characterized by increased osteoclast and osteoblast activity and excessive woven bone, high bone turnover, increased quantity of unmineralized bone matrix (osteoid).

The clinical manifestations include muscle weakness, bony pain, fractures with minor trauma, and valgus and varus deformities of long bones. Slipped femoral epiphysis, bowing of lower extremities, soft tissue calcification, rachitic rosary, and Harrison sulcus may be present. Pathophysiology of osteodystrophy is depicted in **Flowchart 17.5**.

Short stature is the sequelae of childhood CKD (30–60% of children with *end-stage kidney disease* may grow up to become stunted adults). The causes include protein and calorie malnutrition, fluid and electrolyte disturbances, renal osteodystrophy, end organ hyporesponsiveness to growth hormone, and anemia. Growth failure is severe in children who develop kidney insufficiency in the first 2 years of life as children normally attain one-third of their final adult height during this period.

Flowchart 17.5: Pathophysiology of renal osteodystrophy

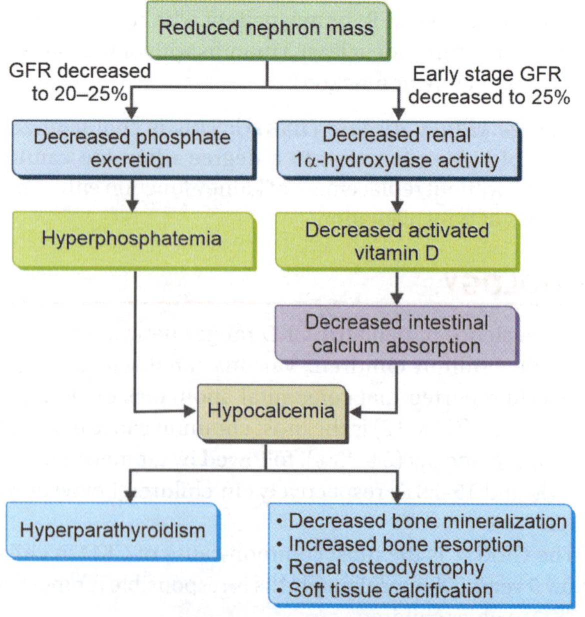

(GFR: glomerular filtration rate)

INVESTIGATIONS

Renal Functions

The first and most important step in evaluation is calculation of eGFR (mL/min/1.73 m^2) of the patient (by modified Schwartz formula: 0.413 × height (cm)/serum creatinine. Initial evaluation includes complete blood count, peripheral blood smear, serum creatinine, urea, electrolytes, calcium, phosphorus, alkaline phosphatase, iPTH, 25 (OH) vitamin D, total protein/albumin, uric acid, cholesterol, triglycerides, TSH, serum iron, percentage saturation of transferrin, serum ferritin, reticulocyte count, vitamin B12, folate levels, and arterial blood gases. Urine analysis should look for hematuria, proteinuria (protein/creatine ratio of >0.2 mg/mg), casts, and specific gravity.

For diagnosis of anemia in children with CKD, KDIGO recommended hemoglobin level <11 g/dL in 6 months–5 years, <11.5 g/dL in 5–12 years, <12 g/dL in 12–15 years, transferrin saturation (TSAT) <20%, and serum ferritin <100 ng/mL. Complete blood count, reticulocytes, ferritin and TSAT testing are to be done annually in CKD G3, twice in a year in CKD G4 and every 3 monthly in CKD G5 or G5D.

Imaging

X-rays of wrist, long bones, chest, and spine should be done every 6 months in children with CKD. KDIGO suggests use of bone mineral density measurement to assess risk of fracture and evidence of CKD-bone mineral disease.

Early radiographic findings are features of osteopenia (thinning of cortices and trabeculae gives ground glass appearance), salt and pepper skull, epiphyseal thickening, and fraying of metaphysis but no cupping, late epiphyseal ossification, and slipped epiphysis.

Late radiological features are secondary to hyperparathyroidism and include subperiosteal cortical resorption of distal phalanx, end of clavicle, ischium, pubis, sacroiliac joints, metaphyseal-diaphyseal junction of long bones, lucent metaphyseal bands, bowing of long bones, rugger jersey spine, brown tumor of ribs and jaw.

The USG of KUB should also be done for kidney size, hydronephrosis, calculi, cystic and solid lesions of kidney, and anatomy of ureters and bladder.

Others

Decreased serum calcium, increased phosphate, increased alkaline phosphatase, and increased iPTH level are usual findings in children with renal osteodystrophy. Kidney biopsy can be undertaken to demonstrate the underlying glomerular pathology, but should not be performed in small and contracted kidneys.

TREATMENT Chronic Kidney Disease

The aim of treatment is to replace absent/diminished kidney functions which progressively deteriorate in parallel with the progressive loss of GFR and slow the progression of kidney dysfunction. Hyperkalemia is usually not observed until GFR decreases to <10 mL/min/1.73 m^2. Management of hyperkalemia, acidosis, and hypertension should be done as already described in **Table 17.17**.

Nutritional Therapy

Poor nutritional status in children with CKD is due to anorexia, altered taste, frequent illnesses, and dietary restriction. Dietary changes are required when GFR is <30 mL/min/1.73 m^2.

Usually, children with CKD should have energy intake of 100% of recommended dietary allowance (RDA) required as per age, body mass index (BMI), and physical activity. Protein intake should be 100–140% RDA, 100–120% RDA in G4 and G5 CKD, and 100% + allowance for dialysis loss in G5D. Vitamins and trace elements are to taken 100% RDA. About 50% of energy should be from carbohydrate, 35–40% from fat, and rest proteins. The recommended allowance of protein is 2.2 g/kg/day in children <6 months and 0.9–1.9 g/kg/day for older one. Patients who are on hemodialysis should be given additional protein of 0.4 g/kg/day, whereas those on PD; additional 0.7–0.8 g/kg/day for losses because of larger surface area of peritoneum. Proteins of high biological values such as eggs, milk, meat, and fish are recommended.

Fat-rich diet should be given but "heart healthy fats" (corn oils, safflower, soy, olive, peanut oils) should be consumed. Omega-3 fatty acids have beneficial effect on cardiovascular status in patients of CKD. Therapeutic dose is 3–8 g/day in the form of fish oil supplements.

Weight, height, head circumference, and mid-arm circumference should be measured every 3–6 months to look for nutritional status and detect growth retardation in children, especially below 5 years. Hypertensive children of more than 2 years old should consume <1.5 g/day of salt. Recommended intake of phosphate in CKD is 600–800 mg/day, when phosphate binders are started. Low phosphate containing foods are animal flesh proteins; while eggs, dairy products, legumes have higher phosphate protein ratio. Calcium supplements if given with meals bind phosphate but empty stomach increases calcium absorption.

Hypertension

As per KDIGO guidelines, BP monitoring once a year with ambulatory blood pressure monitoring (ABPM) and every 3–6 monthly with standardized auscultatory office BP should be done and 24-hour mean arterial pressure (MAP) by ABPM should be lowered to ≤50th percentile for age, gender and height. When ABPM is not available, it is reasonable to target manual auscultatory office systolic BP to 50th-75th percentile for age, gender, and height. ACE inhibitors are preferred due to its antiproteinuric effect. They should be avoided if GFR <30 mL/min/1.73 m^2, may cause fall in GFR and can also lead to hyperkalemia. In such patients, calcium channel blocker (Amlodipine) and/or alpha blocker (Prazocin) and beta blocker (Atenolol/Metoprolol/Carvedilol) given to have target blood pressure control.

Dyslipidemia

The treatment of uremic dyslipidemia is one of the methods of renoprotective measure. Approach should focus on treatment of malnutrition, metabolic acidosis, hyperparathyroidism, and anemia. In addition, diet, exercise, and weight reduction in obese CKD patients should also be advised. Statins have been recommended in adults with CKD but has not been evaluated in children.

Treat Anemia

The management of anemia includes recombinant human erythropoietin (rHuEPO) and iron therapy. rHuEPO is started when hemoglobin falls below 10 g/dL. It may be given subcutaneously (half-life 14–25 hours) and intravenously (half-life 5.6–7.5 hours).

The initial dose for subcutaneous rHuEPO receiving PD is 100 units/kg/week in two divided doses and may be increased to 150 units/kg/week in severe anemia. Dose for intravenous administration is 150 units/kg/week in three divided doses and may be increased to 200–300 units/kg/week in severe anemia in children <5 years old. The goal is to increase hemoglobin by 1–2 g/dL per month and it is maintained between 11 and 12 g/dL

Another preparation such as Darbepoetin alfa (0.45 μg/kg) can be given once in a week and long acting Mircera once per month. Dose relationship of rHuEPO of 2,000 units is equivalent to 10 micrograms of Darbepoetin alfa and 30 micrograms of Mircera. Complications of recombinant erythropoietin therapy include iron deficiency, hypertension, seizures, and pure red cell aplasia.

Oral iron and folic acid should be given along with erythropoietin. The dose of iron is 3–6 mg/kg/day in children not on hemodialysis and intravenous iron in CKD patients on hemodialysis. Parenteral iron can maintain hemoglobin levels and reduce the need for erythropoiesis-stimulating agents (ESAs). Patients on erythropoietin and iron therapy, TSAT should be maintained >20% and serum ferritin >100 ng/mL. Cases with hypothyroidism should receive L-thyroxine therapy also to correct anemia. Use of new class of oral agents called hypoxia-inducible factor-prolyl hydroxylase inhibitors (HIF-PHD inhibitors), have been found to correct anemia in CKD. However, long-term safety profile and data on children are awaited.

Correct Acidosis

Children with CKD should receive sodium bicarbonate 2–3 mEq/kg/day to target serum bicarbonate levels at 20–22 mEq/L.

Manage Growth Failure

Gradual loss of standard height must be expected in children and adolescents on long-term dialysis. General measure of treatment is adequate calorie and protein intake, dialysis, and hormonal replacement therapy. There is variable response for starting to catch up growth after kidney transplantation and depend on impairment of kidney function and glucocorticoid dosage.

Hormonal treatment includes calcitriol and growth hormone. The administration of growth hormone markedly increases systemic (mainly hepatic) and local insulin-like growth factor 1 (IGF-1) production (in growth cartilage) in children with CKD who remain <3rd centile for height or growth velocity <2 SD despite optimal medical support.

The dose of recombinant human growth hormone (rHuGH) is 0.05 mg/kg/day, subcutaneously with periodic adjustment of dose to achieve normal height velocity. Daily dosing is more effective than three times administration per week. The response of growth hormone depends on residual kidney function, target height, initial target height deficit, duration of treatment, and age at start of treatment (younger age more response). The adverse effects of rHuGH are pseudotumor cerebri, hyperinsulinemia, increased risk of atherosclerosis, and accelerated progression of kidney failure.

Management of Renal Osteodystrophy

The dietary management includes limitation of foods such as milk, cheese, nut, chocolate, and organ meat. Low phosphorus formula milk (Similac PM 60/40) and fresh or frozen breastmilk pretreated with sevelamer are recommended for infants with renal osteodystrophy. Though phosphate is easily dialyzable but efficacy of removing phosphate is limited because of concomitant intake of calcitriol (0.25–0.50 microgram or 5–10 ng/kg/day) and phosphate binders, which result in 50% absorption.

Initial treatment restricts dietary phosphorus intake when phosphate or parathyroid hormone (PTH) levels begin to rise. Serum phosphorus levels should be maintained between 2.7 and 4.6 mg/dL in patients with G3a–G4 CKD, and between 3.5 and 5.5 mg/dL in individuals with G5 CKD. KDIGO suggests that individual values of calcium and phosphorous are evaluated rather than their product in patients with CKD G3a–G5D. Target should be to lower serum phosphorous and maintain calcium in the normal range.

Calcium-based binders: Calcium acetate, carbonate, and phosphate have limited phosphate binding capacity and prolonged administration leads to hypercalcemia. Hence, it should be given with meals. Calcium acetate binds more phosphate; improved phosphate control and has decreased incidence of hypercalcemia. Calcium carbonate has fewer gastrointestinal side effects.

Sevelamer hydrochloride: It is a hydrogel of polyallylamine and efficient phosphate binders. It is resistant to digestive degradation and hypercalcemia occurs less frequently. It also acts as bile acid sequestrant and decreases total cholesterol and LDL cholesterol. Dose is 100 mg/kg/day orally in three divided doses with meals and adjusted as per serum phosphate level.

Vitamin D therapy: It is indicated in vitamin D level below the established range for child's age or in child with PTH level above target for that stage. In a patient with severe vitamin D deficiency (25-OH-vitamin D <5 ng/mL), vitamin D_3 is given 60,000 IU/week for 4 weeks, followed by 60,000 IU every other week for 3 months. Moderate deficiency (25-OHD 5–15 ng/mL) can be treated with 60,000 IU every other week for 3 months. Mild vitamin D deficiency (25-OHD 16–30 ng/mL), should be treated with 60,000 IU every 4 weeks for 3 months. However, if secondary hyperparathyroidism persists despite vitamin D2 therapy, calcitriol (5–10 ng/kg/day) is also recommended.

Kidney Support Therapy

The initiation of dialysis should be considered when GFR is <15 mL/min/1.73 m^2. PD is indicated in all patients <2 years. In children above 5 years, hemodialysis/hemodiafiltration is performed. Differences between the two are summarized in **Table 17.21**. Hemodiafiltration is preferred over hemodialysis as the later involves principles of both convection and diffusion and removes both small (urea, creatinine, phosphate) and large (β_2 microglobulin, cytokines) molecules and results in better appetite, growth, reduce cardiovascular co-morbidity, and results in better bone turnover.

Kidney transplantation is the ultimate goal as it provides most normal lifestyle and possibility for rehabilitation for the child and family.

Immunization

All children with CKD should receive standard immunization according to schedule. Live vaccines to be withheld in CKD related to children with glomerulonephritis on immunosuppressive medications. All children should receive MMR, varicella, and pneumococcal vaccines before kidney transplantation. They should also receive yearly influenza vaccine.

PROGNOSIS

Early diagnosis (antenatal screening), treatment of etiology, reduction of proteinuria, control of blood pressure, correction of anemia, acidosis, maintenance of calcium, phosphorus, and

Table 17.21 Peritoneal Dialysis versus Hemodialysis

Peritoneal dialysis	*Hemodialysis/hemodiafiltration*
Daily sessions are required	Usually three per week required
Less restrictive diet	More restriction on fluid and dietary intake
Can be done at home and technically easier	Hospital setting required
Complications	*Complications*
Malfunction of catheter, infection of exit site, peritonitis, negative body image	Thrombosis, stenosis of access, and catheter sepsis

iPTH in normal range and modification of drug doses based on eGFR are some of the factors that may retard the progression of CKD and improve the prognosis.

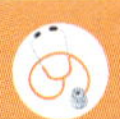

CASE STUDY **Chronic Kidney Disease (CKD)**

A 4-year-old male child presented with not growing well, looking pale, decreases appetite, and urinary stream abnormality in the form of dribbling of urine. There is history of previous recurrent febrile UTIs treated by Pediatrician. On examination, child has weight 14 kg, height 89 cm, pulse rate 84/min, respiratory rate 38-minute, blood pressure 124/86 mm Hg, and moderate anemia. There were no clinical features of rickets. Abdominal examination revealed bilateral kidney lump and bladder is also palpable.

What is the likely diagnosis?

In view of presence of recurrent UTI, urine stream abnormality, presence of anemia, short stature (weight 1–2 SD, height <3 SD) , hypertension (>99th percentile) and palpable kidneys and bladder, the likely diagnosis is obstructive uropathy with CKD grade 5 D (eGFR 10.5 mL/min/1.73 m^2). Since patient is a male child, possibility of PUV should be considered.

Enumerate the relevant investigations to be undertaken?

Hemogram revealed hemoglobin of 7 g/dL, total leukocyte count of 6,500/mm^3, polymorphs 55%, lymphocytes 40%, eosinophils 3%, and monocytes 2%. Serum urea 134 mg/dL, creatinine 3.5 mg/dL, sodium 132 mEq/L, K 5.8 mEq/L, Ca 8.5 mg/dL, phosphate 6.5 mg/dL, alkaline phosphate 445 IU/L, and iPTH 350 pg/mL. Arterial blood gas showed pH of 7.25, HCO_3 13 mEq/L, ionic Ca 0.8 mEq/L, K 5.8 mEq/L, and Cl 101 mEq/L.

Ultrasonography of abdomen showed right kidney 9.5 cm, left kidney 9.4 cm with dilated pelvicalyceal system. Bladder showed thickened wall and significant residual urine volume (75 mL). MCU showed bilateral grade IV VUR with spinning top appearance of bladder and dilated posterior urethra.

What is the final diagnosis?

Posterior urethral valve with bilateral VUR, hydronephrosis, and CKD grade 5 D, metabolic acidosis, and renal anemia.

Outline the management of this patient?

Medical: Correction of acidosis by oral sodabicarbonate, anemia correction initially-oral iron and folic acid, followed by rHEPO therapy blood pressure control by Amlodipine, supplementation of oral calcium, vitamin D3 and 1,25-dihydroxy cholecalciferol and phosphate binder as calcium acetate/sevelamer. Further monitoring of blood pressure, hemoglobin, kidney function test, Ca, PO_4, iPTH, and growth of child. Parent should be counseled for start of maintenance hemodialysis (three times per week) and plan for the kidney transplantation.

Surgical: Immediate bladder catheterization to relieve the obstruction, followed by fulguration of PUV.

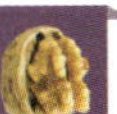

IN A NUTSHELL

Chronic Kidney Disease (CKD)

1. CAKUT is the most common cause of CKD in children below 5 years while chronic glomerulonephritis is the main etiology above 5 years of age.
2. Hypertension, proteinuria, and acidosis are the independent risk factors for progression of CKD.
3. Anemia, growth retardation, hypertension, azotemia, and features of renal osteodystrophy are diagnostic features of CKD.
4. Medical management includes correction of anemia, control of proteinuria, hypertension, acidosis, hyperphosphatemia, and vitamin D and calcium carbonate supplementation.
5. Dialytic therapy (peritoneal/hemodialysis/hemodiafiltration) and kidney transplantation has improved survival in these children.

Cheung AK, Chang TI, Cushman WC, et al. Executive summary of the KDIGO 2021 Clinical Practice Guideline for the Management of Blood Pressure in Chronic Kidney Disease. Kidney Int. 2021;99(3):559-69.

Gutiérrez OM. Treatment of iron deficiency anemia in CKD and End-Stage Kidney Disease. Kidney Int Rep. 2021;6(9):2261-9.

Kidney Disease: Improving Global Outcomes (KDIGO) CKD Work Group. KDIGO 2024 Clinical Practice Guideline for the Evaluation and Management of Chronic Kidney Disease. Kidney Int. 2024;105(4S): S117-S314.

Kidney Disease: Improving Global Outcomes (KDIGO) CKD-MBD Update Work Group. KDIGO 2017 Clinical Practice Guideline Update for the Diagnosis, Evaluation, Prevention, and Treatment of Chronic Kidney Disease–Mineral and Bone Disorder (CKD-MBD). Kidney Int Suppl. 2017;7:1-59.

Kidney Disease: Improving Global Outcomes (KDIGO) CKD Work Group. KDIGO 2012 Clinical Practice Guideline for the Evaluation and Management of Chronic Kidney Disease. Kidney Int Suppl. 2013;3:1-150.

Poustie VJ, Smyth RL, Watling RM. Oral protein calorie supplementation for children with chronic disease. Cochrane System Rev. 2010;(3): CD001914.

Roderick PJ, Willis NS, Blakeley S, et al. Correction of chronic metabolic acidosis for chronic kidney disease patients. Cochrane System Rev. 2007;2007(1):CD001890.

Shroff R, Smith C, Ranchin B, et al. Effects of hemodiafiltration versus conventional hemodialysis in children with ESKD: The HDF, Heart and Height Study. J Am Soc Nephrol. 2019;30:678-91.

17.11 Wilms Tumor

PE 20.7

INTRODUCTION

Wilms tumor is the most common renal tumor in younger children; however, beyond 14 years of age, renal cell carcinoma (RCC) is more common. Bilateral disease is seen in 5–7% patients. Occasionally nephrogenic rests may be seen in the other kidney. Congenital malformations are seen in approximately 10% of children with Wilms tumor, which may be isolated or part of a syndrome. The syndromes commonly associated with Wilms

Table 17.22 Syndromic Associations with Wilms Tumor

Condition	*Locus*	*Clinical constellation*	*Risk of Wilms tumor*
WAGR syndrome	11p13, *WT1* gene	Wilms tumor, aniridia, genitourinary abnormalities, renal failure	30%
Beckwith–Wiedemann syndrome	11p15, *WT2* gene (dysregulation of imprinted gene IGF 2)	Hemihypertrophy, macroglossia, omphalocele, neonatal hypoglycemia, large for dates at birth	5%
Fraser syndrome	11p13, *WT1* gene	Pseudohermaphroditism, focal segmental glomerulosclerosis	8%
Denys–Drash syndrome	11p13, *WT1* gene	Ambiguous genitalia, diffuse mesangial sclerosis	>90%
Li-Fraumeni syndrome	17p13, *TP53* gene	More common in anaplastic histology as compared to favorable histology Wilms tumor. There may be a family history suggesting the diagnosis of Li-Fraumeni	• Somatic mutations in *TP53* seen in 75% • Anaplastic WT

tumor are listed in **Table 17.22**. Approximately 7% children with Wilms tumor have an underlying syndrome.

ETIOPATHOGENESIS

Wilms tumor is linked closely to early nephrogenesis. While unilateral disease is more likely to be sporadic, patients with multifocal disease or bilateral disease have a higher incidence of underlying syndromes associated with overgrowth or genitourinary malformation. However, all patients with these syndromes do not necessarily develop the malignancy. While the genetic factors leading to Wilms tumor are known, the sporadic factors are not well recognized.

Wilms tumor along with retinoblastoma, was one of the tumors used to develop the two-hit oncogenic transformation hypothesis by Knudson. However, multiple genes are implicated in the pathogenesis of Wilms tumor, unlike retinoblastoma, where a single *Rb* gene is implicated. Molecular studies are being carried out to understand the landscape of WT, and several cancer genes, apart from those involved in nephrogenesis have been implicated in the pathogenesis of the tumor. The genes involved may be mutated, or epigenetically altered, and include *WT1* on chromosome 11p13, *WTX* gene on chromosome X, *WT2* gene at 11p15 locus, *TP53*, and *CTNNB1*, among others.

Typically, Wilms tumor is a triphasic tumor, consisting of elements from (1) blastema, (2) stroma, and (3) epithelium. High-risk histopathological features include presence of focal or diffuse anaplasia, predominance of blastemal element, or pathology like clear cell sarcoma or rhabdoid tumor of the kidney. Both latter entities are now no longer classified as subtypes of Wilms tumor but as separate renal tumors of the childhood.

CLINICAL FEATURES

The median age at diagnosis is 3 years. Most of the children present with an incidentally detected lump in the flank, felt by the mother while bathing or dressing the child **(Fig. 17.12)**. Occasionally, there may be presence of frank hematuria, though microscopic hematuria is more common. Fever, pain in the abdomen, and hypertension are other manifestations, with hypertension being present in about 25% patients. Occasionally, hypertension may be severe enough to lead to end organ damage like encephalopathy. The reason for hypertension is increased renin production. Rarely, patients may present with an acute abdomen due to tumor rupture. All the manifestations improve with treatment of primary disease. Wilms tumor typically involves the other kidney in about 7%. There may be local vascular invasion in 4–10% patients with involvement of the renal veins, or the inferior vena cava with rare tumor invasion up to the right atrium. The typical sites of metastasis of Wilms tumor are lungs, liver, bone, and brain, in that sequence.

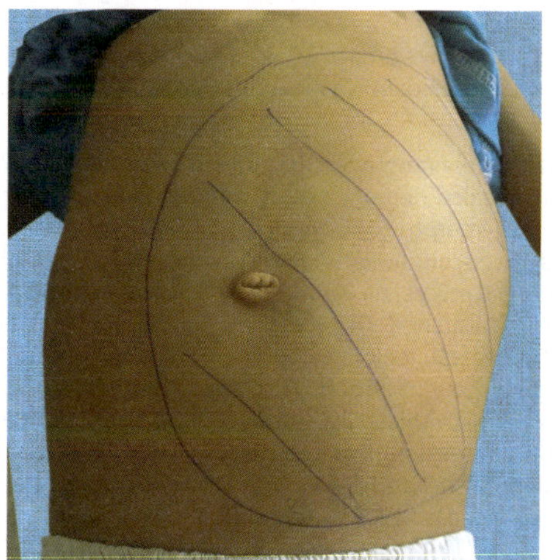

Fig. 17.12: Well-looking child with incidentally discovered left-sided flank mass. Tissue diagnosis confirmed the presence of Wilms tumor

INVESTIGATIONS AND STAGING

In a child with abdominal mass, an ultrasound of the abdomen is the initial investigation, and will yield information to confirm the organ of origin, cystic versus solid nature of mass, extend of local spread and involvement of other organs like liver and lymph nodes. A contrast computed tomography of the abdomen (**Fig. 17.13**) may have a specific *claw sign* in the involved kidney.

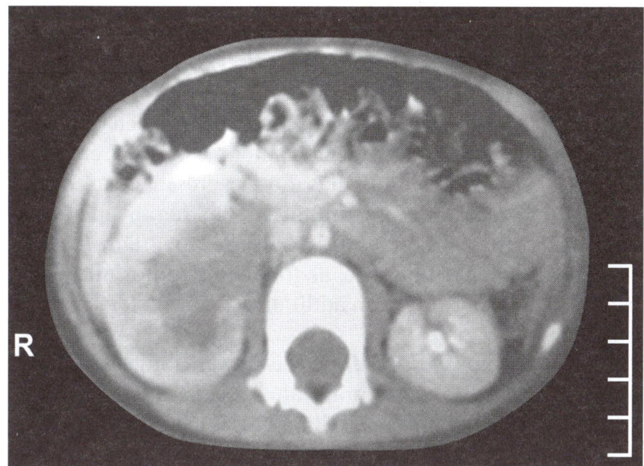

Fig. 17.13: A contrast-enhanced CT of the abdomen with a large Wilms tumor replacing the entire right kidney. A normal left kidney can be seen

Abdominal imaging will also confirm about the anatomy and involvement of the other kidney. Additionally, contrast excretion from the contralateral kidney confirms that it is functioning.

A computed tomography scan of the chest is required to check for presence of metastasis to the lungs, and a chest radiograph is not considered adequate for this purpose any longer. There is no role of positron emission tomography (PET) as an imaging modality in Wilms tumor. Staging in Wilms tumor is mentioned in **Box 17.8**.

Tissue Diagnosis

There is a divided opinion on need for tissue diagnosis in the form of core biopsy in a renal tumor. In a small tumor, a biopsy may not be done, and primary nephrectomy may be performed. On the other hand, in a large extensive tumor, or in presence of distant metastasis, it is better to confirm the diagnosis by a core biopsy enabling the administration of neoadjuvant chemotherapy. This will make surgical resection easier subsequently.

Box 17.8 Staging of Wilms Tumor (National Wilms Tumor Study Group)

- *Stage I:* Tumor is limited to the kidney and is excised completely. Capsule surface intact; no tumor rupture and no residual tumor apparent beyond margins of excision
- *Stage II:* Tumor extends beyond the kidney but is excised completely. Regional extension of tumor, vessel infiltration, tumor biopsied, or local spillage of tumor confined to the flank. No residual tumor apparent at or beyond margins of excision
- *Stage III:* Residual nonhematogenous tumor confined to abdomen lymph node and/or involvement of hilus, periaortic chains or beyond; diffuse peritoneal contamination by tumor spillage, peritoneal implants of tumor, tumor extends beyond surgical margins microscopically or macroscopically and tumor not completely removable because of local infiltration into vital structures
- *Stage IV:* Deposits beyond stage III (e.g., lung, liver, bone, and brain)
- *Stage V:* Bilateral renal involvement at diagnosis

TREATMENT Wilms Tumor

Wilms tumor is a curable disease, with survival rates in the excess of 90%. Treatment is typically multimodality, with chemotherapy and surgery both required for most patients. Radiotherapy is required occasionally in the presence of certain high-risk histological features like anaplasia, stage III disease, or in the presence of metastatic disease persisting after neoadjuvant chemotherapy. Chemotherapeutic agents used typically include vincristine and actinomycin D. For higher stage disease, doxorubicin, etoposide, and platinum agents may be required. Usually, nephrectomy is performed after a few cycles of neoadjuvant chemotherapy to enable complete and easy resection. Duration and drugs required for adjuvant chemotherapy, as well as decision to give radiotherapy is based on the extent of resection and histological features of the resected tumor. In a small tumor, upfront nephrectomy may be done without any preoperative chemotherapy, but most children in our country present with large tumors requiring neoadjuvant chemotherapy.

Guidelines of treatment as per recommendation of International Society of Pediatric Oncology (SIOP) according to the UMBRELLA protocol for Wilms tumor ***(Table 17.23)****:*

- Treatment with preoperative chemotherapy to all stage I, II, and III tumors for 4 weeks.
- Treatment with preoperative chemotherapy for 6 weeks for all stage IV tumors.
- Surgery after 4 weeks of therapy in stage I–III tumors or after 6 weeks of therapy in stage IV tumor.
- Surgery may be radical nephrectomy with lymph node dissection. In selected cases, nephron sparing surgery may be considered.
- Staging and histological risk-assessment in the postoperative specimen.
- Radiotherapy to all patients with stage II disease with anaplasia, stage III disease, and if presence of residual metastasis in stage IV disease after preoperative chemotherapy.
- Postoperative chemotherapy with two drugs (vincristine and actinomycin D) to stage I–III disease, with either low or intermediate risk histology; for stage I disease, postoperative therapy for 4 weeks, and for stage II–III disease, for 26 weeks.
- For high-risk disease or for stage IV disease, 3–4 drugs for 26–34 weeks will be required. The drugs include etoposide, doxorubicin, carboplatin, and cyclophosphamide.

Table 17.23 Preoperative Chemotherapy for Stages I to IV of Wilms Tumor

Preoperative chemotherapy for stage I, II, and III of Wilms tumor			
Week 1	*Week 2*	*Week 3*	*Week 4*
Vincristine Actinomycin D	Vincristine	Vincristine Actinomycin D	Vincristine
Preoperative chemotherapy for stage IV of Wilms tumor			
Week 1	*Week 2*	*Week 3*	*Week 4*
Vincristine Actinomycin D Doxorubicin	Vincristine	Vincristine Actinomycin D	Vincristine
Week 5	*Week 6*		
Vincristine Actinomycin D Doxorubicin	Vincristine		

COMPLICATIONS

The complications associated with Wilms tumor can be manifold. They can be classified as complications related to the tumor, and complications related to the treatment.

The tumor per se, can lead to specific complications. These include formation and extension of tumor thrombosis into the inferior vena cava in approximately 6–8% cases. The thrombus, in rare cases, can extend into the right atrium. Rarely, a large tumor may rupture, and lead to an acute abdomen, requiring an emergency surgery. Relapse of the disease is a well-known complication and may be observed in 15–20% of the cases. The relapse typically occurs within the initial 2 years of diagnosis.

Assessment for therapy related complications require a long-term follow-up in patients with Wilms tumor. One of the most significant long-term complications is development of cardiac toxicity secondary to treatment with anthracyclines, and in children requiring lung irradiation in case of metastases to lung. Other long-term complications may include ototoxicity secondary to platinum use, and development of secondary malignant neoplasm postradiotherapy. Long-term risk of gonadal dysfunction remains in females who received abdominal radiotherapy. Renal failure needs to be assessed for in the long-term, due to presence of a single functioning kidney. This risk increases significantly in children who have syndromic Wilms tumor like Denys-Drash, Frazier, or WAGR syndrome, with an intrinsic risk of renal failure.

Acute complications of treatment include risk of developing cytopenia, like neutropenia, anemia and thrombocytopenia. This may need transfusion support with packed red blood cell and platelets. Patients with neutropenia are at a heightened risk of febrile neutropenia, and would require intravenous antibiotics. Additionally, a rare but life-threatening complication is the development of sinusoidal obstruction syndrome secondary to use of actinomycin D, and rarely cyclophosphamide **(Table 17.24)**.

Table 17.24 Complications Associated with Wilms Tumor

Acute/short-term complications	*Tumor-related complications:* • Tumor thrombus in IVC • Tumor thrombus extending to the right atrium • Hypertension • Tumor rupture • Relapse *Therapy-related complications:* • Cytopenia (anemia, thrombocytopenia) • Febrile neutropenia • Sinusoidal obstruction syndrome • Vincristine neuropathy
Long-term complications	• Development of ESRD (more likely in syndromic WT) • Cardiotoxicity secondary to radiotherapy/ anthracyclines • Vincristine neuropathy • Ototoxicity (platinum compounds) • Ovarian dysfunction (radiotherapy)

(ESRD: end-stage renal disease; IVC: inferior vena cava; WT: Wilms tumor)

OTHER RENAL NEOPLASMS

- ***Clear cell sarcoma of the kidney (CCSK):*** It used to be classified as an aggressive variant of Wilms tumor previously. However, it was realized subsequently that the cell of origin, genetics, behavior, and metastatic potential of CCSK are quite different from Wilms tumor. It is more aggressive than Wilms tumor, but is curable using multimodality therapy including chemotherapy, surgery, and radiotherapy. The staging investigations are the same, as for Wilms tumor and bone scan is usually performed in addition as bone metastasis may be seen.
- ***Rhabdoid tumor of the kidney:*** It is now no longer classified as a subtype of Wilms tumor, but as a separate tumor. It is usually seen in the first year of life. This is a highly aggressive malignancy and is at times associated with atypical teratoid-rhabdoid brain tumor. Prognosis in a metastatic disease is dismal. Even in nonmetastatic disease, the outcome with multimodality therapy is relatively poor.
- ***Renal cell carcinoma:*** It is uncommon in young children, and its incidence increases with age. The primary modality of treatment is surgery, with poor response to chemotherapy.

CASE STUDY Wilms Tumor

A 2-year-old boy was brought to the outpatient department (OPD) by his mother because she felt a mass on the right side of his abdomen while bathing him. He was otherwise well and playful. Examination revealed hypertension (blood pressure >95th centile for age). There was a firm immobile lump in the right lumbar region, palpable bimanually. Other systemic examination was normal. Ultrasound abdomen confirmed the presence of a solid mass replacing the right kidney. A possibility of Wilms tumor was considered and diagnosis was confirmed by a fine needle aspiration of the tumor. A staging computed tomography of the chest and abdomen showed a relatively large right renal tumor, with abdominal lymphadenopathy. The other kidney was normal. Antihypertensive was started (amlodipine) and preoperative treatment with vincristine and actinomycin was initiated, and surgery was done after 4 weeks of chemotherapy. Postoperatively, based on the surgical findings and the histological report, the child was staged as intermediate risk, stage III disease. He required radiotherapy to the abdomen in addition to further chemotherapy in view of lymph node involvement. He is currently off therapy, and well for the last 5 years.

What do we learn from this case study?

1. Most children with Wilms tumor are well looking and otherwise healthy.
2. Blood pressure examination is essential in a child with a renal mass.
3. Ultrasound is the initial investigation to confirm the origin of the mass.
4. Needle aspiration or biopsy are the investigations of choice to establish the diagnosis of Wilms tumor.
5. Metastatic work up (CECT of chest and abdomen) is essential prior to initialing therapy.
6. Evaluation of the other kidney is mandatory.
7. It is preferable to give neoadjuvant chemotherapy to shrink the tumor before surgery.
8. Detailed histological evaluation of the resected specimen helps in accurate staging and further therapy decisions.
9. Wilms tumor usually has an excellent outcome.

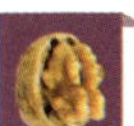

IN A NUTSHELL

Wilms Tumor
1. Wilms tumor is the second most common renal malignancy in children.
2. Wilms tumor classically presents as a unilateral abdominal mass, it is bilateral in 5–7% cases. Other manifestations include hematuria and hypertension.
3. Radical nephrectomy is treatment of choice for unilateral diseases, preceded by chemotherapy. Radiotherapy is required in high-risk cases.
4. Overall survival is 90%.

Armstrong AE, Daw NC, Renfro LA, Geller JI, Kalapurakal JA, Khanna G, et al. Children's Oncology Group AREN0321 and AREN03B2 Study Committees. Treatment of focal anaplastic Wilms tumor: A report from the Children's Oncology Group AREN0321 and AREN03B2 studies. Cancer. 2025;131:e35713.
Dome JS, Graf N, Geller JI, et al. Advances in Wilms tumor treatment and biology: Progress through international collaboration. J Clin Oncol. 2015;33:2999-3007.
Godzinski J, Graf N, Audry G. Current concepts in surgery for Wilms tumor—the risk and function-adapted strategy. Eur J Pediatr Surg. 2014;24:457-60.
Irtan S, Ehrlich PF, Pritchard-Jones K. Wilms tumor: "State-of-the-art" update, 2016. Semin Pediatr Surg. 2016;25:250-6.
Kieran K, Shnorhavorian M. Pediatric Urologic Oncology Series—late effects after treatment for Wilms Tumor and Other Pediatric Renal Neoplasms. Urology. 2025:S0090-4295(24)01226-3.
Kieran K, Davidoff AM. Nephron-sparing surgery for bilateral Wilms tumor. Pediatr Surg Int. 2015;31:229-36.
Pater L, Melchior P, Rübe C, et al. Wilms tumor. Pediatr Blood Cancer. 2021;68(Suppl 2):e28257.
Spreafico F, Fernandez CV, Brok J, et al. Wilms tumour. Nat Rev Dis Primers. 2021;7:75.
User IR, Ekinci S, Kale G, et al. Management of bilateral Wilms tumor over three decades: The perspective of a single center. J Pediatr Urol. 2015;11:118.e1-6.
Weil BR, Murphy AJ, Liu Q, et al. Late health outcomes among survivors of Wilms tumor diagnosed over three decades: A Report From the Childhood Cancer Survivor Study. J Clin Oncol. 2023 Jan 24:JCO2202111.

17.12 Referral and Parent Education for Kidney Disease

Salient points to be kept in mind while referring the child or counseling the parents for kidney disease are summarized in **Table 17.25**.

Table 17.25 Referring the Child or Counseling the Parents for Kidney Disease

Clinical condition	*Guidelines for referral*	*Parental counseling*
1. *Hematuria* • Passage of red colored urine, confirmed by presence of ≥5 red blood cells (RBCs) per high power field in a fresh centrifuged urine sample • Painful or painless, gross, or microscopic, first episode or recurrent gross hematuria • Renal biopsy needed in cases with deranged kidney function test (KFT), nephrotic range proteinuria and presence of systemic features	• Recurrent episodes of gross hematuria • Family history of hematuria, renal stones, or renal failure • Systemic complaints such as fever, rash, arthritis, and hemoptysis • Associated with hypertension, edema, deranged KFT, and nephrotic range proteinuria • Requirement of renal biopsy • Urologist referral in consultation with pediatric nephrologist in cases with renal calculi, structural renal malformation, tumor, hydronephrosis or no obvious cause identified even after extensive evaluation	• Anxiety of the parents should by allayed by explaining that red colored urine is not all blood and as little as 1 mL of blood is sufficient to turn a liter of urine red • Site of bleeding as glomerular or extraglomerular and its implications on immediate as well as long-term outcome should be explained • Children with glomerular hematuria should be followed up in outpatient department (OPD) because of increased risk of progression to chronic kidney disease (CKD) • Parents of children with isolated microscopic hematuria in absence of proteinuria, hypercalciuria, hypertension and normal kidney function should be reassured about the transient nature of this condition and often a good prognosis • However, a long-term follow-up is recommended for early detection of proteinuria, hypertension, which may be suggestive of Alport syndrome or IgA nephropathy that may require further evaluation and treatment

Clinical condition	*Guidelines for referral*	*Parental counseling*
2. *Nephrotic syndrome (NS)* • Presence of edema in association with oliguria, 3+/4+ proteinuria, hypoalbuminemia, and hyperlipidemia	• Children with following conditions should be referred to a pediatric nephrologist • *Steroid resistant nephrotic syndrome (SRNS):* Failure to achieve remission even after 4 weeks of daily prednisolone in adequate dose (2 mg/kg/day) • Frequently relapsing or steroid dependent NS • Features of steroid toxicity; such as cushingoid features, cataract or glaucoma, hypertension, etc., and need to start a steroid sparing agent	• Parents should be taught to maintain a diary for daily urine protein monitoring and to bring the child for consultation if urine dipstick shows 3+/4+ proteinuria for ≥3 days having child been in remission before • Parents should be counseled regarding chronicity of the disease and relapses these children will have, especially during an episode of infection • SRNS children who fail to achieve remission with cyclosporine are at risk of developing CKD and kidney failure
3. *Urinary tract infection (UTI)* • Growth of significant number of organisms (≥10^5 CFU/mL) of a single species in an appropriately collected urine sample in presence of clinical symptoms	• Recurrent UTI (≥2 episodes of febrile UTI during childhood) • Complicated UTI (fever >39°C, systemic toxicity, persistent vomiting, renal angle tenderness, and raised creatinine) • Underlying urological abnormalities on ultrasonography (USG) of kidney, ureter, and bladder (KUB) or vesicoureteric reflux on micturating cystourethrogram (MCU) • Clinical features suggestive of voiding dysfunction; lower urinary tract symptoms (urgency, frequency), holding maneuvers, urinary incontinence	• Child should be encouraged to maintain a good genital and anal hygiene • Parents should ensure a proper voiding habit by the child by asking him/her to empty the bladder completely and not holding the urine for a long time • Avoid constipation • Repeat urine culture is not required to document clearance of infection, if child shows improvement with antibiotic therapy • Recurrent UTI can be associated with underlying urological abnormalities or bladder bowel dysfunction, so these children need to undergo thorough evaluation • As recurrent episodes of febrile UTI may result in renal scarring and CKD, each febrile episode without an obvious focus in children with previous UTI should be evaluated by taking a urine sample for culture before starting antibiotic therapy
4. *Acute glomerulonephritis (AGN)* • Edema, oliguria, gross or microscopic hematuria, hypertension, and acute kidney injury	Child should be referred to a pediatric nephrologist if AGN is associated with rapidly deteriorating kidney function requiring dialysis, nephrotic range proteinuria, persistence of gross hematuria >2 weeks, hypertensive crisis, or presence of any systemic clinical features; such as fever, rash, arthritis, and hemoptysis	• Majority of cases of acute poststreptococcal glomerulonephritis recover completely with excellent long-term outcome • Those with rapidly progressing course requiring dialysis or with systemic clinical features are at increased risk of progression to CKD
5. *Congenital abnormalities of kidney and urinary tract (CAKUT)* • An important cause of chronic kidney disease in children, frequently detected with antenatal USG • Common CAKUT are pelvi-ureteric junction obstruction, posterior urethral valve, renal dysplasia, cystic kidney disease, ectopic kidney, and vesicoureteric reflux	• All antenatally detected hydronephrosis cases should be referred to a pediatric nephrologist/urologist soon after birth for detailed evaluation and follow up • Male child with antenatally detected bilateral hydroureteronephrosis and bladder wall abnormalities may have underlying posterior urethral valve (PUV) and should be referred to a urologist urgently • Children with polycystic kidney disease should be referred to a pediatric nephrologist	• Antenatally detected unilateral hydronephrosis, unilateral multicystic dysplastic kidney disease and unilateral renal agenesis generally have a good long-term outcome as other kidney is functioning normal • Unilateral hydronephrosis of any severity does not warrant early delivery or fetal intervention • One-third of children with PUV may progress to end stage renal disease before 10 years of age
6. *Refractory rickets* • Failure to respond (no radiological healing or biochemical improvement) to adequate doses of vitamin D3 • Causes of refractory rickets are vitamin D dependent rickets type 1 and 2, hypophosphatemic rickets, renal tubular acidosis, and chronic kidney disease	• All cases with refractory rickets should be referred to a pediatric nephrologist for a detailed evaluation and specific therapy • Most of the cases with refractory rickets have marked bony deformity and should be referred to an orthopedic surgeon for corrective osteotomy	• Many of the cases of refractory rickets are hereditary in nature and there are chances of recurrence of disease in future pregnancy • These children require lifelong treatment

Contd...

Contd...

Clinical condition	*Guidelines for referral*	*Parental counseling*
7. *Acute kidney injury (AKI)* • Sudden decrease in kidney function characterized by retention of nitrogenous wastes and acid-base and electrolyte imbalances • AKI is defined as increase in serum creatinine by 50% or more from the baseline and/or decrease in urine output by <0.5 mL/kg/h for 6 hours	• Children with anuria >12 hours or serum creatinine >2–3 times from the baseline, severe hyperkalemia, clinical features of fluid overload, like pulmonary edema or congestive heart failure, uremic encephalopathy and severe metabolic acidosis should be referred to a center with dialysis facility	• Parents should be explained that dialysis will not alter the course of the disease and will only support the kidney function till its recovery • Those requiring dialysis are at increased risk of progression to CKD and becoming dialysis dependent, so these children require long-term follow-up with periodic test for serum creatinine, urine examination, and blood pressure monitoring
8. *Chronic kidney disease (CKD)* • Clinical condition with eGFR of <60 mL/min/1.73 m^2 or eGFR >60 mL/min/1.73 m^2 with structural damage or other markers of kidney dysfunction like persistence of proteinuria for >3 months	• All children with CKD should be referred to a pediatric nephrology unit with kidney replacement therapy (KRT) facility • Children with CKD with eGFR <15 mL/min/1.73 m^2 should be offered the option of kidney transplantation and if the parents are willing should be referred to a center with kidney transplantation facility	• Parents should be offered the options of both dialytic modalities: continuous ambulatory peritoneal dialysis and hemodialysis • Parents should be explained about kidney transplantation as the most effective mode of RRT in children with end-stage renal disease • Dialysis will only work as a bridge therapy till the time of kidney transplantation is performed • Even after kidney transplantation, child will have to take combination of immunosuppressive agents to prevent rejection
9. *Hypertension* Defined as blood pressure more than 95th percentile for age, gender, and height or >130/80 mm Hg in children >13 years of age by an auscultatory method	• A child with hypertensive emergency should be referred urgently to a pediatric nephrologist for appropriate blood pressure management and detailed evaluation to find out the cause of hypertension • A child with hypertensive emergency should be ideally managed in a pediatric intensive care unit • An endocrinologist and a pediatric surgeon referral to be made in presence of an abdominal mass • A cardiologist referral for echocardiography in children with hypertensive emergency or suspected coarctation of aorta	• Parents should be counseled regarding the role of healthy lifestyle measures in the prevention and treatment of hypertension • Children should adopt a healthy lifestyle measure consisting of a healthy diet (low in salt, sugar, and saturated fat and high in fruits, vegetables, poultry, fish, and whole grains), good sleep and moderate to vigorous physical activity at least 3–5 days per week (30–60 minutes per session)
10. *Phimosis* • Common clinical condition in children where foreskin cannot be retracted over the glans penis • "Physiological phimosis" is normal where prepuce is naturally adherent to the glans penis • "Pathological phimosis" results from prepucial scarring due to recurrent balanoposthitis (inflammation of the glans or prepuce)	• Should be referred to a urologist for release of prepucial adhesions if prepuce remains nonretractile by 3 years of age and there is a difficulty or pain during micturition • For circumcision in case of pathological phimosis	• Physiological phimosis is normal in most of the children and do not require any treatment except gentle daily retraction of the prepuce and cleaning with soap and water • Forcible retraction of the prepuce should be avoided
11. *Undescended testis* • A common condition in a male child where testis fails to reach its normal position into the scrotum. It can be unilateral or bilateral • Cryptorchidism or hidden testis is a clinical condition, where testis is not present along its normal path from abdomen to the scrotum	• A child with undescended testis by 3 months of corrected gestational age should be referred to a pediatric surgeon • Bilateral undescended testes with hypospadias or bifid scrotum should be referred to a pediatric surgeon with the suspicion of disorders of sex development • Pain with or without erythema should raise the suspicion of testicular torsion and be referred to a pediatric surgeon urgently • Should be referred to an endocrinologist if associated with ambiguous genitalia with a possibility of congenital adrenal hyperplasia	• Parents should be counseled regarding increased risk of infertility, more with bilateral undescended testes • Children with undescended testis are at risk of developing testicular malignancy, risk is higher if it is in the abdomen than in the groin and when both testes are undescended

Flynn JT, Kaelber DC, Baker-Smith CM, et al. Subcommittee on Screening and Management of High Blood Pressure in Children. Clinical Practice Guideline for Screening and Management of High Blood Pressure in Children and Adolescents. Pediatrics. 2017;140(3):e20171904.

Hari P, Meena J, Kumar M, et al; Indian Society of Pediatric Nephrology. Evidence-based clinical practice guideline for management of urinary tract infection and primary vesicoureteric reflux. Pediatr Nephrol. 2024;39(5):1639-68.

Kallash M, Rheault MN. Approach to persistent microscopic hematuria in children. Kidney360. 2020;1(9):1014-20.

Sinha A, Bagga A, Banerjee S, et al.; Expert Group of Indian Society of Pediatric Nephrology. Steroid Sensitive Nephrotic Syndrome: Revised Guidelines. Indian Pediatr. 2021;58(5):461-81.

Srivastava RN, Bagga A. Pediatric Nephrology, 7th edition. New Delhi: Jaypee Brothers Medical Publishers (P) Ltd; 2024.

Vasudev AS, Ugra D, Mehta K, et al. IAP Specialty Series on Pediatric Nephrology, 3rd edition. New Delhi: Jaypee Brothers Medical Publishers (P) Ltd; 2019.

Vedula R, Iyengar AA. Approach to diagnosis and management of hematuria. Indian J Pediatr. 2020;87(8):618-24.

OP Mishra, Rajniti Prasad [Anatomy and Physiology of Kidney (online content), Edema, HUS, AKI, CKD]; Bobbity Deepthi, Sriram Krishnamurthy (Evaluation of Genitourinary System); Shilpa Sharma, Ankur Bhardwaj (Cystic Kidney Disease) (online content); Kirtisudha Mishra (UTI); R Ganesh (Hematuria); Kanika Kapoor (Glomerulonephritis); Sudarsan Krishnasamy, Sriram Krishnamurthy (Proteinuria); Sriram Krishnamurthy, Sudarsan Krishnasamy (Nephrotic Syndrome); Richa Jain (Wilms Tumor); Anup Mohta (Genitourinary Malformations) (online content); and Manish Kumar (Referral and Parent Education for Kidney Disease)

18 CHAPTER Rheumatological and Immune System Disorders

AS PER NMC COMPETENCIES

PE21.1	Enumerate the common rheumatological problems in children. Discuss the clinical approach to recognition and referral of a child with rheumatological problem.	*Ch 18.1*
PE21.2	Describe the etiopathogenesis, diagnosis and management of Henoch-Schoenlein purpura.	*Ch 18.4, Ch 18.6*
PE21.3	Describe the etiopathogenesis, diagnosis and management of Kawasaki disease.	*Ch 18.4, Ch 18.5*
PE21.4	Describe the etiopathogenesis, diagnosis and management of SLE.	*Ch 18.3*
PE21.5	Describe the etiopathogenesis, diagnosis and management of JIA.	*Ch 18.2*

Topics available online: ***Juvenile Dermatomyositis***

18.1 Evaluation of Rheumatic Diseases *PE 21.1*

INTRODUCTION

Rheumatic diseases are complex multisystemic diseases with potential to affect any part of the body. Juvenile idiopathic arthritis (JIA) has predominant joint manifestations whereas systemic lupus erythematosus (SLE) and vasculitis are multisystemic. Juvenile dermatomyositis (JDM) though multisystemic, has predominant manifestations involving skin and muscles.

JOINT PAIN

Joint pain is the most common symptom of rheumatological diseases, although it can also occur in many nonrheumatological diseases. Pediatric gait, arms, legs and spine (pGALS) examination is a good screening tool for children presenting with musculoskeletal complaints. Videos are available free at *http://www.arthritisresearchuk.org/health-professionals-and-students/video-resources/pgals.aspx*. This should be followed by a detailed examination of joints. All physicians must incorporate this examination in their routine clinical practice.

After taking history and examination, one should be able to answer three questions:

1. Whether the pain is really because of joint problem?
2. Whether there is arthritis?
3. How many joints are involved, for how long, and what are the other symptoms?

The scheme is also depicted in **Flowchart 18.1**.

Flowchart 18.1: Causes of musculoskeletal pain

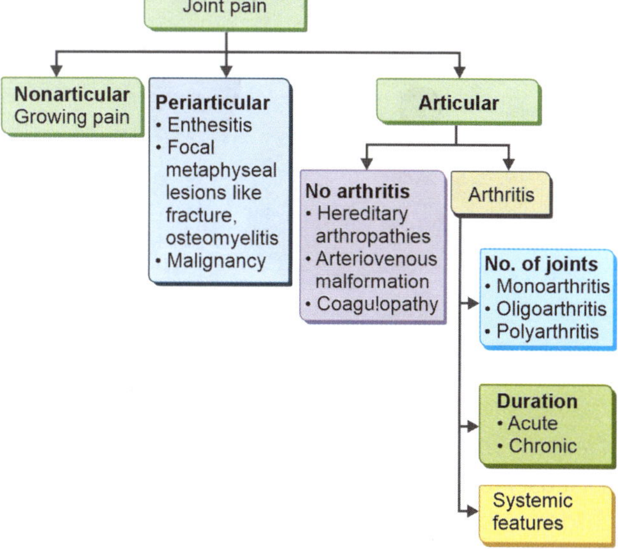

1. Whether the Pain is due to Joint Problem or is it Extra-articular?

In diseases related to joints, pain tends to be across the joint line (line across which joint movement occurs) whereas extra-articular pain is pinpoint and around the joint.

Nonarticular Pains

Typical prototype is "*growing pains*", which is a benign condition seen in children between the ages of 3 and 12 years. The pain is intermittent, usually bilateral and localized to shin, calves, thighs, and popliteal fossa. The child is absolutely well in between the episodes. Such children do not need any investigations. Parents need to be counseled regarding benign nature of the complaints and symptomatic treatment suffices.

Periarticular Pains

Around the joints, one can have pain due to enthesitis, fractures, and osteomyelitis in the metaphyseal region **(Figs. 18.1 and 18.2)**.

- ***Enthesitis*** is defined as inflammation at the insertion of tendons or ligaments to bone. It can present as localized pain or tenderness and/or swelling at these insertion sites.
- ***Focal lesions like fractures or osteomyelitis in metaphyseal region*** can cause pinpoint tenderness and swelling.
- *Hematological conditions:* Malignancies like acute lymphoblastic leukemia can present with only musculoskeletal complaints. Red flag features include night pains, significant disability, pallor, bleeds, bone tenderness, and hepatosplenomegaly **(Box 18.1)**. Less commonly, neuroblastoma can present with diffuse bone pains. Hematological conditions such as sickle cell disease and thalassemia can present with bone pains and arthralgia.

Articular Pain

Articular pain can be due to inflammation of joint (arthritis) or noninflammatory causes. If there is no doubt about articular pain, one should try to answer whether there is arthritis.

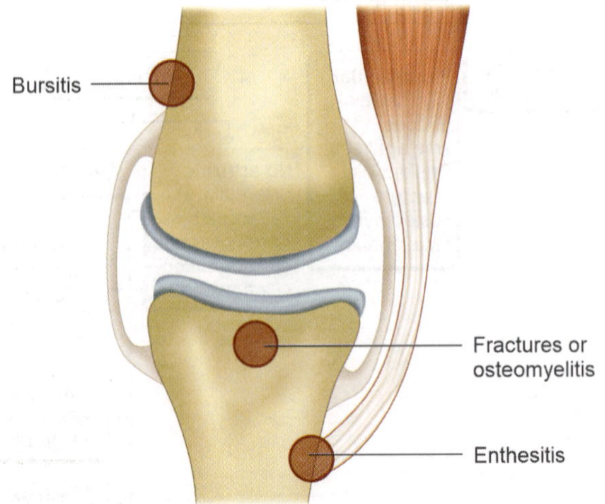

Fig. 18.1: Causes of periarticular pain

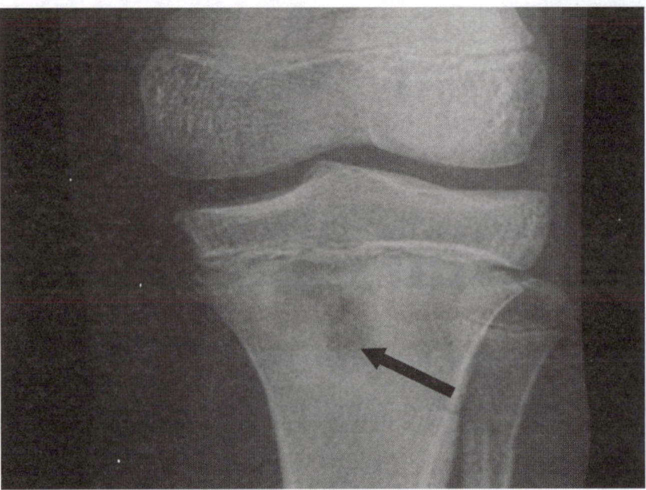

Fig. 18.2: Radiograph showing metaphyseal osteomyelitis in tibia

Box 18.1 Red Flags in a Child with Joint Pain

A. *Clinical:*
1. Not able to walk or bedridden
2. Nocturnal pain
3. Bone tenderness
4. *Systemic features:* Pallor, bleeds, hepatosplenomegaly

B. *Investigations:*
1. Leukopenia or leukocytosis with lymphocytic predominance
2. Thrombocytopenia (leukemia, SLE)
3. Isolated raised lactate dehydrogenase (leukemia)

2. Whether there is Arthritis?

Arthritis is defined as presence of swelling or presence of at least of two of three signs of inflammation namely redness, warmth, and diminished range of motion.

- Redness over the joint is hardly ever seen in inflammatory arthritis except septic arthritis.
- Early morning stiffness and gelling indicate inflammatory cause of joint pain. Early morning stiffness refers to pain and difficulty in moving the joint for ≥30 minutes after getting up from sleep. Gelling is similar to this, but tends to happen after prolonged rest during day.
  Absence of these signs indicates noninflammatory conditions, e.g., Perthes disease (avascular necrosis of femoral head). Here pain is worse in evenings unlike in arthritis where pain is worse after a prolonged period of rest.
- Pain worsening during sleep points to an alternative diagnosis like malignancy.

If there is no doubt about arthritis, one should look for number of joints involved, duration of arthritis, and associated systemic features.

3. Number of Joints Involved, Duration of Arthritis, and Associated Systemic Features

Number of Joints Involved

Single joint arthritis is called *monoarthritis* whereas involvement of more than four joints with arthritis is called *polyarthritis*.

Involvement of less than five joints is called oligoarthritis. Certain etiologies (septic arthritis, tubercular arthritis) involve only single joints.

Acute versus Chronic Arthritis

Arthritis of <6 weeks duration is called *acute arthritis* whereas arthritis persisting beyond 6 weeks is called *chronic arthritis*.

Acute arthritis: Acute arthritis can occur due to multiple etiologies. Short history with single joint involvement suggests a possibility of "septic arthritis". Septic arthritis should be considered as a differential for any sick looking febrile and toxic child with acute monoarthritis. Typically, large joints are involved. The involved joint is extremely tender, warm, and swollen.

In contrast, multiple joints are involved in rheumatic fever and rheumatological conditions. Arthritis in rheumatic fever involves large joints and is typically migratory. A brisk response to nonsteroidal anti-inflammatory drugs (NSAIDs) is diagnostic. Arthritis can also be seen in association with many rheumatological diseases such as SLE, juvenile dermatomyositis (JDM), and vasculitis.

Chronic arthritis: Chronic arthritis can occur due to infectious as well as rheumatological conditions. Tuberculosis can present with chronic monoarthritis involving large joints. Chronic rheumatological conditions such as SLE and vasculitis can present with arthritis, but usually these patients have multisystemic involvement. JIA is the most common idiopathic cause of chronic arthritis in children, but it is important to remember that it is a diagnosis of exclusion.

Systemic Features

All children with arthritis should be examined for systemic features. Following clinical features may give a clue to underlying etiology:

- Presence of extra-articular features except uveitis and systemic features of systemic juvenile idiopathic arthritis (sJIA) goes against a diagnosis of JIA.
- Malar rash **(Fig. 18.3)** and oral ulcers point to SLE.

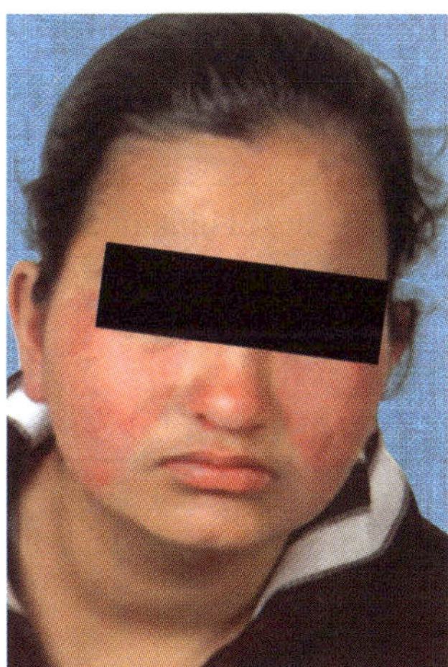

Fig. 18.3: Malar rash

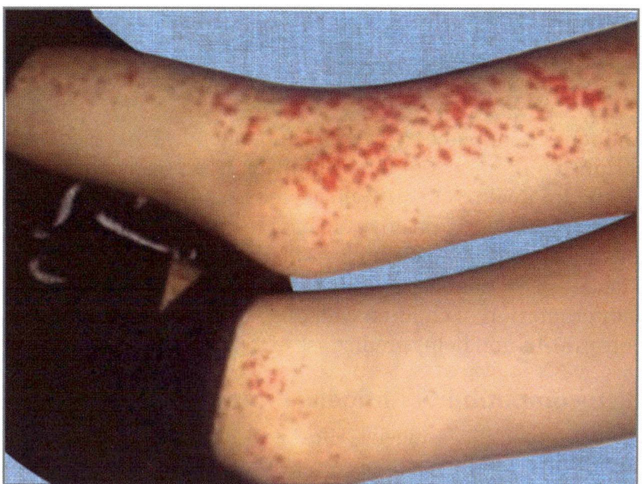

Fig. 18.4: Raised purpuric rash over lower limbs in Henoch-Schönlein purpura

- High grade quotidian fever with rash appearing at the peak of fever, lymphadenopathy, and hepatosplenomegaly point to sJIA.
- Palpable purpuric rash **(Fig. 18.4)** along with joint pain points toward Henoch-Schönlein purpura (HSP).
- ***Skin rash*** may be associated with (sJIA), collagen vascular disease, vasculitis, and psoriasis.
- ***Gastrointestinal features*** (diarrhea, constipation, pain abdomen, hepatitis, and pancreatitis) are seen in inflammatory bowel diseases, collagen vascular disease, systemic vasculitis, and reactive arthritis.
- ***Ocular involvement*** (uveitis) is typical of oligoarthritis and enthesitis related arthritis (ERA).
- ***Hypertension*** can be seen in SLE and vasculitis.
- ***Muscular involvement*** with arthritis suggests a possibility of JDM.
- ***Cardiac involvement*** can occur in rheumatic fever and SLE.
- ***Pulmonary involvement*** as pleuritis is observed in SLE and systemic vasculitis.
- ***Renal involvement*** presenting with hematuria and proteinuria is characteristic of SLE and vasculitis.

LABORATORY INVESTIGATIONS

Acute Phase Reactants

Acute phase reactants are increased as a response of the body to the inflammation. These include ESR, C-reactive protein (CRP), and fibrinogen. These are nonspecific markers and are not diagnostic of rheumatological conditions.

The CRP is a reliable marker of inflammation as it rises within 24 hours of inflammation and falls rapidly on resolution of inflammation.

Rheumatoid Factor

Rheumatoid factor (RF) is not diagnostic of JIA as only 5–10% of children with JIA are positive for RF. It is used to classify polyarthritis. It is nonspecific and can be positive in many infections and rheumatological conditions.

Antinuclear Antibodies

Antinuclear antibodies (ANA) are autoantibodies that react with various components of the cell nuclei. It is positive in nearly all children with SLE, but can also be seen in 2–5% of healthy children. If ANA is positive, special tests need to be done to look for specific autoantibodies such as antibodies to double-stranded deoxyribonucleic acid (DNA). ANA is positive in a significant proportion of children with oligoarthritis and RF negative polyarthritis and helps predict risk of uveitis in these children.

Histocompatibility Antigens Typing

Histocompatibility antigens (HLA) are controlled by genes that are localized to the sixth chromosome. HLA-B27 is used as a diagnostic criterion for ERA and exclusion criteria for systemic onset and polyarticular JIA.

Anticardiolipin Antibodies

These antibodies are directed against phospholipids and are associated with increased risk of arterial and venous thrombosis. These antibodies can be documented in SLE.

Markers of Complement Activation

The complement system is a group of proteins that react sequentially to mediate inflammation. In children with SLE, one may find low levels of C3 and C4 indicating consumption of complement. Total serum hemolytic complement (CH50) level is low in children with active lupus nephritis.

Synovial Fluid Examination

A normal joint contains small amount of synovial fluid (<2 mL in knee joint), that is transparent, viscous, and shows good mucin clot. It contains <200 cells/mm^3, majority being lymphocytes.

- In *septic arthritis*, synovial fluid is turbid and has poor mucin clot formation; cell count is >100,000/mm^3 with >80% neutrophils.
- *Hemorrhagic synovial fluid* is typical of a child with hemarthrosis.
- It plays no role in identifying specific etiology in a child with inflammatory arthritis.

Tissue Biopsy

Biopsy of the involved tissue such as skin, muscle, and kidney can provide valuable information. Skin biopsy is advised for HSP only when some atypical features are present. Muscle biopsy is recommended in patients with suspected JDM when the clinical diagnosis is uncertain. On the other hand, renal biopsy is a must for a child with lupus nephritis for its diagnostic and prognostic value.

Others

The biochemical tests tell us about the involvement of various organ systems. Raised antistreptolysin O (ASO) titer may help to reach a diagnosis of acute rheumatic fever. Bone marrow examination may be necessary to rule out a neoplastic process. Cardiac evaluation is needed to exclude carditis in rheumatic fever.

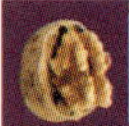

IN A NUTSHELL

Evaluation of Rheumatic Diseases

1. Rheumatological diseases are often multisystemic with a potential to involve any organ-system.
2. Musculoskeletal pain is one symptom which is seen more frequently in rheumatological diseases.
3. All physicians should include pGALS as a screening tool for evaluation of children with musculoskeletal complaints.

Berard R. Approach to the child with joint inflammation. Pediatr Clin North Am. 2012;59(2):245-62.
Sen ES, Clarke SL, Ramanan AV. The child with joint pain in primary care. Best Pract Res Clin Rheumatol. 2014;28(6):888-906.

18.2 Juvenile Idiopathic Arthritis (JIA)

PE 21.5

INTRODUCTION

Juvenile idiopathic arthritis (JIA) is the most common autoimmune disease in children. It is the most common cause of chronic arthritis in children. It has a prevalence rate of 1 in 1,000 children under the age of 16 years.

DEFINITION

For the diagnosis of JIA, it is important that the child has all of the following three criteria:

1. Arthritis persisting for longer than 6 weeks (chronic arthritis).
2. Arthritis beginning before 16 years of age (juvenile onset).
3. Exclusion of other conditions associated with or mimicking arthritis.

PATHOGENESIS

Synovium is the primary site of inflammation. Inflamed synovium becomes thick and hyperemic and protrudes into joint space. It causes destruction of underlying articular cartilage and bones by proteolytic enzymes.

CLINICAL FEATURES

Main clinical feature of JIA is persistent joint swelling in the absence of any defined cause, which begins before the age of 16 years. Other features of inflammation in joint may be:

- ***Pain*** is common but not consistent. It is frequently absent in preschool children who cannot describe their symptoms. In such children, parents may notice limp if lower limb joints are involved.

- ***Stiffness:*** Early morning stiffness is a variable feature. Stiffness improves with movement and is helped by a warm bath or shower.
- ***Redness over joint:*** This is an unusual feature of JIA and is hardly ever seen.
- ***Diminished range of movements***.
- ***Systemic features*** may also be seen in a subset of JIA. High-grade fever, transient skin rash, hepatosplenomegaly, and lymphadenopathy are seen in patients with systemic arthritis.
- Uveitis is frequently seen in patients with oligoarthritis.

CLINICAL PATTERNS OF JUVENILE IDIOPATHIC ARTHRITIS

The JIA is not a single disease, rather a group of heterogenous diseases. It has been classified into following categories by International League of Associations for Rheumatology (ILAR). Definition and differentiating features are summarized in **Tables 18.1** and **18.2**.

1. ***Polyarthritis*** (>4 joints in first 6 months of disease), ***rheumatoid factor positive***
2. ***Polyarthritis, rheumatoid factor negative***
3. ***Oligoarthritis***
   - Persistent (<5 joints in the first 6 months of disease and throughout the disease course)
   - Extended (onset is oligoarticular but >4 joints affected after the first 6 months of disease)
4. ***Systemic arthritis***
5. ***Psoriatic arthritis***
6. ***Enthesitis-related arthritis***
7. ***Unclassified arthritis***

TYPES OF JUVENILE IDIOPATHIC ARTHRITIS

Systemic Arthritis

Systemic arthritis (sJIA) begins in early childhood with prominent extra-articular features. High-grade quotidian (daily) fever is a prominent clinical feature. Typically, child is well in between two spikes of fever. Rash is erythematous, evanescent, maculopapular, and obvious only at the height of the fever. It is usually confined to the axillary region, anterior chest wall, and inside both thighs. There may be generalized lymphadenopathy and hepatosplenomegaly.

The systemic features may resolve after a few months but may also last indefinitely. The pattern of arthritis is variable, ranging

Table 18.1 International League of Associations for Rheumatology Classification Criteria for Juvenile Idiopathic Arthritis

ILAR category	*Definition*	*Exclusion criteria*
Systemic arthritis	Arthritis with or preceded by daily fever of at least 2 weeks that is documented to be daily ("quotidian") for at least 3 days and one or more of the following: • Evanescent (nonfixed) erythematous rash • Hepatomegaly and/or splenomegaly • Generalized lymphadenopathy • Serositis	a, b, c, d
Oligoarthritis	Arthritis affecting 1–4 joints during the first 6 months of disease Subcategories • *Persistent oligoarthritis:* Affecting <5 joints throughout the disease course • *Extended oligoarthritis:* Affecting a total of >4 joints after the first 6 months of disease	a, b, c, d, e
Polyarthritis (RF negative)	Arthritis affecting 5 or more joints during the first 6 months of disease (RF negative)	a, b, c, d, e
Polyarthritis (RF positive)	Arthritis affecting 5 or more joints during the first 6 months of disease (RF positive)	a, b, c, e
Psoriatic arthritis	Arthritis and psoriasis or arthritis and at least 2 of these: Dactylitis, nail pitting or onycholysis, psoriasis in a first-degree relative	b, c, d, e
Enthesitis-related arthritis (ERA)	Arthritis and enthesitis or Arthritis or enthesitis with at least 2 of the following: • Presence of or a history of sacroiliac joint tenderness and/or inflammatory lumbosacral pain • HLA-B27 antigen + • Onset of arthritis in a male over 6 years of age • Acute (symptomatic) anterior uveitis • History of ankylosing spondylitis, ERA, sacroiliitis with inflammatory bowel disease, Reiter syndrome, or acute anterior uveitis in a first-degree relative	a, d, e
Undifferentiated arthritis	Criteria in no category or >1 aforementioned categories	

Exclusion criteria:

a. Psoriasis or a history of psoriasis in the patient or first-degree relative.
b. Arthritis in an HLA-B27 positive male beginning after the 6th birthday.
c. Ankylosing spondylitis, enthesitis-related arthritis, sacroiliitis with inflammatory bowel disease, Reiter syndrome, or acute anterior uveitis, or a history of one of these disorders in a first-degree relative.
d. Presence of IgM rheumatoid factor on at least 2 occasions at least 3 months apart.
e. Presence of systemic JIA.

Table 18.2 Juvenile Idiopathic Arthritis: Classification and Subtypes

	Oligoarthritis	*Polyarthritis*		*Systemic JIA*
		Rheumatoid factor negative	*Rheumatoid factor positive*	
Proportion of all	50–60%	30%	<10%	<10%
Joints involved (no.)	<5	≥5	≥5	Variable
Joints involved	Knees, and ankles	Asymmetric/symmetric large/small joints, and cervical spine	Symmetrical small and large joints	Knees, wrists, cervical spine, ankles, finger, neck, and hips
Age at onset	1–5 years	2–5 years	Teenagers	Any age (most common <5 years)
Female/male ratio	4:1	3:1	9:1	1:1
Rheumatoid factor	Negative	Negative	Positive	Negative
Extra-articular features	Chronic uveitis	Chronic uveitis		Daily high fever, transient nonitchy erythematous rash, lymphadenopathy, hepato-splenomegaly, and serositis
ANA	Positive in 80% of oligoarthritis with uveitis	Positive in 40%	May be positive	Negative
Prognosis	Resolves spontaneously; uveitis must be managed early	Generally good prognosis	Poor prognosis with severe disability	Chronic erosive arthritis in 25%. Most have self-limiting disease
Treatment	NSAID and intra-articular steroids	NSAID and methotrexate	NSAID, and methotrexate	*Biologicals:* Anakinra, tocilizumab, methotrexate for predominant arthritic manifestations

from a few swollen joints to a widespread polyarthritis. Course may be monophasic, polycyclic, or chronic persistent. Those with chronic persistent course have a bad prognosis with severe growth delay, deforming arthritis, and complications of chronic corticosteroid use. Macrophage activation syndrome (MAS) and amyloidosis are most common complications seen in this subtype.

Oligoarthritis

Persistent oligoarthritis: This subtype of JIA affects preschool girls. Knee is the most frequently affected joint, followed by ankle and wrist. These children are at risk of chronic anterior uveitis, which is usually clinically silent and insidiously progressive and may result in visual loss and blindness if not detected and treated early. Hence, these children should be examined periodically for uveitis. ANA is frequently positive and predicts ocular involvement.

Extended oligoarthritis: One-third of children with oligoarthritis (having <5 joint involvement in first 6 months) develop arthritis in more joints thereafter, hence this subgroup is called extended oligoarthritis. Many of these children also develop anterior uveitis. Prognosis in this subtype is similar to RF negative polyarthritis.

Polyarticular Juvenile Idiopathic Arthritis

Polyarthritis (rheumatoid factor negative): This subtype affects preschool girls who develop symmetrical arthritis of upper and lower limbs. Both large and small joints are involved. Risk of chronic anterior uveitis is less than oligoarthritis. ANA may be positive and RF is always negative.

Polyarthritis (rheumatoid factor positive): This subtype is seen in older girls and behaves like rheumatoid arthritis in adults. Arthritis involves both large and small joints and can be rapidly progressive and destructive. RF is always positive.

Others

Psoriatic arthritis: Arthritis may predate the onset of the classic skin findings of psoriasis by many years. The articular involvement is often asymmetrical, and tends to affect both small and large joints. Extra-articular features of psoriasis can be present in first degree relatives. Asymptomatic uveitis can occur.

Enthesitis-related arthritis: ERA begins after the age of 6 years and affects boys more often. Enthesitis which is described as inflammation of the site where a tendon, ligament, or fascia inserts into the bone is one of the typical clinical features. Arthritis involves large joints of lower limb and is often asymmetrical. It may be a precursor illness to ankylosing spondylitis. These children are predisposed to acute recurrent symptomatic uveitis. HLA-B27 antigen is positive in 80% of patients.

INVESTIGATIONS

Diagnosis of JIA is clinical and no single laboratory test helps in diagnosis. Investigations in children with arthritis help in ruling out important differential diagnosis and in classifying JIA.

- ESR and CRP, if raised, are useful but up to a third of JIA patients, especially those with oligoarthritis, have normal CRP and ESR.
- Rheumatoid factor helps to classify polyarthritis.

- Antinuclear antibody helps in determining the risk of chronic anterior uveitis.
- HLA-B27 may be positive in 80% of children with ERA.
- Coagulation studies are useful if there is a suspicion of hemarthrosis.
- Joint radiographs are hardly ever required in a typical case of JIA. However, they do help to rule out differentials such as fracture, avascular necrosis, osteomyelitis, bone tumor, and skeletal dysplasia.
- Synovial fluid aspiration is usually not required, however, it is a must for any child with suspected septic arthritis.
- Synovial biopsy is not indicated for diagnosis.

COMPLICATIONS OF JUVENILE IDIOPATHIC ARTHRITIS

Complications can be classified as articular or extra-articular.

Articular complications: These arise due to prolonged joint inflammation. Contractures, muscle atrophy, and ankylosis can be seen. Asymmetric growth and limb length discrepancy are common in growing children with arthritis. These complications can be reduced with early and aggressive therapy.

Extra-articular complications: Systemic involvement is not seen in children with JIA except sJIA. The only extra-articular features seen in JIA include uveitis, MAS, and amyloidosis. Whereas, MAS and amyloidosis are seen in sJIA, uveitis is most common in oligoarthritis.

- ***Macrophage activation syndrome:*** This is a hyperinflammatory condition seen in children with active sJIA. It is characterized by sudden development of fever, diffuse intravascular coagulation (DIC), hepatosplenomegaly, pancytopenia, abrupt decrease in the ESR (because of low fibrinogen), very high ferritin, and elevated serum levels of liver enzymes and triglycerides. Coagulogram shows fibrin degradation products and hypofibrinogenemia due to consumptive coagulopathy. Bone marrow examination may show active hemophagocytosis by macrophages and histiocytes. MAS must be treated rapidly since it is associated with high mortality. The conventional approach is to administer intravenous methylprednisolone pulse therapy with or without cyclosporine.
- ***Amyloidosis:*** It is seen with uncontrolled systemic arthritis or polyarthritis of many years' duration and is attributed to chronic persistent inflammation.
- ***Chronic anterior uveitis:*** Seen predominantly in oligoarthritis, it is often clinically silent and insidiously progressive. ANA positivity helps in predicting the risk of uveitis. Routine follow-up for eye disease is a must in all children with JIA.

PROGNOSIS

JIA is a diverse group of conditions associated with persistent arthritis. Whereas, children with oligoarthritis tend to do well in terms of arthritis, children with polyarthritis and systemic arthritis may continue to have disease into adulthood.

TREATMENT Juvenile Idiopathic Arthritis

The goal of therapy is to maintain a good quality of life while preserving joint function. Early and aggressive management helps in achieving this goal. Overall management can be divided into two components:

1. *Drug therapy:* NSAID, glucocorticoids, disease-modifying antirheumatic drugs (DMARDs) such as Methotrexate, biologic response modifiers, and miscellaneous drugs such as leflunomide, sulfasalazine, and thalidomide.
2. *Supportive management:* Counseling and education about disease, physiotherapy, and occupational therapy.

Pharmacotherapy

Nonsteroidal Anti-inflammatory Drugs

The NSAIDs, such as naproxen (15–20 mg/kg per day in two divided doses) or ibuprofen are used as adjuncts for symptom control in patients with JIA. Peak anti-inflammatory effect is achieved after 4–8 weeks, hence they must be continued for 4–8 weeks before their efficacy can be ascertained. Adverse effects include abdominal pain, which can be minimized by taking NSAID with food. Mild asthma is not a contraindication to the use of NSAIDs. NSAIDs do not modify the disease course and should not be used as the only therapy in children with JIA.

Glucocorticoids

Intra-articular steroid is most frequently used form of glucocorticoids in JIA. A single injection resolves signs of joint inflammation in most patients for several months. Systemic steroids should be avoided if possible, because of adverse effects. The use of oral prednisolone is limited to short-term and at low doses for children with severe polyarthritis or systemic arthritis (as a bridge therapy to overcome acute severe symptoms).

Methotrexate

Methotrexate is effective in approximately 70–80% of children with polyarthritis. It should be considered early on in all children with polyarthritis and oligoarthritis (with uveitis). It can be administered either orally or subcutaneously once a week at a dose of 10–20 mg/m^2. Effect is seen after 1–3 months. The most common adverse events are nausea, mouth ulcers, abdominal pain, elevated liver enzymes, hair loss, and bone marrow suppression. Oral folic acid supplementation (1 mg/day) helps to reduce side-effects. Methotrexate is not effective in controlling systemic features of sJIA.

Biologic Response Modifiers

Tumor necrosis factor (TNF) inhibitors: TNF inhibitors are more effective if administered early in the disease course. Commonly used drugs are etanercept and adalimumab, a recombinant human anti-TNF agent.

Anti-TNF agents have been associated with an increased risk of tuberculosis infection. Hence, baseline screening and careful monitoring during the course of treatment are mandatory.

Tocilizumab: This is an interleukin-6 (IL-6) receptor inhibitor, and is used both in systemic arthritis and polyarthritis.

Anakinra: This is an IL-1 receptor antagonist and has been used in systemic arthritis.

Supportive Therapy

Parents should be educated about the disease and its likely course. This helps in ensuring compliance. Need for periodic eye evaluation should be emphasized. Physiotherapy and occupational therapy help in maintaining range of movement across joint along with improving strength of periarticular muscles. An exercise program is advised to restore motion and strength of the joint. Proper nutrition, along with iron and vitamin supplements should be advised.

Surgery: Need for surgery to correct contractures and limb length discrepancies has markedly reduced with advent of aggressive disease modifying agents. In children who are treated early and aggressively, one may not see any articular complications.

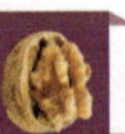

IN A NUTSHELL

Juvenile Idiopathic Arthritis (JIA)

1. Diagnosis of JIA is clinical. It is based on presence of persistent swelling of one or more joints (for >6 weeks), beginning before the age of 16 years, and without any systemic cause.
2. Differential diagnosis includes septic arthritis, neoplasia such as acute lymphoblastic leukemia, rheumatic fever, and nonaccidental injury.
3. No single laboratory test is diagnostic of JIA. Role of investigations lies in excluding differential diagnoses, to classify JIA and to monitor the disease.
4. Drug treatment for JIA begins with NSAIDs and intra-articular corticosteroids, with early use of methotrexate.
5. Biologic disease modifiers have revolutionized management of children with JIA.
6. Physiotherapy and occupational therapy are important supportive therapies to prevent complications.

Martini A, Lovell DJ, Albani S, et al. Juvenile idiopathic arthritis. Nat Rev Dis Primers. 2022;8(1):5.
Sen ES, Ramanan AV. Juvenile idiopathic arthritis-associated uveitis. Clin Immunol. 2020;211:108322.
Zaripova LN, Midgley A, Christmas SE, et al. Juvenile idiopathic arthritis: from aetiopathogenesis to therapeutic approaches. Pediatr Rheumatol Online J. 2021;19(1):135.

18.3 Systemic Lupus Erythematosus

PE 21.4

INTRODUCTION

Systemic lupus erythematosus is a multisystem autoimmune disease. It is described as a disease of young girls and is mostly seen after the age of 8 years.

ETIOLOGY

It is an autoimmune disorder occurring in a genetically predisposed host, and is triggered by certain factors such as drugs, infection, or ultraviolet rays. Childhood SLE has more severe course and poorer prognosis than the adult disease.

CLINICAL FEATURES

The SLE can involve any organ system of the body. Commonly, it presents with fever, fatigue, weight loss, and anorexia. Multisystem involvement is more common, though a single system may be affected at the onset. Skin, musculoskeletal, and renal systems are more commonly involved in childhood SLE. Gastrointestinal disease, liver involvement, and myocarditis are extremely rare.

Mucocutaneous Involvement

- Malar or butterfly rash **(Fig. 18.3)** is the most characteristic cutaneous manifestation. It is typically seen over malar eminences crossing the nasal bridge but spares the nasolabial folds.
- Less common manifestations are discoid lupus lesions (erythematous coin-shaped lesions with central hypopigmentation and peripheral hyperpigmentation and seen on face, ears, and scalp) and vasculitic rashes on digits, pinnae, or nares.
- Oral cavity may show painless ulceration over hard palate **(Fig. 18.5)**.

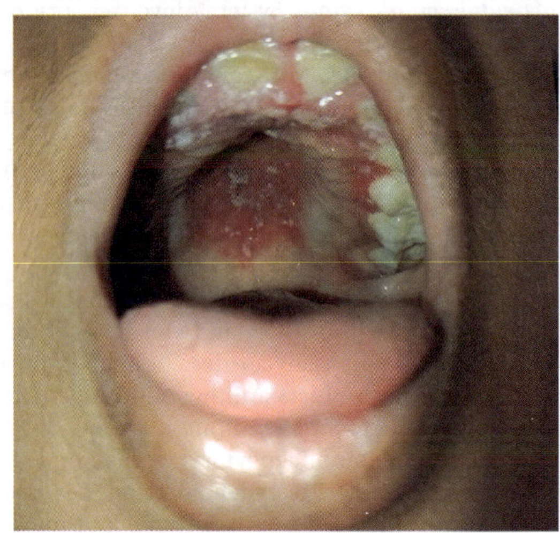

Fig. 18.5: Ulcer over hard palate in a child with systemic lupus erythematosus

- Alopecia may be one of the presenting manifestations of the disease. It occurs classically in the frontal area.
- Photosensitivity is an important feature.

Musculoskeletal Involvement

Arthralgia and arthritis are very common. Arthritis is nonerosive unlike the arthritis of JIA.

Renal Involvement

Renal disease is the most dreaded complication of SLE. Lupus nephritis is present in almost 75% children with SLE. It manifests as proteinuria, microscopic hematuria, hypertension, and elevated blood urea and serum creatinine. Routine urine microscopy, spot urine for protein and creatinine ratio and renal function tests are must for any child at diagnosis and periodically during follow-up. Low complement levels (C3, C4) and elevated anti-double stranded DNA (anti-dsDNA) levels are usual in children with lupus nephritis.

Neuropsychiatric Involvement

Neuropsychiatric involvement occurs in 20–70% of children with SLE and can involve any part of central or peripheral nervous system. Common manifestations include headache, seizures, altered sensorium, psychosis, stroke, and transverse myelitis. Other manifestations include polyneuropathy, myelopathy, cerebellar ataxia, aseptic meningitis, and cranial nerve palsies.

Hematologic Involvement

Anemia, thrombocytopenia, and leukopenia are seen in 50–75% of patients. Anemia can occur due to chronic disease or autoimmune hemolysis. Coombs test may be positive. Thrombocytopenia may be the first presentation of disease presenting as spontaneous mucocutaneus bleeding or menorrhagia. Leukopenia is seen in 20–40% of cases of childhood SLE. Lymphopenia is a sensitive marker of disease activity.

Pulmonary Involvement

Pulmonary involvement can present as pleuritis, pneumonitis, pulmonary hemorrhage, pulmonary hypertension, and pulmonary embolism.

Cardiac Involvement

Symptomatic pericarditis with pericardial effusion is the most common cardiac manifestation. Myocardial and endocardial involvement is less common.

Neonatal Lupus Erythematosus

This syndrome occurs in infants born to mothers with anti-Sjögren's-syndrome-related antigen A (anti-Ro/SSA) and anti-Sjögren's-syndrome-related antigen B (anti-La/SSB) antibodies. Passive transfer of these antibodies to the baby causes neonatal lupus. Mother may have SLE or another connective tissue disorder or may also be asymptomatic. Neonates have photosensitive skin rash and/or congenital heart block. Skin manifestations subside by 6 months of age (because of disappearance of maternally transmitted antibodies), however, congenital heart block is permanent.

INVESTIGATIONS

Role of investigations in SLE lies in confirming the diagnosis, ruling out differential diagnosis, and assessing severity of organ involvement and associated comorbidities. For confirmation of diagnosis, following investigations are required:

- ***Antinuclear antibody*** is positive in >95% patients with SLE. This test should be ordered in an appropriate setting since it can be positive in about 5% of healthy children. If ANA is negative in an appropriate setting, it helps to rule out SLE.
- ***Extractable nuclear antigen panel*** detects autoantibodies to subcellular structures and should be done only if ANA is positive in high titers. Anti-Smith and anti-dsDNA antibodies are highly specific for SLE. Antibodies to dsDNA are present in 70% patients with SLE and indicate active disease and increased risk of nephritis.
- ***Complement (C3 and C4) levels*** are usually reduced in presence of active lupus nephritis.
- ***Antiphospholipid antibodies*** are associated with increased risk of thrombosis in children with SLE.

For assessing organ dysfunction, complete blood count, renal and liver function tests, and urine analysis are required. Direct Coombs test may be needed in children with anemia. Other tests such as renal biopsy and neuroimaging are done as dictated by clinical presentation.

TREATMENT Systemic Lupus Erythematosus

Treatment of SLE is aimed at achieving good control of disease while minimizing side-effects of medications and facilitating growth and development. It is generally decided based on presence or absence of life or organ-threatening complications.

Children with no Significant Life or Organ-threatening Complications

Oral corticosteroids are started at a low dose and then gradually tapered. Hydroxychloroquine (HCQ) is used as adjunct in all patients with SLE. This drug is particularly useful in skin and joint disease and is used at a dose of 5 mg/kg/day. Eye screening is done at baseline and then annually to detect ocular complications associated with HCQ. Low-dose Methotrexate can be added for better control of joint and skin symptoms. Sun protection measures are must for every patient with SLE.

For Patients with Life or Organ-threatening Complications

Aggressive treatment is used to bring disease under control and then to maintain it in that condition. The regimens include combinations of high-dose steroids, steroid sparing agents, and supportive strategies.

- *Induction of remission:* Initial phase is geared to bring disease under control as early as possible and uses aggressive immunosuppression with high-dose steroids such as pulse intravenous methylprednisolone at 30 mg/kg (maximum of 1 g) for 3 consecutive days, in combination with cyclophosphamide or mycophenolate mofetil (MMF). Pulse methylprednisolone is followed by oral steroids. Whereas, cyclophosphamide is used intravenously at 2–4 weekly interval, MMF is used as daily oral therapy.
- *Maintenance of induction:* Lesser degree of immunosuppression is used over longer duration to maintain the induction. Both MMF and azathioprine are used. Azathioprine is started at a low dose and increased slowly to reach a maximum of 2.5 mg/kg/day. Side-effects include nausea, fatigue, alopecia, liver dysfunction, and cytopenias. Oral HCQ and low-dose oral steroids are continued during the maintenance phase.

Table 18.3 2019 EULAR/ACR Classification Criteria for Systemic Lupus Erythematosus

Entry criterion: Antinuclear antibodies at a titer of ≥1:80 on HEp-2 cells or an equivalent positive test (ever)
Additive criteria: As below

Clinical domains and criteria	*Weight*	*Immunological domains and criteria*	*Weight*
Constitutional • Fever	 2	*Antiphospholipid antibodies* • Anticardiolipin antibodies OR • Anti-β2GP1 antibodies OR • Lupus anticoagulant	 2
Hematologic • Leukopenia • Thrombocytopenia • Autoimmune hemolysis	 3 4 4	*Complement proteins* • Low C3 or low C4 • Low C3 and low C4	 3 4
Neuropsychiatric • Delirium • Psychosis • Seizure	 2 3 5	*SLE-specific antibodies* • Anti-dsDNA antibody or • Anti-Smith antibody	 6
Mucocutaneous • Nonscarring alopecia • Oral ulcers • Subacute cutaneous or discoid lupus • Acute cutaneous lupus	 2 2 4 6		
Serosal • Pleural or pericardial effusion • Acute pericarditis	 5 6		
Musculoskeletal • Joint involvement	 6		
Renal • Proteinuria >0.5 g/24 hours • Renal biopsy Class II or V lupus nephritis • Renal biopsy Class III or IV lupus nephritis	 4 8 10		

Total score: Classify as SLE with a score of 10 or more if entry criterion fulfilled.

Note:
- Do not count a criterion if there is a more likely explanation than SLE
- Occurrence of a criterion on at least one occasion is sufficient
- Within each domain, only the highest weighted criterion is counted toward the total score

Source: Aringer M, Costenbader K, Daikh D, et al. 2019 European League Against Rheumatism/American College of Rheumatology classification criteria for systemic lupus erythematosus. Arthritis Rheumatol. 2019;71(9):1400-12.

DIAGNOSIS

The 2019 European League Against Rheumatism (EULAR)/American College of Rheumatology (ACR) classification criteria for SLE are depicted in **Table 18.3**.

PROGNOSIS

The SLE is a disease associated with remissions and flares. Hence, all patients need periodic follow-ups to identify flares and other complications like infections. All patients and parents need to be educated for strict compliance to therapy. Renal, cardiac, and hematological manifestations are the main causes of death. Five-years survival rate in India is 75%.

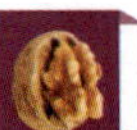

IN A NUTSHELL

Systemic Lupus Erythematosus

1. SLE is a multisystemic autoimmune disease of childhood and can involve any part of the body.
2. Mucocutaneus, renal, and musculoskeletal involvement are frequent in childhood SLE.
3. Diagnosis is based on presence of ANA positivity along with clinical and immunologic criteria.
4. Negative ANA helps in excluding disease. False positive ANA is seen in 5–10% of general population; hence ANA should only be prescribed in an appropriate setting.
5. Management is based on severity of clinical manifestations. Minor organ involvement (mucocutaneous and musculoskeletal) needs low dose steroids and HCQ besides supportive therapy like sun protection measures. Major organ involvement in SLE requires aggressive immunosuppression to save organ and life.
6. The SLE is a disease associated with remissions and flares and a life-long follow-up is mandatory.

Aggarwal A, Srivastava P. Childhood onset systemic lupus erythematosus: how is it different from adult SLE? Int J Rheum Dis. 2015;18(2):182-91.

Trindade VC, Carneiro-Sampaio M, Bonfa E, et al. An update on the management of childhood-onset systemic lupus erythematosus. Paediatr Drugs. 2021;23(4):331-47.

Wenderfer SE, Eldin KW. Lupus nephritis. Pediatr Clin North Am. 2019;66(1):87-99.

18.4 Vasculitis Syndromes

PE 21.2, PE 21.3

INTRODUCTION

Vasculitis is defined as inflammation of vessel wall. Based on the size of vessels involved, vasculitis has been classified in three types **(Table 18.4)**.

PATHOPHYSIOLOGY

Clinical features of vasculitis are attributable to the following pathophysiologic mechanisms:

1. Occlusion of lumen causing distal ischemia.
2. Weakening of vessel wall causing aneurysm formation or rupture.
3. Chronic lesions may be associated with fibrosis of vessel wall leading to further stenosis.
4. Nonspecific features of inflammation such as fever, anorexia, and weight loss.

CLINICAL FEATURES

A. ***Vessel involvement***
   - *Localized:* Involving a few organs like skin, kidney, or lung, etc.
   - *Systemic:* Involving many organs.

B. ***Type of vessel involved***
   - *Large vessel vasculitis:* Absent pulses, claudication, bruits, and hypertension.
   - *Medium vessel vasculitis:* Skin rash, tender nodules, hypertension, abdominal angina, orchitis, gangrene, and mononeuritis multiplex.
   - *Small vessel vasculitis:* Purpura, glomerulonephritis, mucosal ulcers, asthma, symptoms related to ear, nose, and throat.

C. ***Duration of vessel inflammation***
   - Acute, e.g., HSP, Kawasaki disease (KD)
   - Chronic, e.g., Takayasu arteritis

D. ***Etiology***
   - *Primary:* When there is no underlying cause of vasculitis, it is termed as primary vasculitis.
   - *Secondary:* When vasculitis occurs secondary to infections, malignancies, and/or rheumatological conditions like SLE, it is termed as secondary vasculitis. Clinical features of underlying disease are usually present in addition to features of vasculitis.

Organ-specific symptoms and signs depend upon the organ involved **(Box 18.2)**.

Box 18.2 Organ-specific Clinical Features of Vasculitis

1. *Skin:* Palpable purpura, and livedo reticularis
2. *Musculoskeletal:* Myalgia/myositis, and arthralgia/arthritis
3. *Nervous system:* Mononeuritis multiplex, headache, stroke, tinnitus, reduced visual acuity, and acute visual loss
4. *Heart and arteries:* Myocardial infarction, hypertension, absent pulses, and gangrene
5. *Respiratory tract:* Nose bleeds, hemoptysis, and lung infiltrates
6. *Gastrointestinal tract:* Abdominal pain, bloody stool, and perforation
7. *Kidneys:* Glomerulonephritis and renal infarcts

INVESTIGATIONS

Investigations in a child with vasculitis depend on the type of vessel involved and area in which vessels are involved.

A. ***Investigations pointing to inflammation:*** Neutrophilic leukocytosis, thrombocytosis, raised ESR and raised CRP are usual but not specific for any vasculitis.

B. ***Organ-specific clues***
   - *Renal involvement:* Hematuria, proteinuria, and deranged renal functions.
   - *Lung involvement:* Abnormal chest radiographs.

C. ***Diagnosis***
   - *Histopathology:* Demonstration of inflammation in vessel wall on histopathological examination is diagnostic. Various tissue biopsies can be done to demonstrate vessel wall inflammation. This is the method of choice for diagnosis of small vessel vasculitis and medium vessel vasculitis.
   - *Vascular imaging:* Since biopsy from a large vessel is fraught with risk of massive bleeding, diagnosis of large vessel vasculitis depends on vascular imaging, which includes angiography, echocardiography, and ultrasound

Table 18.4 Classification of Vasculitis Syndromes

Category	*Vessels included*	*Prototype disease*	*Primary diagnostic modality*
Large vessel vasculitis	Vessels such as aorta and major branches arising from aorta	*Takayasu arteritis* (aortoarteritis)	Vascular imaging (angiography)
Medium vessel vasculitis	All vessels other than large and small vessels	*Kawasaki disease* (KD)	• Both vascular imaging and histopathology are used for medium vessel vasculitis • KD is a clinical diagnosis which may or may not be supported by vascular imaging
Small vessel vasculitis	Small arteries in tissues, arterioles, capillaries, and venules	*Henoch–Schönlein purpura* (HSP)	Histopathology along with immunofluorescence

Doppler. Vascular imaging is able to demonstrate stenosis, occlusion, and aneurysms. In addition, it may also be able to show vessel wall inflammation. Vascular imaging is also used to support diagnosis of medium vessel vasculitis such as KD but small vessels cannot be seen by imaging.

TREATMENT Vasculitis Syndromes

Management of vasculitis depends on type of vasculitis and will be discussed further with discussion of specific vasculitides.

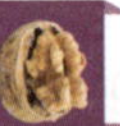

IN A NUTSHELL

Vasculitis Syndromes

1. Vasculitis refers to inflammation of vessel wall.
2. Occlusion of vessel lumen and vessel wall thickening due to inflammation can cause distal ischemia and organ damage. Aneurysm formation may be seen in certain vasculitis and carries a risk of thrombosis.
3. Symptoms and signs vary with the type of vessel involved and the organs involved by vasculitis. Nonspecific features of inflammation may be present.
4. Vascular imaging is used for diagnosis of large vessel vasculitis, whereas histopathology is used for small vessel vasculitis.

Cannon L, Wu EY. Recent advances in pediatric vasculitis. Rheum Dis Clin North Am. 2021;47(4):781-96.
Ozen S, Sag E. Childhood vasculitis. Rheumatology (Oxford). 2020;59(Suppl 3):iii95-iii100.

18.5 Kawasaki Disease

PE 21.3

INTRODUCTION

Kawasaki disease is an acute systemic medium vessel vasculitis of childhood with a predisposition to involve coronary arteries. It was first reported from Japan in early 1960s by Dr Tomisaku Kawasaki as "mucocutaneous lymph node syndrome." It has now been described worldwide and is a leading cause of acquired heart disease in children.

EPIDEMIOLOGY

Japan has a maximum incidence of KD with rates of 240/100,000 children <5 years. Korea and Taiwan have reported the next high incidences. Whereas, the incidence in USA (20 per 100,000 children <5 years) is static over years, Japan has been reporting increasing incidence rates over years. Incidence is not well-known in Indian population.

ETIOLOGY

The exact etiology is unknown. KD appears to be due to a stereotyped pathological immune response to one or a variety of environmental or infectious triggers because of their genetic constitution. About 80% of affected cases are younger than 5 years at diagnosis and there is slight male preponderance.

PATHOGENESIS

The KD is characterized by intensive T cell stimulation with activation of inflammatory cytokines and leukocyte recruitment. This leads to upregulation of proteolytic activity causing elastin degradation and vessel wall damage, which is responsible for characteristic coronary lesions seen in this disease.

CLINICAL FEATURES

The diagnosis is entirely clinical. It presents like an acute febrile illness with features of skin and mucosal involvement. For this reason, it can mimic a viral exanthem.

Characteristic features include fever, polymorphous exanthem, bilateral conjunctival congestion, changes in extremities, changes in lips and oral cavity, and cervical adenopathy.

- ***Fever*** is typically high grade (>39°C) with an abrupt onset and responds transiently to antipyretics. Usually fever persists for >5 days and can persist for >3 weeks, if not treated.
- ***Rash*** is diffuse erythematous maculopapular rash which appears within first 5 days of illness.
- ***Conjunctivitis*** is typically bilateral, nonexudative (no discharge) and spares limbus **(Fig. 18.6)**.

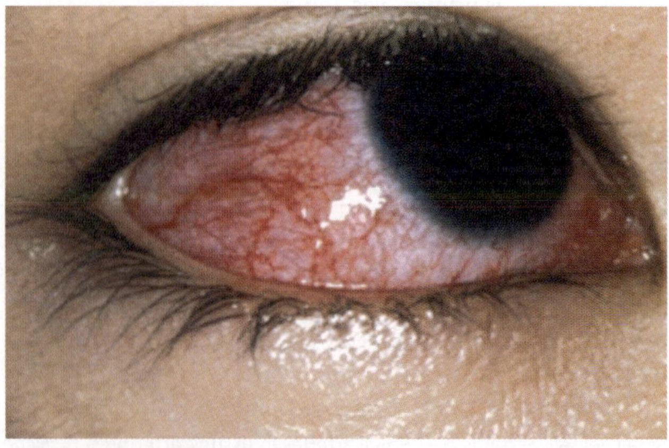

Fig. 18.6: Nonpurulent conjunctivitis sparing limbus

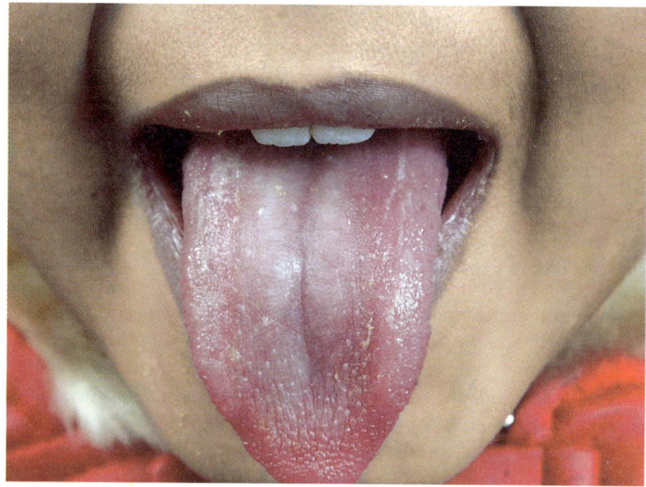

Fig. 18.7: Strawberry tongue with cracked lips in a child with Kawasaki disease

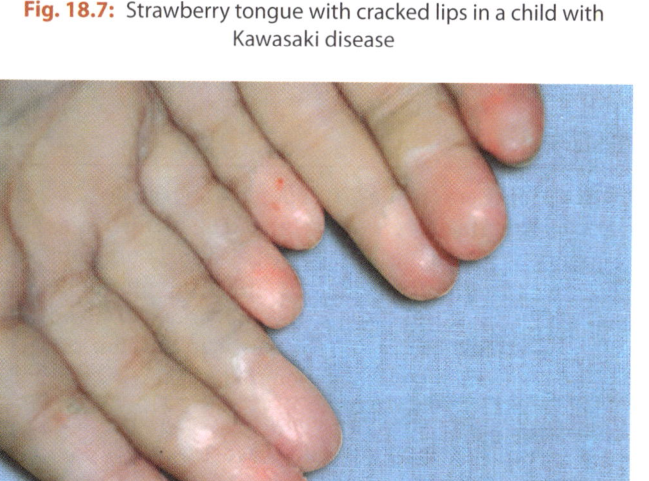

Fig. 18.8: Periungual desquamation

- ***Changes in lips and oral cavity*** include strawberry tongue **(Fig. 18.7)** and cracking of lips.
- ***Changes in extremities*** include diffuse nonpitting edema on the dorsum of hands and feet and characteristic periungual desquamation **(Fig. 18.8)** starting in late second or third week of illness. Perianal desquamation **(Fig. 18.9)** is also characteristic and precedes periungual desquamation.
- ***Cervical adenopathy*** is single, unilateral, and nontender and involves anterior cervical chain.

Box 18.3 describes the American Heart Association Diagnostic Criteria for KD. Besides these, other clinical features may be present and may help or confuse treating physician further. Sometimes, infants are extremely irritable suggesting a possibility of pyogenic meningitis. Aseptic meningitis is common in KD and responds briskly to intravenous immunoglobulins (IVIg). Joint manifestations may include arthralgia and arthritis. Significant right hypochondriac pain can occur due to hydrops of gallbladder. Beau lines, growth arrest lines in nails, are frequently seen in convalescent phase **(Fig. 18.10)**.

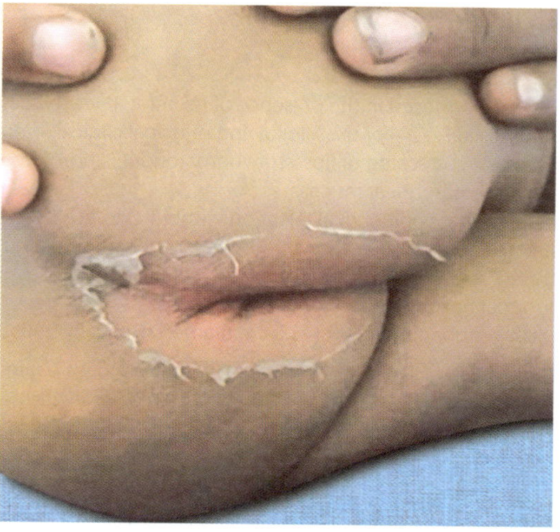

Fig. 18.9: Perianal desquamation

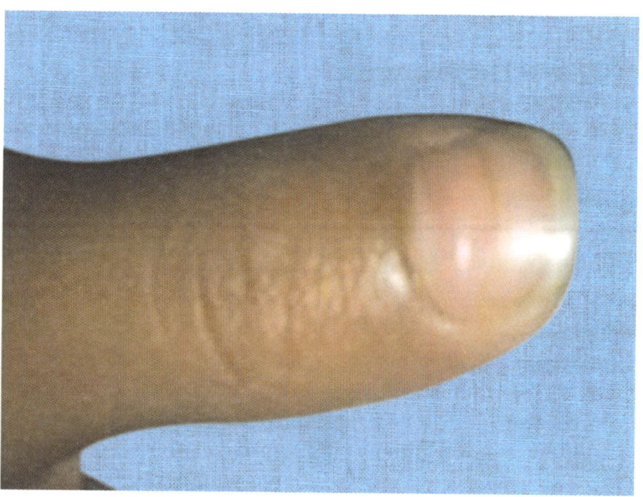

Fig. 18.10: Beau's lines

Incomplete Kawasaki Disease

Incomplete KD is diagnosed if a child presents with fever and fulfills <4 criteria mentioned in **Box 18.3**. Such cases are more common in infancy. Coronary artery involvement on 2D echo can be supportive. Failure to diagnose KD in such a setting carries a significant risk of coronary aneurysms with life-long implications.

INVESTIGATIONS

Diagnosis of KD is clinical and no single investigation is diagnostic.

- During febrile phase, one may see raised markers of inflammation such as neutrophilia, high ESR, high CRP, anemia, hypoalbuminemia, sterile pyuria (due to urethritis), and transaminitis. Cerebrospinal fluid analysis may reveal pleocytosis due to aseptic meningitis. None of these features are specific for KD.
- Thrombocytosis, which is described as a typical feature, is not seen before the end of second week of illness.

Box 18.3 American Heart Association Diagnostic Criteria for Kawasaki Disease

Classic KD is diagnosed in the presence of fever for at least 5 days together with at least 4 of the 5 following principal clinical features:

1. Erythema and cracking of lips, strawberry tongue, and/or erythema of oral and pharyngeal mucosa
2. Bilateral bulbar conjunctival injection without exudate
3. *Rash:* Maculopapular, diffuse erythroderma, or erythema multiforme-like
4. Erythema and edema of the hands and feet in acute phase and/or periungual desquamation in subacute phase
5. Cervical lymphadenopathy (>1.5 cm diameter), usually unilateral

Source: McCrindle BW, Rowley AH, Newburger JW, et al. Diagnosis, treatment, and long-term management of Kawasaki disease: A scientific statement or health professionals from the American Heart Association. Circulation. 2017;135(17):e927-99.

- ***Echocardiography:*** Coronary aneurysms **(Fig. 18.11)** are highly suggestive of KD. ECHO is done at baseline. Another ECHO may be needed in second week of illness in children who do not show response to IVIg or have early coronary involvement. A normal ECHO in first week of illness does not rule out the diagnosis.

There could be other suggestive findings in echocardiography such as perivascular brightness, lack of tapering of vessels, low ejection fraction, mitral regurgitation, and pericardial effusion. These findings may be useful in a child with incomplete KD. A repeat echocardiography at 6–8 weeks of illness helps in picking up residual coronary abnormalities.

DIFFERENTIAL DIAGNOSIS

Since, the clinical features are relatively nonspecific, there are many differential diagnosis of KD. These include viral infections, Stevens–Johnson syndrome, toxin-mediated syndromes, scarlet fever, leptospirosis, and hypersensitivity reactions to drugs. Scarlet fever is not associated with conjunctivitis and shows a brisk response to antibiotics. Visceral involvement and hypotension are frequent in toxin-mediated syndromes.

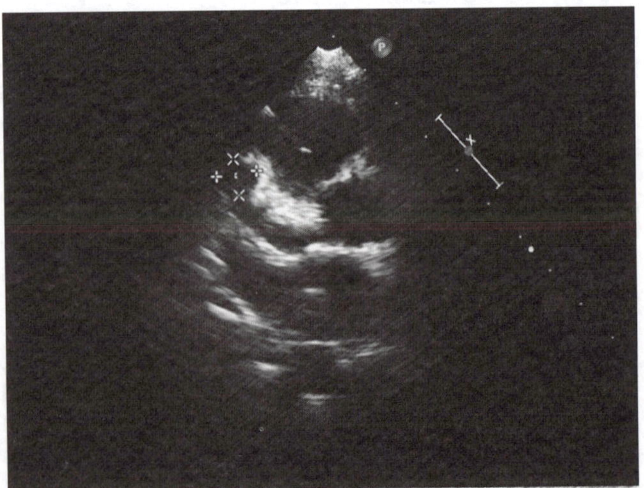

Fig. 18.11: ECHO showing coronary aneurysms

Following five clinical features are not seen in KD and should suggest an alternative diagnosis:

1. Exudative pharyngitis
2. Exudative conjunctivitis
3. Discrete intraoral lesions
4. Bullous or vesicular rash
5. Diffuse lymphadenopathy

TREATMENT Kawasaki Disease

Standard treatment of KD includes administration of IVIg and aspirin.

- *IVIg* is given at a dose of 2 g/kg as a single dose infusion. Most patients show a brisk response with subsidence of fever and general well-being. Inflammatory parameters show gradual improvement. IVIg, when given within first 10 days of illness, has been shown to reduce the risk of coronary abnormalities from 25 to 3–5%.
- *Aspirin* is given at a dose of 30–50 mg/kg/day till subsidence of inflammation. Once the child is afebrile and inflammatory parameters (CRP) show declining trend, dose of aspirin is reduced to antiplatelet doses (3–5 mg/kg/day). Aspirin is discontinued if the follow-up ECHO at 6–8 weeks is normal.

PROGNOSIS

In the pre-IVIg era, about 25% children would go on to develop coronary abnormalities. Use of IVIg has reduced this risk to 3–5%. Coronary abnormalities can persist as ectasia or aneurysms. These aneurysms carry a significant risk of rupture, thrombosis, and stenosis and predispose the individual to myocardial ischemic events. Hence, all patients who develop coronary abnormalities should be on life-long follow-up.

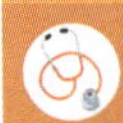

CASE STUDY Kawasaki Disease

A 1-year-old boy was brought with history of fever for 1 week. On examination, he had diffuse maculopapular rash, nontender adenopathy in left jugulodigastric region and red eyes without any discharge. Lips were red and cracked. Oral cavity showed diffuse erythema. With a possibility of KD, he was investigated and found to have raised ESR, raised CRP, and neutrophilic leukocytosis. Ultrasound abdomen to look for gallbladder hydrops was normal. Urine microscopy was not contributory. Echocardiography did not reveal any coronary dilation.

Does normal ECHO rule out possibility of KD?

No, coronary dilation does not occur in all patients. Moreover, it is unusual to see coronary dilation in first week of illness except in very sick patients. Normal ECHO does not rule out KD.

What will be the first line treatment for this child?

This child would need IVIg at a dose of 2 g/kg as single infusion. IVIg is known to reduce the risk of coronary complications. Aspirin is added in anti-inflammatory doses till subsidence of inflammation and then is reduced to antiplatelet doses.

Should I wait for periungual desquamation or thrombocytosis to develop before considering IVIg?

Periungual desquamation and thrombocytosis are usually seen in second and third week of illness. Diagnosis of KD is clinical and this child fulfills AHA criteria for KD. One should not wait for these features before starting treatment as a delay in therapy carries a high risk of coronary aneurysms.

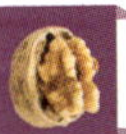

IN A NUTSHELL

Kawasaki Disease

1. Kawasaki disease is an acute systemic vasculitis which should be suspected in a child with fever for >5 days and at least four of the following:
   - Unilateral cervical lymphadenopathy
   - Nonvesicular rash
   - Edema/erythema of hands/feet
   - Nonsuppurative conjunctivitis
   - Lesions of the oropharynx with strawberry tongue
2. Timely recognition and management are important to reduce the risk of coronary complications.
3. No single diagnostic test is useful in the acute phase.
4. IVIg along with aspirin is the standard of care and most patients respond briskly to this treatment.
5. Think of another diagnosis in presence of exudative pharyngitis, exudative conjunctivitis, discrete intraoral lesions, bullous or vesicular rash, and diffuse lymphadenopathy.

McCrindle BW, Rowley AH, Newburger JW, et al; American Heart Association Rheumatic Fever, Endocarditis, and Kawasaki Disease Committee. Diagnosis, treatment, and long-term management of Kawasaki Disease: A scientific statement for health professionals from the American Heart Association. Circulation. 2017;135(17):e927-99.
Rife E, Gedalia A. Kawasaki disease: an update. Curr Rheumatol Rep. 2020;22(10):75.
Tirelli F, Marrani E, Giani T, et al. One year in review: Kawasaki disease. Curr Opin Rheumatol. 2020;32(1):15-20.

18.6 Henoch-Schönlein Purpura (IgA Vasculitis)

PE 21.2

INTRODUCTION

Henoch-Schönlein purpura (HSP), also known as IgA vasculitis, is an acute multisystemic, IgA mediated, small vessel leukocytoclastic vasculitis. Leukocytoclastic vasculitis refers to neutrophilic infiltrate in vessel wall with fibrinoid necrosis and disintegration of neutrophils into fragments. It is one of the most common vasculitis in children and is seen between the ages of 3 and 15 years with a male preponderance. There is a seasonal trend with peak in the months of October and November.

ETIOLOGY

Etiology of HSP is unknown, however, various triggers such as infections, medications, and vaccination have been implicated.

PATHOGENESIS

It is an IgA-mediated disease. Immune complexes tend to deposit in the vessel wall and incite inflammation. The pathognomonic lesion is leukocytoclastic vasculitis and can be easily seen in the dermal capillaries and postcapillary venules, but is not specific. Deposition of IgA is characteristic. Vessel wall inflammation leads to extravasation of blood into the interstitial space resulting in edema and palpable purpura.

CLINICAL FEATURES

The HSP is a clinical diagnosis. It is characterized by a classic tetrad of:

1. Nonthrombocytopenic palpable purpura
2. Arthritis/arthralgia
3. Gastrointestinal involvement
4. Renal involvement

- ***Skin involvement*** is the most common presentation and occurs in the form of purpura, which are palpable **(Fig. 18.12)** and occur in crops over a duration of 4–6 weeks.
  Palpable purpura is characteristic of small vessel vasculitis in contrast to nonpalpable purpura in thrombocytopenia. Purpuric lesions have a predilection for lower limbs. The onset

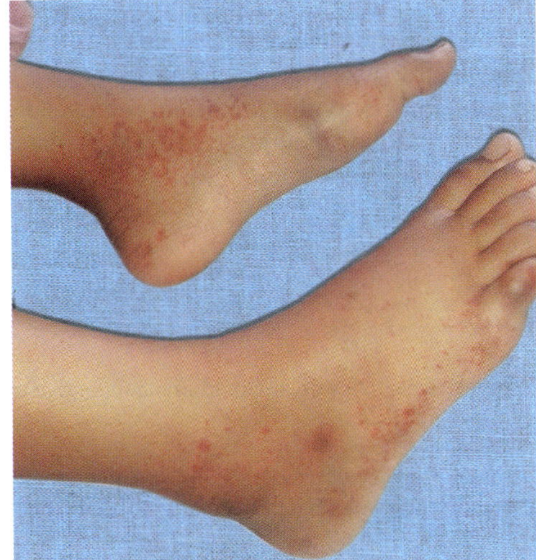

Fig. 18.12: Raised purpuric rash over lower limbs in Henoch-Schönlein purpura

is acute but symptoms may appear sequentially resulting in delay in diagnosis. Involvement of the external genitalia is more common in boys and includes painless scrotal edema, purpura and acute onset edema of the glans penis or prepuce and acute testicular pain mimicking torsion.

- ***Gastrointestinal involvement*** can present as diffuse, acute, colicky abdominal pain. There may also be intussusception and gastrointestinal bleeding, which are most common emergencies in acute phase of disease.
- ***Joints*** may be involved in the form of arthritis (joint swelling or pain with limitation on motion) or arthralgia (joint pain without joint swelling or limitation on motion). Ankles and knees are most commonly affected.
- ***Renal involvement*** can occur in 25–50% cases in the form of hematuria, proteinuria, deranged renal functions, and hypertension. This is the most worrying chronic complication with a potential to cause end-stage renal disease.

DIAGNOSIS

Diagnosis of HSP is largely clinical **(Box 18.4)**. In patients with typical skin lesions, one may not require skin biopsy. Skin biopsy shows leukocytoclastic vasculitis with predominant IgA deposits. In case of renal involvement, renal biopsy may show proliferative glomerulonephritis with IgA deposits.

DIFFERENTIAL DIAGNOSIS

Skin lesions are usually the first manifestation of HSP. Common differential diagnosis for purpuric lesions includes thrombocytopenia, which is associated with nonpalpable purpura.

If gastrointestinal manifestations are the first presentation, one needs to think of common causes of acute surgical abdomen. One should make an effort to undress the child and look for typical skin lesions of HSP in gluteal region and lower limbs.

COMPLICATIONS

- ***Gastrointestinal complications*** are common during acute stage of disease. Plain radiographs may show dilated bowel loops in children with abdominal symptoms. Ultrasound may demonstrate intussusception.
- ***Acute scrotal pain*** is another important complication during acute stage. Ultrasound may help rule out testicular torsion in a child with red tender scrotum.

Box 18.4 Henoch-Schönlein Purpura EULAR/PRINTO/PRES Ankara 2008 Classification

Definition

Purpura or petechiae with lower limb predominance and *at least one of the four following criteria:*

1. Abdominal pain
2. *Histopathology:* Leukocytoclastic vasculitis with predominant IgA deposit or proliferative glomerulonephritis with predominant IgA deposit
3. Arthritis or arthralgia
4. Renal involvement

- ***Renal involvement*** is the most important long-term complication of HSP and is seen within first 6 months of disease. Urine microscopy shows hematuria and proteinuria. Renal function test may show raised blood urea and creatinine. Renal biopsy is required in severe cases.

INVESTIGATIONS

- Hemogram reveals normocytic, normochromic anemia along with leukocytosis. Platelet count and ESR are mildly elevated.
- Biopsy of skin lesion reveals acute leukocytoclastic vasculitis. Immunofluorescence shows perivascular IgA deposition.
- In patients with renal involvement, one may see variable proteinuria, microscopic to gross hematuria, and deranged renal functions. Patients of HSP do not require renal biopsy routinely unless complicated by nephrotic syndrome, acute nephritis with impaired renal function, or rapidly progressive renal failure.

TREATMENT Henoch-Schönlein Purpura (IgA Vasculitis)

HSP is usually a self-limiting illness with remission within 4–6 weeks. Most children require only supportive treatment.

- Analgesics (paracetamol or NSAIDs) are prescribed for pain and swelling associated with joint involvement.
- Steroids are indicated for severe gastrointestinal manifestations, i.e., severe colic, gastrointestinal bleed, or acute abdomen. Oral prednisolone is given at the dose of 1–2 mg/kg per day for 1 week followed by tapering over the 2–3 weeks. Orchitis may also benefit from 2–3 weeks therapy with corticosteroids. Short duration steroids have no role in preventing renal involvement.

Only long-term complication is renal involvement which has the potential to cause end-stage renal disease. Severe renal manifestations including nephrotic syndrome, nephritic syndrome, or rapidly progressive glomerulonephritis may require long-term steroids and immunosuppressive therapy. Children with minor urinary abnormalities (microscopic hematuria or nonnephrotic range proteinuria) should be followed-up for a minimum duration of 1 year to detect any progression.

COURSE AND PROGNOSIS

HSP is generally a benign disease with excellent prognosis. The average duration of disease is 4–6 weeks. Approximately 10–20% patients may have recurrences. Long-term morbidity is due to renal involvement. All patients with HSP should be followed-up for a minimum duration of 6 months to detect renal involvement. A subset of patients with renal involvement tend to progress to end-stage renal disease over 10–25 years.

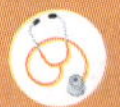

CASE STUDY Henoch-Schönlein Purpura

A 5-year-old boy presented with skin rash for 3 days. There was no history of fever. Examination revealed palpable purpura predominantly in lower limbs and arthritis of left ankle. Rest of the systemic examination was normal.

What investigations will you order in this child?
Hemogram is important as it will show normal or mild elevation in platelet count in HSP and will help rule out thrombocytopenic purpura. Palpable purpura are against a diagnosis of thrombocytopenia. Baseline urine microscopic examination is helpful.

Would this child need a skin biopsy to confirm the diagnosis?
Skin biopsy can show leukocytoclastic vasculitis with predominant IgA deposition on immunofluorescence. However, it is not always required as HSP is usually a self-limiting disease and histopathology and immunofluorescence may not be easily available in all healthcare settings.

How will you counsel the parents and follow-up this child?
Parents are worried because of the skin rash. One must counsel the parents regarding self-limiting nature of this disease. Also, it should be told that this rash can keep on appearing in crops for 4–6 weeks. Parents should be advised to seek urgent medical help in case of abdominal pain, blood in stools or abdominal distension. Periodic urine examination is required in all patients for at least 6 months to pick up renal involvement.

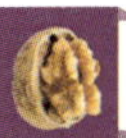

IN A NUTSHELL

Henoch-Schönlein Purpura (IgA Vasculitis)

1. The HSP is an acute small vessel vasculitis predominantly seen in childhood.
2. Diagnosis is clinical based on presence of typical palpable purpura in lower limbs. Other features such as arthralgia/arthritis, gastrointestinal features, and genitourinary features may be present during acute phase.
3. Histopathology from skin lesion shows leukocytoclastic vasculitis with IgA deposition on immunofluorescence.
4. Most children have self-limiting illness and need only supportive therapy.
5. Children with significant gastrointestinal involvement or genitourinary involvement respond briskly to steroids.
6. Steroids in acute phase do not reduce the risk of renal involvement.
7. The HSP nephritis is the most dreaded chronic complication of otherwise innocuous disease.

Fraticelli P, Benfaremo D, Gabrielli A. Diagnosis and management of leukocytoclastic vasculitis. Intern Emerg Med. 2021;16(4):831-41.
Leung AKC, Barankin B, Leong KF. Henoch-Schönlein purpura in children: An updated review. Curr Pediatr Rev. 2020;16(4):265-76.

18.7 Takayasu Arteritis

INTRODUCTION

Takayasu arteritis is a chronic large vessel vasculitis. It was first described from Japan as "pulseless disease" (inability to palpate upper limb vessels) because of involvement of origin of vessels arising from arch of aorta. Pediatric disease accounts for 10–15% of all Takayasu arteritis patients. It is far less common than KD and HSP, but causes significant morbidity due to its chronic course. Usual age at diagnosis is after the first decade and it is more common in girls. This is a chronic vasculitis leading to progressive stenosis of vessel lumen, thus causing distal ischemia.

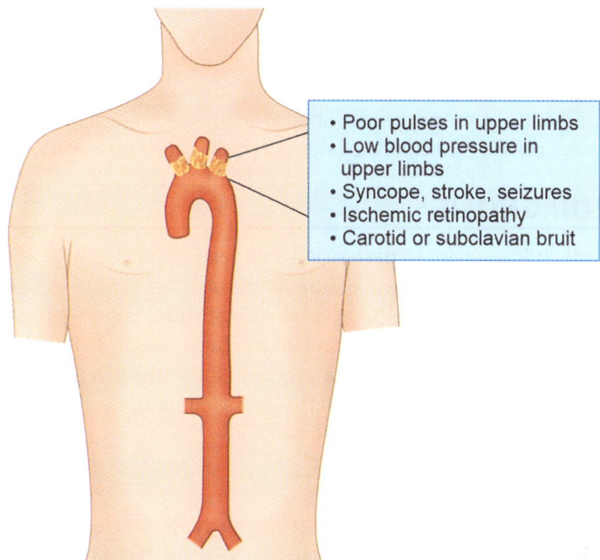

Fig. 18.13: Depiction of symptoms and signs in Takayasu arteritis where origins of arteries in aortic arch are affected

CLINICAL FEATURES

Clinical manifestations depend on the site of vascular involvement and severity of stenosis.

- ***Stenosis of branches of arch of aorta*** leads to features of cerebral and retinal ischemia along with pulselessness of upper limbs **(Fig. 18.13)**. Organ-specific ischemic features may be seen such as stroke, seizures, and visual disturbances. This variant is more common in Japan.
- ***Stenosis of thoracoabdominal aorta*** and its branches like renal artery present with severe hypertension (renal ischemia

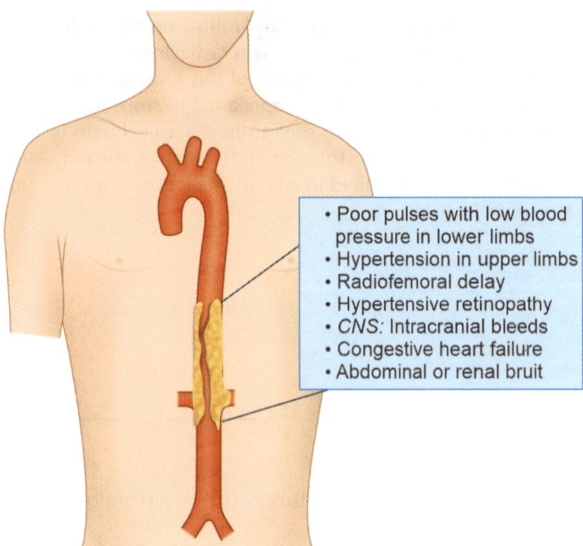

Fig. 18.14: Depiction of symptoms and signs in Takayasu arteritis where descending thoracoabdominal aorta and renal arteries are affected

due to stenosis of renal artery or suprarenal aorta), reduced pulses in lower limbs and congestive heart failure **(Fig. 18.14)**. This variety is more common in Indian children. Typical "pulselessness" in upper limbs is not seen unless branches of aortic arch are also involved. Hypertension is usually severe and may or may not be associated with differential pulses depending on the site involved. Cardiac dysfunction can occur due to severe hypertension and cardiomyopathy.

Symptoms of this disease can be subtle or sometimes alarming such as accelerated hypertension and cerebral ischemia. Nonspecific features such as fever, anorexia, and weight loss are common. Claudication is not a common symptom, probably because children are unable to express this symptom. Bruits can be heard because of irregular flow. Proximal pulses such as brachial, carotid, and femoral arteries should be looked for and reduced or absent pulses are important signs of proximal stenosis.

DIAGNOSIS

In all children with hypertension, congestive heart failure, visual complaints and stroke/seizures/syncope, one must examine pulses in all four limbs as well as carotids. Blood pressure in all four limbs should be taken in these settings. This basic examination is enough to make one suspect this disease.

Diagnosis of Takayasu arteritis is based on the criteria given by EULAR/PRINTO/PRES **(Box 18.5)**.

Angiography

The gold standard for demonstrating typical arterial abnormalities is angiography **(Figs. 18.15A and B)**. Angiography shows occlusion, stenosis (which is usually proximal and ostial), dilation and occasionally aneurysms. Some other useful investigations include ultrasound (to look for kidney size), Doppler (to look for stenosis in carotids, abdominal aorta, or renal arteries) and echocardiography (to look for cardiac dysfunction).

Box 18.5 EULAR/PRINTO/PRES Ankara 2008 Classification

Definition of Takayasu arteritis

Angiographic abnormalities of the aorta or its main branches and pulmonary arteries showing aneurysm/dilatation (mandatory criterion)

Plus one of the five following criteria:

1. Decreased peripheral artery pulse(s) or claudication of extremities
2. Four limb blood pressure (BP) discrepancy
3. Bruits over the aorta or its major branches
4. Hypertension (related to childhood normative data)
5. Acute phase reactants

Source: Ozen S, Pistorio A, Iusan SM, et al. EULAR/PRINTO/PRES criteria for Henoch-Schönlein purpura, childhood polyarteritis nodosa, childhood Wegener granulomatosis, and childhood Takayasu arteritis: Ankara 2008. Part II: Final classification criteria. Ann Rheum Dis. 2010;69(5):798-806.

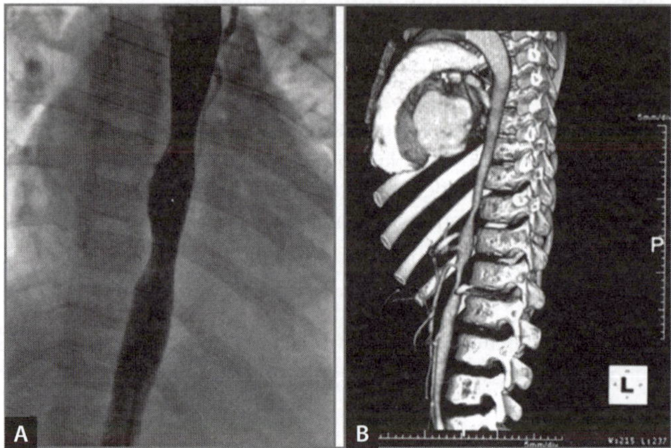

Figs. 18.15A and B: (A) Angiography showing narrowing of vascular lumen in descending thoracoabdominal aorta; (B) CT angiography images showing extensive stenosis of descending thoracoabdominal aorta

DIFFERENTIAL DIAGNOSIS

Coarctation of aorta is a common differential diagnosis and presents with hypertension in upper limbs, decreased pulses in lower limbs and radiofemoral delay. Collaterals are more common because of long duration of illness. Echocardiography and Doppler help in diagnosis. Angiography shows a discrete lesion in aorta in juxtaductal region and poststenotic dilation.

TREATMENT Takayasu Arteritis

Management aims at suppressing vessel wall inflammation and relieving distal ischemia.

- Steroids along with immunosuppression are the mainstay to suppress inflammation.
- Relief of obstruction/stenosis is required in cases with significant distal ischemia and can be achieved by percutaneous or surgical revascularization procedures.

Most patients also need supportive therapy for control of hypertension. Renovascular hypertension is usually severe and needs multiple antihypertensive agents. One must remember not to give angiotensin-converting enzyme inhibitors to control hypertension in a setting of bilateral renal artery stenosis or critical suprarenal aortic stenosis, as this may precipitate renal failure.

PROGNOSIS

It is a chronic disease with relapses and remissions. Adult survival rates of 94–97% at 10–15 years have been achieved with immunosuppression and revascularization procedures. Higher mortality is seen in children because of higher rate of congestive heart failure due both to hypertension and myocardial inflammation.

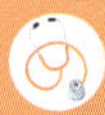

CASE STUDY Takayasu Arteritis

A 12-year-old girl was brought to emergency services with complaints of headache for last 1 week and one episode of seizure 12 hours back followed by unconsciousness. Examination revealed hypertension (BP 180/120 mm Hg in right upper limb), no meningeal signs and no focal neurological signs. Rest of systemic examination was normal. Headache, seizure, and altered sensorium were attributed to severe hypertension and antihypertensive therapy was started as per protocol. Meanwhile certain investigations were ordered to determine the cause of hypertension. Renal function tests were normal and urine dipstick showed 2+ proteinuria. Ultrasound of kidneys was ordered and showed small left kidney with near absent blood flow in left renal artery on Doppler. Ultrasound Doppler also picked up additional blood flow abnormality in suprarenal aorta. Stenosis of suprarenal aorta and left renal artery were confirmed by angiography; thus confirming diagnosis of Takayasu arteritis.

What additional examination should have been done in this child?

Examination for proximal pulses especially carotids, brachials, and femorals could have given a clue. In case of suprarenal aortic stenosis, one may get reduced lower limb pulses. Blood pressure should have been taken in all four limbs. About >10 mm Hg difference in BP between limbs is an important clue to diagnosis. One should also look for bruits over major arteries and may find them over carotids, abdominal aorta, and renal artery.

What precautions should be taken while using antihypertensives in such a child?

Hypertension should be brought under control gradually since abrupt drop in blood pressure can cause ischemia distal to the obstruction. In this child, it could precipitate renal failure.

Angiotensin-converting enzyme inhibitors should not be used because they carry a risk of precipitating renal failure in a setting of bilateral renal artery stenosis or suprarenal aortic stenosis.

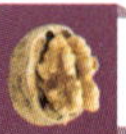

IN A NUTSHELL

Takayasu Arteritis

1. Takayasu arteritis is a chronic large vessel arteritis and leads to progressive stenosis or occlusion of aorta and/or its major branches.
2. Clinical features are related to distal ischemia and effects thereof (renovascular hypertension, cardiac decompensation, seizures, syncope, stroke, and visual manifestations). Claudication is not a common complaint in children.
3. Diagnosis is not difficult if suspected.
4. Conventional angiography is the gold standard for diagnosis.
5. Management is aimed at suppressing vessel wall inflammation and relieving distal ischemia. Inflammation is controlled by steroids and other steroid-sparing drugs. Relief of distal ischemia may need percutaneous or surgical revascularization procedures.

Di Santo M, Stelmaszewski EV, Villa A. Takayasu arteritis in pediatrics. Cardiol Young. 2018;28:354-61.

Seyahi E. Takayasu arteritis: an update. Curr Opin Rheumatol. 2017;29(1): 51-6.

Tombetti E, Mason JC. Takayasu arteritis: advanced understanding is leading to new horizons. Rheumatology (Oxford). 2019;58:206-19.

18.8 Immune System

ORGANS OF IMMUNE SYSTEM

Immune system is a complex network of multiple arms which protects us from pathogens.

Primary Organs

- ***Bone marrow*** is the site of production of all immune cells. B lymphocytes undergo maturation in the bone marrow.
- ***Thymus*** is the site of maturation of T lymphocytes.

Secondary Organs

Immune cells are activated here by various antigens and undergo proliferation and differentiation to become effector cells. Secondary organs include lymph node, spleen, and mucosa associated lymphoid tissue (MALT).

CELLS OF IMMUNE SYSTEM

All cells of immune system are produced from hematopoietic stem cell in bone marrow. They can be divided into two types based on their origin:

1. ***Derived from common myeloid precursor:***
   - *Granulocytes:* Neutrophils, basophils, and eosinophils
   - Macrophages
   - Dendritic cells
   - Mast cells
2. ***Derived from common lymphoid precursor:***
   - T lymphocytes
   - B lymphocytes
   - NK cell (natural killer cells)

LINES OF DEFENSE

Innate Immunity

- ***Barrier defense (acts within 0–4 hours of exposure):*** This includes skin and mucosa and various secretions with antimicrobial properties such as tears, saliva, and gastric juice. This defense is preformed and acts continuously and immediately as we live in an ocean of pathogens around us.
- ***Innate immunity (acts between 4 hours and 4 days of exposure):*** Innate immune system includes phagocytic cells (neutrophils, macrophages, and dendritic cells), complement and cytokines. This response is induced once a pathogen breaches barrier defense and enters the body. This results in inflammation and killing of pathogen at local site. This response is characterized by limited diversity and fixed specificity. Repeat infection by same organism leads to no change in the response.

Adaptive Immunity
(Starts Acting After 4 Days of Exposure)

This system includes T and B lymphocytes. Response is highly specific and diverse. Repeat infection with same pathogen leads to more rapid and effective response.

Table 18.5 depicts important differences between innate and adaptive immunity.

Table 18.5 Differences Between Innate and Adaptive Immunity

Innate immunity	*Adaptive immunity*
Components: • Barriers such as skin and mucosa and their secretions • Cells such as neutrophils, macrophages, and monocytes • Complement proteins	*Components:* • Cell-mediated immunity (T lymphocytes) • Antibody-mediated immunity (B lymphocytes)
First line of defense	Second line of defense
No memory	Memory is present; hence fights recurrence of infection faster and more effectively
No specificity (can fight against a broad range of organisms)	Consists of specific immune responses
Response is quick	Response slower

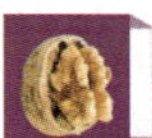

IN A NUTSHELL

Immune System

1. Innate and adaptive immune responses are two important lines of defense against various microbes.
2. Deficiency of any of the pathways in these lines of defense may cause serious defect in immunity.

18.9 Primary Immunodeficiency Disorders

IMMUNE MECHANISMS IN IMMUNODEFICIENCY DISEASES

As we have already seen that immune system is a complex network of various arms which are necessary to tackle different pathogens ranging from viruses to large parasites such as tapeworm. Defect in any one arm of immune system can lead to immunodeficiency (better called "inborn errors of immunity."

Nearly 400 primary immunodeficiency disorders (PIDs) have been described till date with a prevalence of 6–10/100,000 population. The International Union of Immunological Societies (IUIS) has categorized the PID in eight groups **(Table 18.6)**. First three subgroups account for 80% of all PID in general population. Primary antibody deficiencies are the most common.

WHEN TO SUSPECT IMMUNODEFICIENCY?

The usual mode of presentation of PID is *recurrent infections.* Infections occur most frequently at sites which communicate with external environment and such sites include sinuses, respiratory tract, gastrointestinal tract, skin, and draining lymph nodes.

The European Society of Immunodeficiencies (ESID) has suggested *10 warning signs* for suspecting immunodeficiency. PID should be suspected *in a child with* two *or more of the following* warning signs:

1. Four or more new ear infections within 1 year.
2. Two or more serious sinus infections within 1 year.
3. Two or more months on antibiotics with little effect.
4. Two or more episodes of pneumonia within 1 year.
5. Failure of an infant to gain weight or grow normally.
6. Recurrent, deep skin, or organ abscesses.
7. Persistent thrush in mouth or fungal infection on the skin.
8. Need for intravenous antibiotics to clear infections.
9. Two or more deep-seated infections including septicemia.
10. Family history of PID, early deaths, or recurrent infections.

Minor infections such as viral upper respiratory tract infections, recurrent bronchospasm, and recurrent urinary tract infections do not warrant investigations for PID. For recurrent meningitis, local defects (causing exposure of meninges to external environment) should be ruled out before suspecting PID.

Table 18.6 Major Categories of Primary Immunodeficiency Disorders

S. No.	Type of primary immunodeficiency disorders (PIDs)	Examples
1.	Defects affecting cellular and humoral immunity	Severe combined immunodeficiency disease (SCID)
2.	Primary antibody defects	• X-linked (Bruton) agammaglobulinemia (also known as BTK deficiency) • Common variable immunodeficiency (CVID) • Selective IgA deficiency
3.	Congenital defects of phagocyte number, function, or both	• Congenital neutropenia • Chronic granulomatous disease (CGD) • Leukocyte adhesion defect (LAD)
4.	Combined immune deficiencies with associated or syndromic features	• Wiskott–Aldrich syndrome • Ataxia telangiectasia • DiGeorge syndrome • Hyper-IgE syndrome
5.	Diseases of immune dysregulation	Familial hemophagocytic lymphohistiocytosis
6.	Defects in intrinsic and innate immunity	Asplenia
7.	Complement deficiencies	*Neisseria* infections seen in terminal complement deficiencies
8.	Autoinflammatory disorders	• Familial Mediterranean fever • Blau syndrome

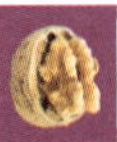

IN A NUTSHELL

Primary Immunodeficiency Disorders (PIDs)

1. Recurrent infections are the most common manifestations of PID.
2. Usual site of infections include respiratory tract, sinuses, gastrointestinal tract, skin and draining lymph nodes.
3. Autoimmune manifestations and malignancy are less common manifestations of PID.

18.10 Approach to Suspected Immunodeficiency

HISTORY

A meticulous history, targeted physical examination, and certain basic investigations can provide important clues to the type of PID. History should include age at onset of infections, type of infections, organism isolated, and response to antibiotics.

Age at Onset

Children with *primary antibody defects* are protected for first 4–6 months because of maternally transmitted antibodies. When maternally transmitted antibodies disappear, these children start developing infections.

Children with *cellular or combined immune defects* and *phagocytic defects* can present with infections any time after birth. Children with severe combined immunodeficiency (SCID) do not survive beyond infancy because of recurrent and chronic infections with unusual organisms.

Site of Infections

- Children with ***primary antibody defects*** present with recurrent pneumonia, otitis media, and sinusitis. Gastrointestinal infections can occur due to *Giardia*.
- ***Phagocytic defects*** present with suppurative infections (lymphadenitis, abscesses) and pneumonia. The only exception is leukocyte adhesion defect (LAD) where no suppuration is seen because of inability of leukocytes to reach the site of infection.
- Children with ***cellular immunodeficiencies*** can present with infection at any site, though pneumonia and recurrent diarrhea are the most common.

Organism Isolated

- Children with *cellular PID* can develop infections due to viruses, bacteria, fungi as well as mycobacteria.
- ***Primary antibody defects*** present with infections due to common community acquired organisms such as *Haemophilus influenzae* and *Streptococcus pneumoniae*.
- ***Chronic granulomatous disease*** (CGD), a phagocytic defect, presents with infections due to signature organisms such as *Staphylococcus aureus, Aspergillus, Nocardia, Serratia* and *Burkholderia*.
- Recurrent or systemic *Neisseria* infections with sepsis or pyogenic arthritis are associated with deficiency of terminal complement pathway.

Response to Antibiotics

Response to antibiotics is quick in children with primary antibody defects because they develop infections with community acquired bacteria. Response is inadequate or may be absent in phagocytic defects and cellular defects because these children frequently develop infections with unusual bacteria, mycobacteria, and fungi.

Family History

Family history of early deaths, recurrent infections, and autoimmune or collagen vascular diseases in past two generations is important. History of consanguinity may provide an important clue to an underlying autosomal recessive condition.

PHYSICAL EXAMINATION

- Children with primary antibody defects such as Bruton's tyrosine kinase (BTK) deficiency (X-linked agammaglobulinemia) typically have absent tonsils **(Fig. 18.16)**, absence of palpable lymph nodes, and absence of palpable liver and spleen. Since infections are usually bacterial and improve with antibiotics, these children may be detected late when bilateral bronchiectasis has already set in.
- Children with CGD present with recurrent suppurative lymphadenitis **(Fig. 18.17)** and pneumonia. They may have generalized lymphadenopathy and hepatosplenomegaly.
- Hepatosplenomegaly may be found in Chédiak-Higashi syndrome and SCID.

Skin and Mucous Membranes

- Petechiae, ecchymosis, and eczema are manifestations of Wiskott-Aldrich syndrome.
- Persistent oral thrush not responding to topical antifungals may be a feature of cellular deficiency.
- Recurrent skin abscesses are a feature of phagocytic defects. These abscesses are deeper in origin and sometimes "cold."

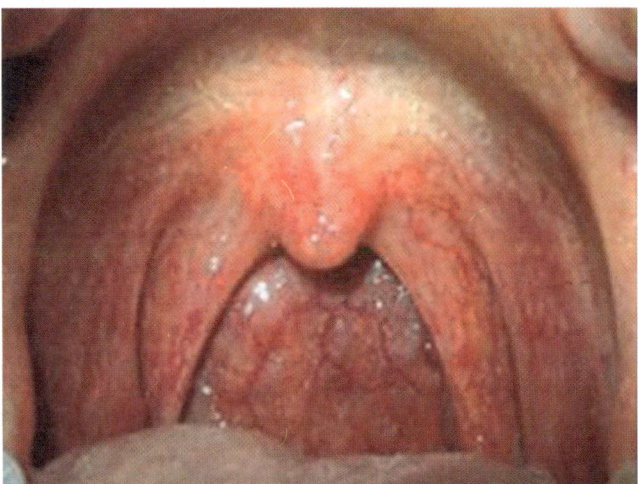

Fig. 18.16: Absent tonsils in a child with recurrent infections point to X-linked agammaglobulinemia

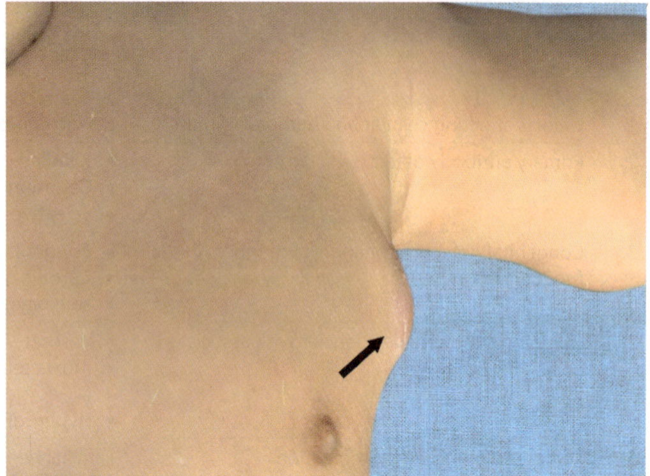

Fig. 18.17: Suppurative lymphadenitis in a child with chronic granulomatous disease

- An eczematoid rash appearing early in infancy and involving scalp, axilla, and trunk is characteristic of hyperimmunoglobulin E (IgE) syndrome. Furuncle, carbuncle, and lung abscess are common accompaniments.
- Telangiectasia can be seen in ataxia telangiectasia. They appear by 2 years of age (rarely delayed up to 9 years).

Other Features

- Coarse facial features may be seen in hyper-IgE syndrome.
- Dysmorphic facies may be noted in DiGeorge syndrome.
- Polyarthritis may occur in hypogammaglobulinemia and other antibody deficiencies.
- Hyperextensible joints are seen in hyper-IgE syndrome.

INVESTIGATIONS

Human immunodeficiency virus (HIV) infection should always be ruled out before starting investigations for PID. Hemogram and immunoglobulin profile (IgG, IgA, and IgM levels) are basic initial investigations. Further work-up may require more sophisticated investigations.

Box 18.6 enlists some screening tests for PID. Abnormalities in serum immunoglobulins and their disease associations are shown in **Table 18.7**.

Hemogram

- ***Lymphocyte count <3,000/mm³*** is abnormal in first 6 months of life. Children with SCID have persistent lymphopenia after birth.
- Hemogram in primary antibody defects does not show significant aberrations.
- ***Severe neutrophilia*** (>50,000 per mm³) (even in absence of infection) is suggestive of leukocyte adhesion defect.
- ***Neutropenia*** (intermittent or persistent) may point to congenital neutropenia.
- ***Persistent thrombocytopenia*** in a boy with eczema and recurrent infections points toward Wiskott-Aldrich syndrome (WAS).

Box 18.6 Laboratory Evaluation for Recurrent Infections

A. *General:*
1. Complete blood count, erythrocyte sedimentation rate
2. Chest X-ray (look for chronic disease and presence of thymus)
3. HIV serology

B. *B-cell defects:*
1. Quantitative immunoglobulins
2. Isohemagglutinin titer
3. Antibody response to vaccine antigens (tetanus, diphtheria, *Haemophilus influenzae, Streptococcus pneumoniae*)
4. B-cell number

C. *T lymphocyte defects:*
1. Absolute lymphocyte count
2. *Candida* skin test
3. T-cell number and in vitro function

D. *Polymorphonuclear leukocyte defect:*
1. Neutrophil count and morphology
2. Nitroblue tetrazolium reduction test
3. Dihydrorhodamine test

E. *Complement deficiency:*
1. CH50 for assessment of classical pathway
2. AH50 for assessment of alternate pathway

- Normal erythrocyte sedimentation rate (ESR) rules out chronic bacterial and fungal infections.

Immunoglobulin Profile

Very low or undetectable IgG, IgA, and IgM levels are seen in X-linked agammaglobulinemia (BTK deficiency). Low immunoglobulins are seen in children with SCID.

Children with phagocytic defects have higher immunoglobulin levels because of immune activation.

Lymphocyte Subsets

Children with SCID typically have lymphopenia and near complete absence of T lymphocytes. B lymphocytes and NK cells may be reduced or normal. On the other hand, children with BTK deficiency have normal T lymphocytes and near absent B lymphocytes, which explains their inability to produce immunoglobulins.

Tests to Assess Phagocytic Activity

- ***Nitroblue tetrazolium (NBT) test:*** Normal neutrophils show formation of formazan granules when mixed with NBT. This effect is greatly enhanced if neutrophils are stimulated to enhance phagocytic activity. In contrast, neutrophils in CGD do not show formation of formazan granules even when stimulated **(Figs. 18.18A and B)**.
- ***Dihydrorhodamine (DHR) test:*** It depends on the principle of oxidation of DHR to rhodamine by stimulated neutrophils. It is diagnostic in CGD.

Table 18.7 Abnormalities in Serum Immunoglobulin Levels

Affected immunoglobulins	*Probable diagnosis*
Low IgG, IgA, and IgM	Agammaglobulinemia
Low IgG with low IgM and/or IgA	Common variable immunodeficiency
Low IgA	Selective IgA deficiency
Low IgG1 or G2 or G3 or G4	IgG subclass deficiency
High IgG, IgA, and IgM	HIV, autoimmune diseases, CGD

(CGD: chronic granulomatous disease; Ig: immunoglobulin; HIV: human immunodeficiency virus)

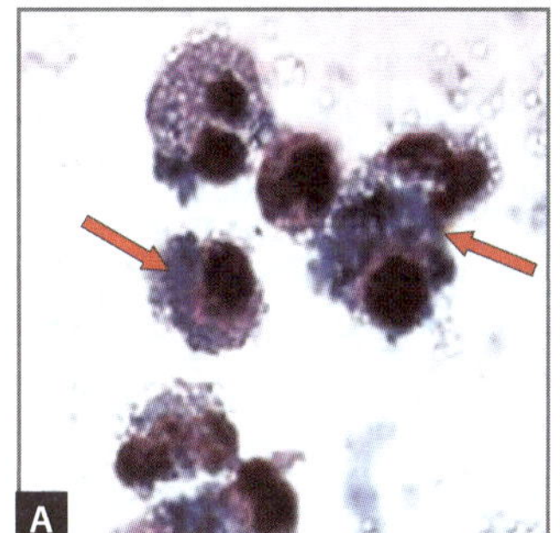

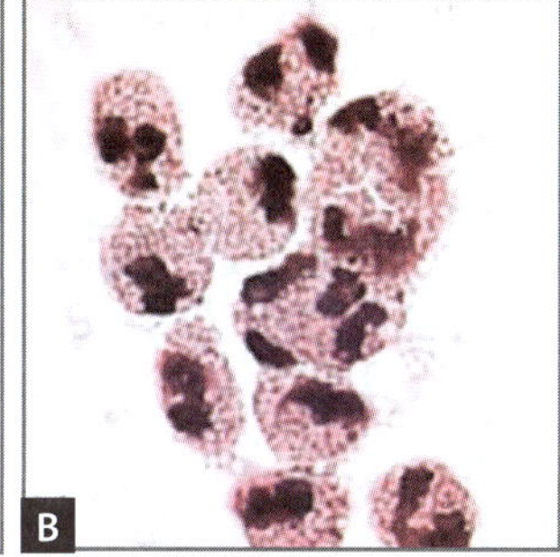

Figs. 18.18A and B: (A) Nitroblue tetrazolium test showing formazan granules (shown with arrows) in control; (B) No granules in a child with chronic granulomatous disease (CGD)

Genetic Tests

Certain advanced tests may be needed to confirm the genetic defect associated with various PIDs. These are especially important for genetic counseling and prenatal diagnosis in next pregnancy. **Table 18.8** depicts major differences in the clinical and investigative profile of these three subgroups.

Table 18.8 Clinical and Investigative Profile of Common Subgroups of Primary Immunodeficiency Disorders

	Defects affecting cellular and humoral immunity	*Primary antibody defects*	*Phagocytic defects*
Prototype	Severe combined immunodeficiency (SCID) [X-linked or autosomal recessive (AR) inheritance]	X-linked agammaglobulinemia (BTK deficiency)	• Congenital neutropenia • Chronic granulomatous disease (CGD) (X-linked or AR) • Leukocyte adhesion defect (LAD)
Age at presentation	Usually early after birth	After 4–6 months of age	Any time after birth

Contd...

Contd...

	Defects affecting cellular and humoral immunity	*Primary antibody defects*	*Phagocytic defects*
Clinical presentation	Recurrent pneumonia, diarrhea, and candidiasis	Sinusitis, otitis media, recurrent diarrhea, absent lymph nodes and tonsils	• Suppurative infections in CGD • Superficial infections without pus formation in LAD **(Figs. 18.19A to C)**
Organisms causing infections	Bacterial, mycobacterial, viral, and fungal	Usually bacterial, *Giardia*, occasionally enteroviruses	• Bacterial (*Staphylococcus aureus, Klebsiella, Burkholderia, Serratia, Nocardia*) • Fungal (*Aspergillus*)
Response to common antibiotics	+/–	+	+/–
Suggestive investigations	• Lymphopenia • Low immunoglobulins • Absent T lymphocytes • Variable B lymphocytes and natural killer (NK) cells • Absent thymic shadow	• Low immunoglobulins • Absent B lymphocytes	• Normal or high immunoglobulins • Neutropenia • Severe neutrophilia in LAD • Defective oxidative burst in CGD
Course	Die early without definitive treatment	Adult survival possible	Adult survival possible
Treatment	Hematopoietic stem cell transplantation	Periodic immunoglobulin replacement	• Antibiotic and antifungal prophylaxis in CGD • Granulocyte colony-stimulating factor (G-CSF) for neutropenia • Definitive therapy depends on type of defect

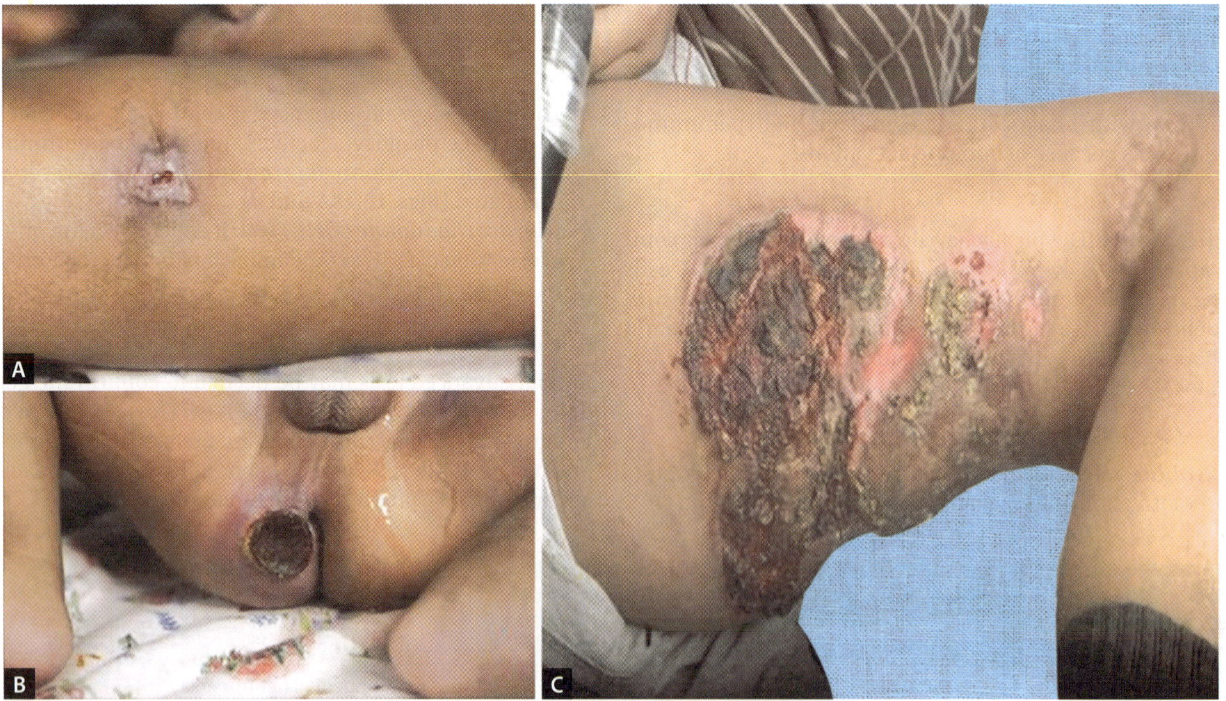

Figs. 18.19A to C: Typical nonhealing ulcers seen in leukocyte adhesion defect (LAD) (Note peculiar absence of purulent discharge)

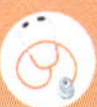

CASE STUDY Severe Combined Immunodeficiency

An 8-week-old boy was hospitalized with cough and respiratory distress for last 2 weeks. Examination revealed tachypnea and mild cyanosis. There was no lymphadenopathy or hepatosplenomegaly. Chest examination was normal. Bacille Calmette-Guérin (BCG) site showed a small papule. Investigations revealed hemoglobin (Hb) 8.9 g/dL, total leukocyte count (TLC) 6,400 (P92, L6, M2, E2), and platelet count 3.5 × 10^5 per mm^3. Blood culture was sterile and chest X-ray showed bilateral interstitial shadows. Thymic shadow was absent in the chest radiograph **(Fig. 18.20)**.

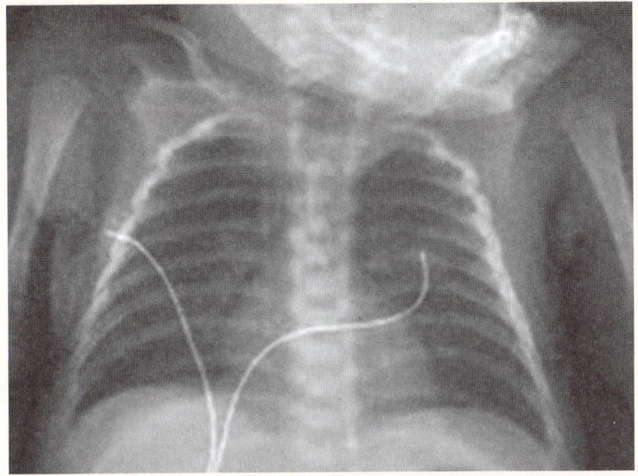

Fig. 18.20: Chest radiograph showing absent thymic shadow and bilateral infiltrates

Are there any clues toward PID in this child?

The history and examination suggest a sub-acute onset severe interstitial pneumonia. Hypoxia disproportionate to chest findings also goes in favor of interstitial pathology. Such a presentation warrants investigations for HIV infection and SCID. A negative HIV serology helps to rule out HIV infection. Lymphopenia (absolute lymphocyte count of 384/mm^3) and absent thymic shadow on chest X-ray support the diagnosis of SCID.

How important is it to isolate an organism?

The SCID patients can have bacterial, mycobacterial, viral, and fungal infections. Hence for appropriate management, it is important to isolate the organism. Since this child has received BCG, disseminated BCG disease may also be responsible for clinical manifestations.

What is the likely outcome in such a child?

Hematopoietic stem cell transplantation is the mainstay of therapy and cures basic defect. Short of that, most children die during infancy.

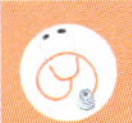

CASE STUDY X-linked Agammaglobulinemia (Bruton's Tyrosine Kinase Deficiency)

A 2-year-old boy was hospitalized with severe pneumonia. He had history of two previous hospitalizations for pneumonia during last 6 months that required intravenous antibiotics. Family history revealed death of a maternal uncle at the age of 3 years with pneumonia.

Would you think of PID in this setting?

Yes, as this child has had three severe infections requiring intravenous antibiotics.

Which group of PID is most likely in this setting?

Combined (cellular and humoral) immunodeficiency is not likely in this setting as age at onset is late at 1.5 years and a good response to antibiotics suggests bacterial infections. This clinical profile fits into primary antibody deficiency.

If you are thinking of primary antibody deficiency in such a young child, would you like to examine him for some specific clues to diagnosis?

Specific clues to primary antibody deficiency would be absent tonsils and absent lymph nodes. Also one should look for features of bronchiectasis as sequelae of repeated lung infections.

Name two tests which will be diagnostic of primary antibody deficiency in this child?

Near absent immunoglobulins (IgG, IgA, and IgM) and absent B lymphocytes would help in diagnosis of BTK deficiency. Genetic analysis would be confirmatory.

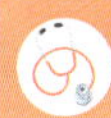

CASE STUDY Chronic Granulomatous Disease

A 3-year-old boy presented with fever and pain abdomen for 2 weeks. He had history of recurrent episodes of suppurative lymphadenitis since early infancy. Investigations led to a diagnosis of pyogenic liver abscess for the present episode. Hemogram showed polymorphonuclear leukocytosis and thrombocytosis. Immunoglobulin profile showed elevated IgG, IgA, and IgM. NBT and DHR tests confirmed the diagnosis of CGD by showing reduced oxidative burst of neutrophils.

What are the clues to a phagocytic defect in this child?

Recurrent suppurative infections in the form of lymphadenitis, pneumonia, and liver abscess suggest the possibility of phagocytic defect.

Is there a difference in clinical profile of patients with CGD from those with congenital neutropenia and LAD?

Infections in LAD are not purulent as there is a defect in transfer of neutrophils from blood vessels to site of infection. This results in severe neutrophilia in blood and paucity of neutrophils in tissues. In children with congenital neutropenia, usual infections are bacterial. Fungal infections can occur if severe neutropenia is prolonged (>5 days).

How will you manage this child?

Isolation of organism is useful in choosing appropriate antibiotics or antifungals. Prolonged course of antibiotics and antifungals are required. Once acute infection is cleared, antibiotic and antifungal prophylaxis is given life-long to prevent further infections. Hematopoietic stem cell transplantation is required, if the child continues to have recurrent infections despite antibiotic and antifungal prophylaxis.

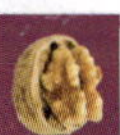

IN A NUTSHELL

Approach to Suspected Immunodeficiency

1. Primary immunodeficiency disorders (PIDs) are a heterogenous group of diseases with propensity to develop recurrent infections; though some patients can present with predominant autoimmunity and malignancy.
2. Clinically one should try to identify a subgroup of disorders based on age at onset and profile of infections.
3. Human immunodeficiency virus (HIV) infection should always be ruled out before investigating for PID.
4. Hemogram can provide vital clues:
   - Lymphopenia in early infancy points toward SCID.
   - Low absolute neutrophil count may point to congenital persistent or cyclic neutropenia.
   - Thrombocytopenia may point to Wiskott–Aldrich syndrome. Platelets are usually small in this disorder.
   - Severe neutrophilia (leukemoid reaction) points to LAD.
   - Moderate neutrophilia can be seen in CGD.
5. Immunoglobulin profile showing panhypogammaglobulinemia (low IgG, IgA, and IgM) points toward primary antibody deficiency (BTK deficiency) or SCID.
6. It is important to diagnose and treat infections early as recurrent infections can lead to sequelae like bronchiectasis. Isolation of organism is useful as the infections can be unusual (such as in SCID, CGD), and polymicrobial. Infections may require prolonged antibiotics to clear infections.
7. Specific management for PID varies with the type.
   - BTK deficiency children do well with immunoglobulin replacement.
   - SCID patients need hematopoietic stem cell transplant.
   - G-CSF (to increase neutrophil counts) is used for neutropenia.
   - Life-long antibiotic and antifungal prophylaxis is used as first line management for CGD.

Aghamohammadi A, Abolhassani H, Mohammadinejad P, et al. The approach to children with recurrent infections. Iran J Allergy Asthma Immunol. 2012;11(2):89-109.
Devonshire AL, Makhija M. Approach to primary immunodeficiency. Allergy Asthma Proc. 2019;40(6):465-9.
Justiz Vaillant AA, Qurie A. Immunodeficiency. In: StatPearls [Internet]. Treasure Island (FL): StatPearls Publishing; 2022.

19 CHAPTER Cardiovascular Disorders

AS PER NMC COMPETENCIES

PE22.1	Describe the hemodynamic changes, clinical presentation, complications and management of acyanotic heart diseases.	*Ch 19.6, Ch 19.7 Ch 19.9, Ch 19.10 Ch 19.11*
PE22.2	Describe the hemodynamic changes, clinical presentation, complications and management of cyanotic heart diseases.	*Ch 19.6, Ch 19.8 Ch 19.12, Ch 19.13*
PE22.3	Explain the etiopathogenesis, clinical presentation and management of cardiac failure in infant and children.	*Ch 19.5*
PE22.4	Explain the etiopathogenesis, clinical presentation and management of acute rheumatic fever in children.	*Ch 19.14*
PE22.5	Describe the etiopathogenesis, clinical features and management of infective endocarditis in children.	*Ch 19.15*
PE22.6	Describe the etiopathogenesis, grading, clinical features and management of hypertension in children.	*Ch 19.16*
PE22.7	Record pulse, blood pressure, temperature and respiratory rate and interpret as per the age.	*Ch 19.3*
PE22.8	Perform independently examination of the cardiovascular system—look for precordial bulge, pulsations in the precordium, JVP and its significance in children and infants, relevance of percussion in pediatric examination, auscultation and other system examination and document.	Ch 19.3
PE22.9	Interpret a chest X-ray and recognize cardiomegaly.	*Ch 19.4*
PE22.10	Interpret pediatric ECG.	*Ch 19.4*
PE22.11	Demonstrate empathy while dealing with children with cardiac diseases in every patient encounter.	*Ch 19.17*

Topics available online: ***Development of Heart; Obstructive Lesions; Pericarditis; Cardiac Arrhythmias; Surgery for Heart Diseases***

19.1 Normal Cardiac Anatomy

Unoxygenated blood from systemic circulation (systemic venous return) enters the right atrium via the superior vena cava and inferior vena cava (**Fig. 19.1**). Right atrium also receives blood from coronary sinus. Right atrium opens into right ventricle via tricuspid valve. Tricuspid valve apparatus attaches both to the ventricular septum and to the right ventricle free wall and is more apically attached than the mitral valve.

Right ventricle is coarsely trabeculated, smoothening toward the outflow tract. The pulmonary valve connects right ventricle to the main pulmonary artery. Pulmonary valve is supported by the subpulmonary infundibulum and sits higher than aortic valve. Normal pulmonary valve is tricuspid and sits left and anterior to the aortic valve. Main pulmonary artery bifurcates into right and left pulmonary arteries, which connect to respective lungs.

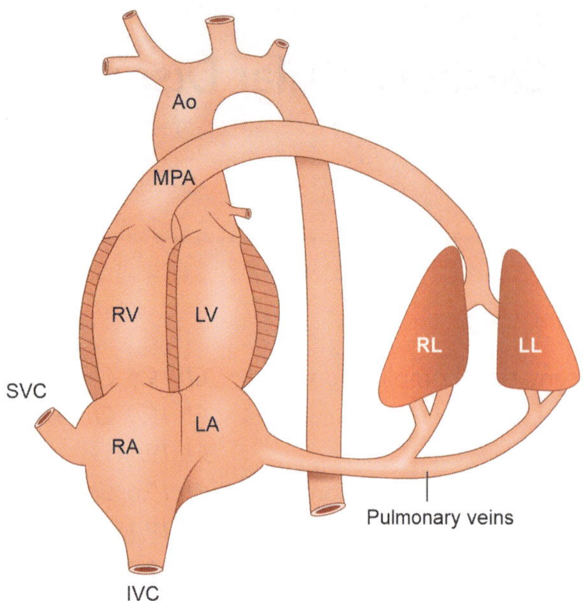

Fig. 19.1: Line diagram depicts course of circulation after birth. Desaturated blood, i.e., systemic venous return (via SVC and IVC) enters right atrium, through tricuspid valve to right ventricle and then to pulmonary arteries. Oxygenated blood, i.e., pulmonary venous return (four pulmonary veins) comes to left atrium and through mitral valve enters left ventricle and then aorta

Right pulmonary artery has a straighter course, crosses posterior to ascending aorta and below the right bronchus (eparterial right bronchus) to join right lung hilum while left pulmonary artery crosses over the left bronchus (left bronchus-hyparterial) before joining left hilum.

Pulmonary blood flow returns to left atrium via four pulmonary veins, two from each lung, and join posterior wall of left atrium. Left atrial appendage is crescent shaped. Left atrium is connected to left ventricle via mitral valve, which is bileaflet, and does not have septal attachment of chordae. The left ventricle is smoothly trabeculated and outflows into the aorta via aortic valve. Aortic valve is tricuspid and sits posterior and right of the pulmonary valve. Right coronary artery arises from right aortic sinus and left coronary artery from left aortic sinus.

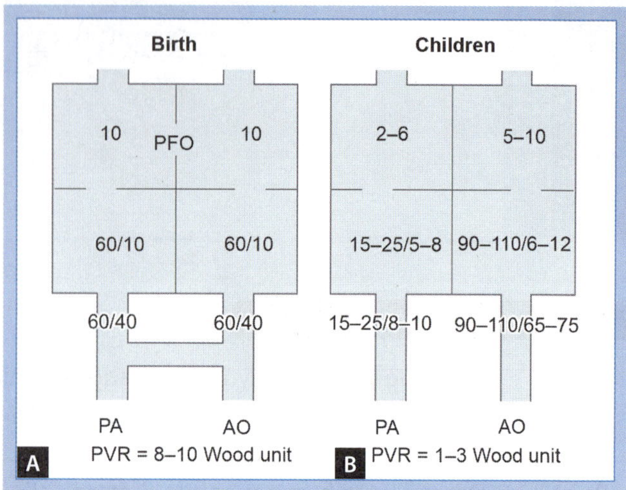

Figs. 19.2A and B: Pressures in cardiac chambers (in mm Hg): (A) At birth; (B) In children

(PFO: patent foramen ovale; PVR: pulmonary vascular resistance)

Both atria are separated by interatrial septum while both ventricles are separated by interventricular septum. Normal pressure range in all cardiac chambers at birth and in childhood is shown in **Figures 19.2A and B.**

Cardiac anatomy and examination of cardiac specimens. In: Allen HD, Shaddy RE, Penny DJ, Feltes TS, Cetta F (Eds), 9th edition. Moss and Adams' Heart Disease in Infants, Children, and Adolescents Including the Fetus and Young Adult. Philadelphia: Lippincott Williams and Wilkins; 2016. pp. 1483-518.

19.2 Fetal Circulation

INTRODUCTION

The heart assumes its normal four-chambered shape by the end of 8 weeks of intrauterine life. After that, changes consist mainly in the growth of the heart as a whole. However, significant differences exist between the fetal circulation and postnatal circulation. Unique aspect of the fetal cardiovascular circulation is its interface with placenta.

Oxygenated blood enters the fetal circulation via placental transfer. Umbilical vein carries oxygenated blood, which enters the fetus at the umbilicus and course through liver to join the portal vein. The ductus venosus provides a low resistance bypass between the portal vein and the inferior vena cava so most of the umbilical venous blood shunts through the ductus venosus to the inferior vena cava. Eustachian valve directs inferior vena cava blood across the foramen ovale to the left atrium. The inferior vena cava blood comprises the streams of hepatic veins, umbilical veins, and that reaching the inferior vena cava directly from lower extremities and kidneys. Deoxygenated blood from upper extremity returns via superior vena cava to right atrium and is preferentially directed to the right ventricle. The right ventricle pumps this blood into pulmonary arteries, and across the patent ductus arteriosus into the descending aorta. Due to this streaming of blood in the fetal heart, coronary and carotid arteries get most oxygenated blood while lower body gets perfused with less oxygenated blood. Oxygen saturation and partial pressure in different chambers during fetal life is given in **Figure 19.3**.

During fetal life, as lungs are relatively high resistance unit, only a small amount of blood from right ventricle flows through the pulmonary arteries and veins. Thus, little of the right ventricular output reaches the left ventricle through the lungs; the rest goes through the ductus arteriosus into the descending aorta. The two ventricles are, therefore, acting together in parallel. The left

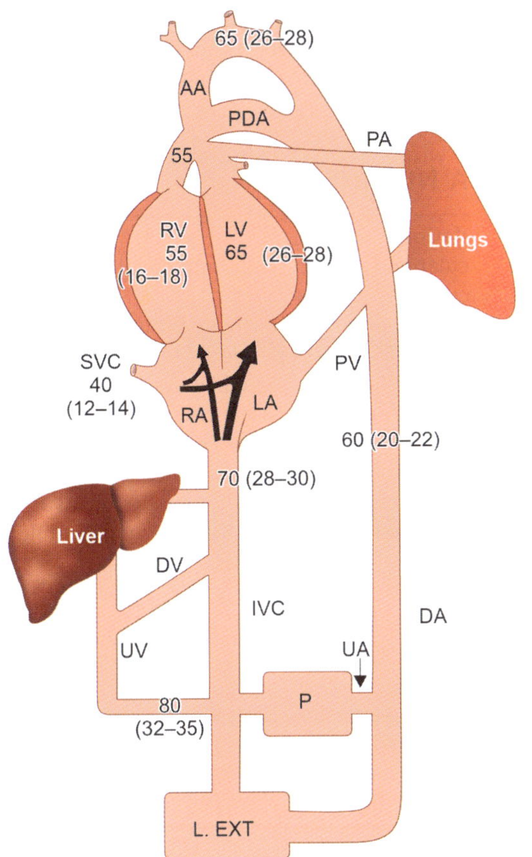

Fig. 19.3: Fetal circulation. The figure indicates oxygen saturation with partial pressure of oxygen in parentheses

(P: placenta; DA: descending aorta; DV: ductus venosus; IVC: inferior vena cava; PA: pulmonary artery; PV: pulmonary vein; SVC: superior vena cava; UA: umbilical artery; UV: umbilical vein)

ventricle supplies the head and upper extremities while the right ventricle supplies the trunk, viscera, and the lower extremities.

The fetal cardiac output is approximately 450 mL/kg/min, the ratio between right ventricular and left ventricular output being approximately 1.3:1. In postnatal life, the two ventricles are connected in series and therefore, the outputs of right and left ventricles are approximately identical.

CIRCULATORY ADJUSTMENTS AT BIRTH

Circulatory adjustments occur immediately following birth and continue to occur for a variable period following birth. This change is brought about because of a shift of the main organ responsible for gas exchange from placenta (in fetus) to lungs (in neonate). A summary of these changes is given below:

Loss of Low-resistance Placental Circulation

Clamping of the umbilical cord results in loss of low resistance placental circulation. This causes a sudden increase in systemic vascular resistance, aortic blood pressure, and the left ventricular systolic pressure. The left ventricular diastolic pressure also rises, causing increase in left atrial pressure.

Closure of Ductus Venosus

Ductus venosus closes because of a sudden reduction of flow, secondary to cessation of placental circulation. The exact pathophysiology is not known. Flow through the ductus venosus disappears by the 7th day of postnatal life.

Closure of Foramen Ovale

The loss of placental flow results in a decrease in the volume of blood returning to the right atrium. The right atrial pressure decreases. The left atrial pressure becomes higher as described above and exceeds the right atrial pressure. As a result, septum primum comes closer to septum secundum to close the flow across foramen ovale (functional closure). This occurs by 3rd month of life. Anatomical closure of the foramen ovale occurs over a period of months to years.

Increased Pulmonary Circulation

Sudden expansion of lungs with the first few breaths causes a fall in pulmonary vascular resistance and an increased flow into the pulmonary trunk and arteries. The pulmonary artery pressure falls due to lowering of pulmonary vascular resistance. The pressure relations between the aorta and pulmonary trunk are reversed so that the flow through the ductus arteriosus is reversed. Instead of blood flowing from the pulmonary artery to aorta, the direction of flow through the ductus arteriosus is from the aorta to pulmonary trunk.

Closure of Ductus Arteriosus

During fetal life, patency of ductus arteriosus is maintained by the combined relaxant effect of low oxygen tension and endogenously produced prostaglandins. In full term neonate, oxygen is the most important factor controlling ductus closure. When PaO_2 of the blood passing through the ductus increases to 50 mm Hg, the ductal wall constricts. This effect of oxygen may be direct or mediated by its effects on prostaglandin synthesis.

In full term neonates the ductus arteriosus closes within 10–21 days. This results in the establishment of the postnatal circulation, which is in series. The ductus arteriosus of preterm baby is less responsive to oxygen. Some functional patency and flow can be demonstrated through the ductus arteriosus for a few days after birth.

APPEARANCE OF MURMUR IN NEONATES WITH HEART DEFECTS

Immediately after birth, the pulmonary pressure and resistance is equal or only slightly lower than the systemic pressure and resistance **(Fig. 19.2A)**. Therefore, even if there is a communication between the two sides, e.g., atrial or ventricular septal defect or patent ductus arteriosus, there is very little flow from left to the right side. Thus, an atrial or ventricular septal defect, or a PDA does not manifest at birth or in first few days after birth.

The pulmonary vascular resistance falls rapidly to reach normal adult levels by 2–3 weeks in normal babies. This results in markedly lower pulmonary pressure as compared to systemic pressure **(Fig. 19.2A)**. The fall in pulmonary vascular resistance and pressure is however slower in the presence of a ventricular septal defect or patent ductus arteriosus and the pulmonary vascular resistance reaches adult values around 6–10 weeks. The ventricular septal defect or patent ductus arteriosus murmurs tend to appear by the middle or the end of the first week of life. They gradually increase in intensity as the pressure and resistance in the pulmonary circuit fall. The maximum shunt becomes apparent only by 6–10 weeks or more, when the pulmonary vascular resistance may have reached its nadir.

In atrial septal defect, the right ventricular hypertrophy, present at birth, prevents a left to right shunt. This right ventricular hypertrophy takes at least 6 months to regress. The shunt of atrial septal defect therefore does not manifest till at least 6 months of life.

Dependent Shunt

The clinical manifestations of atrial, ventricular, or aortopulmonary communication show rapid changes in the first few weeks or months of life, because of their dependency on the fall of pulmonary vascular resistance. These shunts therefore are also known as "dependent" shunts.

Obligatory Shunt

On the other hand, the murmur of obstructive lesions and valvular leaks are audible immediately after birth. Obstructive lesions (aortic or pulmonary stenosis) and valvular leaks (mitral, aortic, pulmonary, or tricuspid regurgitation) would be operative from birth. Some other defects such as left ventricular to right atrial shunt, arteriovenous fistula are also functional from birth as the flow through these defects is not dependent on the fall of pulmonary vascular resistance and these are called "obligatory" shunts.

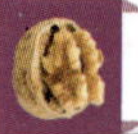

IN A NUTSHELL

Fetal Circulation

1. Fetal circulation is a circulation in parallel while neonatal/adult circulation is in series.
2. Circulatory adjustments at birth are brought about because of a shift from placental dependence for gas exchange in the fetus to pulmonary gas exchange in the neonate.
3. Changes from fetal to neonatal circulation include loss of placental circulation with clamping of the umbilical cord; increase in systemic vascular resistance; closure of ductus venosus, foramen ovale, and ductus arteriosus; fall in pulmonary vascular resistance; and an increased flow into the pulmonary trunk and arteries.

Friedman AH, Fahey JT. The transition from fetal to neonatal circulation: normal responses and implications for infants with heart disease. Semin Perinatol. 1993;17(2):106-21.

Rudolph AM. Congenital cardiovascular malformations and the fetal circulation. Arch Dis Child Fetal Neonatal Ed. 2010;95(2):F132-6.

Sansoucie DA, Cavaliere TA. Transition from fetal to extrauterine circulation. Neonatal Netw. 1997;16(2):5-12.

19.3 Approach to a Child with Heart Disease *PE 22.7, PE 22.8*

HISTORY TAKING

A carefully elicited history and proper clinical examination are crucial in arriving at an accurate diagnosis in >60% of childhood cardiac conditions. Various symptoms, which point toward the presence of heart disease, are described here.

Breathlessness

While eliciting this symptom, emphasis should be laid on the severity of dyspnea, i.e., if it occurs at rest or at activity; and the level of activity, which brings about this symptom. In children, participation in routine activities with peers and ability to attend school properly or ambulate around in house are important pointers. Dyspnea can also occur in respiratory pathologies or anemia and thus further symptoms and signs are employed to differentiate amongst various etiologies.

Feeding Difficulty, Suck-Rest-Cycle, Feeding Diaphoresis

This symptom is described for infantile age group. It is the counterpart of breathlessness on exertion in older children. Breastfeeding is an active energy intensive exercise for infants. Also, the metabolic needs of an infant with a large left to right shunt are higher. Such an infant is in a catabolic state and feeds voraciously, but due to the exertion of feeding, baby gets tired and pauses to catch a breath, and then repeats this *suck-rest cycle*. Thus the *feeding time is prolonged* as compared to healthy infants. Also the sympathetic stimulation during feeding produces sweating over forehead classically known as *feeding diaphoresis*.

Failure to Thrive

Infants with shunt lesions and increased pulmonary blood flow have increased metabolic demands due to excess energy consumed in the effort of breathing. They lag behind in gaining age-appropriate weight and are thin built and marasmic. Although their length gain is age appropriate.

Chest Pain

Chest pain in children is most commonly non-cardiac. It commonly occurs due to musculoskeletal or pleural etiology. Musculoskeletal pain has associated tenderness and pleural pain would aggravate with deep inspiration. Cardiac chest pain can occur due to pericardial or myocardial etiologies. Pericardial pain is relieved by sitting in a stooping forward posture. Myocardial pain characteristically aggravates with exertion and is relieved by rest. It occurs in conditions causing increased myocardial demand such as severe aortic stenosis or severe pulmonary stenosis or in conditions which cause compromise to the coronary blood supply such as ALCAPA (anomalous left coronary artery from pulmonary artery) or coronary stenosis (familial hypercholesterolemia, vasculitis).

Swelling Over Body

Due to increased hydrostatic pressure in conditions, which cause right heart failure, there is transudation of fluid into the dependent parts of body such as feet (in older children) and back (in infants). The swelling generally increases as the day progresses and is least in the morning. The swelling rarely involves the face and periorbital region and it is responsive to diuretics.

Reduced Urinary Output

This is primarily a symptom of renal disease, but in certain cardiac conditions with reduced cardiac output, the renal perfusion pressure is reduced resulting in reduced urinary output. Such conditions include severe left ventricular dysfunction, tight coarctation of aorta, critical aortic stenosis, and other conditions with duct dependent systemic circulation.

Syncope

Syncope is defined as abrupt, transient, complete loss of consciousness with loss of postural tone with rapid and spontaneous recovery. It occurs due to cerebral hypoperfusion to reticular activating system (RAS) that supports consciousness. Important cardiac causes of syncope include critical valvular stenosis (aortic stenosis, mitral stenosis), bradyarrhythmia (sick sinus syndrome, complete heart block), tachyarrhythmia (atrial flutter or fibrillation with fast ventricular rate, ventricular tachycardia).

Cyanotic Spell

Children with cyanotic congenital heart disease with pulmonary stenosis have cyanosis at rest. But during activities such as crying, feeding, defecation, the cyanosis can worsen, and such patients present with cyanotic spells. Cyanotic spells are defined as episodes of hyperpnea associated with deepening of cyanosis that may result in seizures, unconsciousness, coma, or death. Common age of occurrence of such spells is between 6 months to 2 years of age. Mechanism of cyanotic spells is sympathetic stimulation leading to infundibular spasm and tachycardia, which leads to further reduction in pulmonary flow by increasing the right to left shunt. Immature respiratory center responds to desaturation and acidosis by inducing hyperpnea, which further causes increased venous return of hypoxic blood by producing negative intrathoracic pressure. This vicious cycle continues culminating in cyanotic spell.

CLINICAL EXAMINATION

Depending on the presence of above symptoms congenital heart diseases can be classified into the acyanotic and cyanotic categories, further classification is shown in the **Flowchart 19.1**. Clinical examination starts with vital sign assessment, general physical examination, looking for peripheral or systemic signs of heart disease followed by comprehensive cardiovascular systemic examination.

Pulse

Radial pulse should be assessed for pulse rate, rhythm, volume, symmetry, and pulse deficit. Normal pulse rate for age is given in **Table 19.1**. Pulse should be counted for full 1 minute. *High volume pulse* with bounding character is present in lesions with run-off of blood from aorta such as PDA, AP window, aortic

Flowchart 19.1: Classification of congenital heart disease with major symptoms of each sub-group

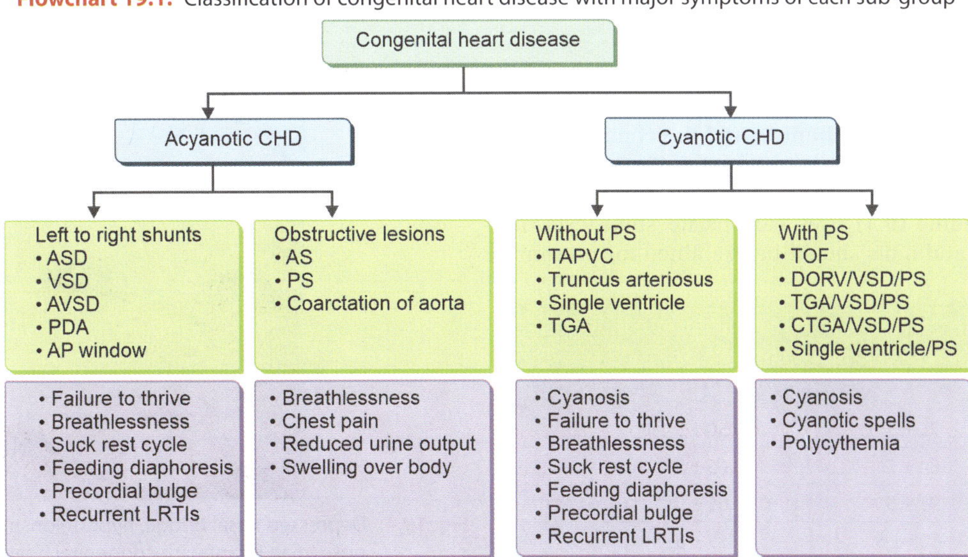

Table 19.1 Normal Range of Age Appropriate Pulse Rate	
Age	*Normal range of resting pulse rate per minute*
Birth–4 weeks Preterm Term	 120–160 100–140
28 days–1 year	100–120
1–5 years	90–110
6–12 years	80–100
Adolescents	60–90

regurgitation, and truncus arteriosus; *low volume pulse* points toward stenotic lesions such as mitral or aortic stenosis or coarctation of aorta. Asymmetry of peripheral pulses is seen in coarctation of aorta.

Blood Pressure

Use the right size of cuff to obtain correct readings. Compare with the normal range for age as shown below (**Table 19.2**). The blood pressure cuff should cover at least two-thirds of the length of the arm and most of the circumference. If the cuff is small, it would give erroneously high reading. Appropriate cuff size for different ages is: infant—2.5 cm; 1 month to 1 year—5 cm; 1-8 years—9 cm; older children—12.5 cm.

In a child suspected to be having heart disease, blood pressure is taken in all the four limbs. Different size cuff should be used to measure arm and leg blood pressure. Hypertension with upper limb blood pressure more than in the legs suggests coarctation of aorta. High blood pressure with wide difference between the systolic and diastolic readings suggests aortic runoff. Severe aortic stenosis would result in narrow pulse pressure.

Respiratory Rate

Infants and children with heart disease have tachypnea with chest retractions. Tachypnea in children is defined as respiratory rate more than expected for that age. **Table 19.3** shows the upper limit of respiratory rate for infants and children.

General Physical Examination

Children with congenital heart disease (CHD) have frequent association with genetic syndromes, and the common ones include Down syndrome, DiGeorge syndrome, Ellis-van Crevald syndrome, William syndrome, Turner syndrome, Rubella syndrome, etc. (**Table 19.4**). Eyes, ears, palate, spine, external genitalia, digits, and nails should be examined for presence of dysmorphism (**Figs. 19.4 to 19.7**). Dental, skin, and joint examination are important in children suspected to have heart disease.

Table 19.2 Normal Range of Age Appropriate Blood Pressure in Children (in mm Hg)		
Age	*Systolic*	*Diastolic*
1–3 months	75 ± 5	50 ± 5
4–12 months	84 ± 5	65 ± 5
1– 8 years	95 ± 5	65 ± 5
9–14 years	105 ± 5	65 ± 5

Table 19.3 Normal Range of Age Appropriate Respiratory Rate in Children	
Age	*Normal range of resting respiratory rate per minute*
Birth to <2 weeks	<60/min
2–12 months	<50/min
1–5 years	<40/min

Table 19.4 Common Syndromes Associated with Heart Defects		
Syndrome	*Heart defect*	*Chromosomal defect*
Goldenhar syndrome	Tetralogy of Fallot	22q11
Congenital rubella syndrome	PDA	20p12 (*Jagged1* gene)
Holt–Oram syndrome	ASD, VSD	12q2
Turner syndrome	Coarctation of aorta	5q35
Trisomy 21	Endocardial cushion defect	21q22
Noonan syndrome	Pulmonary stenosis	12q24
Ellis-van Creveld syndrome	Single atrium	4p16
Williams syndrome	Supravalvular aortic stenosis	7q11 (*elastin* gene)
Marfan syndrome	Mitral valve prolapse	15q21 (*fibrillin* gene)

Cyanosis

Cyanosis is of two types: Central and peripheral. Central cyanosis is present in fingers, toes, and mucous membranes of the mouth

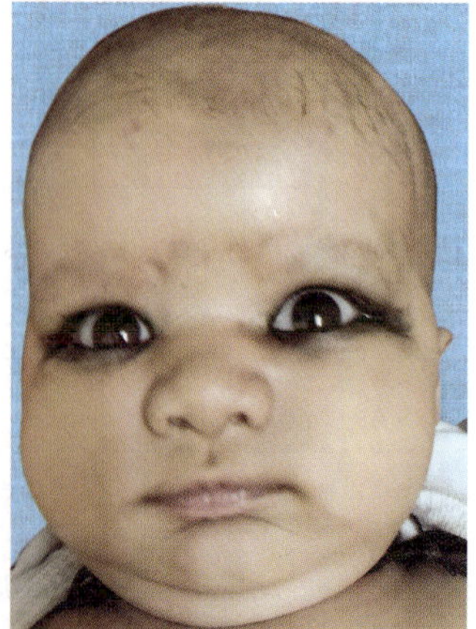

Fig. 19.4: Depressed nasal bridge, hypertelorism, and short stubby nose in an infant with congenital heart defect

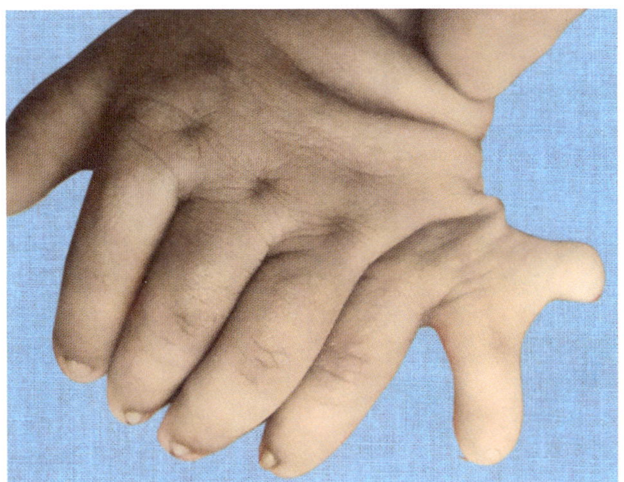

Fig. 19.5: Polysyndactyly in a patient with congenital heart defect

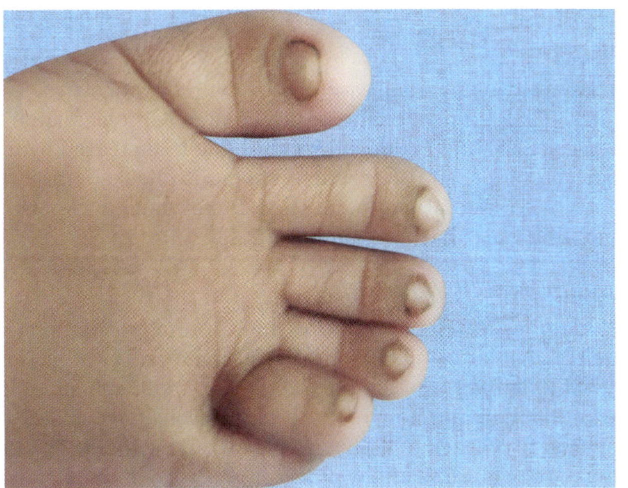

Fig. 19.6: Hypoplastic nails in a patient with Elis-van Creveld syndrome

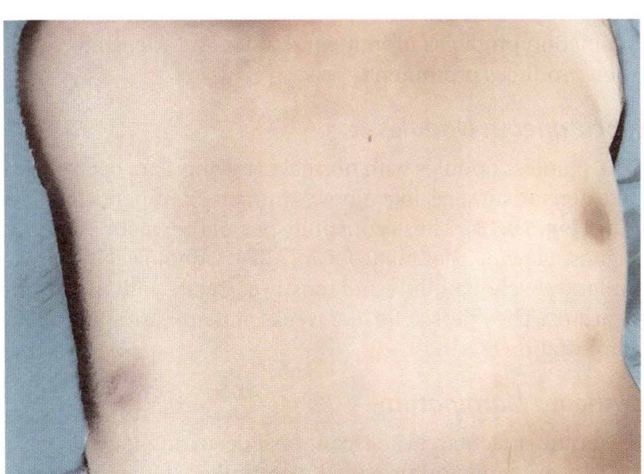

Fig. 19.7: Widely spaced nipples in an infant with congenital heart defect

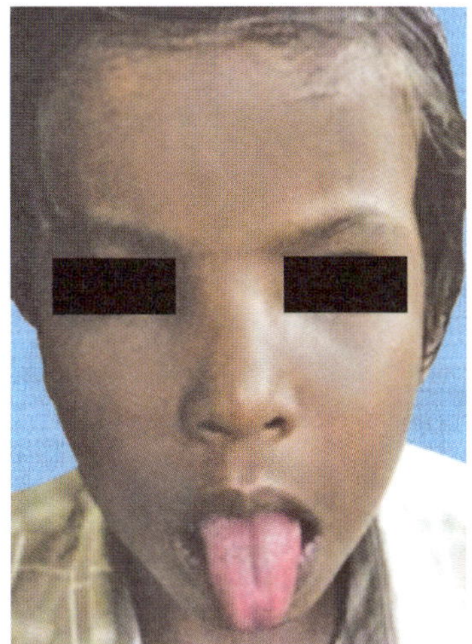

Fig. 19.8: Figure showing cyanosis of tongue in a child with tetralogy of Fallot

and tongue. Presence of central cyanosis implies low systemic arterial oxygen saturation (**Fig. 19.8**). It is frequently associated with polycythemia (**Fig. 19.9**). Peripheral cyanosis is due to peripheral vasoconstriction.

Central cyanosis can occur because of (*i*) inadequate pulmonary blood flow (pulmonary stenosis, right to left shunt); or (*ii*) inadequate oxygenation of pulmonary blood flow (lung pathology). Pulmonary hypoxia also results in *polycythemia* and *clubbing of* fingers and toes. Third cause of central cyanosis is methemoglobinemia, which occurs due to excessive production of methemoglobin following exposure to oxidant drugs, chemicals, or toxins. Methemoglobin cannot bind oxygen, resulting in functional anemia and failure of delivery of oxygen to tissues. However, clubbing does not occur in methemoglobinemia.

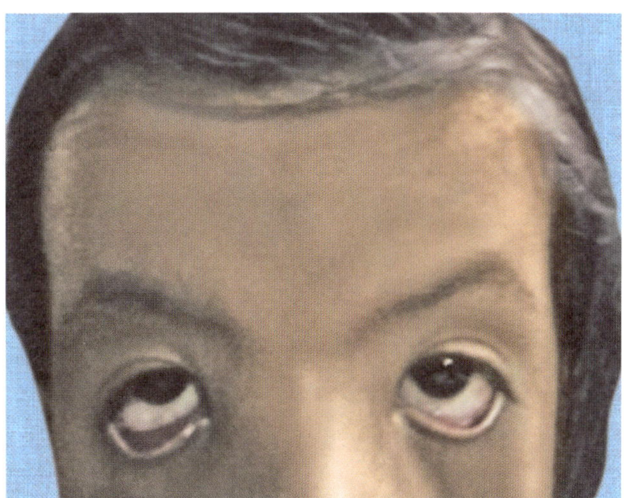

Fig. 19.9: Palpebral conjunctival congestion due to polycythemia in a child with cyanotic congenital heart defect (CHD)

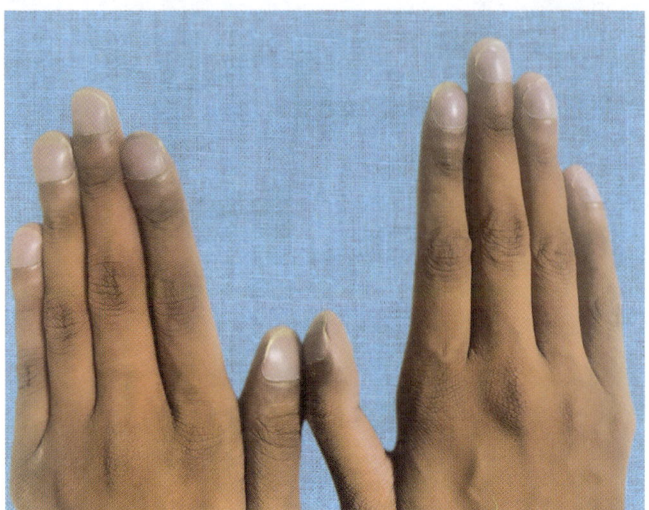

Fig. 19.10: Central cyanosis with clubbing, parrot beak appearance of nail beds

Central cyanosis thus indicates presence of heart disease if methemoglobinemia and lung disease can be ruled out.

Clubbing

It is soft fluctuant swelling of roots of nails, resulting in a visible bulbous prominence of the distal portion of the terminal phalanges of fingers and toes. It is commonly seen in children with cyanotic congenital heart disease and patients with chronic infective endocarditis (**Figs. 19.10 and 19.11**). It occurs due to the entrapment of various growth factors in the capillary network of nail-bed which escape the pulmonary circulation due to intra-cardiac right to left shunt. There are four grades of clubbing starting from softening of nail bed (grade 1), positive Shamroth sign (grade 2), parrot beak appearance (grade 3), hypertrophic osteo-arthropathy (grade 4).

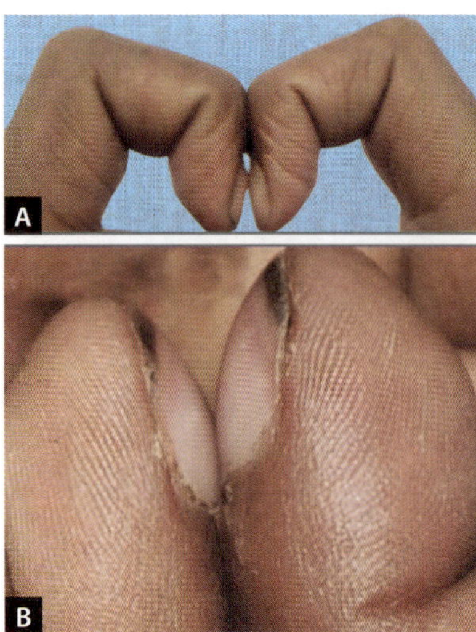

Figs. 19.11A and B: (A) Normal nail-bed angle; (B) Schamroth sign, obliteration of Lovibond angle

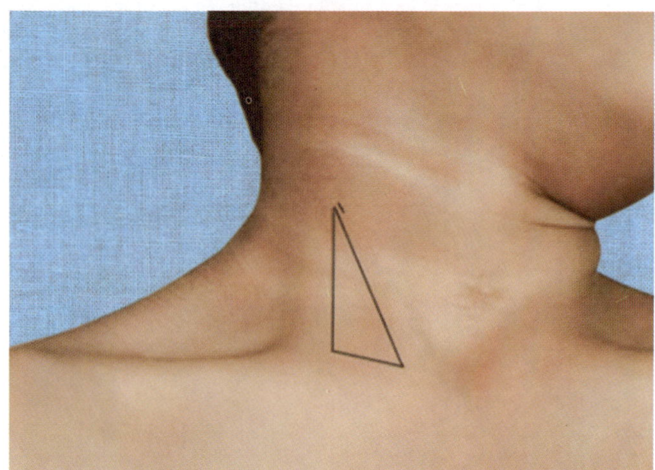

Fig. 19.12: Jugular venous waveform seen between two heads of sternomastoid muscle

Edema

In patients with heart disease, edema denotes congestive heart failure (CHF). It occurs due to sub-cutaneous transudation of intravascular fluid at dependent sites due to increased hydrostatic pressure. The sites where edema is checked are 2 cm superior to medial malleolus, and sacral edema at back in infants because that is the dependent site.

Jugular Venous Waveform

JVP denotes the right atrial pressures and hemodynamics as internal jugular vein is valveless and is in direct continuation with the right atrium. For checking JVP, patient is made to lie in 45° position and height of the venous waveform is noticed between two heads of the sternomastoid muscle (**Fig. 19.12**). There are two waves and two descents. A wave indicates atrial contraction, x descent denotes atrial diastole, V wave denotes atrial filling and y descent denotes atrial emptying due to opening of tricuspid valve. Mean atrial pressures are elevated in patients with CHF so both the waves are tall. RV diastolic dysfunction produces prominent *a* wave, and tricuspid regurgitation produces prominent *v* wave.

Subcutaneous Nodules

Firm, painless nodules with normal overlying skin, occurring on the extensor surfaces like elbow, shin, olecranon, occiput, and spine (**Fig. 19.13**). These constitute one of the major criteria for diagnosing acute rheumatic fever (ARF). Pathologically they are similar to Aschoff nodule and mostly correlate with the severity of carditis. They persist for 1–2 weeks and are rarely an isolated manifestation of ARF.

Erythema Marginatum

It is a pink, macular, evanescent rash occurring for minutes to hours over trunk and proximal extremities. It also constitutes one of the major criteria for diagnosis of ARF, but it is seen only in fair-skinned individuals.

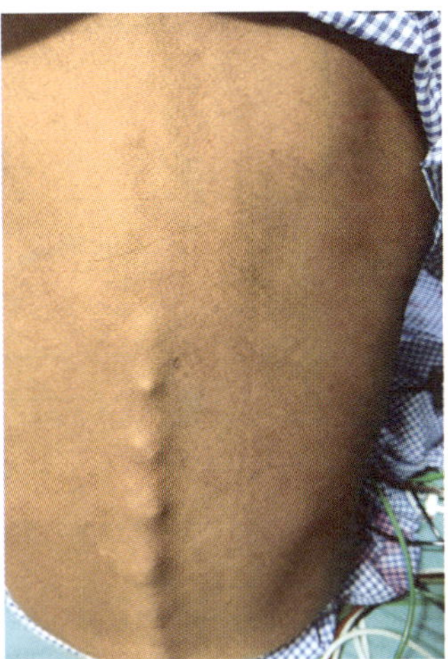

Fig. 19.13: Subcutaneous nodules seen over spinous prominence in a patient with acute rheumatic fever

Osler Nodes

These are cutaneous manifestation of infective endocarditis. They are tender, purple, pink nodules with a pale center and average diameter ranges from 1–1.5 mm. Pathogenesis is micro emboli from heart lodging in the glomus apparatus of dermis. Location is distal fingers and toes (**Fig. 19.14**). They disappear within few days leaving no sequelae.

Janeway Lesions

These are cutaneous manifestation of infective endocarditis. They are irregular, non-tender, erythematous or hemorrhagic macules or papules commonly found on palms and soles. Pathogenesis is cardiac micro emboli producing micro-abscesses in the dermis (**Fig. 19.15**). They last for days or weeks with complete healing.

Arthritis

Migratory polyarthritis is a major criterion to diagnose acute rheumatic fever. The joints are exquisitely painful and tender and the patient winces even with the touch of a bedsheet. There may be overlying erythema and swelling. The large joints are involved with one joint getting better before the involvement of next joint. There is no residual joint deformity once the arthritis heals.

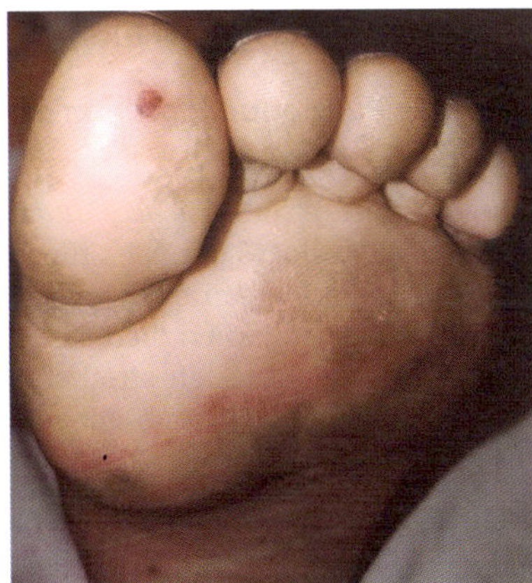

Fig. 19.14: Osler node seen over pulp of big toe in a child with infective endocarditis

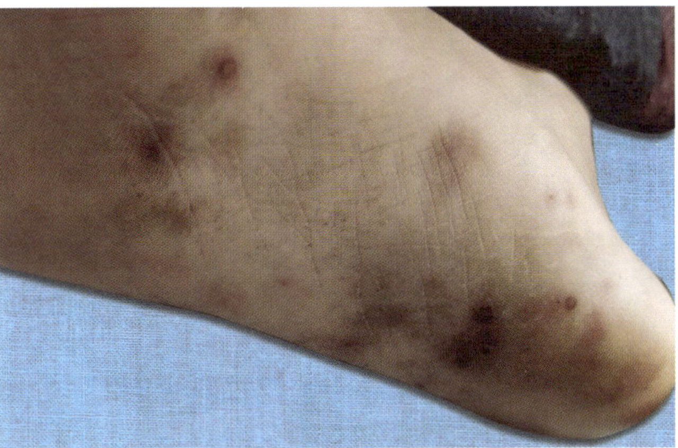

Fig. 19.15: Janeway lesions seen over sole of foot

Chorea

Chorea is major criteria to diagnose acute rheumatic fever. These are quasipurposive, repetitive movements at large joints precipitated with emotional lability. They are primarily seen in children between the ages of 5–15 years. The course of the lines may wax and wane and they generally disappear within 6 months. Few signs which can be elicited in patients with rheumatic chorea include jack-in-the-box tongue (in and out of the mouth movement of tongue when asked to show the tongue), milk-maid grip (rhythmic contractions of closed fist when asked to hold examiner's finger in the fist), pronator sign (pronation of arms when asked to raise the arms overhead), and spooning or hyper-extension of fingers of out-stretched arms.

Dental Examination

Dental examination is very important in evaluating a pediatric patient with heart disease. Infections involving the gingiva, periapical area and root of the tooth including dental caries predispose the patient to infective endocarditis by producing bacteremia during daily dental care such as brushing and flossing. Children with heart disease are generally advised to maintain good dental hygiene (**Fig. 19.16**).

CARDIOVASCULAR SYSTEM EXAMINATION

Inspection, Palpation, Percussion

Normal chest is bilaterally symmetrical. Chest asymmetry is seen in the form of precordial bulge in children with volume overload lesions. Apical impulse is felt as the most prominent and outermost point of maximum impulse. Normal apical impulse lies in fifth intercostal space medial to mid-clavicular line and is felt for first half of systole and produces a gentle lift. In cardiomegaly, the impulse is displaced outwards and downwards. The character of apical impulse is hyperdynamic

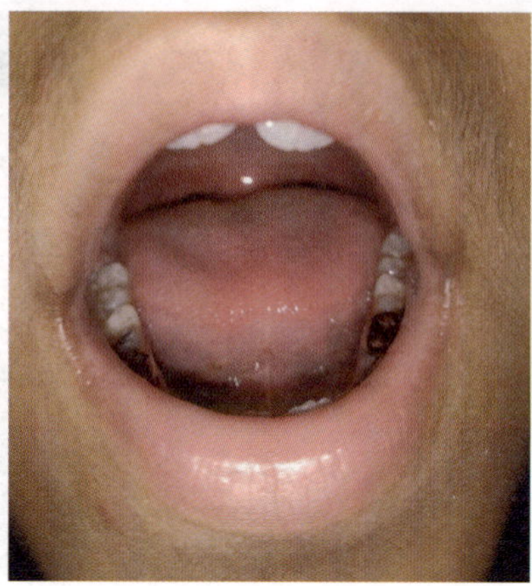

Fig. 19.16: Dental examination showing caries in a child

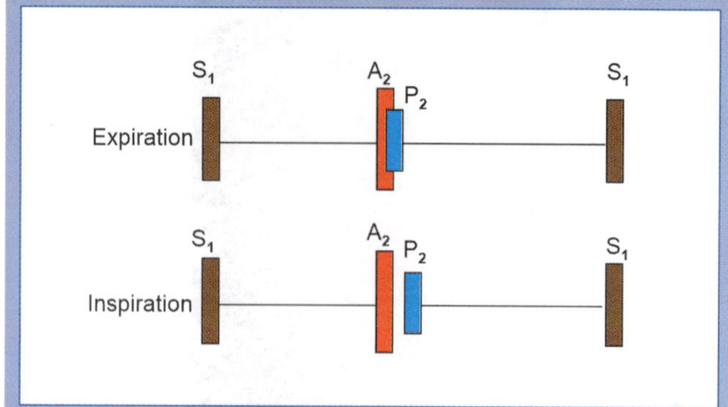

Fig. 19.17: Line diagram showing normal splitting second heart sound (S_2) with respiration, i.e., single second heart sound during expiration and splitting into A_2 and P_2 component during inspiration

in volume overload lesions producing increased amplitude of lift. In pressure overload lesions, the apical impulse is heaving in nature and produces sustained lift lasting >50% of systole duration. Systolic or diastolic thrills can be palpated over the precordium depending on the site of lesions. Heart sounds if very loud, can be palpated over the apex or base of heart.

Precordial Bulge (Frontal Swelling)

In congenital heart diseases with shunt lesions and increased pulmonary blood flow, there is ventricular chamber dilation. In infants and young children, the chest wall is pliable due to softer rib cage, hence the underlying cardiac dilation protrudes the overlying ribcage and produces bulge on the left side, called as precordial bulge or frontal swelling.

Percussion starts with localization of abdominal situs; stomach tympany and hepatic dullness are localized. Right and left heart borders are localized by percussion for cardiac dullness. Left second intercostal space is percussed to look for dilated pulmonary artery.

AUSCULTATION

The first heart sound is produced by closure of atrioventricular valves (mitral and tricuspid) at the onset of systole and normally a single component is audible. Second heart sound is produced due to closure of semilunar valves (aortic and pulmonary) at the end of systole; aortic component occurring before the pulmonary component. Correct evaluation of second heart sound is very crucial in the precise evaluation of heart defects.

Normal second heart sound denotes (i) normal intensity of both components, i.e., aortic closure sound (A_2) and pulmonary closure sound (P_2); and (ii) normal split and variation with respiration.

During expiration, both the components are superimposed on each other and only a single second sound is heard. During inspiration, the aortic component can be heard before the pulmonary component, producing a split sound (**Fig. 19.17**).

Abnormal Second Sound

Abnormalities of the second sound always indicate presence of heart disease. It has been included as a minor criterion only because interpretation of auscultation of second sound is prone to subjective variation.

Abnormalities of the Aortic Component (A_2) of the Second Sound

Intensity: Aortic closure sound may be accentuated or diminished in intensity. A_2 is *accentuated* in conditions where the aortic valve closes against a higher pressure in the left ventricle, as in systemic hypertension, and aortic regurgitation. A_2 is *diminished* in intensity or may be inaudible when the movement of aortic valve is compromised as in fibrosis or calcification, or when the aortic valve is absent.

Timing: Aortic closure sound can occur early or late in timing. A_2 is *delayed* when the left ventricular outflow time is increased resulting in late closure of aortic valve as in aortic stenosis, aortic regurgitation, left ventricular failure, and large patent ductus arteriosus. Another cause of delayed A_2 is left bundle branch block.

Aortic closure sound occurs *early* in conditions where the left ventricle empties earlier than usual. This may occur because of alternative exits for left ventricular outflow as in mitral regurgitation (backflow to left atrium) or ventricular septal defect (shunting of left ventricle flow to right ventricle).

Abnormalities of the Pulmonary Component (P_2) of the Second Sound

Intensity: Pulmonary closure sound is *accentuated* in intensity when the pulmonary valve closes against a higher pressure as in pulmonary arterial hypertension from any cause. P_2 is soft in pulmonary stenosis; but only when there is right ventricular dysfunction, or there is a right to left atrial shunt leading to decreased pulmonary blood flow. P_2 is absent when the pulmonary valve is absent or atretic.

Timing: Pulmonary closure sound is *delayed* in conditions that result in delayed emptying of right ventricle because of outflow obstruction (pulmonary stenosis), increased volume (atrial septal defect and total anomalous pulmonary venous drainage); or right bundle branch block.

Abnormalities in Splitting of the Second Sound (S_2)

- Normally, S_2 is single in expiration and split in inspiration with the louder A_2 preceding the P_2 **(Figs. 19.18A and B)**.
- ***Wide splitting of the second sound is defined*** as splitting during expiration due to an early A_2 or late P_2 that results in an A_2-P_2 interval of 0.3 sec or more during expiration.
- ***Wide and variable split*** refers to a split >0.3 sec during expiration that increases further during inspiration **(Fig. 19.18A)**. It is observed in pulmonary stenosis, mitral regurgitation, and ventricular septal defect with large left to right shunt. In pulmonary stenosis it is due to a delay in P_2 whereas in mitral regurgitation and ventricular septal defect it is due to an early A_2.
- ***Wide and fixed split:*** When A_2-P_2 interval is >0.3 sec but remains unchanged during expiration or inspiration **(Fig. 19.18B)**. This is characteristic of atrial septal defect, right bundle branch block, and total anomalous pulmonary venous connection.
- ***Narrow or absent split:*** This can occur in conditions where A_2 is delayed. A farther delay will result in paradoxically split S_2. Paradoxical split in second sound can be diagnosed when the split is more during expiration, than in inspiration. This is characteristic of critical aortic stenosis, large PDA, and severe aortic regurgitation.
- ***Single S_2:*** A single second sound is either A_2 or P_2 or a combination (overlap) of both. The decision whether it is A_2 or P_2 or a combination of both A_2 and P_2 depends on the overall clinical picture. Truncus arteriosus, pulmonary atresia, and aortic atresia have a single S_2.

Systolic Murmurs

Systolic murmur can be *ejection systolic* or *pansystolic.* A pansystolic murmur is always abnormal irrespective of its intensity. The causes of pansystolic murmur are (*a*) ventricular septal defect, (*b*) mitral regurgitation, and (*c*) tricuspid regurgitation.

An ejection systolic murmur on the other hand may be due to an organic cause or it may be "functional" murmur. An ejection systolic murmur associated with a thrill is always organic. Systolic murmurs less than grade III do not exclude heart disease, *per se.*

- ***Pansystolic murmur:*** A murmur starting with the first heart sound (partially masking it) and ending with the second heart sound without change in character is a pansystolic murmur **(Fig. 19.19A)**. They are usually soft and blowing if due to AV valve regurgitation, and harsh if due to VSD.
- ***Ejection systolic murmur:*** Murmur audible during the phase of ejection, i.e., after the first heart sound and ending with or before the second heart sound is called ejection systolic murmur **(Fig. 19.19B)**. The ejection murmurs are crescendo and decrescendo; the peak may be in the middle of systole or later giving a diamond shape to the murmur. The ejection murmur could be pulmonary or aortic being produced at the respective valves either due to obstruction to the flow or increased flow across the normal valve. A murmur starting with the first heart sound and ending before mid-systole is early systolic murmur and a murmur starting late in systole ending with the second heart sound is late systolic murmur.

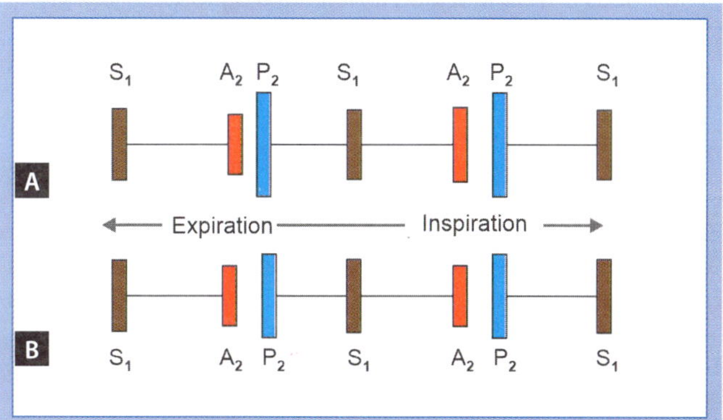

Figs. 19.18A and B: Second heart sound is: (A) Wide and variably split in ventricular septal defect; (B) Wide and fixed split in atrial septal defect with large left to right shunt

Diastolic Murmurs

Presence of a diastolic murmur is almost diagnostic of a heart disease. Rarely one can hear a diastolic murmur, which is not pathological is flow murmur (across tricuspid or mitral valve) in condition of high cardiac output as severe anemia or aortic regurgitation. Diastolic murmur in both these conditions disappears after correcting the underlying cause.

- ***Delayed diastolic murmurs:*** These are low pitched rumbling in character heard after the second heart sound **(Fig. 19.19C)**. They are audible either in tricuspid or mitral area and are due either to obstruction or increased flow across the respective valves. The diastolic murmur heard in the late diastolic phase and ending with the first heart sound is late diastolic or presystolic murmur, this corresponds to atrial systole.
- ***Early diastolic murmurs*** are heard with the aortic or pulmonic component of the second heart sound. They indicate regurgitation of the respective valves.

Continuous Murmurs

A continuous murmur begins in systole and continues without interruption or change in character through the second heart sound into diastole **(Fig. 19.19D)**. It may occupy whole or part of diastole. Causes of continuous murmur include: (*i*) patent ductus arteriosus; (*ii*) coronary arteriovenous fistula; (*iii*) ruptured sinus of Valsalva fistulae into the right side; (*iv*) restrictive aorticopulmonary septal defect; (*v*) systemic arteriovenous fistula over the chest; (*vi*) bronchial collateral murmurs; (*vii*) pulmonary arteriovenous fistula; (*viii*) peripheral pulmonic stenosis; (*ix*) venous hum; and (*x*) small atrial septal defect associated with severe mitral stenosis.

The impression of continuous murmur due to a combination of a pansystolic murmur and regurgitant diastolic murmur occurs most commonly in ventricular septal defect associated with aortic regurgitation. This difficulty may also occur in combinations of mitral and/or tricuspid regurgitation with aortic regurgitation. Combination of aortic stenosis and aortic regurgitation never gives an auscultatory impression of a continuous murmur since a gap between the two murmurs can always be appreciated **(Fig. 19.19E)**. These murmurs are also referred as *to-and-fro murmurs*. Another point of differentiation from continuous murmur is that the character and frequency of the systolic and diastolic components are different in to-and-fro murmurs, but they are similar in a continuous murmur.

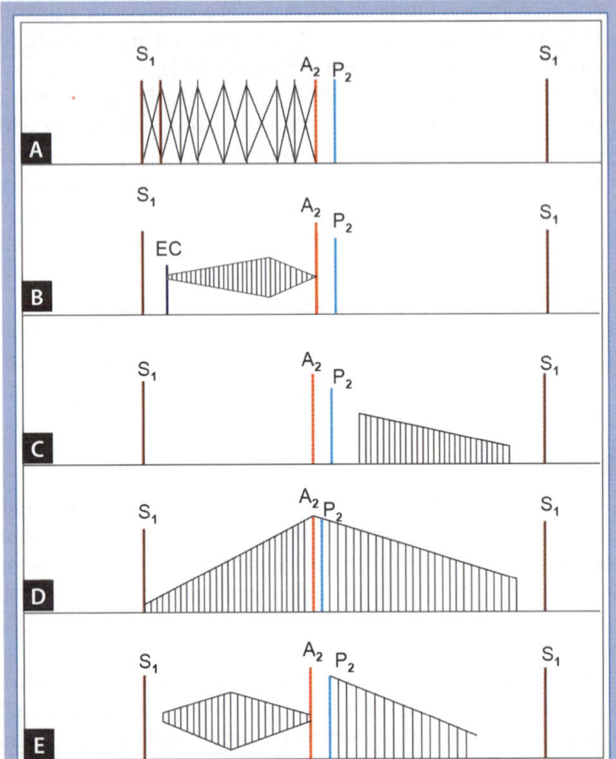

Figs. 19.19A to E: Line diagram representing various types of murmurs: (A) Pansystolic murmur starts with first heart sound (masking first heart sound) and ends with aortic component of second heart sound with same intensity; (B) Ejection systolic murmur starts after first heart sound with a gap, increases in intensity, peaks in later part of systole and then intensity decreases; (C) Delayed diastolic murmur starting with a gap from second heart sound and extending into diastole to variable duration, ends before first heart sound; (D) Continuous murmur in a child with restrictive PDA, starts in systole, peaks in later part of systole and continues into diastole covering second heart sound with same character; (E) Systolic and early diastolic murmur in a patient with aortic stenosis and aortic regurgitation

Additional Sounds

Clicks

High-pitched clicky sounds heard after the first heart sound with the onset of ejection are called ejection clicks.

- If the click does not vary in intensity with the phase of respiration, it is constant ejection click and is associated with aortic valve stenosis or aortic dilatation.
- If the click becomes louder during expiration the click is called *inconstant* and is associated with pulmonary valvular stenosis.
- Some clicks are audible in the middle of systole and are called *mid systolic clicks*. These could be due to mitral valve or tricuspid valve prolapse, and atrial or ventricular septal aneurysm.

Third Heart Sound

Low-pitched sound heard after the second heart sound in early diastolic phase of cardiac cycle is called third heart sound. It could be from right side or left side of the heart. It indicates rapid filling of the respective ventricle, which could be due to high output states, failing ventricles or restrictive filling of ventricles (most of the filling occurring in early diastolic phase).

Table 19.5 Nada's Criteria

Major criteria	*Minor criteria*
1. Systolic murmur grade III or more 2. Diastolic murmur 3. Cyanosis 4. Congestive heart failure	1. Systolic murmur less than grade III in intensity 2. Abnormal second sound 3. Abnormal ECG 4. Abnormal chest X-ray 5. Abnormal blood pressure

Presence of 1 Major or 2 Minor criteria suggests the presence of a heart disease

Fourth Heart Sound

The sound audible at the end of diastole just before the first heart sound, in the phase of atrial filling is called fourth heart sound. The sound may be either right sided or left sided and indicates non-compliant ventricle of the respective side.

Pericardial Rub

This is a low pitch superficial scratchy sound having biphasic or triphasic pattern. The pericardial rub is an evanescent sound and may not be heard at all the times.

NADA'S CRITERIA

In any child with heart murmur the decision should be made whether it is organic or is it the so-called functional murmur. Assessment of child for the presence of heart disease is facilitated by Nada's criteria, which are categorized as *Major* and *Minor* (**Table 19.5**).

This section should serve as a primer and students are advised to refer to "Clinical Methods in Pediatrics" by Piyush Gupta for the detailed aspects of history taking and examination of cardiovascular system.

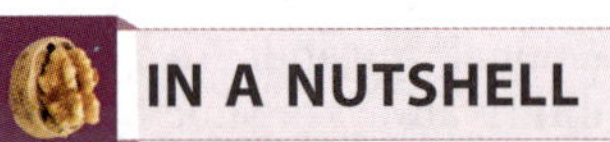

Approach to a Child with Heart Disease

1. Eliciting proper history of the cardinal symptoms of heart disease and exhaustive cardiovascular examination provide fair clues toward reaching a working diagnosis.
2. General physical examination including evaluation of eyes, ears, oral cavity, nails, skin, joints, spine, and oral cavity is essential while assessing a child with suspected heart disease.
3. Combination of a group of symptoms helps in classifying a patient into a physiological category thus facilitating timely management before further diagnostic investigations are carried out.
4. Due to higher heart rates, auscultation of cardiac sounds and murmurs may be cumbersome in children but with practice the auscultation findings can be accurately identified.

Frank JE, Jacobe KM. Evaluation and management of heart murmurs in children. Am Fam Physician. 2011;84(7):793-800.

Gupta P. Clinical Methods in Pediatrics, 5th edition. New Delhi: CBS Publishers and Distributors; 2019.

19.4 Investigations for Heart Disease

PE 22.9, PE 22.10

CHEST X-RAY

Chest X-ray provides information on visceral situs, cardiac size, position and configuration, pulmonary vasculature, pulmonary arterial and venous hypertension, and pulmonary pathology.

What is a Good X-ray Chest?

Proper Centering without any Rotation

If the centering is correct both clavicles should be at the same level. The shadow of the spine should not be rotated. In this position, the right border of the cardiac silhouette is made up by superior vena cava, right atrium, and inferior vena cava; while the left border is made up of aortic knuckle, main pulmonary artery, left atrial appendage if enlarged, and the left ventricle (**Fig. 19.20**).

Correct Exposure

The space between 2nd and 3rd vertebra should be visible if the penetration is adequate. If the whole spine is clearly seen, the chest X-ray is over penetrated and then the vasculature will be underestimated. On the contrary, if the spine is not at all seen the chest X-ray is under penetrated, and this will lead to overestimation of vasculature changes.

Proper Inspiratory Film

A proper inspiratory film should have diaphragm at the level of 9th intercostal space. If the film is taken when the inspiration is not complete the level of the diaphragm will be higher, and the cardiac size will be wrongly overestimated.

Alterations in Cardiac Position

One should always remember to look for extraneous causes to explain the altered cardiac position such as hiatus hernia, pneumothorax or hyperinflation, shifting the heart to opposite side. Collapse or hypoplasia of lung causes shift to the same side. Thymic shadow should be looked for before commenting on abnormal cardiac position, cardiomegaly, or wide mediastinum (**Fig. 19.21**).

Diagnosis of Situs

In normal situs (situs solitus) the gas bubble in stomach is seen on left side and the liver shadow is seen on the right side **(Fig. 19.22A)**. The right dome of the diaphragm being higher than the left dome. If the stomach gas bubble is seen on the right side and the liver shadow with the higher diaphragm is seen on the left side it will indicate that one is dealing with situs inversus (**Fig. 19.22B**). A midline liver indicates asplenia or polysplenia associated with complex heart disease **(Fig. 19.22C)**.

Bronchial division can also give a clue to the situs. The left main bronchus is longer and has a more acute angle with trachea as compared to the right main bronchus. If the right and left bronchi are lateralized normally it indicates normal situs and if vice versa, i.e., inversely lateralized it will indicate situs inversus. If they are identical, it indicates asplenia or polysplenia.

Heart Size

For the assessment of heart size, cardiothoracic (CT) ratio is calculated. The cardiac dimension is measured from middle of the spine to maximum cardiac shadow on right and left side. The thoracic dimension is the widest internal thoracic dimension (**Fig. 19.23**). Cardiothoracic ratio of >60% in neonates, 55% in infants, and 50% in children is taken as cardiac enlargement. While calculating this ratio it is necessary that the chest X-ray is obtained during inspiration and is well-centered. Expiratory film causes false increase in cardiothoracic ratio.

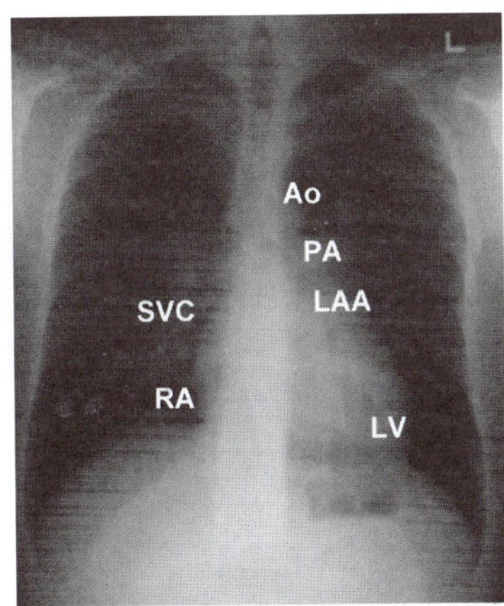

Fig. 19.20: Normal cardiac silhouette

(Ao: aortic knuckle; LAA: left atrial appendage; LV; left ventricle; PA: pulmonary artery; RA: right atrium; SVC: superior vena cava)

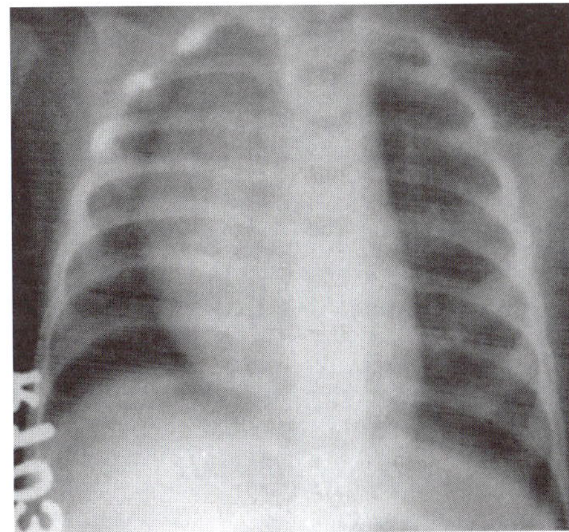

Fig. 19.21: Chest X-ray frontal view of an infant referred as dextrocardia. X-ray showed thymic shadow on right cardiac border giving the impression of dextrocardia. Cardiac size is normal with normal pulmonary vascularity

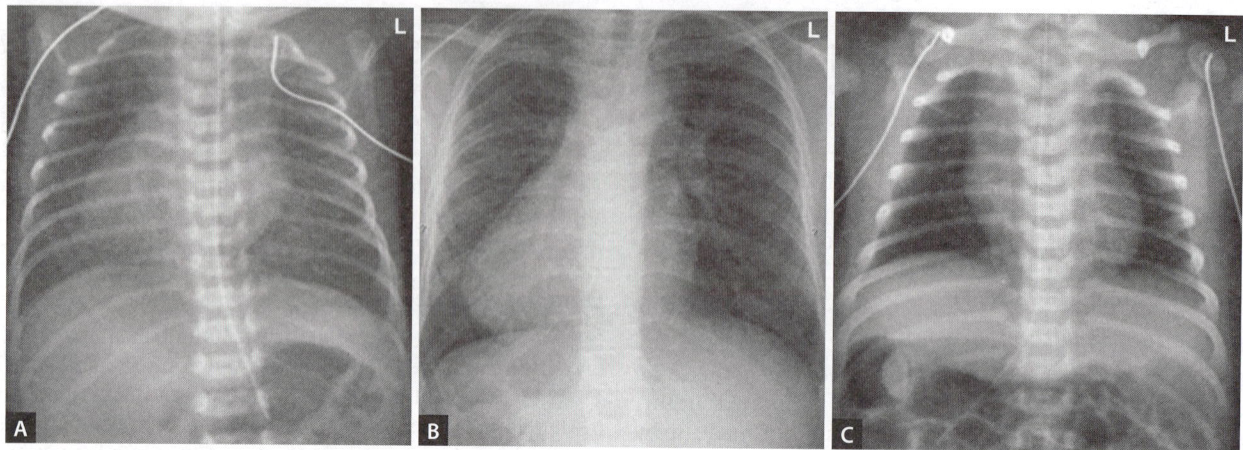

Figs. 19.22A to C: Chest X-rays frontal view with dextrocardia: (A) Situs solitus (gastric bubble on left) with dextrocardia; (B) Situs inversus (gastric bubble on right) with dextrocardia; (C) Isomerism (midline transverse liver) with mesocardia

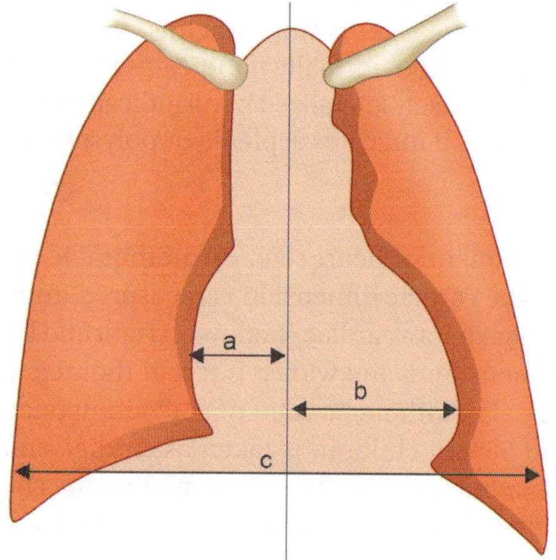

Fig. 19.23: Cardiothoracic ratio: (a +b)/c

Cardiac Configuration

- Left ventricular enlargement results in shifting of the apex of the heart downwards and outwards, evidenced by an obtuse cardiophrenic angle **(Fig. 19.24A)**.
- Right ventricular enlargement is indicated by lifting up of the apex, resulting in an acute cardiophrenic angle **(Fig. 19.24B)**. As right ventricle is an anterior structure, RV enlargement is best characterized in a lateral view film, as obliteration of retrosternal space between pericardium and sternum.
- Enlargement of the right atrium is indicated by an enlarged contour of the right heart border (which is formed by the right atrium) occupying >2½ intercostal spaces.
- Enlargement of left atrium is best judged by seeing the carinal angle. Normally it is <70°. A carinal angle >90° is specific for left atrial enlargement.
- Left atrial enlargement is evidenced by double contour of right heart border. Straightening of left heart border due to dilated left atrial appendage is indirect evidence of LA enlargement.

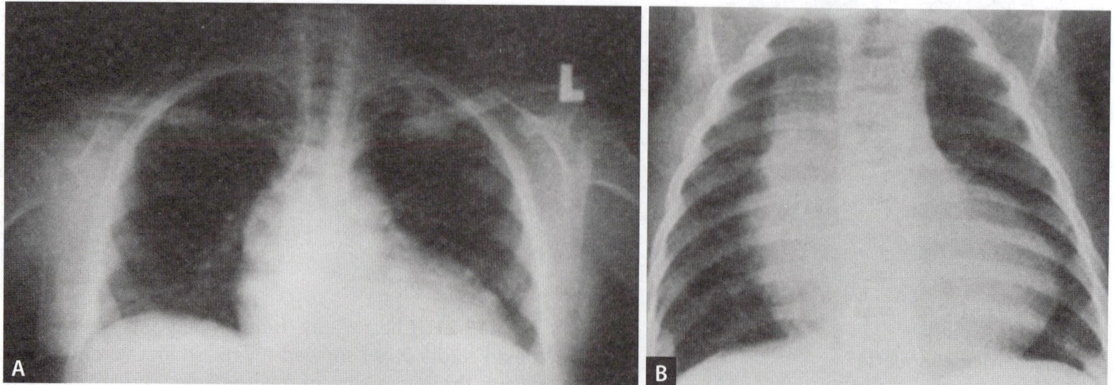

Figs. 19.24A and B: Cardiomegaly with: (A) Left ventricular apex; (B) Right ventricular apex

Vascularity of Lungs

Increased Pulmonary Vascularity

The main pulmonary artery is prominent with normally related great vessels. The hilar pulmonary arteries are also prominent, and the pulmonary arteries can be traced till the lateral third of the lung fields. Additionally, more than four end-on vessels are seen in each lung field (the end on vessel being more than twice the size of accompanying bronchus) **(Fig. 19.25A)**.

Decreased Pulmonary Vascularity

The main pulmonary artery is not prominent and hilar branches appear small. The peripheral pulmonary vessels are thinned out (stringy vasculature). The overall lung fields appear dark **(Fig. 19.25B)**.

Pulmonary Arterial Hypertension

The main pulmonary artery dilates. Right pulmonary artery diameter of more than trachea indicates significant pulmonary arterial hypertension (PAH). If the PAH is severe, with prominent hilar vessels there is sudden tapering of the vessels called pruning. Pruning means that more than a 50% reduction in vessel diameter at any branching level. It is generally clearly seen at the junction of medial and middle third of lung fields.

Pulmonary Venous Hypertension (PVH)

In the initial stages with mild elevation of pulmonary venous pressures the upper lobe vessels dilate with constriction and blurring of the lower zone vessels. With further increase in pulmonary venous pressures the interstitial lung water increases leading to increased lymphatic drainage resulting in cuffing of fluid around bronchi, background haze, Kerley's lines, septal and interstitial edema. Very severe elevation of pulmonary venous pressures results in collection of edema fluid toward the hilum resulting in "Bat's wing" appearance.

BLOOD INVESTIGATIONS

Blood investigations form an integral component of management of children with heart disease. Prior to ordering a blood test, the implication of the expected result should be known. Blanket panel of tests are never done, rather specific blood investigations are done depending on the suspicion of a specific kind of cardiac illness. **Table 19.6** broadly describes the investigations that are carried out according to the suspected cardiac illness. The utility of investigations has been described in the sections associated with the specific disease.

Table 19.6 Blood Investigations in Children with Heart Disease

Acyanotic and cyanotic CHDs	Hemoglobin level
Cyanotic CHDs	Platelet count, PT/INR/APTT
Acute rheumatic fever	• CRP, ESR, ASLO • Throat swab
Infective endocarditis	CBC, ESR, CRP, blood cultures (3 set)
Pericardial effusion	TLC/DLC, CRP, ESR, blood culture, ADA level, thyroid function test
Dilated cardiomyopathy	CPK, troponin, LDH, plasma PCR for viral etiology, Ionized calcium level, vitamin D level, LFT, RFT
Restrictive cardiomyopathy	Iron studies (hemochromatosis), S. ACE level (sarcoidosis), DLC and absolute eosinophil count (Loeffler cardiomyopathy), enzyme studies (lysosomal storage disorder, Gaucher, Hurler, Fabry disease)
Hypertrophic cardiomyopathy	Enzyme study (Pompe disease)
Kawasaki disease	Platelet count, CRP, ESR

(CRP: c-reactive protein; ESR: erythrocyte sedimentation rate; ASLO: anti-streptolysin O; TLC: total leucocyte count; DLC: differential leucocyte count; CPK: creatine phosphokinase; LDH: lactate dehydrogenase; PCR: polymerase chain reaction)

ELECTROCARDIOGRAM

Electrical Conduction in Heart

Cardiac conduction system consists of the following components:

1. SA node (sinoatrial node)
2. AV node (atrioventricular node)

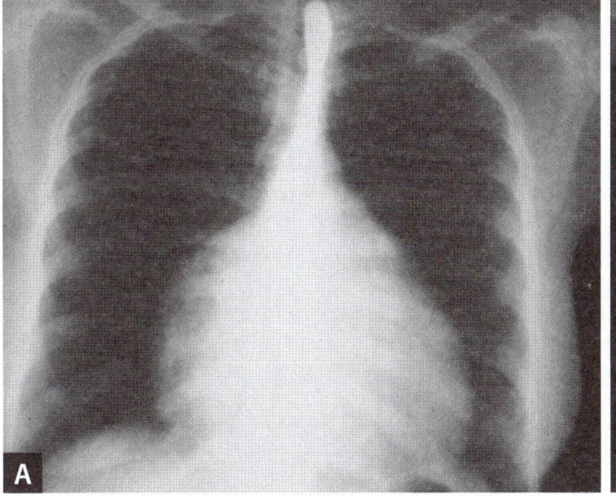

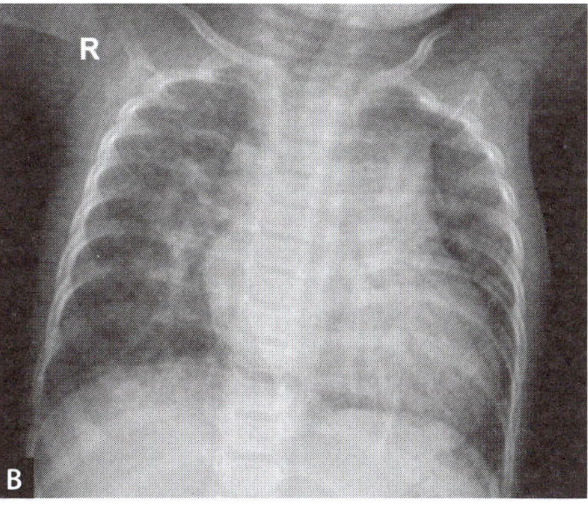

Figs. 19.25A and B: Pulmonary vasculature: (A) Plethora; (B) Oligemia

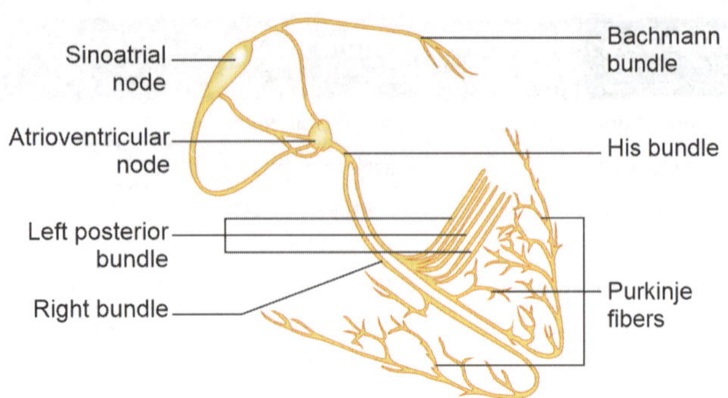

Fig. 19.26: Cardiac conduction system

3. Bundle of His with right and left bundle branches
4. Purkinje fibers.

Sinoatrial node is known as pacemaker of heart and is in right atrium. Electrical activity arises in pacemaker cells of SA node, travels through the wall of atria and internodal fibers and reaches AV node. SA nodal activation causes contraction of atria. From AV node, impulse travels along *bundle of His* lying in the interventricular septum and goes to right and left ventricle through right and left bundle branches. Ultimately the electrical impulse spreads diffusely to the myocardium through Purkinje fibers (**Fig. 19.26**).

Electrical activity is followed by mechanical events in the myocardium. When electrical impulse reaches AV node, there is a period of delay (0.12 sec) before the impulse is transmitted to ventricles. Hence, there is a time gap between atrial contraction and ventricular contraction. Electrocardiogram (ECG) is primarily used to detect abnormalities of cardiac conduction, arrhythmias, and chamber (atrial or ventricular) hypertrophy.

Normal Electrocardiogram

Normal ECG has five waves in following sequence P, Q, R, S, and T wave (**Fig. 19.27**). P wave depicts atrial depolarization. Next three waves occur together forming QRS complex, which depicts ventricular depolarization. T wave depicts ventricular repolarization. Atrial repolarization merges with the QRS complex, hence is not seen as a distinct wave (**Fig. 19.28**).

Major abnormalities and their causes are listed below:

P Wave

- ***Absent P wave:*** Sinoatrial block, atrial fibrillation
- ***Tall P wave (>3 mm):*** Right atrial enlargement
- ***Prolonged P wave duration (wide and often notched):*** Left atrial enlargement

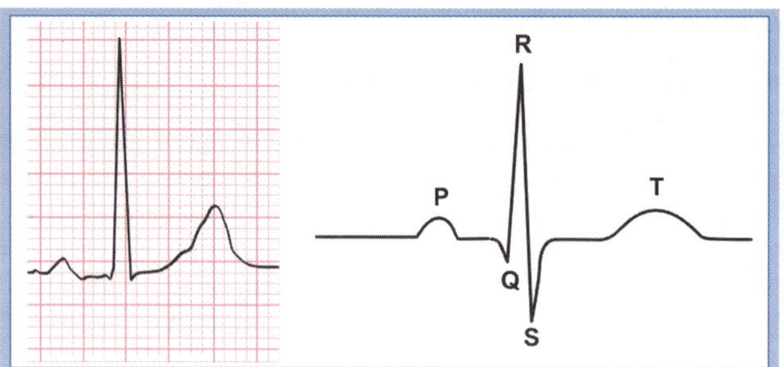

Fig. 19.27: Depicting waveforms in ECG

PR Interval

- ***Short PR interval:*** Delta wave-Wolff–Parkinson–White (WPW) syndrome, Pompe disease
- ***Prolonged PR interval:*** Atrial septal defect, Ebstein anomaly, toxicity of digitalis or quinidine, hyperkalemia, profound hypoxia, myocarditis (rheumatic, viral, diphtheria)
- ***Variable PR interval:*** Mobitz type I second degree atrioventricular block.

Mean Frontal Plane QRS Axis

Normal at birth: Around 120°; By age of 1 year: between +60° and +90°; Adults: +30° to +60°. Transition from +120° to between +30° and +60° may occur somewhat early or late but presence of QRS axis beyond +120° after the age of 6 months is possibly abnormal, and beyond the age of 1 year it should always be considered abnormal and is suggestive of right ventricular hypertrophy.

If the value for the mean vector of QRS complex falls outside the range of normal values for age, then there is deviation of QRS. The commonest cause of right axis deviation in children is right ventricular hypertrophy. The most common causes of left axis deviation in childhood are related to abnormal intraventricular conduction associated with atrioventricular septal defect, or tricuspid atresia. Concentric left ventricular hypertrophy generally does not cause left axis deviation.

QRS Amplitude

Low voltage QRS complex is defined as QRS amplitude <5 mm in all limb leads and <10 mm in all precordial leads (**Fig. 19.29**). It is a nonspecific finding that may be seen in myocarditis, pericardial effusion, myxedema, and generalized edema.

Normal newborn ECG may show low voltage QRS complexes due to vernix caseosa fat being a poor conductor.

Ventricular hypertrophy: The right ventricle forces are directed anteriorly (height of R wave in V1) and to the right (depth of S wave in lead V6). Conversely the posterior forces generated by

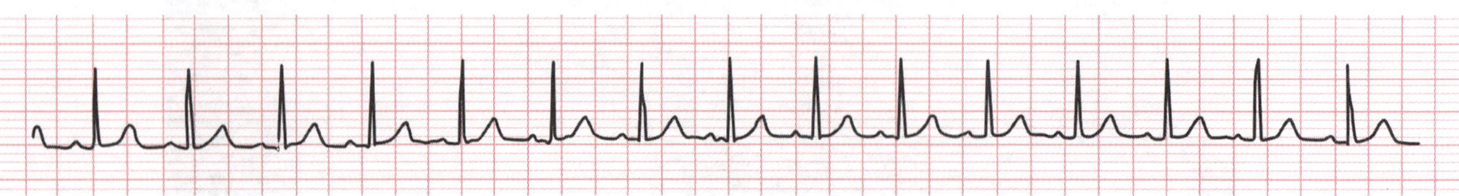

Fig. 19.28: ECG of a 3-year-old child showing normal sinus rhythm

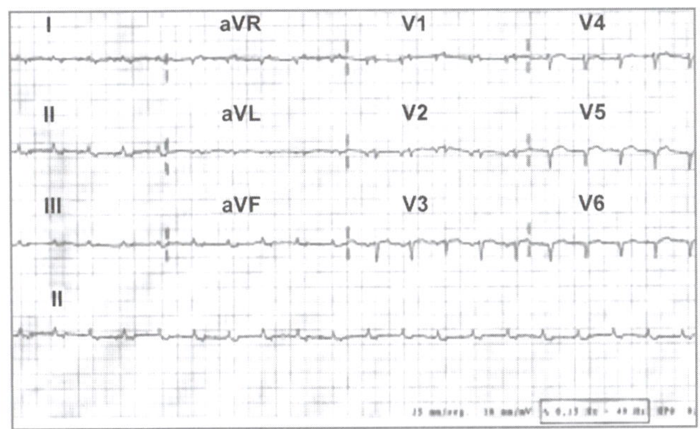

Fig. 19.29: ECG from 12-year-old girl with thiamine deficiency presented with severe ventricular dysfunction, pericardial and pleural effusion and ascites. ECG showing sinus tachycardia (HR-124/min) and generalized low voltage QRS complexes

left ventricle are reflected by depth of S wave in V1 while the leftward forces are reflected by the height of the R wave in V6.

QT Interval

- ***Prolonged QTc interval:*** QTc should not exceed 0.44 sec, except in infants <6 months, QTc up to 0.49 sec may be normal. Causes of prolonged QTc include hypocalcemia, long QT syndrome, and antiarrhythmic drugs—quinidine, procainamide, and amiodarone.
- ***Short QT interval:*** Hypercalcemia, digitalis effect.

Atrial Enlargement

Criteria for atrial enlargement will not be valid with ectopic atrial rhythm.

- ***Right atrial enlargement:*** Tall, peaked P wave in lead II (>3 mm), or biphasic or tall P wave in V1.
- ***Left atrial enlargement:*** Broad notched P wave (P wave > 0.10 sec in children, >0.08 sec in infants) in lead II, or deep, slurred biphasic P wave in V1.

Ventricular Hypertrophy

Criteria for an ECG determination of ventricular hypertrophy are based on whether QRS voltages in specific leads exceed normal values. Right ventricle is anterior, superior and to the right, so that the increased forces are to right, anterior and superior suggest right ventricular hypertrophy (RVH). Left ventricle is to left, posterior, and inferior and increased forces directed to the left, inferior and posterior suggest left ventricular hypertrophy (LVH). Leads V1 and V2 may be used to judge anteroposterior forces, while leads V5 and V6 to judge left-right forces and lead aVF to judge inferior-superior forces.

Left Ventricular Hypertrophy

- ***R wave:*** Greater than 98th percentile for age in V6, S wave greater than 98th percentile for age in V1.
- ***Tall R wave in aVF:*** This may also be present in RVH, in the absence of RVH this criterion is helpful in supporting a diagnosis of LVH.
- ***T wave abnormality:*** A left ventricular strain pattern consists of inverted T wave in inferior leads (II, III, aVF) and left precordial leads (V5,V6), or a wide QRS-T angle (>100°).
- ***Deep Q wave in V5, V6:*** More in favor of volume overloaded left ventricle. Deep Q waves are not seen in severe left ventricular hypertrophy.

Right Ventricular Hypertrophy

- R wave >98th percentile for age in V1
- S wave >98th percentile in V6
- R/S ratio in V1 abnormally high; and in V6 abnormally low

ECHOCARDIOGRAPHY

Echocardiography provides description of all the segments of heart including, cardiac position, systemic and pulmonary venous connections, atrioventricular connections, ventriculo-atrial connections, both the great vessels, coronary arteries, function of cardiac valves, and systolic and diastolic function of heart. It provides information about the intracardiac defects with their location, size, and direction of shunts, along with presence or absence of volume overload of cardiac chambers. It also provides information about the severity of stenosis or regurgitation in cardiac valves. All this information can be used to determine the anatomical defect, its hemodynamic significance, and the need and timing of any intervention if required (**Figs. 19.30 to 19.32**). It is also useful in following up a child with heart disease, during difficult cardiac surgery, in immediate postoperative period, and during catheter intervention as balloon atrial septostomy, device closure, and pericardiocentesis, etc.

- ***Two-dimensional echocardiography:*** It provides a real-time image of cardiac structures with the use of several standard views and has replaced cardiac angiography for the preoperative diagnosis of many of the heart defects.
- ***M-mode echocardiography:*** It is used mostly for the measurements of cardiac chambers, wall thickness, and cardiac function. It also provides information about motion of valves and interventricular septum.

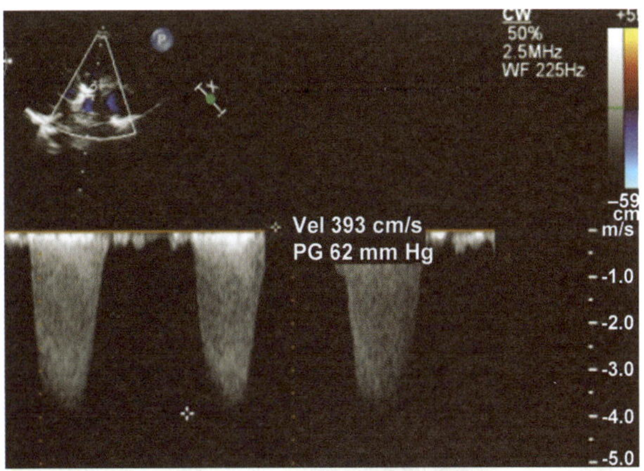

Fig. 19.30: Continuous wave Doppler showing severe pulmonary stenosis with gradient of 62 mm Hg

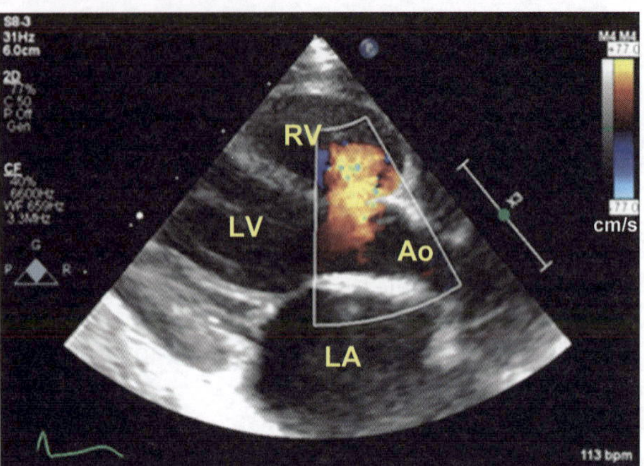

Fig. 19.31: Echocardiogram showing a large subaortic ventricular septal defect with blood flow from left to right ventricle across it (red flow on color Doppler)

- ***Doppler echocardiography:*** It is used to assess the flow velocities across various valves and communications.
- ***Three-dimensional echocardiography:*** It has been used for measurements of volume and ejection fraction of unusual ventricular geometries; visualization of device placement; and simulation of intraoperative preoperative anatomy.

CARDIAC CATHETERIZATION

In past, cardiac catheterization was carried out in all cases of congenital heart disease to confirm the diagnosis and acquire hemodynamic data. But due to advancement in noninvasive imaging techniques use of diagnostic cardiac catheterization is limited to a few indications. However, therapeutic cardiac catheterization has evolved and many interventions are now done by percutaneous route, which were earlier in the ambit of surgical domain. Indications of cardiac catheterization in the current era are as follows:

1. In patients with unclear diagnosis.
2. In large left to right shunts with pulmonary hypertension, for accurate assessment of pulmonary artery pressure and pulmonary vascular resistance, to decide about safety and feasibility of shunt closure.
3. For anatomical delineation in complex CHDs which aids in interventional and surgical management.
4. For carrying out therapeutic interventions such as device closure of left to right shunts [viz., atrial septal defect (ASD), VSD, PDA device closure] balloon dilation of stenotic valves (pulmonary or aortic valve balloon dilation), stenting of stenosed blood vessels (coarctation of aorta stenting), creation of shunts (balloon atrial septostomy).

Limitations and Risks

Cardiac catheterization produces a two-dimensional image, hence the anatomic orientations in complex malformations may not be very well appreciated. Also, it is an invasive procedure and requires access into the various chambers of the heart via arterial or venous puncture culminating in a risk of arterial occlusion or deep vein thrombosis. Also, there is a risk of tachyarrhythmia and bradyarrhythmia or heart block due to catheter manipulations inside the heart. There is risk of infective endocarditis if optimal antibiotic prophylaxis is not observed.

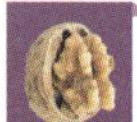

IN A NUTSHELL

Investigations for Heart Disease

1. Chest radiograph is the basic first line investigations done in all children suspected to have heart disease, which supplements the provisional clinical diagnosis.
2. Electrocardiogram (ECG) is the diagnostic investigation to identify cardiac chamber hypertrophy and rhythm assessment.
3. Anemia is an additional hemodynamic burden. Hence hemoglobin should be measured in all children with heart disease. Other blood investigations are done as per the specific diagnosis.
4. ECG is the diagnostic investigation for reaching a final morphological diagnosis. It also provides details of ventricular function and pericardial effusion.
5. Sometimes for planning further management, cardiac catheterization is carried out in certain patients with heart disease, which provides hemodynamic as well as anatomical details. In certain patients catheterization can be therapeutic, involving device closure of defects or balloon dilation of stenotic lesions.

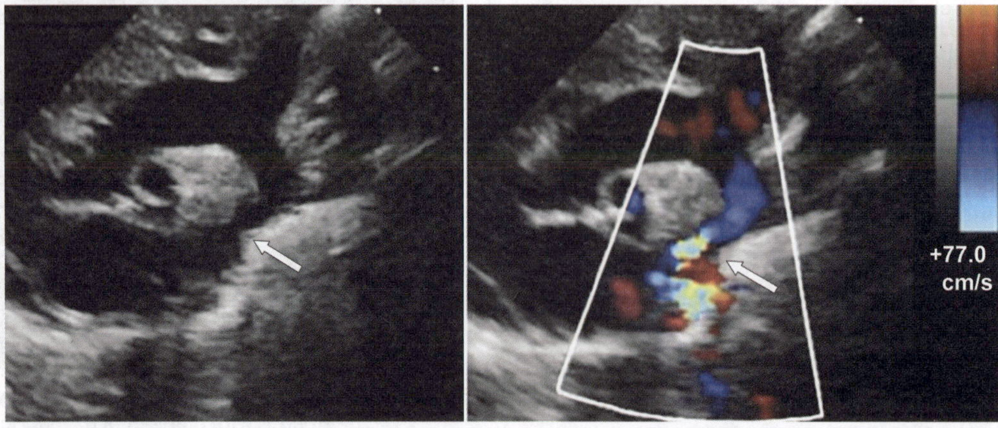

Fig. 19.32: Two-dimensional imaging and color flow mapping across the arch of aorta showing coarctation of aorta (pointer)

Sachdeva S, Gupta SK. Imaging modalities in congenital heart disease. Indian J Pediatr. 2020;87(5):385-97.
Somerville J, Grech V. The chest X-ray in congenital heart disease 4. Images Paediatr Cardiol. 2011;13(3):19-20.
Surawicz B, Childers R, Deal BJ, et al. AHA/ACCF/HRS recommendations for the standardization and interpretation of the Electrocardiogram. Circulation. 2009;119:e235-40.

19.5 Congestive Heart Failure

PE 22.3

INTRODUCTION

Congestive heart failure refers to a clinical state of systemic and pulmonary congestion resulting from inability of the heart to maintain effective circulation. The defect may lie in (*i*) pumping of blood from heart into the systemic circulation (systolic failure); or (*ii*) receiving the blood from peripheral circulation into the heart (diastolic failure).

Systolic failure is more common than diastolic failure. The latter is characteristically seen is constrictive pericarditis, hypertrophic cardiomyopathy, and restrictive heart disease.

PATHOPHYSIOLOGY

Heart failure may result from (*a*) an excessive volume overload (left to right shunt, regurgitation); (*b*) pressure overload on normal myocardium (left or right sided outflow obstruction), or (*c*) ventricular dysfunction (anomalous origin of left coronary artery from pulmonary artery, electrolyte imbalance, myocarditis, cardiomyopathy). Arrhythmias, pericardial diseases, and combination of various factors can also result in CHF.

The resultant decrease in cardiac output triggers physiological responses aimed at restoring perfusion of the vital organs, i.e., (*i*) renal retention of fluid; (*ii*) renin-angiotensin mediated vasoconstriction; and (*iii*) sympathetic overactivity.

- Excessive fluid retention increases the cardiac output by increasing the end diastolic volume (preload), but also results in symptoms of pulmonary and systemic congestion. Clinically this manifests as edema and pulmonary edema.
- Vasoconstriction (increase in afterload) tends to maintain flow to vital organs, but it is disproportionately elevated in patients with CHF and increases myocardial work. This causes cardiomegaly, hepatomegaly, raised jugular venous pressure, and poor peripheral perfusion.
- Similarly, sympathetic over-activity results in increased contractility, peripheral vasoconstriction, which also increases myocardial requirements. Clinically, this manifests in marked tachycardia and S_3 gallop.

An understanding of the interplay of the four principal determinants of cardiac output—preload, afterload, contractility, and heart rate is essential in optimizing the therapy of congestive heart failure.

ETIOLOGY

Congestive Heart Failure during Fetal Life

Restricted foramen ovale and restricted ductus arteriosus during fetal life, fetal heart block or tachyarrhythmias, severe tricuspid regurgitation, myocardial dysfunction, and twin to twin transfusion can initiate CHF in fetal life that may present at birth.

CHF on First Day of Life

Myocardial dysfunction secondary to asphyxia, hypoglycemia, hypocalcemia, or sepsis is usually responsible for congestive heart failure on the first day of life, rather than a structural heart defect. Significant tricuspid regurgitation secondary to hypoxia induced papillary muscle dysfunction or Ebstein anomaly of the tricuspid valve; atrioventricular septal defect with AV regurgitation; and cerebral arteriovenous fistula can also result in congestive failure. CHF with Ebstein anomaly/tricuspid regurgitation improves as the pulmonary artery pressure falls over the next few days.

Congestive Heart Failure in First Week of Life

Congestive heart failure in the first week of life is often precipitated by the closure of the ductus arteriosus leading to catastrophic deterioration in the seemingly healthy neonate. These disorders (**Box 19.1**) can be life-threatening yet they are potentially curable, implying a need for early diagnosis and management. Important tips follow:

- Peripheral pulses and oxygen saturation (by a pulse oximeter) should be checked in both the upper and lower extremities. A lower saturation in the lower limbs means right to left ductal shunting and occurs due to severe pulmonary hypertension. Lower pressure in lower limbs occurs with coarctation of aorta.
- An atrial or ventricular septal defect does not lead to failure in the early neonatal period. Therefore, we should look for additional cause [e.g., aortic stenosis, coarctation of aorta, AV regurgitation, multiple sites of shunt, transposition or obstructed (total anomalous pulmonary venous connection) TAPVC].

Box 19.1 Causes of CHF in First Week of Life

Structural heart defects
- *Critical left sided obstructive lesions:* Aortic stenosis; coarctation of aorta, hypoplastic left heart syndrome
- *Critical right sided obstructive lesion:* Pulmonary stenosis with intact ventricular septum
- *Regurgitant lesions of valves:* Ebstein anomaly, AV septal defect, mitral regurgitation, aortic regurgitation
- Obstructed total anomalous pulmonary venous connection
- d-Transposition of great vessels

Myocardial dysfunction: Sepsis, electrolyte imbalance, asphyxia, hypocalcemia, glycogen storage disease, endocrine disorders
Arrhythmias: Tachyarrhythmias, congenital heart block

- Premature infants have a poor myocardial reserve and there is precipitous fall in pulmonary vascular resistance, and a shunt lesion as patent ductus arteriosus (PDA) may result in CHF in the first week in them.
- Metabolic disorders as glycogen storage disorder, adrenal insufficiency due to enzyme deficiencies, or neonatal thyrotoxicosis could also present with CHF in the first few days of life.

Congestive Heart Failure Beyond First Week of Life

Structural Heart Defects

Shunt lesions manifest with CHF during this period, and the most common cause of CHF is a ventricular septal defect that presents around 6–8 weeks of age. This is because the volume of the left to right shunt increases as the pulmonary resistance falls. Although a murmur of VSD is apparent by 1 week, the full-blown picture of CHF occurs around 6–8 weeks. CHF can appear in the 1st week of life if there are multiple sites of shunt or associated obstructive or regurgitant lesions. Other left to right shunts as PDA, and aortopulmonary window present similarly. Single ventricle, transposition of great vessels with VSD, truncus arteriosus present with mild cyanosis and CHF. The fall in pulmonary vascular resistance is delayed in presence of hypoxic lung disease and at high altitude this could somewhat alter the time course accordingly.

Anomalous left coronary artery arising from the pulmonary artery (ALCAPA), a rare disease, presenting in this age group merits separate mention, since it is curable and often missed. As the pulmonary artery pressure decreases in the neonatal period, these babies suffer from episodes of excessive crying with sweating (angina equivalent) and myocardial infarction. The electrocardiogram may show pathologic "q" wave or left ventricular hypertrophy with or without ST-T changes. These infants are often misdiagnosed as having "dilated cardiomyopathy" due to associated myocardial dysfunction.

Others

1. ***Arrhythmias:*** Tachyarrhythmias, complete heart block
2. ***Metabolic and endocrinal causes:*** Hypocalcemia, glycogen storage disease, hyperthyroidism

Causes of Congestive Heart Failure in Older Children

1. Rheumatic fever and rheumatic heart disease
2. Congenital heart disease complicated by anemia, infection, endocarditis, or development of other valvular lesions such as aortic regurgitation
3. Hypertension
4. Myocarditis and primary myocardial disease

CLINICAL MANIFESTATIONS

The clinical picture of CHF results from a combination of "relatively low output" and compensatory responses to increase it.

Diagnosis of CHF in small children and infants is difficult and needs a high index of suspicion. The most common symptom is feeding difficulty. Mother complains that the baby does not suck the breast continuously for a longer period. He/she sucks for some time and then stops feeding. After some time, he/she is again ready for sucking. This occurs because the baby gets breathless after sucking at the breast as the process involves effort. This situation is similar to "effort intolerance" in older children. Due to poor feeding, the child fails to gain weight. The child may also have excessive sweating especially on forehead associated with feeding. On examination, these children are also found to have tachycardia, gallop rhythm, hepatomegaly, and cardiomegaly.

Congestive heart failure in older children is characterized by tachypnea, tachycardia, gallop rhythm, pedal edema, decreased urinary output, raised jugular venous pressure, poor peripheral pulses, hepatomegaly, cardiomegaly, and basal crepitations (**Table 19.7**).

TREATMENT Congestive Heart Failure

The treatment of CHF includes general supportive measures, management of the precipitating events, control of the congested state, and identification and treatment of the cause.

General Measures

- *Position and nursing:* Nursing the infant with head end elevated, judicious use of sedation, and temporarily denying oral intake to avoid aspiration in the distressed infant are useful practices.
- *Nutrition:* Infants with CHF require high caloric feeds (120–150 kcal/kg/day). Nasogastric feeding may be required. Salt intakes need to be minimized in older children.
- *Oxygen:* Role of oxygen should be cautiously considered as oxygen may sometimes worsen the CHF in patients with left to right shunts due to its pulmonary vasodilating and systemic vasoconstrictor effects. Similarly, it may constrict PDA in neonates and may be detrimental to patients with ductus arteriosus dependent lesions. However, in patients with pulmonary edema and hypoxia, raising alveolar PO_2 by oxygen supplementation is required and regularly used.

Treatment of the Precipitating Events

Almost always, the worsening in clinical state of a patient with CHF can be traced to a precipitating event. These factors include infection, anemia, electrolyte imbalances, arrhythmia, rheumatic activity, infective endocarditis, pulmonary embolism, drug interactions, drug toxicity, or non-compliance, and other system disturbances. Treatment of underlying precipitating event leads to considerable improvement.

Treatment of Congested State

Conventional medical management of congestive heart failure includes three main approaches:

1. Reducing the pulmonary or systemic congestion
   Diuretics: Frusemide, chlorthiazide, aldactone, etc.
2. Increasing myocardial contractility
   Inotropes: Digoxin, other inotropes, and other measures
3. Reducing the disproportionately elevated afterload
   Vasodilators: ACE inhibitors, etc.

Diuretics

Diuretics afford quick relief in pulmonary and systemic congestion. Frusemide (1 mg/kg) is the agent of choice. For chronic use, 1–4 mg/kg of frusemide or 20–40 mg/kg of chlorothiazide in divided dosage are used. It is important to monitor body weight, blood urea, serum electrolytes (at least twice weekly initially).

Table 19.7 Manifestations of Congestive Heart Failure

Neonate	*Infant*	*Older child*
1. Persistent tachycardia (>160/min) 2. Tachypnea (>60/min) 3. Hepatomegaly (>3 cm) 4. Feeding difficulty 5. Poor peripheral perfusion 6. Presence of S_3 7. Cardiomegaly on chest X-ray	1. Poor weight gain 2. Feeding difficulty 3. Tachycardia 4. Tachypnea with grunting and intercostal retraction 5. Hepatomegaly 6. Excessive sweating 7. Poor peripheral perfusion 8. Presence of S_3, gallop rhythm	1. Tachycardia 2. Tachypnea 3. Gallop rhythm 4. Pedal edema 5. Raised JVP 6. Hepatomegaly 7. Cardiomegaly 8. Chest crepitations

Hypokalemia is one of the major concerns in children on frusemide therapy. However, potassium supplementation is usually not required with <2 mg/kg of frusemide or equivalent doses of other diuretics. A daily supplementation of 1–1.5 mEq/kg of potassium may be required if there is significant hypokalemia. Secondary hyperaldosteronism does occur in infants with CHF and addition of spironolactone 1 mg/kg single dose conserves potassium.

Metabolic alkalosis, hypomagnesemia and hyponatremia are the other problems. Infants tolerate hyponatremia much better than adults. The treatment for hyponatremia is rarely required even when serum sodium is as low as 120 mEq/L. Reducing the dose of diuretics, restriction of free water intake, and liberalizing salt for a short period would restore the serum sodium except in patients with a very low cardiac output.

In refractory failure, a combination of diuretics having different sites of action should be tried and intravenous rather oral preparation should be used. Dopamine in a renal vasodilating dose (2–5 mg/kg/min) may be useful as a diuretic although scientific data are limited.

Digoxin

Despite some controversy regarding the use of digoxin in patients with left to right shunt, it remains the mainstay of treatment of CHF in infants and children. Rapid digitalization (over 24 hours) should be resorted to in babies with severe CHF. A total dose of 30–40 µg/kg body weight orally (intravenous doses—75% of the oral dose) would digitalize term infants and children. For most other circumstances, starting with an oral maintenance dose (8–10 µg/kg/day in two divided doses) with no loading dose is adequate. Prolongation of PR interval can be an early feature of digitalis toxicity.

It is the physician's responsibility to ensure that the patient receives the correct dosages, simply because the mistakes in this regard can prove fatal. Nausea and vomiting are commonest signs of toxicity but severe toxicity may be present without these. If the child regurgitates a dose, it may be prudent to give the next dose 12 hours later. Bradycardia and blocks are commoner in children than ectopy during toxicity. The individual tolerance varies, but the safety margin is not high. Digoxin should be avoided in patients with myocarditis.

Vasodilators

Vasodilators include arteriolar dilators (hydralazine), venodilators (nitroglycerine, nitrates), and combined arteriovenodilators (ACE inhibitors, angiotensin receptor blockers, calcium channel blockers). The last group of drugs is used most frequently.

Angiotensin Converting Enzyme Inhibitors

These drugs mainly act by reducing the afterload. However, they may also decrease the preload and increase plasma potassium level. These, therefore, can be combined well with a diuretic; and in this case potassium supplements are not needed. ACE inhibitors are especially useful in the presence of hypertension, mitral, or aortic regurgitation. In children with left to right shunts, ACE inhibitors have been found useful in patients with large shunts or in those with an elevated systemic vascular resistance. These drugs should not be used in patients with stenotic lesions. ACE inhibitors can lead to severe hypotension in volume-depleted patients hence diuretics may have to be reduced initially. A test dose (one-fourth of the usual dose) should be given first, as some patients react with exaggerated hypotension to the initial dose. Patients with pre-existing renal failure (serum creatinine >1.5 mg/dL) should not receive ACE inhibitors. ACE inhibitors precipitate renal failure in bilateral renal arterial stenosis. Dry cough may occur in some cases, angioedema rarely occurs. Optimal dosages are variable. Enalapril in an oral dose from 0.1–0.5 mg/kg/day has been used in children. Captopril is used in a dosage of 0.2–2 mg/kg/dose 8 hourly.

Angiotensin Receptor Blockers

Losartan, candesartan, irbesartan, and valsartan have been extensively used in adults. Data in children are limited. In an open-label study conducted to characterize the pharmacokinetics and antihypertensive response to irbesartan in children, it was well tolerated and may be a treatment option for pediatric hypertensive patients. However, there is no report of its use in CHF in the pediatric age group.

- *Nitroglycerin:* Intravenous nitroglycerin is safe and very effective therapy for pulmonary edema. It is predominantly a venodilator and a weak arteriolar dilator. The blood pressure needs to be monitored frequently. The addition of an ionotrope such as dobutamine may be required if the child develops hypotension (systolic BP <90 mm Hg). With careful noninvasive monitoring, nitroglycerin may be administered with a micro drip set, although the use of an infusion pump is preferable. Dosages are titrated from 0.5–4.0 µg/kg/min.
- *Sodium nitroprusside:* A potent arterial dilator, sodium nitroprusside requires careful monitoring of intra-arterial pressure. It is rapid acting and severe hypotension may occur within minutes. Careful titration is required. The dosage ranges from 0.5–1 µg/kg/min. The infusion fluid needs to be protected from sunlight. Renal failure enhances its toxicity. It is most useful for treatment of acute left ventricular failure in presence of hypertension and for acute mitral or aortic regurgitation in postoperative patients.
- *Nifedipine:* This calcium channel blocker causes peripheral vasodilation and is useful in patients with coarctation of aorta or pulmonary arterial hypertension. The advantages are a rapid onset of action, safety, and sublingual administration. It can be used in infants also in a dose of 0.1–0.3 mg/kg/dose sublingual 6 hourly.
- *Hydralazine:* It is an infrequently used vasodilator for the treatment of CHF now. Chronic use results in tachyphylaxis. The dosage is 1–7 mg/kg/day in divided doses.

Inotropes

Inotropes other than digoxin are used for short-term support of circulation or to tide over the crisis. Their long-term use is not associated with improved long-term survival. Dopamine is currently the most widely used inotrope for acute support in pediatric practice. It has the advantages of peripheral vasoconstriction and raising blood pressure at moderate to high doses (6–10 µg/kg/min). At higher doses (20 µg/kg/min), intense vasoconstriction raises blood pressure but it is counterproductive as it increases myocardial work. Dopamine also increases pulmonary vascular resistance and causes tachycardia. Both these factors may be detrimental to some patients (e.g., mitral stenosis). For hypotension in the preterm neonate, dopamine is particularly effective at low dosage.

Dobutamine is a synthetic sympathomimetic agent and causes increase in contractility with relatively less tachycardia or rise in blood pressure. It is compatible with dopamine in the same infusion and often a combination of dopamine and dobutamine is used to provide inotropic support. The individual variations are wide and dosages of 5–20 µg/kg/min are generally used.

Epinephrine, norepinephrine, and isoprenaline are potent, naturally occurring sympathomimetics used during postoperative low output only. Isoprenaline, a beta stimulant is a pulmonary and systemic vasodilator and causes tachycardia. Rarely, nor-epinephrine has been found effective in septic shock unresponsive to other treatment.

Phosphodiesterase Inhibitors (Milrinone)
This phosphodiesterase inhibitor inotropic agent, used in refractory failure, also has pulmonary vasodilating properties. Dose is 0.3–0.7 µg/kg/min in children, mainly in postoperative or refractory failure. Thrombocytopenia and hepatic dysfunction limit its use. It should not be mixed in dextrose containing solutions or with frusemide.

Miscellaneous
Beta blockers: Paradoxically, some patients with dilated cardiomyopathy may respond to beta-blockers. The rationale relates to downgrading of beta receptors due to chronic catecholamine stimulation. The therapy is best undertaken in hospital as careful monitoring is required. Carvedilol, a nonselective beta blocker with alpha-1 blocking and antioxidative properties has proven to be beneficial in most adult patients with congestive heart failure. Although the experience from adult patients may be extrapolated to older children, symptomatic infants remain a subset for whom dosage, safety, and efficacy need to be established in larger studies. It has been recently reported that carvedilol is well tolerated in infants with dilated cardiomyopathy and there is significant improvement in their functional status. Optimal timing of starting therapy, dosage, and long-term effects need to be investigated with multi-institutional trials. A recent multi-center study has suggested carvedilol as an adjunct to standard therapy for pediatric heart failure. It improves symptoms and left ventricular function. Side effects are common but well tolerated. Further prospective studies are required to determine the effect of carvedilol on survival and to clearly define its role in pediatric heart failure therapy.
L Carnitine: Metabolic cardiomyopathy associated with carnitine deficiency responds to replacement with L-carnitine in a dosage of 50–100 mg/kg/day in divided doses. Its role in other cardiomyopathies is not proved.
Prostaglandins E1: As described earlier, neonates with duct dependent lesions as transposition of great arteries, coarctation of aorta, aortic stenosis in failure or hypoplastic left heart syndrome etc. improve remarkably with prostaglandin E1 (PGE1) infusion. The therapy is initiated at 0.05 µg/kg/min if an adequate response is seen; the dose may be reduced subsequently. Apnea may occur during the infusion and ventilatory support should be available. Irritability, seizures, hypotension, and hyperpyrexia are rare.

OTHER OPTIONS

Extracorporeal membrane oxygenation (ECMO) was initially developed for respiratory failure. Its use, however, has evolved into an excellent method of preoperative and postoperative support in the treatment of infants and children with acquired and congenital heart disease. Along with ECMO, the left ventricular assist device (LVAD), and the intra-aortic balloon pump (IABP) have also found a place in the management of children with heart failure. There is a 74% survival rate and the long-term outcome has been excellent in most cases.

A combination of external implantable pulsatile and continuous-flow external mechanical support now can be used to bridge pediatric patients with end stage cardiomyopathy to orthotopic heart transplantation. Such a combination has been found to complement each other to significantly extend the lives of a wide range of pediatric patients with severe cardiomyopathies and myocarditis.

Biventricular pacing: Biventricular pacing therapy is an innovative therapy for improving cardiac output in adult patients with severe heart failure. However, recently this technique had been used in a 6-month young infant with tetralogy of Fallot and atresia of the left pulmonary artery in whom biventricular stimulation led to improved left ventricular function and successful weaning from extracorporeal circulation.

Cardiac transplantation: Pediatric heart transplantation has become an accepted method of treatment for certain pediatric heart diseases in western countries. Pediatric heart transplantation can provide good intermediate term survival for selected pediatric patients. Cardiac transplantation has since become a standard therapeutic option for certain disorders in which poor cardiac output without other surgical options exists in the face of maximized medical therapy. The most common disorder requiring transplantation is dilated cardiomyopathy, other forms of cardiomyopathy (i.e., restrictive cardiomyopathy, arrhythmogenic right ventricular dysplasia/cardiomyopathy, and hypertrophic cardiomyopathy with poor ventricular function), and hypoplastic left heart.

Treatment of the Cause

It is extremely important, particularly for infants with persistent CHF in the first few months of life to arrive at an accurate early diagnosis for the cause of CHF and planning definitive measures.

Survival is determined by early correction of treatable cause as infection, electrolyte imbalance, arrhythmias, structural heart defects as shunt lesions, complete transposition of great vessels, anomalous origin of left coronary artery from pulmonary artery and critical left or right-sided obstructive lesions. Timely intervention is crucial and the results of catheter and surgical intervention are excellent for structural defects.

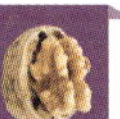

IN A NUTSHELL

Congestive Heart Failure

1. Congestive heart failure (CHF) may occur due to ventricular systolic dysfunction, diastolic dysfunction, or abnormal ventriculoarterial coupling. They are associated with an exaggerated, inappropriate, or abnormal afterload on a normal myocardium.
2. An underlying structural heart disease must be carefully looked for in children with heart failure.
3. Diagnosis of heart failure in children is largely clinical. The cause can be usually confirmed on echocardiography.
4. Conventional drug therapy includes digoxin, frusemide, spironolactone, and inotropes. Adjunctive therapy includes ACE inhibitors (captopril/enalapril) and beta-blockers (carvedilol).

Amdani S, Conway J, George K, et al. Evaluation and management of chronic heart failure in children and adolescents with congenital heart disease. A Scientific Statement from the American Heart association. Circulation. 2024;150:e33-50.
Bautista-Hernandez V, Sanchez-Andres A, Portela F, et al. Current pharmacologic management of pediatric heart failure in congenital heart disease. Curr Vasc Pharmacol. 2011;9:619-28.
Chaturvedi V, Saxena A. Heart failure in children: clinical aspect and clinical evaluation, diagnostic testing, and initial medical management. Eur J Pediatr. 2010;169:269-79.
Chaturvedi V, Saxena A. Heart failure in children: clinical aspect and management. Indian J Pediatr. 2009;76:195-205.
Frobel AK, Hulpke-Wette M, Schmidt KG, et al. Beta-blockers for congestive heart failure in children. Cochrane Database Syst Rev. 2009;1:CD007037.
Hoffman TM. Newer inotropes in pediatric heart failure. J Cardiovasc Pharmacol. 2011;58:121-5.
Hsu DT, Pearson GD. Heart failure in children: part II: diagnosis, treatment, and future directions. Circ Heart Fail. 2009;2:490-8.
Jefferies JL, Hoffman TM, Nelson DP. Heart failure treatment in the intensive care unit in children. Heart Fail Clin. 2010;6:531-58.
Kantor PF, Mertens LL. Clinical practice: heart failure in children. Part II: current maintenance therapy and new therapeutic approaches. Eur J Pediatr. 2010;169:403-10.
Loss KL, Shaddy RE, Kantor PF. Recent and upcoming drug therapies for pediatric heart failure. Front Pediatr. 2021;9:681224.
Madriago E, Silberbach M. Heart failure in infants and children. Pediatr Rev. 2010;31:4-12.
Margossian R. Contemporary management of pediatric heart failure. Expert Rev Cardiovasc Ther. 2008;6:187-97.
O'Connor MJ, Rosenthal DN, Shaddy RE. Outpatient management of pediatric heart failure. Heart Fail Clin. 2010;6:515-29.
Penny DJ, Vick GW 3rd. Novel therapies in childhood heart failure: today and tomorrow. Heart Fail Clin. 2010;6:591-621.

19.6 Congenital Heart Disease

PE 22.1, PE 22.2

INTRODUCTION

The incidence of CHD is 8/1,000 live births, excluding patent ductus arteriosus in preterm, bicuspid aortic valve, and mitral valve prolapse. The incidence is higher in stillborn, abortuses, and premature babies. **Table 19.8** shows relative frequency of congenital heart defects.

AGE AT PRESENTATION

Most of the congenital heart defects are well tolerated during the intrauterine life. This is due to the parallel circulation in fetus in contrast to circulation in series after birth. Lesions that can cause problems during fetal life include atrioventricular valve regurgitation (mitral/tricuspid regurgitation), aortic valve regurgitation, restriction of foramen ovale, restriction of ductus arteriosus, and cardiomyopathies.

Transposition, hypoplastic left heart syndrome, Fallot tetralogy, and coarctation of aorta are the most common lesions presenting within first 2 weeks after birth.

ETIOLOGY

Most cases of congenital heart disease have multifactorial etiology and result from a combination of genetic and environmental stimulus. In some there is definite association with chromosome abnormalities, including trisomy of chromosome 21, 18, and 13, Turner syndrome and microdeletions of chromosome 22q11. Almost 90% of children with trisomy 18 have heart disease. In

Table 19.8 Prevalence of Congenital Heart Defects

Lesion	*Relative prevalence (%)*
Ventricular septal defect (VSD)	16–50
Atrial septal defect (ASD)	8–10
Patent ductus arteriosus (PDA)	6–8
Tetralogy of Fallot (TOF)	3.36–9.7
Complete transposition of great vessels (d-TGA)	5–7
Pulmonary stenosis (PS)	5.8–11.6
Valvular aortic stenosis (AS)	3.7–7.6
Atrioventricular septal defect (AVSD)	4
Hypoplastic left heart syndrome (HLHS)	3.4
Peripheral pulmonary stenosis (PPS)	2–3
Tricuspid atresia	1.2
Total anomalous pulmonary venous connection (TAPVC)	0.8–1.5
Ebstein anomaly	0.38–1

trisomy 21, 50% of children have heart disease—commonest being atrioventricular septal defect in 40%.

Known teratogens, such as maternal insulin-dependent diabetes, rubella, and drug exposure, can be implicated in others. CHD may be associated with specific dysmorphic features suggesting a syndrome, which may show monogenic inheritance (e.g., William, Marfan, Noonan, etc.). However, in the majority of cases of isolated CHD, no single underlying cause can be identified. A list of some syndrome associated with heart defects has been provided in **Table 19.4**.

CLASSIFICATION

Group I: Acyanotic heart disease

- ***Left to right shunts (volume overload):*** Ventricular septal defect (VSD), atrial septal defect (ASD), patent ductus arteriosus (PDA), aortopulmonary window
- ***Obstructive lesions:*** Aortic stenosis, coarctation of aorta, pulmonary stenosis (PS)

Group II: Cyanotic heart disease

- ***Decreased pulmonary blood flow:*** Tetralogy of Fallot (TOF), tricuspid atresia with PS, single ventricle with PS, double outlet right ventricle with PS, transposition of great arteries (TGA) with VSD with PS.
- ***Increased pulmonary blood flow:*** d-Transposition of great arteries (d-TGA), truncus arteriosus, total anomalous pulmonary venous connection (TAPVC), single ventricle without PS.

CLINICAL FEATURES

A heart disease is likely to be congenital in origin in presence of one or more of the following:

1. Presentation in neonatal period or infancy
2. Presence of central cyanosis
3. Presence of parasternal murmur
4. ***Associated extracardiac anomalies:*** Specially of ear, kidneys, and skeleton.

Presentations of congenital heart disease according to the type of defect are detailed below.

Left-to-Right Shunts

The three common left-to-right shunts are VSD, ASD, and PDA. Their presentation is quite similar, yet the age at onset of symptoms varies. VSD and PDA may present in infancy while ASD presents in later childhood. Children with left to right shunts are characterized by absence of cyanosis. They are prone to have frequent chest infections and land up in congestive heart failure. Examination reveals a precordial bulge, and hyperkinetic precordium. Chest X-ray will demonstrate cardiomegaly and plethoric lung fields.

Obstructive Lesions

These lesions are also acyanotic. There is no history of frequent chest infections. Precordial bulge is absent, and the apex beat is forcible or heaving due to concentric hypertrophy of the respective ventricle without cardiac enlargement. There is no cardiomegaly on chest X-ray and pulmonary vasculature is normal.

Obstructive lesions can be right sided (pulmonary stenosis) or left sided (aortic stenosis or coarctation of aorta). ECG can help in differentiating between a right or left sided obstruction; and also helpful in indicating the severity of the obstruction.

Right-to-Left Shunts

Right-to-left shunts are characterized by presence of cyanosis, clubbing, and polycythemia. These children can be categorized into two groups: (*i*) Those with decreased pulmonary blood flow; and (*ii*) those with increased pulmonary blood flow. Children with increased pulmonary blood flow are mildly cyanotic; those with normal or diminished pulmonary blood flow are moderately to severely cyanotic.

Right-to-left shunt with decreased pulmonary blood flow is seen in tetralogy of Fallot and is due to pulmonary stenosis (and other conditions with similar physiology, i.e., good mixing at ventricular level and PS). These children may have a typical history of hypercyanotic spell and squatting episodes. There is no CHF, no cardiomegaly, a quiet precordium, and no chest infections. Chest X-ray shows oligemic lung fields.

Increased pulmonary blood flow with cyanosis is seen in d-TGA, secondary to reversed origin of great vessels; TAPVC, and truncus arteriosus. These children do not have hypercyanotic spells but are characterized by presence of CHF, recurrent chest infections, and cardiomegaly. On chest X-ray, pulmonary vascularity is increased and pulmonary arteries are dilated, along with cardiomegaly.

RISK OF RECURRENCE

- Incidence of congenital heart disease in general population is 0.6–0.8%.
- Incidence in second pregnancy after a child with heart disease is 2–6%.
- Risk further increases if previous two children have the heart disease.
- Recurrence risk with left sided obstructive lesions is higher than other heart defects.
- The recurrence rate of CHD in offspring of either parent with a heart disease is variable, ranging from 3–5%. A higher recurrence risk when the mother rather than the father is affected has raised the possibility of mitochondrial inheritance in some cases.
- Diseases with a single gene disorder and/or chromosomal abnormalities are associated with a high recurrence rate. In Marfan, Noonan, and Holt-Oram syndromes, there is a 50% risk of recurrence in offspring.
- Risk is also higher if 1st degree relatives have a congenital heart disease.

In the above situations, fetal echocardiography is recommended at 16–18 weeks of gestation. However, a negative study cannot guarantee the absence of congenital heart disease.

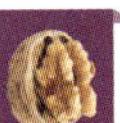

IN A NUTSHELL

Congenital Heart Disease

1. Acyanotic heart diseases consist of left-to-right shunts and obstructive lesions. Left-to-right shunts include ventricular septal defect (VSD), atrial septal defect (ASD), and patent ductus arteriosus (PDA). All of them have increased pulmonary blood flow, cardiomegaly, congestive heart failure (CHF), and repeated chest infections.
2. Common obstructive congenital heart diseases are coarctation of aorta, pulmonary stenosis, and aortic stenosis. Severe pulmonary stenosis, however may present with cyanosis.
3. Cyanotic children are classified into (a) those with decreased pulmonary blood flow (PBF), e.g., tetralogy of Fallot; and (b) those with increased pulmonary blood flow, e.g., transposition of great arteries (TGA), total anomalous pulmonary venous connection (TAPVC).

Rao PS. Diagnosis and management of cyanotic congenital heart disease: part I. Indian J Pediatr. 2009;76:57-70.
Saxena A, Relan J, Agarwal R, et al. Indian guidelines for indications and timing of intervention for common congenital heart diseases: revised and updated consensus statement of the Working group on management of congenital heart diseases. Ann Pediatr Cardiol. 2019;12(3):254-86.
Syamasundar Rao P. Diagnosis and management of cyanotic congenital heart disease: part II. Indian J Pediatr. 2009;76:297-308.

Acyanotic Congenital Heart Diseases

19.7 Ventricular Septal Defect

PE 22.1

INTRODUCTION

Ventricular septal defect (VSD) refers to an abnormal communication between the two ventricles present since birth. Time of clinical manifestation depends on the size and location of defect. Ventricular septal defects are classified into four types:

1. ***Perimembranous ventricular septal defects:*** These are the commonest type of ventricular septal defects, located in the membranous part of the interventricular septum. Some of the perimembranous ventricular septal defects have a tendency for spontaneous reduction in size or at times to get closed by attachment of the septal leaflet of the tricuspid valve to the defect. Less commonly, aortic valve cusp gets prolapsed into the defect, causing restriction of the defect but at the risk of distortion of aortic valve leading to development of aortic regurgitation.
2. ***Doubly committed or subpulmonary ventricular septal defects:*** These defects involve the infundibular septum and so are committed to both aortic and pulmonary outflows. As the right coronary cusp of the aortic valve remains unsupported, chances of developing aortic regurgitation are higher than in perimembranous septal defects.
3. ***Trabecular defect (muscular defect):*** These defects can be single or multiple and may occur in isolation or in association with defects in other locations. These types of defects have the highest tendency toward spontaneous reduction of size and closure.
4. ***Inlet ventricular septal defects:*** These defects occur in inlet part of the ventricular septum. There may be loss of normal offsetting of the atrioventricular valves. Inlet VSDs never close naturally.

SIZE OF DEFECT

Anatomically, ventricular septal defects are classified as large if the defect is larger than two-thirds of the aortic orifice diameter, moderate if the size of the defect is less than two-third but larger than one-third of the aortic orifice diameter; and small if its size is less than one-third of the aortic orifice diameter. Depending on the pressure gradient between the two ventricles, ventricular septal defects are classified as:

- ***Restrictive (small):*** Gradient between two ventricles 64 mm Hg and above.
- ***Moderately restrictive:*** Gradient between two ventricles between 25–64 mm Hg.
- ***Non-restrictive (large):*** No significant pressure gradient between the two ventricles (<25 mm Hg).

HEMODYNAMICS

Because of communication, a pressure gradient between the two ventricles, and the different vascular resistances in the systemic and pulmonary circuits; shunting of oxygenated blood occurs from left ventricle to right ventricle.

Large Non-restrictive Defect

Due to a large defect, the pressure between the two ventricles equalizes very early in systole. Thus, shunting of blood from left to right ventricle produces a short systolic murmur. Pressure increases in the right ventricle due to additional flow coming from the left ventricle. Due to transmission of increased right ventricular flow and pressure to pulmonary artery, P_2 becomes loud, and its closure is delayed. On the other hand, aortic valve

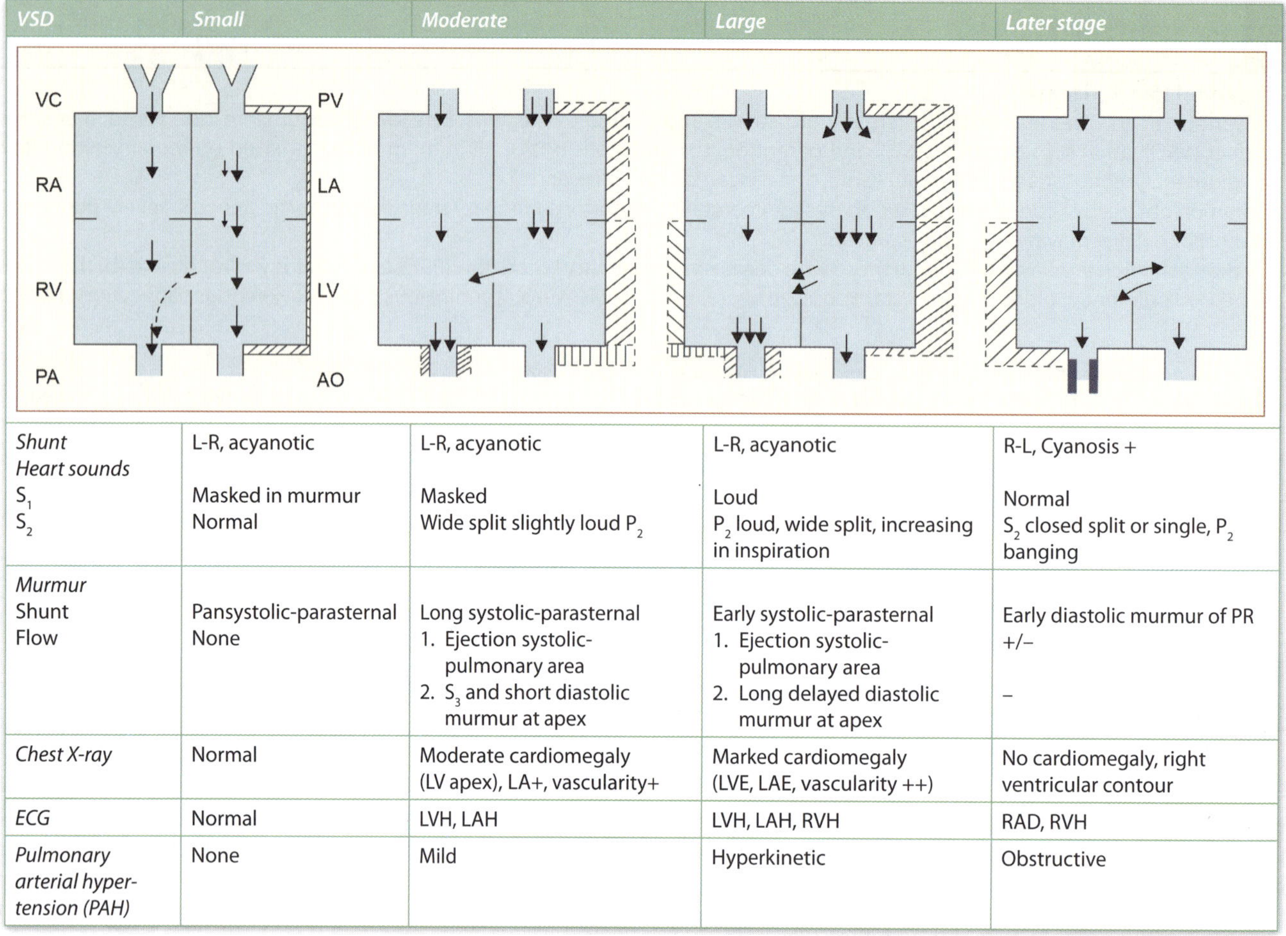

VSD	Small	Moderate	Large	Later stage
Shunt	L-R, acyanotic	L-R, acyanotic	L-R, acyanotic	R-L, Cyanosis +
Heart sounds				
S_1	Masked in murmur	Masked	Loud	Normal
S_2	Normal	Wide split slightly loud P_2	P_2 loud, wide split, increasing in inspiration	S_2 closed split or single, P_2 banging
Murmur				
Shunt	Pansystolic-parasternal	Long systolic-parasternal	Early systolic-parasternal	Early diastolic murmur of PR +/–
Flow	None	1. Ejection systolic-pulmonary area 2. S_3 and short diastolic murmur at apex	1. Ejection systolic-pulmonary area 2. Long delayed diastolic murmur at apex	–
Chest X-ray	Normal	Moderate cardiomegaly (LV apex), LA+, vascularity+	Marked cardiomegaly (LVE, LAE, vascularity ++)	No cardiomegaly, right ventricular contour
ECG	Normal	LVH, LAH	LVH, LAH, RVH	RAD, RVH
Pulmonary arterial hyper-tension (PAH)	None	Mild	Hyperkinetic	Obstructive

Fig. 19.33: Hemodynamics of ventricular septal defect

closes early due to faster emptying of left ventricle. This result in a widely split second heart sound that remains variable with respiration. Increased flow across the pulmonary valve also results in an ejection systolic murmur at the pulmonary area. Large pulmonary flow translates into a larger pulmonary venous return into left atrium and subsequently increased flow across the mitral valve, passing through the normal mitral valve, the large volume of blood (pulmonary blood flow: systemic blood flow ratio >2:1) results in a delayed diastolic murmur at the apex. If the degree of shunt is >1.5: 1 but <2:1, then only a third heart sound (left ventricular S_3) will be audible. In lesser degree of shunts, there is no diastolic sound at apex (**Fig. 19.33**).

Restrictive (Small) Defects

The left ventricle starts contracting before the right ventricle, the flow of blood from left to right ventricle starts very early in systole and a high-pressure gradient will be maintained between the two ventricles throughout the systole. The murmur thus starts early partially masking the first sound and continuing through the systole. This is heard as a parasternal pansystolic murmur, best over 3rd–4th left intercostal space.

CLINICAL PRESENTATION

Large/Non-restrictive Ventricular Septal Defect

The pressures in both ventricles are equal soon after birth but with fall in pulmonary vascular resistance (PVR), which occurs by 6–10 weeks of age, left to right shunt increases and the child becomes symptomatic having features of congestive cardiac failure. Features of a large shunt such as fast breathing, feed intolerance, failure to gain weight, excessive sweating, and recurrent chest infections appear.

Examination shows failure to thrive, hyperkinetic precordium, cardiomegaly, tachycardia, tachypnea, systolic murmur at left 4th intercostal space, wide and variable second heart sound with loud pulmonary component, ejection systolic murmur at left upper sternal border, and delayed diastolic murmur at apex.

Large left to right shunts are usually associated with pulmonary arterial hypertension (PAH), characterized by loud P_2 and ejection systolic murmur at pulmonary area; caused by increased blood flow through the pulmonary bed. This is known as the *hyperkinetic* variety of PAH. With passage of time, sustained increased pulmonary blood flow leads to irreversible changes in pulmonary vascular bed. Pulmonary vascular changes result in increased resistance to pulmonary blood flow. This chain of events suggests the onset of *obstructive pulmonary arterial hypertension.* Ultimately, pulmonary vascular resistance exceeds the systemic vascular resistance. The flow across the shunt now operates from right ventricle to left ventricle. This is known as "*reversal of shunt.*" Clinically, there is a forcible parasternal heave, S_2 becomes single, P_2 is very loud, and mitral murmur disappears. Cyanosis appears due to right to left shunt across the VSD (*Eisenmenger syndrome*).

Restrictive (Small/Moderate) Ventricular Septal Defect

Small ventricular septal defects are asymptomatic and are detected only on routine examination. Moderate size left to right shunt can be present if pulmonary flow is more than twice the systemic flow (Qp/Qs >2:1).

NATURAL COURSE

Untreated patients of ventricular septal defects have a variable course:

1. ***Spontaneous closure or reduction in size:*** Overall, approximately 60–70% of VSDs either decreases in size or close spontaneously. Muscular defects are the commonest type of defects to close or reduce in size spontaneously. Next most common type of defects to do so are the perimembranous ventricular septal defects.
2. ***Pulmonary stenosis:*** Development of right ventricular outflow tract stenosis due to infundibular hypertrophy occurs in about 9% of patients with ventricular septal defects. Right ventricular outflow tract obstruction is more common in patients who have right aortic arch with ventricular septal defects.
3. ***Development of pulmonary vascular obstructive disease:*** Reports show that pulmonary vascular disease occurs in 12.4% of long-term survivors with moderate ventricular septal defects, while it occurs in *majority* of the patients with *non-restrictive* ventricular septal defects, sometimes occurring as early as 2 years of age.
4. ***Development of aortic valve prolapse and aortic regurgitation:*** Prolapse of right coronary cusp of aortic valve is 10 times more common with doubly committed ventricular septal defects than defects of the perimembranous septum. The reasons for prolapse of right coronary cusp are loss of support for the cusp and also the distortion of the cusp due to suction effect of the jet through the septal defect.
5. ***Bacterial endocarditis:*** The incidence of infective endocarditis is 0.9% per year. The risk is small, therefore, restrictive ventricular septal defects with normal pulmonary artery pressure and normal left ventricular dimensions, without pulmonary stenosis or aortic valve prolapse, are not considered as an indication for surgery.

DIAGNOSIS

Electrocardiography

- ***Small ventricular septal defect:*** Normal ECG
- ***Moderate shunts:*** Left ventricular hypertrophy and left atrial overload pattern
- ***Large shunts with hyperkinetic pulmonary artery hypertension:*** Biventricular hypertrophy (**Fig. 19.34**).

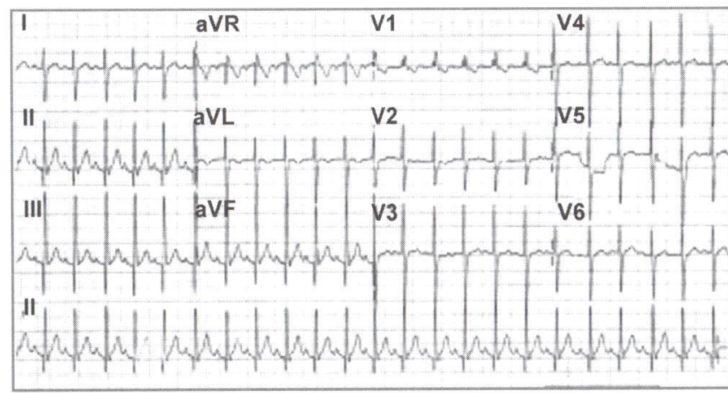

Fig. 19.34: ECG from 6 months old child with nonrestrictive perimembranous ventricular septal defect showing normal "P" wave axis, sinus tachycardia (HR-150/min), right axis deviation (QRS + 160°), biventricular hypertrophy (chest leads in ½ voltage)

- ***Large shunt with severe obstructive pulmonary vascular disease:*** Severe right ventricular hypertrophy.

CHEST X-RAY

The magnitude of changes depends upon the degree of shunt. With small shunt, chest X-ray will be normal. Moderate shunts produce left ventricular type of cardiomegaly. Presence of left atrial enlargement and pulmonary plethora indicates increased pulmonary blood flow and a large left to right shunt (**Fig. 19.35**).

ECHOCARDIOGRAPHY

Echocardiography shows the site of defect, number of defects, assessment of pulmonary artery pressure, left atrial and left ventricular dimensions, associated pulmonary stenosis, condition of aortic valve, coarctation of aorta, etc.

CARDIAC CATHETERIZATION

With availability of echocardiography, cardiac catheterization is rarely done for VSD. Indications for cardiac catheterization include the following:

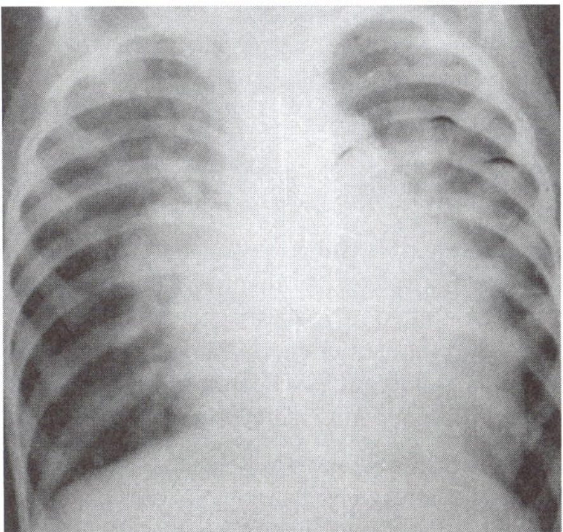

Fig. 19.35: X-ray chest from a patient with large ventricular septal defect; at the age of 5 months showing cardiomegaly (LV type apex) with enlargement of main pulmonary artery segment. Pulmonary vasculature is markedly increased. The aortic shadow is not prominent

- ❖ Large VSD with severe PAH if there is an issue of operability to assess pulmonary vascular resistance and pulmonary vasculature reactivity with vasodilators.
- ❖ Small VSD but clinical findings not correlating with echocardiography
- ❖ Multiple VSDs
- ❖ Device closure of VSD

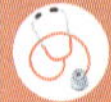

CASE STUDY Ventricular Septal Defect

A 4-month-old girl was brought to emergency department with complaints of fast breathing, poor feeding, fever, and cough for three days. She was born at term gestation with birth weight of 2.8 kg. She was doing well till 2 months of age, when mother noticed feeding problems in form of suck-rest-suck cycle and sweating over forehead while feeding. Mother was also concerned about her poor growth.

On examination, the child looked thin and weighed 3 kg. She was febrile and had tachypnea (RR 65/min with sub-costal and intercostals retractions) and tachycardia (HR 170/min). Pulse volume was low and all the peripheral pulses were felt. Blood pressure was 66/48 mm Hg in right arm. SpO_2 was 98% in all four limbs. Neck veins were dilated. Precordial examination revealed hyperdynamic left ventricular apex outside the mid-clavicular line in 6th intercostal space. First heart sound was normal; P_2 component of second heart sound was loud; S_3 gallop was heard at apex. Grade 3/6, pansystolic murmur was heard in left lower parasternal region with radiation to entire precordium. Short mid diastolic murmur was heard at apex. Liver was felt 4 cm below right costal margin. Respiratory system examination revealed crepitations in bilateral infraclavicular and axillary areas.

What is the most likely diagnosis?

This child has acyanotic congenital heart disease. According to Nada's criteria, presence of CHF and systolic murmur grade 3 (both major criteria), abnormal S_2, abnormal chest X-ray, abnormal ECG (all minor criteria), indicate a cardiac condition. She has feeding problems and has presented with CHF (evidenced by suck-rest-suck cycles, tachypnea, tachycardia, weak pulses, cardiomegaly, prominent neck veins, and hepatomegaly) and lower respiratory tract infection. There was no cyanosis. This favors left to right shunt physiology. Size of the shunt is large as suggested by presence of CHF, S_3 gallop, and mid-diastolic murmur at apex. Presence of pan-systolic murmur indicates a ventricular septal defect.

Describe the findings in X-ray and ECG of this child, shown on next page.

Chest X-ray shows cardiomegaly with cardiothoracic ratio 0.7. The apical contour is left ventricular type. There is increased pulmonary blood flow. Areas of consolidation are visible in both lung fields. ECG characteristically shows large equidiphasic QRS complexes in mid-precordial chest leads indicating biventricular enlargement due to large VSD. This is called *Katz–Wachtel phenomenon*.

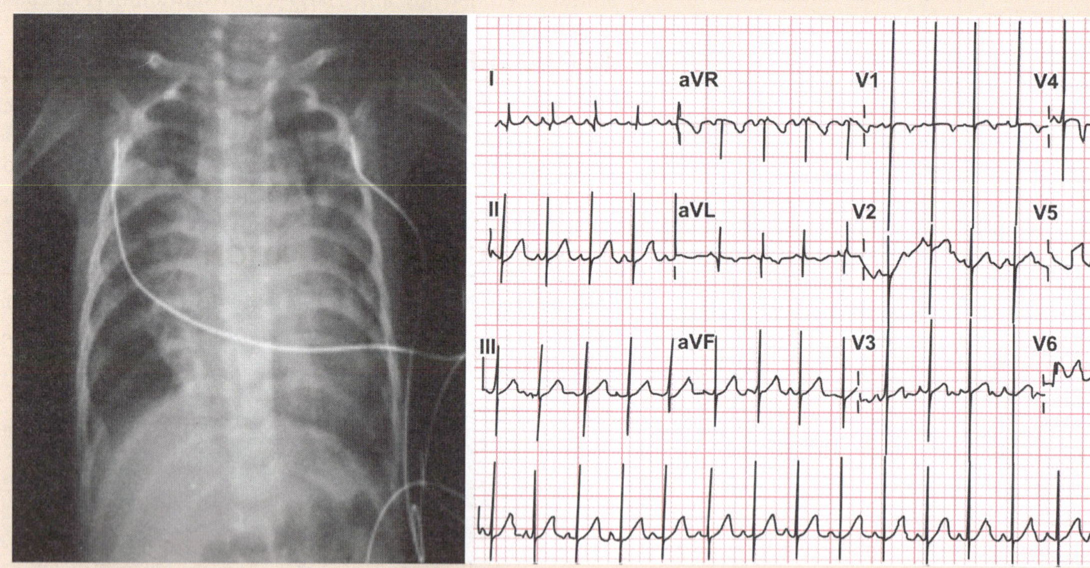

How will you manage this child?

Acute management involves treatment of respiratory infection and control of CHF. Oxygen should be started to relieve respiratory distress. IV fluids and antibiotics need to be started. Injection furosemide and oral spironolactone will be required. Calorie dense feeds are to be given initially by nasogastric (NG) tube till oral intake improves. Iron supplementation for treatment or prevention of anemia must be initiated after control of infection. Echocardiography will confirm the diagnosis. Surgery involving patch closure of VSD is indicated soon after the chest infection is controlled. In the interim period diuretics should be continued.

Is there no role of digitalis/enalapril?

Role of digoxin in patients with heart failure due to left to right shunts is not well defined. It is not used in current pediatric cardiology practice. Angiotensin converting enzyme inhibitors (enalapril) reduce the systemic vascular resistance (blood pressure) hence help in reducing afterload of failing left ventricle. This helps in improving the cardiac output and also reduces the shunt fraction. Hence enalapril can be added as a third line agent if combination of furosemide and spironolactone does not control the symptoms of heart failure. Remember, definite treatment is surgery.

TREATMENT Ventricular Septal Defect

Medical Management

The medical treatment consists of control of congestive cardiac failure. This includes administration of digoxin, diuretic, ACE inhibitors, and control of anemia and infections. Digoxin is indicated only for ventricular dysfunction. Adequate high caloric diet is essential to sustain growth in face of increased demands. Follow-up is needed for development of pulmonary stenosis, pulmonary arterial hypertension, or aortic regurgitation.

Surgical Management

Early surgical treatment (before 6 months) is indicated in large defects and if CHF is not controlled by medical management. Association of aortic regurgitation is also indication for surgery, irrespective of the size of defect.

- *Operative treatment* consists of closure of the ventricular septal defect with the use of a Dacron or pericardial patch. It is being done for >4 decades with very good results and <1% risk.
- *Percutaneous device closure* **(Figs. 19.36A and B)** is indicated in children weighing >10 kg with muscular VSD, or residual VSD after surgery, with good results.

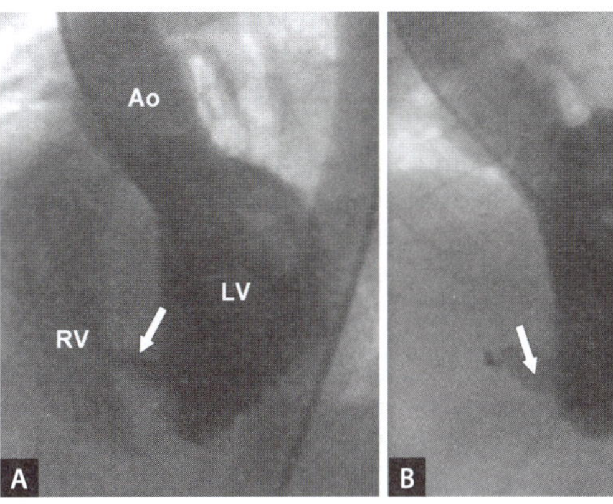

Figs. 19.36A and B: Left ventricular angiography in long axial oblique view: (A) Angiogram showing muscular VSD (arrow) filling right ventricle; (B) LV angiogram after device closure of muscular VSD showing device in situ (arrow), no residual flow

Aguilar NE, Eugenio Lopez J. Ventricular septal defects. Bol Asoc Med P R. 2009;101(4):23-9.
Danford DA, Martin AB, Fletcher SE, et al. Children with heart murmurs: can ventricular septal defect be diagnosed reliably without an echocardiogram? J Am Coll Cardiol. 1997;30(1):243-6.
Saxena A, Relan J, Agarwal R, et al. Indian guidelines for indications and timing of intervention for common congenital heart diseases: Revised and updated consensus statement of the Working group on management of congenital heart diseases. Ann Pediatr Cardiol. 2019;12(3):254-86.

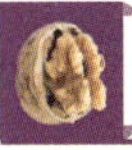

IN A NUTSHELL

Ventricular Septal Defect

1. Ventricular septal defect (VSD) is an acyanotic heart disease with left to right shunt.
2. Moderate to large sized VSD present after 6 weeks of age, with feeding difficulties, suck-rest-suck cycle, and repeated respiratory infections.
3. Clinical examination reveals a pansystolic murmur in left parasternal region, along with a wide split P_2 varying with respiration.
4. Small VSD is asymptomatic and may close spontaneously. Moderate to large VSD will require closure.

19.8 Eisenmenger Syndrome

PE 22.2

INTRODUCTION

Eisenmenger syndrome is characterized by severe, non-reactive, pulmonary vascular obstructive disease resulting in a right to left shunt at the atrial, ventricular, or pulmonary arterial level. The condition develops secondary to long standing pulmonary arterial hypertension associated with left to right shunt lesions (VSD, PDA, AP window and less commonly ASD).

These children present with cyanosis, clubbing, fatigue, effort intolerance, dyspnea, history of chest infections in childhood, parasternal impulse, palpable P_2, and pulmonary ejection click. Differential cyanosis (where the fingers remain pink and the toes show cyanosis and clubbing) is diagnostic of pulmonary artery hypertension with patent ductus arteriosus. There is no significant flow murmur. Pulmonary regurgitation murmur may be audible. In patients with ASD, murmur of tricuspid regurgitation may be audible.

Electrocardiogram reveals right axis deviation and right ventricular hypertrophy. Chest X-ray shows prominent pulmonary artery at hilum and oligemic lung fields.

TREATMENT Eisenmenger Syndrome

Heart lung transplant is the only surgical treatment for these patients. Medical treatment consists of treating congestive heart failure and supportive management. Children should be advised to maintain adequate hydration, iron supplementation, and avoid going to high altitude. Children with severe polycythemia (hematocrit >60%) get symptomatic relief after phlebotomy. Intermittent use of oxygen may help.

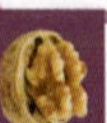

IN A NUTSHELL

Eisenmenger Syndrome

1. Long standing large left to right shunt defects lead to development of non-reactive changes in pulmonary vascular bed leading to shunt reversal called as Eisenmenger syndrome.
2. Prevention of its occurrence by timely treatment of the CHDs should be the goal.
3. Treatment involves pharmacological therapy in the form of pulmonary vasodilators and heart lung transplant.

Beghetti M, Tissot C. Pulmonary arterial hypertension in congenital heart diseases. Semin Respir Crit Care Med. 2009;30:421-8.
Berman EB, Barst RJ. Eisenmenger's syndrome: current management. Prog Cardiovasc Dis. 2002;45:129-38.
Moons P, Canobbio MM, Budts W. Eisenmenger syndrome: a clinical review. Eur J Cardiovasc Nurs. 2009;8:237-45.

19.9 Patent Ductus Arteriosus

PE 22.1

INTRODUCTION

In adult circulation, blood flows from right ventricle to lungs *via* pulmonary artery for oxygenation. Since the fetus does not use the lungs (oxygenation is provided through the mother's placenta), flow from the right ventricle needs an outlet. The ductus arteriosus is a normal fetal structure between pulmonary artery and aorta, allowing the right ventricular outflow to bypass the pulmonary circulation. It shunts the left pulmonary artery flow to the aorta just beyond the origin of the left subclavian artery. Exposure to the high levels of oxygen at birth causes the ductus to close within 24 hours. Persistence of this fetal structure beyond 10 days of life in a term baby is considered abnormal.

EPIDEMIOLOGY

Patent ductus arteriosus represents 5–10% of all congenital heart diseases, excluding those in premature infants. It occurs in approximately eight of 1,000 live births. Females are 2–3 times more likely than males to have patent ductus arteriosus.

HEMODYNAMICS

Patent ductus arteriosus results in a left to right shunt from the aorta to the pulmonary artery (contrary to right-to-left shunt that operates in fetal life). *The flow from aorta to pulmonary artery occurs both during systole and diastole, as a pressure gradient is present throughout the cardiac cycle between the two great arteries.* This leads to overloading of the pulmonary circulation.

1. The flow of blood from aorta to pulmonary artery results in a continuous murmur, which starts in systole after the first sound, reaches a peak at the second sound, and continues in diastole without change in character. Murmur may diminish in intensity and is audible during only a part of the diastole.
2. Shunt results in increased flow to the pulmonary circulation.
3. Left atrium receives a large volume of blood from overloaded pulmonary circulation. Transfer of this volume to left ventricle across a normal mitral valve results in a mitral diastolic murmur (preceded by S_3) along with a loud S_1. Intensity of this murmur is directly proportional to the size of left-to-right shunt across the ductus.
4. The large volume of blood in the left ventricle causes a prolongation of the left ventricular systole and an increase in the size of the left ventricle to accommodate the extra volume. The prolonged left ventricular systole results in *delayed closure of the aortic* valve and a late A_2. With large left-to-right shunts the S_2 *may be paradoxically split* **(Fig. 19.37)**.
5. The large left ventricular volume ejected into the aorta results in *dilatation of the ascending aorta and arch of aorta.* A dilated ascending aorta results in an *aortic ejection click.*
6. Greater volume burden is placed on the left side of the heart, causing both left atrial and left ventricular enlargement.

CLINICAL FEATURES

Children with large patent ductus arteriosus present with congestive cardiac failure at around 6–10 weeks of age. Mild to moderate defects present after infancy with frequent chest infections, effort intolerance, and palpitation. Large defects may be associated with pulmonary arterial hypertension.

- Pulse is high volume and bounding in character. Pulse pressure is wide due to continuous leak of systemic flow from aorta to pulmonary artery.
- Inspection of the precordium reveals prominent carotid pulsations, and a hyperkinetic precordium. Apex is shifted down and out due to left ventricular overload.
- Palpation may reveal a thrill at the second left interspace. P_2 component of second sound may be palpable in large size shunts.

Heart Sounds

The first sound is accentuated. The second heart sound is split normally, or single, or paradoxical split, depending on the size of the shunt. A large shunt causes paradoxical split due to marked delay in emptying of left ventricle (thus causing delayed A_2, after P_2).

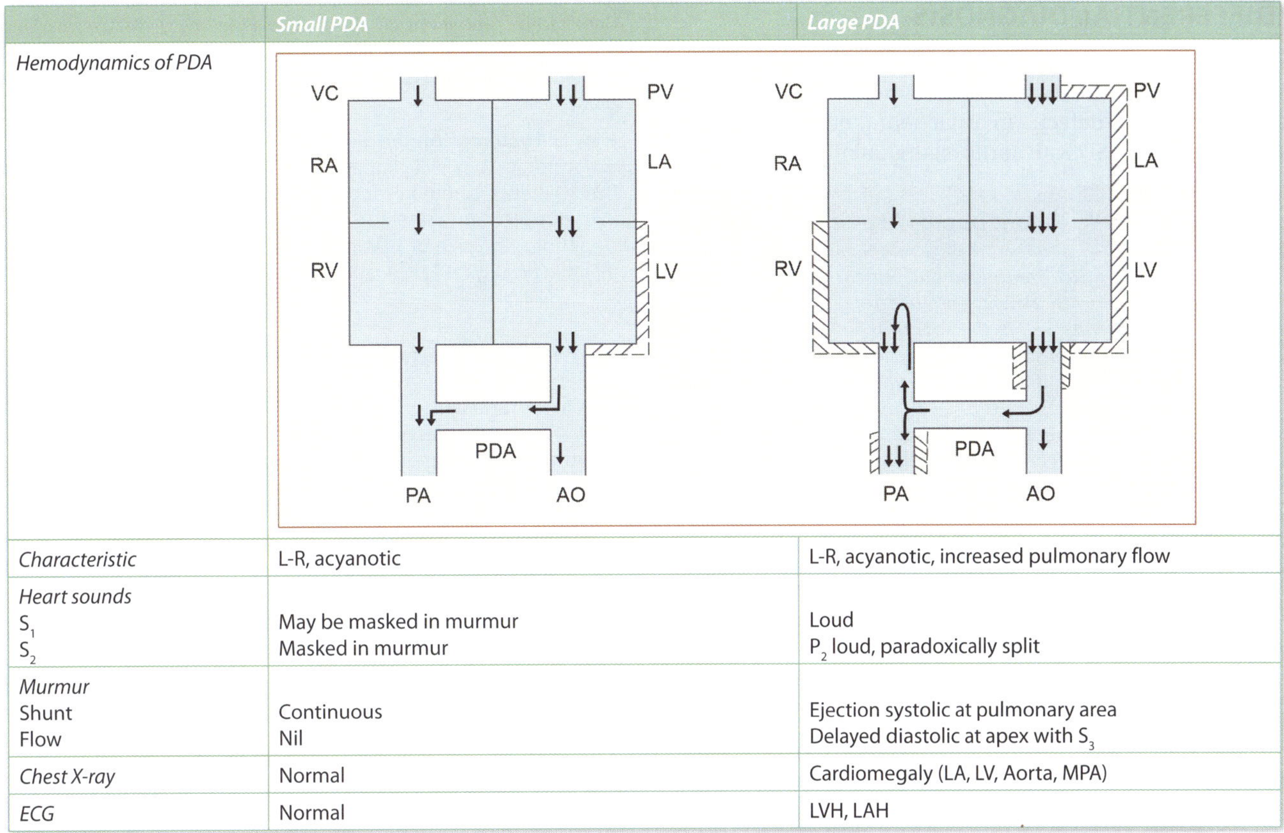

	Small PDA	Large PDA
Hemodynamics of PDA		
Characteristic	L-R, acyanotic	L-R, acyanotic, increased pulmonary flow
Heart sounds S_1 S_2	 May be masked in murmur Masked in murmur	 Loud P_2 loud, paradoxically split
Murmur Shunt Flow	 Continuous Nil	 Ejection systolic at pulmonary area Delayed diastolic at apex with S_3
Chest X-ray	Normal	Cardiomegaly (LA, LV, Aorta, MPA)
ECG	Normal	LVH, LAH

Fig. 19.37: Hemodynamics of patent ductus arteriosus

Murmurs

Continuous murmur: It is a hallmark of PDA. It indicates presence of difference in pressure between the aorta and pulmonary artery during both systole and diastole. The murmur starts after the first sound, overlaps the second sound and continues into diastole without any change in the character. Therefore, it may be difficult to assess the second sound, being masked by continuous murmur. The continuous murmur is best heard below the left clavicle.

Ejection systolic murmur: Patent ductus arteriosus with significant shunts result in markedly increased pulmonary flow and subsequent pulmonary artery hypertension. Thus, pressure gradient between aorta and pulmonary circulation diminishes during diastole, causing disappearance of the diastolic component of the continuous murmur. Presence of ejection systolic murmur instead of a continuous murmur thus indicates a larger size shunt. In these cases, evaluation of S_2 is possible because of its distance from the murmur.

Apical diastolic murmur: Large shunts also result in a delayed diastolic murmur at apex due to increased flow through mitral valve along with a third heart sound.

Obstructive Pulmonary Arterial Hypertension

This results in reversal of shunt (Eisenmenger syndrome) across the PDA and the flow murmurs disappear. Second heart sound remains normally split with very loud pulmonary component. These patients are considered inoperable. Right-to-left shunt through the PDA causes differential cyanosis with cyanosis in toes but not in fingers.

INVESTIGATIONS

Electrocardiography: Left ventricular dominance or hypertrophy is the most common finding. Associated aortic stenosis or coarctation of aorta should be suspected if the ECG shows LVH out of proportion to the degree of the shunt or if the ECG shows ischemic changes in the left precordial leads.

Hyperkinetic pulmonary arterial hypertension (PAH) results in biventricular hypertrophy while obstructive PAH manifests with severe right ventricular hypertrophy.

Chest X-ray: There is cardiomegaly with a left ventricular apex. Left atrium is also enlarged depending on the degree of shunt. Lung fields are plethoric. Aorta is prominent.

Echocardiography: Echocardiography can define PDA size, direction of shunt, pressure gradient across PDA to assess pulmonary artery pressure, evidence of volume overload, and any associated heart defect.

Cardiac catheterization and angiography are useful in adolescents and adults to assess anatomy and pulmonary vascular resistance.

DIFFERENTIAL DIAGNOSIS

Continuous murmur can also be produced by (*i*) AV fistula, (ii) bronchial collaterals, (*iii*) venous hum, (*iv*) small aorto-pulmonary septal defect, (*v*) atrial septal defect with mitral stenosis, and (*vi*) VSD with aortic regurgitation.

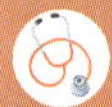

CASE STUDY Patent Ductus Arteriosus

An 8-month-old boy was brought to out-patient department with complaints of poor growth. He was born at term gestation with birth weight of 2.4 kg. He was well in the neonatal period. He developed feeding problems in form of suck-rest-suck cycle and prolonged feeding time in second month of life. During 3rd and 5th month of age he was hospitalized with complaints of fever, reduced oral acceptance, cough, and fast breathing. On examination child looked thin and weighed 4.8 kg. He was afebrile and had tachypnea and tachycardia. Heart rate was 140/min, respiratory rate was 50/min and sub-costal retractions were present. Pulses were bounding in character and all the peripheral pulses were easily felt. Blood pressure was 90/40 mm Hg in right arm. SpO_2 was 98% in all four limbs.

There was no cyanosis. Precordial examination revealed hyperdynamic left ventricular apex outside the mid-clavicular line in 6th intercostal space. First heart sound was normal; P_2 component of second heart sound was loud; S_3 gallop was heard at apex. A continuous murmur without thrill was heard in left infraclavicular region. A short mid-diastolic murmur was heard at apex. Liver was felt 2 cm below right costal margin. Other systemic examination was normal. Chest X-ray of the patient is shown here.

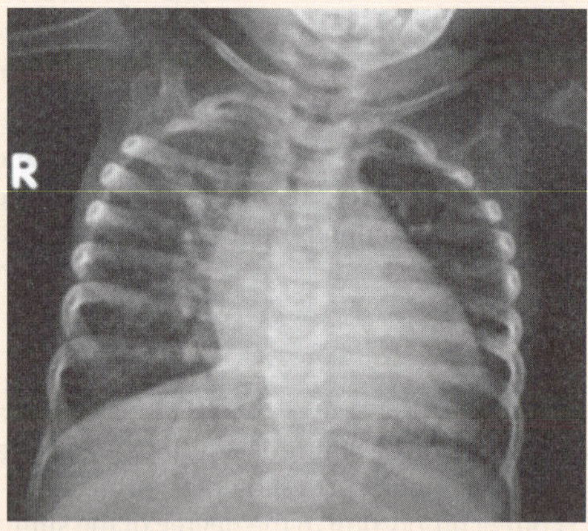

What is the likely diagnosis?

This boy has acyanotic congenital heart disease. According to Nadas criteria, presence of murmur (one major criteria), abnormal S_2, abnormal blood pressure, abnormal chest X-ray (three minor criteria), diagnosis of CHD is justified. He has feeding problems and two episodes of lower respiratory tract infections requiring hospitalization. This favors left to right shunt physiology. Size of shunt is large as suggested by presence of S_3 gallop and mid-diastolic murmur at apex. Presence of continuous murmur at left infra-clavicular area along with bounding pulses and wide pulse pressure indicates patent ductus arteriosus. The child also has failure to thrive.

What does the X-ray depict?

Chest X-ray shows cardiomegaly (cardiothoracic ratio 0.65). The apical contour is left ventricular type. The structures forming left heart border are prominent and merging with each other. Aortic knuckle and pulmonary artery shadow are prominent with a shadow occupying the space between them, this is ductal shadow. Left atrial dilation is depicted by prominent LA appendage. Pulmonary vascular markings are present till the outer 1/3 of lung fields and there are multiple dilated end-on vessels visible. This indicates increased pulmonary blood flow.

How will you confirm the diagnosis and treat?

Echocardiography will confirm the diagnosis. Treatment is closure of PDA. Diuretics, commonly furosemide is started to control symptoms. Iron supplementation for treating anemia should be started. Depending on size of PDA, either transcatheter device closure is planned or surgical PDA ligation is carried out.

TREATMENT Patent Ductus Arteriosus

PDA in Preterm Baby

- *Medical therapy:* Intervene if baby is in heart failure. Indomethacin, a prostaglandin synthetase inhibitor is administered orally (0.1 mg/kg/dose, 12 hourly for three doses) to close the ductus. Indomethacin is contraindicated if the neonate is having renal or hepatic insufficiency or bleeding tendency. Ibuprofen can also be used as an alternative therapy (10 mg/kg 1st dose followed by 5 mg/kg/dose 2 doses at 12-hourly intervals orally).
- *Surgical ligation:* If above drugs fail or are contraindicated.

PDA in Term/Older Child

Initial treatment is directed at control of congestive heart failure. Small PDA in full term baby may close till 3 months of age. Large ductus would require surgical closure at appropriate time.

- *Large/moderate* PDA, with congestive heart failure, pulmonary arterial hypertension—early closure by 3–6 months.
- *Moderate* PDA, no congestive heart failure: 6 months–1 year; if failure to thrive, closure can be accomplished earlier.
- *Small* PDA—at 12–18 months.
- *Silent* PDA diagnosed only on echocardiography without any auscultatory findings: closure not recommended.

Mode of closure can be individualized. Options available include device closure, coil occlusion **(Figs. 19.38A and B)**, or surgical ligation. While surgical ligation is preferred in children <6 months of age, or those with very large PDA; device or coils are preferred in older children.

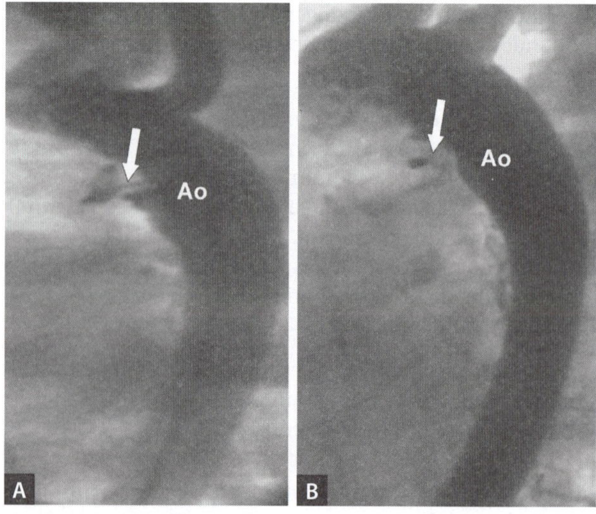

Figs. 19.38A and B: Descending aortogram: Post coil closure of PDA showing: (A) Coil in situ (arrow); (B) Device in situ (arrow), no residual flow

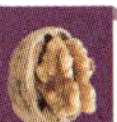

IN A NUTSHELL

Patent Ductus Arteriosus

1. Patent ductus arteriosus (PDA) refers to a communication between the proximal descending thoracic aorta and the main pulmonary artery. It is essential in fetal life and closes within the first few hours to days in all neonates after birth.
2. Persistent patency of the ductus arteriosus (DA) leads to a wide range of hemodynamically significant problems.
3. Continuous murmur peaking around the second sound is characteristic of PDA. Second sound may be paradoxically split.
4. Most preterm ducts are managed by conservative medical therapy.
5. Spontaneous closure of PDA in term babies is rare. PDA usually always needs to be closed. Definitive treatment involves transcatheter closure or surgical closure.

Gillam-Krakauer M, Reese J. Diagnosis and management of patent ductus arteriosus. Neoreviews. 2018;19(7):e394-e402.
Saxena A, Relan J, Agarwal R, et al. Indian guidelines for indications and timing of intervention for common congenital heart diseases: revised and updated consensus statement of the Working group on management of congenital heart diseases. Ann Pediatr Cardiol. 2019;12(3):254-86.

19.10 Atrial Septal Defect

PE 22.1

INTRODUCTION

Atrial septal defect (ASD) is an abnormal communication between the two atria and is classified into five types:

1. ***Ostium secundum atrial septal defect:*** It is the commonest type of atrial septal defect, comprising two-thirds of all atrial septal defects. This type of defect occurs in the central part of the atrial septum and involves whole or part of the flap of foramen ovale.
2. ***Sinus venosus, superior vena cava (SVC) type atrial septal defect:*** The defect lies in the posterosuperior portion of the atrial septum. The anatomical components of this defect are overriding and straddling of the superior vena cava, and anomalous drainage of right pulmonary veins to right atrium.
3. ***Sinus venosus, inferior vena cava (IVC) type atrial septal defect:*** This type of defect occupies the posteroinferior part of the atrial septum and is associated with straddling and overriding of inferior vena cava, and may be associated with anomalous drainage of right lower pulmonary vein to right atrium.
4. ***Coronary sinus type ASD:*** The coronary sinus is unroofed, the left superior vena cava drains directly into the left atrium and opening of the coronary sinus into the right atrium acts as the site for atrial shunting.
5. ***Ostium primum ASD:*** The defect occupies the lower most part of the atrial septum. It is a part of atrioventricular septal defect and frequently associated with deformities of the mitral or tricuspid valves or a small VSD.

HEMODYNAMICS

The hemodynamics of the atrial septal defect is characterized by overloading of right atrium, right ventricle, and pulmonary artery. With normal pulmonary artery pressure, the shunt at atrial level is dominantly left to right (during systole) with small phasic right to left shunting during diastole. However, the atrial shunt remains silent as the pressure gradient between the two atria is not enough to cause turbulent flow.

Right atrium enlarges to accommodate extra blood coming from the interatrial left to right shunting. Increased flow from right atrium to right ventricle across a normal tricuspid valve results in a diastolic murmur at the left lower sternal border. Right ventricle also enlarges to accommodate increased volume coming to it. Volume overload of the right ventricle results in an increased pressure and flow across the pulmonary valve to the pulmonary artery and lungs. An ejection systolic (**Fig. 19.39**) murmur is thus produced by increased flow across a normal pulmonary valve. Pulmonary valve closure is delayed due to increased time taken for emptying of right ventricle. P_2 is thus delayed. On the left side, A_2 occurs early because of siphoning of the systemic flow through interatrial shunt and a relatively lesser volume of oxygenated blood flowing to left ventricle and subsequently aorta. This results in wide spilt second heart sound. The split however does not increase in inspiration as

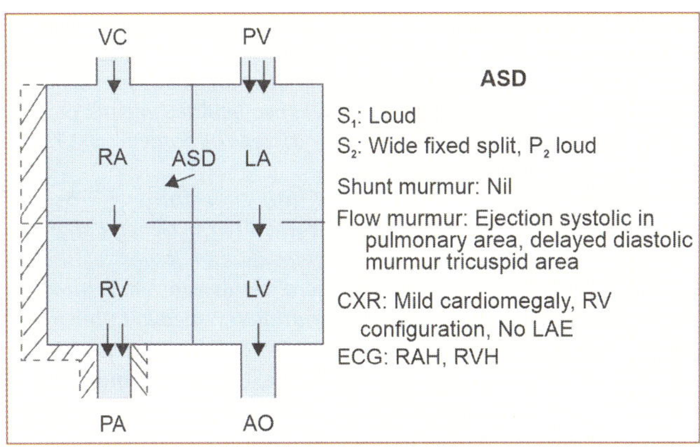

Fig. 19.39: Hemodynamics of atrial septal defect

right atrium is already overloaded and cannot accommodate extra venous return during inspiration. With phasic variations in respiration, the quantum of left-to-right shunt across the atrial septal defect changes but there is no net increase in right sided flow with inspiration. The split of second sound is thus wide and fixed (**Fig. 19.39**).

CLINICAL FEATURES

Most patients with atrial septal defects usually remain asymptomatic with murmur detected on routine evaluation. Some of them present with exertional dyspnea, palpitation, or poor weight gain. In a rare subset, the patients with atrial septal defect develop congestive heart failure; in some series 5–10% of cases of isolated ASDs can develop CHF in infancy. ASD usually presents in adolescent and adulthood with exercise intolerance, rhythm abnormalities, or features of pulmonary hypertension.

Inspection of precordium may reveal a parasternal impulse. Palpation may reveal mild cardiomegaly and a systolic thrill in <10% patients. First heart sound is loud due to loud tricuspid components and second is widely split and does not vary during respiration. P_2 is accentuated. An ejection systolic murmur at second left intercostal space and a delayed diastolic murmur at tricuspid area is audible.

Around 10–15% of patients with large atrial septal defects develop pulmonary arterial hypertension usually by the 3rd or 4th decades of life, more so in female patients. With the development of pulmonary arterial hypertension, (*i*) cardiomegaly persists; (*ii*) flow murmurs across the right ventricular outflow and tricuspid valve disappear; (*iii*) second heart sound remains wide and either fixed or variable split; P_2 becomes louder, and (*iv*) murmurs of tricuspid regurgitation and pulmonary regurgitation may appear.

Associated mitral valve disease has been demonstrated in 20–30% of patients. Presence of pansystolic murmur of mitral regurgitation in a patient with atrial septal defect may point to cleft mitral valve, mitral valve prolapse, or rheumatic mitral valve disease.

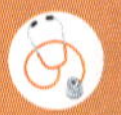

CASE STUDY Atrial Septal Defect

An 8-year-old boy was brought to outpatient department for complaints of not gaining weight as compared to peers. He was a term born neonate with birth weight of 2.9 kg. He did well in his neonatal and infantile period. Presently he is studying in 4th standard and fared well academically. There were no school absences for sick-leave.

On observation he was active and cheerful with normal intellect. Weight was 15 kg and height was 125 cm. General physical examination was normal. Pulse rate was 86/min, it was regular in rhythm, normal volume, and all peripheral pulses were felt. Saturation was 99% in all four limbs. CVS examination revealed left precordial bulge. Diffuse pulsations were seen and felt at left middle and lower parasternal area. Epigastric pulsations were felt. S_1 was normal. S_2 was wide split without any change during respiration. Grade 3/6 ejection systolic murmur was heard in pulmonary area. Other systemic examination was normal.

What is the characteristic finding in this child that can lead to diagnosis?

Wide and fixed splitting of second heart sound is the auscultatory hallmark of atrial septal defect. The left-to-right shunt happens between left atrium and right atrium. Blood from right atrium is received by right ventricle, which becomes volume overloaded. Already volume overloaded RV cannot further increase its capacity of receiving more blood during inspiration, hence S_2 is wide and fixed split. These children usually present after 5 years of age with failure to gain weight, respiratory infection, or congestive heart failure.

What is the cause of murmur?

Left to right shunt in ASD happens between LA and RA both of which are low pressure chambers. Hence there is no murmur at the level of shunt. The extra volume of blood received by RA traverses the tricuspid and pulmonary valves to reach lungs. Flow through tricuspid valve produces a diastolic murmur, which is difficult to appreciate. Flow through pulmonary valve produces ejection systolic murmur that is heard at pulmonary area.

X-ray of this child is given below. Describe the findings.

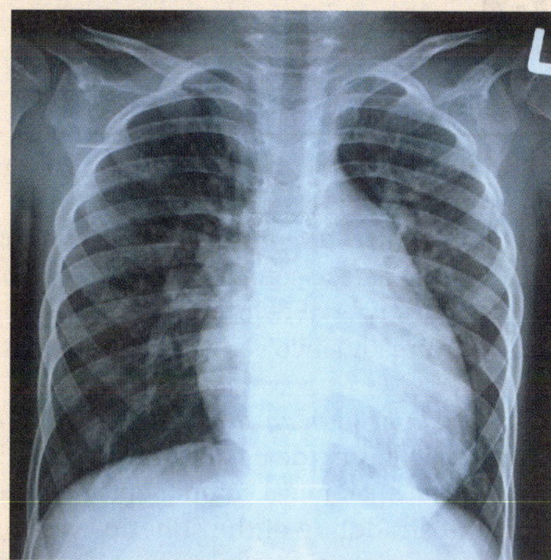

Chest radiograph shows cardiomegaly with CT ratio 0.6. Right atrium is dilated as it occupies more than three intercostal spaces. Cardiac apex is RV type as it forms acute angle with diaphragm. Main pulmonary artery (MPA) segment is dilated and pulmonary vascularity is increased.

How will you manage the patient?

Definitive diagnosis is made by echocardiogram, which shows the location and size of defect. Ostium primum and sinus venosus ASDs need surgical patch closure. Ostium secundum ASD can be closed percutaneously using ASD device provided the rims of the defect are adequate to hold the device.

DIAGNOSIS

Electrocardiography: ECG features in ostium secundum defect include right axis deviation, varying grades of right atrial and right ventricular hypertrophy, and right bundle branch block (RBBB) pattern. Left axis deviation (-30° to -60°) suggests an ostium primum ASD (**Fig. 19.40**).

Left axis deviation of >-60° suggests a complete atrioventricular canal defect. SVC type of sinus venosus ASD may cause abnormal P axis.

Presence of significant right ventricular hypertrophy suggests associated pulmonary arterial hypertension or pulmo-

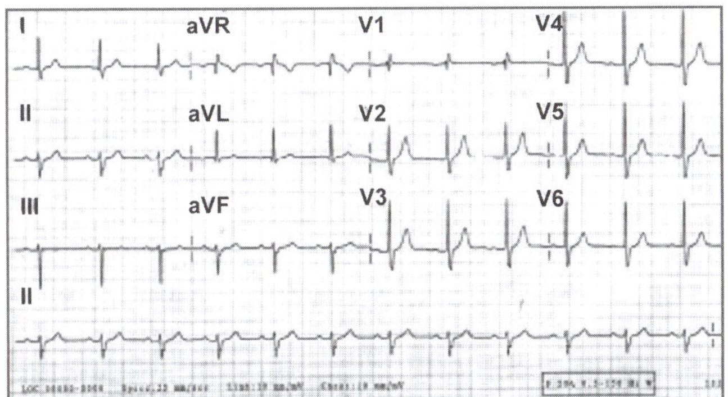

Fig. 19.40: ECG from a 16 years old adolescent with ostium primum ASD, cleft mitral valve, and moderate mitral regurgitation. ECG shows sinus rhythm, normal "P" wave axis, PR interval (0.20 sec), and QRS axis in left upper quadrant (minus 45°), incomplete RBBB

(RBBB: right bundle branch block)

nary stenosis. On the other hand, if the ECG shows additional left ventricular hypertrophy, one should carefully evaluate for mitral regurgitation, which could be caused by an associated mitral valve prolapse, rheumatic mitral valve disease, or cleft mitral leaflet.

Chest X-ray: X-ray is normal with small left to right shunt. With larger shunt, there will be cardiomegaly, right atrium and right ventricle enlargement, prominent pulmonary artery, and increased pulmonary vascularity (**Fig. 19.41**).

Echocardiography: Echocardiography is helpful in complete evaluation of ASD—the type and size of ASD, degree of shunt, pulmonary arterial pressures, and associated defects.

TREATMENT Atrial Septal Defect

Elective closure of ostium secundum ASD in patients with right ventricular overload is advised by age of 2–4 years. Indications for surgery at an earlier age include persistent CHF or evidence of pulmonary arterial hypertension. For fossa ovalis ASD, there are two treatment options:

- ***Percutaneous device closure:*** This modality can be offered only in fossa ovalis ASD with adequate rims in children above 10 kg and size of ASD being not very large for the patient.
- ***Surgery:*** Surgery is the only treatment option for large fossa ovalis ASD or with deficient rims, sinus venosus ASD, and ostium primum ASD. It is a well-established mode of closure with minimal risk (<1%).

Prophylaxis for infective endocarditis is not advised as bacterial endocarditis is rare in patients of isolated ostium secundum atrial septal defect, unless there is associated mitral valve disease.

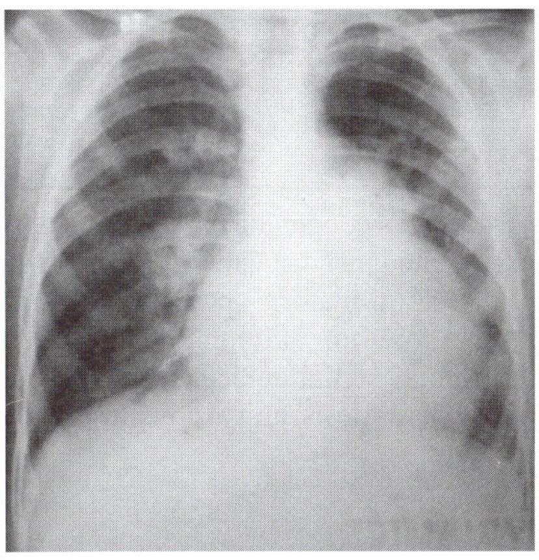

Fig. 19.41: X-ray chest PA view from a child with atrial septal defect with large left-to-right shunt. The X-ray chest shows moderate cardiomegaly, right atrial enlargement and dilated MPA. Also notice prominent hilar PA with evidence of increased pulmonary blood flow indicative of large shunt at atrial level

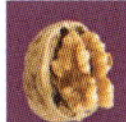

IN A NUTSHELL

Atrial Septal Defect

1. Most atrial septal defects are secundum ASD (75%) and occur in central part of atrial septum in fossa ovalis; 20% are primum ASD (20%) and occur in the region of the endocardial cushion.
2. The classical hallmark of ASD is wide fixed splitting of the second heart sound. CHF occurs only in later childhood.
3. Most children are asymptomatic. A total of 25% of patients with ASD die by 30 years, 50% by 37 years, 75% by 50 years, and 90% by 60 years. Most adults develop heart failure.
4. Enlarged right atrial size leads to atrial arrhythmias especially (atrial flutter or fibrillation). Half of patients aged 40 years have paroxysmal or permanent atrial fibrillation.
5. Secundum ASD can be managed with nonsurgical trans-catheter repair. Open heart surgical correction is required for primum defects.

Butera G, Biondi-Zoccai G, Sangiorgi G, et al. Percutaneous versus surgical closure of secundum atrial septal defects: a systematic review and meta-analysis of currently available clinical evidence. EuroIntervention. 2011;7:377-85.

Johri AM, Rojas CA, El-Sherief A, et al. Imaging of atrial septal defects: echocardiography and CT correlation. Heart. 2011;97:1441-53.

Saxena A, Relan J, Agarwal R, et al. Indian guidelines for indications and timing of intervention for common congenital heart diseases: revised and updated consensus statement of the working group on management of congenital heart diseases. Ann Pediatr Cardiol. 2019;12(3):254-86.

19.11 Coarctation of Aorta

PE 22.1

INTRODUCTION

Coarctation of aorta is a congenital narrowing of aorta. The most common site is located just distal to the origin of left subclavian artery. The indentation in aorta spares the medial wall. Associated defects are common and include bicuspid aortic valve (60–80%), ventricular septal defects (40%), associated valvar and subvalvar aortic stenosis, and atrioventricular valve abnormalities.

HEMODYNAMICS

The narrowing of the aorta obstructs the systemic blood flow through the constricted segment of the aorta; thus increasing left ventricular pressure and workload. Collateral vessels develop, between the branches of the subclavian and intercostal arteries, bypassing the coarct segment of the aorta and supplying circulation to the lower extremities. Coarctation also results in systemic hypertension, the exact pathophysiology of which is not known.

CLINICAL FEATURES

The clinical presentation of coarctation of aorta generally follows one of the three patterns: (*1*) an infant with congestive cardiac failure; (*2*) a child or adolescent with arterial hypertension; or (*3*) a child with a heart murmur.

When coarctation presents in infancy, it often presents as a catastrophic event. After birth as ductus closes, baby presents with congestive cardiac failure and shock. Multiorgan failure, particularly renal failure and necrotizing enterocolitis and subsequent death occur rapidly unless appropriate management is urgently provided.

Severe lesions present in infancy with poor feeding, growth failure, tachypnea, edema, acidosis, and congestive heart failure. A child or adolescent usually presents with intermittent claudication, pain and weakness of legs, and exertional dyspnea. Femoral pulses are weak and delayed as compared to brachial arterial pulses. Carotid pulse is prominent. Arterial pulsations can be felt in the suprasternal notch. Blood pressure measurement reveals hypertension. Characteristically, the blood pressure in upper extremities is more than that in the lower limbs, exactly opposite to what one would expect in a normal child. Degree of hypertension correlates with the severity of coarctation.

The heart size is normal with a left ventricular forcible or heaving apex. A systolic thrill may be palpable in the suprasternal notch. S_1 is loud and followed by an ejection click. S_2 is normally split with a loud A_2. Auscultation reveals a non-specific ejection murmur along the left sternal border which may also be heard over the back in the interscapular region. Collateral circulations in the chest wall may produce faint continuous murmurs and palpable collaterals over back.

DIAGNOSIS

Electrocardiogram shows left ventricular hypertrophy. In newborn period and infancy, the ECG may show right ventricular hypertrophy. Associated ST and T wave changes on left sided leads indicate associated aortic stenosis or endocardial fibroelastosis.

Thoracic roentgenogram shows a normal sized heart. Ascending aorta and the aortic knuckle are prominent. Aortic segments proximal and distal to the site of coarctation are dilated resulting in a typical "3" sign **(Fig. 19.42A)**. Barium swallow shows the characteristic "E" sign and confirms the site of coarctation **(Fig. 19.42B)**. The characteristic notching of the lower borders of the ribs (3–8) **(Fig. 19.42C)** tends to appear only after the age of 4–5 years. Rib notching will be unilateral if origin of subclavian artery is stenosed or it arises distal to the site of coarctation.

Echocardiography and Doppler studies can determine the site and severity of obstruction.

TREATMENT Coarctation of Aorta

Medical management consists of control of congestive heart failure and systemic hypertension. Definitive treatment consists of surgical repair for infants <6 months of age; balloon dilatation or surgery for children >6 months of age **(Figs. 19.43A and B)**; and balloon dilatation with stent deployment in children >10 years of age.

TIMING OF INTERVENTION

1. With left ventricular dysfunction/congestive heart failure or severe upper limb hypertension (for age)—*immediate intervention.*
2. Normal left ventricular function, no congestive heart failure and mild upper limb hypertension—*intervention beyond 3–6 months of age.*

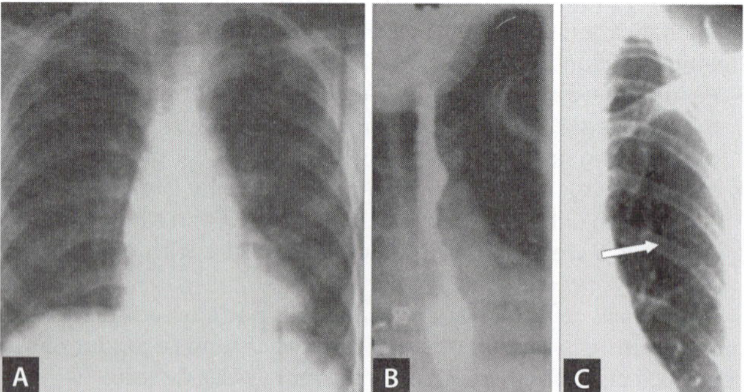

Figs. 19.42A to C: Characteristic radiologic findings in patient with coarctation of aorta: (A) X-ray chest showing characteristic "3" sign (arrow at the site of coarctation); (B) Barium swallow showing "E or reversed 3" sign; (C) Findings of rib notching (arrow) in presence of long standing coarctation of aorta

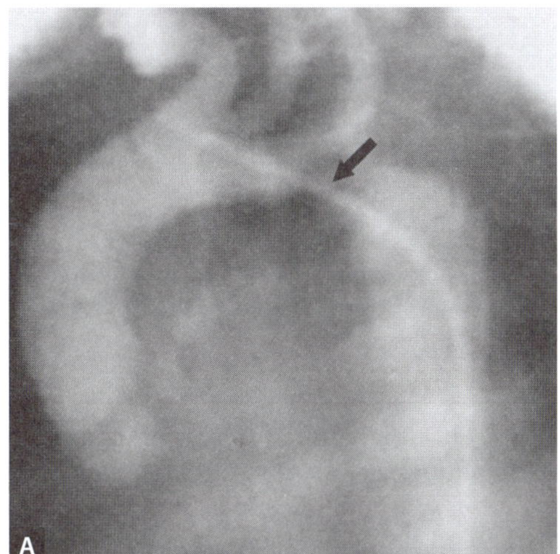

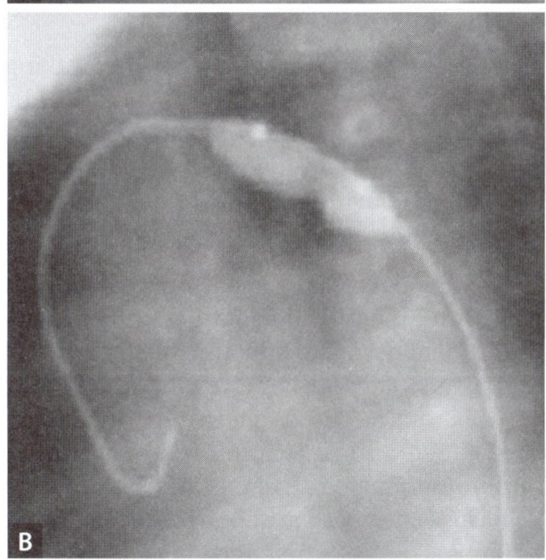

Figs. 19.43A and B: (A) Aortogram from a patient with severe juxtaductal coarctation of aorta (arrow); (B) Percutaneous balloon dilatation of coarctation of aorta is being done under fluoroscopic guidance

3. No hypertension, no heart failure, normal ventricular function—*intervention at 1-2 years of age.*

Systemic hypertension can persist following relief of obstruction if the obstruction is relieved late and re-coarctation of aorta can also occur. Re-coarctation is amenable to treatment by balloon angioplasty.

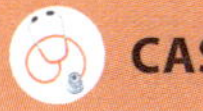

CASE STUDY Coarctation of Aorta

A 15-year-old adolescent boy was detected to have high blood pressure during a school health camp. He was growing well and participated in all activities without any symptom. There was no family history of hypertension. On examination, pulses in bilateral radial and brachial arteries were well felt. However, the femoral pulses and dorsalis pedis were feeble. Four limb blood pressures are mentioned below. JVP was normal. Apex was felt in fourth left intercostal space in mid-clavicular line. Heart sounds were normal and there were no precordial murmurs. A continuous murmur was however heard over back at interscapular area, bilaterally.

Right arm: 170/90 mm Hg; Right leg: 110 systolic; Left arm: 170/90 mm Hg; Left leg: 110 systolic.

What is the diagnosis?

Patient is suffering from coarctation of aorta. The presence of upper limb hypertension with feeble lower limb pulses and radiofemoral delay leads to the diagnosis. Due to the presence of obstruction between arch of aorta and descending aorta there is systolic blood pressure difference between arm and leg. Upper limb blood pressure is higher and pulse volume is good compared to the lower limbs. Very severe coarctation limits blood flow to descending aorta. Blood supply to lower part of body is maintained by collateral blood vessels arising from branches of subclavian arteries. Intercostal arteries have major role in collateral circulation, which dilate and produce notching at the lower border of ribs seen on chest X-ray. These collateral vessels produce continuous murmur which is heard at back.

What is the importance of four limb blood pressure recording?

The diagnosis of coarctation can be easily missed if pulses are not examined in all four limbs. While evaluating a patient with hypertension, it is crucial to take blood pressure measurement with appropriate size cuff in both upper limbs and at least one lower limb. Different size cuff should be used for arm and leg blood pressure recording.

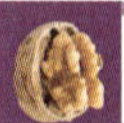

IN A NUTSHELL

Coarctation of Aorta

1. Coarctation of aorta indicates a narrowing along the course of the aorta at some point.
2. There is no cyanosis. Neonates and infants can present with congestive heart failure (CHF), cardiovascular collapse, renal failure, and acidosis. Children and adolescents may present with hypertension, or an incidental murmur.
3. Arterial pulses below the coarctation are diminished in amplitude and delayed in timing compared with the proximal pulses (radiofemoral delay).
4. Systolic blood pressure is elevated proximal to the coarctation, and a systolic pressure gradient is present between the arm and leg (difference >20 mm Hg).
5. Investigations reveal rib-notching (chest X-ray), E-shaped indentation on barium esophagogram, and LAD and LVH on electrocardiogram (ECG).

Abbruzzese PA, Aidala E. Aortic coarctation: an overview. J Cardiovasc Med. 2007;8:123-8.

Hager A. Hypertension in aortic coarctation. Minerva Cardioangiol. 2009;57:733-42.

Kanter KR. Management of infants with coarctation and ventricular septal defect. Semin Thorac Cardiovasc Surg. 2007;19:264-8.

Kenny D, Hijazi ZM. Coarctation of the aorta: from fetal life to adulthood. Cardiol J. 2011;18:487-95.

Tomar M, Radhakrishanan S. Coarctation of aorta—intervention from neonates to adult life. Indian Heart J. 2008;60(4 Suppl D):D22-33.

Cyanotic Heart Diseases

19.12 Tetralogy of Fallot

PE 22.2

INTRODUCTION

Tetralogy of Fallot (TOF) is one of the commonest cyanotic congenital heart diseases, comprising up to 3.5–9.0% of total patients with congenital heart disease. It has following anomalies:

1. Pulmonary stenosis
2. Ventricular septal defect (large and malaligned)
3. Overriding of aorta over the septal defect
4. Right ventricular hypertrophy

HEMODYNAMICS

The most characteristic and hallmark feature of this entity is the subpulmonary stenosis resulting in right ventricular outflow obstruction (**Fig. 19.44**). Pulmonary stenosis causes concentric right ventricular hypertrophy. The right ventricle effectively decompresses into the left ventricle through a large ventricular septal defect and, therefore, there is no cardiomegaly. For the same reason, congestive heart failure does not occur. The child develops congestive heart failure only if there is anemia, infective endocarditis, hypertension, or myocarditis. There is no shunt murmur at the level of the ventricular septal defect, as right and left ventricular pressures are identical.

Flow from right ventricle into pulmonary artery across the stenosed right ventricular out flow produces an ejection systolic murmur. With increasing severity of obstruction, the flow to the pulmonary artery decreases with concomitant decrease in the duration and intensity of the murmur and increase in the degree of cyanosis. Thus, the severity of pulmonary stenosis is directly proportional to the degree of cyanosis and inversely proportional to the loudness of the pulmonary ejection murmur in TOF. Right ventricular outflow obstruction also results in delayed soft P_2, which is usually inaudible.

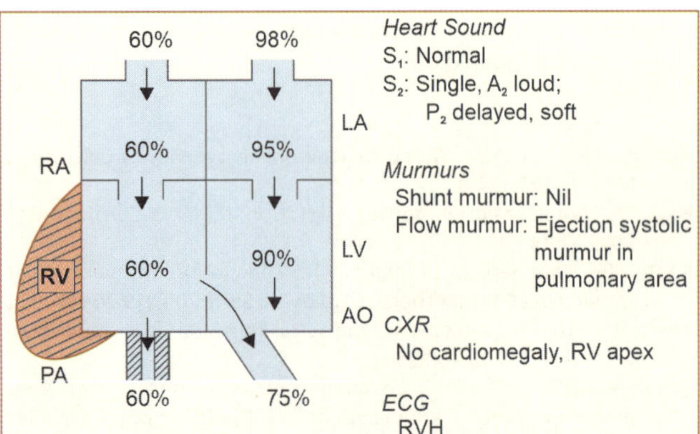

Fig. 19.44: Hemodynamics of tetralogy of Fallot. There is VSD and severe PS. Right-to-left shunt is at the level of VSD leading to systemic arterial desaturation. Values shown are oxygen saturation (%) in different cardiac chambers

CLINICAL FEATURES

Child can present at any time after birth depending on the severity of the pulmonary stenosis. Symptomatology includes central cyanosis, exertional dyspnea, and effort intolerance. During infancy and early childhood, cyanotic/anoxic spells may be the main presenting feature.

Cyanotic spells: These spells usually occur after waking up from sleep or after exertion, feeding, excessive crying, or defecation. Spells are defined as deepening of cyanosis associated with tachypnea, tachycardia, and followed by lethargy or at times unconsciousness or convulsions. Sometimes minor spells occur in the form of unprovoked, inconsolable cry followed by sleep.

Squatting: Children with TOF usually present with a history of getting relief with assuming a squatting (knee-chest) posture following exertional dyspnea. Squatting helps to abort spell by many mechanisms. There is compression of abdominal aorta and kinking of femoral arteries, which leads to increased systemic vascular resistance and thus improves blood flow through stenosed pulmonary valve. There is compression of femoral veins, which causes decrease in venous return of hypoxic blood from lower limbs. This leads to reduction in tachypnea, which is an important part of vicious cycle culminating in a cyanotic spell.

Physical examination reveals following findings:

- ***Cyanosis with clubbing, absence of CHF, and normal sized heart***. In some children, infundibular stenosis is less severe so that cyanosis never develops (*pink tetralogy*).
- Mild parasternal lift.
- Systolic thrill in 2nd, 3rd left intercostal spaces in 30% of cases.
- Normal first heart sound, single second sound (only A_2 is heard; P_2 is inaudible due to decreased pulmonary blood flow).
- An ejection systolic murmur in pulmonary area that ends before the second heart sound.
- Occasionally a constant ejection click may be present (due to dilated aorta).
- An inconstant ejection click may be present rarely if pulmonary stenosis is predominantly at the valvular level.

Features of congestive cardiac failure are absent in TOF as right ventricle is decompressed into the left ventricle through a large ventricular septal defect. Only few conditions can result in cardiac failure in TOF: (*i*) anemia; (*ii*) infection; (*iii*) aortic regurgitation due to dilated aortic root or secondary to infective endocarditis; (*iv*) pulmonary regurgitation in association with "absent pulmonary valve syndrome"; or (*v*) functionally restrictive (small) ventricular septal defect, which occurs in <5% of patients with TOF. As the right ventricle is not effectively decompressed via the septal defect, the chances of right ventricular failure increase with increasing severity of the pulmonary stenosis.

An early diastolic murmur in a child with a diagnosis of TOF may be attributed to aortic or pulmonary regurgitation.

TOF PHYSIOLOGY

Certain cardiac lesions have same pathophysiology as of TOF; i.e., restriction to the pulmonary blood flow and good intracardiac mixing. Children with these lesions have presentation similar to TOF and are grouped as TOF physiology. These conditions are as follows:

1. Double outlet right ventricle (DORV) with pulmonary stenosis.
2. Complete or corrected transposition of great vessels with VSD and pulmonary stenosis.
3. Tricuspid atresia with pulmonary stenosis
4. Single ventricle with pulmonary stenosis.
5. Atrioventricular septal defect with pulmonary stenosis.

DIAGNOSIS

ECG: There is right axis deviation and right ventricular hypertrophy. P waves may be peaked, and tall in 30% cases. Extreme right axis deviation suggests DORV with pulmonary stenosis (PS); or TGA with VSD-PS (**Fig. 19.45**).

Chest X-ray: Cardiac size is normal and lung vascularity is decreased. Aortic knuckle is prominent and there is absence of main pulmonary artery (pulmonary bay). The apex is upturned because of right ventricular hypertrophy and with absence of main pulmonary artery segment may give an appearance of *"Boot shaped heart"* (**Fig. 19.46**). In tetralogy, 30% of the cases may have right aortic arch.

Echocardiography: It is essential to document ventricular septal defect with aortic override, pulmonary outflow obstruction, and right ventricular hypertrophy. Cardiac catheterization and angiography are required only when echocardiographic evaluation is not satisfactory, or for better delineation of collateral vessels and coronary arteries.

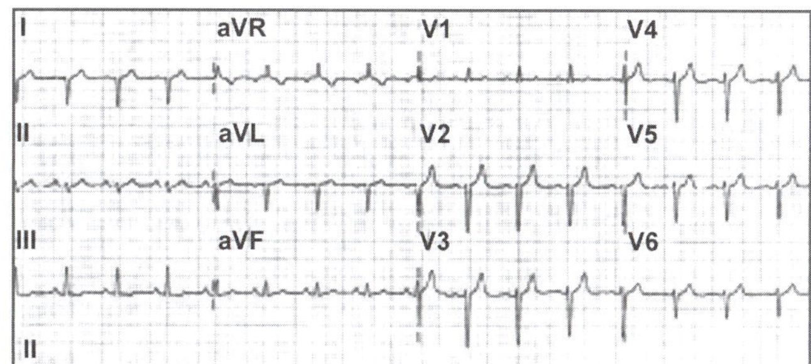

Fig. 19.45: ECG from an 8-year-old child with tetralogy of Fallot showing sinus rhythm, normal "P" wave axis, right axis deviation, right ventricular hypertrophy (chest leads in ½ voltage), early transition from "R" in V1 to rS in V2

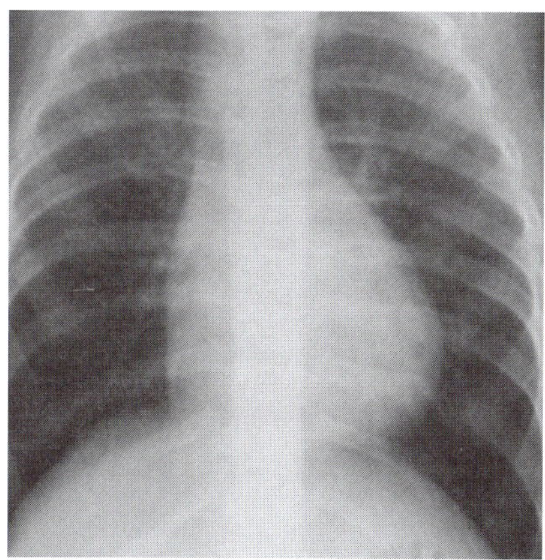

Fig. 19.46: X-ray chest in tetralogy of Fallot showing normal heart size, RV type apex, and presence of pulmonary bay and diminished pulmonary vascular markings. Right aortic arch is also seen

COURSE AND COMPLICATIONS

The pulmonary stenosis increases in severity with age with resultant increase in cyanosis and exercise intolerance, considerably limiting the child's activities. Severity and frequency of cyanotic spells increase and may even prove fatal. Anemia, by decreasing the oxygen carrying capacity further precipitates cyanotic spells and also increases the chances for heart failure, and as the microcytic red blood cells are more prone for sludging, there are higher chances for cerebrovascular accidents.

Neurological complications may occur in patients with TOF as a result of (*i*) anoxic infarction during anoxic spells or due to anemia; (*ii*) paradoxical embolism as there is a right to left shunt; (*iii*) higher chances for venous thrombosis due to sluggish circulation because of polycythemia; and (*iv*) brain abscess.

TREATMENT Tetralogy of Fallot

Cyanotic Spells

While managing a cyanotic spell, care should be taken not to agitate the child further. This is possible by doing all the following measures in a least invasive manner.

1. *Check and maintain airway:* Administer inhaled oxygen.
2. If possible, keep in *knee-chest position*, or at least with legs flexed.
3. *Inject morphine* 0.1 mg/kg body weight. If needed, infusion of 10–60 µg/kg/h can be given.
4. *Correct metabolic acidosis* by giving 1 mL/kg of 7.5% sodium bicarbonate 1:1 dilution, slow intravenous.
5. *Correct anemia* and hypovolemia.
6. *Administer beta blocker:* Heart rate and blood pressure must be carefully monitored while giving beta blockers. Beta blockers act by several mechanisms:
   - Decrease heart rate thus reducing myocardial oxygen consumption;
   - Relieve infundibular spasm, allows more blood to lungs;
   - Beta blockers also cause overactivity of alpha receptors leading to increase in systemic vascular resistance. Subsequently right to left shunt across the VSD decreases and pulmonary blood flow increases;

- Shift oxygen dissociation curve to right, relieving more oxygen at tissue level; and
- Reset respiratory center by reducing hyperpnea reflex.
- Injection metoprolol is the agent of choice given 0.1 mg/kg over 5 minutes. Repeat every 5 minutes for a maximum of three doses. It can also be given in 1–5 µg/kg/min infusion. This is to be followed by oral metoprolol 0.25–0.5 mg/kg/dose, 6 hourly. The traditional alternative is IV propranolol, 0.1 mg/kg IV (during spell). This is followed by oral propranolol (2–4 mg/kg/day 6–8 hourly) for long term use.

7. *Vasopressors:* Injection methoxamine (0.1–0.2 mg/kg/dose) IV/IM.
8. Persistent spells may need general anesthesia, or mechanical ventilation.

After managing the spell, a complete diagnosis should be made by doing a systematic Echo Doppler evaluation. Precipitating factors should be looked for. If after treatment of precipitating factors, the spells subside, surgical intervention can be appropriately planned. If the spells are not controlled, palliation with shunt surgery (modified Blalock–Taussig, i.e., connection between the subclavian artery and pulmonary artery on either side) or balloon dilation of the right ventricular outflow tract should be contemplated urgently if patient is not suitable for total correction.

Surgery

Palliative treatment: It consists of creating a communication between systemic and pulmonary circulation, to increase the pulmonary blood flow. Blalock–Taussig shunt creates an anastomosis between the subclavian and right or left pulmonary artery with interposition of graft.

Definitive treatment: This consists of closure of VSD, and resection of infundibular stenosis, resulting in total correction. *Ideal management plan* for a patient with TOF is as follows:

- *Stable, minimally cyanosed:* Total correction around 6–9 months of age or earlier according to the institution policy.
- *Significant cyanosis (SaO_2 <70%) or history of spells despite therapy:* Age <3 months: Systemic to pulmonary artery shunt. Age >3 months: Shunt or correction depending on anatomy and surgical center's experience. Children having undergone palliation in infancy should be evaluated 1 year later electively for total correction.
- Children with additional large aortopulmonary collaterals need percutaneous coil closure of these collaterals before total correction.

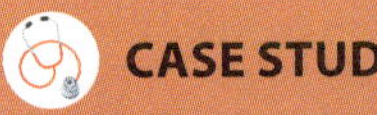

CASE STUDY Tetralogy of Fallot

A 1-year-old girl was brought to emergency room with complaints of excessive cry followed by unconsciousness for last 10 minutes. She had such episodes almost thrice in last 3 months. She had cyanosis and had grade II pan-digital clubbing. There was conjunctival suffusion. She was diagnosed to have congenital heart disease at 4 months of age when evaluated for cyanosis. Saturation was 75% in all four limbs. After stabilization, examination revealed RV type of diffuse apex. S_1 was normal, S_2 was single. A grade 3/6 ejection systolic murmur was heard at left upper parasternal border. Her weight and length were normal for age. Her chest X-ray is shown below.

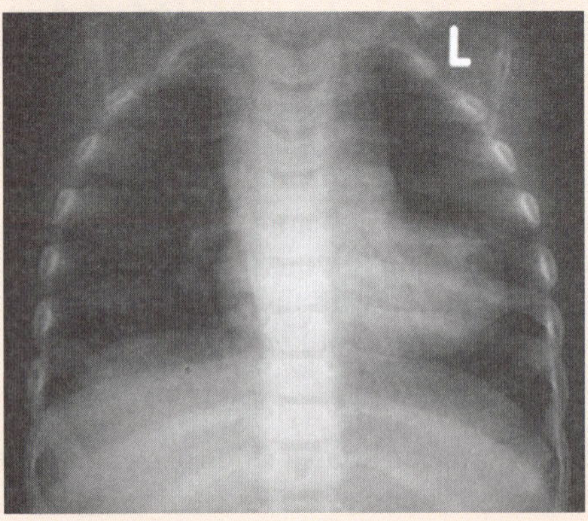

What is the diagnosis?

The child was brought in a cyanotic spell. This indicates a congenital cyanotic heart disease with decreased pulmonary blood flow. Differential diagnoses will include TOF or TOF variants such as DORV/VSD/PS, tricuspid atresia, single ventricle PS, or TGA/VSD/PS. Ejection systolic murmur in pulmonary area occurs due to blood flowing through stenotic pulmonary valve. Chest X-ray shows boot-shaped heart because right ventricle forms the apex and pulmonary bay is concave due to small pulmonary artery. There is pulmonary oligemia as seen by absence of vascular markings beyond medial third of lung fields.

What is a cyanotic spell?

A cyanotic spell is characterized by episodic deepening of cyanosis associated with hyperpnea due to sudden decline in pulmonary blood flow, leading to limpness, syncope, seizure, stroke, or death. An infant may present with excessive cry.

How will you manage this child, now?

- Keep the child in knee-chest position, preferably on mother's shoulder.
- Administer oxygen by hood/face-mask.
- Inject morphine 0.1 mg/kg subcutaneously or intramuscular to calm the child and reduce hyperpnea.
- Secure an intravenous (IV) line and inject fluid bolus 10 mL/kg normal saline.
- Inject sodium bicarbonate 1 mEq/kg to correct acidosis.
- Inject propranolol 0.1 mg/kg to reduce heart rate and counter infundibular contraction.

Most children come out of spell at this stage, but if it does not improve, further treatment includes phenylephrine, ketamine, or general anesthesia with intubation. Emergency Blalock–Taussig shunt may be required in resistant cases.

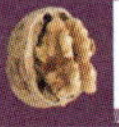

IN A NUTSHELL

Tetralogy of Fallot

1. Tetralogy of Fallot (TOF) is the most common cyanotic form of CHD.
2. TOF is characterized by four abnormalities, infundibular pulmonary stenosis (PS), large non-restrictive subaortic ventricular septal defect (VSD), overriding aorta, and right ventricular hypertrophy (RVH).
3. Severe cyanosis may result in a cyanotic spell, which may be life-threatening.
4. Pulmonary blood flow is reduced. Typically, there is no cardiomegaly, CHF, or recurrent respiratory infections.
5. Open heart surgery for intracardiac repair is the definite treatment.
6. In neonates and young infants, a palliative systemic to pulmonary artery shunt (Blalock–Taussig) may have to be performed before a total repair can be undertaken.

Bailliard F, Anderson RH. Tetralogy of Fallot. Orphanet J Rare Dis. 2009;4:2.
Duro RP, Moura C, Leite-Moreira A. Anatomophysiologic basis of tetralogy of Fallot and its clinical implications. Rev Port Cardiol. 2010;29:591-630.
Fox D, Devendra GP, Hart SA, et al. When 'blue babies' grow up: What you need to know about tetralogy of Fallot. Cleve Clin J Med. 2010;77:821-8.
Saxena A, Relan J, Agarwal R, et al. Indian guidelines for indications and timing of intervention for common congenital heart diseases: revised and updated consensus statement of the Working group on management of congenital heart diseases. Ann Pediatr Cardiol. 2019;12(3):254-86.
Tubbs RS, Gianaris N, Shoja MM, et al. "The heart is simply a muscle" and first description of the tetralogy of "Fallot". Early contributions to cardiac anatomy and pathology by bishop and anatomist Niels Stensen (1638-1686). Int J Cardiol. 2012;154:312-5.
van Roekens CN, Zuckerberg AL. Emergency management of hypercyanotic crises in tetralogy of Fallot. Ann Emerg Med. 1995;25:256-8.
Zhao K, Wang H, Han H, et al. Staged procedures versus primary repair for tetralogy of Fallot and small left ventricle. Heart Surg Forum. 2012;15:E37-9.

19.13 Transposition of Great Arteries

PE 22.2

INTRODUCTION

When the aorta arises from the right ventricle and the pulmonary artery arises from the left ventricle, the malformation is known as "*complete transposition of great arteries*" (d-TGA). It is a condition with *ventriculoarterial discordance* and atrioventricular concordance. The defect clinically presents with both cyanosis and congestive heart failure in infancy. Transposition of great arteries (d-TGA) accounts for 5–7% of all congenital cardiac malformations, with male predilection. Increased prevalence is noted in infants of diabetic mothers, and with prenatal exposure to sex hormone therapy.

Physiologically corrected transposition of great arteries (l-TGA) is characterized by atrioventricular as well as ventriculoarterial discordance. Left atrium is connected to morphological right ventricle, which is then connected to aorta. Right atrium flow, on the other side opens up into pulmonary artery through the morphologic left ventricle. As the route of blood flow is corrected physiologically, hemodynamics, and clinical presentation in corrected transposition of great arteries are determined by other associated cardiac defects (VSD, PS, Ebstein anomaly, and complete heart block), which are present in up to 98% of these children.

HEMODYNAMICS OF COMPLETE TRANSPOSITION

The right atrium receives systemic venous blood (deoxygenated) and empties into the right ventricle, from which the aorta arises. On left side, the left atrium after receiving pulmonary venous (oxygenated) blood empties into left ventricle from which the pulmonary artery arises. This arrangement is compatible with life only if there is a mixing between the two circulations through a shunt, which can be at the level of atria, ventricle, or great arteries. Clinical variants are described below.

CLINICAL FEATURES

Complete Transposition of Great Arteries with Intact Ventricular Septum (Fig. 19.47)

The mixing between the systemic and pulmonary circulation occurs through a patent foramen ovale, atrial septal defect, or patent ductus arteriosus. Patent foramen ovale, being too small, does not ensure adequate mixing of the two circulations. Consequently, these babies present within the first week of life with fast breathing, severe hypoxia, and cyanosis. Another site of mixing could be through a patent ductus arteriosus. Mixing occurs at high pressure, so the baby will present early with signs of cardiac failure. Rarely, bronchopulmonary collaterals can also be a site for mixing.

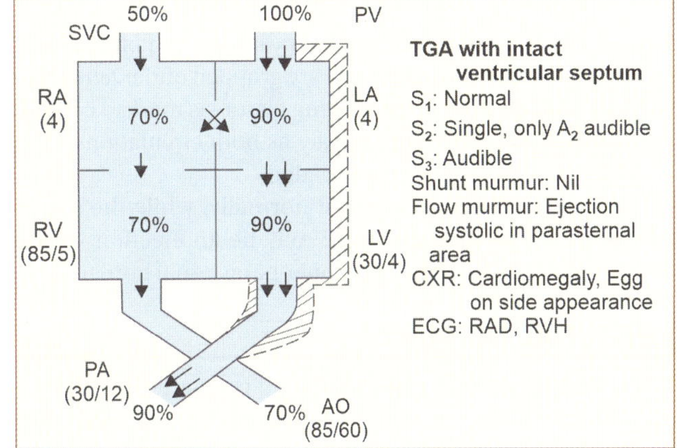

Fig. 19.47: Hemodynamics in an infant of complete transposition of great vessels with large ASD. There is bidirectional shunt at the level of ASD. Values given are oxygen saturation (%) in different cardiac chambers

Physical examination reveals severe cyanosis, features of congestive cardiac failure, normal first heart sound, single second heart sound (as pulmonary arteries are posterior to aorta so pulmonary component is not audible), and S_3 gallop. Murmurs are not significant; a short ejection systolic murmur in parasternal area is the most common.

Complete Transposition of Great Arteries with Ventricular Septal Defect

Without Pulmonary Stenosis (TGA + VSD without PS)

Presence of large ventricular septal defect results in mixing between the two circuits. As the pulmonary vascular resistance falls after birth, due to presence of a large ventricular septal defect, the pulmonary blood flow increases markedly. With increase in pulmonary blood flow there is greater pulmonary venous return, resulting in a rise in the left atrial pressure if atrial communication is restrictive. Therefore, such babies become symptomatic in the first 10–15 days of life with features of a large shunt, congestive cardiac failure, and pulmonary venous congestion. Marked cyanosis may not be a feature in these children. In presence of a large atrial septal defect which is *not* usually the case, the child presents at the age of 4–6 weeks with features of congestive failure and mild cyanosis that increases on crying.

On examination there may be mild cyanosis, cardiomegaly, signs of congestive cardiac failure, normal first heart sound, and single or normally split second heart sound with a loud pulmonary component. S_3 gallop may be present. One may hear an ejection systolic murmur grade 2/6 in the left parasternal area and a delayed diastolic murmur at the mitral area.

With Pulmonary Stenosis (TGA + VSD with PS)

These children present with marked cyanosis from birth without any congestive cardiac failure and are grouped under *tetralogy of Fallot physiology*. The differentiating feature is marked cyanosis since birth with mild cardiomegaly as both circulations in the complete transposition are overloaded.

The first heart sound is heard normally, while the second heart sound is single, and there may be an ejection systolic murmur grade 2–3/6 at the left upper parasternal border.

NATURAL HISTORY

Untreated patients of d-transposition of great arteries have very high mortality: 30% die within the first week of life; 50% within the first month of life; 70% within 6 months, and 90% succumb within the 1st year of life.

Development of pulmonary vascular obstructive disease occurs early in d-transposition, more commonly with ventricular septal defect or associated large patent ductus arteriosus. Children with patent ductus arteriosus who have Eisenmenger physiology show differential cyanosis. Cyanosis is less in the lower limbs than the upper limbs, since blood of higher oxygen saturation from pulmonary artery is shunted to descending aorta.

DIAGNOSIS

Electrocardiography reveals right axis deviation with right ventricular hypertrophy. Patients with d-TGA with VSD show biventricular hypertrophy. *Chest X-ray* shows mild to moderate cardiomegaly. The great vessels are transposed giving the configuration of "egg on side" due to narrowing of pedicle. There is associated pulmonary plethora (**Fig. 19.48**). *Echocardiography* is required to reveal the detailed anatomy.

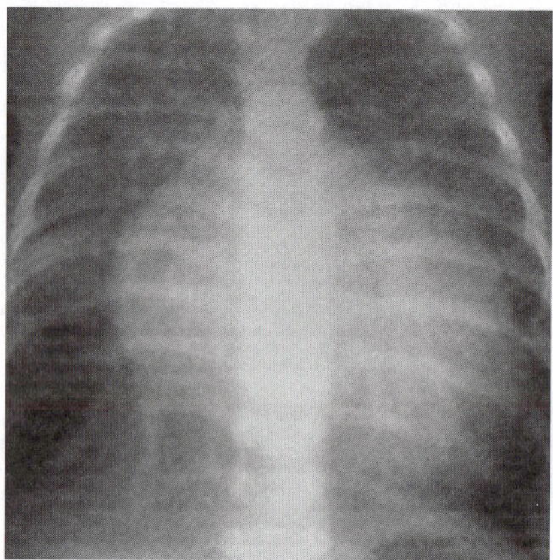

Fig. 19.48: Characteristic "Egg on side" appearance in complete transposition of great arteries with large VSD. Note presence of cardiomegaly with narrow pedicle and increased pulmonary vascular markings. Right side of egg is formed by dilated right atrium and left side of egg is formed by dilated right ventricle. There is narrow pedicle because aorta and pulmonary artery are placed anterior and posterior to each other. Also there is thymic hypoplasia which reduces the width of superior mediastinum

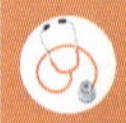

CASE STUDY Transposition of Great Arteries

A 4-month-old infant was brought to emergency room with complaints of bluish discoloration of lips and nails since birth. His birth weight was 4.0 kg. There was history of gestational diabetes in mother, which was controlled on insulin. The baby was sick looking. The mother also complained of feeding difficulties, recurrent episodes of fever with cough and suck-rest-suck cycles. There was tachycardia (HR 160/min), tachypnea (RR 70/min) with deep central cyanosis. Pulses were felt in all four limbs. SpO_2 was 65% in all four limbs. Diffuse left parasternal pulsations and epigastric pulsations were felt. S_1 was normal. S_2 was loud and single. There was an ejection systolic murmur over left parasternal border. Respiratory system examination revealed bilateral basal crepitations.

What is the clinical diagnosis?

The child was born as large for gestational age to a mother with gestational diabetes mellitus. He has presented with features of increased pulmonary blood flow (evidence of respiratory infections + CHF), and right ventricular dominance. This presentation indicates presence of transposition of great arteries (TGA). Presence of murmur indicates a shunt, most probably a VSD. The diagnosis is TGA with VSD.

How will you manage the patient?

We will confirm the diagnosis by echocardiography. Medications for control of heart failure are started. Iron supplementation is initiated. Patient is taken for surgery as soon as possible. Definitive treatment is arterial switch operation (ASO) with VSD patch closure.

TREATMENT Transposition of Great Arteries (TGA)

The first step is to control the congestive heart failure. It is important to maintain hydration, temperature, and electrolyte and sugar levels. In neonates, it may help to keep the ductus open by infusion of prostaglandins. However, this is only a short-term measure. Rashkind Balloon atrial septostomy should be attempted as soon as possible if the saturations are low and the interatrial communication is small.

Jatene arterial switch: This procedure should be performed with in the first 4 weeks of life. The pulmonary artery is shifted to RV above the aortic valve; and the aorta and coronary arteries are shifted to LV above the pulmonary valve. If the age at presentation is >8 weeks, assess left ventricle by echocardiography carefully before recommending the arterial switch operation.

- *If the left ventricle is regressed:* Senning/Mustard atrial switch at 3–6 months or a rapid two-stage arterial switch where the left ventricle is prepared by pulmonary artery banding and BT shunt followed by arterial switch.
- If a ventricular septal defect is there, it can also be closed at the same time.
- For corrected transposition, the surgical options vary with the associated lesions.

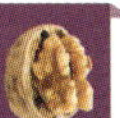

IN A NUTSHELL

Transposition of Great Arteries

1. When the aorta arises from the right ventricle and the pulmonary artery arises from the left ventricle, the malformation is known as "complete transposition of great arteries" (d-TGA). TGA is the most common cardiac cause for neonatal cyanosis.
2. This arrangement is compatible with life only if there is a mixing between the two circulations through a shunt, which can be at the level of atria (ASD), ventricle (VSD), or great arteries (PDA).
3. TGA with a shunt presents in early infancy with severe cyanosis, features of congestive cardiac failure, normal first heart sound, single second heart sound, a short ejection systolic parasternal murmur, and S_3 gallop.
4. Egg-on-side cardiac silhouette on chest X-ray is diagnostic of TGA.
5. Arterial switch operation, done in the first few weeks of life is the benchmark of present-day care in TGA. In good centers this surgery carries <5% mortality.
6. Balloon atrial septostomy (BAS) is performed if arterial switch operation is not being done immediately.

Graham TP Jr, Markham L, Parra DA, et al. Congenitally corrected transposition of the great arteries: an update. Curr Treat Options Cardiovasc Med. 2007;9:407-13.
Hazekamp M, Portela F, Bartelings M. The optimal procedure for the great arteries and left ventricular outflow tract obstruction. An anatomical study. Eur J Cardiothorac Surg. 2007;31:879-87.
Hornung TS, Calder L. Congenitally corrected transposition of the great arteries. Heart. 2010;96:1154-61.
Martins P, Castela E. Transposition of the great arteries. Orphanet J Rare Dis. 2008;3:27.
Prifti E, Crucean A, Bonacchi M, et al. Early and long term outcome of the arterial switch operation for transposition of the great arteries: predictors and functional evaluation. Eur J Cardiothorac Surg. 2002;22:864-73.
Squarcia U, Macchi C. Transposition of the great arteries. Curr Opin Pediatr. 2011;23:518-19.
Warnes CA. Transposition of the great arteries. Circulation. 2006;114:2699-709.

19.14 Acute Rheumatic Fever

PE 22.4

INTRODUCTION

Acute rheumatic fever occurs in 5–15 years age group and is more common in children from poor socioeconomic background.

ETIOLOGY

This is most likely an immunological response resulting in damage to the heart by antibodies. These antibodies are produced in response to a primary infection of the throat by group A beta hemolytic streptococci. A history of preceding sore throat may be present. However, >50% children with rheumatic fever do not have a definite history of sore throat.

Following untreated streptococcal sore throat, there is a latent period that may last from 10 days to several weeks. During this period, antibodies form to the streptococcal antigen. These antibodies have the capacity to react with human connective tissue specially the cardiac muscle. This antigen antibody reaction results in rheumatic fever.

Although the inciting bacterial agent is well known, susceptibility factors remain unclear. The location of the streptococcal infection seems to play an important role. The clinical syndrome typically follows a streptococcal pharyngitis, but streptococcal cellulitis has never been implicated. Genetics may contribute, as evidenced by an increase in family incidence. No significant association with class I human leukocyte antigens (HLA) has been found, but an increase in class II HLA antigens DR2 and DR4 has been found in black and white patients, respectively. Evidence suggests that elevated immune-complex levels in blood samples from patients with acute rheumatic fever are associated with HLA-B5.

INCIDENCE

The incidence of an acute rheumatic fever episode following streptococcal pharyngitis is 0.5–3%. The peak age is 5–15 years. Most major outbreaks occur under conditions of poverty and overcrowding where access to antibiotics is limited. Rheumatic heart disease used to account for 25–50% of all cardiac admissions in India. Regions of major public health concern include the Middle East, the Indian subcontinent, and some areas of Africa and South America. As many as 20 million new cases occur each year. The introduction of antibiotics has been associated with a rapid worldwide decline in the incidence of acute rheumatic fever.

No general clear-cut sex predilection has been reported, but its manifestations seem to be sex variable. For example, certain clinical manifestations (i.e., chorea and tight mitral stenosis) are predominant in females, while males are more likely to develop aortic regurgitation.

CLINICAL FEATURES

The earliest and most common presentation is of fever and migratory joint pains, following streptococcal sore throat. Large joints such as knees, ankles, elbows, or shoulders are typically affected. Another subset of children may present with fever, tachypnea, tachycardia and palpitation, suggestive of heart involvement. Carditis (with progressive congestive heart failure, a new murmur, or pericarditis) may be the presenting sign of unrecognized past episodes and is the most lethal manifestation. Sydenham chorea is the least common presentation that manifests with gradual onset of abnormal choreoathetoid movements. Acute attacks usually resolve within 12 weeks.

Guidelines for the clinical diagnosis of acute rheumatic fever originally suggested by Dr T Duckett Jones, were subsequently revised by the American Heart Association in 1965 and updated in 1992. The latest revision of Jones criteria has been published in 2015.

The disease is diagnosed based on the presence of major, minor, and essential criteria, as follows:

- *Major criteria:*
  - Carditis
  - Polyarthritis
  - Subcutaneous nodules
  - Chorea
  - Erythema marginatum
- *Minor criteria:*
  - *Clinical*
    - Fever
    - Arthralgia
    - Previous rheumatic fever or rheumatic heart disease
  - *Laboratory*
    - *Acute phase reactants:* Leukocytosis, elevated sedimentation rate, and elevated C reactive protein.
    - Prolonged PR interval in the electrocardiogram
- *Essential criteria:*
  - *Evidence for recent streptococcal infection*
    - Increased antistreptolysin "O" titer
    - Positive throat culture
    - Recent scarlet fever

"2 Major" or "1 Major and 2 Minor" criteria are required in the presence of "Essential criteria" to diagnose acute rheumatic fever.

2015 Modifications to Jones Criteria

- According to revised Jones criteria (2015), population has been divided into low risk and moderate/high risk categories based on incidence of acute rheumatic fever (ARF) in school aged children (>2/lac/year) and prevalence of rheumatic heart disease (RHD) in population (>1/1,000).
- To increase the sensitivity of diagnostic criteria, monoarthritis, and polyarthralgia have been included as major criteria and monoarthralgia as minor criteria for moderate/high risk population.
- Subclinical carditis diagnosed by echocardiography as pathological mitral regurgitation and aortic regurgitation, in the absence of clinical carditis, has been included as major criteria in new revised Jones criteria.

Carditis

Carditis occurs in 50–70% of all children with acute rheumatic fever. It can occur as the first manifestation of rheumatic fever in a previously healthy child or can recur in a child who already has an established rheumatic heart disease. It involves all the three layers of the heart, i.e., pericardium, myocardium, and endocardium (*pancarditis*).

- ***Pericarditis*** is suggested by presence of chest pain and a pericardiac friction rub on auscultation. The pericardial effusion is never massive and therefore lacks signs of tamponade or passive venous congestion.
- ***Myocarditis*** presents with tachycardia, cardiomegaly, and congestive failure. In the past, much attention was paid to Carey Coombs murmur, a delayed diastolic murmur best heard at the apex. It was supposed to be a marker of inflammation of the mitral valve papillary muscle complex and due to associated mitral regurgitation. However, we realize now that myocarditis occurs due to interstitial tissue involvement and not due to myocyte damage.
- ***Endocarditis:*** Endocardial involvement is indicated by valvular murmurs. There may be appearance of new murmur or change in the character or intensity of pre-existing murmurs. Mitral, aortic, and tricuspid valves are involved, in that order of frequency. Pulmonary valve is very rarely involved. Endocarditis of the involved valves results in acute regurgitant lesion of the respective valve. Mitral regurgitation is present in 95% children with carditis; of these, one-fourth also has associated aortic regurgitation. Isolated aortic regurgitation occurs in only 5% children. Tricuspid regurgitation does not occur in isolation, though it may be associated with aortic or mitral regurgitation in 10–30% children.

Arthritis

Arthritis usually involves multiple large joints, particularly the knees, ankles, elbows, and wrists. Hips and smaller joints of hands and feet are rarely involved. Typically, a series of painful joints is followed by another series of painful joints. Involved joints become swollen, red, hot, and painful. Migratory polyarthritis is usually associated with a febrile illness. There is no residual damage to the joints, after the arthritis subsides.

Western literature reports joint involvement in 80% of affected children; corresponding data from India indicate arthritis or arthralgia in only 30–50% children with acute rheumatic fever.

Subcutaneous Nodules

Subcutaneous nodules appear on bony prominence such as elbows, shins, occiput, and spine and are non-tender. Nodules of rheumatic fever are better seen than palpated. They measure between a few millimeters to a centimeter. Lesions appear late, 6–8 weeks after onset of acute rheumatic fever. They occur in about 5–20% of cases of rheumatic fever in India. Children who have subcutaneous nodules almost always have carditis. Nodules usually last from a few days to weeks; persistence up to 1 year has been reported.

Chorea

Sydenham chorea or chorea minor (referred to as Saint Vitus Dance) is a disease characterized by rapid, uncoordinated, non-

Table 19.9 Physical Signs of Sydenham Chorea

Procedure	Result
Ask the child to lift the arms and stretch the hands above the head	Forearms tend to pronate
Ask the child to stretch the arms and hands forwards towards you	Wrist is flexed and fingers are hyperextended
Ask the child to grip your fingers tightly	Unable to do so. There is alternate relaxation and tightening of the grip (milk maid grip)
Ask the child to protrude out the tongue	Unable to maintain tongue outside the mouth. It keeps going in and out (darting)

repetitive, involuntary jerking movements affecting primarily the face, fingers, feet, and hands. The child is clumsy and drops things because of a poor grip. Handwriting is badly affected. Movements disappear during sleep. Diagnosis can be confirmed by physical examination, as tests detailed in **Table 19.9**. It is reported to occur in 20–30% of patients with acute rheumatic fever. The disease is usually latent, occurring up to 6 months after the acute infection, but may occasionally be the presenting symptom of rheumatic fever. Sydenham chorea is more common in females than males.

Erythema Marginatum

Erythema marginatum rash is reddish, macular, and non-itching, serpiginous, predominantly observed on trunk. It is very rarely observed in Indian children.

ESSENTIAL CRITERIA

Demonstration of antistreptococcal antibodies is preferred over antigens, as the essential criteria for evidence of recent streptococcal infection, because of several reasons. Firstly, Group A streptococcal antigen detection tests are specific but not very sensitive. In contrast, antistreptococcal antibodies usually reach a peak titer (in Todd units) at the time of onset of rheumatic fever and are more useful. Moreover, specific antibodies to streptococcal antigens also indicate true infection rather than mere carriage of the organism. However, children without acute rheumatic fever may have an isolated positive antistreptolysin O (ASO) titer. This may also be found in children with certain related diseases such as rheumatoid arthritis and Takayasu arteritis. Therefore, rising ASO titers should be combined with a careful clinical evaluation and the discovery of other antistreptococcal antibodies to support the diagnosis of acute rheumatic fever.

Antistreptococcal antibodies include ASO, anti-deoxyribonuclease B (anti-DNAse B), antistreptokinase, and anti-hyaluronidase. These antibodies target extracellular products produced by streptococci. Although age, geographic location, and season affect the titers, an elevated titer of at least one of these antibodies indicates streptococcal infection in 95% of patients. ASO is found in 80–85% of children with acute rheumatic fever. For comparison, the sensitivity of ASO titer (adults with >240 Todd U and children with >320 Todd U) is 80%. The sensitivity increases if multiple antibody titers or paired sera are tested.

The sensitivity of throat culture as evidence of recent streptococcal infection is only 25–40%.

COURSE OF THE DISEASE

The cardiac involvement may result in a permanent damage to the valves. This causes a long-lasting heart lesion (aortic or mitral regurgitation, mitral stenosis, tricuspid regurgitation), that is classically referred to as "Rheumatic Heart Disease".

A child who develops rheumatic heart disease is prone to have recurrent episodes of acute rheumatic fever if the streptococcal focus is not eradicated. Fresh bout of rheumatic fever on a pre-existing rheumatic heart disease may result in further damage to the already diseased valves or involvement of other valves, which were hitherto normal.

TREATMENT Acute Rheumatic Fever

Restriction of Activity

All patients should be restricted to bed rest and monitored closely for carditis. When carditis has been documented, a 4-week bedrest is recommended. Immobilization may have to be continued for longer time especially in the presence of congestive failure. As soon as the signs of acute inflammation subside, patients should resume active ambulation as tolerated.

Diet

Restrict salt intake only if features of congestive heart failure are present, otherwise give normal nutritious diet rich in iron to prevent anemia.

Penicillin

One of the primary goals of treating acute rheumatic fever is to eradicate streptococci from the pharynx. Penicillin is the drug of choice in persons who are not at risk of allergic reaction. A single parenteral injection of benzathine benzyl penicillin (1.2 mega units) or 10 days course of oral Penicillin-V or injectable procaine penicillin (4 lac units IM, twice a day) is considered adequate therapy. Oral cephalosporins, rather than erythromycin, are recommended as an alternative in children who are allergic to penicillin. However, be cautious of the 20% cross-reactivity of the cephalosporins with penicillin.

By promptly treating streptococcal pharyngitis in susceptible hosts, repetitive exposure to pathologically reactive antigens can be avoided. However, management of the current infection will probably not affect the course of the current attack and does not alter the course, frequency, or severity of cardiac involvement.

Suppressive Therapy

Aspirin and steroids are used to suppress activity in acute rheumatic fever. These agents need to be given for the entire duration of rheumatic activity, which is approximately 12 weeks in 80% of the patients. Aspirin is the preferred drug to treat isolated arthritis, while steroids are preferred for treatment of carditis. Consensus Guidelines on Pediatric Acute Rheumatic Fever and Rheumatic Heart Disease Working Group Cardiology Chapter of Indian Academy of Pediatrics has advocated the following regimes for treating acute rheumatic fever in children.

Arthritis ± Mild Carditis (Aspirin Preferred)

Regime I: Aspirin is started in a dose of 100 mg/kg/day for 2–3 weeks. Once symptoms start resolving, taper dosages to 60–70 mg/kg/day, for next 9 weeks. For older children 50 mg/kg/day.

Regime II: Aspirin 50–60 mg//kg/day for 12 weeks. Children who do not tolerate aspirin should be treated with naproxen 10–20 mg/kg/day. Switch over to steroids, if there is no response to aspirin in 4 days.

Moderate to Severe Carditis (Steroids Preferred)

Regime I: Start prednisolone (2 mg/kg/day, maximum 80 mg/day) till erythrocyte sedimentation rate (ESR) normalizes-usually 2 weeks. Taper over next 2–4 weeks, reduce dose by 2.5–5 mg every 3rd day. Start aspirin 50–75 mg/kg/day simultaneously, to complete total 12 weeks of therapy.

Regime II: Prednisolone same doses × 3–4 weeks, taper slowly to cover total period of 10–12 weeks.

Non-responders should be given a trial of intravenous methyl prednisolone (30 mg/kg/day for 3 days), if there is no response to oral steroid therapy. Steroids are a more potent suppressive agent as compared to aspirin. However, there is no proof that the use of steroids results in less cardiac damage as compared to aspirin. It is known that steroids act faster and are superior—at least in the initial phases.

Management of Chorea

Chorea is a late manifestation of rheumatic fever and by the time a patient presents with chorea, the sedimentation rate as well as the anti-streptolysin O (ASLO) may be normal. The patient as well as the parents should be reassured about the self-limiting course of the disease. Protracted Sydenham chorea has responded to haloperidol. Complete physical and mental rest is essential because the manifestations of chorea may be exaggerated by emotional trauma. Recently, glucocorticoids have been used for treating chorea considering this as a sign of acute rheumatic fever. Because chorea disappears with sleep, adequate sedation should be provided. Chorea requires long-term penicillin prophylaxis, even if there are no other manifestations of rheumatic fever. Long-term studies have shown that over a follow-up for 10 years, 10% may develop mitral stenosis; and after 20 years follow-up, 20% may develop mitral stenosis.

PREVENTION OF RHEUMATIC FEVER

For rheumatic polyarthritis, prophylaxis should be continued for 5 years after the last episode or till 18 years of age, whichever is later. Prophylaxis needs to be given till at least the age of 35 years in patients with rheumatic heart disease. Ideally, this should continue lifelong. The principles of treatment include the following:

- The risk of rheumatic fever recurrence is greatest during the first 3–5 years following the attack.
- Prophylaxis must continue indefinitely in children with established heart disease or in those frequently exposed to streptococci.
- Treatment for an indefinite period is required among patients with frequent exposure to streptococci or for those who are difficult to monitor.
- Drug regimens for prophylaxis of rheumatic fever are given in **Table 19.10**.

The decision to withdraw the antibacterial drugs should be individualized after carefully assessing the risk of repetitive exposures.

DIAGNOSIS OF RHEUMATIC FEVER (IN ESTABLISHED RHD)

For the diagnosis of activity, one must go back to the Jones criteria.

- Presence of cardiac involvement cannot be used as a major criterion since it may be the result of a previous attack of rheumatic fever.
- Presence of a pericardial friction rub is evidence of active carditis.
- If the patient has well documented cardiac findings, then the appearance of a new murmur or a significant increase in a pre-existing murmur is very suggestive for active rheumatic fever.
- History of arthralgia or arthritis within a period of <12 weeks is suggestive of active rheumatic fever specially if associated with elevated sedimentation rate, C reactive protein and antistreptolysin "O" titer.
- Elevated antistreptolysin "O" titer goes in favor of active rheumatic fever. If initial titer is low, then a rising titer in repeat sample indicates rheumatic activity.

Table 19.10 IAP Drug Regime for Rheumatic Fever Prophylaxis*

Drug	*Dose*	*Sore throat treatment (duration)*	*Secondary prophylaxis (interval)*
Benzathine Penicillin G	1.2 million unit (>27 kg) (deep IM injection) after sensitivity test 0.6 million unit (<27 kg) (after sensitivity test) *Contraindication:* Penicillin allergy	Single dose Single dose	Every 21 day Every 15 days
Penicillin-V (oral)	*Children:* 250 mg QID *Adult:* 500 mg TID *Contraindication:* Penicillin allergy	10 days 10 days	Twice a day Twice a day
Azithromycin (oral)	12.5 mg/kg/day once daily	5 days	Not recommended
Cephalexin (oral)	15–20 mg/kg/dose BID	10 days	Not recommended
Erythromycin (oral)	20 mg/kg/dose max 500 mg	Not recommended	Twice a day

*Consensus Guidelines on Pediatric Acute Rheumatic Fever and Rheumatic Heart Disease Working Group on Pediatric Acute Rheumatic Fever and Cardiology Chapter of Indian Academy of Pediatrics 2008

RHEUMATIC HEART DISEASE

The sequels of rheumatic fever consist of mitral, aortic and tricuspid valve disease and very rarely pulmonary valve involvement. Other manifestations are atrial arrhythmias, thromboembolism, and cardiac hemolytic anemia. Postinflammatory scarring is presumed to be responsible for delayed sequel. Postrheumatic scarring is more prevalent in girls, with male-to-female ratio of approximately 0.4:1.

Chronic valvular deformities occurring because of rheumatic carditis may cause congestive heart failure. In pediatric age group, the mitral valve involvement manifests predominantly as mitral regurgitation and much less commonly as mitral stenosis while aortic valve involvement presents exclusively with regurgitation. Tricuspid valve involvement usually results in regurgitation but rarely stenosis can occur. Rheumatic aortic stenosis has never been described in children.

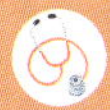

CASE STUDY Acute Rheumatic Fever

A 13-year-old boy was brought to out-patient department with breathlessness for 2 days. He was an active school going student who was faring well in his studies. About 10 days back, he had high grade fever with sore throat followed by pain in right ankle. This later involved the left knee, elbow, and right knee over next 3–4 days. This was not associated with swelling over the joints. The pain subsided after taking treatment from local practitioner. Since last 2 days the boy started having, breathlessness and mild abdominal distension. He was 4th in birth order and lived in a joint family under overcrowded conditions.

On examination he was thin built and sick looking. He was afebrile but has tachycardia (HR 120/min) and tachypnea (RR = 40/min). Pulse was normal volume and all peripheral pulses were felt. The child had pedal edema and JVP was raised. Apical impulse was hyperdynamic and felt in 6th intercostal space just outside the mid clavicular line. S_1 and S_2 were normal. S_3 gallop and pericardial rub were present. Grade 3/6 pansystolic murmur was heard at apex. Respiratory system examination was normal. Liver span was 11 cm.

What is the clinical diagnosis? Justify.

Suspected diagnosis is acute rheumatic fever. The present case fulfils one major (carditis) and two minor (polyarthralgia and fever) criteria for diagnosis of ARF. Carditis is supported by presence of pericardial rub (indicating pericarditis) pedal edema, S_3 gallop, tachypnea, tachycardia, raised JVP (due to myocarditis) and a regurgitant (systolic) murmur of mitral valve (due to endocarditis). Throat swab culture and antistreptococcal antibody titers should be done to document supportive evidence of antecedent Group A beta hemolytic streptococcal infection.

How will you manage this child?

- *Immediate management*
  - We will advise bedrest, prop-up the child, administer oxygen by face mask, and administer IV fluids (2/3 of normal maintenance). These supportive measures will have to be accompanied with administration of IV diuretics to reduce afterload.
  - The child will need to be started on steroids (prednisolone 2 mg/kg/day) in 2–3 divided doses for 3 weeks, after which they can be tapered. Aspirin will have to be started once we start tapering steroids (60–80 mg/kg/day) and continued for 9 weeks. Thus, total of 12 weeks of anti-inflammatory therapy is needed.
- *Eradication of streptococci*
  - One dose of I/M benzathine penicillin 12 lac IU after sensitivity testing
  - Alternatively oral or I/V penicillin can be administered for 10 days
- *Secondary prophylaxis*
  - 12 lac IU benzathine penicillin administered I/M every 3 weekly
  - He should be under regular follow-up to evaluate residual valvar lesion and thus decide for duration of prophylaxis

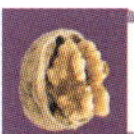

IN A NUTSHELL

Acute Rheumatic Fever

1. Acute rheumatic fever is an inflammatory autoimmune disorder that affects several organs of the body characterized by arthritis, carditis, chorea, rheumatic nodules, erythema marginatum and fever caused by Group A beta hemolytic streptococci.
2. Peak incidence is seen between ages 5–15 years.
3. Diagnosis is based on revised Jones criteria 2015 and confirmation of streptococcal infection.
4. Carditis is the leading cause of valvular involvement. Mitral and aortic valves are mostly involved.
5. Acute rheumatic fever is treated with aspirin and/or steroids depending on the presence of carditis.
6. Primary prevention consists of appropriate treatment of all episodes of streptococcal sore throat.
7. Children with residual heart disease require lifelong prophylaxis with penicillin.

De Rosa G, Pardeo M, Stabile A, et al. Rheumatic heart disease in children: from clinical assessment to therapeutical management. Eur Rev Med Pharmacol Sci. 2006;10:107-10.

Gewitz MH, Baltimore RS, Tani LY, et al. Revision of the Jones criteria for the diagnosis of acute rheumatic fever in the era of Doppler echocardiography: a scientific statement from the American Heart Association. Circulation. 2015;131:1806-18.

Gordon N. Sydenham's chorea, and its complications affecting the nervous system. Brain Dev. 2009;31:11-4.

Kumar RK, Antunes MJ, Beaton A, et al. Contemporary diagnosis and management of rheumatic heart disease: Implications for closing the gap: A scientific statement from the American Heart Association. Circ. 2020;142:e337-e357.

Lee JL, Naguwa SM, Cheema GS, et al. Acute rheumatic fever and its consequences: a persistent threat to developing nations in the 21st century. Autoimmun Rev. 2009;9:117-23.

Lennon D, Kerdemelidis M, Arroll B. Meta-analysis of trials of streptococcal throat treatment programs to prevent rheumatic fever. Pediatr Infect Dis J. 2009;28:e259-64.

Mayosi BM. Protocols for antibiotic use in primary and secondary prevention of rheumatic fever. S Afr Med J. 2006;96:240.

Saxena A. Diagnosis of rheumatic fever: current status of Jones Criteria and role of echocardiography. Indian J Pediatr. 2000;67:283-6.

Saxena A. Diagnosis of rheumatic fever: current status of Jones Criteria and role of echocardiography. Indian J Pediatr. 2000;67:S1-4.

Soudarssanane MB, Karthigeyan M, Mahalakshmy T, et al. Rheumatic fever and rheumatic heart disease: primary prevention is the cost effective option. Indian J Pediatr. 2007;74(6):567-70.

Working Group on Pediatric Acute Rheumatic Fever and Cardiology Chapter of Indian Academy of Pediatrics. Consensus guidelines on pediatric acute rheumatic fever and rheumatic heart disease. Indian Pediatr. 2008;45:565-73.

19.15 Infective Endocarditis

PE 22.5

INTRODUCTION

Infective endocarditis is a microbial infection of the endocardial surface of the heart. It should be considered in any child presenting with (*a*) prolonged fever and (*b*) one of the following—congenital or rheumatic heart disease, postoperative cardiac surgery, indwelling lines, pathological murmur, and embolic phenomenon.

PATHOGENESIS

An underlying structural heart disease, or iatrogenic manipulation of heart (surgery, central catheter) may result in denudation of endocardial epithelium; this exposed raw area serves as a nidus for platelet and fibrin deposition. This initial insult is known as non-bacterial thrombotic endocarditis, that on exposure to bacteremia, subsequently manifests as infective endocarditis.

ETIOLOGY

The most common agent is *Streptococcus viridans*, followed closely by *Staphylococcus aureus*, and enterococci (*Streptococcus bovis, Streptococcus faecalis*).

Uncommon organisms causing infective endocarditis include: *Streptococcus pneumoniae, Haemophilus influenzae, Staphylococcus epidermidis, Coxiella burnetii, Neisseria gonorrhoeae, Brucella, Chlamydia psittaci, Chlamydia trachomatis, Chlamydia pneumoniae, Pasteurella multocida, Campylobacter fetus*, and HACEK (*Haemophilus species, Aggregatibacter species, Cardiobacterium hominis, Eikenella corrodens, and Kingella species*) group of organisms.

Fungal endocarditis should be suspected in sick neonates, immunosuppressed, and those on prolonged antibiotic or steroid therapy. *Aspergillus* and *Candida* are the common etiological agents.

Culture negative endocarditis contributes to approximately 10% of all cases.

CLINICAL MANIFESTATIONS

There is a history of preceding dental, urinary, intravenous, or cardiac procedure in a child with underlying congenital or rheumatic heart disease. Typically, the child will have prolonged low grade fever, fatigue, chest pain, arthralgia, myalgia, body ache, dyspnea, malaise, night sweats, weight loss, or neurological manifestations (stroke, seizures, and headache).

Examination reveals elevated temperature (90%), murmur (100%), tachycardia, and tachypnea. Embolic phenomena can present as Roth spots in eye, hemiparesis (CNS), hematuria (kidney), petechiae, splinter nail bed hemorrhages, Osler nodes in skin, septic pulmonary embolism, and distant infection as arthritis, meningitis, or splenic abscess. Other important clinical findings include clubbing, Janeway lesions, and splenomegaly.

DIAGNOSIS

Essential investigations include three blood cultures taken from three different sites over a period of 3 hours, ESR, hemoglobin, C-reactive protein, urine microscopy, chest X-ray, ECG; and echocardiography for evidence of valve vegetations, prosthetic valve dysfunction or leak, or myocardial abscess.

DUKE CRITERIA FOR THE DIAGNOSIS OF BACTERIAL ENDOCARDITIS

- ***Major criteria:***
  - *Positive blood culture*
    - Typical microorganism for infective endocarditis from two separate blood cultures *Streptococci viridans, Streptococci bovis*, HACEK group, *Staphylococcus aureus* or community acquired enterococci in the absence of a primary focus, Or
    - Persistently positive blood culture, defined as recovery of a microorganism consistent with infective endocarditis from at least three blood cultures drawn >12 hours apart, or all of three or a majority of four or more separate blood cultures, with first and last drawn at least 1 hour apart; Or
    - Single positive blood culture for *Coxiella burnetii* or antiphase 1 IgG antibody titer >1:800.
  - *Evidence of endocardial involvement*
    - *Positive echocardiogram:* Oscillating intracardiac mass, on valve or supporting structures, myocardial abscess, or new partial dehiscence of prosthetic valve or patch.
    - New valvular regurgitation.
- ***Minor criteria***
  - *Predisposition*: Predisposing heart condition or intravenous drug use.
  - Fever >38.0°C (100.4°F)
  - *Vascular phenomena:* Major arterial emboli, septic pulmonary infarcts, mycotic aneurysm, intracranial hemorrhage, conjunctival hemorrhages, Janeway lesions.
  - *Immunological phenomena:* Glomerulonephritis, Osler nodes, Roth's spots, rheumatoid factor.
  - *Microbiological evidence:* Positive blood culture but not meeting major criterion.

Definitive Infective Endocarditis

Pathological Criteria

Microorganism: Demonstrated by culture or histology in a vegetation or in an intracardiac abscess or pathological lesions: vegetation or intracardiac abscess present, confirmed by histology showing active carditis

Clinical Criteria

Two major or one major and three minor or five minor

Possible Endocarditis

One major and one minor or three minor criteria

TREATMENT Infective Endocarditis

Antibiotics are the mainstay of management, aimed at eradication of the micro-organism in vegetations. Decongestive medication (digitalis, salt restriction, and diuretic therapy) and avoidance of physical exertion is required when patient is in congestive cardiac failure. The child should be started on empirical antibiotic therapy on a strong suspicion that can be changed depending upon clinical response and the reports of blood cultures **(Table 19.11)**. Surgical intervention is indicated for:

- Severe aortic or mitral valve regurgitation with intractable heart failure, not stabilizing on medical treatment;
- Dehiscence of an intracardiac patch, rupture of aortic sinus or rarely, a mycotic aneurysm requires an emergency operation; and
- Other surgical indications include failure to sterilize the blood despite adequate antibiotic levels, a myocardial abscess, recurrent emboli, and failure of medical management.

Table 19.11 Treatment of Infective Endocarditis

Etiologic agent	*Drug*	*Route*	*Duration of therapy (weeks)*
Streptococcus viridans, S. bovis (minimal inhibitory concentration [MIC] <0.1 mg/mL)	Penicillin G *or* penicillin G plus gentamicin	IV IV IV	4–6 2–4 2
S. viridans, S. bovis (MIC >0.1 mg/mL)	Penicillin G plus gentamicin	IV IV	4–6 2
S. viridans or enterococci (*S. bovis* or *S. faecalis*) (MIC >0.5 mg/mL)	Penicillin G *or* ampicillin plus gentamicin	IV IV IV	4–6 4–6 4–6
S. viridans, S. bovis (penicillin allergy)	Vancomycin plus gentamicin if resistant	IV IV	4–6 4–6
Staphylococcus Aureus	Nafcillin *or* oxacillin plus optional gentamicin	IV IV	6–8 2
S. aureus (methicillin resistant) (penicillin allergy)	Vancomycin plus optional trimethoprim— sulfamethoxazole	IV IV, PO	6–8 4–8
S. aureus (with prosthetic device, methicillin-sensitive)	Nafcillin/oxacillin plus gentamicin plus rifampin IV/PO	IV IV at least 6	At least 6 2
S. aureus (with prosthetic device, methicillin-resistant)	Vancomycin plus gentamicin plus rifampin	IV IV IV/PO	At least 6 2 at least 6
S. epidermidis	Vancomycin plus optional rifampin	IV IV/PO	6–8 6–8
Haemophilus species	Ampicillin plus optional gentamicin	 IV	4–6 2–4
HACEK Group	Ceftriaxone or ampicillin—sulbactam or ciprofloxacin	IV	4 4 4
Culture negative Native valve	1. Ampicillin—sulbactam plus gentamicin 2. Vancomycin plus gentamicin plus ciprofloxacin	IV IV	4–6 4–6 4–6 4–6 4–6
Prosthetic valve (early-less than or equal to 1 year)	Vancomycin plus gentamicin plus cefepime plus rifampin	IV IV/IM IV IV/PO	6 2 6 6

Drug doses:

Injection aqueous crystalline penicillin 200,000–300,000 U/kg/24 h every 4–6 hourly, not to exceed 20 million U/24 h; Injection gentamicin 3 mg/kg, 3 divided doses IV /IM; Injection ceftriaxone 100 mg/kg /24 h IV/IM once daily; Injection vancomycin 40 mg/kg/day in 2–3 divided doses IV; Injection nafcillin/oxacillin 200 mg/kg/day in 4–6 equally divided doses IV; Injection ampicillin sodium 300 mg/kg/day in 4–6 equally divided doses IV; rifampicin 20 mg/kg/day 3 divided doses IV/oral; Injection ampicillin-sulbactam 300 mg/kg/day 4–6 equally divided doses IV; Injection ciprofoxacin-20–30 mg/kg/day IV/oral 2 divided doses

Removal of vegetations and in some instances, valve replacement may be lifesaving, and sustained antibiotic administration will most often prevent reinfection.

Fungal endocarditis is difficult to manage and has a poor prognosis regardless of treatment. The drugs of choice are amphotericin B and 5-fluorocytosine. Surgery to excise infected tissue is occasionally attempted, usually with limited success.

Endocarditis Prophylaxis

Prophylactic antibiotics should be given as a single dose 30–60 minutes before dental procedures, tonsillectomy, or adenoidectomy in all children having a congenital heart disease, prosthetic cardiac valves, or previous infective endocarditis. Ampicillin, cephalexin, clindamycin, or azithromycin can be used.

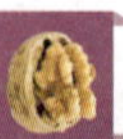

IN A NUTSHELL

Infective Endocarditis

1. The diagnosis of infective endocarditis (IE) is based on clinical findings (prolonged fever and splenomegaly in a child with an underlying heart disease or having immune compromised status), positive blood cultures, laboratory results, and an echocardiogram. The modified Duke criterion is the most commonly used diagnostic criteria for IE.
2. Common blood culture isolates in IE include *Staphylococcus aureus, Streptococcus viridians*, enterococci, and coagulase-negative staphylococci.
3. Principles of management include prolonged antimicrobial therapy, monitoring for complications, and timely surgical intervention if needed.

Akpunonu BE, Bittar S, Phinney RC, et al. Infective endocarditis and the new AHA guideline. Geriatrics. 2008;63:12-9.
Baltimore RS, Gewitz M, Baddour LM, et al. Infective endocarditis in childhood: 2015 update: a scientific statement from the American Heart Association. Circulation. 2015;132:1487-515.
Hoyer A, Silberbach M. Infective endocarditis. Pediatr Rev. 2005;26:394-400.
Kohli V. Infective endocarditis. Indian J Pediatr. 2002;69:333-9.
Milazzo AS Jr, Li JS. Bacterial endocarditis in infants and children. Pediatr Infect Dis J. 2001;20:799-801.
Nishimura RA, Carabello BA, Faxon DP, et al. ACC/AHA 2008 guideline update on valvular heart disease: focused update on infective endocarditis: a report of the American College of Cardiology/American Heart Association Task Force on Practice Guidelines endorsed by the Society of Cardiovascular Anesthesiologists, Society for Cardiovascular Angiography and Interventions, and Society of Thoracic Surgeons. Catheter Cardiovasc Interv. 2008;72:E1–12.

19.16 Hypertension *PE 22.6*

INTRODUCTION

Hypertension is a relatively uncommon finding in children as compared to adults, yet the numbers identified seems to be increasing. The causes for increase in blood pressure are attributed to obesity, change in dietary habits, decreased physical activity, and increasing stress. Overall, 1–5% children suffer from this condition while the prevalence increases up to 24.8% amongst obese adolescents. Incidence in healthy newborn is low 0.3–3% while in high-risk newborns it increases to 9%.

FACTORS AFFECTING BLOOD PRESSURE

- Blood pressure is considerably lower in childhood and increases steadily as the growth and maturation occurs.
- There is a direct association between weight and blood pressure and this is evident as early as 5 years of age. Height or stature is independently related to blood pressure at all ages.
- The blood pressure is slightly higher in boys as compared to girls in the first decade of life and this difference widens after onset of puberty. Therefore, the norms of blood pressure in the pediatric age group are specific for age, gender, and height.
- Children with a family history of hypertension tend to have higher blood pressure.
- LBW has been identified as a risk factor for hypertension in later life. Other factors such as postconceptual age and maternal factors too affect blood pressure recordings during newborn period and infancy.

PRIMARY VERSUS SECONDARY HYPERTENSION

Hypertension is classified as *primary* (essential) or *secondary* to a renal, cardiovascular, or endocrine disorder. Most children with sustained, severe, or symptomatic hypertension have an underlying etiology, and are at risk for acute and chronic complications. There is an emerging consensus that primary or essential hypertension is a multifactorial disorder resulting from an interaction of various genetic and environmental factors and tends to track into adulthood.

DEFINITIONS

According to the 2017, American Academy of Pediatrics (AAP) update report on hypertension in children, hypertension is defined as a systolic or diastolic blood pressure exceeding the 95th percentile for age, gender, and height, on at least three separate occasions, 1–3 weeks apart for children *below 13 years*.

- ***Elevated blood pressure*** (previously known as prehypertension) is defined as systolic or diastolic blood pressure between the 90th and 95th.
- Hypertension is further classified as Stages 1 and 2.
  - *Stage 1* hypertension is defined as systolic or diastolic blood pressure values exceeding the 95th percentile and up to 95th percentile +12 mm Hg.
  - *Stage 2* hypertension is defined as systolic or diastolic blood pressure values >95th percentile + 12 mm Hg.

For children *above the age of 13 years*

Elevated BP is defined as between *120 and 129 systolic/<80 mm diastolic mm Hg* and Stage 1 hypertension *as systolic blood pressure 130–139 mm Hg and diastolic blood pressure between 80 and 89 mm Hg.*

Stage 2 hypertension is defined as blood pressure *>140/90 mm Hg.*

Simplified definitions for detection of hypertension in children and adolescents are provided in **Table 19.12**.

The recordings of high blood pressure should always be repeated on at least three occasions, weeks apart (hypertensive emergency being an exception). Also the recording should be repeated at the same visit after 5–10 minutes of rest if found to be elevated. The subsequent readings tend to normalize in borderline cases due to accommodation of the child to the measurement procedure. It is important to recognize *white coat hypertension*, which is a transient rise of blood pressure in response to medical environment or the observer recording the blood pressure. Repeated readings in a quiet or home environment especially with an ambulatory measuring device helps in excluding white coat hypertension.

TABLE 19.12 Definitions of Childhood Hypertension (Based on 2017 Update)

Classification	*Children aged 1–12 years*	*>13 years age*
Normotensive	<90th percentile*	<120/80 mm Hg
Elevated BP (previously called prehypertension)	90th percentile to <95th percentile	BP-120–129 systolic/<80 mm diastolic mm Hg
Stage 1 hypertension	90th percentile to <95th percentile + 12 mm Hg	130/80–139/89 mm Hg
Stage 2 hypertension	>95th percentile + 12 mm Hg	>140/90 mm Hg

*For that age, gender and height

MEASUREMENT OF BLOOD PRESSURE

Which Device to Use?

Standard mercury-based sphygmomanometer is not used any more due to the environmental toxicity of mercury. Digital and aneroid manometers are more frequently used nowadays. Most monitors and automatic devices are based on the principle of oscillometry and measure the mean pressure while systolic and diastolic values are back calculated based on the device algorithm. While oscillometric devices are easy to use they often tend to overestimate systolic and diastolic blood pressures.

An appropriate sized blood pressure cuff should be used for the measurement. It is recommended that the bladder width of the cuff should be at least 40% of the mid-arm circumference and its length should be 80% of the arm circumference (width to length ratio of 1:2). Use of a small-sized cuff may lead to overestimation of the blood pressure. An approximate size of various blood pressure cuffs to be used at different ages is given in **Table 19.13**. The blood pressure tables are based on auscultatory measurements hence the preferred method of measurement is auscultation using an aneroid/digital manometer. Blood pressure in children should be measured with a standard clinical sphygmomanometer, using a stethoscope placed over the brachial artery pulse, proximal, and medial to the cubital fossa. Systolic blood pressure is the point when Korotkoff sounds are first heard (K1) and disappearance of sounds (K5) is the diastolic pressure. For younger children and infants auscultatory method is difficult hence automatic oscillometric devices can be used. The tables of normative blood pressure data provided in the 2017 update on pediatric and adolescent hypertension should be referred to for categorization blood pressure based on age, gender, and height percentile.

In whom should the Blood Pressure be Measured?

Children over the age of 3 years who are seen in medical care settings should have their blood pressure measured at least once during every healthcare episode. Children under age of 3 should have their blood pressure measured in special circumstances that include history of prematurity, nursery stay, congenital heart disease, genitourinary structural lesions, UTIs, or having received

TABLE 19.13 Appropriate Cuff Sizes for Blood Pressure Measurement

Age	*Cuff width (cm)*	*Cuff length (cm)*
Newborn	4	8
Infant	6	12
Child	9	18
Adolescent	10	24
Adult	13–16	30–38
Thigh cuff	20	42

drugs known to cause hypertension (steroids, phenylepherine, etc.). Also blood pressure should be measured in every overweight and obese child.

ETIOLOGY

Hypertension in children is usually secondary and related to an identifiable and treatable cause. Almost 70–90% cases are due to renal parenchymal and renovascular causes. However, the distribution of causes varies with age. In infancy, coarctation of aorta and renal vessel thrombosis constitute a major group, while renal causes prevail beyond first year of life. Hypertension can occur due to the use of certain drugs (steroids), while central nervous system lesions, and endocrine disorders (pheochromocytoma, Cushing syndrome, hyperthyroidism) are relatively uncommon causes.

Essential hypertension is being recognized more frequently in children beyond 10 years of age (especially in obese).

Transient causes of raised blood pressure such as acute glomerulonephritis, drug therapy, and raised intracranial tension should always be ruled out before starting a detailed evaluation.

Some causes of persistent hypertension are given in **Box 19.2**.

EVALUATION OF HYPERTENSION

History and Examination

- ***Symptoms:*** Irritability, excessive crying, failure to gain weight, poor feeding, low-grade fever are the only symptoms in children younger than 2–3 years. In older children presence of abdominal pain, hematuria, swelling, nocturia may suggest *renal parenchymal disease.*
- A recent or recurrent history of edema, hematuria and hypertension suggests *renal glomerular disorders.*
- Presence of anemia, short stature, rickets and poor growth are pointers toward CKD.
- History of palpitations, headache, sweating and weight loss is present with *neuroendocrine tumors* (pheochromocytoma).
- Hypertension associated with muscle cramps and weakness occurs in conditions of *primary mineralocorticoid excess.*
- Onset around adolescence occurs in some varieties of congenital adrenal hyperplasia (11-hydroxysteroid dehydrogenase and 11-hydroxylase enzyme deficiencies).
- Joint pains, rashes, photosensitivity and swelling occur in connective tissue disorders especially systemic lupus erythematosus and vasculitis.
- Presence of *fundal changes* in the eye and cardiac left ventricular hypertrophy (target organ damage) are indicative of long standing disease.
- A *positive family history* may be present in essential hypertension, polycystic kidney disease, neurofibromatosis, and glucocorticoid remediable hypertension.

Box 19.2 Causes of Sustained Hypertension in Children

- *Renal parenchymal diseases:*
  - Chronic glomerulonephritis
  - Reflux nephropathy
  - Obstructive uropathy
  - Polycystic kidney disease, renal dysplasia
- *Renovascular hypertension:*
  - Idiopathic aortoarteritis (Takayasu disease)
  - Renal artery stenosis
  - Renal artery/vein thrombosis
- *Cardiovascular disease:*
  - Coarctation of aorta
- *Endocrine disorders:*
  - Pheochromocytoma
  - Cushing syndrome
  - Congenital adrenal hyperplasia
  - Primary hyperaldosteronism
- *Tumors:*
  - Wilms tumor
  - Neuroblastoma
- *Essential hypertension*

Source: Adapted from—Bagga, Jain R, Vijayakumar M, et al. Evaluation and Management of Hypertension. Indian Pediatr. 2007;44:103-21

Investigations

A diagnostic evaluation workup is outlined in **Box 19.3**. Phase I investigations are recommended for all hypertensive children while Phase II investigations should be done

Box 19.3 Evaluation for a Hypertensive Child

- *Phase I evaluation (essential):*
  - Complete blood counts
  - Blood urea, serum creatinine, sodium, potassium, calcium, uric acid, lipid profile, Hb1AC
  - Urine routine microscopy
  - Chest X-ray, echocardiography for coarctation/LVH
  - Fundus examination for hypertensive changes
  - Renal ultrasound
- *Phase II (depending upon initial evaluation):*
  - Doppler ultrasound of kidneys for renal artery stenosis
  - Diethylenetriamine penta-acetic acid (DTPA) scan
  - Dimercaptosuccinic acid (DMSA) scan for renal scarring
  - Micturating cystourethrogram (MCU) to rule out reflux/obstruction
  - Urinary catecholamines for pheochromocytoma
  - Magnetic resonance imaging (MRI) abdomen/CT angiography
  - Metaiodobenzylguanidine (MIBG) scan for pheochromocytoma
  - ASLO, C3 for acute glomerulonephritis
  - ANA, dsDNA for lupus nephritis
  - p-ANCA and c-ANCA for vasculitis
  - Renal biopsy in persistent proteinuria and hematuria
  - Renal angiography for renal artery stenosis
  - T3, T4, TSH for hyperthyroidism
  - Plasmacortisol, ACTH for steroid/catecholamine mediated hypertension
  - Plasma renin activity, plasma aldosterone for mineralocorticoid disorders

selectively depending upon the clinical clues and results of initial evaluation. Long-standing hypertension can cause changes in kidney that may manifest as CKD. On the other hand structural abnormalities of the kidney also can result in hypertension. Investigations such as the fasting blood sugar levels, Hb1AC, and the lipid profile should be done for all obese patients.

The most common causes of pediatric hypertension are renal parenchymal and renovascular hence initial investigations should be aimed at ruling out conditions such as acute PSGN, renal artery stenosis, and chronic glomerulonephritis. Some of the useful investigations are:

- ***Ultrasonography:*** Congenital abnormalities of the kidneys and urinary tract (CAKUT) can be identified with a good renal ultrasound. An ultrasound can identify abnormal location, kidney size, shape, and corticomedullary differentiation. Abnormalities of bladder such as neurogenic bladder and bladder outlet defects like PUV too can be identified with sonography.
- In a child with hematuria, proteinuria, and hypertension elevated ASLO titers with low complement C3 levels are diagnostic of PSGN.
- ***Ultrasound Doppler:*** This can be used for screening of renal artery stenosis; the renal resistive index (peak systolic velocity-end diastolic velocity/peak systolic velocity) is measured at the main renal arteries of each kidney and at the interlobar and arcuate arteries of each pole. However, the sensitivity of ultrasound Doppler for identification of artery stenosis is low.
- ***Magnetic resonance angiography*** of abdominal aorta and renal vessels can easily identify renal artery stenosis in almost all cases and has replaced conventional angiography. However, in younger patients CT angiography may be preferred over MRI.
- ***Echocardiography:*** An ECHO can identify left ventricular hypertrophy (concentric hypertrophy) that may occur due to long-standing hypertension (target organ damage) or coarctation of aorta. Also other structural abnormalities of heart can be detected.

ESSENTIAL HYPERTENSION

Primary or essential hypertension is emerging as an important cause especially in adolescents and obese children. Its pathophysiology though not well-understood appears to be multifactorial. Genetic predisposition, environmental factors, lifestyle, and fetal factors appear to influence blood pressures. Obesity and stress among school going children is an important cause of borderline or raised recordings in older children. Obesity is primarily a lifestyle disease and seems to be catching on children worldwide, due to the ever-increasing modern household gadgets and lack of physical activity in addition to the readily available packaged and junk foods. Obesity acquired during childhood, to some extent tracks into adult life. The BMI of a hypertensive child should always be calculated and tables referred for the centiles. The values of >95th centile for that age and gender are diagnostic of obesity. However, before labelling a young child with essential hypertension, reasonable efforts should be made to rule out secondary causes.

TREATMENT Hypertension

Principles of Therapy

The goal of treatment for hypertensive children is directed at reducing the blood pressure to below 95th centile. In patients with concurrent diseases, the blood pressure should be lowered below 90th centile. The KDIGO 2024 guidelines for management of CKD recommend that in children with CKD the 24-hour mean arterial pressure (MAP) by ambulatory blood pressure monitoring (ABPM) should be lowered to <50th percentile for age, sex, and height. In children with CKD, if ABPM is not available, it is reasonable to target manual auscultatory office systolic blood pressure between 50th–75th percentile for age, sex, and height.

Patients with severe hypertension (stage 2 or more) or with target organ damage should be started on antihypertensives immediately and all efforts should be made to identify an underlying cause.

Patients with blood pressure between 90th and 95th centile or >95th centile without target organ damage should be managed with nontherapeutic measures initially for 3–6 months and if these measures are insufficient, antihypertensives should be considered.

Patients with stage 2 hypertension are at risk for hypertensive crises, which are classified as *emergencies* or *urgencies,* based on the respective presence or absence of end organ damage (e.g., hypertensive encephalopathy, intracerebral bleeding, acute left ventricular failure, and acute kidney injury). These complications are related to the rate of rise and duration of hypertension, rather than absolute blood pressure values. In such situations the blood pressure should be reduced in a controlled manner.

Nonpharmacological Methods

Dietary Changes

Salt restriction (maximum 1 g/day for 4–8 year and 1.5 g/day for older children) is recommended for all hypertensive patients; a "no added salt diet" is often sufficient to achieve this. Intake of food products high in sodium (processed and canned foods, fast foods) should be avoided. Increased potassium intake, through vegetables and fruits, is associated with modest reduction of systolic and diastolic blood pressure in adults with essential hypertension. An increased intake of fresh vegetables and fruits, whole grains, and nonfat dairy products is recommended. These foods are low in sodium and saturated fats and are rich in minerals (potassium, calcium, magnesium) and fiber. The family should be motivated to change food dietary habits in general.

Lifestyle Changes

Weight reduction is recommended for those with obesity (BMI >95th centile for that age and gender). Regular physical activity and exercise of 30-60 minutes/day for at least 4 days per week is recommended for all hypertensive children.

Drug Therapy

Step 1

Angiotensinogen convertase enzyme (ACE) inhibitors or angiotensin receptor blockers (ARB's): ACE inhibitors (enalapril, lisinopril, ramipril) or ARB's (losartan, irbesartan, telmisartan) should be considered as the first line drugs in patients with renal parenchymal diseases such as chronic glomerulonephritis, lupus, and CKD (stages 1–3). Besides reducing blood pressure, this class of drug also has a role in modifying the progression of renal disease. Enalapril can be given in doses of 0.2–0.6 mg/kg/day. However, ACE inhibitors and ARB's should be avoided till a renovascular cause has been sufficiently ruled out.

Diuretics: Frusemide (2–6 mg/kg/day) and thiazides (hydrochlorothiazide in doses of 2–3 mg/kg/day) can be used for patients with renal conditions associated with fluid retention such as nephrotic syndrome, acute glomerulonephritis, and CKD.

Patients with transient hypertension like PSGN can be managed with diuretics like frusemide (2–6 mg/kg/day) alone.

Step 2
If the hypertension is not controlled on ACE inhibitors/ARB's and diuretics, *calcium channel blockers* like amlodipine (0.1–0.5 mg/kg/day) or *beta blockers* like atenolol (1–2 mg/kg/day) can be added. Nifedipine, because of its short duration of action should not be used for management of chronic hypertension. It can be used for control of blood pressure in hypertensive urgency without target organ damage. Since it is given sublingual in emergency situations, it should not be used in patients with hypertensive encephalopathy as it may cause an unpredictable fall in blood pressure.

Step 3
If the hypertension is not controlled on maximum doses of these drugs consider *peripheral alpha-receptor blocker* like prazosin (0.005–0.1 mg/kg/dose in 6–8 hourly doses) or *central adrenergic agonist* like clonidine (5–10 µg/kg/day in 6–8 hourly doses). Rarely minoxidil can also be added at doses of 0.1–0.2 mg/kg/day.

Hypertensive Emergency
Hypertensive emergency can be managed with intravenous labetalol at doses 0.4–1 mg/kg/hour as continuous infusion. The aim should be to reduce blood pressure gradually, one-third of the planned reduction over first 6 hours, next third over 12–36 hours, and the last third over 36–72 hours. Rapid reduction of blood pressure can worsen perfusion to critical organs such as heart and brain. Other drugs that can be used in an emergency situation are listed in **Table 19.14.** Intravenous sodium nitroprusside can be used in situations where labetalol is not available. After the first 48 hours oral antihypertensives should be added with the aim of reducing and stopping intravenous drug preferable before 96 hours.

TABLE 19.14 Antihypertensives for Hypertensive Emergencies

Drug class	*Dose, route*	*Comments*
Most useful Esmolol (ß-blocker)	100–500 pg/kg per min intravenous (IV) infusion	Very short-acting; constant infusion preferred. May cause profound bradycardia
Labetalol (α- and ß-blocker)	*Bolus:* 0.2–1.0 mg/kg per dose up to 40 mg/dose infusion; 0.25–3.0 mg/kg per hours, IV bolus or infusion	Asthma and overt heart failure are relative contraindications
Nicardipine (calcium channel blocker)	0.5–5 µg/kg per minute, IV infusion	May cause reflex tachycardia
Sodium nitroprusside (vasodilator)	0.5–10 µg/kg per minute, IV infusion	Monitor cyanide levels with prolonged use (>72 hours) or in AKI/CKD
Hydralazine (vasodilator)	0.2–0.6 mg/kg per dose, IV, IM	Should be given every 4 hours when given IV bolus

Other drugs that can be used: IV fenoldopam, oral clonidine, isradipine, minoxidil, though these drugs are used rarely.

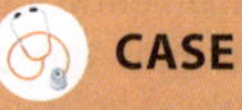

CASE STUDY Hypertension

A 4-year-old boy, being evaluated for short stature and anemia, was found to be hypertensive. His weight was 8 kg and height 88 cm.

What history would you elicit from this child to identify the cause of hypertension?
This case scenario points to a CKD. I would like to ask for any symptoms of difficulty in passing urine or dribbling to rule out urinary obstruction such as PUV, neurogenic bladder; and also ask the history of repeated episodes of fever, pyuria, urinary hesitancy, or frequency for recurrent UTI. History of painful hematuria should be elicited to identify renal stone disease.

What initial investigations would you like to do to identify the cause?
A urinalysis for proteinuria and pyuria should be done. Blood urea, creatinine, Na, K, Ca, P, alkaline phosphatase, and venous blood gas would help in identifying the severity of renal disease. A hemogram should be done to identify the type of anemia. An ultrasound of the KUB region identifies structural abnormalities of the kidney.

How will you identify target organ damage?
A fundus examination would help in identifying constriction in retinal vessels. Any retinal bleeds due to hypertensive emergency can be identified. An ECHO should be done to detect left ventricular hypertrophy due to long-standing hypertension.

Ultrasonography shows bilateral hydronephrosis and a distended bladder with thickened walls. The child has a serum creatinine of 4 mg/dL. What further investigations should be planned?
The child has structural abnormality of the renal tract. Since the bladder is abnormal, a MCU should be done to rule out PUV or a neurogenic bladder.

What is the diagnosis? Which antihypertensive should be used in this child?
The child has a CKD. The child has a calculated eGFR of 12.1 mL/min/1.73 m^2 by modified Schwartz formula which categorizes him as CKD stage. Since the GFR is low, a safe antihypertensive would be calcium channel blocker like amlodipine in doses of 0.5 mg/kg/day as two divided doses. If the blood pressure is not controlled on this drug then a beta-blocker like atenolol can be added. Diuretic like frusemide can be added if there is a decrease in urine output, edema or ECHO findings of left ventricular hypertrophy. ACE inhibitors such as enalapril, ramipril, and receptor blockers such as losartan, irbesartan should be avoided below a GFR of 30 mL/min/1.73 m^2 as their use at low GFR is associated with significant hyperkalemia.

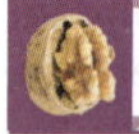

IN A NUTSHELL

Hypertension

1. Hypertension in children is defined as systolic or diastolic BP >95th centile for that age, gender, and height measured on three separate occasions 1–3 weeks apart.
2. Renal parenchymal and renovascular diseases are the most common causes of hypertension in children.
3. An appropriate sized blood pressure cuff should be used for measurement of blood pressure in children.
4. Angiotensinogen convertase enzyme (ACE) inhibitors and ARBs are the preferred antihypertensives except in situations where the renal functions are moderately deranged.

Bagga A, Jain R, Vijaykumar M, et al. Evaluation and management of hypertension. Indian Pediatr. 2007;44:103-21.
Flynn JT, Kaelber DC, Baker-Smith CM, et al. Subcommittee on screening and management of high blood pressure in children. Clinical Practice Guideline for Screening and Management of High Blood Pressure in Children and Adolescents. Pediatrics. 2017;140(3):e20171904.
Munter P, He J, Cutler JA, et al. Trends in blood pressure among children and adolescents. JAMA. 2004;291:2107-13.
Haseler E, Sinha MD. Hypertension in Children and Young Adults. Pediatr Clin North Am. 2022 Dec;69(6):1165-80.
Kidney Disease: Improving Global Outcomes (KDIGO) CKD Work Group. KDIGO 2024 Clinical Practice Guideline for the Evaluation and Management of Chronic Kidney Disease. Kidney Int. 2024;105(4S):S117-S314.

19.17 Parental Counseling

PE 22.11

INTRODUCTION

Parental counseling forms an integral part of the comprehensive care for children with congenital or acquired heart disease. Heart is a mechanical pump and the gross structure and functioning of heart is easily explained to parents with the help of basic morphologic diagrams and basic knowledge of primary level science. Apart from explaining the structural and functional aspects, parental participation is of utmost value in nutritional wellbeing of the child suffering from heart disease. Completion of immunization, need of special vaccines and hygienic practices to avoid recurrent infections also deserve special attention. Timing of interventions, outcome of interventions, need of further interventions in future have to be explained to the family. Also, the expected quality of life and life expectancy should be informed to the parents as a part of counseling. Measures for prevention of recurrence of congenital heart disease in the next gestation also should form an important component of parental counseling. Each CHD needs individualized care and thus counseling is also individualized.

EXPLAINING THE DISEASE ANATOMY AND PHYSIOLOGY

Heart has basic gross structure, and its morphology can be explained very well to the parent with the use of diagrams and pictures. Even individualized 3D models can be employed to explain the detailed anatomy of a particular defect to the family. Knowledge of the anatomical defect helps in understanding, equitable participation and shared decision making about the timing and mode of intervention.

TIMING OF INTERVENTION AND FOLLOW-UP

Certain disease subsets need urgent or early intervention. Therefore, family is counseled about the same and possible consequences or natural history if the intervention is not carried out within stipulated time. Certain defects need medical follow-up and interventions are required at certain point of time later in life, and the same has to be explained to the family depending upon the defect. Many families are lost to follow-up and turn up when the disease has progressed to an advanced stage or has become inoperable. Hence, the parents must be made aware about the expected course of the disease with and without treatment as this would help in better decision making on the family's part.

INFORMATION ABOUT THE OUTCOME OF INTERVENTION

Parents should be made aware about the CHDs needing surgical or catheter intervention and the outcomes of such interventions. The compilations which can arise during the interventions are explained and the measures taken to prevent and treat them are also detailed. Despite good results of the intervention, the lessons can recur or progress later and thus need of future interventions is discussed according to the individual's lesion.

NUTRITIONAL COUNSELING

Children, with diseases having large left to right shunts, have enhanced energy requirements and high BMR. These children need higher kilocalorie intake per day and iron rich diet to avoid catabolic state and anemia. Parents are advised to give energy dense feeds and iron supplementation to these children. Similarly, children with cyanotic heart defects have higher erythropoietic needs and need iron supplementation. Avoidance of foods having excessive salt like packed juices, pickles, chocolates, chips, and packed savory items is also advised while counseling.

GOOD COMPLIANCE WITH MEDICATIONS

Children who are kept on medical follow-up or those who are awaiting interventions or surgery should be advised to have good drug compliance. Parents are informed about the proper dosage and timing of medications and the role of each medicine in symptom control should be explained so that they are into confidence and provide the drugs timely. Many drugs are available as tablets and not as liquid formulations; hence there are chances of overdosing or underdosing. Such errors can be avoided by making powdered sachets for the same.

PREVENTION AND EARLY TREATMENT OF INFECTIONS

Children with left to right shunts are at risk of recurrent respiratory infections and once acquired, the infection take longer time to cure. Therefore, parents should be counseled to maintain strict hygienic practices, such as avoiding contact with individuals having symptoms of fever or respiratory infection; good household ventilation; avoid smoke exposure; and use of air purifiers. Routine immunization as per the national schedule must be completed on scheduled time. Additional vaccination such as pneumococcal and influenza vaccination may be advised. In older children, dental hygiene maintenance is important as dental infections can lead to infective endocarditis. Infective endocarditis prophylaxis is advisable for children with untreated or palliated cyanotic CHDs and after surgery or intervention for 6 months in all other CHDs.

PREVENTION OF FUTURE RECURRENCE

Incidence of CHD is slightly higher in families with a previous sibling with CHD. Hence, advise on preconceptional folate supplementation and utilization of fetal echocardiography in early second trimester is explained to the family.

PSYCHOLOGICAL COUNSELING

Although described above, this is the most important aspect while counseling the family of an infant with CHD. New parents are already coping with learning about childcare and the addition of special care needs as well as added financial burden for the child may be emotionally and psychologically devastating for some parents. Therefore, apart from the scientific aspect of communicating about the disease and the methods of treatment and care, parents should be humanely dealt with providing due importance to the emotional front.

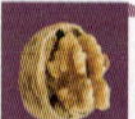

IN A NUTSHELL

Parental Counseling

1. Diagnosis of a congenital heart disease in a child is a sudden shocker to all families.
2. Technical aspects about the disease anatomy, its prognosis, proposed treatment methods, timing of treatment, medical therapy, and nutritional needs of the child should be communicated with clarity to the parents.
3. Congenital heart disease (CHD) diagnosis in a child can be psychologically stressful for vast majority of parents, hence, emotional aspect should be taken care of utilizing effective communication.

Menahem S. Counselling strategies for parents of infants with congenital heart disease. Cardiol Young. 1998;8:400-7.

Utens EMWJ, Callus E, Levert EM, et al. Multidisciplinary family-centred psychosocial care for patients with CHD: consensus recommendations from the AEPC Psychosocial Working Group. Cardiol Young. 2018;28:192-8.

Sakshi Sachdeva, Munesh Tomar, Piyush Gupta; and Mukta Mantan (Hypertension)

20 CHAPTER

Diarrheal Diseases

AS PER NMC COMPETENCIES

PE23.4	Define diarrhea (acute diarrhea, chronic diarrhea, persistent diarrhea). Discuss etiology, risk factors, clinical features, complications, investigations and treatment (according to WHO guidelines) of acute gastroenteritis.	*Ch 20.1, 20.7, 20.8*
PE23.5	Discuss the causes, clinical presentation and management of dysentery in children.	*Ch 20.5*
PE23.6	Discuss the physiological basis of ORT, types of ORS and the composition of various types of ORS. Discuss composition of fluids used in management of diarrhea. Discuss the role of antibiotics, antispasmodics, anti-secretory drugs, probiotics, antiemetics in acute diarrheal diseases.	*Ch 20.3, Ch 20.4*
PE23.7	Elicit history pertaining to diarrheal diseases. Assess for signs and symptoms of dehydration, shock, prerenal AKI, electrolyte disturbances, document and present.	*Ch 20.2, Ch 20.6*
PE23.8	Perform and interpret stool examination including hanging drop, interpret RFT and electrolyte report in the context of diarrhea.	*Ch 20.6*

20.1 Acute Watery Diarrhea *PE 23.4*

INTRODUCTION

Diarrhea is defined as passage of unusually loose or watery stools, at least three times within a 24-hour period. In diarrhea, stool can be more frequent or more liquid, or the amount of stool can be more than usual, but the most characteristic feature of diarrhea is the recent change in consistency of the stool (as per mother's interpretation in case of young children). Daily stool volume exceeding 10–20 mL/kg for children up to 2 years, and >200 g for children over 2 years is considered diarrhea. Dehydration and dyselectrolytemia are the two most dreaded complications of diarrhea, which can also be fatal.

CLASSIFICATION

- ***Acute diarrhea:*** Diarrhea of <2 weeks duration is known as acute diarrhea.
- ***Dysentery:*** A loose stool along with passage of visible blood, abdominal cramps, and fever is defined as dysentery.
- ***Persistent diarrhea:*** A diarrheal episode lasting for >2 weeks. Persistent diarrhea carries a much higher risk for mortality, and leads to malnutrition and malabsorption of nutrients.
- ***Chronic diarrhea:*** A diarrheal episode lasting for >2 weeks, usually having an insidious onset and lasting for months.

What is not Diarrhea?

- Frequent (8–10) semi-loose or pasty stools per day in an exclusively breastfed infant is not diarrhea.
- Frequent passage of formed stools in an older child is not diarrhea.
- Passage of motions immediately following a meal is often due to gastrocolic reflex and should not be taken as a sign of "upset stomach" or diarrhea.

- Passage of frequent loose stools on 3rd, 4th days of life (*transitional stools*) in otherwise well neonates is normal, and should not be considered as diarrhea.

EPIDEMIOLOGY

Globally, diarrheal diseases are one of the leading causes of childhood morbidity and mortality in children under 5 years of age. According to the latest WHO report, every year there have been ~2 billion cases of diarrhea in children globally. In 2019, 370,000 diarrheal deaths were reported in under-5 children. As per the fifth National Family Health Survey (NHFS-5) data, 7.3% children in India had diarrhea in the 2 weeks preceding the survey. The two main dangers of diarrhea are malnutrition and death, where malnutrition is another major cause of death in under-5 children.

ETIOLOGY

Acute diarrhea in children is caused by viral, bacterial and parasitic infections. Most cases are caused by viral infection, and the course is self-limited, but it can be complicated due to very high losses in the stools. Rotaviruses are the most common cause of acute diarrhea in children younger than 2 years. In India, rotavirus accounts for 5–10% of total diarrheal episodes in children. However, the rotavirus is isolated more frequently (25–40%) in children hospitalized with dehydrating diarrhea. With the commencement of the rotavirus vaccination programs, there has been substantial reduction in the rotavirus diarrhea associated hospitalizations across the globe; such reductions are yet to be reported in India, probably because of the rotavirus vaccine being introduced only recently in the National Immunization Program (NIP). Other viruses causing diarrhea in children are adenoviruses, enteroviruses, norovirus and astroviruses.

Shigella and enterotoxigenic *E. coli* are the most common bacterial pathogens causing diarrhea in under-5 children. Other common bacterial agents causing diarrhea include other forms of diarrheagenic *E. coli* such as enteroinvasive *E. coli* (EIEC), enterohemorrhagic *E. coli* (EHEC), localized adherent *E. coli* (LA-EC), diffusely adherent *E. coli* (DA-EC), aggregative adherent *E. coli* (Agg-EC), *Campylobacter*, and *Salmonella*. In endemic areas, possibility of cholera (caused by *Vibrio cholerae*) should always be considered.

Cryptosporidium is increasingly being recognized as a cause of acute and persistent diarrhea in children, and is now considered as one of the four most common causes of moderate-to-severe diarrhea in under-5 children. *Entamoeba histolytica* and *Giardia duodenalis* are the other parasites which can cause diarrhea.

In addition, systemic infections such as pneumonia, meningitis, and urinary tract infections can also cause diarrhea in children.

PATHOGENESIS

Severity and mechanism of diarrhea depends on the response generated by the intestinal mucosa against the infecting organisms. Enteropathogens such as rotavirus, enterotoxigenic *Escherichia coli* (ETEC) and *V. cholerae* cause *noninflammatory diarrhea* by stimulating fluid secretion. Release of bacterial enterotoxins such as cholera toxin and heat-stable enterotoxin leads to the alteration in the intracellular levels of second messenger molecules such as cAMP, cGMP, and Ca^{2+}. These signals to the key channels that drive fluid absorption and secretion, leading to activation of the chloride channel CFTR and inhibition of Na^+ exchanger NHE3, resulting in a massive secretory diarrhea.

Inflammatory diarrhea is caused by the pathogens such as *Salmonella* and *Shigella*, which can directly invade the enterocytes or produce cytotoxins generating a tissue inflammatory response by recruitment of immune cells and release of cytokines, resulting in intracellular Ca^{2+} signaling, leading to alterations in channel protein expression, with consequent impaired Na^+ and Cl^- absorption and diarrhea.

Mode of Transmission

The spread occurs mostly by fecal-oral route (either with contaminated food or water). Hands contaminated with fecal matter and flies may also spread the organisms (**Fig. 20.1**).

Environmental Factors

Diarrheal illnesses are more common in summers and rainy season. Inadequate water supply, lack of sanitary facilities, poor personal and domestic hygiene, improper food preparation and storage, poor weaning practices, early stopping of breastfeeding, and practice of bottle feeding contribute to diarrhea.

Malnutrition

Diarrhea is more common in malnourished children. On the other hand, diarrhea leads to decreased absorption and

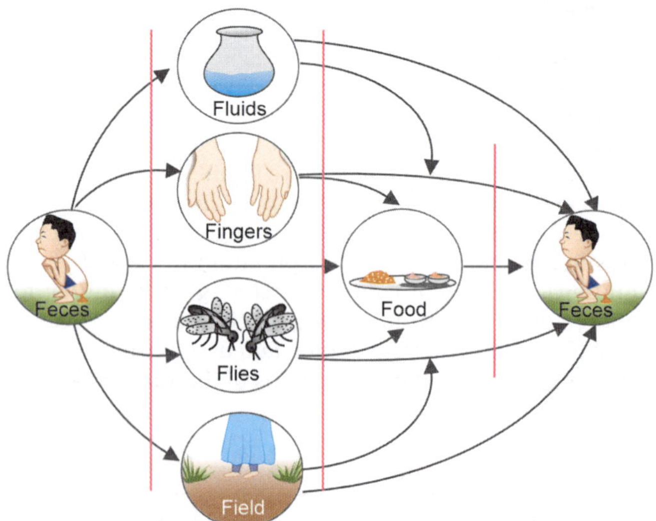

Fig. 20.1: Transmission of diarrheal infection

Source: National Health Mission. (2019). Intensified Diarrhea Control Fortnight Tool Kit, Child Health Division, Ministry of Health and Family Welfare, Government of India. [online] Available from: https://nhm.gov.in/index1.php?lang=1&level=5&sublinkid=1310&lid=691. [Last accessed November, 2022]

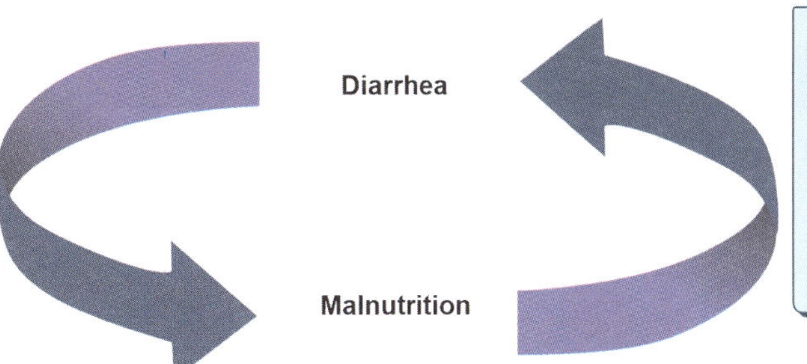

Fig. 20.2: Diarrhea–malnutrition cycle

increased loss of nutrients, decreased appetite and improper feeding during episode, all contributing to malnutrition. A vicious cycle of malnutrition-diarrhea-malnutrition is thus established (**Fig. 20.2**). Malnourished children have more chances to develop persistent diarrhea and are at 15–20 times higher risk for diarrhea related mortality. Diarrhea in malnourished children is more likely to be associated with a systemic infection such as septicemia or meningitis.

CLINICAL PRESENTATION

Most of the clinical features of diarrhea in children are either related to the gastrointestinal and systemic manifestations in response to the infection, or to the volume loss in stools leading to manifestations of dehydration. Child may present with loose stools alone or loose stools with associated nausea, vomiting, fever and abdominal cramps (e.g., *Salmonella* infection). During early stages of infection or in "some dehydration" child is thirsty and irritable, able to accept orally. With the continuation of diarrhea, as dehydration worsens, the child becomes more irritable, skin appears wrinkled (**Fig. 20.3**), eyes appear sunken and dry, and urination is reduced. Young children can have depressed anterior fontanel, if open. Children with severe dehydration may develop acidotic breathing, abdominal distension (due to hypokalemia) and shock, which can be fatal if not treated promptly.

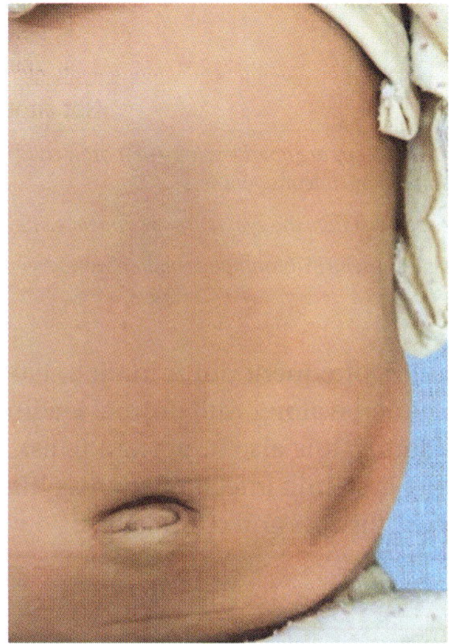

Fig. 20.3: Delayed skin pinch in a child with severe dehydration

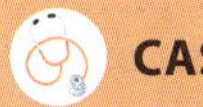

CASE STUDY **Acute Watery Diarrhea**

A 30-month-old girl, belonging to a daily wage laborer family, resident of a slum cluster presents to you with a 3-day history of watery diarrhea and vomiting. There is no history of fever or any other complaints. There is history of similar illness in many children of neighborhood. On asking mother, child has passed urine two times in last 12 hours.

On examination, the child looks irritable, weighs 9.5 kg and is thirsty. Her height is 86 cm. Vitals are normal and systemic examination is noncontributory.

Enumerate all possible risk factors of diarrhea in this child.

The child has an acute onset diarrhea with the occurrence of similar illness in neighborhood suggesting an infectious etiology through a common source. The possible risk factors include:

1. Poor sanitation
2. Unhygienic source of drinking water
3. *Malnutrition:* The expected (50th percentile) weight for height of 86 cm for a girl is 11.6 kg as per WHO growth standards. Thus, this child's weight-for-height is lying between –2 *Z*-score (9.8 kg) and –3 *Z*-score (9.0 kg), classifying her as having moderate wasting.
4. Regarding her vaccination status, we have to check with her parents.

20.2 Assessing a Child with Diarrhea and Dehydration *PE 23.7*

HISTORY TAKING

A careful history taking is essential to decide whether the reported episode is actually diarrhea, and to differentiate between acute, persistent, and recurrent diarrhea. The type of stools passed is important to know to have an idea of possible etiology. For example, rice watery stools are passed in cholera and bloody stools are a feature of dysentery. Other important information to be asked in history includes number of stools passed per day, volume of each stool, number of episodes and

Table 20.1 Assessment of Dehydration

Look and feel	*Signs*	*Dehydration*	*Treatment plan*
• *General condition:* ▪ Lethargic or unconscious* ▪ Restless and irritable	• *Two of the following signs:* ▪ Lethargic or unconscious ▪ Sunken eyes ▪ Not able to drink or drinking poorly ▪ Skin pinch goes back very slowly	Severe	Plan C
• Look for sunken eyes**			
• *Offer the child fluid:* ▪ Not able to drink or drinking poorly ▪ Drinking eagerly (thirsty)			
• *Skin pinch on abdomen:**** ▪ Goes back slowly ▪ Goes back very slowly	• *Two of the following signs:* ▪ Restless, irritable ▪ Sunken eyes ▪ Drinks eagerly, thirsty ▪ Skin pinch goes back slowly	Some	Plan B
	Not enough signs to classify as some or severe dehydration	No	Plan A

**Being lethargic and sleepy are not the same. A lethargic child is not simply asleep: The child's mental state is dull and the child cannot be fully awakened; the child may appear to be drifting into unconsciousness*

***In some infants and children, the eyes normally appear somewhat sunken. It is helpful to ask the mother if the child's eyes are normal or more sunken than usual*

****The skin pinch is less useful in infants and children with severe malnutrition, edema or obesity*

volume of vomiting, frequency of urination, type and amount of fluids taken at home along with normal feeding pattern, and immunization status. It is also important to ask for symptoms indicative of any systemic infection such as high grade fever, cough, respiratory distress and convulsions.

EXAMINATION

- ***State of dehydration:*** Any child reporting with diarrhea must be assessed for presence of dehydration. Simple clinical signs are very useful to classify the state of dehydration as *no* dehydration, *some* dehydration or *severe* dehydration **(Table 20.1)**.
- ***State of nutrition:*** As discussed earlier, the state of nutrition has important bearing on the management and outcome of diarrhea. Therefore, the nutritional status of the child should be assessed by anthropometry.
- ***Signs of systemic infections:*** Look for the presence of any systemic infection, especially in young infants and malnourished children. The following features could be useful to provide a clue for the presence of systemic infection in a child suffering from diarrhea:
  - Fever preceding the onset of diarrhea
  - Fever persisting for >72 hours after the onset of diarrhea
  - General condition of the child is poorer than his/her state of dehydration permits
  - Presence of specific findings such as crepitations, bulging fontanel, meningeal signs.
- ***Signs of complications:*** Look for the pointers suggestive of complications secondary to excessive uncorrected volume loss in stool. The presence of the following on history or examination indicates the presence of complications secondary to dehydration:
  - Tachycardia, weak and thready pulse, cold-clammy extremities, and lethargy/altered sensorium suggest hypovolemic shock. It could be associated with coexisting sepsis.
  - Persistent low urinary volume could be associated with pre-renal acute kidney injury (AKI).
  - Altered sensorium/seizures could be associated with dyselectrolytemia. In cases with systemic infection, the possibility of coexisting meningitis is to be kept.

INVESTIGATIONS

Laboratory investigations do not have much role in the management of acute diarrhea. Stool microscopy is not required in most of the cases. It may be useful when there is suspicion of cholera (to confirm the diagnosis by hanging drop test of fresh stool), a history of mucus in stools (to suspect invasive bacterial diarrhea if finding of pus cells) or if the child does not respond to therapy in dysentery (to find out amebiasis as a cause of dysentery, which requires a different class of antimicrobials). Estimation of kidney function tests and quantification of urine output are helpful in cases with acute kidney injury. Serum electrolytes should be measured when the child has altered sensorium, seizures, abdominal distension, or marked irritability. Children having features suggestive of systemic infection may need tests such as complete blood count, blood culture, urine routine and microscopy, urine culture, chest radiography and CSF evaluation.

20.3 Fluid Therapy for Dehydration

PE 23.6, PE 23.9

ORAL REHYDRATION THERAPY

Oral rehydration therapy (ORT) is the mainstay of management of diarrhea. It includes:

- WHO (reduced osmolarity) oral rehydration salt (ORS) solution **(Table 20.2)**
- Home-made sugar-salt solution
- Food based fluids (rice water + salt, *lassi* + salt)
- Culturally acceptable home fluids (coconut water, lemon water, plain water, *dal* water, soups)

Administration of glucose water without salt, aerated beverages, and tea does not constitute ORT.

Physiological Basis of ORS

In diarrhea, body water, sodium, and potassium are lost in the stools, causing dehydration and electrolyte deficit. Oral administration of glucose electrolyte solution helps to replace this deficit, provide ongoing maintenance, and also replaces the ongoing losses of fluid and electrolytes in diarrheal stools. Water, sodium and potassium in the ORS solution correct the corresponding losses; bicarbonate corrects the acidosis, while glucose facilitates sodium absorption simultaneously providing some nutrition in form of calories. The glucose linked enhanced sodium absorption in the small intestine remains largely intact during acute diarrhea.

The initial standard ORS developed had an osmolarity of 311 mmol/L, and due to poor response in stool output and the need for IV fluids in many cases, reduced osmolarity ORS was developed.

The new ORS with an osmolarity of 245 mmol/L (WHO reduced osmolarity ORS) is now the standard recommended ORS for all ages (**Table 20.2**). Reduced osmolarity ORS has many additional advantages. Apart from preventing and treating dehydration, it reduces stool output, decreases incidence of vomiting, and also reduces the need for unscheduled intravenous fluids. Reduced osmolarity ORS works equally well for dehydration following diarrhea, dysentery, or cholera but there is a risk of asymptomatic hyponatremia in cholera. Reduced osmolarity ORS should be the first choice for correction of dehydration in all diarrheal illnesses.

For the management of dehydration in children with severe malnutrition, World Health Organization (WHO) guidelines recommend oral rehydration with ReSoMal (rehydration solution for severely malnourished children). It has lower sodium (45 mmol/L) and higher potassium (40 mmol/L) content than WHO ORS, and various minerals. The composition of ReSoMal was designed specifically to address theoretical risks of sodium overload and potential under-treatment of severe hypokalemia with rehydration using standard ORS **(Table 20.2)**.

FLUID MANAGEMENT

Treatment Plan A for Prevention of Dehydration

Children without any signs of dehydration also require fluids to prevent dehydration. In such children, feeding should be continued and ORT should be given in form of home available fluids, sugar-salt solution and food-based solutions. ORS should be given to replenish the fluids lost in stools. The amount of ORS required is as follows:

- ***<2 years:*** 50–100 mL for every loose stool
- ***2–10 years:*** 100–200 mL for every loose stool
- ***>10 years:*** As much as desired by the child

Mother should be trained to prepare and give ORS at home and she should be asked to report appearance of danger signs (repeated vomiting, eating or drinking poorly, blood in stools, convulsions, lethargic or unconscious).

Treatment Plan B (for Some Dehydration)

All children showing signs of some dehydration should be treated at health care facility. These children require increased fluids for: (1) correction of dehydration; (2) replacement of ongoing losses; and (3) maintenance.

TABLE 20.2 Composition of Various Oral Rehydration Salt (ORS) Formulations

	Reduced osmolarity WHO oral rehydration salt (ORS)			*ReSoMal*	*Standard ORS*
Salt	*By weight*	*Electrolyte*	*By osmolarity*	*By osmolarity*	*By osmolarity*
Sodium chloride	2.6 g	Sodium	75 mmol/L	45	90
Potassium chloride	1.5 g	Potassium	20 mmol/L	40	20
Trisodium citrate	2.9 g	Citrate	10 mmol/L	7	10
Glucose	13.5 g	Glucose	75 mmol/L	125	111
		Chloride (from NaCl and KCl)	65 mmol/L	76	80
		Magnesium		3	
		Zinc		0.3	
		Copper		0.045	
Water	To 1 liter	**Total**	**245 mmol/L**	**300 mmol/L**	**311 mmol/L**

Table 20.3 Composition of Various Intravenous Fluids used in Dehydration Correction

Intravenous fluid	Na+	K+	Ca	Cl-	Lactate	Dextrose	Osmolarity
	mEq/L				g/L		mOsm/L
0.9% NaCl	154			154			308
Ringer lactate	130	4	3	109	28		275
5% dextrose in lactated Ringer solution	130	4	3	109	28	50	525

Administer 75 mL/kg ORS in the first 4 hours. If the child wants more ORS than the calculated amount, give more. ORS should be given by a teaspoon in children <2 years of age and by frequent sips from a cup in case of older children. If the child vomits, wait for a few minutes and give ORS more slowly. Feeding should be continued. Mother should be instructed to give ORT at home after discharge and asked to return to the health facility, if she notices any danger signs.

Treatment Plan C (for Severe Dehydration)

Severe dehydration should be corrected by intravenous fluids. If intravenous access cannot be obtained, a nasogastric (NG) tube should be placed and fluids given through it.

Ringer lactate with 5% dextrose, normal saline and/or plain ringer lactate are the most commonly used intravenous fluids for correction of dehydration (**Table 20.3**). The total amount of fluid to be given is 100 mL/kg divided as follows:

- ***<1 year old:*** 30 mL/kg in first hour and 70 mL/kg in next 5 hours
- ***>1 year old:*** 30 mL/kg in first 30 minutes and rest in next 2.5 hours

Oral rehydration salt and feeding should be started as soon as the child can drink without difficulty. The child should be frequently monitored for signs of dehydration and the following danger signs:

Danger Signs in Diarrhea

1. Repeated vomiting
2. Eating or drinking poorly
3. Blood in stools
4. Convulsions
5. Lethargy/unconsciousness

Administering ORS through Nasogastric Tube

Rehydration by administering ORS through nasogastric tube is required in situations when the child is in severe dehydration and intravenous line is not established. In children presenting with shock, fluid can be administered through the NG tube by the time intraosseous or intravenous line is established. The steps of NG tube insertion are mentioned here:

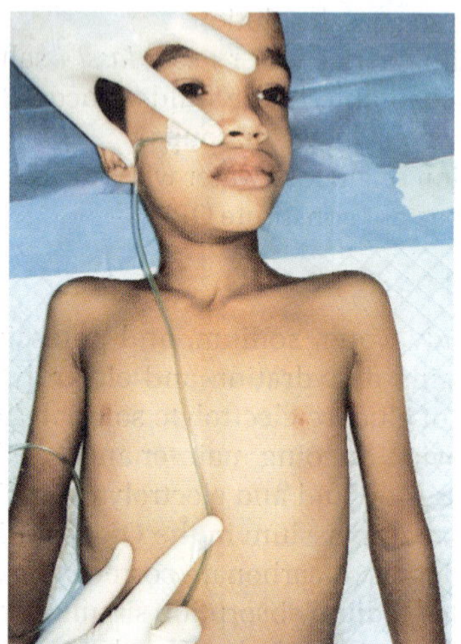

Fig. 20.4: Measurement of the nasogastric tube length

1. Child should be lying supine with the head end elevated.
2. Measure the length of the tube to be inserted: from the tip of the child's nose to the tragus and then to the xiphoid process (**Fig. 20.4**). Mark the tube at this point with a piece of tape.
3. Apply the lubricant at the distal end of the tube.
4. With the neck slightly hyperextended, pass the tube into the nose along the floor of the nose straight backward. If, the child gags when the tube goes beyond oropharynx, flex the neck and have him/her take sips of water, if possible.
5. Advance the tube till mark is reached, and then check its position by pushing air into the tube and simultaneously auscultating over the abdomen to listen for the rush of air.
6. Secure the tube to the nose with the adhesive tape.

20.4 Therapy for Acute Diarrhea *PE 23.6*

INTRODUCTION

The correction of dehydration and replacement of ongoing losses by oral rehydration therapy/intravenous fluids, form the mainstay of diarrhea treatment. Other measures can be divided into pharmacological and nonpharmacological measures.

PHARMACOLOGICAL MEASURES

Zinc for Diarrhea

Zinc is important for various immune mechanisms in the body and modulates the host response to infection. Meta-analyses of randomized trials have demonstrated that zinc supplements

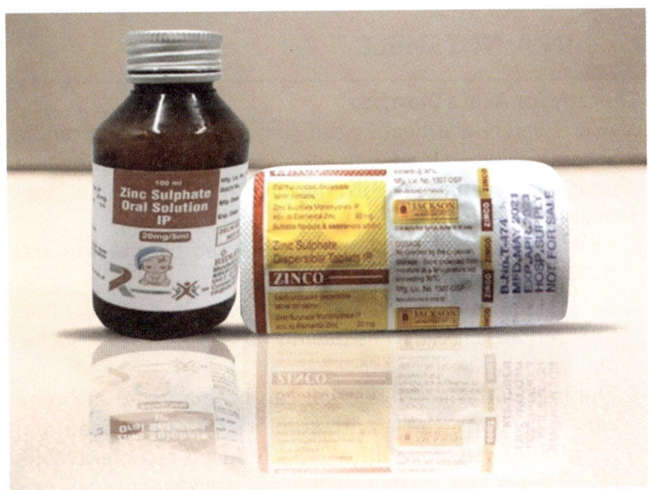

Fig. 20.5: Syrup and tablets of zinc

given during an episode of acute diarrhea reduce the duration and severity of the episode and if given for 14 days, also lower the incidence of diarrhea in the next 3 months (**Fig. 20.5**).

WHO, UNICEF, and IAP therefore recommend daily 20 mg zinc supplement for 14 days for children (6 months to 5 years) with acute diarrhea, and 10 mg per day for infants under 6 months of age, to curtail the severity of the episode and prevent further occurrences in the ensuing 3 months. Zinc (zinc sulfate, gluconate, or acetate) can be given either in form of syrup containing 20 mg of elemental zinc per 5 mL, or dispersible tablets of zinc sulfate, zinc gluconate, or zinc acetate containing 10 mg/20 mg of elemental zinc.

Antimicrobial Therapy

As discussed earlier, most of the diarrheal episodes in children are self-limiting and antibiotics are not indicated. Indications for administration of antimicrobials include (1) dysentery (blood in stools), (2) diarrhea due to *Vibrio cholerae, Cryptosporidium, Giardia*, or *E. histolytica*, (3) associated systemic infections (pneumonia, septicemia, meningitis, etc.), and (4) diarrhea in a severely malnourished child.

Other Drugs

Antimotility agents, such as loperamides are contraindicated for childhood diarrhea as these increase the risk of ileus. The role of probiotics and antisecretory agents such as racecadotril is also unclear and these are not recommended for routine use in childhood diarrhea. Antiemetics can be helpful in cases where the child is having incessant vomiting.

NONPHARMACOLOGICAL MEASURES

Diet in Diarrhea

Nutritional management is a very important aspect in management of diarrhea.

- ***Do not stop feeding:*** Most nutrients are well absorbed during diarrhea. This is an erroneous belief that rest to the bowel promotes early recovery.
- ***Give more food:*** A considerable quantity of nutrients is lost in the diarrheal stools. The dietary intake should be increased to compensate for losses and to promote rapid nutritional recovery.
- ***Continue breastfeeding*** during an attack of diarrhea. Breastmilk contains viable phagocytes and other protective substances, such as secretory IgA and specific IgM, which protect against diarrhea.
- ***Do not stop milk:*** Transient lactose intolerance lasting for 3–5 days may occur during acute diarrhea. This is self-limiting and does not require dilution of milk or stopping it altogether.
- ***Give easily digestible and nutritionally balanced diet.*** The diet should contain adequate amount of concentrated foods, so that enough nutrients are absorbed from a small quantity of food. Milled cereals are preferred to whole cereals. A well-cooked gruel of rice and lentil (*khichri*) is usually well tolerated. Mashed bananas are also good. The diet should be iso-osmolar. These foods should be started within 4–6 hours of starting the treatment.
- Carbonated drinks, sugar sweetened beverages and fruit juices with high sugar content should be avoided during diarrhea.
- Food should be offered in smaller quantities at shorter intervals.
- Contrary to the popular belief, most children tolerate small quantities of fats and oils, which are rich sources of energy, and the diarrhea does not worsen.

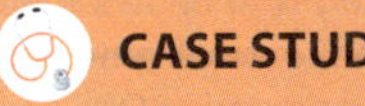

CASE STUDY Therapy for Acute Diarrhea

A 30-month-old girl, belonging to a daily wage laborer family, resident of a slum cluster presents to you with a 3-day history of watery diarrhea and vomiting. There is no history of fever or any other complaints. There is history of similar illness in many children of neighborhood. On asking mother, child has passed urine two times in last 12 hours. On examination, the child looks irritable, weighs 9.5 kg and is thirsty. Her height is 86 cm. Vitals are normal and systemic examination is noncontributory Her investigation reports revealed blood urea of 50 mg/dL and serum creatinine of 0.6 mg/dL.

Assess and classify dehydration in this child.

The child has an acute onset diarrhea. The assessment required in this child would include assessment for dehydration, nutritional status, and presence of any other coexisting illness.

Assess Hydration

Assessment for dehydration should include evaluation of four signs: (1) general condition, (2) skin pinch, (3) intake of fluids or thirst and (4) presence of sunken eyes. This child is irritable and thirsty suggesting two signs of "some" dehydration. Other examination should include examination for sunken eyes and skin pinch. Presence of both "skin pinch going back very slow" and sunken eyes will upgrade the dehydration to *"severe"* as two of the criteria of severe dehydration would be satisfied. If sunken eyes are not present, or the skin pinch goes back slowly but not very slowly, hydration status would still be *"some* dehydration" as two defining criteria for severe dehydration would not be satisfied. Even if both the signs are absent, i.e., skin pinch does not go back slowly and no sunken eyes; the hydration status would be classified as "some dehydration" as two defining criteria for this are already met. For further discussion, let us assume that the child did not meet the criteria for having severe dehydration and is classified as having "some dehydration".

Plan fluid and nutritional therapy for this child.

Assess Nutrition

Next step is to evaluate the nutritional status. The expected (50th percentile) weight for height of 86 cm for a girl is 11.6 kg as per WHO growth standards. Thus, this child's weight-for-height is lying between −2 *Z*-score (9.8 kg) and − 3 *Z*-score (9.0 kg), classifying her as having moderate wasting.

Classifying nutritional status is important for management as severely malnourished children require a different approach to fluid therapy (*see* Chapter 9) and also antibiotics might be needed assuming infection. However, this child is not having severe malnutrition. The child's history does not suggest any other coexisting infection as it is a short duration diarrhea and there is no fever or any other signs suggesting infection. A stool hanging drop examination and culture may be needed if cholera is prevalent in the area and program guidelines need reporting for this illness.

Plan Fluid

Thus, this child is *classified* as having "acute *watery diarrhea with some dehydration*", the fluid therapy for this child would be "Plan B", i.e., oral correction of dehydration with ORS.

The ORS packet should be dissolved in one liter of clean water and kept covered. The child needs 750 mL (75 mL/kg) of this solution in next 4 hours. The child should be given sips of ORS from a glass or a spoon. Do not give too much ORS at one time as it might induce vomiting. Even if the child vomits, ORS should be continued and it should be given more slowly. Preferably, the rehydration should be completed in the health facility itself checking the amount taken by child and state of her hydration hourly. Breastfeeding can be continued during this period if the child is breastfed and sips of plain water are also allowed.

After correction of dehydration, normal feeding is to be resumed and mother instructed to give her energy-rich foods in small amounts frequently. Mother should be trained in mixing and preparing ORS and should be counseled to give the child ORS and other home-available fluids at home till diarrhea continues. Nutritional counseling is to be done to improve the dietary intake once the child gets well, in order to prevent persistence or worsening of malnutrition. Also, counsel the mother about steps to prevent future diarrheal episodes.

Drug Therapy

You also need to decide about any other treatment needed in this child besides correction of dehydration and nutritional status. Antimicrobial treatment is not indicated in this child as there is no dysentery, child is not severely malnourished and there is no sign of any other infection. Zinc (in form of oral tablets or suspension) should be given in dose of 20 mg per day to be continued for 14 days to reduce the severity of diarrheal episode and also to prevent future episodes. The child may be sent back from health facility after correction of dehydration and training of mother in giving ORS and medications. Mother should be instructed to bring back the child in case of danger signs such as convulsions, lethargy, not taking anything orally or vomiting everything.

Interpret the renal function test report of this child.

Ans. The normal range of the renal function parameters in children is 8–20 mg/dL for blood urea and 0.5–1.2 mg/dL for creatinine. As in the present case the values of creatinine are within normal range, while the values of the blood urea are high, suggestive of azotemia. Intravascular hypovolemia cause renal hypoperfusion which can lead to the azotemia, like in the present case where the child has some dehydration on examination. This is likely to improve with fluid replacement. Children with severe dehydration and shock can have the onset of acute kidney injury suggested by high values of both blood urea and creatinine along with oliguria or anuria.

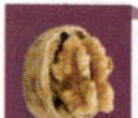

IN A NUTSHELL

Therapy for Acute Diarrhea

1. Acute watery diarrhea is a self-limiting disorder and can be successfully managed with ORT, zinc supplementation and continued feeding. It subsides within 5–7 days in a large majority of cases.
2. Acute diarrhea is most frequently caused by rotavirus and *E. coli*.
3. Dehydration is the primary cause of death in acute diarrhea. Children are classified as having *no, some,* or *severe dehydration.*
4. Children with *no dehydration* can be managed at home with oral fluids; those with some dehydration need oral rehydration therapy with WHO's reduced osmolarity ORS (75 mL/kg in 4 h); and those with *severe dehydration* need intravenous fluids (Ringer lactate or normal saline 100 mL/kg).
5. Antibiotics have no role in acute watery diarrhea except in dysentery, cholera, and children with severe malnutrition or coexisting systemic infections.

Dabas A, Shah D, Bhatnagar S, Lodha R. Epidemiology of *Cryptosporidium* in pediatric diarrheal illnesses. Indian Pediatr. 2017;54:299-309.

Ghosh K, Chakraborty AS, Mog M. Prevalence of diarrhoea among under five children in India and its contextual determinants: a geo-spatial analysis. Clin Epidemiol Global Health. 2021;12:100813.

Guarino A, Lo Vecchio A, Dias JA, et al. Universal recommendations for the management of acute diarrhea in nonmalnourished children. J Pediatr Gastroenterol Nutr. 2018;67(5):586-93.

Huang R, Xing HY, Liu HJ, et al. Efficacy of probiotics in the treatment of acute diarrhea in children: a systematic review and meta-analysis of clinical trials. Transl Pediatr. 2021;10:3248-60.

ICMR. Standard treatment workflow (STW) for the management of Acute Diarrhea ICD-10-R19.7. [online]. Available from: https://www.icmr.gov.in/icmrobject/uploads/STWs/1725952338_paediatrics_diarrhea.pdf. [Last accessed January, 2025].

Lo Vecchio A, Conelli ML, Guarino A. Infections and chronic diarrhea in children. Pediatr. Infect. Dis. J. 2021;40(7):e255-e258.

Ministry of Health and Family Welfare., Govt. of India. National Family Health Survey (NFHS-5). Compendium of fact sheets—key indicators. Available at: https://mohfw.gov.in/sites/default/files/NFHS-5_Phase-II_0.pdf. [Last accessed January, 2025]

Yachha SK, Sarma MS, Mohan N, et al. Indian Academy of Pediatrics Consensus Guidelines for Probiotic Use in Childhood Diarrhea. Indian Pediatr. 2022;59(7):543-51.

WHO. Diarrhoeal disease: factsheet. [online] Available from: https://www.who.int/news-roo m/fact-sheets/detail/diarrhoeal-disease. [Last accessed January, 2025].

20.5 Acute Dysentery

PE 23.5

INTRODUCTION

Dysentery is characterized by the presence of blood in the loose watery stools. Gross blood in the stools is the most reliable sign. It does not include blood streaks on surface of formed stool, blood detected only by microscopic examination, or biochemical tests and passage of digested blood (melena) in stools. Children having dysentery presents with complaints of passage of visible blood in the stools with or without mucus, fever and abdominal cramps which gets relieved with the passage of stools "tenesmus". They can also have signs of variable degrees of dehydration and its complications such as acidosis, oliguria, dyselectrolytemia and shock.

Most important and most frequent cause of acute dysentery is *Shigella* spp., especially *S. flexneri* and *S. dysenteriae*. Other causes include *Campylobacter jejuni, Salmonella* spp.,

Flowchart 20.1: WHO algorithm for treatment of dysentery

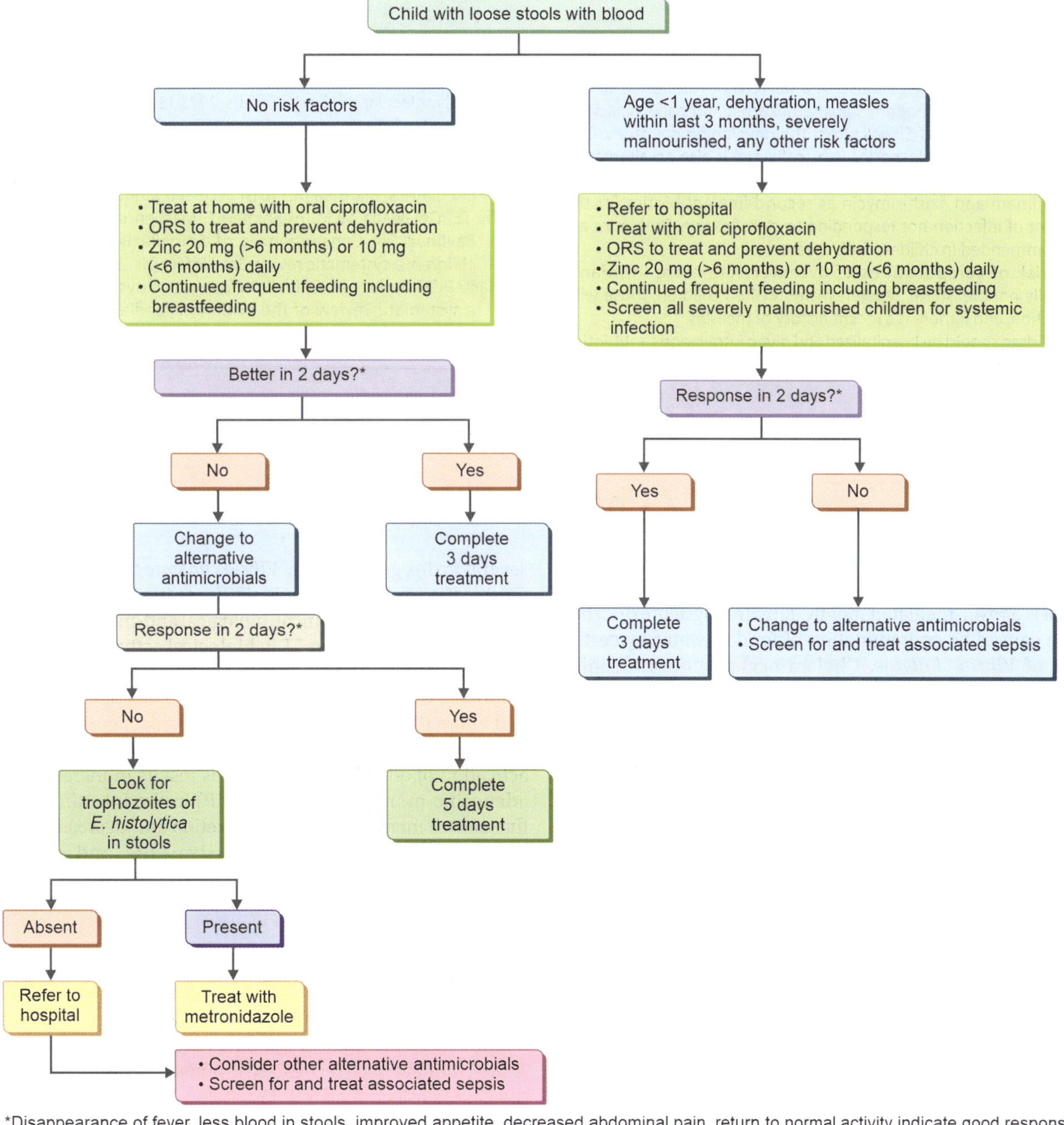

enteroinvasive *E. coli* (EIEC), *enterohemorrhagic E. coli* (EHEC), *Yersinia enterocolitica*, and *Clostridium difficile*. *Entamoeba histolytica* is an uncommon cause of dysentery in children responsible for <5% of cases. Recent studies have reported that the majority of children with *Shigella* infection presents with watery diarrhea rather than bloody diarrhea, and is associated with continued diarrhea and linear growth faltering.

TREATMENT Acute Dysentery

Assessment of state of dehydration and its correction by oral rehydration therapy/intravenous fluids along with the zinc supplementation as mentioned in the management of acute diarrhea should be done. Antipyretic agents such as paracetamol should be given for the fever.

Drug Therapy

Ciprofloxacin is the first-line drug recommended by WHO for the treatment of dysentery because of a pattern of resistance to the other drugs, i.e., trimethoprim sulfamethoxazole and nalidixic acid in a majority of isolates of *Shigella* from the developing countries. Oral third generation cephalosporins (e.g., cefixime) is also an alternative to ciprofloxacin in clinical practice. The WHO recommends ceftriaxone, pivmecillinam and azithromycin as second-line antibiotics for the treatment of infection not responding to ciprofloxacin. Probiotics are not recommended in children with dysentery.

The risk of complications of dysentery are more in infants (especially nonbreastfed), severely malnourished children, those with dehydration, and if there is a recent history of measles.

Such children should be hospitalized and given intravenous antibiotics. **Flowchart 20.1** provides the recommended algorithm for treatment of dysentery.

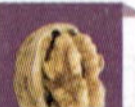

IN A NUTSHELL

Acute Dysentery

1. Bloody diarrhea is referred to as dysentery. *Shigella* is the most common causative organism. Ciprofloxacin is the drug of choice; nonresponders are given cefixime. Serious hospitalized patients are treated with ceftriaxone.
2. Risk of complications of dysentery is more in nonbreastfed infants, severely malnourished children, those with dehydration, and recent history of measles. Such children should be hospitalized.
3. All children with diarrhea or dysentery should be given zinc supplementation for 14 days.

Bansal P, Shah D, Meena RK, et al. Shigella as a cause of diarrhea hospitalization in children under five: evaluation by conventional and molecular methods. Cureus. 2023;15(12):e50546.

ICMR. Standard treatment workflow (STW) for the management of Acute Diarrhea ICD-10-R19.7. [online]. Available from: https://www.icmr.gov.in/icmrobject/uploads/STWs/1725952338_paediatrics_diarrhea.pdf. [Last accessed January, 2025].

Libby TE, Delawalla MLM, Al-Shimari F, MacLennan CA, Vannice KS, Pavlinac PB. Consequences of Shigella infection in young children: a systematic review. Int J Infect Dis. 2023;129:78-95s.

Williams PCM, Berkley JA. Guidelines for treating dysentery (shigellosis): a systematic review of the evidence. Paediatr Int Child Health. 2018;38:S50-S65.

20.6 Cholera

PE 23.7, PE 23.8

INTRODUCTION

Cholera is a toxin-mediated rapidly dehydrating acute diarrheal disease caused by contamination of food or water by certain strains of *Vibrio cholerae*. Cholera occurs more in tropical countries across the globe and more during warm months. Environmental factors such as poverty, overcrowding, and lack of adequate sanitation and safe drinking water also play a role. In developed countries, consumption of raw shellfish or moist grains has been observed to be associated with the disease spread. In endemic areas, possibility of cholera (caused by *Vibrio cholerae*) should always be considered. According to the latest estimates, approximately 50 countries in Africa and South and Southeast Asia have endemic cholera.

ETIOPATHOGENESIS

There are over 200 serogroups of *V. cholerae,* but only two serogroups (O1 and O139) are associated with outbreaks of severe disease in man. Short incubation period and virulence of O1 and O139 is responsible for the high fatality. Cholera enterotoxin called choleragen (CT) is the major toxin among the several toxins generated by *Vibrio cholerae* that are responsible for the disease. Choleragen is similar to heat labile toxin (LT) of *E. coli* in structural, chemical, biological and antigenic properties but far more potent than LT in biological activity.

On entry into the gut through contaminated food, the vibrio colonizes the small intestinal epithelium. Following binding and internalization of the toxin into enterocytes, it catalyzes the ADP-ribosylation of a GTP-binding protein, leading to persistent activation of adenylate cyclase. This results in increased cyclic adenosine monophosphate (cAMP) in the intestinal mucosa that causes increased chloride secretion and decreased sodium absorption, producing the massive fluid and electrolyte loss characteristic of cholera. CT may also lead to increased prostaglandin production, which adds to gastrointestinal loss of water and electrolytes.

CLINICAL FEATURES

The incubation period of *V. cholerae* is very short, ranging from 2 hours to 5 days. Man is the only natural host, but free-living *V. cholerae* have been recognized in aquatic environment. Usually, the case is infectious for 3 days before the onset of symptoms (incubatory carrier period) and 7–10 days thereafter. The ratio of severe cases to subclinical cases is around 1:10. These subclinical cases continue to harbor the bacteria in their feces for 7–14 days after infection and shed back the bacilli into the environment, potentially infecting other people. Asymptomatic cases serve to maintain the infection in the community. Temporary convalescent carriers may continue to excrete *V. cholerae* for 3–4 weeks.

Most patients (75%) infected with toxigenic *V. cholerae* serogroup O1 or O139 are asymptomatic. Only 20% have only a mild to moderate diarrheal illness and approximately 5% develop the classic symptoms and signs of severe cholera (*cholera gravis*). Diarrhea is usually abrupt, painless and profuse. The stools are voluminous (10–20 mL/kg up to 1 liter per stool), isotonic, and rice watery, with flecks of suspended mucus. This is associated with profound vomiting of clear watery fluid. The natural course runs for 2–7 days.

If fluid losses are not corrected rapidly, child becomes apathetic and lethargic that progresses rapidly to obtundation, hypotension, renal failure and hypovolemic shock. Loss of bicarbonate in stool and lactic acidosis from poor perfusion may result in Kussmaul breathing. Muscle cramping and weakness are common due to loss of potassium and calcium. In children, depletion of glycogen stores and inadequate gluconeogenesis can lead to symptoms of severe hypoglycemia or even coma. The purge rate is usually very high (10–20 mL/kg/h up to 1,000 mL/h) and if untreated proves fatal. Death may be attributed to hyponatremic shock, acidosis, and renal failure. Rare complications include aspiration pneumonia and septicemia.

DIAGNOSIS

It is important to identify cholera because of the potential for a widespread outbreak. According to WHO:

- Cholera should be suspected if:
  - A patient older than 2 years develops severe dehydration from acute watery diarrhea (usually with vomiting); or
  - Any person presenting with or dying from acute watery diarrhea in an area where there is an outbreak of cholera, especially patients who pass the *rice watery* stool typical of cholera.
- A case of cholera is confirmed when: *Vibrio cholerae* O1 or O139 is isolated from any patient with diarrhea.

Whenever such cases are suspected and confirmed, reporting to health officials becomes mandatory.

Routine Investigations

Findings of the routine investigations are suggestive of volume loss and its effects, like in complete blood counts there is a rise in hematocrit with leukocytosis without leftwards shift. In biochemistry reports, there is hyponatremia (serum sodium <135 mEq/L), deranged renal function tests, increase in serum specific gravity, and elevation of serum total proteins and metabolic acidosis due to hemoconcentration secondary to enormous intravascular volume loss. Initially potassium remains normal due to exchange with hydrogen ions at the distal tubules but later hypokalemia (serum potassium <3.5 mEq/L) develops, causing paralytic ileus, muscle weakness, and neck flop.

Stool Examination

Bedside diagnosis rests on the presence of rice water stools coupled with demonstration of darting motility in wet mounts of the stools (*hanging drop preparation*) identified under a dark field microscope at 400X magnification. The sensitivity of the motility detection method is increased with the use of specific *V. cholerae* O1 antisera where, the addition of polyvalent antisera against *V. cholerae* O1 results in the cessation of motility, as observed by either dark-field or phase-contrast microscopy, the test is considered positive. Freshly collected liquid ("rice-water") stool is the specimen of choice for the dark-field procedure. If stool is liquid but not rice-water in nature, it should be dilute 1:1 with saline before direct testing. If freshly collected stool is negative, perform a 6- to 8-hour enrichment in media and retest the enrichment broth. Isolation and identification of *V. cholerae* serogroup O1 or O139 by culture of a stool specimen remains the gold standard for the laboratory diagnosis of cholera. Commercially available rapid test kits are available to identify an epidemic outbreak especially in resource poor settings. Immunofluorescence, latex agglutination, and coagglutination methods have been introduced but seldom used due to expenses involved and a low specificity.

Differential Diagnosis

All causes of acute watery diarrhea including rotavirus, *Cryptosporidium* and ETEC can present with similar manifestations.

TREATMENT Cholera

Management of Dehydration and Electrolyte Imbalance

Rehydration is the mainstay of therapy. Rehydration therapy reduces the risk of mortality from 10 to 0.5%. Patients are treated as per WHO guidelines for acute watery diarrhea. For details please see section **20.3**.

Children with cholera are at a great risk for hyponatremic dehydration and the appropriate choice of fluid used for rehydration is crucial. Ringers lactate is preferred for fluid correction once initial boluses have been administered for features of hypovolemic shock as it contains both potassium and bicarbonate, which are lost in stools. Fluid replacement in cholera may reach up to 200–350 mL/kg over the first 24 hours. Rice-based ORS is also proven to be equally efficacious to the standard ORS for rehydration in cholera.

Antimicrobial Treatment

Though the mainstay of management of cholera is effective fluid therapy, appropriate antibiotics are essential in the management of moderate to severe cholera cases as it reduces the volume of rehydration fluids needed by almost 50%, the duration of symptoms and time spent in hospital, as well as the length of *V. cholerae* excretion in the feces to 1–2 days, thereby reducing the risk of transmission. Antibiotic options include tetracyclines, fluoroquinolones and macrolides.

The recommended antibiotic of choice for cholera is single dose doxycycline (6–8 mg/kg) for all patients, including adults, children and pregnant women. Azithromycin or ciprofloxacin and/or erythromycin are alternatives in situations where there is doxycycline resistance or no clinical response. No chemoprophylaxis is needed for contacts. Drug treatment of cholera is summarized in **Table 20.4**.

Table 20.4 Antimicrobials for Treating Cholera

Antimicrobial	*Dose*
Doxycycline	4–6 mg/kg single dose <15 years, 200 mg stat >15 years
Tetracycline	12.5 mg/kg/dose (up to 500 mg/dose) 4 times/day for 3 days
Ciprofloxacin	15 mg/kg per dose (up to 1 g/day) 2 times/day for 3 days
Erythromycin	12.5 mg/kg/dose (up to 500 mg/dose) 4 times/day for 3 days
Azithromycin	20 mg/kg (up to 1 g) single dose

Zinc Supplementation

Oral zinc supplements (10 mg/day for children <6 months and 20 mg/day for those between 6 months and 5 years) for 14 days shortens the duration of illness, decreases the stool volume, decreases the purge rate, and reduces further episodes as in other watery diarrhea. It also has a direct inhibitory action on the CT toxin. However, role of zinc in children older than 5 years with cholera is yet to be proven.

Cholera Vaccine

"Currently, three WHO pre-qualified oral cholera vaccines (OCV) are available: Dukoral®, Shanchol™, and Euvichol®. All three vaccines require two doses for full protection. Euvichol® is approved for use in individuals above 1 year age."

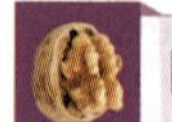

IN A NUTSHELL

Cholera

1. Cholera is a toxin mediated rapidly dehydrating acute diarrheal disease caused by *V. cholerae*, two serogroups (O1 and O139) are associated with outbreaks of severe disease.
2. Cholera toxin increases cyclic adenosine monophosphate (cAMP) in the intestinal mucosa leading to chloride secretion and decreased sodium absorption, causing massive fluid and electrolyte loss.
3. Fluid losses if not corrected rapidly, can lead to renal failure, hypovolemic shock and death.
4. Demonstration of darting motility in wet mounts of the stools (*hanging drop preparation*) is a bedside test for diagnosis.
5. Rehydration is the mainstay of therapy, along with antibiotics (doxycycline/azithromycin) and zinc supplementation.

Bourgeat L, Pacini L, Serghei A, et al. A protocol to measure slow protein dynamics of the cholera toxin B entamers using broadband dielectric spectroscopy. STAR Protoc. 2022;3(3):101561.

Chen Y, Ai X, Yang Y. Vibrio cholerae: a pathogen shared by human and aquatic animals. Lancet Microbe. 2022;3(6):e402.

Chowdhury F, Ross AG, Islam MT, McMillan NAJ, Qadri F. Diagnosis, management, and future control of cholera. Clin Microbiol Rev. 2022;35(3):e0021121.

Kanungo S, Azman AS, Ramamurthy T, Deen J, Dutta S. Cholera. The Lancet. 2022;399(10333):1429-40.

Kaushik JS, Gupta P, Faridi MM, et al. Single dose azithromycin versus ciprofloxacin for cholera in children: a randomized controlled trial. Indian Pediatr. 2010;47:309-15.

Williams PCM, Berkley JA. Guidelines for the management of paediatric cholera infection: a systematic review of the evidence. Paediatr Int Child Health. 2018;38:S16-S31.

Saif-Ur-Rahman KM, Mamun R, Hasan M, Meiring JE, Khan MA. Oral killed cholera vaccines for preventing cholera. Cochrane Database Syst Rev. 2024;1(1):CD014573.

World Health Organization. Cholera. [online] Available from: https://www.who.int/news-room/fact-sheets/detail/cholera. [Last accessed January, 2025].

20.7 Persistent Diarrhea

PE 23.4

INTRODUCTION

Diarrhea starting as an acute episode and lasting for more than 14 days is labeled as persistent diarrhea. Stools are often watery and may lead to dehydration. Persistent diarrhea is more common in children below the age of 2 years and in malnourished children.

Persistent diarrhea needs to be differentiated from *chronic diarrhea* which occurs due to an underlying pathology such as celiac disease, tropical sprue, and congenital and metabolic diseases. Chronic diarrhea is more insidious in onset continuing for months, stools are not watery and do not usually lead to dehydration. For chronic diarrhea please see sections 21.4 and 21.5.

PATHOPHYSIOLOGY

Diarrhea starts as an acute episode due to infection with a microorganism. Most often, the illness subsides in a period of about 5–7 days. However, sometimes the diarrhea continues because of:

- Persistent infection because of poor nutritional status or impaired immunological defenses;
- Presence of systemic infection such as urinary tract infection, pneumonia or protracted septicemia; or
- Malabsorption, particularly of carbohydrates and fats due to loss of intestinal brush border, and associated enzymatic dysfunction.

Nutritional losses further contribute to malnutrition and a vicious cycle is set up. Thus, the child is not able to recover from diarrhea. Infrequently, protein intolerance may also develop. Faulty feeding practices and overuse of antibiotics compound the problem.

CLINICAL FEATURES

Growth faltering, worsening of malnutrition, and *death* are the major consequences of persistent diarrhea. Despite passage of frequent loose stools, the hydration usually remains good. Dehydration may develop if purge rate is high or when oral intake is inadequate because of associated systemic infection. Continued diarrhea may worsen the preexisting malnutrition, predispose to systemic infections and may result in death.

INVESTIGATIONS

Send stool specimen for microscopic examination (especially for pus cells, RBCs, and trophozoites or cysts of *E. histolytica, Cryptosporidium,* or *Giardia*) and culture. Obtain stool pH to determine lactose intolerance (suggested by the stool pH of <5.5 on two separate occasions). Screen for other systemic infections, especially urinary tract infections.

TREATMENT Persistent Diarrhea

Children with persistent diarrhea should be admitted if they are <4 months of age, are dehydrated or having severe malnutrition or a systemic infection. Assess the child for dehydration as described in the Section on acute diarrhea and manage as per Plan A, B or C. The mainstay of management is dietary therapy.

Dietary Therapy

- *Breastfeeding:* Encourage exclusive breastfeeding in infants <6 months of age. Continue breastfeeding in older infants and children up to 2 years of age.
- *Diet A—Reduced lactose diet:* Initially, put the child on a reduced lactose diet. Limit the quantity of top milk to 50 mL/kg/day; it need not be stopped altogether or diluted with water. The feeds may be given in the form of a milk rice gruel, milk *sooji* gruel, rice with curds or *dalia*. Offer 6–7 feeds per day. The total caloric intake should be 150 kcal/kg/d. If oral intake is not satisfactory, feed through a naso-gastric tube. About 60% children will improve on this diet alone.
- *Diet B—Lactose free diet:* If the child does not respond to Diet A, they are shifted to a lactose free diet. This does not contain any milk. Milk protein is replaced by chicken or egg. Cereals are allowed. A typical diet providing 90 kcal and 2.5 g of protein per 100 g of portion can be prepared by mixing egg white (½ egg), puffed rice powder (3 tsp), glucose (1½ tsp), oil (1½ tsp) and water (120 mL).
- *Diet C—Monosaccharide-based diet:* 10% children with persistent diarrhea may not respond either to Diet A or B. These children are given a monosaccharide-based diet that is free of cereals and is largely based on egg/chicken. Besides it contains oil, glucose and water. No milk is allowed.
- *Vitamins and minerals:* Provide vitamin A (200,000 units to those >8 kg and 100,000 units to those weighing <8 kg) as a single dose. Start daily zinc supplementation (10–20 mg/day). Give all other vitamins and minerals in twice the recommended daily allowance. Introduce iron only when diarrhea stops.
- *Monitoring:* Record weight, stool frequency and signs of dehydration daily.
- *Antimicrobials:* Start them as indicated by presence of blood in stools, associated systemic infection or as per reports of urine and stool microscopy and culture. All severely malnourished children would also require treatment with antibiotics.

PROGNOSIS

Though only about 5–10% of episodes of diarrhea in under-5 children last for >14 days, persistent diarrhea is responsible for one-third to one-half of diarrhea related mortality. The case fatality rate of persistent diarrhea is about 20 times higher than that of acute diarrhea; the prognosis being poorer in severely malnourished children, and in those with persistent dysentery.

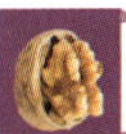

IN A NUTSHELL

Persistent Diarrhea

1. Diarrhea starting as an acute episode and lasting for >14 days is labeled as persistent diarrhea.
2. Persistent diarrhea needs to be differentiated from *chronic diarrhea* which usually occurs due to an underlying pathology such as celiac disease, tropical sprue, and congenital and metabolic diseases.
3. *Growth faltering, worsening of malnutrition* and *death are* the major consequences of persistent diarrhea.
4. Children with persistent diarrhea should be hospitalized if they are <4 months of age, are dehydrated or having severe malnutrition or a systemic infection.
5. The mainstay of management is the dietary therapy. Three diets are primarily used: Diet A: reduced lactose diet; Diet B: lactose-free diet; and Diet C: monosaccharide-based diet.

Bernaola Aponte G, Bada Mancilla CA, Carreazo NY, et al. Probiotics for treating persistent diarrhea in children. Cochrane Database Syst Rev. 2013;8:CD007401.

Das JK, Padhani ZA, Bhutta ZA. Persistent diarrhea in children in developing countries. In: Guandalini S, Dhawan A (Eds). Textbook of Pediatric Gastroenterology, Hepatology and Nutrition. Springer, Cham; 2022.

Gupte S. Persistent diarrhea in childhood: issues and concerns. Gastroenterol Hepatol Int J. 2016;1:000107.

Lo Vecchio A, Conelli M, Guarino A. Infections and chronic diarrhea in children. Pediatr Infect Dis J. 2021;40:e255-8.

Naqvi SK, Zubairi MBA, Ali AA, et al. Antibiotics for acute watery or persistent with or without bloody diarrhoea in children: A systematic review and meta-analysis. J Glob Health. 2024;14:04211.

Rahman AE, Moinuddin M, Molla M, et al. Childhood diarrhoeal deaths in seven low- and middle-income countries. Bull World Health Organ. 2014;92:664-71.

Shankar S, Rosenbaum J. Chronic diarrhoea in children: A practical algorithm-based approach. J Paediatr Child Health. 2020;56(7):1029-38.

20.8 Prevention of Diarrhea

PE 23.4

Diarrhea can be prevented to a large extent by improving poor dietary habits and hygiene, as discussed here.

DIET

- Exclusive breastfeeding should be given for first 6 months.
- Complementary feeding with energy-rich food mixtures containing adequate amounts of nutrients such as balanced amounts of proteins, fats, iron and vitamins should be introduced soon after 6 months of age while continuing breastfeeding (till at least 2 years of age).

HYGIENE (FIG. 20.6)

- Wash hands before preparation or administration of food, and after defecation or cleaning the child.
- Protect food from contamination during preparation, storage or at the time of administration.
- Mothers should be guided to use clean containers, avoiding exposure of food to dust, flies or cockroaches.
- Water given to the child or used for preparing feeds should be clean and potable, preferably boiled during epidemics.
- Vegetables and fruit should be washed and peeled before these are fed to the child.

ENVIRONMENTAL FACTORS (FIG. 20.7)

- Proper sewage disposal
- Potable water supply
- Proper excreta/toilet facilities

VACCINE

Rotavirus vaccine is now a part of the national immunization schedule. Rotavirus vaccine is to be given as 5 drops per oral at 6, 10, and 14 weeks' age, and can be given up to 1 year of age as a part of catch-up vaccination. Rotavirus vaccines will not prevent diarrhea because of other causes; emphasis of prevention should also be on hand washing and general hygiene measures.

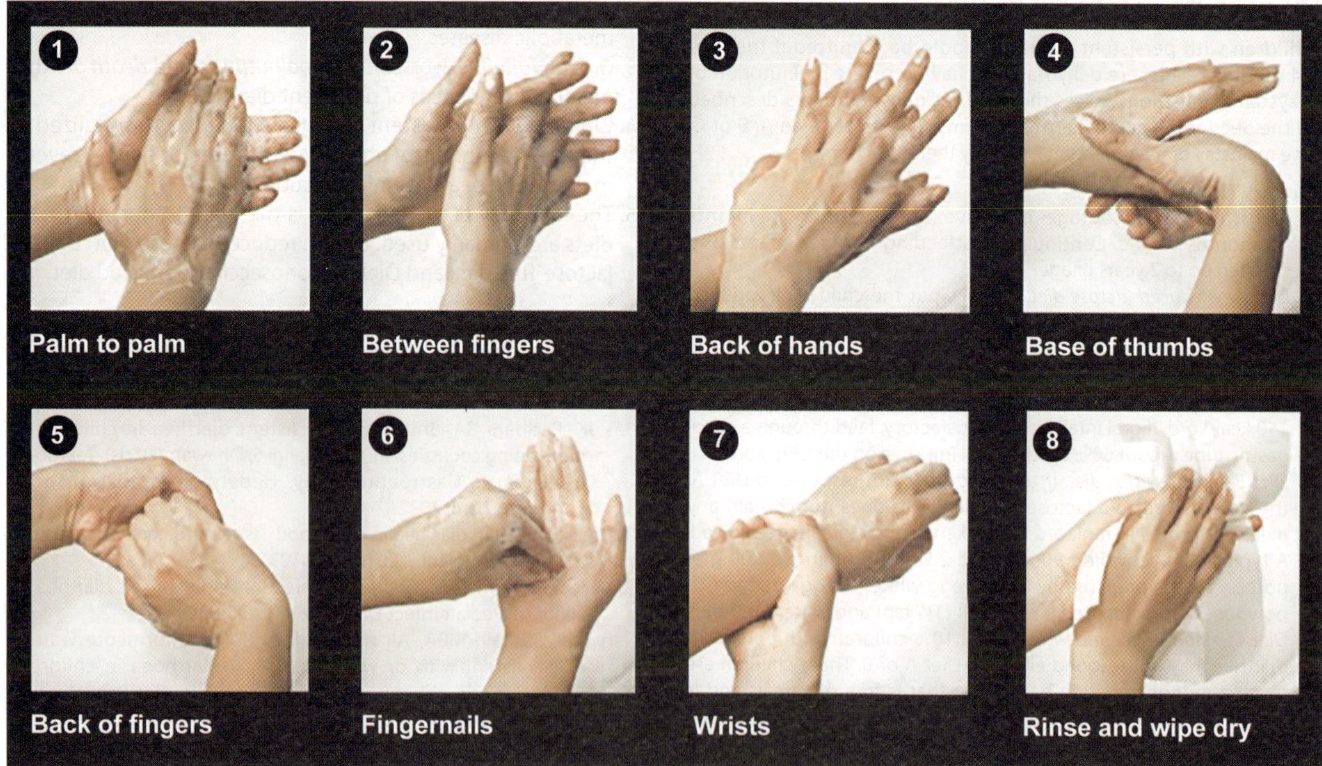

Fig. 20.6: Steps of handwashing

Source: National Health Mission. (2019). Intensified Diarrhoea Control Fortnight Tool Kit, Child Health Division, Ministry of Health and Family Welfare, Government of India. [online] Available from: https://nhm.gov.in/index1. php?lang=1&level=5&sublinkid=1310&lid=691. [Last accessed January 2025]

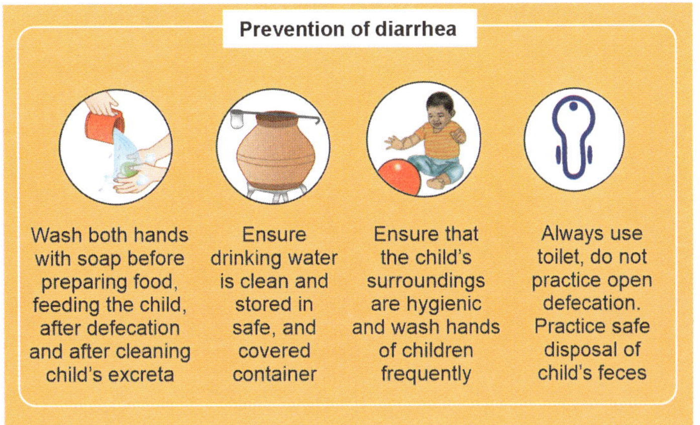

Fig. 20.7: Different ways to prevent diarrhea

Source: National Health Mission. (2019). Intensified Diarrhoea Control Fortnight Tool Kit, Child Health Division, Ministry of Health and Family Welfare, Government of India. [online] Available from: https://nhm.gov.in/index1. php?lang=1&level=5&sublinkid=1310&lid=691. [Last accessed January 2025]

21 CHAPTER

Gastrointestinal and Hepatobiliary Disorders

AS PER NMC COMPETENCIES

PE23.1	Define vomiting, discuss causes, evaluation and management of vomiting in children.	*Ch 21.1*
PE23.2	Define constipation discuss causes, evaluation and management of constipation in children.	*Ch 21.1*
PE23.3	Discuss the causes, evaluation and management of abdominal pain in children.	*Ch 21.1*
PE 23.12	Discuss the etiopathogenesis, clinical presentation and management of malabsorption in children and its causes including celiac disease.	*Ch 21.3, Ch 21.4, Ch 21.5*
PE23.13	Discuss the etiopathogenesis, clinical features and management of acute hepatitis in children.	*Ch 21.6, Ch 21.10*
PE23.14	Discuss the etiopathogenesis, clinical features and management of fulminant hepatic failure in children.	*Ch 21.7, Ch 21.10*
PE23.15	Discuss the etiopathogenesis, clinical features and management of chronic liver diseases in children.	*Ch 21.8*
PE23.16	Discuss the etiopathogenesis, clinical features and management of portal hypertension in children.	*Ch 21.9*
PE23.17	Elicit, document and present the history related to diseases of gastrointestinal system.	*Ch 21.1*
PE23.18	Identify external markers for GI and liver disorders, e.g., jaundice, pallor, gynecomastia, spider angioma, palmar erythema, ichthyosis, caput medusa, clubbing, failing to thrive, vitamin A and D deficiency.	*Ch 21.2*
PE23.19	Perform examination of the abdomen, demonstrate organomegaly, ascites, etc.	*Ch 21.2*
PE23.20	Interpret liver function tests, viral markers, ultrasonogram report.	*Ch 21.1*
PE23.21	Enumerate the indications for upper GI endoscopy.	*Ch 21.9*

Topics available online: ***Physiology of Absorption and Common Surgical Problems***

21.1 Presentation and Diagnostic Approach to Common Gastrointestinal Disorders

PE 23.1, PE 23.2, PE 23.3, PE 23.17, PE 23.20

INTRODUCTION

Gastrointestinal system is a large organ system that can be involved in multiple conditions. Symptoms which arise from gastrointestinal tract (GIT) should be assessed in detail as many symptoms related to the abdomen may not be due to involvement of gastrointestinal system but arise due to pathology in other organ systems. The common symptoms of gastrointestinal disorders are given here.

VOMITING

Vomiting is the sudden forceful oral expulsion of gastric contents, caused by the violent contraction of the abdominal and chest wall musculature. Reflux of the small amount of bile into stomach gives the usual slight yellowish tinge to the vomitus, presence of larger amount of bile into stomach makes the vomitus bright yellow or green in color (bilious) indicating presence of intestinal obstruction or dysmotility distal to the second part of duodenum. Presence of blood in the vomitus indicates gastrointestinal bleed.

Etiology

Vomiting is a common symptom of many disease conditions, its severity can range from a mild self-limiting physiological phenomenon like regurgitation of feeds or overfeeding in an infant to infective conditions such as gastroenteritis, urinary tract infection, to severe life-threatening conditions like raised intracranial pressure due to meningitis/intracranial space occupying lesion. The cause of vomiting in children varies with the age of the child. Congenital anatomic, genetic, and metabolic disorders are more commonly seen in infancy. Peptic, infectious, and psychogenic causes are more prominent with increasing age **(Box 21.1)**.

Pathogenesis

The neural pathways involved in initiating vomiting include the abdominal vagal afferents (evoked by mechanical or chemosensory pathways triggered by food toxins, cytotoxic drugs, mucosal irritation, and overdistention), area postrema also known as chemoreceptor trigger zone located in the floor of fourth ventricle containing receptors for the chemical mediators of vomiting, vestibular system (motion associated vomiting), and amygdala (in response to physical or emotional stress). Signals from these lead to the sudden contraction of abdominal and chest muscles with relaxation of stomach and retrograde peristalsis of intestines. Multiple episodes of vomiting can lead to complications such as dehydration, dyselectrolytemia, and metabolic alkalosis.

Box 21.1 Causes of Vomiting in children

A. *Anatomical/structural defects of gastrointestinal tract:*
1. Hypertrophic pyloric stenosis
2. Malrotation
3. Volvulus
4. Intussusception
5. Intestinal obstruction
6. Hirschsprung disease
7. Gastroesophageal reflux
8. Gastrointestinal motility and functional disorders

B. *Infections and inflammations:*
1. Acute gastroenteritis
2. Pyelonephritis
3. Hepatitis
4. Pancreatitis
5. Cholecystitis
6. Peritonitis
7. Typhoid fever

C. *Central nervous system (CNS) causes:*
1. CNS infections
2. Intracranial space occupying lesions
3. Benign intracranial hypertension
4. Hydrocephalus
5. Extradural/subdural/intracranial bleed

D. *Toxic and metabolic causes:*
- Food poisoning
- Other poisonings
- Uremia
- Diabetic ketoacidosis
- Inborn errors of metabolism
- Drug toxicities

E. *Others:*
1. Milk protein intolerance
2. Psychogenic

Gastroesophageal Reflux

Gastroesophageal reflux (GER) refers to the spontaneous effortless movement of gastric contents proximally into the esophagus. Episodes of transient relaxation of lower esophageal sphincter allowing gastric contents to reflux into the esophagus, is the predominant mode of GER in infants and older children. When the reflux is high enough to be visualized, it is called *regurgitation.*

The GER is extremely common during infancy, in majority of the children this gets resolved within 6–12 months age without any long-term effects. Many times, parents/caregiver perceives regurgitation as vomiting which makes them rush to the hospital.

When the reflux or regurgitation results in complications (e.g., failure to thrive, swallowing difficulties, apnea, pneumonia, reactive airway disease) or contributes to tissue damage or inflammation (e.g., esophagitis), it is called *gastroesophageal reflux disease* (GERD).

APPROACH TO A CHILD WITH VOMITING

The underlying cause of vomiting can be determined by detailed history and physical examination. History should include the details regarding the onset, progression, and pattern (acute, chronic, or recurrent) of vomiting, color, consistency, and volume of the vomitus along with the associated symptoms such as fever, diarrhea, abdominal pain (suggestive of infection), abdominal distension, abdominal pain, inability to pass stool, bilious vomitus (suggestive of obstruction), headache, photophobia, bulging fontanelle (suggestive of central nervous system (CNS) infection/raised intracranial pressure), colicky pain in flanks (suggestive of urinary cause), decreased urine output, lethargy, altered sensorium, and seizures (suggestive of complications). History must include details regarding recent intake of food items, ingestion of drugs/contact with any toxic substances. Presence of recurrent vomiting episodes with failure to thrive, developmental delay with or without seizures can be associated with inborn errors of metabolism. Children with GER can also have associated symptoms such as heartburn and gastrointestinal blood loss.

Clinical Features

Presence of tachycardia and tachypnea could be associated with the fever or depleted volume status. During the general examination, a child must be assessed for signs of dehydration, signs of distress (e.g., lethargy, irritability, inconsolable crying, and altered sensorium). Detailed systemic examination, especially that of abdomen and CNS, can help in detecting the cause of vomiting. Abdominal examination should note distension; presence and quality of bowel sounds (e.g., high-pitched, normal, absent); tenderness and any associated guarding, rigidity, or rebound (peritoneal signs); and presence of organomegaly or mass. CNS examination should focus on signs of infection (e.g., bulging anterior fontanelle, neck rigidity, positive Kernig's and Brudzinski's sign), raised intracranial tension, and focal neurological deficits. Electrolyte disturbances, metabolic alkalosis, shock are the complications which can occur in cases with multiple vomiting.

Children with GER can have nutritional problems such as failure to thrive and anemia. Esophagitis caused by the reflux of gastric acid results in heartburn, irritability, and abnormal posturing (Sandifer-Sutcliffe syndrome).

Investigations

A child with prolonged or repetitive vomiting should have the following investigations: complete blood count, serum electrolytes, blood urea nitrogen, and urinalysis. Specific indications from history and physical examination may help in obtaining other tests such as upper gastrointestinal imaging, abdominal ultrasound, computed tomography (CT) scan or magnetic resonance imaging (MRI) of the head, tests of liver function, serum amylase, toxicology screen, serum ammonia, and urinary organic acids. **Flowchart 21.1** outlines the clinical and investigative approach to the diagnosis in a child with vomiting.

- ***Upper gastrointestinal contrast series*** should be performed to diagnose or exclude hypertrophic pyloric stenosis, esophageal webs, GER, and malrotation in a young child having prolonged or repetitive vomiting associated with failure to thrive.
- ***Ultrasound*** is a sensitive tool to diagnose hypertrophic pyloric stenosis, in children having a palpable pyloric mass.
- ***Endoscopic examination*** of the esophagus, stomach, and duodenum is sometimes helpful if peptic disease, esophagitis, or anatomic abnormality are suspected. The presence of intraepithelial eosinophils along with other inflammatory cells in the distal esophageal mucosal biopsy suggests the diagnosis of esophagitis secondary to GERD.
- ***Manometric evaluation*** of the esophagus, stomach, and duodenum is occasionally helpful in defining primary or secondary motor abnormalities causing emesis.
- ***24-hour esophageal pH*** monitoring with a pH probe is the most sensitive and specific investigation for diagnosis of GER.
- ***Radionuclide studies*** with technetium 99m (^{99m}Tc) are also useful in children with GERD and carry the advantage of being noninvasive and low in radiation.

Flowchart 21.1: Clinical and diagnostic approach to a child with vomiting

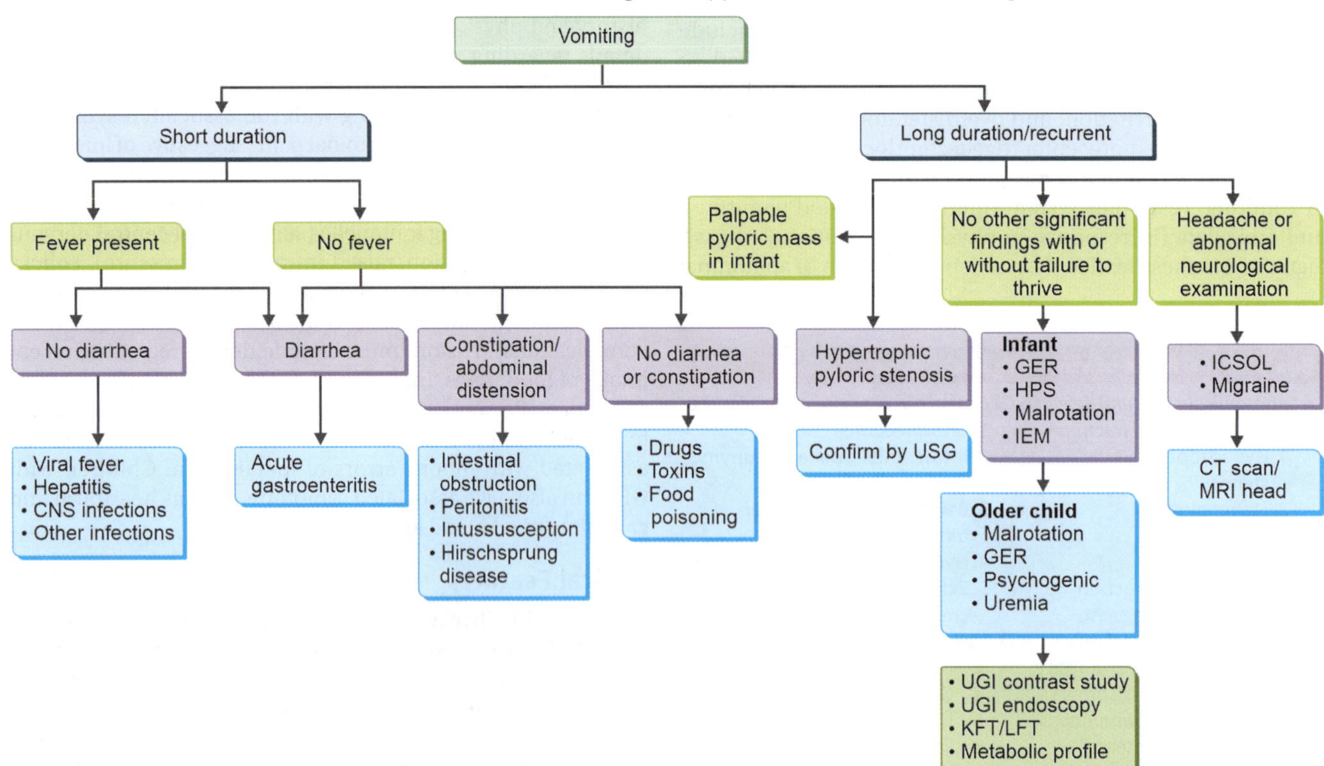

(CT: computed tomography; CNS: central nervous system; GER: gastroesophageal reflux; HPS: hypertrophic pyloric stenosis; IEM: inborn error of metabolism; ICSOL: intracranial space occupying lesion; KFT: kidney function test; LFT: liver function test: MRI: magnetic resonance imaging; UGI: upper gastrointestinal; USG: ultrasonography)

TREATMENT Child with Vomiting

Treatment of children who have vomiting is based on two steps:

1. *Supportive treatment:*
   - Correction of dehydration
   - Correction of the dyselectrolytemia
   - Blood transfusion in hematemesis
   - *In GER:* Elevation of head end and chest, small frequent feeds, and thickening of feeds might benefit.
2. *Definitive treatment:* Treatment of the underlying condition forms the mainstay of the definitive treatment. This includes:
   - Antibiotics for infective conditions
   - Medications such as H2 antagonists or proton pump inhibitors (PPIs) and prokinetic agents for GERD
   - Surgical intervention for conditions such as anatomical/structural defects of GIT, hydrocephalus, and severe GERD.

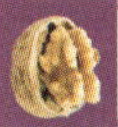

IN A NUTSHELL

Approach to a Child with Vomiting

1. Vomiting is a common symptom of many gastrointestinal and extra-gastrointestinal disease states.
2. Gastroesophageal reflux (GER) refers to the spontaneous effortless movement of gastric contents proximally into the esophagus.
3. Majority of children with vomiting also have other symptoms related to the underlying condition.
4. Gastroesophageal reflux disease (GERD) refers to symptomatic GER. Common symptoms include growth failure, respiratory disease, apnea, or esophagitis.
5. Child with prolonged or repetitive vomiting needs evaluation.
6. Treatment of children who have vomiting is two steps based—(1) Supportive and (2) Definitive.

Benninga MA, Faure C, Hyman PE, et al. Childhood functional gastrointestinal disorders: neonate/toddler. Gastroenterology. 2016;150:1443-55.

Campbell C, Slater Y. Approach to the vomiting child. Paediatr Child Health. 2018;28(11):500-6.

Irwin S, Barmherzig R, Gelfand A. Recurrent gastrointestinal disturbance: abdominal migraine and cyclic vomiting syndrome. Curr Neurol Neurosci Rep. 2017;17(3):21.

Kleinman RE, Goulet O, Mieli-Vergani, et al. Walker's Pediatric Gastrointestinal Disease, 6th edition. USA: People's Medical Publishing House; 2015.

Mier M, Nelson A, Finkel L. Vomiting children: it's not always gastroenteritis. Pediatr Ann. 2020;49(5):e233-41.

Samprathi M, Jayashree M. Child with vomiting. *Indian J Pediatr.* 2017;84(10):787-791.

Shields TM, Lightdale JR. Vomiting in children. Pediatr Rev. 2018;39(7): 342-58.

ABDOMINAL PAIN

Abdominal pain is a very common symptom in pediatric age group. There are mainly three mechanisms by which abdominal pain is perceived, and the perception may be modified by a child's level of tolerance. Psychogenic and environmental factors augment or inhibit the perception of pain to varying degrees in different individuals.

Anatomical Correlates of Abdominal Pain

- ***Autonomic sensory pathways from the abdominal viscera:*** Visceral pain tends to be experienced in the dermatome from which the affected organ receives innervations. It is a dull aching sensation generally perceived in one of the three regions: (1) The periumbilical, (2) epigastric, or (3) suprapubic midline area.
  - Painful stimuli originating in the liver, pancreas, biliary tree, stomach, or upper bowel are felt in the *epigastrium.*
  - Pain from the distal small bowel, cecum, appendix, or proximal colon is felt at the *umbilicus.*
  - Pain from the distal large bowel, urinary tract, or pelvic organs is usually *suprapubic.*

  An example of the visceral pain is the initial pain of appendicitis which is usually felt in the periumbilical area.
- ***Somatic sensory pathways from the parietal peritoneum, abdominal wall, or retroperitoneal skeletal muscles:*** Somatic pain is usually well localized and intense (often sharp) in character. An intra-abdominal process will manifest somatic pain if an inflammatory process affecting a viscus touches a somatic organ (i.e., the anterior parietal peritoneum or abdominal wall). An example of somatic pain is the localized pain of acute appendicitis in the right iliac fossa due to the inflammation affecting the nearby peritoneum.
- ***Referred pain:*** Referred pain may occur from extra-abdominal sites which share central projections with sensory pathways from the abdominal wall. The classic example of referred abdominal pain is the shared central projections of the parietal pleura of the lung and the abdominal wall, such that abdominal pain may be the initial presentation of pneumonia.

Pain in abdomen can be acute, chronic, or recurrent, and the site of localization might indicate the involvement of different organs. As with the symptom of "vomiting," pain in abdomen can be because of non-gastrointestinal or nonabdominal causes. Acute abdominal pain, or "acute abdomen," refers to abdominal pain of recent onset that triggers an urgent need for prompt diagnosis and active treatment. It can be caused by a variety of conditions ranging from mild and self-limiting to life-threatening diseases **(Table 21.1)**.

Chronic abdominal pain (CAP) refers to pain that has been present continuously, or occurring at least on a weekly basis when intermittent, for a minimum period of 3 months. Recurrent abdominal pain is defined as three or more episodes of abdominal pain, over a period of 3 or more months, severe enough to affect the activities. Term "recurrent abdominal pain" is a description of the condition rather than a diagnosis. CAP can be organic or functional in nature. When there is an underlying medical/surgical cause of the pain it is labeled as *organic abdominal pain*, and if the abdominal pain cannot be fully explained by a medical condition after appropriate evaluation, it is labeled as *functional abdominal pain.* Various causes of CAP in children are listed in **Table 21.2**.

TABLE 21.1: Causes of Acute Abdominal Pain in Children

	0–6 months	*6 months–5 years*	*5–18 years*
Surgical conditions	1. Incarcerated inguinal hernia 2. Malrotation and volvulus 3. Intestinal obstruction 4. Intussusception 5. Hypertrophic pyloric stenosis 6. Hirschsprung disease	1. Appendicitis 2. Malrotation and volvulus 3. Intussusception 4. Hirschsprung disease	1. Appendicitis 2. Testicular torsion 3. Acute cholecystitis 4. Small bowel obstructions and adhesions 5. Obstructed inguinal hernia 6. Complicated inflammatory bowel disease 7. Gallstones 8. Ectopic pregnancy, ovarian torsion 9. Intestinal volvulus 10. Foreign body
Medical conditions	1. Sepsis/bacteremia 2. Gastroenteritis with dehydration 3. UTI 4. Gastroesophageal reflux disease 5. Infantile colic 6. Constipation	1. Pneumonia/otitis media 2. Strep throat/tonsillitis 3. Infective gastroenteritis/colitis/hepatitis 4. UTI 5. Constipation 6. DKA 7. Sickle cell crisis 8. Ureteric calculi 9. Acute pancreatitis 10. Lactose intolerance	1. Pneumonia/otitis media 2. Streptococcal pharyngitis/tonsillitis 3. Infective gastroenteritis/colitis/hepatitis 4. UTI 5. Viral gastroenteritis/viral syndrome 6. Constipation 7. DKA 8. Sickle cell crisis 9. Acute pancreatitis 10. Complicated PUD 11. Hemolytic-uremic syndrome 12. Renal vein thrombosis 13. Mononucleosis 14. HSP 15. Mesenteric adenitis 16. Gastroduodenitis, PUD 17. Tubo-ovarian disease, ovarian cyst/menstrual pain, pelvic inflammatory disease, sexually transmitted disease

(DKA: diabetic ketoacidosis; HSP: Henoch–Schönlein purpura; PUD: peptic ulcer disease; UTI: urinary tract infection)

TABLE 21.2 Causes of Chronic Abdominal Pain in Children

Organic causes	*Functional causes*
A. Gastrointestinal: 1. Chronic constipation 2. Celiac disease 3. Parasitic infections (e.g., amoeba, giardia) 4. Dietary intolerance (e.g., lactose) 5. Gastroesophageal reflux disease 6. Inflammatory bowel disease 7. *Helicobacter pylori* infection 8. Chronic pancreatitis 9. Hepatitis 10. Peptic ulcer gastritis 11. Gallbladder calculi 12. Chronic appendicitis *B. Urinary tract:* 1. Urinary tract infection 2. Urinary calculi 3. Pelviureteric junction obstruction *C. Gynecological:* 1. Ovarian cyst 2. Endometriosis 3. Pelvic inflammatory disease *D. Miscellaneous:* 1. Abdominal epilepsy 2. Physical, emotional, and sexual abuse	1. Functional constipation 2. Functional dyspepsia 3. Irritable bowel syndrome 4. Functional abdominal pain syndrome 5. Abdominal migraine 6. Aerophagia

APPROACH TO A CHILD WITH ABDOMINAL PAIN

In a child presenting with abdominal pain, a detailed history should elicit the characteristics of the pain, precipitating and relieving factors, appetite, dietary intake, relation with meals and stool history. Functional constipation is common in childhood, and this diagnosis should be considered with a history of infrequent stools, encopresis, retentive posturing and painful or hard bowel motions. History must elicit the impact of abdominal pain on the child's day-to-day function by asking about school absenteeism, cessation of normal activities, and reduced social interactions. Also, the home management strategies must be noted. Information on diet, social and emotional status, and family should also be obtained. Anxiety, depression, family dysfunction, and child abuse can all present with the somatic symptoms of abdominal pain. Check for a family history of celiac disease, inflammatory bowel disease (IBD), peptic ulcer disease, irritable bowel syndrome, and constipation. History of abuse, stress, psychological disorders, and poor sleep also to be noted. The familiar occurrence of migraine headaches, anxiety/depression, atopy, and food intolerances should also be noted.

Examination should focus on the child's general appearance. Detailed anthropometry must be done to assess the growth of the child. Children with functional abdominal pain syndromes look well and examination findings are within normal limits. Abdominal palpation may reveal a fecal mass due to collection of feces in case of chronic constipation which can be associated with encopresis. Presence of "red flags" in history or examination is the indicator for the presence of underlying organic disease as the cause of CAP (**Table 21.3**).

Acute Abdominal Pain

Although most children with acute abdominal pain have self-limiting conditions, the pain may herald a serious medical or surgical emergency. Therefore, a major challenge is to make a timely *diagnosis of the acute surgical abdomen.* **Flowchart 21.2** outlines the clinical approach for delineating the etiology of acute abdominal pain in a child.

TABLE 21.3 Red Flags in History and Examination of Chronic Abdominal Pain

"Red flags" on history	*"Red flags" on physical examination*
1. Localized pain away from the umbilicus 2. Pain awakening the child at night 3. Pain associated with changes in bowel habits, dysuria, rash, arthritis 4. Occult bleeding 5. Repeated vomiting, especially bilious 6. Delayed puberty 7. Constitutional symptoms such as recurrent fever, loss of appetite, lethargy 8. Family history of inflammatory bowel disease, celiac disease, or peptic ulcer disease	1. Loss of weight or growth retardation 2. Organomegaly 3. Localized abdominal tenderness, particularly away from the umbilicus 4. Joint swelling, tenderness, or heat 5. Pallor, rash, hernias of the abdominal wall

Flowchart 21.2: Clinical approach to a child with acute abdominal pain

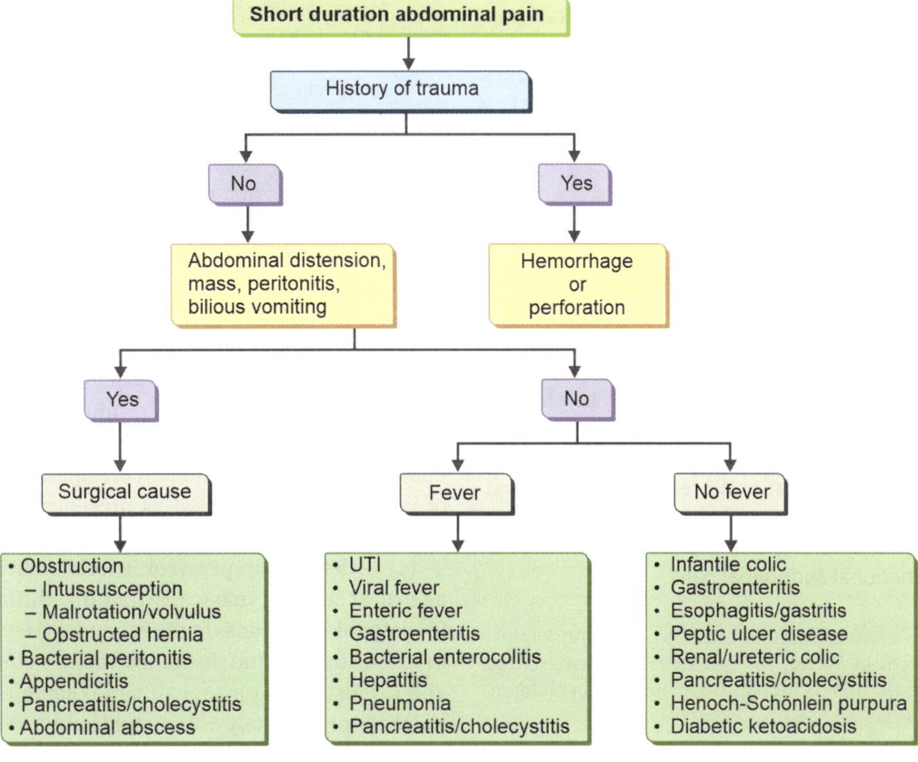

Flowchart 21.3: Clinical approach to a child with chronic/recurrent abdominal pain

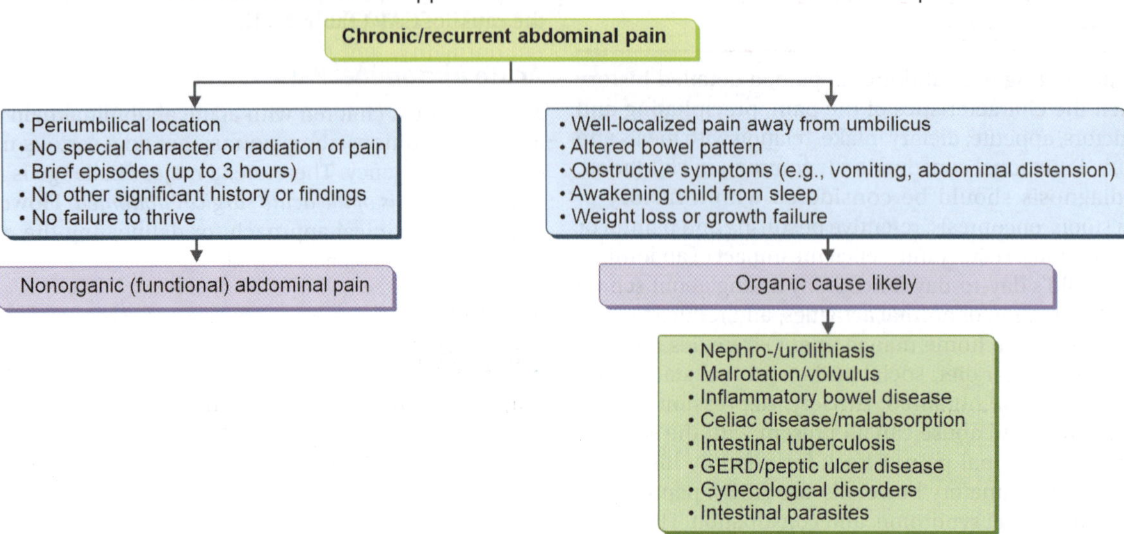

(GERD: gastroesophageal reflux disease)

Chronic Abdominal Pain

Chronic abdominal pain can be *organic* (disease related) or *functional*. Functional abdominal pain disorders, which include irritable bowel syndrome (CAP along with alteration in bowel movements), functional dyspepsia (pain or discomfort in upper abdomen), abdominal migraine (pain associated with nausea, anorexia, vomiting or pallor), and functional abdominal pain—not otherwise specified, are the most common causes of recurrent abdominal pain in children.

Other differential diagnoses of recurrent abdominal pain include a heterogeneous group of anatomic, infectious, noninfectious, inflammatory, and biochemical disorders. Approach to etiological diagnosis of a child with CAP is summarized in **Flowchart 21.3**.

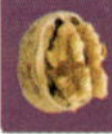

IN A NUTSHELL

Approach to a Child with Abdominal Pain

1. Abdominal pain is a very common symptom in pediatric age group.
2. Psychogenic and environmental factors augment or inhibit the perception of pain to varying degrees.
3. Pain persisting >3 months duration is known as chronic abdominal pain, it can be organic (disease-related) or functional.
4. Differential diagnoses of chronic and recurrent abdominal pain include a heterogeneous group of anatomic, infectious, non-infectious, inflammatory, and biochemical disorders along with the functional abdominal pain.

American Academy of Pediatrics Subcommittee on Chronic Abdominal Pain, North American Society for Pediatric Gastroenterology Hepatology, and Nutrition. Chronic abdominal pain in children. Pediatrics. 2005;115(3):e370-81.

Chakraborty PS, Daniel R, Navarro FA. Non-pharmacologic approaches to treatment of pediatric functional abdominal pain disorders. Front Pediatr. 2023;11:1118874.

Friesen C, Colombo JM, Deacy A, Schurman JV. An update on the assessment and management of pediatric abdominal pain. Pediatric Health Med Ther. 2021;12:373-93.

Gomez-Suarez R. Difficulties in the diagnosis and management of functional or recurrent abdominal pain in children. Pediatr Ann. 2016;45(11):e388-93.

Rasquin A, Di Lorenzo C, Forbes D, et al. Childhood functional gastro-intestinal disorders: child/adolescent. Gastroenterology. 2016; 130(5):1527-37.

Smith J, Fox SM. Pediatric abdominal pain: an emergency medicine perspective. Emerg Med Clin N Am. 2016;34(2):341-61.

Thapar N, Benninga MA, Crowell MD, et al. Paediatric functional abdominal pain disorders. Nat Rev Dis Primers. 2020;6(1):89.

Zia JK, Lenhart A, Yang PL, et al. Risk factors for abdominal pain disorders of gut-brain interaction in adults and children: a systematic review. Gastroenterology. 2022;163(4):995-1023.e3.

CONSTIPATION

Constipation is the infrequent passage of stools with difficulty. The peak incidence of constipation occurs between 2 and 4 years of age, when the toilet training starts. Constipation could be organic or functional in nature. The majority of children with constipation have functional constipation, accounting for 95% of cases, which is defined as presence of two or more of the following for a minimum duration of 1 month:

(1) ≤2 defecations per week in a child having a developmental age of at least 4 years, (2) painful, difficult to pass stools, (3) palpable fecal mass in the rectum, (4) fecal incontinence due to insensitivity of the distended rectum at least once per week, and (5) history of passage of large diameter stools obstructing toilet. Approximately 5% of children have organic diseases as

TABLE 21.4 Causes of Constipation in Children

Inorganic causes	
• Functional constipation of childhood • Psychosocial issues • Dietary (low dietary fluid and fiber intake) • Improper toilet training, exaggerated parental interventions	
Organic causes	
Motility related	Hirschsprung disease, myopathy, spinal cord trauma, tethered cord, congenital megacolon
Congenital anomalies	Rectosigmoid stenosis, anal stenosis, anteriorly located anus, spinal cord anomalies (meningomyelocele, myelomalacia, spina bifida), sacral teratoma
Neurological	Cerebral palsy, intellectual disability
Endocrine/ metabolic	Hypothyroidism, renal tubular acidosis, diabetes insipidus, hypercalcemia
Drugs	Anticonvulsants, antipsychotic, codeine containing formulations, antacids
Others	Celiac disease, Cow's milk protein allergy

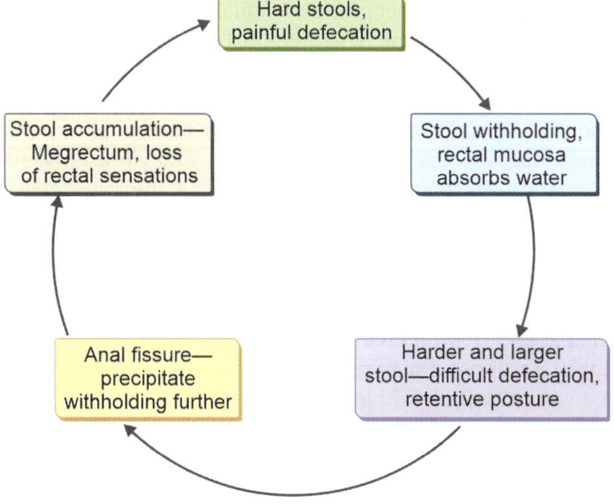

Fig. 21.1: Pathophysiology of constipation in children

the cause of constipation. These children usually have other clinical features suggestive of the relevant underlying organic disease. Organic diseases presenting as isolated constipation are rather uncommon. **Table 21.4** enlists the various causes of constipation in children.

The pathophysiology of constipation in children is multifactorial and is associated with the complex interactions of many risk factors. **Figure 21.1** depicts the pathophysiology of constipation in children.

APPROACH TO A CHILD WITH CONSTIPATION

The chief complaints and their duration should be noted. A note should be made of the nature of toilet training, medications and compliance, and diet and fluid intake. Any psychosocial factors or problems in family or school should be evaluated. Obtain history suggestive of neurological disorders (convulsions, mental subnormality, and tone abnormalities). History of delayed passage of meconium, onset of constipation in the first few months, episodes of severe unexplained diarrhea, and marked abdominal distension suggest possibility of Hirschsprung disease.

On examination, look for any abdominal distension/masses or fissures. Per rectal examination can be useful to confirm impaction and suggest or exclude Hirschsprung disease and anal stenosis. Neurological evaluation should include examinations of spine and perineum, ankle jerk, etc. Presence of abnormal physical findings such as failure to thrive, lack of lumbosacral curve, sacral agenesis, flat buttock, anteriorly displaced anus, tight and empty rectum, gush of liquid stool and air on withdrawal of finger, absent anal wink, and cremasteric reflex are suggestive of an underlying organic cause of constipation. Coarse facies, hoarseness of voice, umbilical hernia, and developmental delay suggest hypothyroidism. **Table 21.5** enlists the red flag signs in history and examination suggesting an underlying organic cause of the constipation.

Investigations are usually unnecessary unless there is some clue toward secondary constipation. X-ray of spine is required if examination suggests tone/tendon reflex abnormalities in lower limb or if neurogenic bladder is also present. T3, T4, and thyroid-stimulating hormone (TSH) needs to be done if clinical features suggest hypothyroidism. Rectal biopsy is indicated for suspected Hirschsprung disease.

TREATMENT Child with Constipation

The explanation of the condition is most important and takes time. It cannot be rushed and must be directed both at parents and the child. Go through the mechanism with parents and the child using pictures and diagrams. Emphasize that withholding a stool or soiling is not deliberate. It takes a long time to get into this state and may take a long time to resolve.

- The bowel needs to be emptied. A clear-out may be more difficult to manage than the previous state of incomplete bowel emptying, e.g., cramps, urgency, or perhaps more soiling. Parents and the child need to be warned of this.
- When the bowel is completely cleared, it then needs to be kept empty with maintenance treatment or it will very quickly fill back.

TABLE 21.5 Red Flag Signs in a Child with Constipation

History	*Examination*
1. Delayed passage of meconium 2. Onset of constipation in early infancy 3. Passage of ribbon or pellet stools 4. Bilious vomiting 5. Uniform abdominal distension 6. Recurrent lower respiratory infections 7. Cold intolerance	1. Coarse facies 2. Failure to thrive 3. Gush of stools on digital rectal examination 4. Anal malformations 5. Presence of myelocele meningomyelocele, tuft of hairs in lower back 6. Neurodevelopmental delay or regression, abnormal neurological examination

It is desirable that a clear-out is achieved before maintenance treatment can be started. A clear-out is done using laxatives like senna, picosulfate or osmotic laxatives like polyethylene glycol (PEG). Colonic lavage might be done in hospitalized children. All children needing bowel clear-out will need maintenance treatment, usually long-term. This should not be suddenly stopped. Misinformation about long-term laxatives causing "lazy" bowels or physical dependence should be addressed. The medications used for maintenance in chronic constipation include lactulose, liquid paraffin, milk of magnesia, and polyethylene glycol (PEG). PEG (0.5–1.0 g/kg/day) has a distinct advantage over other medications in being more effective over long-term with minimal adverse effects.

The most common explanation for "intractable constipation" is the prescription of inadequate therapy or nonadherence to the prescribed regimen. A period of supervised treatment may therefore be necessary. The child should be monitored closely to determine the nature of the problem in their case. This is done using (1) history and stool charts, and (2) abdominal and rectal examination to ascertain that there are no masses or distension. If unsuccessful, try a different option, and consider the psychological and behavioral aspects. Involve a psychologist, if appropriate.

Children must have a clear toilet training regime. They need to know that this is essential, and that they may not initially feel a recognizable desire to defecate. Children with severe constipation usually have diminished or absent rectal sensation due to chronic rectal distension and are therefore unaware of the need to defecate. A supervised visit to sit on the toilet and try to go twice per day is reasonable. A reward system such as a star chart can be helpful in some children but must be very simple.

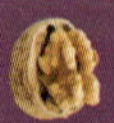

IN A NUTSHELL

Approach to a Child with Constipation

1. Constipation is the passage of hard stools with difficulty.
2. Constipation can be severe, persistent, or recurrent.
3. Severe cases can present with bleeding per rectum due to fissure-in-ano, fecal impaction, encopresis, and secondary enuresis.
4. During the evaluation of cases of constipation, dietary history and per rectal examination are two most important points.
5. Inadequate therapy or nonadherence to the prescribed regimen are the two most common causes of intractable constipation.
6. Treatment involves—medications (disimpaction and maintenance phase with the laxatives) and counseling regarding diet and compliance to the therapy.

Maselli KM, Shah NR, Speck KE. Approach to constipation in children: recommendations for evaluation and management. Adv Pediatr. 2024;71(1):195-211.

Tran DL, Sintusek P. Functional constipation in children: what physicians should know. World J Gastroenterol. 2023;29(8):1261-1288.

Vernon-Roberts A, Alexander I, Day AS. Systematic review of pediatric functional gastrointestinal disorders (Rome IV Criteria). J Clin Med. 2021;10(21):5087.

Wallace C, Sinopoulou V, Gordon M, et al. Probiotics for treatment of chronic constipation in children. Cochrane Database Syst Rev. 2022;3(3):CD014257.

Yachha SK, Srivastava A, Mohan N, et al. Management of Childhood Functional Constipation: Consensus Practice Guidelines of Indian Society of Pediatric Gastroenterology, Hepatology and Nutrition and Pediatric Gastroenterology Chapter of Indian Academy of Pediatrics. Indian Pediatr. 2018;55:885-92.

Zeevenhooven J, Koppen IJ, Benninga MA. The New Rome IV criteria for functional gastrointestinal disorders in infants and toddlers. Pediatr Gastroenterol Hepatol Nutr. 2017;20(1):1-13.

Zuar LR, Thompson LA. What parents should know about constipation in children. JAMA Pediatr. 2023;177(2):216.

DIARRHEA

It is a common presenting symptom in children. Majority of the cases present with acute diarrhea due to gastrointestinal infection. Others can also present as dysentery, persistent diarrhea, or chronic diarrhea. Sometimes, children can also present with complications secondary to dehydration. For details please see **Chapter 20**.

GASTROINTESTINAL BLEEDING

Gastrointestinal bleeding is one of the life-threatening events in childhood. Gastrointestinal bleeding is divided into two major clinical forms—(1) Upper gastrointestinal bleeding and (2) Lower gastrointestinal bleeding. Ligament of Treitz, also known as the suspensory ligament of the duodenum is the anatomic landmark that separates the site of upper and lower gastrointestinal bleeds. Upper bleeding originates from any site between upper parts of the esophagus to the ligament of Treitz, usually presents either as hematemesis or melena. Hematemesis is the regurgitation/vomiting of blood alone or blood mixed with the contents of stomach. Melena is the passage of black tarry stools that typically has a strong characteristic odor caused by the activity of digestive enzymes and intestinal bacteria on hemoglobin. Hematochezia is the passage of bright red blood per anus, usually it occurs due to the diseases of colon or rectum. However, it can also occur with large volume upper GI bleeding or with accelerated Intestinal transit time where digestive enzymes and intestinal bacteria do not get adequate time to modify the hemoglobin. The causes of gastrointestinal bleeding in children are listed in **Table 21.6**.

APPROACH TO CHILD WITH GASTROINTESTINAL BLEEDING

History

Detailed history regarding the following points is important in a child with gastrointestinal bleeding:

- Color of the bleed, amount, frequency of the episodes including any history of previous episodes of gastrointestinal bleeding.
- ***Symptoms associated with bleeding:***
  - Painless in coagulopathy, Mallory-Weiss tear, polyp, Meckel's diverticulum, vascular malformations, esophageal varices, and portal hypertensive gastropathy (PHG).
  - Painful in gastritis, esophagitis, foreign body ingestion, and anal fissure.
  - Preceding forceful emesis or retching—Mallory-Weiss tear

TABLE 21.6 Causes of Gastrointestinal Bleeding in Children

Presentation	Neonate/infant	Older children
Upper gastrointestinal bleeding	1. Swallowed maternal blood 2. Hemorrhagic disease (vitamin K deficiency) 3. Coagulopathy associated with infection 4. Cow's milk protein allergy 5. Vascular anomaly	1. Mallory–Weiss tear 2. Gastritis 3. Esophageal varices, portal hypertensive gastropathy 4. Esophagitis 5. NSAIDs 6. Foreign body 7. Gastroduodenal ulcer 8. Crohn disease 9. Gastrointestinal duplication 10. Vascular anomaly 11. Coagulopathy 12. Hemobilia
Lower gastrointestinal bleeding	1. Infectious colitis 2. Necrotizing enterocolitis 3. Intussusception 4. Rectal prolapse 5. Anal fissure 6. Cow's milk protein allergy 7. Hemorrhagic disease of newborn 8. Coagulation disorders 9. Hirschsprung enterocolitis 10. Vasculitis 11. Meckel diverticulum	1. Infectious colitis 2. Rectal polyp or polyposis syndrome 3. Fissure 4. Amebiasis 5. Pseudomembranous colitis 6. Solitary rectal ulcer syndrome 7. Neutropenic colitis 8. Henoch–Schönlein purpura 9. Inflammatory bowel disease 10. Coagulation disorders 11. Meckel diverticulum 12. Hemorrhoids 13. Rectal varices 14. Ateriovenous malformations 15. Cytomegalovirus (CMV) enterocolitis

(NSAIDs: nonsteroidal anti-inflammatory drugs)

Note: Causes are arranged in order of frequency of occurrence

- ***Feeding:*** Bleeding in a neonate on formula feeds with abdominal distension indicates necrotizing enterocolitis (NEC), while in an infant on top feeds especially cow milk is suggestive of cow milk protein allergy (CMPA).
- ***Abdominal distension:*** A sick neonate with bleeding, abdominal distension, refusal to feeds and hemodynamic instability points toward sepsis induced coagulopathy and NEC. Bleeding in a hemodynamically stable neonate or infant with history of home delivery indicates the possibility of vitamin K deficiency bleeding. Localized abdominal distension, abdominal pain, vomiting and passage of redcurrant jelly stools is seen in intussusception.
- ***Stool:*** Frequency, volume, and consistency of stool, as frequent loose stools with blood, mucus, and crampy abdominal pain toward infectious colitis. Infrequent passage of hard stools with streaking of stools points toward anal fissure seen in chronic constipation cases.
- ***Extraintestinal manifestations*** such as aphthous ulcer, joint pain, fever, weight loss, hepatitis, and skin lesions points toward IBD.
- ***Drug:*** History of intake of contributory or confounding medications (nonsteroidal anti-inflammatory drugs, anticoagulants, antiplatelet agents, bismuth, iron), antibiotic intake before the onset of the bleeding points toward pseudomembranous colitis.
- ***Recurrent infections:*** History suggestive of congenital or acquired immunosuppression can lead to cytomegalovirus (CMV) enterocolitis and polymicrobial typhlitis.
- Past medical history relevant to potential bleeding sources [e.g., varices, portal hypertension, intake of nonsteroidal anti-inflammatory drugs (NSAIDs), gastric/duodenal ulcers, *Helicobacter pylori* infection, and IBD].

Examination

In a child with gastrointestinal bleeding, check for signs of hemodynamic instability which manifests as resting tachycardia, weak thread pulse with low blood pressure. Poor growth during anthropometry indicates systemic causes such as IBD and portal hypertension. In general, physical examination there might be presence of anemia, clubbing, oral ulcers (IBD), orobuccal pigmentation (Peutz-Jeghers syndrome), and palpable purpura on lower limbs (Henoch-Schönlein purpura). Detailed abdominal examination to look for presence of organomegaly (splenomegaly in portal hypertension), any sausage shape mass (intussusception), and left iliac fossa mass (constipation) is important. Examination of the perianal region to look for the presence of fissure and anal tags (Crohn disease), per rectal examination to look for rectal polyps and rectal prolapse is important.

Investigations

Plan them according to possible etiology based on the history and examination findings.

- ***Complete blood count:*** Raised leukocyte counts in infections, microcytic anemia, and thrombocytosis. Raised erythrocyte sedimentation rate (ESR) in inflammatory conditions.
- ***Coagulation profile:*** International normalized ratio (INR), prothrombin time, and activated partial thromboplastin time
- Liver function tests
- ***Stool examination:*** For trophozoites, assay for *Clostridioides difficile* toxin and stool culture.
- ***Ultrasonography:*** For intussusception, features of portal hypertension.
- ***Inflammatory markers:*** C-reactive protein (CRP), peri-nuclear antineutrophil cytoplasmic antibodies (pANCAs) are raised in children with ulcerative colitis (60–80%) and Crohn disease (10–27%). *Anti-saccharomyces cerevisiae* (ASCA) antibodies are commonly found in with Crohn disease.
- ***Gastrointestinal endoscopy:*** Can be diagnostic and therapeutic. It also allows the visualization of the upper GIT

(typically including from the oral cavity up to the duodenum)/ allows visualization of the lower GIT (including the colon and terminal ileum), and treatment with injection therapy, thermal coagulation, or hemostatic clips/bands application, polypectomy/biopsy for histology.

- ***CT angiography:*** In cases with vascular malformations.
- ***Gastrointestinal contrast studies:*** Upper gastrointestinal contrast examination with small bowel follow through may show ulcerations, thickened and nodular folds, or narrowing of the lumen of the bowel (Crohn disease).
- ***99-m Tc pertechnetate scan:*** In Meckel's diverticulum or intestinal duplication.

TREATMENT Child with Gastrointestinal Bleeding

While managing a child with gastrointestinal bleed, first and foremost thing is to assess the severity of bleeding and stabilize the patient with provisions for adequate oxygen delivery, intravascular fluid resuscitation (with normal saline or lactated Ringer solution) to maintain the intravascular volume, and any life-threatening electrolyte or metabolic disturbance. Transfusion of blood components to maintain hemoglobin (Hb) levels, platelet levels or correct coagulation abnormalities. In upper gastrointestinal bleeding, gastric lavage by saline through nasogastric tube to remove fresh blood or clots to facilitate endoscopy.

Medical Management

- Proton pump inhibitors for suppression of acid production.
- Vasoactive medications such as somatostatin or its analog octreotide can be used to treat variceal bleeding by visceral vasoconstriction.
- Antibiotics for cases with sepsis, NEC, infectious colitis, *H. pylori* infection, and immunocompromised state.
- Sengstaken-Blakemore tube can be placed in patients with hemodynamic instability/massive gastrointestinal bleeds in the setting of known esophageal varices.
- *Endoscopy therapy:* Polypectomy, treatment with injection of epinephrine and sclerosants, elastic band ligation can be considered in actively bleeding focal lesion or with a lesion at high risk rebleeding.
- Surgery is reserved for bleeding uncontrollable by less invasive interventions, nonreducible intussusception or a vascular anomaly, etc.

When choosing a specific therapy, factors such as the severity active bleeding; the medical condition of the patient; the quality of endoscopic, radiologic, and surgical resources; and the predicted behavior of an identified lesion must be considered beforehand.

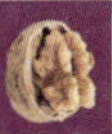

IN A NUTSHELL

Approach to Child with Gastrointestinal Bleeding

1. Bleeding in children can occur due to multiple causes ranging from infections, inflammatory conditions, food allergies, liver disorders, and vascular malformations.
2. Detailed history and clinical examination are helpful in planning the investigations.
3. Management includes stabilization of the patient and treatment of the underlying condition.

Baker RD, Baker SS. Gastrointestinal bleeds. Pediatr Rev. 2021;42(10): 546-57.

Luoto TT, Pakarinen MP. Evolving management of paediatric portal hypertension. Arch Dis Child. 2021;106(10):939-40.

Novak I, Bass LM. Gastrointestinal bleeding in children-current management, controversies, and advances. Gastrointest. Endosc. Clin N Am. 2023;33(2):401-21.

Piccirillo M, Pucinischi V, Mennini M, et al. Gastrointestinal bleeding in children: diagnostic approach. Ital J Pediatr. 2024;50:13.

Thirumal P, Sumathi B, Nirmala D. A clinical entity often missed-solitary rectal ulcer syndrome in children. Front Pediatr. 2020;8:396.

JAUNDICE

Jaundice is the yellow discoloration of the sclera, skin, and mucous membranes, and occurs due to rise in serum levels of bilirubin (hyperbilirubinemia).

- Clinically apparent jaundice in neonates occurs when the bilirubin rises to >5 mg/dL.
- Older children and adults become icteric when the serum concentration of bilirubin reaches 2–3 mg/dL.
- Jaundice is better appreciated by examining the child in daylight rather than under artificial lighting.

Bilirubin Forms and Types of Hyperbilirubinemia

Measurement of the total serum bilirubin concentration allows quantification of jaundice. Bilirubin occurs in plasma in four forms:

1. Unconjugated bilirubin tightly bound to albumin.
2. Free bilirubin (the form responsible for kernicterus, because it can cross cell membranes).
3. Conjugated bilirubin (the only fraction to appear in urine).
4. Delta (δ) fraction which is conjugated bilirubin that is covalently bound to albumin. This form can represent a major proportion of serum bilirubin in children who have had conjugated hyperbilirubinemia for a time. The δ fraction permits conjugated bilirubin to persist in the circulation and delays resolution of jaundice.

Unconjugated Hyperbilirubinemia

Rise in unconjugated bilirubin indicates increased production of bilirubin, hemolysis, reduced hepatic removal, or altered metabolism of bilirubin. Causes are enumerated as follows:

- ***Increased production:***
  - *Hemolysis:* Rh incompatibility, ABO incompatibility, minor blood group incompatibilities, hereditary spherocytosis, G6PD deficiency, sickle cell anemia, thalassemia, sepsis, and drugs.
  - Enclosed hematoma, e.g., cephalhematoma
  - Polycythemia
- ***Decreased bilirubin uptake:***
  - Breastmilk jaundice
  - Hypothyroidism
  - Hypoxia
- ***Decreased conjugation:***
  - Physiological neonatal jaundice
  - Crigler–Najjar syndrome, types I and II
  - Gilbert disease

- ***Increased enterohepatic circulation:***
  - Pyloric stenosis, duodenal atresia, intestinal obstruction, and Hirschsprung disease.

Conjugated Hyperbilirubinemia

Conjugated bilirubinemia (defined as >20% of total bilirubin level) reflects decreased excretion by damaged hepatic parenchymal cells or disease of biliary tract, which may be due to sepsis, endocrine or metabolic disease, inflammation of the liver, or obstruction in the hepatobiliary tree **(Box 21.2)**.

Box 21.2 Causes of Conjugated Hyperbilirubinemia

A. Infections:
1. Acute viral hepatitis
2. Chronic viral hepatitis
3. Septicemia
4. Typhoid fever
5. Kala-azar
6. Leptospirosis
7. Brucellosis
8. Cholangitis
9. Infectious mononucleosis
10. Disseminated tuberculosis

B. Autoimmune:
1. Autoimmune hepatitis
2. Systemic lupus erythematosus
3. Sclerosing cholangitis

C. Infiltrative disorders:
1. Lymphoma
2. Leukemia
3. Histiocytosis
4. Hepatic metastasis

D. Metabolic and storage disorders:
1. Lipid storage disorders (Gaucher and Niemann-Pick disease)
2. Wilson disease
3. α_1-Antitrypsin deficiency
4. Cystic fibrosis
5. Mitochondrial disorders

E. Toxic:
1. Hepatotoxic and cholestatic drugs (e.g., INH, valproate)
2. Snake envenomation

F. Extrahepatic diseases:
1. Sclerosing cholangitis
2. Bile duct obstruction due to stones, worms
3. Mass (neoplasia, lymph nodes)

G. Miscellaneous:
1. Indian childhood cirrhosis
2. Ischemic hepatopathy (associated with shock and hypoperfusion)
3. Parenteral nutrition
4. Neonatal and infantile cholestasis syndromes

The terms direct and indirect bilirubin (measured by traditional diazo methods of bilirubin estimation) are used equivalently with conjugated and unconjugated bilirubin, respectively. However, this is not quantitatively correct, because the direct fraction includes both conjugated bilirubin and δ bilirubin, while the indirect fraction includes the unconjugated bilirubin only. Newer methods of bilirubin measurement such as Ektachem slide method allow more accurate measurement of conjugated, unconjugated, and δ bilirubin levels separately.

APPROACH TO A CHILD WITH JAUNDICE

History

Detailed history includes onset, progression, and duration of jaundice. Onset during neonatal period on day two or later is suggestive of physiological jaundice—normal transitional phenomenon. Onset on first day of life or persistent beyond 14 days is suggestive of pathological jaundice.

In infants, history must include the color of the urine, diaper staining, and color of stool (cholestasis), any history for fever, recurrent vomiting, reduced activity, seizures, developmental delay (metabolic conditions), mothers and baby blood group (ABO, Rh incompatibility).

In older children, history about associated symptoms such as fever, pain abdomen, vomiting, anorexia, loose stools (suggestive of infective etiology—acute viral hepatitis, malaria, enteric fever, and leptospirosis); abdominal colic and worm infestation (obstructive cause), pallor, recent drug intake (hemolysis, drug induced liver injury) must be asked.

Details regarding the similar episodes in the past, poor growth, involvement of joints, eyes, blood transfusions, and bleeding disorder indicate toward the possibility of chronic liver disease (autoimmune, Wilson disease, alpha 1 antitrypsin deficiency, cystic fibrosis, chronic infective hepatitis). Family history must include similar episodes in the siblings, any deaths related with jaundice, source of water, sewage disposal, and vaccination status.

Examination

On examination, anthropometry, vitals and general physical examination must be done to look for extent of jaundice, features of acute bilirubin encephalopathy (high pitched cry, abnormalities of tone, lethargy, opisthotonos posturing) in a neonate, while for any signs of growth failure, chronic liver disease, anemia in older children. Ophthalmological evaluation must be done to look for cataract, signs of congenital infections. On abdominal examination, presence of organomegaly, ascites, features of portal hypertension must be noted.

Investigations

Plan according to the possible etiology based on the history and examination findings. Liver function tests and their interpretation are most important.

- ***Serum bilirubin:*** Values of total, direct as well as indirect bilirubin levels are important. Raised indirect bilirubin levels are predominantly seen in conditions associated with hemolysis, while raised direct fraction can be predominantly seen in liver pathologies.
- ***Serum aminotransferase:*** Alanine aminotransferase (ALT) is primarily present in liver, while aspartate aminotransferase (AST) is also present in other tissues such as heart, kidney, skeletal muscle, and brain along with liver. Serum aminotransferase levels are elevated in all liver disease, and the rise in the enzymes levels may reflect the extent of injury to the liver cells. Severe rise in values (>20 times of upper limit of normal) is seen in severe form of acute viral hepatitis, toxin

induced liver injury, and shock. Moderate values [3–20 times upper limits of normal (ULN)] are seen in acute hepatitis, autoimmune hepatitis, neonatal hepatitis, chronic hepatitis, drug induced liver injury, and acute biliary tract obstructions. Mild elevations (<3 times ULN) are seen in conditions such as sepsis induced hepatitis, extrahepatic biliary atresia (EHBA), fatty liver, cirrhosis, drug toxicity, myositis, and Duchenne muscular dystrophy. Usually ALT is more frequently increased as compared to AST and the AST to ALT ratio is <1 except in chronic liver disease and Wilson disease where it is >2.

- ***Serum alkaline phosphatase:*** Alkaline phosphatase originates from liver or bone and the values vary with the age. ALP levels are relatively high in childhood and puberty, and lower in middle age and higher again in old age. High levels are seen in conditions associated with intra- and extrahepatic obstruction of bile flow such as in EHBA, cholestatic phase of Hepatitis A, and hepatic tumors.
- ***Total proteins and serum albumin:*** Liver parenchymal cells are the major site for synthesis of proteins such as albumin, fibrinogen, and other coagulation factors in the body. Serum albumin levels are the most useful indicator of synthetic function of the hepatocytes. As the half-life of the albumin is 20 days, its levels tend to be normal in acute conditions such as acute viral hepatitis, drug related liver injury, and obstructive jaundice. Serum albumin <3 g/dL in hepatitis should raise the suspicion of presence of chronic liver disease. Hypoalbuminemia is not specific for liver disease, and can also occur in malnutrition, nephrotic syndrome, and protein losing enteropathies.
- ***Prothrombin time and INR:*** As liver is the main site of synthesis of various coagulation factors. Prothrombin time or INR is one of the ways to assess the status of the synthetic function of liver. Though deranged prothrombin is not specific of liver disease, it can also be seen in congenital deficiency of coagulation factors, sepsis with disseminated intravascular coagulation (DIC) and use of certain drugs. But it acts as a prognostic marker for both acute and chronic liver diseases.

Other Investigations

General Investigations

- ***Complete hemogram with peripheral smear:*** To look for hemoglobin levels and for presence of hemolysis.
- ***Coombs test:*** For hemolysis.
- ***Ultrasonography:*** To look for echotexture, size of liver, and features of portal hypertension.

Special Investigations

- Toxoplasma, other agents, rubella, cytomegalovirus, and herpes simplex virus (TORCH) profile
- Ultrasonography (USG) skull to look for congenital infections
- Tandem mass spectrometry, urinary gas chromatography-mass spectrometry (GCMS)
- Viral markers for hepatitis A, E, HBs Ag, and anti-hepatitis C virus (anti-HCV)
- High performance liquid chromatography (HPLC) for hemoglobinopathy
- Serum ceruloplasmin levels, 24-hour urinary copper levels
- ***Markers for autoimmune hepatitis:*** Anti-liver-kidney microsome (anti-LKM), anti-smooth muscle antibody (anti-SMA), antinuclear antibody (ANA), and immunoglobulin G (IgG) levels
- Liver biopsy

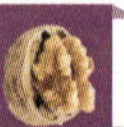

IN A NUTSHELL

Approach to a Child with Jaundice

1. Jaundice in children is a common symptom related to a variety of conditions—hepatic/extrahepatic.
2. Jaundice can be due to acute, chronic, or acute on chronic liver disorder.
3. Detailed history and clinical examination are helpful in planning the investigations to look for the cause.
4. Treatment depends on the underlying condition.

Alam S, Abqari S. Approach to a child with jaundice. Indian J. Pract Pediatr. 2011;13(2):185-92.
Ansong-Assoku B, Shah SD, Adnan M, et al. Neonatal Jaundice. In: StatPearls [Internet]. Treasure Island (FL): StatPearls.
Chee YY, Chung PH, Wong RM, et al. Jaundice in infants and children: causes, diagnosis, and management. Hong Kong Med J. 2018;24(3):285-92.
Jaundice in the newborn. Gastrointestinal and Hepatobiliary Tract and Nutrition. Clinical Protocols -2023. Available from: https://newbornwhocc.org/pdf/Jaundice-in-the-Newborn.pdf [Last accessed January, 2025].
Lala V, Goyal A, Minter DA. Liver Function Tests. In: StatPearls. Treasure Island (FL): StatPearls Publishing; 2022.
Thapa BR, Walia A. Liver function tests and their interpretation. Indian J. Pediatr. 2007;74(7):663-71.

ABDOMINAL DISTENSION

Abdominal distension can be localized or generalized. The cause of the localized distension can be delineated by the organ situated in that particular quadrant of the abdomen, while in cases with generalized abdominal distension, presence of systemic features gives clue about the underlying cause. Also the onset, progression, duration of distension gives the hint about the etiology. **Table 21.7** enlists the various causes of abdominal distension in children.

APPROACH TO HEPATOSPLENOMEGALY

Hepatosplenomegaly with Fever and Anemia

- ***Enteric fever:*** History of high fever for 1–3 weeks, toxic look, mild and soft enlargement of spleen.
- ***Malaria:*** Short or recurrent history of fever, history of chills and rigors, firm and tender enlargement of spleen.
- ***Leishmaniasis:*** Firm and massive spleen enlargement, residence in endemic area.

TABLE 21.7 Causes of Abdominal Distension in Children

Localized distension	
Epigastrium	Duodenal atresia, pyloric stenosis, gastric outlet obstruction, malrotation, bezoar
Umbilical	Jejunal atresia, malrotation, intestinal obstruction, pancreatic pseudocyst
Right hypochondrium	Hepatomegaly, hepatic tumors, choledochal cyst, hydrops of gallbladder
Left hypochondrium	Splenomegaly, splenic cyst
Right and left lumbar	Hydronephrosis, polycystic kidney, Wilms tumor, nephroblastoma, renal vein thrombosis
Hypogastrium	Distended urinary bladder, fecal mass, presacral teratoma, urachal cyst, hematocolpos, hydrometrocolpos, enlarged uterus
Right inguinal	Appendiceal mass, appendiceal abscess, ovarian mass, Crohn disease, lymph nodes
Left inguinal	Ovarian mass, fecal mass, Hirschsprung disease
Generalized distension	
	Septic ileus, toxic megacolon, nephrotic syndrome, hypokalemia, malnutrition, rickets, congestive heart failure, ascites, and malignancy

- ***Leukemia:*** Bleeding spots, lymphadenopathy, and sternal tenderness.
- ***Lymphoma:*** Lymphadenopathy.

Hepatosplenomegaly with Anemia, No Fever

- ***Hemolytic anemia:*** History of blood transfusions, hemolytic facies, and predominant enlargement of spleen.
- ***Chronic liver disease:*** Firm and irregular enlargement of liver, nodular surface of liver. Presence of splenomegaly and ascites indicates associated portal hypertension. Jaundice may be present in decompensated disease.
- ***Intrauterine infections:*** Low birth weight, onset in infancy, microcephaly or hydrocephalus, and mental retardation.
- ***Lysosomal storage disorders:*** Gaucher disease and Niemann- Pick disease.

Hepatosplenomegaly with Jaundice

- ***Acute hepatitis:*** Presence of low grade fever, jaundice, anorexia, clay-colored stools, tender hepatomegaly, and mild enlargement of spleen.
- ***Decompensated chronic liver disease:*** Firm and irregular enlargement of liver, nodular surface of liver, and ascites.
- ***Hemolytic anemia:*** History of blood transfusions, hemolytic facies, predominant enlargement of spleen, and mild jaundice without dark-colored urine.
- ***Neonatal and infantile cholestasis syndromes:*** Seen in infants.

21.2 Clinical Markers of Gastrointestinal and Liver Disorders

PE 23.18, PE 23.19

EXTERNAL MARKERS

Icterus is better appreciated in a broad day light or white light. Most common site to look for icterus is sclera **(Fig. 21.2)**, but it can also be observed at the palate, under surface of tongue, tip of the nose, and palms and soles.

Pallor (paleness) of skin or mucous membrane occurs primarily due to anemia but may also be a manifestation of shock. Pallor should be examined for in the lower palpebral conjunctiva, palm **(Fig. 21.3)**, plantar creases, skin, nails, and dorsum of tongue. In severe pallor, the palmar creases become faint and pale.

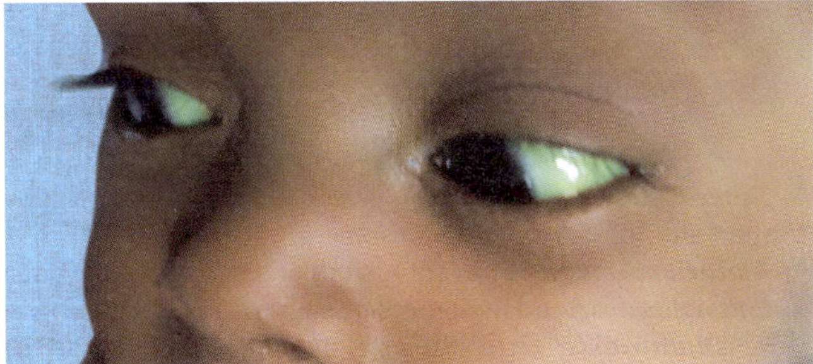

Fig. 21.2: Icteric sclera in an infant

Clubbing: Clubbing is characterized by proliferation of distal soft tissues of fingers and toes especially the nail beds, resulting in thickening and widening of distal phalanges and abnormally curved nails. It occurs due to opening of the anastomotic channels in the nail bed due to anoxic stimuli.

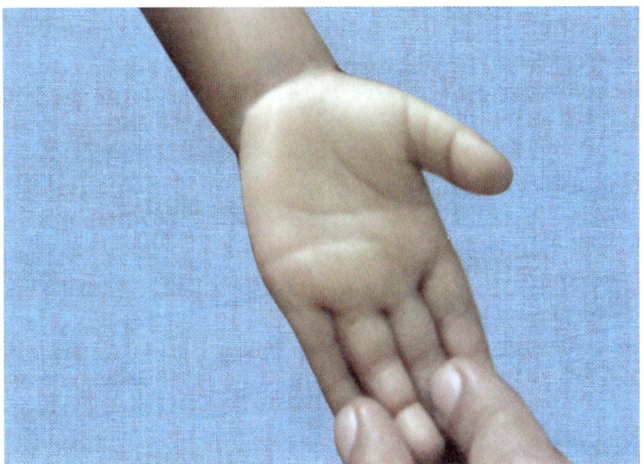

Fig. 21.3: Palmar pallor

Gynecomastia: Gynecomastia is the benign enlargement of male breast glandular tissue **(Fig. 21.4)** and is the most common breast condition in males. Alteration in the estrogen catabolism in chronic liver disease results in excess estrogen in the body and imbalance between estrogen and androgen effects, leading to the enlargement of glandular breast tissue and adipose tissue.

Spider angioma: It is a cutaneous vascular lesion characterized by a dilated central arteriole with its outward radiating thin-walled capillaries **(Fig. 21.5)**. It is also known as spider nevus or spider telangiectasia. The presence of multiple spider angiomas is characteristic of advanced stage of chronic liver disease. Spider angiomas are mostly found on the neck and upper extremities in children.

Palmar erythema: Palmar erythema is redness involving the heel of the palm and occasionally the fingers **(Fig. 21.6)**. It is due to increased dilatation of surface capillaries in the hand caused by hyperestrogenemia in liver cirrhosis.

Caput medusa: Caput medusa is system of visible, prominent abdominal wall veins with centrifugal blood flow **(Fig. 21.7)**. Seen in children with portal hypertension, it is the result of an attempt to divert the portal blood flow via the paraumbilical veins into the caval system.

Nutritional deficiencies: Failure to thrive **(Figs. 21.8A and B)** and deficiency of fat-soluble vitamins (vitamin A, vitamin D) should be looked for **(Figs. 21.9A and B)**.

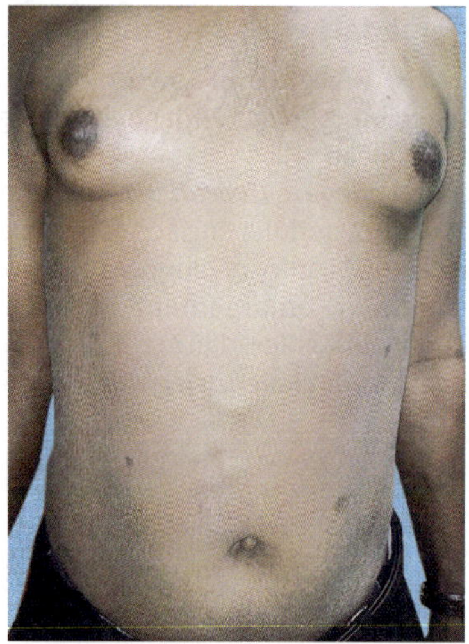

Fig. 21.4: Gynecomastia

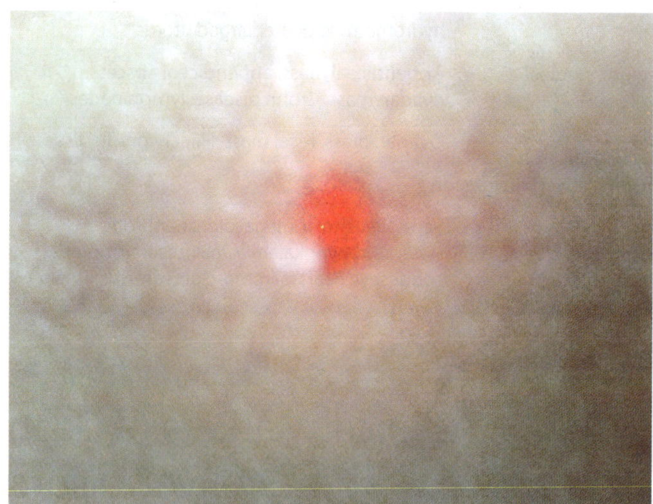

Fig. 21.5: Spider angioma

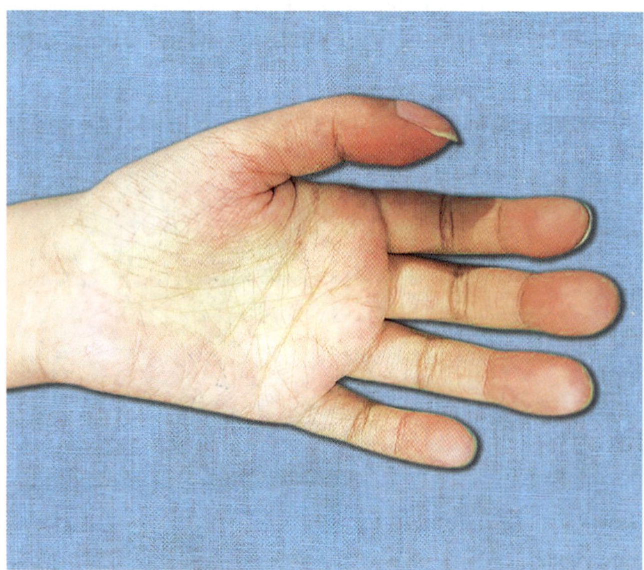

Fig. 21.6: Palmar erythema

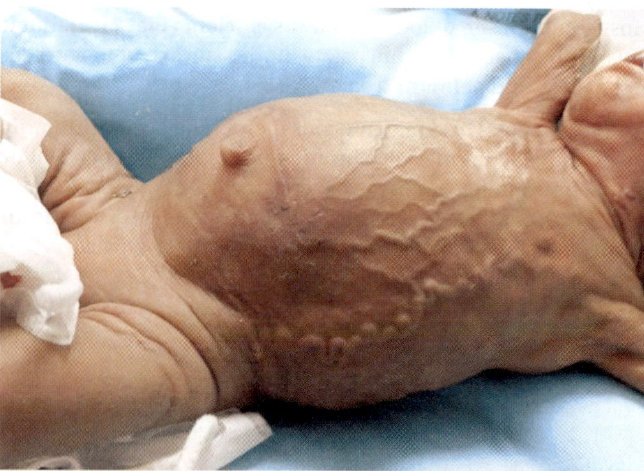

Fig. 21.7: Caput medusae

Source: Reproduced with permission from Editors-in-Chief, Indian Pediatrics and IP Cares. Published in: Ahmed J, Balasubramanian H, Ansari V, Kabra N. Inferior vena cava agenesis-associated thrombosis in a neonate. Indian Pediatr Case Rep. 2021;1:36-9

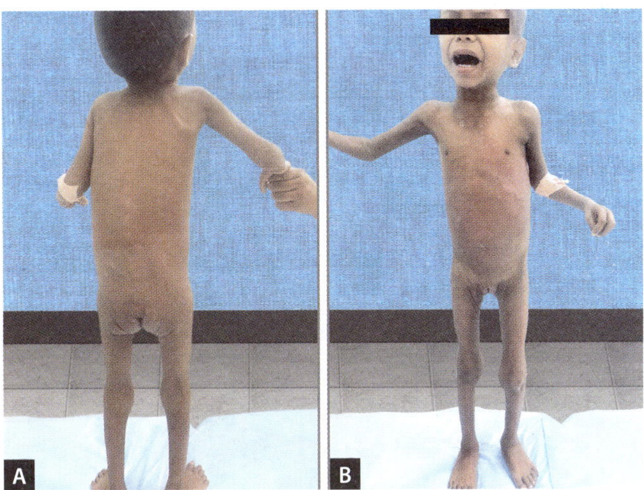

Figs. 21.8A and B: Failure to thrive (note the poor muscle mass, loose folds of skin in axilla, and gluteal region)

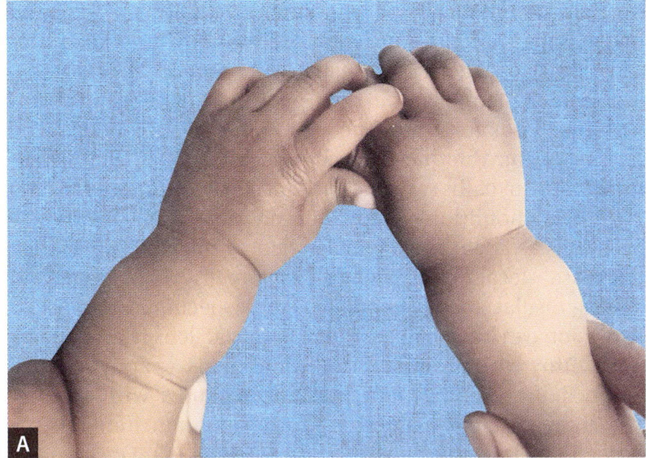

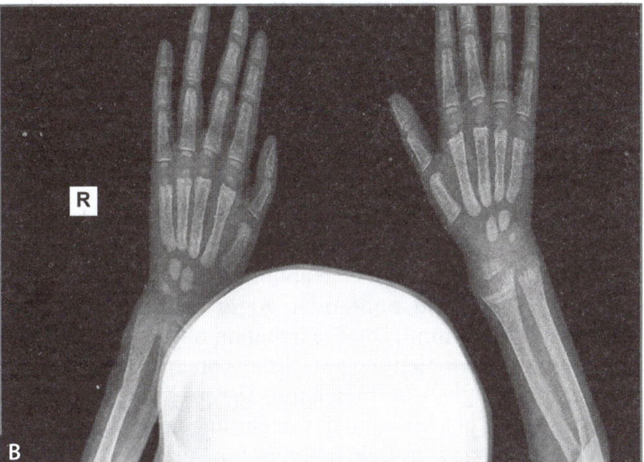

Figs. 21.9A and B: Sign of vitamin D deficiency: (A) Wrist widening; (B) X-ray wrist showing presence of cupping and fraying at distal ends of radius and ulna, suggestive of rickets

EXAMINATION OF THE ABDOMEN

For the purpose of examination, abdomen is divided into nine quadrants by a pair of vertical and horizontal lines. By using these quadrants, it becomes easier to describe the site of abnormality, and to point out the organ which might be involved. The two vertical lines are drawn passing through the tips of both 9th costal cartilages above and the femoral arteries below. These lines also correspond to the midclavicular line. Upper horizontal line is drawn between the lowest points of both costal margins. The lower horizontal line is drawn to join the upper borders of two iliac crests. The contents of these nine quadrants are as shown in **Figure 21.10**.

Inspection

It is the first step of abdominal examination, young children can be examined in the mother's lap as they are too apprehensive to lie down on examination couch. Young infants and older children are to be examined on the couch. During inspection,

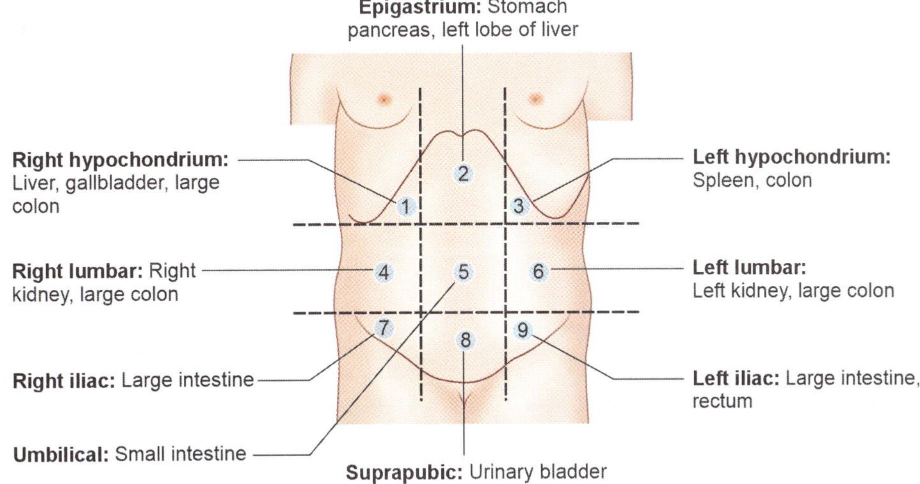

Fig. 21.10: Quadrants of the abdomen and the organs located in the quadrants

the child should ideally be lying supine with arms by side and lower limbs should be flexed at the hip joint to relax abdominal muscles. Inspect the shape, symmetry of the abdomen, and position of umbilicus in both erect and supine (lying down) positions. Look for any fullness or visible swelling. Localized distension may be due to organomegaly/tumor/fecal mass/ hernia and usually restricted to one or two quadrants only (right hypochondrium—hepatomegaly, left hypochondrium—splenomegaly, right or left lumbar region—enlarged kidneys, left iliac fossa—fecal mass), giving an asymmetric appearance and causing displacement of umbilicus on inspection. Generalized distension can be due to gas/fluid/paralytic ileus (skin appears tense shiny with prominent intestinal loops—paralytic ileus, septic ileus; predominant fullness in flanks with smiling umbilicus—ascites; hypotonia—rickets, malnutrition; visible peristalsis—intestinal obstruction) **(Fig. 21.11)**. Observe the movement of the abdomen. All nine regions should move with respiration. Note the skin scars, dilated superficial veins, peristalsis, pulsations, and any other abnormality such as hernia **(Fig. 21.12)**.

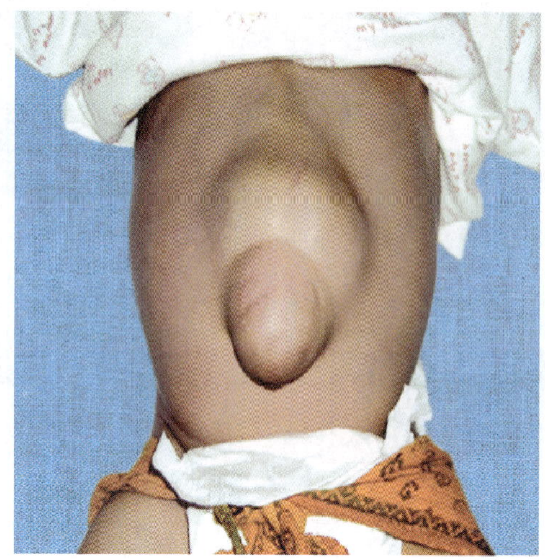

Fig. 21.12: Pathological umbilical hernia. Note the localized distension, abdominal asymmetry with displacement of umbilicus

Palpation

It is the next step of examination to confirm the findings of inspection. Palpate with warm hands. Start with light (superficial) palpation to see how the abdomen feels like. A normal abdomen is soft and nontender. Rigid abdomen suggests perforation or peritonitis due to irritation of the parietal peritoneum. Tense abdomen suggests distension due to gas or fluid. Light palpation gives an idea about the presence of tenderness in any part of abdomen, this needs to be examined in last during deep palpation. Deep palpation by dipping the hands into the abdomen is done for palpating liver, spleen, and kidneys.

Liver: For palpating the liver start from the right iliac fossa by placing fingers parallel to the ribs and ask the patient to take deep breaths, feel for the descending liver striking the lateral border of index finger. Gradually proceed upward till you feel the edge of the liver. At this point the size of liver below right costal margin, surface (smooth/nodular), consistency (hard/firm/ soft), margins (smooth/sharp), and presence of tenderness, if any, must be noted. Enlarged left lobe is palpable in epigastrium suggests chronic hepatomegaly **(Fig. 21.13)**.

Spleen: For palpating the spleen start from the right iliac fossa by placing fingers pointing toward the left subcostal margin and ask the patient to take deep breaths, try to feel for splenic tip as comes and strikes with your fingers during peak of inspiration. Gradually proceed upward till fingertip reaches left subcostal margin. A small spleen can be palpable in right lateral by supporting the left lower ribcage by left hand and dipping the right hand under the subcostal margin **(Fig. 21.14)**. Once spleen has been identified, note its size, consistency, and presence of tenderness.

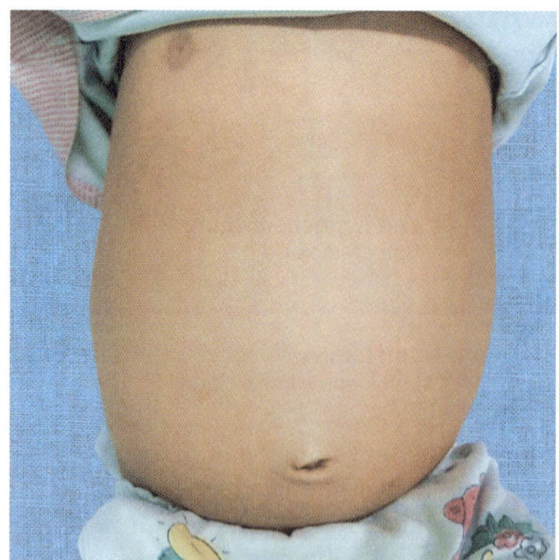

Fig. 21.11: Abdominal distension due to ascites. Note the generalized distension, fullness in bilateral flanks, and the stretched umbilicus

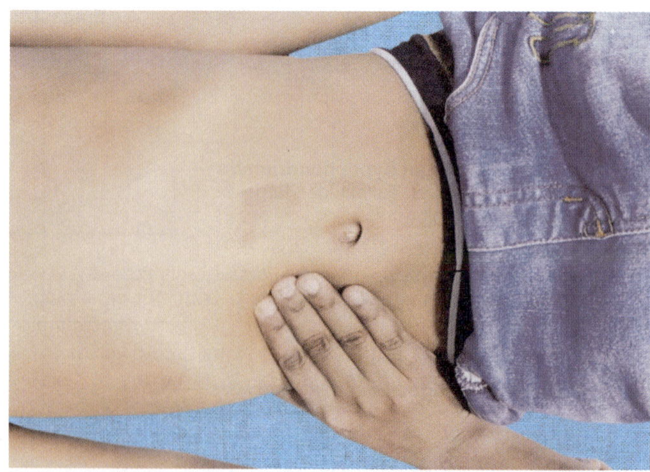

Fig. 21.13: Palpation of the liver by keeping the fingers parallel to the right subcostal margin

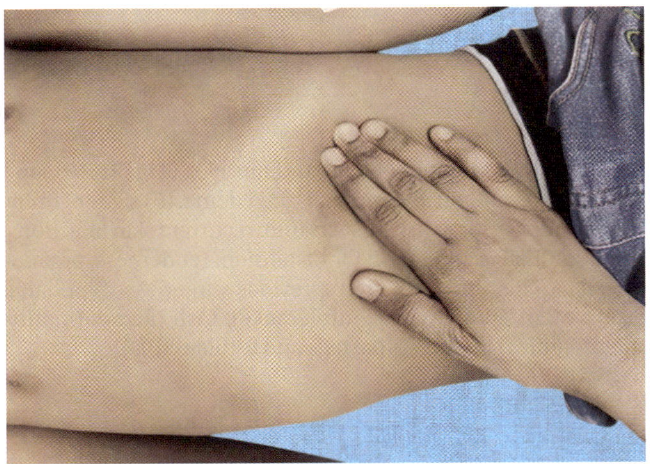

Fig. 21.14: Palpation of the spleen by keeping the fingers toward the left subcostal margin

Kidneys: These are palpated bimanually; to palpate right kidney, keep the right hand over right lumbar region and the left hand behind the right loin to the renal angle. Press the right hand deep into the abdomen to push the kidney posteriorly during expiration, and with left hand push it anteriorly try to feel for the lower pole of kidney as patient takes deep breath. Kidney is felt as smooth rounded swelling. Same way left kidney can also be palpated. If any lump is there then size, shape, surface, margins, consistency, mobility, and ballotability must be noted to get an idea about its origin along with the presence of any signs of inflammation.

Percussion

Abdominal percussion confirms the findings of palpation. It should be done in supine position with lower limbs flexed at hip joints. In a case with abdominal distension percussion helps in detecting the cause of distension (resonant or tympanic note suggestive of gaseous distension, masking of liver dullness on percussion indicates intestinal perforation, and dull note suggestive of ascites). Presence of fluid in peritoneal cavity can be detected by eliciting puddle sign (minimal ascites), shifting dullness (moderate ascites), or by fluid thrill (moderate to large volume ascites). Percussion also helps in demarcating the size of liver and spleen by defining the upper border of these organs.

Auscultation

Auscultate the abdomen by placing stethoscope on the lower abdomen to listen to bowel sounds. There appear as gurgling sounds. Usually, they appear with a frequency of five per minutes. Absent or diminished bowel sounds suggests paralytic items while exaggerated (increased) bowel sound in suggestive of intestinal obstructions. Other sounds which can be auscultated over abdomen are renal bruit which indicates renal artery stenosis and venous hum over liver or spleen suggestive of presence of vascular tumors.

21.3 Malabsorption Disorders and Chronic Diarrhea *PE 23.12*

Malabsorption disorders are associated with decreased intestinal absorption of one or more dietary nutrients, characterized by presence of chronic diarrhea, abdominal distension, and failure to thrive.

Chronic diarrhea is the direct consequence of malabsorption, which results in malnutrition and failure to thrive. Chronic diarrhea here refers to primarily conditions associated with "abnormal stools" which continues or recurs over several months.

ETIOLOGY

Malabsorption disorders can be divided into two groups—(1) malabsorption of specific nutrient, or (2) malabsorption of multiple nutrients—based on the extent of the mucosal affection. Chronic diarrhea can be categorized into one or more of the three major pathophysiologic mechanisms, i.e., (1) impaired intraluminal digestion, (2) intestinal malabsorption, and (3) fermentation.

- ***Chronic diarrhea due to impaired intraluminal digestion*** is seen in conditions such as cystic fibrosis, lipase deficiency, deficiencies of other pancreatic enzymes, and bile duct atresia. Stools are loose and pasty, obviously greasy with undigested fat oozing like oil when it is passed in a pot. The oil may float on the surface of the water in the toilet with an offensive cheesy smell.
- ***Chronic diarrhea due to intestinal malabsorption*** occurs because of mucosal changes in the intestinal wall. The most important of these changes is the villous atrophy. This occurs in celiac disease, cow milk protein allergy (CMPA), giardiasis, immunodeficiency, and malnutrition. Stools are loose or liquid, often with an acidic smell, and rarely greasy. These children have modest steatorrhea, abnormal d-xylose test, and abnormal intestinal histology. Intestinal biopsy is usually necessary for exact diagnosis.
- ***Chronic diarrhea due to fermentation*** is seen in congenital deficiencies of certain mucosal enzymes digesting mono- or disaccharides. Stools are acidic (pH <5.5) and often passed with flatus, and its volume is variable, roughly proportionate to the amount of malabsorbed carbohydrate that has been ingested.

21.4 Approach to a Child with Malabsorption Disorders and Chronic Diarrhea

PE 23.12

HISTORY

In a case of malabsorption disorder/chronic diarrhea, history must include details regarding the—(1) nature, frequency, consistency and presence of blood/mucus/visible oil in stools, and presence of nocturnal diarrhea; (2) age at the time of onset of symptoms is important as various illnesses present in different age groups (**Table 21.8**); (3) association with diet is also important both in physiological conditions such as passage of stools only after eating is suggestive of gastrocolic reflex, and in pathological conditions such as CMPA, celiac disease, pancreatic insufficiency where the symptoms are related to exposure to a particular food; (4) history suggestive of poor growth and nutrient deficiencies, such as anemia, rickets, vitamin B complex deficiency, indicates generalized mucosal involvement; (5) history of recurrent infections at multiple sites in immunodeficiency, recurrent respiratory infections in cystic fibrosis, atopic dermatitis/asthma in food allergy, joint pain/red eye/oral ulcers in IBD suggests the systemic disease; and (6) past history of abdominal surgery point toward blind loop, bacterial overgrowth or short gut.

PHYSICAL EXAMINATION

Important points to be noted during examination are: (1) anthropometry to assess the growth (**Fig. 21.15**), (2) signs of dehydration, (3) signs of wasting of body fat and muscles (**Fig. 21.16**), and deficiency of vitamin and minerals, (4) edema, (5) signs of immunodeficiency—oral thrush, scars from recurrent skin infections, (6) abdominal examination for distension, tenderness, organomegaly, ascites and scars from previous surgeries, (7) perianal region excoriation (lactose intolerance), rash (acrodermatitis enteropathica), fissures, anal tags and fistulae (IBD).

INVESTIGATIONS

Following investigations are important to make a diagnosis of site of involvement as well as for etiology in a child suspected to have chronic diarrhea and malabsorption:

- Complete blood count helpful in picking up cases with infections, inflammation, allergy, and iron deficiency
- Serum electrolytes and renal function tests—abnormal electrolytes and complications of diarrhea
- C-reactive protein and erythrocyte sedimentation rate—inflammatory diarrhea
- Repeated stool examination, especially for *Giardia, Clostridium difficile*
- Stool electrolytes and pH in cases with intractable diarrhea, lactase deficiency
- Fecal fat excretion studies for evidence of fat malabsorption
- D-xylose test (blood levels and urinary excretion) and/or hydrogen breath tests for carbohydrate malabsorption

Table 21.8 Causes of Chronic Diarrhea in Children

Age <1 year	*Age >1 year*
Common causes: • Cow's milk protein allergy (CMPA) • Toddler's diarrhea • Lymphangiectasia • Acquired lactase deficiency • Celiac disease • Infections, e.g., giardiasis • Immunodeficiency states • Cystic fibrosis • Hirschsprung enterocolitis	*Common causes:* • Celiac disease, CMPA, irritable bowel syndrome • Infections, e.g., giardiasis • Toddlers diarrhea • Lymphangiectasia, tropical sprue • Inflammatory bowel disease (ulcerative colitis and Crohn disease) • Gastrointestinal tuberculosis • Immunodeficiency (both congenital and acquired) • Pancreatic insufficiency (cystic fibrosis, chronic pancreatitis) • *Drug-induced:* Antibiotics (including *C. difficile*), laxatives, antacids, etc.
Uncommon causes: • *Intractable diarrhea of infancy:* Microvillus inclusion disease, tufting enteropathy, autoimmune enteropathy • *Congenital enzyme defects:* Glucose galactose malabsorption, sucrose isomaltase deficiency, congenital lactase deficiency, etc. • Cholestasis (intra- or extrahepatic) • Acrodermatitis enteropathica • Abetalipoproteinemia • Shwachman-Diamond syndrome • Drug induced	*Uncommon causes:* • Hyperthyroidism • Anatomical defects, e.g., blind loop, fistula • Hypoparathyroidism • Addison disease • Immune proliferative small intestinal disease (IPSID) • Zollinger Ellison syndrome • Abetalipoproteinemia • VIPoma, carcinoid • Shwachman-Diamond syndrome • Cholestasis intra- or extrahepatic

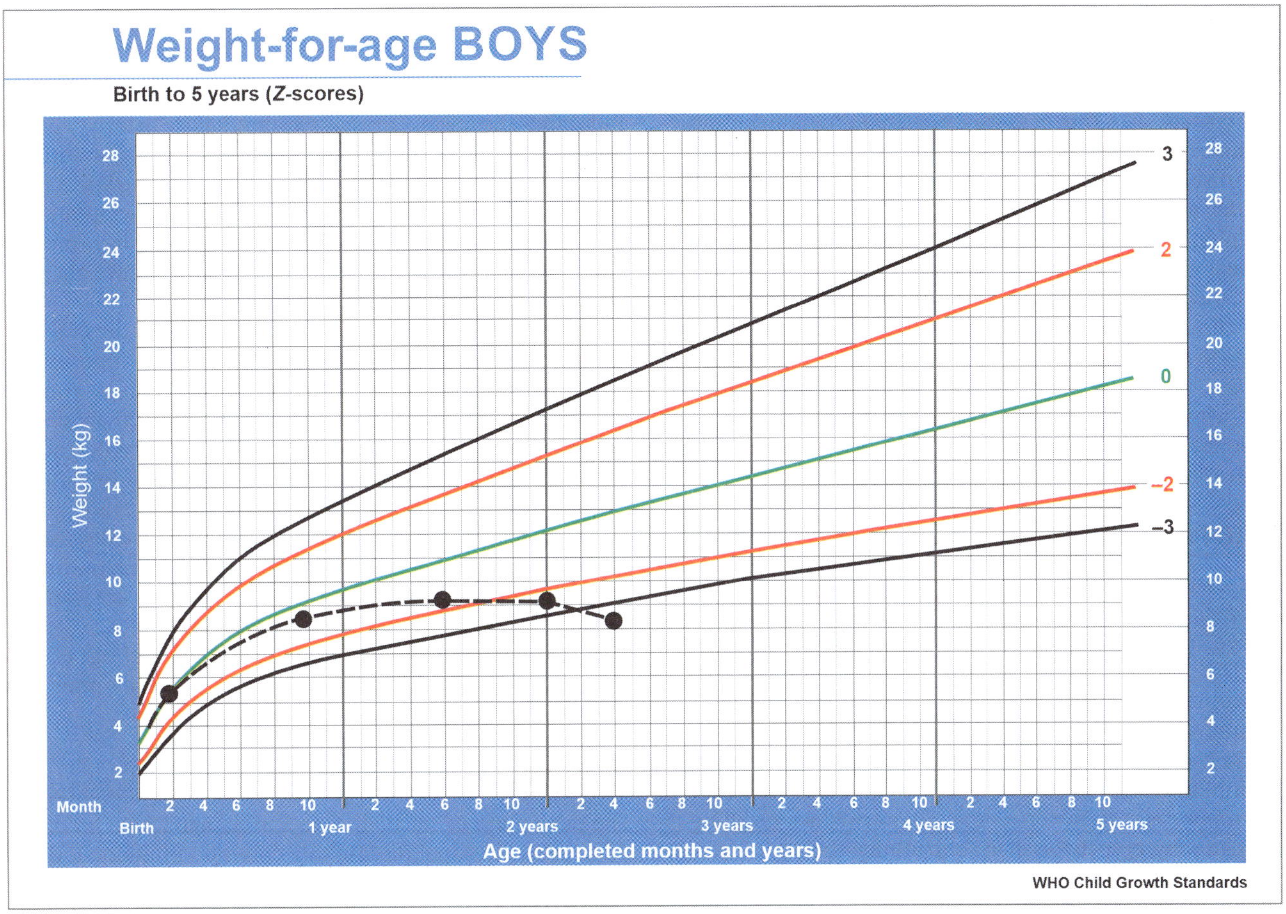

Fig. 21.15: Weight-for-age growth chart of a boy indicating failure-to-thrive (Note the growth faltering depicted by the dotted line, especially after 1 year of age)

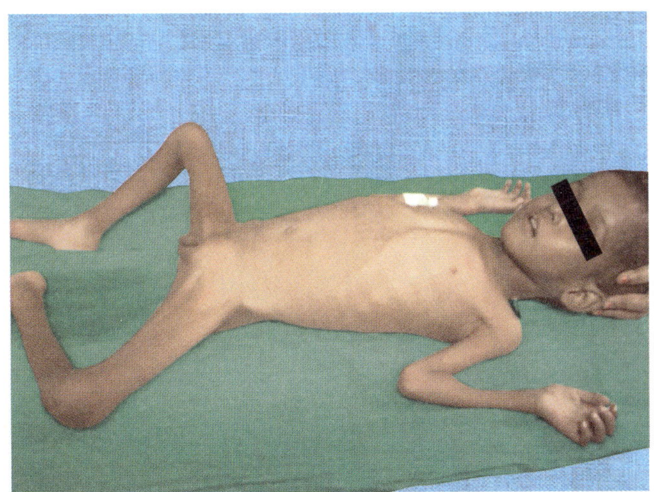

Fig. 21.16: Failure-to-thrive in a 2-year-old child (note the poor muscle mass and loose folds of skin)

- Estimation of fecal α_1-antitrypsin levels and fecal elastase levels
- Intestinal biopsy, celiac disease, inflammatory bowel disease
- Specific tests, e.g., sweat chloride for cystic fibrosis, exocrine pancreatic function tests; and serology for celiac disease and HIV

MANAGEMENT OF CHRONIC DIARRHEA

The principles of management of chronic diarrhea in children involve accurate and timely diagnosis and specific treatment of the underlying cause. Correction of dehydration and treatment of complications is the most important initial step, followed by the definitive management depending on the underlying etiology, which involves dietary modifications (like in celiac disease, lactose intolerance, cow milk protein allergy), specific drug therapy (for conditions like intestinal infection, inflammatory bowel disease, pancreatic insufficiency), and parenteral nutrition in children with functional or anatomical defects.

21.5 Celiac Disease *PE 23.12*

Celiac disease, also known as *gluten enteropathy*, is an immune-mediated enteropathy triggered by gluten and related prolamins. Celiac disease is a lifelong condition, which can present *at any age after* a child starts consuming wheat and other gluten-containing products. It presents with malabsorption, recurrent diarrhea, short stature, growth failure, and micronutrient deficiencies, including anemia. Removal of gluten from the diet leads to full clinical remission and restoration of the small intestinal mucosa to normal.

Celiac disease is common worldwide, with documented global prevalence of 1.4% and 0.6% in the Asian region. Its prevalence is higher in northern India (~1%), a predominantly wheat eating region, in comparison to southern India.

ETIOPATHOGENESIS

Celiac disease is a T-lymphocyte-mediated small intestinal enteropathy induced by gluten (a protein found in wheat, barley, oats, rye, and triticale) in genetically predisposed individuals (HLA-DQ2, HLA-DQ8 positive). Tissue transglutaminase (TTG), an enzyme present in the intestinal epithelium deamidates the gliadin (peptide present in the gluten) and generates negatively charged residues of glutamic acid which stimulates the lymphocytes. Activated lymphocytes generate interferon-γ, IL-4, tumor necrosis factor-α, and other cytokines resulting in villous atrophy, crypt hyperplasia and intraepithelial and lamina propria infiltration of inflammatory cells leading enterocyte damage. In the long term, the chronic stimulation of T cells in celiac disease, sometimes results in T-cell lymphoma of the gut (**Fig. 21.17**).

CLINICAL PRESENTATION

Celiac disease is known for its variable clinical presentation. In a *typical* case, the common features include: chronic diarrhea, abdominal distension, muscle wasting, failure to thrive, anemia, vomiting, anorexia and irritability. Onset occurs after introduction of wheat in the diet, but there might be a long latent period between introduction of wheat and the onset of symptoms. The child may pass foul greasy and bulky stools or may have recurrent episodes of diarrhea. The appetite decreases and weight gain is inadequate.

In *atypical* cases, diarrhea is not present but iron therapy resistant anemia, short stature and/or constipation are prominent findings. Apart from these, other less common manifestations include attention deficit hyperactivity disorder (ADHD), seizures, psychiatric disorders, etc. The diagnosis in these children usually gets delayed because of low index of suspicion of celiac disease by the treating physicians.

There is a high degree of association of celiac disease with other autoimmune disorders such as type 1 diabetes mellitus and autoimmune thyroiditis; and screening tests are warranted for these disorders in children with celiac disease.

A first-degree relative (parent, child, and sibling) of celiac disease patient has a higher (10%) risk of developing celiac disease.

DIAGNOSIS

The perception of celiac disease has changed from an uncommon gastrointestinal disease to a common multiorgan disease strongly dependent on the haplotypes human leukocyte antigen (HLA-DQ2 and HLA-DQ8).

Detection of circulating antibodies to gliadin, reticulin, endomysium, and/or TTG, suggests the diagnosis. IgA anti-endomysial antibody (EMA), IgA antigliadin antibody, and IgA-TTG antibodies characteristically occur in children with untreated celiac disease. Estimation of IgA-TTG antibodies is the most frequently used serological test for screening of celiac disease in children.

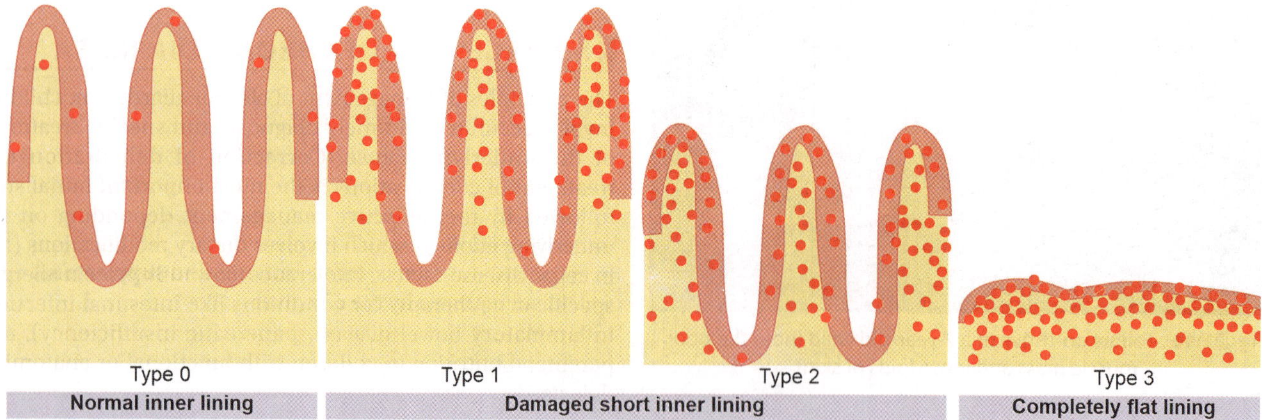

Fig. 21.17: Progressive damage to the inner lining of the gut in celiac disease (CD)

The diagnosis of celiac disease is based upon the demonstration of an abnormal small intestinal mucosa with features characteristic of celiac disease (villous atrophy, crypt elongation, increased intraepithelial lymphocytes) in a biopsy specimen from small intestine (duodenum). Although duodenal biopsy is required for confirmation of diagnosis of celiac disease, and should be done in all cases before starting gluten-free diet, it can be avoided in few patients in which IgA-TTG levels are raised more than 10 times the upper limit of normal, along with positive antiendomysial antibody (done by sampling on a separate occasion) and compatible HLA phenotype (DQ2 or DQ8).

Finally, it is crucial to demonstrate a clinical response to the withdrawal of gluten from the child's diet, in terms of relief of symptoms and significant weight gain. Repeat duodenal biopsy to document resolution of atrophic changes is not routinely required in children who respond well to the dietary management.

TREATMENT Celiac Disease

Stop all gluten containing foods. Gluten is a collective term used to describe the elastic protein component of the cereal grains: wheat, rye, barley, and triticale. A strict gluten-free diet is the cornerstone of management of celiac disease. A gluten-free diet should not contain any detectable source of gluten in it. To manage this, it requires a lot of care in terms of avoiding unintentional consumption of gluten and cross contamination with foods containing gluten.

Wheat contains the greatest amount of gluten, and therefore, *chapattis*, breads, cakes, biscuits, breakfast cereals, etc., are the most significant source of gluten in Indian diet. The starch derived from these cereal grains may also contain small amount of gluten, and should therefore be avoided. These starches are used as thickeners, binders, fillers, stabilizers in many types of processed foods and drinks available in the market.

In celiac disease, rice and maize are the main cereals to be consumed as wheat substitutes. *Chapattis* and breads can be made from mixture of other flours such as gram flour (*besan*), soya flour, maize flour or dried water chestnut (*singhara*) flour. It is best to make these flours at home as commercially available unlabeled flours or flours made in local mills are likely to be contaminated with wheat flour made in the same grinding machine. Commercially available gluten-free flours are acceptable and convenient, but expensive.

A list of common foods which are allowed or forbidden in a child with celiac disease is given here. The clinical response to gluten withdrawal is dramatic. Diarrhea stops, and the growth velocity improves rapidly. A lifelong strict gluten free diet is mandatory.

What is Permitted in Celiac Disease?

- Rice, rice flour, South Indian foods such as *Dosas, Vadas,* and *Uttapams* (except *Rawa/Sooji* preparations such as *Rawa Idli, Rawa Dosa, Upma*)
- Maize, maize flour, corn, bajra, millets, ragi
- Pulses, and flour made out of them (*besan*, soya flour, *moong* dal flour)
- Fresh fruits, fruit juices, salads
- Vegetables and tubers (e.g., potato)
- Home cooked meat, fish, poultry, eggs
- Milk and homemade milk products
- Nuts (not coated/roasted) and dry fruits
- Ghee, butter and oils

What is to be Avoided?

- *Grains:* Items made of wheat, barley, maida, *sooji* such as *roti, poori*, samosa, bhature, etc.
- *Breakfast items:* Bread, bread-rolls, oatmeal, all bakery items, commercial breakfast cereals, seviyan, upmas, etc. (*Note:* All bakery products are likely to contain wheat or traces of wheat gluten)
- *Snacks:* Patty, burger, kulcha, *naan*, biscuits, cutlets, cakes, samosa, mathri, pizza, bread crumbs, soup-sticks, etc.
- *Commercially prepared:* Noodles, pasta, and vermicelli.
- *Beverages:* Barley water, hot chocolate, commercial preparations for enhancement of taste/nutrient content of milk (e.g., Complan, Horlicks, Boost, Bournvita, Protinex), soup cubes, or soup made of a powder mix.
- *Fruits:* Processed fruits and commercial sweets made of fruit extracts, and commercial juices.
- *Sweets/Indian mithai:* All sweets prepared in the market are unsafe to be consumed in celiac disease.
- *Nonvegetarian items:* All nonvegetarian food prepared/available in the market may contain wheat or *maida*. For example, meat kebabs, steak, sausages, etc. Boiled eggs available on the roadside become unsafe when combined with bread kept along with them.
- Readymade ice creams. Some ice creams such as plain vanilla and strawberry flavors may be safe, especially if labeled as gluten-free.

COUNSELING AND FOLLOW-UP

Counseling is important for the family to understand the basis of the disorder and its management, so that they can help the child in dealing with the situation. Parents and other family members may need to go gluten-free too sometimes, for a short while so that the child does not feel left out. Day care attendants and school teachers should be informed and made aware of the child's problem and the need for gluten-free diet (GFD). Plan in advance for special occasions so that child does not feel left out by keeping some nonperishable gluten-free food with the teacher. Adolescents must be encouraged to take the responsibility of their health and diet.

Follow-up and monitoring by the pediatrician/pediatric gastroenterologist/dietitian is a crucial and critical component of celiac disease management.

First visit: Generally, after a week, the comprehension and acceptance of GFD by parents is tested by giving them a structured or verbal questionnaire. The food diary is checked to assess the frequency and the adequacy of the GFD.

Second visit: Done a month later, and the following issues are assessed:

- Child's condition and height/weight charting
- Adequacy of GFD/food diary review
- Need and duration of micronutrients and supplements
- Difficulties faced by the caregiver
- Status of sibling and parent screening

Subsequent visits: The child can now be called for a 3-monthly review for a year followed by 6-monthly/yearly reviews later.

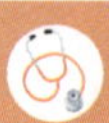

CASE STUDY Celiac Disease

A 5-year-old boy belonging to a middle-income North Indian family has been visiting the pediatric clinic for last 1 year with nonspecific abdominal pain, poor appetite and inadequate weight gain. On one such visit, his records were examined in detail.

He was noted to have microcytic hypochromic anemia on several occasions and thus received iron containing medications every time for varying periods. He had history of several episodes of diarrhea subsiding on its own or on receiving medications. His examination revealed pallor and a slightly protuberant abdomen. On asking, mother reported that the child often develops abdominal fullness after meals. The child's weight was 12 kg and height was 91 cm. Other systemic examination was noncontributory.

A diagnosis of short stature and anemia was made and celiac disease was suspected to be a cause of the child's problems.

What made clinician think of celiac disease?

In this child, presence of short stature and refractory anemia along with GI symptoms such as recurrent diarrhea and protuberant abdomen made the clinician suspect celiac disease.

The mode of presentation of celiac disease may be quite variable. Though many children with celiac disease have a history of diarrhea, it may not always be typical greasy, bulky and foul smelling stools. Associated short stature (child's height is 83% of expected for age signifying severe stunting but weight for height is 92% signifying no wasting) suggests some chronic disease. Also, presence of anemia despite receiving hematinics several times suggests ongoing malabsorption.

Though this child had GI symptoms classifying him as having a "typical" presentation of celiac disease, any child whose rate of growth is slow, accompanied by recurrent or refractory iron deficiency anemia, irrespective of presence of GI symptoms, should be investigated for presence of celiac disease.

Discuss the investigations required to confirm or refute the diagnosis.

Diagnosis of celiac disease requires demonstration of IgA antiendomysial antibodies or IgA-TTG antibodies along with demonstration of mucosal changes (such as total or subtotal villous atrophy) in intestinal biopsy.

Serology is useful as initial test and both antiendomysial antibodies and TTG antibodies have comparable sensitivity and specificity. However, these alone should not be relied on for final diagnosis for the purpose of instituting therapy because false negative as well as false positive tests are known to occur. Small intestinal endoscopy and biopsy should be done while the child is still consuming a gluten containing diet is mostly required for establishing the diagnosis. Other investigations such as thyroid function tests and blood glucose should be done to exclude other autoimmune disorders, once celiac disease is confirmed.

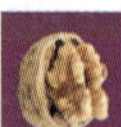

IN A NUTSHELL

Malabsorption Disorders

1. Malabsorption disorders are characterized by chronic diarrhea, abdominal distension, and failure to thrive.
2. Chronic diarrhea can be caused by—(1) impaired intraluminal digestion, (2) intestinal malabsorption, or (3) fermentation.
3. Detailed history and examination play an important role in diagnosing the cause.
4. The management of chronic diarrhea mainly depends on the underlying etiology.
5. Celiac disease, also known as gluten enteropathy, is induced by gluten (a protein found in wheat). It is a lifelong disorder.
6. Onset of celiac disease occurs after introduction of wheat in the diet, but there might be a long latent period between introduction of wheat and the onset of symptoms.
7. Presentations of celiac disease include diarrhea, short stature, and nonresponsive anemia.
8. Detection of circulating antibodies to gliadin, reticulin, endomysium, and/or tissue transglutaminase, suggests the diagnosis of celiac disease. Intestinal biopsy is diagnostic.
9. Removal of gluten from the diet leads to full clinical remission of celiac disease.

Bolia R, Thapar N. Celiac disease in children: a 2023 update. Indian J Pediatr. 2024;91(5):481-9.

Jimenez J, Loveridge-Lenza B, Horvath K. Celiac disease in children. Pediatr Clin North Am. 2021;68:1205-19.

Lal SB, Venkatesh V, Aneja A, et al. Clinical spectrum and changing presentation of celiac disease in Indian children. Indian J Med Res. 2023;158(1):75-84.

Lau MS, Sanders DS. Optimizing the diagnosis of celiac disease. Curr Opin Gastroenterol. 2017;33:173-80.

Lo Vecchio A, Conelli ML, Guarino A. Infections and chronic diarrhea in children. Pediatr Infect Dis J. 2021;40(7):e255-e258.

Sahin Y. Celiac disease in children: A review of the literature. World J Clin Pediatr. 2021;10(4):53-71.

Shankar S, Rosenbaum J. Chronic diarrhoea in children: A practical algorithm-based approach. J Paediatr Child Health. 2020;56(7):1029-38.

Singh P, Arora A, Strand TA, et al. Global prevalence of celiac disease: Systematic review and meta-analysis. Clin Gastroenterol Hepatol. 2018;16:823-836.e2.

Sivaramakrishnan VM. Approach to chronic diarrhea in children. Indian J Pract Pediatr. 2024;26(2):177-84.

Thiagarajah JR, Kamin DS, Acra S, et al. Advances in evaluation of chronic diarrhea in infants. Gastroenterology. 2018;154:2045-2059.e6.

Tripathi PR, Srivastava A. Approach to a child with chronic diarrhea. Indian J Pediatr. 2024;91(5):472-80.

Zuvarox T, Belletieri C. Malabsorption syndromes. Treasure Island (FL): StatPearls Publishing; 2022.

21.6 Acute Hepatitis

PE 23.13

INTRODUCTION

Acute hepatitis is a clinical syndrome characterized by abrupt onset of jaundice associated with conjugated hyperbilirubinemia and elevation of hepatic enzymes. Although acute hepatitis may occur alone or as a part of systemic disease, the most common cause in children is infection—usually by one of the five hepatotropic viruses (hepatitis A to E).

ETIOLOGY

Hepatitis A Virus

The hepatitis A virus (HAV) infections occur most often in developing countries with almost all children demonstrating evidence of past infection by the age of adolescence. The risk of infection is more in contacts of infected persons, child-care centers, and travelers to endemic areas. Transmission of HAV is almost always by person-to-person contact. Spread is predominantly by the fecal-oral route (through contaminated food or water) and maternal-neonatal transmission is not recognized.

Hepatitis A virus causes only acute hepatitis syndrome and does not lead to chronicity or cirrhosis. Most infections in children younger than 5 years of age are asymptomatic or have mild, nonspecific manifestations; the illness is much more likely to be symptomatic in older children and adults.

Hepatitis B Virus

The major route of transmission in children is from mother-to-child (perinatal transmission). Other important modes include blood products, unsafe injections, sexual contact, institutional care, and contact with carriers. No risk factors are identified in about 40% of cases.

Hepatitis B virus (HBV) infection may present as asymptomatic infection, acute hepatitis syndrome, or chronic hepatitis. The risk of chronicity is related inversely to age; the older the age of acquisition, the lower the risk of chronic disease. Chronic carrier stage of hepatitis B predisposes to hepatocellular carcinoma. Infection during pregnancy does not influence the maternal or fetal outcome adversely.

Hepatitis C Virus

The risk factors for transmission are exposure to contaminated blood products, sexual contact, and unsafe injections. Perinatal transmission is uncommon.

Most acute infections are clinically silent, <25% of children become icteric. Clinically apparent acute infections are mild and progression to fulminant hepatitis is exceedingly rare. Hepatitis C virus (HCV) is the most likely hepatotropic virus to cause chronic infection with about 85% of cases becoming chronic.

Hepatitis D Virus

The hepatitis D virus (HDV) cannot produce infection without HBV as a helper virus. HDV can cause an infection at the same time as the initial HBV infection (coinfection), or can infect a person who is already infected with HBV (superinfection). The routes of transmission are same as that for HBV.

Acute hepatitis is common with coinfection and is usually much more severe than for HBV alone. In superinfection, acute illness is rare and chronic hepatitis is common. However, the risk of fulminant hepatitis is highest in superinfection.

Hepatitis E Virus

Hepatitis E virus (HEV) infection occurs through fecal-oral route usually contracted through contaminated water. It occurs in outbreaks or as sporadic cases in endemic areas. The highest attack rate of overt disease occurs in adolescents and adults. HEV infection is associated with a very high mortality rate among infected pregnant women.

Drugs

Most drug-induced liver disease is cytotoxic. Some drug-induced liver disease, however, is predominantly cholestatic. Acute hepatotoxic injuries develop over a relatively short time and cause a lesion without any features of chronicity.

The most common drugs associated with hepatotoxicity in children are isoniazid, valproate, paracetamol, azathioprine, and halothane.

Autoimmune Hepatitis

Though mostly associated with chronic liver disease, 25–30% of children with autoimmune hepatitis, particularly children, the illness may mimic acute viral hepatitis. Acute liver disease may also be associated with other immune-mediated disorders such as systemic lupus erythematosus (SLE), IBD, and celiac disease.

Metabolic Diseases

Wilson disease may present as acute self-limited hepatitis or as fulminant hepatic failure. Alpha-1-antitrypsin deficiency may also rarely presents as acute hepatitis.

Other Infections

Diseases such as typhoid fever, kala azar, leptospirosis, scrub typhus, and brucellosis can also cause acute hepatitis like state. Though asymptomatic elevation of hepatic enzymes is most frequently seen, frank jaundice is sometimes present.

CLINICAL FEATURES

Acute viral hepatitis is ordinarily an acute self-limited illness. The incubation period is about 4 weeks for HAV and 4 months for HBV. In infants and young children, the infection may be entirely asymptomatic or manifest by a nonspecific gastroenteritis-like syndrome with no icterus.

In older children and in adults, there may be a prodromal period of several days in which fever, headache, and malaise predominate, followed by the onset of jaundice, abdominal pain, nausea, mild vomiting, and anorexia. Pruritus may accompany the jaundice. Over the next several days, as the jaundice peaks, the systemic symptoms wane. In hepatitis B infection, a serum sickness like state consisting of arthralgia or arthritis, urticaria or angioedema, and a maculopapular rash might occur. The arthritis is migratory and symmetric and subsides when jaundice begins.

On examination, marked jaundice is present with a mildly enlarged, tender liver. Occasionally, splenomegaly is noted. Mild-to-moderate ascites may be present in some cases especially with HAV infection. Jaundice and other symptoms usually resolve by 2–4 weeks after onset. In some cases, the disease progressively worsens to hepatic failure manifesting as encephalopathy and coagulopathy. Progression to fulminant hepatic failure is not seen with HCV and extremely rare with HEV except in pregnant women.

COMPLICATIONS

Acute liver failure: Discussed in the next Section 21.5.

Others

Chronic hepatitis: HCV, HBV, HDV superinfection, and autoimmune hepatitis.

Cirrhosis and portal hypertension: HCV, HBV, HDV superinfection, Wilson disease, and autoimmune hepatitis.

Hepatocellular carcinoma: HBV and HCV.

DIAGNOSIS

Evidence of Jaundice and Hepatic Dysfunction

Acute hepatitis is suspected clinically in any child with a short history of jaundice associated with other nonspecific symptoms such as anorexia, vomiting, fever, and abdominal pain. The serum bilirubin may only be mildly elevated especially in younger children, or it becomes very high. The conjugated fraction is typically raised to >20% of total levels. Serum aminotransferase (ALT and AST) values usually peak around the time that jaundice occurs; values are often 20–100 times the upper limit of normal. Prolongation of prothrombin time indicates the need for hospitalization.

Evaluation of Cause

A detailed history is taken regarding exposure to persons having similar disease, history of travel to endemic areas, or similar cases in neighborhood for possible fecal-oral mode of transmission. Details of any blood transfusions, sexual contact/abuse, and unsafe injections are to be noted. A record of the medications recently used should be made for possible drug-induced liver damage. Family history of jaundice or neurological illness should be asked for possibility of Wilson disease presenting as acute hepatitis.

Wilson disease and autoimmune hepatitis need to be considered if tests for the viral antibodies are negative. Salmonellosis, leptospirosis, scrub typhus, and brucellosis also need to be considered as a cause of acute hepatitis like illness, especially if fever is persistent.

The diagnosis of viral etiology is usually made serologically. Presence of following markers is required for diagnosis of acute infection with the respective viruses:

- ***Acute hepatitis A:*** IgM anti-HAV positivity.
- ***Acute hepatitis B:*** IgM anti-HBcAg along with hepatitis B surface antigen (HBsAg) positivity.
- ***Acute hepatitis C:*** Detection of HCV ribonucleic acid (RNA) in serum by either polymerase chain reaction (PCR) or branched deoxyribonucleic acid (DNA) amplification technique (anti-HCV, the most commonly available serological test for HCV may become positive only after 2 months of acute infection and thus not useful in diagnosing acute hepatitis because of HCV).
- ***HDV coinfection:*** IgM anti-HDV positivity along with HBsAg positivity.
- ***Acute hepatitis E:*** IgM anti-HEV positivity.

TREATMENT Acute Hepatitis

Treatment for acute hepatitis is purely supportive, and most children recover fully.

- Adequate rest should be ensured till the acute symptoms start resolving.
- Further liver insult should be prevented by avoiding hepatotoxic drugs.
- Adequate fluid intake should be ensured to avoid dehydration due to vomiting.
- Good nutritious diet, rich in carbohydrates and with adequate proteins is to be given. Fat restriction may be advised in initial stages to minimize vomiting but is not essential if nausea and vomiting is not marked.
- Wilson disease and autoimmune hepatitis if presenting as acute fulminant hepatitis carry grave prognosis and usually require liver transplantation.

IN A NUTSHELL

Acute Hepatitis

1. Acute hepatitis is characterized by jaundice, conjugated hyperbilirubinemia, and raised liver enzymes.
2. Viral hepatitis caused by five hepatotropic viruses (hepatitis A to E) is the most common cause.
3. Hepatitis A, E are spread by feco-oral route while hepatitis B, C, D have parenteral transmission. Hepatitis B is also transmitted from mother to the newborn (vertical transmission).
4. Hepatitis A, E infections are acute; while hepatitis B, C, may become chronic.
5. Drugs, autoimmune hepatitis, and metabolic diseases (Wilson disease) are other common causes of hepatitis in children.
6. Acute viral hepatitis is an acute self-limited illness. Treatment is supportive. Acute liver failure is the most dreaded complication.

Ncdc.gov.in. Viral Hepatitis: The silent disease. Prevention, control and treatment guidelines 2016. [online] Available from: https://ncdc.gov.in/linkimages/guideline_hep20158117187417.pdf [Last accessed January, 2025].
Nnhcp.gov.in. National guidelines for diagnosis and management of viral hepatitis 2018. [online] Available from: https://www.nvhcp.ogv.in/common_libs/diagnosis-management-viral-hepatitis.pdf [Last accessed January, 2025].
Sathiyasekaran M, Ramaswamy G. Diagnosis and management of Hepatitis B and Hepatitis C infections in children. Pediatr Infect Dis. 2020;2:12-8.

21.7 Acute (Fulminant) Liver Failure

PE 23.14

DEFINITION

Acute liver failure (ALF), also known as fulminant hepatic failure, is rare but most important complication of acute hepatitis in children. The definition of ALF in children is different from that of adults due to difficulty in accurately assessing the presence and stage of encephalopathy in infants and children. The currently accepted definition of ALF in children has three components, (1) acute onset of liver disease without evidence of chronic liver disease, (2) biochemical evidence of severe liver injury, (3) presence of coagulopathy (defined as INR >1.5 in presence of encephalopathy or INR >2 in absence of encephalopathy) not corrected by vitamin K administration. There is severe hepatic dysfunction affecting liver's synthetic, detoxification, and metabolic function. HAV, HBV, HDV superinfection, Wilson disease, autoimmune hepatitis, drugs (e.g., paracetamol) and toxins (e.g., poisonous mushrooms) are common causes of ALF.

CLINICAL FEATURES

Clinical features vary with the stage of the disease from mild nonspecific features of fatigue, malaise, nausea, and abdominal pain in early stage to increasing jaundice, abdominal distension, gastrointestinal bleeding, shock, fever, and worsening of neurological status (confusion, poor attentiveness, irritability, altered sensorium, and coma) with the advancement of the disease.

TREATMENT Acute Liver Failure

Acute liver failure should be managed in intensive care setting, preferably in a center having facilities for liver transplantation. The prognosis with conservative management is generally poor with survival rates not exceeding 50%. Poor prognostic factors are: INR >5, rapid decrease in liver size without clinical improvement, Wilson disease, and deeper stages of encephalopathy. Liver transplantation is indicated in cases where risk of mortality is high with only medical management.

Conservative management of ALF involves following:

- *Fluid and electrolyte balance:* Intravenous fluids containing glucose to prevent and correct hypoglycemia and dehydration. Strict input/output charting should be done.
- *Correction of coagulopathy and bleeding* by repletion of injection vitamin K by intravenous route, in cases having active bleeding transfusion of fresh frozen plasma, platelet concentrates and blood can be considered.
- *Cerebral edema* should be managed by keeping the head elevated by 30°, administration of Mannitol or hypertonic saline. Endotracheal intubation and hyperventilation may be required in children having coma.
- *Administration of H2 blockers* (ranitidine 1–2 mg/kg/dose 8–12 hourly) to prevent gastric bleeding.
- *Oral lactulose* (5–40 mL) every 2–4 hourly initially till diarrhea, then titrate the dose so that the child passes 2–4 semi-loose acidic stools per day. This results in reduction of ammonia production by gut bacteria, by reducing their load.
- *Broad-spectrum antibiotics* (e.g., cefotaxime and cloxacillin) may be given empirically as coexistent bacterial infection is present in almost 50% of cases. Oral administration of nonabsorbable antibiotics such as neomycin also helps to clear the gut of bacteria thus decreasing ammonia production.
- *Renal care:* Associated renal failure is managed by dialysis and a careful fluid administration titrated to the urine output.
- *Diet:* In children taking orally or during recovery, protein intake should be restricted.

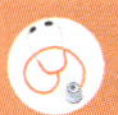

CASE STUDY Acute (Fulminant) Liver Failure

A 10-year-old girl weighing 25 kg suffering from jaundice for last 15 days is brought to the hospital with complaints of repeated vomiting and agitated behavior since last night. On examination, deep icterus is present and there are large ecchymotic patches over buttocks. She appears confused and deep tendon reflexes are exaggerated.

What investigations need to be done in this child?

Tests for hepatocellular dysfunction: The first step would be to confirm whether this jaundice is hepatocellular or hemolytic. Children with cerebral malaria can have CNS involvement in presence of hemolytic jaundice, which will be indirect type. Presence of direct hyperbilirubinemia (direct bilirubin >20% of total) and elevated liver enzymes suggest hepatocellular involvement. Liver enzymes especially ALT will be raised manifold (20–50 times) if it is acute hepatitis due to hepatotropic viruses. Prothrombin test must be done in all cases. Prothrombin raised beyond 15 seconds (INR >1.5) will suggest ALF as there is clinical evidence of encephalopathy. If prothrombin is deranged, test should be repeated after giving vitamin K (5 mg intravenously) injection. Prothrombin >60 seconds (INR >5) will suggest a grave prognosis, and the child should be referred to a center having facility for liver transplantation in that case.

Investigations for likely cause: IgM HAV, IgM HEV, and HBsAg should be done to rule out acute hepatitis due to hepatitis A, hepatitis E, and hepatitis B, respectively. If HBsAg is positive, IgM HBcAg should be done to confirm presence of acute hepatitis B as Australia antigen positivity alone could be incidental. If these viral markers are negative, investigations for Wilson disease (serum ceruloplasmin, 24 hours urinary copper, and slit-lamp examination for Kayser–Fleischer ring) and autoimmune hepatitis (total immunoglobulins, antinuclear antibody, anti-smooth muscle antibody, anti-liver-kidney-muscle I antibody) should be done, as these disorders can occasionally present as acute hepatitis. History of drug or toxin ingestion should be recorded. If fever is a prominent symptom, tests for malaria (peripheral smear for malaria parasite, malaria antigen test), typhoid fever (blood culture, serum widal), scrub typhus (Weil–Felix test, immunofluorescence), and leptospirosis (leptospiral antibodies, immunofluorescence) should also be undertaken.

Investigations for other complications: Blood sugar should be done to rule out hypoglycemia. Platelet count should be done as child has ecchymotic patches. Kidney function tests (serum urea and creatinine) should be done to find any evidence of hepatorenal syndrome. Serum electrolytes should be done to diagnose any electrolyte disturbances (e.g., hyponatremia, hypokalemia). Blood culture and urine culture should be taken to guide therapy for any coexistent infection.

Outline the management protocol

- Shift the child to intensive care unit after explaining the nature of disease, its severity, and its likely course to the parents. Explain possible need of blood product transfusion, and possible need of hepatic transplantation (if available) or referral to a higher center.
- Administer intravenous fluids (N/4 10% dextrose) and prevent/treat hypoglycemia or any electrolyte disturbance.
- Put a nasogastric tube for early diagnosis of any upper gastrointestinal bleeding, and also for giving lactulose and oral medications in case the child is not accepting orally.
- Lactulose 10–20 mL 2 hourly. Increase dose if required till the child starts passing clear liquid stools. Reduce frequency of administration to 6–8 hourly thereafter.
- Start broad spectrum antibiotics (cefotaxime + gentamicin) to treat any coexistent infections.
- Administer ranitidine 25 mg intravenous 8 hourly.
- Send sample for cross matching. Administer fresh frozen plasma (FFP) if gastric contents are hemorrhagic or if there is bleeding from any site.
- Monitor input/output, vital parameters, and CNS status. Intubate and hyperventilate if child slips into coma.

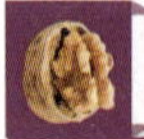

IN A NUTSHELL

Acute Liver Failure

1. Acute Liver failure is the most important complication of acute hepatitis in children.
2. Characterized by severe hepatic dysfunction affecting liver's synthetic, detoxification, and metabolic function.
3. Acute liver failure should be managed in intensive care setting, preferably in a center having facilities for liver transplantation.
4. The prognosis with conservative management is generally poor with survival rates not exceeding 50%.

Bhatt H, Rao GS. Management of acute liver failure: a pediatric perspective. Curr Pediatr Rep. 2018;6:246-57.

Larson-Nath C, Vitola B. Pediatric acute liver failure. Crit Care Clin. 2022;38(2):301-15.

Lal BB, Khanna R, Sood V, et al. Diagnosis and management of pediatric acute liver failure: consensus recommendations of the Indian Society of Pediatric Gastroenterology, Hepatology, and Nutrition (ISPGHAN). Hepatol Int. 2024;18:1343-81.

Shanmugam N, Dhawan A. Acute liver failure in children. Pediatric Hepatology and Liver Transplantation. 2018;145-53.

Squires JE, Alonso EM, Ibrahim SH, et al. North American Society for Pediatric Gastroenterology, Hepatology, and Nutrition Position Paper on the Diagnosis and Management of Pediatric Acute Liver Failure. J Pediatr Gastroenterol Nutr. 2022;74:138-58.

21.8 Chronic Liver Disease *PE 23.15*

INTRODUCTION

Chronic liver disease is long-term liver damage resulting from continuing inflammatory, infiltrative, metabolic, congestive, or obstructive process with a potential to lead to irreversible change in the structure of the liver and the complications of cirrhosis.

Cirrhosis refers to diffuse involvement of liver with evidence of fibrosis and regenerative nodules.

Neonatal cholestasis is defined as prolonged elevation of conjugated bilirubin in serum, beyond the first 14 days of life. However, the onset of problem can be anytime during the infancy depending on the clinical condition causing cholestasis. If not treated this can result in the development of chronic liver disease.

ETIOLOGY

Hepatotropic viruses including hepatitis B, C, and D viruses which can cause chronic liver disease and cirrhosis because of persistent hepatic inflammation. The risk of developing chronic HBV infection, defined as being positive for HBsAg for >6 months or being negative for IgM anti-HBC and positive for HBsAg, is related inversely to age; the older the age of acquisition, the lower the risk of chronic disease. Almost 90% children acquiring the hepatitis B infection perinatally become chronic carriers.

Other than viruses, chronic liver disease is caused by metabolic disorders such as Wilson disease, Alpha-1-antitrypsin deficiency, hemochromatosis, and inborn errors of metabolism. Autoimmune hepatitis (Type I, II, and III) is also important cause of chronic liver disease in older children.

Cholestasis in a newborn or infant may be due to a variety of abnormalities giving rise either to (1) mechanical obstruction of bile flow; or to (2) functional impairment of hepatic excretory function and bile secretion. The causes of neonatal and infantile cholestasis can be broadly categorized into intrahepatic and extrahepatic, listed in **Box 21.3**. Cholestasis, defined physiologically as a reduction in canalicular bile flow, is caused by intrahepatic or extrahepatic obstruction. If the process predominantly involves hepatocytes or intrahepatic bile ducts, it

Box 21.3 Causes of Neonatal and Infantile Cholestasis

Intrahepatic disorders

A. *Cholestasis associated with infections:*
   1. Sepsis with possible endotoxemia* [Gram-negative sepsis or urinary tract infections (UTI)]
   2. Syphilis*
   3. Toxoplasmosis
   4. Perinatal viral infections [cytomegalovirus (CMV)*, rubella, herpes simplex, hepatitis B virus (HBV), hepatitis C virus (HCV)]

B. *Metabolic and endocrine disorders:*
   1. Galactosemia
   2. Tyrosinemia
   3. α_1-antitrypsin deficiency
   4. Niemann-Pick disease
   5. Gaucher disease
   6. Glycogen storage disease, Type IV
   7. Zellweger syndrome (cerebrohepatorenal syndrome)
   8. Cystic fibrosis
   9. Hypothyroidism

C. *Anatomic and structural defects:*
   1. Intrahepatic bile duct paucity* (Alagille syndrome)
   2. Persistent familial intrahepatic cholestasis (PFIC)
   3. Benign recurrent intrahepatic cholestasis
   4. Hereditary cholestasis with lymphedema (Aagenaes disease)
   5. Caroli disease

D. *Toxic:*
   1. Parenteral nutrition related
   2. Drugs

E. *Others:*
   1. Idiopathic neonatal hepatitis*
   2. Gestational alloimune liver disease

Extrahepatic disorders

1. Extrahepatic biliary atresia*
2. Choledochal cyst
3. Bile duct stricture
4. Mass (neoplasia, stone)

*Relatively common causes

results in intrahepatic obstruction and if the process predominantly involves extrahepatic bile ducts, it results in extrahepatic biliary obstruction.

Despite extensive investigations, a significant proportion of children having chronic liver disease are found to be having no obvious cause and are labeled as having idiopathic or cryptogenic chronic liver disease.

CLINICAL PRESENTATION

Acute Hepatitis-like Presentation

- Chronic liver disease should be suspected whenever an episode of acute hepatitis-like illness continues for a prolonged period (usually 3 months) or when there is a relapse of apparent acute hepatitis.
- However, this cut-off period of 3 months is not strict and chronic liver disease may be suspected earlier than 3 months if there is a history suggestive of chronic liver disease or if examination or investigations suggest otherwise **(Box 21.4)**.

Box 21.4 Features Suggesting Chronicity of Liver Disease

A. *History:*
   1. Relapsing disease
   2. Clinical or biochemical features of hepatitis persisting >12 weeks
   3. History of neonatal/infantile cholestasis
   4. Past history of acute hepatitis
   5. Family history of chronic liver disease
   6. History of some etiological disorder, e.g., known HBsAg or anti-HCV positivity, Wilson disease, autoimmune disease or cystic fibrosis

B. *Examination:*
   1. Small liver
   2. Enlarged left lobe of liver
   3. Hard/irregular liver
   4. Firm splenomegaly
   5. Moderate to massive ascites
   6. Edema
   7. Growth failure/muscle wasting

C. *Cutaneous features:*
   1. Portosystemic shunts
   2. Spider angiomas
   3. Facial telangiectasia
   4. Palmar erythema

D. *Investigations:*
   1. Low serum albumin
   2. Raised prothrombin despite vitamin K therapy
   3. High serum gamma globulins
   4. Ultrasound
      - Nodular/heterogeneous liver parenchyma
      - Impaired portal vein flow velocity
      - Flat venous forms in hepatic veins
      - Increased hepatic artery pulsatility

- Continuing abnormality of liver function after an apparent acute hepatitis also suggests chronic liver disease.
- Some children with an apparent acute hepatitis but clinical examination or investigations suggest chronic liver disease.

Chronic/Insidious Presentation or Presentation with Complications

- Most children will present with bleeding varices, ascites, or hypersplenism—known complications of previously undiagnosed portal hypertension.
- Some children present with nonspecific symptoms such as failure to thrive with or without prolonged/recurrent episodes of jaundice.
- Examination findings of firm/hard liver, firm splenomegaly, or ascites in any child with nonspecific symptoms should alert the clinician toward possibility of chronic liver disease.
- Jaundice is not an essential feature for diagnosis of chronic liver disease and would be present only in decompensated or cholestatic disease.
- Neonatal cholestasis often presents as persistence of jaundice in the neonatal period beyond the limit for physiological jaundice (14 days). This is accompanied with passage of dark-colored urine and there might be passage of pale or clay-colored stools. Hepatomegaly is often present. Spleen may

also be enlarged because of the primary disorder itself or because of portal hypertension in later stages.

Asymptomatic Elevation of Liver Enzymes

Occasionally, the condition is discovered in children with no current or past evidence of liver disease, when liver function tests are performed as part of a routine medical examination or for complaints unrelated to the liver. Findings of raised liver enzymes, prolonged prothrombin time, or low serum albumin suggest possibility of chronic liver disease.

ASSOCIATED PROBLEMS

Cholestasis

Cholestasis refers to impairment of bile flow. Involvement of liver in a chronic disease process often leads to some amount of cholestasis. This manifests as jaundice, pruritus, and acholic stools. Malnutrition and vitamin deficiencies also may occur because of malabsorption related to cholestasis.

Portal Hypertension

Involvement of the portal system in the fibrosis process leads to obstruction of portal flow leading to portal hypertension. Spleen invariably enlarges in portal hypertension and hypersplenism may occur resulting in pancytopenia. Variceal bleeding and ascites are other features of portal hypertension.

Hepatocellular Impairment

The hepatocellular function usually remains intact in chronic liver disease except in later stages when decompensation occurs. Features suggesting decompensation in chronic liver disease are: (1) jaundice; (2) edema; (3) coagulopathy not responding to vitamin K; (4) pedal edema; (5) low serum albumin; (6) massive ascites; and (7) encephalopathy.

Nutritional Problems

Malnutrition and failure to thrive are usually seen in chronic liver disease because of cholestasis, anorexia leading to low caloric intake, and presence of chronic disease state.

INVESTIGATIONS

The aims of investigating a child suspected to be having chronic liver disease are (1) to document evidence of hepatic dysfunction and to evaluate the extent of damage; (2) to detect or rule out associated complications; and (3) to establish an etiological diagnosis.

Assessment of Hepatic Dysfunction

- ***Serum bilirubin (direct and indirect):*** Presence of conjugated hyperbilirubinemia usually suggests decompensation. Presence of unconjugated hyperbilirubinemia suggests coexisting hemolysis (e.g., Wilson disease, autoimmune hemolytic anemia in autoimmune hepatitis).
- ***Enzymes*** [ALT, serum glutamic-pyruvic transaminase (SGPT)] typically shows a mild rise (2–5-fold increase) as against 20–100-fold rise usually seen with acute viral hepatitis. Other enzymes such as alkaline phosphatase and γ-glutamyl transpeptidase (GGT) may also be raised.
- ***Serum albumin*** is low because of impairment of synthetic function of liver and also due to malnutrition.
- ***Prothrombin time*** is raised because of impairment of synthesis of coagulation factors by liver or because of cholestasis associated vitamin K deficiency. In the latter case, the correction of prothrombin occurs following vitamin K administration whereas in the former, prothrombin does not normalize after vitamin K therapy.
- ***Liver biopsy:*** A percutaneous liver biopsy should be done in all children with chronic liver disease to (1) define severity of morphological changes and for evidence of chronic active hepatitis; and to (2) establish the etiological diagnosis, e.g., alpha-1-antitrypsin deficiency, infiltrative disorders. Biochemical and genetic analysis on liver tissue can also be done for diagnosis of some disorders such as Wilson disease and some inborn errors of metabolism.
  Prothrombin time and platelet count must be done before liver biopsy and biopsy should be deferred if INR >1.3 or platelet count is $<70 \times 10^9$/L. In these situations, if the cause is identified and treatable (such as Wilson disease, hepatitis B, or autoimmune hepatitis), start specific therapy and reattempt liver biopsy when there is no coagulopathy. Otherwise, liver biopsy may be done under cover of transfusions (fresh frozen plasma, platelets, and whole blood) if there is a dire need.

Liver Biopsy

Position: Liver biopsy is to be done under sedation after placing the infant or child in the supine position. A rolled towel is to be placed under the right upper back to push the liver forward and stabilize the position.

Site of biopsy: Liver biopsy can be performed percutaneously by intercostal or subcostal approach, under ultrasound guidance or in a blind manner. In intercostal approach, biopsy is done at the level of 8th or 9th intercostal space in midaxillary line. However, when the liver is enlarged the biopsy can be performed below the costal margin in midaxillary line (subcostal approach).

Other approaches for performing liver biopsy are transvenous (transjugular or transfemoral) biopsy and laparoscopic biopsy. Transvenous approach is useful in patients with clinically demonstrable ascites; a known or suspected hemostatic defect; a small, hard, cirrhotic liver; morbid obesity while laparoscopic biopsy is useful in cases when liver is noted to be abnormal in appearance prior to planned surgery or at the time of surgery

Procedure

- All medications that increase the risk of bleeding, must be stopped 5–7 days prior to the procedure.
- The child is kept nil per oral for at least 5 hours prior to the procedure.
- Site of biopsy must be marked beforehand, if doing the procedure blindly.
- Platelet count, prothrombin, INR should be measured prior to the procedure.

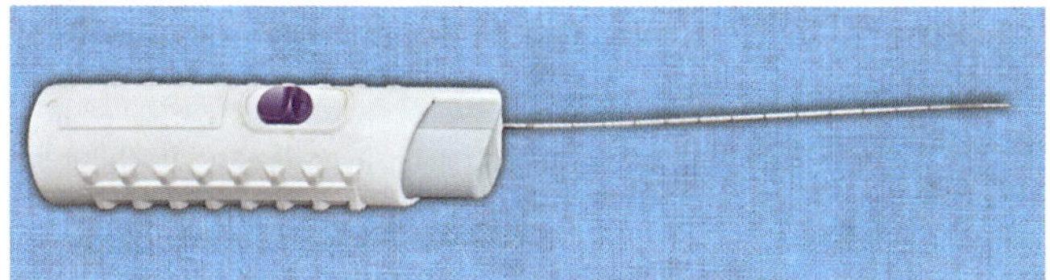

Fig. 21.18: Liver biopsy gun

- Place an intravenous access for appropriate sedation and analgesia.
- Desired area is cleaned with spirit, povidone iodine followed by spirit and draped with sterile linen.
- The skin, subcutaneous tissue, intercostal muscles are anesthetized with 1–2% lignocaine.
- A small incision in the skin can be made to facilitate the entry of biopsy needle.
- The patient is asked to hold his breath at the end of expiration.
- Tru-cut biopsy needle (23 gauge) **(Fig. 21.18)** is inserted perpendicular to the skin at the marked site till a sudden feel of resistance is felt once the needle enters the liver. The position of the needle is confirmed by the movement of the needle with respiration.
- The outer sheath of the needle is held firmly, the cutting needle inserted quickly. The outer sheath is advanced rapidly over the cutting needle and thereafter the entire device is withdrawn.
- The biopsy specimen is placed in 10% neutral buffered formalin for histopathological examination. An ideal sample is 10–20 mm in length.
- Local pressure must be applied for few minutes and pressure dressing is done.
- Monitor vital signs and watch for bleeding for next 24 hours.

Detection of Complications of Chronic Liver Disease

- *Full blood count, serum urea, and electrolytes:* To detect associated abnormalities—anemia, pancytopenia, infection, and electrolyte disturbances.
- Upper gastrointestinal endoscopy for evidence of varices.
- Hepatic and portal venous studies by ultrasound Doppler to detect portal hypertension.
- Ascitic fluid analysis is required in suspected spontaneous bacterial peritonitis.

For Etiological Diagnosis

- ***Viral markers:*** HBsAg, HBeAg, anti-HBe, HBV DNA; anti-HCV, HCV PCR.
- ***Markers for autoimmune hepatitis:*** Presence of raised levels of IgG suggests diagnosis of autoimmune hepatitis. Antinuclear antibodies (ANA) and/or anti-SMA are present in type I autoimmune hepatitis. Antibodies to anti-LKM antigen-1 are present in type II autoimmune hepatitis where ANA and anti-SMA would be absent. If these three antibodies are absent but diagnosis of autoimmune hepatitis is strongly suspected, antibodies to soluble liver antigen (anti-SLA) should be detected which are raised in the rare type III variety of autoimmune hepatitis.
- ***Markers for Wilson disease:*** Slit-lamp examination for Kayser–Fleischer ring should be done in all suspected cases but a negative test does not rule out Wilson disease. Serum ceruloplasmin and 24-hour urinary copper excretion studies should be done. Copper content in liver biopsy should be estimated for definitive diagnosis.
- ***Imaging:*** Ultrasound and Doppler studies can detect choledochal cyst, Budd–Chiari syndrome, and extrahepatic portal hypertension.
- ***Alpha-1-antitrypsin*** phenotype for diagnosis of Alpha-1-antitrypsin deficiency. This diagnosis is also suggested if there are Periodic acid–Schiff (PAS) positive, diastase resistant granules on microscopic examination of liver biopsy specimen.
- ***Sweat chloride test*** for cystic fibrosis.
- ***Others:*** Fasting blood sugar, lactate, and screening for inborn errors of metabolism.

DIFFERENTIAL DIAGNOSIS

Extrahepatic Portal Hypertension

This diagnosis should be strongly considered in a child having portal hypertension and splenomegaly. The liver is not enlarged; liver functions are normal with a normal liver biopsy. The child is well preserved, and there is no evidence of cholestasis.

Constrictive Pericarditis

Constrictive pericarditis can cause firm enlargement of liver and massive ascites and thus can mimic chronic liver disease. In constrictive pericarditis, jugular venous pressure would be elevated and associated cardiac complaints such as chest pain and discomfort might be present. Electrocardiogram (ECG), chest X-ray, and cardiac catheterization can help in ruling out constrictive pericarditis.

Infiltrative Disorders

Lymphoma, histiocytosis, and leukemia can mimic chronic liver disease clinically. Infective disorders such as kala-azar and chronic malaria can also cause a chronic liver disease like presentation. The enlargement of liver in these cases is usually regular with a smooth surface. Aspiration of bone marrow/lymph nodes can detect evidence of infiltration (lymphoma, leukemia, etc.) or infection (kala-azar, chronic malaria).

TREATMENT Chronic Liver Disease

Symptomatic Therapy

- *Diuretics:* Spironolactone and furosemide are used if ascites is massive and causing distress to the child.
- *Stop bleeding:* Coagulopathy should be corrected by giving vitamin K 5 mg intravenously and by transfusions of fresh frozen plasma if decompensation is present. Variceal bleeding is to be managed by sclerotherapy and giving transfusions.
- *Cholestasis:* The choleretic agent ursodeoxycholic acid may be particularly useful in children with predominant biliary features such as itching and cholestasis.

- *Nutrition:* Adequate nutritional intake should be ensured by making food calorie dense. Fat-soluble vitamins are required in 5–10 time the recommended doses. In cases with neonatal cholestasis, fats should be given in the diet in the form of medium chain triglycerides (MCT) as they do not require bile salts for absorption. Coconut oil is a good source of MCT.
- *Vitamins:* Supplementation with fat-soluble and water-soluble vitamins (vitamin A 5,000–15,000 IU daily or 50,000 IU weekly; vitamin D 2,500–5,000 IU daily or 30,000 IU weekly; vitamin E 50–400 IU/day; vitamin K 2.5–5 mg twice a week; water-soluble vitamins twice the recommended daily allowance) is required to prevent or treat deficiency states.
- *Psychological support* should be given to the child and family while the child is being worked up and also if there is progression to irreversible cirrhosis.

Specific Therapy

Specific therapy can be offered in viral hepatitis due to HBV or HCV, autoimmune hepatitis and Wilson disease. Corticosteroid therapy, with or without low doses of azathioprine, improves the clinical, biochemical, and histologic features in most children with autoimmune hepatitis and prolongs survival in most children with severe disease.

In neonatal cholestasis cases treatment depends on the underlying causes of cholestasis, some of the treatable conditions are:

- *Congenital syphilis:* Treat with crystalline penicillin for 10–14 days.
- *Galactosemia:* Lactose free formula feeding.
- *Choledochal cyst or other obstructive lesions:* Surgical removal.
- *Extrahepatic biliary atresia:* All children suspected of having biliary atresia should undergo exploratory laparotomy and direct cholangiography to determine the presence and site of obstruction.
- If the cholangiogram indicates that the biliary tree is patent but of diminished caliber, cholestasis is not due to biliary tract obliteration but because of intrahepatic disease. In these cases, transection of or further dissection into the porta hepatis should be avoided.
- For children in whom EHBA is confirmed, the hepatoportoenterostomy procedure of Kasai can be carried out. The success rate for this surgery is much higher (90%) if performed before 8 weeks of life. Therefore, it is very important to refer the suspected cases early to a suitable center.
- If no treatable cause is found or if the disease has already progressed to irreversible cirrhotic stage, liver transplantation may be the only alternative.

A diagnostic and therapeutic approach in a child with chronic liver disease is presented in **Flowchart 21.4**.

Abou-Taleb A, Ahmed A, El-Hennawy A. Pediatric chronic liver diseases: a clinicopathological study from a tertiary care center. Int J Pediatr. 2019;7: 9305.

Dhole SD, Kher AS, Ghildiyal RG, et al. Chronic liver diseases in children: clinical profile and histology. J Clin Diagn Res. 2015;9(7):SC04-7.

Gupte GL, Srivastava A. Chronic liver disease in children: from diagnosis to liver transplantation. Indian J Pediatr. 2024;91:260-1.

Fernando M, van Mourik I, Wassmer E, et al. Wilson disease in children and adolescents. Arch Dis Child. 2020;105(5):499-505.

Mouzaki M, Bronsky J, Gupte G, et al. Nutrition Support of Children With Chronic Liver Diseases: A Joint Position Paper of the North American Society for Pediatric Gastroenterology, Hepatology, and Nutrition and the European Society for Pediatric Gastroenterology, Hepatology, and Nutrition. J Pediatr Gastroenterol Nutr. 2019;69: 498-511.

Ravindranath A, Yachha SK. An approach to investigations of chronic liver disease. Indian J Pediatr. 2024:91:262-9.

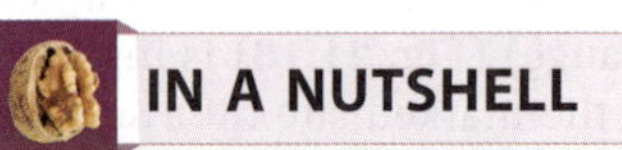

Chronic Liver Disease

1. Chronic liver disease is long-term liver damage that may lead to *cirrhosis.*
2. It should be suspected whenever an episode of acute hepatitis-like illness continues for a >3 months.
3. Common causes include hepatitis B, C, and D virus infections, Wilson disease, autoimmune hepatitis, and other metabolic disorders.
4. Untreated neonatal cholestasis can lead to development of chronic liver disease.
5. Most children will present with prolonged/recurrent jaundice, bleeding varices, ascites, or hypersplenism. Jaundice is not an essential feature for diagnosis of chronic liver disease.
6. Investigations include liver function tests, prothrombin time, liver biopsy, viral marker studies, antibodies for autoimmune hepatitis, and markers of Wilson disease.
7. Treatment is symptomatic. Specific therapy can be offered in viral hepatitis due to HBV or HCV, autoimmune hepatitis, and Wilson disease.

Flowchart 21.4: Algorithmic approach toward management of chronic liver disease

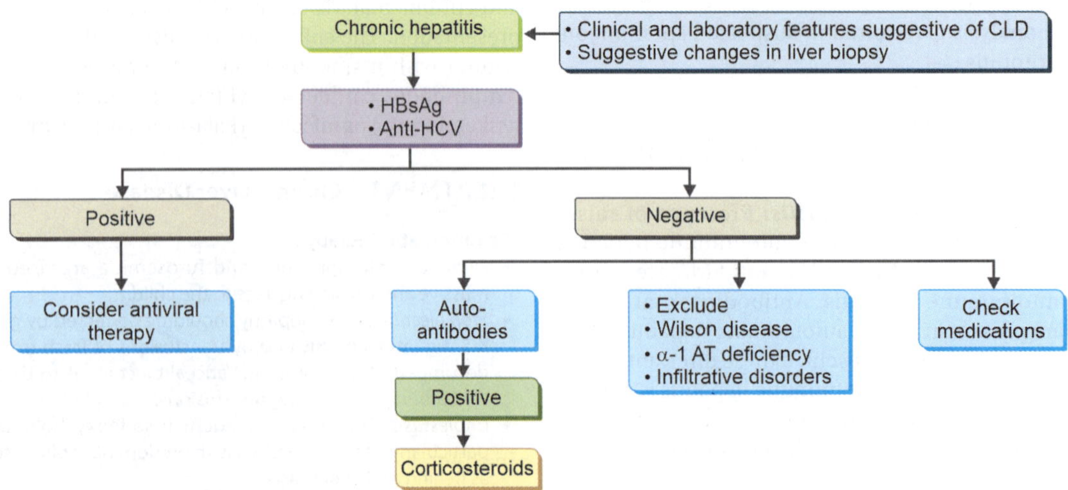

(AT: antitrypsin; CLD: chronic liver disease)

21.9 Portal Hypertension, Upper Gastrointestinal Bleed, and Ascites

PE 23.16, PE 23.21

DEFINITION

Portal hypertension is a clinical condition characterized by the pathological increase in the pressure in the portal venous system (>10–12 mm Hg).

ETIOPATHOGENESIS

The causes of portal hypertension can be divided into intrahepatic and extrahepatic, extrahepatic causes can be further divided into prehepatic and posthepatic (**Table 21.9**). The underlying causes of portal hypertension in children from developed countries are different from developing countries, as intrahepatic causes (~50% cases) are more common in the former and extrahepatic causes (~60–75% cases) in the later. In India, extrahepatic portal vein obstruction is the most common cause followed by chronic liver disease. Portal hypertension is the most common cause of gastrointestinal bleeding in children of India. The mortality after index hematemesis in variceal bleeding is 30% and after recurrent variceal bleeding is as high as 70%.

CLINICAL FEATURES

The age of presentation in extrahepatic portal vein obstruction (EHPVO) cases range from 12 months to adulthood (mean age 5–6 years). Majority of the patients present with upper gastrointestinal (UGI) bleed in the form of hematemesis with or without melena due to esophageal or gastric variceal bleeding. Splenomegaly is almost universal in patient with EHPVO. It can be present as early as 1 month of age and is usually seen before 3 years of age. These children have poor growth in comparison to their siblings. They usually do not develop encephalopathy even after massive gastrointestinal bleeding and on abdominal examination ascites is absent. They have normal liver function.

Children having portal hypertension secondary to chronic liver disease leading to cirrhosis have jaundice, ascites, hepatosplenomegaly and UGI bleeding. In Budd–Chiari syndrome cases massive ascites with isolated hepatomegaly along with the tortuous prominent veins are the main findings. Persistent or massive ascites in children with EHPVO should doubt about the diagnosis or suggests the possibility of presence of coexistent cirrhosis.

Upper gastrointestinal endoscopy is an important investigation for evaluation of UGI bleeding in children. The various indications of UGI endoscopy are enumerated in **Table 21.10**.

Table 21.9 Causes of Portal Hypertension in Children

Location of lesion	*Condition*
Intrahepatic	• Biliary atresia • Progressive familial intrahepatic cholestasis • Primary sclerosing cholangitis • Cystic fibrosis-related liver disease • Autoimmune hepatitis • Chronic viral hepatitis B • Chronic viral hepatitis C • Nonalcoholic fatty liver disease • Congenital hepatic fibrosis • Caroli disease
Prehepatic	• Portal vein thrombosis • Tumor (infiltration by hepatoblastoma, hepatocellular carcinoma, or compression by large focal nodular hyperplasia) • Drug therapy (6-thioguanine and azathioprine)
Posthepatic	• Budd–Chiari syndrome • Inferior vena cava obstruction • Congestive heart failure • Veno-occlusive disease (sinusoidal obstruction syndrome)

Table 21.10 Indications of Upper GI Endoscopy in Children

Diagnostic indications	*Therapeutic indications*
• Hematemesis • Hematochezia • Caustic ingestion • Dysphagia or odynophagia • Recurrent vomiting of unknown cause • Unexplained chronic diarrhea • Unexplained anemia	• Esophageal varices • Percutaneous endoscopic gastrostomy placement • Foreign body removal • Dilatation of esophageal stricture • Achalasia • Percutaneous jejunostomy placement

UPPER GASTROINTESTINAL BLEEDING

Upper gastrointestinal bleeding in children usually manifests as *hematemesis* (fresh blood in vomitus), *melanemesis* (altered blood leading to brownish "coffee ground" vomitus), or *melena* (black, tarry stools).

The minimum quantity of blood required to produce melena is 50–100 mL. Melena may persist for 3–5 days after acute gastrointestinal bleed and cannot be used as an indicator of ongoing bleeding. Melena may be seen very rarely in lower gastrointestinal bleeding if bleeding is very slow or if the child is constipated. Sometimes, massive gastrointestinal bleed may present as *hematochezia* (passage of unaltered blood in stools) due to rapid transit of blood through the gut.

ETIOLOGY

Table 21.11 enumerates the age-specific causes of UGI bleeding in children.

Table 21.11 Etiology of Upper Gastrointestinal Bleeding in Children

Newborn	*Infant*	*Child/adolescent*
• Swallowed maternal blood • Hemorrhagic disease of newborn • Stress gastritis or ulcer • Vascular anomaly • Coagulopathy • Milk protein sensitivity • Malrotation	• Stress gastritis • Gastroesophageal reflux disease (GERD) • Mallory-Weiss tear • Vascular anomaly • Gastrointestinal duplication • Esophageal/gastric varices • Bowel obstruction and webs	• Esophageal/gastric varices • Acid peptic disease • Mallory-Weiss tear • Caustic ingestion • Vasculitis (Henoch-Schönlein purpura) • Crohn disease • Bowel obstruction

- ❖ Hematemesis on first or second day of life in a well-appearing child is most commonly due to swallowed maternal blood.
- ❖ On 3rd to 7th days, bleeding in a well-child is usually due to vitamin K deficiency bleeding (VKDB).
- ❖ In a sick-appearing neonate, UGI bleeding is usually the result of stress bleed or DIC.
- ❖ In infants, GERD may cause small amount of UGI bleed.
- ❖ Streaks of blood in vomitus following forceful vomiting are usually due to Mallory-Weiss tear.
- ❖ Variceal bleeding is the most common cause of severe UGI bleeding in children. The varices are secondary to either cirrhotic portal hypertension or more commonly because of extrahepatic portal hypertension.

EVALUATION OF A CHILD WITH UPPER GASTROINTESTINAL BLEEDING

A prioritized diagnostic and therapeutic approach to the child with suspected gastrointestinal blood loss is critical to avoid a delay in diagnosis. Important clues to the diagnosis are obtained with a careful history, physical examination, and knowledge of the potential causes of UGI bleeding in infants and children.

History and Examination

- ❖ Treatment with drugs like aspirin or other NSAIDs suggests drug-induced gastritis or ulcer as a cause.
- ❖ History of umbilical sepsis or catheterization in neonatal period is suggestive of extrahepatic portal hypertension due to portal/splenic vein thrombosis.
- ❖ History of recurrent pain abdomen, regurgitation, and retrosternal burning is suggestive of GERD or peptic ulcer.
- ❖ Presence of jaundice, firm hepatomegaly, shrunken liver, or cutaneous stigmata (palmar erythema, spider nevi, gynecomastia) is suggestive of variceal bleed due to cirrhosis.
- ❖ Presence of splenomegaly suggests portal hypertension as a cause. However, spleen may regress after massive hematemesis to reappear again only after child is stabilized with volume resuscitation and transfusions.

Investigations

- ❖ Send the blood sample immediately for grouping and cross-matching. A complete blood count, electrolytes, and liver function test (LFT) should be done.
- ❖ ***UGI endoscopy*** is the preferred method to evaluate the UGI tract for a source of bleeding. Any child with significant UGI bleed should be stabilized by volume resuscitation, transfusions, and medical therapy and thereafter referred to an endoscopist experienced with children. Endoscopy is performed under intravenous sedation or general anesthesia. UGI endoscopy is best avoided if the child is clinically unstable, such as in shock or profound anemia and every effort should be made to stabilize the child first by conservative management.
- ❖ ***Abdominal ultrasound*** is useful in assessment of chronic liver disease and portal hypertension. Doppler flow studies can identify portal blood flow dynamics.

TREATMENT Upper Gastrointestinal Bleeding

Initial Assessment and Stabilization

Any child who presents with hematemesis or malena should be considered a potential emergency. The initial goal in the treatment of any child with UGI bleeding is to provide hemodynamic stability including oxygen delivery, fluid and blood resuscitation, and correction of coagulopathy, and metabolic or electrolyte abnormality. Presence of significant tachycardia suggests that the child has lost about 20% of blood volume whereas presence of shock indicates about 40% blood loss.

- Make a quick assessment of child's vitals including heart rate, blood pressure, and oxygen saturation.
- Establish a venous line and draw blood samples for counts, grouping, and cross-matching.
- Start crystalloid infusion with Ringer's lactate or normal saline till blood transfusion can be given.
- Give oxygen if shock or hypoxemia is present.
- Pass a Ryle's tube and give gastric lavage with normal saline and then maintain continuous drainage to assess amount of continuing blood loss.
- Monitor vitals including pulse rate, blood pressure, respiration, and oxygen saturation. Urine output and fluid intake/output should be measured if shock is present.

Pharmacological Treatment

- *Octreotide:* This is synthetic analogue of somatostatin and can be given as a bolus or by infusion. This is the drug of choice. A loading dose of 1 μg/kg is given as an intravenous infusion over 30 minutes followed by continuous infusion at the rate of 0.5 μg/kg/h which can be titrated up to 2 μg/kg/h.
- *Vasopressin:* It acts by causing splanchnic vasoconstriction, thus decreasing the blood supply to the portal vein and the varices. It is used in dose of 0.33 units/kg in 20 minutes, followed by intravenous infusion of 0.33 units/kg/h.

- *Somatostatin:* It also acts by causing splanchnic vasoconstriction but has a very short half-life. In adults, it is given in the dose of 250 µg, intravenous bolus, followed by continuous infusion of 250 µg/h.
- *Antacids:* H2 blockers (ranitidine) and PPIs (omeprazole, pantoprazole) decrease gastric acid secretion and thus prevents clot lysis by inhibiting activation of pepsinogen.

Endoscopic Treatment

Endoscopic sclerotherapy and endoscopic variceal ligation are effective for controlling esophageal variceal bleeding. The commonly used sclerosants are ethanolamine oleate and alcohol. Variceal ligation is safer than sclerotherapy but requires special equipment and expertise.

Mechanical Methods

Sengstaken–Blakemore tube stops bleeding mechanically by balloons that compress esophageal and gastric varices (mechanical tamponade). It is very effective in controlling hemorrhage but is associated with high incidence of rebleeding once the tube is removed.

Surgical Methods

Emergency surgical methods such as portosystemic shunting, esophageal transaction, and liver transplantation are associated with high morbidity and mortality and should be reserved for the most refractory cases.

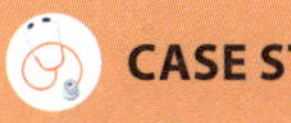

CASE STUDY Upper Gastrointestinal Bleeding

A 7-year-old boy weighing 20 kg presents with bouts of hematemesis and passage of black tarry stools for last 6 hours. He has weak peripheral pulses, severe pallor, and marked tachycardia. He had reported to outpatient department about a week back with vague abdominal pain and discomfort where the doctors detected a spleen enlargement of 5 cm without any other abnormality. His blood tests, including liver function tests were found to be normal at that time, and he was advised to continue follow-up for investigations.

Identify the likely cause of bleeding.

This boy has massive hematemesis resulting in circulatory failure. The most likely cause is portal hypertension as massive hematemesis in children is almost always due to variceal bleeding. Another pointer toward portal hypertension in this child is detection of splenomegaly on a previous outpatient visit. Remember that spleen regresses during episode of massive bleeding, and may be absent on examination at this time. The cause of portal hypertension is likely to be extrahepatic (prehepatic) as his clinical examination and liver function tests were normal.

Outline the emergency treatment required to control bleeding.

- Establish an intravenous line.
- Send blood sample for cross matching, and arrange whole blood. Transfuse blood as early as possible. This child will need two units of blood immediately as he would have lost about 40% of his blood volume. Meanwhile, administer crystalloids (e.g., Ringer lactate, normal saline) and colloids (e.g., dextran) to restore intravascular volume.
- Administer oxygen as there would be hypoxia due to severe anemia and circulatory collapse.
- Put a nasogastric tube to estimate the ongoing bleed.
- Give octreotide 20 µg as intravenous infusion over 30 minutes. Start octreotide infusion 10–20 µg/h through infusion pump. (*Referring the child for endoscopy at this stage would be dangerous as child is in circulatory failure*).
- Administer ranitidine 20 mg intravenously 8–12 hourly to take care of any associated portal gastropathy.
- Monitor vital parameters and record amount of ongoing bleed. Titrate the blood transfusions as per the estimated loss, and vital parameters of the child.
- Once the child is stabilized, he should be referred for endoscopy to directly visualize the varices.
- Endoscopic variceal banding or endoscopic sclerotherapy should be done preferably in that sitting itself.
- Child should be well sedated/anesthetized before the procedure.

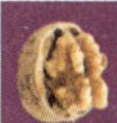

IN A NUTSHELL

Upper Gastrointestinal Bleeding

1. Upper gastrointestinal bleeding in children usually manifests as hematemesis (fresh blood in vomitus) or melena (black, tarry stools).
2. Esophageal or gastric varices (secondary to portal hypertension) are the most important causes of severe UGI bleeding.
3. Presence of splenomegaly suggests portal hypertension as a cause.
4. Upper gastrointestinal endoscopy is done to find the source of bleeding.
5. The initial goal in the treatment of any child with upper gastrointestinal bleeding is to provide hemodynamic stability, including oxygen, fluid, and blood transfusion.
6. Octreotide is the drug of choice for stopping the bleed. Other alternatives include vasopressin and somatostatin.
7. Endoscopic sclerotherapy and endoscopic variceal ligation are effective for controlling esophageal variceal bleeding.

Di Giorgio A, D'Antiga L. Portal hypertension in children. In: Guandalini S, Dhawan A (Eds). Textbook of Pediatric Gastroenterology, Hepatology and Nutrition. Springer, Cham. 2022.

Grama A, Pirvan A, Sîrbe C, et al. Extrahepatic portal vein thrombosis, an important cause of portal hypertension in children. Journal of Clinical Medicine. 2021;10(12):2703.

Grammatikopoulos T, McKiernan PJ, Dhawan A. Portal hypertension and its management in children. Arch Dis Child. 2018;103:186-91.

Kassam AF, Goddard GR, Johnston ME, et al. Natural course of pediatric portal hypertension. Hepatol Commun. 2020;4:1346-52.

Novak I, Bass LM. Gastrointestinal bleeding in children-current management, controversies, and advances. Gastrointest Endosc Clin N Am. 2023;33(2):401-21.

Piccirillo M, Pucinischi V, Mennini M., et al. Gastrointestinal bleeding in children: diagnostic approach. Ital J Pediatr. 2024;50:13.

ASCITES

Collection of serous fluid within the peritoneal cavity is termed ascites. Excessive fluid in the peritoneum could be a part of generalized edema (anasarca) or it may be the sole or predominant site of fluid accumulation.

ETIOLOGY

In children, hepatic, renal, and cardiac diseases are the most common causes of ascites. Common causes are listed as follows:

- ***Ascites with no edema or ascites out of proportion to peripheral edema:***
  - *Hepatic causes:* Cirrhosis, congenital hepatic fibrosis, portal vein obstruction, and Budd-Chiari syndrome.
  - Constrictive pericarditis
  - Urinary ascites (perforation or leakage from urinary tract)
  - Chylous ascites
  - Peritoneal tuberculosis
  - Acute pancreatitis
  - *Intra-abdominal malignancies:* Lymphoma and neuroblastoma.
- ***Ascites with generalized edema:***
  - *Renal causes:* Nephrotic syndrome, acute glomerulonephritis, and renal failure
  - *Cardiac causes:* Congestive heart failure and constrictive pericarditis.
  - *Polyserositis:* Systemic lupus erythematosus, dengue fever, and sepsis.
  - Severe malabsorption

CLINICAL FEATURES

The clinical hallmark of ascites is abdominal distension, but this may also be caused by other conditions, including gaseous distension, fecal retention, abdominal masses, and obesity. History of generalized and progressively increasing abdominal distension usually suggests ascites. The physical signs suggesting ascites are fullness of flanks, fluid thrill, shifting dullness, and umbilical herniation. Small amount of fluid may be detectable only by ultrasonography.

EVALUATION OF CAUSE

The causes of ascites differ according to whether it is a part of generalized edema or it is the predominant or sole manifestation. When the ascites is disproportionately more in relation to edema, hepatic, peritoneal, or intra-abdominal causes are more likely.

Age: Ascites in a neonate usually suggests urinary ascites or chylous ascites as a cause. In the later neonatal period and infancy, cholestatic syndromes are important causes of ascites.

Clinical evaluation: Findings suggestive of an underlying liver disorder (jaundice, firm hepatomegaly, shrunken liver, cutaneous stigmata) indicate chronic liver disease (with or without portal hypertension) as a cause of ascites. History of contact with tuberculosis and associated pulmonary findings suggest tuberculosis as the cause of ascites. Presence of significant lymph nodes suggests tuberculosis or lymphoma as possible diagnosis.

Ascitic fluid analysis: Diagnostic paracentesis is helpful in delineating the underlying cause of ascites. Serum-ascites albumin gradient (SAAG) is the best single test for classifying ascites into portal hypertensive (SAAG >1.1 g/dL) and non-portal hypertensive (SAAG <1.1 g/dL). Low SAAG ascites is seen with tuberculosis, malignancies, and infections whereas high SAAG ascites is seen with chronic liver disease and when ascites is a part of generalized edema (anasarca).

Ascitic fluid should also be sent for cytologic examination, gram stain, and cultures especially if infection is suspected. A neutrophil count ≥250 cells/mm^3 is highly suggestive of bacterial peritonitis. Lymphocytic pleocytosis is seen with tuberculosis and a predominant polymorphic response is obtained in bacterial peritonitis. Hemorrhagic ascites is seen with pancreatitis, malignancies, and rarely in tuberculosis. Milky fluid is obtained in chylous ascites.

IMAGING AND BIOCHEMISTRY

Ultrasound examination estimates quantity of fluid and is also helpful to diagnose the etiology. Intra-abdominal lymph nodes are enlarged in tuberculosis and lymphoma. Coarsening of hepatic echotexture suggests chronic liver disease. Portal venous Doppler studies may suggest presence of portal hypertension. CT scan of the abdomen may be required to assess intra-abdominal malignancies or cysts.

Liver function tests and ***UGI endoscopy*** are required to assess presence of chronic liver disease and portal hypertension.

Chest X-ray and ***Mantoux** test* are done for assessment of tuberculosis as a cause of ascites.

TREATMENT Ascites

- Low salt diet
- Diuretics such as spironolactone and furosemide
- Intravenous albumin (0.5–1 mg/kg/day) in refractory cases
- Repeated large volume paracentesis with volume expansion to minimize risks of hypovolemia.
- Treatment of the cause:
  - Antitubercular therapy ± steroids for peritoneal tuberculosis
  - Antibiotics if spontaneous bacterial peritonitis is present
  - Treatment of cause of chronic liver disease (e.g., interferons for HBV, HCV; steroids for autoimmune hepatitis)
  - Portal hypertension is controlled by medications (e.g., propranolol) or surgical methods (e.g., portosystemic shunting)
- In liver disease, diuretics as monotherapy or dual therapy and salt restriction form the mainstay of treatment in children with mild to moderate ascites.

Liver transplantation may be the only alternative if hepatic decompensation, cirrhosis, and portal hypertension are present.

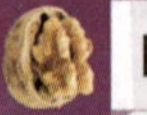

IN A NUTSHELL

Ascites

1. Collection of serous fluid within the peritoneal cavity is termed as ascites.
2. Hepatic, renal, and cardiac diseases are the most common causes of ascites in children.
3. To differentiate transudate from exudates, the preferred method is determination of serum-ascitic albumin gradient.
4. Low salt diet, diuretics, albumin transfusion and treatment of the cause are the mainstay of treatment.

Aithal GP, Palaniyappan N, China L, et al. Guidelines on the management of ascites in cirrhosis. Gut. 2021;70:9-29.
Bavdekar A, Thakur A. Ascites in children. Indian J Pediatr. 2016;83:1334-40.
Karnsakul W, Ingviya T, Seaberg E, et al. Ascites in children: a single-center experience of 27 years. J Pediatr Gastroenterol Nutr. 2017;64:83-8.
Karnsakul W, Wasuwanich P, Ingviya T, et al. Clinical usage of serum albumin to ascitic fluid albumin gradient and ascitic fluid total protein in pediatric ascites. Clin Res Hepatol Gastroenterol. 2021;45(3):101549.
Vadlapudi SS, Srivastava A, Saini N, Sen Sarma M, Poddar U, Yachha SK. Aetiology and diagnostic utility of serum ascites albumin gradient in children with ascites. Dig Liver Dis. 2024;56(9):1537-43.

21.10 Parent Education for Liver Diseases

PE 23.13, PE 23.14

REGARDING THE ILLNESS

- Jaundice is only a symptom (like cough) and not a disease, its level rises in the conditions which affect functioning of liver. There are many causes of the malfunctioning of liver but viral infections are the common cause in children.
- Hepatitis A virus and HEV are common, spread by ingestion of contaminated food and water. In majority the infection is self-limiting and it improves without complications and does not progress to chronicity.
- Hepatitis B virus and HCV are less common, spread by transfusion of infected blood and blood products. Other sources of transmission are the use of injection syringes without disposable needles, tattoos, intravenous drug abuse, earlobe boring, blood transfusions without screening, and mother-to-child transmission. Infection with these two viruses can progress to chronic liver disease, cirrhosis, end-stage liver disease, and liver cancer leading to death.
- Most children with acute viral hepatitis (AVH) can be managed at home, without the need of any investigations. A child with AVH should be hospitalized, if any of the following symptoms are present:
  - Persistent vomiting
  - Swelling of feet
  - Persistent fever
  - Deepening jaundice
  - Poor intake of food
  - Repeated jaundice
  - Drowsiness
  - Severe abdominal pain
  - Decreased urine output
  - Red/black colored vomiting and/or stools
- During the illness there is no restriction on the diet, child can take plenty of liquids, fruits, and home-based regular diet of cereals, fruits, vegetables, and dal depending on the appetite. Improvement of appetite is indicator of convalescence period.
- Use of herbal medications are not safe and there are reports of hepatitis following herbal drugs, better to avoid them.
- ***Follow up:*** Children diagnosed with HAV and HEV infection do not need any follow-up. But children diagnosed with hepatitis B or HCV infection need follow-up to check whether the body has cleared the virus. Biochemical tests such as SGPT and serum glutamic oxaloacetic transaminase (SGOT) are done as surrogate markers to check liver status. Those children who have elevated values even 6 months following illness need further tests to detect hepatitis B surface antigen/HCV RNA detection. Positive reports suggest that development of chronic HBV infection/chronic hepatitis C infection requires evaluation and treatment.

REGARDING THE PREVENTION

Viral hepatitis can be prevented.

Hepatitis A and E: These two viruses are spread by the orofecal route. They can be prevented by following good and strict hygiene and ensuring proper sanitaton. Washing hands before eating, drinking boiled water, taking food from home or in hygienic places, washing hands with soap and water after defecation.

To prevent infections in siblings avoid sharing utensils for eating and drinking. The toilet seat should be cleaned and disinfected before use.

Hepatitis B and C: These two viruses are spread by the parenteral route. They can be prevented by avoiding unnecessary injections using reusable needles, unsafe ear boring, and tattooing, and shared intravenous drug abuse.

Proper screening for hepatitis B and hepatitis C in all blood banks before blood transfusion.

Screening of children born to mothers who are hepatitis B or HCV positive.

Vaccines: Safe and effective vaccines are available for the prevention of hepatitis A and hepatitis B infection.

Rajesh Kumar Meena and Dheeraj Shah

22 CHAPTER Respiratory Disorders

AS PER NMC COMPETENCIES

PE25.1	Describe the etiopathogenesis, clinical features and management of acute otitis media (AOM).	*Ch 22.2*
PE25.2	Describe the etiopathogenesis, clinical features and management of epiglottitis.	*Ch 22.7*
PE25.3	Explain the etiopathogenesis, clinical features and management of acute laryngotracheobronchitis.	*Ch 22.8*
PE25.4	Describe the etiology, clinical features and management of stridor in children.	*Ch 22.6*
PE25.5	Describe the types, clinical presentation, and management of foreign body aspiration in infants and children.	*Ch 22.9*
PE25.6	Describe the etiopathogenesis, diagnosis, clinical features, management and prevention of lower respiratory infections including bronchiolitis, wheeze associated LRTI pneumonia and empyema.	*Ch 22.10, Ch 22.11, Ch 22.12, Ch 22.13, Ch 22.14*
PE28.1	Describe the etiopathogenesis, clinical signs, management and prevention of allergic rhinitis in children.	*Ch 22.5*
PE28.2	Explain the etiopathogenesis, clinical types, presentations, management and prevention of childhood asthma.	*Ch 22.15*
PE28.3	Develop a treatment plan for Asthma appropriate to clinical presentation and severity.	*Ch 22.15*
PE28.4	Enumerate the indications for PFT.	*Ch 22.15*
PE28.5	Observe administration of nebulization.	*Ch 22.15*

Topics available online: ***Examination of Ear, Nose and Throat; Making a Diagnosis in a Child with ENT Symptoms; and Imaging in Respiratory Disorders***

22.1 Anatomy and Physiology of the Respiratory Tract

CLASSIFICATION OF THE RESPIRATORY SYSTEM

- ***Anatomical division:*** The respiratory system can be subdivided into two areas depending on the location within or out of the thorax. The upper respiratory tract includes those structures that are external to the thorax, i.e., the nasal cavity, pharynx, and larynx. The lower respiratory tract includes structures that lie within the thorax. This includes the respiratory tract from trachea downwards.
- ***Functional division:*** The conductive zone does not participate in the gaseous exchange. This area includes the respiratory tract up to the terminal bronchioles. The respiratory zone is where gas exchange takes place. This includes respiratory bronchioles, alveolar ducts, and the alveoli.

STRUCTURE OF THE RESPIRATORY TRACT (FIG. 22.1)

The atmospheric air first enters the nose. The nose consists of a nasal septum and two lateral walls that have three turbinate or conchae. The air then flows into the pharynx. It connects the back of the nostrils to the throat and mouth. Next comes the larynx which is like a sphincter that carries the air from the pharynx into the trachea. The larynx is protected by leaf-like cartilage called epiglottis which prevents the swallowed food and water from entering the respiratory tract. In the middle part of the laryngeal cavity, there is Glottis, which is a V-shaped opening surrounded by the vocal cords. Below the vocal cords lies the subglottic space which down toward the trachea.

Tracheobronchial Tree

The trachea can be surface marked anteriorly from the cricoid cartilage to the sternal angle and posteriorly from the spinous process of the sixth cervical vertebrae to that of the fourth thoracic vertebra. Thereafter, the trachea divides into two main bronchi. The tracheobronchial tree has 23 generations.

- ***Conducting airways:*** This includes the airway up to the terminal bronchioles (i.e., up to the 15–16th generation). As discussed previously, there is no gas exchange here. The volume of air that fills these airways comprises the anatomic dead space. In general, around 30% volume of tidal breath is taken up by these conducting airways (approximately 150 mL in adults).
- ***Gas exchange units (acinus):*** The terminal bronchioles (16th generation) divide into respiratory bronchioles (17–19th generation). These have occasional alveoli on their walls. The respiratory bronchioles further divide into alveolar ducts (20–22nd generation) which are completely lined by alveoli.

Lungs

Lobes: The right lung is anatomically divided into three lobes (upper, middle, and lower) whereas the left lung has only two lobes (upper and lower). However, there is an inferior projection of the left upper lobe which is an anatomically parallel part of right middle lobe.

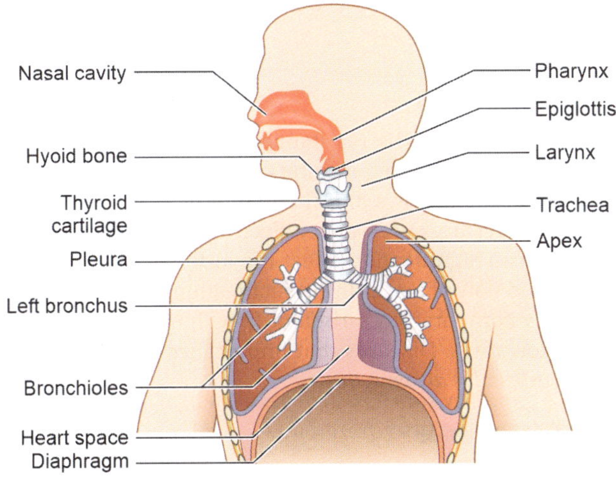

Fig. 22.1: Anatomy of the respiratory tract

Bronchi: In each lobe, the lobar bronchi are divided into segmental or tertiary bronchi. The portion of the lungs supplied by each segmental bronchi and its associated vessel is referred to as a bronchopulmonary segment. There are ten bronchopulmonary segments in each lung. However, in the case of the left lung, some of the segments may fuse together, leading to overall eight or nine segments (**Fig. 22.2**).

Lung parenchyma: It is made up of respiratory bronchioles, alveolar ducts, and alveoli. The alveoli are lined by two types of epithelial cells:

- ***Type I alveolar epithelial cells*** are extremely broad, thin cells that cover about 95% of the alveolar area. They can transport electrolytes (Na^+ and Cl^-), thus contributing to the absorption of fluids from the airways.
- ***Type II alveolar epithelial cells*** are much larger than type I cells, but they occupy only about 5% of the total alveolar area. These cells are involved in the production of surfactant.

Surface Landmarks of Lung and Pleura (Fig. 22.3)

Anterior margin: The anterior margin of the lung is different on each side and corresponds to the parietal pleural reflection. It begins at the apex of the lung on both sides that extend about 3 cm above the medial third of the clavicles. It then descends to the sternoclavicular joint and reaches the fourth costal cartilage on each side. From here, the right pleura continues straight reaching the xiphisternum whereas the left pleura arches out by 3–5 cm and then moves inferiorly to cross the anterior end of the sixth rib (cardiac notch).

Inferior margin: Conventionally, the inferior margin of the lung on both sides lies at the level of T6 in the mid-clavicular line, T8 in the mid-axillary line, and the level of T10 adjacent to the vertebral column. At each of these points, the parietal pleural reflections lie further inferiorly by approximately two ribs, i.e., at the level of T8, T10, and T 12 respectively. Recent data from CT findings have suggested some variations.

Posterior margin: The lung margin moves upward from the tenth thoracic vertebrae to the apex while the pleural margins start a little lower from the twelfth thoracic vertebrae and reach the apex on both sides.

Development of Lung and Respiratory Tract

Lung development begins as early as 3 weeks of gestation. There are five major stages of development, with each stage focused on the growth and development of specific structures (**Fig. 22.4**).

PULMONARY MECHANICS

The lungs maintain adequate oxygen supply to the tissues and remove excess of carbon dioxide from the blood. Various factors can affect this gaseous exchange—the air reaching the alveoli through the respiratory tract, the working of muscles of respiration and rib cage, the nature of alveoli—capillary interface, and neuromuscular control of respiration.

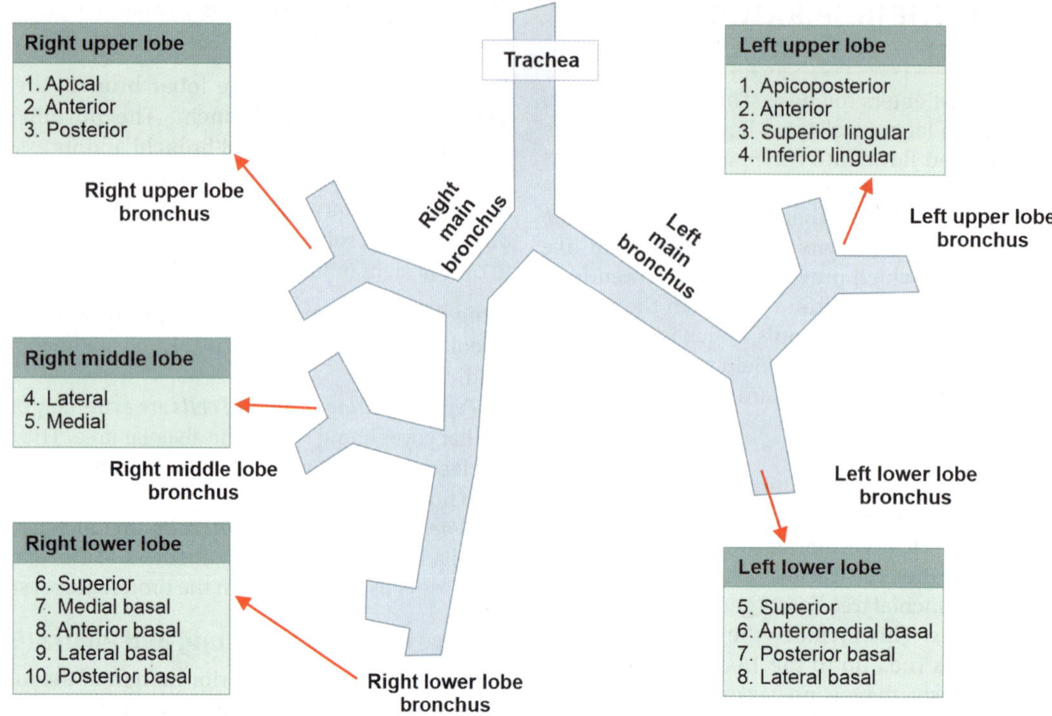

Fig. 22.2: Bronchopulmonary segments

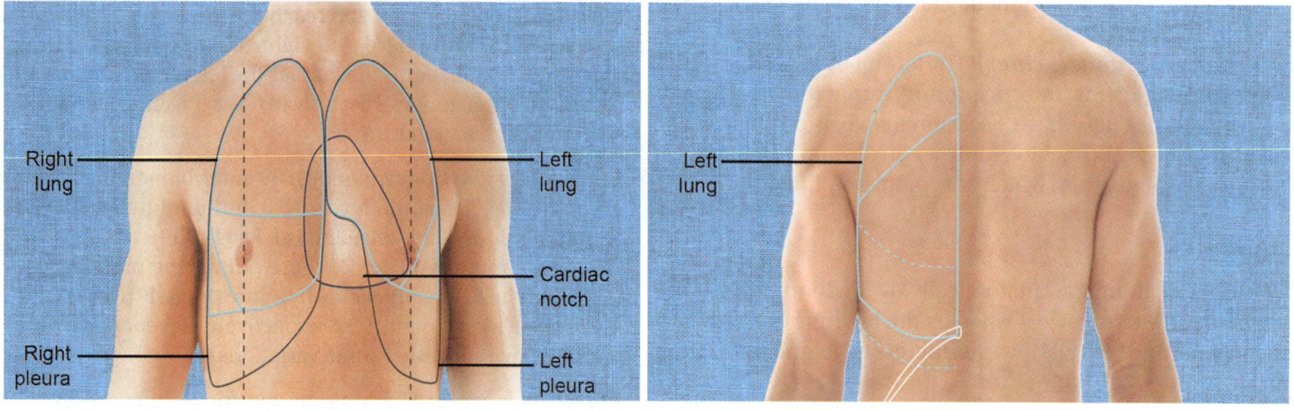

Fig. 22.3: Surface marking of lung and pleura

Inspiration and Expiration

Air enters the lungs when the intrathoracic pressure reaches below the atmospheric pressure. This negative intrathoracic pressure is created by contraction and thereby lowering of diaphragm during inspiration. During exercise and in certain disease states, the accessory muscles of respiration help to raise and enlarge the rib cage. This further increases the pressure difference between the atmosphere and thorax. Exhalation is generally a passive process. The use of certain abdominal and respiratory muscles is limited to active exhalation.

Lung Volumes and Capacities

These are defined and depicted in **Figure 22.5**.

Airway Resistance

Airway resistance is the resistance offered by the respiratory tract to flow of air during inspiration and expiration. Both the diameter of the airways and the nature of airflow have been shown to affect airway resistance. Even a small change in airway diameter can significantly affect the airflow. The laminar or streamlined flow of air during quiet breathing faces less airway resistance compared to turbulent flow that is observed with higher flow rates. Diseases that impact airway resistance are called *obstructive airways disease.*

Lung Compliance

Lung compliance is the measure to which the lungs will expand for each unit change of transpulmonary pressure. Processes

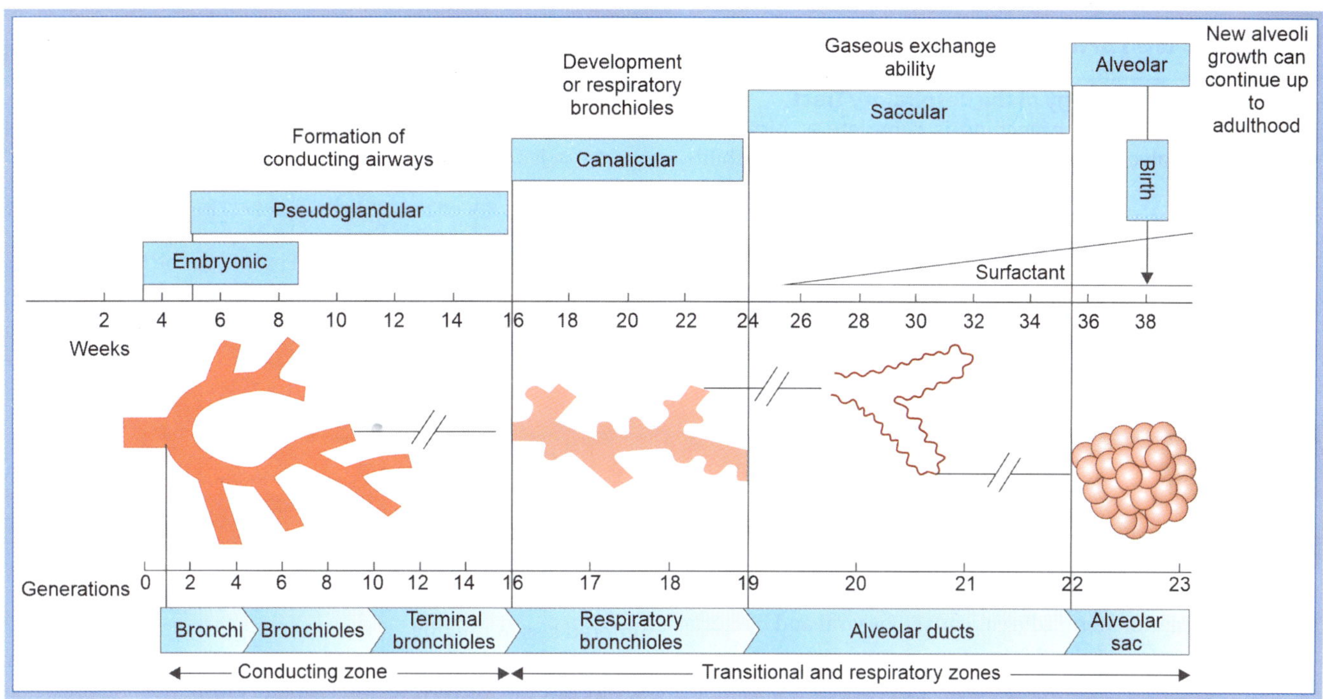

Fig. 22.4: The tracheobronchial tree: Branching and stages of development

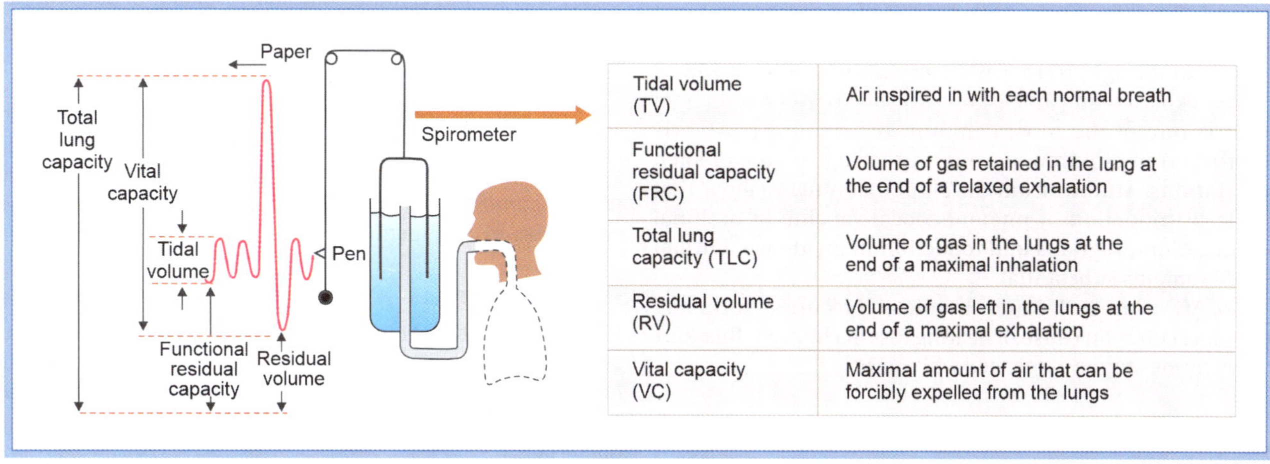

Tidal volume (TV)	Air inspired in with each normal breath
Functional residual capacity (FRC)	Volume of gas retained in the lung at the end of a relaxed exhalation
Total lung capacity (TLC)	Volume of gas in the lungs at the end of a maximal inhalation
Residual volume (RV)	Volume of gas left in the lungs at the end of a maximal exhalation
Vital capacity (VC)	Maximal amount of air that can be forcibly expelled from the lungs

Fig. 22.5: Lung volumes

associated with a decrease in lung compliance may lead to *restrictive lung disease* (such as surfactant deficiency, pulmonary edema, pleural effusion, and respiratory muscle weakness).

Respiratory Gas Exchange

The ventilation of the alveoli, the capillary blood flow to the alveoli, and the diffusion of gases across the alveolar-capillary interface—all can affect the exchange of gases.

The exchange of carbon dioxide is shown to be primarily determined by alveolar ventilation, whereas the transport of oxygen is influenced predominantly by the matching of alveolar ventilation with alveolar blood flow in different lung regions. There are five major disease processes associated with hypoxemia (**Table 22.1**).

Table 22.1 Causes of Hypoxemia

Causes	*Examples*
Ventilation—perfusion mismatch (most common)	Pneumonia, atelectasis, bronchopulmonary dysplasia
Hypoventilation	Neuromuscular diseases, apnea
Shunt	Cyanotic heart diseases, arteriovenous malformations
Low FiO_2	High altitude
Diffusion impairment	Pulmonary fibrosis

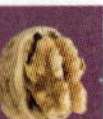

IN A NUTSHELL

Anatomy and Physiology of the Respiratory Tract

1. Even though airway branching is complete at birth, the number of alveoli continue to increase throughout childhood.
2. In obstructive airway disease, the resistance to airflow increases, whereas in restrictive airway disease the pulmonary compliance is reduced.
3. Ventilation-perfusion mismatch is the most important cause of hypoxemia in children.

Albertine KH. Anatomy of the Lungs. In: Broaddus VC, Mason RJ, Ernst JD, King TE, Lazarus SC, Murray, JF, Nadel JA, Slutsky AS, Gotway MB (Eds). Murray and Nadel's Textbook of Respiratory Medicine: Volume 1,2, 7th edition. Elsevier Saunders; 2021. pp. 3-21.

Ochs M, O'Brodovich H. The structural and physiologic basis of respiratory disease. In: Wilmott RW, Chernick V, Boat TF (Eds). Kendig and Chernick's Disorders of the Respiratory Tract in Children, 8th edition. Philadelphia, PA: Elsevier Saunders; 2012. pp. 35-74.

West JB, Luks AM. West's Respiratory Physiology: The Essentials, 11th edition. Baltimore, MD: Lippincott Williams and Wilkins; 2020. pp. 1-30.

22.2 Acute Otitis Media

PE 25.1

INTRODUCTION

Acute middle ear infection or acute otitis media (AOM) is an acute inflammation of middle ear caused by viral and bacterial agents.

EPIDEMIOLOGY

Estimated incidence of AOM worldwide is 11%, translating to around 709 million cases each year. Half of these estimated cases occur in children <5 years of age. AOM is most common in the age group of 6–24 months with almost 75% of children experiencing at least one episode of AOM by school age. It is one of the most common reasons for antibiotic prescription in children, accounting for up to 25% of such prescriptions. Studies from developed countries show that despite introduction of pneumococcal vaccine in national immunization programs and reduction in incidence, burden of AOM remains substantial.

Also, AOM can evolve into chronic and recurrent form and is the most common cause of hearing loss in children. **Box 22.1** defines various terms associated with AOM.

ETIOPATHOGENESIS

Microbiology

Microorganisms isolated from middle ear fluid in children with otitis media include both bacterial and respiratory viruses. The three most common bacterial agents causing AOM include *Streptococcus pneumoniae*, non-typeable *Haemophilus influenzae* and *Moraxella catarrhalis*. *Streptococcus pyogenes*, *Staphylococcus aureus* and gram-negative organisms are encountered less frequently.

S. pneumoniae has been reported to cause early and more severe disease with greater inflammatory response and presentation with high grade fever, more intense otalgia and potential for more complications such as mastoiditis. *H. influenzae* causes less severe disease but is more commonly isolated in bilateral AOM and often associated with concurrent conjunctivitis. *S. aureus* and gram-negative bacteria are found more commonly in neonates and young infants requiring hospitalization.

Viral isolates are frequently found in middle ear fluids in AOM. Most frequently isolated viruses include respiratory syncytial virus, rhinovirus, influenza, adenovirus and human metapneumovirus. These viruses may be found alone or more commonly in conjunction with bacterial pathogens.

Box 22.1 Definition of Terms Associated with Acute Otitis Media (AOM)

- *Uncomplicated AOM:* AOM without otorrhea
- *Severe AOM:* AOM with moderate/severe otalgia or fever ≥39°C
- *Nonsevere AOM:* AOM with mild otalgia and temperature below 39°C
- *Recurrent AOM:* Three or more documented episodes of AOM in preceding 6 months or 4 or more episodes in preceding 12 months with at least one episode in last 6 months

Pathogenesis

Pathogenesis of AOM is multifactorial involving complex interaction between host (anatomical, immunological, and genetic); environment (frequent exposure to viral infection in day care, pollution/smoking, feeding practices) and pathogen (viral/bacterial).

Eustachian tube dysfunction/obstruction either due to preceding viral infection (intraluminal inflammatory obstruction) or other causes such as adenoid hypertrophy (extraluminal obstruction) impairs middle ear drainage causing accumulation of secretions and fluid stasis. Colonization of this fluid with bacterial/viral pathogens leads to AOM.

Risk Factors

Various risk factors, both modifiable and nonmodifiable, have been identified that predispose to development of AOM.

- ***Nonmodifiable risk*** factors include young age, male gender, having siblings in day care, premature birth, atopy, family history of otitis media, underlying immunodeficiency, anatomical factors such as craniofacial abnormalities/cleft palate.

- ❖ ***Modifiable risk factors*** include day care attendance, lack of breastfeeding, bottle feeding, use of pacifiers, exposure to passive smoking/pollutants and obesity.

CLINICAL FEATURES

Symptoms

Acute otitis media is often preceded by a viral upper respiratory tract infection. Presenting symptoms are nonspecific and include cold, fever, irritability and difficult sleeping.

Older children can complain of ear pain and young nonverbal children can manifest otalgia with rubbing/tugging ear. Otalgia can be absent in 50% children <2 years of age and almost 35% of those over 2 years of age. Also, otalgia may just indicate tympanic membrane inflammation due to viral infections. Otalgia of AOM needs to be differentiated from that of otitis externa (pain on movement of tragus and ear canal inflammation).

New onset ear discharge due to tympanic membrane perforation can occur in 15–20% children.

Otoscopic evaluation: As symptoms of AOM are nonspecific, direct observation of tympanic membrane by otoscopy is essential both for diagnosis and defining severity of AOM. Various signs of AOM include signs of TM inflammation: intense hyperemia or yellow color (due to translucency of purulent material in middle ear); middle ear effusion (bulging TM, reduced/absent mobility of TM) and TM perforation (**Figs. 22.6A to D**). **Box 22.2** outlines the essential criteria for diagnosis of AOM. **Box 22.3** outlines the signs that are insufficient for a certain diagnosis of AOM.

TREATMENT Acute Otitis Media

Acute otitis media is a self-limiting infection with most children getting better in 3 days. Antibiotic treatment may hasten the resolution of symptoms but have associated side effects and promote colonization with drug-resistant microbes. Mainstay of AOM treatment is symptomatic treatment for otalgia with or without antibiotics.

- *Pain management:* Adequate pain relief should be provided with either paracetamol (15 mg/kg/dose, up to 4 times daily) or ibuprofen (10 mg/kg/dose up to 3 times daily).
- Topical analgesics/anesthetics/natural extracts: 2022 update of National Institute for Health and Care Excellence (NICE) guidelines recommend topical analgesics/ anesthetics ear drops if immediate oral antibiotic is not given and

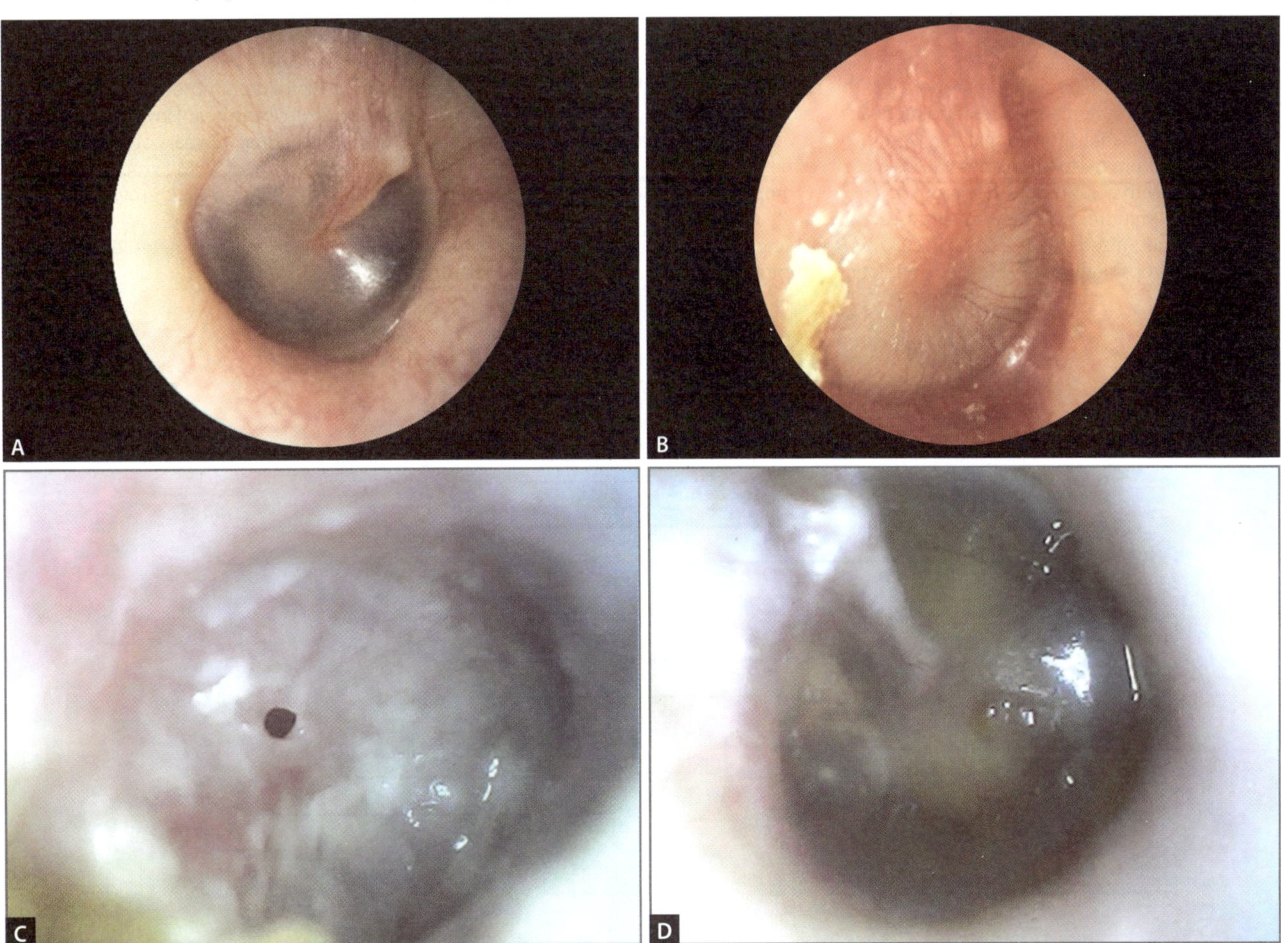

Figs. 22.6A to D: Tympanic membrane (TM) otoscopic view: (A) Normal TM; (B) Congested and bulging TM; (C) Congested TM with perforation and purulent fluid in middle ear/ear canal; (D) Middle ear effusion with amber TM without congestion (otitis media with effusion)

Source: (Figs. A and B) Michael Hawke MD, CC BY 4.0 <https://creativecommons.org/licenses/by/4.0>, via Wikimedia Commons

Box 22.2 Diagnostic Criteria for Acute Otitis Media (AOM)

For a certain diagnosis of AOM, all of the following should be present:

1. Acute onset of symptoms associated with middle ear inflammation (e.g., otalgia, tugging/pulling ear, irritability, disturbed sleep, fever)
2. Signs of tympanic membrane (TM) inflammation (intense hyperemia/yellow color due to collection of purulent material in middle ear)
3. Presence of middle ear effusion (bulging TM/reduced or absent mobility of TM/otorrhea due to TM perforation)

Note: Sole presence of otorrhea (not due to otitis externa) associated with spontaneously perforated TM is a certain objective sign of AOM in itself

Box 22.3 Signs Inadequate for a Certain Diagnosis of Acute Otitis Media (AOM)

1. TM hyperemia alone (frequent finding in URTI, in young children after prolonged crying, following manipulation of ear canal for cerumen removal)
2. Loss of TM landmarks alone
3. TM retraction
4. Air fluid level in middle ear

Points 2 to 4 may point toward otitis media with effusion

(TM: tympanic membrane; URTI: upper respiratory tract infection)

there is no eardrum perforation or otorrhea. This recommendation was based on a systematic review and meta-analysis of randomized controlled trials that showed that in children aged 3 years and over without eardrum perforation, these drops increased the proportion of children with a 50% and a 25% reduction in pain compared with placebo, 10 minutes after having eardrops (low quality evidence). Another randomized controlled trial in children (1–10 years) showed that these drops significantly reduced antibiotic consumption at day 8 compared with usual care, i.e., no or delayed antibiotic prescription (2.6% vs. 29.0%; moderate quality evidence) and were associated with significant reduction in parent-reported pain scores at day 2 (low quality evidence). However, no other guideline recommends topical analgesic/anesthetic ear drops.

- *Antibiotics:* Current guidelines agree on initial observation and delayed antibiotic treatment in children more than 2 years of age with non-severe disease without otorrhea. However, guidelines differ about antibiotic usage in children <2 years of age. **Table 22.2 and Flowchart 22.1** outline treatment of AOM as recommended by Indian Academy of Pediatrics (IAP). **Table 22.3** provides details of antibiotics choice.
- *Other treatments:* There is no role of antihistamines, decongestants (systemic/local), or steroids.

Table 22.2 Indian Academy of Pediatrics (IAP) Guidelines for Management of AOM

Age <2 years	*Age >2 years*
• Adequate analgesia ▪ Paracetamol/ibuprofen ▪ Paracetamol in appropriate dose as good as ibuprofen • Antibiotic in all cases with confirmed diagnosis of AOM irrespective of severity of illness	• Adequate analgesia—mainstay of treatment • *Antibiotics:* ▪ *Severe AOM:* Antibiotics for 7 days ▪ *Nonsevere AOM:* - No urgency to start antibiotics - Wait and watch for 48–72 hours - Start antibiotics if worsening/ nonresolution of symptoms

Note: Severe AOM: severe otalgia not responding to analgesics, high grade fever ≥39°C, and toxic appearance

Flowchart 22.1: Management of acute otitis media

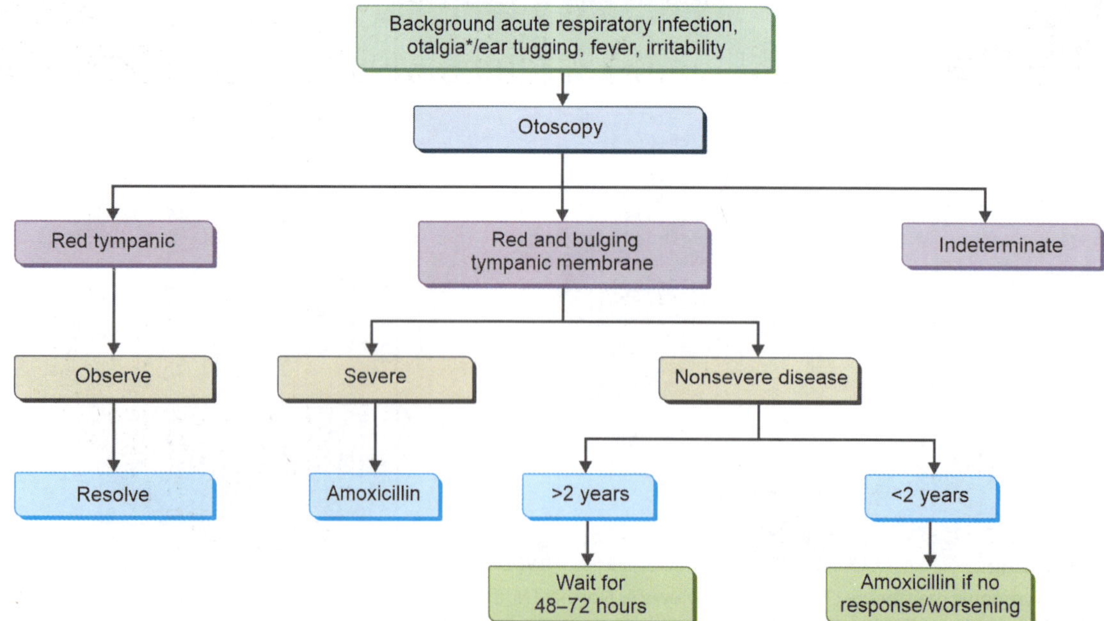

*Severe AOM—severe otalgia not responding to analgesics, high grade fever ≥39°C, toxic appearance

Table 22.3 Antibiotic Selection for AOM as per Indian Academy of Pediatrics (IAP)

Initial management with antibiotics (<2 years, severe AOM in >2 years)[#]	Antibiotics after 48–72 hours of observation (>2 years with nonsevere AOM)[#]	Treatment failure at 48–72 hours after initial management with antibiotics
Amoxicillin (40 mg/kg/day in 3 divided doses)	Amoxicillin (40 mg/kg/day in 3 divided doses)	Amoxicillin-clavulanate* Ceftriaxone**

**Amoxicillin-clavulanate can be used as first-line treatment if child has received amoxicillin in past 30 days or those who have otitis media with conjunctivitis*

**Use Amoxicillin-clavulanate as second line if amoxicillin was used as first-line drug and ceftriaxone if amoxicillin-clavulanate was used as first line

Other alternatives:
- *Type 1 penicillin allergy:* Azithromycin, Clarithromycin, Clindamycin
- *Nontype 1 allergy:* Cefdinir, Cefpodoxime, Cefuroxime

 # Duration of antibiotic treatment:
- Amoxicillin, amoxicillin-clavulanate, oral cephalosporin, clarithromycin and clindamycin: children <2 years—10 days, children >2 years—5–7 days
- Azithromycin—5 days
- Ceftriaxone—one to three doses, depending on symptom persistence

Failure of second-line treatment: Tympanocentesis plus clindamycin

COMPLICATIONS

Complications of AOM may result due to spread of infection to nearby structures or development of chronicity and can be divided as intratemporal or intracranial complications.

Intratemporal Complications

- Infectious dermatitis of external auditory canal
- ***TM perforation:*** Most of the time TM perforation due to AOM heals spontaneously after treatment. Persistent TM perforation beyond 3 months requires referral to ENT specialist for further management
- ***Otitis media with effusion (OME):*** It may occur as a sequel to AOM or due to Eustachian tube dysfunction. It refers to presence of fluid in middle ear and does not represent acute/ongoing infection. It needs to be distinguished from AOM and does not require antibiotic treatment.
- ***Chronic suppurative otitis media (CSOM):*** It refers to persistent middle ear infection and otorrhea through a perforated TM and is diagnosed if there is persistent purulent ear discharge for 2–6 weeks. It may lead to hearing loss and requires referral to ENT specialist for further management.
- ***Others:*** Acute mastoiditis, petrositis, labyrinthitis, facial nerve palsy, and bezold abscess.

Intracranial Complications

- Meningitis
- Epidural abscess, subdural abscess; and brain abscess
- Sigmoid sinus thrombosis

PREVENTION

Preventive strategies for AOM include reduction of modifiable risk factors such as avoiding exposure to passive smoke, limiting exposure to indoor/outdoor pollutants, exclusive breastfeeding for 6 months, discouraging use of pacifiers/bottle feeding, reducing daycare attendance in first year of life, keeping track of body weight, and pneumococcal and influenza vaccination. There is no role of antibiotic prophylaxis, vitamin D supplementation, probiotics, xylitol for prevention or recurrence of AOM.

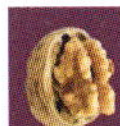

IN A NUTSHELL

Acute Otitis Media

1. Direct observation of tympanic membrane by otoscopy is essential for making accurate diagnosis and starting appropriate management in acute otitis media (AOM).
2. Diagnosis of AOM requires: (i) acute onset of symptoms; (ii) inflammation of tympanic membrane; and (iii) middle ear effusion.
3. Recent onset otorrhea (in absence of otitis externa) associated with TM perforation, alone, is also diagnostic for AOM.
4. Adequate analgesia should be provided by giving adequate doses of paracetamol/ibuprofen.
5. Amoxicillin is the antibiotic of choice for children requiring antibiotics. Children >2 years of age with nonsevere AOM do not require immediate antibiotics.

Chinnappa J, Trivedi C, Dutta S. Acute Otitis Media. In: Remesh Kumar, Vinod Ratageri, Piyush Gupta. IAP Standard Treatment Guidelines. New Delhi. Jaypee Brothers Medical Publishers; 2023.

Hu T, Podmore B, Barnett R, et al. Incidence of acute otitis media in children <16 years old in Germany during 2014–2019. BMC Pediatr. 2022;22:204.

Le Saux N, Robinson JL. Canadian Pediatric Society, Infectious Diseases and Immunization Committee. Management of acute otitis media in children six months of age and older. Paediatr Child Health. 2016;21(1):39-50.

Mohanty S, Podmore B, Cuñado Moral A, et al. Incidence of acute otitis media from 2003 to 2019 in children ≤17 in England. BMC Public Health. 20213;23:201.

National Institute for Health and Care Excellence. Otitis media (acute): antimicrobial prescribing. NICE guidelines [NG91]. London: NICE; 2018. Last updated: 11 March 2022

Ovnat Tamir S, Shemesh S, Oron Y, et al. Acute Otitis Media guidelines in selected developed and developing countries: uniformity and diversity. Arch Dis Child. 2017;102:450-7.

Suzuki HG, Dewez JE, Nijman RG, Yeung S. Clinical practice guidelines for acute otitis media in children: a systematic review and appraisal of European national guidelines. BMJ Open. 2020;10(5):e035343.

22.3 Approach to a Child with Upper Respiratory Symptoms

INTRODUCTION

Respiratory disorders are very common cause of significant mortality and morbidity in the pediatric age group. Respiratory tract infection (RTI) such as rhinitis or common cold, sore throat, cough, and sinusitis are frequent cause for the hospital visit. Most of them are caused by viruses and are self-resolving. A careful history and examination are vital in making diagnoses and approaches to disorders of the upper respiratory tract.

For example: *History taking in a child with a cough*

- ***Duration:*** Persistent productive cough can be a sign of bronchiectasis
- ***Onset:*** Acute in URTI, foreign body aspiration. Chronic in CHF, asthma, pertussis
- ***Character:*** Dry irritating suggestive of pharyngeal etiology while harsh, repetitive with stridor suggestive of laryngeal etiology. Ask about the diurnal and postural variation of cough.
- Enquire about the associated symptoms such as wheeze, breathlessness, fever.

CONGENITAL ABNORMALITIES OF THE UPPER RESPIRATORY TRACT

- ***Choanal atresia:***
  - Due to persistent buccopharyngeal membrane and can be unilateral or bilateral.
  - The newborn with bilateral choanal atresia presents with severe breathing difficulty and cyanosis, which is relieved by crying.
  - The screening for choanal atresia should be done in all newborns. The failure of passage of nasogastric tube down through the nose is diagnostic clue.
  - The CT scan and nasal endoscopy may help for confirmation and assessment of disease severity.
- ***Laryngomalacia:***
  - It is one of the common congenital anomalies of the larynx which is associated with collapse of the supraglottic structures during inspiration.
  - Laryngomalacia manifests with intermittent low-pitched, inspiratory stridor, during the early neonatal period.
  - The loudness of stridor is high during initial 3–8 months of age and resolves by 11–18 months.
  - It is confirmed with flexible fiberoptic laryngoscopy.
  - The management depends upon the severity. In most of the healthy children, laryngomalacia is resolves spontaneously.
- ***Tracheomalacia:***
  - Tracheomalacia refers to diffuse or seg mental tracheal weakness that results in amplified widening during inspiration and luminal narrowing during expiration.
  - Clinical manifestations are dyspnea, cough, and sputum retention. Wheezing or stridor may also exist.
  - In a suspected child, we need to do the dynamic CT and bronchoscopy with forced exhalation maneuvers to evaluate the degree of tracheomalacia. Both tests are necessary because either test alone may underestimate the degree of tracheomalacia.
  - Asymptomatic patients generally do not require therapy, whereas therapy may be warranted for symptomatic patients.
- ***Hemangioma of airways:***
  - The abnormal vessels can obstruct the larynx and manifest as stridor.
  - Diagnosis by direct evaluation by bronchoscope.
  - There are various invasive (surgical removal of the lesion) and noninvasive treatment options (laser therapy) are available.

COMMON UPPER RESPIRATORY TRACT INFECTIONS

Upper respiratory tract infections (URTIs) can be secondary to viral (majority of the cases) or bacterial etiology. The common clinical conditions are common cold, acute pharyngitis and tonsillitis, acute otitis media (AOM), and acute sinusitis. The incidence is low in older children, and it reaches its peak between 1 and 5 years of age.

Majority of the URTIs in children are due to underlying viral infections which requires only analgesic/antipyretic medications (**Table 22.4**).

Evaluation of Upper Respiratory Tract Infection

Choice of therapy should made after proper clinical evaluation. The evaluation aims at the following:

- Ensuring an accurate diagnosis
- Assessing disease severity
- Identifying complications
- To rule out the severe conditions such as pneumonia, and sometimes bacterial infections (e.g., meningitis and sepsis)

Investigations in Upper Respiratory Tract Infection

The complete blood count (CBC) may be normal in most of cases associated with viral infection. Lymphocytosis, lymphopenia and atypical lymphocytes may be seen in some viral infection. If child has epistaxis, we must look for thrombocytopenia in CBC.

Blood investigations such as blood culture, ESR, and CRP are not recommended routinely during OPD visits. ASO titers are not recommended routinely. It is good to do the blood culture in a hospitalized child.

Throat culture is a gold standard for streptococcal pharyngitis. Negative throat culture has a very high negative predictive value. However positive results do not distinguish between infection

Table 22.4 Etiology and Symptoms of Common Upper Respiratory Tract Infections

	Common cold	*Pharyngitis and tonsillitis*	*Acute bacterial sinusitis*	*Acute otitis media*
Viruses	• Rhinoviruses • Influenza • Parainfluenza • RSV • Coronaviruses	• Rhinoviruses • Influenza • Parainfluenza • RSV • Coronaviruses • HSV types 1 and 2 • Epstein-Barr virus • Cytomegalovirus • Coxsackievirus		• Rhinoviruses • Influenza • Parainfluenza • *Enteroviruses* • Rhinoviruses • Cytomegalovirus • Adenovirus
Bacteria		• Group A *Streptococcus* • Anaerobes • Diphtheria	• *Pneumococcus* • Nontypeable *Haemophilus* • Group A *Streptococcus*	• *Pneumococcus* • Nontypeable *Haemophilus* • Group A *Streptococcus*
Symptoms	Fever—more common in young children and usually only short-lived (2 or 3 days) at the start of the illness. The persistent fever is unusual, and requires prompt reassessment and suspicion of secondary bacterial infection	• Tender lymph node enlargement and lymphadenitis • Fever • Conjunctivitis • Scarlet fever rash or viral exanthema	• Persistent fever • Purulent nasal discharge • Facial tenderness and periorbital edema may be present	• Unilateral or bilateral erythematous bulging tympanic membranes • Fever • Purulent aural discharge
Typical duration in children	<10 days	7–10 days	14–21 days	4–5 days

and carriage. *Rapid antigen detection tests* have good specificity but poor sensitivity.

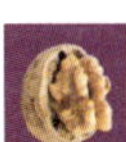

IN A NUTSHELL

Approach to a Child with Upper Respiratory Symptoms

1. Upper respiratory tract infection (URTI) such as common cold or rhinitis, sore throat, cough, and sinusitis are frequent cause for the hospital visit.
2. Differentiating URTI due to viral or bacterial etiology is important to prevent the unnecessary antibiotics use.
3. The screening for choanal atresia should be done in all newborns soon after birth.

Ministry of Health & Family Welfare Government of India. (2016). Management of common Respiratory Infections in Children in India [The Clinical Establishments (Registration and Regulation) Act, 2010]. [online] Available from: https://clinicalestablishments.mohfw.gov.in/ [Last accessed August, 2025].

Nagaraju K, Shah R, Ganapathy S, et al. Practical Approach for the Diagnosis, Prevention, and Management of Recurrent Upper Respiratory Tract Infection in Children: Report from an Expert Closed-group Discussion. Pediatr Inf Dis. 2021;3(3):105-12.

Short S, Bashir H, Marshall P, et al. Institute for Clinical Systems Improvement. Diagnosis and Treatment of Respiratory Illness in Children and Adults. ICSI; 2017. pp. 1-77.

22.4 Nasopharyngitis and Tonsillopharyngitis

NASOPHARYNGITIS

Nasopharyngitis is the inflammation of the nasal passages and the pharynx, or throat. It is another name for the common cold and manifests as mild infection. It is estimated to occur an average of 2-5 times for adults and 6-10 times for children each year in the general healthy population.

Etiology

More than 200 viruses can cause nasopharyngitis. Rhinovirus is the most common cause and accounts for 10–40% of colds followed by coronaviruses (10–15% of colds) and influenza viruses (5–15% of colds). Other cold viruses such as respiratory syncytial virus are responsible for much flu-like illness. Parainfluenza, Adenovirus, Coxsackievirus A and Human Metapneumovirus are other causative agents.

Pathogenesis

The symptoms of URTIs are triggered in response to the viral infection of the upper airway and immune response to infection rather than damage to the airway. The surface of the macrophage exhibits toll-like receptors that combine with the components of the virus and trigger the production of cytokines. The cytokines act to recruit other immune cells, trigger inflammation, and generate systemic symptoms such as fever. A complex mix of proinflammatory cytokines and mediators are released with bradykinin leading to local symptoms like sore throat and nasal congestion; and cytokines leading to systemic symptoms.

Clinical Features

After the virus enters the body, symptoms start within 1–3 days. Typical symptoms include sneezing, runny or stuffy nose, sore throat, and coughing. Affected children may also experience mild fever, headache, weakness, and joint pain.

Postnasal drip may develop due to rhinitis that causes fluid to flow from the sinus system through the back of the nose down to the back of the throat. The fluid causes causing throat congestion, sore throat, cough, and itching in throat. Nasopharyngitis can also cause diarrhea and vomiting.

Course of the Disease

It is usually a self-limiting disease with symptoms lasting for 10–14 days. Cough may continue up to 2–3 weeks. Fever, if present, generally lasts only 24–48 hours.

The nasopharyngitis virus can affect a child's sinuses, throat, bronchial passages, and ears leading to secondary complications like otitis media, sinusitis, and exacerbation of asthma. Secondary infections include pneumonia, croup, and bronchiolitis may also follow, rarely.

TREATMENT Nasopharyngitis

Treatment is symptomatic. There is no role of antibiotics or antivirals. Paracetamol may help in discomfort due to fever. There is no proven role of vitamin C, zinc, garlic, etc. Decongestants can adversely affect blood pressure and thyroid disease. Aspirin may cause Reye syndrome, so best avoided. Warm fluids may help.

Prevention

Children can reduce their likelihood of catching a cold by washing the hands frequently, staying away from the sick, and avoid touching the mouth, eyes, and nose with unwashed hands.

Affected children can lower the risk of transmitting the cold to others by staying at home; moving away from people before coughing or sneezing; avoiding close contact with others, such as hugging or shaking hands; sneezing or coughing into a tissue and then throwing it away; and washing the hands after sneezing or coughing.

TONSILLOPHARYNGITIS

Tonsillopharyngitis is characterized by fever, sore throat, and tonsillar or pharyngeal exudates.

Etiopathogenesis

In children younger than 2 years, most pharyngitis is of viral origin. In older children, Group A beta hemolytic streptococci (GABHS) are the most common cause. The peak prevalence of GABHS pharyngitis is in children 5–10 years. Untreated GABHS pharyngitis may lead to rheumatic fever. Common causes of tonsillopharyngitis in children are listed in **Table 22.5**.

Table 22.5 Etiology of Tonsillopharyngitis in Children

Causes	*Organisms*
Viral pharyngitis	*Enterovirus*, SARS-CoV-2, adenovirus, Epstein-Barr virus (EBV), herpes simplex virus types 1 and 2 (HSV 1 and 2), influenza A and B, *Cytomegalovirus* (CMV)
Bacterial pharyngitis	Group A beta-hemolytic *Streptococcus* (GABHS), *Fusobacterium necrophorum* and other anaerobic bacteria, *Neisseria gonorrhoeae*, group C and G *Streptococcus*, *Arcanobacterium haemolyticum*, *Mycoplasma pneumoniae*, *Chlamydia pneumoniae*, *Francisella tularensis*, *Corynebacterium diphtheriae*

Group A Beta-hemolytic Streptococcus Tonsillopharyngitis (GABHS)

Group A beta-hemolytic streptococci, are the most common cause of bacterial pharyngitis in children and adolescents. Most cases occur in winter. Spread among close contacts is frequent.

Clinical Features

Transmission of GABHS results from contact with respiratory tract secretions of infected individuals. The incubation period is 2–5 days. During this time the infection can be transmitted to others.

Symptoms include throat pain, fever, headaches, and chills. Other symptoms are abdominal pain, nausea, and vomiting. Children with GABHS sore throat do not present with cough, coryza, or conjunctivitis which are specific for viral infection. In older children it has an abrupt onset with fever, sore throat, headache, abdominal pain, nausea, and vomiting.

Examination findings include exudative tonsillopharyngitis, enlarged erythematous tonsils, enlarged tender anterior cervical lymph nodes, palatal petechiae, and inflamed uvula.

Most cases of GAS pharyngitis resolve without complications.

Serious nonsuppurative and suppurative complications may occur if left untreated.

Complications

- ***Nonsuppurative complications:*** Acute rheumatic fever, rheumatic heart disease, poststreptococcal glomerulonephritis and pediatric autoimmune neuropsychiatric disorders associated with *Streptococcus* (PANDAS).
- ***Suppurative complications:*** Necrotizing fasciitis, bacteremia, peritonsillar abscess, and retropharyngeal abscess, sinusitis, mastoiditis, and otitis media.

Timely and appropriate treatment of GABHS in children is essential to prevent suppurative/nonsuppurative complications, especially acute rheumatic fever. It also helps in preventing disease transmission and reducing the duration and severity of symptoms.

Diagnosis

Throat Culture

Culture of a specimen obtained by throat swab is required for the microbiologic confirmation of Group A streptococcal pharyngitis. If taken appropriately, a single throat swab has a sensitivity of 90–95% in detecting Group A streptococci.

Obtain the throat swab specimen by vigorous swabbing of both tonsils and posterior pharynx. Avoid touching the tongue or oropharynx to avoid contamination. Even with appropriately collected specimens, false-negative results may be obtained if patient receives antibiotics prior to specimen collection.

Culture of the diphtheria bacilli from the swab obtained from the larynx or the pharynx is necessary for confirmation of pharyngeal diphtheria.

Rapid Antigen Detection Tests

Rapid antigen detection tests (RADTs) have been developed for the identification of Group A streptococci directly from throat swabs, as throat swab cultures are time consuming with delays in diagnosis. This rapid identification and treatment can reduce the spread of Group A streptococci and speed up clinical improvement. Currently available RADTs have specificity of 95% or greater as compared to cultures; the sensitivity varies between 80 and 90%. Enzyme immunoassays are better than latex agglutination tests.

Streptococcal antibody tests such as anti-streptolysin O (ASO) and antideoxyribonuclease B (anti-DNase B) have no role in the diagnosis or treatment of acute streptococcal pharyngitis as these reflect past and not present immunologic events. It takes several weeks for them to become positive.

Newer Tests

Molecular tests based on PCR and nucleic acid amplification techniques are widely available for etiology testing. Many respiratory pathogen panels including combination of viruses, bacteria, etc., are available are popular. High sensitivity, higher costs and inability to differentiate carrier and commensals with pathogens are limitations of routine use of these tests.

TREATMENT Acute Pharyngitis

Specific Treatment

Antimicrobial therapy is indicated for documented streptococcal infection, either by throat culture or RADT. Early initiation of antimicrobial therapy results in shortening of the clinical course of illness. The goals of pharmacotherapy are to reduce the morbidity and to prevent complications. A 10-day treatment with penicillin is the preferred option. Amoxicillin is a widely used alternative. Therapeutic options are detailed below:

1. *Oral penicillin V children:* 250 mg twice or thrice daily for 10 days.
2. *Oral amoxicillin* 30–40 mg/kg/day for 10 days.
3. *Intramuscular single dose benzathine penicillin G* 1.2 mU (patients >27 kg); 0.6 mU (patients <27 kg).
4. *Oral erythromycin* 40–50 mg/kg/day for 10 days.
5. *Oral azithromycin* 12 mg/kg/day once a day for 5 days.
6. *Oral cephalexin* 50 mg/kg/day for 10 days.

Pharyngeal diphtheria requires oral or parenteral penicillin for 14 days along with administration of antitoxin. Three negative cultures at 24-hour intervals should be obtained before the patient is declared free of the organism. Bedrest for 2–3 weeks is recommended for all patients to reduce the risk of cardiac complications.

Treatment for viral pharyngitis is mainly supportive.

Supportive Management

Warm fluids or gargling may have a soothing effect on the throat. Antipyretics (paracetamol 15 mg/kg/dose) and analgesics are used for relief of pain or pyrexia. First generation antihistaminics; i.e., chlorpheniramine, and promethazine may relieve rhinorrhea by 25–30% due to anticholinergic action. Routine use of cough suppressants (dextromethorphan, codeine) and expectorants (guaifenesin, ammonium citrate, and ambroxol, etc.) is of no value and may be harmful.

RECURRENT STREPTOCOCCAL PHARYNGOTONSILLITIS

Recurrence of tonsillitis requires the management of each episode as an acute episode. Tonsillectomy is indicated only under the following circumstances:

1. More than 7 episodes of tonsillitis in last 1 year (*true bacterial tonsillitis and not mere sore throat or URI*) *or* 5 or more episodes per year over a 2-year period.
2. Enlarged tonsils that create significant upper airway obstruction.
3. An abscess in the tonsils.

Following tonsillectomy, the incidence of pharyngitis is reduced significantly for 1–2 years.

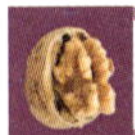

IN A NUTSHELL

Pharyngitis

1. Self-limiting viral infections are the most common cause of upper respiratory infections. Group A *Streptococcus* (GAS) is the most common bacterial cause of acute pharyngitis.
2. Clinical distinction between viral and bacterial etiology of pharyngitis is difficult.
3. Throat swab culture and rapid diagnostic tests are recommended if there is clinical suspicion of GAS pharyngitis.
4. Penicillin (for 10 days) is the first-line treatment of GAS pharyngitis.
5. Antibiotics given within 9 days of onset of symptoms can prevent acute rheumatic fever.

Alderaro A, Buttrini M, Farina B, et al. Respiratory Tract Infections and Laboratory Diagnostic Methods: A Review with A Focus on Syndromic Panel-Based Assays. Microorganisms. 2022;10(9):1856.

Hedin K, Thorning S, van Driel ML. Different antibiotic treatments for group A streptococcal pharyngitis. Cochrane Database Syst Rev. 2023;11(11):CD004406.

Kenealy T, Arroll B. Antibiotics for the common cold and acute purulent rhinitis. Cochrane Database Syst Rev. 2013;6:CD000247.

Krüger K, Töpfner N, Berner R, et al. Guideline group. Clinical Practice Guideline: Sore Throat. Dtsch Arztebl Int. 2021;118:188-94.

Multifaceted Pediatric Infection Cycles. Influenza Other Respir Viruses. 2024;18(11):e70037.

Mustafa Z, Ghaffari M. Diagnostic Methods, Clinical Guidelines, and Antibiotic Treatment for Group A Streptococcal Pharyngitis: A Narrative Review. Front Cell Infect Microbiol. 2020;10:563627.

22.5 Allergic Rhinitis

PE 28.1

INTRODUCTION

Allergic rhinitis (AR) or hay fever is one of most common allergic diseases worldwide, caused by an IgE-mediated inflammation to outdoor or indoor allergens (such as house dust mites, pollens, cockroaches, fungus, pets, etc.). In India, the burden of allergic rhinitis constitutes about 55% of all allergies, most of which are underdiagnosed and undertreated.

Allergic rhinitis not only troubles the nose, but may also affect the sinuses, speech, CNS function, cognitive ability and constitutional issues such as behavior, irritability, anger, sleep, lethargy, fatigue and school performance.

Around 40% of allergic rhinitis cases progress to asthma and around 80% of asthmatics have concurrent AR. Effective and adequate treatment can improve their quality of life (QoL).

DEFINITION

Allergic rhinitis is defined as type 1 hypersensitivity inflammation of nasal mucosa, induced by exposure to allergenic substance, having at least two cardinal nasal symptoms (sneezing, nasal congestion, nasal pruritus, and rhinorrhea) present for >1 hour per day for ≥2 weeks in a year.

CLASSIFICATION

Based Upon Duration

- ***Intermittent:*** Symptoms will appear at irregular intervals (<4 days/weeks and/or <4 consecutive weeks)
- ***Persistent:*** Symptoms will continue to exist over a prolonged period (>4 days/weeks and >4 consecutive weeks)

Based Upon Severity

- ***Mild:*** Normal sleep; no impairment of daily activities, sports, attending school/work; no bothersome symptoms
- ***Moderate to severe:*** Disturbed sleep pattern; impairment of daily activities, sports and absence from school/work; some bothersome symptoms

Based Upon Symptoms

- ***Runners:*** Running nose is the predominant symptom
- ***Sneezers:*** Sneezing is the predominant symptom
- ***Blockers:*** Nose block is the predominant symptom

Based Upon Occurrence

- ***Seasonal:*** Symptoms predominant during one specific season (summer/rainy/winter)
- ***Perennial:*** Symptoms present throughout the year on most days
- ***Perennial with seasonal exacerbations:*** Symptoms present throughout the year and becoming severe in one specific season

ETIOPATHOGENESIS

The innate or nonspecific immune system of our body is the first line of defense against any microbial pathogens by detecting the molecules (e.g., lipopolysaccharides, peptidoglycans, flagellins, etc.) on the surface of microbes known as pathogen-associated molecular patterns (PAMPs) with help of pattern recognition receptors (PRRs). Allergic rhinitis is a type I (immediate) hypersensitivity reaction to allergen cascading the mechanism through PAMPs and T cells [decrease in Th1 (protective) and increase in Th2 (proallergic) response]. In PAMP deficient children, there is more Th2 expressions as compared to Th1, ultimately resulting in allergy **(Flowcharts 22.2A and B)**.

Flowcharts 22.2A and B: Pathogenesis of allergic rhinitis in (A) PAMP rich child; (B) PAMP deficient child

A. In a PAMPs rich child

On first exposure, allergen enters nasal epithelium by APC#
↓
Allergen then transported by APC to naïve T cell
↓
Release of IL-2, IL-12, IFN-α and naïve T cell converted to Th1
↓
Immunological tolerance develops by release of IL-10 and IFN-γ
↓
No reaction during second exposure of same allergen

B. In a PAMPs deficient child

On first exposure, allergen enters the nasal epithelium by APC#
↓
Allergen then transported by APC to naïve T cell
↓
Release of IL-4 and naïve T cell converted to Th2
↓
Th2 cell converted into B (plasma) cell and releases IL-4, IL-5, IL-13 and TNF-α
↓
B cell secrets IgE in response to the allergen which attaches on the surface of mast cell
↓
On second exposure with same allergen, it directly binds with attached IgE on surface of mast cell
↓
This Ag–Ab interaction leads to degranulation of mast cells resulting in release of histamine which causes clinical manifestations of AR

(APC: antigen presenting cells; IL: interleukin; IFN: interferon; PAMP: pathogen-associated molecular patterns)

CLINICAL FEATURES

Symptoms are listed in **Table 22.6**. Signs are pictorially depicted in **Table 22.7**. Differentiating features of allergic rhinitis and common cold are shown in **Table 22.8**.

DIAGNOSIS

- Mostly clinical; investigations are needed only for support where history is inconclusive
- Eosinophil count >4% in peripheral smear (poor marker) and >10% in nasal smear (Hansel stain)
- Absolute eosinophil count >400/mm^3 and total eosinophil count >1,500/mm^3 is indicative but may not be useful
- Total IgE is nonspecific (>100 IU/mL indicative of possible atopic condition)
- Skin prick test (SPT) with standardized allergen extracts

Table 22.6 Symptoms of Allergic Rhinitis

Cardinal symptoms	*Associated symptoms*	*Other symptoms*
1. Sneezing 2. Nasal congestion 3. Nasal pruritus 4. Rhinorrhea	1. Hyposmia/anosmia 2. Snoring 3. Aural congestion or pruritus 4. Sore throat/halitosis 5. Headache 6. Cognitive impairment	1. Ocular/pharyngeal pruritus 2. Wheezing/cough 3. Nasal stifling 4. Sleep difficulty 5. Fatigue
Psychosocial symptoms		
1. Tiredness 2. Depression 3. Embarrassment		

Table 22.7 Signs of Allergic Rhinitis

Sign	*Location*
Allergic shiners	Bluish-black discolorations under lower lid

Looks like

Sign	*Location*
Allergic line	Dark line between cartilaginous and bony septum

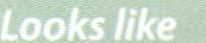

Looks like

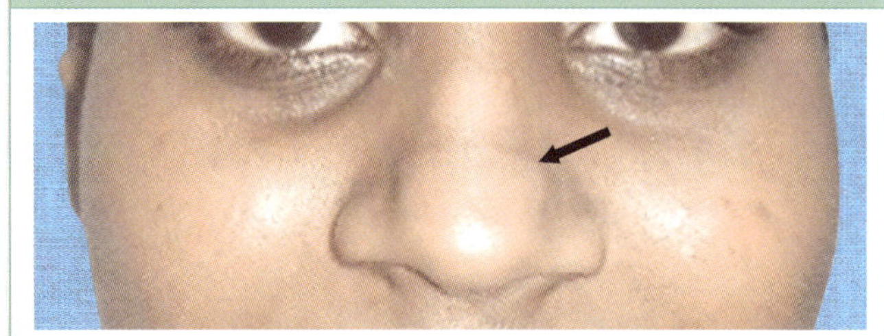

Sign	*Location*
Dennie Morgan folds	Creases in lower eyelid

Looks like

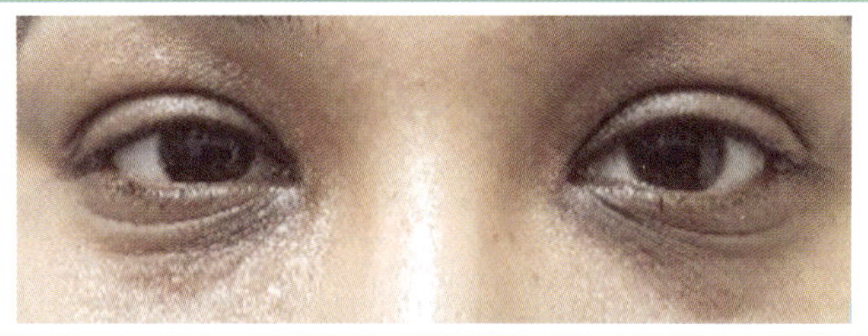

Sign	*Location*
Allergy mannerism	Facial grimaces like nose and mouth wrinkling

Looks like

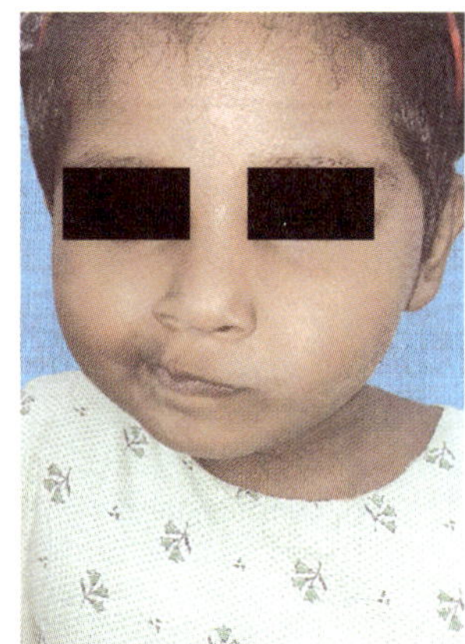

Sign	*Location*
Allergy salute	Done to relieve itching and free the edematous turbinate from septum

Looks like

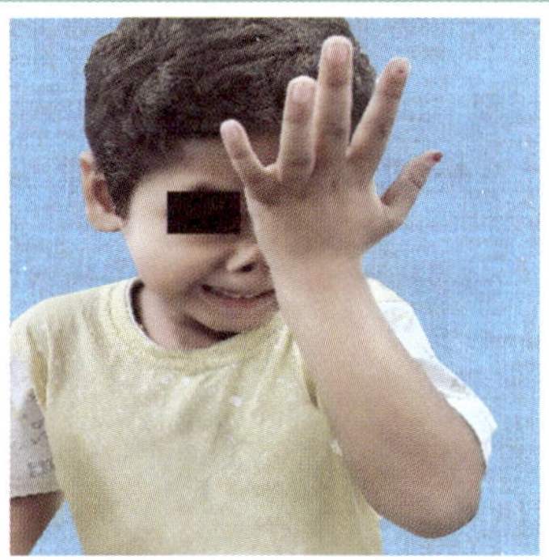

Contd...

Contd...

Sign	Location
Cobble stoning of oropharynx	Follicular hypertrophy in posterior pharyngeal wall
Looks like	
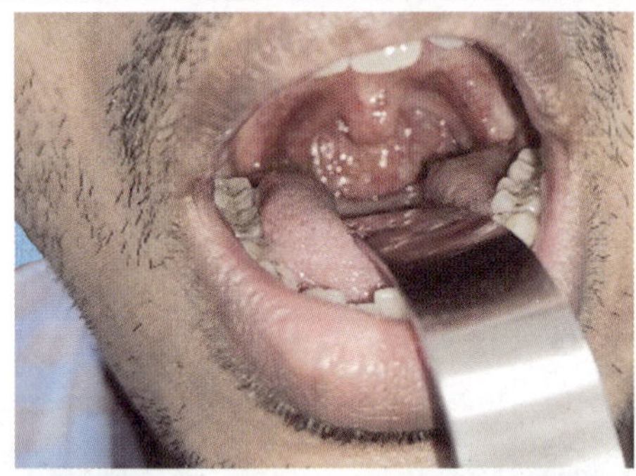	
Sign	**Location**
Allergic conjunctivitis	Redness of eyes due to histamine induced conjunctival vasodilation
Looks like	
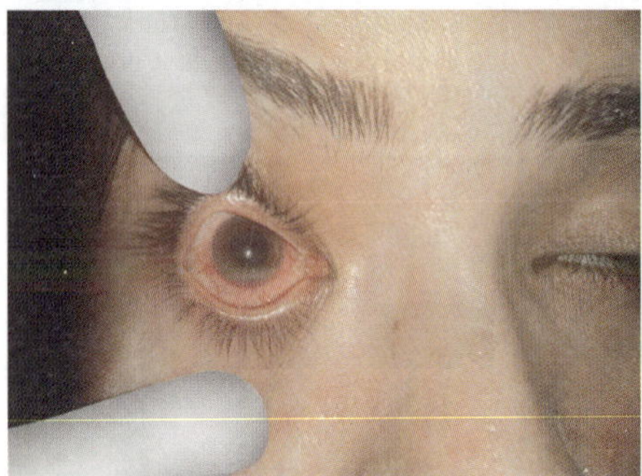 *Courtesy:* Dr Payal Gupta	
Sign	**Location**
Ear fingering	Manipulating the external auditory canal to relieve the Eustachian tubal block
Looks like	
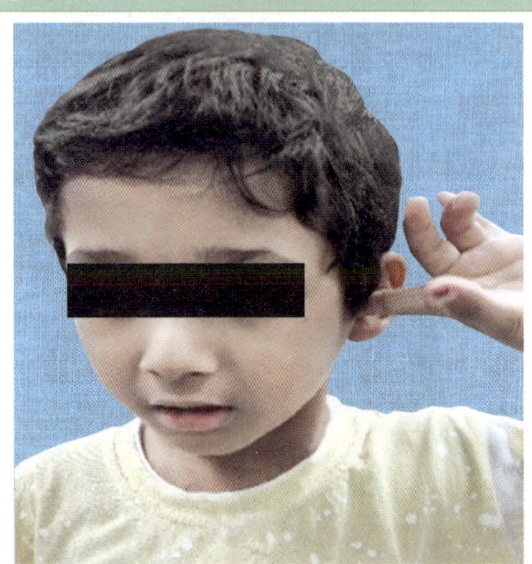	

Contd...

Contd...

Sign	Location
Hypertrophied inferior turbinates	Enlarged and externally visible inferior turbinates
Looks like	
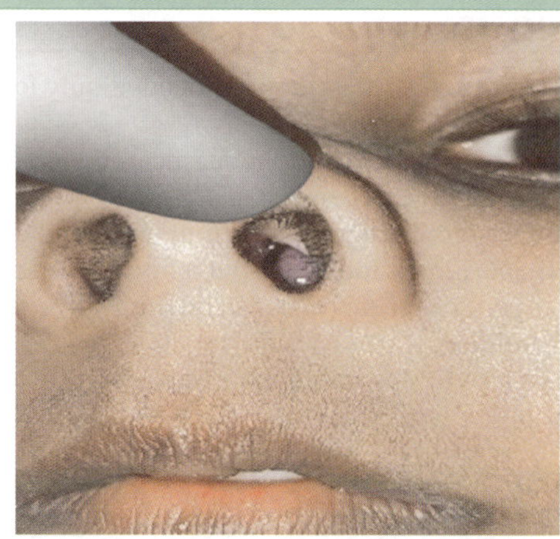	
Sign	**Location**
Allergy gape	Due to nasal block, the child will breathe by mouth
Looks like	
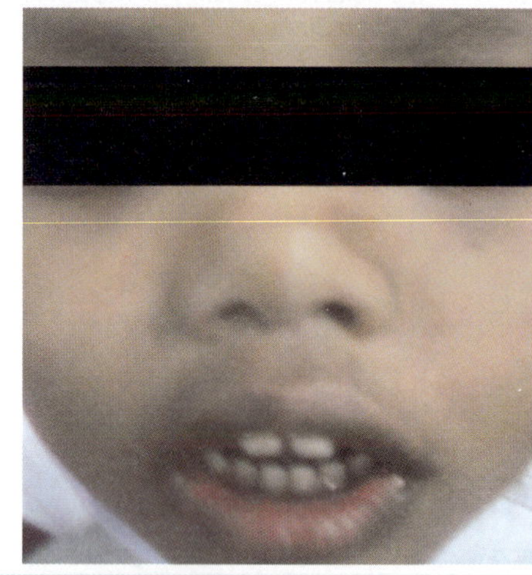	
Sign	**Location**
Enlarged tonsils	Lymphoid hypertrophy at oropharynx
Looks like	
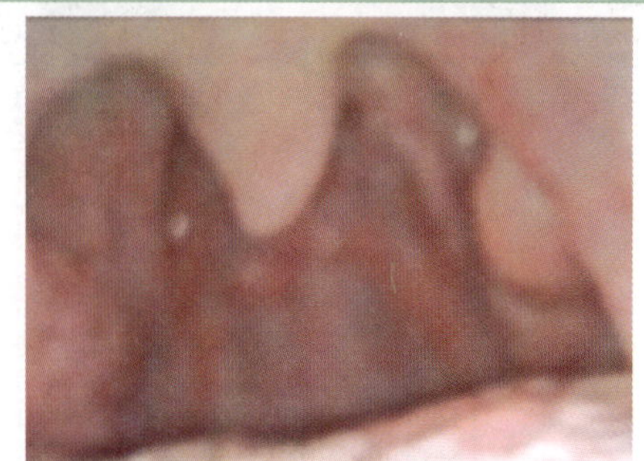	

Contd...

Contd...

Sign	*Location*
Atopic dermatitis	Dry, itchy and scaly skin over flexural aspects of extremities
Looks like	
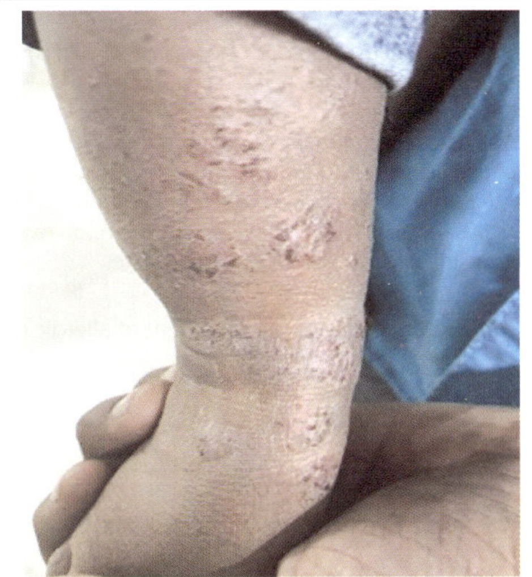	
Sign	*Location*
Urticaria	Wheal with rash with itching on body surface
Looks like	
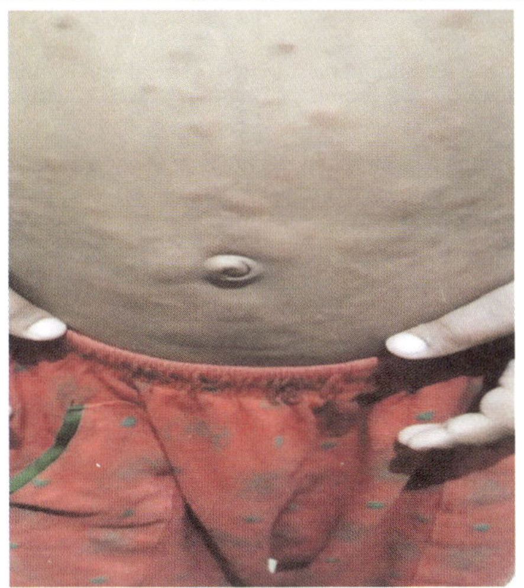	
Respiratory sounds associated with allergic rhinitis	
Clearing of throat	Sound as if there is something in the throat and patient is trying to clear it
Allergic click	Between roof of pharynx and tongue due to itching
Sniffling	Breathing quickly and repeatedly through nose, like crying
Hypernasality of voice	Voice seems to come from nose (nasal twang)
Wheezing	Externally audible musical sound due to bronchoconstriction, if AR is associate with asthma

Table 22.8 Differentiating Allergic Rhinitis from Common Cold

Features	*Allergic rhinitis*	*Common cold*
Duration	>10 days	<10 days
Onset	Sudden	Gradual
Constitutional symptoms	Absent	Present
Nature of discharge	Clear	Mucoid
Treatment	Antihistamines	Symptomatic

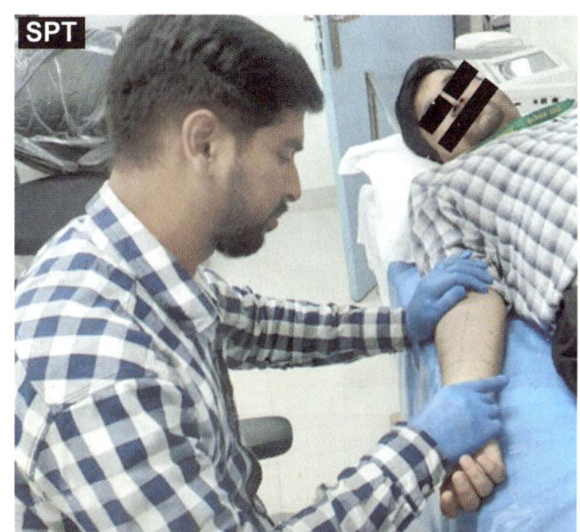

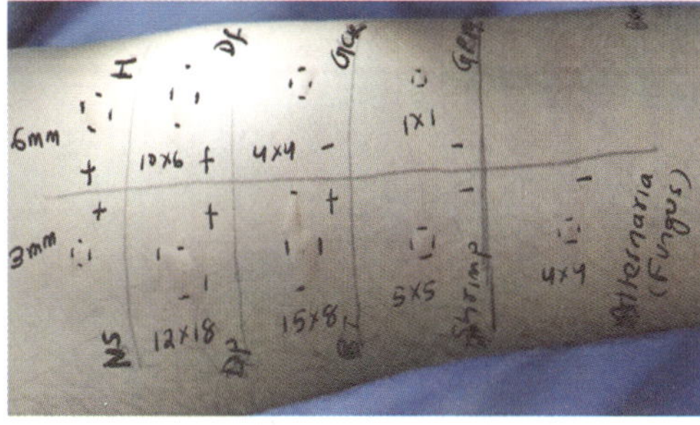

- ❖ Nasal allergen provocation test (NAPT) is gold standard, but available at selected centers only
- ❖ Serum specific IgE (by ImmunoCAP method only); nasal specific IgE at selected centers only
- ❖ Nasal endoscopy to rule out polyp/turbinate hypertrophy/septal deviation/sinusitis
- ❖ Peak nasal inspiratory flow meter (PNIF) to assess the degree of nasal blockage (to access treatment efficacy)

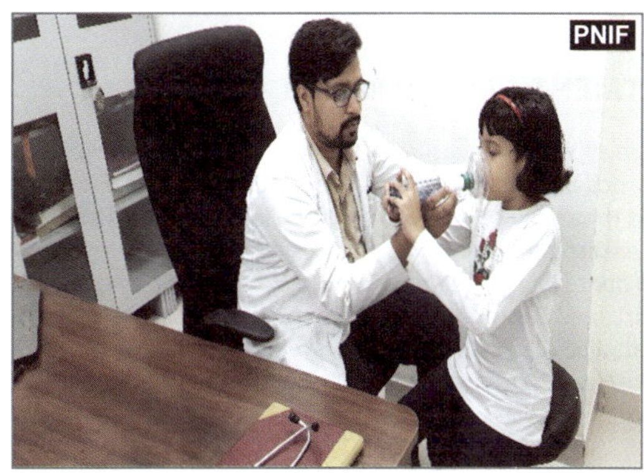

- Radiographic studies (X-ray/CT/MRI of nose and paranasal sinuses) to rule out structural abnormalities.
- Spirometry/impulse oscillometry/forced oscillation technique (FOT) to rule out associated asthma

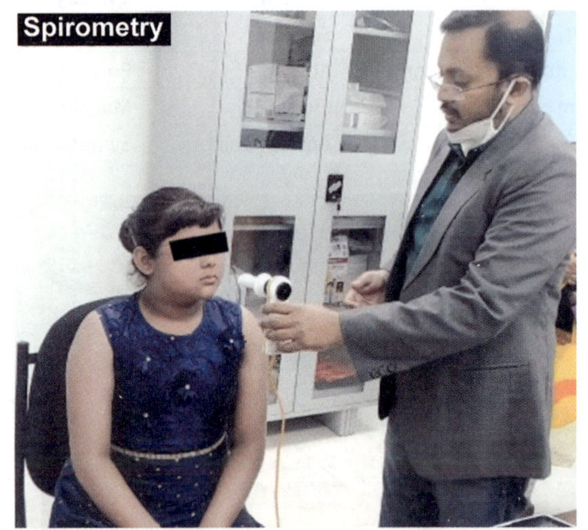

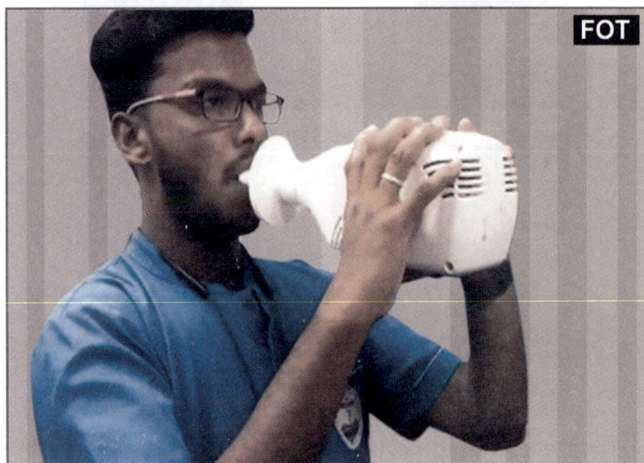

- ***Recent advances:*** Component resolved diagnosis (CRD), common carbohydrate determinants (CCD) and molecular allergen testing by microarray technique are some of the newer modalities for diagnosing offending allergens. Eosinophilic cationic protein, exhaled nitric oxide, and histamine releasing factor assays are newer modalities to identify ongoing eosinophilic inflammation.

TREATMENT Allergic Rhinitis

Allergen avoidance measures (for house dust mites, cockroach, fungal spores, pollens, and pet animals) are listed in **Box 22.4**. **Flowchart 22.3** depicts the stepwise management of allergic rhinitis. Drugs and their doses are listed here.

- *Oral nonsedating second generation H_1 antihistamines:* Fexofenadine, Cetirizine, Desloratadine (6 months), Ebastine Levocetirizine, Loratadine (2 years), Bilastine (>6 years).
- *Nasal H_1 antihistamines:* Azelastine (0.1%) and Olopatadine (0.6%) for children >5 years

Box 22.4 Allergen Avoidance Measures

1. *Avoidance of house dust mites:*
   - Expose beddings to sunlight at least once a week
   - Washing bedding linen weekly in water >130°F (55°C); maintaining humidity <45%
   - Use high efficiency particle arresting (HEPA) filters in vacuum cleaners; regular wet mopping of floor for dust
2. *Avoidance of cockroach:* Keep food and trash in closed containers; use boric acid/cypermethrin chalks, baits, and traps
3. *Avoidance of fungus:* Fix water leaks, wash water coolers and change AC filters regularly; cleaning bathroom surfaces regularly
4. *Avoidance of pollens:* Keep windows and doors closed; stay indoors in pollen season; use spectacles/mask during outdoor visit
5. *Avoidance of pets:* Clean pet with water and shampoo regularly; avoid pets inside bedroom

Flowchart 22.3: Stepwise management of allergic rhinitis

Step 1: Parental education, avoidance of trigger/allergen exposure, skin prick test, serum IgE
↓
Step 2: Nonsedating 2nd generation H_1 antihistamines
↓
Step 3: Intranasal steroids (INS)
↓
Step 4: INS + Nasal/oral H_1 antihistamines
↓
Step 5: Nasal saline irrigation with INS + Nasal/oral H_1 antihistamines
↓
Step 6: Intranasal ipratropium, Montelukast (when associated with asthma), eye drops (AHs/steroids) if associated with conjunctivitis
↓
Step 7: Allergen-specific immunotherapy, omalizumab if associated with severe asthma

- *Oral decongestants:* Phenylephrine, Pseudoephedrine
- *Nasal decongestants (if needed, for maximum 5–7 days):* Oxymetazoline (0.05%), Xylometazoline (0.1%)
- *Intranasal steroids (INS):* Mometasone furoate 50 µg for children >2 years or fluticasone furoate 27.5 µg for children >4 years—moderate to severe variety or not responding to H_1 antihistamines
- *Oral steroids:* Prednisolone (<7 days, in severe, nonresponding AR)
- *Leukotriene receptor antagonist (LTRA):* Montelukast, if AR associated with asthma, to be prescribed by pediatric allergist only.
- *Anti-IgE antibody Omalizumab:* If AR associated with severe asthma, to be prescribed by pediatric allergist only.
- *Anti IL-4/IL 13 antibody Dupilumab:* Above 6 years atopic dermatitis with AR, above 12 years moderate to severe asthma with AR
- *Intranasal ipratropium (0.06 % w/v):* For rhinorrhea among children >5 years
- *Intranasal chromones (2% Nedocromil):* Decreases degranulation of mast cell in children >2 years
- *Nasal saline irrigation:* For thick and profuse secretions
- *Surgery:* For nasal polyp, deviated septum

Acknowledgment: Authors acknowledge contribution from Department of Pediatrics, SCB Medical College, Cuttack; Departments of Pediatrics, Dermatology, and ENT of AIIMS, Kalyani, West Bengal; and Dr Ashik Majumder.

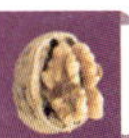

IN A NUTSHELL

Allergic Rhinitis

1. AR is the most common chronic respiratory disease among children.
2. Diagnosis is primarily clinical, based upon symptoms and signs.
3. First-line treatment consists of second generation nonsedating H_1 antihistamines in milder variety.
4. Intranasal steroids (INS) are indicated only for moderate to severe and persistent variety.
5. Allergen specific immunotherapy is effective in nonresponders to INS.
6. If not treated early in life, it may lead to development of asthma.

Barne M, Singh S, Mangal DK, et al. Global Asthma Network Phase I, India: Results for allergic rhinitis and eczema in 127,309 children and adults. J Allerg Clin Immunol: Global. 2022;1(2):51-60.

Nagaraju K, Kasyapi VN. Treatment of Allergic Rhinitis. In: Nagaraju K (Ed). Manual of Pediatric Allergy, 2nd edition. New Delhi: Jaypee Brothers Medical Publishers (P) Ltd; 2022. pp. 185-204.

Nagaraju K. Clinical Features and Diagnosis of Allergic Rhinitis. In: Nagaraju K (Ed). Manual of Pediatric Allergy, 2nd edition. New Delhi: Jaypee Brothers Medical Publishers (P) Ltd.; 2022. pp. 169-84.

Muluk B, Cingi C. Biologics in allergic rhinitis. European Review for Medical and Pharmacological Sciences. 2023;27(5 Suppl):43-52.

22.6 Approach to Stridor

PE 25.4

DEFINITION

Stridor is a high-pitched, harsh, respiratory sound generated due to turbulent airflow through a partially obstructed airway. Often it can be heard without a stethoscope, although loudness does not correlate with the severity of obstruction. It is commonly seen in children of different age groups. All the cases must be evaluated for underlying cause.

ETIOPATHOGENESIS

Etiology of stridor is listed in **Box 22.5**.

Mechanism of Stridor

Stridor can occur due to pathology at the level of the glottis and above or below it. It may occur during any respiratory phase, as shown in **Figure 22.7**. The phase of respiration associated with stridor gives the clue about the site of etiology:

- The inspiratory phase stridor suggests airway obstruction above the glottis.
- The expiratory phase stridor suggests obstruction in the lower trachea.
- Biphasic (both inspiratory and expiratory) stridor suggests glottic/subglottic lesion.

CLINICAL FEATURES

Acute Onset Stridor

- ***Laryngotracheobronchitis (Croup):***
  - Common cause of acute stridor in children
  - Usual age of presentation from 6 months to 2 years
  - Child may have low-grade fever
  - Child may have barking cough which worsens during night
- ***Aspiration of foreign body:***
  - Secondary to inhalation of edible (e.g., nuts, popcorn, and hard candy) and nonedible items (e.g., button, coin).
  - History of sudden onset coughing and choking prior to the development of respiratory symptoms.
  - The most common site is right lower bronchus.

Box 22.5 Etiology of Stridor

A. *Congenital causes:*
1. Laryngeal web
2. Laryngomalacia
3. Vocal cord paralysis
4. Subglottic stenosis
5. Abnormal tongue
6. Hemangioma
7. Craniofacial anomalies

B. *Acquired causes:*
1. *Febrile:*
   - Acute laryngitis
   - Diphtheria
   - Infectious mononucleosis
   - Peritonsillar abscess
   - Epiglottitis
   - Laryngotracheitis
2. *Afebrile:*
   - Foreign body
   - Local trauma
   - Adenotonsillar hypertrophy
   - Laryngeal edema
   - Papillomatosis

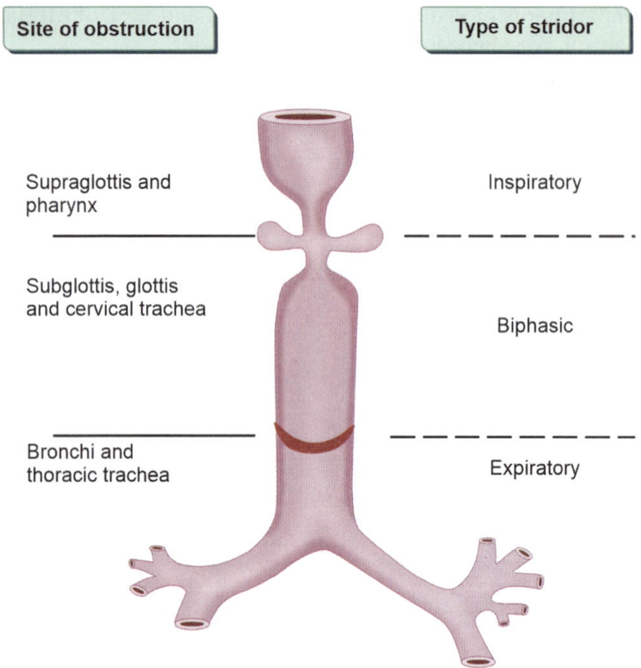

Fig. 22.7: Anatomical sites of stridor

- ***Retropharyngeal abscess:***
  - Complication of bacterial pharyngitis, usually age <6 years
  - Sudden onset of high-grade fever, refusal to feed, difficulty swallowing, sore throat, respiratory distress.
- ***Bacterial tracheitis:***
  - Uncommon cause of stridor, presents in <3 years of age
  - Develops due to secondary infection (mostly due to *S. aureus*) following a viral infection (e.g., croup or influenza)
- ***Peritonsillar abscess:***
  - Commonly seen during the preadolescents and adolescent period
  - Infection in the peritonsillar space (space between the tonsil and superior constrictor muscle)
  - The child presents with severe throat pain, and difficult swallowing or speaking
- ***Allergic reaction (i.e., anaphylaxis):***
  - A serious acute life-threatening condition. Presents with itching eyes, sneezing, nasal congestion, and dysphagia.
  - Other signs and symptoms include urticaria, hoarseness, wheezing, inspiratory stridor.
- ***Acute spasmodic laryngitis (spasmodic croup):***
  - Mostly seen in children aged 1–3 years
  - May have similar clinical presentation like anaphylaxis and croup
- ***Epiglottitis:***
  - Mainly caused by *H. influenzae* type B infections.
  - A serious life-threatening condition, mostly seen in children between 2 and 7 years.
  - The affected child presents with sudden onset high-grade fever, dysphagia and sore throat.

Chronic Stridor

- ***Laryngomalacia:***
  - Most common cause of inspiratory stridor (around 75% of all cases) during the early infancy and neonatal period.
  - The laryngeal structures are soft and floppy and that fall over the airway opening and block it.
  - Stridor may be aggravated by crying or feeding
  - Mostly resolved by 18–20 months of life.
- ***Subglottic stenosis:***
  - Child may have inspiratory or biphasic stridor. It can be congenital or acquired.
  - Congenital subglottic stenosis occurs due to partial canalization of the subglottic and cricoid rings.
  - Acquired is caused by prolonged intubation.
- ***Vocal cord dysfunction:***
  - Vocal cord paralysis may involve either unilateral or bilateral vocal cord. Unilateral dysfunction is due to some congenital or acquired causes such as trauma during birth or cardiac or intrathoracic surgery.
  - Spontaneously improvement can be seen in unilateral cord paralysis.
  - The child with bilateral vocal cord paralysis presents with high-pitched stridor, aphonia, and severe respiratory distress.
- ***Others:*** Laryngeal webs, laryngeal cysts, and laryngeal hemangiomas.

Figure 22.8 depicts various causes of stridor in different age groups. Risk stratification in a child with stridor as per IMNCI guidelines is shown in **Figure 22.9.**

TREATMENT Stridor

The child presents with stridor requires prompt evaluation and determination of respiratory distress severity. The treatment should be aimed at treating the underlying cause.

Supportive Treatment

- The child presents with stridor should be differentiated into acute or chronic disease.
- The ABC (airway, breathing, circulation) should be established immediately in a child with severe respiratory distress. Avoid agitating the child and minimize the interventions.
- Oxygen, intravenous fluid, suction, and aerosol treatment (3% NaCl, epinephrine), according to the severity and underlying disease.
- Monitor for signs and symptoms of rapid deterioration (tachypnea, tachycardia/bradycardia, sensorium, breathing efforts)

Specific Treatment

- Consider flexible/rigid bronchoscopy for foreign body diagnosis/removal.
- In suspected croup; nebulization with adrenaline, consider IV/IM dexamethasone.
- In acute onset stridor secondary to anaphylaxis, treat with injection epinephrine.
- Consider adding IV antibiotics in a suspected case of bacterial tracheitis or secondary bacterial infection.
- Discharge the child from hospital when there is no respiratory distress and stridor at rest, afebrile, and taking orally well.

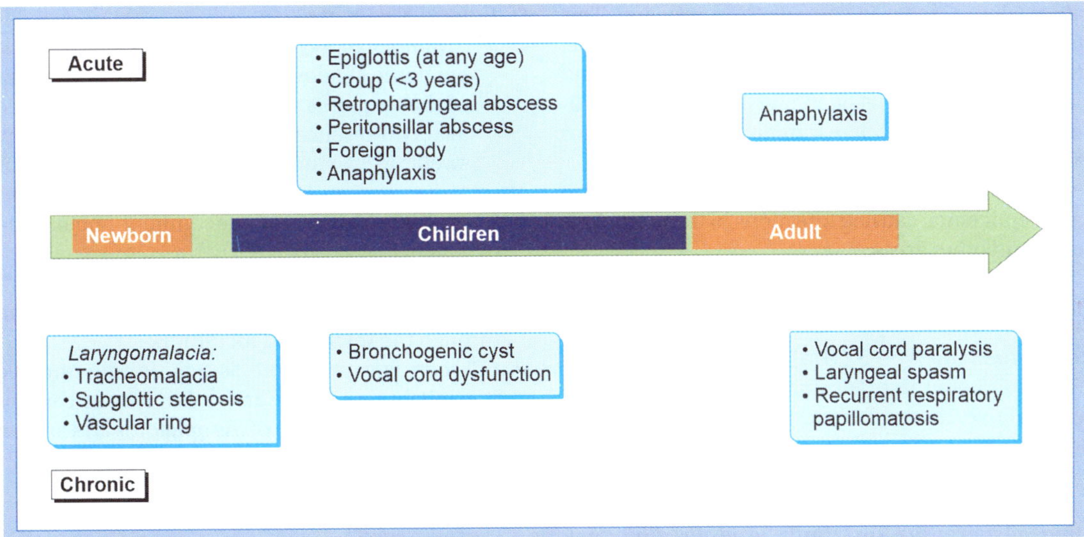

Fig. 22.8: Etiology for the stridor in different age groups

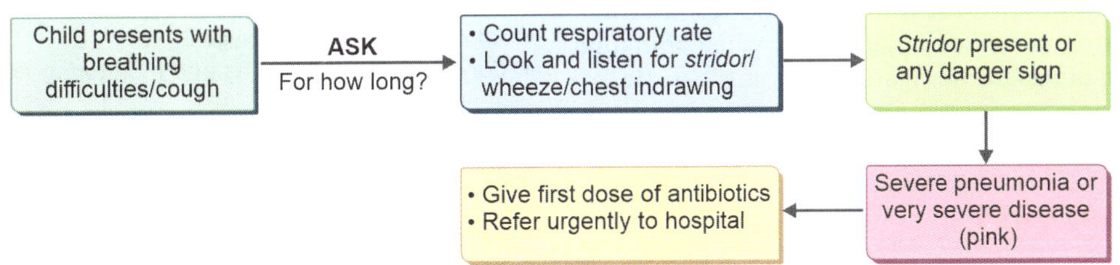

Fig. 22.9: Risk stratification in a child presenting with stridor as per IMNCI guidelines

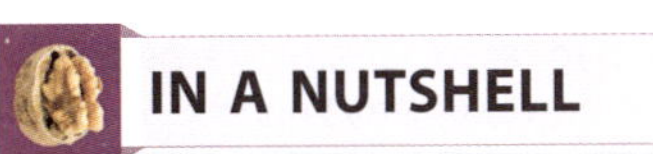

IN A NUTSHELL

Approach to Stridor

1. Stridor secondary to congenital anomalies become symptomatic soon after birth
2. Important to know the age-specific etiology
3. The most common cause of congenital stridor is laryngomalacia and mostly associated with spontaneous resolution (80%) without need for intervention
4. Severe cases require early identification and urgent treatment.

Boudewyns A, Claes J, Van de Heyning P. Clinical practice: an approach to stridor in infants and children. Eur J Pediatr. 2010;169(2):135-41 .

Iicari V, Zabbo CP. Stridor. In: StatPearls [Internet]. Treasure Island (FL): StatPearls Publishing; 2022.

Rodrigues K, Roosevelt G. Acute inflammatory upper airway obstruction (croup, epiglottitis, laryngitis, and bacterial tracheitis). In: Kligeman R, St Geme III J (Eds). Nelson Textbook of Pediatrics, 21st edition. Philadelphia: Elsevier; 2020. pp. 2202-5.

Sicari V, Zabbo CP. Stridor in Children. [Updated 2023 Nov 12]. In: StatPearls [Internet]. Treasure Island (FL): StatPearls Publishing; 2025 Jan-. Available from: https://www.ncbi.nlm.nih.gov/books/NBK525995/ [Last accessed August, 2025]

22.7 Acute Epiglottitis

PE 25.2

INTRODUCTION

Acute epiglottitis is a potentially life-threatening disorder as it might result in laryngospasm and airway compromise. It is an infection and edema of epiglottis and the surrounding structures including arytenoids, aryepiglottic folds and vallecula. Subglottic structures are spared.

PATHOGENESIS

For epiglottitis to occur, posterior nasopharynx is the most common source of pathogen and it is predisposed to by microscopic trauma to epithelial surface (either following viral infection or due to food), which manifests as cellulitis of the epiglottis, aryepiglottic folds and other tissues.

Inflammatory edema results in supraglottic narrowing. This is further compounded by Venturi effect and Bernoulli principle, increasing the obstruction. Also, due to increase in weight and mass of epiglottis with the inherent pliancy of the cartilage, a ball-valve effect may occur where each inspiration pulls edematous epiglottis over laryngeal airway, resulting in laryngeal spasm.

Bacteria spreading beyond mucosal barriers can lead to bacteremia and septicemia, causing infections in the meninges, skin, lungs, ears, and other areas.

ETIOLOGY

Haemophilus influenzae type B (Hib) is the most common cause, however, with better immunization coverage, incidence of alternative infective causes has increased. Other infective causes include *Streptococcus pyogenes, S. pneumoniae, S. aureus* and viruses (including influenza A and B, parainfluenza type 3, EBV, herpes simplex and COVID-19). In immunocompromised patients, fungi (*Aspergillus* spp. and *Candida albicans*), *Pseudomonas aeruginosa, Serratia, Enterobacter* and anerobic flora can be causative.

Noninfectious *causes* include traumatic injuries, thermal injuries as inhalation of heated objects, e.g., when smoking illicit drugs, or use of electronic cigarettes/vaping, caustic, or foreign body ingestion. Epiglottic injuries of this type should be especially suspected in patients with mental disorders.

CLINICAL FEATURES

The onset is sudden and the child appears toxic (agitation, restlessness and irritability). The diseases is characterized by high fever, sore throat, character of voice change (muffled, "hot potato" voice), stridor, and 3 Ds (drooling, dysphagia, and distress/dyspnea).

Children often assume characteristic posture of sitting up and leaning forward, neck hyper-extended and chin thrust forward (tripod position) in order to enhance airflow. General malaise and a globus sensation may precede presentation. Epiglottitis can also be observed in adults, with up to 10% requiring airway intervention, and about half of them are in Friedman severity stage 3 at presentation.

With a good history and examination, other causes of acute upper airway obstruction as laryngotracheitis (croup), bacterial tracheitis, uvulitis, foreign body, retropharyngeal abscess, diphtheria, thermal and caustic injury, peritonsillar abscess, angioedema, and congenital anomalies (e.g. laryngeal web, laryngomalacia), must be excluded.

All students should be warned never to use a tongue blade or depressor to examine a child's throat with suspected epiglottitis as it may lead to acute complications as laryngospasm.

DIAGNOSIS

- In young children with imminent complete airway obstruction, laboratory studies should not be done till airway is secured, as pain induced agitation can potentially precipitate sudden respiratory arrest. Swabbing the epiglottis is potentially dangerous in patients who are not intubated.
- ***Lateral X-rays of neck:***
  - "*Thumb sign*" is visible due to the rounded thickening of the epiglottic shadow. It is indicative of severe inflammation of the epiglottis with potential for irrevocable loss of the airway. Presence of both epiglottic and aryepiglottic fold swelling gives an appearance of the double thumb sign.
  - *Vallecula sign:* Absence of a deep, well-defined vallecula
- Chest X-ray may reveal concomitant pneumonia in 10–15% of patients.
- ***Ultrasonography*** reveals an "alphabet P sign" in a longitudinal view: investigation of epiglottis by a longitudinal view through the thyrohyoid membrane.
- ***CT scan*** is rarely done as positioning and sedation may precipitate respiratory arrest. But if done can reveal marked edema and thickening of the epiglottis and aryepiglottic folds with narrowing of the airway.

TREATMENT Acute Epiglottitis

General Management

- This condition should be treated as a pediatric and airway emergency.
- The treating doctor must take care not to agitate the patient.
- Administer humidified oxygen.
- Continue vital monitoring and monitoring for features of upper airway obstruction.
- Allow the child to choose the position in which he is most comfortable.
- The treating team must be prepared for sudden worsening of clinical status. ENT and anesthesia team should be alerted for possibility of difficult intubation, and tracheostomy set kept ready.
- All nonintubated patients must be admitted for observation, with ENT/anesthesia team on stand-by and a tracheostomy tray must be available at the bedside.

Intubation

Most important aspect of treatment is to secure the airway especially if patient has signs of advancing upper airway obstruction.

- Tracheal intubation of a patient with epiglottitis must be regarded as a potentially difficult procedure.
- It should be done in strict monitored conditions, i.e., in the operating room, while maintaining spontaneous ventilation.
- Forcing the child/patient into a supine position may precipitate acute airway obstruction.
- Further management after intubation should be done in ICU.
- Tracheal extubation should be preceded by a cuff leak test with a deflated cuff and, usually, a second look by direct laryngoscopy with deep sedation or general anesthesia. Intubation and appropriate antibiotic management for 2–3 days is usually necessary before extubation can be done.

Antibiotics

Empiric antimicrobials should be initiated. Ampicillin or cephalosporins as cefuroxime, ceftriaxone, and cefotaxime should be started immediately. Once culture and sensitivity results are available, the regimen should be adjusted. If epiglottic swelling persists beyond 72 hours, further optimization of antibiotic regimen and development of complications as epiglottic abscess must be kept in mind.

COMPLICATIONS

Complications of acute epiglottitis may include deep neck space infection, epiglottic abscess, Ludwig angina type submental infection, recurrent illness and vocal granuloma, cervical adenitis, cellulitis, epiglottic abscess, and Ludwig angina-type submental infection. It may progress to sepsis (which may progress to shock), respiratory failure, requirement of prolonged ventilation and tracheostomy and may even result in death if not managed adequately.

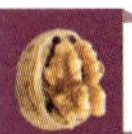

IN A NUTSHELL

Acute Epiglottitis

1. Acute epiglottitis is a life-threatening pediatric and airway emergency.
2. In case of advancing upper airway obstruction emergent intubation in operating room by ENT and anesthetic team is required.
3. Presenting features include high grade fever, stridor, drooling, dysphagia, and distress/dyspnea.
4. Airway management and antibiotics are the mainstay of management.

Booth AWG, Pungsornruk K, Llewellyn S, et al. Airway management of adult epiglottitis: a systematic review and meta-analysis. BJA Open. 2024;9:100250.
Guerra AM, Waseem M. Epiglottitis. Treasure Island (FL): StatPearls Publishing; 2022.
Lee J, Loh J, Lee TS. Double thumb sign in a case of epiglottitis. Radiol Case Rep. 2021;(16):1810-4.
Sutton AE, Guerra AM, Waseem M. Epiglottitis. [Updated 2024 Oct 5]. In: StatPearls [Internet]. Treasure Island (FL): StatPearls Publishing; 2025 Jan-. Available from: https://www.ncbi.nlm.nih.gov/books/NBK430960/ [Last accessed August, 2025]
Woods CR. Epiglottitis (supraglottitis): Clinical features and diagnosis. UptoDate. Updated: 20.12.2023. Accessed: 5.2.2025

22.8 Acute Laryngotracheobronchitis (Croup) *PE 25.3*

INTRODUCTION

Laryngotracheobronchitis is the inflammation of the larynx, trachea, and bronchi. Cases of laryngotracheobronchitis can be more severe than laryngotracheitis (as the former extends into the lower airway). The term "croup" colloquially describes both laryngotracheobronchitis and laryngotracheitis. It is a common childhood illness, which primarily affects those between the ages of 6 months and 3 years of age (peak annual incidence in 2nd year of life).

The infective organism (usually viral) causes inflammation and edema of the upper airway, manifesting in abrupt onset barking cough, hoarseness, inspiratory stridor and respiratory distress due to features of upper airway obstruction.

ETIOLOGY

- ***Viral:***
  - Human parainfluenza virus (types 1 and 3) is the most common pathogen: Type 1 is the most common cause of croup, type 2 is the mildest, and 3 is the most severe type
  - *Influenza A and B viruses:* Tend to have longer hospitalization periods
  - Other viruses include rhinovirus, coronavirus, human metapneumovirus, adenovirus respiratory syncytial virus, metapneumovirus, measles, adenovirus, and mycoplasma.
- ***Bacterial (laryngeal diphtheria, bacterial tracheitis):*** Bacteria are responsible for tracheitis, diphtheria, laryngotracheobronchopneumonitis. The common bacterial causes are *Staphylococcus aureus*, *Streptococcus pneumoniae*, *Haemophilus influenzae*, and *Moraxella catarrhalis*.

PATHOGENESIS

The viral infection in acute laryngotracheitis and laryngotracheobronchitis (LTB) begins in the nasopharynx and spreads to the respiratory epithelium of the larynx and trachea. As it spreads to the laryngeal mucosa, it leads to inflammation, edema, and hyperemia. *This leads to narrowing of the subglottic region*. This results in dynamic obstruction at or below the cartilaginous ring, manifesting as stridor.

As the upper airway obstruction worsens, the compliant chest wall starts drawing inwards during inspiration (paradoxical breathing), if untreated, it will result in hypoxia/hypercapnia, respiratory failure and finally arrest. Also, extension of the infection into the bronchi, as occurs with laryngotracheobronchitis, can lead to wheezing, crackles, air trapping, and increased tachypnea. This clinical picture needs to be differentiated from asthma (**Flowchart 22.4**).

CLINICAL FEATURES

Clinical Presentation

The illness usually starts like a common cold with symptoms of rhinorrhea, cough, sore throat, and fever. Features of upper airway obstruction, i.e., high pitched inspiratory stridor, hoarseness of voice, and barking or seal like cough develop over next 2–3 days. In most cases, symptoms usually resolve within a week. A few children develop symptoms of severe airway obstruction characterized by intercostal recession, tachypnea, irritability, lethargy, and cyanosis; and need hospitalization. These symptoms usually occur due to inflammation of larynx, trachea, and bronchus (hence the term

Flowchart 22.4: Pathogenesis of respiratory distress in acute laryngotracheobronchitis

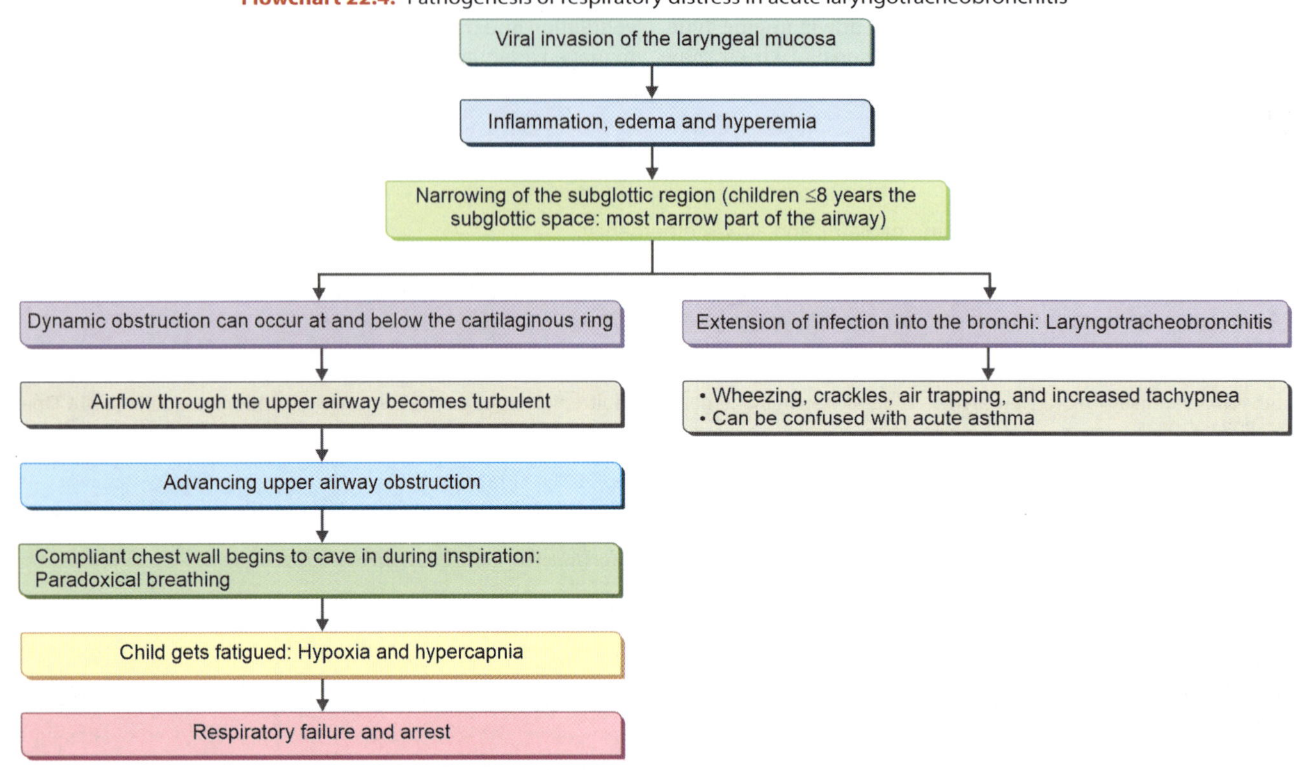

laryngotracheobronchitis). However, it is specifically the subglottic inflammation and resultant swelling that compromises the airway and results in stridor and difficult breathing.

It is imperative to rule out other entities such as acute epiglottitis, bacterial tracheitis, foreign body, spasmodic cough, and laryngeal diphtheria because the management would differ in each case.

Assessment of the Severity

- ***General appearance:*** Agitation, restlessness, head nodding, hypotonia, and lethargy are the signs of hypoxia due to severe airway obstruction. Examination should preferably be done in attendant's lap or position of comfort, in order to avoid agitation and further airway narrowing.
- ***Degree of respiratory distress:*** Stridor at rest, intercostal or subcostal indrawing, tachypnea, and pulses paradoxus indicate moderate to severe obstruction.
- ***Stridor:*** The loudness of stridor is not a good indicator of severity of obstruction. However, presence of biphasic stridor indicates fixed obstruction (like foreign body, subglottic stenosis, or hemangioma).
- ***Cyanosis or extreme pallor:*** Either of the two indicates severe obstruction.
- ***Oxygen saturation:*** Falling saturation is a late and unreliable sign to assess the degree of respiratory distress and not a good substitute for clinical assessment.
- ***Croup severity score:*** Westley croup score **(Table 22.9)** can help deciding admission, and treatment modality. Subsequent scoring can identify treatment response.

RADIOLOGICAL SIGNS

X-ray Neck: Frontal View

It shows steeple sign (also called the inverted V sign) (similar to church steeple). It occurs due to narrowing of upper trachea but denotes only subglottic edema, and can be absent in croup and present in other inflammatory conditions of the upper airway. Hence, the absence of this sign does not rule out croup (**Fig. 22.10**).

X-ray Soft Tissue Neck: Lateral View

It may reveal narrowing of the subglottic region and overdistention (ballooning) of the hypopharynx. It can also help differentiate from acute epiglottitis and retropharyngeal abscess (**Fig. 22.11**). Retropharyngeal soft tissues should be less than the anteroposterior width of a cervical vertebral body. When thickened, the retropharyngeal soft tissues bow anteriorly and displace the airway.

DISEASE COURSE AND PROGNOSIS

On an average, 5–10% of children with croup presenting to the emergency room require hospitalization and only 1% require admission to the PICU. More than 85% of children present with mild disease; severe croup is rare and mortality is usually low. Uncommon complications may include pneumonia, pulmonary edema, and bacterial tracheitis.

Further evaluation, admission and observation are needed in children with stridor at rest, having a rapid progression of symptoms (upper airway obstruction signs within 12 hours of

Table 22.9 Westley Croup Score for Laryngotracheobronchitis

Name of score	*Number of components*	*Range*	*Scoring components*
Westley croup score (Wesley, 1978)	5 (stridor/retractions/cyanosis/level of consciousness/air entry)	0–17	• Stridor (0 = none, 1 = with agitation only, 2 = at rest) • Retractions (0 = none, 1 = mild, 2 = moderate, 3 = severe) • Cyanosis (0 = none, 4 = cyanosis with agitation, 5 = cyanosis at rest) • Level of consciousness [0 = normal (including asleep), 5 = disorientated] • Air entry (0 = normal, 1 = decreased, 2 = markedly decreased)
Westley score			*Severity*
0–2			**Mild croup:** Occasional barking cough; no stridor at rest; and no-to-mild suprasternal, intercostal indrawing
3–5			**Moderate croup:** Frequent barking cough, easily audible stridor at rest, and suprasternal and sternal wall retraction at rest, but no or little distress or agitation
6–11			**Severe croup:** Frequent barking cough, prominent inspiratory and, occasionally, expiratory stridor, marked sternal wall retractions, decreased air entry on auscultation, and significant distress and agitation
>11			**Impending respiratory failure:** Barking cough (often not prominent), audible stridor at rest (can occasionally be hard to hear), sternal wall retractions (may not be marked), usually lethargic or decreased level of consciousness, and often dusky complexion

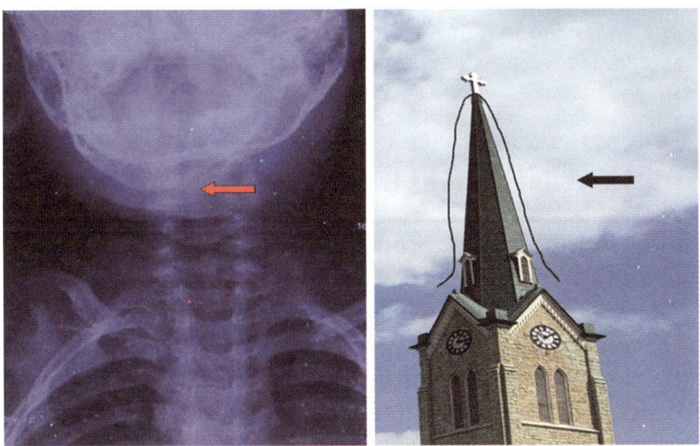

Fig. 22.10: Steeple sign, bears resemblance to a church steeple which is a tall tower on a building, topped by a spire and often incorporating a belfry and other components

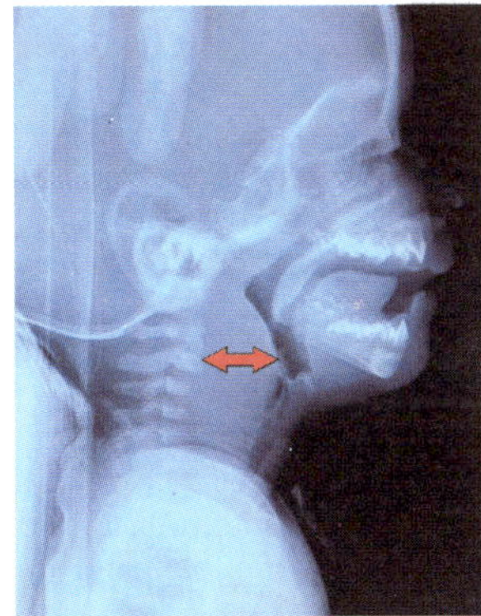

Fig. 22.11: Retropharyngeal abscess: Lateral neck radiograph shows thickening of the retropharyngeal soft tissues. In a normal person, the anteroposterior width of the retropharyngeal soft tissues should be less than the AP width of a cervical vertebral body. When thickened; the retropharyngeal soft tissues bow anteriorly and displace the airway

onset), inability to tolerate oral fluids, associated known airway abnormality (e.g., subglottic stenosis, subglottic hemangioma, previous intubation), associated medical conditions that predispose to respiratory failure (e.g., neuromuscular disorders or bronchopulmonary dysplasia or heart disease), previous episodes of moderate to severe croup/recurrent croup, parental concern that cannot be relieved by reassurance, and if the child has prolonged symptoms (>3 days) or has an atypical course (this may need a re-consideration of diagnosis). These children can have a poor outcome.

Discharge can be considered when there is no stridor at rest, maintaining vitals including normal SpO_2, good air exchange, normal color and level of consciousness, child has demonstrated ability to tolerate fluids by mouth, and the caregivers understand the indications for return to care and would be able to return if necessary.

Normally croup is self-limiting, however, atypical croup is considered if there is:

- Severe manifestations necessitating definitive airway management
- Child has prolonged, symptoms persisting ≥7 days despite appropriate medical therapy
- Atypical age of presentation: <6 months or older than 6 years
- Caused by atypical pathogen
- Presenting with an airway lesion other than the classically findings
- >4 recurrent episodes or ≥2 or more episodes necessitating inpatient care

DIFFERENTIAL DIAGNOSIS

Depends upon the clinical signs and symptoms and may include bacterial tracheitis, epiglottitis, foreign body aspiration, hemangioma, peritonsillar/parapharyngeal or retropharyngeal abscess, neoplasm, retropharyngeal abscess, smoke inhalation, subglottic stenosis, vocal cord paralysis, vascular ring, foreign body aspiration, anaphylaxis, and asthma.

TREATMENT Acute Laryngotracheobronchitis (Croup)

The goal of treatment is to decrease airway obstruction. Children with moderate to severe croup are usually administered both epinephrine and corticosteroids concurrently.

- *Supplemental oxygen* via blow by or nasal cannula can also be used for hypoxic patients with croup. In case of work of breathing, discuss with PICU consultant and consider HHHFNC. Be ready for intubation in case of progressive respiratory deterioration, with the help of airway experts. Endotracheal intubation is rarely required in croup.
- *Monitoring:* Monitor for the vitals (including SpO_2), mental status, hydration status, chest auscultatory findings, worsening stridor, work of breathing (chest wall/subcostal retractions, nasal flaring, sitting in a sniffing position, suprasternal retractions, grunting, accessory muscle use), and serial Wesley croup scores.
- *Fluids:* Fever and tachypnea increase fluid requirement and insensible losses, and lethargy and disease severity limits oral intake. Watch if the child can take oral fluids, otherwise start IV fluids as per clinical status.
- *Fever:* Give antipyretics as needed.
- *Comfort:* Try to avoid unnecessary interventions. Encourage caregiver to hold and comfort the child, to avoid agitation in the child especially in moderate to severe croup. Avoid sedatives as this can lead to respiratory depression.
- *Steroids:* Corticosteroids, such as dexamethasone results in faster resolution of symptoms, decreased return to medical care, and decreased length of stay. The standard dose of dexamethasone is 0.6 mg/kg, but doses as low as 0.15 mg/kg have been studied in randomized trials (maximum of 10 mg as a one-time dose). Dexamethasone has comparable or superior efficacy for treatment of croup compared with other glucocorticoids that have been evaluated. Dexamethasone can be given IM, IV, or orally, as per patient's condition and treating physician's assessment. Oral or intramuscular route corticosteroids is as efficacious or superior to the nebulized form of medication, and adding inhaled budesonide to oral dexamethasone was not found to provide extra benefit in children admitted with croup.
- *Nebulized epinephrine:* Nebulized epinephrine is associated with clinically significant transient reduction of symptoms of croup 30 minutes post-treatment. It has an onset of effect within 10 minutes and waning of effect between 1 and 2 hours. L-epinephrine: 0.5 mL/kg per dose (maximum of 5 mL) of a 1 mg/mL (1:1000) preservative-free solution, administered over 15 minutes by nebulizer. Consider admission of patients requiring more than one or two doses of nebulized epinephrine in the emergency department, without improvement or worsening.
- *Hospitalization:* Consider admission for children with severe croup (Westley croup score ≥8); stridor at rest, marked retractions with agitation, lethargy, cyanosis, persistent respiratory signs and symptoms after two or more treatments with epinephrine, worsening symptoms, altered consciousness, toxic appearance (suggesting secondary bacterial infection), need for supplemental oxygen, and dehydration. Also, consider admission for children less than 6 months, those requiring recurrent emergency visits less than 24 hours, when the treating doctors doubt the ability of the parents/caregiver to comprehend instructions regarding red flag deterioration features/signs, or in conditions when there is a suspicion that the caregivers may not be able to come back (either due to distance, etc.).
- *Intubation:* Intubation is reserved for severe cases of croup not responding to medical treatment. The endotracheal tube size should be smaller than typical for the patient's age and size to avoid trauma to the already edematous airway.
- *Antibiotics:* Croup is most commonly a viral disease. Antibiotics are reserved for cases when primary or secondary bacterial infection is suspected.

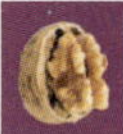

IN A NUTSHELL

Acute Laryngotracheobronchitis (Croup)

1. Croup is manifested by abrupt onset barking cough, hoarseness, inspiratory stridor, and respiratory distress due to features of upper airway obstruction.
2. Parainfluenza virus is the most common cause of viral croup.
3. Corticosteroid (dexamethasone) and nebulized adrenaline are the mainstay of therapy in moderate to severe croup.
4. Exclude other life-threatening causes of upper airway obstruction.

Alsaeed RA, Aljehani NA, Alabdali AF, et al. Evaluation of recent updates regarding diagnosis and management of croup in children. Arch Pharm Pract. 2019;10(1):11-4.

Aregbesola A, Tam CM, Kothari A, et al. Glucocorticoids for croup in children. Cochrane Database Syst Rev. 2023;1(1):CD001955.

Bjornson CL, Johnson DW. Croup in children. CMAJ. 2013;185(15):1317-23.

Darras KE, Roston AT, Yewchuk LK. Imaging acute airway obstruction in infants and children. Radio Graphics. 2015;35:2064-79.

Donaldson D, Poleski D, Knipple E,et al. Intramuscular versus oral dexamethasone for the treatment of moderate-to-severe croup: a randomized, double-blind trial. Acad Emerg Med. 2003;10(1):16-21.

Ernest S, Khandhar PB. Laryngotracheobronchitis. [Updated 2023 Jun 26]. In: StatPearls [Internet]. Treasure Island (FL): StatPearls Publishing; 2025 Jan-. Available from: https://www.ncbi.nlm.nih.gov/books/NBK519531/ [Last accessed August, 2025]

Hanna R, Lee F, Drummond D, Yunker WK. Defining atypical croup: A case report and review of the literature. Int J Pediatr Otorhinolaryngol. 2019;127:109686.

Johnson DW. Croup. BMJ Clin Evid. 2014;2014:0321.

Ortiz-Alvarez O. Acute management of croup in the emergency department. Paediatr Child Health. 2017;22(3):166-73.

Toward Optimized Practice (TOP) Working Group for Croup. 2008. Diagnosis and Management of croup., Edmonton, AB: toward Optimized Practice

Westley CR, Cotton EK, Brooks JG. Nebulized racemic epinephrine by IPPB for the treatment of croup: a double-blind study. Am J Dis Child. 1978;132(5):484-7.

Woods, CR. Croup: Management. UpToDate. Updated: Mar 05, 2024.

22.9 Foreign Body Aspiration

PE 25.5

INTRODUCTION

A child aspirating a foreign body (FB) into the lower airways is one of the common emergencies in daily practice. If the FB blocks the large airways, it may be associated with impaired ventilation and oxygenation, and can be life-threatening. A missed/forgotten foreign body can lead to chronic respiratory problems, and thus a high index of suspicion is required for the diagnosis of foreign body aspiration when a typical history is not forthcoming.

EPIDEMIOLOGY

Majority (80%) of foreign body aspiration occur under 3 years, with the peak incidence being between 1 and 2 years of age, as at this age most children can stand and explore their world. They put small things in the mouth, while they lack the molars necessary for adequate chewing. Older siblings also tend to insert food in their sibling's mouth. There is a male preponderance of approximately 2:1.

The features of foreign bodies that make them dangerous are round, smooth, and slippery surface and compressibility (**Box 22.6**). Certain drugs such as iron and potassium cause severe inflammation and stenosis by tending to dissolve in the airways, and hence early diagnosis and definitive treatment is essential.

Most of the aspirated foreign bodies tend to locate in the right lung (**Box 22.7**). The laryngotracheal foreign bodies are usually large or irregular; and are associated with increased mortality than those that lodged in the bronchi.

CLINICAL FEATURES

In 50–75% of children, foreign body aspirations present within 24 hours of the episode. The symptoms and signs depend on the age of the child, nature of the FB, location, and degree of blockage of the airways, and time elapsed.

Box 22.6 Common Foreign Bodies

Vegetable foreign bodies (around 80%)—usually toddlers:
- Groundnuts and Bengal gram (approximately 50%)
- Other nuts and seeds (such as watermelon seeds, betel nut, pea nut kernel, walnut, almond, rajma, tamarind seed, maize seed, etc.)
- Popcorn, crumpled potato chips, coconut, etc. **(Figs. 22.12A and B)**

Inorganic foreign bodies—older children and adolescents:
- Plastic (such as pen cap, pen head, small parts of toys, whistle, button)
- Metallic foreign bodies (such as clips, nails, screw, nut bolt, pins, jewelry, etc.) **(Figs. 22.13 and 22.14)**

Others:
- Glass beads, marbles, charcoal piece, cane straw, etc.
- Balloon-like materials (such as gloves or condoms)—may be fatal

Box 22.7 Common Areas of Localization of Foreign Bodies

- Right lung—60% (approximately 52% in the bronchus intermedius)
- Left lung—23%
- Trachea—13%
- Larynx—3%
- Bilateral—2%

- A history of choking, defined as a sudden onset of cough, with or without dyspnea or cyanosis, in a previously healthy child, is present in only around 50% of children.
- In case of a complete airway obstruction or reflex laryngospasm following an acute choking episode, there can be immediate death due to suffocation.
- Most children, however, enter a temporary symptom-free period after the acute episode, which may last for seconds to minutes, which is followed by persistent symptoms.
- Late onset symptoms include unexplained dyspnea, recurrent wheeze and cough; or suppurative complications such as pneumonia, lung abscess and bronchiectasis.

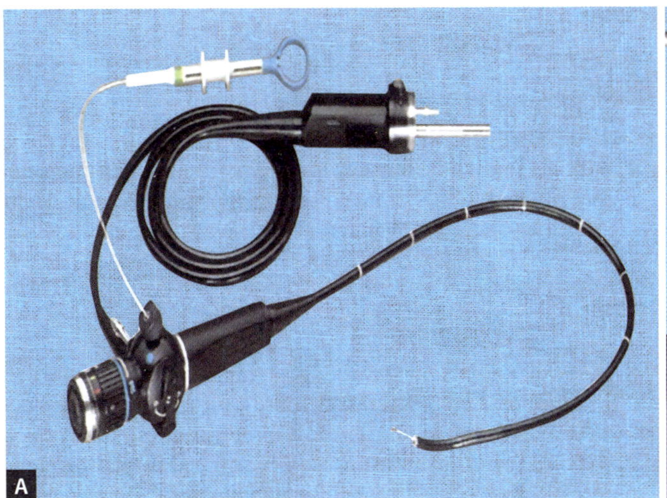

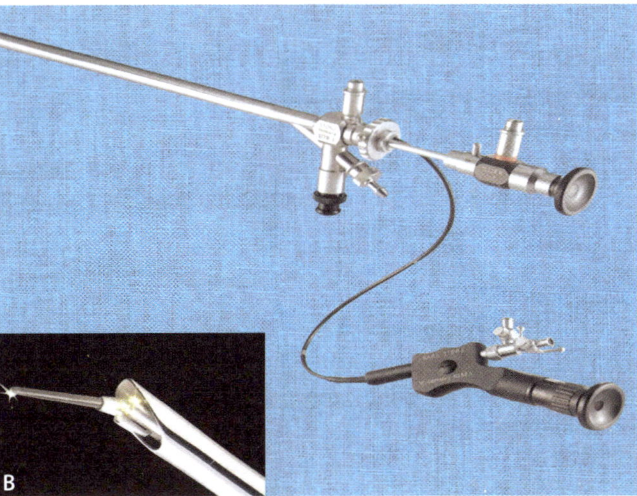

Figs. 22.12A and B: (A) Fiberoptic bronchoscope; (B) Rigid bronchoscope

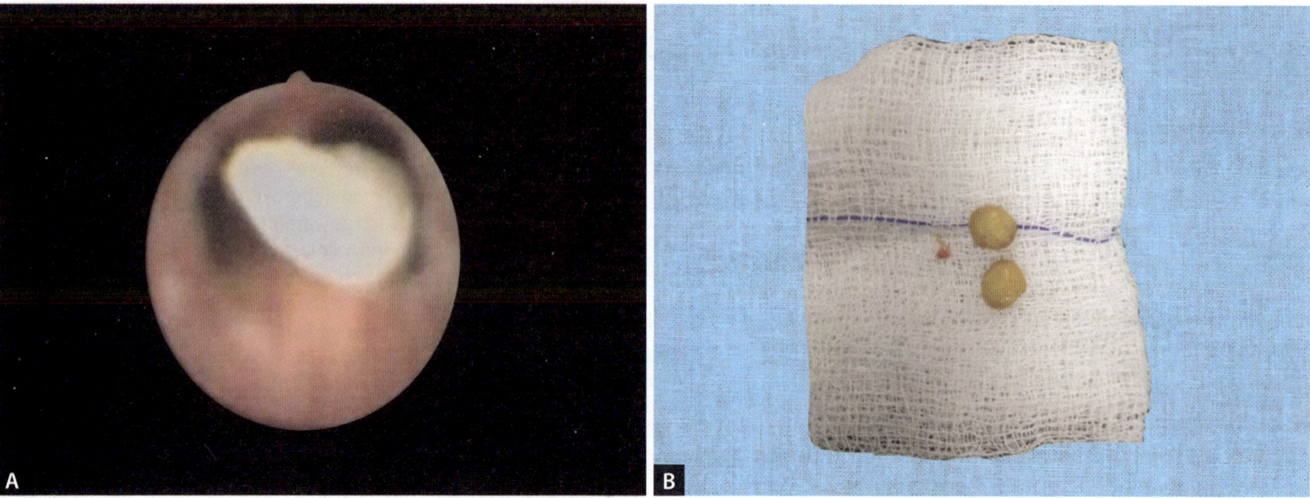

Figs. 22.13A and B: (A) Vegetable foreign body; (B) Extracted vegetable foreign body

Courtesy: Dr Anindya Chattopadhyay

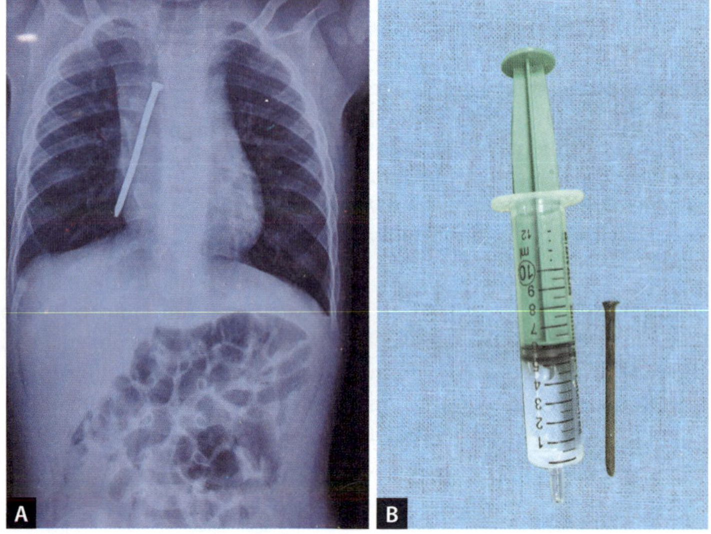

Figs. 22.14A and B: (A) Metal foreign body right main bronchus; (B) Extracted metal foreign body

Courtesy: Dr Anindya Chattopadhyay

- The classic triad of cough, localized wheeze, and decreased breath sounds is present in about 57% of children and has a high sensitivity but a low specificity.

Site of Foreign Body

Symptoms and signs vary according to the site of the foreign body.

- In the *central airways*, they are usually life-threatening and present with stridor, difficulty in breathing, hoarseness and sometimes dysphagia (in case of large penetrating foreign bodies).
- The foreign bodies in the *large bronchi* present with cough, wheeze, dyspnea, cyanosis, and decreased breath sounds.
- Foreign bodies in the *lower airways* are usually the ones that present with a delayed diagnosis with fever and chest infiltrates on the X-ray that do not resolve or recur.

DIAGNOSIS

In cases of a suspected FBA and an asymptomatic child, a plain chest X-ray is performed, preferably in both inspiration and expiration (or left lateral decubitus, if expiratory film is not possible). The usual findings are hyperinflation, atelectasis, mediastinal shift away from the FB and consolidation. Late manifestations include bronchiectatic changes and abscess. If this is normal (approximately in 30% of cases), and the suspicion

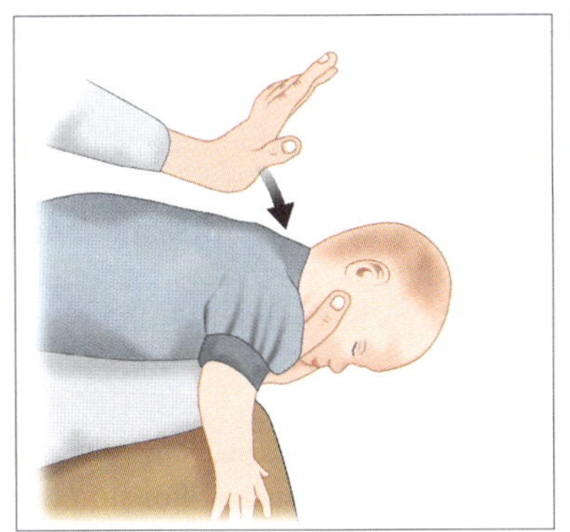

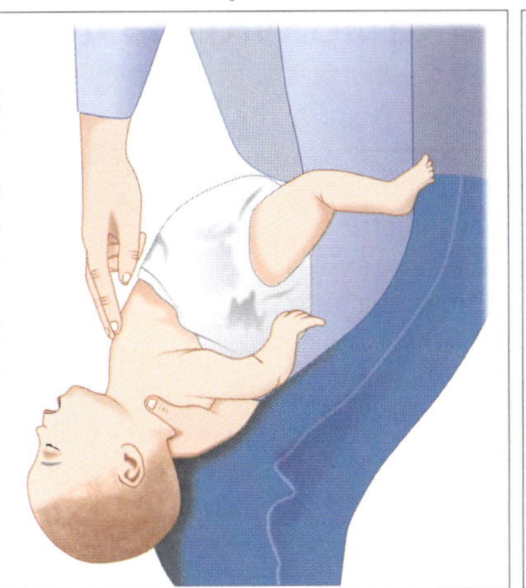

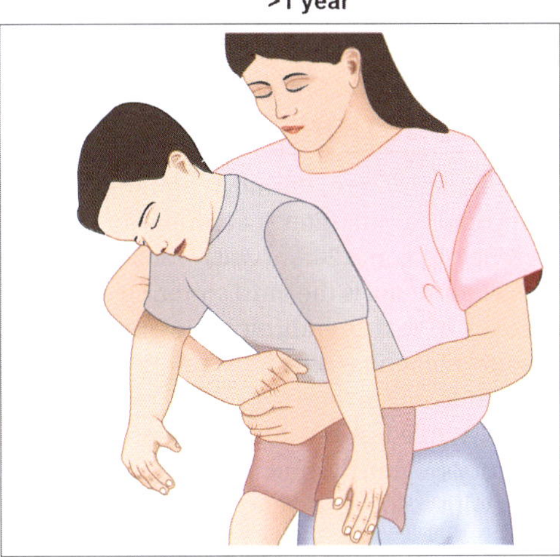

Fig. 22.15: Management of complete laryngotracheal obstruction

is very high, a flexible bronchoscopy or a CT scan of the chest is performed for diagnosis, the former being more definitive.

TREATMENT Foreign Body Aspiration

Immediate Management

In a life-threatening FBA, where the child has a complete obstruction of the airway, dislodgement should be attempted. In infants below 1 year, 5 slaps on the back in the head low position with 5 chest thrusts; while in kids above 1 year, 5 abdominal thrusts (Heimlich maneuver), is recommended **(Fig. 22.15)**.

Foreign Body Removal

Blind finger-sweep', should be avoided in children who are able to cough or speak, as they may convert a partial obstruction to a complete obstruction.

Though the American Thoracic Society recommends only rigid bronchoscopy, some centers with high expertise use the flexible bronchoscope for removal of foreign bodies **(Figs. 22.12A and B)**. In case of a prolonged retained FB, it may be difficult to remove it at one sitting and may require a second bronchoscopy after a course of antibiotics and steroids.

COMPLICATIONS

Death rates have come down over the years where individual studies show rates between 0.21 and 0.94%. Approximately one-third of these present with a hypoxic arrest while another one-third suffer an arrest during the removal procedure. Other major complications include severe laryngospasm or bronchospasm that may require intubation or tracheostomy, and air-leaks like pneumothorax or pneumomediastinum.

PREVENTION

The American Academy of Pediatrics suggests some guidance to be provided to all caregivers at 6 months of age regarding foreign body aspiration. These include avoidance of marbles, balloons, coins, and toys with small parts; feeding of solid food in infants only by adults, and supervised feeding in older children sitting only in the upright position, and not during other activities such as playing, running, crying, or laughing; or when administering chewable medications after 3 years of age and hard round foods above 4 years of age. All child caregivers, teachers, and parents should take a course in Basic Life Support.

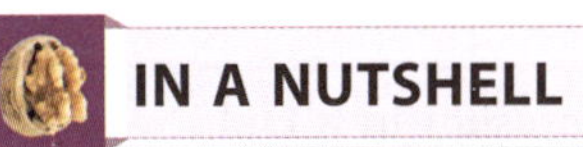

IN A NUTSHELL

Foreign Body Aspiration

1. Majority of foreign body aspirations occur below 3 years of age, the peak incidence being between 1 and 2 years.
2. Most common symptom is acute onset of cough in the absence of other signs of upper respiratory infection.
3. A normal chest X-ray does not exclude foreign body aspiration; two-thirds cases have indirect radiological evidence such as overinflation or atelectasis, depending on the site and degree of obstruction.
4. Rigid bronchoscopy is the management of choice, though recently flexible bronchoscopy is being used more frequently for the same.

Cohen S, Avital A, Godfrey S, et al. Suspected foreign body aspiration in children:what are the indications for bronchoscopy? J Pediatr. 2009; 155:276-80.

Doull I. Foreign body aspiration. In: Eber E, Midulla F (Eds). ERS Handbook of Pediatric Respiratory Medicine, 2nd edition. Switzerland: European Respiratory Society; 2022. pp. 563-8.

Eber E, Antón-Pacheco JL, Blic Jd, et al. ERS Statement: interventional bronchoscopy in children. Eur Respir J. 2017;50:1700901.

Gang W, Zhengxia P, Hongbo L, et al. Diagnosis and treatment of tracheobronchial foreign bodies in 1024 children. J Pediatr Surg. 2012;47:2004-10.

Singh V, Parakh A. Tracheobronchial foreign body aspiration. In: Piyush Gupta (Ed). PG Textbook of Pediatrics, 3rd edition. New Delhi: Jaypee Brothers Medical Publishers (P) Ltd.; 2022. pp. 2246-7.

22.10 Approach to a Child with Fast Breathing

PE 25.6

INTRODUCTION

Fast breathing is one of the most common complaints of children seeking medical attention. It accounts for nearly 10% of pediatric emergency visits and 20% of visits of children younger than 2 years of age. Pneumonia is the most common cause of fast breathing.

Causes of fast breathing are usually reversible, however, failure to recognize and treat underlying cause may lead to adverse outcome in form of cardiac arrest, hypoxic brain damage or death. While fast breathing commonly reflects pathology of respiratory system, dysfunction in other organ systems may also present with respiratory rates higher than usual.

CLINICAL FEATURES

- Fast breathing is defined as respiratory rates higher than >60/min (0–2 months), >50/min (2 months to 1 year), >40/min (1–5 years).
- The higher the respiratory rate above the cut-off, greater is the degree of respiratory distress.
- Fast breathing is also a compensatory mechanism for hypoxia, hypercapnia and acidosis, and can also occur with pain, fever or anxiety.
- Fever increases respiratory distress by up to 10 breaths per degree above the normal.
- Other features that may be present in a child with fast breathing are:
  - Use of accessary muscles of respiration
  - Hypoxemia
  - Grunting
  - Cyanosis
  - Head bobbing
  - Stridor
  - Audible wheeze

Severe Respiratory Distress

Following symptoms/signs suggest severe respiratory distress:

- Inability to feed or drink
- Convulsions
- Excessive sleepiness or lethargy
- Stridor in a calm child
- Cyanosis

DIFFERENTIAL DIAGNOSIS

In addition to primary respiratory illnesses, disease or dysfunction of other organ system may result in fast breathing by either compromising respiratory system or by stimulating compensatory respiratory mechanism.

Respiratory Causes

Fast breathing in a child may be caused by upper or lower airway obstruction or by disorders involving lung parenchyma or interstitium. Upper airway obstruction includes congenital causes such as choanal atresia, laryngomalacia, laryngeal web or stenosis, vocal cord paralysis in neonates; and croup, retropharyngeal abscess, foreign body, epiglottitis, and adenotonsillar hypertrophy in older children.

- ***Lower airway obstruction:*** It may be caused by inflammation and/or bronchospasm and causes include asthma, allergy/anaphylaxis, and bronchiolitis.
- ***Disorders of the alveoli and interstitium:*** These include fluid or pus collection, collapse and structural or functional abnormalities. Pneumonia is the most common causes of respiratory distress in children involving lung parenchyma.

Neurological Causes

Disorder of central nervous system may result in hypo- or hyperventilation, loss of protective airway reflexes or loss of pharyngeal tone. Disorders of peripheral neuromuscular system may result is muscle weakness or paralysis resulting in weak cry, hoarse voice, suppressed cough and gag reflexes, shallow or irregular respiratory pattern.

Cardiovascular Causes

Congenital or acquired heart diseases may result in respiratory distress from congestive heart failure, decreased cardiac output, or reduced oxygen saturation. Manifestation of cardiac involvement may include poor feeding, failure to thrive, feeding diaphoresis, edema, palpitations, and easy fatigability.

Gastrointestinal Causes

Abdominal distension results in impaired diaphragmatic movements and may result in respiratory distress. Massive ascites, intestinal perforation, gaseous bowel distension or any mass in abdomen may cause abdominal distension severe enough to cause respiratory discomfort. Gastroesophageal reflux can cause recurrent aspiration pneumonitis.

Metabolic Causes

Metabolic disturbances can manifest as compensatory alteration in respiratory status. While metabolic acidosis results in rapid and deep breathing, hyperammonemia causes stimulation of respiratory center to result in tachypnea. Blood gas analysis and serum electrolyte estimation can be used to confirm the diagnosis.

Hematological Causes

Low hemoglobin results in decreased oxygen delivery to tissues. Patients with extremely low level of hemoglobin may present with features of congestive heart failure. Polycythemia, on the other hand, leads to sluggish blood flow resulting in impaired tissue oxygenation.

EVALUATION

History Taking

A brief history should be obtained while resuscitating the child. Information regarding onset and progression of symptoms,

Table 22.10 Diagnostic Tests for Evaluation of Fast Breathing in a Child

Radiology	*Invasive tests*
1. Chest X-ray 2. Ultrasound chest 3. CT chest 4. Echocardiogram 5. Barium swallow 6. Chest angiography	1. Bronchoscopy 2. Thoracocentesis
Blood investigations	***Miscellaneous***
1. Arterial blood gas 2. Blood culture 3. Serum electrolytes	1. ECG 2. Pulse oximetry 3. Pulmonary function test 4. Capnography 5. Sputum culture 6. Tuberculin skin sensitivity test

possible precipitating factors, history of recent travel, past history of similar illness, environmental exposure and history of any chronic underlying medical conditions must be obtained.

Physical Examination

The physical examination should focus on quick assessment of degree and likely cause of fast breathing.

- General appearance, vital signs, work of breathing, oxygenation status and level of consciousness should be documented.
- Respiratory rate should be counted for full 1 minute as neonates and young infants may have periodic breathing.
- Once the child is stable, more detailed respiratory examination should be conducted.
- Always examine the cardiovascular and neurological systems to rule out their involvement.

Investigations

Diagnostic tests should be performed selectively to confirm the findings of history and examination. Chest radiography is an important tool to determine the site, extent and possible etiology of fast breathing. Ultrasound chest is an emerging modality used to assess pulmonary status. Ultrasonography is real time, free of radiation and can be performed bedside quickly and repeatedly. Bronchoscopy can be used for both diagnostic and therapeutic indications. A list of various diagnostic tests used in evaluation of respiratory distress in a child is shown in **Table 22.10**.

TREATMENT Fast Breathing

The approach to a child with fast breathing begins with assessment of airway, breathing and circulation (**Flowchart 22.5**). This is followed by establishing the diagnosis. Simultaneously assess the severity of respiratory distress and start supportive treatment as given below.

Patients with severe respiratory distress and/or impending respiratory failure are better managed in intensive care units. Patients suspected to have infectious disease (influenza, COVID-19, tuberculosis, etc.), should be isolated.

For patients with mild to moderate distress, the initial focus is on maintenance of adequate hydration and oxygenation. Arterial blood gas and chest X-ray are the first-line investigations.

- Blood cultures should be obtained in all cases of suspected sepsis but should not lead to delay in administration of antibiotics in a sick child.
- Patient suspected to have a foreign body aspiration should undergo urgent bronchoscopy.
- Tension pneumothorax or massive pleural effusion must be decompressed immediately.
- A nasogastric tube must be placed in patients with abdominal distension to decompress the abdomen.
- Metabolic derangements should be corrected through appropriate measures. AND, finally treat for the cause.

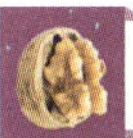

IN A NUTSHELL

Approach to a Child with Fast Breathing

1. Fast breathing is one of the most common complaints of children seeking medical attention.
2. Dysfunction in other organ systems may also present with respiratory rates higher than usual.
3. The higher the respiratory rate above the normal, greater is the degree of respiratory distress.
4. Management of airway, breathing and circulation is always a priority while taking care of a child with fast breathing.

Erickson S. Practical Approach to the Child with Rapid Breathing. In Textbook of Rapid Response Systems: Concept and Implementation. Cham: Springer Nature Switzerland; 2025. pp. 555-70.

Ginsburg AS, May S. Fast-breathing vs chest-indrawing childhood pneumonia: Baseline characteristics. Int J Infect Dis. 2021;104:361-2.

World Health Organization. Revised WHO classification and treatment of childhood pneumonia at health facilities: evidence summaries. Geneva: WHO; 2018.

World Health Organization. Revised WHO classification and treatment of childhood pneumonia at health facilities: Evidence Summaries. [online] Available from: https://www.who.int/publications/i/item/9789241507813. [Last accessed August, 2025].

World Health Organization. Integrated management of childhood illness: chart booklet. Geneva: WHO; 2020.

World Health Organization. Integrated Management of Childhood Illness. [online] Available from: http://apps.who.int/iris/bitstream/handle/10665/104772/9789241506823_Chartbook_eng.pdf?sequence=16. [Last accessed August, 2025].

Flowchart 22.5: Approach to a child with fast breathing

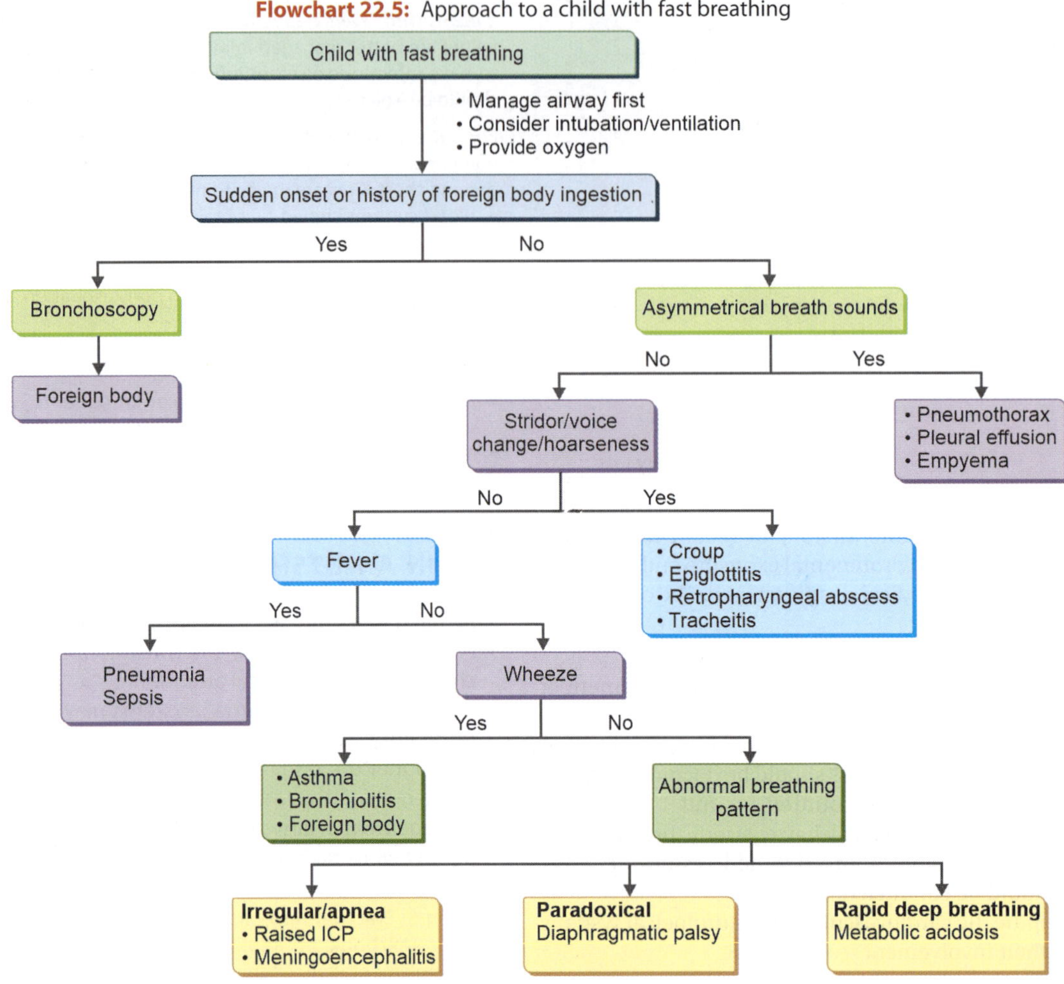

22.11 Pneumonia

PE 25.6

INTRODUCTION

Pneumonia is an important cause of morbidity and mortality in children below 5 years of age. There were 0.7 million deaths due to pneumonia under the age of 5 in the year 2019, which accounted for 14% of all deaths in children under 5 years. Deaths due to pneumonia were highest in South Asia and sub-Saharan Africa.

Pneumonia is an acute inflammation of lung parenchyma usually caused by infection. It can be classified based on anatomical location, the source of infection, and etiological agents. **Box 22.8** provides the classification of pneumonia.

Box 22.8 Types of Pneumonia

- *Anatomical location:*
  - Lobar pneumonia
  - Bronchopneumonia
- *Source of infection:*
  - Community-acquired pneumonia
  - Hospital-acquired pneumonia
- *Etiology:*
  - Bacterial, viral, fungal, parasitic, atypical

ETIOLOGY

The etiology of pneumonia chiefly depends on age. The leading cause of pneumonia in India and developing countries is *Streptococcus pneumoniae* followed by *H. influenzae* type *B. Staphylococcus aureus* and *Klebsiella*. In the first 2 months of life, gram-negative organisms such as *E. coli* and *Klebsiella* are the most important and common causes of pneumonia. Atypical organisms such as *Mycoplasma* and *Chlamydia* usually cause pneumonia in older children and adolescents. However, they are also emerging as pathogens leading to pneumonia in preschool children. **Table 22.11** shows the etiological agents according to various age groups.

Table 22.11 Etiological Agents for Pneumonia	
Age group	*Common causes of pneumonia*
0–2 months	• *Klebsiella* • *E. coli* • Other gram-negative bacteria • *Staphylococcus aureus* • *S. pneumoniae* • *H. influenzae* • Viruses
2 months to 5 years	• *S. pneumoniae* • *H. influenzae* • *Staphylococcus aureus* • Viruses
>5 years	• *S. pneumoniae* • *Mycoplasma* • *Chlamydia* • Viruses

Viruses (mainly RSV) are the most common cause of pneumonia in children in the Western world. They account for up to 50% of cases of pneumonia in children younger than 5 years of age. However, in developing countries, bacterial agents are still the most common cause of pneumonia in children <5 years of age.

PATHOGENESIS

Predisposing Factors

Pneumonia is caused by a combination of risk factors related to the host, environment, and infections. The risk factors for pneumonia in children include low birth weight, malnutrition, vitamin A deficiency, lack of immunization, lack of breastfeeding, passive smoking, large family size, advanced birth order, overcrowding, younger age, and air pollution.

Stages of Pneumonia

Pneumonia is due to an invasion of the lower respiratory tract, below the larynx by pathogens either by inhalation, aspiration, respiratory epithelium invasion, or hematogenous spread. The lower respiratory tract air spaces fill with inflammatory cells, leading to an exudative process that impairs oxygenation. There are four stages of pneumonia:

1. The *first stage* of pneumonia is known as *congestion* and occurs within 24 hours. It is characterized by alveolar edema and vascular congestion.
2. The *second stage is red hepatization* which is characterized by neutrophils, red blood cells, and desquamated epithelial cells.
3. The *third stage* of pneumonia is known as *gray hepatization* which is characterized by hemosiderin and hemolysis of red cells with the replacement of neutrophils by macrophages.
4. The *fourth stage* is the *stage of resolution* in which cellular infiltrates are resorbed, and the pulmonary architecture is restored. If the healing is not proper, then it may lead to parapneumonic effusions and pleural adhesions.

CLINICAL FEATURES

History

The usual symptoms of pneumonia are fever, cough, and fast breathing. In severe cases, the child may present with an inability to tolerate feeds, with grunting or apnea. The uncommon manifestations of pneumonia in infants include refusal to accept feeds, diarrhea, vomiting, and while older children may sometimes complain of pain in the chest or upper abdomen.

Children with atypical pneumonia usually have gradual onset with headache, malaise, nonproductive cough, systemic manifestations, and low-grade fever.

Examination

Pneumonia is characterized by fast breathing and signs of respiratory distress. The child may have nasal flaring, chest retraction, hypoxia on room air, or cyanosis. The physical findings depend on the severity, stage, and complication of pneumonia.

- On auscultation during the early stage of pneumonia crackles may be present on the affected side. Wheezing is usually not a feature of bacterial pneumonia but it may present in viral pneumonia and atypical pneumonia.
- During the late stage of pneumonia or the development of complications such as pleural effusion, there may be dull note on percussion with diminished or absent breath sound during auscultation.

During the physical examination, one should also assess the general well-being of the child including hydration status. The respiratory rate should be counted for a full 1 minute when the child is not crying. The pattern of respiration should be observed. The other systems should also be examined for associated infections or complications.

DIAGNOSIS

WHO Clinical Definition

Pneumonia is a clinical diagnosis. Tachypnea is the most consistent and useful sign for the diagnosis of pneumonia. The World Health Organization (WHO) uses age-specific criteria for tachypnea for making diagnoses and referrals of pneumonia at the community level in the developing world. The WHO criteria for diagnosis and referral of pneumonia are given in **Table 22.12**.

Table 22.12 WHO Classification of Pneumonia in Children 2 Months to 5 Years with Cough or Difficulty in Breathing	
Signs and symptoms	*Classification*
No fast breathing/chest indrawing	*No pneumonia*
Fast breathing* and/or chest indrawing *RR ≥50/min (infant 2–11 months) RR ≥40/min (children 12–59 months)	*Pneumonia*
General danger signs# #Not able to drink, persistent vomiting, convulsions, lethargic or unconscious, stridor in a calm child, or severe malnutrition	*Severe pneumonia*

Chest X-ray

A routine chest X-ray is not required to confirm the diagnosis of pneumonia in children. Indications for the chest X-ray are given in **Box 22.9**. The chest X-ray may be normal during the early course of pneumonia.

Box 22.9	Indications for Chest X-ray in Children with Pneumonia

1. Severe pneumonia
2. A recurrent or prolonged course of illness despite treatment
3. Infants aged 0–3 months
4. Suspected complications such as pleural effusion or pneumothorax
5. Children with atypical presentation
6. Children not responding after 48 hours of treatment

- In viral pneumonia, the chest X-ray shows interstitial infiltrates, bronchial wall thickening, and patchy atelectasis (**Fig. 22.16**).
- The homogeneous opacity with an air bronchogram suggests bacterial pneumonia. Confluent lobar consolidation suggests pneumococcal pneumonia (**Fig. 22.17**).
- Pneumonia due to staphylococcal infection shows areas of breakdown with the air-filled thin-walled cysts (pneumatoceles) (**Fig. 22.18**).

Ultrasound and CT Lung

Lung ultrasound is an emerging modality to diagnose pneumonia in a pediatric emergency. High-resolution chest CT is reserved only for patients who require more extensive imaging or clarification of radiographic findings.

Other Investigations

Routine blood and microbiological tests are not required. Acute phase reactants such as total leukocyte counts, C-reactive protein (CRP), procalcitonin, etc., are not very helpful for diagnosis; however, may be useful for monitoring the treatment. Moreover, these tests do not distinguish between viral and bacterial etiology. The blood culture may be positive in 10–15% of patients with bacterial pneumonia. Nasopharyngeal aspirates can be used for the detection of viruses by using polymerase chain reaction (PCR) technology. Atypical organisms can be confirmed by PCR-based assay on respiratory specimens or raised IgG or IgM in blood.

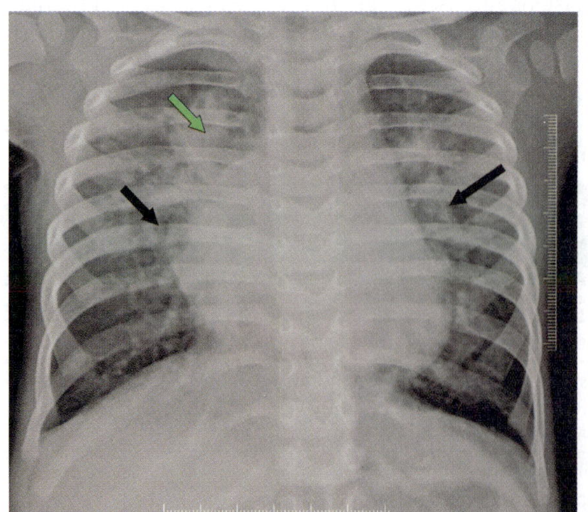

Fig. 22.16: X-ray chest showing bilateral diffuse interstitial infiltrates (black arrows) and bronchial wall thickening (green arrow)

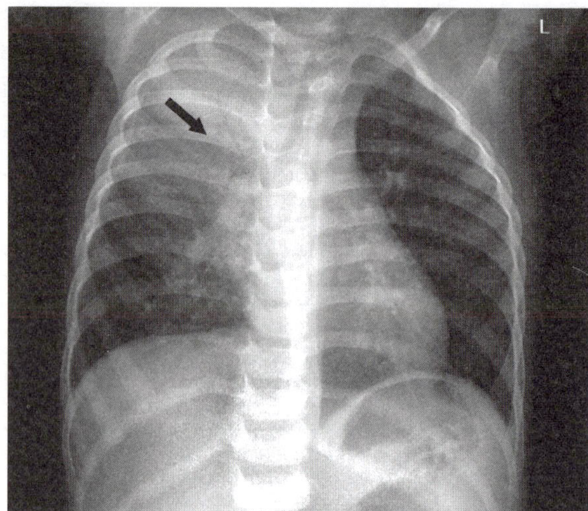

Fig. 22.17: X-ray chest showing lobar consolidation of right upper lobe (arrow)

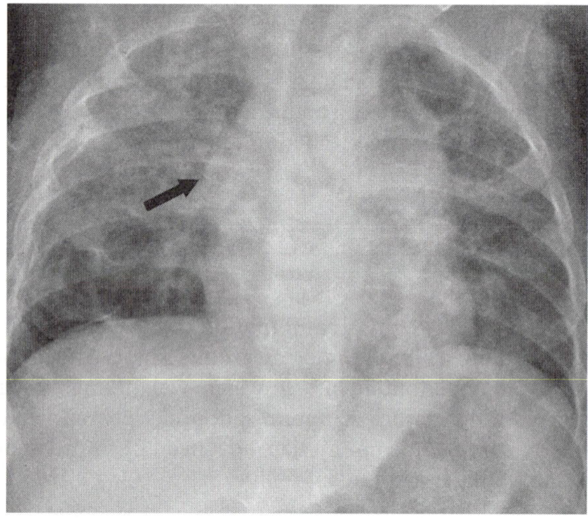

Fig. 22.18: X-ray chest showing bronchopneumonia with pneumatoceles (arrow)

TREATMENT Pneumonia

The management of bacterial pneumonia in children includes specific antibiotic therapy and symptomatic and supportive treatment.

Specific Antibiotic Therapy

Start the antibiotics as early as possible to prevent complications and death due to pneumonia. Empiric antibiotic therapy is based on the knowledge of the most prevalent microorganisms in the community, the patient's age, the severity of illness, and the presence of risk factors. The risk factors associated with poor outcomes of pneumonia include young age, severe malnutrition, unimmunized, receiving antibiotics in the past 2–4 weeks, underlying illnesses such as congenital heart disease, immunodeficiency, chronic respiratory diseases, etc.

Nonsevere Pneumonia

All children aged >2 months with nonsevere pneumonia and without risk factors can be managed at the domiciliary level. The choice of antibiotics for nonsevere pneumonia without risk factors is given in **Table 22.13**. Oral amoxicillin is the preferred first-line antibiotic.

The first-line antibiotics should be given for 5 days while the second-line antibiotics may be given for 5–7 days. The child should be followed up after 48 hours to see the response to therapy. The clinical response comprises the absence of fever and improvement in breathing. In case of nonresponse to antibiotics therapy or clinical deterioration, one should look for alternative diagnoses and complications. In case of clinical deterioration and/or complications the child should be given second-line antibiotics and require hospital admission.

Severe Pneumonia

A child with severe pneumonia and the presence of the risk factors mentioned above should be managed in the hospital with parenteral ampicillin and gentamycin.

- The second line of therapy consists of injectable third-generation cephalosporins preferably ceftriaxone.
- In all HIV-infected children less than 1 year with severe pneumonia, additionally, empirical co-trimoxazole has to be added.
- In case of suspected or proven staphylococcal pneumonia either co-amoxiclav or a combination of ceftriaxone with cloxacillin should be used.
- The duration of treatment for uncomplicated staphylococcal pneumonia is 2 weeks. For methicillin-resistant or complicated staphylococcal pneumonia, the treatment should be given for 4–6 weeks.

Viral Pneumonia

The treatment of viral pneumonia is largely symptomatic and supportive. There is no role for antibiotics in the case of viral pneumonia. However, it is very difficult to distinguish it from bacterial pneumonia at the community level. Therefore, at the community level where no facilities are available to differentiate viral pneumonia from bacterial pneumonia, WHO and National Policy recommend treating all children as bacterial pneumonia.

Symptomatic and Supportive Treatment

Supplemental oxygen should be given for hypoxia. It should be guided by pulse oximetry and signs of respiratory difficulty. Antipyretics for fever and fluids for dehydration should be given. Currently, the available data do not support the use of chest physiotherapy and corticosteroids in pneumonia.

PREVENTION OF PNEUMONIA

Prevention of pneumonia is a key policy to prevent under-5 mortality in children.

Immunization: Routine immunization against tuberculosis, measles, pertussis, *Haemophilus*, and *Pneumococcus*, is the most essential way to prevent pneumonia. After the introduction of the Hib and pneumococcal vaccine, the mortality due to pneumonia has significantly decreased. These vaccines should be routinely administered to all children.

Nutrition: A balanced diet with micronutrients is an important component to improve the natural defense mechanism of the child. Exclusive breastfeeding for 6 months is effective in preventing pneumonia and also in reducing the length of illness.

Air pollution: It is also important to address environmental risk factors such as indoor air pollution since smoke and biomass are found to be an important risk factor for the development of pneumonia. The indoor air pollution can be taken care of by providing liquid petroleum gas (LPG) for cooking and adequate ventilation. Improve hand hygiene and avoidance of crowded places also reduce the risk of pneumonia.

Early diagnosis: It is also important to identify and treat pneumonia as early as possible to reduce pneumonia-related death. One should follow the WHO guidelines for pneumonia and for starting antibiotics at a community level. Healthcare workers may play an important role in the prevention and early identification of pneumonia.

Global Action Plan for Pneumonia and Diarrhea

World Health Organization and UNICEF have launched an integrated Global Action Plan for Pneumonia and Diarrhea (GAPPD) which aims to hasten pneumonia control. This program combines the intervention to protect against pneumonia by providing exclusive breastfeeding for 6 months, preventing pneumonia by providing routine immunization, and treating pneumonia by providing access to health care for every sick child so that appropriate and right care is provided. The child should get early antibiotics and other supportive measures such as oxygen if required. It is important to reduce child mortality by ending preventable diarrhea and pneumonia-related deaths to meet the Sustainable Development Goal (SDG) targets for SDG 3.2.1.

SAANS (Social Awareness and Actions to Neutralize Pneumonia Successfully)—initiative to raise awareness about childhood pneumonia, improve early identification, and promote proper treatment across India. The program also promotes the use of PCV under Universal Immunization Program. The goal of the program is to reduce mortality from childhood pneumonia to less than 3 per thousand live births by the year 2025.

Table 22.13 Choice of Antibiotics for Non-severe Pneumonia without Risk Factors

Age	First line	Dose	Second line	Dose
≤5 years	Amoxicillin	40–50 mg/kg/day, may need to increase to 80 mg/kg/day if there is high resistance to penicillin	• Co-amoxiclav • Cefuroxime • Macrolides*	• 40–50 mg/kg/day • 20–30 mg/kg/day
>5 years	Amoxicillin	40–50 mg/kg/day	Macrolides* Co-amoxiclav Cefuroxime	 40–50 mg/kg/day 20–30 mg/kg/day

*Erythromycin: 30–40 mg/kg/day, Clarithromycin: 15 mg/kg/day, Azithromycin: 10 mg/kg day

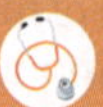

CASE STUDY 1 Pneumonia

A 10-month-old male child, weighing 10 kg presented with a history of cough and difficulty in breathing for 3 days. On examination, his temperature and hydration are normal while his respiratory rate is 56/min. He is accepting orally well and there was no cyanosis.

What is your diagnosis?
List the investigations you should ask for.
How will you manage this child?

1. This child has a cough and fast breathing. His RR is >50/min as per the WHO cut-off for the age. The child has no danger signs. Therefore, the diagnosis is pneumonia (nonsevere).
2. Usually, no investigations are required for nonsevere pneumonia.
3. This child can be treated on an outpatient/domiciliary basis. Start syrup/tablet Amoxicillin 250 mg BD for 5 days. Ask the parents to maintain hydration and provide paracetamol at a dose of 10–15 mg/kg if the child develops a fever. Ask the child to come for a follow-up after 48 hours, and assess for fast breathing and danger signs. If the child is improving then ask the parents to complete 5-day course of antibiotics.

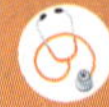

CASE STUDY 2 Pneumonia

A 6-month-old female child presented to you with a history of fever, cough, and difficulty breathing for 2 days. The child is not able to accept orally and vomits everything. On examination, her temperature is raised and the child is lethargic. Her respiratory rate is 64/min with severe chest indrawing. The child also has pyoderma on the trunk.

What is your diagnosis?
What is the probable etiology?
List the investigations you should ask for?
How will you manage this case?

1. The child has a cough and fast breathing with general danger signs including lethargy, and not being able to accept orally. Therefore, the diagnosis is severe pneumonia.
2. The child has pyoderma on the trunk which points toward staphylococcal etiology.
3. Pulse oximetry and complete blood count should be done. Since the child has severe pneumonia, a chest X-ray should also be done.
4. The child should be started on intravenous antibiotics. Since we suspect a staphylococcal infection, we should start either IV co-amoxiclav or third-generation cephalosporin with cloxacillin for a total duration of 7 days.
5. The child should also be started on IV fluid to maintain hydration. Oxygen therapy should be given based on saturation and respiratory distress. Paracetamol should be given for fever.

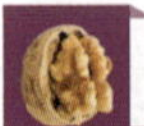

IN A NUTSHELL

Pneumonia

1. Pneumonia is an important cause of morbidity and mortality in children below 5 years of age.
2. Pneumonia may be caused by viruses, bacteria, or fungi. In developing countries, bacteria are still the most common cause of pneumonia.
3. Diagnosis of pneumonia is essentially clinical. Tachypnea is the most useful sign for the diagnosis of pneumonia.
4. Non-severe pneumonia can be managed at the domiciliary level with oral amoxicillin.
5. Severe pneumonia requires hospitalization and parenteral antibiotics.
6. Pneumonia can be prevented by exclusive breastfeeding, routine immunization, and addressing environmental risk factors.

Dean P, Florin TA. Factors associated with pneumonia severity in children: a systematic review. J Pediatric Infect Dis Soc. 2018; 7:323-34.

Goyal JP, Kumar P, Mukherjee A, et al. Acute Respiratory Infection Treatment Unit Study Group. Risk Factors for the Development of Pneumonia and Severe Pneumonia in Children. Indian Pediatr. 2021;58:1036-9.

Grief SN, Loza JK. Guidelines for the Evaluation and Treatment of Pneumonia. Prim Care. 2018;45:485-503.

Kumar P, Medigeshi GR, Mishra VS, et al. Etiology of Acute Respiratory Infections in Infants: A Prospective Birth Cohort Study. Pediatr Infect Dis J. 2017;36:25-30.

Kumar V, Abbas AK, Aster JC. Robbins Basic Pathology, 10th edition. Elsevier-Health Sciences Division; 2020.

Lodha R, Kabra SK, Pandey RM. Antibiotics for community-acquired pneumonia in children. Cochrane Database Syst Rev. 2013;2013(6):CD004874.

Qazi S, Aboubaker S, MacLean R, et al. Ending preventable child deaths from pneumonia and diarrhoea by 2025. Development of the integrated Global Action Plan for the Prevention and Control of Pneumonia and Diarrhoea. Arch Dis Child. 2015;100(Suppl 1):S23-8.

Revised WHO classification and treatment of pneumonia in children at health facilities: evidence summaries; 2014.

World Health Organization. (2016). Pneumonia (Fact sheet No. 331). [online] Available from: https://www.who.int/health-topics/pneumonia#tab=tab_1. [Last accessed August, 2025].

22.12 Empyema Thoracis

PE 25.6

INTRODUCTION

A collection of fluid in the pleural space is referred to as pleural effusion. The nature of fluid can be serous, pus, blood, or chyle.

- ***Parapneumonic effusion*** (PPE) is the common cause of fluid in the pleural space which is commonly associated with pneumonia in the children and resolves with treatment. A small proportion may get complicated and develop into an empyema.
- ***Empyema thoracis*** is an accumulation of pus in the pleural space.

About 40% of bacterial pneumonia is complicated by PPE and among this 10% developed empyema.

ETIOLOGY

Staphylococcus aureus is the most common organism causing empyema, followed by *S. pneumoniae*. Gram-negative organisms (*Pseudomonas aeruginosa* and *Klebsiella*) and fungi (*Candida*) are important etiological agents in immunocompromised children. Setting of pneumonia can have different bacterial flora; community acquired has *Streptococcus pneumoniae* and hospital acquired has *Staphylococcus aureus* (methicillin resistant) and *Pseudomonas aeruginosa*. Anaerobic infections can also cause empyema.

PATHOPHYSIOLOGY

The pleura has two layers—parietal layer that covers the inner surface of mediastinum, thoracic cage and diaphragm; and visceral layer, which covers the entire surface of lung. Both layers are continuous at the hilum of the lung. The pleural space contains 0.3 mL/kg body weight of pleural fluid and fluid turnover is estimated to be approximately 0.15 mL/kg/h. The biochemistry of fluid is pH 7.60, protein 1.5 g/dL and WBCs 1,700 cells/mL (macrophages 75%, lymphocyte 23% and mesothelial cells 2%). Pleura continuously secrets fluid which is absorbed by microvilli, capillary membranes, and lymphatics. The movement of fluid is determined by the equilibrium between filtration and reabsorption.

- The elevated systemic or pulmonary hydrostatic pressure (cardiac failure) or decreased plasma oncotic pressure (nephrotic syndrome or cirrhosis) can affect balance between filtration and reabsorption and lead to accumulation of *transudative fluid*.
- Altered pleural surface and increased capillary permeability (infection) can lead to *exudative fluid*, which meets at least one of the following criteria given by Light:
  - Pleural fluid-to-serum protein ratio >0.5
  - Pleural fluid LDH level (V/L) >200
  - Pleural fluid-to-serum LDH ratio >0.6

  The application of Light criteria should be in context of clinical setting because it was not validated in pediatric population.

PATHOGENESIS

A focus of parenchymal infection leads to increased pulmonary interstitial fluid, which crosses the visceral pleura. Further invasion and multiplication of bacteria in pleural space increases the cellular response, fibrin deposition, and suppuration. The evolution of empyema thoracis can be described under three stages—(1) *exudative*, (2) *fibrinopurulent*, and (3) *organizational*.

Stage I (*Exudative Phase, 1–3 Days*)

Increased pulmonary interstitial fluid, secondary to parenchymal infection, crosses the inflamed visceral pleura and accumulates in pleural space. The fluid is thin, sterile, has low white cell count and free flowing fluid without any septations. The biochemistry of fluid is pH >7.3, glucose >60 mg/dL and LDH <1,000 IU/L and pleural fluid Gram stain and culture is negative. This is parapneumonic effusion.

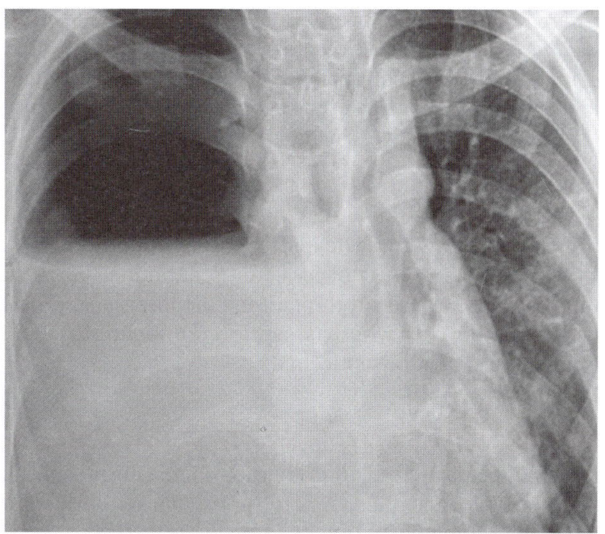

Fig. 22.19: X-ray chest PA view showing air fluid level with homogeneous opacity and obliteration of costophrenic angle on right side

Stage II (*Fibrinopurulent, 4–14 Days*)

This stage is characterized by formation of fibrinous strands in the pleural fluid leading to septations and loculation. The biochemistry of fluid is pH <7.2 (increased lactic acid production), glucose <40 mg/dL (increased glucose utilization by bacteria) and LDH >1,000 IU/L (dead leukocytes). Gram stain shows bacteria ± positive culture.

The fibrin is deposited as continuous sheets that cover both the layers of pleura and thickening of the parietal pleura. If underlying pus is not released, it may travel through the pleura into lung parenchyma producing bronchopleural fistula and pyopneumothorax (**Fig. 22.19**). Rarely, the pus dissects through the chest wall (*empyema necessitans*).

Stage III (*Organizational, After 14 Days*)

In this stage, the fibroblasts grow into the exudate from both the visceral and the parietal pleural surfaces to produce an inelastic membrane "the peel" that entraps lung and prevent expansion.

CLINICAL MANIFESTATIONS

The child with a PPE/empyema usually presents with classical symptoms of pneumonia (cough, dyspnea, fever, malaise, loss of appetite), and may have pleuritic chest pain. The clues which suggest empyema in a case of pneumonia are—rapid worsening of distress or failure to respond after 48–72 hours of initiation of appropriate antibiotic therapy. Child may lie on affected side of hemithorax to splint for symptomatic relief.

On inspection empyema is suggested by unilateral bulging of intercostal space or localized chest wall edema, tenderness, decreased chest expansion and splinting of chest wall to relieve pain. *Palpation* will reveal shifting of trachea and apex beat to opposite side with decreased chest wall movement and tactile vocal fremitus on affected side. Stony dullness is demonstrated on *percussion*. Breath sounds are decreased or absent on *auscultation*. There may be pleural rub in early course of effusion and increased sound conductance in the slightly collapsed area under the fluid may manifest as egophony (examiner hears an "a" sound when patient is saying "e").

COMPLICATIONS

Empyema may be complicated by bronchopleural fistulas pyopneumothorax, purulent pericarditis, pulmonary abscesses, peritonitis from extension through the diaphragm, and osteomyelitis of the ribs whereas septic complications can be meningitis, arthritis, or septicemia.

DIAGNOSIS

Empyema is suspected when there is increasing respiratory distress, persistence of fever, no response to appropriate antibiotics, shift of mediastinum, dull percussion notes, decreased breath sound and vocal resonance on affected side. Imaging, pleurocentesis, and culture can confirm the diagnosis.

Complete Blood Count, Acute Phase Reactant, Electrolytes and Blood Culture

Complete blood count (CBC), CRP and erythrocyte sedimentation rate (ESR) cannot differentiate between pneumonia with or without empyema or PPE or complicated PPE, however, leukocytosis and elevated CRP and or ESR may be found. Syndrome of inappropriate antidiuretic hormone secretion (SIADH) can be suggested by electrolyte estimation. Blood culture is recommended for identification of organism and its yield is low (10–20%) but higher yield than culture of pleural fluid.

Pleural Fluid Cytology, Biochemistry and Culture

Pleurocentesis may be indicated if measured distance between the inside of the chest wall and the outside of the lung is ≥1 cm on a lateral decubitus X-ray. The pleural fluid should be sent for total and differential count, Gram and AFB stains, culture and biochemistry (pH, protein, sugar, and LDH). Features suggestive of empyema are thick pus or gross pus, pH <7.2, glucose <40 mg/dL, LDH >1,000 IU/L and Gram stain showing bacteria ± positive culture.

Complicated PPE is characterized by thin pus (>50,000 WBCs/μL, pH <7.2, glucose <40 mg/dL, LDH >1,000 IU/L) and Gram stain showing bacteria ± positive culture. Pleural fluid culture has low yield. PCR has a better yield.

Imaging

X-ray Chest

X-ray chest findings range from obliteration of costophrenic angle to complete opacification of the hemithorax with shift of mediastinum to opposite side (**Figs. 22.20A to C**). Lateral decubitus radiograph shows fluid occupying between inside of the chest wall and the outside of the lung.

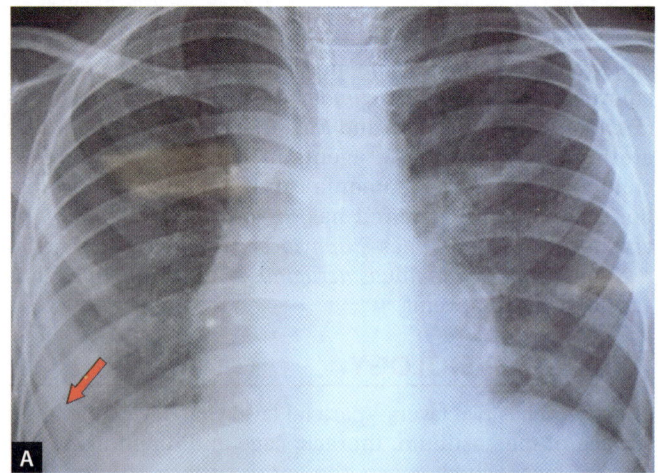

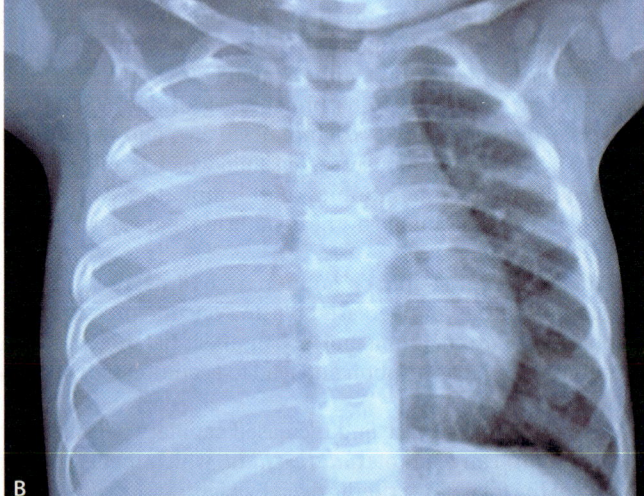

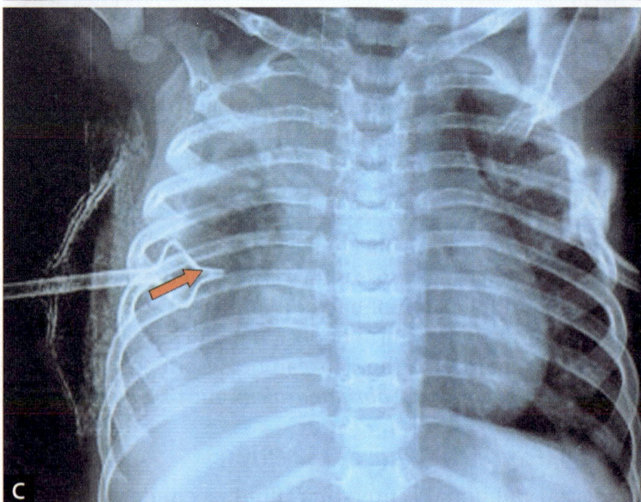

Figs. 22.20A to C: X-ray chest PA view showing: (A) Obliteration of costophrenic angle (red arrow); (B) Complete homogeneous opacity in right hemithorax; (C) Intercostal drainage malecot (orange arrow)

The amount of fluid has different appearance in the different view; a minimum of 250 mL of fluid leads to obliteration of costophrenic angle in an upright chest radiograph. Even 10 mL of fluid can be detected in lateral decubitus radiograph. Free flowing effusion can be identified by shifting of fluid location with change in position of patient (upright to lateral view) or concave meniscus sign paralleling the chest wall or layering of fluid on lateral decubitus radiograph.

- Loculated effusion is characterized by absence of shifting of fluid location with position or pleural collection having a lenticular shape with internal convexity.
- The presence of empyema on X-ray chest may be suggested by presence of lung abscess, cavitary pneumonia adjacent to pulmonary alveolar consolidation, or loculated effusion.
- Radiological resolution of empyema takes time, it ranges from 3 months to 1.5 years. Therefore, chest X-ray has limited role in follow-up of empyema.

Ultrasonography

Ultrasonography of chest can detect small PPE to large loculated effusion. It can measure size of effusion, differentiate between free flowing and loculated effusion, detect echogenicity of the fluid, and demonstrate plural thickening. Ultrasonography is helpful in staging of effusion:

- Anechoic fluid
- Echoic fluid with septations
- Fibrinous septations and
- Septations with solid appearing components comprising more than one-third of effusion. Septations and debris are well identified on ultrasound than CT scan and site of pleurocentesis can be marked by ultrasound.

Chest Computed Tomography

CT chest is indicated when an alternative diagnosis (pulmonary abscess) or mediastinal pathology needs clear delineation or prior to open thoracotomy/thoracoscopy.

TREATMENT Empyema Thoracis

The objective of empyema treatment is sterilization of pleural fluid and restoration of normal lung function. The outcome of treatment depends on early diagnosis and appropriate intervention, stage of effusion, and availability of surgical intervention. Treatment is broadly categorized into medical and surgical which includes appropriate antibiotics, chest tube drainage and instillation of fibrinolytics in the pleural cavity, video-assisted thoracoscopy surgery (VATS) and open decortications.

It is advisable to document the stage of pleural effusion before selecting the most appropriate intervention for better clinical outcome.

- Stage I effusion (PPE or exudative phase) is treated with antibiotics and close monitoring for deterioration, if effusion is increasing, intercostal drainage (ICD) will required.
- Stage II effusion is treated with antibiotics, ICD and instillation of fibrinolytics in pleural cavity, however VATS has clinically equivalent outcome when compare with ICD and fibrinolytics.
- Stage III effusion is treated with VATS or open thoracotomy.

Medical Treatment

Antibiotics

A combination of cloxacillin and aminoglycoside is preferred for initiating therapy. Alternative combination is third generation cephalosporin and cloxacillin. If Gram stain is suggestive of gram-negative bacilli, a combination of third generation cephalosporin and aminoglycoside would be the choice. Later, the culture report will guide the choice, duration, and tailoring of antibiotics.

The common practice is to give intravenous therapy till resolution of fever or removal of ICD followed by oral antibiotics for 1–4 weeks. Recommended duration of antibiotics for empyema caused by *S. pneumoniae* and *H. influenzae* is 7–10 days whereas for *S. aureus* is about 4–6 weeks. Almost 6–12 weeks may be required for empyema caused by anaerobic organisms.

Antibiotics available for methicillin resistant *S. aureus* (MRSA) include vancomycin, linezolid, and teicoplanin.

Supportive Care

Fever should be treated with paracetamol and homeostasis is maintained by proving fluid and electrolyte. Oxygen supplementation is given by nasal prongs or high-flow nasal cannula, CPAP, or BiPAP as per severity of distress. Respiratory physiotherapy is recommended to increase pleural fluid drainage and to restore pulmonary functions.

Intercostal Drainage

The indication of ICD placement are thick/gross pus or thin pus (>50,000 WBCs/μL). Repeated needle thoracentesis is not recommended in case of empyema.

The selection of size of chest tube does not impact of fluid drainage when used with fibrinolytics and published literature demonstrated that equivalent success rate either using small bore or large bore ICD. Ultrasound-guided small bore drains are better than large bore drains inserted by blunt dissections.

Daily monitoring of ICD output is required, and removal of ICD is recommended when fluid output is <50 mL or 1 mL/kg/day for 3 days with sign of improvement in X-ray/ultrasound and clinical well-being.

Fibrinolytics

The available fibrinolytics are streptokinase (SK), urokinase (UK) and alteplase (tPA) with different mechanism of actions. The use of fibrinolytics agent in early stage of effusion (7–10 days) increases fluid drainage, relief fever, shorten hospitalization, decrease need of surgical intervention, and prevents complications (pleural thickening and fibrosis). However, late instillation beyond 14 days with more doses also show response and are effective. Controlled trials comparing effect of saline and fibrinolytics agents demonstrated that fibrinolytics are superior. The choice of fibrinolytic agents are depend on it availability and dose of agents are not standardized; SK-15000 U/kg in 50 mL saline once daily over 1 hours with dwell time of 4 hours for 3 days, UK-40000 U/kg in 40 mL saline (>1 year) or 10000 U/kg in 10 mL saline (<1 year) twice a day for 3 days with dwell time of 4 hours and (tPA)-0.1 mg/kg in 30 mL saline with dwell time of 1 hour three times a day for 3 days or 4 mg in 40 mL saline with dwell time of 1 hour once in day for 3 days. All fibrinolytic agents can be associated with intrapleural bleeding and allergic or anaphylaxis is seen with streptokinase; chest discomfort during intrapleural instillation. The contraindication of fibrinolytic therapy is bronchopleural fistula and bleeding diathesis. There is ongoing debate on VATS versus intrapleural fibrinolytic therapy; however available randomized controlled trials and meta-analysis suggested that both are clinically equivalent and fibrinolytic therapy is cost effective, less invasive and can be performed in conscious sedation. The factors associated with poor response to agents are pleural thickening, lung abscess and use after VATS.

Surgical Management

Indication of surgery include antibiotic therapy failure, ineffective chest drainage, or inadequate response to fibrinolytics. The surgical modalities include VATS, mini-thoracotomy, and open thoracotomy with decortication.

- VATS is least invasive and is the preferred option. Organized empyema, bronchopleural fistula, pyopneumothorax and significant loculated empyema require VATS/mini-thoracotomy. Early VATS (within 48 hours of hospitalization) significantly decreases the length of hospitalization.
- In case of significant pleural thickening or when VATS is not available, open thoracotomy with decortication would be the choice. The other indication of surgery is failure of medical therapy.

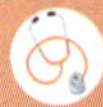

CASE STUDY Empyema Thoracis

A 3-year-old girl weighing 12 kg presented to the hospital emergency with history of fever, cough, vomiting and decreased appetite for 15 days. She had received some oral drugs for 10 days but her symptoms continued to persist. She had developed difficulty in breathing and left-sided chest pain for the last 2 days. She is taking rapid but short breaths. She prefers to lie on the left side. Her pain increases on coughing.

Outline the differential diagnoses based on history. Justify your approach.

The symptoms of fever, cough and chest pain indicate respiratory illness, which has been progressive (chest pain and breathing difficulty for 2 days) and of a long duration with significant severity (decreased oral acceptance and breathing difficulty), therefore, the most probable diagnosis would be *severe pneumonia*. Difficulty in breathing and chest pain on left side indicate either synpneumonic effusion or pneumothorax on left side. Tuberculosis should also be kept as a differential diagnosis, since it may also present with similar features in highly endemic areas.

On examination, she was lethargic, had a temperature of 39°C, pulse rate of 120/min and the blood pressure was 96/50 mm Hg. The respiratory rate was 58/min and SpO_2 was 85%. Child had nasal flaring, with significant chest indrawing. Trachea was shifted to right. The left side of the chest appeared bulging when inspected from the foot end of the patient lying supine. The chest movements were decreased on the left side and it was stony dull to percussion. Auscultation revealed decreased breath sounds with decreased vocal resonance on left side. The heart sounds were better heard on the right side of the chest suggesting a shift of the mediastinum.

What is the most probable diagnosis? Justify.

The shifting of mediastinum to right side, increased left hemithoracic volume (bulge) with decreased chest movements, suggests that the lesion is on the left side. On percussion, the left side was stony dull and auscultation revealed ipsilateral decrease in breath sounds. All these findings suggest a left-sided pleural effusion. Looking at the poor general condition of the patient and features of severe respiratory distress (tachypnea, chest indrawing, hypoxia and lethargy) there is a high likelihood of pyogenic infection.

List the investigations required to confirm the diagnosis, in order of priority:

- Chest skiagram in erect posture.
- *Pleural tap and fluid examination:* Gross and microscopic examination. Gram staining, bacteriological culture; and biochemical examination.
- Complete hemogram including differential leukocyte count.
- Blood culture.

Describe the initial management of this child.

This child has significant respiratory distress and hypoxemia. She should be admitted and immediately put on oxygen supplementation to maintain SpO_2 above 92%. She will need supportive therapy in form of antipyretics such as paracetamol and maintenance intravenous fluids. Further specific treatment shall be guided by the pleural fluid examination.

On pleural tapping, frank thick pus was aspirated and sent for microbiological testing.

Outline the specific therapeutic plan for this child.

This child has empyema. The pus in the pleural cavity should be drained with an intercostal thoracostomy tube using an under water drainage. She should be given injectable antibiotics covering for staphylococcal infection, e.g., a combination of cloxacillin/amoxy clavulanic acid with an aminoglycoside (gentamicin or amikacin). Antibiotic therapy shall need to be given for 4–6 weeks, of which initial 10–14 days therapy should be intravenous. Chest tube can be removed when the drainage is <50 mL per day for 3 consecutive days and there is no suggestion of a bronchopleural fistula. A nutritious diet with high protein is given.

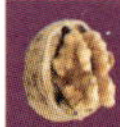

IN A NUTSHELL

Empyema Thoracis

1. Empyema is mostly a complication of bacterial pneumonia.
2. *Staphylococcus aureus* is the most common causative pathogen.
3. Very young children may present with predominantly abdominal signs and symptoms.
4. Ultrasonography is a better modality than CT scan to differentiate free from loculated fluid.
5. Thoracocentesis is ultimately required for differentiation of uninfected parapneumonic effusion from empyema.
6. Initial therapy consists of IV cloxacillin and gentamicin. Total duration of treatment is 4–6 weeks.
7. Intercostal drainage with a chest tube is the mainstay of therapy.

Buonsenso D, Cusenza F, Passadore L, et al. Parapneumonic empyema in children: a scoping review of the literature. Ital J Pediatr. 2024;50(1):136.

Fernandez Elviro C, Longcroft-Harris B, Allin E, et al. InsightScope Team. Conservative and Surgical modalities in the management of Pediatric Parapneumonic Effusion and Empyema: a living systematic review and network Meta-analysis. Chest. 2023;164(5):1125-38.

Forster J, Paul P, Liese J. Current management of Pediatric Parapneumonic Pleural effusions and Pleural Empyema. Pediatr Infect Dis J. 2023;42(11):e407-10.

Zuccatosta L, Piciucchi S, Martinello S, et al. Is there any role for medical thoracoscopy in the treatment of empyema in children? Clin Respir J. 2023.

22.13 Approach to a Child with Wheeze

PE 25.6

INTRODUCTION

Wheeze is a whistling and/or musical adventitious sounds that are produced due to lower airway obstruction. These are heard most commonly but not exclusively during expiration. Common causes of wheezing in children are asthma and bronchiolitis.

Wheezing is a common presentation in children, with approximately 20% of children having an episode of wheezing in the first year of life. Almost 50% of children have at least one episode of wheeze by the age of 6 years. Recurrent wheeze is seen in one-third of children of preschool age and causes significant morbidity, decreased quality of life and economic burden on family.

- ***Polyphonic wheezing:*** It refers to musical sounds of varied pitch, due to widespread but variable narrowing of the airways as seen in bronchiolitis, bronchitis, and bronchial asthma.
- *Monophonic wheezing:* It refers to a single-pitch sound produced during expiration, due to localized obstruction of the larger airways, as in foreign body or extraluminal compression of the airway, e.g., due to enlarged lymph node or vascular rings, etc.

PATHOPHYSIOLOGY

Obstruction to airflow is the underlying mechanism of wheezing in all cases, irrespective of the etiology. Obstruction to the airway may be anatomic or physiological and is usually caused by either intraluminal obstruction or extraluminal compression (**Figs. 22.21A to C**). In airway malacia, the tracheal or bronchial wall abnormally collapses during expiration. Airway edema, bronchiolar constriction and intraluminal blockage due to secretion may occur simultaneously in asthma, leading to severe manifestations. Intrinsic airway narrowing is more likely to result in predominately expiratory wheeze, while biphasic wheeze is usually caused by extrinsic airway compression.

Risk Factors Associated with Early or Preschool Wheezing

These include influences of certain genes (*ORMDL3* and *GSDMB* genes on chromosome 17q21), prenatal environment (uncontrolled maternal asthma or maternal smoking); and postnatal environment (rapid weight gain in early infancy, exposure to tobacco smoke or traffic-related particles, endotoxins, paracetamol, day care attendance and older siblings). Having older siblings or attending day care increases the chances of respiratory viral infections [(respiratory syncytial virus (RSV) and human rhinovirus being the most common viruses], thus increasing the risk of preschool wheezing.

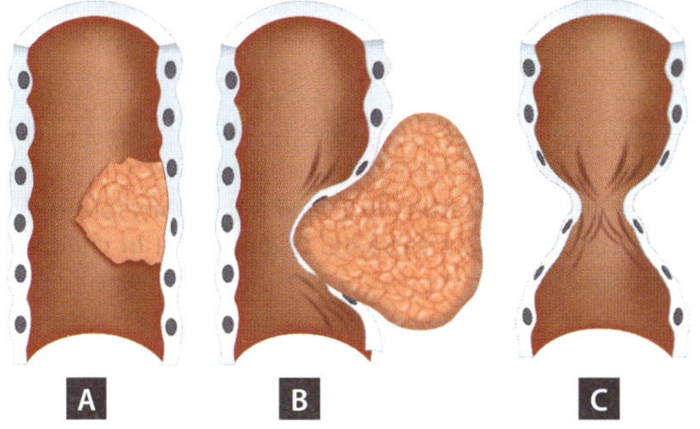

Figs. 22.21A to C: Modes of airway compression: (A) Intraluminal compression; (B) Extrinsic compression; (C) Malacia

Box 22.10 Life-threatening Causes of Wheeze in Children

1. Status asthmaticus
2. Severe bronchiolitis
3. Foreign body aspiration
4. Pulmonary hemorrhage
5. Congestive heart failure
6. Chemical pneumonitis
7. Anaphylaxis
8. Smoke inhalation

ETIOLOGY

Wheeze can be caused by variety of diseases in children, however few conditions are seen more commonly than others. Life-threatening causes of wheeze (**Box 22.10**) should be recognized and managed appropriately.

Most wheezing in infants is caused by infection (generally bronchiolitis), but many other entities can manifest with wheezing, as listed here:

- Infection
  - *Viral:* RSV, parainfluenza virus, influenza virus, rhinovirus C, and human metapneumovirus
  - *Bacterial: Streptococcus pneumoniae, Chlamydia trachomatis, Mycoplasma,* tuberculosis
- Asthma
- Anatomic abnormalities
  - *Central airway abnormalities*: Laryngomalacia, tracheomalacia, bronchomalacia
  - *Extrinsic airway anomalies resulting in airway compression:* Mediastinal lymphadenopathy from tuberculosis or tumor, vascular ring or sling, mediastinal mass or tumor, duplication cyst, and esophageal foreign body
- ***Mucociliary clearance disorders:*** Cystic fibrosis, primary ciliary dyskinesias, bronchiectasis
- ***Aspiration syndromes:*** Gastroesophageal reflux disease (GERD)
- ***Others:*** Congenital heart disease with left-to-right shunt (increased pulmonary edema), foreign body.

PHENOTYPES OF WHEEZERS

The most common phenotype seen in children is "*episodic viral wheeze*" where viral respiratory infection results in wheezing and respiratory distress, but there are no interval symptoms. The other phenotype is labeled as *multitrigger wheeze* (preschool asthma). Children with this phenotype have clinical behavior similar to asthma and they have exacerbations in response to multiple triggers (viral infections, cold air, crying, exercise). They also have interval symptoms and commonly have family history of atopy.

CLINICAL ASSESSMENT

- ***Triggers:*** Viral infections of the respiratory tract are the most common predisposing factors leading to airway obstruction and wheeze. This phenomenon of wheeze-associated respiratory infection is not uniquely associated with viral infections; and can also be seen with bacterial infections of lower respiratory tract. All these disorders used to be collectively termed as wheeze-associated lower respiratory tract infections (WALRIs). Other triggers include running, laughing, crying, cold weather, fumes, and dust, etc. (usually seen in asthma).
- ***Type of cough:*** A spasmodic cough which is more at night or in early morning, is characteristic of wheezy disorders. In a few cases, isolated spasmodic cough may be the only indication of a wheezy disorder (cough variant asthma).
- ***Age of onset and duration of wheezing:*** Onset of wheezing in infancy indicates bronchiolitis, WALRI, GERD, or congenital heart disease. While children with severe and persistent asthma can present early, yet any child with infantile onset should be diligently assessed for asthma mimickers such as congenital airway malformations, vascular ring, GERD, and cystic fibrosis. Asthma is, however, the most frequent cause of recurrent wheezing in children after 5 years of age.
- ***Associated symptoms:*** Vomiting/regurgitation of feeds suggests GERD. History of atopy, eczema, or rhinitis should alert to possibility of asthma.
- ***Birth history:*** Need for prolonged ventilation or oxygen therapy in neonatal period can predispose to chronic lung disease of infancy which can present with tachypnea with crackles and wheeze.
- ***Past history:*** Recurrent respiratory tract infections, malabsorption, failure to thrive suggest immunodeficiency or mucociliary disorders including cystic fibrosis or alpha-1 antitrypsin deficiency.
- ***Family history:*** Ask for history suggestive of asthma, cystic fibrosis, tuberculosis in siblings, parents, and grandparents.
- ***Social history:*** Parental smoking habits, overcrowding at home, presence of pets, molds, cockroaches should be enquired for.
- ***Physical examination:*** Record vitals, oxygen saturation (SpO_2), signs of respiratory distress including character of wheeze, pulsus paradoxus, and timing and presence of stridor. Look for signs of atopy: Dermatitis, sneezing, hives, boggy turbinates, etc.
- ***Presence of atypical features*** such as clubbing, recurrent multisystemic infections, chronic diarrhea, failure to thrive, feeding difficulties, recurrent or persistent radiological shadows, localized monophonic wheeze, etc., should alert to a possibility of nonasthmatic wheezing.

DIFFERENTIAL DIAGNOSIS

In the first 2 years of life, wheezing is mostly caused by acute viral respiratory infections such as bronchiolitis and WALRI. After first 2 years of age, wheezing is often due to asthma particularly if the child has a definite history of afebrile episodes. Sometimes children with pneumonia present with wheeze. It is important to consider pneumonia as an alternative diagnosis, particularly in the first 2 years of life. The differential diagnoses of the common causes of wheezing and their salient features are detailed here:

- ***Asthma:***
  - History of recurrent wheeze, some unrelated to coughs and colds
  - Family or personal history of asthma/eczema/hay fever
  - Hyperinflation of the chest and prolonged expiration
  - Reduced air entry (if very severe airway obstruction)
  - Good response to bronchodilators
- ***Bronchiolitis:***
  - First episode of wheeze in a child aged <2 years
  - Wheeze episode at time of seasonal bronchiolitis
  - Hyperinflation of the chest and prolonged expiration
  - Reduced air entry (if very severe, airway obstruction)
  - Poor/no response to bronchodilators
- ***Wheeze associated with lower respiratory infection:***
  - Wheeze always related to coughs and colds
  - No family or personal history of asthma/eczema/hay fever
  - Prolonged expiration
  - Good response to bronchodilators
- ***Foreign body:***
  - History of sudden onset of choking or wheezing
  - Wheeze may be unilateral
  - Air trapping with hyper-resonance and mediastinal shift
  - *Signs of lung collapse:* Reduced air entry and impaired percussion note
  - No response to bronchodilators
- ***Pneumonia:***
  - Fever
  - Cough with fast breathing
  - Lower chest wall indrawing
  - Crackles or bronchial breathing on auscultation

EVALUATION OF A CHILD WITH WHEEZING

History

Age of onset, duration and course of illness, aggravating or relieving factors and associated clinical features must be asked in every patient. A history of response to medication, especially bronchodilators may point toward reversible hyper-reactive airway disease. A family history of asthma, atopy and smoking should be asked. While sudden onset of disease point toward foreign body inhalation or anaphylaxis, a gradual onset is seen in conditions such as chronic lung disease or tuberculosis. Persistent wheeze is seen in mechanical airway obstruction like vascular ring or external airway compression.

Physical Examination

One must differentiate the actual wheeze from other causes of noisy breathing such as stridor, stertor and conducted

Flowchart 22.6: Approach to a child with wheeze

Recurrent wheezer

Symptoms based

- Episodic (viral) wheeze*
- Multitrigger wheeze**

Time-trend based

- **Transient wheeze** Symptoms begin and end before the age of 3 years
- **Persistent wheeze** Symptoms begin before the age of 3 years and continue beyond the age of 6 years
- **Late-onset wheeze** Symptoms begin after the age of 3 years

*Wheezing during specific time period (during URTI), absence of symptoms in between episodes

**Episodic wheezing with symptoms along with symptoms in between episodes (e.g., during sleep or with triggers like activity, laughing, exercise, crying, smoke or cold air)

sounds. Wheezing is a high pitch, polyphonic, whistling sound, heard mostly during expiration. The intensity of wheeze correlates with degree of airway obstruction, however it must be noted that critically narrowed airways may present with a "silent chest".

Apart from respiratory system examination, one must look for other associated features or signs of complication such as clubbing, cardiomegaly, hepatomegaly, pedal edema, lymphadenopathy, eczema, conjunctivitis, or allergic rhinitis.

An algorithm is presented in **Flowchart 22.6** for elucidating cause of wheezing in a child.

INVESTIGATIONS

Most children with wheezing do not require any investigations and diagnosis can be made on history itself. Chest X-ray is usually done to rule out any serious pathology, but not routinely recommended in every patient with wheeze. High resolution computed tomography (HRCT) may be needed in patients with bronchiectasis or chronic lung disease. Pulmonary function test with documentation of reversible airflow obstruction is required to make a diagnosis of asthma. Rarely, genetic testing may be required in some cases such as cystic fibrosis or alpha-1 antitrypsin deficiency. Bronchoscopy may be needed for suspected foreign body. Recent GINA (Global Initiative for Asthma) guidelines advocate the use of peak expiratory flow (PEF) measurements for the diagnosis of asthma.

TREATMENT Child with Wheeze

Treatment depends on underlying etiology. However, irrespective of the cause, a trial of bronchodilator must be given in a child with wheeze. The response to bronchodilator can be unpredictable, especially in young infants but patients with asthma usually show an excellent response. Steroids may be indicated in asthma or anaphylaxis or in patients with history of atopy including eczema and food allergy.

In children younger than 5 years of age, distinguishing between viral-induced episodes, seasonal variation or allergen-triggered asthma can be very challenging. Short acting bronchodilators can be used intermittently. However, If SABA (short acting beta-2 agonist) use exceeds twice weekly on average over a month, a trial of low-dose ICS is recommended for at least 3 months.

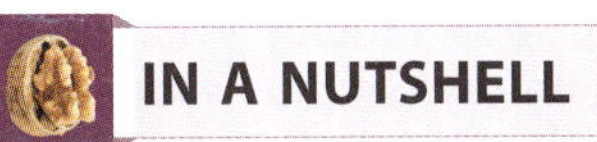

Approach to a Child with Wheeze

1. Wheezing in children could be a sign of diverse clinical conditions.
2. History alone can establish the diagnosis in majority of cases.
3. Every wheeze is not asthma, and other causes must be excluded wherever needed.
4. Bronchodilators and steroids are the mainstay of treatment in a child with wheezing, but response is unpredictable.

Ahmed H, Turner S. Severe asthma in children—a review of definitions, epidemiology, and treatment options in 2019. Pediatr Pulmonol. 2019;54(6):778-87.

Al-Shamrani A, Bagais K, Alenazi A. Wheezing in children: approaches to diagnosis and management. Int J Pediatr Adol Med. 2019;6(2):68.

Ardura-Garcia C, Stolbrink M, Zaidi S. Predictors of repeated acute hospital attendance for asthma in children: a systematic review and meta-analysis. Pediatr pulmonol. 2018;53(9):1179-92.

Fainardi V, Santoro A, Caffarelli C. Preschool wheezing: trajectories and long-term treatment. Front Pediatr. 2020;8:240.

Global Initiative for Asthma. 2024 GINA Main Report. Global strategy for asthma management and prevention. Accessed on Feb 07, 2024. Available from: https://ginasthma.org/2024-report/

22.14 Bronchiolitis

PE 25.6

INTRODUCTION

Bronchiolitis is a viral lower respiratory infection which occurs in infants and children under 2 years of age, usually in the first year of life, with a peak incidence between 3 and 6 months of age.

Bronchiolitis is seasonal, predominantly occurring in autumn/winter; it accounts for approximately 15% of hospitalizations and emergency department presentations in children under 2 years.

ETIOPATHOGENESIS

Bronchiolitis is commonly caused by respiratory syncytial virus (RSV), which has two antigenic strains (RSV-A and RSV-B). These strains often have an alternating dominance annually, but RSV-A is associated with higher morbidity. RSV infection accounts for approximately 50% of hospital admissions in children under 6 months with bronchiolitis.

The pathology is characterized by increased secretion of pro-inflammatory cytokines which result in acute airway inflammation, edema, epithelial cells damage, and increased mucus production. Together these features result in bronchospasm (**Fig. 22.22**).

Risk factors for bronchiolitis are listed in **Box 22.11**.

Box 22.11 Risk Factors for Bronchiolitis

1. Premature birth, particularly under 32 weeks
2. Chronic lung disease of prematurity (including bronchopulmonary dysplasia)
3. Hemodynamically significant congenital heart disease
4. Age (under 3 months)
5. Neuromuscular disorders including those who have difficulty swallowing or clearing mucus secretion
6. Immunodeficiency

CLINICAL FEATURES

Symptoms usually begin with a viral upper respiratory tract infection including rhinorrhea, with or without fever, for a 1 or 2 days followed by lower respiratory symptoms including cough, tachypnea, increased work of breathing, grunting or nasal flaring. One-third may have a high temperature of 39°C lasting 1–3 days, followed by persistent cough and poor feeding typically after 3–5 days of illness. Cough resolves in 90% of infants within 3 weeks.

Findings on examination include tachypnea and/or chest recession associated with either wheeze and/or crackles on chest auscultation. Presentation varies by age; young infants may present with apnea while older children present with wheeze.

INVESTIGATIONS

- ***Blood tests*** should not be performed routinely in the assessment of a baby or child with bronchiolitis.
- ***Chest X-ray*** is not routinely performed in suspected bronchiolitis because changes may mimic pneumonia and should not be used to determine the need for antibiotics. Consider chest X-ray if diagnostic doubt, e.g., congenital cardiac disease, lobar pneumonia, high fever, in a child who has failed to improve within the expected time frame, or grossly asymmetric findings on examination.
- ***Nasopharyngeal aspirate*** should be taken to detect causal viruses by qPCR including RSV, influenza A&B, parainfluenza, metapneumovirus, adenovirus, rhinovirus and parechovirus.
- ***Blood gas*** should only be done in a child with respiratory failure who is deteriorating and may need high dependency of intensive care support.

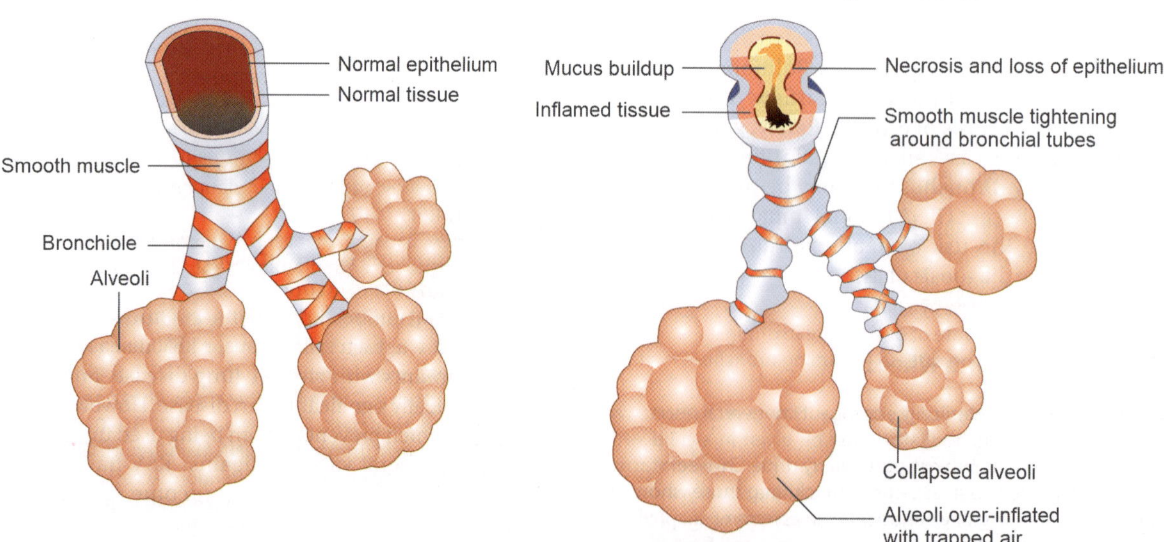

Fig. 22.22: Pathophysiology of bronchiolitis

DIFFERENTIAL DIAGNOSIS

Pneumonia should be considered if there is a high fever (over 39°C) and/or persistently focal crackles. Viral-induced wheeze or early-onset asthma is likely, rather than bronchiolitis, in older children with persistent or episodic wheeze without crackles, or with a personal or family history of atopy.

TREATMENT Bronchiolitis

The mainstay of management remains supportive. Respiratory support may be needed for infants that require admission. This ranges from oxygen therapy alone to positive airway pressure therapies. The other main consideration is nutritional support and hydration. Infants may need admission because of poor oral intake secondary to increased respiratory distress and work of breathing (**Box 22.12**). In this case nasogastric feeding may be needed, or if severe, intravenous fluids may be required. **Table 22.14** summarizes the guidelines on various therapeutic interventions in the management of bronchiolitis.

Oxygen Therapy

Supplemental oxygen therapy must be given to maintain oxygen saturations at >94%. There is no evidence of benefit of supplemental oxygen in infants who do not have hypoxia. Oxygen may be administered via nasal cannulae, or face mask. If supplemental oxygen alone is insufficient to maintain normal oxygen saturations, then additional support may be required.

High-flow nasal cannula (HFNC) oxygen therapy is indicated in moderate-to-severe bronchiolitis. CPAP should be considered in children with increasing evidence of respiratory failure.

Intubation and mechanical ventilation is indicated in infants with progressive respiratory failure despite support with noninvasive positive pressure ventilation.

Hydration Support

Infants with bronchiolitis can have difficulty feeding because of nasal congestion or hypoxemia related to lower airway disease and increased respiratory distress. If the child is unable to maintain sufficient oral hydration, nasogastric fluids are recommended and preferred over intravenous fluids. There is no evidence of benefit of intravenous hydration over nasogastric hydration, with no increase in aspiration episodes or adverse events associated with nasogastric hydration. One of the risks of intravenous hydration includes hyponatremia, so only isotonic intravenous fluids must be used.

Box 22.12 Indications for Hospitalization in Bronchiolitis

1. Feeding <50% normal volume or who appear to be clinically dehydrated
2. Infants younger than 3 months of age are at greatest risk of getting bronchiolitis because their lungs and immune systems are not yet fully developed
3. Saturations persistently <92% in air
4. Children with a respiratory rate of over 60 breaths/min
5. All children with chronic lung disease (including broncho-pulmonary dysplasia)
6. All children with hemodynamically significant congenital heart disease
7. All children born premature birth, particularly under 32 weeks
8. All children with neuromuscular disorders including those who have difficulty swallowing or clearing mucus secretion
9. Children with immunodeficiency

Table 22.14 Recommended Use of Interventions in Management of Bronchiolitis: Summary of NICE (UK) Guidelines (2015)

Treatment/ intervention	*NICE recommendation*
Beta agonists	Not recommended
Corticosteroids	Not recommended
Adrenaline	Not recommended
Nebulized hypertonic saline	Not recommended
Antibiotics	Not recommended
Suctioning	• Do not perform routinely • Upper airway suction in those with respiratory distress or difficulty feeding because of increased secretions
Chest physiotherapy	• Not to be done routinely • May be indicated in the presence of comorbidities such as spinal muscular atrophy, tracheomalacia, underlying chest disease
Supplemental oxygen	Use to maintain normal oxygen saturations >94%
Heated humidified high-flow oxygen or air via nasal cannula	Can be used and may be beneficial to help maintain saturations. Although current evidence insufficient to suggest *must* be used. Most evidence suggests it may be helpful in mild to moderate bronchiolitis in alleviating respiratory distress
CPAP	Should be considered in children as a noninvasive measure to support children with impending respiratory failure
Monitoring and pulse oximetry	Intermittent pulse oximetry and monitoring to be used in all children admitted to hospital. May need to escalate to continuous monitoring as the need for respiratory support increases to either high-flow oxygen or CPAP
Hydration and nutrition	• Preferred and first line—nasogastric or orogastric fluids in those unable to maintain adequate oral fluid intake • Isotonic intravenous fluids in children unable to tolerate nasogastric feeds, and those with worsening respiratory distress or impending respiratory failure • The ideal volume of intravenous fluids to initiate is unknown, can start with between 60 and 100% maintenance

PREVENTION

Immunoprophylaxis is currently only available against RSV infection. The only licensed preventive strategy for RSV infection is the monoclonal antibody palivizumab, which is administered to infants who are at high risk of severe RSV disease. This includes premature infants with chronic lung disease, and infants with hemodynamically significant heart disease. However, palivizumab is expensive which prevents it from being used universally.

Although several vaccines against RSV have been trialed, none to date have met primary outcome criteria. The most promising has been a maternal vaccine, but only showed benefit for secondary trial endpoints.

LONG-TERM SEQUELAE OF SEVERE BRONCHIOLITIS

- Infants who have had a severe episode of bronchiolitis especially those that have had infection with RSV or rhinovirus C are at risk of recurrent episodes of lower respiratory tract infections and wheezing in the subsequent 2–3 years, during preschool age.
- Approximately one-fourth of those with recurrent wheeze may also progress to develop asthma at school age. Up to one-fourth of children with an episode of bronchiolitis requiring mechanical ventilation may progress to develop asthma at age 6–12 years.
- A rare, long-term sequela of viral bronchiolitis, affecting <1%, is postinfectious bronchiolitis obliterans. The most common etiological pathogen is adenovirus. It is usually only seen after a very severe illness involving a prolonged period of mechanical ventilation.

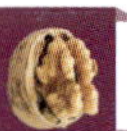

IN A NUTSHELL

Bronchiolitis

1. Bronchiolitis is a clinical syndrome in children <2 years of age characterized by fever, cough, cold, tachypnea and/or wheezing.
2. Bronchiolitis is primarily caused by respiratory syncytial virus.
3. Risk factors for severe disease and/or complications include gestational age <37 weeks, age <12 weeks, chronic pulmonary disease, congenital and anatomic defects of the airways, congenital heart disease, immunodeficiency and neurologic disease.
4. Bronchiolitis is diagnosed clinically. Chest radiographs and laboratory tests are not routinely indicated.
5. Management is supportive. Bronchodilators may work in some patients.

Dalziel SR, Haskell L, O'Brien S, et al. Bronchiolitis. Lancet. 2022;400:392-406.
Franklin D, Babl FE, Schlapbach LJ, et al. A randomized trial of high-flow oxygen therapy in infants with bronchiolitis. N Engl J Med. 2018;378:1121-31.
Kepreotes E, Whitehead B, Attia J, et al. High-flow warm humidified oxygen versus standard low-flow nasal cannula oxygen for moderate bronchiolitis (HFWHO RCT): an open, phase 4, randomised controlled trial. Lancet. 2017;389: 930-9.
Zar HJ, Nduru P, Stadler J, et al. Early-life respiratory syncytial virus lower respiratory tract infection in a South African birth cohort: epidemiology and effect on lung health. Lancet Glob Health. 2020;8:e1316-e1325.

22.15 Bronchial Asthma

PE 28.2, PE 28.3, PE 28.4, PE 28.5

INTRODUCTION

Bronchial asthma (BA) is a heterogeneous disease characterized by chronic airway inflammation and hyper-responsiveness. The prevalence of bronchial asthma in children varies widely from 2 to 20% in India.

The typical presentation of BA is cough, wheezing, and breathing difficulty. Symptoms can be controlled with appropriate management.

Global Initiative for Asthma (GINA) Definition

"Asthma is a heterogeneous disease usually characterized by chronic airway inflammation. It is defined by the history of respiratory symptoms (e.g., wheeze, cough, etc.) that vary over time and in intensity together with variable expiratory airflow limitation".

ETIOPATHOGENESIS

The exact etiology of asthma is not known. It is postulated to be multifactorial in origin. A close interaction between host and environmental factors is responsible for the inception of bronchial asthma (**Flowchart 22.7**). In genetically susceptible children, any breach in the respiratory epithelium leads to a cascade of immunological reactions. It activates helper T (Th2) cells which in turn release many cytokines and chemokines, leading to eosinophilic inflammation (IL-5), IgE production

Flowchart 22.7: Risk factors and pathogenesis of asthma

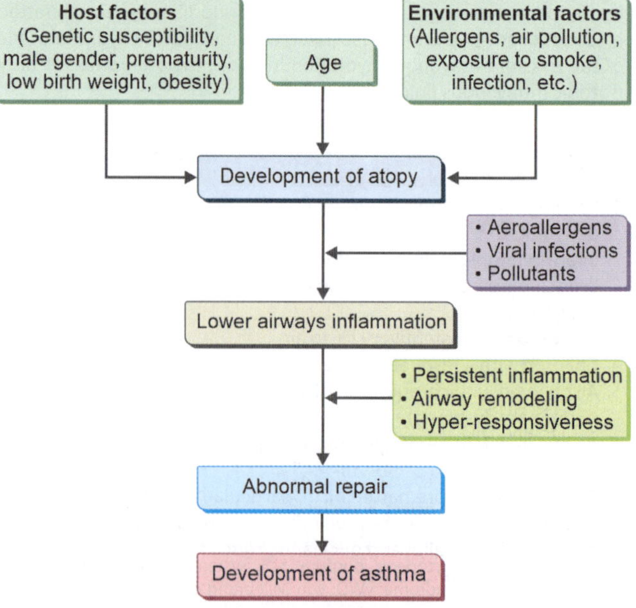

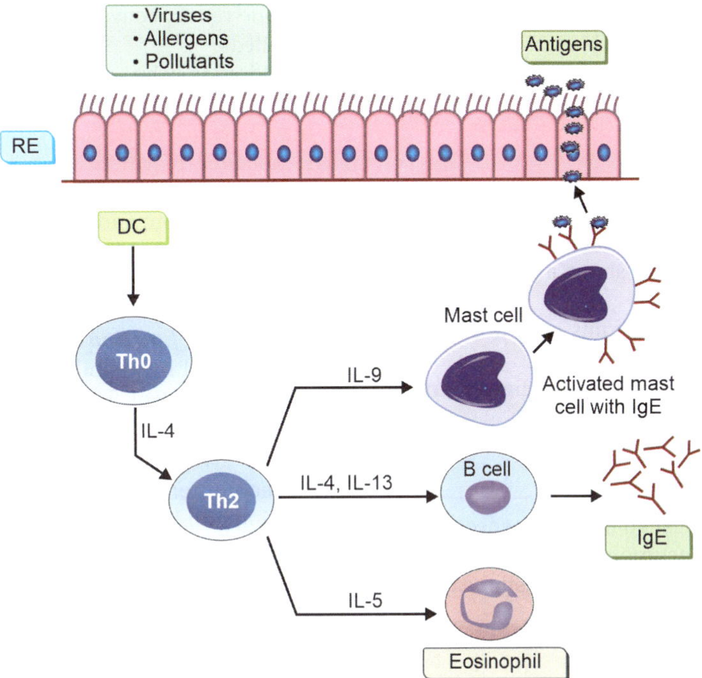

Fig. 22.23: Etiopathogenesis of asthma. Exposure to viruses, allergens or pollutants causes injury to the respiratory epithelial (RE) barrier. Antigens enter through injured RE and present to dendritic cells (DC). DC activates naïve T-cells (Th0) which in the presence of IL-4 activate helper T2 (Th2) cells. Th2 cells activate mast cells, B cells and eosinophils. B cells form IgE which binds to the mast cells. Subsequent antigen exposure binds to IgE on the mast cells surface to result in its degranulation and release several chemokines and growth factors

(IL-4, IL-13), and mucus overproduction (IL-13) (**Fig. 22.23**). In addition to an inflammatory reaction, structural change in airways (airway remodeling) is also seen which also causes asthma symptoms.

Airway narrowing is the common final pathophysiology of BA, resulting in asthma symptoms and variable airflow limitation. The underlying mechanism of airway narrowing is smooth muscle contraction, airway edema, thickening, and mucus hypersecretion. Airway hyper-responsiveness is another mechanism of airway narrowing in response to external (e.g., air pollution, smoke, etc.) or internal (e.g., emotional stress, etc.) stimuli and is responsible for intermittent asthma symptoms. Furthermore, the circadian rhythm of circulating hormones leads to increased airway inflammation and narrowing at night, which is responsible for increased asthma symptoms at night.

Precipitating Factors

There are two types—(1) external and (2) internal. *External factors* are viral infection, irritants (dust, *agarbatti*, dust, mosquito repellent, etc.), allergens (pollens, animal dander, pets, molds, etc.), and weather changes. *Internal factors* are exercise, emotional stress (laughing, crying), and puberty.

CLINICAL FEATURES

The most common symptoms in children are recurrent episodes of cough and wheezing. The cough is usually dry. These symptoms are often associated with shortness of breath, chest tightness, and exercise intolerance. The characteristic feature of asthma is that more than one symptom is present and varies with time and intensity (**Table 22.15**). These symptoms often worsen at late night or in the early morning. Symptoms often worsen with exercise, laughter, viral infection, exposure to cold air, allergens, and seasonal variation. Initially, the severity of asthma was labeled at the time of diagnosis; however, now it is done retrospectively, a step at which symptoms are well controlled.

Table 22.15 Characteristics Pattern of Asthma Symptoms

Symptoms characteristics of asthma	*Symptoms not characteristics of asthma*
More than one symptom should be present: • Cough • Wheezing • Shortness of breath • Chest tightness	*When present in isolation:* • Only cough or chronic wet cough • Shortness of breath associated with dizziness • Exertional dyspnea • Chest pain

The child may have the clinical features of associated comorbidities such as sneezing, itching, nasal discharge and block (*allergic rhinitis*), rash, itching (*atopic dermatitis*), redness, discharge and itching of the eyes (*vernal conjunctivitis*), snoring, and interruption of sleep (*obstructive sleep apnea, adenoid hypertrophy*), nausea or vomiting, nocturnal cough (*gastroesophageal reflux*) and obesity.

CLINICAL PHENOTYPES

It is a recognizable clinical or demographic pattern of asthma. It is of the following types:

- ***Allergic asthma:*** It is common during childhood asthma. There is often a family or personal history of allergy (e.g., nasal, skin, or eye allergy). It responds well with inhaled corticosteroid (ICS) therapy.
- ***Nonallergic asthma:*** It is not associated with allergy. It is common in adult-onset asthma. It shows a poor response to ICS therapy.
- ***Exercise-induced asthma:*** Symptoms only occur during exercise.
- ***Asthma with obesity:*** This is an emerging asthma phenotype with variable response to ICS therapy.

DIAGNOSIS

The diagnosis of asthma is established in the presence of characteristics clinical features, and documentation of expiratory flow limitation. A diagnostic approach to childhood asthma is shown in **Flowchart 22.8**.

Clinical History and Examination

A detailed clinical history and physical examination are carried out to elicit characteristic patterns of symptoms. Children often have a history of atopic dermatitis and allergic rhinitis. One should also look for lead points for another differential diagnosis. In the past, the severity of asthma was made at diagnosis; now, it is done retrospectively, the step at which symptoms are well controlled.

Children may be completely normal during physical examination. The most common sign is expiratory wheeze; however, it may be heard in both inspiration and expiration or absent. The absence of wheezing may be an indication of severe exacerbation. Other findings are barrel-shaped chest, tachypnea, diffuse crepitation, and chest retraction. The child may present in severe respiratory distress and may have cyanosis, arrhythmia, and pulsus paradoxus. The presence of clubbing, localized chest finding, or failure to thrive indicates an alternative diagnosis.

Pulmonary function test (PFT) is needed to document flow limitation and reversibility. It can be performed either with spirometry or a peak flow meter.

Spirometry

It is recommended test for the documentation of airflow limitation and bronchodilator reversibility. The indication for spirometry in children is shown in **Box 22.13**.

Box 22.13 Indications for Spirometry in Children

1. Knowing the pattern of lung disease, i.e., obstructive vs. restrictive
2. Diagnosis of asthma
3. Classifying severity of the disease
4. Monitoring response to therapy
5. Monitoring the progression of the disease
6. To assess preoperative risk

Flowchart 22.8: Approach to diagnosis of asthma

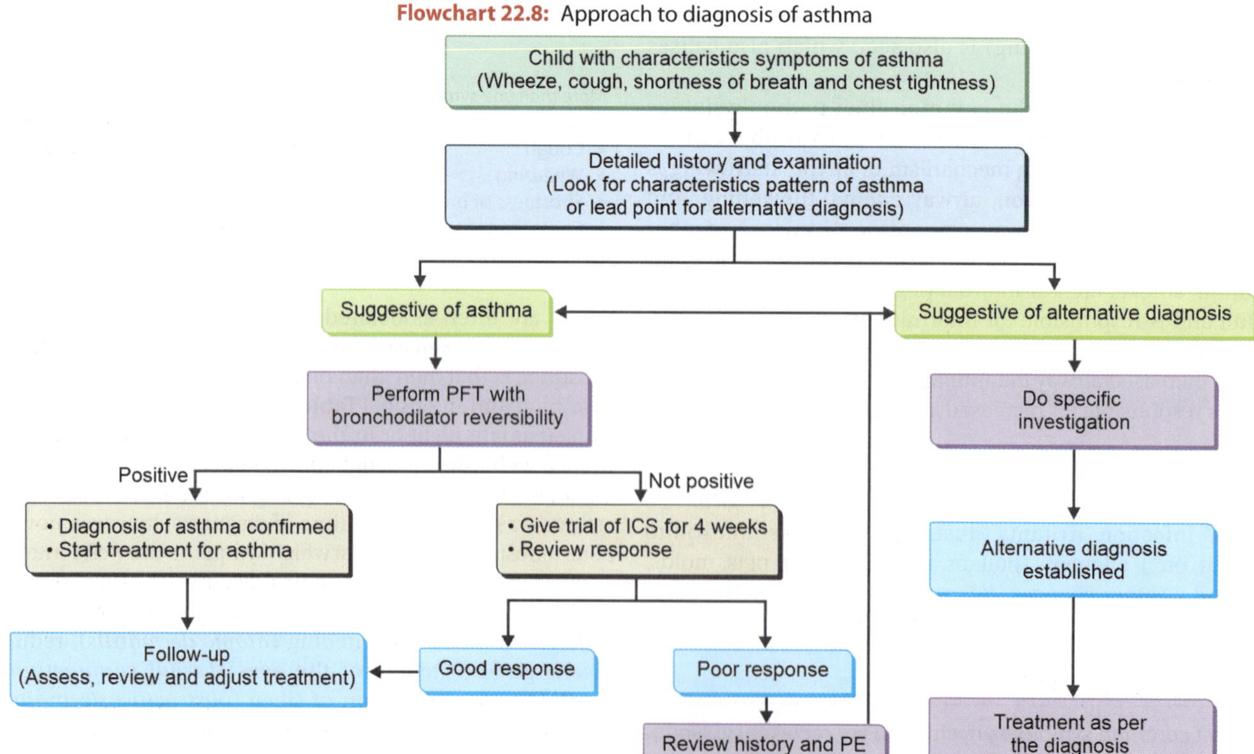

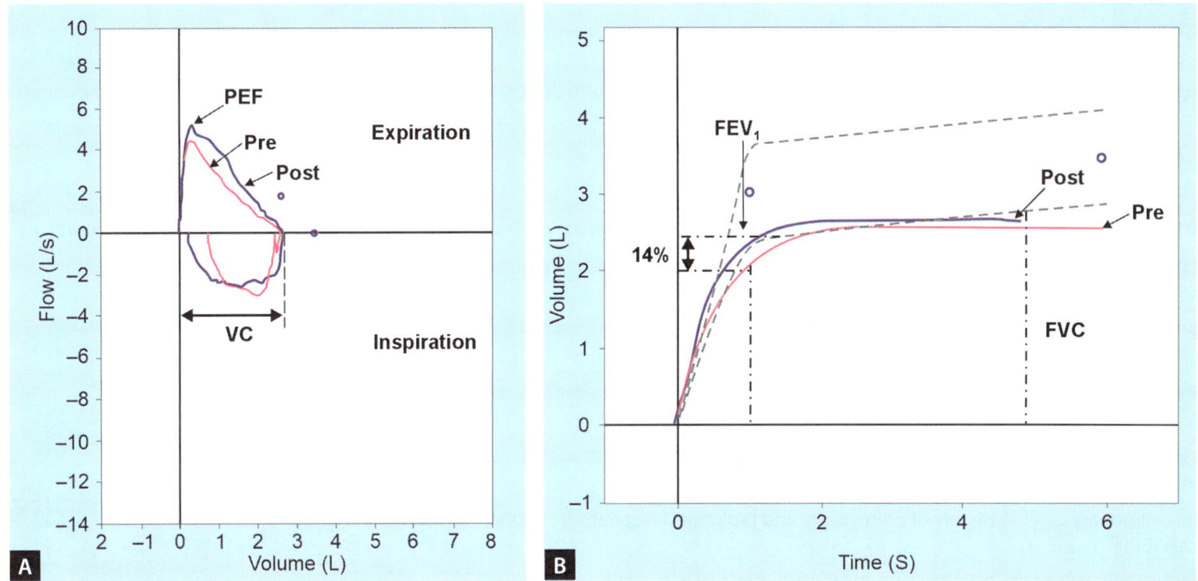

Figs. 22.24A and B: Typical spirometry graphs. Spirometry from 8-year-old child: (A) Flow-volume loop; (B) Volume-time graph [PEF: peak expiratory flow; FEV_1: forced expiratory volume in one second; FVC: forced vital capacity; VC: vital capacity. Postbronchodilator (purple), there is a 14% increase in FEV_1 from the prebronchodilator value (pink)]

The child is asked to inhale maximally in this procedure, followed by fast and forceful expiration. It gives rise to two types of graph: (1) flow-volume loop and (2) flows time graph (**Figs. 22.24A and B**). The test is accepted if it is free from errors (e.g., cough, premature cessation, etc.). The procedure is repeated three times, and the highest value is taken. Since it is an effort-dependent maneuver, the children should be given prior instruction to get acceptable and reproducible results.

Interpretation

Spirometry provides several parameters, the commonly used are forced expiratory volume in one second (FEV_1), forced vital capacity (FVC), the ratio of FEV_1/FVC, and forced expiratory flow between 25 and 75 (FEF_{25-75}) of expiration. Their result is compared with the predicted value derived from the population study based on age, sex, and height and expressed in percentage. In asthma, all these parameters are decreased. For bronchodilator reversibility, the test is repeated 10–15 minutes after administration of 2–4 puffs (200–400 µg) of meter dose inhaler (MDI) or 0.15 mg/kg of nebulized salbutamol. It is recommended to withhold short-acting beta-2 agonist (SABA) for 4 hours, long-acting beta-2 agonist (LABA) for 12 hours, and ICS for 24 hours before spirometry. The spirometry criteria for the diagnosis of asthma in children are summarized in **Table 22.16**.

Peak flow meter: A peak flow meter is a simple and inexpensive device that measures peak expiratory flow. It is useful when spirometry is unavailable, or a child cannot perform it. Its value is compared with patients' previous value taken during the asymptomatic period (personal best). It is repeated three times, and the highest value is taken. Postbronchodilator ≥15% change in PEF is considered a positive change.

Table 22.16 **Spirometry Criteria for the Diagnosis of Childhood Asthma**

Parameters	*Diagnostic criteria*
Expiratory flow limitation	FEV_1 or FEV_1/FVC <90% of predictive value
Positive bronchodilator responsiveness (BDR)	≥12% change in FEV_1 or ≥15% change in PEF

(FEV_1: forced expiratory volume in one second; FEV_1/FVC: ratio of FEV_1 to forced vital capacity (FVC); PEFR: peak expiratory flow rate)

OTHER INVESTIGATIONS

There is no role of other investigations in the diagnosis of asthma; however, they can help to exclude other differentials or evaluate a child whose symptoms are not controlled with adequate therapy.

Hemogram: Eosinophils count may be increased (≥3% or ≥400/mm³). However, it may be within normal range or elevated due to other causes (e.g., parasitic infection). Therefore, it is not required to make a diagnosis of asthma. If present, it predicts an excellent response to ICS.

Serum IgE: It is also not specific to asthma and is not recommended for the diagnosis of asthma.

Chest X-ray: It is not routinely required to make a diagnosis of asthma. If performed, it is usually normal or may show bilateral hyperinflation (air trapping) with increased bronchovascular marking. However, when the diagnosis is unsure or has atypical findings (e.g., unilateral findings), it may help exclude other diagnoses.

Sputum analysis: It may help to document eosinophilic or neutrophilic inflammation; however, there is currently insufficient evidence to recommend it for asthma diagnosis in children.

Table 22.17 Differential Diagnosis of Asthma in Children

Differential diagnosis	*Lead point in history and examination*
Foreign body (FB)	History of FB aspiration, a sudden bout of cough during eating or playing, unilateral or localized chest findings
Tuberculosis (TB)	History of fever for ≥2 weeks with or without a history of cough, weight loss, and positive history of contact
Congenital airway malformations	• Onset since early infancy, noisy breathing • No response to bronchodilator therapy
Aspiration	History of nausea, vomiting, burning sensation or chest pain in relation to food intake, abnormal posturing
Cystic fibrosis	• History of recurrent respiratory tract infection, large bulky stool, poor weight gain • History of similar illness in other siblings
Primary ciliary dyskinesia (PCD)	History of neonatal respiratory distress in term baby, frequent pneumonia, ear infection, or sinusitis. Presence of dextrocardia or situs inversus
Immunodeficiency	• Early onset, recurrent infection at multiple sites (e.g., skin, lung, intestine, ear, etc.) • History of sibling death
Hypersensitivity pneumonitis (HP)	History of worsening with exposure to inciting agents
Bronchopulmonary dysplasia (BPD)	History of prematurity and prolonged respiratory support, symptoms since birth
Congenital heart disease	In the examination, cardiac murmur

Testing for allergic sensitization: It helps recognize asthma triggers in a child. It does not necessarily indicate the cause of asthma. It is performed using two methods: a skin prick test or a specific serum IgE level. It is not recommended as an initial investigation; however, it may be helpful in severe asthma with no response to adequate therapy.

Fractional exhaled nitric oxide (FeNO): Its value may be elevated in eosinophilic asthma; however, many other conditions such as allergic rhinitis, eczema, etc., may have elevated value. It is not recommended to diagnose asthma in children in the general population.

DIFFERENTIAL DIAGNOSES

Many common childhood conditions may mimic asthma presentation. However, a careful history and physical examination can help diagnose asthma. **Table 22.17** describes the common differential diagnosis and their lead points in history and examination.

TREATMENT Bronchial Asthma

The primary goals of asthma management are (1) good symptom control and (2) risk reduction of future exacerbation, fixed airflow limitation, and medication side effects. **Box 22.14** lists the risk factors for future exacerbations in children.

Box 22.14 Risks of Future Exacerbation

1. Uncontrolled asthma symptoms
2. Poor adherence to therapy
3. Presence of comorbidities
4. Exposure to smoke
5. FEV_1 <60% of predicted
6. Major psychological and socioeconomic problems
7. Severe exacerbation/or required hospitalization in the last year
8. Ever intubated or PICU admission

The success of asthma management depends on the active participation of parents and/or children. They must be counseled regarding the nature of the disease, available treatment options, duration of therapy, and possible adverse effects. Asthma comorbidities should also be recognized and adequately treated. The treatment of asthma is both pharmacological and nonpharmacological.

Pharmacological Therapy

There are two types of pharmacological therapy—(1) *reliever* and (2) *controller* therapy. Reliever therapy is given as and when needed, whereas controller therapy is taken daily in prescribed doses. The dose of controller therapy is adjusted on follow-up based on the level of asthma control. Another drug group is add-on therapy, which is added to the existing controller therapy whenever needed.

Drugs used in Asthma Management

1. *Short-acting β_2-adrenergic agonist (SABA):* Used as a reliever therapy. Recent guidelines do not recommend SABA alone treatment for asthma management in children ≥12 years of age. It has an essential role in the management of acute exacerbation of asthma.
2. *Inhaled corticosteroid (ICS):* Steroids are the most effective anti-inflammatory drug for the treatment of asthma. It reduces asthma symptoms, exacerbation, and hospitalization and improves PFT and quality of life. It is the first line of treatment for asthma management, irrespective of the severity. It is usually well tolerated in children with minimal adverse effects. They are mainly local, such as pharyngeal candidiasis or dysphonia, which can be minimized by using a spacer and rinsing the mouth after using ICS. The major concern for long-term use of ICS is its effect on growth (1–2 cm). However, recent evidence has shown that children recover growth and ultimately attain the predicted height. Budesonide is the most used in children. Other salts are beclomethasone and fluticasone.
3. *Oral corticosteroid (OCS):* Oral steroids not routinely used for asthma management. It has an essential role in managing moderate to severe asthma exacerbation.
4. *Long-acting β-adrenergic agonist (LABA):* It should always be used in combination with ICS. It has steroid-sparing and a synergistic effect with ICS. Its onset of action is 30–60 minutes and has a prolonged effect (12–24 hours). Due to safety and efficacy, it is recommended in children ≥4 years of age. Formoterol is the most common salt used in children.

5. *Leukotriene receptor antagonists (LTRA):* These are weak anti-inflammatory agents. Currently, they have a limited role in asthma management. It is used either as alternative controller therapy in step 2 or as add-on therapy in severe asthma (steps 4 and 5). It is also helpful in the presence of AR. Montelukast is the most commonly used LTRA in children.
6. *Muscarinic receptor antagonist:* Ipratropium bromide has a short-acting role in asthma exacerbation. Tiotropium long-acting is used as add-on therapy in children ≥12 years of age with severe asthma.
7. *Biological therapy:* There is increasing evidence of biological treatment in children with severe asthma. In children, Omalizumab (anti-IgE), Mepolizumab (anti-IL-5), Dupilumab (anti-IL-4), and anti-thymic stromal lymphopoietin (anti-TSLP) are safe. The first three drugs are approved in children ≥6 years, while the last one is only approved in ≥12 years.
8. *Theophylline:* It has no role in routine asthma management in children except in severe asthma exacerbation.
9. *Allergy immunotherapy (AIT):* There is no routine recommendation for AIT. It is only indicated in severe asthma as add-on therapy in step 5 under specialist supervision. It can be administered subcutaneously or sublingually.

Inhalation Technique

There are many inhalation devices with their advantages and disadvantages. The selection of an appropriate inhaler device is mandatory for optimal delivery of asthma medication. These are listed below and shown in **Figures 22.25A to F**:

- *Pressurized metered-dose inhaler (pMDI):* It is a small portable device. The drug is suspended in hydrofluoroalkane (HFA) propellant. The major advantage is that the drug can be effectively delivered on tidal breathing. However, it needs skill and training for proper inhalation in children. It must be used with a spacer in children ≥4 years and with a spacer with a face mask in children <4 years. Studies have shown that the effectiveness of pMDI is the same or even better than nebulizers. The steps for the correct use of MDI are shown in **Box 22.15**.
- *Dried powder inhaler (DPI):* In this device, the drug is in powder form contained in a capsule. These are breath-activated devices that require forced inspiration to generate sufficient inspiratory flow. It can be used in children >4–5 years of age.
- *Nebulizer:* In this device, a liquid drug is broken into a small aerosol that can be inhaled. The disadvantages are that medication is required in a higher dose, takes prolonged time (10–15 minutes), produces noise, and requires electricity. The major advantage is that it does not require one respiratory effort and can be given during severe exacerbation.

Initial Therapy

Currently, stepwise management is recommended. The guide to choosing the initial step of therapy is shown in **Table 22.18**. Once the treatment is started, the child is continuously assessed, reviewed, and adjusted to the treatment **(Fig. 22.26)**.

Stepwise Asthma Management in Children ≥12 years

The treatment in children ≥12 years is similar to the adult population **(Fig. 22.27)**. Recent GINA guideline do not recommend SABA alone therapy for mild asthma (step 1) due to the increased risk of severe exacerbation. Therefore, low-dose ICS must be used whenever SABA is taken. In steps 1 and 2, the preferred controller therapy is a low-dose ICS-formoterol combination. Maintenance controller and reliever therapy (MART) is the preferred controller therapy in steps 3–5. The preferred reliever therapy is ICS-formoterol combination therapy in all the steps. In severe asthma (step 5), a long-acting muscarinic antagonist (LAMA) such as tiotropium may be added if symptoms are not controlled with a maximum dose of ICS-formoterol. Biological therapy (omalizumab, mepolizumab, dupilumab, and anti-TSLP) may be considered an add-on therapy under specialist supervision.

Stepwise Asthma Management in Children 6–11 Years

The treatment in this age group is slightly different from older children **(Fig. 22.28)**. The preferred controller therapy in step 1 is low-dose ICS whenever SABA is taken. In steps 2–5, the preferred controller therapy is daily ICS with or without LABA. In this age group, SABA is the preferred reliever therapy in all the steps. The evidence for MART therapy is not robust in this age group. In severe asthma (step 5). Tiotropium can be added whenever needed. Biological therapy may be considered an add-on therapy under specialist supervision.

MONITORING OF ASTHMA CONTROL

Once the treatment is started, the child is frequently monitored. Parents may be asked to maintain a symptoms diary. At each visit, the child is assessed for compliance with therapy, inhalational technique, symptom control, and adverse effects. GINA asthma symptom control tool is simple, quick, and widely used for the assessment (**Table 22.19**). It classifies asthma control into three groups: (1) well-controlled, (2) partly controlled, or (3) uncontrolled. In addition, validated questionnaires, e.g., asthma control test (ACT), asthma control questionnaire (ACQ), etc., can be used to assess asthma control.

Parents are counseled at each visit and are encouraged to bring their inhaler devices. The first follow-up is after 2 weeks, then every 4 weeks for the first 3 months, and after that, every 3 months. If available, PFT should be performed at diagnosis, after 3–6 months of starting treatment, and then every 1–2 years. If symptoms are well controlled for 2–3 months, the therapy may be tapered gradually (every 2–3 months) until a minimum effective dose is achieved.

ASTHMA IN PRESCHOOL CHILDREN (<5 YEARS)

Recurrent wheezing is common in preschool children. Diagnosing asthma in preschool children is challenging as wheezing in this age group is highly heterogeneous. In addition, preschool children cannot perform PFT to document expiratory flow limitation.

Classification

Preschool wheezing has been classified into two groups: (1) episodic viral wheeze and (2) multitrigger wheeze. Episodic wheezing occurs only with a viral respiratory infection, while multitrigger wheeze can also be triggered by exertion, laughter, cold, and food. However, this classification is not absolute and it may switch to either side. Recently, GINA has given a probability-based approach that depends upon the frequency and duration of symptoms, interval of symptoms, and history of atopy (**Table 22.20**).

TREATMENT Asthma in Preschool Children (<5 Years)

Children with a high probability of asthma are candidates for starting controller therapy. Low-dose ICS is the preferred controller therapy, and as-needed SABA is a reliever with the appropriate device. LTRA is an alternative controller therapy, though it is less effective than ICS.

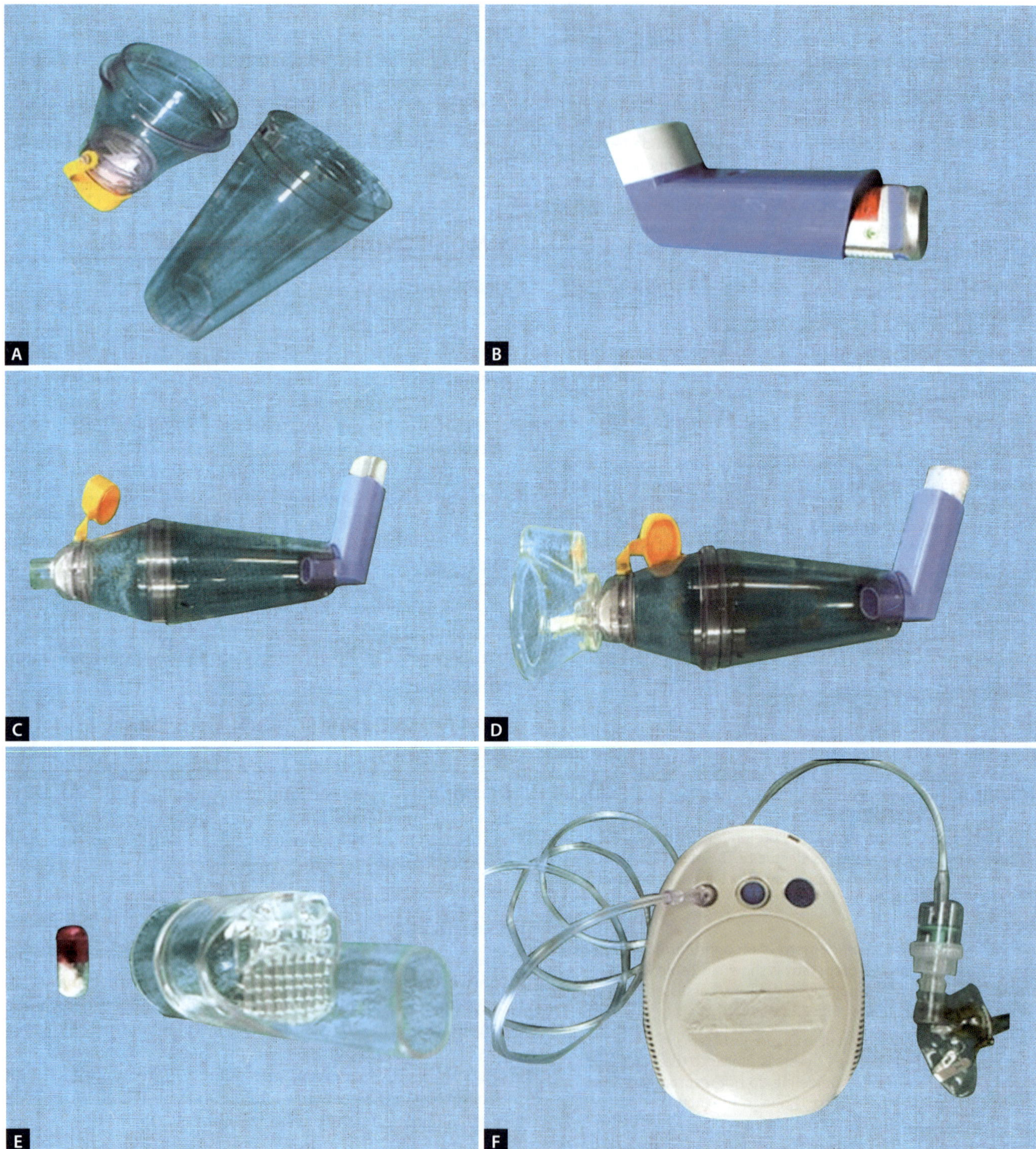

Figs. 22.25A to F: Different types of inhalation devices commonly used in children: (A) Spacer; (B) Pressurized meter dose inhaler (pMDI); (C) pMDI with spacer (assembled); (D) pMDI with spacer with mask; (E) Dried powder inhaler (Rotahalar) with capsule for use; (F) Nebulizer with face mask

Box 22.15 Steps for Proper Use of Pressurized Metered-Dose Inhaler (pMDI)

1. Assemble the spacer ± face mask and pMDI
2. Remove the cap of pMDI
3. Hold the pMDI in an upright position and shake it well 4–5 times
4. Stand or sit straight
5. Place the mouth-piece between teeth and close lips without leaving any gaps
6. Ask the patient to inhale and exhale into the spacer
7. Actuate the pMDI in spacer
8. Take 5–10 tidal breaths
9. Wait for at least 60 seconds before the next puff and repeat steps 3–8
10. Gargle/rinse the mouth after taking steroid-containing pMDI

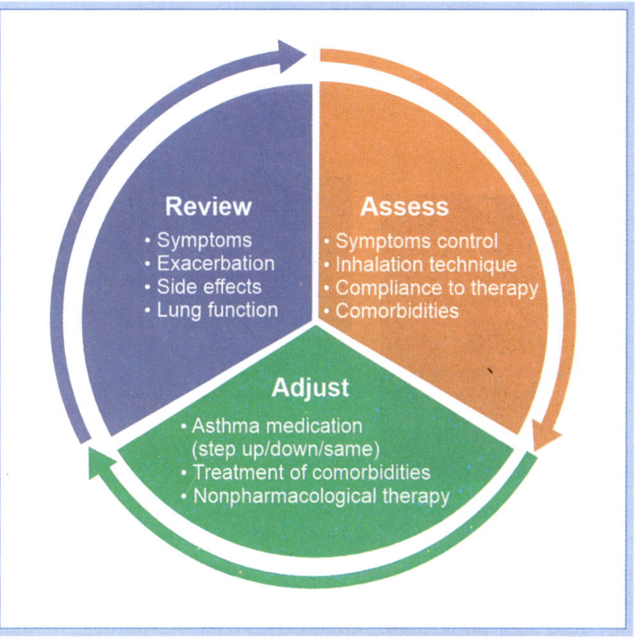

Fig. 22.26: Continuum cycle of asthma management

Source: Adapted from Global Strategy for Asthma Management and Prevention (GINA) 2024. www.ginasthma.org

Table 22.18 Guide to Choosing the Initial Step of Therapy

Frequency of symptoms	*Step of therapy*
Infrequent symptoms <2 episodes/month	I
Symptoms ≥2 episodes/month but not daily	II
Symptoms almost daily with night symptoms ≥1/week	III
Daily symptoms with night symptoms ≥1/week and low lung function	IV
Severely uncontrolled symptoms even on step-IV therapy	V

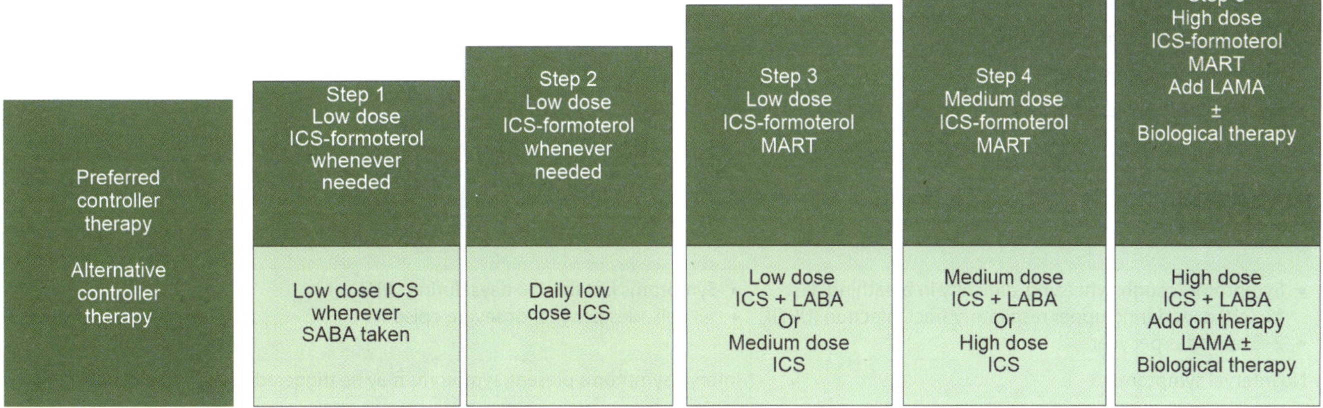

Fig. 22.27: Stepwise management of asthma in children ≥12 years [ICS: inhaled corticosteroid; SABA: short-acting beta agonist; LABA: long-acting beta agonist; MART: maintenance and reliever therapy; LAMA: long-acting muscarinic antagonist, low dose ICS (200–400 µg/day), medium dose (>400–800 µg/day), and high dose (>800 µg/day), low dose ICS-formoterol: Bud/form (200/6)]

Source: Adapted from Global Strategy for Asthma Management and Prevention (GINA) 2024. (www.ginasthma.org)

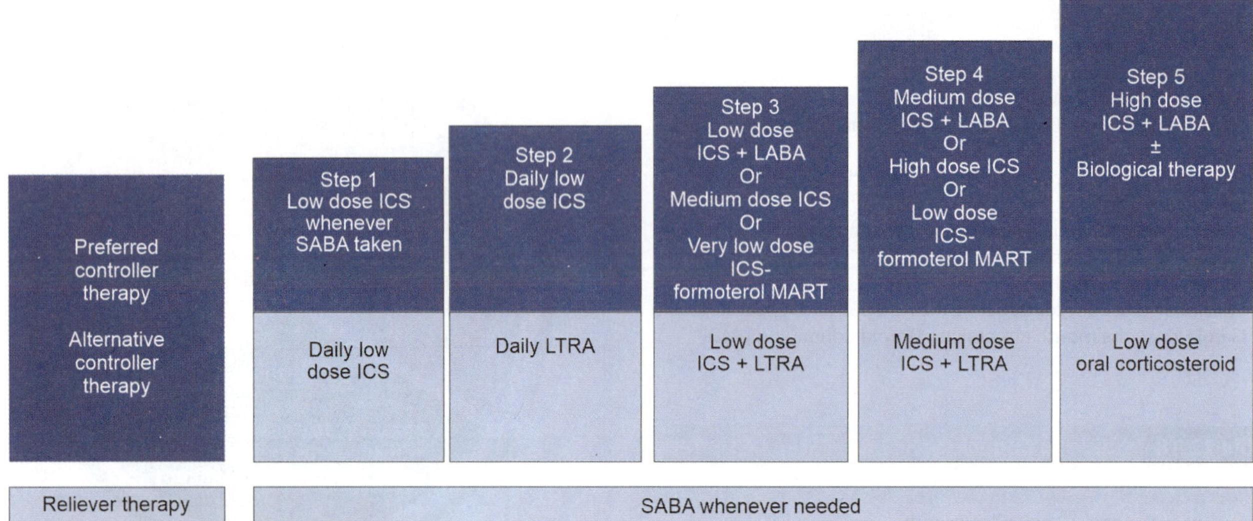

Fig. 22.28: Stepwise management of asthma in children <12 years [ICS: inhaled corticosteroid; SABA: short-acting beta agonist; LTRA: leukotriene receptor antagonist; LABA: long-acting beta agonist; MART: maintenance and reliever therapy [very low lose Bud/form (100/6), low dose Bud/form (200/6)], low dose ICS (200–400 µg/day), medium dose (>400–800 µg/day), and high dose (>800 µg/day)]

Source: Adapted from Global Strategy for Asthma Management and Prevention (GINA) 2024. www.ginasthma.org

Table 22.19 GINA Assessment of Symptom Control in Children

In the last 4 weeks, has any of the following?	*Level of asthma control*		
	Well-controlled	*Partly-controlled*	*Uncontrolled*
Daytime asthma symptoms, more than twice/week?	None	1–2	3–4
Any night awakening due to asthma?			
Reliever* for symptom control more than twice/week?			
Any limitation of activity due to asthma?			
Short-acting β_2-agonist (SABA)			

Source: Adapted from Global Strategy for Asthma Management and Prevention (GINA) 2024. (www.ginasthma.org)

Table 22.20 Probability of Asthma in Preschool Children

Low probability	*High probability*
• Symptoms (cough, wheezing, difficulty in breathing) last for <10 days during upper respiratory tract infection (URTI) • 2–3 episodes per year	• Symptoms last for >10 days during URTI • >3 episodes per year or severe episodes
No interval symptoms	Interval symptoms present; symptoms may be triggered by play, crying, or laughing
No family or personal history of atopy	Family or personal history of atopy present

Source: Adapted from Global Strategy for Asthma Management and Prevention (GINA) 2024. (www.ginasthma.org)

After starting treatment, the child is reviewed for the response after 2–3 months. ICS can be abruptly stopped if a child improves and is kept on follow-up. If a child does not improve, refer to specialist care to exclude other etiology. If symptoms recur, they are treated with daily ICS as per the older children with asthma. Moreover, no intervention has been shown to prevent or change the natural course of asthma.

ASTHMA ACTION PLAN

A written asthma action plan should be given to parents or caretakers of every child with BA. It includes:

- How to recognize worsening symptoms?
  - It is usually identified by an increase in cough, wheezing, or shortness of breath.

- What action should they take during such a condition?
  - They should start reliever (SABA) more frequently.
- If there is no response to reliever therapy or worsening symptoms, what will be the next action?
  - Parents should start the first oral steroid dose (1-2 mg/kg, maximum 40 mg) and immediately visit nearby health care facilities.

ACUTE EXACERBATION OF ASTHMA

It is an acute worsening of asthma symptoms from the normal state. The term *"status asthmatics"* is coined for severe exacerbation that does not respond to repeated or continuous administration of SABA in an emergency setting. Asthma management should begin at home as per the written asthma action plan. If the symptoms do not improve or worsen, the child should be brought to healthcare facility. The severity of asthma should be clinically assessed as it guides further management. The pulmonary index score (PIS) is a commonly used clinical score for asthma severity in children (**Table 22.21**). An overview of asthma exacerbation management at a healthcare facility is shown in **Flowchart 22.9**.

Table 22.21 Pulmonary Index Score (PIS)

Sore	Respiratory/ min (<6 years)	Respiratory/ min (>6 years)	Wheezing	Accessory muscle use/ retraction
0	<30	<20	None	None
1	31–45	21–35	End expiratory	Questionable
2	46–60	36–50	Full expiration	Apparent
3	>60	>50	Both inspiration and expiration or silent	Maximal

Interpretation: Mild: 0–3, Moderate: 4–6, Severe: >6

Mild-to-moderate Exacerbation

Administration of salbutamol with MDI 4-10 puffs every 20 minutes for 1 hour is the most effective therapy.

- ***In mild exacerbation***, a child can be sent home after stabilization and follow-up in 1-2 weeks.
- ***In moderate exacerbation***, a short course of steroids (prednisolone 1-2 mg/kg, maximum 40 kg/day, for 3-5

Flowchart 22.9: Approach to asthma exacerbation in children

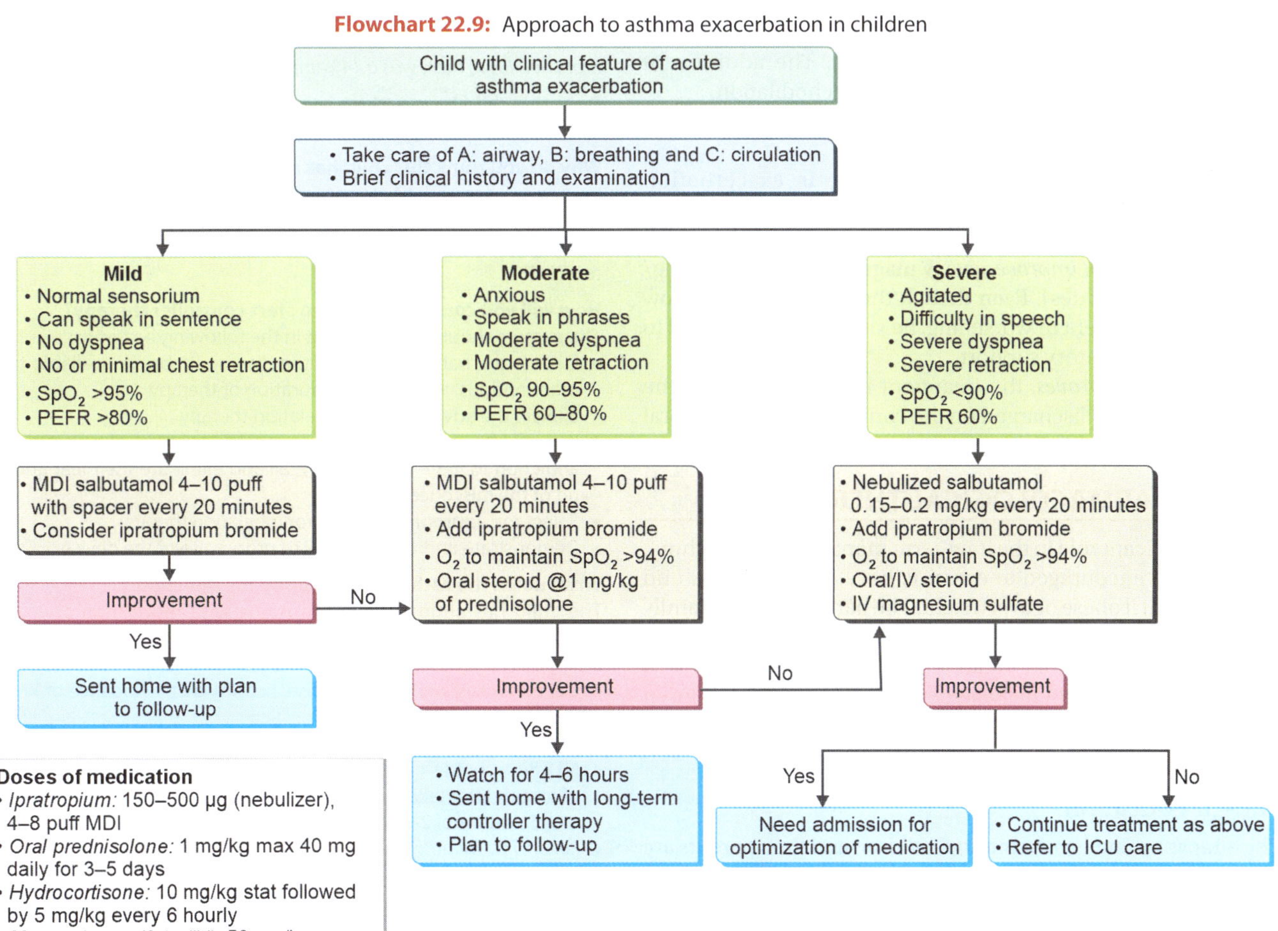

Box 22.16 Indications for Referral in Children with Asthma

1. Diagnosis of asthma in doubt
2. A child does not respond to adequate controller therapy—requires add-on therapy
3. Poor compliance with outpatient treatment
4. Risk factors for uncontrolled disease
5. Moderate exacerbation not responding with home care
6. Severe exacerbation
7. Require oxygen/respiratory support
8. Need ICU care
9. Drug overdose/adverse effects

days) is given as it reduces the need for hospitalization. Oxygen therapy is titrated to maintain SpO_2 >94%. Children are monitored for 4–6 hours and, if they remain stable, discharged, and followed up in 2–7 days. Controller therapy is started if the child is not on any treatment.

Severe Exacerbation

In severe exacerbation, the first step is identifying and managing life-threatening conditions, viz. cyanosis, silent chest, altered sensorium, poor respiratory efforts, and hypoxia. The indications for hospital referral in children are shown in **Box 22.16**.

- Intramuscular adrenalin is administered when there is associated anaphylaxis or angioedema. The addition of ipratropium to salbutamol improves bronchodilation.
- Steroid is given either orally or IV as per the clinical status within 1 hour of presentation.
- Routine use of antibiotics has no role in exacerbation management until there is a strong suspicion of bacterial infection.

If a child does not improve, give IV magnesium sulfate (50 mg/kg over 30–60 minutes). Even though the child does not show signs of improvement or worsening, he should be transferred to ICU care for respiratory support.

If the child improves, the treatment is optimized until the child is stable and discharged on the controller, SABA, and oral steroid. Follow up in 2–7 days.

NONPHARMACOLOGICAL THERAPY

It has a significant role in the long-term management of asthma. Children are encouraged to exercise, have a healthy diet, and reduce weight if obese or overweight. The parents or other family members should discuss stopping smoking at home. Recent evidence has shown that breathing exercises and yoga have a beneficial impact on BA management. Avoiding food in children is not recommended unless there is a documented allergy to some food or chemicals.

Patient Education

The education and involvement of children and their parents are critical factors in managing asthma. They should understand:

- Nature of disease, its course, and available treatment option
- There is no cure, but symptoms can be controlled
- Monitors symptoms diary
- Learn to administer inhaler therapy
- Written asthma action plan
- Maintenance and cleaning of the device

PREVENTION

Currently, no intervention can prevent asthma development in children. The beneficial strategies are preventing exposure to smoke during pregnancy and early life, promoting vaginal delivery, avoid broad-spectrum antibiotics during infancy. Though breastfeeding does not prevent asthma, it should be encouraged for general health. Routine immunization is encouraged. There is insufficient evidence of supplementation of vitamin D_3, vitamin E, fish oil, and probiotics in asthma prevention.

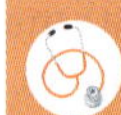

CASE STUDY 1 Asthma in an 8-year-old

An 8-year-old boy (weight 25 kg) presented with c/o recurrent episodes of cough, wheezing, and difficulty breathing for the last 3 years. Initially, he had symptoms 1–2 episodes/month, but for the past 3 months, he had almost daily symptoms and night symptoms once a week. The symptoms worsen after playing for a while and during the winter season. He also has nasal itching and block >4 days/week. There was a family history of asthma in his grandmother. A diagnosis of asthma was suspected, and PFT was performed, which showed FEV_1 was 75%, and post-bronchodilator, there was a 14% improvement in FEV_1.

Does this child have asthma?

Yes, this child has asthma.

Why do you think this child has asthma?

He has a characteristic symptom pattern (more than one symptom which varies in time and intensity, worsens with exertion, seasonal variation), expiratory flow limitation (FEV_1 75%) and a positive BDR test (14%).

How will you counsel parents to start controller therapy?

The parents should be counseled in the following headings:

- Discuss the natural course of the disease (in brief), available treatment options, and expected duration of therapy
- Explain the advantages of inhalation therapy
- Parents often have a fear of adverse effects and risk of developing an addiction to ICS—explain in detail and eliminate their fear and get rid of the misconception
- Select the appropriate device for inhalation therapy
- Demonstrate and train the skill of proper use of the device

Write down the asthma prescription for this child.

The child has almost daily symptoms with more than one-night symptoms/week. Step 3 treatment will be started.

Diagnosis: Asthma with allergic rhinitis

- General measures (daily exercise, healthy diet, avoidance of known allergens)
- Maintain asthma diary
- MDI Budesonide + Formoterol (100/6) 2 puff BD with spacer. (Rinsing of mouth after taking ICS)
- MDI Salbutamol 2–10 puffs with spacer as and when required
- *For allergic rhinitis:* Tablet cetirizine one tablet at HS for 1 week
- Write and explain the asthma action plan
- Review in 2 weeks (please bring your medication and device)

Write down the asthma action plan for this boy.
- Start pMDI Salbutamol 4–10 puffs with a spacer, and give three doses at an interval of 15–20 minutes whenever there is an increase in cough, wheezing, or difficulty in breathing
- If symptoms do not improve or worsen, start tablet prednisolone 30 mg stat and visit a nearby healthcare facility/use a telemedicine facility
- Continue reliever therapy during visits to a healthcare facility

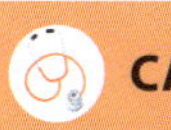

CASE STUDY 2 Wheezing in a 3-year-old

A 3-year-old girl (weight 10 kg) presented with c/o recurrent cough episodes and wheezing since infancy. Symptoms worsen at night. She has one episode every month, and each episode lasts for weeks. There was a history of improvement with nebulization. In between the child also developed symptoms with crying, laughing, and play. She has a history of atopic dermatitis. Her grandmother has asthma.

Does she have asthma? How to diagnose asthma in preschool children?
She has preschool wheeze, which has a frequent and prolonged course. We cannot say with certainty that she has asthma, as many childhood conditions may have wheezing, and we cannot perform spirometry in this age group. However, going through the GINA probability-based approach, she has a high probability of asthma.

Is she a candidate for controller therapy?
Since she has a high probability of asthma, controller therapy should be given to her as it helps control symptoms and improves her quality of life.

Is treatment in preschool children similar to older children?
No. In preschool children, ICS is given in low doses. Formeterol is not recommended in this age group. Furthermore, they require a facemask attached to a spacer for proper drug delivery. The treatment may be stopped in 2–3 months if it improves by then.

Write down the prescription for this child.
Diagnosis: Preschool wheeze with a high probability of asthma
- General measures (daily exercise, healthy diet, avoidance of known allergens)
- Maintain asthma diary
- MDI Budesonide (100 µg) 2 puff BD with spacer and mask. (rinsing of mouth after taking ICS)
- MDI Salbutamol 2–10 puff with spacer and mask as and when required
- *For atopic dermatitis:*
    - Keep the area moist with emollient
    - If symptoms disturb daily activity, apply low-strength local steroid Flutivate for LA twice a day
- Review in 2 weeks (please bring your medication and device)
- Write and explain the asthma action plan

Will ICS therapy prevent the future development of asthma in her?
No. No intervention will change the natural course of preschool wheeze.

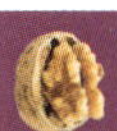

IN A NUTSHELL

Bronchial Asthma
1. Asthma is a heterogeneous disease characterized by chronic airway inflammation and hyper-responsiveness.
2. Asthma is diagnosed in the presence of characteristic symptoms (cough, wheeze, difficulty in breathing) and documentation of expiratory flow limitation and reversibility.
3. Stepwise therapy is recommended in children; inhaled corticosteroid with the proper device is the first line of treatment.
4. The child should be frequently monitored, assessed, reviewed, and adjusted to the therapy. A written asthma action plan should be given to the parents.

Global Initiative for Asthma. Global Strategy for Asthma Management and Prevention, 2024. Wisconsin: GINA; 2024.

IAP. Asthma training module (ATM), revised version 2022. IAP National Respiratory Chapter. Mumbai: IAP; 2022.

National Heart, Lung and Blood Institute. 2020 Focused Updates to the Asthma Management Guidelines: A Report from the National Asthma Education and Prevention Program Coordinating Committee Expert Panel Working Group. Bethesda, MD: NIH; 2020

National Institute of Health Care Excellence (NICE), British Thoracic Society (BTS), and Scottish Intercollegiate Guidelines Network (SIGN) Guideline. Asthma: diagnosis, monitoring and chronic asthma management; 2024.

22.16 Parental Counseling for Prevention of Respiratory Disorders

INTRODUCTION

Education programs, focused on prevention of respiratory infections are cost-effective measures that reduce hospital visits and improve health outcomes in children.

Parental counseling: Good communication between patient/caregiver and doctor encompasses listening skills, checking understanding about basic facts/causes triggers and then providing information regarding preventive measures of respiratory diseases.

STRATEGIES FOR PREVENTION OF RESPIRATORY DISEASE

Parental education: Regarding prevalence, course of respiratory infections risk factor modification, measures for its control.

Respiratory hygiene: It comprises cough etiquette and hand hygiene.

Cough Etiquette

Parents can guide their child's behavior by showing the child how it is done (**Fig. 22.29**).

- ***Cover your cough:*** This prevent the spread of germs from coughing
- Best way is coughing into your elbow or sneezing into your elbow instead of directly onto their hands. This decreases the number of germs that you get onto your hands and decreases the risk of spreading them to other people.
- Cover your mouth and nose with a tissue when coughing or sneezing.

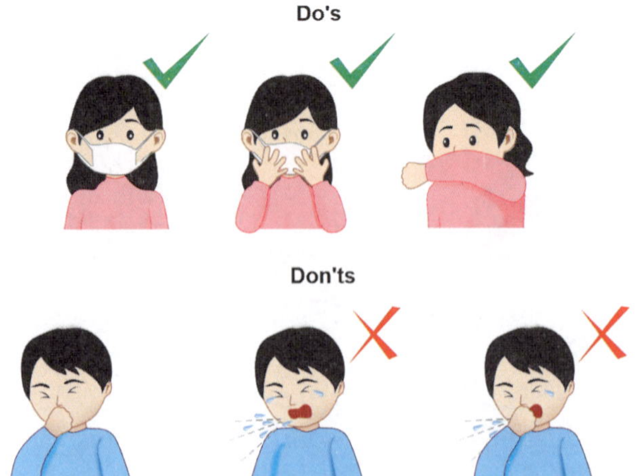

Fig. 22.29: Cough etiquette

- Use in the nearest waste receptacle to dispose the tissue after use.
- Teach your child to stay healthy by encouraging them to wash their hands frequently.

COVER YOUR COUGH AND SNEEZE

Hand Hygiene

- Perform hand hygiene (e.g., handwashing with non-antimicrobial soap and water, alcohol-based hand rub, or antiseptic handwash) after having contact with respiratory secretions and contaminated objects/materials
- ***Always wash your hands with soap and water after:***
  - Blowing your nose, coughing or sneezing
  - Before and after preparing food
  - Touching an animal, animal feed or waste
  - If your hands are visibly dirty
- Maintaining hand hygiene can cut the respiratory infection rate by up to 25%.

For ensuring hygiene/cough etiquette in waiting areas of schools/public places:

- Tissues and no-touch receptacles for tissue disposal should be used
- Ensure conveniently located dispensers of alcohol-based hand rub; where sinks are available, ensure hand washing with soap and water

Good Practices

- ***Vaccinate your child:*** It has a role in reducing the burden of respiratory diseases
- Appropriate breastfeeding practices
- No bottle feeding
- Avoid unnecessary antibiotic therapy (overuse)
- Encourage mask use and physical distancing during outbreaks.

Other Control Measures for Respiratory Diseases

Avoid:

- Poorly ventilated spaces and crowds
- Smoking and exposure to environmental tobacco smoke during pregnancy and early childhood
- Damp housing conditions causing indoor air pollution
- Exposure to indoor allergens/volatile organic compounds
- Touching your eyes, nose, and mouth with unwashed hands.
- Visual alerts may be used in healthcare settings/schools/public places which create awareness of cough etiquette and hand hygiene.

Protection from COVID-19

- Wearing a mask
- Get vaccinated-COVID-19 vaccines are highly effective at preventing severe illness, hospitalizations, and death
- Social distancing
- Hand washing

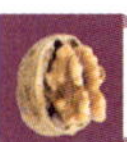

IN A NUTSHELL

Parental Counseling for Prevention of Respiratory Disorders

1. Burden of respiratory disease in children is high and strategies to prevent it play a pivotal role.
2. Parental counseling should be done regarding *respiratory hygiene*.
3. It includes cough etiquette and hand hygiene.
4. Good practices such as vaccination, breastfeeding, avoiding antibiotic overuse should be encouraged.

CDC (2025). Preventing Respiratory Illnesses. [online]. Available from https://www.cdc.gov/respiratory-viruses/prevention/index.html. [Last accessed September, 2025]

Ladomenou F, Moschandreas J, Kafatos A, et al. Protective effect of exclusive breastfeeding against infections during infancy: a prospective study. Arch Dis Child. 2010;95(12):1004-8.

Mihrshahi S, Oddy WH, Peat JK, Kabir I. Association between infant feeding patterns and diarrhoeal and respiratory illness: a cohort study in Chittagong, Bangladesh. Int Breastfeed J. 2008;3:28.

Rabie T, Curtis V. Handwashing and risk of respiratory infections: a quantitative systematic review. Trop Med Int Health. 2006;11(3):258-67.

Satvik C Bansal (Anatomy and Physiology of the Respiratory Tract); Vinod Kumar (Examination of ENT, Approach to Child with Upper Respiratory Symptoms, Making a Diagnosis in a Child with ENT Symptoms, Approach to Stridor) (Online only); Satnam Kaur (Examination of ENT, AOM); Hema Gupta Mittal, Sarika Gupta (Nasopharyngitis and Tonsillopharyngitis); Nihar Ranjan Mishra, Narayan Prasad Modi (Allergic Rhinitis, Approach to Child with Wheeze); Romit Saxena {Acute Epiglottitis, Acute Laryngotracheobronchitis (Croup)}; Pallab Chatterjee (FB Aspiration); Vikram Bhaskar (Approach to a Child with Fast Breathing, Approach to a Child with Wheeze); Jagdish P Goyal (Pneumonia); Sunil Kumar Rao (Empyema Thoracis); Sejal Saglani, Arvind Shah (Bronchiolitis); Prawin Kumar (Bronchial Asthma); Nitin Dhochak, Rakesh Lodha (Imaging in Respiratory Disorders) (Online only); Shetanshu Srivastava (Parental Counseling for Prevention of Respiratory Disorders)

23 CHAPTER

Hematological Disorders

AS PER NMC COMPETENCIES

PE26.1	Explain the etiopathogenesis, clinical features, classification and approach to a child with anemia.	*Ch 23.3*
PE26.2	Describe the etiopathogenesis, clinical features and management of Iron Deficiency anemia.	*Ch 23.4*
PE26.3	Describe the etiopathogenesis, clinical features, and management of VITB12, folate deficiency anemia.	*Ch 23.5*
PE26.4	Explain the etiopathogenesis, clinical features and management of hemolytic anemia, thalassemia major, sickle cell anemia, hereditary spherocytosis, autoimmune hemolytic anemia and hemolytic uremic syndrome.	*Ch 23.6, Ch 23.7, Ch 23.8, Ch 23.9, Ch 23.10, Ch 23.11*
PE26.5	Describe the National Anemia Control Program.	*Ch 11.3*
PE26.6	Describe the cause of thrombocytopenia in children: Describe the clinical features and management of Idiopathic Thrombocytopenic Purpura (ITP).	*Ch 23.13*
PE26.7	Explain the etiology, classification, pathogenesis, and clinical features of hemophilia in children.	*Ch 23.14*
PE26.8	Explain the etiology, clinical presentation and management of acute lymphoblastic leukemia in children.	*Ch 23.15*
PE26.9	Explain the etiology, clinical presentation and management of lymphoma in children.	*Ch 23.16*
PE26.10	Perform examination of the abdomen, demonstrate organomegaly.	*Ch 23.2*
PE26.11	Interpret CBC, LFT.	*Ch 23.2*
PE26.12	Perform and interpret peripheral smear.	*Ch 23.2*
PE26.13	Explain the indications for hemoglobin electrophoresis and interpret report.	*Ch 23.7, Ch 23.8*
PE26.14	Demonstrate, performance of bone marrow aspiration in manikin.	*Ch 23.18*
PE26.15	Enumerate the referral criteria for hematological conditions.	*Ch 23.17*
PE26.16	Counsel and educate patients about prevention and treatment of anemia.	*Ch 23.19*
PE26.17	Enumerate the indications for splenectomy and precautions.	*Ch 23.9*

Topics available online: ***Bone Marrow Failure, Red Blood Cell Enzyme Defects,***

23.1 Components and Physiology of Blood

INTRODUCTION

Red blood cells (RBCs) or erythrocytes, white blood cells (WBCs) or leukocytes, and platelets or thrombocytes, constitute the cellular part of blood. The plasma is the river in which the blood cells travel. It carries not only the blood cells but also dissolved gases (carbon dioxide and oxygen), nutrients (such as sugars, amino acids, fats, and minerals), waste products (such as lactic acid and urea), antibodies, clotting proteins (called clotting factors), chemical messengers such as hormones and proteins including enzymes that help maintain the body's fluid balance. Blood also serves to maintain normal body temperature and body's pH balance (normally between 7.35 and 7.45).

HEMATOPOIESIS

Hematopoietic stem cells (HSCs) in the bone marrow differentiate into progenitor cells, which under the influence of various hematopoietic growth factors mature into erythrocytes, thrombocytes, monocytes, macrophages, lymphocytes, neutrophils, eosinophils, and basophils **(Fig. 23.1)**.

- ***Erythropoiesis*** leads to differentiation of a progenitor cell into a red blood cell under the influence of erythropoietin (EPO). Normoblasts and reticulocytes are different stages in the process of maturation. In the process the red cell size decreases, the nucleus is extruded, and hemoglobinization of the cell takes place.
- ***Lymphopoiesis*** is the process of maturation of progenitor cells into lymphocytes.
- ***Granulopoiesis*** is the process of maturation of myeloblasts into different types of granulocytes, i.e., basophils, neutrophils, and eosinophils under the influence of granulocyte and monocyte colony stimulating factor (GM-CSF), G-CSF, and M-CSF.
- ***Monocytopoiesis*** is the process of maturation of myeloblasts into monocytes. The monocytes further mature as macrophages.
- ***Megakaryocytopoiesis*** is the hematopoiesis of platelets. Thrombopoietin is the growth factor responsible for regulating the maturation of megakaryocytes into mature platelets (thrombopoiesis).

Once the progenitor cells have differentiated into mature cells they are released into the blood.

LOCATION OF HEMATOPOIESIS

These cells are produced in the body at different sites depending upon the stage of life. Hematopoiesis starts by the 2nd week of

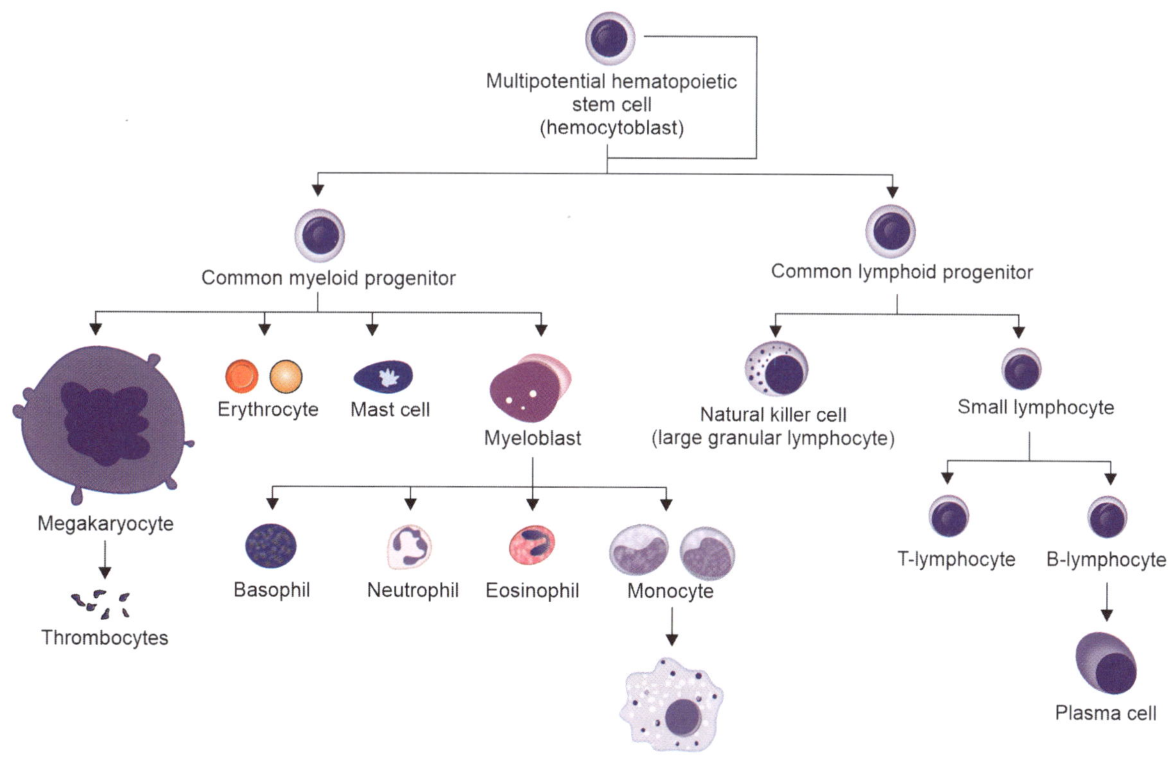

Fig. 23.1: Hematopoiesis

Table 23.1 Hematological Values in Different Age Groups

Age	Hb (g/dL) mean	PCV (%) mean	R/C (%) mean	MCV (fL) lower limit	TLC (/mm³) range	N (%) mean	L (%) mean
Cord blood	17	55	5	110	9,000–30,000	60	30
2 weeks	16	50	1	90	5,000–21,000	40	65
3 months	12	35	1	77	6,000–18,000	30	50
6 months to 6 years	12	37	1	70	6,000–15,000	45	50
7–14 years	13	38	1	80	4,000–13,000	55	40
>14 years • Girls • Boys	 14 16	 42 48	1.5	80	5,000–10,000	55	35

(Hb: hemoglobin; L: lymphocyte; MCV: mean corpuscular volume; N: neutrophil; PCV: packed cell volume; R/C: reticulocyte count; TLC: total leucocyte count)

gestation in the yolk sac; this function is gradually taken over by the liver. The spleen and lymph nodes also start contributing to a lesser extent. By the fifth month of gestation the bone marrow becomes active; and from 7th month of gestation onward it remains the main site of hematopoiesis.

In children, hematopoiesis occurs in the marrow of the long bones such as the femur and tibia. In adults, it occurs mainly in the medulla of flat bones such as pelvis, cranium, vertebrae, and sternum. Maturation and some proliferation of lymphoid cells occur in lymph nodes, spleen, and thymus. Sometimes, liver, thymus, and spleen may resume their hematopoietic function (extramedullary hematopoiesis), if necessary.

NORMAL VALUES

Hematological parameters including hemoglobin, total leukocyte count, differential counts, and red blood indices such as mean corpuscular volume, etc., vary with age **(Table 23.1)**.

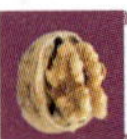

IN A NUTSHELL

Components and Physiology of Blood

1. Blood comprises 55% plasma and 45% as cellular components (99% erythrocytes and 1% as leukocytes and thrombocytes).
2. Leukocytes can be categorized as *agranulocytes* (lymphocytes and monocytes) and granulocytes (neutrophils, basophils, and eosinophils).
3. Hematopoiesis starts by the 2nd week of gestation in the yolk sac and this function is gradually taken over by the liver. By the 5th month of gestation, the bone marrow becomes active; and from 7th month of gestation onward it remains the main site of hematopoiesis.

Fanni D, Angotzi F, Lai F, et al. Four stages of hepatic hematopoiesis in human embryos and fetuses. J Matern Fetal Neonatal Med. 2018; 31(6):701-7.

Sachdev HP, Porwal A, Acharya R, et al. Haemoglobin thresholds to define anemia in a national sample of healthy children and adolescents aged 1-19 years in India: a population-based study. Lancet Glob Health. 2021;9:e822-31.

Sieff CA, Daley GQ, Zon LI. Anatomy and Physiology of Hematopoiesis. In: Orkin SH, Fisher DE, Look T, et al (Eds). Nathan and Oski's Hematology and Oncology of Infancy and Childhood, 8th edition. Philadelphia: WB Saunders; 2015. p. 3.

World Health Organization. Haemoglobin concentrations for the diagnosis of anemia and assessment of severity. Vitamin and Mineral Nutrition Information System. [Online] Available from: http:// www.who.int/vmnis/indicators/haemoglobin.pdf. [Last accessed March, 2025].

23.2 Evaluation of a Child with Suspected Hematological Disorder

PE 26.10, PE 26.11, PE 26.12

INTRODUCTION

Child presenting with paleness (anemia) and poor growth is a commonly encountered scenario during outpatient clinic. History and clinical examination can guide the clinician toward the possible etiology and differential diagnosis. The initial laboratory tests, particularly a complete blood count (CBC) and peripheral smear examination are especially important to narrow the diagnostic possibilities and guide further testing.

HISTORY TAKING

It is important to assess the child for complaints of paleness, fatigue, weakness, bleeding from any site (skin bleeds, epistaxis, hematemesis, hematuria, malena, and menorrhagia), fever, lump in the body, and jaundice, all of which may be related to the underlying blood disorders.

Age of onset is especially important; thalassemia often presents at 6–12 months of age and nutritional anemias are common in toddlers and adolescents.

- ***Family history of bleeding disorders*** is relevant in inherited clotting factor or platelet defects. Family history of regular blood transfusion is also relevant in thalassemia syndromes/hemoglobinopathies. X-linked diseases affect males and maternal side relatives (e.g., hemophilia). Asymptomatic parents with affected siblings suggest an autosomal recessive inheritance.
- ***A history of pica*** is important in children with suspected irondeficiency anemia.
- ***Neonatal history*** such as jaundice can point to hemolysis due to hereditary spherocytosis and enzyme deficiencies. Congenital factor deficiencies can manifest with bleeding in the newborn period. Dietary history must be taken to assess sources of iron, vitamin B_{12} and folic acid in children with nutritional anemia. Vegans are more predisposed to vitamin B_{12} deficiency.
- A child with hematological malignancy is likely to present in acutely ill condition with bleeding, organomegaly, fever, and anemia requiring blood transfusion.
- ***History of chronic and systemic illnesses,*** like chronic kidney disease or inflammatory bowel disease, may present with anemia (anemia of chronic disease) which is unlikely to respond to iron therapy. Sickle cell disease is a hemolytic anemia that can affect multiple systems and present with musculoskeletal, pulmonary, hepatic, and neurological complications in addition to anemia.
- In a bleeding child, it is important to assess if the child has had a mucosal bleed or deep bleed as it can give a clue to underlying pathology. **Flowchart 23.1** provides a clinical approach to a bleeding child and **Flowchart 23.2** provides a clinical approach to a bleeding child with suspected coagulation disorder.

EXAMINATION

The general physical examination must include assessment for pallor, icterus, lymphadenopathy, mucositis, glossitis (seen in nutritional anemia), hyperpigmentation (seen in vitamin B_{12} deficiency) and nail changes (koilonychia and platynychia). Systemic examination should include evaluation for organomegaly (hepatomegaly and splenomegaly). While hepatosplenomegaly could be seen in hemolytic anemia, malignancies, or nutritional anemia, absence of organomegaly

Flowchart 23.1: Approach to child with bleeding disorder

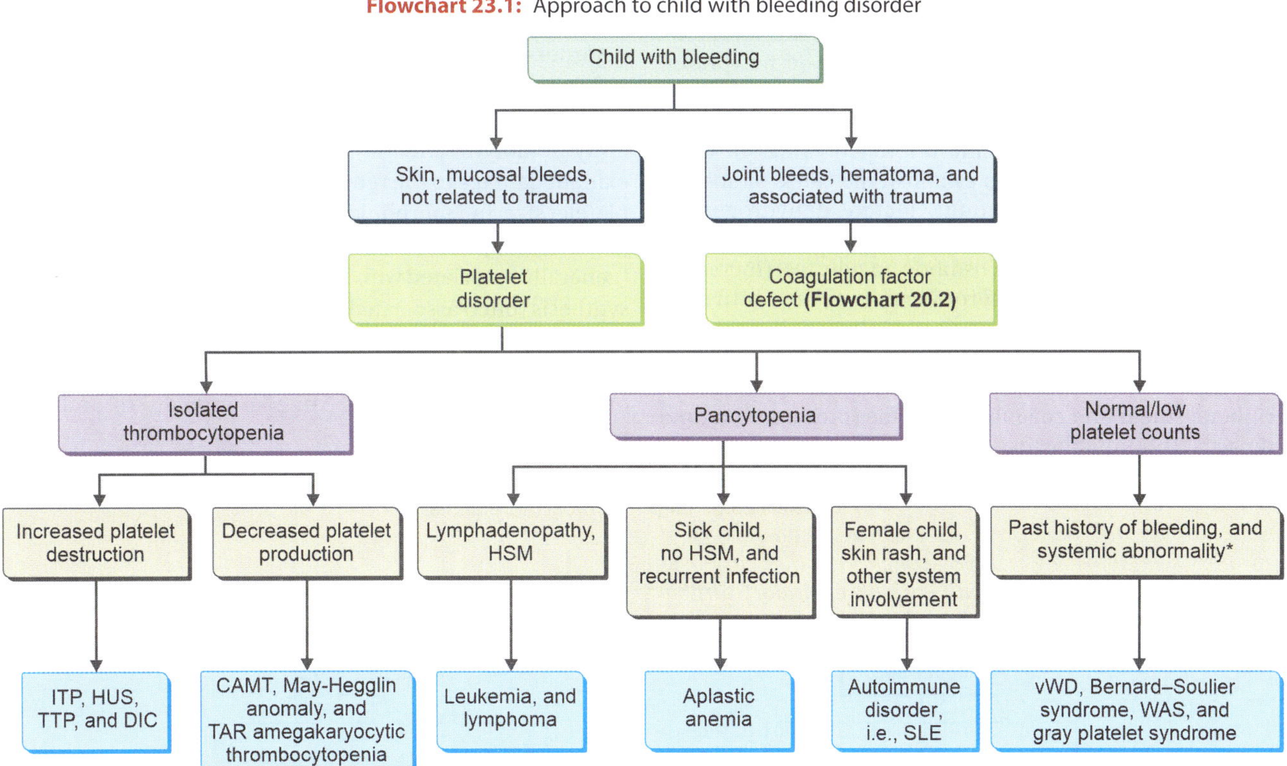

*Loss of hair color, vision defect, and albinism

(CAMT: congenital amegakaryocytic thrombocytopenia; DIC: disseminated intravascular coagulation; HSM: hepatosplenomegaly; HUS: hemolytic uremic syndrome; ITP: immune thrombocytopenic purpura; SLE: systemic lupus erythematosus; TAR: thrombocytopenia absent radius; TTP: thrombotic thrombocytopenia purpura; WAS: Wiskott Aldrich syndrome; vWD: von Willebrand disease)

Flowchart 23.2: Approach to child with suspected coagulation factor defect

Coagulation factor defect

- Sick child, jaundice, ascites, edema PT and aPTT prolonged → Liver disease and DIC
- Prolonged antibiotic exposure, newborn child PT and aPTT prolonged → Vitamin K deficiency and warfarin
- Repeated history of bleeding, male child, family history in male sibling, PT normal and aPTT prolonged → Hemophilia A and B

(aPTT: activated partial thromboplastin time; DIC: disseminated intravascular coagulation; PT: prothrombin time)

with pancytopenia points to aplastic anemia and bone marrow failure syndromes. Additionally, examination of cardiovascular and respiratory system is needed to exclude congestive cardiac failure which needs emergency management. Locomotor system may need to be assessed in patients with coagulopathy who have joint or muscular bleeds. Inherited bone marrow failure syndromes are commonly associated with musculoskeletal abnormalities (absent radius) as well as dysmorphism and short stature. Refer to **Flowchart 23.3** for a clinical approach to a child with anemia. For details on examination procedures, refer to the textbook on clinical methods.

LABORATORY WORKUP

Detailed laboratory workup of a child with suspected hema tological disorder includes a CBC and a good peripheral smear examination, along with relevant investigations depending upon the suspected underlying disorder. **Table 23.1** has shown the agespecific reference values of CBC. These investigations can help establish the cause of anemia and include: reticulocyte count, lactate dehydrogenase (raised levels in hemolysis), Coombs test (positive in immune hemolytic anemias), osmotic fragility test (increased fragility in hereditary spherocytosis), serum bilirubin (raised in hemolysis), hemoglobin electrophoresis (in hemoglobinopathies), red blood counts (RBC) enzyme assay, and cytogenetics (in leukemias). In a bleeding child CBC with peripheral smear and coagulation profile (prothrombin time and partial thromboplastin time) are basic tests, while factor assays and platelet flow cytometry are confirmatory tests. Details and relevance of each of these tests is explained in subsequent sections in this chapter.

PERIPHERAL SMEAR EXAMINATION

Examination of the peripheral blood smear is an inexpensive but powerful diagnostic tool in both children presenting with suspected blood disorders. When used in conjunction with clinical history and examination, it is invaluable to establish a diagnosis. The smear offers a window into the functional status of the bone marrow. Morphology of blood cells is particularly useful in certain conditions such as suspected hemolytic anemias, nutritional anemias, white blood disorders such as leukemias and thrombocytopenias. The red cell morphology can help delineate the etiology of RBC destruction (e.g., the presence of bite cells points to a Heinz body hemolytic anemia) and the ultimate diagnosis (e.g., oxidant damage to the red cell secondary to drugs). Likewise, platelet size and morphology can sometimes suggest whether thrombocytopenia is due to increased platelet consumption (generally associated with larger platelets) or reduced platelet synthesis (often associated with smaller platelets or abnormal platelet morphology). Abnormal distribution of white blood cells (WBCs) like increased neutrophils or eosinophils, or atypical looking WBCs can also indicate to underlying pathology.

Flowchart 23.3: Clinical approach to anemia

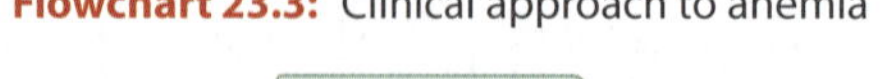

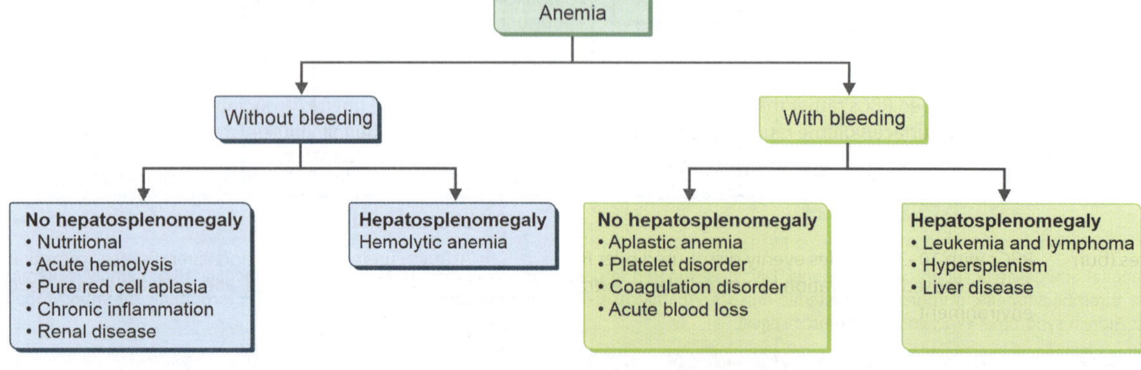

Slide Preparation

The thin peripheral smear is prepared using wedge technique on a clean glass slide using a single drop of blood which is not allowed to clot **(Fig. 23.2A)**. The smear is allowed to air dry and then stained using special stains (Wright's stain). The dried smear is viewed under a low power microscope to determine the optimal area to view. A good smear is tongue shaped with a tail **(Fig. 23.2B)**. It has both thick and thin areas with gradual transition. In the optimal area, red cells will be more or less evenly spaced, and central pallor will be appreciated; mostly RBCs will not abut on each other unless there is rouleaux formation due to conditions such as cold agglutinin disease. Normally, RBCs are round and have a smooth contour with about one-third of the central pallor. Specific RBC abnormalities to be looked for in peripheral smear are depicted in **Table 23.2**. A spectrum of mature leukocytes including lymphocytes (30–40%), neutrophils (30–60%), eosinophils (<5%), basophils (1%), and monocytes is normally seen. Left shift of granulocytes (i.e., abundant band forms, metamyelocytes, and myelocytes) may be due to severe infection/sepsis or chronic myeloid leukemia (CML), while the presence of significant number of blasts suggests acute leukemia; occasionally, blasts can be seen with extreme inflammation or bone marrow stimulation. Döhle bodies and toxic granulations suggest an infectious or inflammatory process. Eosinophilia and or basophilia accompanying neutrophilia may be due to allergic conditions, parasitic or helminthic infections, malignancies, or inflammatory conditions like autoimmune disorders. Hypersegmentation of neutrophils is seen in megaloblastic anemia.

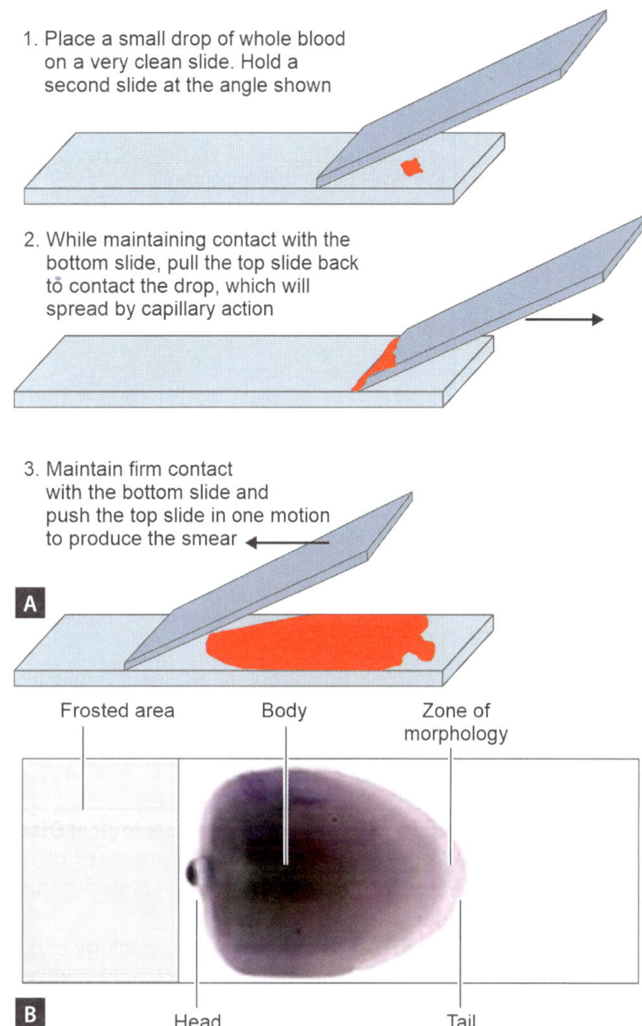

Figs. 23.2A and B: (A) Making a good peripheral blood smear; (B) A good peripheral blood smear

TABLE 23.2 Specific Red Cell Morphologic Abnormalities

Abnormality	*Description*	*Causes*
Anisopoikilocytosis	Red cells of varying sizes (anisocytosis) and shapes (poikilocytosis)	Nutritional anemia, severe thalassemia
Target cells	Abnormal form of RBC which appear to have a dark center (a central and hemoglobinized area) surrounded by a white ring (an area of relative pallor), followed by dark outer (peripheral) second ring containing a band of hemoglobin like a shooting target with bull's eye	Alpha and beta thalassemia, hemoglobin C disease, hemoglobin E (homozygous or heterozygous)
Sickle cells	Crescentic or boat shaped cells	Homozygous Hb S, Hb SD disease, Hb SC disease
Spherocytes	Sphere-shaped RBCs rather than biconcave disk-shaped with decreased surface/volume ratio, and raised MCHC	Hereditary spherocytosis, immune hemolytic anemia, and fragmentation of RBCs (microangiopathy and burns)
Acanthocytes (spur cells)	RBCs with 5–10 spicules of varying length with wide bases	Liver disease, disseminated intravascular coagulation (DIC), postsplenectomy, vitamin E deficiency, and abetalipoproteinemia
Echinocytes (burr cells)	RBCs with 10–30 spicules evenly distributed over RBC surface caused by alteration in intracellular or extracellular environment	Artifact, uremia, dehydration, liver disease, immediately following RBC transfusion, and pyruvate kinase deficiency

Contd...

Contd...

Abnormality	Description	Causes
Schistocytes (helmet cells)	Helmet or triangular shaped RBCs or fragmented RBCs	DIC, severe hemolytic anemia, microangiopathic hemolytic anemia, hemolytic uremic syndrome (HUS), burns, purpura fulminans, and renal vein thrombosis
Elliptocytes	Elliptical RBCs and normochromic	Hereditary elliptocytosis, iron deficiency, megaloblastic anemia, leukoerythroblastic reaction, and malaria
Tear drop cells	Shape of drop, usually microcytic, often hypochromic	Newborn, thalassemia major, and myeloproliferative disorders
Nucleated RBCs	Immature RBCs not normally seen in peripheral blood beyond neonatal period	Neonate (up to 7 days of life), intense bone marrow stimulation as in hemolytic anemias, acute bleeding, hypoxia, postsplenectomy, leukoerythroblastic reaction, and megaloblastic anemia
Basophilic stippling	Coarse/fine punctate basophilic inclusions (aggregates of ribosomal RNA)	Hemolytic anemia, iron-deficiency anemia, and lead poisoning
Howell–Jolly bodies	Small, well-defined, round, densely stained inclusions, eccentric in location, and 1 mm in diameter	Postsplenectomy, newborn, megaloblastic anemia, and dyserythropoietic anemia
Bite/blister cells and Heinz bodies	Red cells show indentation in the border, Heinz bodies are rounded masses adjacent to red cell membrane visible only on supravital staining	G6PD deficiency, oxidant induced hemolysis
Polychromasia	Red cells show variable colour due to presence of bluish reticulocytosis	Newborn, hemolysis

(DIC: disseminated intravascular coagulation; MCHC: mean corpuscular hemoglobin concentration; RBCs: red blood cells; RNA: ribonucleic acid)

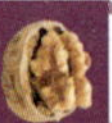

IN A NUTSHELL

Evaluation of a Child with Suspected Hematological Disorder

- A detailed clinical history including family history of bleeding or blood transfusions, and completed physical examination for signs and symptoms compatible with a bleeding disorder, are mandated before laboratory workup of a child with suspected bleeding disorder.
- History should be focused to determine the etiology of bleeding: (1) the most common site and type of bleeding (coagulation defects are commonly associated with articular or deep muscle while platelet defects are commonly associated with skin and mucocutaneous bleeds), (2) bleeding on hemostatic challenge such as surgeries or trauma, (3) family history of bleeding, (4) age on onset of bleeding (acquired causes for bleeding disorders have later age of onset).
- Basic laboratory tests in a child with suspected hematological disorder include a complete blood count with peripheral smear examination along with coagulation profile (prothrombin time and activated partial thromboplastin time).

23.3 Anemia *PE 26.1*

INTRODUCTION

Anemia is defined as a reduction in the red cell mass or blood hemoglobin concentration two standard deviations under neath the expected values for age and sex. The World Health Organization (WHO) cut-off values of hemoglobin for defining anemia in children are as follows:

- ***Neonates:*** <13 g/dL
- ***6–23 months:*** <10.5 g/dL
- ***24–59 months:*** <11 g/dL
- ***5–11 years:*** <11.5 g/dL
- ***12–14 years:*** <12 g/dL

Severity of anemia as defined by World Health Organization (WHO) based on hemoglobin cut-offs for age is depicted in **Table 23.3**.

ETIOLOGY

Normal RBC values represent a balance between RBC synthesis and their destruction. Usually, RBCs circulate in the blood for about 120 days before they are sequestered in the spleen. Hence, anemia may occur when there is:

- Excessive RBC loss (as occurs with hemorrhage)
- Premature RBC destruction (hemolysis)or
- Insufficient RBC production

However, anemia may be physiological in children aged 2–3 months (physiological anemia of infancy). Likewise, transient erythroblastopenia in children may occur in children aged 3 months to 6 years, especially following viral infections. These conditions usually do not require much treatment and are not a cause for concern. **Table 23.4** enlists the etiology of anemia.

TABLE 23.3 Hemoglobin Thresholds (g/dl) to Define Anemia and its Severity as per the World Health Organization

Age group	*Nonanemic*	*Mild*	*Moderate*	*Severe*
6–23 months	≥10.5	9.5–10.4	7–9.4	<7
24–59 months	≥11	10–10.9	7–9.9	<7
5–11 years	≥11.5	11–11.4	8–10.9	<8
12–14 years	≥12	11–11.9	8–10.9	<8

TABLE 23.4 Etiology of Anemia

Mechanism of anemia	*Clinical condition*
Blood loss	• *Acute:* Hemorrhage • *Chronic:* Worm infestation and cow's milk allergy
Decreased production of RBCs	• Deficiency of iron, vitamin B_{12}, folic acid, zinc, or other micronutrients • Aplasia or hypoplasia of bone marrow (aplastic anemia) • Impaired erythropoietin production as in chronic kidney failure, hypothyroidism, or hypopituitarism • Infiltration of the bone marrow as in leukemias and storage disorders • Chronic inflammatory conditions (lupus and rheumatic illness), and chronic infections (tuberculosis)
Increased RBC destruction (hemolytic anemia)	• Corpuscular defects ▪ RBC membrane defects (spherocytosis and elliptocytosis) ▪ RBC enzyme defects [pyruvate kinase deficiency and glucose-6-phosphatase deficiency (G6PD)] ▪ Hemoglobin defects (thalassemia, sickle cell anemia) • Extracorpuscular defects ▪ Immune (autoimmune hemolytic anemia, lupus, drug-induced, hemolytic disease of the newborn, incompatible blood transfusion, etc.) ▪ Nonimmune (mechanical fragmentation—cardiac or microangiopathic hemolysis, hypersplenism, infections such as malaria, gram-negative sepsis, leishmaniasis, *Clostridia*, toxoplasmosis, *Cytomegalovirus*, and lead poisoning)

PATHOPHYSIOLOGY

Anemia leads to decreased oxygen carrying capacity of the blood, which causes signs and symptoms depending upon the severity of anemia. In response to a decrease in hemoglobin levels, the body tries to increase the red cell production by secreting more erythropoietin. Erythropoietin stimulates the bone marrow, which becomes more active and hypercellular resulting in the release of more immature red cells into the peripheral circulation. This results in increased number of nucleated red blood cells (normoblasts) and reticulocytes in the peripheral blood.

The body also compensates for the decreased oxygen carrying capacity of blood by increasing the cardiac output. This is achieved by increasing the stroke volume, heart rate, and shunting of blood toward vital organs. All this leads to a high output state and a flow ejection systolic murmur can be heard in chronic cases. The body also tries to increase the oxygen delivery to tissues by shifting the oxygen dissociation curve to right. However, compensatory mechanisms become insufficient with progress of anemia and the child becomes symptomatic.

CLINICAL FEATURES

Anemia manifests as pallor, fatigue, loss of appetite, irritability, tachypnea, dyspnea, tachycardia, and finally the child develops congestive cardiac failure. The most important sign is pallor, which is visible in the palpebral conjunctiva, lips, tongue, nails, palms, and soles.

A simple way to grade the severity of anemia is palmar pallor. If palms are pale but creases are pink, it indicates moderate anemia. If creases are also pale, it usually means severe anemia. A rapid fall in hemoglobin results in more severe symptoms at a higher hemoglobin level than a slow gradual fall in hemoglobin level because there is not sufficient time for the compensatory mechanisms to operate fully.

MORPHOLOGICAL CLASSIFICATION OF ANEMIA

A peripheral smear examination is needed for classifying anemia according to the morphology of red blood cells. The important things to be observed are the size of the red blood cell and pattern of staining. Other important features that also need attention are shape of RBC, any inclusion bodies, morphology, and number of leukocytes and the platelets **(Table 23.2)**.

Microcytic Anemia

The mean corpuscular volume (MCV) is less than the lower limit of normal for age. Up to 2 years of age, MCV < 70 fL is considered microcytosis. Thereafter between 2 and 10 years age, MCV < [70 + age (y)] fL is regarded as microcytosis and beyond 10 years, MCV < 80 fL is microcytosis. This is also associated with decrease in mean corpuscular hemoglobin (MCH) and decrease in mean corpuscular hemoglobin concentration (MCHC) also called *hypochromia*. In this type of anemia there is defect in the RBC formation mainly affecting the hemoglobin synthesis; other cellular components are spared. The important causes of microcytic anemia are listed here.

- ***Iron-deficiency anemia***
  - Nutritional
  - Posthemorrhagic
- ***Ineffective erythropoiesis***
  - Thalassemia
  - Anemia of chronic disease
  - Pyridoxine responsive (sideroblastic) anemia

- Dyserythropoietic anemia
- Lead poisoning

Macrocytic Anemia

The MCV of RBCs in patients with macrocytic anemia is more than the upper limit of normal for that age. In children aged up to 10 years, MCV >84 + [0.6 × age (years)] fL and, in children aged ≥10 years MCV >90 fL, is defined as macrocytosis. The defect lies in the deoxyribonucleic acid (DNA) synthesis instead of hemoglobin synthesis and therefore also affects other cell lines. The red blood cells are usually normochromic, i.e., MCH and MCHC are normal. The presence of hypersegmented neutrophils (≥5 lobed nuclei in >5% of neutrophils) and leukopenia are commonly seen in nutritional etiology of macrocytic anemia. It is usually associated with a megaloblastic bone marrow, i.e., the erythroid precursors are also larger in size than normal. However, macrocytosis is not synonymous with megaloblastosis as a macrocytic peripheral blood picture may be associated with a normoblastic bone marrow picture. Spuriously high MCV can be due to red cell agglutination associated with the cold type of autoimmune hemolytic anemia. Important causes of macrocytic anemia are listed here.

- ***Megaloblastic erythropoiesis***
  - *Nutritional*
    - Vitamin B_{12} deficiency
    - Folate deficiency
  - *Toxic*
    - *Drug-induced:* Antifolate compounds (e.g., metho trexate and trimethoprim), anticonvulsant (e.g., phenytoin).
  - *Malabsorption*
    - Pernicious anemia
    - Postgastrectomy and ileal resection
    - Human immunodeficiency virus (HIV) enteropathy
  - Increased demands including hemolysis, and leukemia
- ***Nonmegaloblastic erythropoiesis***
  - *Chronic hemolytic anemia:* Peripheral smear shows macrocytic erythrocytes due to relative folate deficiency resulting from increased compensatory erythropoiesis.
  - Liver diseases
  - Hypothyroidism
  - Down's syndrome
  - Inherited marrow failure syndromes: Fanconi anemia and Diamond–Blackfan anemia (hypocellular marrow)

Normocytic Anemia

The MCV is within normal limits along with the MCH and MCHC so the RBCs are also normochromic.

- ***Impaired cell production*** (reticulocyte count is low)
  - *Leukocytes and platelets are normal*
    - Physiological anemia of infancy
    - Infections
  - *Leukocytes and platelets are normal or decreased*
    - Chronic renal and liver disease
    - Hypothyroidism
  - *Leukocytes and platelets are reduced*
    - *Aplastic anemia*
    - *Myeloproliferative disorders:* Leukemia
- ***Hemolytic anemia*** (reticulocyte count is high)
  - **Red cell enzymopathy**
  - Red cell membranopathy
  - Warm type autoimmune hemolysis

CLINICAL APPROACH TO ANEMIA

Relevant history such as the age of onset, progression, blood loss, jaundice, bleeding tendency, blood transfusion, and family history are very important and will give some clue to the cause. A detailed examination from head to toe is important especially regarding the degree of pallor, icterus, petechiae, ecchymotic patches, presence of lymphadenopathy, enlarged liver and spleen, and bony tenderness. Association of anemia with bleeding and the presence or absence of hepatosplenomegaly are important in making a differential diagnosis **(Flowchart 23.3)**.

- ***Age of onset:*** Nutritional anemias usually manifest between 6 months and 3 years of age. Alpha thalassemia presents with anemia or hydrops *in utero* or just after birth. Beta thalassemia usually presents after 6 months of age when fetal hemoglobin (HbF) starts decreasing. A congenital bone marrow hypoplasia may present soon after birth. Anemia in a neonate will mostly be due to hemorrhage, hemolysis (Rh or ABO isoimmunization) (usually with indirect hyperbilirubinemia) or rarely due to failure of RBC production (Diamond–Blackfan anemia).
- ***Neonatal jaundice*** with or without anemia can be seen in Rh/blood group incompatibility between mother and baby, RBC enzyme defects, and hereditary spherocytosis.
- ***Family history of blood transfusions indicates an inherited*** cause such as thalassemia, enzyme defects (G6PD deficiency), or membrane defects (hereditary spherocytosis). In addition to anemia; recurrent jaundice, cholecystectomy before 40-years of age, and splenectomy in family members may also suggest congenital hemolytic anemia.
- Repeated history of blood transfusions usually indicates a nonnutritional anemia such as hemoglobinopathy, thalassemia, or bone marrow hypofunction.
- ***Community*** G6PD deficiency is more common in *Parsis* and *Sindhis*. Thalassemia is seen more in *Punjabis* and *Sindhis*. Sickle cell anemia is more common in Central Indian states such as Madhya Pradesh, Gujarat, Chattisgarh; Tamil Nadu, Kerala, and Andhra Pradesh. Hemoglobin E beta thalassemia is mostly seen in Indians residing in North Eastern states, West Bengal, Odisha, and Andaman and Nicobar.
- ***Dietary history:*** A child with predominantly milk-based diet with minimal or no complementary feeding is more likely to suffer from nutritional anemia. History of pica suggests an iron-deficiency anemia. A child on goat's milk is predisposed to folic acid deficiency due to its poor folate content. Vegan diet and food fads can cause vitamin B_{12} deficiency.
- ***History of passage of worms, blood in stools or melena*** for a long time leads to chronic blood loss and anemia.

- ❖ ***History of skin bleeds (petechiae or ecchymosis) or bleeding from any other site:*** This suggests a platelet or a hepatic involvement. Chronic liver disease could be a cause of anemia that will also affect the coagulation factors and lead to bleeding manifestations. Skin bleeds associated with anemia suggests hypoplasia or infiltration of the bone marrow.
- ❖ ***History of fever*** with sudden appearance of pallor suggests malaria.
- ❖ ***Facies:*** A typical hemolytic facies is characteristic of thalassemia.
- ❖ ***Jaundice:*** The presence of mild jaundice without passage of high colored urine indicates a process of hemolysis whereas the presence of conjugated hyperbilirubinemia indicates primary hepatic pathology.
- ❖ ***Malnutrition and wasting*** may be associated with nutritional anemia.
- ❖ ***Hepatosplenomegaly:*** Presence of significant hepatosplenomegaly with lymphadenopathy is highly suggestive of malignancy (leukemia and lymphoma). Significant hepatosplenomegaly without lymphadenopathy sug gests hemolytic anemia, e.g., thalassemia, or infective pathology (malaria). HIV/acquired immunodeficiency syndrome (AIDS) should also be ruled out in presence of hepatosplenomegaly.
- ❖ ***Presence of associated anomalies*** such as skeletal deformities, hyperpigmentation, hypopigmentation, renal anomalies, and eye and ear malformations point toward a possibility of inherited pancytopenia such as Fanconi anemia or dyskeratosis congenita or Diamond–Blackfan anemia.

INVESTIGATIONS IN ANEMIA

- ❖ ***Hemoglobin:*** Estimation of hemoglobin to confirm anemia, and assess its severity to decide for the need of packed red blood cell transfusion.
- ❖ ***Red blood cell indices:*** Hematocrit (packed cell volume), mean corpuscular volume (MCV), mean corpuscular hemoglobin (MCH), mean corpuscular hemoglobin concentration (MCHC), and red cell distribution width (RDW) are helpful in indicating the type of anemia **(Flowchart 23.4)**. Increased

Flowchart 23.4: Laboratory approach to anemia

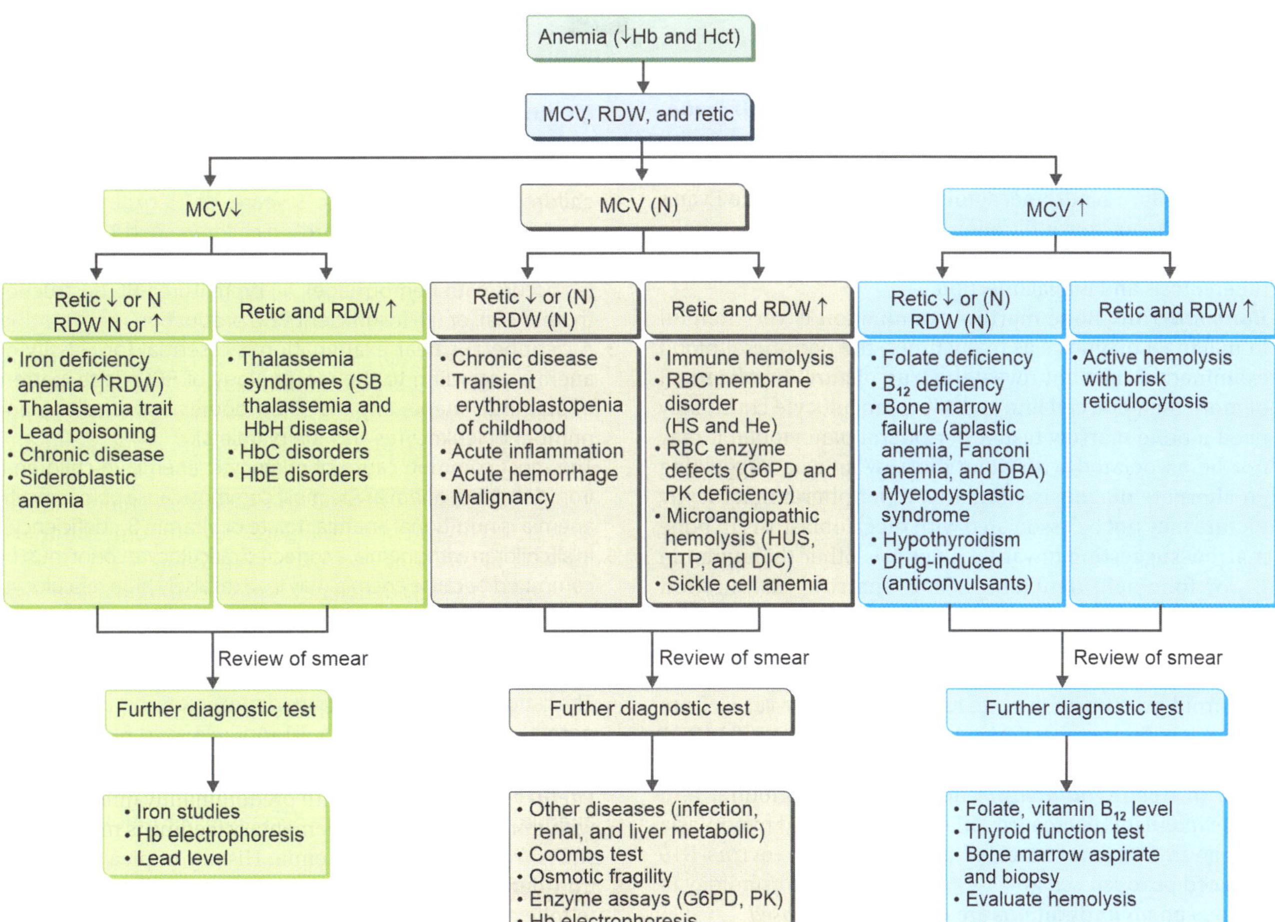

(DBA: Diamond–Blackfan anemia; DIC: disseminated intravascular coagulation; G6PD: glucose-6-phosphate dehydrogenase; Hb: hemoglobin; Hct: hematocrit; HUS: hemolytic uremic syndrome; MCV: mean corpuscular volume; PK: pyruvate kinase; RBC: red blood cell; Retic: reticulocyte count; RDW: red cell distribution width; TTP: thrombotic thrombocytopenic purpura).

MCHC is seen in hereditary spherocytosis. RDW indicates the variation in red blood cell size. Increased RDW indicates presence of anisocytosis as seen in iron-deficiency anemia and folate/vitamin B_{12} deficiency (nutritional anemia). A normal RDW (12–14%) indicates not much variation in size of the red blood cells as in thalassemia, anemia of chronic disease, hemorrhage, hereditary spherocytosis, and aplastic anemia. RDW when used together with MCV can aid in diagnosing the cause of anemia.

- ***Reticulocyte count:*** Number of reticulocytes in the blood reflects the bone marrow activity and is expressed as the percentage of the total red blood cell count. If the bone marrow is hyperactive as in cases of hemolytic anemia or following hemorrhage, the reticulocyte count increases. The reticulocyte count is decreased in patients with bone marrow hypoplasia or aplasia, malignancies, infections especially Parvovirus B_{19} infection and in nutritional anemia.
- Anemia *per se* results in increased bone marrow activity to compensate for decreased hemoglobin, leading to falsely high reticulocyte count. Therefore, correction should be made for the existing severity of anemia. This is done as follows:

Corrected reticulocyte count =

$$\text{Observed reticulocyte count} \times \frac{\text{Patient hematocrit}}{\text{Normal hematocrit}}$$

- ***Anemia associated with leukopenia and/or thrombocytopenia*** vitamin B_{12}/folate deficiency can present with bi/pancytopenia. Other causes include congenital bone marrow failure syndrome, autoimmune etiology (like Evan's syndrome), marrow infiltration in malignancy or metabolic disorder (Gaucher's disease), or chronic infection such as tuberculosis and fungal infection.
- ***Bone marrow:*** Bone marrow examination is very helpful in making a diagnosis as many times, the peripheral blood examination may not reveal the true picture. Involvement of more than one cell line and a low reticulocyte count may need a bone marrow test. A peripheral pancytopenia may not be associated with bone marrow aplasia suggesting an alternate diagnosis. Similarly, a peripheral macrocytic picture may not be associated with megaloblastosis in bone marrow suggesting toward a diagnosis other than vitamin B_{12} or folic acid deficiency. Bone marrow examination can be diagnostic in aplastic anemia and leukemia. It is important to ascertain the cellularity and the myeloid to erythroid ratio (M:E ratio) in marrow. The ratio of myeloid to erythroid precursors in bone marrow normally varies from 2:1 to 4:1. An increased M:E ratio may suggest infections or chronic myeloid leukemia. Erythroid hyperplasia is seen in hemolytic anemia, megaloblastic anemia, and hypersplenism (decreased M:E ratio). Erythroid hypoplasia is seen in Diamond Blackfan anemia and Parvovirus-B19 induced pure red cell aplasia. Bone marrow morphology in various anemic conditions are as follows:
  - *Normal:* Irondeficiency anemia (Perls stain in the marrow shows iron stores), infection, malignancy, renal disease, connective tissue disorders, and hemolytic anemia.
  - *Megaloblastic:* Vitamin B_{12} deficiency, folate deficiency, congenital/acquired disorders in DNA synthesis, and druginduced (methotrexate and phenytoin).
  - *Rare anemias:* Ringed sideroblasts can be seen in sideroblastic anemia due to genetic or acquired (Copper deficiency, drug induced) causes. Congenital dyserythropoietic anemias can demonstrate peculiar features such as multinucleate erythroblasts and internuclear chromatin bridging.
- ***Other investigations:*** Specific investigations for etiological diagnosis include serum iron studies, serum folate and vitamin B_{12} levels for deficiency anemias; hemoglobin electrophoresis, high performance liquid chromatography for hemoglobinopathies and thalassemia; osmotic fragility and eosin-maleimide binding in hereditary spherocytosis, enzyme level assays in red cell enzymopathies, and direct Coombs test for autoimmune hemolytic anemia Genetic studies such as beta-globin gene sequencing in beta-thalassemia and clinical exome sequencing in hemolytic anemias are important in congenital anemias for diagnostic confirmation and to offer antenatal counselling and diagnosis in the next pregnancy for the parents.

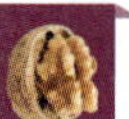

IN A NUTSHELL

Anemia

1. Anemia is a reduction in the red cell mass or blood hemoglobin concentration, 2 standard deviations below the expected values for age and sex. The WHO cut-off values of hemoglobin for defining anemia in children are <11 g/dL in children aged 6 months to 5 years, <11.5 g/dL in children aged 5–11 years, and <12 g/dL in children aged 12–14 years.
2. Anemia may occur when there is—(i) excessive RBC loss (as occurs with hemorrhage), (ii) premature RBC destruction (hemolysis), or (iii) insufficient RBC production.
3. A peripheral smear examination is essential for classifying anemia according to the morphology of RBCs (size, pattern of staining, shape, any inclusion bodies, morphology and number of leukocytes and the platelets).
4. The most common cause of microcytic anemia in children is iron-deficiency anemia. The most common cause of macrocytic anemia is nutritional anemia (folate or vitamin B_{12} deficiency).
5. In all children with anemia, a corrected reticulocyte count must be computed because anemia may lead to falsely high reticulocyte count. Reticulocyte count increases in cases of hemolytic anemia or following hemorrhage, and decreases in patients with bone marrow hypoplasia or aplasia, malignancies, and infections.
6. The ratio of myeloid to erythroid precursors in bone marrow normally varies from 2:1 to 4:1. An increased M:E ratio may suggest infections or chronic myeloid leukemia. Erythroid hyperplasia is seen in hemolytic anemia, megaloblastic anemia, and hypersplenism (decreased M:E ratio).

GENERAL MANAGEMENT

All children should be regularly dewormed as hookworm infestation is a very common cause of anemia especially in children from lower socioeconomic strata. For nutritional anemia, specific supplementation needs to be started once the diagnosis is made. Treatment of nutritional anemia (iron, vitamin B_{12}, and folate deficiency) is described in respective sections ahead in this chapter. Apart from medication, proper dietary advice needs to be given regarding which food is rich in the deficient nutrient. All children with fever in the endemic zone for malaria should be treated with antimalarials unless there is some other known cause for fever.

Emergency Management

A child in congestive cardiac failure should be managed promptly and aggressively. The child should be nursed in a propped-up position, i.e., head and chest elevated above the rest of the body, to decrease the venous return and alleviate the symptoms. Oxygen should be supplemented and a diuretic administered to decrease the pulmonary edema. Fluid should be restricted to decrease preload. Packed red blood transfusion 10–15 mL kg must be given at a rate of 3–5 mL/kg/h. Whole blood should not be transfused as it increases the chances of fluid overload. Intravenous furosemide should be given during transfusion in a dose of 1–2 mg/kg to avoid circulatory overload. **Box 23.1** enlists the indications for packed cell transfusion in anemia in children.

Box 23.1 Indications of Packed Red Cell Transfusion in Children >4 Months

- Blood loss >15% of total blood volume
- *Hb <9 g/dL:* Severe cardiopulmonary disease
- *Hb <7 g/dL:* Severe infection, perioperative period, marrow failure, symptomatic chronic anemia, signs of hypoxia, and congestive cardiac failure
- Hb <4 g/dL

Brugnara C, Oski FA, Nathan DG. Diagnostic approach to the anemic patient. In: Orkin SH, Fisher DE, Look T, et al (Eds). Nathan and Oski's Hematology and Oncology of Infancy and Childhood, 8th editon. Philadelphia: WB Saunders; 2015. p. 293.
Dixit S, Jha T, Gupta R, et al. Practical approach to the interpretation of complete blood count reports and histograms. Indian Pediatr. 2022;59(6):485-91.
Gallagher PG. Anemia in the pediatric patient. Blood. 2022;140 (6):571–93.
Pabón-Rivera S, Flores RR, Frei-Jones M. The complete blood count: a practical tool for the pediatrician. Pediatr Rev. 2023;44(7):363–82.
Valentine SL, Bembea MM, Muszynski JA, Cholette JM, Doctor A, Spinella PC, et al. Pediatric Critical Care Transfusion and Anemia Expertise Initiative (TAXI); Pediatric Critical Care Blood Research Network (BloodNet), and the Pediatric Acute Lung Injury and Sepsis Investigators (PALISI) Network. Consensus Recommendations for RBC Transfusion Practice in Critically Ill Children From the Pediatric Critical Care Transfusion and Anemia Expertise Initiative. Pediatr Crit Care Med. 2018;19(9):884-898.

23.4 Iron-deficiency Anemia

PE 26.2

INTRODUCTION

Nutritional deficiency of iron is the most common cause of anemia in children. The most vulnerable age is 6–24 months. The rapid growth seen in children increases the demand of iron substantially for hemoglobin synthesis and any deficiency in the diet leads to anemia.

Apart from nutritional deficiency, other factors that may lead to iron-deficiency anemia (IDA) are (i) poor iron body stores at birth as seen in preterm infants and due to iron deficiency in the mother; (ii) worm infestations; and (iii) impaired absorption from intestine as seen in celiac disease. IDA may also be seen in children from across socioeconomic strata due to improper complementary feeding after the first 6 months of exclusive breastfeeding, food fads and unhealthy eating practices. Excessive phytates in diet can impair iron absorption. Chronic blood loss due to peptic ulcer, Meckel diverticulum, gastrointestinal polyps or hemangiomas, and irritable bowel disease can also cause of iron deficiency. In infants, cow milk allergy may lead to occult gastrointestinal blood loss. In developing countries, infestation with hookworm, *Trichuris trichiura*, *Plasmodium* parasite, and *H. pylori* can contribute to blood loss.

In the initial stages of iron deficiency, the body stores of iron are mobilized for hemoglobin synthesis. When the stores are all used up, the hemoglobin synthesis is decreased, and the affected child becomes pale and symptomatic.

IRON METABOLISM

Stores

Iron is present in the body in three forms: Hemoglobin, plasma iron, and tissue iron. Hemoglobin iron constitutes a major part of body iron which gets released into plasma when the RBCs get lysed. The plasma iron is reutilized for synthesis of hemoglobin. The tissue iron is present as ferritin and hemosiderin in liver, spleen, and bone marrow; and myoglobin in muscles and cellular enzymes. Of the available storage forms, ferritin is normally predominant.

Serum ferritin levels vary with age and sex and body iron stores. It may be falsely elevated in conditions such as infection, inflammation, malignancy, and liver disease even in the presence of iron deficiency. Iron, when absorbed by the mucosal cells, binds to form ferritin which is released as and when required into the plasma. This ferritin stored in the mucosal cells gets excreted when the mucosal cells are exfoliated once in 2–3 days.

Transport

Iron is carried from the intestines to the tissue stores, from storage sites to bone marrow, and from one storage site to another with the help of transferrin. Transferrin carries iron to the site of storage as well as utilization. When it reaches the desired site, transferrin attaches itself to the transferrin recep tors and iron is released into the cells.

The transferrin present in the serum can bind to a maximum of 47–70 μmol/L of iron. This is known as the total ironbinding capacity (TIBC). Percentage of total transferrin present in the serum to which iron is bound is called *percentage saturation of transferrin*. Under normal conditions, 33% of transferrin is bound to iron and rest is free.

Absorption

Absorption of iron mainly takes place in the duodenum and the proximal jejunum. This mechanism can be up or down regulated through a feedback system depending upon the iron stores. Iron is best absorbed when taken on an empty stomach with water or fruit juice about one or two hours after meals. The bioavailability of iron through normal diet is 10%. Phytates in diet interfere with absorption of dietary iron, while vitamin C enhances iron absorption. The body absorbs iron from animal sources (such as meats), i.e., heme iron, better than iron from plant sources, i.e., nonheme iron.

Requirements

One mg/day of iron should be absorbed by the body to meet the physiological demands of iron. Since, only 10% of dietary iron is ultimately absorbed, 10–15 mg/day iron is needed.

CAUSES OF IRON DEFICIENCY

Iron deficiency results whenever there is an imbalance between supply and demand. Three major reasons for a negative balance are (i) increased physiological demands of iron, (ii) pathological blood loss, and (iii) inadequate intake of iron. Main reasons are given here:

- ***Decreased intake***
- ***Increased demand:*** Prematurity, twins, multiple gestation, infancy, adolescence, and cyanotic congenital heart disease.
- ***Chronic blood loss:*** Worm infestation (hookworm and *Trichuris trichiura*), *Plasmodium* infections, esophageal varices, cow's milk protein intolerance, hemorrhoids, rectal polyp, and peptic ulcer.
- ***Impaired absorption:*** Celiac disease, inflammatory bowel disease, postgastrectomy, and severe prolonged diarrhea impair iron absorption. Intake of large amounts of antacids or a diet rich in phytates also decrease absorption of dietary iron. Large amounts of tea or coffee consumed with a meal (the polyphenols bind the iron) can impair absorption of iron.

PATHOGENESIS

Increased Demand

A child born with normal iron stores (200–300 mg at birth) can meet the increased physiological demand till 4–6 months of age. Iron deficiency results, if the body stores are poor at the time of birth because of prematurity, low birth weight, or perinatal hemorrhage from cord, fetofetal, or fetomaternal hemorrhage. Children have higher growth rates and so demand is always high and they are at risk of iron-deficiency anemia especially during later half of infancy till 24 months or by 6–8 weeks of age in a premature baby. Adolescent girls are especially prone to irondeficiency anemia (IDA) due to adolescent growth spurt (increased demand) and menstrual losses (chronic blood loss).

Inadequate Intake

It is the most common cause of IDA especially in developing countries like India. Inappropriate dietary practices result in a negative iron balance. Babies who remain on predominant milk diet are prone to IDA. Breastmilk as well as cow milk, are poor sources of dietary iron (1 mg/L). Though, bioavailability of breastmilk iron is 2–3 times more than that from cow milk, both are inadequate to meet the nutritional dietary needs of the body. Infants, in whom appropriate complementary feeding is not started by 6 months age, may develop iron deficiency.

Chronic Blood Loss

It also causes depletion of the body iron stores, e.g., abnormal bleeding from gut as in worm infestation, esophageal varices, hemorrhoids, cow milk protein intolerance, and Meckel diverticulum.

CLINICAL FEATURES

The manifestations are insidious in onset. The child may stop eating well, becomes irritable, gets tired easily and becomes lethargic. There is failure to thrive. Pallor gradually increases in severity. Often the parents may not notice paleness of the body till the anemis is severe. There may be other associated signs of malnutrition and vitamin deficiencies. The child may just lose interest in studies or the school performance may go down. Some children with irondeficiency anemia have a history of pica (craving for nonedible things such as chalk, mud, and paper) and pagophagia (desire to eat ice). There may be history of dyspnea on exertion.

On examination, the most striking finding is pallor of varying degree. Iron deficiency leads to certain epithelial tissue changes especially if deficiency is long standing. The fingernails become thin, brittle and lusterless and flat (platynychia) or even spoon-shaped (koilonychias) **(Fig. 23.3)**. There is atrophy of the tongue papillae resulting in a smooth looking tongue.

Tachycardia may be present along with cardiomegaly and a functional systolic murmur due to hyperdynamic circulation. If the child is in congestive cardiac failure; pedal edema, increased jugular venous pressure, congestive hepatomegaly, and basal crepitations in the chest can be documented.

The nutritional status of the child may vary. In India, most of these children are malnourished with multivitamin deficiency. But the nutritional status may be normal or some children may even be obese.

INVESTIGATIONS

- ***Assessment for type and severity of anemia:*** A peripheral smear will show microcytic and hypochromic anemia when the hemoglobin level is below 10 g/dL **(Fig. 23.4)**.

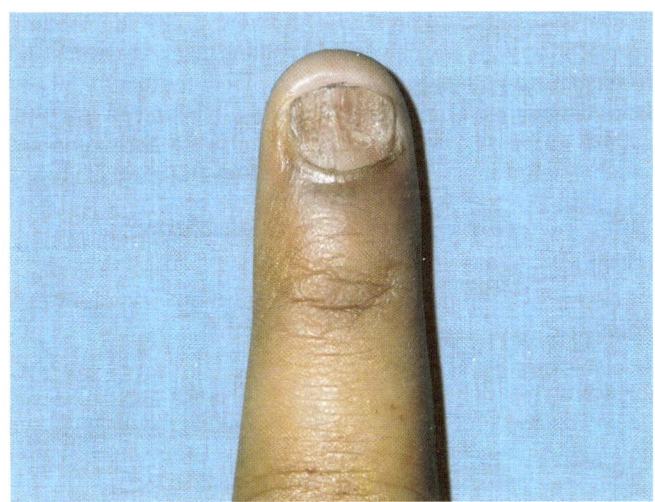

Fig. 23.3: Koilonychia seen in iron-deficiency anemia

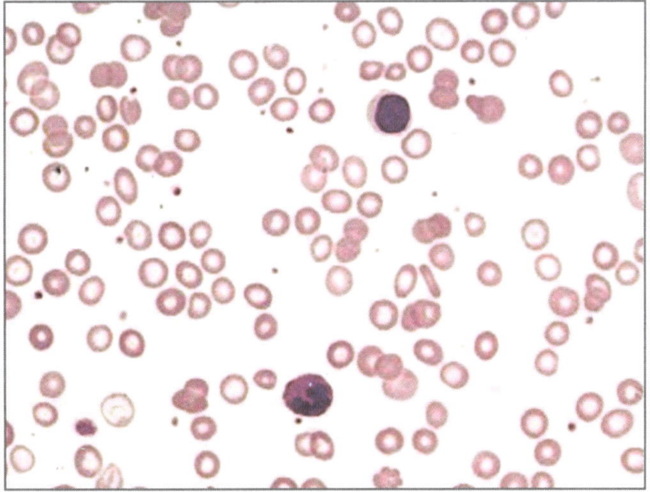

Fig. 23.4: Peripheral smears showing microcytic hypochromic red blood cells (RBCs) in a child with iron-deficiency anemia

Anisopoikilocytosis and pencil cells can be seen in the blood smear. Red blood cell indices can confirm this; MCV < 70 fL in under two children and MCV < 70 + age (in years) in children between 2 and 10 years, MCH < 27 pg, MCHC < 30%. Other cells lines are usually not affected. Thrombocytosis is frequently seen in IDA, though severe IDA may be rarely associated with thrombocytopenia.

- ***Assessment of iron status:*** Serum iron <10 µmol/L, low serum ferritin (SF) and transferrin saturation <16% are suggestive of iron deficiency. SF <12 µg/L in children under-five years of age and SF <15 µg/L in individuals over 5 years of age in the absence of any active inflammation are suggestive of IDA. In the presence of infection or inflammation, SF <30 µg/L is suggestive of IDA in children. Total iron binding capacity (TIBC) and free erythroid porphyrin (FEP) on the contrary increase (TIBC > 350 µg/dL, FEP > 70 mg/dL) as now more transferrin and porphyrin are free. Other tests in iron deficiency include elevated soluble transferrin receptor >27.3 nmol/L, decreased reticulated hemoglobin < 29 pg, and increased percentage of hypochromic red cells > 5%. A bone marrow test is not recommended for diagnosing IDA, but if done for another indication Perls Prussian blue stain can illustrate the iron store.

The sequence of events is usually as follows: Decreased serum ferritin → decreased serum iron → decreased % saturation of transferrin → increased TIBC → increased FEP → microcytic hypochromic anemia → increased red cell distribution width (RDW).

DIFFERENTIAL DIAGNOSIS

Although microcytic hypochromic anemia is usually caused by iron-deficiency anemia, several other conditions may have similar peripheral blood picture. The most common alternative causes include α- and β-thalassemia and hemoglobinopathies, including hemoglobin E and C.

- Iron studies and red cell distribution width are normal in microcytic hypochromic anemia secondary to thalassemia trait. Individuals with thalassemia trait have a lower MCV and a normal to RBC count. A Mentzer index (calculating by dividing MCV by RBC count in million/microlitre) < 13 favors thalassemia trait over iron-deficiency.
- The anemia of chronic disease is usually normocytic but can be microcytic sometimes. Serum iron is also low in anemia of chronic diseases, but associated with normal or increased serum ferritin, and decreased total iron-binding capacity.
- Lead poisoning can also cause microcytic anemia, but more commonly IDA leads to pica which results in lead intoxication.
- ***Other disorders associated with microcytic anemia include:*** Sickle cell thalassemia, hemoglobin SC disease, lead poisoning, chronic infections, copper deficiency, hereditary orotic aciduria, sideroblastic anemia, malignancy, hypo- or atransferrinemia, and congenital defect of iron transport to red cells.

TREATMENT Iron-deficiency Anemia

Iron Supplementation

Oral iron supplementation is the route of choice, administered at the dose of 3–6 mg/kg/day of elemental iron (2–3mg/kg/day has also shown to be effective). The expected rise in the hemoglobin is ≥ 1 g/dl by 14 days of compliant iron therapy. To achieve best results, iron preparations should be given on empty stomach. Dairy products, tea, coffee, antacids, proton pump inhibitors, and calcium supplement should not be administered at the same time as iron therapy. In patients with gastrointestinal intolerance to iron, it may be given 1-2 hours after dinner. Deworming with albendazole should be ensured if not done already.

The elemental iron content in the various chemical oral iron preparations commonly available is: Ferrous fumarate (33%), ferrous sulphate (20%), and ferrous gluconate (12%) are the commonest formulations. Ferrous lactate (19%), anhydrous (desiccated) ferrous sulfate (37%), ferrous carbonate (16%), ferrous succinate (35%) and iron-amino acid chelates, ferrous gluconate (12%), ferric ammonium citrate (15.5%), iron polymaltose complex, and colloidal iron are other available preparations. Ferric compounds should be avoided as these are heavily chelated and so poorly absorbed.

The intake of oral iron is associated with side effects like metallic taste, constipation or loose stools, nausea, vomiting, staining of teeth, and dark-colored stools. Ferrous sulfate has the best iron absorption but the incidence of gastrointestinal side-effects is greater compared to other iron preparations like ferrous fumarate, ferrous lactate and ferrous gluconate. Simultaneous intake of vitamin C enhances iron absorption, when given empty stomach or in between meals. The phytates in cereals and phosphates in milk impair iron absorption. The supplementation should continue for at least 8 weeks after the hemoglobin levels have returned to normal to replenish the depleted body stores. The first sign of improvement is an increase in the activity and appetite. A rise in the reticulocyte count indicating the bone marrow response can be demonstrated after 2–3 days of supplementation; it peaks at day 5–7 of therapy. A rise of hemoglobin is seen by the end of the first week. The iron stores are replenished after 2–3 months of therapy.

Failure of response should be investigated by looking for following causes: (i) inadequate dose; (ii) poor compliance; (iii) malabsorption; (iv) wrong diagnosis; (v) continuing blood loss especially occult gastrointestinal bleeding; (vi) concurrent folate or vitamin B_{12} deficiency, (vii) concurrent infection, (viii) iron refractory iron deficiency anemia due to congenital defects in iron metabolism (IRIDA).

Parenteral iron therapy is not used frequently for nutritional iron deficiency. It can be used for patients with malabsorption, severe intolerance, ongoing significant blood loss, chronic kidney disease, and IRIDA. Formulations include iron sucrose, ferric gluconate, iron dextran, and ferric carboxy maltose.

Blood Transfusion

Transfusion of packed red blood cells is needed if the anemia is severe (Hb < 4 g/dL), or the child is in congestive cardiac failure, or there is associated superimposed severe infection which can interfere with the response to supplementation.

Diet

Apart from therapeutic interventions the child's diet needs to be modified. Diet rich in iron should be advised. Sources rich in iron include animal products such as liver, red meat, egg yolk, green leafy vegetables (spinach, cabbage, mustard leaves, drumstick leaves), tubers (turnip, sweet potato), radish, gooseberry, tomato; fruits such as orange, pomegranate, guava, watermelon, and apple; and dry fruits (dates, walnuts, etc.). Jaggery is rich in iron. Cooking food in iron utensils can increase the iron content of the food. Milk is a poor source of iron. It is important to ensure timely introduction of healthy complementary feeds at 6 months of age.

Inhibitors of iron absorption such as phytates, phosphates, and tea should be restricted in diet, while vitamin C which facilitates iron absorption should be included.

Identify and Treat the Underlying Cause

Hookworm infestation, chronic infection, or celiac disease, or any other underlying cause of anemia needs to be treated.

PREVENTION

To prevent IDA, supplementary foods rich in iron should be initiated as soon as complementary feeding is started, preferably at 6 months of age. Pulses, green leafy vegetables and beans must be included in diet. Vulnerable groups like preterm low birth weight infants need to be supplemented with iron in a dose of 2–4 mg/kg/day starting from 4 to 6 weeks age. Diet of girls attaining menarche should be fortified with iron. Iron supplements are also necessary during adolescence for preventing anemia of puberty. Hookworm infestation should be curbed by regularly deworming children every 6 months and by encouraging them to not walk bare feet. Another important intervention that can augment iron stores in infants after birth is to delay umbilical cord clamping after birth by at least 3 minutes (not before 1 minute) or till cord pulsations stop.

Weekly Iron and Folic Acid (IFA) Supplementation (WIFS) Program

Government of India has implemented the Weekly Iron and Folic Acid Supplementation (WIFS) program since January 2013, under the National Rural Health Mission (NRHM) in government/aided and municipal schools (nationwide) and *aaganwadi* centers across all states in India to combat anemia amongst adolescents. Weekly prophylactic supplementation of iron is as effective as daily supplementation.

Iron Fortification

The Government of India is implementing fortification of common salt with iron to control IDA in community. The National Institute of Nutrition has successfully fortified the common salt with iron (ferrous sulfate: 3.2 g, sodium acid sulfate: 5 g, and orthophosphoric acid: 3.2 g in 1 kg of common salt).

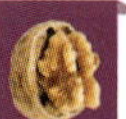

IN A NUTSHELL

Iron-deficiency Anemia

1. Nutritional deficiency of iron is the most common cause of anemia in children.
2. A child with IDA manifests with pallor, nail changes like koilonychias and platynychia, bald tongue, pica, and irritability. Laboratory diagnosis includes presence of microcytic hypochromic RBCs on peripheral smear with low reticulocyte count and raised RDW. Serum iron, serum ferritin, and percent saturation of transferrin are reduced to <10 µmol/L, <12 ng/mL (or 15 ng/mL in children > 5 years), and <16%, respectively. TIBC is increased (>350 µg/dL).
3. Common differential diagnosis of microcytic hypochromic anemia includes IDA, thalassemia trait, hemoglobinopathies, sideroblastic anemia, copper deficiency, and anemia of chronic disease.
4. Treatment of IDA includes deworming, oral iron supplementation and dietary modification (dietary sources of iron include animal products liver, meat, egg yolk, green vegetables, fruits, and jaggery).

Chandra J, Dewan P, Kumar P, Mahajan A, Singh P, Dhingra B, et al. Diagnosis, treatment and prevention of nutritional anemia in children: Recommendations of the Joint Committee of Pediatric Hematology-Oncology Chapter and Pediatric and Adolescent Nutrition Society of the Indian Academy of Pediatrics. Indian Pediatr. 2022;59(10):782-801.

Fletcher A, Forbes A, Svenson N, Thomas DW. A British Society for Haematology Good Practice Paper. Guideline for the laboratory diagnosis of iron deficiency in adults (excluding pregnancy) and children. Br J Haematol. 2022;196(3):523-9.

23.5 Megaloblastic Anemia

PE 26.3

INTRODUCTION

Megaloblastic anemia is characterized by ineffective erythropoiesis associated with macrocytic anemia {up to 10 years, MCV > 84 + [0.6 × age (years)] fL and children aged ≥10 years MCV > 90 fL} in the peripheral smear and megaloblasts in the bone marrow. Deficiency of vitamin B_{12} and folic acid are the most common causes in children. Deficiency of vitamin B_{12} and/or folic acid results in defective DNA synthesis leading to cytological and functional abnormalities in peripheral blood and bone marrow.

Megaloblasts are abnormal nucleated red blood cell pre cursors, which are larger than normal. They result in abnormal mature red blood cells, which are also larger in size known as macrocytes **(Fig. 23.5)**. There is an asynchrony between nuclear and cytoplasmic maturation. The nuclear maturation is delayed. There is an increased erythrocyte production but early cell death. The maturation of myeloid and platelet precursors is also affected. There is an associated thrombocytopenia and leukopenia. Neutrophils are characteristically hyperlobated (>5 lobes).

ETIOLOGY OF MEGALOBLASTOSIS

- Vitamin B_{12} deficiency
- Folate deficiency
- ***Disorders of DNA synthesis***
- ***Congenital:*** Orotic aciduria, thiamine-responsive megaloblastic anemia, inborn errors of B_{12}/folate metabolism, congenital dyserythropoietic anemia, Lesch– Nyhan syndrome.
- ***Acquired:*** Liver disease, sideroblastic anemia, leukemia, aplastic anemia, Di Guglielmo disease, and refractory megaloblastic anemia.

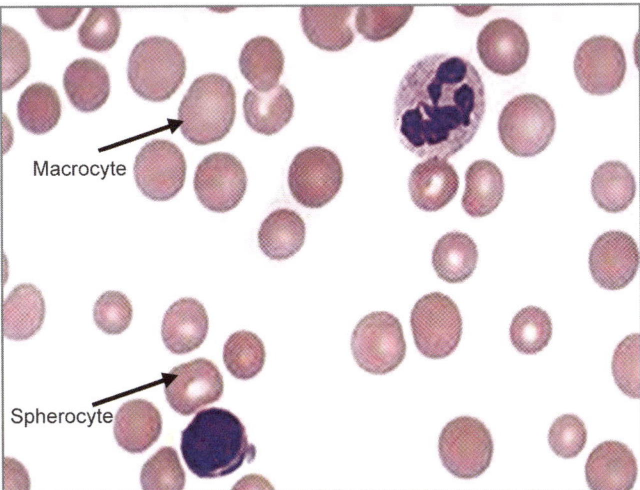

Fig. 23.5: Hypersegmented neutrophil with macrocytes and sphercocytes

- ***Drug-induced:*** Methotrexate, 6mercaptopurine, azathio prine, thioguanine, 5-fluorouracil, valproate, lithium, pyrazinamide, cytosine arabinoside, hydroxyurea, pheny toin, and nitrous oxide.

Vitamin B_{12} Deficiency

Vitamin B_{12} (cobalamin/extrinsic factor) acts as a cell coenzyme in chemical reactions affecting the synthesis of DNA and plays a crucial role in cell metabolism. Humans obtain vitamin B_{12} third hand, either by eating animals that have ingested the bacteria that synthesize cobalamin or by eating animal products such as milk, cheese, and eggs. Cobalamin binds to the intrinsic factor derived from gastric parietal cells and this complex is endo cytosed by the ileal cells after which it is further activated to methylcobalamin and adenosylcobalamin.

The recommended daily allowance of vitamin B_{12} is 1–2 µg in childhood and 0.5 µg in infants. It plays a significant role in hematopoiesis and maintenance of the integrity of nervous system.

- Foods rich in vitamin B_{12} are mostly of animal origin, e.g., meat, shellfish, heart, liver, kidney, and eggs. A little amount is present in milk, cheese, mushrooms, and curds.
- Vitamin B_{12} is largely stored in the liver in the form of adenosylcobalamin.

Causes of Vitamin B_{12} Deficiency

- ***Inadequate dietary intake (<1 µg/day):*** Nutritional deficiency is the most common cause of vitamin B_{12} deficiency. Vegetarianism/veganism and malnutrition are commonly associated with vitamin B_{12} deficiency.
- ***Defective vitamin B_{12} absorption:***
  - ***Failure to secrete intrinsic factor:*** Pernicious anemia (intrinsic factor deficiency), congenital deficiency, and gastric mucosal disease (postgastrectomy and corrosives).
  - Failure of intestinal absorption (malabsorption syndromes), abnormal intrinsic factor, abnormal ileal uptake, ingestion of EDTA and phytates, small-bowel bacterial overgrowth, and *Diphyllobothrium latum* infestation
- ***Defective vitamin B_{12} transport*** deficiency of transcobalamin I and II.
- ***Disorders of vitamin B_{12} metabolism:*** Specific in ability to form or transport adenosylcobalamin (vitamin B_{12} responsive methylmalonic acidemia), defect in methyl malonyl-CoA mutase apoenzyme (vitamin B_{12} nonresponsive methylmalonic acidemia), failure to form both adenosyl cobalamin and methylcobalamin (methylmalonic acidemia), and abnormality of N5methylenetetrahydrofolate homo cysteine methyltransferase apoenzyme.

Folic Acid Deficiency

Folic acid also plays a crucial role in cellular metabolism. But contrary to vitamin B_{12}, it is present in abundance in plants. Rich sources are liver, kidneys, fruits like lemons, bananas, oranges, mango, lady's fingers, beetroot, and green leafy vegetables. The vitamin is labile and gets destroyed on cooking or heating (boiling can lead to 40% loss of dietary folate). Milk is not a good source of folic acid. Goat milk is particularly deficient in folate. Inadequate intake is the most common cause of folic acid deficiency. The absorption of folic acid occurs throughout the small intestine. Recommended daily allowance of folic acid is 100–250 µg/day.

Malnutrition, exclusive goat milk consumption, and faulty cooking methods such as overcooking can lead to reduced intake. Absorption of folic acid can be impaired in chronic diarrhea, celiac disease, inflammatory bowel disease, and anticonvulsant therapy with phenytoin and phenobarbitone. Methotrexate, pyrimethamine, and tri-methoprim also have antifolic acid activity. Secondary folic acid deficiency can be precipitated by increased demand as in premature babies, hemolytic anemia, inflammatory diseases, leukemia, and lymphoma. Inborn errors of folate metabolism include methylene tetrahydrofolate deficiency, dihydrofolate deficiency, and methionine synthase deficiency.

The metabolism of folate and vitamin B_{12} is interlinked. Folate and vitamin B_{12} are involved in the DNA synthesis and in addition vitamin B_{12} has a role in myelin synthesis, hence a deficiency of vitamin B_{12} also produces neurological manifestations in addition to features of macrocytic anemia.

CLINICAL FEATURES

The deficiency is mostly seen in children <5 years of age with median age of presentation being 1.5–2 years, both of which are poor in vitamin B_{12} and folic acid. Adolescents may also develop vitamin B_{12} deficiency due to poor eating habits.

The clinical features of vitamin B_{12} and folate deficiency are identical, difference being in the neurological dysfunction, which occurs with vitamin B_{12} deficiency. Folate deficiency has a rapid evolution (weeks or months) and is usually associated with signs of other vitamin deficiencies. Vitamin B_{12} has a slow onset (years) and is usually a purer deficiency state because of the usual specificity of cobalamin malabsorption. The most important clinical finding is anemia with its associated symptoms. Some children have a characteristic hyperpigmentation of the hands, feet, or face, and presence of glossitis (beefy red tongue). Vitamin B_{12} deficiency also leads to peripheral neuropathy, and subacute combined degeneration of spinal cord. These children can present with neurological symptoms such as paresthesia, sensory deficits, hypotonia, seizures, and developmental delay. Neurological features may be present without any anemia. Vitamin B_{12} deficiency in infants may present with developmental delay, tremors, hypotonia and even seizures. Infantile tremor syndrome has been associated with vitamin B_{12} deficiency. Mild hepatosplenomegaly may be seen with megaloblastic anemia.

INVESTIGATIONS

Peripheral Smear

The red blood cells are macrocytic **(Fig. 23.5)** and normochromic. This may be associated with the presence of hypersegmented neutrophils (>5 lobes) in > 5% of cells **(Fig. 23.6)**. There may also be associated neutropenia and thrombocytopenia, which are usually asymptomatic. Reticulocyte count is decreased. Howell-Jolly bodies may be seen **(Fig. 23.7)**.

Macrocytic anemia of vitamin B_{12} and folic acid deficiency is characterized by increased red cell width (RDW). A normal RDW should alert to other causes of macrocytic anemia; such as hemolytic anemia, posthemorrhagic anemia, acute leukemia, aplastic anemia, liver disease, bone marrow infiltration, and hypothyroidism.

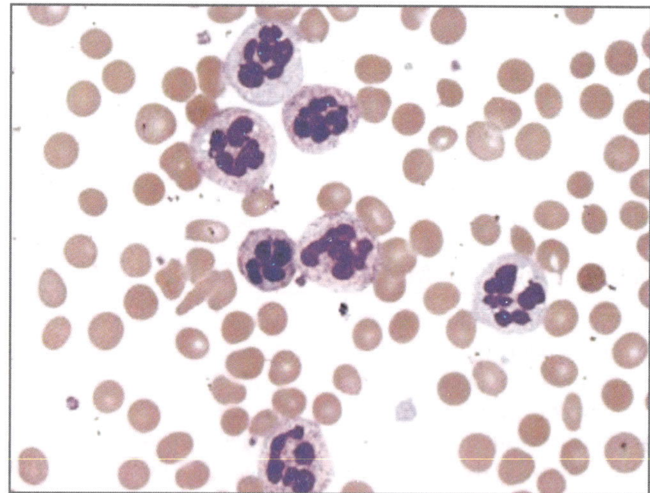

Fig. 23.6: Hypersegmented neutrophils in peripheral blood smear of megaloblastic anemia

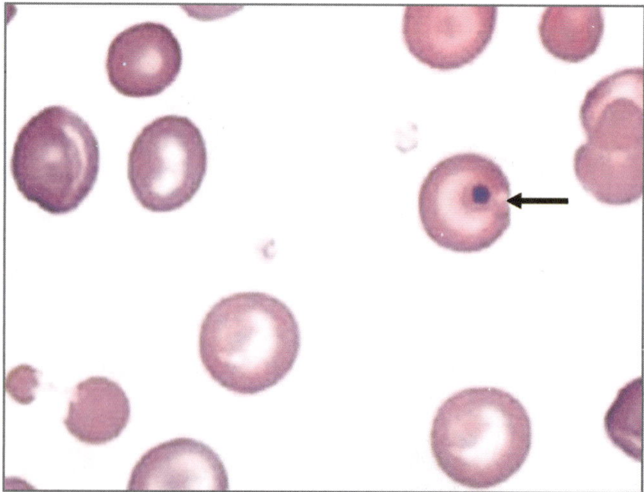

Fig. 23.7: Howell–Jolly bodies

Bone Marrow

A bone marrow is typically not required if there is a predisposing factor for B_{12}/folate deficiency and the CBC and smear demonstrate typical findings. The marrow smear demonstrates megaloblastic changes in all the stages of red cells **(Fig. 23.8)**. The marrow is hypercellular with erythroid hyperplasia and M:E ratio of 1:1. The leukocyte precursors are also abnormal and large in size. Macrocytosis is not synonymous with megaloblastosis. Macrocytic anemia with a normoblastic marrow is suggestive of other causes of macrocytosis, as outlined earlier.

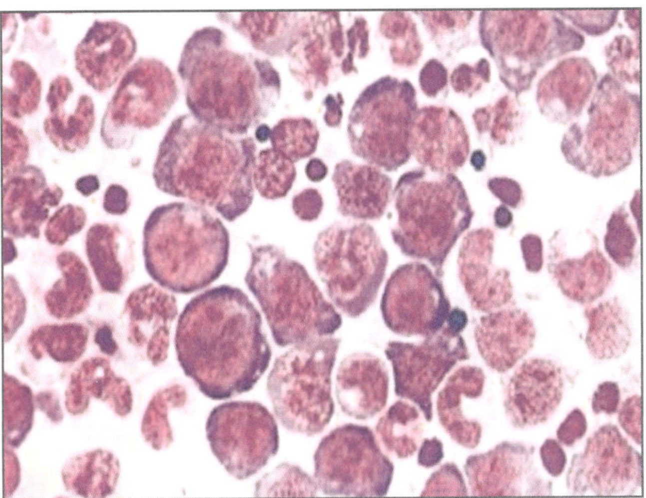

Fig. 23.8: Megaloblastic red cell precursors in bone marrow

Serum Levels

Serum levels of folic acid and vitamin B_{12} can be assessed to confirm the deficiency. Normal levels of folic acid are 5–20 ng/mL and <4 mg/mL suggests deficiency. Red cell folate level (150–640 ng/mL) is a better indicator of the folate status during the entire 120 days of RBC life span and <100 ng/mL suggests folate deficiency. Serum B_{12} levels > 300 pg/mL are normal, 200–300 pg/mL is borderline, and <200 pg/mL is suggestive of cobalamin deficiency. Holotranscobalamin assay <35 pmol/L is a more sensitive but sparsely available test for B_{12} deficiency. Although low levels of B_{12}/folate corroborate the diagnosis of deficiency, normal levels in a patient with typical features do not rule out the diagnosis as they may be affected by several factors such as drug exposure, concomitant deficiencies, and recent blood transfusions.

Serum Methylmalonic Acid (MMA) and Serum Homocysteine (Hcy)

Accuracy of serum vitamin B_{12} and/or folate levels alone has limitations. It is therefore recommended to evaluate for functional folate or vitamin B_{12} deficiency with tests like serum MMA or Hcy level, to confirm a diagnosis of vitamin B_{12} and/or folate deficiency where the diagnosis is doubtful. The normal range of plasma MMA is 70–270 nmol/L and of homocysteine is 5-15 µmol/L. Serum MMA > 750 nmol/L as indicative of vitamin B_{12} deficiency and Hcys above 15 mol/L could be indicative of folate deficiency. Elevation of both MMA and Hcys is seen in B_{12} deficiency, while elevated Hcy with a normal MMA suggests folate deficiency.

Flowchart 23.5 depicts diagnostic approach to a child with vitamin B_{12} and folate deficiency.

TREATMENT Megaloblastic Anemia

Folic acid is orally supplemented in the dose of 1–5 mg/day for 3–4 months. Infants require lower doses of 50 µg/day. Even in apparently isolated folate deficiency, concomitant vitamin B_{12} supplementation is advised, to avoid neurological worsening secondary to masked B_{12} deficiency. Vitamin B_{12} can be administered orally at a dose of 500 µg in infants and 1000 µg in older children daily for a week, followed by decreasing frequency to alternate days for a week, twice weekly for a week, then weekly for the first month; once in two weeks for the second month; and then once a month for a total of 3-4 months duration. Due to a danger of hypokalemia in young children, and in children with severe anemia, and malnutrition; parenteral vitamin B_{12} is recommended to be administered at lower doses of 25–50 µg/day for 3 days, then 100 µg/day for 7 days, then 100 µg on alternate days for one more week, followed by 1000 µg weekly for 1 month. IM route is preferred, while deep SC and IV routes are also acceptable. In case of neurological manifestations or doubtful absorption, parenteral administration of vitamin B_{12} is recommended for 6 months. In case of pernicious anemia, lifelong treatment with parenteral vitamin B_{12} administered monthly (1 mg intramuscular) is needed. Dietary advice is important apart from supplementation.

Response to Treatment

Administration of either vitamin B_{12} or folate influences manifestations of nutritional megaloblastic anemia. Symptoms improve within a day with a sense of well-being and glossitis improves by second day. The reticulocyte count improves in 2-3 days, MCV reduces and hypersegmented neutrophils disappear by 2 weeks, and the CBC normalizes by 6-8 weeks.

Symptomatic and Supportive Treatment

Blood transfusions may be needed to tide over initial crisis if the patient is in congestive heart failure. Other conditions such as achlorhydria and fish tapeworm infestation may need specific management. Celiac sprue may need gluten-free diet apart from vitamin replacement. Broad spectrum antibiotics may be needed in tropical sprue.

Flowchart 23.5: Diagnostic approach to a child with suspected vitamin B12 and folate deficiency

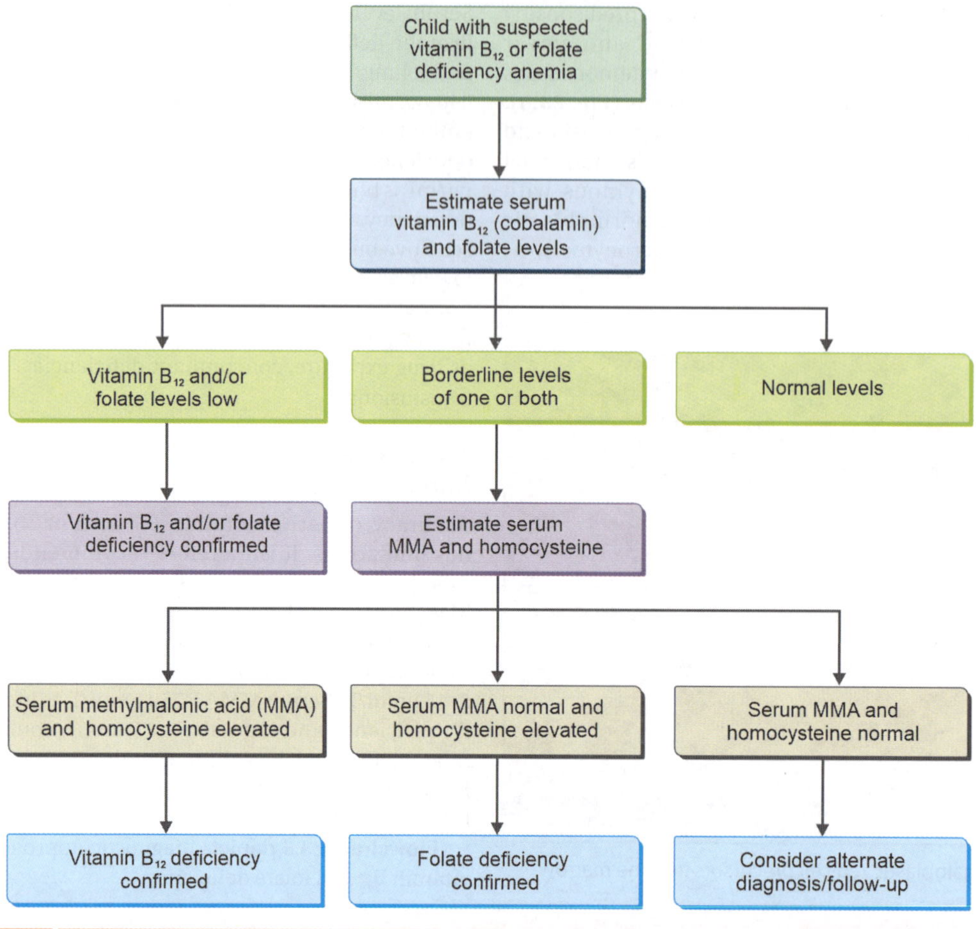

CASE STUDY Dimorphic Anemia

A 5-year-old boy was brought to the outpatient department by his mother. She noticed that the child had been listless and tired easily for the past 3 months. She also noticed that the child had been complaining of perianal itching and has passed small worms in his stools on several occasions.

Dietary history of the child revealed that he was a vegetarian. He consumed about half a liter of cow's milk every day. Examination revealed moderate pallor with no lymphadenopathy. The child's weight was 15 kg and height was 111 cm. Other systemic examination was noncontributory.

Laboratory examination revealed: *Hemoglobin 9 g/dL, total leukocyte count 4,300 cells/mm^3, platelet count 200,000/mm^3. Peripheral smear showed hypochromic red blood cells with presence of both microcytes and macrocytes. Stool microscopy showed ova of hookworm. The child was started on oral iron preparation at 15 mg/day. After 3 months of treatment, the child showed no clinical improvement.*

What is the diagnosis?

The child is suffering from "dimorphic anemia with hookworm infestation." The presence of both microcytes and macrocytes on the peripheral smear was suggestive of dimorphic anemia due to combined deficiency of iron and folic acid in diet. The child was a vegetarian and had been consuming mainly cow milk which is a poor source of iron, vitamin B_{12}, and folic acid. High concentration of phytates, calcium salts, and fiber in vegetarian diet also leads to impaired absorption of dietary iron. Hookworm infestation leads to occult blood loss in stools which further predisposes to iron deficiency. Pallor is the most common sign. Symptoms include lassitude, fatigability, anorexia, and failure to thrive. Mild splenomegaly is seen in only 15% of cases. Bald tongue and koilonychia may be seen in iron-deficiency anemia while hyperpigmented extensor surfaces characterize megaloblastic anemia due to vitamin B_{12} or folate deficiency.

What was wrong with his treatment?

The child was misdiagnosed as iron-deficiency anemia and started on only iron supplementation. In addition, the dose of iron prescribed was inadequate to treat anemia. Iron should be given in a dose of 3 mg/kg/day for a period of about 3 months instead of 1 mg/kg/day that was prescribed for him in this case. He should have also been given folic acid in a dose of 1–5 mg/day to correct the folate deficiency. In addition, at least 1 mg of vitamin B_{12} should be given to ensure adequate hematological response.

He should also have been dewormed with antihelminthics to reduce the occult blood loss because of hookworm infestation. Dietary modification in the form of increasing intake of animal products liver, meat, egg yolk, green vegetables, fruits, and jaggery should be asserted to correct the underlying deficiency of iron. Green leafy vegetables and sprouted pulses can help provide dietary folate.

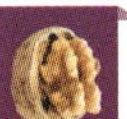

IN A NUTSHELL

Megaloblastic Anemia

- Megaloblastic anemia is characterized by ineffective erythropoiesis associated with macrocytic anemia (up to 10 years, MCV > 84 + [0.6 × age (years)] fL and children aged ≥10 years MCV > 90 fL) and hypersegmented neutrophils in the peripheral blood smear and megaloblasts in the bone marrow. Deficiency of vitamin B_{12} and folic acid are the most common causes of megaloblastic anemia in children.
- Vitamin B_{12} deficiency is commonly seen in vegetarians as its sources are mostly of animal origin (e.g., meat, heart, liver, kidney, and eggs). Pernicious anemia (intrinsic factor deficiency), gastric mucosal disease (postgastrectomy and corrosives), and malabsorption (e.g., small bowel bacterial overgrowth, *Diphyllobothrium latum* infestation) are other common causes of vitamin B_{12} deficiency.
- Folate deficiency can occur due to over-cooking, poor intestinal absorption (chronic diarrhea and celiac disease), anticonvulsant therapy (phenytoin), drug-induced (methotrexate, pyrimethamine, and trimethoprim) and in conditions with increased demand (e.g., hemolytic anemia).
- Serum levels of folic acid and vitamin B_{12} can be assessed to confirm the deficiency. Normal levels of folic acid are 5–20 ng/mL. Red cell folate level (150–640 ng/mL) is a better indicator of the folate stores and it is decreased in case of megaloblastic anemia due to folate deficiency. Serum B_{12} levels < 200 pg/mL are suggestive of cobalamin deficiency.
- Clinical manifestations of vitamin B_{12} and folate deficiency are nearly identical (pallor, hyperpigmented extensors, and glossitis) except that neurological manifestations can occur with vitamin B_{12} deficiency.
- Treatment of folic acid deficiency should be initiated only after excluding coexisting vitamin B_{12} deficiency.

Carmel R, Watkins D, Rosenblatt DS. Megaloblastic anemia. In: Orkin SH, Fisher DE, Ginsburg D, et al (Eds). Nathan and Oski's Hematology and Oncology of Infancy and Childhood, 8th edition. Philadelphia: Elsevier Saunders; 2015. pp. 308-43.

Chandra J, Dewan P, Kumar P, et al. Diagnosis, Treatment and Prevention of Nutritional Anemia in Children: Recommendations of the Joint Committee of Pediatric Hematology-Oncology Chapter and Pediatric and Adolescent Nutrition Society of the Indian Academy of Pediatrics. Indian Pediatr. 2022;59(10):782-801.

23.6 Hemolytic Anemia

PE 26.4

INTRODUCTION

All red blood cells are destroyed once their lifespan of 90–120 days is over. But in certain conditions the cells get lysed earlier; the lifespan of RBCs is reduced leading to increased red blood cell destruction (hemolysis). There is compensatory bone marrow hyperplasia, which increases the red cell production manifold to maintain normal hemoglobin levels. Hemolytic anemia results when this bone marrow hyperplasia is unable to keep up the hemoglobin levels to normal.

Bone marrow hyperplasia also leads to increased release of immature red cells in the blood, elevating the reticulocyte count. Erythropoietin induced erythroid hyperplasia leads to expansion of medullary spaces. Extramedullary erythropoiesis also starts in the liver and spleen leading to hepatosplenomegaly.

ETIOLOGY

Common causes of hemolytic anemia are listed here:

- ***Intracorpuscular defects (within RBC)***
  - *Membrane defects:* Hereditary spherocytosis, hereditary elliptocytosis, and hereditary stomatocytosis.
  - *Hemoglobin defects:* Thalassemia, sickle cell anemia, and other hemoglobinopathies (HbC, HbD, HbE, HbH, and HbM).
  - *Enzyme defects:* Glucose6phosphate dehydrogenase deficiency and pyruvate kinase deficiency.
- ***Extracorpuscular defects (outside RBC):***
  - *Immune mechanism:* Autoimmune hemolytic anemia, incompatible blood transfusion, hemolytic disease of the newborn, and drug-induced.
  - *Non-immune mechanism:* Hemolytic uremic syndrome, disseminated intravascular coagulation, and paroxysmal nocturnal hemoglobinuria.
  - *Others:* Druginduced, infection (malaria, *Salmonella*, leishmaniasis, clostridial infections, and grampositive infections), burns, lead poisoning, hypersplenism, Wilson disease.

Most of the hemolytic anemias encountered are extravascular. The causes of intravascular hemolysis in children include G6PD deficiency, burns, clostridial infections, incompatible blood transfusion, black water fever, and paroxysmal nocturnal hemoglobinuria.

POINTERS TO THE DIAGNOSIS OF HEMOLYTIC ANEMIA

- A family history of repeated blood transfusion, death due to severe anemia, early onset of gallstones, and need for splenectomy suggests a congenital hemolytic anemia.

- Neonatal jaundice may be the first presentation of certain congenital hemolytic anemias such as hereditary spherocytosis or G6PD deficiency.
- A long-standing anemia with multiple transfusions suggests a chronic hemolytic anemia.
- Jaundice due to unconjugated hyperbilirubinemia, with anemia, and a palpable spleen comprise the classical triad of hemolytic anemia. However, jaundice may not be clinically evident in all patients with hemolytic anemia.
- In extravascular hemolysis, hyperbilirubinemia can cause a high colored urine. In intravascular hemolysis the urine is typically dark or cola-colored due to hemoglobinuria,
- Hemolytic facies characterized by frontal bossing, depressed nasal bridge, and maxillary prominence, prominent malar eminences and malformed teeth is seen typically in thalassemia. (**Figs. 23.9A and B**). Due to ineffective erythropoiesis and marrow expansion, there is widening of the diploic spaces with medulla getting less dense and development of trabeculae giving the typical haironend appearance in the skull (**Fig. 23.10**). Widening of the marrow cavity and decreased density of the medulla is evident in tubular bones of the extremities
- Extravascular hemolytic anemias such as hereditary spherocytosis typically have splenomegaly as the spleen is the predominant site of hemolysis. In thalassemia where the bone marrow is ineffective, prominent hepatosplenomegaly is common due to extramedullary hematopoiesis.
- Platelets and coagulation factors are not affected except in microangiopathy hemolytic anemias such as HUS and TTP
- Peripheral smear RBCs are microcytic and hypochromic in thalassemia; and normocytic or macrocytic and normo chromic in acute hemolysis. Hemolysis in peripheral smear is evidenced by presence of tear drop cells, fragmented RBCs, increased number of reticulocytes, nucleated RBCs, and characteristic cell morphology such as spherocytes and elliptocytes (**Fig. 23.11**).
- Reticulocytosis is prominent with the reticulocyte count increasing to 5–20% against a normal of 0.5–2%. Nucleated red blood cells (normoblasts) are also seen commonly in the peripheral blood. Nucleated red blood cells can cause a spuriously high white blood cell count.
- Osmotic fragility of RBCs is increased in hereditary spherocytosis, i.e., they demonstrate an enhanced tendency to lyse in hypotonic saline. The spherocytes swell in the presence of hypotonic saline and get lysed more easily than normal biconcave cells. In contrast, in thalassemia, the osmotic fragility of RBCs is decreased.
- *Hemoglobin electrophoresis or high-performance liquid chromatography:* Detects the presence of abnormal hemoglobins such as HbS and HbH or HbE or variation in different types of hemoglobin, i.e., HbA1, HbA_2, and HbF as in thalassemia (**Figs. 23.12A and B**).
- Special investigations such as sickling test, G6PD levels, and Coombs test are required according to the disease being suspected.

LABORATORY EVIDENCE OF HEMOLYSIS

- ***Evidence of increased hemoglobin breakdown***
  - Unconjugated hyperbilirubinemia
  - Decreased haptoglobin and hemopexin
  - Increased plasma lactate dehydrogenase
- Evidence of intravascular hemolysis
  - Hemoglobinemia
  - Hemoglobinuria
  - Decreased serum haptoglobulin
- ***Evidence of erythroid hyperplasia in the bone marrow***
  - Increased reticulocyte count, nucleated RBCs
  - M:E ratio changes from 3 to 4:1 to 1:1
  - Bone marrow biopsy showing hypercellularity with sheets of erythroid cells (bone marrow test is not necessary for establishing diagnosis of hemolysis)

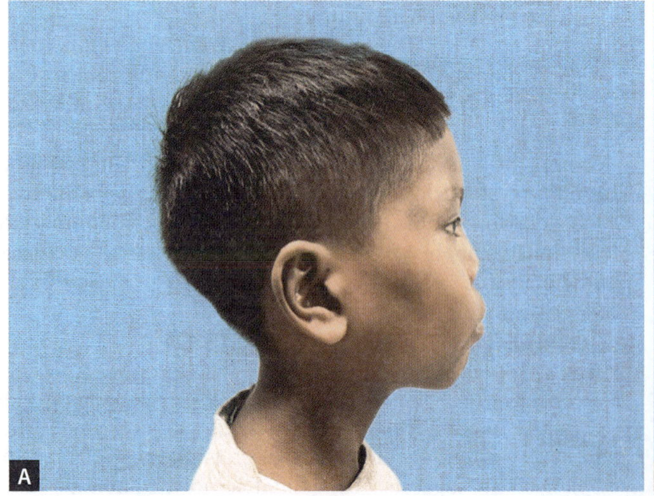

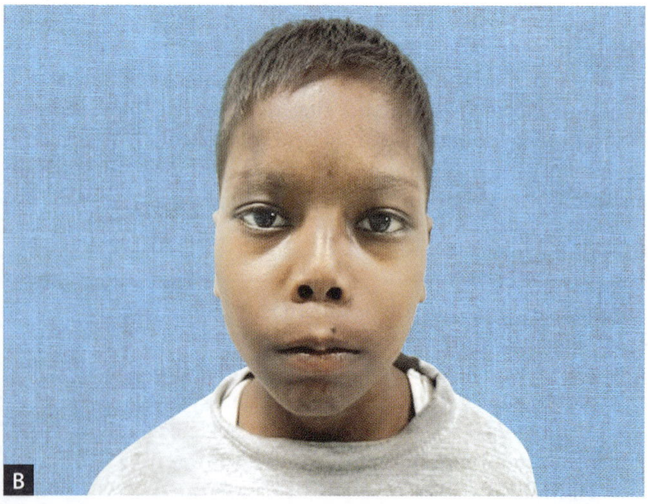

Figs. 23.9A and B: Hemolytic facies in a child with thalassemia characterized by frontal bossing and maxillary/malar prominence

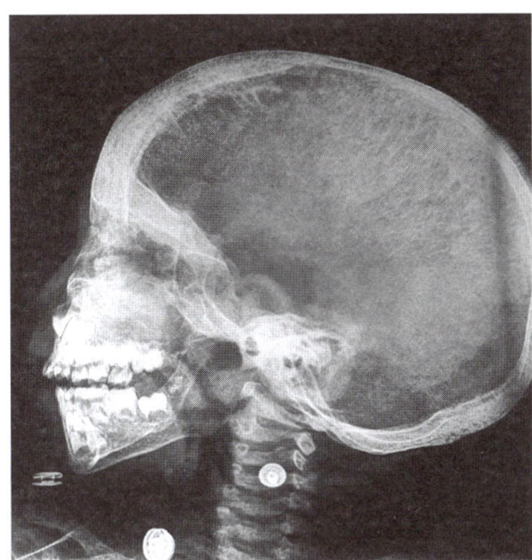

Fig. 23.10: 'Hair on end' appearance in skull X-ray of child with thalassemia.

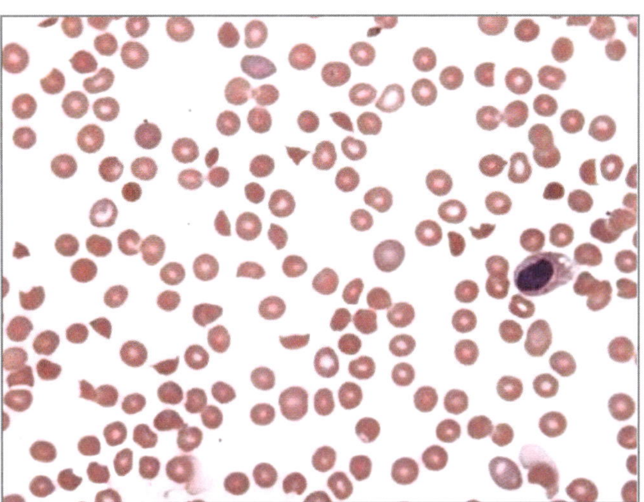

Fig. 23.11: Peripheral blood smears in a child with hemolytic anemia showing spherocytes, helmet cells, and fragmented cells

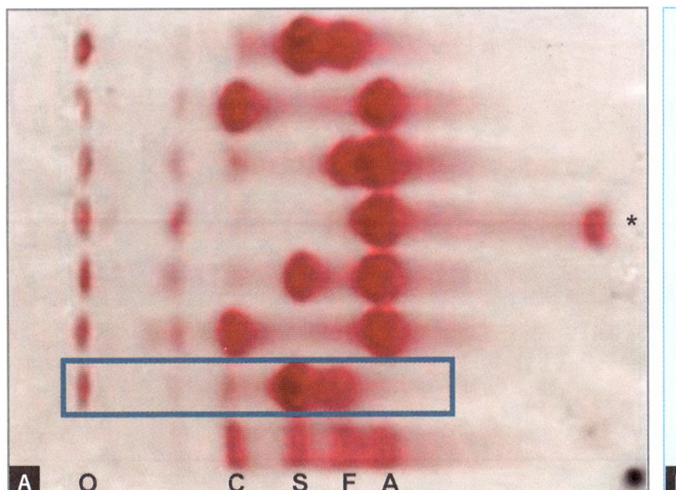

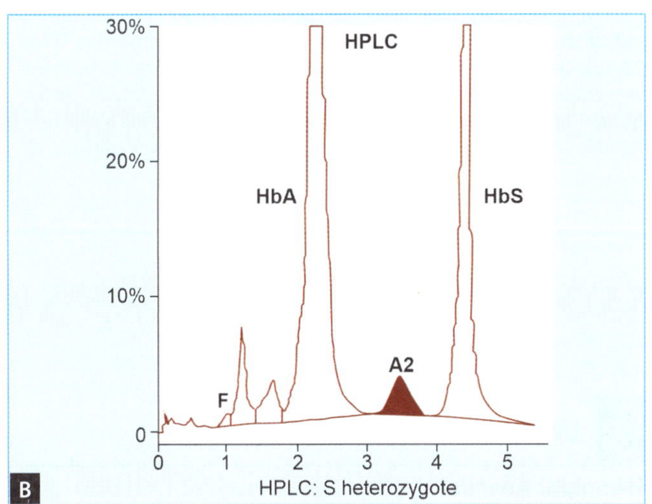

Figs. 23.12A and B: Hemoglobin electrophoresis (A) and HPLC (B) pattern in HbS heterozygote showing two peaks in HbA and HbS region (HbA: hemoglobin A; HbS: sickle hemoglobin; HPLC: high-performance liquid chromatography)

CASE STUDY Hemolytic Anemia

A mother brings her 10-month-old girl child to the emergency with increasing pallor and difficulty in feeding for last 1 month. There was no history of fever, swelling over the body, bleeding from any site, or jaundice. The baby had been started on appropriate complementary feeds at 6 months of age. Examination revealed marked pallor, no lymphadenopathy or petechial rash. Systemic examination revealed HR = 180/m, RR = ejection systolic murmur over the precordium with marked tachycardia, abdominal examination = liver palpable 5 cm below costal margin with moderate splenomegaly.

Laboratory investigations revealed Hb 3 g/dL, TLC 4,500/mm^3, platelet count: 500,000/mm^3. Peripheral smear showed microcytic hypochromic red cells with target cells and tear drop cells, reticulocyte count 20%. Serum iron 96 µg/dL, TIBC 250 µg/dL. Hemoglobin electrophoresis suggests β-thalassemia major.

Outline the expected abnormalities on hemoglobin electrophoresis in β-thalassemia.

Beta thalassemia occurs due to impaired production of beta chains in the hemoglobin. The genes for β-chain production are present on the short arm of chromosome 11. The presence of β-*thal*^{0} gene results in absent β-chains while presence of β-*thal*+ gene results in decreased beta chains. Hemolysis occurs due to imbalance in production of α and β-chains. Since β-chain synthesis is impaired, the excess of α-chains produces α-tetramers which get precipitated in red cells. Hemoglobin electrophoresis reveals raised fetal hemoglobin ($\alpha_2\gamma_2$), HbA_2 ($\alpha_2\delta_2$), and decreased HbA ($\alpha_2\beta_2$).

What are the major sites of extramedullary hematopoiesis?

The liver and spleen are the chief sites of extramedullary hematopoiesis in children with thalassemia.

Describe in brief the options for chelation therapy in this child.

Children with thalassemia require periodic blood transfusions to sustain life. Since the human body lacks a mechanism to excrete excess iron, the iron from the transfused red cells accumulates in the body. This iron overload leads to end organ damage in the heart, liver, and endocrine organs. Deferoxamine (DFO), deferiprone (DFP), and deferasirox (DFX) are the commonly used iron chelating agents in thalassemia. Deferoxamine is administered as continuous subcutaneous infusion in a dose of 25–50 mg/kg/day over a period of 8–12 hours during night using microinfusion pumps (5–6 nights/week). Vitamin C should be administered along with DFO to facilitate iron excretion. Deferiprone is given orally in a dose of 75–100 mg/kg/day in 2–3 divided doses. Deferasirox can be given orally in a daily dose of 20–40 mg/kg. It has a half-life of 8–16 hours thereby allowing once a day dosing.

TREATMENT Hemolytic Anemia

Packed Red Cell Transfusions

Repeated regular packed red cell transfusions are the mainstay of the treatment in most congenital hemolytic anemias. The frequency of transfusion depends upon the severity of the disease. Ideally extended red cell typing and cross matching should be performed with issue of leukodepleted packed cells to minimize the development of antibodies against antigen on leukocytes and platelets, and to reduce transfusion-related viral infections. Leukocytes can also be filtered out at the time of transfusion by using bedside microfilters **(Fig. 23.13).** Use of blood products donated by first degree relatives must be avoided as it can precipitate transfusion associated graft versus disease. Irradiation of blood is recommended if the patient is planned for or is undergoing an allogeneic hematopoietic stem cell transplant.

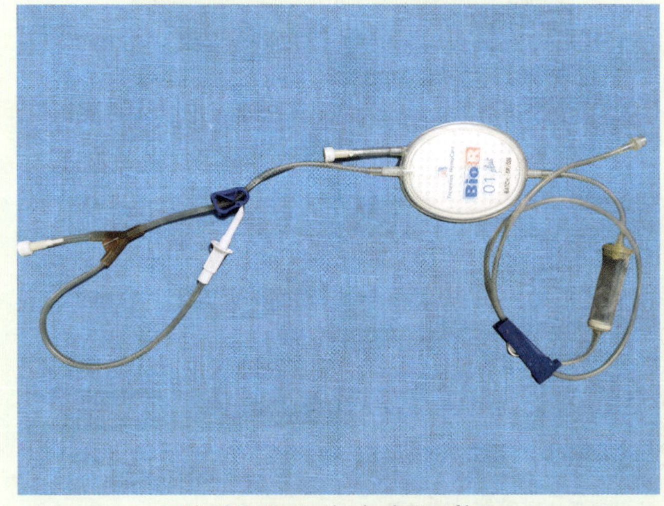

Fig. 23.13: Leukodepleting filter

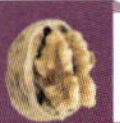

IN A NUTSHELL

Hemolytic Anemia

1. Hemolytic anemia is characterized by a reduction in the lifespan of the circulating RBCs (normal red cell lifespan 90–120 days).
2. Bone marrow hyperplasia in hemolytic anemias leads to increased release of immature nucleated RBCs and reticulocytes in peripheral blood. Erythroid hyperplasia leads to expansion of medullary spaces and extramedullary erythropoiesis in the liver and spleen leading to hepatosplenomegaly.
3. Hemolytic anemia may be due to defects in the RBCs (intracorpuscular defects—hemoglobinopathies, red cell enzyme defects, RBC membrane defects) or outside the RBCs (extracorpuscular—immune-mediated, drug-induced infections, metabolic conditions such as Wilson disease, DIC, and hemolytic uremic syndrome).
4. The presence of free hemoglobin and methemoglobin in blood and detection of hemoglobin and hemosiderin in urine indicates intravascular hemolysis which is seen in conditions such as incompatible blood transfusion, black water fever, and paroxysmal nocturnal hemoglobinuria.
5. Chronic hemolytic anemias are characterized by characteristic hemolytic facies, mild jaundice, hepatosplenomegaly, and history of regular blood transfusions.

Blackall D, Dolatshahi L. Autoimmune hemolytic anemia in children: laboratory investigation, disease associations, and treatment strategies. J Pediatr Hematol Oncol. 2022;44(3):71-8.

Chueh HW, Hwang SM, Shim YJ, et al. Korean RBC Disorder Working Party. Korean clinical practice guidelines for the diagnosis of hereditary hemolytic anemia. Blood Res. 2022;57(2):86-94.

Weli M, Ben Hlima A, Belhadj R, et al. Diagnosis and management of autoimmune hemolytic anemia in children. Transfus Clin Biol. 2020;27(2):61-4.

23.7 Hemoglobin Disorders

PE 26.4, PE 26.13

NORMAL HEMOGLOBIN

Normal hemoglobin (Hb) is a protein consisting of two pairs of polypeptide chains to each of which heme is attached. The different types of hemoglobin differ in the globin chains. Hemoglobin A (HbA) consists of two alpha (α) and two beta (β) chains and comprises 97% of adult hemoglobin. HbA has two alpha and two delta (δ) chains and is the minor hemoglobin; normal values are up to 3.5% in adults. HbF or fetal hemoglobin comprises two (α) alpha and two (γ) gamma chains and is the major hemoglobin in the fetal and neonatal period comprising 70–90% of the total hemoglobin in a term child. It falls rapidly thereafter to 25% at 4 weeks and ~5% at 6 months. HbF is <1% in adults. HbA_2 is increased in β-thalassemia traits but decreased in iron-deficiency anemia and α-thalassemia. HbF is elevated in many hemoglobin defects.

HEMOGLOBIN VARIANT ANALYSIS

Hemoglobin variants can be analysed by high performance liquid chromatography (HPLC) or hemoglobin electrophoresis. Electrophoresis is a technique based upon the separation of hemoglobin molecules in an electric field because of differences in total molecular charge. Any change in amino acid sequence in hemoglobin molecule alters the charge thereby affecting its motility in electric field; different hemoglobins migrate at varying speeds. HPLC uses a stationary phase and mobile phase with differing Ph and ionic strengths. Hemoglobin variants elute at different times based on their ionic interactions and their retention times are used to distinguish and quantify them. Hemoglobin variant analysis is used to diagnose hemoglobinopathies and to detect hemoglobin variants. Indications of hemoglobin electrophoresis in children are mentioned below:

- ❖ Suspected hemoglobinopathy such as thalassemia, sickle cell anemia, and HbC, HbE, and HbD
- ❖ Premarital hemoglobin electrophoresis to prevent inherited hemoglobinopathy
- ❖ For screening asymptomatic children with family history of hemoglobinopathy for carrier status
- ❖ To detect presence of abnormal hemoglobin, i.e., hereditary persistence of fetal hemoglobin
- ❖ Inherited bone marrow failure syndrome, i.e., Diamond-Blackfan anemia (to detect increased HbF)
- ❖ To measure HbA1c levels for diagnosis and monitoring of diabetes mellitus (high performance liquid chromatography)
- ❖ Evaluation of unexplained hemolytic anemia

Electrophoresis patterns of different hemoglobinopathies is described **Table 23.5**.

Figure 23.14 depicts the HPLC test of a patient with βthalassemia major which shows HbF > 90%, absent HbA and HbA_2 < 3.5%.

DEFECTS OF HEMOGLOBIN

Defects of hemoglobin can be categorized into two groups:

1. Hemoglobinopathies in which there is production of structurally abnormal hemoglobin due to abnormalities of the formation of globins moiety, e.g., HbS (sickle cell disease), HbC, HbD, or HbE disease.
2. Thalassemia in which there is a reduced rate of production of normal hemoglobin due to absent or decreased synthesis of the globin chains, e.g., α (alpha)- and β (beta)-thalassemia.

Hemoglobinopathies thus refer to qualitative defect of hemoglobin (resulting in abnormal or variant hemoglobin, while thalassemia is a result of quantitative defects of hemoglobin.

Hemoglobinopathies

Abnormal hemoglobin arises due to some genetic defect affecting the synthesis of a specific pair of polypeptide chain. The common abnormal hemoglobins are HbS, HbC, HbE, and HbD. These are all βchain variant hemoglobins, in which there is defect in the synthesis of β–chains.

TABLE 23.5 Electrophoresis Patterns in Hemoglobinopathies

Electrophoresis pattern	*Hemoglobinopathy/variant*
• HbA 92–95% • HbA_2 <3.5% • HbF <1%	Normal adult hemoglobin
• HbF—high (>90%) • HbA_2—variable • HbA—absent or very low	Beta thalassemia major
• HbA_2 >3.5% • HbA_2—normal/low • HbF—low/absent	Beta thalassemia minor/trait
• HbS >90% • HbA_2 <3.5% • HbA—absent	Sickle cell disease
• HbS 35–40% • HbA_2 <3.5% • HbA 60–65%	Sickle cell trait
• HbS >80% • HbA_2 >3.5% • HbA—absent • HbF often elevated	Sickle cell—β-thalassemia
• HbS >60% • HbA_2 >3.5% • HbA 5–30% • HbF often elevated	Sickle cell—β^+-thalassemia
• HbS—50% • HbC—50%	Hemoglobin sickle cell disease
• HbF >90% • HbA_2 <3.5% • HbA <10%	Hereditary persistence of fetal hemoglobin

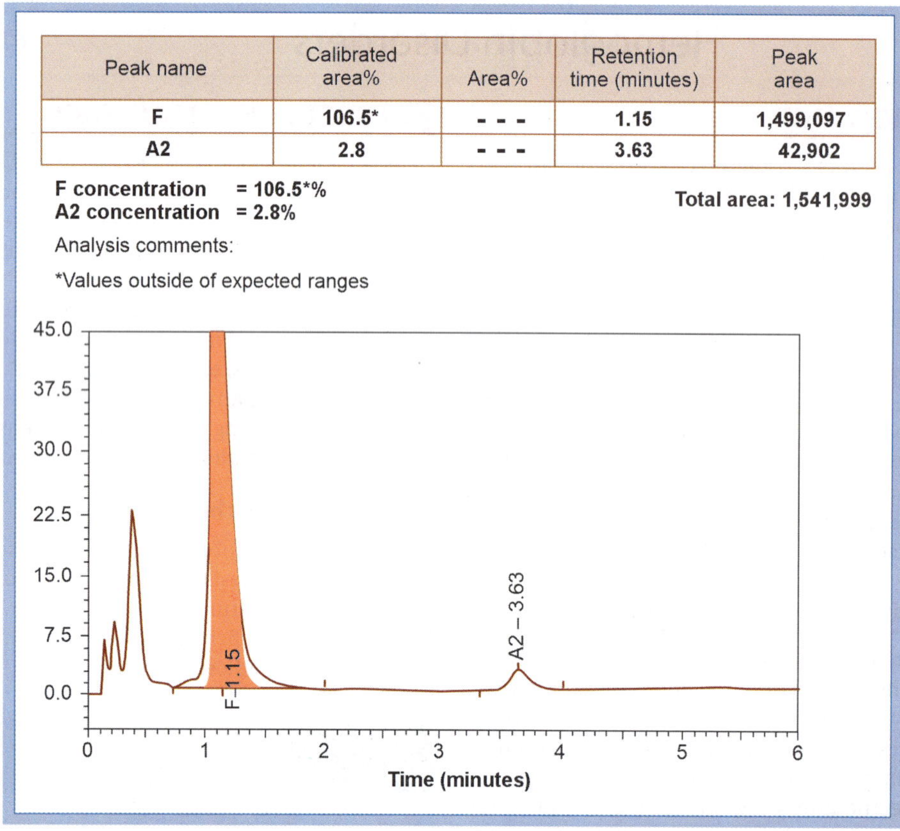

Peak name	Calibrated area%	Area%	Retention time (minutes)	Peak area
F	106.5*	- - -	1.15	1,499,097
A2	2.8	- - -	3.63	42,902

F concentration = 106.5*%
A2 concentration = 2.8%

Total area: 1,541,999

Analysis comments:

*Values outside of expected ranges

Fig. 23.14: High performance liquid chromatography pattern of a patient with β-thalassemia major showing absence of HbA, HbA_2 <3.5% and HbF >90%

Thalassemia

Thalassemia are a genetic group of disorders in which there is a decreased synthesis of one or more types of polypeptide chains and are autosomal recessive in inheritance. The Hb in which the affected globin and polypeptide chain is incorporated is reduced. α and β are the two main types of globin chains used. Thalassemia can be categorized as—(i) α-thalassemia in which production of αchains are reduced, β-thalassemia in which β-chains are reduced.

Alpha thalassemia occurs most often in people from Southeast Asia, the Middle East, China, and in those of African descent. Beta thalassemia occurs most often in people of Mediterranean origin. To a lesser extent, Chinese, other Asians, and African Americans can be affected. Thalassemia is one of the most common genetic hematological disorders in India with over 10,000 children of thalassemia major born each year. It is more common in north-west India. The case rate can be as high as 5–15% in some ethnic groups of north India (Punjabis and Sindhis).

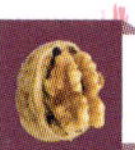

IN A NUTSHELL

Hemoglobin Disorders

1. Normal hemoglobin (Hb) is a protein consisting of two pairs of polypeptide chains to each of which hem is attached. The different types of hemoglobin differ in the globin chains. Hemoglobin A (HbA) consists of two alpha (α) and two beta (β) chains, HbA_2 has two alpha and two delta ($\alpha_2\delta_2$) chains, and HbF or fetal hemoglobin comprises two α and two γ ($\alpha_2\gamma_2$) chains.
2. Normal adult hemoglobin comprises 97% HbA, up to 3.5% HbA_2 and <1% HbF. HbA_2 is increased in β-thalassemia trait (minor) but decreased in iron-deficiency anemia. HbF is elevated in many hemoglobin defects like thalassemia major.
3. Hemoglobinopathies occur when there is production of structurally abnormal hemoglobin molecules due to abnormalities of the formation of globins moiety, e.g., HbS (sickle cell disease), HbC, HbD, or HbE disease.

Agarwal AM, Rets AV. Advances in hemoglobinopathies and thalassemia evaluation. Clin Lab Med. 2024;44(3):441-53.
Kaur G, Chatterjee T, Ahuja A, Sen A. Challenges in diagnosis of thalassemia syndromes. Med J Armed Forces India. 2024;80(6):632-7.
Munkongdee T, Chen P, Winichagoon P, et al. Update in laboratory diagnosis of thalassemia. Front Mol Biosci. 2020;7:74.

23.8 Thalassemia Major

PE 26.4, PE 26.13

INTRODUCTION

Thalassemia major, now referred to as transfusion-dependent thalassemia, is the most severe form of the disease resulting from a complete or major suppression of βchain synthesis.

ETIOPATHOGENESIS

A genetic mutation leads to decreased rate of synthesis of βchain. The main hemoglobin beyond 6 months of age is adult hemoglobin A (HbA). Therefore, there is a decrease in amount of HbA (α_2, β_2) in the affected children. A decrease in the β-chains triggers a compensatory increase in production of fetal hemoglobin and αchains. This leads to an increase in HbF (α_2, γ_2) or HbA_2 (α_2, δ_2). The excess of uncombined αchains results in their accumulation and precipitation to form tetramers (α4) in the RBCs and normoblasts. These intracytoplasmic inclusions lead to increased destruction of normoblasts and RBCs in the marrow, rendering the erythropoiesis as ineffective. As a result, the maturation and function of RBCs is affected and hemolysis occurs.

A complete absence of beta chain synthesis is known as β^0thalassemia and an incomplete suppression is known as β^+-*thalassemia*. Based on the clinical severity, thalassemia is categorized as thalassemia major (transfusion dependent thalassemia), minor, and intermedia (non transfusion dependent thalassemia).

CLINICAL FEATURES

Age at Presentation

Newborns with βthalassemia major are asymptomatic at birth. The high level of fetal hemoglobin at birth, which does not require the βchains, protects these children till 4–6 months of age. The clinical features of thalassemia major start manifesting usually after 6 months of age.

Signs and Symptoms

Anemia is the first and most prominent manifestation. There is associated failure to thrive and anorexia. Anemia becomes severe if regular blood transfusions are not given. There is hepatosplenomegaly due to extramedullary hematopoiesis; and spleen progressively increases in size. Mild jaundice may be present. Gradually there is a development of typical hemolytic facies if the child is not initiated on regular transfusions to suppress the marrow expansion **(Figs. 20.13A and B)**.

Routine screening of blood and blood products for HIV, hepatitis B, and hepatitis C has significantly brought down the incidence of these transfusion-transmitted infections. Psychosomatic changes such as depression, poor self-esteem, and poor school performance frequently accompany this chronic disease.

Natural History

These children are transfusion-dependent and require packed red cell transfusion every 3–4 weeks. Untreated children may not survive beyond 3–4 years of age. All the complications and manifestations depend on how regular the transfusions are; and how well the child is chelated to prevent the iron overload.

Children on irregular transfusions or those on regular transfusion but poor chelation have more complications. These children usually die in the second decade of life due to cardiac complications. The ongoing endogenous hemolysis as well as repeated red cell transfusions leads to release of excess of iron which gets deposited in heart, liver, pancreas, and endocrine glands affecting their function. Compromise of cardiac and endocrine functions results in hypothyroidism, gonadal failure, hypoparathyroidism, and diabetes mellitus. There is a delayed puberty and bronze discoloration of the skin because of iron overload. Hepatic iron overload contributes to hepatic fibrosis and cirrhosis, and even hepatocellular carcinoma. Non transfusion dependent thalassemia can also be associated with iron overload due to increased gastrointestinal iron absorption. Pulmonary hypertension, leg ulcers, and gall stones are other chronic complications.

Children who receive regular transfusions and proper chelation therapy have significantly prolonged survival and better quality of life. In the last two decades, with the advent of blood component therapy and improved chelation therapy, thalassemia major has evolved from an invariably fatal genetic disorder into a chronic disease that permits normal or at least prolonged survival.

LABORATORY INVESTIGATIONS

Peripheral Blood Picture

The RBCs are microcytic and hypochromic with marked anisocytosis and poikilocytosis. Target cells and tear drop cells are seen. Reticulocytes and nucleated RBCs are increased. Howell-Jolly bodies, basophilic nuclear remnants, or remnants of DNA, may be seen in the cytoplasm of RBCs. Granular cytoplasmic inclusion bodies representing the alpha chains are visible in normoblasts or reticulocytes. Pappenheimer bodies and erythrocytic inclusions containing iron that are usually located at the periphery of the cell and stain with Prussian blue may be seen in multitransfused thalassemia patients. The white cells and platelets are normal unless there is hypersplenism which leads to leukopenia and thrombocytopenia.

Bone Marrow

Examination of the bone marrow is usually not indicated in a suspected case of thalassemia. Marrow shows erythroid hyperplasia with a little effect on WBCs and platelets. Staining for iron deposits (Prussian blue staining) reveals increased hemosiderin deposits in bone marrow.

Biochemical Indicators

- ***Serum bilirubin:*** Bilirubin levels are mildly elevated due to hemolysis and production of bilirubin along with compromised function of the liver due to iron deposition.
- ***Indicators of iron overload:*** Serum ferritin levels are raised (normal levels: 10–200 ng/mL). Total iron binding capacity is reduced (normal: 250–400 µg/dL) and % saturation of transferrin is increased (normal: 20–45%).
- ***Hemoglobin electrophoresis or HPLC:*** Hemoglobin electrophoresis at alkaline pH or HPLC can enable quantification of HbA_2 and HbF. At birth, HbF is the predominant hemoglobin amounting to 95–98% of the total hemoglobin. HbA_2 amounts to ~2% and adult hemoglobin HbA is in traces **(Table 23.6)**.

Hb electrophoresis of the parents may establish them as carriers (raised HbA_2, >3.5%) and thereby provide supportive evidence to diagnose thalassemia in the child. It will also help the parents to plan future pregnancy and plan antenatal diagnosis in case of the next child. **Figure 23.15** illustrate the inheritance pattern in βthalassemia.

TABLE 23.6 Hemoglobin Electrophoresis Profile of β-thalassemia

	Hemoglobin (%)		
Type	*HbA*	*HbA_2*	*HbF*
β-thalassemia minor	90–95	3.5–7.0	1–5
β-thalassemia major			
β+	10–90	1–4	10–90
β0	0	1–2	98

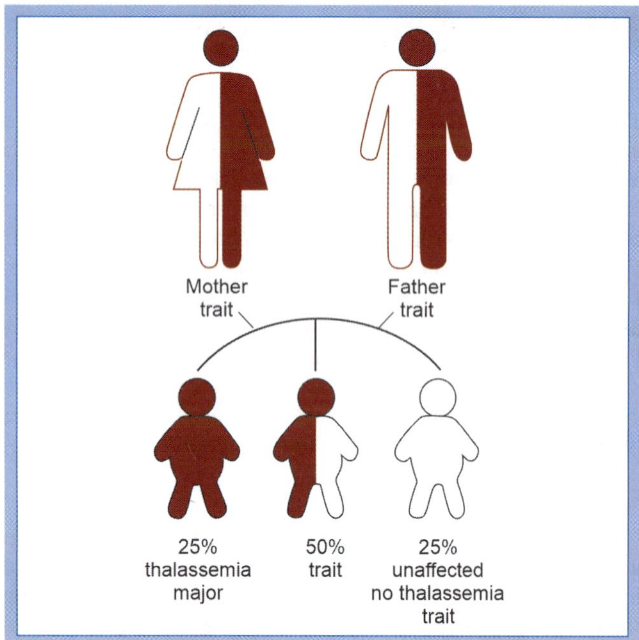

Fig. 23.15: Genetics of β-thalassemia major.

Diagnostic tests in a child with thalassemia should not be performed after a recent blood transfusion. An ideal gap of 3 months from transfusion is required but may not be possible in a child with transfusion dependent thalassemia. Testing can be done just before the next blood transfusion.

TREATMENT β-thalassemia

Packed Red Blood Cell Transfusion

Repeated lifelong transfusions are the backbone of the treatment. The aim is to maintain a pretransfusion hemoglobin of 9.5-10.5 g/dL. Most children require a transfusion at every 3–4 weeks interval. A higher target of 10-11 g/dL is preferred in patients with cardiac disease and significant extramedullary hematopoiesis. Ideally, leukoreduced RBCs should be transfused after extended red cell typing and cross matching to reduce the side effects of transfusion. Otherwise, bedside leukofilters should be used. The problems associated with repeated transfusions include alloimmunization, risk of transmission of hepatitis B, HIV, hepatitis C infections, and iron overload. Increased absorption of iron from gut due to chronic anemia, and ongoing hemolysis both add to the state of iron overload.

Chelation Therapy

Apart from repeated transfusions to take care of symptoms due to chronic anemia, adequate chelation is essential to prevent transfusion-related hemosiderosis. Serum ferritin level is a useful marker for screening and assessing the iron stores but ideal is to measure the iron stores in the liver by doing a liver biopsy.

When to Start?

Chelation therapy should be started when serum ferritin levels rise above 1,000 ng/mL and child has received 10-20 transfusions to date. The chelators bind with iron allowing its excretion in urine and stool. Children with thalassemia on chelators should be periodically monitored for serum ferritin levels which should be maintained below 1,000 ng/mL. Previously liver biopsies were used to quantify liver iron concentration. However MRI techniques like T2* have made it possible to evaluate cardiac and liver iron load in a non-invasive manner. T2*MRI should be performed at 8-10 years and repeated annually. A T2* > 20 msec is desirable.

Choice of Chelating Agent

- *Deferoxamine (DFP):* It was the first iron chelator used and is very effective but has a disadvantage that it has to be administered subcutaneously with a pump over 10–12 hours, 5–6 days in a week. It is given in a dose of 30–60 mg/kg/day (5–7 times a week) through a microinfusion pump which is strapped to the child's body. This agent is excreted in bile and urine, resulting in red discoloration. It readily chelates iron from ferritin and hemosiderin, but not from transferrin. This is an ototoxic drug and also affects the retina. It also affects the linear growth with evidence of cartilaginous dysplasia of long bones and spine. It is the only drug effective in established heart disease due to cardiac iron overload where it is administered intravenously as a continuous infusion.
- *Deferiprone (DFP):* It is taken orally and so compliance is better. It is given 2–3 times/day at a dose of 75–100 mg/kg/day. Adverse effects include arthropathy, agranulocytosis, and hepatotoxicity. Patients on deferiprone should be monitored for complete blood count every 2–3 weeks and for liver functions every month. Using DFO in combination with DFP increases the quantity of iron excreted from the body (additive effect). Using DFO 2–5 days per week with DFP can lead to negative iron balance in most patients.

- ***Deferasirox (DFX):*** It is an effective oral iron chelator that needs to be given in the dose of 20–40 mg/kg/day once daily. Adverse effects include gastrointestinal disturbances such as nausea, vomiting, diarrhea, abdominal, pain, and skin rash. The adverse effects are usually mild and transient. Patients on DFX should undergo monthly evaluation of liver and renal function as the drug can lead to elevated transaminases, creatinine, and proteinuria. A film-coated tablet is available now which is better tolerated and administered at 70% of the usual dose of DFX.

Curative Therapy

Allogenic hematopoietic stem cell transplantation (HSCT) is the most commonly available curative modality. It is expensive and available at few centers. Availability of a matched HLA donor is another limiting factor. Hema topoietic stem cell transplantation is cost effective if compared to the cost of lifelong transfusions, chelation therapy, and treatment of other complications apart from the psychological trauma. Best results after stem cell transplantation are expected in younger children who have mild or no hepatomegaly, minimal hepatic fibrosis, and good iron chelation.

Splenectomy

Splenectomy is indicated for hypersplenism or when the requirement of blood exceeds 200–250 mL/kg/year. It should be avoided before 6 years of age because of higher chances of sepsis in younger age. Children should be vaccinated against encapsulated bacteria such as pneumococcus, *Haemophilus influenzae* B, and *Neisseria meningitidis* at least 3–4 weeks before splenectomy and started on antibiotic (penicillin) prophylaxis for at least 2 years after splenectomy or till 6 years of age, whichever is later. In an ideal situation, prophylaxis should be given lifelong. Episodes of infections should be treated promptly with broad- spectrum antibiotics and children should be hospitalized. Patient should receive influenza vaccine every year prior to start of flu season, one booster dose of pneumococcal polysaccharide vaccine 5 years after the first dose, and a booster dose of meningococcal group A, C, W-135 and Y conjugate vaccine (MenACWY vaccine) every 5 years.

Diet and Nutrition

Folic acid, 1 mg should be given daily to prevent folate deficiency. Drinking tea and avoiding vitamin C rich foods during meals may help to reduce iron absorption through the intestinal tract. Thalassemia patients should consume a wholesome diet as nutritional deficiencies are common in them. Calcium and vitamin D supplements should be administered guided by the musculoskeletal status and serum levels in the patients.

Novel Therapies

- *Gene therapy:* After successful phase 3 trials gene therapy using a lentiviral vector based addition of normal beta-globin gene to hematopoietic stem cells has been approved by the FDA for transfusion dependent thalassemia. Other forms of gene therapy include gene editing and increasing the HbF production.
- *Luspatercept:* This is a TGF-β inhibitor that promotes erythropoiesis and increases hemoglobin and reduces transfusion requirement.

GENETIC COUNSELING

Carrier Detection

Carrier detection should be attempted in parents of affected children (retrospective diagnosis) and those belonging to high risk communities (prospective screening programs). As the mode of inheritance is autosomal recessive, if both the parents have thalassemia trait, the risk of having an affected child with thalassemia major is 25%, chances of an unaffected child would be 25% and that of having a child with thalassemia trait would be 50%. The target population for screening would include couples in high-risk communities at the time of marriage, preconception, or early pregnancy. Carrier detection is done by simple hematological tests such as a low MCV in a complete blood count followed by a HPLC or Hb electrophoresis that confirms HbA2 of > 3.5% levels. Beta thalassemia is characterized by a mutation in the β-globin (*HBB*) gene located on the short arm of chromosome 11. More than 200 disease-causing mutations have been so far identified; majorities are single nucleotide substitutions, deletions, or insertions of oligonucleotides leading to frameshift. The five common mutations—(1) IVS-1→ 5(G → C), (2) IVS 1 → 1 (G → T). (3) Codon 41/42 (-TCTT), (4) Codon 8/9, and (5) the 619 bp deletion account for over 90% of the mutations in β-thalassemia patients. IVS15 (G → C) is the most common β-thalassemia allele in the Indian population. *Sindhis* and *Lohanas* especially from Gujarat show high prevalence of the 619 bp deletion mutation. A classic case of thalassemia trait will have an elevation of the RBC count, decrease in the MCV and MCH, a normal RDW and Mentzer index (MCV/RBC) below 13. Establishing genetic diagnosis in patients with thalassemia is essential so that antenatal diagnosis can be offered for the next pregnancy,

Naked Eye Single Tube Red Cell Osmotic Fragility Test: Screening Test

If the facility for automated cell counter is not available, then naked eye single tube red cell osmotic fragility test (NESTROFT) is highly sensitive for mass screening and detection of thalassemia carrier. NESTROFT is performed using 2 mL of 0.36% buffered saline solution in a tube (10 cm × 1 cm diameter) and 2 mL distilled water taken in another tube. A drop of blood is added to each tube and they are left undisturbed for half an hour at room temperature. Both the tubes are then shaken and held against a white paper on which a thin black line is drawn. The line is clearly visible through the contents of the tube containing distilled water. If the line is similarly visible through the contents of the tube with the buffered saline, the test is considered negative. If the line is not clearly visible, the test was considered positive. A positive test indicates lowered red cell osmotic fragility, suggestive of thalassemia trait. Measurement of HbA_2 levels (>3.5%) is also used for carrier detection.

Prenatal Diagnosis

Prenatal diagnosis is done in the first trimester of pregnancy by chorionic villous sampling (8–10 weeks of gestation) and analysis of fetal DNA by polymerase chain reaction (PCR) based methods. Information should be provided about the mode of transmission, available tests for antenatal diagnosis, carrier detection and their reliability and treatment options to the parents. Explanatory booklets are very useful. Emphasis should be laid on details of fetal testing, i.e., sampling procedure, risk to the fetus, failure and misdiagnosis. The predicted natural course of the disease based on the genotype should be discussed.

Detection of the carrier state in the parents and early detection of the disease in the fetus will help the parents in handling the situation and decide about the fate of the unborn child. Finally, the information regarding risks to their relatives should be given with recommendation to inform them so that they can choose to take the test as well.

NON-TRANSFUSION-DEPENDENT THALASSEMIA (THALASSEMIA INTERMEDIA)

Severity of the disease lies inbetween the major and minor thalassemia. It does not fit into the clearly defined major and minor thalassemia. It includes a range of mutations in different thalassemia genes resulting in a milder defect in globin chain synthesis and so a milder clinical picture.

The children have microcytic, hypochromic anemia which is less severe Hb > (7 g/dL) and these children are not trans fusiondependent. They need packed red cell transfusion occasionally. The splenomegaly is moderate and all the features and complications are less severe. Hemoglobin electrophoresis reveals increased fetal hemoglobin (10–90%), decreased adult hemoglobin (10–90%), and normal HbA_2. Hydroxyurea is a drug that increases HbF level and gives good outcomes in patients with non transfusion dependent thalassemia. Monitoring of iron overload and administering iron chelation is necessary in these patients too.

THALASSEMIA MINOR

This is the asymptomatic heterozygous form of thalassemia in which there is only mild to moderate suppression of the globin chain. There is compensatory increase in the delta chains. These children usually remain undiagnosed as anemia is mild Hb (~10 g/dL) and may never require a transfusion. They may be picked up on a routine hematological examination. The spleen is not palpable and the complications and features of thalassemia are not seen. They lead normal lives and life expectancy is normal. They are usually treated for iron-deficiency anemia but failure of the hemoglobin to rise despite iron supplementation should raise the suspicion of thalassemia minor.

Microcytosis is more marked in thalassemia minor and anisocytosis is more marked in irondeficiency anemia (RDW is increased in IDA and normal in thalassemia trait). The two conditions may also be differentiated based on red cell counts which are decreased in IDA and increased in thalassemia trait.

Serum iron profile will be normal in thalassemia minor and Hb electrophoresis reveals elevated HbA_2 (3.5–7%), a near normal HbF (1–5%) and HbA (90–95%).

Current classification of thalassemia is clinically based on requirement of blood transfusions. Children who require regular lifelong transfusions are classified as "transfusion-dependent thalassemia (TDT)" and children who seldom require or do not require transfusion are considered as "nontransfusion dependent thalassemia (NTDT)." This definition embraces all types of thalassemia including αthalassemia, HbE/βthalas semia, HbE, HbC, etc. TDT children usually present with anemia before 2 years of age. They commonly have baseline hemoglobin <7 g/dL, hepatosplenomegaly and retarded growth and height.

ALPHA THALASSEMIA

This is a disorder where there is absence or deficiency of α-globin chains. Since the αchain is essential for all the three types of hemoglobin, i.e., fetal, adult, and A2, the levels of all these are decreased. There is a resultant excess of uncombined β- and γ-chains. The excess of β-chains form tetramers (β4) known as HbH and γ-chains form Hb Bart (γ4). HbH is beta tetramer and is milder variant. Hb Bart is γ-tetramer and is more severe and fatal. The α-thalassemias have a high incidence in Asian, Filipinos, and Saudi Arabian populations. It is seen in four different clinical variants **(Table 23.7)**.

Hydrops fetalis—is the most severe form characterized by a total absence of alpha chain synthesis. Hemoglobin A is absent and instead only hemoglobin Bart, high oxygen affinity hemoglobin, is formed. Hemoglobin Bart holds onto oxygen and resists delivering oxygen to the tissues and the resultant anemia is severe and usually leads to stillbirth or spontaneous abortion.

Hemoglobin H—disease is the next most severe condition wherein scant hemoglobin A is produced and a new hemoglobin H is formed, which represents 5–40% on alkaline electrophoresis. Individuals with hemoglobin H disease have lifelong anemia with variable splenomegaly and bone changes.

Alpha thalassemia trait (two-gene deletion state) and the silent carrier (one-gene deletion state) are relatively asymptomatic conditions.

TABLE 23.7 Clinical Classification of α-Thalassemia

Conditions	Genotype	Clinical features
Silent carrier	aa/a_	Clinically and hematologically normal
Thalassemia trait	aa/_ _a_/a_	Microcytosis, hypochromia, and mild anemia
HbH disease	_ _/a_	Moderate to severe microcytic hypochromic chronic hemolytic anemia, mild jaundice, and moderate hepatosplenomegaly
Hb Barts/hydrops fetalis syndrome	_ _/_ _	Severe anemia, generalized anasarca, ascites, hepatosplenomegaly, skeletal and cardiovascular abnormalities, and fatal at birth

CASE STUDY Thalassemia Trait

A 14-year-old girl was started on oral iron therapy as her blood counts indicated iron-deficiency anemia, with MCV of 75 fL, Hb 10 g/dL, Hct 33%, and RBC 5.8 × 1,012/L. She had complaints of fatigue and lethargy. But 3 weeks later her laboratory results were virtually the same.

Her HPLC revealed HbA2 of 4.2% confirming a β-thalassemia carrier status. The parents were counselled that the condition did not require any active intervention or medical management. However, it was emphasized to the parents that at the time of marriage the partner should be screened for hemoglobin variants as if he is a carrier too, there would be a 25% chance of thalassemia in the progeny.

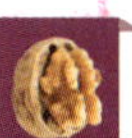

IN A NUTSHELL

Thalassemia Major

1. *Hemoglobin A (HbA):* Two globin α-chains and two globin beta chains ($\alpha_2\beta_2$)
2. *Hemoglobin F (HbF):* Two globin α-chains and two globin gamma chains ($\alpha_2\gamma_2$)
3. *Hemoglobin A_2 (HbA_2):* Two globin α-chains and two globin delta chains ($\alpha_2\delta_2$)
4. Thalassemia are hereditary (autosomal recessive) hemolytic anemias in which there is reduced rate of production of normal adult hemoglobin (HbA) due to absent or decreased synthesis of the α- or β-globin chains. Imbalances of globin chains cause hemolysis and impair erythropoiesis.
5. Alpha thalassemia is characterized by a reduced production of α-chains and β-thalassemia has reduced β-chain production.
6. Alpha thalassemia is less common. Silent carriers of alpha thalassemia and persons with alpha thalassemia trait are asymptomatic. Alpha thalassemia intermedia or hemoglobin H disease causes hemolytic anemia. Alpha thalassemia major with hemoglobin Bart usually results in fatal hydrops fetalis.
7. Beta thalassemia major (Transfusion dependent thalassemia) is a severe transfusion-dependent anemia and necessitates regular iron chelation therapy (subcutaneous deferoxamine injections, or oral deferiprone, or oral deferasirox) to remove iron introduced in excess with transfusions. Hematopoietic stem cell transplantation (HSCT) is the only permanent cure for β-thalassemia major.
8. Non-transfusion-dependent thalassemia (NTDT) is suspected in individuals who present at a later age with similar but milder clinical findings. Individuals with NTDT require episodic blood transfusion but may later require frequent blood transfusions.
9. Thalassemia minor is the mildest variety and a heterozygous form in which there is only mild to moderate suppression of the β-globin chain. There is compensatory increase in the delta (δ) chains with consequently increased HbA_2 on electrophoresis.
10. Prenatal diagnosis of β-thalassemia major can be done in the first trimester of pregnancy by chorionic villous sampling (8–10 weeks of gestation) and analysis of fetal DNA by PCR-based methods.

Which inherited hematological condition can show a clinical picture similar to iron-deficiency anemia?

The case illustrates problem in the management of patients with microcytic anemia. In this case the girl was offered a trial of oral iron supplementation based on her red cell indices and iron profile was not ordered. However, failure to respond should make the physician consider thalassemia trait which can present with mild to moderate lifelong microcytic hypochromic anemia. Such patients may be asymptomatic or may become symptomatic during pregnancy, adolescence (menstrual losses), or during illnesses which could worsen anemia.

What laboratory test can aid the differentiation of this condition from IDA?

Thalassemia trait can be confirmed by performing hemoglobin electrophoresis as HbA_2 will be raised (5–8%) in such cases. Moreover, unlike IDA, these patients have high RBC counts with normal RDW.

Colah RB, Seth T. Thalassemia in India. Hemoglobin. 2022;46(1):20-26.
Musallam KM, Cappellini MD, Porter JB, Farmakis D, et al. TIF Guidelines for the Management of Transfusion-Dependent β-Thalassemia. Hemasphere. 2025;9:e70095.
Taher AT, Musallam KM, Cappellini MD. Guidelines for the Management of Non-Transfusion-Dependent β-Thalassaemia [Internet]. 3rd ed. Nicosia (Cyprus): Thalassaemia International Federation; 2023.

23.9 Sickle Cell Disease

PE 26.4, PE 26.17

INTRODUCTION

This hemoglobinopathy may manifest as (i) sickle cell trait (heterozygous state, AS); (ii) sickle cell anemia (homozygous state and SS), or (iii) in compound heterozygous states for HbS with hemoglobin C, D, E, or other structural variants and the combination of the sickle cell gene with different forms of thalassemia (sickle cell anemia and compound heterozygous sickle hemoglobinopathies together constitute sickle cell disease). Sickle cell disease (SCD) is more common in the central belt of India extending from Gujarat, Maharashtra, and Madhya Pradesh to Chhattisgarh and Odisha. In addition, the Nilgiri hills region of South India is also an endemic region. Aboriginal (scheduled tribe) communities are particularly affected in India, although other communities are involved too. It is also seen in African populations near areas endemic for malaria including Central and West Africa, parts of the Mediterranean and Asia, and in the Caribbean islands of America.

ETIOPATHOGENESIS

Sickle cell hemoglobinopathy is a group of hereditary disorders in which the red cells contain abnormal hemoglobin, i.e., HbS. This hemoglobin consists of two alpha and two β-chains, however, the β-chain in HbS contains valine instead of glutamic acid in the sixth position from N terminal end.

The HbS is less soluble compared to HbA when it is in the deoxygenated state leading to sickling (assuming a crescent shape) of the red blood cells. The cells assume a normal shape in the oxygenated state. The sickling can also be precipitated by dehydration, fever, and acidosis. This phenomenon of sickling of RBCs has two major effects:

- Sickled cells are rigid and distorted; they lead to sluggish blood flow and blockage of capillaries causing ischemia and infarction. Infarction can occur in any organ including liver, spleen, bones, and brain.
- The sickled cells adhere to the endothelium and cause endothelial inflammation and injury.
- Repeated sickling unsickling of the cells makes the RBCs fragile leading to excessive hemolysis. Seventy per-cent of the hemolysis is extravascular in the reticuloendothelial system and 30% is intravascular. Free hemoglobin and scavenging of nitrix-oxide following hemolysis cause further oxidative damage

The above mechanisms thus contribute to acute complications such as vas-occlusive painful crises, acute chest syndrome, hepatic or splenic sequestration, and infections. Further, chronic tissue hypxoxia leads to end organ damage, particularly in the brain, lungs, spleen, kidney, and heart.

CLINICAL FEATURES

Most of the children present after 6 months of age because till that age the presence of fetal hemoglobin prevents sickling of cells. Varying degree of anemia is seen due to RBC lysis. All the children have hepatosplenomegaly initially but the spleen undergoes recurrent infarction and atrophies with time and by 7–8 years most of the children do not have a palpable spleen. This is also referred to as autosplenectomy. There may be mild jaundice. These children have growth retardation and delayed puberty. Other features are detailed here:

- ***Infections:*** All children with sickle cell disease are prone to infections especially by encapsulated bacteria such as pneumococcus or *H. influenzae B* because of functional asplenia and defective opsonization. Bacterial sepsis is the one of the most common causes of morbidity and death in these children. It is notable that in India *Staphyloccus aureus, Escherichia coli, Klebsiella pneumoniae* and are more common causal organisms than encapsulated bacteria.
- ***Hand and foot syndrome (dactylitis):*** This is due to micro infarction of the medulla of the carpal and tarsal bones symmetrically due to vaso-occlusive crisis. This leads to swollen and tender dorsum of hands and feet. This is an extremely painful condition.
- ***Vaso-occlusive episodes:*** These extremely painful episodes may affect any part of the body involving the chest, abdomen, and extremities more commonly. A stressful condition such as physical stress, dehydration, hypoxia, and exposure to cold can precipitate these painful episodes due to compromised blood flow leading to ischemia.
- ***Acute chest syndrome:*** Acute manifestation with cough, dyspnea, and other lower respiratory tract signs with new pulmonary infiltrates on radiology characterize acute chest syndrome. Fever and middle lobe involvement are common in children with SCD.
- ***Splenic sequestration:*** This is characterized by acute pooling of blood in the spleen, hypovolemia, shock and sudden increase in the splenic size. This is a potentially fatal condition.
- ***Hepatobiliary complications:*** Gallbladder and bile duct stones, and hepatic sequestration crisis can occur.
- ***Aplastic crisis:*** This is precipitated by parvovirus B19 infection which causes erythroid hypoplasia and reticulocytopenia.
- ***Hyperhemolytic crisis:*** During painful crises there may be a marked increase in the rate of hemolysis with a fall in the hemoglobin level.
- ***Other features:*** These include chronic leg ulcers, gallstones, neurological complications such as stroke and seizures, priapism, pulmonary complication, renal and retinal involvement, and the skeletal changes including osteonecrosis secondary to chronic erythroid hyperplasia.

LABORATORY INVESTIGATIONS

Peripheral Smear

It reveals varying degree of anisocytosis and poikilocytosis. Typical sickle-shaped cells may be present but are not universal **(Fig. 23.16)**. Reticulocytes are increased in number and may go up to 10–20%.

Sickling Test

This test demonstrates the tendency of RBCs to "sickle" in hypoxic state. Sickling occurs because of distortion of red cells containing HbS, which undergoes polymerization. When HbS gets deoxygenated, it undergoes a pronounced decrease in solubility. Deoxy HbS polymers in the cells exist as highly ordered fiber aggregates which fill the cell and distort it into the classic sickle shape. This is demonstrated by adding sodium meta bisulphite to the blood of the patient following which the RBCs rapidly change to sickle shape.

Sickle Solubility Test

The solubility test is the most common screening test for sickle cell or presence of HbS. When anticoagulated blood is mixed with a

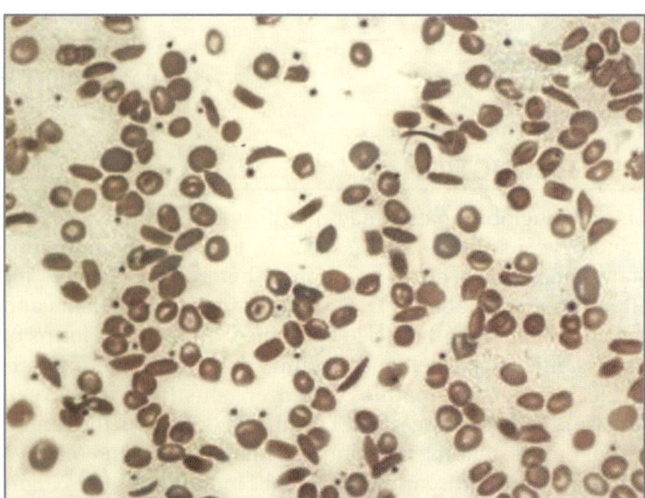

Fig. 23.16: Peripheral blood smears showing sickle cell red blood cells (RBCs).

reducing agent like sodium dithionite, the red cells will lyse due to the presence of saponin and the hemoglobin in the red cells will be released. If HbS is present, it will give a cloudy or turbid appearance to the solution due to poor solubility. If HbS is not present, the solution will appear clear. The solubility test cannot differentiate sickle cell disease (HbSS) from sickle cell trait (HbAS).

Hemoglobin Variant Analysis

Definite diagnosis can be made only on hemoglobin electrophoresis or high-performance liquid chromatography that reveals the presence of HbS. Parents and asymptomatic siblings should be tested for carrier status and offered antenatal and premarital counselling, respectively. Similar to thalassemia, there will be 25% risk of the disease in each child born to carrier parents.

TREATMENT Sickle Cell Anemia

Treatment is by and Large Supportive.

- *Transfusion:* Anemia and all the other complications in these patients need specific management. Packed red cell transfusions are required to treat chronic anemia. An urgent blood transfusion may be required in conditions such as splenic sequestration and aplastic crisis.
- *Infections need to be identified early and managed aggressively:* All children diagnosed with sickle cell anemia should be started on penicillin prophylaxis (oral penicillin V 125 mg BD) to prevent *Streptococcus pneumoniae* infection till at least 5 years of age. After 5 years of age the dose of oral penicillin V is 250 mg BD. If compliance is a problem, monthly injections of 600,000 units of benzathine penicillin IM can be used. However, these injections are painful, and the effectiveness of the injection for the later half of the month is questionable. Amoxicillin 20 mg/ kg/day is an alternative to penicillin. For patients who are allergic to penicillin, erythromycin 125 mg twice daily is given to children younger than 5 years of age, and erythromycin 250 mg twice daily is given to children 5 years of age or older. Children older than 5 years may discontinue their penicillin prophylaxis provided they have not had previous pneumococcal infection or functional asplenia. Prevention of infection by encapsulated bacteria can be done by immunizing the child with pneumococcal and meningococcal vaccine.
- ***Table 23.8*** summarizes the recommendations for managing acute and chronic complications of sickle cell disease.
- Dehydration should be prevented and managed aggressively by intravenous fluids.
- Hydroxyurea, 5-azacytidine, and butyrates have been used to stimulate HbF production and decrease the levels of HbS. Hydroxyurea is recommended to be started as early as 9 months of age in children with sickle cell anemia regardless of symptomatology and has been demonstrated to reduce complications such as pain crises and acute chest syndrome, and improve hemoglobin. The starting dose is 10-20 mg/kg/day.
- In the presence of a fully HLA-matched donor an allogeneic hematopoietic stem cell transplant can be curative in patients with severe SCD.
- Red cell HbS concentration reducing agents such as nifedipine, verapamil, and DDAVP have been used.
- Novel therapies include crizanlizumab which is a P-selectin inhibitor that can reduce vaso-occlusive crises.
- And gene therapy where viral vectors are used to transduce the normal beta-globin gene to hematopoietic stem cells. L-glutamine has been added to treatment to reduce oxidative injury.

Table 23.8 Management of Acute Complications and Surveillance of Chronic Complications of Sickle Cell Disease

Complication	*Recommendation*
Vaso-occlusive crisis	Analgesia should be started within 30 minutes of triage. Paracetamol and NSAIDs can be used for mild to moderate pain. Severe pain should be managed with opioids titrated to achieve round the clock analgesia. Hydration of the patient must be ensured and patient should be kept warm.
Acute chest syndrome	Supplemental oxygen should be started to target a spo2 of >95%. A combination of intravenous cephalosporin and oral macrolide is started. A simple red cell transfusion can be given if the baseline Hb has dropped by ≥1 g/dL. If spo2 continues to drop to <90% on oxygen, an exchange transfusion may be necessary.
Priapism	Aggressive hydration and analgesia, surgical consultation if persistent, transfusion avoided for immediate management
Retinopathy	Annual retinal examination from 10 years of age
Renal disease	Annual spot urine testing for proteinuria from 10 years of age
Stroke	Annual transcranial doppler from 2 to 16 years of age. Consider long term transfusion if finding is ≥200 cm/second

SCREENING OF POPULATION

Screening procedures for adults include the dithionite solubility, a solubility test based on the principle that hemoglobin S precipitates in high molarity buffered phosphate solutions. The end point is easy to read as a turbid solution in the presence of hemoglobin S and a clear solution if hemoglobin S is not present.

Neonatal screening involves collection of newborn blood samples by heel prick onto a dried filter paper. The samples are then analyzed by hemoglobin electrophoresis at either alkaline or acid pH or both, isoelectric focusing, or high-performance liquid chromatography. If electrophoretic techniques are used, two bands, hemoglobin F and hemoglobin S, will be seen in patients with sickle cell anemia because hemoglobin F is predominant in neonates. The healthy neonate will show two bands at hemoglobin A and hemoglobin F, while the individual with sickle cell trait will show three bands: One at F, one at A, and one at S.

In 2023 the Government of India launched the National Sickle Cell Anemia Elimination Mission (NSCAEM). The NSCAEM includes screening of individual in high prevalence areas and confirming diagnosis; providing sickle status identity cards which can be matched at the time of marriage planning; antenatal screening for carrier status followed by free screening of spouses of carriers and offering antenatal diagnosis if both parents are carriers; newborn screening using dried blood spot cards; and comprehensive management with folic acid and penicillin prophylaxis, hydroxyurea, and pneumococcal vaccination.

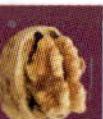

IN A NUTSHELL

Sickle Cell Disease

1. Sickle cell hemoglobin (HbS) results from an autosomal recessively inherited mutation in which the 17th nucleotide of the *β-globin* gene is changed from thymine to adenine, and the amino acid glutamic acid is replaced by valine at position 6 in the beta globin chain.
2. Sickle solubility test can be used as a screening test for detecting HbS.
3. Hemoglobin electrophoresis is needed to confirm the diagnosis of sickle cell disease (no HbA, 80–95% HbSS, and 2–20% HbF).
4. Sickle cells have a reduced deformability and are easily distorted, causing occlusion of the microcirculation and a chronic hemolytic anemia.
5. Clinical severity of sickle cell disease is very variable. Some have few complications and remain largely asymptomatic; majorities have intermediate forms; and a few have severe complications (vaso-occlusive crisis, aplastic crisis, sepsis, acute chest syndrome, splenic sequestration, stroke, and priapism).
6. Hydroxyurea therapy initiation in all patients, penicillin prophylaxis and pneumococcal vaccination in children < 5-years can prevent complications

Gupta K, Krishnamurti L, Jain D. Sickle cell disease in India: the journey and hope for the future. Hematology Am Soc Hematol Educ Program. 2024;2024(1):1-9.

Jain D, Gupta M, Madkaikar M, Jena RK, et al. Sickle cell disease in India: current status and progress. Lancet Haematol. 2024;11(5):e322-e323.

Pecker LH, Lanzkron S. Sickle cell disease. Ann Intern Med. 2021;174(1):ITC1-ITC16.

23.10 Hereditary Spherocytosis

PE 26.4

INTRODUCTION

Hereditary spherocytosis is an autosomal (autosomal dominant inheritance in 75% and autosomal recessive in 25%) defect of the red cell membrane, resulting in chronic hemolytic anemia. The disease is characterized by anemia, icterus, moderate splenomegaly, and presence of micro-spherocytes in the peripheral smear.

ETIOPATHOGENESIS

There is a molecular defect of the red cell membrane proteins such as ankyrin, band-3, α-spectrin, β-spectrin, and protein 4.2 which are responsible for RBC shape. Deficiency of any of the proteins results in change of RBC shape from biconcave to spherical. A spherical RBC is more rigid and cannot be deformed easily; it is thus prone to hemolysis while passing through the spleen. This is associated with an increased permeability to sodium and increased glycolysis by the cell.

CLINICAL FEATURES

The age of presentation depends upon the severity of the disease. It may present in the neonatal period as hyperbilirubinemia and anemia warranting phototherapy or exchange transfusion. It may also present later in life as mild to moderate anemia, moderate splenomegaly, mild jaundice, fatigue, and gallstones. Complications of bone marrow hyperplasia evident in the skeletal system are less marked than β-thalassemia major. They are also prone to aplastic crisis resulting from parvovirus infection like sickle cell disease. Though autosomally inherited, up to 25% of patients may not have a family history of the disease.

Many children may go undetected and remain asymptomatic till adulthood.

LABORATORY DIAGNOSIS

- Peripheral smear shows anemia with microspherocytosis.
- Reticulocyte count is increased. MCV is normal but the MCHC may be raised.
- Red cell distribution width (RDW) is increased in HS.
- Osmotic fragility of the red cells is increased **(Figs. 23.17A and B)**, due to increased permeability of the cell membrane to sodium, leading to increased absorption sodium and water when exposed to hypotonic saline. The spherical cells swell up and lyse more readily than the normal concave cells. However, increased osmotic fragility is not pathognomonic of hereditary spherocytosis and can be seen in other hemolytic anemias as well.
- Serum bilirubin levels are mildly elevated.
- Eosin-5'-maleimide (EMA) binding test is the most specific test for HS. This flow cytometric test with fluorescent EMA dye allows for the detection of RBCs with plasma membrane deficiency.
- Sodium dodecyl sulfate polyacrylamide gel electrophoresis (SDS-PAGE) can identify abnormal plasma membrane proteins but has limited availability
- Molecular tests allow for identification of the genetic mutation within genes encoding plasma membrane proteins, the deficiency of which leads to HS. The genetic defects confirmed to cause HS include the *SPTA1* gene encoding alpha spectrin, *SPTB* gene encoding beta spectrin, *ANK1*

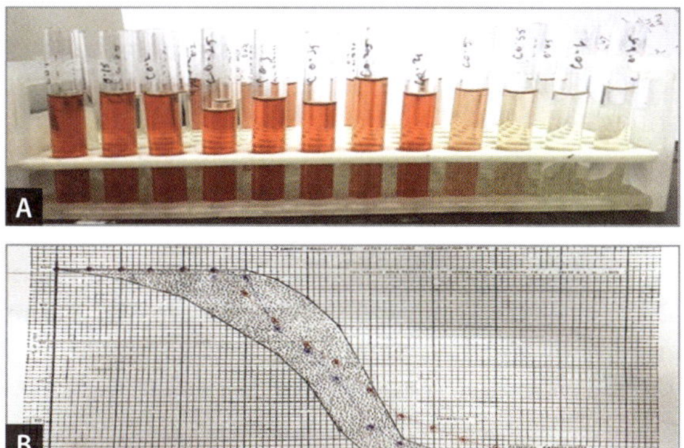

Figs. 23.17A and B: Osmotic fragility test showing red cells added to increasingly hypotonic saline concentrations in the left hand image and a shift of curve (blue line–normal and red line–patient) to right on the right hand image showing increased osmotic fragility.

gene encoding ankyrin, *SLC4A1* gene encoding band 3 protein, and/or *EPB42* gene encoding protein 4.2.

TREATMENT Hereditary Spherocytosis

All patients require life long folic acid supplementation at a dose of 1–5 mg daily. Packed red cell transfusion may occasionally be required. Regular transfusions are not required except in severe cases. Splenectomy is reserved for patients with severe disease which is characterized by a Hb of <8 g/dl, reticulocyte count of >10%, recurrent transfusion requirement, and growth failure. As the spleen is the site for lysis of cells, the anemia and associated symptoms improve following splenectomy. The reticulocyte count goes down and there is almost a complete and sustained remission of the disease. All modalities to prevent infection as described earlier should be adopted before and after splenectomy, including vaccination for encapsulated organisms 3–4 weeks before splenectomy, and penicillin prophylaxis post splenectomy. Splenectomy is performed typically after the age of 6 years to avoid an increased risk of sepsis. Cholecystectomy may be required for symptomatic choledocholithiasis.

HEREDITARY ELLIPTOCYTOSIS

It is a genetically determined, uncommon RBC disorder that varies markedly in severity and is characterized by elliptical red cells in the peripheral smear. The disorder is transmitted as an autosomal dominant trait and is prevalent in malaria endemic areas such as West Africa. Compared to hereditary spherocytosis where the vertical links in the red cell membrane are affected, horizontal linkages (spectrin dimer interaction or spectrin-actin-protein 4.1 complex are affected). Clinical symptoms vary from asymptomatic carrier state to severe hemolytic anemia. Members of the same family may show different clinical severity and an individual's frequency and severity of symptoms may change with time. Splenectomy can reduce severity of disease in severely affected patients.

Other rare disorders of RBC membrane are ovalocytosis, pyropoikilocytosis, xerocytosis, and acanthocytosis. It is important to note that splenectomy is contraindicated in the overhydrated variant of hereditary stomatocytosis as there is an unacceptably high risk of thromboctic complications.

IN A NUTSHELL

Hereditary Spherocytosis

1. Red cell membrane disorders are inherited diseases due to mutations in various membrane or skeletal proteins, resulting in decreased red cell deformability, reduced lifespan, and premature removal of the erythrocytes from the circulation.
2. The red cell membrane disorders include hereditary spherocytosis (HS), hereditary elliptocytosis, hereditary ovalocytosis, and hereditary stomatocytosis.
3. Hemolytic anemia in HS can range from compensated to severe, sometimes requiring exchange transfusion at birth and/or repeated blood transfusions, variable jaundice, splenomegaly, and cholelithiasis.
4. Osmotic fragility test is used for screening patients with HS as the osmotic fragility of the red cells is increased in HS.

Bolton-Maggs PH, Langer JC, Iolascon A, Tittensor P, King MJ. Guidelines for the diagnosis and management of hereditary spherocytosis—2011 update. Br J Haematol. 2012;156(1):37-49.

Polizzi A, Dicembre LP, Failla C, Matola TD, Moretti M, Ranieri SC, et al. Overview on hereditary spherocytosis diagnosis. Int J Lab Hematol. 2025;47(1):18-25.

Turpaev K, Bovt E, Shakhidzhanov S, Sinauridze E, Smetanina N, Koleva L, et al. An overview of hereditary spherocytosis and the curative effects of splenectomy. Front Physiol. 2025;16:1497588.

23.11 Autoimmune Hemolytic Anemia *PE 26.4*

INTRODUCTION

Autoimmune hemolytic anemia (AIHA) is an uncommon group of disorders characterized by destruction of red blood cells by autoantibodies. It can occur at any age and has a predilection for female sex. While, in most cases no cause can be ascertained, it may sometimes be associated with disorders such as systemic lupus erythematosus (SLE), Crohn's disease, rheumatic illnesses, and lymphoproliferative disorders. Rarely, it may follow the use of certain drugs such as penicillin or certain viral infections.

ETIOPATHOGENESIS

It is of two types:

1. ***Warm antibody hemolytic anemia:*** The autoantibodies (usually IgG type and polyclonal) attach to and destroy red blood cells at temperatures equal to or in excess of normal body temperature. The hemolysis is extravascular.
2. ***Cold antibody hemolytic anemia:*** The autoantibodies (usually IgM type) become most active and attack red blood cells only at temperatures well below normal body temperature. The hemolysis is mostly intravascular.

- *Paroxysmal cold hemoglobinuria:* (Donath-Landsteiner syndrome) It is a rare type of cold antibody hemolytic anemia. An IgG antibody binds to the P antigen on red blood cells at low temperatures and causes destruction of red blood cells within arteries and veins after warming. It occurs most often after a viral illness or in otherwise healthy people, although it occurs in some people with syphilis.
- *Cold agglutinin syndrome:* It is a type of cold antibody (IgM mediated) hemolytic anemia, seen more frequently in older age group and characterized by C3 mediated hemolysis. IgM antibodies bind to the i/I antigen on RBCs in cold conditions and cause agglutination followed by complement activation and intravascular hemolysis.

CLINICAL FEATURES

Warm AIHA usually presents acutely with severe and symptomatic anemia, and jaundice. Congestive failure may occur with severe anemia. A mild to moderate splenomegaly is often present. Cold AIHA typically occurs after 1–2 weeks of a viral infection such as EBV or after mycoplasma infection.

DIAGNOSIS

The hemoglobin is around 4–7 g/dL with normal red cell indices. A spuriously high MCV can occur due to red cell agglutination in cold AIHA. The reticulocyte count is typically elevated. Spherocytes are seen in peripheral smear especially in warm autoimmune hemolytic anemia. Pancytopenia may also be seen. Coombs test can aid the diagnosis. Direct antiglobulin test (DAT) or direct Coombs test detects increased amounts of autoantibodies attached to red blood cells while the indirect antiglobulin or indirect Coombs test can detect their presence in serum. DAT is positive in 95% of warm AIHA. By performing a polyspecific DAT, IgG and C3d coated red cells can be differentiated. Warm AIHA is always IgG positive while cold AIHA shows only C3d positivity. Presence of IgM in serum suggests cold AIHA. Cold agglutinin titers will be elevated in cold agglutinin disease. Secondary work up such as viral serology (HIV, HBSAg, and anti-HCV), ANA (for lupus erythematosus), and serum immunoglobulin levels (for primary immunodeficiency) can be considered based on the clinical presentation.

TREATMENT Autoimmune Hemolytic Anemia

Glucocorticoids are the first-line therapy for warm-reactive AIHA. Glucocorticoids are preferred over other therapies because the response is generally more rapid, short-term side effects are manageable. High doses are used at first, followed by a gradual reduction of the dose over many weeks or months. Intravenous methylprednisolone 0.5–1 mg/kg/dose every 6–8 hours for the first 24–72 hours (after which they are transitioned to oral prednisone. Occasionally, pulse high-dose methylprednisolone (30 mg/kg with maximum dose of 1 g once daily for 3 days) may be warranted for the most severely affected patients, such as those with rapidly evolving and severe hemolysis. Once an adequate response has been achieved (i.e., hemoglobin >9–10 g/dL), which typically occurs within 2–4 weeks, the steroid dose can be tapered to a single daily dose as tolerated over 2–3 months. When people do not respond to corticosteroids or when the corticosteroid causes intolerable side effects, rituximab or immunosuppressants like cyclosporine or azathioprine or intravenous immune globulin (IVIG) can be given. Splenectomy can be offered in refractory cases. When red blood cell destruction is severe, blood transfusions are sometimes needed, but they do not treat the cause of the anemia and provide only temporary relief. The best treatment for paroxysmal cold hemoglobinuria is avoidance of exposure to cold. Rituximab or plasmapheresis is the recommended treatment for severe cold agglutinin (IgM-mediated) AIHA. Blood and fluids can be warmed in cold type of AIHA.

Blackall D, Dolatshahi L. Autoimmune hemolytic anemia in children: laboratory investigation, disease associations, and treatment strategies. J Pediatr Hematol Oncol. 2022;44(3):71-78.
Voulgaridou A, Kalfa TA. Autoimmune hemolytic anemia in the pediatric setting. J Clin Med. 2021;10(2):216.

23.12 Bleeding and Coagulation Disorders *PE 26.7*

INTRODUCTION

Abnormalities in platelets, vessel wall, or clotting factors can prevent hemostasis resulting in hemorrhage. The following is a basic classification of bleeding disorders:

- ***Primary hemostatic pathway defects:*** Thrombocytopenia, platelet function defects, and von Willebrand disease
- ***Coagulation disorders:*** Congenital or acquired deficiency of clotting factors
- ***Vascular disorders:*** Henoch-Schönlein purpura, scurvy, and Ehlers-Danlos syndrome.

HISTORY

- Features of abnormal bleeding such as prolonged bleeding after minor trauma, epistaxis not relieved by 15 minutes of pressure along the entire side of the nose, menstrual periods lasting longer than 7 days with passage of clots, and ecchymotic patches inconsistent with degree of trauma, should lead to suspicion of a bleeding or coagulation disorder.
- Family history of bleeding is especially relevant for identifying the inheritance pattern, e.g., X-linked inheritance in

hemophilia and autosomal recessive inheritance in other factor deficiencies and platelet function defecys.

- ***Type of bleeding:*** Mucosal membrane bleeding, petechiae, and bruising are associated with qualitative or quantitative platelet disorders and von Willebrand disease (vWD). Spontaneous, deep muscle, and joint bleeding are commonly seen with coagulation factor deficiency such as hemophilia.
- ***Time of onset of syndrome:*** Acute onset over a period of days to weeks is suggestive of acquired disorders like immune thrombocytopenic purpura (ITP) or vitamin K deficiency. Bleeding following trauma in which there is a good initial hemostasis followed by persistent oozing due to failure to form a firm clot is suggestive of a factor XIII deficiency and disorders of fibrinolytic pathway.
- ***General condition of the patient (sick/well appearing):*** A healthy-looking child with petechiae or ecchymotic patches without significant anemia is most probably a case of ITP. A sick patient is likely to suffer from aplastic anemia, or malignant disorder, or liver disease, or DIC.
- ***Neonatal history:*** severe congenital bleeding disorders can manifest in the newborn period with cephalhematomas and intracranial hemorrhage. Umbilical stump bleeding and delayed fall can occur in deficiency of factor XIII.

PHYSICAL EXAMINATION

The following clinical features need to be checked for: Presence of petechiae, mucosal bleeds, hematoma, joint mobility and swelling, retinal bleeding, hematuria, jaundice and presence of anemia, hepatomegaly, splenomegaly, and lymphadenopathy. **Table 23.9** depict differences between coagulation factor deficiencies and platelet or vessel wall abnormalities.

- The presence of significant anemia along with thrombocytopenia and lymphadenopathy or hepatosplenomegaly suggests underlying leukemia or lymphoma.
- Anemia and thrombocytopenia without any other significant finding is suggestive of aplastic anemia or immune mediated pathology (Evans syndrome).
- Patients with platelet or vessel abnormality usually have spontaneous and superficial bleeds such as petechiae, ecchymosis, hematomas, and epistaxis.

TABLE 23.9 Clinical Features to Distinguish Bleeding and Coagulation Disorders.

Clinical sign/ symptom	*Platelet/vascular abnormality*	*Coagulation factor deficiency*
Ecchymosis	Small and superficial	Large and deep
Petechiae	Frequent	Never
Mucosal hemorrhage	Frequent	Uncommon in hemophilia and acquired defects
Muscle/joint or internal bleeding	Uncommon	Frequent hemorrhage
Bleeding following trauma/ surgery	Immediate. Stops with pressure	Delayed oozing. Does not stop with pressure

- Children with coagulation factor deficiencies do not develop petechiae but may have superficial bleeds like ecchymotic patches or subcutaneous hematoma and they characteristically manifest with deep bleeding into the muscle or joints.
- Patient with abnormal collagen matrix and vessel wall may have loose joints and lax skin associated with easy bruising.

LABORATORY EVALUATION

- ***Platelet count:*** A healthy child has a platelet count of 150–400 × 10^9/L. Accurate results are obtained by electronic counts but an experienced pathologist can also comment on the adequacy of platelets on a peripheral smear. A normal peripheral smear shows platelets in clumps. Thrombocytopenia is defined as a reduction in number of platelet (<150 × 10^9/L). Defect in platelet function is known as *thrombasthenia*.
- Thrombocytopenia due to decreased platelet production is associated with a decreased number of megakaryocytes in the bone marrow. Presence of coexisting abnormalities in leukocytes and erythrocytes indicates involvement of the bone marrow. Presence of coexisting abnormalities in coagulation, suggests consumptive coagulopathy including DIC.
- Mean platelet volume is normally 7–11 fL. Small platelets are typical of Wiskott-Aldrich syndrome and large platelets are seen in Bernard-Soulier syndrome, MYH9 defects, and immune thrombocytopenia.
- ***Peripheral smear examination:*** This is important to evaluate rule out to the involvement of other cell lines especially in cases of leukemia and aplastic anemia.
- ***Bleeding time:*** It is the time required for the cessation of bleeding from a puncture site. The normal range is 4–7 minutes. The bleeding time is prolonged if the circulating platelets are reduced in number as in idiopathic thrombocytopenic purpura (ITP) or if there is a functional intrinsic platelet defect leading to platelet deficiency even if the number is normal, e.g., Glanzmann thrombasthenia.
- ***Prothrombin time (PT):*** This indicates the integrity of the extrinsic and common pathway of coagulation **(Fig. 23.18)**. The normal value is 12 seconds, but it should always be assessed in relation to a control done from a normal person simultaneously. Prothrombin time is prolonged in deficiency of factors II, V, VII and X **(Table 23.10)**.
- ***Activated partial thromboplastin time (APTT):*** This demonstrates the intrinsic and common pathways of coagulation. The normal values are 25–40 seconds but should be compared with a control value. APTT is prolonged in deficiency of factors V, VIII, IX, X, XI, and XII.
    - An increase in PT with normal APTT indicates deficiency of factor VII.
    - A normal PT with increased APTT indicates factor VIII, IX, XI, XII deficiency.
    - Both PT and APTT are deranged in acquired disorders such as vitamin K deficiency, liver disorder, and disseminated intravascular coagulation (DIC), or inherited defects of the common pathway such as deficiencies of factors II, V, X, and fibrinogen.

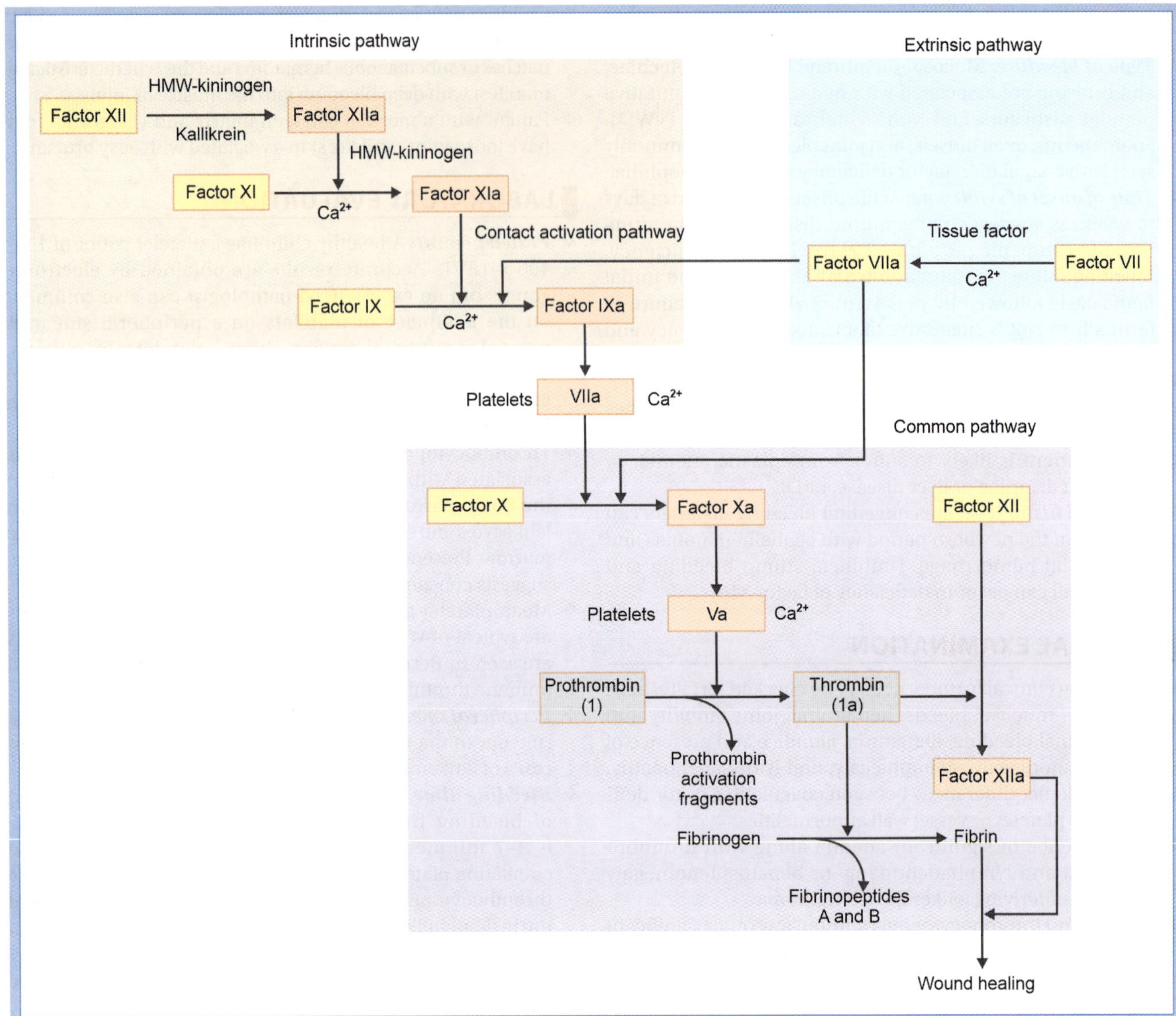

Fig. 23.18: Coagulation cascade

TABLE 23.10 Approach to a Child with Bleeding Disorder

GC	*BT*	*PT*	*APTT*	*P/C*	*Probable diagnosis*
Well	N	N	↑	N	Hemophilia A or B
Well	N	↑	N	N	Factor VII deficiency
Well	N	↑	↑	N	Vitamin K deficiency
Sick	↑	↑	↑	↓	DIC, liver disease
Well	↑	N	N	↓	ITP
Sick	↑	N	N	↓	Aplastic anemia, leukemia
Well	↑	N	N	N	Qualitative platelet defects, factor XIII deficiency, vWD

(APTT: activated partial thromboplastin time; BT: bleeding time; GC: general condition; PT: prothrombin time; P/C: platelet count; vWD: von Willebrand disease)

- ***Factor assay:*** It can be done to diagnose isolated factor deficiencies.
- ***Platelet function:*** It can be analyzed using a platelet function analyzer which can test the adhesion and aggregation properties of platelets. Platelet function defects can also be diagnosed with flow cytometry where the deficient platelet antigens can be identified.
- ***Genetic confirmation:*** Genetic conformation of the mutation in inherited bleeding disorders such as hemophilia is important for offering antenatal diagnosis in the next pregnancy.

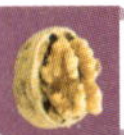

IN A NUTSHELL

Bleeding and Coagulation Disorders

1. Thrombocytopenia is defined as a reduction in number of platelet (<150 × 10^9/L). Defect in platelet function leading to bleeding is known as thrombasthenia.
2. Superficial and mucosal bleeding are usually associated with qualitative or quantitative platelet disorders and von Willebrand disease (vWD).
3. Spontaneous, deep muscle and joint bleeding are commonly seen with coagulation factor deficiency.
4. Presence of significant anemia along with thrombocytopenia and lymphadenopathy or hepatosplenomegaly suggests underlying leukemia, or lymphoma.
5. Prothrombin time (PT) indicates the integrity of the extrinsic and common pathway of coagulation and is prolonged in deficiency of factors II, V, VII, and X.
6. Activated partial thromboplastin time (APTT) demonstrates the intrinsic and common pathways of coagulation and is prolonged in deficiency of factors II, V, VIII (hemophilia A), IX (hemophilia B), X, XI, and XII.
7. Both PT and APTT are deranged in generalized disorders such as vitamin K deficiency and liver disorder or disseminated intravascular coagulation (DIC). They are both prolonged in deficiencies of common pathway factors such as fibrinogen, II, V, and X.

Bansal D, Oberoi S, Marwaha RK, et al. Approach to a child with bleeding in the emergency room. Indian J Pediatr 2013;80:411-20.
Branchford B, Di Paola J. Approach to a child with suspected bleeding disorder. In: Orkin SH, Fisher DE, Ginsburg D, et al. (Eds). Nathan and Oski's Hematology of Infancy and Childhood, 8th edition. Philadelphia: Saunders; 2015. pp. 999-1009.e2.

23.13 Thrombocytopenia

PE 26.6

INTRODUCTION

Defects of platelets can be either in terms of absolute number or in terms of their function, resulting in defective hemostasis causing bleeding manifestations. The common causes are enumerated here:

- Immune thrombocytopenia (ITP)
- ***Drug-induced thrombocytopenia:*** Heparin, valproate, phenytoin, quinine, penicillin, cephalosporins, NSAIDs, gold salts, procainamide, chemotherapy, digoxin, rifampicin, ethambutol, vancomycin, and clindamycin.
- Marrow infiltration, e.g., leukemia and storage disorders
- Aplastic anemia
- Hypersplenism
- ***Infections:*** Parvovirus, rubella, mumps, varicella, hepatitis C, Epstein-Barr virus (EBV), malaria, HIV, and septicemia.
- Megaloblastic anemia
- Liver disease
- Massive blood transfusion
- Disseminated intravascular coagulation
- Connective tissue disorders, e.g., SLE
- von Willebrand disease
- Hemolytic uremic syndrome

Sometimes the platelet count is normal but the child continues to bleed. The defect herein may lie in the platelet function or the clotting cascade **(Fig. 23.18)**.

IMMUNE THROMBOCYTOPENIC PURPURA (ITP)

Etiopathogenesis

This is the most common cause of thrombocytopenia in children and characterized by isolated destruction of platelets due to antiplatelet antibodies (usually IgG) produced by the body. These antibodies are directed against platelet surface glycoproteins GP (glycoprotein) 2b/3a and GP1b.

The autoimmune phenomenon is usually seen 2–4 weeks after viral infection. Because of the similarity between the viral antigen and the platelets, the antibodies produced against the virus binds with the platelets and cause their destruction. The antibodyplatelet complex attaches to the Fc receptors on the macrophages in the reticuloendothelial system especially the spleen and the platelets are destroyed. There is a compensatory increase in the number of immature megakaryocytes in the bone marrow.

Clinical Features

Immune thrombocytopenia may be acute, persistent, chronic, or recurrent.

- ***Newly diagnosed (or acute):*** *ITP* refers to all new cases at diagnosis up to 3 months duration.

- ***Persistent:*** *ITP* refers to ITP between 3 and 12 months from diagnosis.
- ***Chronic:*** *ITP* refers to thrombocytopenia persisting longer than 12 months.
- ***Recurrent:*** *ITP* refers to return of thrombocytopenia after at least 3 months of remission, sustained without treatment.

Acute ITP is the usual presentation in children, while chronic ITP occurs mainly in adults. ITP may be labeled as primary in the absence of an underlying disorder or secondary ITP where a specific etiology has been identified like SLE. Peak prevalence of ITP in children occurs in the age group 2–4 years. Spontaneous remission occurs in >80% of cases in children but is uncommon in adults.

Newly Diagnosed ITP

The incidence is equal in both boys and girls. There is sudden and spontaneous onset of mucocutaneous bleeds including petechiae, gum bleed, or epistaxis. History of antecedent viral infection may be present in some patients. Skin is only site of bleeding in majority of patients. Petechiae are usually pinpoint to pinhead sized skin bleeds which are macular and not blanchable **(Fig. 23.19)**. They are numerous and may be present over any part of the body. Epistaxis and gum bleeds are less common. Some children may have hematuria, menorrhagia and melena. Intracranial bleed is rare and may be fatal.

The child is otherwise well without significant anemia. There is remarkable absence of any physical sign apart from the skin bleeds. of anemia out of proportion to the severity of blood loss, significant splenomegaly, hepatosplenomegaly, or significant lymphadenopathy should arouse the suspicion of an alternate diagnosis such as leukemia.

The disease is usually self-limiting and majority of the patients recover within 6 months of onset of symptoms. Treatment seems to have a little effect on the course or duration of the disease.

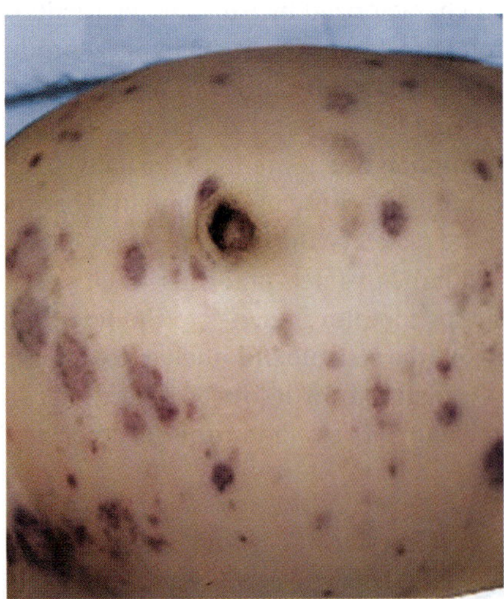

Fig. 23.19: A child with immune thrombocytopenic purpura (ITP) showing skin bleeds.

Diagnosis

Thrombocytopenia is universal with counts being $<20 \times 10^9$/L in many children. The RBCs and leukocytes are normal. Hemo globin may decrease in cases of severe bleeding. The bone marrow examination shows normal erythroid and myeloid series with normal or increased number of megakaryocytes, which are morphologically normal. Bone marrow examination is not warranted in a typical case of ITP (a welllooking child with sudden appearance of petechiae all over the body and no other physical finding, with isolated thrombocytopenia in the complete blood count, and a normal peripheral smear). Bone marrow should be examined to rule out the suspicion of leukemia, or aplastic anemia, or when 'red flag' signs are present. Other tests such as Coombs test, antinuclear antibody tests, serology for hepatitis B and C and HIV, antiphospholipid antibody, and serum immunoglobulin levels may be considered in patients with persistent ITP.

TREATMENT Immune Thrombocytopenic Purpura

Majority of the children do not require any treatment. Proper counseling of the parents about the self-limiting and benign nature of the disease is of utmost importance. Any kind of therapy is not beneficial in mild to moderate symptoms and 70–80% of children with acute ITP improve spontaneously. About 55–75% of these patients recover within 4 weeks and 90% improve within 4–6 months.

Therapeutic intervention has only shown to probably rapidly increase the platelet counts to a relatively safe level. The time to remission and severity remains unaffected by treatment. Treatment may be offered in circumstances where follow-up is difficult or child stays in a remote location.

Decision to intervene or start pharmacotherapy should be based on the clinical picture of the child rather than the platelet count alone. Isolated skin bleed do not warrant any definitive treatment. Treatment is indicated in presence of nonmajor mucosal bleeding, significant mucosal or internal bleeding; or suspected intracranial bleed, irrespective of the platelet count. Remember that you need to treat the patient and not his platelet count.

First-line Therapy includes Corticosteroids, Anti-D, and IVIG.

- *Corticosteroids:* Corticosteroids raise the platelet count to a safe level by several mechanisms—(i) inhibition of phagocytosis and antibody synthesis, (ii) improved platelet production, (iii) increased endothelial stability. Prednisolone is given in a dose of 2–4 mg/kg/day for 4–7 days. Intravenous or oral methylprednisolone has also been used. Prednisolone or methylprednisolone is preferred over dexamethasone. Usually, the initial response takes 2-7 days.
- *IVIG:* Intravenous immunoglobulin raises the platelet count rapidly in 90–95% of children within 1–2 days. . It helps by decreasing the phagocytosis of antibody coated platelets in spleen by binding to the Fc receptors. It is given in a single dose of 0.8–1 g/kg. The therapy is expensive.
- Side effects include flu-like symptoms, and rarely anaphylaxis (more so in IgA deficient patients), or aseptic meningitis.
- *Anti-D globulin:* This is effective only in Rh-positive individuals in a dose of 50–70 µg/kg intravenously. It is as effective as IVIG and much cheaper. The anti-D antibody binds to the Rh-positive RBCs and this complex goes and binds to the Fc receptors and blocks them. This prevents Fc receptor-mediated destruction of the platelets. Although a cheap and effective option, there is a risk of hemolysis.

- *Splenectomy:* Splenectomy is reserved for children >4 years of age as the last resort with life-threatening bleeding not responding all other modalities, the child shows intolerance to other drugs and quality of life is impaired.
- *Platelet transfusion:* Platelet transfusion has no role in most patients. Whatever new platelets are transfused, they are rapidly destroyed by circulating autoantibodies. It may be rarely be indicated in patients with severe life-threatening bleed to immediately raise the platelet count and tide over of the crisis for a very short duration of time.
- *Supportive:* Restriction of physical activity, avoidance of contact sports, use of helmets and knee/elbow caps while playing are advisable to prevent trauma which can precipitate bleeding. Use of antiplatelet drugs such as aspirin and nonsteroidal antiinflammatory drugs should be avoided.
- *Antifibrinolytic agent:* Tranexamic acid is a good adjunct to the management of mucosal bleeding. It is avoided in hematuria.

CHRONIC ITP

About 15–20% of the children with acute ITP continues to have thrombocytopenia beyond 12 months. These children have a more insidious onset of symptoms. Chronic ITP is common in children above 10 years of age. Girls are affected 2–3 times more often than boys. Other causes of thrombocytopenia such as SLE, HIV, and von Willebrand disease must be ruled out.

These children are managed by medical therapy (IVIG, steroids, anti-D) as and when required depending upon the bleeding manifestations. Rituximab and thrombopoietin receptor agonists (TPORAs) are preferred over splenectomy in children with chronic ITP. Rituximab is a chimeric monoclonal antibody (mAb) directed against the B cell surface protein CD20 and decreases plasma cells via apoptosis, antibody-dependent cyto-toxicity, and complement-mediated lysis. TPO-RAs, also called *thrombopoietin (TPO) mimetics*, include small molecule peptide and nonpeptide agents. These act by stimulating the production of megakaryocytes and ultimately platelets in the bone marrow by binding to and activating the TPO receptor.

These include romiplostim (subcutaneous injection) and eltrombopag (oral) which are both approved for the use in children more than 1-year of age with persistent ITP that has poor response to steroids and IVIg. Possible risks include increased risk for thrombosis and increased reticulin in bone marrow.

Children not going into remission and having repeated significant bleeding manifestation for >1–2 years may benefit from splenectomy.

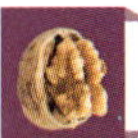

IN A NUTSHELL

Immune Thrombocytopenic Purpura

1. Immune thrombocytopenia (ITP) is most common cause of thrombocytopenia in children and is characterized by isolated destruction of platelets due to antiplatelet anti-bodies.
2. ITP may be newly diagnosed (thrombocytopenia up to 3 months duration), persistent (3–12 months duration), chronic (>12 months duration), or recurrent.
3. A child with ITP appears otherwise well without significant anemia and has usually superficial bleeding.
4. Bone marrow may be examined to rule out the suspicion of leukemia or aplastic anemia.
5. Spontaneous remission occurs in >80% of cases of ITP in children. Treatment is indicated in presence of nonmajor mucosal bleeding, significant mucosal or internal bleeding; or suspected intracranial bleed, irrespective of the platelet count. First line therapy includes corticosteroids, anti-D, and intravenous immunoglobulin (IVIG). Rituximab or TPO-Ras are used in chronic ITP. Splenectomy is best avoided.
6. Platelet transfusion has no role in most patients.

Gotesman M, Shear M, Raheel S, Procassini M, Panosyan EH. Pediatric immune thrombocytopenia. Adv Pediatr. 2024;71(1):229-240.
Neunert C, Terrell DR, Arnold DM, et al. American Society of Hematology 2019 guidelines for immune thrombocytopenia. Blood Adv. 2019;3(23):3829-66.
Singh G, Bansal D, Wright NAM. Immune thrombocytopenia in children: consensus and controversies. Indian J Pediatr. 2020;87(2):150-7.
Thakur Y, Meshram RJ, Taksande A. Diagnosis and management of immune thrombocytopenia in paediatrics: a comprehensive review. Cureus. 2024;16:e69635.

23.14 Congenital Coagulation Disorders

PE 26.7

HEMOPHILIA

Hemophilia A occurs more commonly, i.e., 1 in 10,000 male births, than hemophilia B which has an incidence of 1 in 40,000 male births. Approximately 1 woman in 5,000 is a carrier for hemophilia A, and 1 in 20,000 is a carrier of hemophilia B.

Etiology

Hemophilia is characterized by prolonged bleeding especially in a male child, often with a family history, with a normal prothrombin time, and prolonged partial thromboplastin time. Coagulation defect is—(i) either due to deficiency of factor VIII (hemophilia A), (ii) deficiency of factor IX (hemophilia B), or (iii) deficiency of factor XI (hemophilia C). Hemophilia A and B are inherited as X-linked recessive disorders; affecting only the males, and females are carrier. Hemophilia C is inherited in an autosomal recessive manner.

Classification

Individuals with <1% active factor are classified as having severe hemophilia, those with 1–5% active factor have moderate hemophilia, and those with mild hemophilia have between 5 and 40% of normal levels of active clotting factor.

Pathogenesis

Factor VIII gene is located in the most distal band (Xq28) of the long arm of the X chromosome. Factor VIII deficiency in hemophilia A results due to one of the following defects in this gene—(i) gross gene rearrangements, (ii) deletions or insertions of genetic sequence of a size varying from one base pair up to the entire gene, and (iii) single DNA base substitutions resulting in either amino acid replacement "missense," premature peptide chain termination ("nonsense" or stop mutations), or mRNA splicing defects. Factor IX gene is located in the X chromosome at Xq27.1. The majority of defects are point mutations, followed by small insertions or deletions, splice site mutations, large deletions or insertions, and mutations in the promoter region which results in factor IX deficiency or defects.

Clinical Features

Hemophilia A and B cannot be differentiated clinically. Mild deficiency may go unnoticed till adolescence or adulthood, as there is no spontaneous bleed. Moderate deficiency usually presents after infancy as severe bleeding following trauma or surgery; spontaneous bleed is occasional. The diagnosis is only made when these children have heavy bleeding following a surgery, dental procedure, or accident. Children with severe disease have spontaneous bleeding in the joints and muscles with onset in infancy.

- The symptoms can present right from the neonatal period. Circumcision can lead to excessive bleeding in the neonatal period. Some neonates may present with large cephalohematoma following a difficult or instrumental delivery.
- In most children, manifestations start appearing in the latter half of the infancy when the child starts crawling or walking, and are prone to falls and injuries. These children bleed profusely for days, following minor cuts and injuries.
  There is no other significant finding apart from the ecchy motic patches.

Formation of an intramuscular hematoma following an intramuscular injection may be the first symptom of hemophilia.

- Hemarthrosis bleeding into joints is the most characteristic feature of severe hemophilia **(Fig. 23.20)**. Knee joint is the most common joint to be involved, followed by elbow and ankle joints. There is progressively increasing swelling of the joints after a trivial trauma. Repeated bleeding into the same joint (target joint) leads to destruction of the joint and bones leading to physical disability and restriction in joint movements. The swelling is initially painful but the pain disappears in 3–4 days and swelling may take months to subside. In patients with severe recurrent bleeding there can be formation of contractures. Isolated hemarthrosis may be confused with rheumatic, idiopathic, or septic arthritis.
- Intracranial bleed can be fatal and is not uncommon in severe hemophilia.

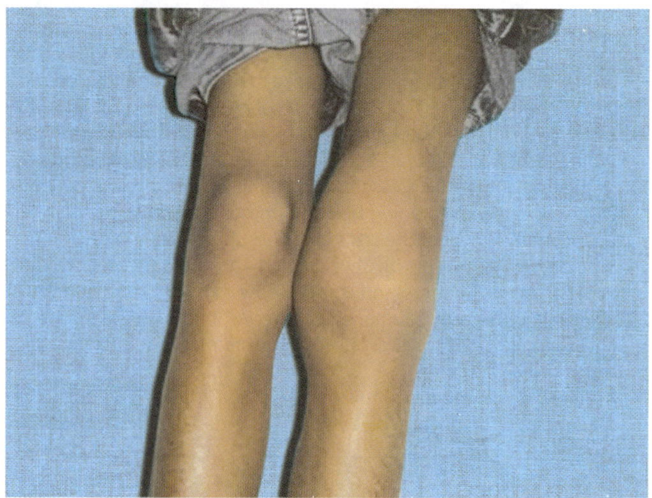

Fig. 23.20: Left knee hemarthrosis in a child with hemophilia A.

Investigations

Complete blood count (CBC) is usually normal in persons with hemophilia. However, the activated partial thromboplastin time (aPTT) is prolonged. aPTT may be prolonged due to deficiency of factors VIII, IX, XI, or XII. Therefore, mixing studies need to be done to identify the deficient clotting factor. If mixing with normal plasma corrects the aPTT, it suggests an underlying factor deficiency, but if it remains prolonged, it could be due to presence of inhibitors of clotting cascade such as lupus or any acquired inhibitor. Prothrombin time (PT) will be normal among people with hemophilia A and B. Diagnosis is usually established by bioassay of the factor VIII or IX.

TREATMENT Hemophilia

The goal of treatment is to prevent life-threatening bleeding and avoid chronic damage to joints. Trauma and injury should be avoided especially in infants and toddlers. Injury can be avoided by use of elbow and knee pads; using furniture with rounded instead of sharp margins; avoidance of contact sports; and use of helmet while cycling. Parents should be counseled about the disease and first aid required for bleeding.

Control Bleeding

Bleeding can be controlled by replacement of the deficient factor, using their concentrates derived from plasma or recombinant technique; or appropriate blood products (plasma, cryoprecipitate, and whole blood) **(Table 23.11)**.

- *Local measures:* Protection (splinting), optimal loading, ice, compression, and elevation (POLICE) for hemarthrosis, topical hemostatics.
- *Non-specific measures:* Tranexamic acid, epsilon-aminocaproic acid (EACA), or desmopressin can be used for minor mucocutaneous bleeding in children with mild hemophilia A. Desmopressin 0.3 mg/kg diluted in 50 mL of normal saline is infused intravenously in hemophilia A patients as it causes release of factor VIII from stores. It can also be given subcutaneously or intranasally.
- Levels of factor VIII should be raised to at least 30% in hemarthrosis or muscle bleed. It should be raised to 100% for a life-threatening intracranial bleed.

- *One unit of the specific:* Factor concentrate per kg body weight increases the plasma concentration of factor VIII by 2%, and factor IX by 1%. Cost of the factor concentrates and development of antibodies against these recombinant factors because of repeated administration are the limiting factors.

Storing Concentrates

Factor concentrates can be stored in a refrigerator for quite long periods (up to 6 months). However, they should not be frozen. Factor VIII is available in vials of 250, 500, and 1,000 IU. Factor IX is available in vials of 300 and 600 IU.

Blood Products

If factor concentrates are not available, it is possible to use fresh frozen plasma (FFP) (for hemophilia A and B), cryoprecipitate (for hemophilia A), whole blood, or prothrombin complex concentrates (for hemophilia B) as an alternative life-saving option. However, their administration entails a high risk for acquiring infections like HIV, hepatitis B and C, and CMV.

- A bag of cryoprecipitate made from one unit of FFP (200–250 mL) may contain 70–80 units of FVIII in a volume of 30–40 mL.
- One bag of FFP contains 200 IU of factor VIII and IX.

Treatment of Specific Hemorrhages

In case of large internal hemorrhage, hemoglobin should be checked and corrected while other measures are being planned. Ensure hemodynamic stability while factor replacement therapy is initiated. The dose of the factor used and the duration of therapy to treat the bleeding episode vary according to the nature and site of bleeding. Administer the appropriate dose of factor concentrate to raise the patient's factor level suitably as enumerated in **Table 23.11.**

The use of viral inactivated, plasma-derived, or recombinant concentrates is recommended for treating bleeding episodes in hemophiliacs.

In the absence of an inhibitor, each unit of FVIII per kilogram of body weight infused intravenously will raise the plasma FVIII level approximately 2 IU/dL. The half-life of FVIII is approximately 8–12 hours. The dose is calculated by multiplying the patient's weight in kilograms by the desired rise in factor level in IU/dL, multiplied by 0.5.

In absence of an inhibitor, each unit of FIX per kilogram of bodyweight infused intravenously will raise the plasma FIX level approximately 1 IU/dL. The half-life is approximately 18–24 hours.

To calculate dosage, multiply the patient's weight in kilograms by the desired rise in factor level in IU/dL.

Factor concentrates should be infused by slow IV injection at a rate not to exceed 100 units/min in young children.

Prophylactic Therapy

Early prophylactic use of clotting factors with severe hemophilia is gaining acceptance to prevent pain and morbidity associated with bleeding disorders. Regular administration of factor concentrates can aid in maintaining the factor levels above 5%. The indications for prophylactic therapy are recurrent hemarthrosis and an episode of intracranial bleed. Non-steroidal anti-inflammatory drugs (NSAIDs) should be avoided in hemophiliacs.

TABLE 23.11 Factor Replacement Therapy for Bleeding Episodes in Hemophilia (for Resource-Poor Countries)

	Hemophilia A		*Hemophilia B*	
Type of bleed	*Desired level (IU/dL)*	*Duration (days)*	*Desired level (IU/dL)*	*Duration (days)*
Hemarthrosis*	10–20	1–2	10–20	1–2
Superficial muscle bleed (without compromise)	10–20	2-3	10–20	2-3
Iliopsoas bleed or deep muscle bleed (with compromise)* • Initial • Maintenance	20–40 10–20	3–5 (or longer)	15–30 10–20	3–5 (or longer)
Central nervous system (CNS) bleed • Initial • Maintenance	50–80 30–50 20–40	1–3 4–7 8–14	50–80 30–50 20–40	1–3 4–7 8–14
Renal	20–40	3–5	20–40	3–5
Deep laceration	20–40	5–7	20–40	5–7
Major surgery • Preoperative • Postoperative	50–70 30–40 20–30 10–20	1–3 4–6 7–14	50–70 30–40 20–30 10–20	1–3 4–6 7–14
Minor surgery • Preoperative • Postoperative	40–80 20–50	1–5	40–80 20–50	1–5
Gastrointestinal bleeding • Initial • Maintenance	30–50 10–20	1–3 4–7	30–50 10–20	1–3 4–7
Renal	20–40	3–5	15–30	3–5

*Prednisolone may be added for 1–3 days as adjunctive treatment

Carrier Status and Prenatal Testing

Since hemophilia has X-linked inheritance **(Fig. 23.21)**, men with the genetic mutation will have hemophilia, therefore a male who does not have the condition cannot be a carrier of the disease. A woman who has two or more sons with known hemophilia, or is a daughter of a man with hemophilia, or has one son with hemophilia and one more relative who has hemophilia or is a carrier; is termed an obligate carrier, and no testing is needed to establish that she is a carrier of hemophilia. Women whose carrier status is unknown can be evaluated either by testing for the clotting factors or by methods to characterize the mutation in the DNA. The DNA screening methods are generally the most reliable. A hemophilia gene test can be done during pregnancy by chorionic villus sampling (CVS) test. A simple factor assay can also help ascertain carrier status. A woman who is a hemophilia carrier is likely to have low levels of factor VIII or IX. Estimation of factor VIIIC: F VIII Ag is useful; ratio <0.6 is suggestive of carrier state in hemophilia A.

Table 23.12 exhibits the laboratory findings which may enable us to differentiate a bleeding episode due to the various coagulation defects and platelet defects, described previously.

DEVELOPMENT OF ANTIBODIES (ACQUIRED HEMOPHILIA)

About 33% of patients with severe hemophilia A and 3% of patients with hemophilia B develop antibodies against factor VIII/IX. It should be suspected whenever patients fail to respond to adequate replacement therapy. Inhibitors can be estimated by Bethesda assay. Treatment of acquired hemophilia may be done with high doses of factors VIII and IX, porcine factor VIII, activated prothrombin complex, activated factor VII, factor eight inhibitor bypassing agents, use of immunosuppressive agents, and recombinant factor VIII or IX. Recently, emicizumab has been used for adults and children with hemophilia A, with or without factor VIII inhibitors. Emicizumab exerts its action by performing the function of the coagulation factor VIII without presenting a structural homology. It presents a dual specificity which allows it to bind to both the factor IXa and factor X, performing the required bridging activity for the launch of the coagulation cascade. Other novel agents in hemophilia include fitusiran which suppresses antithrombin, and concizumab and marstacimab which are antibodies to tissue factor pathway inhibitor. Gene therapy has also shown successive outcomes in trials in hemophilia.

VON WILLEBRAND DISEASE

von Willebrand disease is an autosomal disorder that occurs due to a mild (Type 1) or severe (Type 3) deficiency, or a qualitative defect (Type 2) of von Willebrand factor (vWF). vWF is present in platelets, endothelial cell, and in plasma along with F VIII. Children with vWD present with mucosal bleeding and symptoms akin to hemophilia A. Laboratory investigations reveal prolonged bleeding time with decreased F VIII levels. Activated partial thromboplastin time may be prolonged in severe disease. Management is similar to hemophilia with von Willebrand factor replacement or cryoprecipitate infusion.

TABLE 23.12 Laboratory Findings in Bleeding Due to Coagulation or Platelet Disorders.

Condition	*Prothrombin time*	*Partial thromboplastin time*	*Bleeding time*	*Platelet counts*
Von Willebrand disease	Unaffected	Prolonged	Prolonged	Unaffected
Vitamin K deficiency or warfarin	Prolonged	Normal or mildly prolonged	Unaffected	Unaffected
Thrombocytopenia	Unaffected	Unaffected	Prolonged	Decreased
Liver failure	Prolonged	Prolonged	Prolonged	Unaffected
Hemophilia	Unaffected	Prolonged	Unaffected	Unaffected
Glanzmann thrombasthenia	Unaffected	Unaffected	Prolonged	Unaffected
Factor X deficiency	Prolonged	Prolonged	Unaffected	Unaffected
Factor V deficiency	Prolonged	Prolonged	Unaffected	Unaffected
Disseminated intravascular coagulation	Prolonged	Prolonged	Prolonged	Decreased
Congenital afibrinogenemia	Prolonged	Prolonged	Prolonged	Unaffected
Bernard–Soulier syndrome	Unaffected	Unaffected	Prolonged	Normal or decreased
Aspirin	Unaffected	Unaffected	Prolonged	Normal
Warfarin	Prolonged	Unaffected/prolonged	Prolonged	Normal
Heparin	Unaffected/prolonged	Prolonged	Prolonged	Normal/low (immune-mediated)

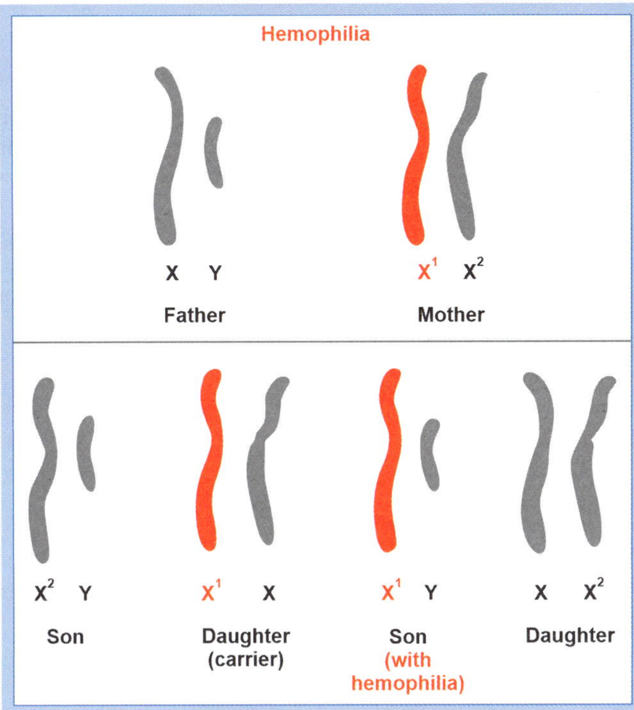

Fig. 23.21: Inheritance pattern in hemophilia.

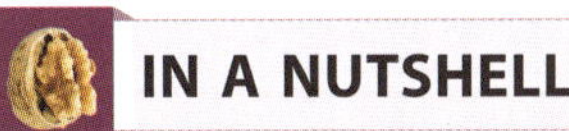

IN A NUTSHELL

Hemophilia

1. Hemophilia A and B are X-linked recessive disorders characterized by prolonged bleeding especially in a male child, often with a family history, with a normal prothrombin time, and prolonged partial thromboplastin time.
2. Diagnosis of hemophilia is confirmed by assays of factor VIII and IX.
3. Bleeding into joints is the most characteristic feature of severe hemophilia.
4. Bleeding can be controlled by replacement of the deficient factor, using their concentrates derived from plasma or recombinant technique; or appropriate blood products (plasma, cryoprecipitate, whole blood). The use of viral-inactivated, plasma-derived, or recombinant concentrates are recommended for treating bleeding episodes in hemophiliacs. One unit of the specific factor concentrate per kg body weight increases the plasma concentration of factor VIII by 2%, and factor IX by1%.
5. Local measures such as protection, optimal loading, ice, compression, and elevation (POLICE), topical hemostatics, and splinting are important in management of acute bleeds.
6. *Non-specific measures:* Tranexamic acid, epsilon-aminocaproic acid (EACA), or desmopressin can be used for minor mucocutaneous bleeding.
7. Early prophylactic use of clotting factors with severe hemophilia to maintain the factor levels above 5% is gaining acceptance as a way to prevent pain and morbidity associated with bleeding disorders.

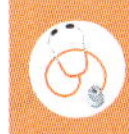

CASE STUDY Hemophilia

A 4-year-old boy was brought by his mother to the emergency department with complaints of sudden onset weakness in both lower limbs following trivial trauma. There was no associated fever, rash, headache, vomiting, seizures, or recent vaccination. The mother gave a history of easy bruisability and repeated hemarthrosis noticed since infancy in her son. His younger brother also had similar complaints of repeated skin bleeds, though his older sister was normal. Laboratory investigation revealed: Hemoglobin: 10.4 g/dL, TLC: 4,600, platelet count: 2.13 lac/mm³, with an essentially normal peripheral smear, PT = 12s (C = 14s), PTTK = 84s (C = 32s) and a normal bleeding time. CECT (spine) revealed an extradural collection suggestive of a hematoma, extending from D7–D11.

What is the probable diagnosis?

The child is probably suffering from hemophilia, as his partial thromboplastin time is deranged suggesting a defect in the intrinsic pathway (factors XII, XI, IX, or VIII deficiency). Hemophilia A is due to the deficiency of clotting factor VIII, hemophilia B is due to the deficiency of factor IX, and hemophilia C is due to the deficiency of factor XI. Hemophilia has an X-linked recessive inheritance.

How will you confirm the diagnosis?

Specific factor assays viz., factor VIII and factor IX should be done to confirm this condition. Mixing studies should be done to rule out the presence of inhibitor of factor VIII or factor IX in the plasma.

What is the specific treatment of this disorder?

Specific therapy, i.e., replacement therapy in the form of recombinant or plasma derived factor VIII or IX concentrates or fresh frozen plasma (containing factor VIII and factor IX) or cryoprecipitate (containing factor VIII, von Willebrand factor and fibrinogen) can be given for managing bleeding seen in patients of severe hemophilia. One unit of factor VIII raises the factor VIII level by 2% (t1/2 of factor VIII 8–12 hours) while one unit of factor IX raises the factor IX level by 1% (t1/2 of factor IX 18–24 hours). There is a risk of blood transfusion associated infections such as HIV, hepatitis B and C, Cytomegalovirus) with use of blood products. Hence factor concentrates should be used as far as possible. Antifibrinolytic drugs like epsilon-aminocaproic acid (EACA) or tranexamic acid, and desmopressin (intranasal or intravenous) can be given in mild or moderate hemophilia A.

Sachdeva A, Gunasekaran V, Ramya HN, Dass J, Kotwal J, Seth T, et al; 'Consensus in Diagnosis and Management of Hemophilia' Committee*, Indian Academy of Pediatrics. Consensus Statement of the Indian Academy of Pediatrics in Diagnosis and Management of Hemophilia. Indian Pediatr. 2018;55(7):582-590.

Srivastava A, Santagostino E, Dougall A, et al. WFH Guidelines for the Management of Hemophilia, 3rd edition. Haemophilia 2020; 26(Suppl 6): 1-158.

23.15 Acute Lymphoblastic Leukemia

PE 26.8

INTRODUCTION

Acute lymphoblastic leukemia (ALL) represents clonal expansion and arrest at a specific stage of lymphoid hematopoiesis. ALL contributes to 25–30 % of pediatric malignancies and 80% of all childhood acute leukemia.

ETIOLOGY

Etiology of acute leukemia is related to acquisition of a series of genetic events, most of which are somatic in origin. Ionizing radiation, chemical exposure, and alkylating drugs are implicated in the pathogenesis of acute leukemia. Genetic conditions which increase the risk of acute leukemia are: Down syndrome, Bloom syndrome, Fanconi anemia, ataxia telangiectasia, Li-Fraumeni syndrome, neurofibromatosis, ata xia telangiectasia, Shwachman-Diamond syndrome, etc.

CLINICAL FEATURES

Child can present with systemic features such as fever, lassitude, and pallor. Bone marrow involvement may result in anemia which causes fatiguability, pallor, dyspnea, and sometimes congestive cardiac failure. Neutropenia can result in fever, and infection. Petechiae, ecchymosis, easy bruisability, bleeding from mucous membrane and sometimes internal bleeding can be presenting features due to thrombocytopenia. Child may have lymphadenopathy, and abdominal distension due to liver and spleen enlargement. Sometimes, patient presents with features of CNS involvement, skin involvement or renal involvement, etc. Testicular enlargement may be seen infrequently.

DIAGNOSIS

- ***Blood counts, coagulation profile, and peripheral smear:*** Complete blood count may reveal anemia, thrombocyto penia, leucopenia or leukocytosis. Peripheral smear examination may show presence of blasts. Coagulation profile may be deranged in some patients presenting with high white blood cell counts.
- ***Biochemical studies:*** Baseline renal and liver function should be assessed. Lymphoblasts may lyse spontaneously or with treatment releasing their intracellular contents. This can precipitate an oncological emergency called tumor lysis syndrome comprised of hyperkalemia, hyperuricemia, hyperphosphatemia, hypocalcemia, and elevated serum creatinine.
- ***Bone marrow aspiration:*** This is the most important diagnostic investigation to detect the presence of blasts. Immunophenotyping by flow cytometry is useful in determining the type of acute leukemia. Cytogenetics using karyotype and molecular studies are helpful in further classification and determining prognosis.
- ***Chest radiograph:*** It is useful to detect mediastinal mass especially in children with T ALL
- ***Cerebrospinal fluid examination:*** It is mandatory to look for blasts by cytospin.
- ***Cardiac function:*** Echocardiography is recommended to demonstrate normal cardiac function before starting anthracycline chemotherapy.
- ***Infectious disease profile:*** Human immunodeficiency virus antibody, hepatitis B surface antigen, hepatitis C antibody, and hepatitis B antibody screening.

Prognostic Factors

Children with ALL are risk stratified based on prognostic factors.

Table 23.13 enlists the prognostic factors in childhood ALL.

TABLE 23.13 Prognostic Factors in Children with Acute Lymphoblastic Leukemia (ALL)

Factor	*Favorable*	*Less favorable*
Age (years)	1–9	<1, >10
Initial white blood cells	$<50 \times 10^9$/L	$>50 \times 10^9$/L
Immunophenotype	B cell	T cell
Genetics	• Hyperdiploidy >50 chromosomes or DNA index >1.16 • Trisomy 4 and 10 • t(12;21)/ETV6-RUNX1	• Hypodiploidy <44 chromosomes or DNA index <0.81 • MLL rearrangements • t(9;22)/BCR-ABL1 • Ph-like/BCR-ABL like • iAMP21
CNS involvement	Absent	Present
Minimal residual disease (MRD)	B cell ALL—end of induction MRD <0.01%	B cell ALL—end of induction MRD >0.01% T cell ALL—positive MRD at end of consolidation >0.1%

(CNS: central nervous system; iAMP: intrachromosomal amplification; Ph: Philadelphia chromosome)

TREATMENT Acute Lymphoblastic Leukemia

The general supportive care of newly diagnosed case of acute leukemia requires prevention and management of tumor lysis syndrome and febrile neutropenia. There are many successful treatment regimens for curative treatment of ALL which are based on similar treatment elements and principles. These include—remission induction, consolidation (intensification of remission), extra compartmental therapy [prevention of central nervous system (CNS) leukemia], and maintenance therapy. A complete remission is obtained usually after 1 month of treatment—which is defined as—resolution of symptoms attributable to disease, no physical findings related to disease, normal blood counts, moderately cellular regenerating bone marrow with <5% blasts and normal cerebrospinal fluid examination. Chemotherapeutic agents with different mechanism of action and mechanism of resistance are used to intensify the remission during consolidation. Common chemotherapeutic agents used are anthracyclines, vinca alkaloids, steroids, L-asparaginase, alkylating agents, purine analogs, and antimetabolites. Extra compartmental therapy commonly includes high dose methotrexate, intrathecal therapy and cranial radiation. Maintenance chemotherapy is continued for approximately two years to eradicate residual low-level disease. Prevention and treatment of complications of therapy and disease is also an important aspect of treatment. Contemporary protocols also use immunotherapies either in first line or recurrent treatment regimens. With this combination chemotherapy regimen 5 years survival has exceeded 90% for B cell ALL and ranges from 75 to 93% for T cell ALL.

Relapse

Despite intensive treatment of ALL, 10–20% children relapse. Relapse may occur during or after therapy for ALL. The relapse may be in the bone marrow or extramedullary at sites such as CNS and testes.

Treatment Modalities in Relapsed ALL

- *Chemotherapy:* Intensive chemotherapy incorporating combination of agents with different mechanism of actions is used to bring disease in remission before proceeding for hematopoietic stem cell transplant (HSCT). Chemotherapy alone can be curative in certain relapse groups with good prognosis.
- *HSCT:* Allogenic HSCT is the only curative modality of treatment for majority of the children with relapsed disease. It involves administration of high dose chemotherapy sometimes along with radiation followed by donor stem cell infusion.
- *Immunotherapy:* Currently different immunotherapy agents are being tried in pediatric relapsed ALL patients to bring the disease in remission before the HSCT. The common agents being used are blinatumomab, inotuzumab, ozogamicin, and chimeric antigen receptor T cell therapy. They have less toxicity and better efficacy as compared to chemotherapy.

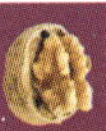

IN A NUTSHELL

Acute Lymphoblastic Leukemia

1. Childhood acute lymphoblastic leukemia (ALL) is the most common cancer in children characterized by clonal proliferation of immature lymphocytes (lymphoblasts) in bone marrow.
2. Prognosis depends upon age of the child, extent of disease, type of clone, and genetic mutations.
3. Therapy includes chemotherapy, radiation therapy, chemotherapy with stem cell transplant, targeted therapy, and immunotherapy.
4. A child with acute lymphoblastic leukemia may relapse after/during treatment. Site of relapse include bone marrow, testes, or central nervous system.

Inaba H, Pui CH. Advances in the diagnosis and treatment of pediatric acute lymphoblastic leukemia. J Clin Med. 2021;10(9):1926.
Pillai P, Carrol W. Acute lymphoblastic leukemia. In: Fish J, Lipton J, Lanskowsky P (Eds). Lanzkowsky's Manual of Pediatric Hematology and Oncology, 7th edition. London, United Kingdom: Elsevier; 2022.

23.16 Lymphoma

PE 26.9

INTRODUCTION

Lymphomas are the third most common group of cancers in children and adolescents in the West, accounting for 10–15% of all newly diagnosed cancers in this age group. In India, lymphomas are the second most common malignancy in children ahead of CNS tumors, especially in males. Lymphomas are broadly classified into two groups: (1) Hodgkin and (2) Non Hodgkin lymphoma **(Table 23.14)**.

HODGKIN LYMPHOMA

Hodgkin lymphoma (HL, formerly known as *Hodgkin disease*) was named after Thomas Hodgkin, who first described the disease and its associated abnormalities in the lymph system in 1832.

Epidemiology

The incidence of HL is bimodal with regard to age. In developed countries, the early peak occurs in young adults (20–34 years), followed by a late rise in the elderly (55–74 years).

Risk Factors

The etiology of HL is believed to be multifactorial and may include the following:

- ***Infectious agents:*** Epstein-Barr virus (EBV) has been associated with HL and is most commonly associated with mixed cellularity and lymphocytedepleted HL subtypes and less frequently with nodular sclerosis HL.

- ***Genetic influences:*** Clustering of cases in families or races suggests a genetic predisposition or exposure to a common infectious agent. The risk is postulated to be 100fold for a sibling of an affected monozygotic twin.
- ***Immune dysregulation:*** Immunodeficiency disorders, either congenital (like ataxiatelangiectasia) or acquired (like HIV infection), are associated with a higher risk of HL.

Pathological Classification

Box 23.2 enumerates WHO classification of Hodgkin lymphoma and **Table 23.14** describes immunophenotype differences between non Hodgkin lymphoma and classical Hodgkin lymphoma.

Clinical Manifestations

Common presenting symptoms and signs of HL in children include contiguous lymphadenopathy and systemic or B symptoms. From 80 to 90% of children with HL usually present with painless, firm (rubbery) lymphadenopathy, usually in volving the cervical or supraclavicular group of lymph nodes **(Fig. 23.22)**. From 15 to 20% of patients have noncontiguous extranodal involvement (stage IV) of lung, liver, bone, and bone marrow. Systemic symptoms classified as B symptoms are considered important in staging. These include fever >38°C for more than three days, weight loss >10% over 6 months, or drenching night sweats. Patients with nodular lymphocyte predominant Hodgkin lymphoma (NLPHL) are usually males

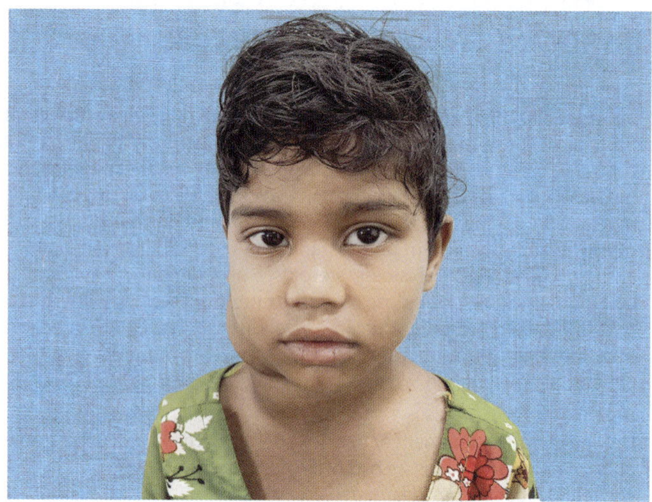

Fig. 23.22: A child presenting with cervical lymphadenopathy.

younger than 10 years and generally present with slow growing, localized, nonbulky disease, usually in the axilla and inguinal regions without any B symptoms.

Box 23.2 WHO Classification of Hodgkin Lymphoma

- Nodular lymphocyte predominant Hodgkin lymphoma
- Classic Hodgkin lymphoma
  - Lymphocyte rich
  - Lymphocyte depleted
  - Nodular sclerosis
  - Mixed cellularity

TABLE 23.14 Comparative Clinical Features of Hodgkin and Non-Hodgkin Lymphoma

Clinical features	*Hodgkin lymphoma*	*Non-Hodgkin lymphoma*
Nodal spread	Contiguous	Discontiguous
Waldeyer ring involvement	Less common	More common
Localized	Usually	Rare
Extranodal disease	Rare	Common
Central nervous system (CNS) disease	Rare	Common
Bone marrow involvement	Rare	Common
B symptoms	Common	Uncommon
Abdominal disease	Uncommon	Common
Cure rates	85–95%	70–90%

Differential Diagnosis

The differential diagnosis includes—(i) *infections*: Typical and atypical mycobacterial infections, HIV, EBV, and CMV, (ii) *other malignancies*: Such as nonHodgkin lymphoma, soft tissue sarcoma, nasopharyngeal carcinoma, germ cell tumor, and Castleman disease, (iii) autoimmune disorders such as systemic lupus erythematosus, (iv) benign lymphadenopathy like Rosai–Dorfman disease.

Evaluation

In addition to a thorough history and physical examination, the workup of a patient with suspected HL includes disease confirmation and staging by the following tests.

Confirmatory Tests

Biopsy: An excisional lymph node biopsy is mandatory for confirmation of diagnosis. Since lymph node architecture is important for histological classification, fine needle aspiration cytology alone is not sufficient and not recommended. Reed-sternberg cells (large multinucleate neoplastic cells with 'owls eye' nucleoli) are seen among a background of inflammatory white blood cells. Immune histochemistry confirms diagnosis by showing positivity for CD15 and CD30 on the malignant cells. Compared to classical Hodgkin lymphoma, the nodular lymphocyte predominant variety has a distinct morphology. CD20 is positive rather than CD15 and CD30 in the latter variant.

Disease Staging

- ***Imaging:*** Chest Xray, computed tomography (CT) scan of neck, chest, abdomen, and pelvis should be obtained. Aggregate nodal (peripheral) mass >6 cm is considered as bulky lymphadenopathy. Bulky mediastinal mass is defined as a transverse mediastinal diameter greater than one- third of maximum intrathoracic diameter on an upright posteroanterior (PA) chest radiograph. On CT scan, volume >200 mL of mediastinal or peripheral lymphadenopathy is considered bulky.

- ***Positron emission tomography (PET) scan:*** Whole body PET scan using 18Ffluorodeoxyglucose activity is a more sensitive radiographic modality than computed tomography (CT) scanning.
- ***Bone marrow aspiration and biopsy:*** It is done for patients with advanced disease (stage III/IV), B symptoms, bony involvement, and abnormal counts. Bone marrow biopsy may be avoided in patients undergoing staging evaluation with PET-CT.

Supportive Investigations

These include complete blood counts, liver function tests, kidney function tests, erythrocyte sedimentation rate (ESR), serum lactate dehydrogenase, serum albumin, and viral markers [HIV, hepatitis B surface antigen (HBsAg), and antiHCV].

Staging and Risk Stratification

The Ann Arbor staging system with Cotswolds modification is the current staging system used for patients with HL **(Table 23.15)**. Most pediatric oncology groups use a risk adapted treatment approach. While the specific definitions of low, intermediate-, and high-risk disease may vary with the group, most stratify patients based on stage, disease bulk, systemic (B) symptoms, and extra-lymphatic organ involvement.

TABLE 23.15 Modified Ann Arbor Classification of Hodgkin Lymphoma

Stages	*Definitions*
I	Involvement of a single lymph node (LN) region (I) or of a single extranodal organ or site (IE) in the absence of any lymph node involvement
II	Involvement of two or more LN regions, on the same side of the diaphragm (II) or localized involvement of an extralymphatic organ or site in association with regional lymph node involvement with or without the involvement of other lymph node regions on the same side of the diaphragm (IIE)
III	Involvement of LN regions on both sides of the diaphragm (III), which may be accompanied by involvement of the spleen (IIIS) or by the involvement of an extra-lymphatic organ in association with adjacent lymph node involvement (IIIE) or both (IIISE)
IV	Diffuse or disseminated involvement of one or more extra-lymphatic organ, with or without associated lymph node involvement or isolated extra-lymphatic organ involvement in the absence of adjacent regional lymph node involvement, but in conjunction with the disease at distant site(s). It also includes any involvement of liver, bone marrow, or lungs (other than by direct extension from another site) or cerebrospinal fluid
Annotations	*Definitions*
A B X E	No B symptoms *At least one of the following within the last 6 months:* Unexplained weight loss >10%, unexplained persistent or recurrent fever >38°C for 3 days, drenching night sweats Bulky disease (>6 cm in diameter or mass >1/3rd of transthoracic diameter) Extension to a single extra-lymphatic organ from contiguous nodal disease

TREATMENT Hodgkin Lymphoma

The treatment of HL in children requires a delicate balance to maximize the treatment efficacy and minimize the risk for late toxicities associated with both radiation therapy (RT) and chemotherapy. While RT acts to control known tumor sites, chemotherapy aims at occult disease outside the radiation field. Contemporary protocols tailor treatment intensity based on response to therapy. Hence, the current standard of care for childhood HL is a risk and response adapted use of combination chemotherapy with or without low-dose involved-field RT (IFRT).

Chemotherapy

The contemporary chemotherapy regimens in HL combine non-cross- resistant agents wherein each agent is individually active against tumor but targets different cellular events to prevent drug resistance and have non-overlapping toxicities, which allows delivery of each agent at the full dose. A few commonly used chemotherapy regimens have been highlighted in **Table 23.16**.

Radiotherapy

Radiation has been used as an adjunct to multiagent chemotherapy, especially in intermediate- or high-risk pediatric HL, to reduce the risk of relapse in initially involved sites and prevent toxicity associated with second-line chemotherapy. Doses of 15–25 Gy are typically used with modifications based on patient's age, presence of bulky or residual (post-chemotherapy) disease. Involved-field radiation therapy is the current standard of care in children in place of total nodal RT.

Follow-up and Late Effects

The current 5-year survival for HL is approximately 90%, with higher rates reported in younger populations. The late complications primarily include impaired growth of bones and soft tissues, thyroid dysfunction, gonadal dysfunction, cardiopulmonary toxicity, and second malignancies. Hence, all children treated with HL should be closely followed for relapse as well as late effects. Imaging is not recommended for routine follow-up, as recent studies have shown that most relapses can be detected based on symptoms, laboratory, and physical findings without any incremental value of imaging.

TABLE 23.16 Commonly Used Chemotherapy Regimens for Children with Hodgkin Lymphoma.	
Name	*Drugs*
COPP	Cyclophosphamide, vincristine, procarbazine, and prednisone
COPDAC	Dacarbazine substituted for procarbazine in COPP
OPPA	Vincristine (Oncovin®), procarbazine, prednisone, and Adriamycin
OEPA	Vincristine, etoposide, prednisone, and Adriamycin
ABVD	Adriamycin, bleomycin, vinblastine, and dacarbazine
COPP/ ABV	Cyclophosphamide, vincristine, procarbazine, prednisone, Adriamycin, bleomycin, and vinblastine
VAMP	Vinblastine, Adriamycin, methotrexate, and prednisone
DBVE	Doxorubicin, bleomycin, vincristine, and etoposide
BEACOPP	Bleomycin, etoposide, Adriamycin, cyclophosphamide, vincristine, prednisone, and procarbazine

NON-HODGKIN LYMPHOMA

Epidemiology

Mature B (Burkitt and diffuse large B cell lymphoma) account for 50% of pediatric NHL, followed by T-lymphoblastic lymphoma which constitutes approximately 1/3 of pediatric NHL. Anaplastic large cell lymphoma (ALCL) is another less frequently encountered type. NHL is uncommon in children <5 years of age. Pediatric NHL is more common in males than females in all age groups (3:1), with the exception of primary mediastinal B-cell lymphoma (PMBCL), in which the incidence is almost equal in males and females.

Etiology

The etiology of pediatric NHL is largely unknown. However, known risk factors are immunodeficiency, both congenital (Wiskott-Aldrich syndrome, Xlinked lymphoproliferative syndrome, ataxiatelangiectasia, and severe combined immunodeficiency) and acquired (HIV) or post-transplant immunodeficiency), which increase the risk of NHL 100-fold as compared with age matched controls. Epstein–Barr virus (EBV) is associated with most cases of NHL seen in the immune deficient population.

Clinical Features

Pediatric NHL is a heterogeneous group of neoplasms with a diverse presentation depending on the histological type, primary site and extent of disease **(Table 23.17)**. Pediatric NHL being aggressive, two-thirds of children will have locally advanced or metastatic disease (Stages III and IV) at time of diagnosis. Being rapidly growing tumors, symptoms develop quickly over a few weeks. Signs and symptoms are usually due to local effects attributable to bulk of tumor mass, regional effects due to compression of surrounding structures, and metastasis (bone marrow and CNS). CNS involvement presents with CNS symptoms such as headaches and/or cranial nerve palsy. Bone marrow involvement may lead to pancytopenia.

Staging of NHL

Pediatric NHL are staged according to revised International Pediatric NHL staging system. Stage is important to decide about treatment and prognosis. **Box 23.3** describes staging system for pediatric NHL.

Diagnosis

It is very common for child with NHL to present with an oncological emergency like tumor lysis syndrome, superior mediastinal syndrome, etc. Child should be admitted immediately and pro phylactic and therapeutic measures for tumor lysis syndrome and other oncological emergencies should be started. Adequate hydration and allopurinol should be started and rasburicase should be considered depending upon clinical and biochemical parameters.

TABLE 23.17 Common Subtypes of Pediatric Non-Hodgkin Lymphoma (NHL)			
Histology	*Pathology immunophenotype*	*Clinical presentation*	*Genetics*
Burkitt/Burkitt-like lymphomas (40%)	"Starry sky appearance" intermediate sized homogenous cells Mature B-cell CD10+, CD20+, sIg+ (surface Ig)	Intra-abdominal mass, tonsillar mass, bone marrow involvement with cytopenias, central nervous system (CNS) involvement, and jaw swelling (endemic)	t(8;14), t(2;8), and t(8;22)
Diffuse large B-cell lymphoma (10–20%)	Large B cell with granular cytoplasm, mature B cell CD10+ or CD10-, CD19+, CD20+, CD22+	Lymph node and abdominal masses, bone swelling primary CNS involvement (when associated with immunodeficiency)	
Lymphoblastic lymphoma (15–20%)	Pre-T cell CD3+, TdT+, CD7+,	Mediastinal mass with respiratory distress, lymph node masses, and bone marrow involvement with cytopenias	t(1;14), t(11;14), t(10;14), and t(7;19) t(1;7)
	Pre-B-cell CD10+, CD79a+	Skin and soft tissue nodules and bone involvement	
Anaplastic large cell lymphoma (10–15%)	T cell or null cell type CD30+ (Ki-1+), EMA +ve, ALK +/–	Skin nodules, lymph node masses, bone swelling, soft tissue mass, and lung	t(2;5)
Primary mediastinal large B-cell (3%)	B cells of medullary thymus CD10+ or CD10–, CD19+, CD20+, CD22+, CD79a+	Mediastinal mass	Del 9q
(EMA: epitherial membrane antigen; ALK: anaplastic lymphoma kinase)			

Box 23.3 International Staging System for Pediatric Non-Hodgkin Lymphoma (IPNHLSS)

Stage I

A single tumor (extranodal) or involvement of a single anatomical area (nodal), with the exclusion of the mediastinum and abdomen

Stage II

- A single tumor (extranodal) with regional node involvement
- Two or more nodal areas on the same side of the diaphragm
- Two single (extranodal) tumors, with or without regional node involvement on the same side of the diaphragm
- A primary gastrointestinal tract tumor (usually in the ileocecal area), with or without involvement of associated mesenteric nodes, that is completely resectable without malignant ascites or local extension

Stage III

- Two single tumors (extranodal) on opposite sides of the diaphragm
- Two or more nodal areas above and below the diaphragm
- Any primary intrathoracic tumor (mediastinal, pleural, or thymic)
- Extensive primary intra-abdominal disease
- Any paraspinal or epidural tumor
- Primary bone lymphoma

Stage IV

Any of the above findings with initial involvement of the central nervous system, bone marrow, or both

- Blood count, serum electrolytes, serum uric acid, blood urea, serum creatinine, serum calcium and, serum phosphate, and lactate dehydrogenase (LDH).
- Chest Xray and ultrasound abdomen.
- Computed tomography scan of neck, chest, abdomen, and pelvis.
- Bone marrow aspiration and biopsy can be diagnostic if marrow is involved by lymphoma and also required as a part of staging investigation.
- In case of pleural or peritoneal effusion, fluid cytology, and flow cytometry of fluid.
- Lymph node biopsy from accessible location if lymphadenopathy present.
- Open/image-guided biopsy of mass in case above investigations do not yield diagnosis
- Magnetic resonance imaging in children with paraspinal mass or suspected CNS infiltration.
- Cerebrospinal fluid analysis.

Differential Diagnosis

- ***Infections:*** Tuberculosis, toxoplasmosis, atypical mycobacterium infections, and EBV infection
- ***Immunological/inflammatory:*** Systemic lupus erythematosus and disorders causing reactive hyperplasia of lymph nodes
- ***Malignancy:*** Hodgkin lymphoma, metastatic adenopathy from other primary tumors (e.g., nasopharyngeal carcinoma and soft tissue sarcoma), germ cell tumor, thymic carcinoma, neuroblastoma, and Castleman disease.
- Benign lymphadenopathy such as Kikuchi disease and Rosai–Dorfman disease
- ***Surgical:*** Appendicitis and intussusception

TREATMENT Non-Hodgkin Lymphoma

Childhood NHL is an extremely chemosensitive disease. Surgery plays a very limited role, mainly for arriving at a diagnosis, or for emergency management of obstruction or perforation. Radiation of primary sites is used very rarely in emergency situations, such as a large mediastinal mass causing airway obstruction. Multiagent chemotherapy directed to the histologic subtype and stage of the disease remains the cornerstone of therapy. Immunotherapy with drugs such as rituximab now has a proven role in advanced stage aggressive B-cell lymphomas. Early stage NHL have a survival of 85-95% with treatment, while survival is 70-90% even in most advanced stage NHL.

IN A NUTSHELL

Lymphoma

1. Painless, progressive, lymphadenopathy is one of the most common presentations of pediatric lymphoma.
2. Other symptoms and signs of lymphoma include unexplained fever, night sweats, loss of appetite or weight loss, coughing or difficulty breathing or abdominal distention (due to organomegaly or lymphadenopathy).
3. Lymphomas are broadly classified into two groups: Hodgkin and (2) non-Hodgkin lymphoma.
4. Lymph node biopsy is the cornerstone of diagnosis of childhood lymphoma. Other tests such as bone marrow aspiration, CT scan, and PET scan help in staging the lymphoma.
5. Pediatric lymphomas are typically chemosensitive and are managed with regimens using multiple chemotherapy drugs with synergistic effect. Radiotherapy is used in adjunct with chemotherapy in selected cases.

Belsky JA, Hochberg J, Giulino-Roth L. Diagnosis and management of Hodgkin lymphoma in children, adolescents, and young adults. Best Pract Res Clin Haematol. 2023;36:101445.

Catueno S, Cuglievan B. Pediatric lymphomas: key concepts and clinical approaches for pediatricians. Pediatr Rev. 2025;46:78-90.

Daw S, Hasenclever D, Mascarin M, et al. Risk and Response Adapted Treatment Guidelines for Managing First Relapsed and Refractory Classical Hodgkin Lymphoma in Children and Young People. Recommendations from the EuroNet Pediatric Hodgkin Lymphoma Group. Hemasphere. 2020;4(1):e329.

23.17 When to Refer a Child with Hematological Disorder?

PE 26.15

Children with following symptoms or laboratory findings should be referred to pediatrician or specialist:

- Unexplained progressive symptomatic anemia (thalassemia and hemolytic anemia)
- Iron deficiency showing suboptimal response to oral iron therapy after a 6–8 weeks trial of iron (thalassemia and hemolytic anemia)
- Anemia in association with—splenomegaly or lymphadenopathy or other cytopenia (suspected leukemia)
- Platelet count 50–100 × 10^9/L in association with other cytopenia (hemoglobin <100 g/L, neutrophils <1 × 10^9/L) splenomegaly, and lymphadenopathy (leukemia or aplastic anemia)
- Platelet count <50 × 10^9/L (immune thrombocytopenic purpura, aplastic anemia, and leukemia)
- Persistent, unexplained thrombocytopenia <100 × 10^9/L (immune thrombocytopenic purpura and aplastic anemia)
- Lymphadenopathy >1 cm persisting for >6 weeks with no obvious infective precipitant (Hodgkin lymphoma, non Hodgkin lymphoma, and leukemia)
- ***Lymphocytosis in association with:*** Anemia, thrombo cytopenia or neutropenia, splenomegaly, painful or progressive lymphadenopathy, "B" symptoms (weight loss >10%, soaking sweats, and unexplained fever)
- Suspected myelodysplastic syndrome (based on blood film report)
- Neutrophil count <1 × 10^9/L (aplastic anemia and leukemia)
- Neutropenia in association with: other cytopenia, lymphadenopathy or splenomegaly (leukemia)

23.18 Bone Marrow Aspiration and Bone Biopsy

PE 26.14

INTRODUCTION

Bone marrow examination is a useful tool in the diagnosis and staging of various hematologic diseases and in the assessment of bone marrow cellularity, cellular morphology, and maturation. Highly specialized testing, such as cytogenetic, immunophenotypic, and molecular analyses, can be performed on these specimens, and have become critically important in establishing certain diagnoses, especially the leukemias and lymphomas. Bone marrow biopsy is particularly important to evaluate the bone marrow cellularity.

INDICATIONS

- Diagnosis and management of acute leukemia, myelodysplastic syndrome, and myeloproliferative neoplasm
- Staging for lymphoma
- Staging for small round cell tumors such as neuroblastoma, rhabdomyosarcoma, and Ewing sarcoma
- Evaluation of pancytopenia
- Evaluation of unexplained anemia, thrombocytopenia, and/or neutropenia
- Fever of unknown origin
- Evaluation of iron metabolism and stores when routine laboratory testing is inadequate
- Evaluation of unexplained splenomegaly
- Confirmation that the bone marrow is normal in a potential allogeneic hematopoietic cell donor.

CONTRAINDICATIONS

- Skin or soft tissue infection at aspiration site
- Osteomyelitis at aspiration site
- Severe hemophilia, severe disseminated intravascular coagulopathy, or other related severe bleeding disorders. Thrombocytopenia is not absolute contraindication provided effective hemostasis can be achieved at procedure site

CHOICE OF SITE

The posterior superior iliac crest and spine is the preferred site of aspiration in children and in most infants. This site also provides the least discomfort to the patient compared with other sites. In premature infants and some full-term infants, the iliac bone has not completely ossified, and the anterior portion of the tibia can be used for aspiration only.

Salah bone marrow aspiration needle with a stylet is used **(Figs. 23.23A and B)**. Jamshidi biopsy needle with stylet and an obturator for removing the biopsy core from the needle without damage to the specimen is recommended **(Fig. 23.24)**. Detailed descriptions of bone marrow aspiration and biopsy procedures are available in "*Clinical Methods in Pediatrics*" by Piyush Gupta.

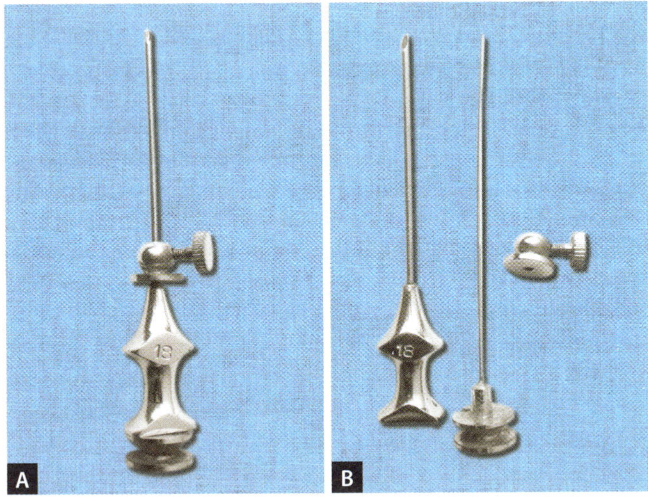

Figs. 23.23A and B: Salah bone marrow aspiration needle with stylet and guard

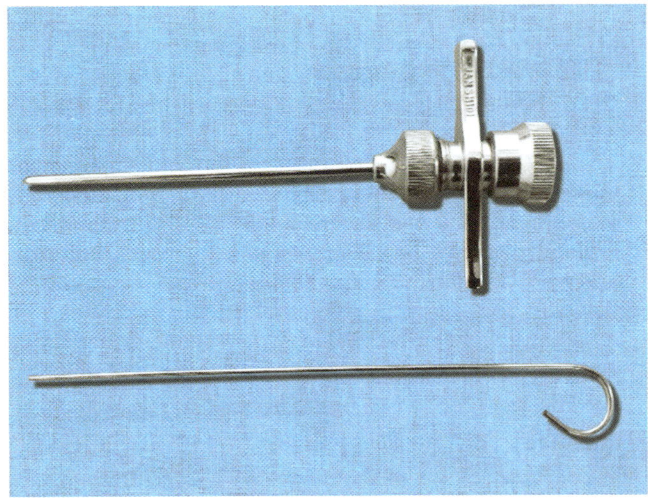

Fig. 23.24: Jamshidi bone marrow biopsy needle

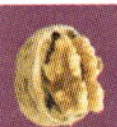

IN A NUTSHELL

Bone Marrow Aspiration and Bone Biopsy

1. Bone marrow examination is useful in the diagnosis and staging of hematologic disease, as well as in the assessment of overall bone marrow cellularity.
2. It is also useful in the assessment of patients with fever of undetermined origin as well as in the diagnosis of various storage and infiltrative disorders.
3. Highly specialized testing such as cytogenetic immuno-phenotypic and molecular analyses, can be performed on bone marrow aspirates and especially in children with suspected lymphoreticular malignancy.
4. The posterior superior iliac crest is the preferred site for bone marrow aspiration.
5. Bone marrow aspiration and/or biopsy is contraindicated patients with severe hemophilia, severe disseminated intravascular coagulation, or other related severe bleeding disorders.

Bhaskar N. Bone marrow aspiration and biopsy in critical pediatric patients: a pathologist's perspective. Cureus. 2021;13(8):e17423.

23.19 Counseling for Prevention of Anemia

PE 26.16

INTRODUCTION

Parents should be given information regarding at risk children for developing anemia, and counseled regarding measures to be taken to reduce the risk of anemia.

INFANTS AND CHILDREN AT HIGHEST RISK OF IRON DEFICIENCY

- Premature or low birth weight infants
- Maternal anemia during pregnancy
- Multiple gestation
- Babies who are started on cow's milk or goat's milk before age of 1 year
- Breast-fed infants who are not given complementary foods containing iron after age 6 months
- Formula-fed infants that is not fortified with iron
- Children who have certain health conditions, such as chronic infections
- Children who do not eat enough iron-rich foods
- Children who are overweight or obese
- Adolescent girls also are at higher risk of iron deficiency because their bodies lose iron during menstruation

COUNSEL TO TAKE FOLLOWING MEASURES TO PREVENT ANEMIA

- Children should be provided foods with added iron. For older children, good sources of iron include red meat, chicken, fish, beans, and spinach. Green leafy vegetables such as amaranth (*chaulai sag/dantu*), spinach (*palak*), turnip leaves (*shalgam ka sag*), mint leaves (*pudina*), and small amounts of tamarind (*imli*) added to the diet daily will together provide the amount of iron recommended.

- Parents should be counseled to start complementary feeding at 6 months with appropriate amount and frequency.
- Children should be given foods from all food groups.
- Child should be given whole grain or enriched breads and cereals.
- Vitamin C increases the absorption of iron. Parents should be encouraged to combine vitamin C foods with iron foods. It is recommended to increase the intake of germinated seeds, fermented cereals, heatprocessed cereals, meats, and fruits and green vegetables rich in vitamin C.
- It is also important to recommend that vegetables rich in vitamin C, folate, and other watersoluble or heatlabile vitamins be minimally cooked in small amounts of water.
- Use cast iron cookware.
- Limit tea and coffee consumption.
- For fully breastfed babies, iron supplements should be started after 3 months.
- For premature infants, iron supplement should be started at age 2 weeks and should be continued until 1 year of age.
- Children should be dewormed using oral albendazole biannually.
- Cow's milk intake should be delayed till 1 year of age if possible.
- Delayed cord clamping must be practised after birth (after cessation of visible cord pulsations or till 120-180 seconds).

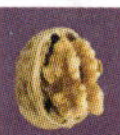

IN A NUTSHELL

Counseling for Prevention of Anemia

1. Infants and children at risk of developing anemia should be identified and parents should be given information about prevention of anemia.
2. Children should be started on complimentary feeding at 6 months of age with appropriate food and frequency.
3. Foods from all the classes should be included in diet along with food rich in iron.
4. All infants should be given iron supplements and deworming should be done biannually.
5. Delayed cord clamping must be practised after birth (after cessation of visible cord pulsations or till 120–180 seconds).

Sidharth Totadri and Pooja Dewan

CHAPTER 24

Neurological Disorders

AS PER NMC COMPETENCIES

PE27.1	Explain the etiopathogenesis, clinical features, complications, management, and prevention of acute bacterial meningitis in children.	*Ch 24.3*
PE27.2	Describe the etiopathogenesis, clinical features, complications, management and prevention of tuberculous meningitis.	*Ch 24.4*
PE27.3	Distinguish bacterial, viral and tuberculous meningitis.	*Ch 24.2, 24.3, 24.4*
PE27.4	Explain the etiopathogenesis, classification, clinical features, complication and management of hydrocephalus in children.	*Ch 24.7*
PE27.5	Explain the etiopathogenesis, clinical features, and management of infantile hemiplegia.	*Ch 24.8*
PE27.6	Explain the etiopathogenesis, clinical features, complications and management of febrile seizures in children.	*Ch 24.9*
PE27.7	Define epilepsy. Discuss the pathogenesis, clinical types, presentation and management of epilepsy in children.	*Ch 24.10*
PE27.8	Define status epilepticus. Discuss the clinical presentation and management.	*Ch 27.8*
PE27.9	Describe the etiopathogenesis, clinical features and management of mental retardation in children.	*Ch 3.1*
PE27.10	Describe the etiopathogenesis, clinical features and management of children with cerebral palsy.	*Ch 24.11*
PE27.11	Enumerate the causes of floppiness in an infant and discuss the clinical features, differential diagnosis and management.	*Ch 24.12* *Ch 24.13*
PE27.12	Explain the etiopathogenesis, clinical features and management of Duchenne muscular dystrophy.	*Ch 24.14*
PE27.13	Interpret and explain the findings in a CSF analysis.	*Ch 24.2*
PE27.14	Perform in a mannequin lumbar puncture. Discuss the indications, contraindication of the procedure.	*Ch 24.2*

Topics available online: ***Ataxia, Central Nervous System (CNS) Tumors, Headache, Microcephaly, Movement Disorders, Neural Tube Defects***

24.1 Neurological History and Examination

INTRODUCTION

In 1885, while facing a patient with complex neuropathology, Dr Jean-Martin Charcot, alongside observing students Josef Babinski, Sigmund Freud, and others, relied on his key resources: a thorough history and a meticulous examination. Even today, neurologic examination, informed by a comprehensive history, remains fundamental to diagnosing neurological conditions. Perhaps now more than ever, the neurologic examination sharpens the diagnostic process and safeguards patients from unnecessary harm.

HISTORY

There is no substitute for a thorough history. Clinical history-taking goals include building rapport and trust with the child and family, pinpointing the anatomical location of neurologic symptoms, and understanding the possible pathological process leading to the symptoms. A proficient clinician can frequently reach a diagnosis by the conclusion of the complete history and uses the examination to validate the diagnosis and assess the degree of impairment. The various components of history include the following.

A. ***Presenting complaint and history of presenting illness:*** The patient or parent starts by explaining their concern, known as the "Presenting complaint(s)." In most history-taking setups, this initial statement rarely exceeds 60 seconds unless interrupted, which, unfortunately, is often done by the physician. Following the presenting complaint, more specific questions are asked about the complaint to understand the onset, duration, and course of the symptoms. This is followed by a history pertaining to the neuraxis to aid in localizing the pathological process. Next, a history of various etiological factors and complications related to the disease is obtained. These questions are designed to develop a differential diagnosis and assess the degree of impairment. **Table 24.1** summarizes the salient features of the history of the presenting illness. The goal is to start broadly and consider all disease categories until a more focused differential diagnosis can be made.

B. ***Antenatal history:*** Reviewing the history from conception is essential in any history taking and often provides critical information for making an appropriate diagnosis, complementing details gathered from the current illness history **(Table 24.1)**.

C. ***Birth history:*** Delivery details are critical **(Table 24.1)**. These are often not fully recalled by parents, so reviewing available birth records is essential. Relevant information includes labor duration, mode of delivery (like normal vaginal delivery, forceps and vacuum extraction, or lower segment cesarean section), presence of meconium, and gestational age; all these impact brain development. The newborn's status right after delivery is significant, including objective information like birth weight, Apgar scores, head circumference, and any neonatal complications.

Table 24.1 Summary of History-Taking in a Child with a Suspected Neurological Disorder

History	*Details*
Presenting complaints	• Patient or parent begins with an explanation of his or her concern, which is the presenting complaint. • It should include the complaint and its duration
History of present illness	• Clarifying the history of the current illness is to answer four basic questions: ▪ Is the process acute or insidious? ▪ Is it focal or generalized? ▪ Is it progressive or static? ▪ At what age did the problem begin? • Typically begins with details about the presenting complaint and includes: ▪ Duration of symptoms ▪ Whether symptoms are constant or episodic (episodic symptoms are characteristic of transient ischemic attack, syncope, seizure, or migraine) ▪ Whether symptoms are static, progressive, or resolving ▪ Whether activities of daily living have been compromised • History to suggest a neuroanatomic localization ▪ Involvement of the cerebral cortex should be suspected in patients with cognitive dysfunction and/or seizures ▪ Symptoms of weakness along with tightness of limbs suggests involvement of corticospinal tract (i.e., upper motor neuron type of disorder) ▪ History suggestive of bizarre twisting movements of limbs (dystonia) or flinging and quasi-purposive movements (chorea) and slow writhing movements (athetosis) suggests involvement of basal ganglia ▪ History suggestive of cranial nerve involvement should be sought [visual acuity (cranial nerve II), malalignment of eyes (cranial nerve III/IV/VI), difficulty in chewing (cranial nerve V), inability to close the eyes while sleeping/drooling from angle of mouth/deviation of angle of mouth (cranial nerve VII), auditory acuity (cranial nerve VIII), nasal regurgitation of liquids and solids (cranial nerve IX and X) and inability to move bolus of food in mouth (cranial nerve XII)]

Contd...

Contd...

History	Details
	▪ History of instability during walking or smearing of face while eating or jerky movements of eyes or slurring of speech is suggestive of cerebellar disorders ▪ History of reduced perception of pain after a fall or impaired temperature perception while handling hot objects (spinothalamic pathway) ▪ History of banging head on the wash basin or losing stability while washing face (dorsal column involvement) ▪ Disorders of the spinal cord may result in dissociation of motor and sensory function below a certain spinal level with/without bowel and bladder dysfunction. This implies lower motor neuron lesion at the level of spinal segment involvement and upper motor neuron lesion below that level ▪ Disorders of the motor unit (anterior horn cells, peripheral nerve, neuromuscular junction, muscle) should be suspected in patients with weakness manifested by inability to climb stairs, raise the arms, grasp, stand, or walk • History to suggest underlying etiology ▪ Antenatal, birth and neonatal details (as below) suggest an intrauterine/perinatal insult ▪ History of traumatic brain injury or febrile encephalopathy or near drowning may suggest post-natal insults to brain ▪ History of episodes of altered sensorium associated with minor febrile events, abnormal body odor, abnormal hair or skin pigmentation may suggest an underlying inborn error of metabolism • History of associated conditions and complications ▪ Sleep impairment related to initiation and duration of sleep ▪ Recurrent respiratory tract infections may suggest impaired deglutition ▪ Tightness of limbs with inability to move across certain joints (for contractures) ▪ Behavioral disorders ▪ Compromise in activities of daily living
Antenatal history	• Mother's age at the time of pregnancy • History of mother's previous pregnancies (gravida, para, miscarriages, and gestational age at the time of miscarriages) • Intake of folic acid before conception and during pregnancy especially first trimester • Fever with rash (intrauterine infections) • Exposure to drugs (methotrexate/antiseizure drugs/chemotherapeutic drugs) • Exposures to toxins such as alcohol, nicotine • Any medical issues encountered during pregnancy like hypertension, diabetes • At what point was fetal movement first noted (i.e., quickening), which should be at approximately 4–5 months of gestation, and did it continue throughout the entire pregnancy?
Birth history	• Gestational age at delivery • Mode of delivery (normal vaginal/instrumental/cesarean and indication) • Presence of meconium at delivery • Need for resuscitation • Birth weight • History suggestive of neonatal encephalopathy including irritability/lethargy/feed refusal/seizures • History of hypoglycemia/delayed cry at birth/hyperbilirubinemia • History of NICU admission/respiratory support • Age at which breast feedings were established and age of discharge from hospital
Development history	• The clinician should record the child's age at acquisition of developmental milestones, such as social smiling, developing adequate head control, cooing, reaching out for objects, rolling over, being able to maintain a sitting position, coming to a sitting position independently, crawling, walking independently, babbling, and using first words, phrases, and sentences. These should be clubbed under following domains: gross motor/fine motor/socio-cognitive/language. • Specific history for loss of previously attained milestones should be obtained (for regression)
Family history	• History of consanguinity • History of similar or related neurological issues in other family members • A pedigree chart is often helpful
Socioeconomic history	• History related to financial status/earning members • Number of members staying in household • Status of water supply

D. ***Development history:*** Development history should include all major developmental domains (gross motor, fine motor, socio-cognitive, and language). Documenting the attainment of milestones in these domains allows for the characterization of a child's developmental progress compared with age-based norms. These should be categorized as normal, delayed attainment of milestones but progressively gaining, or regression of milestones (i.e., losing previously attained milestones). This information is essential for the diagnosis of static or progressive neuropathology.

E. ***Family history:*** Family history helps in narrowing down the possible genetic etiologies. Begin by asking about consanguinity and if any family members suffer from similar complaints. The same genetic disorder can have different phenotypes; hence, a history of different phenotypes among family members should be obtained (intellectual disability, epilepsy, and early childhood deaths can be different phenotypes of the same underlying genetic underpinning). Consanguinity refers to the relationship between individuals who share a common ancestor. It indicates a genetic relationship where two people have a blood relation, which can be established through direct lineage. Consanguinity is often categorized by degrees, such as first-degree relatives (parents, siblings), second-degree relatives (grandparents, aunts, uncles), and third-degree (relation beyond the second degree).

Autosomal-dominant traits can appear in consecutive generations, though their expressiveness can differ. In contrast, autosomal-recessive traits typically skip generations but may be observed in siblings. Consanguinity should be taken into account when considering autosomal recessive disease as part of the differential diagnosis, even if it does not emerge from interviewing the parents. X-linked recessive conditions typically manifest in male siblings, male first cousins, and maternal uncles. Mitochondrial diseases are typically inherited through the transmission of maternal DNA. Trinucleotide repeat diseases such as fragile X syndrome may show genetic anticipation manifested by increasing severity through generations.

F. ***Social history:*** A child's cognitive and behavioral development is shaped by their home environment. Social history can reveal risk factors like family's economic and affordability status, violence, parental depression, or bullying. In addition, parental occupation may suggest exposure to toxins like lead.

EXAMINATION

The neurologic examination reveals essential and distinctive information that cannot be obtained in other ways. This information remains consistent across all age groups and includes mental status, cranial nerve function, motor evaluation, deep tendon reflexes, sensory function, and cerebellar testing. However, the methods for obtaining this information vary significantly with age. The neurologic examination starts during the interview. Observing the child's appearance and movements indirectly provides important clues regarding any underlying disorders. For example, it might be apparent if the child displays dysmorphic features, has an unusual posture, shows signs of motor function abnormalities such as hemiparesis or gait issues, or exhibits abnormal behavior.

The examination must take place in a welcoming, child-friendly environment. Children should have the option to sit in a comfortable spot, whether on a parent's lap or on the floor of the examination room. The physician should approach gradually, postponing any invasive, painful, or uncomfortable tests until the end (for instance, head circumference measurement or gag reflex assessment). Ultimately, if the examination feels more like a game, the child is likely to cooperate better.

Table 24.2 highlights the clues in general examination specific to a child with a neurological disorder. The neurological exam should be customized and frequently conducted in a non-linear manner to foster trust between the child and the examiner throughout the process. Older, collaborative children can be assessed like adults, following a specific sequence and with careful attention, while expecting them to comprehend and adhere to the instructions provided. The summary of details of the neurological examination is highlighted in **Table 24.3**. These may have to be tailored to the chronological and developmental age of the child.

Table 24.2 Specific General Physical Examination of a Child with a Suspected Neurological Disorder

Examination	*Details*
Appearance and behavior	• The examination should begin with a statement of child's general appearance, behavior and any obvious abnormalities noted, which may be described in detail later
Vital signs	• Pulse: Bradycardia along with hypertension may suggest raised intracranial pressure • Blood pressure: Determining the blood pressure in both arms is useful in patients with suspected cerebrovascular disease. Significant asymmetries may reflect extracranial cardiovascular occlusive disease. Measuring the BP with the patient supine, seated, and upright may be necessary to detect orthostatic hypotension which may suggest autonomic insufficiency
Anthropometry	• Head circumference should be measured and plotted to categorize the head size as normal, microcephalic or macrocephalic • Anterior fontanelle (size and pulsatility)
Neurocutaneous markers	• Café-au-lait macules (neurofibromatosis Type 1, McCune-Albright syndrome) • Ash leaf macules (tuberous sclerosis) • Facial angiofibromas (tuberous sclerosis) • Periungual fibromas (tuberous sclerosis) • Shagreen patch (tuberous sclerosis) • Hemangioma/port wine stain (Sturge-Weber syndrome) • Angiokeratomas (Fabry's disease)
Dysmorphism	• Facial features ▪ Prominent ears (Fragile X) ▪ Flat nasal bridge (Down syndrome) ▪ Mongoloid slant (inwards downwards slant of the eye seen with Down syndrome) ▪ Epicanthal folds (Down syndrome) ▪ Hypertelorism (increased distance between the eyes, seen with craniosynostosis like Apert syndrome) ▪ Corneal clouding (mucopolysaccharidosis) • Body morphology ▪ Short stature (Turners syndrome) ▪ Polydactyly (presence of extra digits, seen with Dow syndrome) ▪ Syndactyly (presence of fused digits, seen with trisomy 13 and 21, Fanconi anemia, VACTERL) ▪ Clinodactyly (finger, usually the fifth finger bending inwards towards the fourth finger, seen with Down syndrome)

Contd...

Contd...

Examination	*Details*
Others	• Shape of head along with ridging of sutures for craniosynostosis • Cranial bruit for cranial AVM • Abnormal body odor/hair or skin pigmentation (suggestive of inborn error of metabolism) • Congenital cataract (congenital rubella infection, galactosemia) • Transillumination may be used in infants with suspected hydrocephalus • Kayser-Fleischer rings (Wilson's disease) • Tortuous conjunctival vessels (ataxia telangiectasia) • Signs of micronutrient deficiency (Bitot spots, conjunctival xerosis, angular stomatitis, cheilitis, glossitis, frontal bossing, widened wrists, rachitic rosary)

Table 24.3 Neurological Examination Summary

Examination	*Details*
Mental status examination	A. General behavior and appearance ▪ Behavior: Normal, hyperactive, agitated, quiet, or immobile ▪ Appearance: Dressed in accordance with age, peers, sex B. Stream of talk ▪ Does the patient converse normally? ▪ Is the speech lacking spontaneity, tangential, or unable to reach the conversational goal. C. Mood and affective responses ▪ Is the child euphoric, agitated, inappropriately happy or silent, weeping, or angry. ▪ Is the child emotionally labile or overtly depressed? D. Content of thought: Does the child have illusions, hallucinations, delusions, misinterpretations, and obsessions. E. Intellectual capacity: Is the child bright, average or intellectually disabled. F. Sensorium ▪ Consciousness ▪ Orientation for time, place and person ▪ Memory ▪ Attention span ▪ Fund of information ▪ Insight ▪ Calculation
Speech	• Comprehension (ability to understand speech) • Articulation (enunciation of words and phrases) • Phonation (production of vocal sounds) • Prosody (rhythm, intonation, stressing certain parts and pauses during speech) • Naming • Repetition • Reading • Writing

Contd...

Contd...

Examination	*Details*
Cranial nerves	• I: May be challenging to test in children; aromatic, nonirritating substance can be used to test each nostril separately with patients' eyes closed. • II: Visual acuity, color vision, field of vision, fundoscopy and pupillary reflex (has optic nerve as afferent and oculomotor as efferent) • III, IV, VI: Test range of ocular movements and smoothness of pursuit as the child's eyes follow your finger through all fields of gaze • V: Inspect the masseter and temporalis muscle bulk and palpate masseter muscles when the child bites for the motor component of trigeminal nerve. For the sensory component, corneal reflex and touch, pain and temperature are tested over the three divisions • VII: Test forehead wrinkling, eyelid closure, loss of buccolabial fold, deviation of angle of mouth, whistling or puffing out of cheeks • VIII: Assess threshold and acuity by noting the Pt's ability to hear conversational speech and to hear a tuning fork, a watch tick, or finger rustling • IX, X: Listen for phonation, articulation (labial, lingual, and palatal sounds) and check swallowing and palatal elevation. Due to inconsistencies associated with gag reflex and also the associated risks, it can be avoided. • XI: Inspect sternocleidomastoid and trapezius contours and test strength of head movements and shoulder shrugging • XII: Inspect for atrophy, and fasciculations; and midline protrusion, lateral movements.
Motor system	• *Inspection* ▪ Posture of limbs (scissoring suggests hypertonia, external surfaces of limbs touching the bed suggests hypotonia) ▪ Voluntary movements if present ▪ Involuntary movements including tremors or extrapyramidal movements. • *Gait assessment* should include stance, free walk (heel to toe or toe first; stride length), arm swing during walking, executing a turn, tandem walking, toe walking and heel walking ▪ *Spastic gait:* Toe walking with buckling of knees and hip flexion; legs may scissor as they walk ▪ *Hemiparetic gait:* Associated with spasticity and circumduction of the leg, and decreased arm swing on the affected side ▪ *Cerebellar ataxia:* Results in a wide-based gait like that of a drunk person/walking in a moving train ▪ *Sensory ataxia:* Results in high-steppage gait where the patient lifts the legs up higher than usual in the swing phase and then slaps the foot down. ▪ *Myopathic or waddling gait:* Associated with hip girdle weakness. Affected children walk with side-to-side movement of pelvis and torso and often develop a compensatory lordosis.

Contd...

Contd...

Examination	Details
	• *Palpation* ▪ Bulk of muscles measured bilaterally at equivalent points ▪ Tone is assessed as per - Posture (inspected as above) - Feel of muscles - Passive movements across joints and assessing resistance to movements and range of movements - Maneuvers like vertical suspension, horizontal suspension, rolling the limb and sudden jerk across the ankle joint and assessing the fall • *Power:* Should be across all the muscle groups in upper and lower limbs, and trunk. It should be graded as per the MRC scale from 0 to 5 • *Reflexes* ▪ *Deep tendon jerks* should be assessed and grade from 0 to 3 and designated as clonic, where applicable - Jaw jerk (CrN V afferent; CrN V efferent) - Biceps reflex (C5–6) - Brachioradialis reflex (C5-6) - Triceps reflex (C7–8) - Quadriceps reflex (knee jerk; L2–4) - Ankle jerk (S1–2) ▪ *Superficial reflexes* - Abdominal reflex (upper quadrants T8–9; lower quadrants T11–12) - Cremasteric reflex (afferent L1; efferent L2) - Anal pucker reflex (S4–5) - Plantar reflex (Babinski's maneuver; afferent S1; efferent L5–S1–2) • *Percussion of muscle:* Percuss the thenar eminence for percussion myotonia and test for a myotonic grip • *Abnormal movements:* Like seizures, extrapyramidal movements (dystonia, chorea, athetosis, ballismus), tremors, fasciculations • *Primitive reflexes:* Primitive reflexes (Moro, palmar grasp, asymmetric tonic neck reflex, Landau, parachute) appear and fade at specific developmental stages, and their absence or persistence beyond these periods indicates CNS dysfunction.
Sensory system	• Superficial sensations ▪ Light touch ▪ Temperature discrimination ▪ Pain perception • Deep sensory modalities ▪ Vibration ▪ Position sense ▪ Astereognosis ▪ Directional scratch test ▪ Romberg test
Cerebellar	• Finger-to-nose • Heel to shin

Contd...

Contd...

Examination	Details
	• Rapid alternating hand movements (dysdiadokokinesia) • Dysmetria • Hypotonia • Ataxia • Dysarthria • Pendular knee jerk
Signs of meningeal irritation	• Nuchal rigidity • Brudzinski • Kernigs
Developmental assessment	• Developmental examination should be carried out using age-appropriate tests. At the end of developmental assessment, developmental age in each of domains (motor, socio-cognitive and language) should be determined.

A. ***Mental status:*** Careful observation of the patient during the assessment can help gauge the emotional well-being, memory, intellect, observational skills, character, and personality of the child. Following the mental status examination, the examiner should be able to summarize the findings as appearance, behavior, stream of talk, mood, content of thought, intellectual capacity and sensorium. Sensorium assessment is significant and is further subdivided into consciousness (conscious, minimally conscious, vegetative, or comatose), orientation to time, place, and person, memory (recent and remote), attention span, fund of information, insight, and calculation. Consciousness signifies awareness of self and environment.

B. ***Speech:*** Communicative speech comprises words organized according to the rules of grammar and syntax, enhanced by prosody. Basically, there are four levels of disturbed speech production: dysphonia, dysarthria, dysprosody, and dysphasia.
   - *Dysphonia* is a disturbance in or a lack of, the production of sounds in the larynx.
   - *Dysarthria* is a disorder that involves abnormalities in articulating speech.
   - *Dysprosodies* consist of scanning speech (cerebellar), plateau speech (basal motor nuclei/parkinsonian), and stuttering, and absence of emotional inflections (cerebral).
   - *Dysphasia* means a disturbance in the understanding or expression of words as symbols for communication.

C. ***Cranial nerves:*** Examining cranial nerves is an integral part of neurological assessment. It aids in the localization of the lesion and determining the likely differential diagnosis. Testing for olfactory nerve is challenging among children. The optic nerve (cranial nerve II) extends from the retina posteriorly through the optic chiasm, where it separates into two optic tracts. Each optic tract comprises two sets of axons. One set of axons comes from the ipsilateral temporal half of the retina, while the other set of axons comes from the contralateral nasal half of the retina. These two groups of axons connect the right and left visual half-fields from each eye. The visual field defects associated with lesions involving various parts of visual pathway are depicted in **(Fig. 24.1)**. The extraocular movements and associated impact of muscle paresis has been illustrated in **(Fig. 24.2)**.

D. ***Motor system:*** The tone, bulk, and strength of the skeletal muscles should be determined during the examination of the motor system.

- *Muscle bulk* is assessed through gentle palpation and observation. Abnormalities include atrophy and fasciculations associated with anterior horn cell disease, as well as muscle hypertrophy, particularly of the gastrocnemius and deltoid muscles linked to Duchenne muscular dystrophy and other dystrophies, along with myotonia congenita. Muscle tenderness, nerve tenderness, and nerve hypertrophy can also be assessed by palpation.
- *Muscle tone* is assessed when the child is relaxed, allowing for an observation of resistance to passive movement. In addition to evaluating the passive movement of limbs at joints, the examiner checks the extensibility of muscles by gently shaking the limbs and measuring their range of motion. Often, multiple muscles are involved in the movement. Therefore, when testing the strength of selected muscles, the examiner should observe and palpate the surrounding muscles to identify any substitution of action by other muscles.
- *Muscle strength* is graded according to the Medical Research Council scale **(Table 24.4)**. Deep tendon reflexes are easily elicited with a reflex hammer while the child sits quietly. The response to the elicitation of deep tendon reflexes can be characterized as follows:
    - 0 = Absent
    - 1 = Hyporeflexia (elicited only with reinforcement)
    - 2 = Normal
    - 3 = Hyperreflexia
    - 4 = Unsustained clonus
    - 5 = Sustained clonus

The motor system examination should aid in determining whether the lesion is related to upper or lower motor neurons **(Table 24.5)**.

E. ***Sensory system:*** Sensory system evaluation involves the assessment of lateral column (crude touch, pain, and temperature) and dorsal column sensations (light touch, proprioception, vibration, stereognosis, graphesthesia) and cortical sensations (like two-point discrimination).

F. ***Cerebellar function assessment:*** Cerebellar functions are crucial for the coordination of voluntary movements, balance, and posture. Cerebellar dysfunction is usually associated with hypotonia, intention tremors, dysdiadokokinesia, dysmetria, ataxia, nystagmus, and dysarthria.

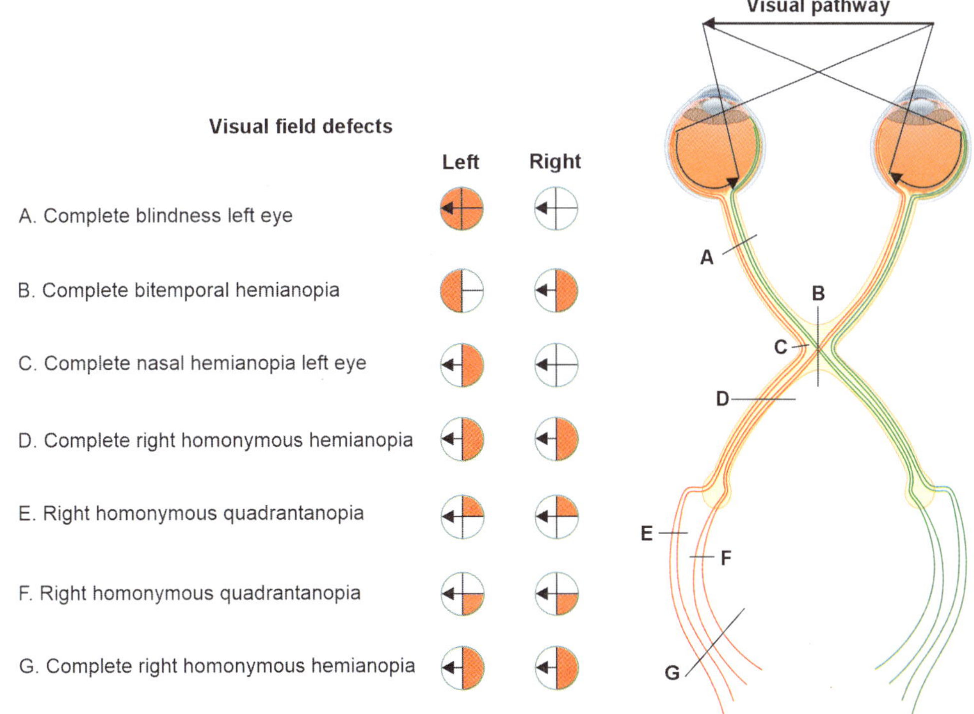

Fig. 24.1: The visual pathway has been depicted. The optic nerve runs from the retina posteriorly to the optic chiasm where it divides into two optic tracts. Each optic tract contains two sets of axons. One set of axons comes from the ipsilateral, temporal half of the retina. A second set of axons comes from the contralateral, nasal half of the retina. These two groups of axons unite the right and left visual half fields from each eye. The lesions and the associated visual field deficits have been highlighted in the figure

Source: Created in BioRender. Sondhi, V. (2025) https://BioRender.com/6obdtc6"

A. Extraocular movements and involved muscles

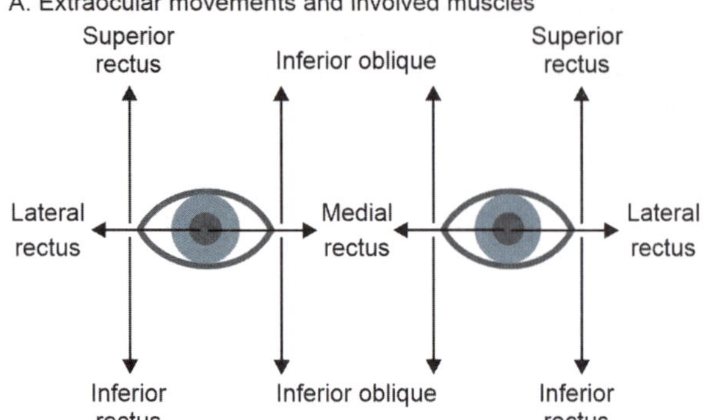

B. Impact of extraocular muscle paresis

Cranial nerve	Muscle involved	Eye deviation
III	Inferior oblique	Down and out
III	Inferior rectus	Up and in
III	Medial rectus	Laterally
III	Superior rectus	Down and in
IV	Superior oblique	Upward and outward
VI	Lateral rectus	Medially

Fig. 24.2: The role of extraocular muscles in various movements of the eye have been depicted. Table illustrates the paretic extraocular muscle and related eye deviation

Source: Created in BioRender. Sondhi, V. (2025) https://BioRender.com/ia2tw65"

Table 24.4 Medical Research Council Grading of Muscle Power

Grade	*Description*
5	Normal power
4	Inability to maintain position against moderate resistance
3	Inability to maintain position against gravity
2	Active movement with gravity eliminated
1	Trace or flicker of contraction
0	No contraction of muscle

Table 24.5 Characteristics of Upper and Lower Motor Neuron Lesions

Upper motor neuron lesion	*Lower motor neuron lesion*
Disuse atrophy (later in the course)	Significant atrophy of muscles
Hypertonia (spasticity)	Hypotonia
Loss of power is less compared to LMN lesion	Significant loss of power and weakness
Deep tendon reflexes are exaggerated	Deep tendon reflexes are lost
Plantar response is extensor	Plantar response is flexor

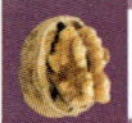

IN A NUTSHELL

Neurological History and Examination

1. A thorough history and examination are crucial for determining the neuroanatomic localization, related etiologies, and differential diagnosis for any child with a neurological disorder.
2. These modalities are irreplaceable and guide further diagnosis and management.

24.2 Investigations in Neurology *PE 27.3, PE 27.13, PE 27.14*

INTRODUCTION

When evaluating a child with suspected neurological disorders, a comprehensive assessment is essential. The selection of investigations will depend on the history, clinical examination findings, and the specific neurological symptoms present. To accurately perform and interpret the investigations detailed in this chapter, it is essential to have a clear grasp of the different clinical signs and symptoms of neurological conditions in children, as well as a solid understanding of normal neuroanatomy and its changes during various disease processes.

SPINAL FLUID EXAMINATION

The cerebrospinal fluid (CSF) offers buoyancy and physical protection to the brain by absorbing stretching and compressive forces from regular/deceleration/rotational head movements, thereby reducing the impacts of forces. Additionally, the CSF serves a protective role by redistributing itself in response to acute changes in other intracranial components, helping to keep intracranial pressure stable. It also facilitates the expulsion of metabolites through the absorption of interstitial fluid from the brain and spinal cord. This "sink action," along with the various methods that maintain the CSF composition, indicates that it plays a crucial role in normal physiology and in compensating for pathological conditions.

Anatomy

Cerebrospinal fluid (CSF) is obtained for analysis through a lumbar puncture (LP). In this procedure, a styletted needle is inserted between the interspinous processes of the lumbar vertebrae, passing through the supraspinal and intraspinal ligaments, ligamentum flavum, dura mater, and arachnoid mater, until it reaches the subarachnoid space. CSF is subsequently collected for sampling.

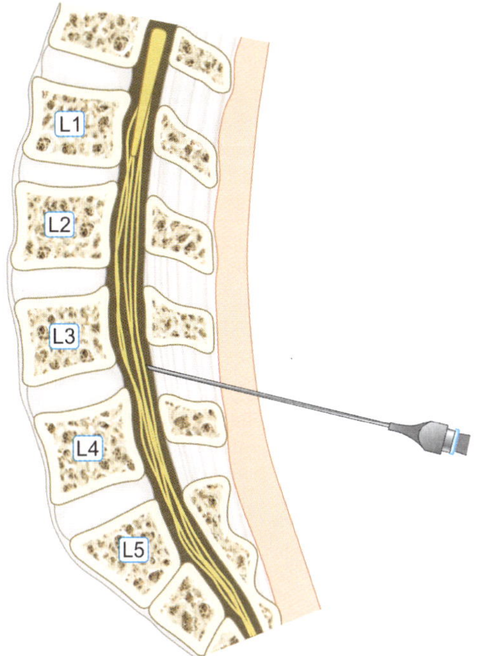

Fig. 24.3: Lumbar puncture should be performed distal to the inferior most part of spinal cord (conus medullaris). Among older children, this can be safely performed below the L2-L3 intervertebral space

Source: Created in BioRender. Sondhi, V. (2025) https://BioRender.com/7xsw7co

Table 24.6 Indications and Contraindications of Performing a Lumbar Puncture

A. **Indications of performing lumbar puncture**
1. Suspected central nervous system infection
2. Suspected autoimmune encephalitis
3. Suspected subarachnoid hemorrhage
4. Measurement of opening pressure and removal of CSF for the diagnosis and treatment of idiopathic intracranial hypertension
5. Guillain-Barré syndrome
6. Acquired demyelination disorders (multiple sclerosis)
7. Inborn errors of metabolism (like GLUT-1 deficiency, mitochondrial disorders)
8. Leptomeningeal carcinomatosis
9. Pediatric neurotransmitter diseases
10. Instillation of chemotherapy for intrathecal treatment or prevention of CNS malignancy
11. Spinal anesthesia
B. **Contraindications of performing lumbar puncture**
1. Children with clinical suspicion for elevated intracranial pressure (CSF should be performed after neuroimaging to prevent herniation)
2. Children with respiratory compromise may become hypoxemic or apneic while undergoing LP, especially in the lateral recumbent position
3. Hemodynamic instability
4. Soft tissue infection at the puncture site
5. Bleeding disorder (platelet counts <20,000/microL; international normalized ratio >1.4)

LP should be performed distal to the inferior most part of spinal cord (conus medullaris), specifically at the level of the cauda equina **(Fig. 24.3)**. At birth, the spinal cord's inferior tip aligns with the L3 vertebra. The vertebral column grows faster than the spinal cord, resulting in the tip of the spinal cord reaching the inferior border of L1 in adulthood. For older children, LP can be safely performed from the L2-L3 intervertebral space to the L5-S1 intervertebral space, as these areas are below the conus medullaris. In children under 12 months, LP must be conducted below the L2-L3 intervertebral space. An imaginary line joining the two posterior-superior iliac crests intersects the spine around the fourth lumbar vertebra. This aids in identifying the L3-L4 intervertebral space above this line and the L4-L5 space below it.

Indications and Contraindications

Alterations in CSF composition are linked to numerous neurological disorders. **Table 24.6** summarizes the salient indications and contraindications for performing LP. The interpretation of CSF analysis has been summarized in **Table 24.13** in the chapter on meningoencephalitis.

NEUROIMAGING

A. Cranial Ultrasound

During the prenatal and perinatal period, real-time sonography is the most commonly used neuroimaging technique. Since its introduction for clinical use in the 1950s, ultrasound has developed into a potent diagnostic tool for examining fetal and neonatal conditions. The anterior fontanel, which usually remains open until 15–18 months, provides an excellent window for evaluating the underlying brain and CSF. After birth, sonography plays a crucial role in assessing hypoxic-ischemic encephalopathy, germinal matrix/intraventricular hemorrhage, screening for intrauterine infections, and identifying the cause of an increasing or enlarged head size. While ultrasound can evaluate ischemic white matter injury, periventricular leukomalacia, and cystic encephalomalacias, it may not fully capture the extent of the injuries. For preterm neonates born at <30 weeks of gestational age, routine cranial ultrasonography screening is recommended once during the first week of life, followed by a repeat between 7–14 days of age to detect intraventricular hemorrhage. Additionally, ultrasound should be conducted again between 36–40 weeks of corrected gestational age to screen for periventricular leukomalacia, ventriculomegaly, and intrauterine infections. Additionally, sonography serves as a screening tool for myelodysplasia in early infancy, helps identify the conus medullaris level, and assesses newborns who may have closed spinal dysraphism.

B. Computed Tomography (CT) Scan

Since its introduction in the 1970s, the CT scan has been the most common neuroimaging technique used in emergencies. Its ability to be conducted in minutes makes it well-suited for urgent situations. The digital tomographic image consists of a

Table 24.7 Summary of Density Spectrum in a CT Scan of the Head

Bright (hyperdense)	Bone, calcifications, contrast-enhanced areas, acute blood
Dark (hypodense)	Air, fat, cerebrospinal fluid, areas of edema
Intermediate	Brain tissue, some tumors, chronic blood collections

matrix of voxels (volumetric pixels created by the tomogram's thickness). Each voxel is assigned a numeric value known as a CT number, which correlates with tissue density. Typically, these CT numbers are measured in Hounsfield units, with water as the reference point assigned a value of zero. Other tissues are evaluated according to their densities compared to this reference.

In a CT scan of the head, different tissues and structures appear with varying densities, which result in different levels of brightness (radiopacity). How these structures appear depends largely on their composition and the X-ray attenuation properties of the tissues. Here's a breakdown of which structures typically appear bright and which ones appear dark **(Table 24.7)**:

1. **Structures that appear bright (hyperdense) on a CT scan:**
   - *Bone:* The skull, which is composed of dense cortical bone, appears very bright due to its high density and ability to attenuate X-rays effectively.
   - *Calcifications:* Calcified structures such as granulomas and neoplasms (such as pheochromocytomas and meningiomas) may appear bright.
   - *Contrast media:* If contrast material is used, areas where the contrast has been concentrated will appear bright (hyperdense). This is often used to visualize blood vessels, certain tumors, or areas of inflammation.
   - *Acute blood:* Fresh hemorrhages (such as epidural or subdural hematomas) appear bright due to the density of clotted blood.
2. **Structures that appear dark (hypodense) on a CT scan:**
   - *Air:* Sinuses (e.g., frontal and maxillary) appear very dark due to the low density of air.
   - *Fat:* Fatty tissues (e.g., subcutaneous fat or fat within the orbits) also appear dark because of their lower density compared to other soft tissues.
   - *CSF:* The ventricles and subarachnoid spaces filled with CSF typically appear dark because of the low density of the fluid compared to brain tissue.
   - *Brain edema:* In cases of brain edema or specific pathologies (e.g., tumors, strokes), affected areas can appear darker (hypodense) than normal brain tissue.
3. **Intermediate densities:**
   - *Brain tissue:* Normal brain tissue has a moderate density and appears with intermediate brightness on a CT scan, generally being brighter than CSF but darker than bone.
   - *Pathologies*:
     - Chronic hematomas (older bleeds) may appear less bright than acute hemorrhages, often demonstrating intermediate densities.
     - Certain tumors: Depending on the type of tumor (e.g., gliomas may present as hypodense lesions, while other types may be hyperdense due to calcifications), their appearance can vary.

Table 24.8 Highlights of Different MRI Sequences

Sequence	*Tissues highlighted*	*Characteristics*	*Clinical uses*
T1 weighted	Fat, anatomy	Fat bright, water dark, good anatomical detail	Anatomical details pre- and post-contrast imaging
T2 weighted	Water, edema	Fluid bright, fat dark	Assesing edema, tumors, demyelination
FLAIR	Edema, lesions	CSF dark, edema bright	Demyelinating diseases, subtle lesions
Diffusion weighted	Ischemic changes	Bright in acute stroke (suggests restricted diffusion)	Acute ischemic stroke, tumor density
T1 contrast	Tumors, inflammatory lesions	Highlights abnormal vascularity and lesions	Tumor evaluation, inflammation

C. MRI Brain

MRI is increasingly recognized as the most powerful neuroimaging modality for both adults and children. It does not involve ionizing radiation, unlike CT, nor does it require an acoustic window, which restricts cranial ultrasound to the infancy period before the fontanels close. MRI offers multiplanar imaging with excellent resolution without the need to reposition the patient or the machine. However, MRI has less tolerance for patient movement compared to CT or ultrasound, making sedation necessary for most young children.

Distinguishing between different MRI sequences used in brain imaging is fundamental for interpreting images accurately and for making correct diagnoses **(Table 24.8)**. Each MRI sequence highlights different tissue characteristics, and understanding these distinctions can aid clinicians in their assessment **(Figs. 24.4A to D)**.

ELECTROPHYSIOLOGY

A. Electroencephalography (EEG)

EEG serves as a crucial diagnostic tool for assessing patients with suspected epilepsy. In a standard EEG procedure, electrical activity is captured from specific sites on the scalp, following the international 10–20 system for electrode placement **(Fig. 24.5)**. The EEG output is reliant on differential amplification, meaning it is always represented as the difference between two inputs, visualized in a tracing referred to as a channel. Generally, a montage displays 21 or more channels, which form

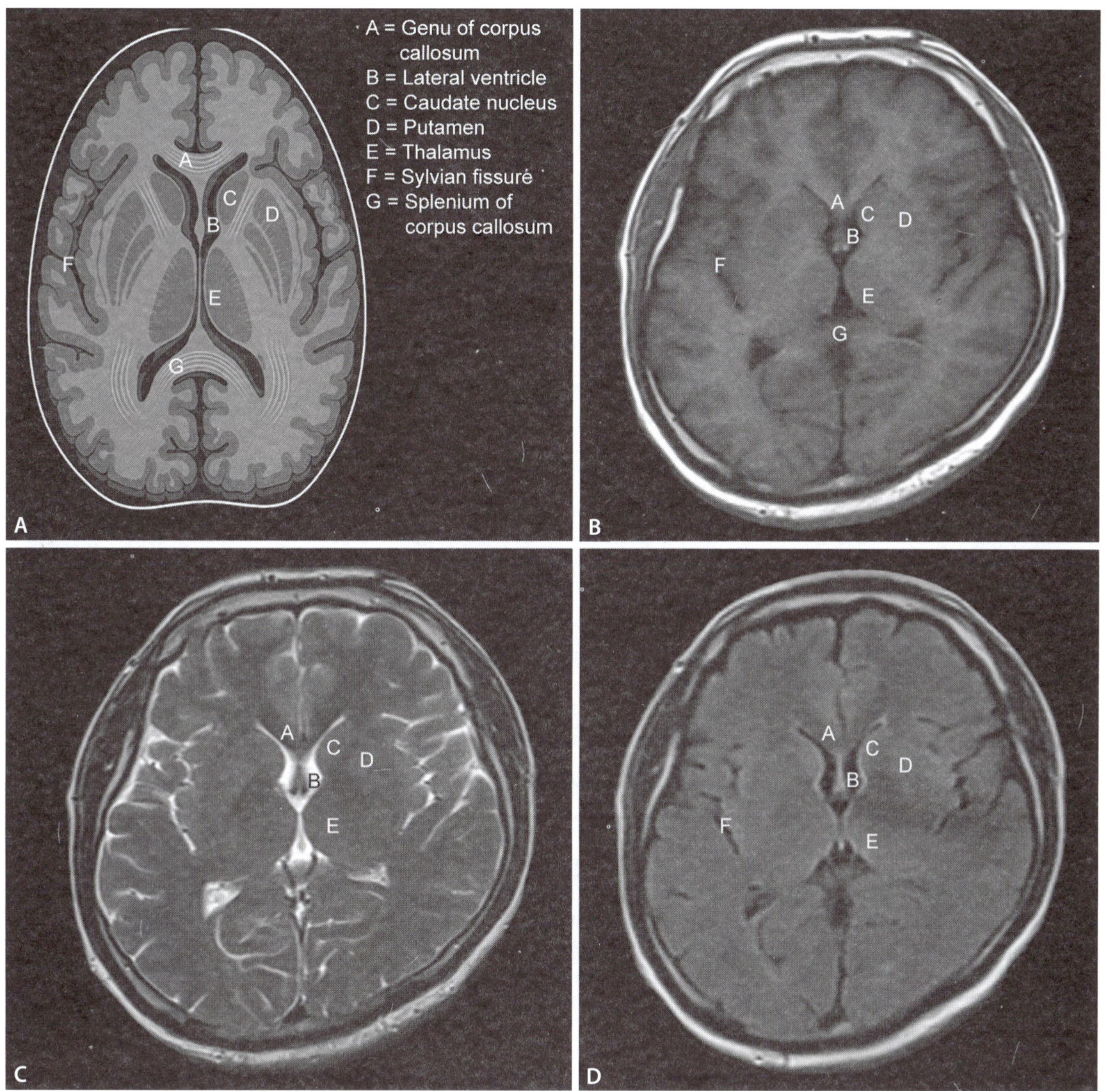

Figs. 24.4A to D: Different sequences of MRI in the axial section are depicted: (A) depicts a cartoon representation; (B) T1 sequence, while (C and D) are T2 and FLAIR sequences, respectively. The anatomical landmarks have been highlighted by alphabets from A to G

Source: Created in BioRender. Sondhi, V. (2025) https://BioRender.com/olj3wcd.

the foundation for interpreting EEG results. With the advent of modern digital EEG technology, electroencephalographers can virtually endlessly fine-tune the montages and various technical parameters for each recording, enhancing both interpretation and analysis.

EEG waveforms are classified based on their frequency ranges as delta (1–4 Hz), theta (4–8 Hz), alpha (8–12 Hz), and beta (12–30 Hz) activities (**Fig. 24.6**). Age, alertness level, medications, and any underlying neurological disorders or dysfunctions affect these waveforms. In awake EEG recordings, the alpha rhythm is observed in the posterior or occipital electrodes (posterior dominant rhythm). During sleep, EEG recordings in children reveal typical sleep markers such as sleep spindles, vertex waves, and K complexes. It is essential to always correlate EEG results with clinical findings.

B. Electromyography (EMG) and Nerve Conduction Studies (NCS)

EMG involves the clinical examination of the electrical activity generated by motor units and their muscle fibers, both individually and together. EMG usually assesses electrical activity when the muscle is at rest and during voluntary contraction periods. NCS play a crucial role in assessing peripheral nervous system function, dysfunction, and disease. They are valuable for identifying both focal conditions, such as entrapment neuropathies, and general conditions, like

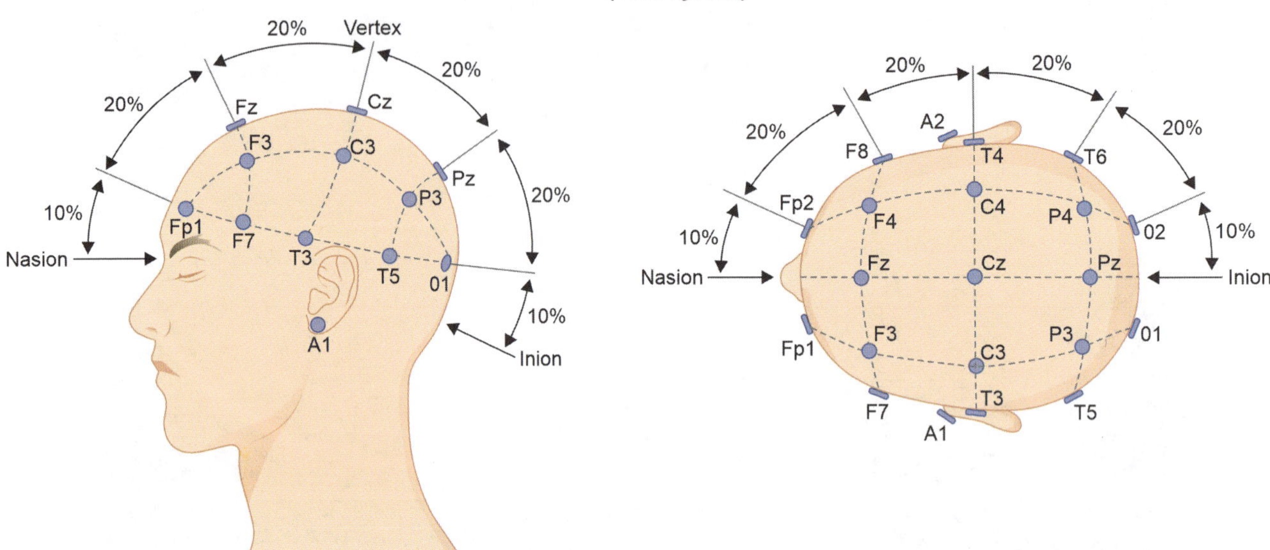

Fig. 24.5: The International 10-20 System is a standardized method for placing electrodes on the scalp for electroencephalographic (EEG). The distances between electrodes are specified in terms of percentage, i.e., 10% and 20% of the total distance measurements are used to define the placement sites. Distances are measured from standardized anatomical landmarks on the skull, including the nasion and the inion. Electrode placements are identified by letters corresponding to the scalp's location, followed by numbers indicating the position in relation to the midline (odd numbers denote left, even numbers denote right, and "z" denotes midline)

Source: Created in BioRender. Sondhi, V. (2025) https://BioRender.com/s7n9oa1.

polyneuropathies. Additionally, NCS helps evaluate the extent of axonal damage in comparison to demyelination. The sensory nerve action potential (SNAP) and compound muscle action potential (CMAP) reflect the combined electrical activity of individual nerve fibers that are activated simultaneously during nerve stimulation.

C. Brainstem Evoked Response Audiometry

The auditory brainstem response (ABR) test [also be known as auditory brainstem evoked response (ABER), brainstem evoked response audiometry (BERA), or brainstem auditory evoked response (BAER)] uses click and tone burst stimuli ranging from loud (80 or 90 dB) to soft (0 to 20 dB) to stimulate responses from the auditory pathway. Electrodes placed on the child's head and ears record these responses. Delayed or absent waves may indicate cochlear or neurologic issues. Additionally, patterns of normal hearing or conductive hearing loss can be identified.

D. Visual Evoked Potential

Visual evoked potential (VEP), also known as visual evoked response (VER), is a neurophysiological test that assesses the electrical activity in the brain in response to visual stimuli. VEPs are particularly useful for evaluating the visual pathways from the retina, through the optic nerve, and into the occipital cortex of the brain. VEPs can help in diagnosing various conditions affecting vision, including optic neuritis, demyelination, lesions compressing optic nerve, and neoplasms.

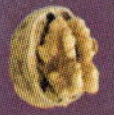

IN A NUTSHELL

Investigations in Neurology

1. Investigations can be a helpful tool in establishing diagnosis in neurological disorders but they can only "aid" after a thorough history and examination have helped in narrowing down the differential diagnosis. They are not a substitute for clinical evaluation.
2. CSF helps establish a diagnosis in cases of suspected meningitis, encephalitis, subarachnoid hemorrhage, intracranial hypertension, leptomeningeal carcinomatosis, pediatric neurotransmitter diseases, and neurodegenerative diseases.
3. Cranial ultrasonography utilizing anterior fontanelle is useful in neonates for detecting intracranial hemorrhage, periventricular leukomalacia, and ventriculomegaly.
4. A CT scan of the head is extremely helpful in emergency situations. Edema and infarctions look dark (hypodense) on CT scan, while hemorrhage and calcifications look bright (hyperdense).
5. MRI is the most powerful neuroimaging modality. In brain MRI, T1 imaging excels in visualizing neuroanatomy, while T2 imaging is effective for identifying pathological lesions. On T2 images, edema and infarctions appear bright (hyperintense).

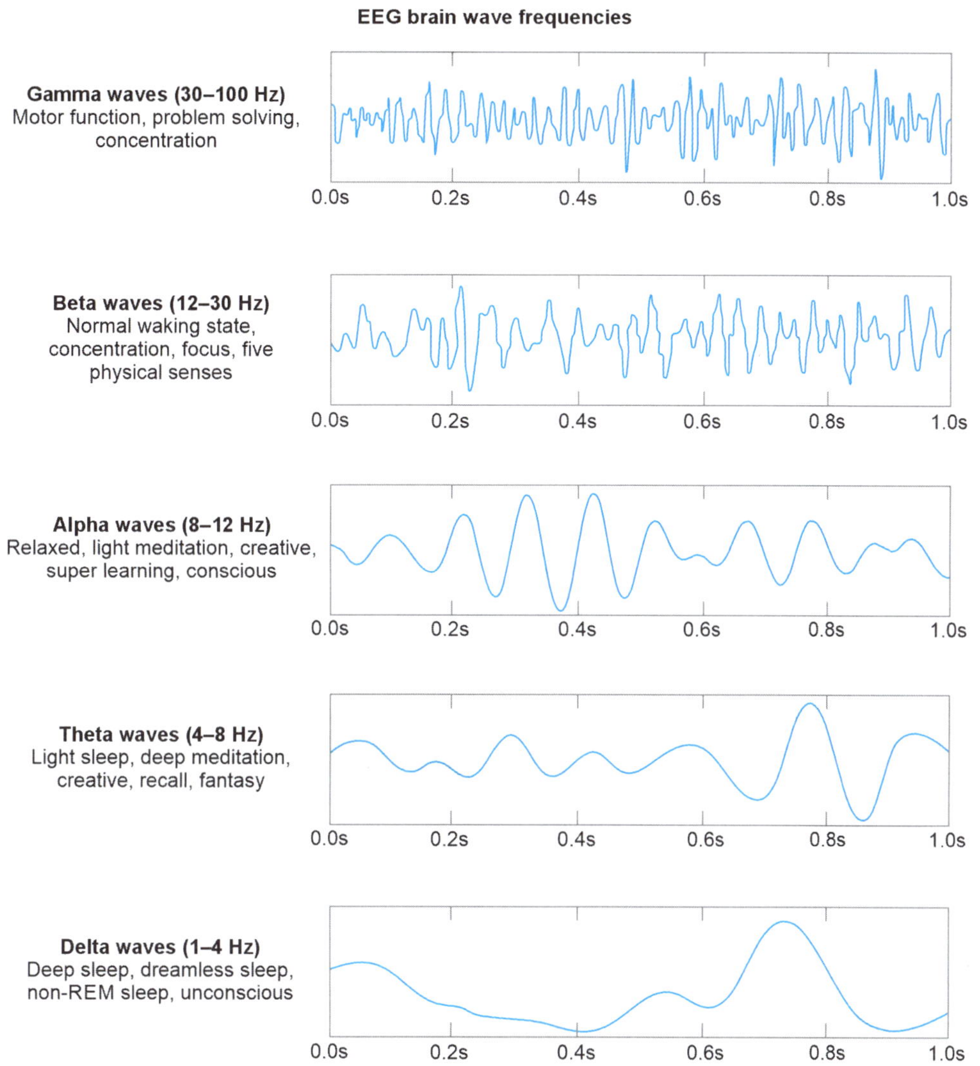

Fig. 24.6: Different EEG waveforms have been depicted

Source: Created in BioRender. Sondhi, V. (2025) https://BioRender.com/wklukfa.

Abdelhalim AN, Alberico RA. Pediatric neuroimaging. Neurol Clin. 2009;27:285-301.
Chiappa KH. In: Evoked Potentials in Clinical Medicine. 3rd ed. Philadelphia: Lippincott–Raven; 1997.
Kapoor KG, Katz SE, Grzybowski DM, et al. Cerebrospinal fluid outflow: an evolving perspective. Brain Res Bull. 2008;77(6): 327-34.
Wezel-Meijler Gv, de Vries LS. Cranial ultrasound—optimizing utility in the NICU. Curr Pediatr Rev. 2014;10:16-27.

24.3 Pyogenic Meningitis *PE 27.1, PE 27.3*

INTRODUCTION

Infections of the CNS are a significant cause of morbidity and mortality in children. The mortality rate for untreated bacterial meningitis is nearly 100%. Despite treatment, complications and death may occur; neurologic issues are common in survivors. Infections of the CNS primarily involve two interrelated entities: meningitis and encephalitis. Meningitis refers to the primary inflammation of the meninges, while encephalitis indicates inflammation of the brain's parenchyma. However, during infection/inflammation, the anatomical distinction between these two may become unclear, with many patients exhibiting clinical or imaging signs of both meningeal and parenchymal involvement. **The term meningoencephalitis may more accurately describe widespread infections of CNS.**

This chapter primarily details the evaluation and management of bacterial meningitis among children.

Table 24.9 Terminologies Related to CNS Infection and Inflammation	
Terminology	*Description*
Meningitis	Meningitis refers to the inflammation of the leptomeninges (the pia mater, arachnoid, and associated subarachnoid space). It presents with an increased white blood cell count in the CSF. The inflammation is typically due to infection but can also occur due to other inflammatory disorders like neoplasms.
Encephalitis	Encephalitis is characterized by inflammation of the encephalon (brain tissue), presenting with neurological manifestations such as altered sensorium, behavioral disorders, personality changes, sensory or motor deficits, speech abnormalities, development of movement disorders, focal motor deficits, and sensory phenomenon like paresthesias. The inflammation is typically due to infection but can also occur due to other inflammatory disorders like autoimmune dysfunction.
Meningoencephalitis	Meningoencephalitis refers to the inflammation/infection of the meninges, and the brain's parenchyma manifesting with features of involvement of both
Myelitis	Myelitis is a condition characterized by spinal cord inflammation, leading to flaccid paralysis with diminished or absent reflexes at the level of lesion and upper motor neuron signs below the level, and sphincter abnormalities characterized by flaccid/spastic bladder and anal incompetence.
Aseptic meningitis	Aseptic meningitis refers to the clinical condition of meningeal inflammation where routine bacterial cultures are negative in a patient who has not received antibiotics prior to lumbar puncture.
Pyogenic meningitis	Pyogenic meningitis also known as bacterial meningitis, is the bacterial infection of leptomeninges, typically characterized by neutrophil dominated white blood cell pleocytosis in the CSF and demonstration of the offending bacteria in culture, Gram stain or molecular tests.

The common terminologies related to CNS infection/ inflammation are listed in **Table 24.9.**

ETIOLOGY

The epidemiology and etiology of the causative pathogens of bacterial meningitis differ with age and geographic location. Additionally, specific infections may be more prevalent based on the mode of transmission and individual host characteristics. The common agents associated with meningitis in children are highlighted in **Table 24.10**. The risk factors associated with the occurrence of meningitis are listed in **Table 24.11**.

Table 24.10 Etiological Agents Associated with Bacterial Meningitis	
Age	*Common causes*
Less than one month	• *Streptococcus agalactiae* • *Listeria monocytogenes* • *E. coli* • Gram-negative bacilli [*Escherichia coli, Klebsiella pneumoniae, Citrobacter, Acinetobacter* (coccobacillus)]
1–3 months	• *Streptococcus agalactiae* • *Listeria monocytogenes* • *Streptococcus pneumoniae* • *Neisseria meningitidis* • *Haemophilus influenzae* Type B • Gram-negative bacilli [*Escherichia coli, Klebsiella pneumoniae, Citrobacter, Acinetobacter* (coccobacillus)]
3 months to 21 years	• *Streptococcus pneumoniae* • *Neisseria meningitidis* • *Haemophilus influenzae* Type B • Gram-negative bacilli [*Escherichia coli, Klebsiella pneumoniae, Citrobacter, Acinetobacter* (coccobacillus)]

Table 24.11 Risk Factors Predisposing to Bacterial Meningitis in Children	
Risk factors	*Examples*
Immunodeficiency	• Congenital immunodeficiency ▪ Asplenia (functional asplenia with sickle cell disease) ▪ Complement deficiency ▪ Hypogammaglobulinemia • Acquired immunodeficiency ▪ HIV ▪ Immunosuppressants like glucocorticoids/ chemotherapeutic agents ▪ Diabetes mellitus
Congenital malformations	• Cranial or spinal dermoid sinus • Mondini dysplasia
Acquired anatomic defects	• Basilar skull fractures
Medical devices/ neurosurgery	• CSF shunts • Ventriculostomy • Cochlear implant
Parameningeal infections	• Otitis media • Mastoiditis • Sinusitis
Exposure	• Contact with a person with meningitis

PATHOGENESIS

The primary mechanisms contributing to the development of meningitis have been illustrated in **Figures 24.7A and B**. These include:

A. ***Colonization of the nasopharynx, followed by bloodstream invasion and subsequent CNS invasion:*** Most instances

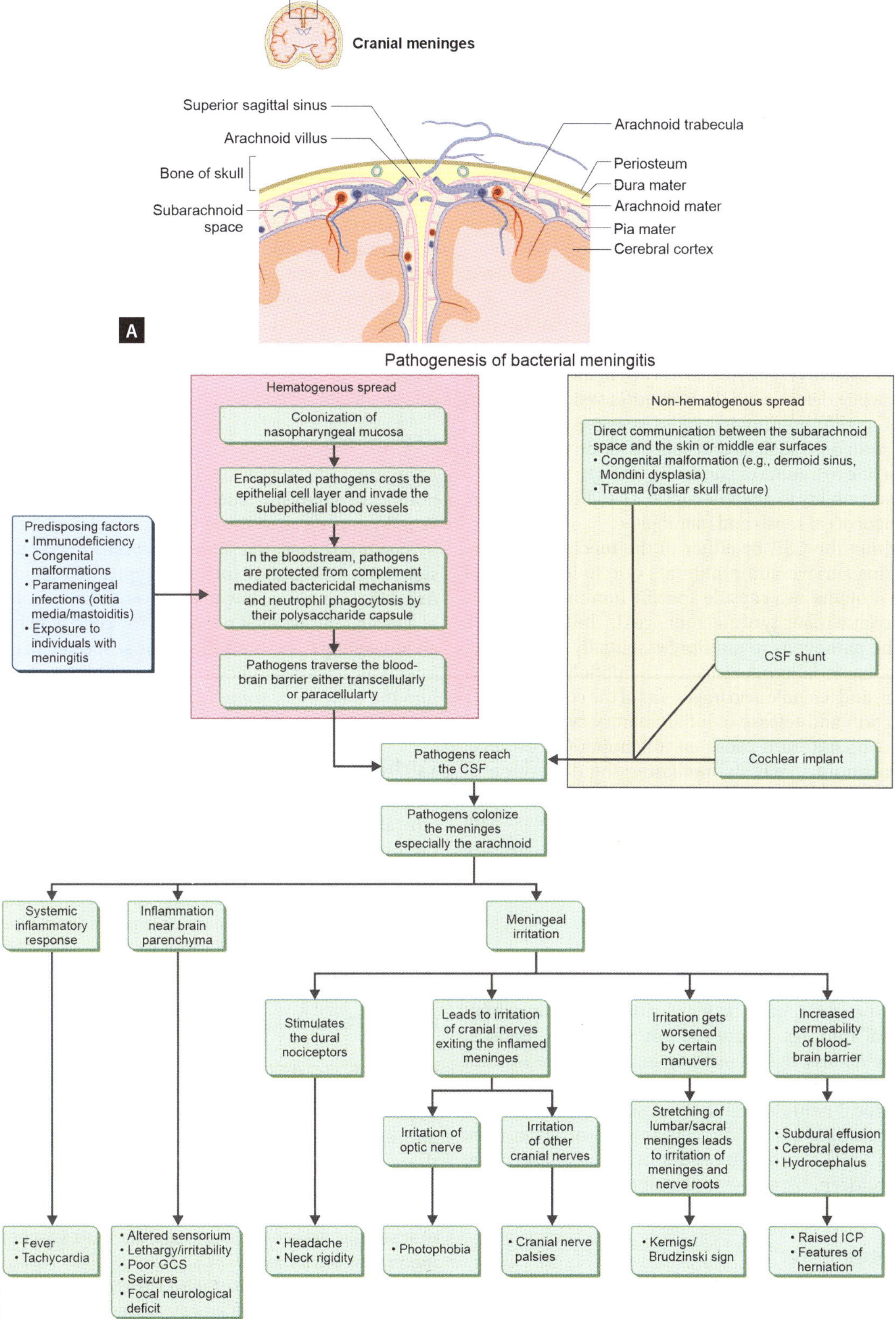

Figs. 24.7A and B: Diagrammatic representation of meninges (A) and pathogenesis of meningitis (B), along with the underlying pathways involved in the occurrence of various signs and symptoms of meningitis, have been highlighted

Source: Created in BioRender. Sondhi, V. (2025) https://BioRender.com/5myi8y8

of bacterial meningitis probably result from bacteremia, which occurs when the pathogen enters the bloodstream after colonizing the nasopharyngeal mucosa. Most bacterial meningitis pathogens spread from person to person via the respiratory route.

B. ***Direct entry of organisms into the CNS from any of the following:*** (a) Contiguous infection (e.g., sinusitis, mastoiditis); (b) trauma, neurosurgery, cerebrospinal fluid (CSF) leak (due to basilar skull fracture), and congenital defects (like dermal sinus, meningomyelocele); and (c) medical devices (e.g., CSF shunts, cochlear implants).
C. ***CNS invasion*** occurring after bacteremia from a localized infection source (e.g., infective endocarditis).
D. ***Immune dysfunction:*** Some children may have bacteremia from immune defects. For example, deficiencies in the complement system (C5-C8) lead to recurrent meningococcal infections, while defects with the properdin system heighten the risk of severe meningococcal disease. Additionally, splenic dysfunction, such as that seen in sickle cell anemia, or asplenia due to trauma or congenital defects, is linked to a greater susceptibility to pneumococcal, *H. influenzae* type b, and meningococcal sepsis and meningitis.

After reaching the CSF, by either of the mechanisms, the microorganisms survive and proliferate due to low levels of complement proteins and capsule specific immunoglobulins, as well as the relative paucity of macrophages in the CSF. Overall, this causes the pathogens to multiply essentially unchecked. The release of bacterial products, such as lipopolysaccharide, peptidoglycan, and teichoic acid fragments of the cell wall, leads to the production and release of inflammatory cytokines and chemokines, which in turn cause an inflammatory response in the subarachnoid space. By mediating the disruption of the blood-brain barrier and triggering cytokines, matrix metalloproteases aid in the inflammatory process. The complicated pathophysiologic changes in the CNS and the clinical signs of bacterial meningitis are mostly caused by the growing cycle of cytokine-promoted granulocytic inflammation **(Figs. 24.7A and B)**.

CLINICAL FEATURES

Regardless of the cause, most patients with meningitis exhibit similar clinical findings. These include headache, nausea, vomiting, appetite loss, light sensitivity, and altered sensorium with lethargy and irritability. Common signs include fever, neck rigidity, focal neurological deficits, seizures, and altered sensorium, including coma. The classic triad of fever, neck rigidity, and altered sensorium occurs in a small percentage of affected children. The essential components of clinical evaluation are summarized in **Table 24.12**.

Neonatal Meningitis

A high index of suspicion is required because the clinical signs of bacterial meningitis in neonates can be very subtle. Neonatal meningitis is divided into two categories: early-onset infection, which occurs within the first 72 hours of life, and late-onset infection, which occurs between one week and three months of life. Pregnancy and perinatal risk factors like chorioamnionitis, prolonged rupture of the membranes, or obstetric trauma may be more common in those with an early onset. More often than not, early-onset disease presents with non-specific, non-neurologic symptoms, primarily associated with respiratory distress and sepsis. Aside from altered sensorium, other symptoms may include respiratory distress (including apnea), poor feeding, vomiting, diarrhea, and temperature dysregulation.

Seizures, focal neurologic deficits (such as paresis of limbs and cranial neuropathies), and other previously described nonspecific signs are more likely to be present in late-onset neonatal meningitis. A bulging anterior fontanel in appropriate settings increases the risk of bacterial meningitis by three to five times. Although neck rigidity or features of meningeal irritation are rare in the first year of life, they should not be disregarded if they do occur.

CSF Shunts

As many as 5–10% of CNS shunts get infected. Although a number of organisms, such as gram-negative bacteria and other skin flora, can cause shunt infections, the majority are caused by coagulase-negative *Staphylococcus* or *S. aureus*. Clinical signs of a CNS shunt infection typically include lethargy or irritability, vomiting, low-grade fever, and other clinical features of elevated intracranial pressure. Any child who has a fever and an indwelling CNS shunt should be suspected of having a shunt infection. Because infected ventriculoperitoneal shunts drain into the abdomen, some children with these shunt infections may present with peritonitis or abdominal pain.

Cochlear Implants

Patients with severe to profound sensorineural hearing loss are typically treated with cochlear implantation. The electrode of the neural stimulator implant is surgically positioned in the cochlea's lumen, close to the auditory nerve. With the implants being manufactured currently, the risk of meningitis is the highest in the first two years post-procedure. The mechanism of meningitis in these children involves the entry of bacteria through the middle ear following an episode of otitis media. The two most prevalent offending pathogens are *S. pneumoniae* (about 80%) and *H. influenzae* (~16%).

INVESTIGATIONS

Bacterial meningitis is diagnosed based on the clinical suspicion and definitive findings on CSF examination. Antimicrobial therapy should be started as soon as possible and not postponed due to delays in conducting investigations such as lumbar puncture (LP) or CT scan. The details of investigations that should be conducted in a child with suspected bacterial meningitis are as below.

A. ***Complete blood count with differential:*** Leukocytosis with neutrophil predominance is suggestive of bacterial infection
B. ***Blood culture:*** About 60–85% of children with bacterial meningitis have positive blood cultures.

Table 24.12 Clinical Evaluation of a Child with Suspected Meningitis or Encephalitis

History		
Age	Specific etiologic agents which are more likely in different age groups have been highlighted in **Tables 24.10**.	
Symptoms	*Infants* • Fever or hypothermia • Lethargy/irritability • Altered mental status • Poor feeding • Seizures • Respiratory distress • Bulging fontanel • Vomiting • Diarrhea • Jaundice	*Children and adolescents* • Fever • Headache • Neck stiffness • Altered mental status • Seizures • Photophobia • Nausea/vomiting • Confusion • Lethargy/irritability
History of predisposing factors	• Recurrent infections in past (may suggest immunodeficiency) • Anatomic defects (to consider direct seeding of CNS with pathogens) • Prior neurosurgery • Medical devices (e.g., CSF shunt, cochlear implant) • Exposure to someone with bacterial meningitis • Recurrent transfusions (sickle cell anemia with functional asplenia) • Purulent ear discharge with retroauricular pain (mastoiditis) • Rash, conjunctivitis, herpangina, pharyngitis (may suggest an underlying viral illness)	
Vaccination history	Specifically for vaccination against HiB, pneumococcus and meningococcus	
Examination		
General appearance	Children with meningitis are usually toxic looking	
Vitals	• Fever is usually present at presentation • Tachycardia and hypotension are suggestive of depleting volume status and help in detection of shock • Systemic hypertension, bradycardia, and respiratory depression, collectively known as Cushing's triad, serves as a late indicator of elevated ICP	
Head to toe evaluation	• Bulging anterior fontanelle in an infant is suggestive of raised intracranial pressure • Petechiae and purpura (purpura fulminans) are seen with meningococcal infection	
Signs of meningeal irritation	• Neck rigidity • Kernig's sign (flexion of the hip 90 degrees with subsequent pain upon extension of the leg) • Brudzinski sign (involuntary flexion of the knees and hips after passive flexion of the neck while supine)	
Neurological examination	• Altered mental status: Glasgow Coma Scale (GCS) should be charted for all patients. Patients who are obtunded, semicomatose, or comatose tend to experience worse outcomes. • Seizures • Fundus examination to check for papilledema • Cranial nerve palsies may be present. Presence of pupillary asymmetry and lateral rectus palsy may suggest raised intracranial pressure with (impending) herniation. Facial nerve palsy may exist as part of primary disease or as a complication • Motor system examination for any focal neurological deficits should be conducted. These may include hemiparesis, quadriparesis, asymmetric or absent deep tendon reflexes, abnormal plantar reflexes. Children who have these findings are more likely to have a poor outcome	
Other systemic examination	• Arthritis (meningococcal) • Pneumonia (HiB, pneumococcus, influenza) • Sinusitis/otitis media (HiB, pneumococcus)	

C. ***Inflammatory markers:*** Elevations of C-reactive protein, erythrocyte sedimentation rate, and procalcitonin may be observed in both bacterial and viral meningitis.

D. ***Biochemistry:*** Serum electrolytes, blood urea nitrogen, and creatinine are important for evaluating volume status and guiding fluid administration. Additionally, the serum glucose level plays a critical role in calculating the CSF-to-blood glucose ratio.

E. ***Lumbar puncture (LP):***

a. Performing an LP to collect CSF for Gram stain and culture is crucial for diagnosing meningitis.

b. Test the CSF for neutrophilic pleocytosis, elevated protein levels, and/or reduced glucose concentrations suggests bacterial meningitis.

c. Immediate LP is contraindicated in cases of (a) signs of increased intracranial pressure [bulging fontanel, focal

Table 24.13 Interpretation of CSF Results

Condition	Pressure (cm H_2O)	WBC count (mm^3)	Protein (mg/dL)	Glucose (mg/dL)	Others tests
Normal	<28	<5 In neonates:<20	20-45	>50 (or >2/3rd of blood glucose)	
Acute bacterial meningitis	Elevated	100–10,000 or more Neutrophils predominate	Usually 100–500	Decreased, usually <40 (or <50% of serum glucose)	Organisms usually identified on Gram stain or culture or PCR
Partially treated bacterial meningitis	Normal or elevated	5–10,000; Usually neutrophil dominate, but lymphocytes/ mononuclear cells may predominate if pretreated for extended period	Usually 100–500	Normal or decreased	Pretreatment may render CSF sterile and organisms may not be seen on gram stain. PCR-based assays may detect bacterial DNA
Viral meningitis or meningoencephalitis	Normal	5–100 Lymphocytes predominantly	50–300	Normal May be decreased with mumps	Most viruses can be identified by CSF PCR analysis
Tuberculous meningitis	Elevated	10–500; neutrophils early, but lymphocytes predominate through most of the course	100–3,000	Usually <50	*Mycobacterium tuberculosis* can be detected by PCR of CSF

neurological deficits, third or sixth cranial nerve palsies in patients with a diminished level of consciousness, or the Cushing reflex (characterized by hypertension, bradycardia, and respiratory irregularities)]; (b) severe cardiopulmonary distress that necessitates urgent resuscitation; (c) skin infection at the LP site; and (d) features of bleeding diathesis (thrombocytopenia or coagulopathy). If the procedure is postponed, then blood culture should be obtained, and empiric antibiotic treatment should be started immediately.

d. *Tests to perform on the CSF include:* (a) Cell count and differential; (b) glucose and protein concentration; (c) Gram stain and culture (± special stains as indicated clinically); and (d) molecular testing like PCR amplification for detection of pathogen nucleic acid. It is beneficial to reserve a tube of CSF for additional testing, which may be required if the patient does not improve as anticipated. The interpretation of CSF results has been summarized in **Table 24.13**.

F. ***Neuroimaging:*** CT scans of the head are not routinely recommended before a LP unless the patient has clinical signs or is at risk for elevated ICP, such as papilledema, focal neurological findings, coma, a history of hydrocephalus, or previous neurosurgical procedures, including shunt placement. If a CT scan is required prior to an LP, antimicrobial therapy should not be delayed.

TREATMENT Pyogenic Meningitis

Prompt recognition, diagnostic testing, and timely initiation of appropriate antimicrobial therapy are essential for improving clinical outcomes in patients with bacterial meningitis (**Fig. 24.8**). Delays in starting antimicrobial therapy, even by a few hours, are significantly linked to adverse clinical outcomes and increased mortality.

Since CSF is a site of impaired humoral immunity, a fundamental principle in the treatment of bacterial meningitis is that antibiotics must exert a bactericidal effect within the CSF to ensure optimal microbiologic cure. The various antimicrobial agents used in the management of bacterial meningitis are listed in **Table 24.14**.

Initial Antibiotic Therapy

The suggested empirical antibiotic treatment for suspected bacterial meningitis beyond the neonatal period includes a *third-generation cephalosporin (ceftriaxone) combined with vancomycin.*

In cases where the patient is immunocompromised and gram-negative bacterial meningitis is suspected; initial treatment may involve cefepime or meropenem. Once culture results are available, treatment should be adjusted based on the specific pathogen isolated from CSF and/or blood cultures.

In scenarios where distinction from encephalitis is not feasible, the initial empiric treatment may include acyclovir and artesunate, which can be stopped after the CSF results and assessment of rapid diagnostic tests for malaria.

Duration of therapy

- The treatment duration for uncomplicated *S. pneumoniae* meningitis is 10–14 days; for *N. meningitidis*, it is 5–7 days.
- Uncomplicated *H. influenzae* type b meningitis requires 7–10 days of treatment.
- Patients who received antibiotics before LP and lack identifiable pathogens but show bacterial meningitis evidence in their CSF profile and PCR should be treated for a minimum of 7–10 days; however, the decision to continue or discontinue empiric antibiotic therapy is individualized based upon the clinical status of the child and level of clinical concern for bacterial meningitis.

A repeat LP before discontinuation of antibiotics for typical bacterial meningitis is not recommended.

Corticosteroids

Intravenous dexamethasone 0.15 mg/kg/dose given every 6 hours for 2 days has been shown to reduce hearing loss associated with *H. influenzae* type b meningitis in children over 6 weeks of age. Corticosteroids seem to provide the greatest benefit when administered 1–2 hours prior to the initiation of antibiotics, which can be challenging to implement; however, they may also be effective when given concurrently with or shortly after the first dose of antibiotics.

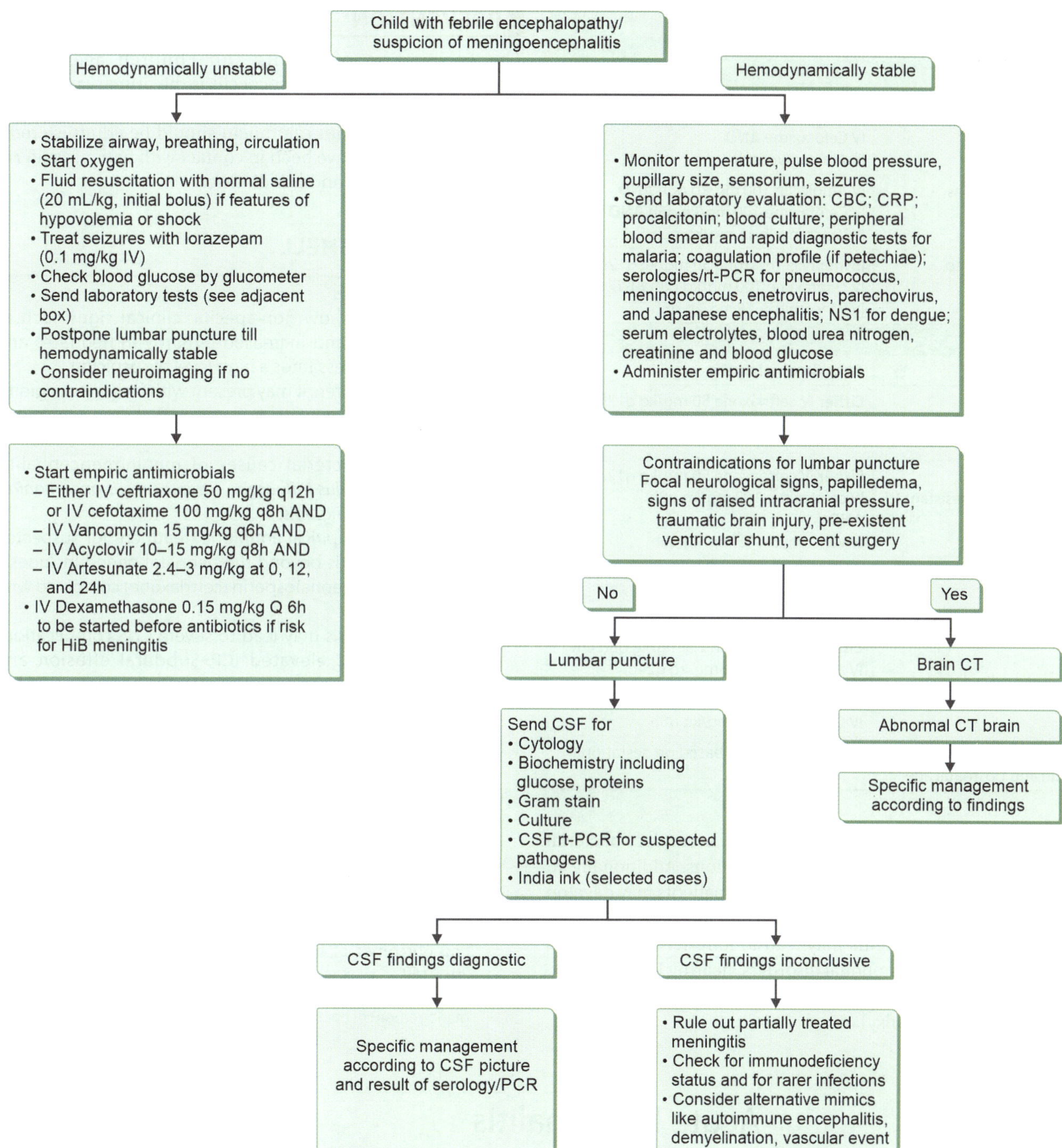

Fig. 24.8: An algorithmic approach to a child with suspected meningoencephalitis. The approach needs to be tailored to the individual child based on clinical manifestations and results of laboratory and neuroimaging investigations

COMPLICATIONS AND LONG-TERM SEQUELAE

Bacterial meningitis may lead to severe CNS complications such as seizures, elevated ICP, subdural effusion and empyema, cranial nerve palsies, stroke, herniation of the cerebrum or cerebellum, SIADH, brain abscess, and cerebral venous sinus thrombosis.

Fever associated with bacterial meningitis typically subsides within 5–7 days following the start of treatment. However, around 10% of patients may experience prolonged fever lasting more than 10 days. This extended fever is often associated with

Table 24.14 Antimicrobial Agents Used in a Child with Bacterial Meningitis

Empiric antibiotics	
Age: <1month*	IV Ampicillin **AND** IV Cefotaxime **AND** IV Aminoglycoside
Age: 1–3 months	IV Ampicillin 100 mg/kg q6h **AND** IV Cefotaxime 100 mg/kg q8h **AND** IV Vancomycin 15 mg/kg q6h
Age: 3 months to 21 years	**Either** IV ceftriaxone 50 mg/kg q12h **or** IV cefotaxime 100 mg/kg q8h **AND** IV Vancomycin 15 mg/kg q6h
Pathogen Specific Antibiotics	
Pathogen	**Antimicrobial agent**
Streptococcus pneumoniae (sensitive to beta lactams)	**Either** IV ceftriaxone 50 mg/kg q12h **or** IV cefotaxime 100 mg/kg q8h
Streptococcus pneumoniae (resistant to beta lactams)	**Either** IV ceftriaxone 50 mg/kg q12h **or** IV cefotaxime 100 mg/kg q8h **AND** IV vancomycin 15 mg/kg q6h
Haemophilus influenzae	**Either** IV ceftriaxone 50 mg/kg q12h **or** IV cefotaxime 100 mg/kg q8h
Listeria monocytogenes	IV ampicillin 100mg/kg q6h **AND** **Either** IV Gentamicin 2.5 mg/kg q8h **OR** IV amikacin 15–22.5mg/kg q24h
Streptococcus agalactiae	IV Cefotaxime 100mg/kg q8h **AND** IV Gentamicin 2.5 mg/kg q8h

* Drug dosages during the neonatal period are based on gestational age and postnatal age

concurrent viral infections, nosocomial or secondary bacterial infections, thrombophlebitis, or drug reactions. Additionally, in cases of meningitis due to *N. meningitidis*, patients may develop pericarditis or arthritis during their treatment.

In addition, meningitis may lead to long-term disabilities like behavioral and emotional disorders, hearing loss, epilepsy, vision impairment, cognitive impairment, and motor disability (including cerebral palsy).

PREVENTION

The vaccination of infants and children against Hib, pneumococcus, and meningococcus is the primary method for reducing the occurrence of bacterial meningitis. Additionally, chemoprophylaxis with rifampicin should be administered to all individuals who have been in contact with patients suffering from meningococcal and Hib diseases.

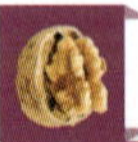

IN A NUTSHELL

Pyogenic Meningitis

1. Meningitis may show non-specific clinical signs such as irritability, fever, and increased lethargy in neonates and infants, which necessitates a high level of suspicion.
2. Among older children, it may present with fever, neck rigidity, focal neurological deficits, seizures, and altered sensorium, including coma.
3. The common bacterial causes of meningoencephalitis include *Haemophilus influenzae, Streptococcus pneumoniae,* and *Neisseria meningitidis.*
4. The suggested empirical antibiotic treatment for suspected bacterial meningitis beyond the neonatal period includes a third-generation cephalosporin (ceftriaxone) combined with vancomycin.
5. Bacterial meningitis may lead to severe CNS complications such as seizures, elevated ICP, subdural effusion and empyema, cranial nerve palsies, stroke, herniation of the cerebrum or cerebellum, SIADH, brain abscess, and cerebral venous sinus thrombosis.

Curtis S, Stobart K, Vandermeer B, et al. Clinical features suggestive of meningitis in children: a systematic review of prospective data. Pediatrics. 2010;126:952.

Oordt-Speets AM, Bolijn R, van Hoorn RC, et al. Global etiology of bacterial meningitis: a systematic review and meta-analysis. PLoS One. 2018;13:e0198772.

Ouchenir L, Renaud C, Khan S, et al. The epidemiology, management, and outcomes of bacterial meningitis in infants. Pediatrics. 2017;140.

Tunkel AR, Hartman BJ, Kaplan SL, et al. Practice guidelines for the management of bacterial meningitis. Clin Infect Dis. 2004;39:1267.

24.4 Acute Encephalitis

PE 27.2, PE 27.3

INTRODUCTION

Inflammation of the brain parenchyma, accompanied by neuroimaging, and/or laboratory, and clinical signs of neurologic dysfunction, is known as encephalitis. This chapter primarily focuses on the infectious causes of encephalitis. Inflammatory processes linked to autoimmune, paraneoplastic, neoplastic, or collagen vascular diseases can cause noninfectious forms of encephalitis, which are not discussed here. The terminologies related to encephalitis are described in **Table 24.15**.

Acute Encephalitis Syndrome (AES)

This is defined by the World Health Organization (WHO) as an illness that can affect a person of any age at any time of year and is characterized by an acute onset of febrile illness, altered sensorium, and/or new onset seizures, excluding simple febrile seizures. Japanese encephalitis (JE) surveillance has been done using this definition. A consensus definition of presumed infectious or autoimmune encephalitis was presented by the International Encephalitis Consortium in 2013. In accordance

Table 24.15 Terminologies Related to Encephalitis

Terminology	*Definition*
Encephalopathy	A disturbance in brain function that does not result from a direct inflammatory process in the brain parenchyma is known as encephalopathy. It presents with altered mental status, manifesting as confusion, disorientation, behavioral changes, or other cognitive impairments. This can be due to metabolic disturbances, hypoxia, ischemia, drugs, intoxications, organ dysfunction, or systemic infections.
Encephalitis	Encephalitis is characterized by inflammation of the encephalon (brain tissue), presenting with neurological manifestations such as altered sensorium, behavioral disorders, personality changes, sensory or motor deficits, speech abnormalities, development of movement disorders, focal motor deficits, and sensory phenomenon like paresthesias. The inflammation is typically due to infection but can also occur due to other inflammatory disorders like autoimmune dysfunction.
Rhombencephalitis	Rhombencephalitis is also known as brainstem encephalitis. Its manifestations include tremors, ataxia, involvement of the cranial nerve, autonomic instability, respiratory abnormalities, shock, and coma.
Acute encephalitis syndrome	In 2006, WHO introduced the term "acute encephalitis syndrome" in context for the syndromic surveillance of Japanese encephalitis. This is clinically defined as any individual, regardless of age or season, experiencing an acute onset of fever accompanied by altered mental status (which may include confusion, disorientation, coma, or speech difficulties) and/or new onset of seizures (excluding simple febrile seizures).

with this definition, the diagnosis of encephalitis requires major and minor criteria **(Table 24.16)**.

ETIOLOGY

In nearly half of encephalitis cases, the cause remains unidentified despite thorough diagnostics. Viruses are the most identified infectious causes of encephalitis. Enteroviruses, arboviruses, and herpesviruses are the most frequent viral causes of encephalitis (**Table 24.17**).

Various other infectious agents, such as bacteria, fungi, and parasites, can cause encephalitis, but they are less frequent than viruses. Beyond acute infections, encephalitis can also arise from an immune-mediated response in the CNS (post-infectious/para-infectious autoimmune encephalitis), which typically occurs days to weeks after the initial symptoms of the infection appear.

Table 24.16 International Encephalitis Consortium Definition of Encephalitis

Major criteria (mandatory criteria)	*Minor criteria*
Patients presenting with altered mental status (defined as decreased or altered level of consciousness, lethargy or personality change) lasting ≥24 hours with no alternative cause identified.	1. Fever >38°C (100°F) 2. Generalized or focal seizures not fully attributable to a preexisting seizure disorder 3. New focal neurological findings 4. CSF pleocytosis with >5 cells/mm^3 5. Neuroimaging showing brain parenchymal changes 6. Electroencephalography findings consistent with encephalitis
Definitions A. **Definite acute encephalitis syndrome:** Requires presence of major criteria with ≥3 minor criteria and one of the following: 1. Pathological confirmation of encephalitis-like brain inflammation 2. Documented pathological, microbiological, or serological evidence of acute infection with a pathogen closely associated with encephalitis from an appropriate clinical specimen; or 3. Laboratory evidence of an autoimmune disorder closely associated with encephalitis.	
B. **Probable acute encephalitis syndrome:** Presence of major criteria with three or more minor criteria	
C. **Possible acute encephalitis syndrome:** Presence of major and two minor criteria	

Table 24.17 Pathogens Associated with Encephalitis

Viruses	• Enteroviruses
	  ▪ Echovirus
	  ▪ Coxsackievirus A and B
	  ▪ Poliovirus
	  ▪ Other numbered enteroviruses
	• Parechoviruses
	• Herpes simplex virus (type 1 or 2)
	• Human herpesvirus 6
	• Influenza virus
	• Epstein-Barr virus
	• Cytomegalovirus
	• Arboviruses
	  ▪ Dengue virus
	  ▪ Japanese encephalitis virus
	  ▪ Chikungunya
	• Varicella-zoster virus
	• HIV
	• Measles virus
	• Mumps virus
	• Rubella virus
	• Parvovirus B19
	• SARS-CoV-2
	• Tick-borne encephalitis virus

Contd...

Contd...

Bacteria	• *Mycoplasma pneumoniae* • *Bartonella henselae* (Cat Scratch Disease) • *Rickettsia rickettsii* (Rocky Mountain spotted fever) • *Borrelia burgdorferi* (Lyme disease) • *Coxiella burnetii* (Q fever) • *Listeria monocytogenes* • *Mycobacterium tuberculosis* • *Bartonella quintana* ("trench fever")
Fungi	• *Cryptococcus neoformans* • *Coccidioides species* • *Histoplasma capsulatum*
Parasites	• *Plasmodium falciparum* • *Taenia solium (cysticercosis)* • *Toxoplasma gondii* • *Naegleria fowleri* • *Acanthamoeba spp* • *Balamuthia mandrillaris* • *Baylisascaris procyonis* • *Gnathostoma spinigerum* • *Trypanosoma brucei gambiense*

PATHOGENESIS

Most viral pathogens affecting the CNS first infect mucosal surfaces in the respiratory and gastrointestinal tracts, followed by replication in regional lymph nodes. This is followed by primary viremia, indicating illness onset and organ seeding. Aside from neonatal herpes simplex virus infection, most viruses access the CNS during a second viremia after replicating in other organs, especially the liver and spleen.

The pathogenesis of Japanese encephalitis starts with the transmission of the Japanese encephalitis virus via mosquito bites (Culex) into the human bloodstream **(Fig. 24.9)**. Once inside, the virus replicates initially in the skin and local lymph nodes, resulting in primary viremia. A subsequent secondary viremia may occur, potentially leading to a systemic infection and the virus's entry into the CNS. Once in the brain, the Japanese encephalitis virus infects glial cells, such as astrocytes and microglia, which activate a neuroinflammatory response. This response, combined with the direct effects of the virus on neurons, can result in neuronal cell death and damage.

CLINICAL FEATURES

Common symptoms include fever, seizures, altered sensorium (lethargy or irritability, or abnormalities of personality or behavior), focal neurologic deficits (such as pyramidal deficits including motor paresis, extrapyramidal deficits including movement disorders, and cranial nerve palsy).

Neonatal encephalitis: Similar to other infections in neonates, encephalitis often presents with nonspecific clinical manifestations. It should be considered in neonates or young infants exhibiting fever/hypothermia, seizures, feeding difficulties, irritability, or lethargy.

Older children: Encephalitis may manifest with febrile episodes with altered sensorium (stupor, lethargy, coma), psychiatric manifestations, emotional disorders, extrapyramidal

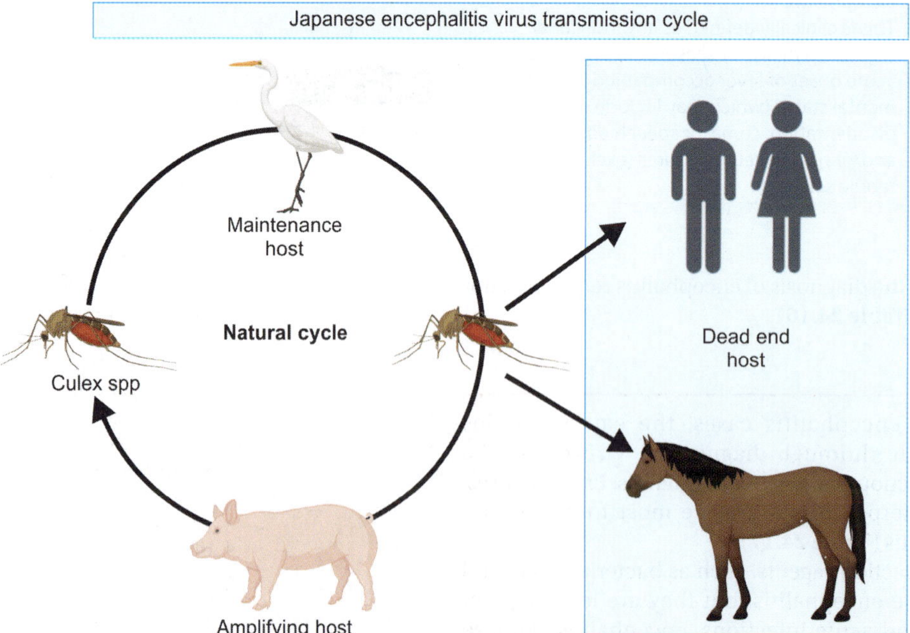

Fig. 24.9: The transmission cycle of Japanese encephalitis virus has been depicted diagrammatically. Japanese encephalitis virus is transmitted through the bite of infected Culex mosquitoes, primarily *Culex tritaeniorhynchus*. The virus cycles between these mosquitoes and vertebrate hosts, mostly pigs (amplifying hosts) and wading birds (maintenance hosts). Humans are considered incidental or dead-end hosts because they don't develop high enough virus levels to infect mosquitoes

Source: Created in BioRender. Sondhi, V. (2025) https://BioRender.com/ead3y31

movements, ataxia, seizures, or focal neurologic changes (including paresis or cranial nerve defects). Severe cases may lead to status epilepticus, cerebral edema, syndrome of inappropriate antidiuretic hormone secretion, or cardiorespiratory failure **(Table 24.18)**. Meningeal irritation symptoms can occur, but they are not a reliable indicator of encephalitis.

With certain viruses, focal brain dysfunction occurs.

- Brainstem encephalitis with an early onset of coma can be brought on by the *West Nile virus.*
- Hemiparesis, aphasia, and seizures are among the focal cortical neurologic deficits that the *herpes simplex virus* frequently causes. Before the patient's level of consciousness

Table 24.18 Clinical Evaluation of a Child with Meningoencephalitis

History		
Age	• Specific etiologic agents are more likely in different age groups ▪ For example, CMV, HSV (type 1 or 2), enteroviruses, parechoviruses, rubella virus are more likely among neonates.	
Travel	• History of travel to areas endemic for mosquito-borne diseases (like Japanese encephalitis, cerebral malaria, dengue)	
Immunization	• History of vaccination against Japanese encephalitis virus • An episode of encephalopathy following a vaccination may suggest acute disseminated encephalomyelitis	
Symptoms	*Infants* • Fever or hypothermia • Lethargy/irritability • Altered mental status • Poor feeding • Seizures • Respiratory distress/apnea • Bulging fontanel • Vomiting • Diarrhea • Jaundice	*Children and adolescents* • Fever • Headache • Altered mental status • Seizures/status epilepticus • Personality change • Psychiatric manifestations • Emotional disorders • Movement disorders • Focal deficits like paresis of limbs or cranial nerve deficits (diplopia)
History of predisposing factors	• History of rash ▪ Vesicular rash (varicella zoster virus) ▪ Erythematous macules with spread from head to toe ± conjunctivitis (measles) ▪ Maculopapular/petechial rash beginning at ankles and wrists (rickettsial infection especially Rocky Mountain spotted fever) • Rash, conjunctivitis, herpangina, pharyngitis (may suggest an underlying viral illness) • History of arthritis/arthralgia (chikungunya, dengue) • History of blood transfusion (HIV, EBV, West Nile virus, CMV) • History of recurrent infections in the past, suggestive of immunodeficiency (HIV) and predisposition to encephalitis with herpes simplex virus, varicella zoster virus, enteroviruses and cryptococcus	
Family and past history	• History of similar episodes in past may suggest a neurometabolic disorder with decompensation during the febrile illness • History of early childhood deaths/similar illness in family suggests inherited disorders associated with encephalopathy	
Examination		
General appearance	• Varying degrees of altered sensorium (stupor to coma) is always present • There may be presence of decerebrate or decorticate posturing among the sicker children	
Vitals	• Fever is usually present at presentation • Tachycardia and hypotension are suggestive of depleting volume status and help in detection of shock • Systemic hypertension, bradycardia, and respiratory depression, collectively known as Cushing's triad, serves as a late indicator of elevated ICP	
Head to toe evaluation	• Bulging anterior fontanelle in an infant is suggestive of raised intracranial pressure • Petechiae and purpurae are seen with dengue, or rickettsial infection (can also occur with meningococcal meningitis) • Presence of eschar suggests a rickettsial infection • Generalized lymphadenopathy may indicate infection with Ebstein-Barr virus, cytomegalovirus, HIV • Oral/genital ulcers suggest HSV infection • Presence of parotid swelling suggests mumps • Palmar-plantar erythema suggests human parechovirus type 3 infection • Conjunctivitis, pharyngitis, rash, herpangina, hand-foot-mouth disease suggests infection with enterovirus or parechovirus	

Contd...

Contd...

Signs of meningeal irritation (*are more commonly associated with meningitis*)	• Neck rigidity • Kernig's sign (flexion of the hip 90 degrees with subsequent pain upon extension of the leg) • Brudzinski sign (involuntary flexion of the knees and hips after passive flexion of the neck while supine)
Neurological examination	• Altered mental status: Glasgow Coma Scale (GCS) should be charted for all patients. Patients who are obtunded, semicomatose, or comatose tend to experience worse outcomes. • Seizures • Fundus examination to check for papilledema • Cranial nerve palsies may be present. Presence of pupillary asymmetry and lateral rectus palsy may suggest raised intracranial pressure with (impending) herniation. Facial nerve palsy may exist as part of primary disease or as a complication • Motor system examination for any focal neurological deficits should be conducted. These may include hemiparesis, quadriparesis, asymmetric or absent deep tendon reflexes, abnormal plantar reflexes. Children who have these findings are more likely to have a poor outcome • Specific findings: ▪ Cerebellar manifestations including ataxia: Enteroviruses, varicella zoster virus, Ebstein-Barr virus, mumps virus ▪ Extrapyramidal manifestations: Japanese encephalitis virus, West Nile virus, Nipah virus ▪ Poliomyelitis-like flaccid paralysis: Japanese encephalitis virus, West Nile virus, tick-borne encephalitis virus, enteroviruses ▪ Rhombencephalitis: Enterovirus 71, herpes simplex virus, west nile virus, *Listeria*
Other systemic examination	• Arthritis (dengue, chikungunya) • Respiratory tract involvement (*Mycoplasma*, influenza, adenovirus) • Hepatosplenomegaly (malaria) • Liver involvement, especially hepatitis (herpes simplex virus, enterovirus)

is reduced, rabies, human herpesvirus-6, or herpes simplex encephalitis can cause noticeable behavioral changes due to involvement of the limbic regions of the brain. When encephalitis affects the cerebral cortex, particularly the limbic system and hippocampus, focal or generalized seizures are more likely to occur.

- Depressed consciousness, hydrophobia, and brainstem-mediated laryngospasm are commonly linked to *rabies*.
- Due to the involvement of spinal cord anterior horn cells, infections with the West Nile virus, poliovirus, rabies virus, and Japanese encephalitis virus can result in focal or asymmetrical weakness with areflexia.

INVESTIGATIONS

The investigations in a child with suspected encephalitis include CSF analysis, neuroimaging (preferably MRI), and EEG. In addition, other supportive laboratory tests are performed to establish the etiology of encephalitis **(Table 24.19)**.

A. ***Complete blood count:*** Neutropenia with lymphocytosis may suggest viral etiology. Thrombocytopenia may be observed in patients with Dengue and rickettsial infections.

B. ***Blood culture:*** Should be taken before initiating antimicrobial therapy.

C. ***Peripheral blood smear and rapid diagnostic tests for Plasmodium spp:*** Rapid diagnostic tests that utilize antigen detection can identify one or more of the following: histidine-rich protein 2 (HRP2; used for detecting *P. falciparum*), *Plasmodium* lactate dehydrogenase (pLDH; for detecting all species or specifically *P. falciparum* and *P. vivax*), and aldolase (for detecting all species).

Table 24.19 Investigations to be Considered in a Child with Suspected CNS Infection

A. **Laboratory tests:** Blood/serum/urine a. CBC b. Peripheral blood smear c. Rapid diagnostic tests for malaria d. Blood glucose e. Kidney function tests: Serum electrolytes, blood urea nitrogen, and creatinine f. Liver function tests including ALT, AST, ALP g. Coagulation profile h. NS1 and IgM for dengue virus i. Blood culture j. HIV k. Hold acute serum and collect convalescent serum 10–14 days later for paired antibody testing
B. **CSF** a. Collect at least 5 cc fluid, if possible; freeze unused fluid for additional testing b. Opening pressure c. WBC count with differential d. RBC count e. Protein f. Glucose (perform a simultaneous blood glucose) g. Gram stain h. Bacterial culture i. PCR for HSV 1 and 2, Japanese encephalitis, CMV, HHV6, influenza, VZV
C. **Imaging** a. MRI preferred, should be done for all patients b. CT scan, if there are features of imminent herniation or the child is hemodynamically unstable c. Chest radiograph (case based, if findings of respiratory tract infection)

Contd...

Contd...

D. **EEG**
E. **Conditional testing, on case-to-case basis** a. Cryptococcal antigen and/or India Ink staining if HIV positive b. *Mycoplasma pneumoniae* serology and throat PCR and CSF PCR (if respiratory features or hemolytic anemia) c. Japanese encephalitis CSF PCR if acute flaccid paralysis d. Rickettsial serology if elevated transaminases or tick exposure e. Listeria PCR; *Brucella* antibody (serum) if brainstem involvement on imaging f. EBV PCR (CSF) and serology if cerebellum involvement on imaging g. Anti-NMDAR antibody (serum, CSF) if psychiatric disorder with movement abnormalities h. Autoimmune limbic encephalitis testing if features of limbic encephalitis

D. ***Blood glucose:*** To rule out hypoglycemia and for ruling out hypoglycorrhachia when performing CSF analysis.

E. ***Kidney Function tests*** (serum electrolytes, blood urea nitrogen, and creatinine): for evaluating for SIADH, which may occur as a complication.

F. ***Liver function tests,*** including ALT, and AST, to rule out hepatitis caused by certain viruses and malaria.

G. ***Coagulation studies:*** to rule out coagulopathy due to multisystem dysfunction. It may also coexist with rickettsial infections.

H. ***CSF analysis:*** The details of performing lumbar puncture have been outlined in the chapter on pyogenic meningitis. If there are no contraindications, lumbar puncture should be performed immediately. This helps establish the diagnosis by distinguishing between viral, bacterial, fungal, and parasitic causes based on the characteristics of the CSF and by identifying the pathogen through next-generation sequencing and culture, thus facilitating early empirical treatment.

I. ***Neuroimaging:*** Before performing a lumbar puncture, neuroimaging should be done immediately if there are indications of an elevated intracranial pressure or imminent herniation (asymmetric pupils, severe obtundation, decorticate or decerebrate posturing, Cheyne-Stokes breathing).

Since CT head is quicker and usually doesn't involve sedation or anesthesia, it is usually done as the first study in this situation. In all other circumstances, MRI should be preferred. Even among patients who have undergone a CT scan, an MRI should be performed.

A typical pattern of herpes simplex virus-related encephalitis involves the temporal lobe and insular cortices and is typically unilateral or asymmetrically bilateral **(Figs. 24.10A and B)**. Lesions in the thalamus and basal ganglia are frequently observed in cases of Japanese encephalitis virus and West Nile virus infection **(Figs. 24.10A and B)**. Brainstem involvement (midbrain, pons, and medulla) is characteristic of enterovirus A71 encephalitis.

Neuroimaging may also reveal alternative diagnoses like acute disseminated encephalomyelitis and neoplastic disorders.

J. ***EEG:*** When determining the kind and frequency of seizures, as well as whether nonconvulsive status epilepticus is present, an EEG can be useful.

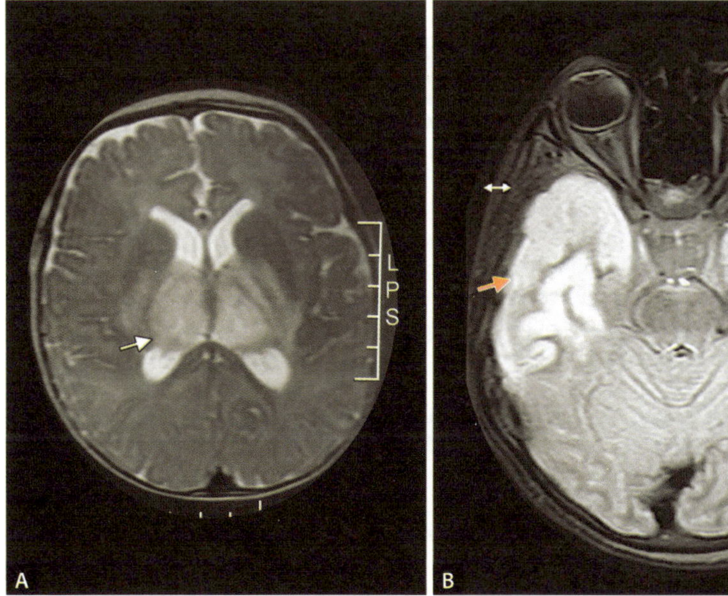

Figs. 24.10A and B: The neuroimaging features of Japanese encephalitis and herpes simplex encephalitis have been illustrated: (A) Depicts the bilateral thalamic involvement (white arrow) on the MRI brain of a child with Japanese encephalitis; (B) Highlights the asymmetrical hyperintensity involving the right temporal lobe (orange arrow) in a child with herpes simplex encephalitis

TREATMENT Acute Encephalitis

Patients with encephalitis should be closely monitored in an intensive care unit or similar setting because their clinical status can quickly deteriorate. The management of encephalitis is as below. An algorithmic approach to a child with suspected CNS infection has been illustrated in **Figure 24.8** in the chapter on Pyogenic Meningitis.

A. **Supportive therapy:**
  a. *Ensuring ABC*: The supportive therapy involves ensuring an open airway with adequate breathing and circulatory efforts. This involves monitoring of pulse, respiratory rate and SpO_2 and blood pressures. Regular monitoring of GCS and pupils should be performed. In addition, endotracheal intubation should be considered for GCS ≤8 or compromised airway.
  b. *Fluid resuscitation*: Fluid resuscitation with normal saline (20 mL/kg, initial bolus) should be performed if there are features of hypovolemia or shock.
  c. *Management of seizures*: It should be done by administration of intravenous lorazepam followed by phenytoin or levetiracetam.
  d. *Management of raised intracranial pressure*: Intracranial hypertension is managed by maintaining a 15–30° elevation of the head, keeping the head in the midline, preventing noxious stimuli, and instituting antiedema measures (mannitol or hypertonic saline).

B. **Empiric antimicrobial therapy:**
  - Until bacterial meningitis and cerebral malaria have been excluded, all children with suspected CNS infection should be managed with antibiotics, antimalarials, and antivirals.
  - The initial empiric treatment should include: (a) a third-generation cephalosporin (ceftriaxone) combined with vancomycin PLUS; (b) intravenous acyclovir PLUS; (c) intravenous artesunate.
  - In addition, empiric treatment may include other diseases based on clinical presentation, such as azithromycin and/or levofloxacin for *Mycoplasma*; oseltamivir for influenza; and doxycycline for *Rickettsia*. The details of antimicrobial agents, including drug dosages, are listed in **Table 24.20**.

PROGNOSIS

The overall risk of death varies from 0% to 7%. Certain pathogens, such as herpes simplex encephalitis, are associated with higher mortality. Children who survive encephalitis are susceptible to long-term neurodevelopmental disabilities, such as learning difficulties, behavioral issues, visual defects, hearing impairment, and developmental delays with motor deficits or cerebral palsy.

PREVENTION

The following are the main preventative steps: Measles, mumps, rubella, varicella, influenza, and, where appropriate, Japanese encephalitis vaccinations should be administered to infants, children, and teenagers regularly. Additionally, controlling insects and preventing exposure to ticks and mosquitoes is important. To avoid neonatal HSV, genital HSV infection during pregnancy should be properly identified, monitored, and treated.

Table 24.20 Antimicrobial Agents Used in a Child with Suspected Encephalitis

Pathogen	*Antimicrobial agent*
Streptococcus pneumoniae (sensitive to beta lactams)	**Either** IV ceftriaxone 50 mg/kg q12h **or** IV cefotaxime 100 mg/kg q8h
Streptococcus pneumoniae (resistant to beta lactams)	**Either** IV ceftriaxone 50 mg/kg q12h **or** IV cefotaxime 100 mg/kg q8h **AND** IV vancomycin 15 mg/kg q6h
Haemophilus influenzae	**Either** IV ceftriaxone 50 mg/kg q12h **or** IV cefotaxime 100 mg/kg q8h
Listeria monocytogenes	IV ampicillin 100mg/kg q6h **AND** **Either** IV gentamicin 2.5 mg/kg q8h **OR** IV amikacin 15–22.5mg/kg q24h
Herpes simplex virus	Age >28 days to <3 months—IV acyclovir 20 mg/kg q8h Age ≥3 months to <12 years—IV acyclovir 10 to 15 mg/kg q8h Age ≥12 years—IV acyclovir 10 mg/kg q8h
Cerebral malaria	Weight ≥20 kg : IV artesunate 2.4 mg/kg at 0, 12 and 24h Weight <20 kg: IV artesunate 3.0 mg/kg at 0, 12 and 24h **OR** IV quinine: Loading dose: 20 mg salt/kg in 5% dextrose over 4 hours; followed by 10 mg salt/kg over 4 hours at q8h
Cryptococcus neoformans	IV liposomal amphotericin B 3 to 4 mg/kg q24h **AND** Oral flucytosine 100 mg/kg/day in four divided doses

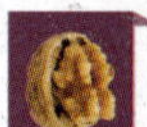

IN A NUTSHELL

Acute Encephalitis

1. Encephalitis refers to the inflammation of the encephalon (brain parenchyma), which clinically manifests with dysfunction of the brain (altered sensorium, focal neurological deficits, seizures) AND evidence of CNS inflammation (as demonstrated by CSF pleocytosis and/or findings aligning with encephalitis in neuroimaging).
2. During the neonatal period and infancy, encephalitis may present with fever, seizures, feeding difficulties, irritability, or lethargy.
3. In older children, it may manifest as a febrile episode with psychiatric manifestations, emotional lability, extrapyramidal movement disorders, ataxia, seizures, altered sensorium, or focal neurological deficits.
4. The mandatory evaluation of a child with suspected encephalitis includes CSF examination, neuroimaging, EEG, and blood tests for malaria and dengue virus.
5. The initial empiric treatment should include: (a) a third-generation cephalosporin (ceftriaxone) combined with vancomycin PLUS; (b) intravenous acyclovir PLUS; (c) intravenous artesunate.

Aneja S, Sharma S. Diagnosis and management of acute encephalitis in children. Indian J Pediatr. 2019;86(1):70–5.
Thompson C, Kneen R, Riordan A, et al. Encephalitis in children. Arch Dis Child. 2012;97:150.
Tunkel AR, Glaser CA, Bloch KC, et al. The management of encephalitis: clinical practice guidelines by the Infectious Diseases Society of America. Clin Infect Dis. 2008;47:303.
Venkatesan A, Tunkel AR, Bloch KC, et al. Case definitions, diagnostic algorithms, and priorities in encephalitis: consensus statement of the international encephalitis consortium. Clin Infect Dis. 2013;57:1114.

24.5 Tubercular Meningitis

PE 27.2, PE 27.3

INTRODUCTION

A central nervous system (CNS) infection caused by *Mycobacterium tuberculosis* (MTB) may manifest as spinal arachnoiditis, tuberculoma, or meningitis. Tuberculous meningitis (TBM) refers to the inflammation of the leptomeninges surrounding the brain and spinal cord due to infection by *M. tuberculosis*. It is associated with high morbidity and mortality if not treated promptly. The common terminologies associated with CNS tuberculosis (CNS TB) have been highlighted in **Table 24.21**.

PATHOPHYSIOLOGY

Mycobacterium tuberculosis initially enters the host through droplet inhalation, infecting the alveolar macrophage. The primary infection is localized in the lungs with dissemination to the lymph nodes. At this stage of the infection, a significant level of bacteremia may seed the entire body. In some patients, dissemination may occur due to late reactivation. Following dissemination, MTB infects the meninges (resulting in TBM) and forms subependymal collections known as Rich foci. These foci can burst into the subarachnoid space, triggering a severe inflammatory response that results in meningitis symptoms. This can result in three prominent pathological changes manifesting clinically.

Table 24.21 Terminologies Associated with CNS TB

Terminology	*Description*
Tubercular meningitis	Tuberculous meningitis is the involvement of the leptomeninges of the brain and spinal cord due to infection by *Mycobacterium tuberculosis*.
Tuberculoma	A tuberculoma is a conglomerate granulomatous focus that develops from coalescing tubercles acquired during disseminated *Mycobacterium tuberculosis* bacillemia.
Spinal arachnoiditis	Spinal tuberculous arachnoiditis is characterized by the breakdown of tuberculous granulomatous foci within the spinal cord or meninges, which results in the encasement of the spinal cord and spinal nerve roots in tuberculous exudates.
Optochiasmatic arachnoiditis	This condition occurs when thick tuberculous exudates envelop the optic nerves and optic chiasma.
Basal exudates	When tubercular bacilli and proteins leak from the Rich focus into the subarachnoid space, it causes a severe hypersensitivity reaction that results in inflammatory changes. This results in a thick gelatinous exudate, particularly prominent at the basal part of the brain which is referred to as basal exudate. It is associated with the encasement of cranial nerves, which clinically manifests as cranial nerve palsies.

A. ***Basal exudates:*** The inflammatory response leads to leakage of proteinaceous fluid and cells (exudates) from the blood vessels into the subarachnoid space, particularly in the basilar cisterns. This response can encase cranial nerves, leading to cranial nerve palsies.
B. ***Vasculitis:*** In response to MTB infection, inflammatory cells (primarily lymphocytes and monocytes) infiltrate meninges and CSF. These inflammatory cells produce inflammatory cytokines (YNF-alpha, IL-1, IL-6) that can damage the vessel walls (vasculitis), particularly in the small and medium-sized cerebral vessels. This can further lead to cerebral ischemia/infarction and encephalopathy. The structures most commonly involved are the basal ganglia, thalamus, and internal capsule.
C. ***Hydrocephalus:*** Hydrocephalus results from inflammatory exudates blocking the CSF flow. When the obstruction is at the level of the arachnoid villi, it results in communicating hydrocephalus. Obstruction at other levels (foramina of Monroe, aqueduct of Sylvius, foramen of Magendie and Luschka) results in obstructive hydrocephalus.

CLINICAL FEATURES

The presentation of patients with TBM typically includes symptoms such as headache, fever, vomiting, and altered consciousness. These symptoms are also frequently observed in bacterial meningitis. However, certain characteristics may facilitate differentiation between TBM and bacterial meningitis. These characteristics include a subacute emergence of symptoms (with symptoms developing over 1–3 weeks for TBM and within a few days for bacterial meningitis), a higher prevalence of cranial nerve palsies in TBM, and an increased occurrence of altered sensorium and coma in TBM **(Table 24.22)**. Based on their neurologic symptoms and mental state, children with TBM can be classified into the following stages.

Table 24.22 Clinical Evaluation of a Child with Suspected Tubercular Meningitis

History	
Onset	Subacute onset, typically over 1–3 weeks
Symptoms	• Headache • Fever • Vomiting • Personality changes • Altered sensorium • Cranial nerve palsies (history suggestive of visual disturbance, lateral rectus palsy, facial nerve palsy) • Hemiparesis • Seizures
History of predisposing factors	• History suggestive of HIV should be sought • History of contact with tuberculosis patient or past history of undergoing treatment for tuberculosis
Vaccination history	BCG has a protective effect of TBM
Examination	
General appearance	Children with TBM are usually toxic looking
Vitals	• Fever is usually present at presentation • Tachycardia and hypotension are suggestive of help in detection of shock • Presence of systemic hypertension, bradycardia, and respiratory depression (Cushing triad) is a late sign of raised intracranial pressure
Anthropometry	• Patients usually are malnourished and may have low weight for age
Head to toe evaluation	• Bulging anterior fontanelle in an infant is suggestive of raised intracranial pressure • Generalized lymphadenopathy • Icterus may suggest disseminated TB or may be a side effect of antitubercular therapy
Signs of meningeal irritation	• Neck rigidity • Kernig's sign (flexion of the hip 90 degrees with subsequent pain upon extension of the leg) • Brudzinski sign (involuntary flexion of the knees and hips after passive flexion of the neck while supine)
Neurological examination	• Altered mental status: Glasgow Coma Scale (GCS) should be charted for all patients. • Seizures • Fundus examination to check for papilledema • Cranial nerve palsies may be present. Presence of pupillary asymmetry and lateral rectus palsy may suggest raised intracranial pressure with (impending) herniation. Facial nerve palsy may exist as part of primary disease or as a complication • Motor system examination for any focal neurological deficits should be conducted. These may include hemiparesis, quadriparesis, asymmetric or absent deep tendon reflexes, abnormal plantar reflexes.
Other systemic signs of disseminated tuberculosis	• Hepatosplenomegaly • Bone/joint lesions • Dermatological findings (scrofuloderma/lupus vulgaris)

A. ***Stage I:*** The individual is alert and oriented, showing no specific neurological features. This initial phase, lasting 1–3 weeks, features a gradual onset of fatigue, lethargy, headaches, mild fever, along with shifts in personality and mood.
B. ***Stage 2:*** This stage of meningitis is marked by the emergence of neurological deficits in individuals. Although they remain conscious, they often exhibit inattention, confusion, and lethargy. Mild focal signs may be present, including cranial nerve palsies or hemiparesis, with a Glasgow coma score ranging from 11 to 15.
C. ***Stage 3:*** Symptoms of this advanced stage include hemiplegia, convulsions, delirium, stupor, coma, multiple cranial nerve palsies, and poor sensorium (Glasgow Coma Score ≤10).

INVESTIGATIONS

The investigations in a child with suspected meningoencephalitis include the following. Antimicrobial therapy should be started as soon as possible and not postponed due to delays in conducting investigations such as lumbar puncture (LP) or CT scan.

A. ***Complete blood count with differential***: Patients may have leukocytosis with lymphocytosis and anemia, suggesting chronic infection.
B. ***Blood culture:*** Blood cultures are positive in approximately 60–85% of patients with bacterial meningitis.
C. ***Inflammatory markers:*** Elevations of C-reactive protein and erythrocyte sedimentation rate, is frequently observed with TBM.
D. ***Serum electrolytes, glucose, blood urea nitrogen, and creatinine:*** These are useful for assessing volume status and planning fluid administration. The serum glucose level is essential for determining the CSF-to-blood glucose ratio.
E. ***Lumbar puncture:*** The opening pressure is generally moderately raised (180–300 mm H_2O). Common CSF characteristics in TBM are lymphocytic pleocytosis, increased protein levels, and decreased glucose levels. The interpretation of CSF results has been summarized in **Table 24.13** of the chapter on meningitis. In addition to routine testing, measurement of the CSF adenosine deaminase (ADA) level may be a useful adjunctive test for diagnosing tuberculous meningitis. Definitive diagnosis of TBM requires identification of MTB in the CSF. The following modalities are used for identifying MTB in CSF:
   - *Ziehl-Neelsen staining:* The sensitivity of acid-fast staining in diagnosing TBM ranges from 30% to 60%. The diagnostic yield improves with greater volumes of cerebrospinal fluid (up to 10–15 mL) and by collecting more CSF specimens (up to four). Additionally, acid-fast bacilli (AFB) smears and cultures can remain positive for several days even after treatment has started.
   - *MTB cultures:* CSF mycobacterium cultures show variable yields, being positive only 40–83% of the time and requiring 6–8 weeks for growth.
   - *Nucleic acid amplification:* The World Health Organization has recommended the use of the Xpert MTB/RIF Ultra assay as an initial diagnostic test for TBM.
   - *Metagenomic next-generation sequencing (NGS)* is a promising diagnostic tool. Preliminary studies indicate

NGS can identify M. tuberculosis in CSF and differentiate TBM from other conditions.

F. ***Neuroimaging***: Brain CT or MRI are used in radiographic evaluation for suspected CNS TB; MRI is better than CT at defining lesions affecting the brainstem, midbrain, and basal ganglia. Hydrocephalus, basilar exudates, periventricular infarcts, and cerebral tuberculomas are common findings in tuberculous meningitis. Tuberculous exudates are seen in the interpeduncular, suprasellar, perimesencephalic, and Sylvian cisterns in patients with optochiasmatic arachnoiditis, which can manifest with vision loss.

G. ***Other tests***: A chest radiograph should be performed to rule out a co-existent pulmonary focus. In addition, HIV testing should be considered based on clinical profile.

TREATMENT Tubercular Meningitis

The management of tuberculous meningitis requires the immediate initiation of antituberculous therapy (ATT) along with glucocorticoids. For those presenting with hydrocephalus, a surgical consultation for the placement of a CSF shunt is necessary. It is critical not to postpone empiric treatment due to the high risk of mortality and complications associated with untreated infections. Patients exhibiting relevant epidemiological factors (such as a history of MTB infection or disease, known or suspected MTB exposure), clinical symptoms, significant radiographic findings, and typical CSF characteristics should promptly receive empiric treatment.

A. ***Antitubercular therapy:*** Typically, the treatment for CNS TB starts with an intensive phase lasting 2 months, where four drugs are administered. This is followed by a prolonged continuation phase, which generally involves two to three drugs over an additional 7–10 months, making the entire treatment duration range from 9 to 12 months. According to NTEP/RNTCP guidelines, every child diagnosed with CNS-TB should undergo 2 months of intensive treatment with four drugs (2HRZE), followed by an extended phase of 8 months utilizing three drugs (8HRE). The drug dosages of ATT have been listed in **Table 24.23**.

Table 24.23 Drug Dosages of Antitubercular Drugs

Drug	*Preparation*	*Dose*	*Maximum dose*
Isoniazide	• Tablets (50 mg, 100 mg, 300 mg) • Elixir (50 mg/5 mL)	10 mg/kg/day	300 mg
Rifampicin	• Capsules (150 mg, 300 mg) • Syrup (100 mg/5 mL)	15 mg/kg/day	600 mg
Pyrazinamide	Tablets (250 mg, 500 mg, 750 mg, 1000 mg)	35 mg/kg/day	2000 mg
Ethambutol	Tablets (100 mg, 200 mg, 400 mg, 800 mg, 1000 mg)	20 mg/kg/day	1500 mg
Streptomycin	Injection (0.75 grams)	20 mg/kg/day	1000 mg

Second line antitubercular therapy includes (in alphabetical order): Amikacin, Bedaquiline, Capreomycin, Clofazimine, Cycloserine, Delamanid, Ethionamide, Imipenem-cilastatin, Kanamycin, Levofloxacin, Linezolid, Meropenem, Moxifloxacin, Para-aminosalicylic acid, Streptomycin

B. ***Corticosteroids:*** In addition to ATT, children with TBM should be administered dexamethasone 0.6 mg/kg/day IV for four weeks, followed by a tapering course over four weeks, or oral prednisone 2 mg/kg daily for 4–6 weeks, which should also be tapered gradually.

C. ***Management of complications:***
- *Hydrocephalus*: Increasing intracranial pressure is a clinical manifestation of progressive ventriculomegaly. Patients with altered sensorium and progressive vision impairment should be assessed for endoscopic third ventriculostomy or ventriculoperitoneal shunt-based CSF diversion.
- *Optochiasmatic arachnoiditis*: In tuberculous meningitis, one of the main causes of vision loss is optochiasmatic arachnoiditis, which is the encasement of optic nerves and optic chiasma by thick tuberculous exudates. There is still uncertainty regarding the best way to handle this issue. Isolated case reports have linked the tumor necrosis factor-alpha inhibitor thalidomide to clinical improvement.

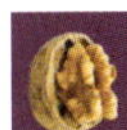

IN A NUTSHELL

Tubercular Meningitis

1. A sub-acute clinical presentation with fever, headache, vomiting, altered sensorium, cranial nerve palsies and raised intracranial pressure should raise suspicion for tubercular meningitis.
2. The diagnosis of tuberculous meningitis may be definitively established in CSF with a positive smear for acid-fast bacilli, a CSF culture positive for *Mycobacterium tuberculosis*, or a positive nucleic acid amplification test. Relevant clinical and epidemiologic factors, along with typical CSF findings (lymphocytic pleocytosis, elevated protein concentration, and low glucose concentration), may lead to a presumptive diagnosis of tuberculous meningitis.
3. Cerebral parenchymal tuberculomas, periventricular infarcts, hydrocephalus, and basilar exudates are classic neuroimaging findings that indicate tubercular meningitis.
4. The course of treatment for CNS TB consists of 2 months of intensive treatment (four medications) followed by 7–10 of continuation treatment (2–3 medications). The entire course of treatment lasts 9–12 months.

Aulakh R, Chopra S. Pediatric tubercular meningitis: a review. J Pediatr Neurosci. 2018;13(4):373-82.

Evans EE, Avaliani T, Gujabidze M, et al. Long term outcomes of patients with tuberculous meningitis: the impact of drug resistance. PLoS One. 2022;17:e0270201.

Israni AV, Dave DA, Mandal A, et al. Tubercular meningitis in children: clinical, pathological, and radiological profile and factors associated with mortality. J Neurosci Rural Pract. 2016;7(3): 400-4.

Jaganath D, Beaudry J, Salazar-Austin N. Tuberculosis in Children. Infect Dis Clin North Am. 2022;36:49.

Wilkinson RJ, Rohlwink U, Misra UK, et al. Tuberculous meningitis international research consortium. Tuberculous meningitis. Nat Rev Neurol. 2017;13(10):581-98.

24.6 Neurocysticercosis

INTRODUCTION

Neurocysticercosis (NCC) is the infestation of the CNS caused by the encysted larval stage of the *Taenia solium* (pork tapeworm), referred to as cysticercus. It is the most common cause of acquired epilepsy in India. Although epilepsy is the most common presentation, NCC can show a range of clinical manifestations, from asymptomatic cases to life-threatening presentations. The terminologies related to NCC have been highlighted in **Table 24.24**.

Table 24.24 Terminologies Related to Neurocysticercosis

Terminology	*Explanation*
Taeniasis	Taeniasis is an intestinal infection caused by tapeworms, including *Taenia solium* (pork tapeworm), *T. saginata* (beef tapeworm), and *T. asiaticus* (Asian tapeworm). The transmission occurs through the fecal-oral route between humans (the definitive hosts) and intermediate hosts: pigs for *T. solium* and *T. asiaticus*, and cattle for *T. saginata*. Human infections stem from consuming the meat of infected animals
Cysticercosis	Cysticercosis is a parasitic infection caused by the larval stage (cysticercus) of the pork tapeworm, *Taenia solium*. It is caused by ingesting *Taenia solium* eggs, which are shed in the feces of infected individuals
Neurocysticercosis	Neurocysticercosis is a parasitic infection of the central nervous system caused by the larval stage (cysticercus) of the pork tapeworm *Taenia solium*

LIFE CYCLE

Development of taeniasis and cysticercosis are two distinct processes involving the same host and nematode **(Fig. 24.11)**. Taeniasis has been discussed in Chapter 14 on Infectious Diseases. Cysticercosis refers to an infestation by cysticercus, which is the larval stage of *T. solium*.

Cysticercosis occurs when *T. solium* eggs are ingested, typically through contaminated food or from infected food handlers. Once

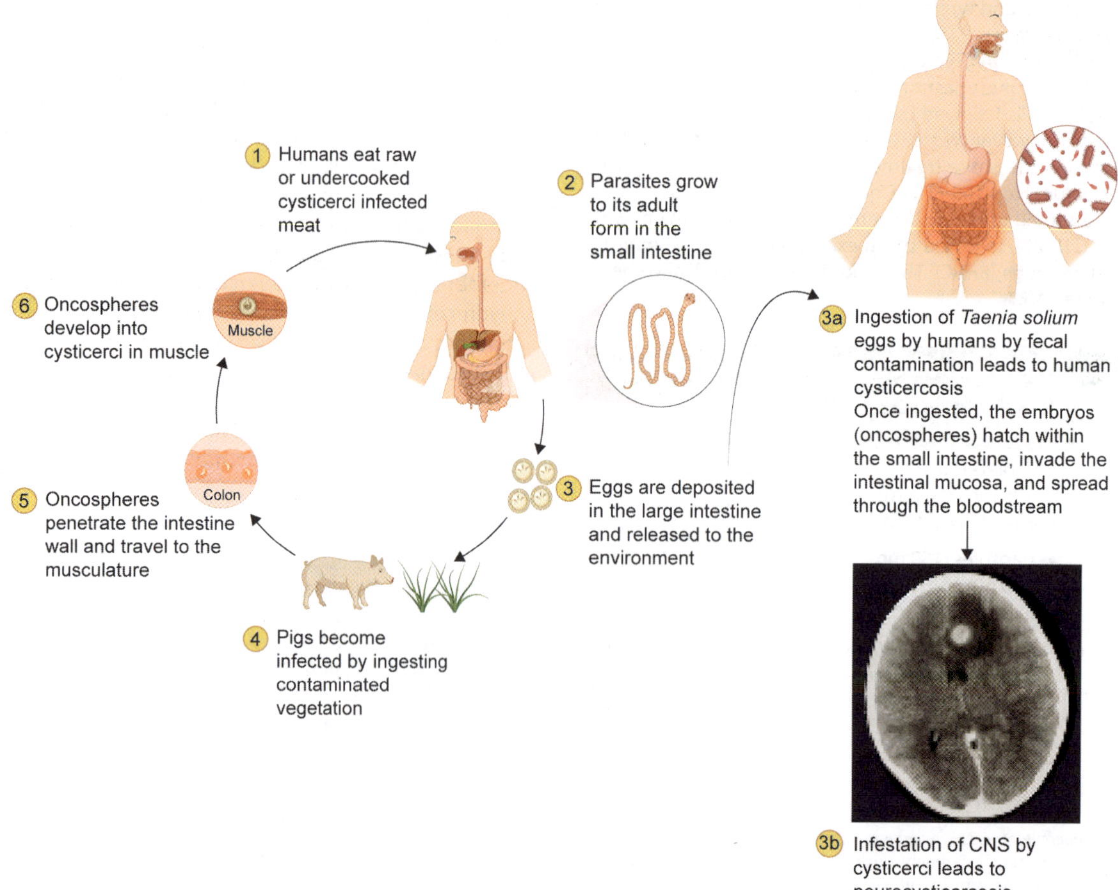

Fig. 24.11: Life cycle of *T. solium* and occurrence of cysticercosis has been illustrated

Source: Created in BioRender. Sondhi, V. (2025) https://BioRender.com/5yzey8p

Table 24.25 Stages of Cysticerci

Stage	Explanation
Vesicular	Viable cyst containing clear liquid, with a thin, semitransparent wall and an eccentric protoscolex appearing as a nodule adjacent to the wall
Colloidal	Degenerative changes in the cyst, with thickening of the cyst wall and the transformation of the clear fluid into a whitish gel
Granular nodular	Host inflammatory response damages the cyst, leading to larval death and forming a granulomatous lesion
Nodular calcified	Degenerated granular tissue is replaced by fibrous tissue which may undergo calcification over course of time

ingested, the embryos (oncospheres) hatch within the small intestine, invade the intestinal mucosa, and spread through the bloodstream to the CNS, eyes, skeletal muscles, subcutaneous tissue, liver, and other tissues. Over 3–8 weeks, tissue cysticerci form, characterized by membranous walls filled with fluid and an invaginated scolex. When this infestation with cysticerci involves the CNS, it is referred to as NCC.

A common misunderstanding is believing that eating infected pork is necessary to contract cysticercosis. Consuming pork infected with cysts results in adult tapeworm infestation (taeniasis), while ingesting *T. solium* eggs leads to cysticercosis.

PATHOGENESIS

Cysticerci develop through four key stages **(Table 24.25)**.

1. The *initial stage* is the live cyst (vesicular stage), where the nematode exists in a clear fluid. This thin-walled cyst contains fluid and a live larva along with *T. solium* head.
2. The *second stage* is characterized by degenerative changes in the cyst, characterized by thickening of the cyst wall and the conversion of the fluid from clear to a whitish colloid (colloidal stage).
3. In the *third stage*, the larva degenerates and dies (granular stage), causing the cyst to fill with caseous material due to damage from an inflammatory response.
4. The degenerated cyst is finally replaced by fibrotic tissue and goes through calcification (calcified nodular stage) in the *fourth stage*.

CLASSIFICATION

Based on their location within the CNS, NCC has been classified as below.

A. ***Intra-parenchymal NCC:*** Parenchymal NCC is the most prevalent type in children, with cysticerci predominantly located at the gray-white junctions. Seizures are the most common manifestation of this category of NCC.
B. ***Intraventricular NCC:*** This category is characterized by cysts present within the CSF. It may coexist with subarachnoid CSF and frequently presents with features of obstructive hydrocephalus/raised intracranial pressure.
C. ***Subarachnoid NCC:*** This rare category is characterized by cysts in the subarachnoid space. The cysts may grow large, forming grape-like structures (racemose) and may present with manifestations of meningitis or intracranial hypertension.
D. ***Spinal NCC:*** These may present either with leptomeningeal involvement or with parenchymal (intramedullary) lesions.
E. ***Ocular cysticercosis:*** Commonly found in the subretina, it may involve other tissues, including the subconjunctival space, anterior chamber, vitreous, retina, and extraocular muscle.

CLINICAL FEATURES

Clinical symptoms can range from no symptoms at all to severe diseases, influenced by the infection's characteristics (such as the number, size, location, and stage of cyst lesions) and the host's immune response. The common clinical manifestations include the following.

A. ***Seizures and epilepsy:*** Seizures are the most frequent manifestation of an intraparenchymal cyst. They typically start as focal seizures but can occasionally evolve into generalized seizures. The characteristics of the seizures correspond with the anatomical location of the parasite.
B. ***Headache:*** Headache often results from elevated intracranial pressure due to extraparenchymal NCC. Additionally, it can manifest as a postictal symptom.
C. ***Raised intracranial pressure:*** Intracranial hypertension arises from various mechanisms, including obstruction of the CSF pathways (such as intraventricular cysts), mass effects from large cysts in the Sylvian or interhemispheric fissures, and chronic conditions like arachnoiditis.
D. ***Impaired vision:*** Ocular cysticerci may present with vision impairment, recurring eye pain, and diplopia. Inflammation caused by degenerating intraocular cysticerci can jeopardize vision by leading to chorioretinitis, retinal detachment, or vasculitis.
E. ***Cysticercal meningitis:*** Patients present with fever and neck rigidity, typical of meningitis. However, eosinophilia in CSF aids in differentiating this entity from bacterial meningitis.
F. ***Cysticercotic encephalitis:*** A rare entity, it is typically seen in adolescent girls and presents with headache, altered sensorium, and can be life-threatening.
G. ***Myelitis:*** Cysticerci in the spinal cord can present with symptoms mimicking transverse myelitis.
H. ***Radiculopathy:*** Cysts located in the intradural extramedullary space lead to symptoms of nerve root involvement, including numbness, tingling, pain, or weakness in the area served by the involved nerve.

DIAGNOSIS

Cysticercosis should be considered in children experiencing seizures or signs of increased intracranial pressure, particularly if there is relevant epidemiological exposure. The differential diagnosis for NCC is listed below.

1. Granulomatous brain lesions a. Tuberculoma b. Fungal infections like cryptococcoma c. Toxoplasmosis d. Langerhans histiocytosis
2. Brain abscess
3. Neoplastic brain lesions
4. Arachnoid cysts

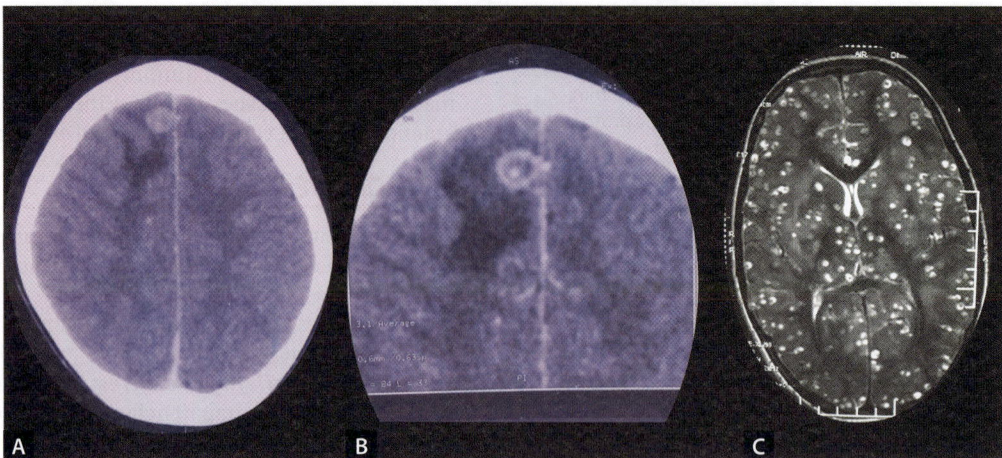

Figs. 24.12A to C: (A and B) Depict the contrast-enhanced CT scan of the brain showing a ring-enhancing lesion with scolex visualized as an internal asymmetric nodule in the cysts ("hole with dot" appearance). Perilesional edema is also observed around these lesions; (C) Highlights the starry sky appearance of multiple neurocysticercoses seen on MRI of the brain

The diagnosis relies heavily on neuroimaging findings, encompassing both computed tomography (CT) and magnetic resonance imaging (MRI), when possible.

- A typical CT finding is a singular, small lesion (less than 20 mm) appearing as a low-density area with ring or disc enhancement, featuring an eccentric scolex that resembles a bright hyperdense nodule **(Figs. 24.12A to C)**.
- Occasionally, multiple lesions, or even numerous ones, may be identified. The presence of several cysts at different developmental stages can create the characteristic "starry sky" appearance, indicative of neurocysticercosis (NCC).
- Additionally, CT scans are beneficial for detecting intracranial calcifications in the nodular calcified stage.
- MRI offers superior imaging for smaller lesions and those near the skull or in the posterior fossa, providing enhanced information about parenchymal inflammation or periventricular effusion in cases of hydrocephalus. It is particularly effective for identifying extraparenchymal lesions.

Neuroimaging aids in differentiating NCC from tuberculomas, which is a common differential diagnosis for all ring-enhancing lesions on neuroimaging **(Table 24.26)**.

Table 24.26 Features Differentiating NCC from Tuberculoma on Neuroimaging

Neuroimaging feature	*Neurocysticercosis*	*Tuberculoma*
Size of lesion	Usually <20 mm	Usually >20 mm
Location of lesion	Grey-white matter junction in parenchymal neurocysticercosis	Basal area of the brain
Number of lesions	Can be single or multiple	Usually multiple and conglomerate
Surrounding edema	Extensive, may or may not have midline shift	Extensive, may have midline shift
T2 image in MRI brain	Core will look hyperintense	Core will look hypointense
MR spectroscopy	Amino acid peak	Lipid peak

TREATMENT Neurocysticercosis

The management of NCC typically involves supportive therapy and definitive anthelminthic therapy **(Fig. 24.13)**.

Supportive Therapy

The initial strategy for managing a patient with NCC should focus on effectively controlling symptoms through antiseizure medications and neuroprotective methods. Steroids may be combined with anthelminthic medication to reduce inflammatory responses, vasculitis, or cerebral edema. Typically, a single antiseizure medication, such as carbamazepine or phenytoin, is employed to manage seizures arising from a solitary lesion of NCC. The likelihood of seizure recurrence is significantly associated with an abnormal CT scan (indicating either lesion persistence or calcification) and an abnormal EEG during the withdrawal of antiseizure medication. Antiseizure medications can be discontinued after a one-year seizure-free period when both the lesion has resolved and the EEG has returned to normal; however, prolonged AED treatment may be necessary for patients with enduring or calcified lesions.

Oral corticosteroids are typically given for a few days, starting 1 or 2 days prior to cysticidal therapy. This timing helps reduce perilesional edema and prevents adverse reactions stemming from the host's inflammatory response. Prednisolone is usually prescribed at a dosage of 1–2 mg/kg for a period of 5–7 days. Alternatively, dexamethasone may be administered at a dose of 0.15mg/kg/dose thrice daily.

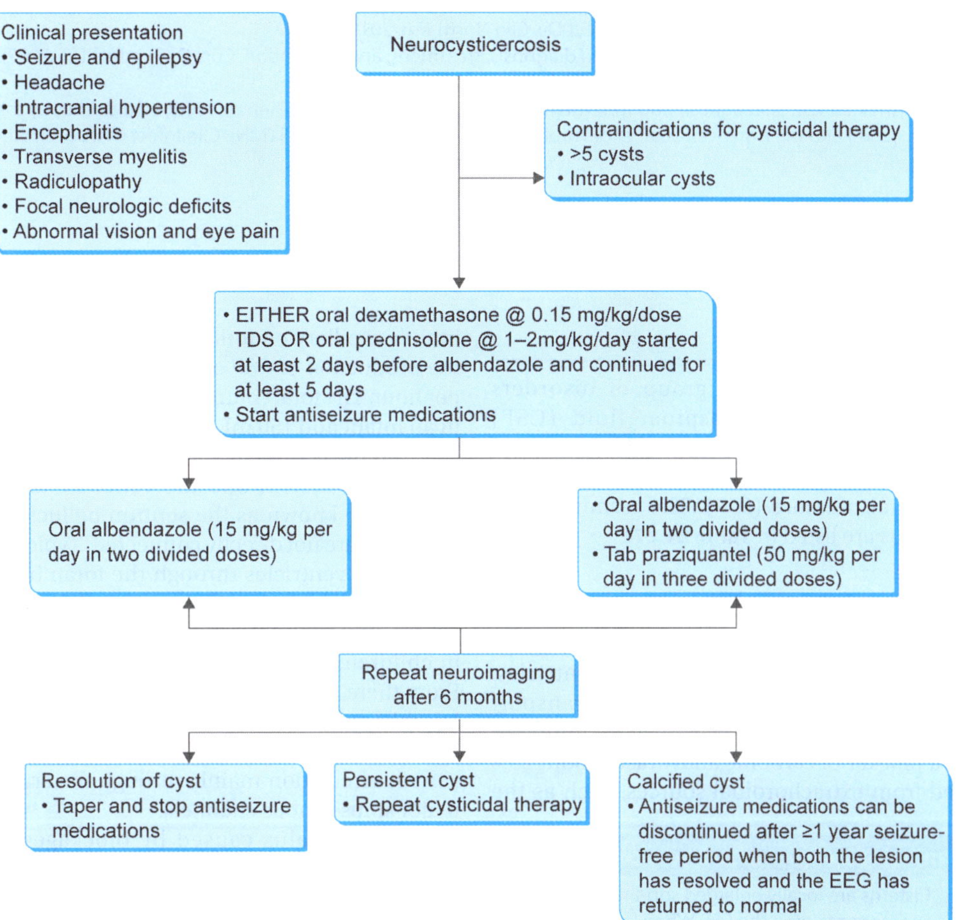

Fig. 24.13: An algorithmic approach to the management of neurocysticercosis has been illustrated along with the common clinical manifestations

Anthelminthic Therapy

Albendazole, 15 mg/kg/d, divided into two doses daily for 10–14 days, taken with food, is the antiparasitic treatment of choice for cysticidal therapy in NCC. Recent studies suggest that combining albendazole with praziquantel (50 mg/kg/d) enhances effectiveness against multiple cysticercal cysts without increasing side effects. For patients with one or two viable and/or degenerating parenchymal cysts, treatment with albendazole is advised. In cases where patients have more than two viable and/or degenerating parenchymal cysts, both albendazole and praziquantel are recommended for treatment. However, there is a possibility of worsened neurological status following antiparasitic treatment due to the host's inflammatory response to dying parasites. Patients with basal subarachnoid NCC require a longer duration of antiparasitic treatment. It is important to note that antiparasitic therapy is contraindicated for those with ophthalmic lesions and severely elevated intracranial pressure. A CT scan is typically performed after 3–6 months to check if the lesions have resolved. For children with persistent lesions, an additional round of cysticidal therapy is often administered.

Those with significantly elevated intracranial pressure and ophthalmic NCC should only receive steroid treatment, as cysticidal therapy may aggravate the situation by triggering an inflammatory response. It is important to note that cysticidal therapy does not affect calcified lesions.

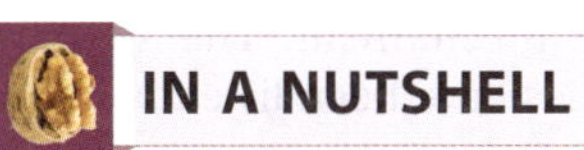

IN A NUTSHELL

Neurocysticercosis

1. NCC results from ingesting *T. solium* eggs. Eating contaminated pork leads to adult tapeworm infections (taeniasis), but does not result in cysticercosis.
2. Consider NCC in patients presenting with seizures and/or signs of increased intracranial pressure.
3. The diagnosis of NCC primarily relies on neuroimaging findings, including cystic lesions, enhancing lesions, and/or calcifications. Identification of a scolex within a cystic lesion is deemed diagnostic for NCC.
4. For patients with one or two viable and/or degenerating parenchymal cysts, treatment with albendazole is advised. In cases where patients have more than two viable and/or degenerating parenchymal cysts, both albendazole and praziquantel are recommended for treatment.

Coyle CM. Neurocysticerosis: an Individualized approach. Infect Dis Clin North Am. 2019;33:153.
Pineda-Reyes R, White AC Jr. Neurocysticercosis: an update on diagnosis, treatment, and prevention. Curr Opin Infect Dis. 2022;35:246.
Singhi P, Suthar R. Neurocysticercosis. Indian J Pediatr. 2015;82:166-71.
White AC Jr, Coyle CM, Rajshekhar V, et al. Diagnosis and Treatment of Neurocysticercosis: 2017 Clinical Practice Guidelines by the Infectious Diseases Society of America (IDSA) and the American Society of Tropical Medicine and Hygiene (ASTMH). Clin Infect Dis. 2018;66:e49.

24.7 Hydrocephalus

PE 27.4

INTRODUCTION

Hydrocephalus represents a diverse group of disorders characterized by abnormal cerebrospinal fluid (CSF) accumulation within the cerebral ventricles and/or subarachnoid spaces, leading to ventricular dilation and an elevation in intracranial pressure (ICP). The terminologies related to hydrocephalus are listed in **Table 24.27**.

PHYSIOLOGY

About 60–80% of CSF is produced by the choroid plexus, which is located in the lateral, third, and fourth ventricles. Choroidal epithelial cells produce CSF via active transport reliant on carbonic anhydrase; this process can be inhibited by acetazolamide, a blocker of carbonic anhydrase. About 25% of CSF is produced from extrachoroidal sources, such as the brain's capillary endothelium parenchyma. In a healthy child, the production of CSF occurs at a rate of approximately 20 mL per hour. The total volume of CSF is estimated to be about 50 mL in an infant and 150 mL in an older child or adult.

CSF flow is driven by the pressure difference between the ventricular system and the venous channels. Because of a membrane known as the septum pellucidum, the two lateral ventricles are not directly connected. Typically, CSF moves from the lateral ventricles through the foramina of Monro into the third ventricle. It then flows through the narrow aqueduct of Sylvius, measuring around 3 mm in length and 2 mm in diameter in children, before entering the fourth ventricle **(Fig. 24.14)**. From there, the CSF exits through the paired lateral foramina of Luschka and the midline foramen of Magendie into the cisterns located at the base of the brain. CSF is absorbed into systemic venous circulation mainly through the arachnoid villi into the major sinus venous channels.

Hydrocephalus caused by blockages in the ventricular system is termed obstructive or noncommunicating hydrocephalus. In contrast, hydrocephalus that arises from the obstruction of the subarachnoid cisterns or malfunctioning arachnoid villi is known as nonobstructive or communicating hydrocephalus.

Table 24.27 Terminologies Related to Hydrocephalus

Term	Description
Cistern	Cisterns are focally enlarged sub-arachnoid spaces containing the CSF. When located at the base of the brain, they are called basal cisterns and those located between the cerebral peduncles in the midbrain are called interpeduncular cisterns
Hydrocephalus	Hydrocephalus is characterized by excessive amount of CSF accumulation within the cerebral ventricles and/or subarachnoid spaces
Obstructive hydrocephalus	Hydrocephalus caused due to structural blockage of CSF flow within the ventricular system (lateral ventricles/third ventricle/fourth ventricle). It is also called as non-communicating hydrocephalus
Communicating hydrocephalus	Hydrocephalus from obstructed subarachnoid cisterns or malfunctioning arachnoid villi is termed nonobstructive or communicating hydrocephalus
Ventriculomegaly	Ventriculomegaly is ventricular enlargement seen on neuroimaging and is found in all forms of hydrocephalus. The ventricle just before the obstruction is maximally dilated
Hydranencephaly	Hydranencephaly is characterized by the complete absence of cerebral hemispheres, and they are represented by thin membranous sacs that are filled with CSF. The mid-brain and brainstem are relatively intact

ETIOLOGY

Hydrocephalus occurs when there is an imbalance between the production and absorption of intracranial cerebrospinal fluid (CSF). This imbalance may arise from obstruction in the circulation of CSF, insufficient absorption, or, rarely, overproduction of CSF. Regardless of the cause, the excessive volume of CSF leads to increased ventricular pressure and results in ventricular dilation.

Hydrocephalus can be congenital or acquired, further classified as obstructive and communicating based on the primary underlying pathogenic mechanism. The specific etiologies related to these categories have been listed in **Table 24.28**.

CLINICAL FEATURES

Hydrocephalus presents with varying clinical features influenced by multiple factors like the age at onset of pathology, type of the lesion causing the obstruction, and the duration and rate of increase of the intracranial pressure. The important clinical features have been highlighted in **Table 24.29**.

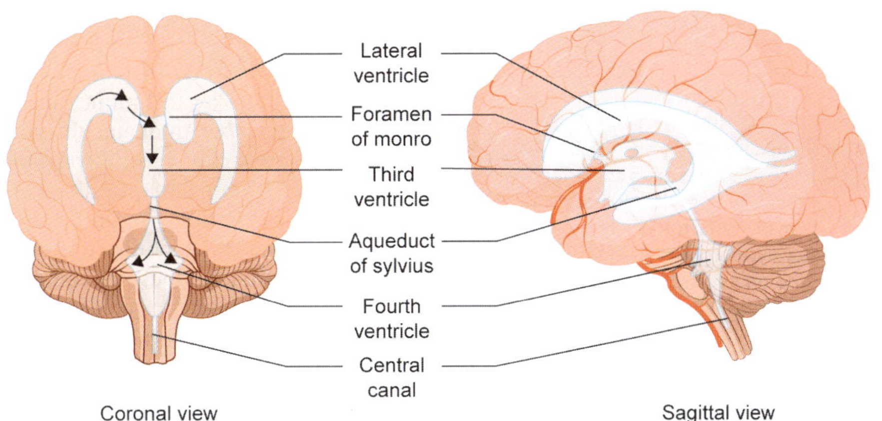

Fig. 24.14: Circulation of cerebrospinal fluid is illustrated in coronal and sagittal views. CSF is produced by the choroid plexus and moves from the lateral ventricles through the foramina of Monro into the third ventricle, then flows through the aqueduct of Sylvius into the fourth ventricle. It exits through the lateral foramina of Luschka and midline foramen of Magendie into the cisterns at the brain's base. CSF is absorbed into systemic circulation mainly through arachnoid villi and into major venous channels. The image has been created in BioRender

Source: (Created in BioRender. Sondhi, V. (2025) https://BioRender.com/zgk0vod)

Table 24.28 Hydrocephalus Etiologies

Congenital hydrocephalus	
Communicating	• Intrauterine infections* (rubella, cytomegalovirus, lymphocytic choriomeningitis, syphilis, and Zika virus) • Choroid plexus papilloma or carcinoma • Syndromic forms like trisomy 13, 18
Obstructive	• Aqueductal stenosis (**commonest**) • Brain malformations ▪ Chiari II malformation ▪ Dandy Walker malformation ▪ Vein of Galen malformation • Intrauterine infections* (rubella, cytomegalovirus, toxoplasmosis, lymphocytic choriomeningitis, syphilis, and Zika virus)
Acquired hydrocephalus	
Communicating	• Posthemorrhagic hydrocephalus with hemorrhage into subarachnoid space like post-traumatic or AV aneurysm • Choroid plexus papilloma or carcinoma
Obstructive	• Complication of CNS infections like tuberculous meningitis, bacterial meningitis (**commonest)** • Posthemorrhagic hydrocephalus with hemorrhage into ventricles like IVH in preterm infants • CNS tumors (particularly posterior fossa medulloblastomas, astrocytomas, and ependymomas) • Achondroplasia

*Intrauterine infections can cause inflammation of the ependymal lining of the ventricular system and/or the meninges in the subarachnoid space. This may result in impaired absorption of CSF and/or obstruction of CSF flow through the aqueduct or basal cisterns, potentially causing both communicating and obstructive hydrocephalus.

Table 24.29 Salient History and Clinical Features in a Child with Hydrocephalus

History	
A. Antenatal history	1. History suggestive of intrauterine infections 2. History of anomalies noted during fetal scans
B. Birth history	1. History of prematurity, ELBW/VLBW status 2. History of birth trauma
C. Developmental history	1. Delayed attainment of milestones especially motor milestones (head holding may be delayed due to large head size) 2. There may be delay in attainment of other milestones too like cognitive and vision
D. History of other symptoms	1. Large head size 2. History suggestive of raised ICP a. Irritability, lethargy, or a significant change in the child's behavior b. Feed refusal c. Vomiting 3. Visual impairment 4. Strabismus 5. In later stages the child can have altered sensorium and seizures
Examination	
A. Vital signs	1. Bradycardia 2. Hypertension 3. Altered respiratory rate and pattern
B. Physical examination of head and spine	1. Macrocephaly 2. Anterior fontanelle may become full or distended 3. Sutures feel more widely split

Contd...

Contd...

	4. "Cracked pot" sound on percussion (Macewen sign) 5. Frontal bossing 6. Prominent scalp veins 7. Spine examination to check for neural tube defects, or their tell-tale signs like hemangioma, tuft of hair 8. Any dysmorphism suggestive of syndromes 9. Cranial bruit heard with vein of Galen malformation
C. Neurological examination	1. Ocular abnormalities a. Compression of the third or sixth cranial nerve may result in extraocular muscle paresis leading to diplopia ± strabismus ± head tilt b. Sun setting sign, characterized by eyes turned downward making the sclera visible above iris. This is caused due to pressure on the midbrain resulting in impairment of upward gaze 2. Fundus a. To evaluate for papilledema b. Chorioretinitis may suggest intrauterine infection 3. Spasticity (due to stretching of the corticospinal fibers from the motor cortex around the dilated ventricles) 4. Abnormal posturing like decerebrate or decorticate posturing will indicate severe compromise with likely herniation

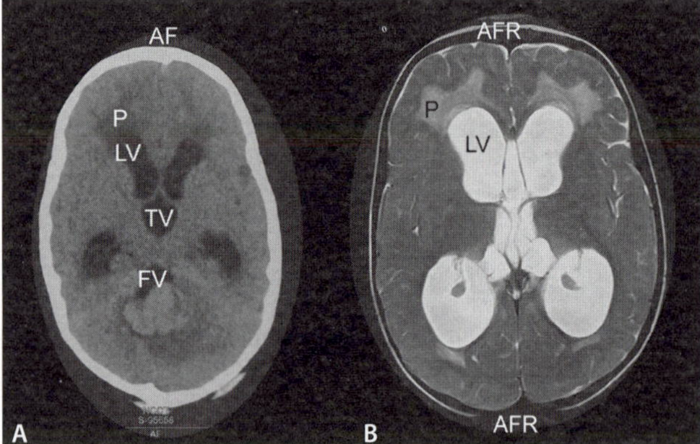

Figs. 24.15A and B: The neuroimaging characteristics have been highlighted. (A) Demonstrates an NCCT brain and (B) Illustrates a T2-weighted sequence of MRI depicting dilated lateral ventricles (LV), and third ventricle (TV) with a normal-sized fourth ventricle (FV), suggesting an obstructive hydrocephalus. Also the periventricular ooze (P) is apparent on both images

INVESTIGATIONS

The diagnosis of hydrocephalus is established with neuroimaging. The key techniques and findings are as below:

A. ***Ultrasonography:*** Antenatal ultrasonography is an effective method for detecting ventriculomegaly during pregnancy. In a newborn or young infant with an open anterior fontanelle, cranial ultrasound is the preferred method for the initial examination. This technique is favored because it avoids ionizing radiation, does not require sedation, and is both readily available and portable.
B. ***CT Scan:*** A CT scan is usually performed in the acute setting when concerns about raised intracranial pressure of uncertain etiology exist. It is fast and can usually be performed without anesthesia. CT scans have disadvantages, such as radiation exposure. Additionally, they offer significantly less information; therefore, children who receive CT scans as their initial assessment and are diagnosed with hydrocephalus typically require further evaluation with an MRI.
C. ***MRI:*** MRI is the preferred imaging method for children with suspected hydrocephalus. With its different sequences, it provides superior visualization of the brain, CSF and related pathologies (**Figs. 24.15A and B**).
D. ***Plain radiograph skull:*** Although seldom used, plain radiograph of skull can reveal separation of the sutures, erosion of the posterior clinoids in an older child, and an increase in convolutional markings (beaten-silver appearance) on the inner surface of the skull with prolonged increased intracranial pressure.

TREATMENT Hydrocephalus

Most children with hydrocephalus will need mechanisms to divert the excess CSF to relieve the raised intracranial pressures. The most effective treatment for most patients is surgical drainage, using a shunt or third ventriculostomy. However, concurrently medical management is also initiated.

A. **Medical management:** The medical management of a child with hydrocephalus involves administration of acetazolamide (50–75 mg/kg/day) in 3–4 divided doses. This drug, acting via carbonic anhydrase inhibition, reduces the CSF production; however, its effect is modest and disappointing. In children with features of raised intracranial pressure, while they are awaiting surgical diversionary procedure, intravenous mannitol or hypertonic saline can be administered to reduce intracranial pressure.
B. **Surgical management:** Most children with hydrocephalus need extracranial shunts, especially a ventriculoperitoneal shunt. Endoscopic third ventriculostomy is viable, with established criteria, but may require repetition for effectiveness. Endoscopic fenestration of the third ventricle floor into the subarachnoid space can be attempted in patients over 6 months with noncommunicating hydrocephalus.

Complications: Hydrocephalus can lead to various complications that may arise from the condition itself or from the treatments used to manage it. These have been illustrated in **Table 24.30**.

Table 24.30 Complications Related to Hydrocephalus

A. Due to underlying disease:
   a. Cognitive impairment
   b. Developmental delays
   c. Seizures/epilepsy
   d. Vision abnormalities ± vision loss
   e. Emotional and behavioral issues
   f. Accelerated pubertal development

B. Shunt related complications:
   a. Shunt infection (usually caused by S. epidermidis)
   b. Shunt occlusion
   c. Over drainage (can cause functional shunt failure with subnormal intracranial pressures)
   d. Intestinal obstruction

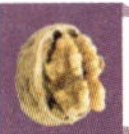

IN A NUTSHELL

Hydrocephalus

1. Hydrocephalus is characterized by the excessive amount of CSF accumulation within the cerebral ventricles and/or subarachnoid spaces. Hydrocephalus caused due to structural blockage of CSF flow within the ventricular system is defined as obstructive hydrocephalus; else it is defined as communicating hydrocephalus.
2. Common causes of congenital hydrocephalus include intraventricular hemorrhage and neural tube defects, including myelomeningocele. Other causes include infection, genetic defects, trauma, tumors, and teratogens.
3. Common clinical features include headaches, irritability, behavior changes, developmental delays, vomiting, and lethargy.
4. Diagnosis is established by neuroimaging. MRI is more useful compared to CT scan as it can delineate posterior fossa.
5. The most effective treatment for most patients is surgical drainage, using a shunt or third ventriculostomy. However, concurrently, medical management with mannitol/hypertonic saline is also initiated.

Dewan MC, Rattani A, Mekary R, et al. Global hydrocephalus epidemiology and incidence: systematic review and meta-analysis. J Neurosurg. 2019;130:1065.
Kirkpatrick M, Engleman H, Minns RA. Symptoms and signs of progressive hydrocephalus. Arch Dis Child. 1989;64:124.
Tully HM, Dobyns WB. Infantile hydrocephalus: a review of epidemiology, classification and causes. Eur J Med Genet. 2014;57:359.
Whitehead WE, Weiner HL. Infantile and Childhood Hydrocephalus. N Engl J Med. 2022;387:2067.

24.8 Infantile Hemiplegia

PE 27.5

INTRODUCTION

Hemiplegia is the paralysis of one side of the body, while *hemiparesis* refers to weakness on one side. These terms are frequently used interchangeably, and both describe motor deficits affecting one-half of the body.

Hemiplegia is often a result of an underlying cerebrovascular accident and is a neurologic emergency. A sudden acute neurological deficit typically indicates a vascular event unless proven otherwise. These events, often referred to as strokes or cerebrovascular event, can be categorized into ischemic and hemorrhagic types based on their underlying pathophysiology.

- The ischemic forms, including arterial ischemic stroke (AIS) and cerebral sinovenous thrombosis (CSVT), occur more frequently than brain malignancies.
- A comparable number of children also experience hemorrhagic strokes (HS) and other types of cerebrovascular diseases.

PATHOPHYSIOLOGY

Arterial Circulation

The arterial blood supply of brain is through two main channels: the "anterior" circulation, which consists of the paired internal carotid arteries, and the "posterior" circulation formed by the paired vertebral arteries that join to create the basilar artery (known as the "vertebrobasilar system") **(Fig. 24.16)**. The anterior and posterior circulations converge at the Circle of Willis. The major cerebral arteries emerging from the Circle of Willis include the anterior, middle, and posterior cerebral arteries **(Fig. 24.17)**. Smaller "perforating arteries" arise from these cerebral arteries to deliver blood to deep brain areas, including the basal ganglia, thalamus, and midline structures of the brainstem. Meanwhile, larger circumferential arteries (the posterior inferior, anterior inferior, and superior cerebellar arteries) deliver blood to the lateral aspect of the

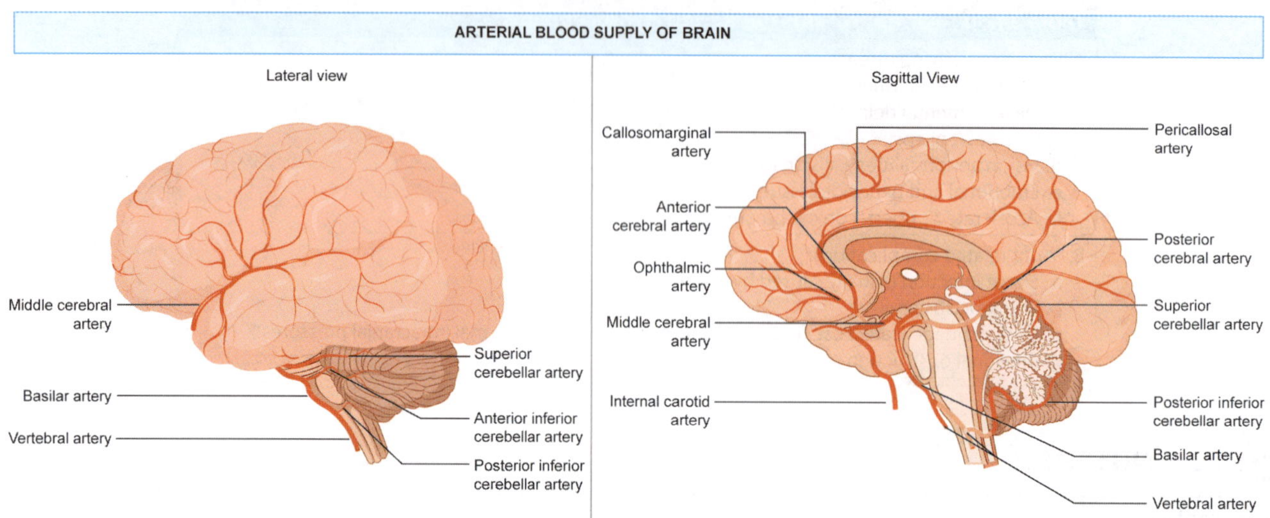

Fig. 24.16: Arterial blood supply of brain is illustrated in the lateral view and midline sagittal section

Source: Created in BioRender. Sondhi, V. (2025) https://BioRender.com/73f4x18

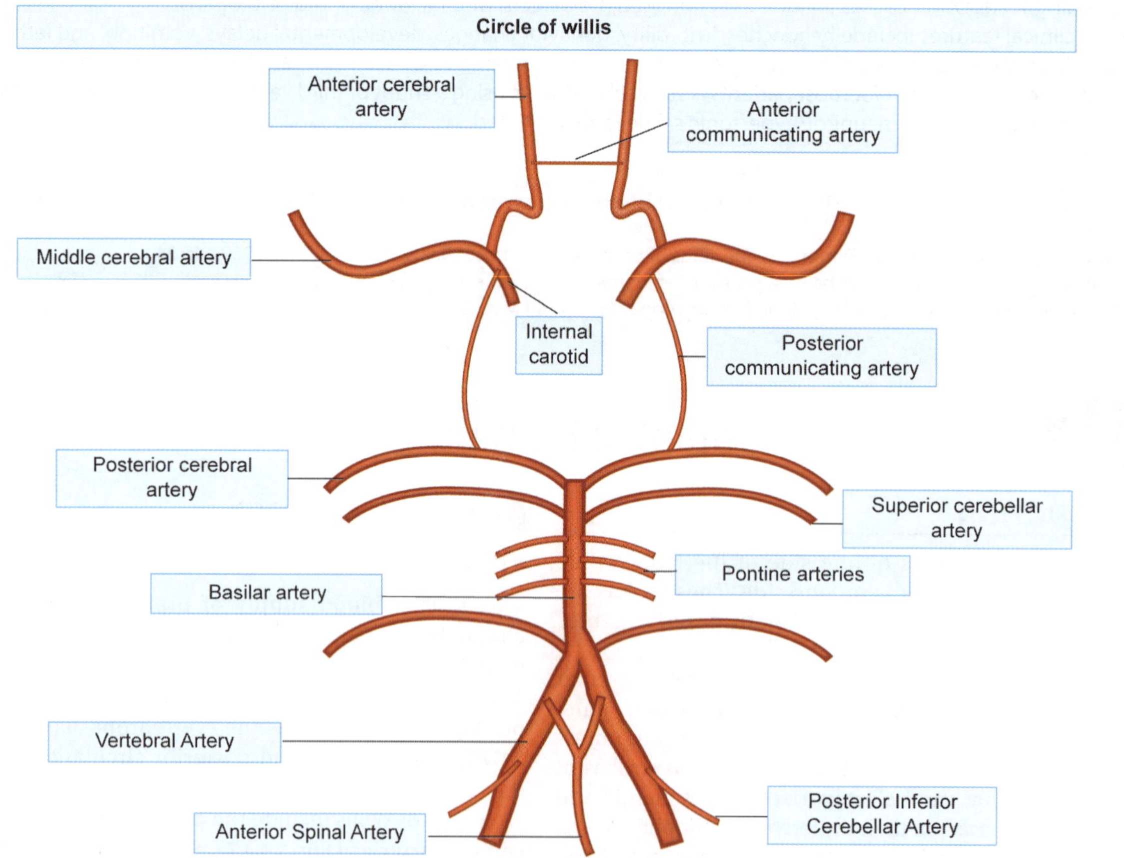

Fig. 24.17: Arterial blood supply to the brain is through the "anterior" circulation, which consists of the paired internal carotid arteries, and the "posterior" circulation formed by the paired vertebral arteries that join to create the basilar artery. The anterior and posterior circulations converge at the circle of willis, which further gives rise to principal arteries that supply the brain

Source: Created in BioRender. Sondhi, V. (2025) https://BioRender.com/gku2um7

brainstem and cerebellum. The circle of Willis and smaller distal leptomeningeal anastomoses provide collateral flow, which may improve brain perfusion during vaso-occlusive strokes.

Most AIS affect the middle cerebral artery, leading to peripheral wedge-shaped lesions that involve the cortical gray matter and subcortical white matter. As end arteries, lenticulostriate lesions lack collateral circulation, increasing the possibility of permanent infarction. Despite their small size, these resultant infarctions often impact vital anatomical areas and functional pathways, like the internal capsule.

Venous Drainage

The drainage of venous blood from the brain occurs via a system of cerebral veins and sinuses, primarily divided into superficial and deep venous systems **(Fig. 24.18)**. The superficial system involves cortical veins that collect blood from the cerebral cortex and relatively superficial subcortical white matter, directing it medially towards the superior sagittal sinus. The deep venous system comprises internal cerebral, medullary, thalamic, and choroidal veins, all converging centrally at the vein of Galen, which subsequently drains into the straight sinus. This system drains the centrally situated basal ganglia nuclei and thalami and the deeper parts of the white matter from both hemispheres. Ultimately, both systems then unite posteriorly at the torcula. The bilateral transverse sinuses drain laterally from the torcula into the sigmoid sinuses, which then drain into the internal jugular veins. This drainage system also includes additional routes that connect at significant locations, including the anterior cavernous and petrosal sinuses.

Sagittal sinus thrombosis frequently leads to bilateral parasagittal infarcts, in which hemorrhagic transformation may or may not co-exist. The bilateral basal ganglia, thalami, and surrounding deep white matter may develop edema and infarction due to thrombosis within the deep venous system.

ETIOLOGY AND RISK FACTORS

Stroke is the leading cause of infantile hemiplegia. It can have multiple risk factors. Common risk factors for pediatric stroke encompass congenital heart disease, meningitis/encephalitis, sepsis, and sickle cell disease. Merely 30% of ischemic and hemorrhagic strokes in children are linked to a recognized risk factor **(Table 24.31)**. Many children presenting with stroke may have a multifactorial etiology.

CLINICAL FEATURES

Stroke should always be considered when a previously healthy child develops a focal neurological deficit (like hemiparesis). The key features of history and examination have been summarized in **Table 24.32**. The differential diagnosis of a child with hemiplegia are listed in **Box 24.1**.

INVESTIGATION

Investigations as guided by history and physical examination are performed to identify underlying etiology of ataxia. These include the following:

- ***Neuroimaging:*** MRI with MRA of head and neck is the imaging technique of choice. It is superior than CT for detecting acute ischemia **(Figs. 24.19A and B)**.
- ***Baseline laboratory testing:*** These include: CBC including platelets, liver function tests, blood glucose, prothrombin time (PT) and international normalized ratio (INR), partial thromboplastin time. These investigations aid to determine

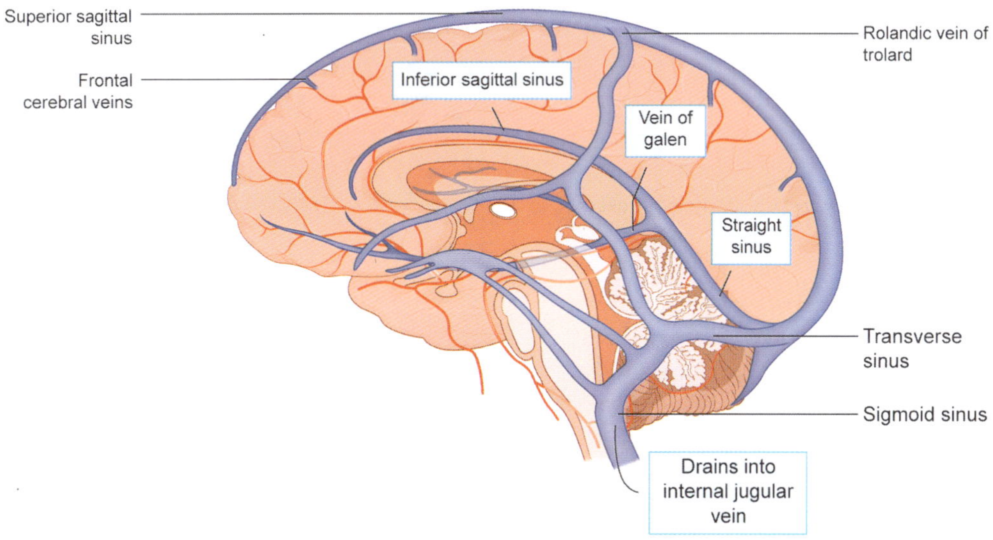

Fig. 24.18: Diagram of cerebral venous drainage systems has been illustrated

Source: Created in BioRender. Sondhi, V. (2025) https://BioRender.com/9zr9zna

Table 24.31 Risk Factors Associated with Stroke Leading to Hemiplegia

A. Cardiac disorders ▪ Arrhythmia ▪ Atrial myxoma ▪ Bacterial endocarditis ▪ Cardiac catheterization ▪ Cardiomyopathy ▪ Cyanotic congenital defects ▪ Mitral valve prolapse ▪ Prosthetic heart valve ▪ Rhabdomyoma ▪ Rheumatic heart disease
B. Hematological disorders ▪ Antiphospholipid antibodies/lupus anticoagulant ▪ Congenital coagulation defects ▪ Disseminated intravascular coagulation ▪ Drug-induced thrombosis ▪ Iron deficiency anemia ▪ Malignancy ▪ Polycythemia ▪ Sickle cell anemia/disease ▪ Thrombocytopenic purpura
C. Cerebrovascular malformations ▪ Arteriovenous malformation ▪ Fibromuscular dysplasia ▪ Sturge-Weber syndrome
D. Trauma ▪ Arterial dissection ▪ Blunt trauma to neck ▪ Intraoral trauma ▪ Vertebral manipulation
E. Vasculitis ▪ Carotid infection ▪ Hemolytic-uremic syndrome ▪ Hypersensitivity vasculitis ▪ Meningitis (**see Ch 24.3**) ▪ Mixed connective tissue disease ▪ Systemic lupus erythematosus ▪ Takayasu arteritis ▪ Varicella infection
F. Vasculopathy ▪ Fabry disease ▪ Homocystinuria ▪ Mitochondrial encephalopathy, lactic acidosis and stroke (MELAS) ▪ Moyamoya disease ▪ Mineralizing angiopathy
G. Prothrombotic state ▪ Factor V Leiden ▪ Prothrombin gene 20210A ▪ Protein C deficiency ▪ Protein S deficiency ▪ Antithrombin III deficiency
H. Miscellaneous ▪ Nephrotic syndrome ▪ Diabetes ▪ Drugs like L-asparaginase, OCPs

Table 24.32 History and Physical Examination in a Child with Ataxia

History	
Onset of symptoms	• Rapid onset/acute nonprogressive: Maximum weakness at onset with gradual improvement is suggestive of embolism, intra cranial bleed • Acute progressive: Gradual increase in the severity/extent of weakness is characteristic of thrombotic stroke • Chronic nonprogressive: Longstanding weakness with no progression is a feature of cerebral palsy or post meningitic/encephalitic sequelae • Chronic progressive hemiplegia are observed with AV malformation and space occupying lesions like brain neoplasms
Associated symptoms	• Focal features: ▪ Hemiparesis and hemifacial weakness ▪ Speech or language disturbance ▪ Visual disturbance ▪ Ataxia • Nonlocalizing features ▪ Headache ▪ Altered mental status ▪ Vomiting • Seizures (if focal can help in localizing) • Early hand preference is indicative stroke in early infancy
History suggestive of underlying etiology	• Cyanosis, cyanotic spells (for cyanotic congenital heart diseases) • Fever, increased fatiguability, breathlessness (for endocarditis) • Trivial trauma (for mineralizing angiopathy) • Intraoral trauma/motor vehicle injury with rapid vertebral movement (arterial dissection) • Pallor, recurrent blood transfusion requirement, painful crisis (sickle cell anemia) • Ear discharge (mastoiditis) • Skin rash (varicella, SLE) • Abnormal urinary odor, consanguinity, recurrent sibling loss, unexplained encephalopathy (inborn errors of metabolism) • Anasarca (nephrotic syndrome) • History of varicella infection in the previous 12 months • Postradiation arteriopathy secondary to head or neck radiation for neoplastic disorders • History of drug intake including oral contraceptives, chemotherapy, sympathomimetics, or illicit drugs (amphetamine, cocaine)

Contd…

Contd...

Physical examination	
Vital signs	• Bradycardia, abnormal respiratory pattern, and hypertension may occur with increased intracranial pressure • Fever is suggestive of an infectious process
General examination	• Bulging of the anterior fontanel may indicate increased intracranial pressure • Auscultation of head and neck for bruits may indicate vasculopathy/dissection • Skin lesions may suggest neurofibromatosis, fabry disease, or PHACES syndrome • Pallor/icterus for hemolytic anemia like sickle cell disease • Cortical thumb/fist • Limb length discrepancy is suggestive of intrauterine/perinatal stroke
Eye examination	• Corneal clouding associated with fabry disease • Fundoscopy may show arteriopathy changes
Neurological examination	• Altered sensorium may be present • Speech deficits • Focal neurological deficits: hemiplegia, facial palsy

Box 24.1 Differential Diagnosis in a Child with Hemiplegia

A. Cerebrovascular accident
B. Seizures
C. Alternating hemiplegia
D. Migraine
E. Neoplasm
F. Demyelination
G. Hypertensive encephalopathy
H. Inborn errors of metabolism
I. Functional neurologic disorders

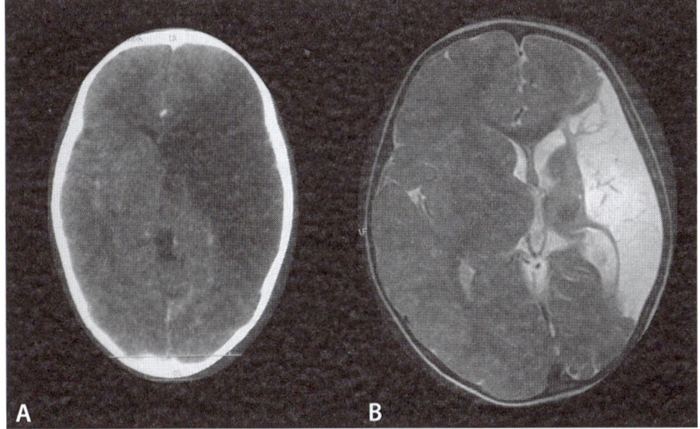

Figs. 24.19A and B: Wedge-shaped infarct conforming to the left MCA territory is depicted as hyper density in CT Scan (A) and as hyperintensity in T2 weighted sequence of MRI (B)

the hydration status and help rule out contraindications to pharmacotherapy.

- ***Investigations to determine underlying risk factor:***
  - *Hemoglobin electrophoresis and a peripheral blood smear* are evaluated to rule out sickle cell disease.
  - *Iron studies* (serum ferritin, serum iron, and total iron binding capacity) are performed to rule out iron deficiency anemia.
  - An *autoimmune profile*, including ANA, anti-dsDNA, Lupus anticoagulant, and ANCA, is performed to assess the autoimmune disorders associated with vasculitis.
  - *Prothrombotic workup* for protein C, protein S and antithrombin III are assessed typically 3 months after the acute episode. Genetic tests for underlying prothrombotic disorders (Factor V Leiden mutation, MTHFR polymorphism) can be performed earlier.
  - *2D-ECHO and Doppler studies* are performed to establish/rule out any underlying cardiac disorder and arterial dissection, respectively.

TREATMENT Infantile Hemiplegia

Overall, pediatric stroke treatment is primarily based on adult stroke protocols. However, in children, there are significant differences in the application of acute anticoagulation and reperfusion therapies, such as intravenous thrombolysis and mechanical thrombectomy. The therapy comprises the following:

A. **Emergency management**

- Initial management should adhere to basic life support guidelines that include stabilization of airway, breathing, and circulation
- Maintenance of euthermia, euglycemia, normal electrolyte levels and normal blood oxygen and carbon dioxide levels
- Hypertension leads to higher mortality rates, while hypotension can reduce blood flow to penumbral tissue. For most patients, maintaining blood pressure at up to 15% above the 90th percentile is advisable. Elevated pressures can be progressively reduced using short-acting antihypertensives such as labetalol, while administering fluids and vasopressor drugs may mitigate relative hypotension to prevent penumbral damage due to hypoperfusion.

B. **Antithrombotic therapy:** There exists a scarcity of data to establish the efficacy and safety of tissue plasminogen activator (tPA) and thrombectomy among children. Hence, thrombolysis and thrombectomy are not routinely recommended for children with AIS. The primary target of medical management is the thrombus (arterial in AIS and venous/sinus thrombus in CSVT). The antithrombotic therapy includes:

- *Anticoagulation*: Anticoagulation involves (a) unfractionated heparin (28 U/kg/h for infants; 18–20 U/kg/h for older children), (b) low molecular weight heparin (1 U/kg/dose q12h), and (c) warfarin (dose titrated to maintain INR between 2 and 3). Rapid and complete reversal of the anticoagulation effects of heparin with protamine offers a potential advantage in situations of increased bleeding risk or impending surgery. In contrast, LMWH offers significantly consistent pharmacokinetics, subcutaneous route of administration, reduced monitoring frequency, and moderately improved safety profiles. Warfarin is typically administered to children who need anticoagulation for usually more than 6 months.
- *Antiplatelet agents*: Management guidelines advocate the use of antiplatelet agents for secondary prophylaxis among children with noncardioembolic AIS. Platelet-mediated thrombosis may be the

main underlying pathophysiology in many patients with childhood AIS, especially those with arteriopathy and moyamoya disease. Aspirin (2–5 mg/kg/day) is the recommended antiplatelet agent.

C. **Management of malignant cerebral edema:** Cerebral edema following a stroke is a serious early complication that can be life-threatening. Supratentorial strokes can cause acute transtentorial brain herniation. In contrast, cerebellar strokes may result in brainstem compression, cerebellar herniation, or blockage of the fourth ventricle, leading to obstructive hydrocephalus. Medical management includes measures to reduce elevated intracranial pressure, including sedation, hypocapnia, and osmotic therapy. In patients not responsive to medical management, decompressive craniectomy should be considered.

D. **Management of underlying etiology:** The underlying cause of ischemia/hemorrhage should be addressed wherever feasible.

E. **Chronic management:** Over 50% of children who survive a stroke experience long-term moderate to severe neurological deficits or epilepsy. The chronic management should include:

- Constraint-induced movement therapy (CIMT) is a treatment method that encourages the functional use of a weakened limb by immobilizing the more capable limb.
- Management of spasticity (as outlined in cerebral palsy chapter)
- Movement disorders need to be managed with anticholinergic (e.g., trihexyphenidyl), antidopamine (e.g., pimozide), or dopamine depleting (e.g., tetrabenazine) agents as well as Botox injections.
- Remote symptomatic epilepsy requires administration of antiseizure medications.

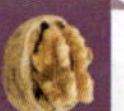

IN A NUTSHELL

Infantile Hemiplegia

1. Hemiplegia and other focal neurological deficits are secondary to a cerebrovascular accident unless proven otherwise.
2. Conditions frequently linked to strokes in children and young adults encompass congenital and acquired heart lesions, arteriopathies, hematological/coagulation disorders, infections, trauma to the head and neck, and genetic disorders. The causes are often multifactorial in many cases situations.
3. Investigations involve neuroimaging (MRI preferably) and workup for underlying etiologies/risk factors.
4. Management involves the use of antithrombotic and antiplatelet agents.

Australian Childhood Stroke Advisory Committee. Guideline for the Diagnosis and Acute Management of Childhood Stroke; 2017. Available from https://informme.org.au/media/typfmgso/damcs-cg2017_web_final.pdf. [Last accessed August, 2025].

Dunbar M, Kirton A. Perinatal stroke: mechanisms, management, and outcomes of early cerebrovascular brain injury. Lancet. 2018;2:666-76.

Ferriero DM, Fullerton HJ, Bernard TJ, et al. On behalf of the American Heart Association: management of stroke in neonates and children: a scientific statement from the American Heart Association/American Stroke Association, Stroke Council, and Council on Cardiovascular and Stroke Nursing. Stroke. 2019;50.

24.9 Febrile Seizures

PE 27.6

DEFINITION

Febrile seizures in simplistic terms refers to seizures with fever, which fulfills the following criteria: (a) seizure with temperature >100.4°F; (b) child aged 6 months to 5 years; (c) absence of CNS infection or inflammation; (d) absence of acute systemic metabolic abnormality that could cause produce seizures; and (e) no prior occurrences of afebrile seizures episodes.

CLASSIFICATION

Febrile seizures are categorized into two types: simple and complex, depending on their clinical characteristics. Simple and complex distinctions impact prognosis, with studies showing that complex features raise the likelihood of recurrent febrile seizures and slightly increase the risk of future nonfebrile seizures. The terminologies associated with febrile seizures have been highlighted in **Table 24.33**.

They occur in about 2–4% of children under five, peaking at 12–18 months. Febrile seizures recur in approximately

Table 24.33 Terminologies Related to Seizure and Epilepsy

Term	Description
Febrile seizure	Febrile seizures are seizures that occur with fever, typically in children aged 6 months to 5 years, without evidence of central nervous system infection or inflammation, and without acute systemic metabolic abnormalities that could lead to convulsions, as well as no history of prior afebrile seizures
Simple febrile seizures	Simple febrile seizures are characterized as generalized seizures lasting under 15 minutes, without recurrence within 24 hours
Complex febrile seizures	Complex febrile seizures are defined by seizure episodes that exhibit a focal onset, last for a duration exceeding 15 minutes, or manifest more than once within a 24-hour timeframe

Table 24.34 Factors Influencing the Likelihood of Febrile Seizure Recurrence and Epilepsy Occurrence

Risk factors associated with febrile seizure recurrence
Major • Age <1year • Duration of fever <24h • Fever 100.4–102.2°F
Minor • Family history of febrile seizures • Family history of epilepsy • Complex febrile seizure • Daycare • Male gender • Lower serum sodium at time of presentation
Risk factors associated with future epilepsy
• Neurodevelopmental abnormality • Complex febrile seizure • Family history of epilepsy • Complex febrile seizures with focal onset • Febrile seizures that occurred within 1 hour of a fever onset

30% of individuals following their initial episode, in 50% after experiencing two or more episodes, and in 50% of infants whose onset occurs before the age of 1 year. The risk factors associated with the recurrence of febrile seizures are detailed in **Table 24.34**. Furthermore, it is noted that five percent of children who experience febrile seizures subsequently develop epilepsy later in life.

Table 24.34 summarizes the risk factors linked to epilepsy development.

RISK FACTORS

Febrile seizures occur in specific age groups and are likely linked to the developing nervous system's heightened sensitivity to fever as well as genetic factors. In addition to age, key risk factors include high fever, viral infections (such as HHV-6 and influenza), and a family history of febrile seizures. A positive family history suggests a genetic predisposition to febrile seizures. In some families, this disorder is inherited as an autosomal dominant trait, with several genes identified. In most cases, however, it appears polygenic, with many predisposing genes still unidentified.

PATHOPHYSIOLOGY

The pathophysiology of febrile seizures remains unclear; however, there is likely an age-specific susceptibility to seizures induced by fever. Recent data indicate that peak temperature, rather than the rate of temperature rise, may be key. The type of illness seems influential, with gastroenteritis linked to a lower likelihood of febrile seizures, whereas infections such as HHV-6, HHV-7, and influenza are strongly associated with febrile seizures.

CLINICAL FEATURES

Diagnosing a febrile seizure requires excluding meningitis, encephalitis, electrolyte imbalances, and other acute neurologic conditions. Clinical evaluation and investigations focus on this exclusion. When evaluating a child with suspected febrile seizures, the clinical assessment should concentrate on two aspects: the history related to the seizure and the history related to fever and its associated causes.

The history pertaining to the seizure should address all aspects highlighted in the chapter on seizures and epilepsy (i.e., preictal, ictal, and postictal phases). An attempt should be made to classify the episode as simple or complex based on this. Simple febrile seizures are generalized, last under 15 minutes, and do not recur in 24 hours. Complex febrile seizures have a focal onset, are prolonged, or recur within 24 hours.

The history and examination related to fever should delineate the following: onset of fever, peak temperature recorded, and the interval between the onset of fever and the occurrence of a seizure episode. Furthermore, a detailed history should focus on underlying causes of fever, such as respiratory tract infections, gastrointestinal infections, or other systemic infections.

Additionally, history related to development (to rule out underlying neurodevelopmental abnormalities), a past history of seizures, and a family history of febrile seizures and epilepsy should be obtained.

Children with febrile seizures often appear well, with postictal drowsiness resolving within 5–10 minutes. Prolonged encephalopathy should raise suspicion of CNS infection or severe systemic infection. A clinical evaluation, including neurologic examination, should assess vital signs, sensorium, meningismus, motor system dysfunctions like abnormalities of power, tone, or spontaneous movements, or any focal neurological deficits. The presence of any of these signs may indicate meningitis or structural abnormalities.

A systemic examination focusing on the respiratory and gastrointestinal systems should be done to rule out any underlying cause of fever.

INVESTIGATIONS

Febrile seizure is a clinical diagnosis. Investigations aim to rule out other factors that can lead to fever and seizures independently. In the absence of red flags during clinical evaluation, laboratory tests like CBC and metabolic profile (electrolytes, glucose) have limited value. The laboratory investigations conducted should be based on the clinical presentation of the febrile illness.

Need for Lumbar Puncture

The primary concern in any child with febrile seizures is deciding whether to conduct a lumbar puncture to exclude meningoencephalitis. A lumbar puncture is usually not needed for the majority of children who look well and have returned to their normal state after the episode. However, it should be conducted in the following scenarios:

a. If there are features suggestive of meningeal irritation, or other indicators pointing to potential meningitis or an intracranial infection;
b. For infants aged 6–12 months especially if they unimmunized for hemophilus influenzae B or pneumococcus;
c. In cases where the child has been administered antibiotics, as such management can obscure the features of meningitis;
d. Seizures that occur after the second day of a febrile episode and the clinician is concerned about possible meningoencephalitis; and
e. Children with febrile status epilepticus.

EEG

An EEG is not needed in cases where a neurologically normal child experiences his/her first simple febrile seizure. An abnormal EEG does not serve as a predictor for the future recurrence of febrile seizures or the onset of epilepsy. Thus, EEGs should be limited to specific situations where epilepsy is strongly suspected, serving primarily to identify the type of epilepsy rather than to forecast its likelihood.

Neuroimaging

Neuroimaging is not advised for assessing a child following their initial simple febrile seizure. An MRI is warranted for children exhibiting unusually large heads, abnormal neurological evaluations, particularly focal deficits, or any features of raised intracranial pressure.

TREATMENT Febrile Seizures

Antipyretic agents do not prevent febrile seizures or recurrence. Prophylactic antiseizure medications should be withheld, as treatment risks outweigh benefits. Managing a child experiencing febrile seizures should involve the following.

A. **Terminating febrile seizure**

- Most febrile seizures are brief, lasting under 5 minutes, and usually do not need treatment.
- If the seizure lasts for more than 5 minutes, domiciliary/prehospital management with intranasal midazolam (0.2 mg/kg) and rectal diazepam (0.3 mg/kg) has proven effective in stopping these seizures.
- In a hospital setting, intravenous diazepam (0.1–0.2 mg/kg) or lorazepam (0.05–0.1 mg/kg) are known to be effective treatment options.

B. **Preventing febrile seizure**

- Antipyretic medications (paracetamol, 15 mg/kg) do not lower the risk of febrile seizures or stop them from recurring. It is essential to recognize the limitations of antipyretics to prevent unnecessary anxiety and guilt in parents.
- Administering benzodiazepines, such as oral clobazam or rectal diazepam, at the start of a febrile illness can decrease the likelihood of a febrile seizure. Nonetheless, this slight reduction in the recurrence of seizures should be considered alongside the potential adverse effects of sedating children whenever they experience a febrile episode.
- Long-term antiseizure medications should not be administered to children with febrile seizures.

C. **Treating underlying cause of fever:** Alongside the management of seizures, treatment should be initiated for the underlying cause of fever based on the focus of infection.

PROGNOSIS

The outcome for children experiencing febrile seizures is generally favorable. Neurologic sequelae, including neurologic impairments, cognitive disabilities, and behavioral issues, are not observed as a result of febrile seizures. However, children who have complex febrile seizures, developmental delay, or a family history of epilepsy face a higher likelihood of developing epilepsy later on.

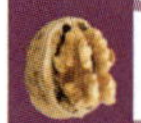

IN A NUTSHELL

Febrile Seizures

1. Febrile seizures occur in children with fever, which is often due to viral infections. These seizures typically affect children between 6 months and 5 years of age with absence of CNS infection or inflammation, and absence of acute systemic metabolic abnormality, and no history of previous afebrile seizures.
2. Simple febrile seizures are characterized by seizures lasting ≤15 minutes, having a generalized onset, and occurring once in 24 hours. Complex febrile seizures are defined by seizures lasting >15 minutes, have focal features, or recur within 24 hours.
3. The initial evaluation should differentiate febrile seizures from other, more serious causes, such as meningoencephalitis
4. In children experiencing febrile seizures lasting more than 5 minutes, treatment with intravenous diazepam or lorazepam should be initiated. Intranasal or buccal midazolam should be used in prehospital setting or when IV access is unavailable.

Knudsen FU. Febrile seizures: treatment and prognosis. Epilepsia 2000; 41:2.

Natsume J, Hamano SI, Iyoda K, et al. New guidelines for management of febrile seizures in Japan. Brain Dev. 2017;39:2.

Steering Committee on Quality Improvement and Management, Subcommittee on Febrile Seizures American Academy of Pediatrics. Febrile seizures: clinical practice guideline for the long-term management of the child with simple febrile seizures. Pediatrics. 2008;121:1281.

Wilmshurst JM, Gaillard WD, Vinayan KP, et al. Summary of recommendations for the management of infantile seizures: Task Force Report for the ILAE Commission of Pediatrics. Epilepsia. 2015;56:1185.

Kaushik JS, Sondhi V, Yoganathan S, et al. Association of child neurology (AOCN) consensus statement on the diagnosis and management of febrile seizures. Indian Pediatr. 2022;59(4):300-6.

24.10 Childhood Epilepsy

PE 27.7

INTRODUCTION

Children and infants with epilepsy differ from adults not only in the clinical manifestations of their seizures but also in unique electroencephalogram (EEG) patterns, causes, and responses to antiseizure medications. The immature brain, especially in neonates and young infants, is different from the adult brain in the fundamental mechanisms of epileptogenesis and seizure propagation, making them more susceptible to seizures. However, seizures among infants and children are more likely to resolve as they grow older.

About 30% of patients experiencing their first afebrile seizure will go on to develop epilepsy; the risk drops to about 20% if neurological examination, EEG, and neuroimaging results are normal. The cumulative lifetime incidence of epilepsy is 3%, with more than half of cases beginning in childhood. The annual prevalence ranges from 0.5% to 1.0%.

The terminologies related to seizures and epilepsy are listed in **Table 24.35**.

TYPES OF SEIZURE AND EPILEPSY AND THEIR CLASSIFICATION FRAMEWORK

The 2017 International League Against Epilepsy (ILAE) has proposed a multilevel framework for classification of seizure/epilepsy. This framework is helpful in establishing and categorizing diagnosis, planning therapeutics, and prognostication of these children. The four levels of this framework are as follows:

Level 1: Seizure Type

This is the first step where the clinician should determine if the event was a true seizure and differentiate it from seizure mimics. If the event was a true seizure, the seizure type should be determined and categorized into one of the following.

- ***Focal seizure:*** A seizure is classified as focal if the first clinical and EEG changes suggest activation of a set of neurons limited to part of one cerebral hemisphere. These were earlier referred to as partial seizure. A seizure is classified as a focal seizure without impaired awareness when the patient remains conscious (aware) during the event (formerly called a simple partial seizure). In contrast, focal seizures with impaired awareness correspond to what were previously referred to as complex partial seizures and are characterized by altered consciousness and awareness of surroundings. Impaired awareness refers to the inability to respond appropriately to external stimuli due to altered consciousness and/or awareness. Focal seizures are further subdivided primarily based upon the clinical signs and symptoms and the EEG localization into motor seizure (tonic, clonic, myoclonic) and nonmotor seizures (sensory, autonomic, cognitive).
- ***Generalized seizure:*** Seizures are categorized as generalized when clinical and EEG changes at onset show synchronous involvement of both hemispheres. This may lead to impaired awareness, which could be the first sign observed. If motor symptoms occur, they appear bilaterally from the beginning. The ictal EEG patterns are also bilateral from the onset.
- ***Unknown onset:*** A seizure is classified as having an unknown onset when there is insufficient clinical information to

Table 24.35 Terminologies Related to Seizure and Epilepsy

Term	Definition
Seizure	A seizure is defined as a sudden and transient occurrence of symptoms ± signs (motor, sensory, autonomic or psychological) caused by abnormal, excessive, or synchronized discharges of neurons in the cerebral cortex
Acute symptomatic seizure	Acute symptomatic seizure also known as provoked seizures occurs due to an acute pathology affecting brain excitability. Examples include dyselectrolytemia, traumatic brain injury, meningoencephalitis
Unprovoked seizure	An unprovoked seizure refers to a seizure that happens without an obvious underlying clinical condition that could be responsible
Reflex seizure	A reflex seizure is triggered by specific sensory stimuli (e.g., light flashes, auditory stimuli like music, bathing in hot water)
Epilepsy	An individual is diagnosed as having epilepsy if any of the following exists: a. At least two unprovoked (or reflex) seizures occurring >24 hours apart b. One unprovoked (or reflex) seizure and a probability of further seizures that is similar to the general recurrence risk after two unprovoked seizures (e.g., ≥60%), occurring over the next 10 years (example following stroke, CNS infection). c. Diagnosis of an epilepsy syndrome
Epileptic syndrome	Epileptic syndrome is defined by one or more seizure types, a distinct age of onset, and a particular prognosis
Epileptic encephalopathy	Epileptic encephalopathy is a type of epilepsy syndrome characterized by severe epilepsy and related EEG abnormalities that lead to cognitive impairment (i.e., encephalopathy)
Developmental encephalopathy	Developmental encephalopathy is defined as a clinical condition in which the underlying etiology, such as a genetic disorder, contributes to developmental delays and cognitive decline, independent of the child's epilepsy and EEG
Developmental and epileptic encephalopathy	Developmental and epileptic encephalopathy is a disorder where both the underlying etiology, such as genetic disorders, alongside epilepsy and EEG abnormalities contribute to the child's developmental delays and cognitive decline

ascertain whether it was focal or generalized at its onset (for example, epileptic spasms).

❖ ***Unclassified:*** If the seizure exhibits unusual clinical characteristics and a determination of onset remains unclear even after thorough evaluation, it may be categorized as unclassified.

Level 2: Epilepsy Type

Based on the type of seizures a child is having, epilepsy is categorized into focal, generalized, focal and generalized, or unknown.

Level 3: Epilepsy Syndrome

At this stage, based on clinical information and supporting investigations (e.g., EEG and/or MRI), the diagnosis of a specific epilepsy syndrome can be made (e.g., juvenile myoclonic epilepsy, West syndrome).

Level 4: Etiology

At this final stage of epilepsy classification, considering the information from all previous levels, a unified diagnosis should be reached with determination of possible underlying etiology(ies) and associated comorbidities.

ETIOLOGY

The causes of epileptic seizures must be evaluated at every level of an epilepsy diagnosis, as previously mentioned. The etiologic categories include:

A. ***Genetic:*** Genetic epilepsy refers to an epilepsy syndrome that directly results from a known or suspected genetic defect, without causing any structural or metabolic brain disorders apart from epilepsy. These include genetic generalized epilepsies like childhood absence epilepsy, juvenile absence epilepsy, and juvenile myoclonic epilepsy, and also include more severe syndromes such as Dravet syndrome (mutation in SCN1A gene).

B. ***Structural:*** Structural epilepsy was previously referred to as symptomatic epilepsy. This is a type of epilepsy syndrome that arises from an underlying structural brain disorder, which may or may not have a genetic component. This includes causes such as cerebrovascular accident, hippocampal sclerosis, cortical dysplasia, hypoxic-ischemic injury, and epilepsy resulting from tuberous sclerosis (which is also genetic due to mutation involving TSC genes).

C. ***Metabolic:*** Numerous metabolic disorders significantly elevate the likelihood of developing epilepsy (examples include glucose transporter deficiency, creatine deficiency syndromes, and mitochondrial cytopathies).

D. ***Immune:*** Immune-mediated epilepsy refers to epilepsies that arise as a result of immune-mediated inflammation in the CNS (examples include autoimmune encephalitis).

E. ***Infectious:*** Infectious epilepsy refers to epilepsy caused by chronic infections like tuberculosis and HIV, as opposed to acute infections like bacterial meningitis or HSV encephalitis. Acute seizures may arise from chemical or inflammatory reactions due to infection (e.g., meningitis, encephalitis, sepsis). These seizures usually resolve with the infection but can lead to epilepsy from brain injury, with seizures potentially reappearing after weeks, months, or years.

F. ***Unknown:*** When the underlying cause of epilepsy could not be deciphered despite clinical and supportive investigations, the epilepsy is described as of unknown cause.

Table 24.36 Pathophysiologic Mechanisms Associated with Epilepsy

Underlying etiology	*Mechanism in example conditions*
Genetic	• Channelopathies: Mutations in channels leading to excessive activation • Down syndrome: Abnormal structure of dendrites and dendritic spines • Angelman syndrome/Juvenile myoclonic epilepsy: Abnormal GABA receptor subunits
Structural	• Cortical dysplasia/hippocampal sclerosis: Altered neuronal circuits; formation of aberrant excitatory connections
Metabolic	• Hypoglycemia: Energy depletion, neurotransmitter imbalance, and hyperexcitability • Hypocalcemia: Hyperexcitability and hypersynchrony • Nonketotic hyperglycinemia: Excess glycine leads to excessive activation of NMDA receptors • Pyridoxine dependent epilepsy: Decreased GABA synthesis
Immune	• NMDA encephalitis: Excessive activation of NMDA receptors
Infectious	• Neuronal hyperexcitability

PATHOGENESIS

The electrical activity that triggers a seizure is the overall result of biochemical processes taking place at the cellular level within extensive neuronal networks.

At the cellular level, two key characteristics of a seizure are neuronal hyperexcitability and hypersynchrony. Hyperexcitability describes the lowered threshold for neuronal firing, which may occur due to an excess of excitatory neurotransmitters, abnormalities in their receptors, or decreased levels of inhibitory neurotransmitters and related receptor issues. Hypersynchrony occurs when neurons in a particular region fire simultaneously.

Thus, a seizure represents dysfunctional activity at both the individual neuron level and within the broader neuronal network. The pathophysiological mechanisms linked to epilepsy are summarized in a **Table 24.36**. Epileptogenesis refers to the process through which neural circuits experience structural or physiological changes that lead to a persistent epileptic state.

CLINICAL FEATURES

Seizures in children can present with a wide variety of clinical features, which may vary based on the type of seizure, the child's age, and underlying causes. The important clinical features have been highlighted in **Table 24.37**.

Table 24.37 Salient History and Clinical Features in a Child with Seizure/Epilepsy	
Preictal	
A. Aura	Some children may experience a preseizure sensation, such as a strange smell, visual disturbances, or feelings of déjà vu, serving as a warning sign. The most common aura experienced by children consists of epigastric discomfort or pain and a feeling of fear. Presence of aura signifies a focal seizure
B. Behavioral change	Changes in behavior may occur before, during, or after a seizure. These can include irritability, decreased responsiveness, or unusual behaviors
Seizure semiology	
A. Generalized seizures	1. Tonic-clonic seizures a. Sudden loss of consciousness followed by stiffness (tonic phase) and rhythmic jerking (clonic phase) b. Possible tongue biting or loss of bladder/bowel control c. Postictal state (confusion, fatigue, muscle soreness) afterward 2. Absence seizures a. Brief episodes of staring or "blanking out," lasting a few seconds b. May be accompanied by subtle eyelid fluttering or automatisms (e.g., lip-smacking) c. No postictal confusion; child usually resumes activity immediately 3. Myoclonic seizures a. Sudden, brief muscle jerks b. May occur in clusters and can happen upon waking 4. Atonic seizures a. Sudden loss of muscle tone, leading to falls or head drops
B. Focal seizures	1. Focal onset seizures with preserved awareness a. Child is aware during the seizure b. Symptoms can include localized twitching, unusual sensations (like tingling), or emotional changes 2. Focal onset seizures with impaired awareness a. Impaired consciousness or awareness during the seizure b. May involve automatisms (e.g., repetitive movements like lip-smacking or hand movements)
Postictal	
C. Postictal phenomenon	Child may have postictal phenomenon like sleep, headache, hemiparesis
Other clinical evaluation	
D. Etiology related	1. Fever (for meningoencephalitis) 2. Head injury (for Traumatic brain injury) 3. Metabolic disturbances 4. Prenatal or perinatal distress/developmental delay (for perinatal structural brain damage) 5. Personality changes or symptoms of increased intracranial pressure (for brain tumors) 6. Cognitive decline (neurodegenerative disorders) 7. Personality changes, psychiatric symptoms, and/or associated movement abnormalities (autoimmune epilepsy) 8. Family history of seizures/epilepsy
E. Examination findings	1. Head circumference (for hydrocephalus/megalencephaly) 2. Dysmorphism (for genetic/chromosomal disorders) 3. Neurocutaneous markers (neurocutaneous syndromes like Sturge-Weber syndrome, tuberous sclerosis) 4. Fundus evaluation (for papilledema, optic neuritis, retinal hemorrhages, uveitis, chorioretinitis) 5. Focal neurological signs like hemiparesis 6. Hepatosplenomegaly (for storage disorders)

INVESTIGATIONS

The cornerstone of diagnosis is a detailed and directed clinical history from the patient and a reliable witness. However, the following investigations aid in diagnosis and underlying etiology.

A. ***Electroencephalogram (EEG):*** EEG is essential for patients with seizures and epilepsy. When performed in between the seizures (called as interictal EEG), it evaluates brain function and identifies epileptiform discharges. The EEG helps determine the epilepsy syndrome and guide antiseizure medication choices. Certain abnormalities indicate specific epilepsy syndromes. For instance, EEG may display hypsarrhythmia in West syndrome or the classic 3-Hz spike wave in generalized absence seizures.

B. ***Neuroimaging:*** Brain imaging is crucial as seizures may be the presenting symptom of brain tumors, stroke, abscess, or other treatable lesions. MRI is preferred for patients with seizures, revealing both major abnormalities and subtle lesions like hippocampal sclerosis. CT scan has a limited role in patients suspected of having trauma, intracranial hemorrhage, or increased intracranial pressure due to its effectiveness for acute conditions. However, a normal CT does not negate the need for an MRI, as many subtle lesions not apparent on CT can be seen on MRI.

C. ***Laboratory investigations:*** Laboratory testing should encompass screening for metabolic disorders such as hyponatremia, hypokalemia, hypocalcemia, and hypoglycemia. If there is a suspicion of an infectious/inflammatory cause, tests should include blood cultures and a lumbar puncture. It's essential to carefully document the patient's medications and note any recent changes, as missing doses of antiseizure medications (ASM) or interactions with newly added or removed drugs can trigger seizures. Consequently, ASM levels may need to be assessed if clinically necessary.

D. ***Targeted testing:*** Targeted investigations are usually individualized based on clinical suspicion. These may include genetic testing, testing for inborn errors of metabolism, testing for neuronal autoantibodies.

TREATMENT Childhood Epilepsy

The management of a child with epilepsy consists of pharmacotherapy with ASMs. Epilepsy surgery may be used in specific scenarios.

A. **Medical management:** A child's initial seizure might stem from an acute illness like a metabolic issue or infectious disease and could either be a one-time event or signal the start of epilepsy. The management of acute symptomatic seizures should be focused on correcting the acute provoking illness or anomaly and preventing its recurrence. These children may require no or short-term ASM depending upon the underlying cause. If no reversible acute cause is identified during assessment, a decision needs to be made regarding the commencement of chronic ASM treatment. The ASM and the type of seizure or epilepsy in which it is most effective have been highlighted in the **Table 24.38**. The mechanism of action of various ASM has been illustrated in **Figure 24.20**.

B. **Epilepsy surgery:** Surgical treatment involves the removal (example cortical dysplasia) or disconnection of the brain area (example corpus callosotomy) that houses the seizure focus.

Table 24.38 Common Antiseizure Medications

Drug	*Mechanism of action*	*Seizures most effective in*	*Starting dose*	*Maintenance dose*	*Adverse events*
Carbamazepine	Voltage-gated sodium channels	Focal and generalized tonic-clonic	10 to 20 mg/kg/day	10 to 35 mg/kg/day	Hyponatremia, rash, pruritus, drowsiness, dizziness, blurred or double vision
Clobazam	GABA receptors	Focal and generalized tonic-clonic	0.5 to 1 mg/kg/day	0.5 to 1 mg/kg/day	Increased salivation, constipation, somnolence, ataxia,
Clonazepam	GABA receptors	Focal and generalized tonic-clonic	0.01 to 0.03 mg/kg/day	0.05 to 0.2 mg/kg/day	
Ethosuximide	Voltage-gated calcium channels	Absence	15 mg/kg/day	15 to 40 mg/kg/day	Sleep disturbance, drowsiness, hyperactivity
Lacosamide	Voltage-gated sodium channels	Focal	2 mg/kg/day	6 to 12 mg/kg/day	Ataxia, headache, diplopia
Lamotrigine	Voltage-gated sodium channels	Focal and generalized tonic-clonic Lennox-Gastaut syndrome	Monotherapy/without valproic acid: 0.3 mg/kg/day	4.5 to 7.5 mg/kg/day	Rash, diplopia, tremors
			Added to valproic acid: 0.15 mg/kg/day	1 to 5 mg/kg/day	
Levetiracetam	Synaptic vesicle protein 2A	Focal and generalized tonic-clonic	20 mg/kg/day	40 to 60 mg/kg/day	Somnolence, agitation, anxiety, irritability, depression
Oxcarbazepine	Voltage-gated sodium channels	Focal	8 to 10 mg/kg/day	30 to 40 mg/kg/day	Hyponatremia, dizziness, vertigo, ataxia, diplopia
Phenytoin	Voltage-gated sodium channels	Focal and generalized tonic-clonic	5 mg/kg/day	4 to 8 mg/kg/day	Gingival hypertrophy, rash, ataxia, diplopia
Phenobarbital	GABA receptors	Focal and generalized tonic-clonic	3 to 4 mg/kg/day	3 to 5 mg/kg/day	Sedation, lethargy, behavioral changes, hyperactivity, ataxia
Topiramate	Voltage-gated sodium channels	Focal and generalized tonic-clonic Lennox Gastaut syndrome	1 to 3 mg/kg/day	5 to 9 mg/kg/day	Weight loss, anxiety, mood problems, tremor
Valproate	Unknown/? Ionotropic glutamate receptors	Focal and generalized tonic-clonic	10 to 15 mg/kg/day	30 to 60 mg/kg/day	Weight gain, hair loss, dizziness, transaminitis
Zonisamide	Voltage-gated sodium channels	Focal and generalized tonic-clonic	1 to 2 mg/kg/day	5 to 8 mg/kg/day	Somnolence, dizziness, ataxia

Mechanism of action of antiseizure drugs

Excitatory synapse
Presynaptic neuron
Propagated action potential
• Phenytoin
• Carbamazepine
• Valproic acid
• Felbamate
•Rufinamide
• Lamotrigine
• Lacosamide
• Topiramate
• Zonisamide
• Oxcarbazepine
Na^+
Voltage-gated Na^+ channel
• Gabapentin
• Pregabalin
Depolarization
$\alpha_2\delta$ subunit of Ca^{2+} channel
Ca^{2+}
Glutamate
Levetiracetam
SV2A
Vesicular release
Felbamate
Topiramate
Ethosuximide
NMDAR
AMPAR/KAR
T-type Ca channel
Na^+, Ca^{2+}
Na^+
Postsynaptic neuron

Inhibitory synapse
Presynaptic neuron
Glutamate
GAD
Vigabatrin
GABA
GABA-T
Succinic semi-aldehyde
Vesicular release
GAT1
Tiagabine
• Benzodiazepines
• Barbiturates
• Felbamate
• Topiramate
• Zonisamide
GABAAR
Cl^-
Postsynaptic neuron

Fig. 24.20: Mechanisms of action of antiseizure medications involve modulation of voltage-activated ion channels, GABA potentiation, and glutamate inhibition. Antiseizure medications can exert their effects on inhibitory (right-hand side) and excitatory (left-hand side) nerve terminals

Source: Created in BioRender. Sondhi, V. (2025) https://BioRender.com/15k5yl7.

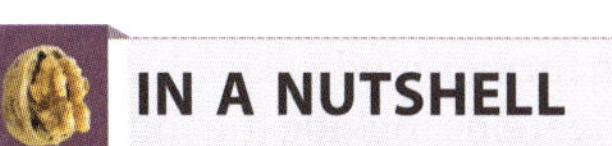

IN A NUTSHELL

Childhood Epilepsy

1. A seizure represents the clinical manifestation of abnormal, excessive, or synchronous discharges of neurons in the cerebral cortex. Epilepsy is a condition characterized by a lasting tendency toward recurrent epileptic seizures, which is based on specific criteria.
2. The International League Against Epilepsy has established a multi-level classification system that categorizes seizures and epilepsy into four levels: seizure type, epilepsy type, epilepsy syndromes, and their etiology.
3. The clinical evaluation of a child with seizure should include a detailed description of preictal, ictal, and postictal events.
4. The investigations of a child with seizure include EEG, neuroimaging and laboratory investigations (blood tests ± lumbar puncture)

Scheffer IE, Berkovic S, Capovilla G, et al. ILAE classification of the epilepsies: Position paper of the ILAE Commission for Classification and Terminology. Epilepsia. 2017;58:512.
Fisher RS, Acevedo C, Arzimanoglou A, et al. ILAE official report: a practical clinical definition of epilepsy. Epilepsia. 2014;55:475.
Pack AM. Epilepsy Overview and revised classification of Seizures and Epilepsies. Continuum (Minneap Minn). 2019;25:306.
Sansevere AJ, Avalone J, Strauss LD, et al. Diagnostic and therapeutic management of a first unprovoked seizure in children and adolescents with a focus on the revised diagnostic criteria for epilepsy. J Child Neurol. 2017;32:774.

24.11 Global Developmental Delay and Intellectual Disability

PE 27.10

INTRODUCTION

Global developmental delay (GDD) and intellectual disability (ID; the preferred term replacing "mental retardation") are interrelated, complementary terms that share both similarities and unique traits. Similar to cerebral palsy, each represents a complex of symptoms that defines a clinically identifiable condition characterized by diverse causes, necessitating specific evaluation, management, and intervention strategies. The terminologies related to GDD and ID are listed in **Table 24.39**.

Table 24.39 Terminologies Related to Global Developmental Delay and Intellectual Disability

Terminology	*Description*
Global developmental delay	• Global developmental delay (GDD) is defined as a significant delay in two or more developmental domains • Two or more out of the following domains should be delayed: (a) gross/fine motor; (b) cognitive; (c) speech/language; (d) personal/social; and (e) activities of daily living • When referring to intellectual and adaptive impairment in infants and young children under five years old, GDD is the preferred term
Intellectual disability	• Intellectual disability is a neurodevelopmental disorder that starts before the age of 18 years and is characterized by limitations in both intelligence and adaptive skills, affecting at least one (but typically all) of the three adaptive domains (conceptual, social, and practical) • This manifests with severe problems in the individual's *capacity* to perform (i.e., impairment), *ability* to perform (i.e., activity limitations), and *opportunity* to function (i.e., participation restrictions)
Syndromic intellectual disability	An individual is diagnosed as syndromic intellectual disability when he/she has intellectual and adaptive impairments alongside identifiable physical or comorbid symptoms recognized as a syndrome (for example, Down syndrome, Fragile X syndrome)
Non-syndromic intellectual disability	When intellectual disability occurs without features of a known syndrome, it's referred to as non-syndromic intellectual disability

CAUSES

The causes of ID primarily fall into two categories: genetic abnormalities and environmental factors.

- ***Genetic abnormalities*** include single gene mutations, copy number variations, or chromosomal changes. These genetic abnormalities may lead to metabolic disorders, neurodevelopmental issues, or neurodegeneration.
- ***Environmental factors*** involve maternal exposure to toxins or infectious agents, maternal medical conditions, delivery-related complications, post-natal trauma, and toxin or infectious agent exposure. The most prevalent and preventable environmental cause of intellectual disability is fetal alcohol syndrome. In contrast, Down syndrome is the leading chromosomal cause, and Fragile X syndrome is the most common genetic cause.

The causes of ID are listed in **Table 24.40**. The clinical features and relevant investigations for common causes of ID are listed in **Table 24.41**.

INVESTIGATIONS

The choice and order of diagnostic tests for children with ID depend on a detailed history, thorough physical and neurologic examinations, evaluation for dysmorphic features, and the availability and cost of tests. The key investigations are as below.

A. Genetic Testing

Genetic testing should be offered to children with unexplained ID because it can provide diagnostic and prognostic information and facilitate informative genetic counseling. Genetic testing may also identify conditions requiring further medical evaluation or management. The various investigations include the following:

- ***First-line genetic tests:*** These include chromosomal microarray, whole exome sequencing, and whole genome sequencing.
- ***Testing for Fragile X syndrome:*** Fragile X syndrome arises from an abnormal expansion of the CGG triplet repeat in the FMR1 gene (over 200 repeats) and is the most common inherited form of intellectual disability. Chromosomal microarray and whole exome sequencing cannot detect the trinucleotide repeat expansions characteristic of Fragile X syndrome. The diagnosis can be established through Fragile X DNA analysis, also known as Fragile X CGG repeat analysis.
- ***Karyotype:*** G-banded karyotype analysis can serve as an initial test for children presenting clinical signs of a common aneuploidy, such as Down syndrome or a sex chromosome aneuploidy.
- ***Metabolic testing:*** Tests for plasma amino acid concentrations, urine organic acids, acylcarnitine profile,

Table 24.40 Causes of Intellectual Disability

Genetic causes	*Non-genetic causes*
Chromosomal disorders • Down syndrome • Klinefelter's syndrome	**Antenatal causes** • Intrauterine infections including TORCH • Teratogens like alcohol, drugs (like antiseizure medications, chemotherapy) • Maternal phenylketonuria • Radiation exposure • Maternal medical conditions like uncontrolled diabetes, hypertension
Deletion, microdeletion, and duplication syndromes • DiGeorge syndrome • William syndrome • Prader-Willi syndrome	**Perinatal causes** • Perinatal asphyxia • Metabolic disturbances like hypoglycemia, hyperbilirubinemia • Prematurity • Intraventricular hemorrhage • Birth trauma • Neonatal sepsis/meningoencephalitis
Single gene disorders • Autosomal dominant conditions include denovo mutations involving many genes including ARID1B, CDK13, STXBP, 1 etc. • Autosomal recessive conditions including inborn errors of metabolism (phenylketonuria, galactosemia) and other genetic conditions involving single genes like ADAT3, CRBN, TANGO2 etc. • X-linked disorders like Fragile X syndrome, MECP2 related disorders (Rett's syndrome) **Mitochondrial disorders** • Leighs disease • MELAS **Imprinting disorders** • Angelman syndrome • Prader-Willi syndrome	**Postnatal causes** • Congenital hypothyroidism • Traumatic brain injury • Febrile encephalopathy • Hypoxia (e.g., near-drowning) • Environmental toxins like lead • Psychosocial deprivation • Malnutrition • CNS malignancy • Demyelination

Table 24.41 Clinical Features and Diagnostic Tests for Common Causes of ID in Children

Cause of ID	*Clinical feature*	*Specific investigation*

Down syndrome	• Dysmorphism
	  ▪ Mongoloid slant (upslanting palpebral fissure)
	  ▪ Epicanthal folds
	  ▪ Incurved fifth finger with hypoplastic middle phalanx
	  ▪ Transverse palmar crease
	  ▪ Sandal gap between first and second toe
	• Cognitive impairment (most have mild to moderate intellectual disability)
	• Hypothyroidism
	• Congenital heart disease and multiple congenital anomalies
		Karyotype

Fragile X	• Males with moderate to severe ID, long and narrow face, macrocephaly, large ears, enlarged testes after puberty, and poor eye contact • Behavioral problems (autism spectrum disorder, inattention, hyperactivity) • Males and females with family history of ID	Measuring the number of repeats in the CGG segment of *FMR1* gene by doing *FMR1* DNA analysis
Rett syndrome	• Females with normal initial development followed by loss of speech, regression to moderate or severe ID • Stereotypic hand movements	MECP2 gene testing
Klinefelter syndrome	• Males with mild intellectual disability, hypogonadism including hypospadias, tall stature, gynecomastia • Delayed puberty • Learning disorders	Karyotype
Prader-Willi syndrome	• Infancy: Hypotonia, feeding difficulties • Older children: Intellectual disability, behavior difficulties, hyperphagia, sleep disorders, obesity, hypogonadism	Methylation analysis to detect abnormal parent-specific methylation imprinting on chromosome 15q11.2–13

Contd...

Contd...

Cause of ID	*Clinical feature*	*Specific investigation*
Inborn errors of metabolism	• Variable severity of intellectual disability • Febrile illness or conditions associated with metabolic stress leading to episodic decompensation • Family history of consanguinity, early childhood deaths, intellectual disability, or confirmed inborn errors of metabolism • Seizures, neuroregression	Metabolic screening including analysis of plasma amino acids, urine organic acids, serum ammonia, and lactate
Congenital hypothyroidism	• Short stature • Cold intolerance • Puffy facies • Macroglossia • Large fontanels • Hypotonia • Dry skin • Prolonged neonatal jaundice	• Serum TSH • Free T4
Lead poisoning	• Mild to moderate intellectual disability • Language delay • Behavior problems • Vomiting • Colicky abdominal pain • Kidney function impairment • Exposure history	Blood levels of lead

ammonia and lactate levels, and serum electrolytes should be considered based on profile of individual patient.

B. Other Laboratory Investigations

- ***Blood lead levels:*** Lead is the most common environmental neurotoxin. Estimation of blood lead levels should be strongly considered in children with persistent mouthing behavior and pica, the use of certain herbal remedies, and specific parental occupations, such as smelting, soldering, and auto body repair.
- ***Thyroid profile:*** All children with unidentified causes of GDD/ID should undergo testing for TSH and Free T4 levels. Congenital hypothyroidism is a treatable cause of GDD/ID and should be sought in all children.

C. Neuroimaging

MRI should be considered for children with seizures, progressive or degenerative neurologic symptoms, microcephaly or macrocephaly, and focal neurologic deficits. Common findings include CNS malformations, white matter abnormalities, and cerebral atrophy.

ASSESSMENT OF DEGREE OF DISABILITY

Assessing the degree of disability in a child with intellectual disability is a comprehensive process that requires a multidisciplinary approach. This involves gathering information from parents and teachers via a detailed history, performing a physical evaluation to understand the co-existing comorbidities, and understanding the specific concerns that prompted the assessment, such as learning difficulties, behavioral issues, or social challenges. The evaluation may also include assessment of motor impairments and associated visual or hearing disabilities that may impact intellectual and adaptive functioning. This is followed by standardized testing for intellectual and adaptive functioning assessment.

As per the Government of India guidelines, among children ≥5 years of age, intelligence quotient should be tested using the Binet Kamat Test (BKT) of Intelligence or the Malins Intelligence Scale for Indian Children (MISIC). The guidelines suggest using the Vineland Social Maturity Scale (VSMS) for adaptive functioning assessment. The details, along with severity grading, are summarized in **Figure 24.21**.

TREATMENT Global Developmental Delay and Intellectual Disability

Improving functioning in the child's everyday environments, such as the home, school, and community, preventing or limiting deterioration, and lessening the impact of disability are the main goals of managing ID. The management is multidisciplinary and involves the following components.

A. **Early interventions**

a. Physical therapy: Physical therapy can enhance mobility, improve motor skills, offer postural support, and other aids for affected individuals.

b. Occupational therapy: Occupational therapy aids in activities of daily living by enhancing hand-eye coordination and other motor skills essential for daily living, schooling, community engagement, and work activities.

c. Speech therapy: Many children with ID experience language-based impairments that can affect their adaptive functioning and daily activities. Engaging in speech and language therapy can enhance a child's communication skills, including language, speech, and articulation, while also fostering additional skill development.

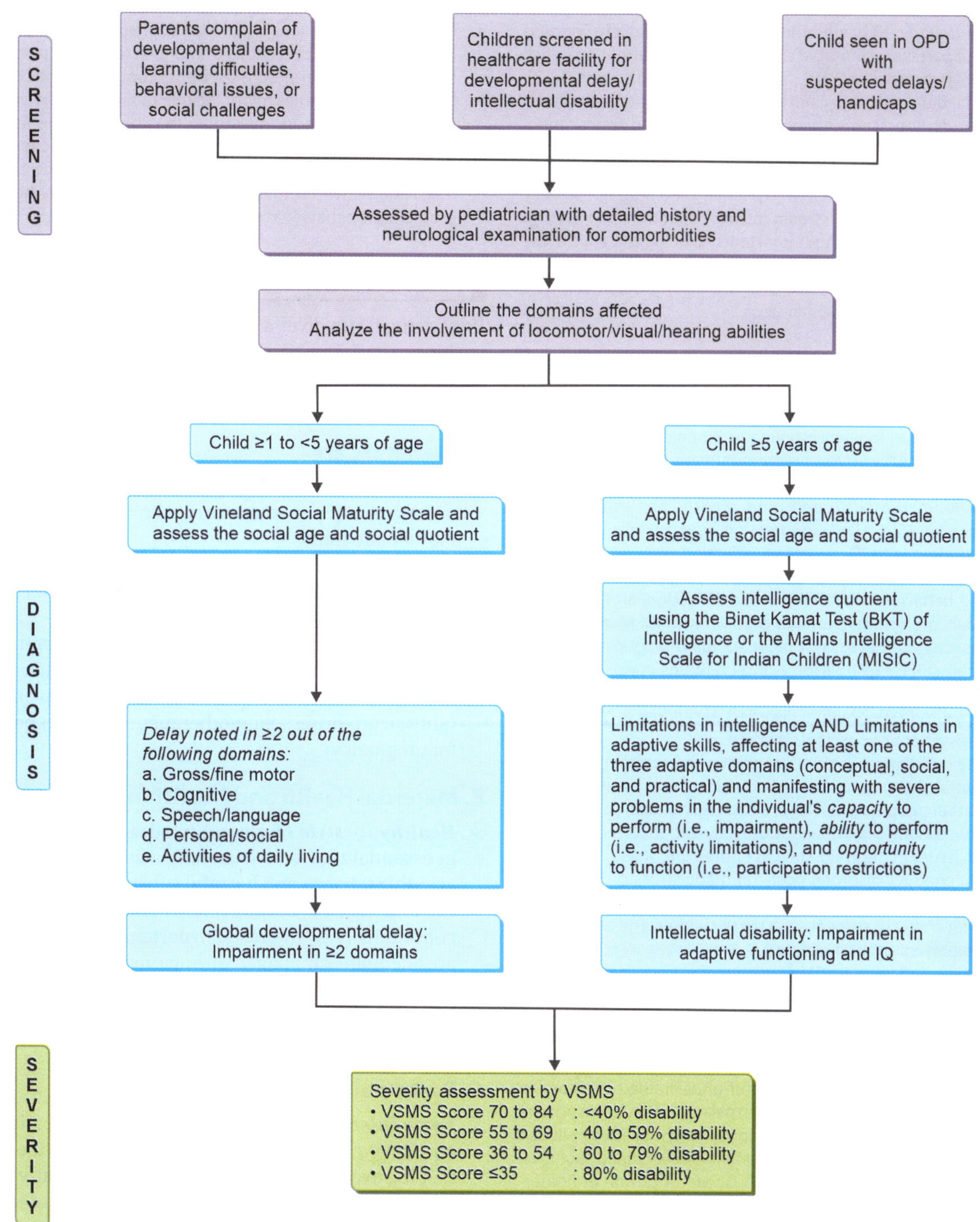

Fig. 24.21: Algorithmic approach to a child with suspected global developmental delay/intellectual disability has been illustrated. The tools depicted for intelligence assessment [using the Binet Kamat Test (BKT) of Intelligence or the Malins Intelligence Scale for Indian Children (MISIC)] and adaptive function assessment [using the Vineland Social Maturity Scale (VSMS)] are in accordance with the Government of India guidelines

d. *Behavioral therapy*: Behavioral interventions target challenging behaviors or particular comorbid conditions, such as attention deficit hyperactivity disorder (ADHD), autism spectrum disorder (ASD), oppositional defiant disorder, anxiety, depression, and sleep issues. These interventions can enhance behavior-related functioning, boost performance, and increase participation in daily activities, as well as other service interventions.

e. *Functional skills*: This entails help with planning and problem-solving. Some tactics used in the classroom include repetition, giving extra time, and preferential seating (for instance, placing the child close to the teacher), minimizing distractions, leveraging interests and strengths to improve weaker skills, and breaking down complex tasks into manageable sequential steps.

B. **Specific management**:

a. *Treatable cause of ID*: The majority of ID causes don't have a particular remedy or intervention. Nonetheless, if a treatable underlying etiology, such as congenital hypothyroidism or a manageable inborn error of metabolism (phenylketonuria or biotinidase deficiency), is recognized, the child must receive prompt treatment to avert further disability.

b. *Neurodevelopmental disorders and mental health problems*: Conditions like ASD, ADHD, depression, and anxiety frequently occur in children with ID, negatively affecting their quality of life, adaptation, and overall functioning. Self-injurious behaviors, self-stimulating behaviors, wandering, suicidal ideation, and substance use disorders are common among children with ID. Many of these conditions may not necessarily meet standard diagnostic criteria, yet they can still be troublesome. Interventions consist of family counseling, educational support, behavioral strategies tailored for particular neurodevelopmental disorders in children (e.g., ADHD or ASD), and psychopharmacologic therapy.

c. *Child abuse and neglect*: A child's cognitive and social impairment, such as literal thinking, a lack of knowledge, and trouble understanding other people's expectations and feelings, can perpetuate a cycle of abuse. Additionally, such abuse may lead to further mood or behavioral issues in the child, such as depression, suicidal thoughts or actions, conduct disorder, post-traumatic stress disorder, and substance use disorders. It is important to have a high index of suspicion for child abuse/neglect in these children and educate the parents/caregivers about the same.

d. *Sleep disorders*: Children with ID frequently suffer from sleep disorders, which can impact their behavior, attention, memory, learning, and cognitive function. Side effects of medication can contribute to this issue. Behavioral interventions should be tailored to each child to promote good sleep hygiene, establish a supportive routine, and prevent unintentional reinforcement of undesirable behaviors. In some instances, pharmacotherapy with melatonin may be an option. Sleep disorders can become more complicated in individuals with an underlying genetic syndrome that leads to intellectual disabilities. For instance, children diagnosed with Down syndrome or Prader-Willi syndrome face an increased risk of obstructive sleep apnea, while those with Smith-Magenis syndrome often experience insomnia. It is typically essential for children with these conditions to undergo a comprehensive assessment by a sleep specialist, including polysomnography.

e. *Behavior intervention*: Many children with intellectual disabilities (ID) benefit from tailored interventions aimed at enhancing their social skills and behavioral performance. It's essential to customize these interventions. Understanding the purpose behind a child's problematic behavior (such as expressing frustration or specific needs), the events that lead up to it, and how others respond to it (like unintentionally reinforcing bad behavior) is crucial. Positive reinforcement should be applied to encourage desirable behaviors, while approaches that are restrictive or punitive should be avoided. Interventions must be appropriate for the child's level of functioning. Strategies might include minimizing known triggers of undesirable behaviors, rewarding the child with positive attention for acceptable behaviors, ignoring inappropriate actions, teaching alternative behaviors that can't coexist with the problematic ones, and swiftly removing the child from activity when a specific problematic behavior arises.

PREVENTION

Preventing ID involves a multifaceted approach that addresses various risk factors before and during pregnancy, as well as early childhood. Here are several strategies that can be implemented:

A. Prenatal Care

- ***Regular medical check-ups:*** Encourage prospective parents to seek regular prenatal care to monitor the health of both the mother and fetus.
- ***Genetic counseling:*** Provide genetic counseling for families with a history of intellectual disabilities to understand risks and options.
- ***Avoiding teratogens:*** Educate expectant mothers about avoiding substances harmful to fetal development, such as alcohol, recreational drugs, and certain medications (antiseizure drugs, chemotherapeutic agents) not approved for pregnancy.

B. Maternal Health and Nutrition

- ***Healthy lifestyle choices:*** Encourage a balanced diet rich in essential nutrients (e.g., folic acid), regular exercise, and avoiding tobacco and harmful substances.
- ***Chronic disease management:*** Ensure that chronic health conditions (e.g., diabetes, hypertension, thyroid disorders) are adequately managed during pregnancy.
- ***Preventing infections:*** Promote vaccinations and hygiene practices to prevent infections (e.g., rubella, toxoplasmosis) during pregnancy.

C. Postnatal Care

- ***Early intervention programs:*** Implement early screening and intervention programs for children identified as at risk, helping to address developmental delays as early as possible.
- ***Parental education:*** Provide resources and support for new parents on child development, nutrition, and effective parenting techniques.

D. Screening and Diagnostic Programs

- ***Newborn screening:*** Implement and maintain comprehensive newborn screening programs to identify metabolic and genetic disorders early.
- ***Developmental screening:*** Conduct routine developmental screening for young children to identify delays early and initiate support services.

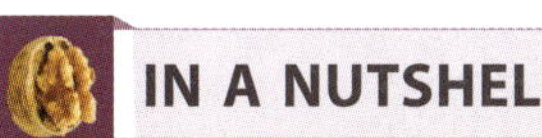

IN A NUTSHELL

Global Developmental Delay and Intellectual Disability

1. Global developmental delay is a term applied to children <5 years of age and is defined as a significant delay in two or more developmental domains. Intellectual disability is a neurodevelopmental disorder that is characterized by limitations in both intelligence and adaptive skills, affecting at least one of the three adaptive domains (conceptual, social, and practical).
2. The causes of ID primarily fall into two categories: genetic abnormalities and environmental factors. Genetic abnormalities may include single gene mutations, copy number variations, or chromosomal changes. Environmental factors can involve maternal exposure to toxins or infectious agents, maternal medical conditions, delivery-related complications, post-natal trauma, and toxin or infectious agent exposure.
3. Key investigations for a child with GDD/ID include neuroimaging, genetic tests, and testing for lead levels and thyroid profile.
4. Children at risk of GDD/ID should be initiated on early intervention, including physical, occupational, speech, and behavior therapy.
5. Treatable causes such as hypothyroidism should be prioritized and managed. Supportive treatment should be provided for other conditions.

Kaufman L, Ayub M, Vincent JB. The genetic basis of non-syndromic intellectual disability: a review. J Neurodev Disord. 2010;2:182.

Siegel M, McGuire K, Veenstra-VanderWeele J, et al. Practice parameter for the assessment and treatment of psychiatric disorders in children and adolescents with intellectual disability (intellectual developmental disorder). J Am Acad Child Adolesc Psychiatry. 2020;59:468.

Smythe T, Zuurmond M, Tann CJ, et al. Early intervention for children with developmental disabilities in low and middle-income countries—the case for action. Int Health. 2021;13:222.

Totsika V, Liew A, Absoud M, et al. Mental health problems in children with intellectual disability. Lancet Child Adolesc Health. 2022;6:432.

24.12 Cerebral Palsy *PE 27.11*

DEFINITION

Cerebral palsy (CP) refers to a diverse set of conditions that involve lifelong motor dysfunction, affecting muscle tone, posture, and/or movement.

The term cerebral palsy has been defined by Rosenbaum et al., as "a group of permanent disorders of the development of movement and posture, causing activity limitation, that are attributed to nonprogressive disturbances that occurred in the developing fetal or infant brain. The motor disorders of cerebral palsy are often accompanied by disturbances of sensation, perception, cognition, communication and behavior; by epilepsy and by secondary musculoskeletal problems".

The condition is described as a nonprogressive disorder (earlier referred to as static encephalopathy), which primarily implies that the insult to the brain is nonprogressive/static. However, the clinical expression of that injury to the brain changes over time as the child grows and the central nervous system matures into adulthood, making the clinical findings dynamic.

ETIOLOGY

CP is the most prevalent neuromotor disorder in children, occurring in approximately 1 to 4 out of every 1,000 live births. The incidence of CP is greater among those born prematurely or with low birth weight. Additionally, it is more common in low- and middle-income communities compared to high-income ones, largely due to differences in access to antenatal and perinatal medical care.

The causes of CP are typically multifactorial and can involve a variety of factors that negatively affect the developing brain of the fetus or neonate. **Table 24.42** illustrates the various factors associated with CP occurrence.

CLASSIFICATION AND EARLY SIGNS

CP results from various genetic, metabolic, ischemic, inflammatory/infectious, and additional influences that contribute to a shared group of neurological issues. Therefore, CP classification emphasizes phenotype over etiology, relying on the type and distribution of motor abnormalities **(Table 24.43)**.

CLINICAL FEATURES

There are three prominent types of CP syndromes: spastic, dyskinetic, and ataxic.

Spastic CP is typically caused by injuries to the cerebral cortex or corticospinal tract, accounting for approximately 80% of cases. It is characterized by a velocity-dependent increase in muscle tone (i.e., when the limb is moved quickly, there is a catch or resistance to movement). Additionally, spasticity may involve hyperreflexia and can be accompanied by clonus and persistence of primitive reflexes.

In extrapyramidal CP, brain injury spares the pyramidal tracts (hence extrapyramidal) and involves the basal ganglia/thalamus and related tracts, thus resulting in disorders of movement, coordination, and balance. The clinical features associated with different types of CP are as below.

A. Spastic CP

Children with spastic CP have features of upper motor neuron lesion including clasp-knife spasticity, brisk deep tendon reflexes

Table 24.42 Etiology/Factors that Increase the Likelihood of Developing Cerebral Palsy

A. **Antenatal**
1. Intrauterine infections (TORCH), Zika
2. Chorioamnionitis
3. Maternal trauma
4. Maternal malnutrition
5. Maternal medical disorders like uncontrolled diabetes, hypertension, preeclampsia causing placental insufficiency
6. Exposure to teratogens like antiepileptic drugs (phenytoin, valproate), smoking, alcohol)

B. **Birth related**
1. Prematurity (periventricular leukomalacia, intraventricular hemorrhage, bronchopulmonary dysplasia)
2. Intrauterine growth restriction
3. Intracranial hemorrhage
4. Hypoxic ischemic encephalopathy
5. Neonatal metabolic disorders like hypoglycemia, hyperbilirubinemia
6. Neonatal sepsis/meningoencephalitis
7. Perinatal stroke
8. Congenital structural abnormalities related to:
   i. Genetic abnormalities (Lissencephaly, schizencephaly)
   ii. Intrauterine infections (like TORCH)
   iii. Toxins (like antiepileptic drugs, nicotine)

C. **Post-neonatal period**
1. Traumatic brain injury
2. Febrile encephalopathy (meningoencephalitis)
3. Stroke
4. Hypoxic events like near drowning
5. Sequelae of status epilepticus

Table 24.43 Classification of Cerebral Palsy, with Neuroimaging Findings and Underlying Etiology

Classification (approximate % of CP cases)	*Neuroimaging findings*	*Etiological/risk factors*
Spastic CP (55–75%)		
Spastic diplegia (15–25%)	Periventricular leukomalacia	Prematurity
Spastic hemiplegia (20–40%)	• Neonatal stroke • Prenatal stroke • Congenital malformations	• Periventricular hemorrhagic infarction • Infection • Thrombophilic disorders • Genetic disorders
Spastic quadriplegia (20–40%)	• Multicystic encephalomalacia • Periventricular leukomalacia • Cortical malformations	• Hypoxic ischemic encephalopathy • Infection • Metabolic disorders (Hypoglycemia) • Genetic disorders
Dyskinetic CP (10–15%)		
Choreoathetoid CP	Scars in globus pallidus	Kernicterus
Dystonic CP	Symmetric scars in thalamus and putamen	• Hypoxia (in a term neonate) • Mitochondrial disorder • Genetic disorders
Ataxic CP (5–10%)	Cerebellar hypoplasia	Genetic disorders

(± clonus), and extensor plantar. The motor abnormalities lead to reduced muscle activity or movement patterns and interfere with function. Thus, these children have slow and effortful voluntary movements and may have persistent primitive reflexes. Topographically spastic CP includes:

- ***Spastic diplegia:*** Spastic diplegia is defined by the presence of bilateral spasticity in the lower extremities, which is more pronounced than that observed in the upper extremities. This condition frequently arises because of periventricular leukomalacia (PVL) or periventricular hemorrhagic infarction (PVHI).
  Children impacted by this may face visual difficulties. Usually, the initial clinical symptom of spastic diplegia becomes apparent when the affected infant begins to crawl. The child typically moves their arms in a normal reciprocal pattern but drags their legs, often called a commando crawl, rather than using the typical crawling method that involves all four limbs. When spasticity is severe, changing diapers can become difficult because of excessive hip adduction. The evaluation reveals the presence of symmetric spasticity in the lower limbs, accompanied by hyperreflexia, ankle clonus, and a bilateral Babinski sign. When the child is lifted by the axillae, the lower extremities are maintained in an extended scissoring posture. The onset of walking may be significantly delayed, with the feet positioned in an equinovarus alignment, and it is not uncommon for the child to ambulate on tiptoes.
- ***Spastic quadriplegia:*** Spastic quadriplegia represents the most severe type of CP, characterized by considerable motor impairment in all limbs and a strong association with multiple comorbidities, including cognitive impairment, epilepsy, communication and visual impairments, and feeding challenges. Swallowing difficulties usually occur due to supranuclear bulbar palsies, which can often lead to aspiration pneumonia and growth failure.
  Clinical evaluation reveals spasticity in all extremities, reduced spontaneous movements, hyperreflexia, and plantar extensor responses. By late childhood, flexion contractures of the knees, elbows, and wrists frequently occur. Children with spastic quadriparesis may also exhibit extrapyramidal symptoms due to the widespread nature of the brain injury.
- ***Spastic hemiplegia:*** Spastic hemiplegia is marked by reduced spontaneous movements on the affected side, with a noticeable preference evident from early infancy. Typically, the arm shows more impairment than the leg. Walking often gets delayed until 18 to 24 months, accompanied by a distinct circumduction gait. Examination of the extremities may reveal unilateral upper motor neuron signs with growth arrest, resulting in shortened limbs and reduced muscle bulk on the affected side.

B. Dyskinetic CP

Dyskinetic CP can be classified into two primary types of: Choreo-athetoid and dystonic. In this form of CP, the injury usually occurs in the subcortical areas, which serve as centers for coordination for movement and balance. While the injury may not lead to weakness, it can result in an inability to control movements voluntarily. Collectively, dystonic CP accounts for nearly 15–20% of all cases of CP.

Patients with dyskinetic CP often show multiple types of involuntary movements. Their limbs commonly become rigid when trying to move or when reacting to emotions, as a result of the simultaneous contraction of both agonist and antagonist muscle groups. Tendon reflexes can either present as normal or may be hard to elicit. Athetoid movements, especially in the toes and particularly the great toe (referred to as the striatal toe), serve as important signs of extrapyramidal dysfunction. Dyskinesia can also be present in specific spastic syndromes. In contrast to children with spastic CP, those exhibiting purely dyskinetic syndromes generally do not develop contractures.

- ***Choreoathetoid CP:*** Children experiencing choreoathetoid CP have rapid, disorganized, and unpredictable contractions of individual muscles or muscle groups, particularly affecting the facial area, bulbar muscles, proximal extremities, and digits. In addition, they demonstrate slow, writhing movements involving distal muscles. Facial grimacing may lead to oropharyngeal complications. Furthermore, primitive reflexes frequently persist into later stages of development childhood.
- ***Dystonic CP:*** This condition involves the co-contraction of both agonist and antagonist muscles. The truncal muscles are typically more impacted than the appendicular, leading to twisted postures and opisthotonus.

C. Ataxic CP

Ataxic CP is the rarest form, and its clinical presentation varies from hypotonia to mild spasticity, along with incoordination, depending on the other systems involved. Walking gait tends to be quite wide and can also be irregular at times. There may be difficulties in controlling eye movements and depth perception. Other causes of ataxia in infancy and childhood, including hydrocephalus, neoplasms, and degenerative disorders, should be ruled out before diagnosing CP.

Associated Conditions

Children with CP frequently experience additional cerebral function disorders motor impairments alongside motor impairments. These associated cerebral disorders can affect various domains, including cognition, vision, hearing, language, sensory processing, attention, and alertness behavior. The common co-morbidities include: intellectual disability, neurobehavioral problems (emotional lability, autistic traits, inattention), epilepsy, visual impairment, hearing and speech impairment, growth failure, gastrointestinal disorders (reflux, constipation), chronic pulmonary disease (due to scoliosis, aspiration pneumonitis), orthopedic disorders (scoliosis, dislocation of hip, foot deformities), dysfunctional voiding, pain and sleep disturbances.

INVESTIGATIONS

Although the diagnosis of CP is made clinically and no specific test can confirm or rule out CP, a diagnostic evaluation should be conducted for all children with CP to identify its underlying cause and to rule out other conditions. Also, some of the investigations are done for diagnosing comorbidities and aid management.

A. ***Neuroimaging:*** A brain MRI is recommended to identify the location and extent of structural lesions or related congenital malformations. An MRI revealing abnormalities consistent with CP supports the diagnosis and raises the level of certainty, but the diagnosis is still clinical. The typical neuroimaging findings have been highlighted in **Table 24.43**.
B. ***Vision assessment:*** Eye evaluation including fundus examination, examination for for strabismus should be done for all children with CP. Additionally visual evoked potential testing should be performed based on clinical evaluation.
C. ***Hearing assessment:*** All children with CP should undergo hearing assessment ± BERA.
D. ***EEG:*** All children with history of seizures should undergo EEG. In addition, EEG should be considered for children whose developmental delay continues to be out of proportion to the insult.
E. ***Metabolic and genetic testing:*** Metabolic and/or genetic testing is indicated in the following scenarios:
   - Perinatal history and clinical examination do not identify an etiology
   - Symptoms are atypical for CP
   - Neuroimaging is not congruent with the insult suggested by history
   - Clinical exacerbation in the setting of a catabolic state

TREATMENT Cerebral Palsy

The optimal treatment strategy for CP is formulated within a multidisciplinary, patient-centered environment, where medical interventions are integrated into a rehabilitation context that accounts for the patient's unique goals. The various strategies utilized are as below:

A. ***Early intervention***: Early intervention refers to initiation of therapeutic interventions soon after the insult. These are typically started in the NICU to enhance functional improvement connected to the neuromuscular plasticity of development brain.
B. ***Physiotherapy and occupational therapy:*** Physiotherapy emphasizes the development of gross motor skills and serves a vital function in improving range of motion, positioning, and coordination, all of which can significantly influence mobility. Occupational therapy emphasizes the development of fine motor skills and includes specific activities like feeding, toileting, dressing, personal hygiene, and hand grasps.
C. ***Constraint-induced movement therapy:*** Constraint-induced movement therapy involves intermittently restraining the unaffected limb and forcing the child to perform therapeutic tasks using the hemiplegic limb. This has been shown to enhance the motor and sensory functions of the affected limb.
D. ***Orthotics and devices to aid functionality:*** Numerous children diagnosed with CP benefit from orthotic devices, which enhance musculoskeletal alignment, promote functional abilities, and delay or prevent the occurrence of joint contractures. Ankle-foot orthotics are the most commonly used, followed by orthotics for the wrist and hand.

E. ***Tone management strategies:*** Pharmacotherapy is often the first-line approach to manage the tone abnormalities seen in CP. Commonly used drugs include baclofen, tizanidine, and benzodiazepines. Medications used to treat dystonia include benzodiazepines, trihexyphenidyl, clonidine, levodopa, and gabapentin. Tetrabenazine is beneficial for hyperkinetic movement disorders, including athetosis and chorea. Focal/segmental spasticity or dystonia includes chemodenervation using targeted injections of botulinum toxin A, phenol, or ethyl alcohol. Of these, botulinum toxin is most commonly used. Neurosurgical options for tone management include intrathecal baclofen, selective dorsal rhizotomy, and deep brain stimulation.
F. ***Surgical interventions:*** Children with CP can develop fixed joint deformities and contractures, which may need surgical procedures like muscle-tendon surgeries or bone surgeries.

PREVENTION

Although CP itself is not preventable or "curable", certain underlying causes, particularly those that predispose to CP, can be prevented.

A. Maternal Health Interventions

- ***Prenatal care:*** Comprehensive prenatal care can minimize risks associated with maternal infections, such as rubella vaccination, that can affect fetal brain development.
- ***Management of chronic conditions:*** Conditions like diabetes and hypertension should be well managed before and during pregnancy to reduce risks. Also, modifying antiseizure medications during pregnancy reduces the associated teratogenicity.
- ***Healthy lifestyle choices:*** Encouraging all the proper habits such as adequate nutrition, avoidance of alcohol and cessation of smoking contribute to healthier pregnancies.

B. Perinatal Care

- ***Premature birth:*** Strategies to prevent preterm labor, such as the use of tocolytics in high-risk women should be used when feasible. If a preterm delivery is likely, then in-utero transfer of fetus should be done to appropriate center equipped for handling premature neonate.
- ***Appropriate delivery practices:*** Monitoring and managing delivery complications (e.g., using proper fetal monitoring) to avoid birth asphyxia.
- ***Immediate neonatal care:*** Ensuring prompt treatment of respiratory distress, jaundice, and infections in newborns to prevent neurological damage. For infants with neonatal asphyxia, therapeutic hypothermia improves survival and neurodevelopmental outcome.

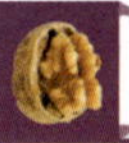

IN A NUTSHELL

Cerebral Palsy

1. Cerebral palsy (CP) refers to a central motor disorder impacting muscle tone, posture, and movement, resulting from non-progressive disturbances in the developing brain of a fetus or infant.
2. Based on patterns/types of tonal abnormalities and anatomical topography, it is classified into spastic diplegia, spastic quadriplegia, spastic hemiplegia, dyskinetic CP and ataxic CP.
3. The motor impairments of CP are often accompanied by other cerebral function disorders that may affect cognition, vision, hearing, and language. These children may have comorbidities including epilepsy, intellectual disability, sleep disturbance, vision and hearing impairment, pain and gastro-esophageal reflux.
4. Though CP is a clinical diagnosis, brain MRI is recommended to identify the location and extent of structural lesions or related congenital malformations. Evaluation of vision, hearing, and EEG are done to determine the comorbidities.
5. Management of a child with CP involves an interdisciplinary team that includes physiotherapy, occupational therapy, tone management, and braces/orthosis.

Gulati S, Sondhi V. Cerebral palsy: an overview. Indian J Pediatr. 2018;85(11):1006-16.
Harber V, Grasshoff U, Sellier E, et al. The role of neuroimaging and genetic analysis in the diagnosis of children with cerebral palsy. Front Neurol. 2021;11:628075.
Rosenbaum P, Paneth N, Leviton A, et al. A report: the definition and classification of cerebral palsy April 2006. Dev Med Child Neurol Suppl 2007;109:8.
Usuba K, Oddson B, Gauthier A, Young NL. Changes in gross motor function and health-related quality of life in adults with cerebral palsy: an 8-year follow-up study. Arch Phys Med Rehabil. 2014;95:2071.

24.13 Acute Flaccid Paralysis *PE 27.11*

DEFINITIONS

The World Health Organization has defined AFP as a syndrome marked by the rapid onset of weakness in any part of the body, including the respiratory and swallowing. This weakness peaks in severity from days to weeks, particularly in children under 15.

"Flaccid" refers to the absence of spasticity, while "paralysis" indicates a lack of muscular contraction due to the disruption of motor inputs from the cortex to muscle fibers.

Initially designed for poliomyelitis, this broad definition aims to capture patients with flaccid weakness due to myelitis,

Guillain-Barré syndrome (GBS), toxic/acquired neuropathy, and muscle pathologies.

The terminologies related to acute flaccid paralysis (AFP). AFP are listed in **Table 24.44**.

ANATOMY AND ASSOCIATED ETIOLOGIES

The lower motor neuron (LMN) is the efferent neuron that connects the central nervous system with the muscle it innervates. The major components of LMN are illustrated in **Figure 24.22**.

Table 24.44 Terminologies Related to Acute Flaccid Paralysis

Terminology	*Definition*
Acute flaccid paralysis	Acute flaccid paralysis is defined to be present in a child/adolescent <15- years-old presenting with weakness, where the following components are fulfilled: • Acute: <4 weeks duration and rapid progression from onset to maximal weakness • Flaccid: Characterized by loss of tone (hypotonia) and absent reflexes • Paralysis: "LMN" weakness
Acute flaccid myelitis	A specific type of AFP that is often associated with a polio-like illness affecting the anterior horn cell of the spinal cord, leading to sudden onset of muscle weakness and loss of reflexes
Lower motor neuron	A lower motor neuron (LMN) is a neuron that has its cell body in the spinal cord's ventral horn (anterior horn cell) or in cranial nerve motor nuclei. It directly innervates skeletal muscles and serves as the final pathway for motor activity. Components of LMN are anterior horn cell, root, peripheral nerve, neuromuscular junction and the muscle fibers
Bulbar palsy	Weakness or paralysis of the muscles involved in swallowing, speech, and facial movements
Tone	Muscle tone is the inherent resistance of skeletal muscles to passive movement. It's a state of partial contraction, even when the muscle is at rest, that helps maintain posture and allows for smooth, controlled movements

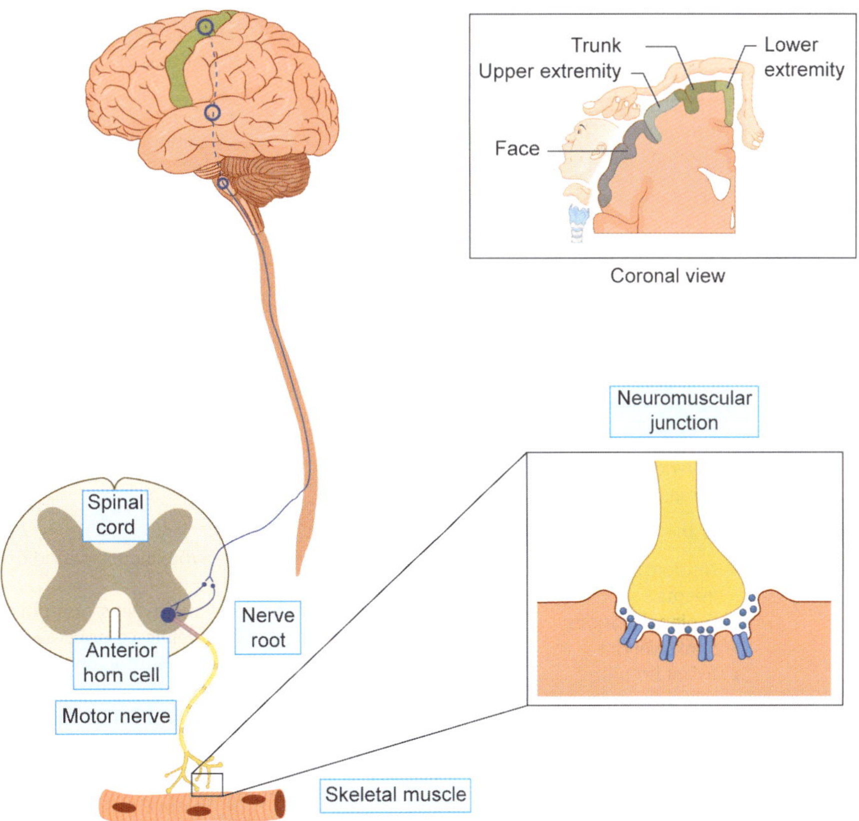

Fig. 24.22: Anatomy of upper and lower motor neuron has been depicted. Upper motor neuron refers to the corticospinal tract from the motor cortex till its point of termination in the spinal segment. Lower motor neuron (motor unit) refers to anterior horn cell, root/nerve, neuromuscular junction, and the associated muscle fibers. The image has been created in BioRender

Source: Created in BioRender. Sondhi, V. (2025) https://BioRender.com/3zegfgp

The various causes of acute flaccid paralysis (AFP) are enumerated in **Table 24.45** based on the site of involvement. As polioviruses and vaccine-derived polioviruses (VDPVs) are nearly eradicated globally, other enteroviruses, mainly enterovirus-D68 (EV-D68) and EV-A71, have become the leading causes of infection-related AFP. Other common entities associated with the syndrome of AFP include GBS, transverse myelitis, and traumatic neuritis.

Table 24.45 Anatomical Sites Related Etiologies of Acute Flaccid Paralysis

Site	*Pathophysiology*	*Etiology*
Spinal cord	Compressive myelopathy	• Trauma • Hematoma • Epidural abscess
	Inflammatory	Transverse myelitis
Anterior horn cell	Vascular	Infarction (anterior spinal artery syndrome)
	Infectious	• Poliomyelitis/VAPP and other non-polio enteroviruses (Coxsackie A and B, Echovirus, Enterovirus 70 and 71) • Japanese encephalitis
	Postinfectious	Acute flaccid myelitis (Enterovirus D68)
Roots/nerves	Immune mediated	• Guillain-Barré syndrome • Vasculitis
	Drugs/toxins	**Drugs:** Amitriptyline, Dapsone, Glutethimide, Hydralazine, Isoniazid, Nitrofurantoin, Nitrous Oxide, Critical illness neuropathy **Toxins:** Acrylamide, Glue sniffing, Fish Toxins, heavy metals (lead, arsenic, mercury, thallium), insecticides, organophosphates, snake venom, diphtheria, tick paralysis
	Trauma	Traumatic neuritis
	Infectious	• Herpesviridae (CMV, HSV Type 2, Varicella Zoster) • Lyme disease
Neuromuscular junction	Immune	Myasthenia Gravis
	Drugs/toxins	• Neuromuscular blocking agents • Aminoglycosides • Snake venom • Infant botulism
Muscle	Inflammatory	• Acute viral myositis • Acute inflammatory myopathies (PM, JDM)
	Drugs/toxins	• Steroid toxicity • Critical illness myopathy
	Metabolic	• Metabolic myopathies • Periodic paralysis • Hypo- or hyperkalemia • Hypomagnesemia

CLINICAL APPROACH

Each patient with AFP is an emergency. Necessitating prompt assessment. A comprehensive clinical evaluation, which includes a detailed medical history and examination, is essential before investigations are undertaken. **Tables 24.46 and 24.47** highlight the key components of history and examination related to a child with AFP.

Table 24.46 Clinical Approach to a Child with Acute Flaccid Paralysis

History	*Possible differential*
Fever at onset	• Poliomyelitis or other enteroviral myelitis; Varicella-Zoster, JE • Transverse myelitis • Epidural abscess • Viral myositis
Trauma	A history of trivial trauma could indicate compressive myelopathy due to fracture/ displacement in patients with vertebral defects or a ruptured AV malformation
Pattern of weakness	Ascending (involving lower limbs before upper limbs): • Guillain-Barré syndrome • Rabies • Ascending myelitis • Varicella Zoster Virus • Tick paralysis • CMV polyradiculoneuropathy (subacute) Descending (involving upper limbs before lower limbs): • Botulism • Diphtheria
Symmetry of weakness	Symmetrical: • Transverse myelitis • Guillain-Barré syndrome • Rabies, Varicella • Botulism • Tick bite Asymmetrical: • Poliomyelitis, non-polio enteroviruses • JE cirus
Progression of weakness: Sudden (postprandial) Hours to days Days to weeks	 • Hypokalemic periodic paralysis • Poliomyelitis, non-polio enteroviruses, transverse myelitis, compressive myelopathy, non-depolarizing drugs, viral myositis, critical illness polyneuropathy/myopathy • Guillain-Barré syndrome
Pain	• Compressive myelopathy, trauma (severe pain) • Transverse myelitis • Epidural abscess • Poliomyelitis and non-polio enteroviruses • Traumatic neuritis • Guillain-Barré syndrome (AMAN>AIDP) • Inflammatory myopathy • Viral myositis

Contd...

Contd...

History	*Possible differential*
Bladder/Bowel involvement	• Transverse myelitis • Epidural abscess • Compressive myelopathy • Non-depolarizing drugs • CMV polyradiculoneuropathy, rabies • Poliomyelitis (rare)
Exposure	• Animal bite: Rabies, snake envenomation, tick paralysis • Heavy metals: Lead, arsenic • Drug intake • Large meal (hypokalemic periodic paralysis) • Honey (in a child <1 year): Botulism • Immunization (Guillain-Barré or Traumatic Neuritis) • Diarrheal illness: Dyselectrolytemia, enteroviral infection, GBS (following *C. jejuni*)
Examination	
Vitals	• Pulse: Rate/rhythm to rule out autonomic instability • Respiration: Rate, and depth of respiration; can be evaluated by single breath count in older child • Blood pressure: Hypotension and hypertension suggesting autonomic instability
General examination	• Exanthem • Insect bite • Abnormal skin/hair pigmentation
Neurological examination	• Assessment of mental functions (drowsiness/irritability) • Cranial nerve examination (especially involvement of cranial nerves VII, IX, X) • Motor system assessment (consisting of bulk, tone, power and deep tendon reflexes) • Sensory examination (touch, pain, vibration, and proprioception) • Meningismus • Autonomic nervous system abnormalities (tachycardia/bradycardia, hypo/hypertension, and bowel and bladder dysfunction)

Table 24.47 Clinical Findings Suggestive of an Anatomic Level of Lesion

Anatomic level	*Clinical findings*
Spinal cord	Early bladder/bowel involvement, sensory level, early reduced/absent deep tendon reflexes, signs of meningeal irritation, spinal tenderness/painful spine movement
Anterior horn cell	Proximal > distal weakness, meningism ±, asymmetry
Roots and nerves	Symmetric findings. GBS may have autonomic instability and facial nerve involvement along with muscular or radicular or back pain
Neuromuscular junction	Fluctuating weakness, fatiguability, ptosis (early and prominent), multifocal (myasthenia)
Muscle	Muscle tenderness preserved deep tendon reflexes. Acute onset neck floppiness can be indicative of hypokalemia

INVESTIGATIONS

The investigations should be individualized based on clinical evaluation and lesion localization.

A. Electrophysiological Studies

Nerve conduction studies (NCS) are essential to establish the diagnosis of GBS. NCS findings can be normal in the initial stages of the disease and become progressively more pronounced 2 weeks after the start of the illness. They also help differentiate acute inflammatory demyelinating polyneuropathy from axonal neuropathy. Single-fiber EMG can be used to demonstrate decremental response and fatiguability in cases of myasthenia gravis. EMG may also be used to diagnose traumatic neuritis.

B. Cerebrospinal Fluid Studies

CSF studies are indicated to exclude diagnoses other than GBS, which may include viral/aseptic meningitis. The hallmark of GBS is elevated protein with normal cell counts (albumino-cytological dissociation), but this is not essential for diagnosis, as only 64% may exhibit it. CSF protein levels rise in the second half of the first week, with only 50% showing elevation by day 3 and 80% by the week's end. Acute flaccid myelitis may show moderate pleocytosis (up to 100 cells/μL) and normal to mildly elevated protein, whereas transverse myelitis usually presents with mild to moderate pleocytosis and normal to slightly elevated protein and IgG index.

C. Contrast-enhanced MRI Spine

A contrast-enhanced MRI of the spine can immensely help in determining the etiology of a suspected spinal cord/anterior horn cell lesion. Epidural abscess, arteriovenous malformations, discitis, and trauma can be easily determined by imaging. In addition, CE MRI of the spine can help differentiate between transverse myelitis (discrete lesions, white ± gray matter), spinal cord stroke (anterior cord lesions, predominantly gray matter involvement), acute flaccid myelitis (extensive hyperintensities in gray matter and edema which may be accompanied by nerve roots enhancement) and GBS (enhancement of intrathecal nerve roots with thickening of cauda equina).

D. Other Tests

- ***Auto-antibodies:*** Anti-acetylcholine receptor (Anti-AChR) antibody and anti-muscle specific kinase (Anti-MuSK) antibody can be used for myasthenia gravis. GBS can exhibit positive anti-ganglioside antibodies (GM1 and GD1a).
- ***Serum potassium:*** Can be decreased (hypokalemic periodic paralysis) or elevated (in addition to myoglobinuria, CKemia and raised creatinine as in metabolic myopathy).
- ***Creatine kinase:*** Elevated in viral myositis and inflammatory myopathy.
- ***Urine for heavy metals*** or porphobilinogen based on clinical suspicion.

SPECIFIC CONDITIONS LEADING TO ACUTE FLACCID PARALYSIS

Infectious Disease (Poliomyelitis and other Infections)

Poliomyelitis is an infection caused by a neurotropic RNA virus from the Picornaviridae family, and it used to be a significant cause of AFP before the implementation of widespread immunization. While the transmission of wild-type Poliovirus has been eradicated, the World Health Organization continues to monitor AFP cases for any occurrences of wild-type or, more critically, vaccine-derived polio virus (VDPV) infections.

VDPV derives from the weakened poliovirus used in the oral polio vaccine (OPV) but has mutated to exhibit behavior like that of the wild strain. VDPVs can be categorized as circulating (resulting from low immunization rates), immunodeficient (from mutations in immunocompromised hosts), or ambiguous (isolated from immunocompetent individuals with no evidence of circulating poliovirus in the community).

Other non-polio enteroviruses have been linked to AFP, such as Coxsackie A and B, Echovirus, and Enterovirus 70 and 71. The clinical symptoms of these infections are similar to those of poliomyelitis. Other neurotropic viruses associated with AFP include paralytic rabies (which involves ascending paralysis, sphincter difficulties, and sensory disruptions), Herpesviridae (including Epstein-Barr virus, Cytomegalovirus, and Varicella, the latter two being capable of inducing polyradiculoneuropathy), and the Japanese encephalitis virus, which causes damage to anterior horn cells.

Guillain-Barré Syndrome

Guillain-Barré syndrome (GBS) is an immune-mediated polyneuropathy acquired following an infection, leading to either demyelination or axonal damage. There are several variants of GBS, including *Miller-Fisher syndrome*, which is marked by ataxia, areflexia, and ophthalmoplegia; *Bickerstaff brainstem encephalitis*; paraparetic variants; and pharyngeal-cervical-brachial weakness. Currently, it stands as the most prevalent acute paralytic neuropathy globally, affecting over 100,000 individuals each year.

Etiopathogenesis

GBS is typically associated with a history of a non-specific illness or vaccination up to 4 weeks before developing neurological symptoms. The organisms typically associated with GBS include those that cause gastro-intestinal manifestations (*Campylobacter, Helicobacter*), respiratory illness (*Mycoplasma*), or other viral illnesses, including EBV, CMV, HIV, West Nile virus and Zika virus. GBS has been reported following influenza, measles, polio, and rabies vaccinations.

Clinical Features

Symptoms begin with tingling, numbness, and paresthesia, followed by increasing irritability and radicular/back pain with myalgia. This is succeeded by a progressive symmetric ascending paralysis with typically proximal weakness being more prominent. The weakness progresses from the lower limbs to involve the upper limbs, the respiratory muscles and finally bulbar weakness and other cranial nerve palsies. The disease progresses over days and if untreated, the maximum severity is attained at ≤4 weeks. 60% of patients experience loss of ambulation, and 50% have bulbar involvement. Rapidly progressive GBS is characterized by prominent respiratory muscle weakness, an inability to handle respiratory and/or oral secretions and facial nerve involvement. Involvement of the vocal cords may lead to hoarseness of voice. Autonomic dysfunction is also characteristic of GBS, with the common features being labile temperature, sweating, tachycardia or bradycardia, fluctuating blood pressure, and postural hypotension.

Investigations

- ***Nerve conduction studies (NCS):*** NCS can help to further classify it into acute inflammatory demyelinating polyneuropathy (AIDP) or acute axonal neuropathy (pure motor—AMAN or motor-sensory—AMSAN). Making a distinction is essential as cases of axonal neuropathy are more challenging to treat (higher chances of treatment-related fluctuations) and higher chances of residual weakness.
- ***CSF:*** CSF may demonstrate albuminocytological dissociation (CSF protein > twice the upper limit of normal, with cells <10 per µL) and will help in ruling out other infectious/inflammatory causes of weakness.
- ***Neuroimaging:*** Contrast MRI of the spine can demonstrate the thickening of the cauda equina and the thickening of the nerve roots.
- ***Serology:*** Recently anti-ganglioside antibodies have also been discovered that are implicated in GBS. In clinical settings, commercially available testing for serum IgG antibodies to GQ1b proves valuable in diagnosing Miller Fisher syndrome, with a sensitivity ranging from 85 to 90%.

Making a Diagnosis

Clinical/laboratory findings that make a diagnosis of GBS less likely include CSF pleocytosis, severe pulmonary dysfunction with little or no limb weakness at onset, severe sensory signs with little or no weakness at onset, bladder/bowel dysfunction at onset, fever at onset, sharp spinal cord sensory level, marked and persistent asymmetry of weakness, and persistent bladder/bowel dysfunction or slow progression of weakness.

TREATMENT **Guillain-Barré Syndrome**

- GBS is an emergency, and patients should be admitted to an ICU/HDU with an initial 2 hours monitoring of progression of weakness, respiratory rate, pattern of respiration ± single breath count (in cooperative children), swallowing difficulties, and autonomic dysfunction.
- The primary treatment options for GBS *are intravenous immune globulin (IVIG)* and *plasma exchange (PLEX)*. IVIG and PLEX should be limited to children with GBS who exhibit any of the following: increasing weakness, deteriorating respiratory muscle weakness or requirement for mechanical support, bulbar weakness, or inability to walk independently. In children, IVIG is favored over PLEX due to its relative safety and ease of administration, though there is no reliable data indicating that one is better than the other.

- IVIG is administered at a dose of 2 g/kg (either 1 g/kg/day for 2 days or 400 g/kg/day for 5 days). The IVIG is likely involved in the suppression of inflammatory and immune processes and neutralization of circulating antibodies. PLEX leads to the removal of antibodies directed against nerves from the circulation. Apart from this, patients with GBS will require respiratory care, physiotherapy, and analgesics for pain.
- Even after the acute phase, patients of GBS may continue to have residual weakness and pain for a prolonged period. About 20% of patients with GBS are unable to walk unassisted 6 months after onset. Maximum improvement in weakness happens in the first year, but patients can show further recovery even after 3 or more years.

Transverse Myelitis

Transverse myelitis (TM) is a rare, acquired inflammatory disorder affecting the spinal cord and presenting with acute-subacute motor, sensory and autonomic features.

Pathogenesis

Immunopathogenesis ranges from idiopathic to disease-associated myelitis. TM is not solely a demyelinating condition; instead, it is a mixed inflammatory disorder impacting neurons, axons, oligodendrocytes, and myelin.

- ***Idiopathic TM*** typically arises as a complication following an infection, likely due to an autoimmune mechanism.
- ***Secondary TM*** may be directly linked to infectious, systemic inflammatory, or multifocal diseases affecting the central nervous system.

Etiology

The most common infections implicated include Enteroviruses, Herpesviridae, HIV, HTLV-1, Zika disease, Lyme disease, and Mycoplasma. TM can also occur as a component of nervous system demyelination syndromes like Multiple Sclerosis or Neuromyelitis Optica Spectrum Disorder.

Clinical Features

The onset of TM is marked by the acute or subacute development of motor, sensory, and/or autonomic dysfunction. The most common first symptoms are sensory change, weakness, and pain followed by bladder and bowel symptoms and balance problems.

Motor symptoms include an acute onset of paraparesis or quadriparesis, depending upon the level of lesion, manifesting initially with flaccidity, followed by spasticity. Flaccidity may persist at the level of spinal cord involvement (i.e., lower motor type of lesion), and upper motor neuron signs appear below the level of the lesion over the subsequent days to weeks.

Typical sensory findings include pain, dysesthesia, and paresthesia with a definite sensory level.

Autonomic symptoms include urinary urgency, sphincter incontinence or difficulty with voiding, and constipation.

Diagnosis

TM should be suspected in cases with clinical localization to the spinal cord, bilateral symptoms and signs, clearly defined sensory level, progression to the nadir between 4 hours–21 days, and MRI images suggestive of T2 WI in the white ± gray matter after excluding compressive myelopathy. There may also be gadolinium enhancement on the MRI with mild to moderate pleocytosis in the CSF with elevated IgG Index.

When inflammatory myelopathy is confirmed, it becomes crucial to differentiate idiopathic TM from TM secondary to disorders including CNS demyelination (NMOSD/MOGAD), infectious myelitis, systemic autoimmune disorders, or paraneoplastic syndromes.

Idiopathic TM is characterized by its occurrence without a definitive etiology, even after comprehensive evaluation. Hence, testing for autoimmune disorders should be individualized and may include all or some of the following: anti-aquaporin 4 antibodies, anti-myelin oligodendrocyte glycoprotein antibodies, antinuclear antibodies, anti-ds DNA, antiphospholipid antibodies, antineutrophil cytoplasmic antibodies, and CSF and serum oligoclonal bands.

TREATMENT Transverse Myelitis

Management includes high-dose methylprednisolone (20–30 mg/kg/day for 5 days) and IVIg (400 mg/kg/day for 5 days). Other therapies may include immunosuppressive drugs, including cyclophosphamide, mycophenolate, and rituximab. Plasmapheresis can also be attempted in cases that do not respond to immunosuppression in the acute stage.

AFP SURVEILLANCE

AFP surveillance involves designated staff visiting health facilities regularly to identify, report, and investigate AFP cases. These staff members are typically external to the healthcare facility and gather data from individual cases, registers, medical records, or logbooks at reporting sites to ensure no cases go unreported. Initially, when the polio eradication initiative started, most countries recorded polio cases as just one among many diseases in their surveillance systems, often reporting annually. This made detecting new polio cases and managing outbreaks challenging, as many diseases can mimic polio. Therefore, a more sensitive system was required to quickly identify, report, and investigate suspected new cases. This need led to the adoption of AFP as the syndrome for reporting, paralleling how the detection and investigation of the "rash and fever" syndrome was utilized during the smallpox eradication campaign. With these efforts, India had its last case of polio in 2011. However, as part of an ongoing policy, the AFP surveillance is ongoing.

Non-polio AFP Indicator

The incidence of non-polio AFP cases in any population is estimated to be one case per 100,000 children under 15 years of age. This statistic serves as a useful indicator for assessing the sensitivity of the surveillance system. Achieving this indicator suggests that the surveillance system is sufficiently sensitive to detect polio cases if they arise. It forms the foundation for evaluating the quality of AFP surveillance.

What Should be Reported?

All children fulfilling definition of AFP mentioned above, including children up to 15 years with facial palsy should be notified the local/regional center in the district.

Protocol

Following reporting of AFP cases, the surveillance staff from nodal center visits the healthcare facility and the patient to note the clinical details and collects two adequate stool samples. Stool samples are called adequate when two specimens are collected at least 24 hours apart, both within 14 days after the onset of paralysis, shipped on ice or frozen packs and arrive in good condition at a WHO-accredited laboratory. The stool samples are then analyzed in the laboratory and reported as "Polio" or "Discarded" (i.e., non-polio). The process of AFP surveillance has been highlighted in **Figure 24.23**. The primary indicator of effective AFP surveillance is a non-polio AFP rate of at least one, along with a specimen adequacy of at least 80%.

CONCLUSION

Acute flaccid paralysis (AFP) is a complex clinical syndrome that necessitates prompt and thorough evaluation of differential diagnoses. Every instance of AFP is an emergency, both clinically and from a public health standpoint, making an accurate understanding of the etiology, the underlying pathophysiological mechanisms, and the anatomical and morphological changes critical for prognosis and treatment options. **Figure 24.24** offers a comprehensive framework that addresses most scenarios associated with AFP.

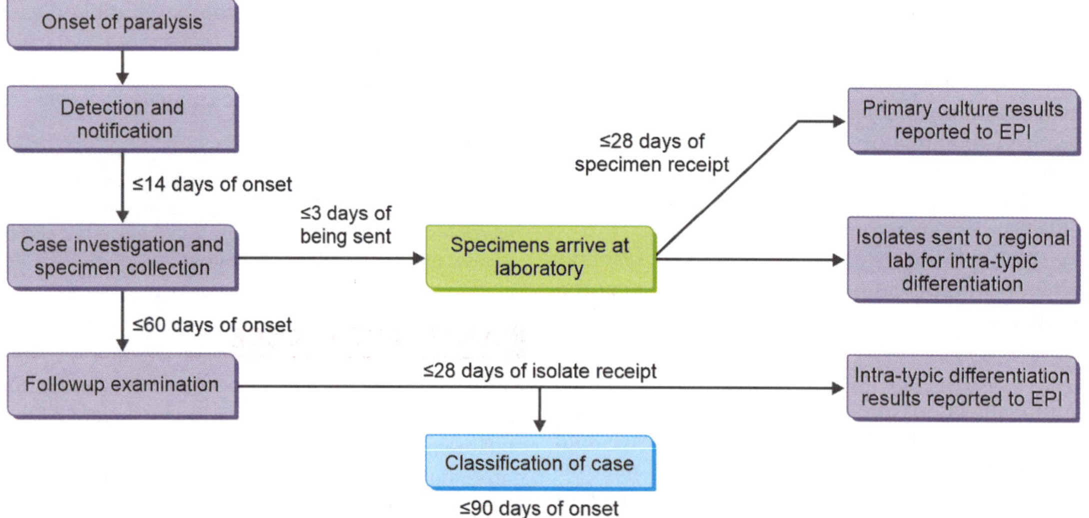

Fig. 24.23: Process of surveillance of a case of acute flaccid paralysis

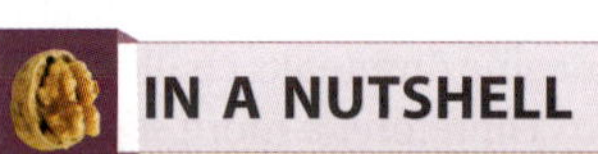

IN A NUTSHELL

Acute Flaccid Paralysis

1. Acute flaccid paralysis (AFP) is defined as any child under 15-years-old who presents with weakness that is acute in onset (<4 weeks), flaccid in nature [characterized by loss of muscle tone (hypotonia) and absent reflexes] and is of the lower motor neuron type.
2. The lower motor neuron is the efferent neuron that connects the central nervous system with the muscle it innervates. The lower motor neuron lesion comprises lesions involving the anterior horn cell, root/nerve, neuromuscular junction and muscle.
3. Common clinical entities associated with the syndrome of AFP include polio/polio like virus infection, Guillain-Barré syndrome (GBS), transverse myelitis, and traumatic neuritis.
4. The investigations in a child with AFP include nerve conduction studies, CSF analysis and contrast enhanced MRI of spine.
5. Management depends on the underlying etiology. GBS is treated with IVIG and/or plasmapheresis. Transverse myelitis is managed with corticosteroids.

Abbassi N, Ambegaonkar G. Guillain-Barré syndrome: a review. Paediatr Child Health. 2019;29(11):459-62.
Chung A, Deimling M. Guillain-Barré syndrome. Pediatr Rev. 2018;39:53.
Shahrizaila N, Lehmann HC, Kuwabara S. Guillain-Barré syndrome. The Lancet. 2021;397(10280):1214-28.
Yuki N, Hartung HP. Guillain-Barré syndrome. New England Journal of Medicine. 2012;366(24):2294-304.

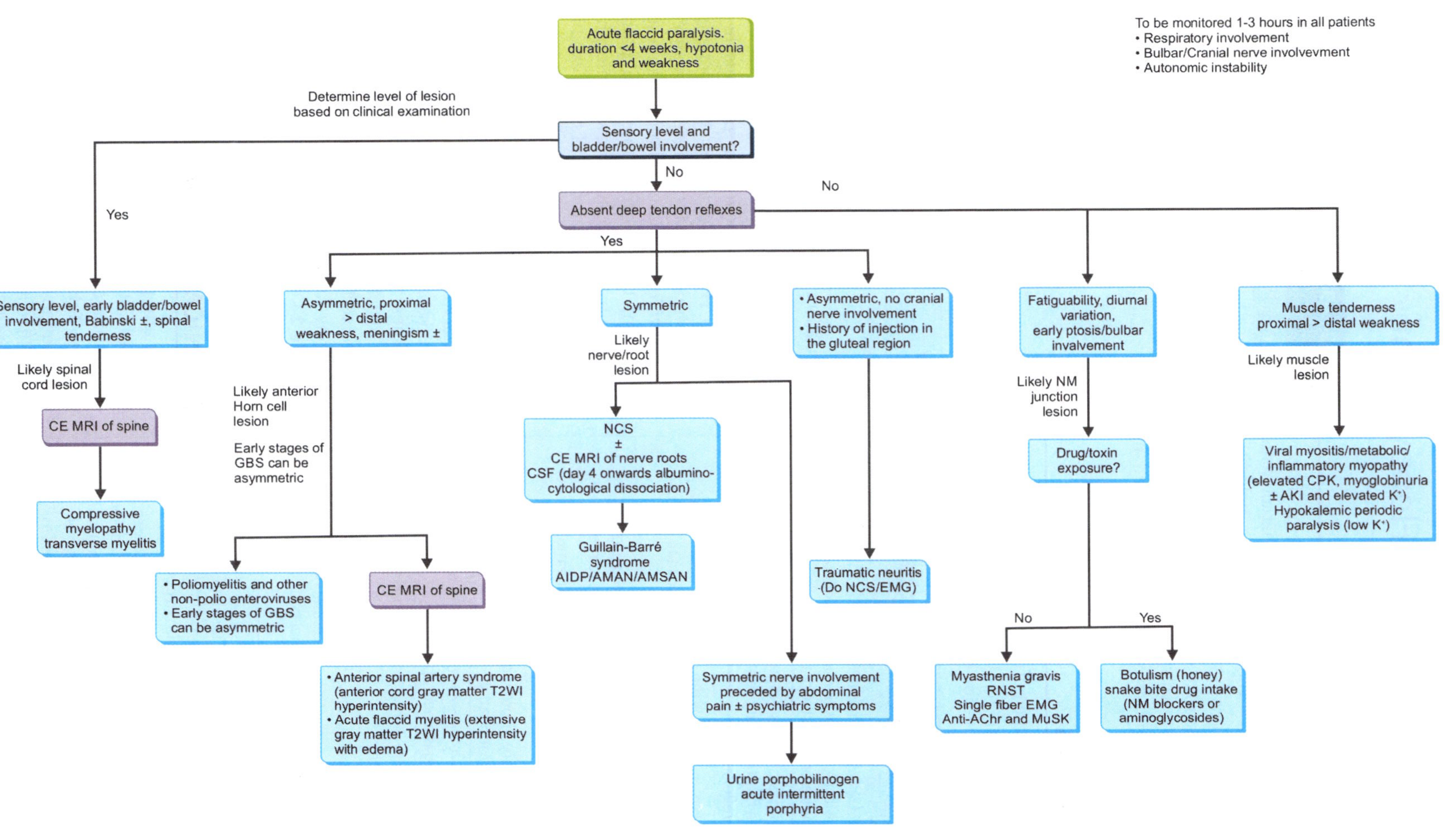

Fig. 24.24: Approach to a child with acute flaccid paralysis

24.14 Floppy Infant

PE 27.12

DEFINITION

Tone is the resistance of muscle to stretch. The term "floppy infant" informally refers to generalized hypotonia, a characteristic observed in various systemic and neurologic diseases, including disorders of the central nervous system (like cerebral palsy), the peripheral nervous system (like neuromuscular disorder), or genetic syndromes (like Down syndrome). The common terminologies associated with this diagnosis are listed in **Table 24.48.**

ETIOPATHOGENESIS

Muscle tone is regulated by the peripheral fusimotor system, with input from the CNS. Any failure within the motor unit components, such as the anterior horn cell, motor neuron, neuromuscular junction, or the muscle itself, can lead to hypotonia. Hypotonia can be central or peripheral. The primary distinguishing factor is the presence or absence of weakness.

- ***Central hypotonia*** is a clinical manifestation of conditions affecting the CNS and supraspinal pathways. Infants with central hypotonia may show dysmorphic features, altered sensorium, or seizures, and might exhibit brisk reflexes and clonus. Older children may have a history of developmental delays that compromise cognitive and motor skills.
- ***Peripheral hypotonia*** is observed in disorders affecting the motor neuron unit are referred to as peripheral hypotonia. Infants with peripheral hypotonia are usually alert and meet cognitive milestones on schedule, but they have significant weakness with limited antigravity movements. Additionally, they may have myopathic facies. This group frequently has characteristics of lower motor neuron lesion, like muscle atrophy, fasciculations, and decreased reflexes.

Table 24.49 illustrates features distinguishing central and peripheral hypotonia. The etiologies related to the syndrome of "floppy infant" are listed in **Table 24.50**.

Table 24.48 Terminologies Associated with Floppy Infant

Terminology	*Definition*
Tone	Muscle tone is defined as a skeletal muscle's inherent resistance to passive movement
Phasic tone	Phasic tone is a rapid contraction in response to a high intensity stretch (example deep tendon reflexes)
Postural tone	Postural tone is the prolonged contraction of antigravity muscles in response to the low intensity stretch of gravity
Power	Muscle power or strength is a muscle's maximum voluntary resistance to movement
Motor unit	One anterior horn cell and all the muscle fibers that it innervates make up a motor unit
Neuronopathy	A primary disorder of the anterior horn cell body is a neuronopathy
Neuropathy	A primary disorder of the axon or its myelin covering is a neuropathy
Myopathy	A primary disorder of the muscle fiber is a myopathy
Central hypotonia	Conditions leading to hypotonia due to primary disorders affecting the central nervous system, and therefore supraspinal pathways, are termed central hypotonia
Peripheral hypotonia	Peripheral hypotonia refers to an infant who exhibits hypotonia as a result of a pathology affecting the motor neuron unit. They usually have weakness along with hypotonia
Spasticity	Spasticity is defined as "a motor disorder characterized by a velocity dependent increase in tonic stretch reflexes (muscle tone) with exaggerated tendon jerks, resulting from hyperexcitability of the stretch reflex, as one component of the upper motor neuron syndrome"

Table 24.49 Features Differentiating Central vs. Peripheral Hypotonia

Variable	*Central hypotonia*	*Peripheral hypotonia*
Cognition	Delayed	Normal/alert
Motor delay	Yes	Yes
Pull to sit	Head lag (more than normal)	Marked head lag
Bulk	Normal or slightly reduced	• Significantly reduced with anterior horn cell disease, neuropathy and myopathy • Can be normal in disorders of neuromuscular junction • Can have pseudohypertrophy with muscular dystrophies
Power	Mild to moderate reduction	Significant reduction (*paralytic*)
Reflexes	Decreased or increased	Absent
Fasciculations	Absent	Present with anterior horn cell disease

CLINICAL APPROACH

History and physical examination are the keys to confirming hypotonia, localizing and classifying it as central/peripheral or combined, and determining the differential diagnosis/etiology. **Table 24.51** summarizes the details of history and examination in the context of a floppy infant. An algorithm with a simplified approach to a child with hypotonia is presented in **Figure 24.25**.

Table 24.50 Etiologies of Floppy Infant

Central hypotonia (upper motor neuron lesion)	*Peripheral hypotonia (lower motor neuron lesion)*	*Mixed (UMN and LMN lesion)*

• Acute cerebral insult
• Cerebrovascular accident
• Hypoxic-ischemic encephalopathy
• Infection (e.g., viral, bacterial, fungal, parasitic)
• Chromosomal abnormality
  ▪ Angelman syndrome
  ▪ Down syndrome
  ▪ Prader-Willi syndrome
• Cerebral palsy
• Metabolic disease (organic acidemia, mitochondrial disorders)
• Traumatic brain injury
• Toxins
  ▪ Bilirubin
  ▪ Phenytoin
	• Anterior horn cell disorder
	  ▪ Spinal muscular atrophy
	  ▪ Poliomyelitis
	• Neuropathy
	  ▪ Hereditary motor-sensory neuropathies
	  ▪ Guillain–Barré syndrome
	• Neuromuscular junction disorder
	  ▪ Myasthenia gravis
	  ▪ Botulism
	• Muscle disorder
	  ▪ Glycogen storage disease (e.g., acid maltase deficiency)
	  ▪ Congenital myopathies
	  ▪ Myotonic dystrophy
	  ▪ Polymyositis
		• Adrenoleukodystrophy
		• Krabbe disease (globoid cell leukodystrophy)
		• Metachromatic leukodystrophy
		• Zellweger syndrome

Table 24.51 Key History and Examination Findings in a Floppy Infant

History	
Antenatal history	• History of polyhydramnios (caused by decreased fetal swallowing), paucity of fetal movements, and malpresentation (breech presentation) may suggest peripheral hypotonia, likely due to a neuromuscular disorder • History of myasthenia gravis in mother • Intrauterine infections or exposure to drugs which can lead to multisystem involvement or CNS involvement leading to central hypotonia • Advanced maternal age at conception may suggest chromosomal disorder
Birth history	• Gestational age because prematurity alone may cause hypotonia in infancy • History of HIE should be sought. HIE may lead to hypotonia early in infancy before manifesting UMN signs. In addition, HIE may be a result of neuromuscular disorders • History of risk factors of HIE should be checked, including maternal hypotension, breech extraction, aberrant fetal heart rate, cord prolapse, or placental abruption
Onset and progression	• Central hypotonia tends to improve with time; if secondary to HIE, it may evolve to hypertonia • Peripheral hypotonia may remain stable or may gradually worsen • Acute onset with sudden deterioration after an uncomplicated pregnancy, delivery, and neonatal course suggests an inborn error of metabolism
Associated symptoms	• Alert child with lack/paucity of limb movements above the plane of bed may suggest peripheral hypotonia especially anterior horn cell disease like spinal muscular atrophy • Following an otherwise uneventful neonatal course, progressive weakness and a history of constipation point to infantile botulism. Consumption of honey or corn syrup should be ruled out in this scenario • Fluctuating weakness, ptosis may be seen with certain congenital myasthenia syndromes • Myasthenic syndromes can cause fatigue when feeding • Seizures typically suggest central hypotonia
Developmental history	• Motor delay (due to hypotonia) • Myotonic dystrophy and central causes are more likely to cause cognitive delay
Family history	• Consanguinity is associated with a higher risk of autosomal recessive disorders (example, spinal muscular atrophy) • History of recurrent abortions in the mother or in family suggests a chromosomal disorder • Malignant hyperthermia in a family member is suggestive of congenital myopathy • Maternal characteristics of myotonic dystrophy, such as arrhythmias, insulin resistance, cataracts, cardiomyopathy, distal muscle weakness, and intellectual disability may suggest myotonic dystrophy in infant • Maternal history of exercise intolerance, migraine headache, diabetes mellitus, retinitis pigmentosum, and sensorineural hearing loss may suggest mitochondrial disorder • A family history of intellectual disability, developmental delay, congenital abnormalities, and skeletal muscle disease should be obtained in every floppy infant

Contd...

Contd...

Examination	
Vital signs	• Abnormalities of respiratory rate, pattern, or diaphragmatic weakness or intercostal weakness may suggest peripheral hypotonia like congenital myopathy • Wek cry suggests weakness of respiratory muscles; high pitched cry may suggest cerebral etiology • Tachycardia/hypotension may be seen with cardiomyopathy (associated with peripheral hypotonia due to fatty oxidation disorders/mitochondrial disorders)
Dysmorphism	• Dysmorphism may be seen with central hypotonia like with chromosomal disorders (e.g., Down syndrome, congenital disorders of glycosylation, peroxisomal disorders) • Myopathic facies (dolicocephaly, long expressionless face, high arched palate and inability to elevate the corners of the mouth)
General examination	• Hyperlaxity of joints may be seen with COL6A related congenital muscular dystrophies • Anomalies of the genitalia, including undescended testis, may be seen with peripheral hypotonia • Joint contractures (suggesting long periods of paucity/absence of movements) may be seen with spinal muscular atrophy, congenital myopathy, and congenital muscular dystrophy
Neurological examination	• Posture: Posture of the infant and spontaneous movements gives a clue about the tone and strength of muscles. A hypotonic infant typically has flaccid extension of upper limbs with abduction of lower limbs along with outer surface of limbs touching the bed. This is typically referred to as "frog-leg" position. • Assessment of tone: Various maneuvers performed for tone assessment include: ▪ Pull to sit for assessing upper limbs and axial tone ▪ Scarf sign for assessing upper limb tone ▪ Popliteal angle for lower limb tone ▪ Vertical suspension for appendicular tone (around shoulders) ▪ Horizontal suspension for axial tone • Power assessment is significant because the peripheral hypotonia is usually a combination of loss of muscle tone and strength, while central hypotonia is associated with relative preservation of muscle strength. Absence of antigravity muscles strongly suggests peripheral hypotonia • Deep tendon reflexes are brisk (or clonus may be present) in upper motor neuron lesion (suggesting central hypotonia). Hyporeflexia/areflexia is characteristic of lesions involving anterior horn cell, peripheral nerves or muscles • Fasciculations are suggestive of anterior horn cell disease (spinal muscular atrophy, polio)

INVESTIGATIONS

Investigations are guided by the clinical findings and distinction between central and peripheral hypotonia. They key investigations include:

A. ***Hematology and biochemistry:***
- Complete blood count and inflammatory markers are performed to rule out underlying sepsis that may contribute to hypotonia
- *Electrolytes* are analyzed to rule out dyselectrolytemia. Hypokalemia, hypocalcemia are manageable causes of hypotonia
- ***Creatine kinase*** is a muscle enzyme that is elevated in muscular dystrophies and metabolic myopathies.
- ***Transaminases*** may act as a surrogate marker of creatine kinase and may be elevated in muscle disorders
- ***Specific metabolic tests*** like arterial lactate, plasma ammonia, tandem mass spectrometry, gas chromatography and carnitine levels may be needed if suspecting mitochondrial disorders or inborn errors of metabolism

B. ***Electrophysiology:*** Nerve conduction study and electromyography are beneficial for evaluating conditions impacting the motor unit (lower motor neuron and innervated muscle fibers). Electromyography is crucial in diagnosing spinal muscular atrophy and neuromuscular junction disorders such as botulism and congenital myasthenia gravis. Additionally, these studies are valuable for diagnosing hereditary motor sensory neuropathies and distinguishing axonal disorders from demyelinating diseases.

C. ***Neuroimaging:*** In infants with central hypotonia, MRI of the brain and spine is useful for detecting structural malformations, defects in neuronal migration, abnormalities in the brain stem and cerebellum, and features indicating potential mitochondrial disorders and inborn errors of metabolism.

D. ***Genetic tests:*** The karyotype is useful for detecting chromosomal duplications, deletions, trisomy such as Down syndrome, and genetic imprinting disorders such as Prader-Willi syndrome. Molecular genetic tests like MLPA help diagnose spinal muscular atrophy (SMN1 gene deletion). Targeted genetic testing and whole-exome sequencing are utilized for congenital myopathies, congenital muscular dystrophies, and congenital myasthenic syndrome.

E. ***Other investigations:*** ECG and ECHO might be needed if Pompe disease is suspected. Those with concurrent aspiration pneumonia may require a chest radiograph and arterial blood gas analysis.

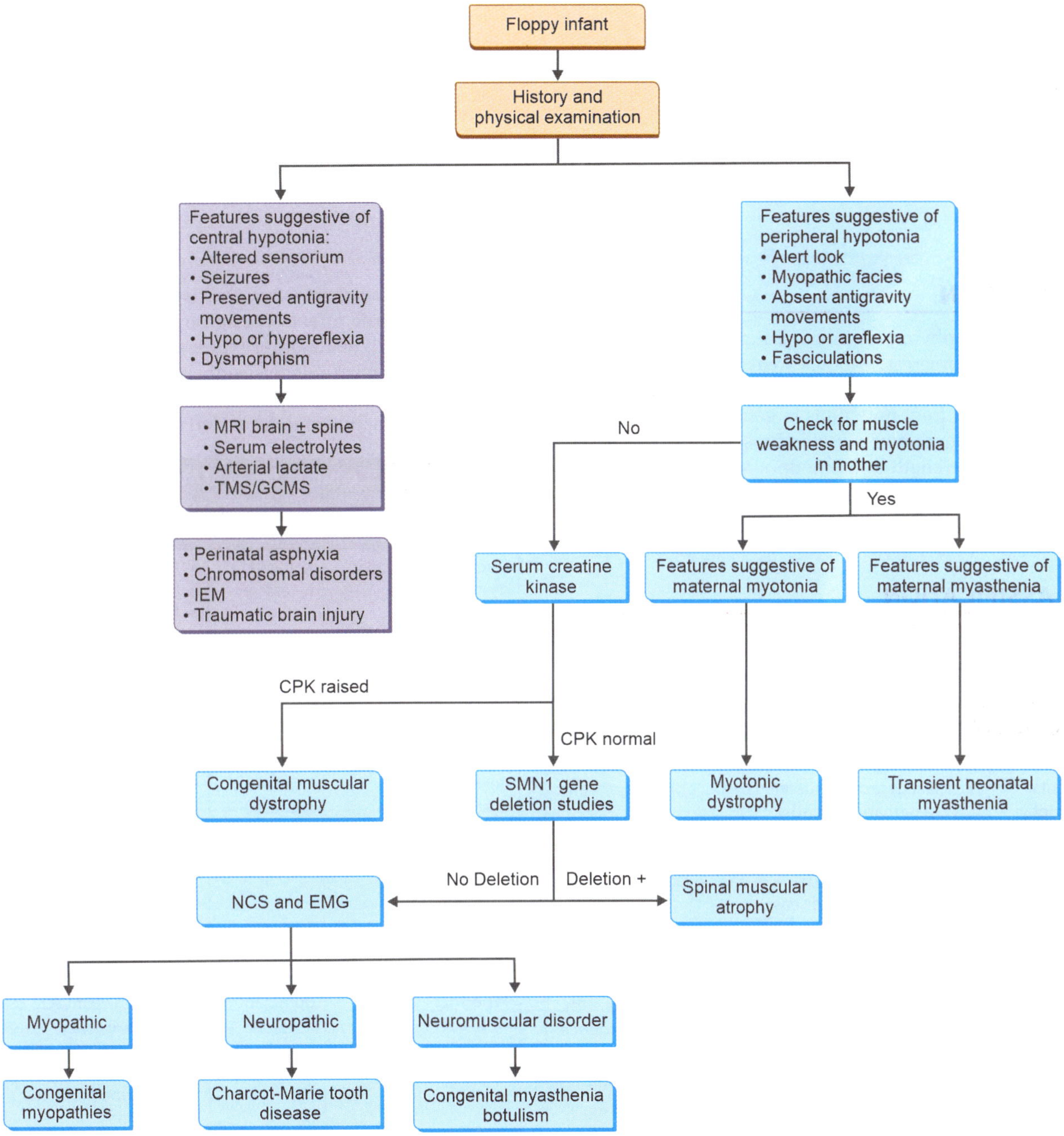

Floppy infant

↓

History and physical examination

↓

Features suggestive of central hypotonia:
- Altered sensorium
- Seizures
- Preserved antigravity movements
- Hypo or hypereflexia
- Dysmorphism

↓

- MRI brain ± spine
- Serum electrolytes
- Arterial lactate
- TMS/GCMS

↓

- Perinatal asphyxia
- Chromosomal disorders
- IEM
- Traumatic brain injury

Features suggestive of peripheral hypotonia
- Alert look
- Myopathic facies
- Absent antigravity movements
- Hypo or areflexia
- Fasciculations

↓

Check for muscle weakness and myotonia in mother

No → Serum creatine kinase
- CPK raised → Congenital muscular dystrophy
- CPK normal → SMN1 gene deletion studies
  - Deletion + → Spinal muscular atrophy
  - No Deletion → NCS and EMG
    - Myopathic → Congenital myopathies
    - Neuropathic → Charcot-Marie tooth disease
    - Neuromuscular disorder → Congenital myasthenia botulism

Yes →
- Features suggestive of maternal myotonia → Myotonic dystrophy
- Features suggestive of maternal myasthenia → Transient neonatal myasthenia

Fig. 24.25: The figure depicts a simplified approach to a floppy infant

(CPK: creatine phosphokinase; EMG: electromyography; NCS: nerve conduction study)

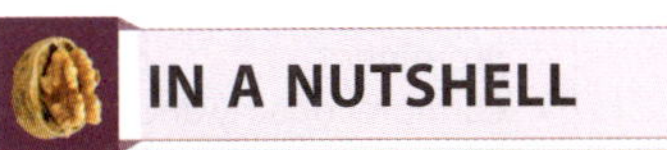

IN A NUTSHELL

Floppy Infant

1. Muscle tone is the intrinsic resistance of skeletal muscles to passive movement.
2. The term floppy infant is used to describe an infant with generalized hypotonia. It is regarded as a clinical feature with varying underlying diagnoses.
3. Hypotonia can be central or peripheral.
4. *Central hypotonia* is characterized by hypotonia with relatively preserved muscle strength and hyperreflexia (UMN lesion).
5. *Peripheral hypotonia* is characterized by hypotonia and weakness (LMN lesion).
6. The investigations are guided by the clinical findings and distinction between central and peripheral hypotonia.

Bodensteiner JB. The evaluation of the hypotonic infant. Semin Pediatr Neurol. 2008;15:10.
Kitamura Y, Kondo E, Urano M, et al. Target resequencing of neuromuscular disease-related genes using next-generation sequencing for patients with undiagnosed early-onset neuromuscular disorders. J Hum Genet. 2016;61:931.
Leyenaar J, Camfield P, Camfield C. A schematic approach to hypotonia in infancy. Paediatr Child Health. 2005;10:397-400.
Paro-Panjan D, Neubauer D. Congenital hypotonia: Is there an algorithm? J Child Neurol. 2004;19:439-42.

24.15 Muscular Dystrophy

PE 27.12

DEFINITION

Muscular dystrophy represents a group of genetic disorders characterized by progressive muscle weakness and degeneration, which significantly impacts mobility and quality of life. These conditions result from mutations in genes responsible for the structure and function of muscle fibers, leading to a gradual loss of muscle strength and function. Muscular dystrophy is not a single disease but encompasses various types, each with distinct genetic causes, patterns of inheritance, and clinical manifestations.

CLASSIFICATION

The common terminologies related to neuromuscular disorders are listed in **Table 24.52**.

Table 24.52 Terminologies Related to Muscular Dystrophy

Terminology	*Description*
Muscular dystrophy	Muscular dystrophy is defined by four obligatory criteria: a. It is a primary myopathy b. It has a genetic basis c. The course is progressive d. Degeneration and death of muscle fibers occur at some stage in the disease.
Congenital muscular dystrophy	Congenital muscular dystrophies are defined as early-onset muscle disorders that are present at birth or manifest in early infancy with muscle weakness, and are characterized by a muscle biopsy compatible with a dystrophic process and lacking histological evidence of another neuromuscular disease.
Congenital myopathy	Congenital myopathy refers to a group of inherited disorders that usually result in muscle weakness at birth and have a static or slowly progressive course. These disorders are marked by muscle weakness and hypotonia caused by structural abnormalities in muscle fibers or defects in muscle function. Unlike muscular dystrophies, congenital myopathies primarily impact muscle cells without the considerable degeneration often associated with muscular dystrophies.
Myositis	Myositis is a term used to describe inflammation of the muscles, which can lead to muscle weakness, pain, swelling, and damage to muscle fibers. Myositis can occur as a result of various underlying conditions, including autoimmune diseases, infections, and exposure to certain medications or toxins.

The most prevalent form, Duchenne muscular dystrophy (DMD), primarily affects young boys and often presents in early childhood, while other types, such as Becker muscular dystrophy and myotonic dystrophy, may have different onset ages and varying degrees of severity. The common types of muscular dystrophy are summarized in **Table 24.53**.

Table 24.53 Common Types of Muscular Dystrophies

Type of muscle dystrophy	*Inheritance*	*Salient clinical features*
Duchenne muscular dystrophy	X-linked recessive	• Onset usually between ages 2–5 • Rapid progression of muscle weakness • Gait changes, falls • Pseudohypertrophy of calf muscles • Cardiac and respiratory complications
Becker muscular dystrophy	X-linked recessive	• Onset typically in later childhood or adolescence • Slower progression than DMD • Muscle weakness primarily affecting proximal muscles • Cardiac involvement is common
Myotonic dystrophy Type 1	Autosomal dominant	• Muscle stiffness (myotonia) • Progressive muscle weakness • Facial weakness and ptosis • Cardiac issues and endocrine problems • Cataracts
Myotonic dystrophy Type 2	Autosomal dominant	• Similar to DM1 but milder • Muscle weakness in proximal muscles • Myotonia, but less prominent • Cardiomyopathy and diabetes may occur
Facioscapulohumeral muscular dystrophy	Autosomal dominant	• Weakness in facial, shoulder, and upper arm muscles • Scapular winging • Typically, a later onset and variable progression

Contd...

Contd...

Type of muscle dystrophy	*Inheritance*	*Salient clinical features*
Limb-girdle muscular dystrophy	Autosomal recessive/ autosomal dominant	• Weakness primarily affecting the hip and shoulder girdle muscles • Symptoms can closely resemble DMD in some variants like sarcoglycanopathy • Onset can vary; progressive muscle weakness • Variable severity and age of onset
Emery-Dreifuss muscular dystrophy	X-linked recessive, autosomal dominant	• Early contractures, usually at the elbows and Achilles tendons • Shoulder and upper arm muscle weakness • Cardiac issues, such as arrhythmias

DUCHENNE AND BECKER MUSCULAR DYSTROPHY

Duchenne muscular dystrophy (DMD) and Becker muscular dystrophy (BMD) stem from a defective dystrophin gene on the X chromosome, which is essential for dystrophin production.

Although they have a shared genetic basis, DMD and BMD differ significantly in the severity and onset of symptoms due to the nature of the mutations and their effects on dystrophin protein.

Etiopathogenesis

A. Genetic Basis

- ***Dystrophin gene:*** The dystrophin gene (DMD), consisting of 79 exons, is approximately 2.4 million base pairs in length. It encodes the **dystrophin** protein, which plays a critical role in maintaining the structural integrity of muscle fibers.
- ***Mode of inheritance:*** Both DMD and BMD are X-linked recessive disorders, primarily affecting males. Females can be carriers and may exhibit mild symptoms or none at all due to one normal allele on the other X chromosome.
- ***Type of mutations:*** The mutations that lead to DMD typically include large deletions, duplications, and point mutations that disrupt the reading frame of dystrophin. This results in a complete absence of functional dystrophin protein in muscle cells. In contrast, BMD is often caused by mutations that allow for some dystrophin production. These may include in-frame deletions or point mutations that retain the reading frame of the gene, resulting in a partially functional dystrophin that is synthesized in lower amounts or with altered properties. The same is depicted in **Figure 24.26**.

B. Consequences at Protein Level

- ***Role of dystrophin:*** Dystrophin is crucial for linking the internal cytoskeleton of muscle fibers to the extracellular matrix (ECM) through a complex known as the dystrophin-associated protein complex (DAPC). This complex includes various proteins, such as sarcoglycans, dystroglycans, and other associated proteins, providing stability and structural support to muscle fibers during contraction.
- ***Pathological consequences:*** In DMD, the complete lack of dystrophin leads to muscle fiber instability. During muscle contraction, the absence of this protein causes damage to the muscle membrane, resulting in myofiber degeneration, inflammation, and, ultimately, fibrosis (replacement of muscle tissue with scar tissue). Muscle fibers gradually weaken, leading to progressive muscle wasting and functional decline. In BMD, even though some dystrophin is produced, it is often structurally or functionally abnormal. The presence of partially functional dystrophin—while it can provide some protection to muscle fibers—still results in muscle cell damage, albeit at a slower rate compared to DMD. Individuals with BMD typically experience milder symptoms, with a later onset and a slower progression of muscle weakness.
- ***Pseudohypertrophy:*** As muscle fibers degenerate and die, they are replaced by adipose tissue and connective tissue. This replacement of muscle tissue with fibrotic tissue contributes to the size increase, creating a rigid and non-functional muscle. Since, there is an apparent increase in size of muscle, without an actual increase in size or number of muscle fibers, it is referred to as pseudohypertrophy (false enlargement) of muscles. The muscles prominently demonstrating pseudohypertrophy include calf muscles (gastrocnemius and soleus), tongue, muscles of the forearm, deltoid, and infraspinatus.

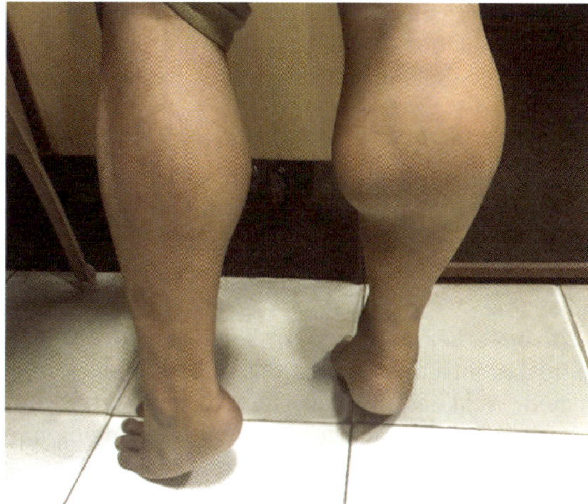

Fig. 24.26: Clinical photograph illustrating (pseudo) hypertropy of calf muscles with contractures of Achilles tendon (illustrated by standing on tip toes) in a boy with DMD

Clinical Features

DMD is associated with severe clinical symptoms and an earlier age of onset compared with BMD. Boys with DMD typically present with symptoms between 2 and 5 years of age. Parents most commonly describe abnormal gait, often as toe walking immediately on gait acquisition, but gait onset may also be delayed. Many of these initial symptoms are recalled by parents in retrospect. The salient clinical features are listed below.

A. Muscle Weakness and Atrophy

- ***Proximal muscle weakness:*** The initial and most prominent symptom of DMD is weakness in the proximal muscles of the pelvis, hips, and shoulders, making activities such as climbing stairs, running, and rising from the floor particularly challenging.
- ***Distal and other muscle groups involvement:*** As the disease progresses into the teenage years, distal muscles become affected. Weakness typically spreads to the arms and legs. Patients may have increased difficulties bringing hands to mouth independently, fatigue with writing, and worsening contractures, including in the hands and fingers. Distinctive facies are not an early feature because facial muscle weakness is a late event; in later childhood, a "transverse" or horizontal smile may be seen.
- ***Muscle atrophy and pseudohypertrophy:*** Over time, affected muscles begin to waste away due to the ongoing cycle of degeneration and regeneration, leading to reduced muscle bulk. Enlargement of the calves (pseudohypertrophy, **Fig. 24.26**) and wasting of thigh muscles are classic features. The enlargement is caused by hypertrophy of some muscle fibers, infiltration of muscle by fat, and proliferation of collagen. After the calves, the next most common site of muscular hypertrophy is the tongue, followed by the muscles of the forearm.

B. Delayed Motor Milestones

Early gross motor skills, such as rolling over, sitting, and standing, are typically achieved at the expected ages, although some may experience mild delays. Walking is often delayed beyond 18 months in about 50% of cases, and subtle hip girdle weakness may manifest subtly as early as the second year.

C. Gait Abnormalities

- ***Waddling gait:*** As proximal muscle weakness becomes pronounced, the child may develop a waddling gait (also known as Trendelenburg gait) due to weak hip muscles, which affect balance and stability.
- ***Gowers' sign:*** A characteristic feature seen in DMD is Gowers' sign, where a child typically abducts their thighs and then uses their hands and arms to "climb" up their body when getting up from the floor, indicating weakness in the hip and thigh muscles.
- ***Ambulation:*** Typically, complete loss of ambulation occurs between the ages of 10 and 14 years in DMD. Over time, the age at which independent ambulation is lost has risen, largely due to corticosteroid use (e.g., prednisone or deflazacort) for boys with DMD.

D. Skeletal Deformities

- ***Spinal deformities:*** Many individuals with DMD develop scoliosis as spinal muscle weakness progresses. This can lead to postural difficulties and also affect pulmonary functions.
- ***Contractures:*** Muscle tightness often leads to joint contractures, particularly in the ankles, knees, and hips, further limiting mobility.

E. Respiratory Complications

- ***Respiratory muscle weakness:*** As DMD progresses, the muscles involved in breathing, such as those in the diaphragm and intercostal muscles, become weakened, which can result in respiratory insufficiency.
- ***Increased risk of infections:*** Weak respiratory muscles can lead to issues with coughing and clearing secretions, increasing the risk of aspiration and respiratory infections.

F. Cardiac Complications

DMD is associated with dilated cardiomyopathy. Symptoms may include shortness of breath, fatigue, and arrhythmia.

G. Cognitive and Behavioral Aspects

- ***Cognitive impairment:*** Cognitive impairment affects most patients, although only 20–30% have an IQ of 70. The severity of intellectual disabilities varies; some individuals need specialized education and struggle with reading and writing, while others may just require a bit of extra help. Additionally, certain patients may exhibit behaviors similar to autism.
- ***Psychosocial challenges:*** Living with a progressive muscle disorder can lead to emotional and psychological challenges, including anxiety and depression.

H. Life Span

Males with DMD often experience death in their late teens to 20s due to respiratory failure during sleep, heart failure, pneumonia, or occasionally aspiration and airway obstruction. Recent care standards have extended survival into the 30s for many patients.

In BMD, symptoms typically emerge after the age of 5 or 7, and most boys retain their ability to walk into adulthood. Similar to DMD patients, they exhibit calf pseudohypertrophy, cardiomyopathy, and elevated serum CK levels. Initial signs may include exercise-induced cramps and myoglobinuria. Due to their higher activity levels, BMD patients might show cardiac symptoms such as tachycardia, shortness of breath, or fatigue earlier than children with DMD.

Symptomatic Females

About 22% of female carriers with a mutated dystrophin gene display noticeable symptom. These symptomatic carriers of DMD show significant variability in both the age at which symptoms appear and the severity of muscle weakness or cardiac issues. The muscle weakness can vary from mild to, in rare cases, resembling a classic DMD phenotype. Serum CK levels are increased in approximately 70% and 50% of female carriers of Duchenne and Becker muscular dystrophy, respectively.

Investigations

The investigations are carried out to confirm the diagnosis, evaluate the extent of muscle involvement, and rule out other conditions. These include:

A. Laboratory

- ***Creatine kinase (CK) levels:*** One of the most critical initial investigations is a blood test to measure creatine kinase (CK) levels. CK is an enzyme released into the bloodstream when muscle fibers are damaged. In DMD, significantly elevated levels of CK (often 10–100 times the normal range) are typically found. A normal CK level makes DMD and BMD unlikely and should prompt an evaluation for alternative diagnoses.
- ***Transaminases:*** Clinicians must recognize that serum aspartate aminotransferase (AST) and alanine aminotransferase (ALT) levels are elevated in dystrophinopathies, as these enzymes exist in both muscle and liver. For unexplained transaminase elevations, serum CK should be checked before liver biopsy.
- ***Genetic testing:*** If elevated CK levels are observed, genetic testing becomes essential. This can involve:
  - *Multiplex Ligation-dependent Probe Amplification (MLPA):* This test detects deletions or duplications in the dystrophin gene, which are commonly seen in DMD.
  - *Next-Generation Sequencing (NGS):* If no mutations are found with MLPA, whole exome sequencing or targeted sequencing may be considered for a more comprehensive genetic evaluation.
- ***Muscle biopsy:*** If genetic testing is inconclusive, a muscle biopsy may be performed to analyze the muscle tissue. The biopsy can reveal the absence of dystrophin protein through immunohistochemical staining, in addition to evidence of necrosis, regeneration, and inflammatory changes.

B. Neurophysiology

Electromyography (EMG) assesses the electrical activity of muscles and can help distinguish between muscle disorders and nerve-related issues. In DMD, EMG typically shows myopathic changes consistent with muscle disease. Serum CK testing should always be done before EMG.

C. Echocardiography

Since boys with dystrophinopathy are at risk for cardiomyopathy, a baseline echocardiogram is often performed to assess heart structure and function. Further it should be evaluated periodically for assessing cardiac functions.

D. Pulmonary Function Testing

As respiratory muscle weakness is a concern in DMD, pulmonary function tests may be conducted to evaluate respiratory capacity, particularly as the child ages.

TREATMENT Muscular Dystrophy

A. **Multidisciplinary approach:** Care for individuals with DMD and BMD should involve a multidisciplinary team, including neurologists, physiotherapists, occupational therapists, orthopedic surgeons, cardiologists, respiratory therapists, nutritionists, genetic counselors, and psychologists/psychiatrists.

B. **Glucocorticoids and disease modifying treatment:**
- *Glucocorticoids*: Glucocorticoids (prednisone and deflazacort) are the cornerstone of pharmacologic treatment for DMD. They are recommended for children with DMD and should be initiated before significant physical decline occurs. For children with DMD aged 4 years or older, whose motor skills have plateaued or begun to decline, daily treatment with glucocorticoids—either oral prednisolone or deflazacort—should be commenced. The typical starting dose of oral prednisone for treating DMD is 0.75 mg/kg per day, while the standard starting dose of oral deflazacort is 0.9 mg/kg per day. For patients who lose their ability to walk and require a wheelchair, the glucocorticoid dosage is reduced to 0.3 mg/kg/day for prednisolone and 0.5 mg/kg/day for deflazacort. Glucocorticoid treatment of DMD using prednisone and deflazacort is advantageous for enhancing motor function, strength, and pulmonary function; minimizing the risk of scoliosis; and postponing the loss of ambulation. Regular monitoring for side effects including weight gain, growth suppression, and osteoporosis is necessary.
- *Gene therapy*: Genetic therapies that involve exon skipping (eteplirsen, casimersen), read-through of premature termination codon (ataluren), or microdystrophin transgenes delivered by adeno-associated virus vectors are approved in some countries for the treatment of DMD. These therapies increase dystrophin expression, but clinical benefit has not been established. Mechanism of action of these therapies has been depicted in **Figure 24.27**.

C. **Rehabilitation:** Patients should engage in physiotherapy to enhance mobility and reduce the likelihood of contractures. Key aspects of physiotherapy involve passive stretching exercises for the ankles, knees, and hips, which are crucial for preventing contractures in the Achilles tendons, iliotibial bands, and hip flexors. Additional helpful interventions include ankle-foot orthoses, long-leg braces, and wrist or hand splints. Early institution of the use of night-time ankle-foot orthoses (AFOs) decreases the development and progression of heel cord contractures. Furthermore, orthopedic evaluations must monitor scoliosis and other potential complications, and surgical procedures should be applied as necessary. Boys with DMD, whether ambulatory or in the early non-ambulatory phase, should partake in regular submaximal (i.e., gentle) aerobic exercise to prevent disuse muscle atrophy, immobility, excessive weight gain, and social isolation.

D. **Bone health:** The approach to monitoring and diagnosis of bone health focuses on identifying the earliest signs of bone fragility. Children should be monitored with serum levels of calcium, phosphate, and alkaline phosphatase. Calcium supplementation (500–1000 mg/day) is suggested for children on steroid therapy. Vitamin D supplementation is indicated if the serum concentration of vitamin D is <30 ng/mL.

E. **Cardiac management:** A baseline assessment of cardiac function, which includes an electrocardiogram and echocardiography, is recommended at the time of DMD diagnosis. For asymptomatic individuals, this cardiac evaluation should be repeated at least once a year. Boys with DMD should begin treatment with an angiotensin converting enzyme (ACE) inhibitor or an angiotensin receptor blocker (ARB) by age 10. If overt heart failure occurs, additional therapies such as diuretics and digoxin will be managed by a cardiologist.

F. **Respiratory support:** Pulmonary insufficiency is a leading cause of mortality. Respiratory therapy, including bilevel positive airway pressure/nocturnal ventilatory support are crucial for increasing life expectancy and enhancing quality of life in DMD patients.

G. **Vaccination:** Children should receive the HiB, pneumococcal, and varicella vaccines if they have not been previously vaccinated, prior to starting steroid therapy. All DMD patients should receive annual vaccination with an inactivated influenza vaccine.

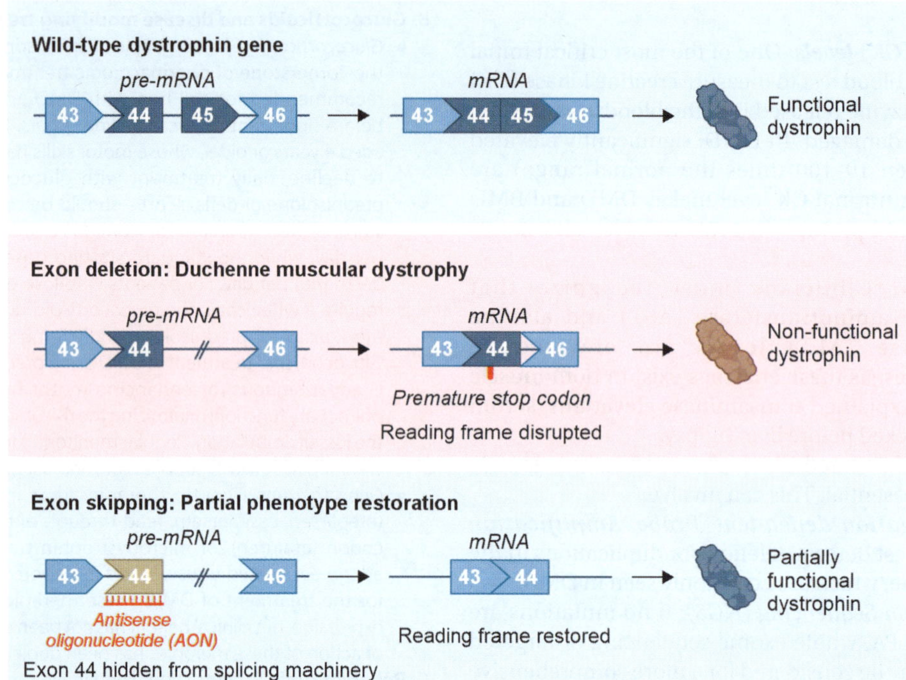

Fig. 24.27: The wild-type dystrophin gene shown in the top panel is the normal gene that produces functional dystrophin protein. A deletion or point mutation in this gene disrupts the reading frame, leading to the production of a dysfunctional protein, which manifests as DMD (middle panel). Gene therapy facilitates exon skipping, resulting in a partial restoration of the reading frame and the production of a partially functional protein (lower panel)

Source: Created in BioRender. Sondhi, V. (2025) https://BioRender.com/bhu26r5

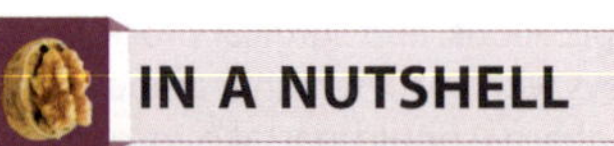

IN A NUTSHELL

Muscular Dystrophy

1. Duchenne and Becker muscular dystrophies (DMD and BMD) result from pathogenic variants in the dystrophin (DMD) gene on the X chromosome, which is responsible for producing dystrophin.
2. DMD typically causes weakness onset between ages two and three, starting with proximal limb muscles before distal ones. Other features include cardiomyopathy, conduction abnormalities, bone fractures, and scoliosis. Affected children often have mild cognitive impairment. Physical exams reveal calf pseudohypertrophy, occasional quadriceps pseudohypertrophy, lumbar lordosis, a waddling gait, shortened Achilles tendons, and weak muscles may show hyporeflexia or areflexia.
3. Serum creatine kinase levels are elevated. A diagnosis is confirmed if a DMD gene mutation is identified.
4. Glucocorticoids are the primary treatment for DMD. Some countries offer genetic therapies like eteplirsen and ataluren, which boost dystrophin expression, but clinical benefits remain unproven.
5. Patients with DMD need multidisciplinary care to coordinate specialized assessments and interventions that maximize function and quality of life. Orthopedic interventions focus on maintaining function and preventing contractures. Cardiac evaluation should include ECG and echocardiography, with ACE-inhibitors or angiotensin receptor blockers introduced as necessary.

Birnkrant DJ, Bushby K, Bann CM, et al. Diagnosis and management of Duchenne muscular dystrophy, part 1: diagnosis, and neuromuscular, rehabilitation, endocrine, and gastrointestinal and nutritional management. Lancet Neurol. 2018;17:251.

Birnkrant DJ, Bushby K, Bann CM, et al. Diagnosis and management of Duchenne muscular dystrophy, part 2: respiratory, cardiac, bone health, and orthopaedic management. Lancet Neurol. 2018;17:347.

Brandsema JF, Darras BT. Dystrophinopathies. Semin Neurol. 2015;35:369.

Emery AE. The muscular dystrophies. Lancet. 2002;359:687.

25 CHAPTER

Genetic and Metabolic Disorders

AS PER NMC COMPETENCIES

PE29.1	Describe the genetic basis, risk factors, clinical features, complications, prenatal diagnosis, management and genetic counseling in Down syndrome.	*Ch 25.3, Ch 25.4, Ch 25.5, Ch 25.6*
PE29.2	Interpret normal karyotype and recognize Trisomy 21.	*Ch 25.1, Ch 25.2*
PE29.3	Counsel parents regarding: (1) Present child, (2) Risk in the next pregnancy.	*Ch 25.3, Ch 25.6, Ch 25.7*
PE29.4	Describe the genetic basis, risk factors, clinical features, complications, prenatal diagnosis, management and genetic counseling in Turner syndrome.	*Ch 25.3, Ch 25.4, Ch 25.5, Ch 25.6*
PE29.5	Describe the genetic basis, risk factors, clinical features, complications, prenatal diagnosis, management and genetic counseling in Klinefelter syndrome.	*Ch 25.3, Ch 25.4, Ch 25.5, Ch 25.6*

Topics available online: ***Congenital Structural Abnormalities; Inborn Errors of Metabolism; Skeletal Dysplasias***

25.1 Genetic Basis of Inheritance *PE 29.2*

INTRODUCTION

Deoxyribonucleic acid (DNA) is the genetic material in human beings and most of the organisms. DNA transmits the genetic information from parents to the offspring and a cell to the daughter cells and is a fundamental molecule of life. Segments of DNA constitute *genes,* which code for various proteins that in turn govern various functions of the body. The genes are located on *chromosomes,* which are formed by histone and non-histone proteins in addition to "DNA."

The Human Genome Project, completed in 2003, has deciphered the sequence of whole genome (constituted of 46 chromosomes) and it is expected that there are about 25,000 genes in humans. Genes also play an important role in non-genetic disorders to variable extent. This is obvious because proteins produced by genes are fundamental to all biological processes.

DEOXYRIBONUCLEIC ACID (DNA)

Deoxyribonucleic acid is a long double-stranded molecule consisting of a series of nucleotides attached to one another. Each nucleotide consists of a deoxyribose sugar, phosphate group, and a nitrogen containing base. The bases are of two types, purines (Adenine—A, Guanine—G) and pyrimidines (Thymine—T, Cytosine—C). The sugar molecules are attached to each other by phosphodiester bond connecting 5th carbon atom of a sugar (5′) to 3rd carbon atom (3′) of the next sugar molecule and this forms a backbone of DNA molecules. Two strands of DNA molecule are wound to form a double helix with bases pointing towards each other. The two strands of DNA run opposite to each other so that one strand run from 5′ end to 3′ end while the other runs from 3′ end to the 5′ end **(Fig. 25.1)**. The bonds between nucleotides on opposing strands bind the

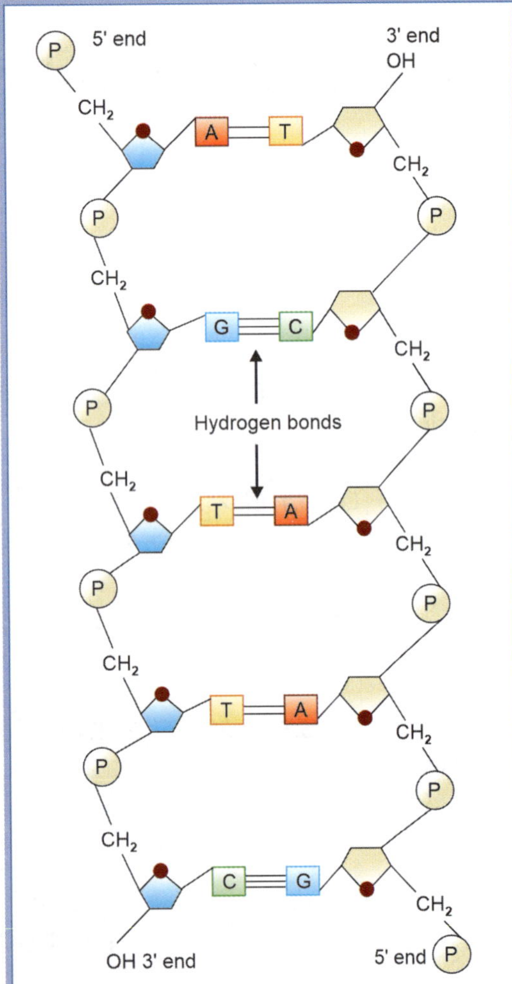

Fig. 25.1: Deoxyribonucleic acid (DNA) molecule. One end of a DNA strand has 5′ end free and not attached to any sugar molecule and the other end has 3′ end free. The other strand has an opposite orientation

two DNA strands to each other; only complementary nucleotides pair with each other, i.e., A with T, and G with C.

Deoxyribonucleic acid is tightly packed in a chromosome. The total length of DNA of a cell [6 billion base pairs (bp)] in a single human cell is 1 meter. It must be packed in a nucleus <10 microns. During interphase most of the DNA is uncoiled and stretched, while during metaphase, the DNA gets tightly coiled onto itself and is packed to get the form of chromosomes.

Extragenic DNA: Only 2% of the nuclear DNA, which consists of roughly 20,000 genes, codes for proteins; the majority of the remaining DNA is repetitive and primarily transcriptionally inactive. Although it is also referred to as "junk DNA," its significance for gene expression is now better understood.

DNA Replication

Deoxyribonucleic acid replication is the process by which genetic information is transmitted from one generation to the next. During nuclear division, the two strands of the DNA double helix are separated by DNA helicase, each DNA strand directing the synthesis of a complementary DNA strand through specific base pairing, resulting in two daughter DNA duplexes that are identical to the original parent molecule. In this way, when cells divide, the genetic information is conserved and transmitted unchanged to each daughter cell. The process of DNA replication is termed semi-conservative, because only one strand of each resultant daughter molecule is newly synthesized.

DNA polymerase is the key in the process of DNA replication, which is initiated at multiple points, forming bifurcated Y-shaped structures known as replication forks. The synthesis of both complementary antiparallel DNA strands occurs in the 5′-3′ direction during the S (synthetic) phase of cell cycle. One strand, known as the *leading strand,* is synthesized as a continuous process. The other strand, known as the *lagging strand,* is synthesized in pieces called Okazaki fragments, which are then joined together as a continuous strand by the enzyme DNA ligase **(Figs. 25.2A and B)**.

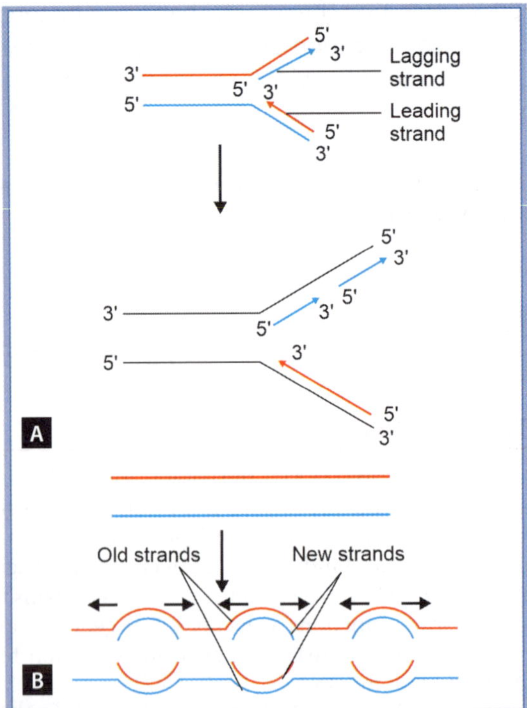

Figs. 25.2A and B: Deoxyribonucleic acid (DNA) replication. (A) Replication fork showing continuous DNA synthesis on the leading stand in 5′-3′ direction and discontinuous synthesis in the lagging stand with formation of Okazaki fragments; (B) Multiple points of origin of DNA replication and semiconservative nature of DNA synthesis

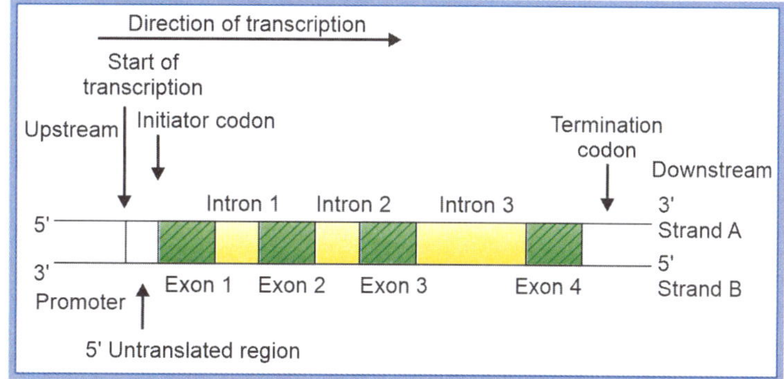

Fig. 25.3: Structure of a gene. Exons are separated by introns. The sequence of strand A represents the sequence of the gene while strand B acts as a template for ribonucleic acid (RNA) synthesis

Gene

A segment of DNA coding for a protein or polypeptide is called a gene. It is continuous with DNA on either side. In addition to the coding sequences, the regulatory elements such as promoters and enhancers of the gene expression are also parts of the gene. These elements are near the 5′ end of the gene but some may be far away from the gene, and some may be on other chromosomes as well.

Information about regulatory elements controlling gene expression is yet far from complete. The sequence of nucleotides decides the sequence of amino acids in the polypeptide. A set of three consecutive nucleotides is called a *codon*. Four nucleotides generate 64 codons, which code for 20 amino acids; and three codons, which code for *stop signals*. Each gene has coding sequences known as "exons," intercepted with non-coding sequences called "intervening sequences" or 'introns' **(Fig. 25.3)**.

CENTRAL DOGMA

The process of the transfer of the genetic information from DNA to *Ribonucleic acid* (RNA) to protein is called the central dogma in genetics.

Transcription

It is the process of making an RNA copy of the DNA sequence. The information stored in the genetic code is transmitted from the respective gene in the DNA segment to *messenger RNA*, or *mRNA*. All the bases in the newly synthesized mRNA molecule are complementary to a corresponding base in the DNA of the gene, except for uracil replacing thymine in mRNA. mRNA is single stranded and is synthesized by the enzyme RNA polymerase II. It adds the appropriate complementary ribonucleotide to the 3′ end of the RNA chain. Before the primary mRNA molecule leaves the nucleus, it undergoes several modifications known as RNA processing. This involves splicing (removal of introns at specific splice sites), 5′ capping (addition of a methylated guanine nucleotide to the 5′ end of the molecule), and polyadenylation (addition of about 200 adenylate residues at the 3′ end). The process of transcription can be affected permanently by both environmental (e.g., hormones) and genetic (cell signaling) factors.

Translation

Translation is the conversion of the genetic information from mRNA to protein. Newly processed mRNA is transported from the nucleus to the cytoplasm, where it associates with the ribosomes, which are the site of protein synthesis. The RNA component of ribosomes, known as *ribosomal ribonucleic acid* (rRNA) catalyzes protein synthesis. Translation involves yet a third type of RNA, *transfer RNA (tRNA)*, which provides the molecular link between the code contained in the base sequence of each mRNA and the amino acid sequence of the protein encoded by that mRNA. Proteins are synthesized from the amino terminus to the carboxyl terminus, which corresponds to translation of the mRNA in a 5′–3′ direction.

Post-translational modification: Many proteins, before they attain their normal structure or functional activity, undergo post-translational modification, which can include chemical modification of amino-acid side chains (e.g., hydroxylation, methylation), the addition of carbohydrate or lipid moieties (e.g., glycosylation), or proteolytic cleavage of polypeptides (e.g., the conversion of proinsulin to insulin). These post-translational modifications help in transport to specific cellular locations (e.g., the nucleus), or secretion from the cell.

CHROMOSOMES

The normal human chromosome number, i.e., 46 was established in 1956. Cytogenetics is the branch of genetics that studies the structure, and inheritance of chromosomes. There are 22 pairs of autosomes present in males and females. In addition, there is a pair of sex chromosomes, namely "X" and "Y" chromosomes. Males have an X and a Y chromosome while females have two X chromosomes and there is no Y chromosome. One set of chromosomes is inherited from the father one set from the mother. Thus, in human beings for every gene there are two copies.

Mutations

A mutation is a permanent change in the nucleotide sequence or the DNA arrangement. Naturally occurring mutations are referred to as spontaneous mutations and arise due to chance errors in chromosomal division or DNA replication. Mutations can also occur due to exposure to mutagenic agents such as ionizing radiation, chemicals such as mustard gas, formaldehyde, benzene, and some basic dyes. Sequence variations can be in the form of single base substitution or insertion/deletion of single or multiple bases. Alteration in DNA arrangement includes inversion of a chromosomal segment or loss or gain of a segment of chromosome, or entire chromosomes. Some mutations cause diseases, while some may be responsible for predisposition to various diseases. Some nucleotide substitutions do not change the amino acid (synonymous mutations) as an amino acid may be represented by more than one codon. The term "mutation" is now being replaced by "variant". For the purpose of interpretation, a variant can be classified as pathogenic (P), likely pathogenic (LP), uncertain significance (VUS), likely benign (LB), and benign (B) as per the American College of Medical Genetics and Genomics (ACMG) guidelines.

Polymorphism

Sequence variations with no obvious disease-causing effect, are known as polymorphisms. When a single nucleotide variation occurs at any position in the DNA sequence, it is known as *single nucleotide polymorphism* or SNP and are found in >1% of the population. In the human genome, an SNP occurs every 500–1,000 bases. SNPs influence health, disease, drug response, and other traits; hence can be utilized for an individual's risk scoring for complex diseases such as cancers, diabetes, ischemic heart disease, etc. SNPs also find application in gene discovery and mapping.

Alleles

The alternate forms of a gene caused due to change in the gene sequence (mutation/polymorphism) are known as *alleles*. If a person has two different alleles of a gene, he or she is called a *heterozygote*. If both the copies of a gene are identical, the person is a *homozygote* or *homozygous* for the allele. The persons may be homozygous for a normal (also known as "wild") allele or a mutated allele.

GENETIC DISORDERS

1. ***Monogenic disorders*** are caused by mutation of a single gene and follow Mendelian patterns of inheritance; hence they are also known as Mendelian disorders.
2. ***Chromosomal disorders*** are caused by gain or loss of a chromosome or a part of chromosome. Chromosomal deletion or duplication detectable under microscope contains a number of genes (5–10 million base pairs) and a loss or gain of even a small part of an autosome usually is associated with multiple malformations and mental retardation. Significant imbalance of genetic material in a conceptus usually leads to spontaneous abortion. The birth defects caused by smaller deletion/duplications of chromosomal segment, and which can be detected only by molecular cytogenetic techniques like microarray or fluorescent in situ hybridization (FISH) are known as *microdeletion/microduplication syndromes.*
3. ***Multifactorial disorders*** are seen more commonly amongst the relatives of a person with a disorder than among the general population but do not follow Mendelian pattern of inheritance. The increase of prevalence of such disorders amongst the relative of an affected person is explained by a model of multifactorial etiology where multiple genes and environmental factors are involved in the causation of the disease. The examples of multifactorial disorder include congenital malformations such cleft lip, Hirschsprung disease, pyloric stenosis, and many common diseases such as hypertension, ischemic heart diseases, autoimmune disorders, and psychiatric illnesses.

IN A NUTSHELL

Genetic Basis of Inheritance

1. The genetic code stored in the deoxyribonucleic acid (DNA) is constituted of a linear sequence of two types of nucleotides, the purines (adenine [A] and guanine [G]) and the pyrimidines (cytosine [C] and thymine [T]), linked by a sugar–phosphate backbone.
2. DNA is made up of two antiparallel strands held in a double helix by hydrogen bonds between the complementary G-C and A-T base pairs.
3. DNA replication is semi-conservative with one strand acting as a template for synthesis of a complementary strand.
4. Transcription is the process of synthesis of a single stranded complementary ribonucleic acid (RNA) copy of a gene's DNA sequence and is known as messenger RNA (mRNA).
5. During mRNA processing, the non-coding portions are removed in the nucleus. This processed mRNA is transported to the nucleus and gets associated with ribosomes for protein synthesis, i.e., translation.
6. Regulation of gene expression is majorly at the level of transcription and is regulated by the 5′ flanking promoter region and also by the general and specific transcription factors.

Alberts B, Johnson A, Lewis J, et al. Molecular Biology of the Cell, 6th edition. London: Garland; 2014.

Nussbaum R, McInnes R, Willard H. Thompson and Thompson Genetics in Medicine, 8th edition. Philadelphia: Elsevier; 2015.

Richards S, Aziz N, Bale S, et al. ACMG Laboratory Quality Assurance Committee. Standards and guidelines for the interpretation of sequence variants: a joint consensus recommendation of the American College of Medical Genetics and Genomics and the Association for Molecular Pathology. Genet Med. 2015.

Strachan T, Read AP. Human Molecular Genetics, 4th edition. London: Garland Science; 2010.

Turnpenny PD, Ellard S, Cleaver R. Elements of Medical Genetics and Genomics, 16th edition. Philadelphia: Elsevier; 2022.

Willard HF. The human genome: a window on human genetics, biology and medicine. In: Ginsburg GS, Willard HF (Eds). Genomic and Personalized Medicine, 2nd edition. New York: Elsevier; 2013.

25.2 Patterns of Inheritance

PE 29.2

INTRODUCTION

Mendel hypothesized "factors" governing various traits from experiments on plants. These "factors" are now known as genes and are primarily identified as causes of several disorders and traits. These disorders are known as monogenic disorders and follow Mendel's laws of inheritance and are also known as *Mendelian disorders.*

PEDIGREE DRAWING

Family history is an important part of clinical information, especially for genetic disorders. A pedigree is a graphical representation of the lineage of a family depicting the relationships and medical data of the individuals in the family. Using the standard symbols **(Fig. 25.4)**, a three generations pedigree needs to be drawn **(Fig. 25.5)**. The person with a disorder who brings the family to notice is known as "proband."

The pedigree helps to decide the mode of inheritance of the disorder in the family. If the mode of disorder in concern is known, then the pedigree can be used to identify probable and obligate (definite) carriers. These carriers can be offered genetic counseling and/or genetic testing.

MENDELIAN INHERITANCE

Diseases inherited in Mendelian fashion are categorized according to whether the gene is on an autosome, or a sex chromosome and the trait is dominant or recessive.

1. Autosomal Dominant Inheritance

These diseases manifest even when only one copy of an autosomal gene is mutated. Thus, the disorders inherited in autosomal dominant fashion manifest in heterozygotes. Homozygotes for the dominant mutant genes may or may not be severely affected. **Figure 25.6** shows a pedigree with autosomal dominant inheritance.

Examples: Holt-Oram syndrome, achondroplasia, Marfan syndrome, Neurofibromatosis, and Waardenburg syndrome.

Characteristics

- Successive multiple generations are affected.
- Both males and females are affected in equal proportion.
- Both males and females can transmit the disease to their offspring.
- The risk of transmission of the disease from an affected parent to the offspring is 50% **(Fig. 25.7)**.

Penetrance and Expressivity

Reduced penetrance and variable expressivity are characteristic of autosomal dominant disorders and affect the risk of recurrence. In some autosomal dominant disorders, a person may be a carrier of a mutation but does not show manifestation. Such a phenomenon is called *incomplete penetrance* which may result in apparent *skipping of a generation* for a dominant genetic disease wherein, in a pedigree an apparently healthy individual has an affected parent and an affected offspring, and he/she constitutes the skipped generation.

Variable expressivity implies variable severity of the disease, variable clinical manifestations, or variable age of onset of the disease, in different members of a family. Mother and the child shown in **Figures 25.8A to C** have different severity of upper limb shortening and finger malformations. Variable expressivity is very common for Waardenburg syndrome. Most of the affected children may have heterochromia iridis, white forelock of hair, and telecanthus (lateral displacement of inner canthi). Deafness is seen in only 50% of patients while some may have only pigmentary changes of eyes and/or hair.

Another classical example of variable severity is tuberous sclerosis. In a family of tuberous sclerosis, different individuals may have only one or two manifestations from the following: seizures, adenoma sebaceum, hypopigmented patches on skin. Some children may have severe form of developmental delay and/or seizure disorder with some of the above-mentioned features.

2. Autosomal Recessive Inheritance

Autosomal recessive inheritance is due to genes located on the autosomes and the disease manifest when both the copies of the gene are mutated. The heterozygotes with one mutated copy of the gene and one normal copy of the gene are called "carriers" of the disease and do not manifest clinically (**Fig. 25.9**).

Examples: Thalassemia major, Sickle cell disease, Wilson disease, Cystic fibrosis, spinal muscular atrophy, Gaucher disease, and ataxia-telangiectasia.

Characteristics

- Both males and females are affected.
- The disorder usually occurs in only one generation, mostly in a single sibship.
- Consanguinity in parents of affected child may be present especially if the disorder is rare. However, consanguinity is not essential.
- Both the parents of a person with autosomal recessive disease are not affected but are always carriers.
- The risk of recurrence of the disorder in the siblings of a child with an autosomal recessive disorder is 25% or 1 in 4. However, it should be noted that in a family, there can be 2, 3 or more consecutively affected children.

Sex-influenced disorders: Some diseases are more common in one sex than the other. An example is gout, which is more common in males than in females. In postmenopausal women

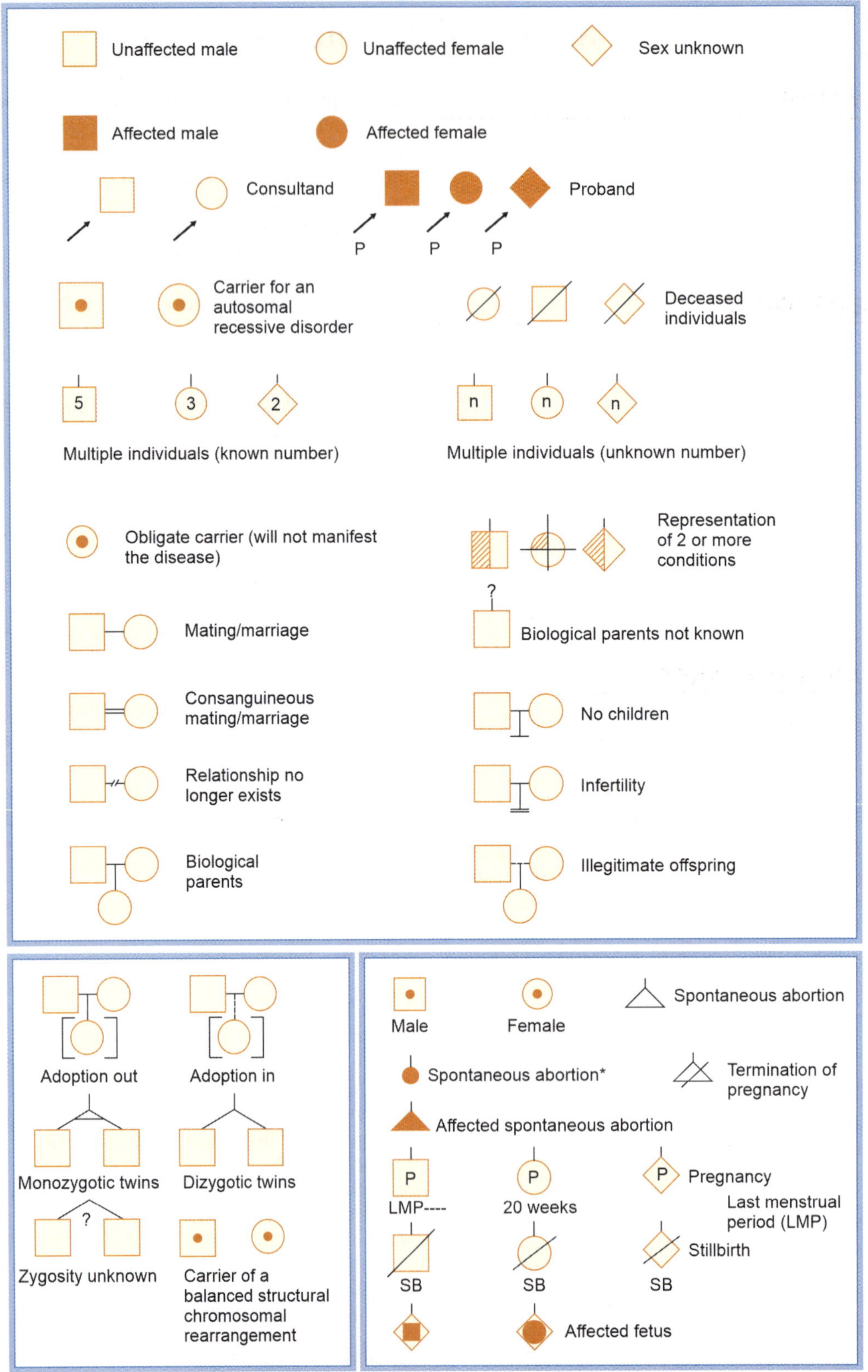

Fig. 25.4: The commonly used symbols for drawing of a pedigree

*This symbol is also used for spontaneous abortion

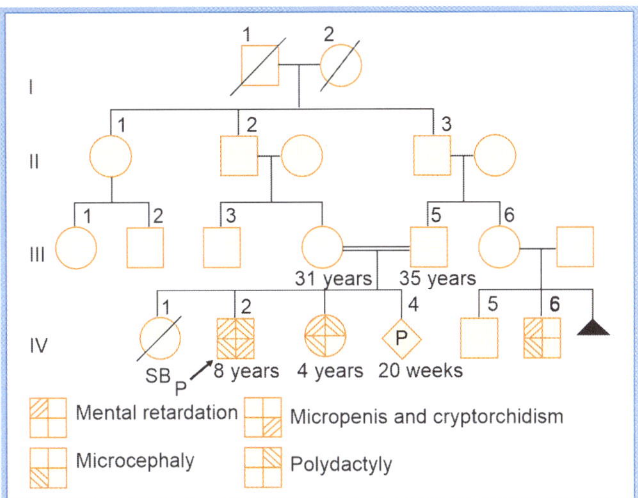

Fig. 25.5: A representative pedigree with consanguineous marriage between individuals III-4 and III-5. They have similarly affected a son and a daughter suggestive of autosomal recessive mode of inheritance. The individual IV-6 may or may not have the same disorder present in individuals IV-2 and IV-3

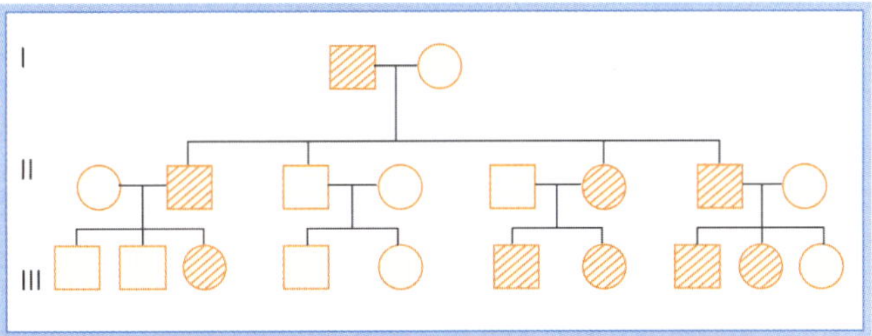

Fig. 25.6: Autosomal dominant inheritance

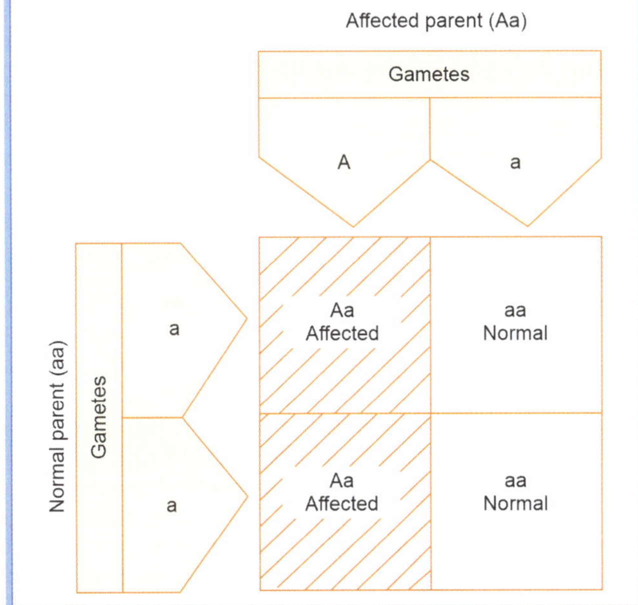

Fig. 25.7: A Punnett square showing the possible gamete combinations for an autosomal dominant disorder in a couple with one normal spouse and one spouse with an autosomal dominant disorder

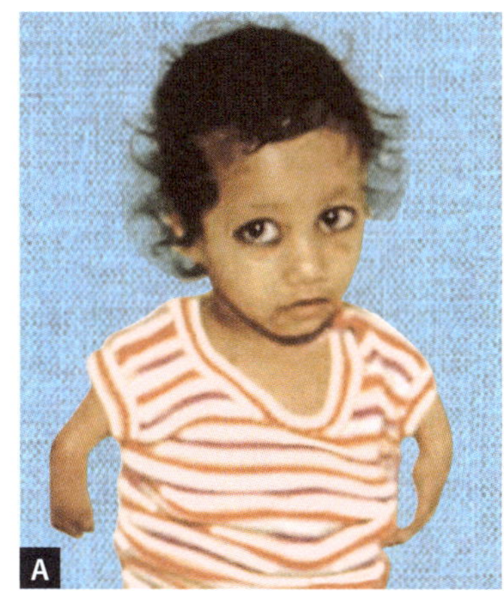

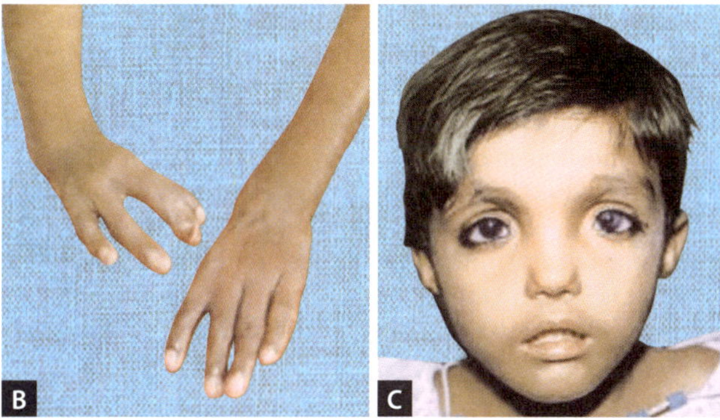

Figs. 25.8A to C: A mother and her daughter with Holt–Oram syndrome. Expression of upper limb abnormality is more severe in the child (A) as compared to the mother (B), and (C) Waardenburg syndrome type I—an autosomal dominant inherited syndrome of deafness

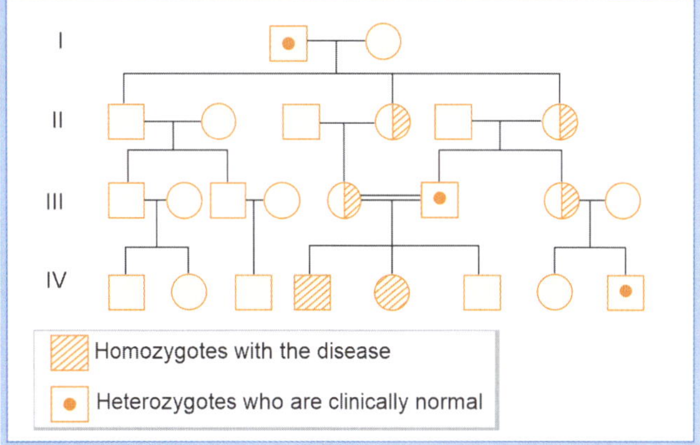

Fig. 25.9: A pedigree showing an autosomal recessive inheritance

the prevalence is similar to that in males, suggesting the protective influence of hormones.

Sex-limited disorders: Disorders of sex organ, though caused by autosomal genes, can occur only in the sex that has that organ; for example, familial testotoxicosis (male limited precocious puberty) occurs only in males though transmitted through females.

3. X-linked Recessive Inheritance

This is conventionally referred to as sex-linked inheritance and is due to the presence of recessive genes on the X chromosome. Males have a single X chromosome and therefore are hemizygous for most of the genes in the X chromosome. Hence, if a male has a mutated gene on the X chromosome, he will be affected. On the other hand, a female with one copy of mutated gene and the other normal copy will usually do not have manifestations of the disease.

Examples: Hemophilia A, hemophilia B, Duchenne muscular dystrophy, Becker muscular dystrophy, X-linked aqueductal stenosis, mucopolysaccharidosis II (Hunter syndrome).

Characteristics

- Males are affected almost exclusively.
- All affected males are related through unaffected female (carrier) relatives.
- Male-to-male transmission is never observed because the X chromosome in a male is always contributed by a female.
- An affected male can pass on the disorder to his grandson through unaffected carrier daughter.
- The risk of transmitting the disease to the sons of a carrier female is 50% and the chance that her daughter will be carrier is 50% **(Fig. 25.10)**. All daughters of an affected male will be carriers **(Fig. 25.11)**.

Duchenne muscular dystrophy (DMD): DMD is a progressive neuromuscular disease, caused by mutation in the dystrophin gene located on the short arm of chromosome X. DMD is inherited in X linked recessive manner but may be sporadic in 30% of cases. Becker muscular dystrophy (BMD) is a milder manifestation of the same disease. Molecular mechanism of pathogenesis is multi-exonic deletion, single nucleotide variants, duplications in DMD gene in 60–70%, 25–35%, and 5–10% males, respectively. Large deletions and duplications abolish the reading frame of the dystrophin gene, which leads to formation of severely truncated protein, which is quickly degraded.

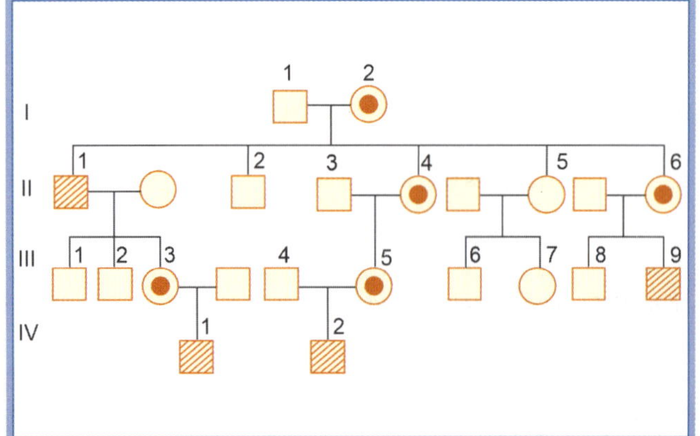

Fig. 25.10: A pedigree of an X-linked recessive disorder. Non-manifesting carrier females are denoted by a dot inside the circle

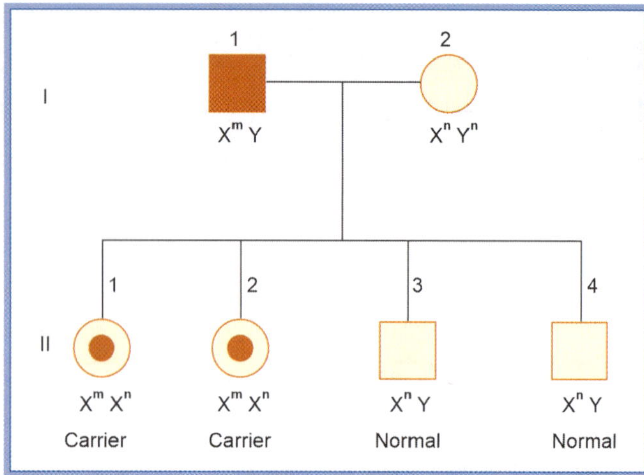

Fig. 25.11: A pedigree showing transmission of mutation of an X-linked recessive disorder from an affected father to his offspring

4. X-linked Dominant Inheritance

This is a less common form of inheritance and is caused by the presence of a *dominant disease-causing allele on an* X chromosome. The pedigree of an X-linked dominant disorder superficially looks similar to that of an autosomal dominant disorder. But the number of females with the disease is more than the number of males with the disease. The disease manifestations in females are milder than in the males and there is no male-to-male transmission.

The classical example is X-linked hypophosphatemic rickets (XLH), also known as vitamin D-resistant rickets caused by mutation in the *PHEX* gene. XLH is characterized by a spectrum of phenotype ranging from isolated hypophosphatemia to severe lower extremity bowing in children and classical signs of rickets.

Some X-linked disorders are so severe in males that the affected males die *in utero* and only affected females are seen. Incontinentia pigmenti is another example of X-linked dominant disorder with lethality in males.

Fragile X mental retardation is usually labeled as *X-linked semi-dominant disorder*, as manifesting females are common.

5. Y-linked Inheritance

Y-linked inheritance implies transmission of Y-linked genes (holandric genes) through a male to his son; thus, in Y linked disorders only sons are affected through their father and daughters are spared. Certain traits such as hairy ears and webbed toes are inherited through the Y chromosome.

The H-Y histocompatibility antigen and genes involved in spermatogenesis are also Y chromosome linked. Deletion/mutation of genes related to spermatogenesis may manifest as infertility due to azoospermia. Male offspring conceived through intracytoplasmic sperm injection in vitro fertilization (or rarely spontaneously) will inherit infertility due to the same mutation/deletion.

Sex-limited expression: Certain disorders caused by autosomal genes may manifest only in a particular sex. This type of manifestation is known as *sex limited expression*. For example, *SRD5A2* gene related androgen insensitivity syndrome manifests only in genetic males as this gene codes for 5α-reductase that converts testosterone to dihydrotestosterone, which is responsible for virilization of the male external genitalia.

Sex-influenced expression: The autosomal dominant disease manifests preferentially in one sex as compared to the other. For example, gout and presenile baldness is more common in males, and hereditary hemochromatosis causes more severe iron overload in males as compared to affected females because of disease attenuation in females due to menstrual blood loss.

NON-MENDELIAN INHERITANCE

Many disorders do not follow Mendelian patterns of inheritance. Advances in molecular genetics have led to the identification of mechanism for these disorders. Non-Mendelian modes of inheritance and their common example are given below:

1. ***Mitochondrial:*** Leber hereditary optic atrophy
2. ***Genomic imprinting:*** Prader–Willi syndrome, Angelman syndrome
3. ***Uniparental disomy:*** Prader–Willi syndrome, Angelman syndrome
4. ***Somatic and germline mosaicism:*** Polyostotic fibrous dysplasia
5. ***Dynamic mutation*** (triplet repeat disorders): Fragile X syndrome, myotonic dystrophy, Friedreich's ataxia
6. ***Digenic/oligogenic inheritance:*** Hirschsprung disease, Bardet–Biedl syndrome.
7. ***Multifactorial inheritance:*** Neural tube defect

1. Mitochondrial Inheritance

A typical human somatic cell contains up to 1,000 mitochondria and each mitochondrion typically contains several copies of mitochondrial DNA (mtDNA). mtDNA is a 16.6 kb long, double stranded circular DNA. The mitochondrial DNA codes for ribosomal RNA, transfer RNA and some protein involved in cellular respiration. These genes are important for function of all cells of the body and hence, mitochondrial diseases can manifest with symptoms of any system of body including eyes, muscles, heart, brain, liver, and endocrine glands.

Mitochondrial disorders should be suspected when multiple systems of body are involved, or the patient has characteristic features of a mitochondrial disorder. Two examples are Kearns–Sayre syndrome (external ophthalmoplegia, retinitis pigmentosa, myopathy), and MELAS (mitochondrial encephalopathy, lactic acidosis, and stroke-like episodes).

- Both males and females can be affected in a mitochondrially inherited disorder however it can be transmitted only through mother as only the ovum contributes mitochondria to the zygote **(Fig. 25.12)**.
- The severity and the extent of involvement vary depending on the load of mutant mitochondria in each tissue. Variability in the number of mutant mitochondria in each cell and each tissue is characteristic of mitochondrial disorder. Unless the number of mutant mitochondria crosses a "*threshold*," symptoms will not appear.
- Both the mutant and the non-mutant (wild) type of mtDNA may be present in the same individual/tissue/cell, or even in the same mitochondrion **(Fig. 25.13)**. This is known as *heteroplasmy*. The percentage of the different mtDNA can vary between 0–100%. Similarly, if only one type of variant (either wild or mutant type) is present in all the

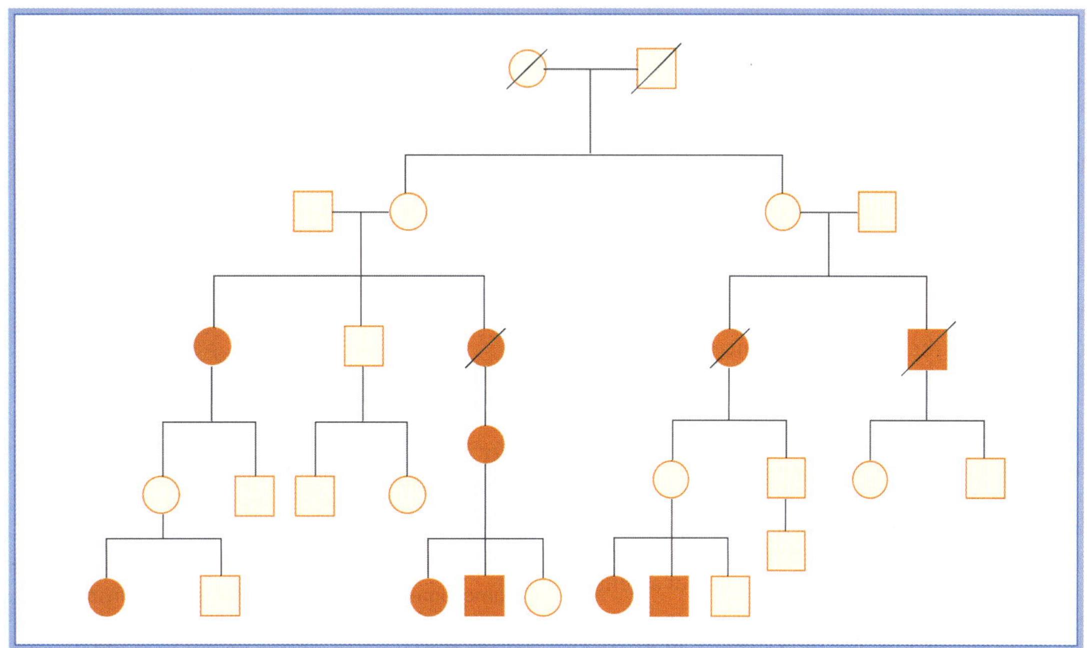

Fig. 25.12: Pedigree showing mitochondrial inheritance

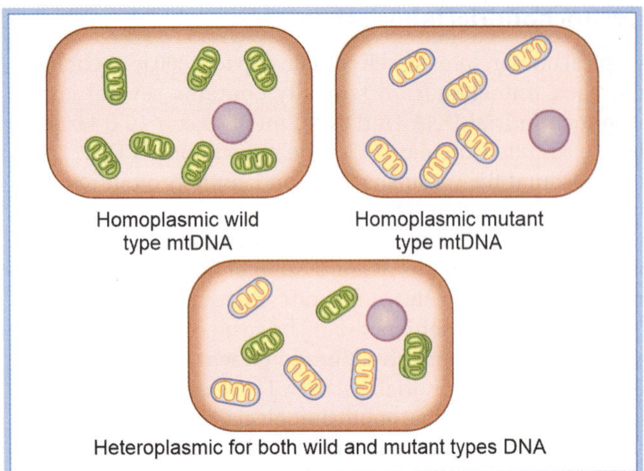

Fig. 25.13: Mitochondrial homoplasmy and heteroplasmy (DNA: deoxyribonucleic acid; mtDNA: mitochondrial DNA)

mitochondria/cell/tissue or individual, then this feature is known as *homoplasmy*.

- In heteroplasmic disorders, the level of mutant mtDNA load may change over time leading to a fall in the level in blood and accumulation in non-dividing cells such as muscles. Hence, respiratory enzyme/mtDNA study on the biopsied sample of the affected organ may be helpful in situation where blood report is negative for any mtDNA mutation.
- A significant variation in the heteroplasmy level in the oocytes leads to variation in the variant load and its type in the offspring. This is explained by the *bottleneck hypothesis,* which states that the number of mtDNA during oogenesis is either relatively small or only few mtDNA have been used as template for amplification. The manifestations in offspring will depend on the number of mutant mitochondria transmitted to the zygote. Hence, the risk of recurrence in the offspring cannot be predicted in mitochondrial disorders.
- Detection of mutation in prenatal sample may not be able to predict the phenotype as the mutant load in the sample tested (chorionic villi/amniotic fluid cells) may be different from that in the various organs of the fetus. Hence, counseling for risk of recurrence in mitochondrial disorders remains a challenge.

2. Genomic Imprinting

In Mendelian disorders, there is no difference between the function of maternally and paternally inherited copies of the gene. However, for some genes, the behaviors of paternal and maternal copies of the gene may be different. This is known as genomic imprinting. This occurs due to heritable modification of the imprinted copy of the gene.

- The imprinted copy is the copy of the gene, which is silenced, i.e., not expressed, though the DNA sequence of the gene is normal. The important mechanism of silencing of a gene is methylation of the gene.
- Methylation of a gene means that the cytosines in the CpG islands (clusters of cytosine and guanine, which occur together near transcription sites of many genes) are methylated at the 5′ position of the pyrimidine ring of the cytosine residues to form 5-methylcytosines. If the maternal allele is inactive or suppressed, the gene is said to be maternally imprinted. In paternally imprinted gene, the paternal copy is silenced. Thus, imprinting results in monoallelic expression of the gene in a parent of origin specific manner. The process of imprinting is reversible as during gametogenesis, the imprint is erased and a new one is established depending upon the parent of origin **(Fig. 25.14)**.
- Examples of disorders occurring due to the imprinted genes include Prader-Willi syndrome (obesity, hypogonadism, and mental retardation) and Angelman syndrome (mental retardation, seizures, bursts of laughter, and ataxic gait). On chromosome 15, a small region has imprinted genes for Prader-Willi syndrome and Angelman syndrome. Prader-Willi syndrome genes are maternally imprinted, and the disease occurs when the active paternal copy of the gene is deleted. In Angelman syndrome, the gene is paternally imprinted and hence, the disorder occurs only when the active maternal copy of the gene is deleted.

3. Uniparental Disomy

The other evidence of imprinting comes from uniparental disomy. Uniparental disomy (UPD) implies that both the homologous chromosomes (thus genes) are inherited from one parent only. This can occur due to various mechanisms. Usually, two events of non-disjunction are required **(Figs. 25.15A to C)**.

- In uniparental disomy, both the homologous chromosomes of a parent (*uniparental heterodisomy*) may be inherited or there may be two copies of one of the homologous chromosomes of a parent (*uniparental isodisomy*). In case of uniparental isodisomy, if there is a mutated gene for a recessive disorder

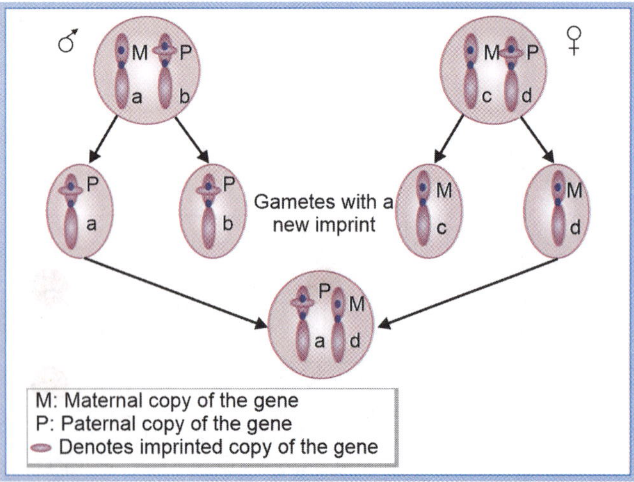

Fig. 25.14: Establishment of new imprint during gametogenesis. Chromosome "a," which was of maternal origin in the father, is passed on as paternal to his offspring. Similarly, chromosome "d," which was of paternal origin in the mother, is transmitted as maternal to her offspring

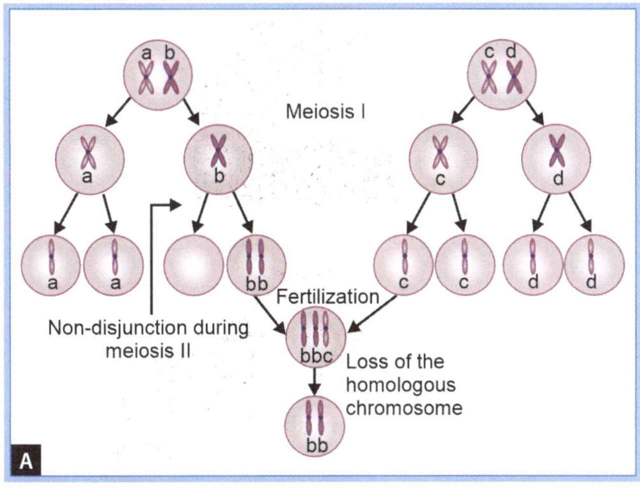

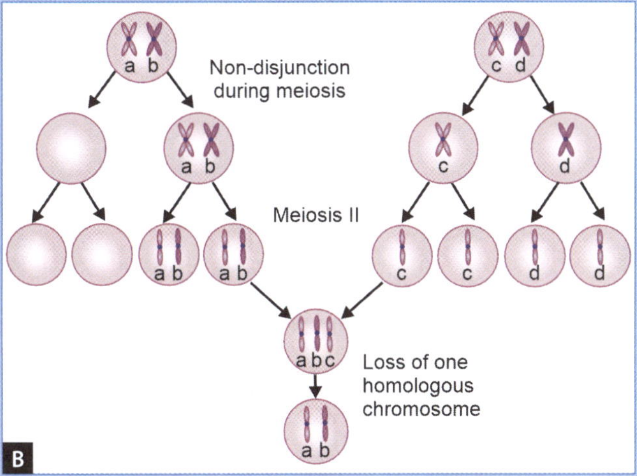

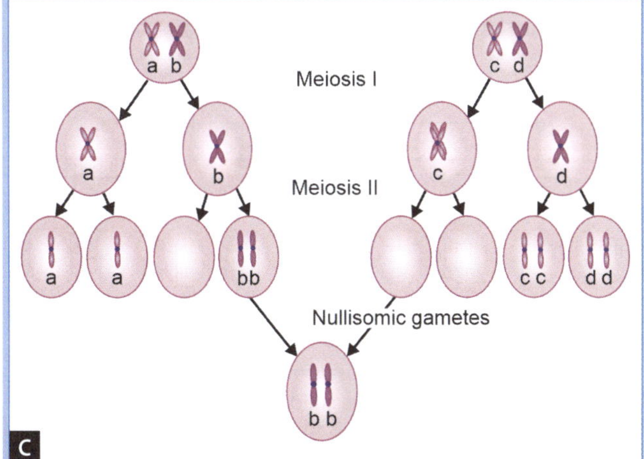

Figs. 25.15A to C: Gametogenesis resulting in uniparental disomy. Two events of non-disjunction are needed for uniparental disomy. "a" and "b" are homologous chromosomes of a parent and "c" and "d" are homologous chromosomes of another parent. (A) Uniparental isodisomy; (B) Uniparental heterodisomy; and (C) Fusion of disomic gamete of a parent with nullisomic gamete from another parent

on that chromosome, the individual will manifest with the recessive disorder.

- If the UPD occurs for a chromosome, which has some imprinted gene, then there may be disease manifestation though there are two copies of genes with normal DNA sequence. Examples are Prader-Willi syndrome and Angelman syndrome. Paternal UPD of chromosome 15 leads to Angelman syndrome (as the active maternal copy of the gene are missing) and maternal UPD of chromosome 15 leads to Prader-Willi syndrome (as the active paternal copy of the gene is missing).

4. Mosaicism

Mosaicism implies presence of two types of cell lines (derived from a single zygote) in an individual, one with the mutation and one without the mutation, which can be a chromosomal abnormality or a single gene mutation. Mosaicism can be of two types—somatic and germline.

- ***Somatic mosaicism*** is a postzygotic event and is associated with presence of more than one cell lineage in the somatic cells of the body. This phenomenon may decrease the severity of the disorder and may manifest with patchy distribution of lesions, e.g., streaky pigmentary abnormalities of skin as in hypomelanosis of Ito **(Fig. 25.16)**, or patchy involvement of bones in McCune-Albright polyostotic fibrous dysplasia. The latter condition is caused by somatic mosaicism for mutation of *GNAS1* gene encoding the alpha-subunit of G-protein.
- Mosaicism that is limited to gonads is known as *gonadal/germ line mosaicism*. This may lead to birth of more than one child with an autosomal dominant or X-linked disorder even if the parent is not a carrier of the disease-causing mutation in the blood. Germ line mosaicism is commonly seen in osteogenesis imperfecta, achondroplasia and Duchenne muscular dystrophy.
- Sometimes, mutation may be present in a proportion of germ cells as well as somatic cells which is known a *gonosomal mosaicism*.

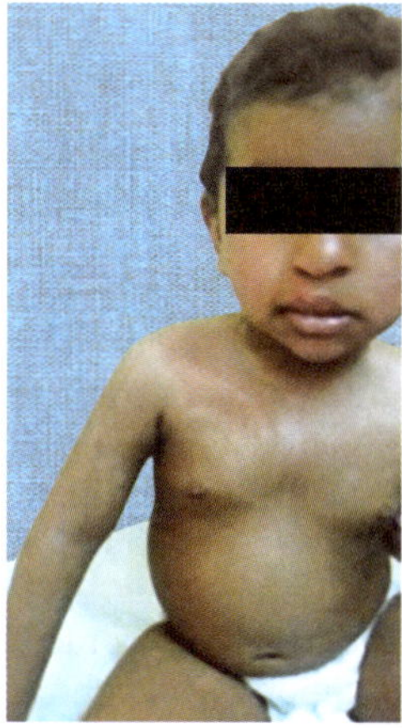

Fig. 25.16: Streak-like hypopigmentation along the lines of Blaschko. It suggests mosaicism for chromosomal or single gene mutation

5. Chimerism

Chimera: It is an organism or tissue that contains at least two or more genetically distinct cell lines, often originating from the fusion of as many different zygotes. There are two types of human chimeras

1. ***Dispermic chimeras:*** Resulting from double fertilization whereby two genetically different sperms fertilize two ova and the resulting two distinct zygotes fuse to form one embryo. If the two zygotes are of different sex, then the fused embryo can be a true hermaphrodite (having both male and female gonads) with a 46,XX/XY mosaicism in blood.
2. ***Blood chimeras:*** Sometimes between non-identical twins, there can be *in utero* exchange of red blood cells via placental circulation. For example, 90% of one twin's cells can have an XY karyotype with red blood cells showing predominantly blood group B, whereas 90% of the cells of the other twin can have an XX karyotype with red blood cells showing predominantly blood group A.

6. Unstable Dynamic Mutation (Triplet Repeat Disorders)

Some disorders are caused by an increase in the number of triplet repeats within or near a gene. The triplet repeats are repeats of three nucleotides occurring in tandem. The examples are CGG repeats in fragile X mental retardation, CTG repeats in myotonic dystrophy, and GAA repeats in Friedreich ataxia. These repeats are usually transmitted stably from one generation to the next.

In a person with higher number of repeats, the number of repeats changes during transmission to the offspring. Increase/expansion above a specific number of repeats leads to manifestation of disease. With a higher number of repeats, there is instability during DNA replication of these units leading to variation in the number of repeats indifferent tissues in an individual, and also amongst different members in a family. The increase in number of repeats over generations leads to increasing severity of manifestations and earlier age of onset, a phenomenon known as *anticipation*. Anticipation is observed in many nucleotide repeat disorders like Huntington chorea and spinocerebellar ataxia.

Fragile X Syndrome

It is the commonest cause of inherited intellectual disability and transmitted in an X-linked fashion. Fragile X syndrome accounts for 1–3% of cases of intellectual disability without obvious cause. Long face with prominent mandible, autistic features, and large testes in post-pubertal boys are features other than intellectual disability **(Fig. 25.17A)**.

Unlike other X-linked recessive disorders, many of the carrier females show manifestations. Thus, the mode of inheritance is described as X-linked semi-dominant or X-linked dominant with incomplete penetrance. The normal allele for the gene for fragile X syndrome—*FMR1* gene has less than 50 CGG repeats **(Fig. 25.17B)**.

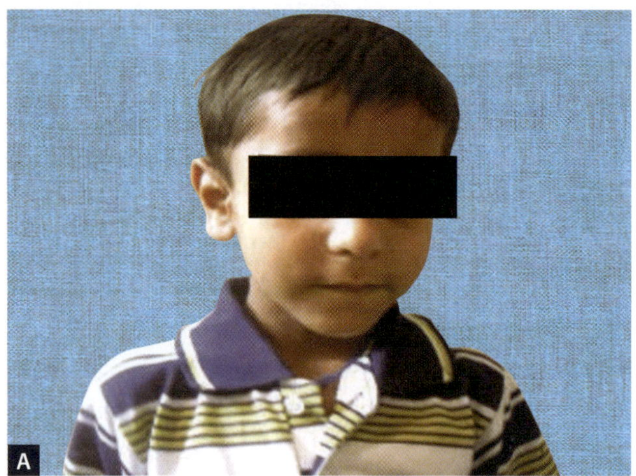

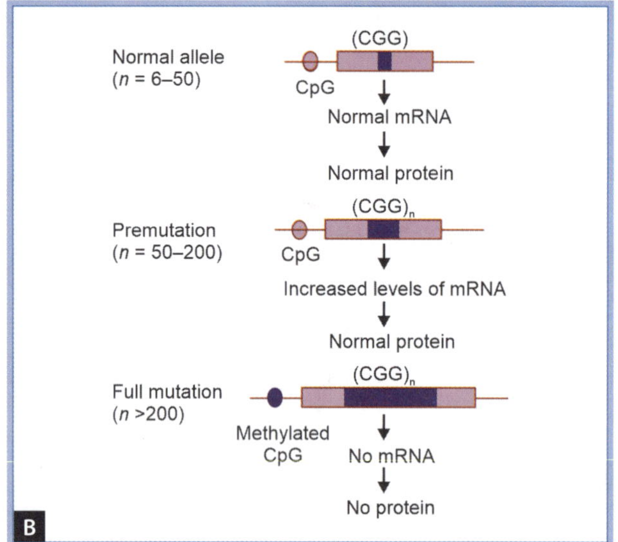

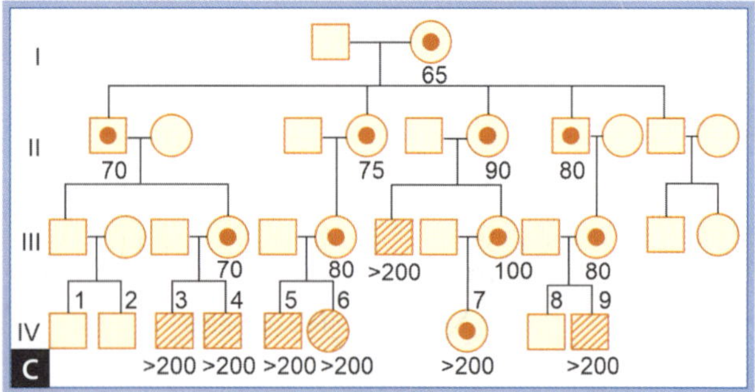

Figs. 25.17A to C: (A) Face of a child with fragile X syndrome. The features are too subtle to be able to diagnose clinically; (B) Normal allele, premutation and full mutation alleles of *FMR-1* gene showing increasing number of CGG repeats and the effect on mRNA and protein synthesis; and (C) A pedigree of fragile X syndrome. The numbers of CGG repeats in carriers are shown below each individual. There is increase in the number of repeats of premutation allele over generations with subsequent conversion to mutation. Obligate carriers are shown by dot (•) inside the symbols. Affected cases are shown by shaded symbols. The number of repeats has not increased when the allele is transmitted by the father

(CGG: cytosine guanine guanine; mRNA: messenger ribonucleic acid)

Children with Fragile X syndrome have >200 repeats (known as full mutation). The alleles with repeats in between 50–200 are called *premutation alleles*. Individuals with premutation do not have mental retardation and other features of Fragile X syndrome but may have ataxia and tremors in old age known as Fragile X-associated tremor/ataxia syndrome (FXTAS) and females may have premature ovarian failure. The premutation allele when transmitted from mother to her offspring expands and the offspring with >200 repeats have Fragile X syndrome.

Some females with full mutation have some features such as long face, learning difficulties, or mild mental retardation. The manifestation in female depends probably on lyonization pattern, i.e., the relative ratio of active X chromosomes with mutation and without mutation. A characteristic pedigree of fragile X syndrome is shown in **Figure 25.17C**.

As the clinical features of fragile X syndrome are not diagnostic, testing all individuals with intellectual disability and developmental delay is important to identify cases. Screening of possible female carriers in the pedigree of an individual diagnosed with fragile X syndrome and offering prenatal diagnosis to the carriers is essential for prevention of recurrences.

7. Digenic and Oligogenic Inheritance

It has now been proved that many genetic disorders that were previously described as monogenic are, in fact, caused by mutations at two or more loci/genes. Such digenic inheritance has been reported in retinitis pigmentosa and Bardet–Biedl syndrome. At least 20 genes are known for Bardet–Biedl syndrome and some pedigrees show that mutations in both copies of *BBS2* gene and in one copy of *BBS6* gene are required to manifest the disease (**Fig. 25.18**). This mechanism of oligogenic inheritance is known as digenic triallelic mutation. In some oligogenic disorders, monoallelic mutation in two genes (digenic diallelic) is needed for the disease to manifest.

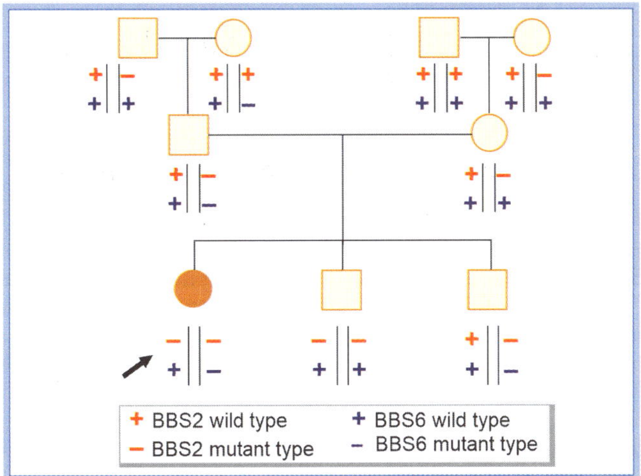

Fig. 25.18: Pedigree showing Bardet–Biedl affected proband with triallelic digenic inheritance

Hirschsprung disease is an important example of oligogenic inheritance. Mutation in *RET* and some other genes are known to be associated with Hirschsprung disease. But not all family members with *RET* gene mutation have Hirschsprung disease, indicating that the mutation in *RET* gene alone does not cause the disease.

The variable expressivity seen amongst family members of Mendelian disorders and incomplete penetrance observed in some autosomal dominant disorders suggest that in addition to mutated gene, functioning of some other genes is also important for the development of phenotype. These genes are called *modifier genes*. Research in identification of modifier genes for various Mendelian disorders may bring up new treatment strategies.

8. Multifactorial Inheritance

Model of multifactorial inheritance was initially developed to explain the high risk of recurrence of some disorders amongst the relatives of an individual with the disorder. The disorder is the combined effect of many genetic variations and environmental factors. Now many of these genetic factors are being identified in reality. This type of inheritance is seen in many congenital malformations such as cleft lip/palate congenital dislocation of the hip, and congenital heart defects and is also implicated in common disorders of adult life, including hypertension, ischemic heart disease, psychiatric diseases, and autoimmune disorders.

Factor V Leiden mutation in cerebral venous thrombosis, DR3 and DR4 alleles at HLA locus in type I diabetes mellitus, and a genetic variant of 5,10-methylenetetrahydrofolate reductase enzyme in neural tube defects, are some of the genetic risk factors identified in multifactorial disorders. Because multifactorial illnesses account for a major health burden; these are the recent thrust areas of research following completion of the human genome project.

9. Polygenic Inheritance

Many common complex diseases such as cardiovascular disease, type 2 diabetes, breast and prostate cancers, and Alzheimer disease, are polygenic in inheritance. This implies that the onset and development of the disease is determined by variation in many genes at different loci, with each variant exerting a small, generally additive effect. Additive means that the influence of each genetic variant on the phenotype is cumulative, not dominant or recessive. For instance, if a variant double the risk for coronary heart disease, compared with homozygous carriers of the low-risk allele, heterozygotes will have a twofold increased risk and homozygotes for the same will incur a fourfold increased risk of heart disease.

Genome Wide Association Study (GWAS): Genome-wide association studies test the numerous genetic variants across many genomes to find those statistically associated with a specific trait or disease. GWAS has revolutionized the field of complex disease genetics over the past decade and has facilitated the concept of precision medicine. Based on relevant GWAS of the individual, a statistical calculation of the cumulative effect of the large number of genomic variants can be done. This summation of risk is known as polygenic risk score (PRS) which estimates the individual's genetic liability to a trait or disease. PRS is becoming increasingly popular as a means of predicting complex trait at an early stage in the life course and subsequently guiding about disease modifying intervention.

IN A NUTSHELL

Patterns of Inheritance

1. Autosomal dominant, autosomal recessive, X-linked, and Y-linked disorders are monogenic disorders and are prototypes of Mendelian inheritance pattern, following the Mendel's laws of heredity.
2. Autosomal dominant and recessive disorders have a 50% and 25% recurrence risk respectively in the offspring.
3. In a typical X linked recessive disorder, there is a recurrence risk of 50% in a male offspring of a carrier mother and a daughter will have a 50% chance of being a carrier.
4. Non-Mendelian disorders include trinucleotide repeat expansion, mitochondrial inheritance, genomic imprinting, uniparental disomy (UPD), mosaicism, oligogenic inheritance, and multifactorial inheritance.

Bennett RL, Steinhaus KA, Uhrich SB, et al. Recommendations for standardized human pedigree nomenclature. Am J Hum Genet. 1995;56:745-52.
Bennett RL, French KS, Resta RG, et al. Practice resource-focused revision: standardized pedigree nomenclature update centered on sex and gender inclusivity: a practice resource of the National Society of Genetic Counselors. Journal of Genetic Counseling. 2022;31:1238-48.
Hall JG. Genomic imprinting: review and relevance to human diseases. Am J Hum Genet. 1990;46:857-73.
Kingston HM. An ABC of clinical genetics, 2nd edition. London: British Medical Association; 1994.
Pyeritz RE, Korf BR, Grody WW. Principles and Practice of Medical Genetics, Foundations, 7th edition. Elsevier; 2018.
Schäffer AA. Digenic inheritance in medical genetics. J Med Genet. 2013;50:641-52.

25.3 Chromosomal Disorders

PE 29.1, PE 29.3, PE 29.4, PE 29.5

CYTOGENETICS AND KARYOTYPE

The study of chromosomes is known as cytogenetics. Traditional cytogenetics needs live dividing cells. The cells are cultured in tubes and the cell division is arrested by adding colchicines, which is a spindle poison. The cells arrested in metaphase stage show chromosomes as discrete bodies. During slide preparation, the chromosomes of one cell are spread in a localized area and can be counted and analyzed. A photograph of a metaphase is taken, and the chromosomes are cut and arranged in pairs. Such an arrangement of chromosomes is called "karyotype" **(Fig. 25.19)**.

Karyotype also denotes the chromosome complement of an individual, i.e., total number of chromosomes, sex chromosomes, and chromosomal abnormality, if any. The smallest chromosomal abnormality detected by traditional karyotype contains at least 5–10 million base pairs (Mb). Now, the analysis of whole genome by microarray based cytogenetic analysis can detect genomic imbalances as small as 10 kilobases (Kb) and has found an important role in evaluation of children with global developmental delay, intellectual disability, and autism.

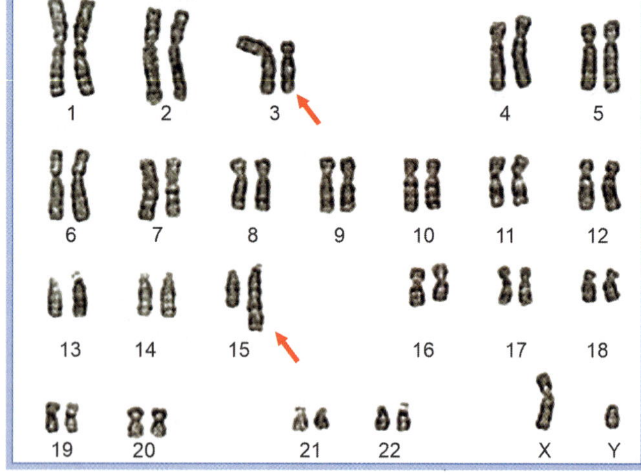

Fig. 25.19: A karyotype of a male showing 46 chromosomes with a balanced translocation between chromosomes 3 and 15. The normal chromosomes are on the left sides of the pairs and the derivatives chromosomes are shown by arrows. Note that each chromosome has different banding pattern which is used to identify chromosomes and to detect chromosomal abnormalities

ABNORMALITIES OF CHROMOSOMES

Abnormalities of chromosomes can be *numerical* or *structural* and may involve autosomes or sex chromosomes. These abnormalities may present at different ages with different problems. Chromosomal abnormalities are usually unbalanced, due to gain or loss of chromosomal material. Embryo with significant chromosomal imbalance is spontaneously aborted; chromosomal anomalies account for about 50% of early spontaneous abortions. Some chromosomal imbalances of autosomes are not embryonically lethal and lead to live-born child with multiple malformations and intellectual disability. Sex chromosomal abnormalities usually lead to hypergonadotropic hypogonadism.

- ***Numerical abnormalities*** of chromosomes can be aneuploidy or polyploidy. Polyploidies are 69,XXX (triploidy); 92,XXYY (tetraploidy) where the total number of chromosomes is an exact multiple of haploid (23) set of chromosomes. The karyotype with number of chromosomes, which is not an exact multiple of 23 is known as aneuploidy. The examples of aneuploidy are trisomy 21 (three copies of chromosomes 21), or monosomy X (only one of the sex chromosomes pair).
- ***Structural abnormalities:*** These include deletion or duplication of a part of chromosome, translocation of a segment from one chromosome to the other (which may be balanced or unbalanced), isochromosome (loss of one arm of a chromosome and duplication of the other), inversion (two breaks), and ring chromosome (breaks in both ends of a chromosome and joining of the sticky ends to form a ring structure).

DISORDERS OF AUTOSOMES

Numerous abnormalities of chromosomes are described in liveborns, stillbirths, and aborted material. The three non-mosaic aneuploidies of autosomes compatible with survival are trisomy 21, trisomy 13, and trisomy 18. Syndromes of other structural abnormalities such as deletions of 4p, 5p, etc., are well delineated. Use of newer techniques to study chromosomes has led to identification of new syndromes associated with microdeletions/microduplications, not visible on routine chromosomal analysis **(Figs. 25.20A and B)**.

Down Syndrome

Down syndrome is the commonest chromosomal abnormality occurring in live births. It accounts for 30% of individuals with mental handicap. The etiology of Down syndrome is an extra copy of chromosome 21 **(Fig. 25.21)**. This may occur due to non-disjunction (free trisomy—95%), translocation (4%), or mosaicism (1%).

Translocation: The extra chromosome 21 is attached to some other chromosome, commonly to 14, 21, or 22. In about 50% of such cases one of the parents is a carrier of such balanced rearrangement **(Fig. 25.22)** and hence, at high risk of giving birth to offspring with trisomy 21. The risk of Down syndrome in the offspring of a female carrier of 14;21 or 21;22 translocation is 10–15%. If such balanced arrangement is seen in a male, the risk of Down syndrome in his offspring is 1–5%.

Clinical Features

Facial features of Down syndrome are characteristic: Flat face, hypertelorism, up slant of eyes, depressed nasal bridge, open

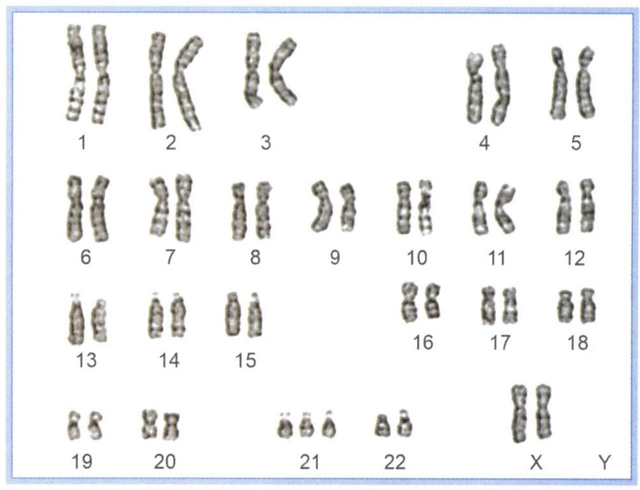

Fig. 25.21: A karyotype of trisomy 21

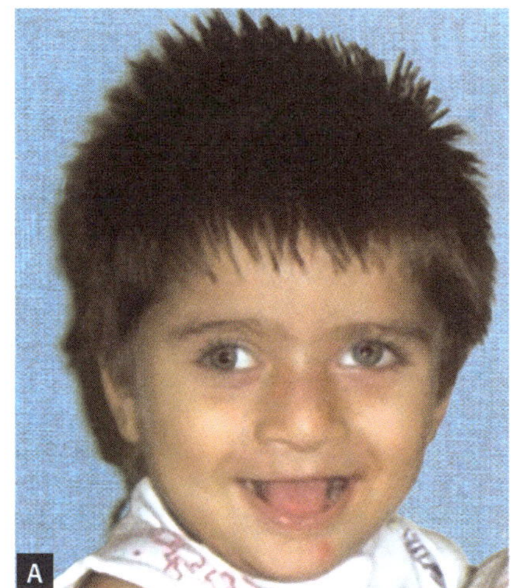

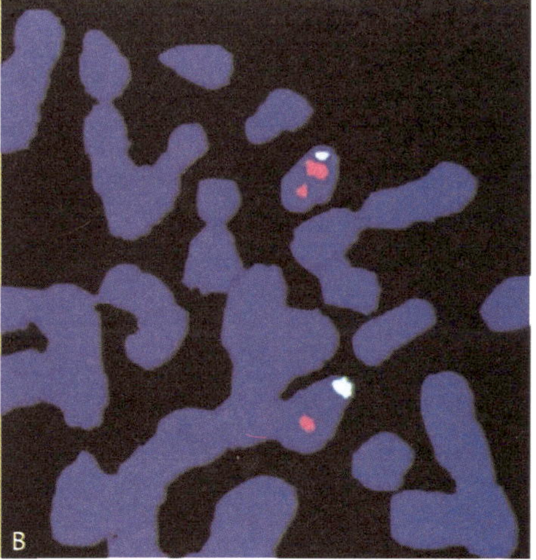

Figs. 25.20A and B: (A) A child with Angelman syndrome. Note happy predisposition and slight prognathism; (B) Fluorescence *in situ* hybridization shows deletion of region for Angelman syndrome on one chromosome 15 (red signal near green signal for the centromere). The green signal is for centromere of chromosome 15 and the distal red signal is a control probe on chromosome 15

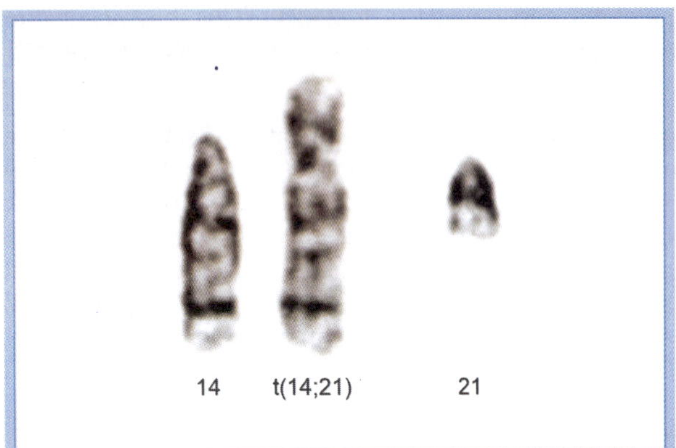

Fig. 25.22: A partial karyotype showing t(14;21). The individual is a balanced carrier as she has deoxyribonucleic acid (DNA) material of 2 chromosomes 21 and 2 chromosomes 14, but the number of total chromosomes is 45 as one 21 and one 14 are joined to each other

mouth, and small ears **(Figs. 25.23A to C)**. Clinical diagnosis may be a little difficult in neonates and preterm babies. Other common features are listed below:

- ***Neonatal period:*** Hypotonia, excess skin fold at the nape of neck.
- ***Craniofacial:*** Increased distance between eyes, epicanthic folds, up slant of eyes, flat face, small ears, depressed nasal bridge, flat occiput, protruding, and fissured tongue.
- ***Limbs:*** Small hands, clinodactyly of fifth finger, simian crease, increased gap between first and second toes.
- ***Major malformations:*** Atrioventricular canal defects and other cardiac malformations, duodenal atresia, tracheo-esophageal fistula, and Hirschsprung disease.
- ***Other problems:*** Short stature, strabismus, obesity, cataract, atlantoaxial joint instability, risk of leukemia, and hypothyroidism.

Intellectual disability is the most important problem associated with Down syndrome. The average IQ of children with Down syndrome is 40–60 and though late, they can talk, walk, do self-care, and lead a happy and useful life under sheltered conditions. Children with Down syndrome communicate well with the family, love the family, and can do repetitive and simple jobs with supervision.

Investigations

Examination and investigations for major malformations are the first steps, whatever may be the age of the child with Down syndrome. Chromosomal analysis (karyotyping) is essential to estimate the risk of recurrence in the family. An extra chromosome 21 (47XX,+21 or 47XY,+21) accounts for 95% children with Down syndrome, and the risk of recurrence of Down syndrome in the sibs of these children is 1%. Karyotypes of the parents of a child with such free trisomy 21 are not needed.

Translocation accounts for 4–5% cases of Down syndrome. In 50% of these cases one of the parents will be carrier of the translocation and hence, karyotypes of the parents need to be studied.

TREATMENT Down Syndrome

At present, there is no curative treatment for Down syndrome, but major malformations need to be surgically treated. Early intervention and stimulation therapies can lead to better outcome with the child developing into a minimally dependent individual. Counseling is a continued process and revisits to provide information and support are needed. The regular surveillance for hearing problem, hypothyroidism, cataract, anemia, and other medical problems is necessary.

Genetic counseling: Break the news to the family as soon as possible in the presence of both parents. A realistic information about prognosis should be given. Stress should be laid on the positive aspects such as ability to lead semi-independent and fruitful life. Rare complication such as risk of leukemia need not be mentioned. Explain the risk of recurrence and need for prenatal diagnosis.

Risk of recurrence: Risk of recurrence after one child with free trisomy 21 is 1%. The risk for inherited translocation is 10–15% if the mother is carrier of balanced translocation and up to 5% if the father is the translocation carrier. A carrier of translocation between two chromosomes 21 [t(21;21)] is rare; but in such case risk of Down syndrome in the offspring is 100% irrespective of which of the parent is the carrier. Risk of recurrence in the sibling, if the child has *de novo* translocation (i.e., the parents' karyotypes are normal) is only 1%.

Prenatal diagnosis during the next pregnancy can be done by karyotyping of prenatal chorionic villi or amniotic fluid samples.

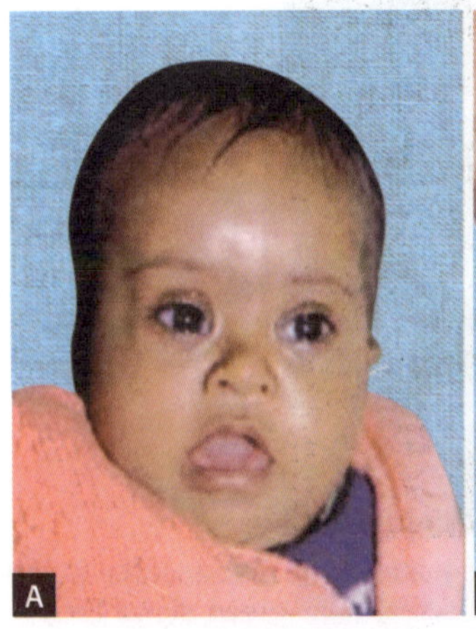

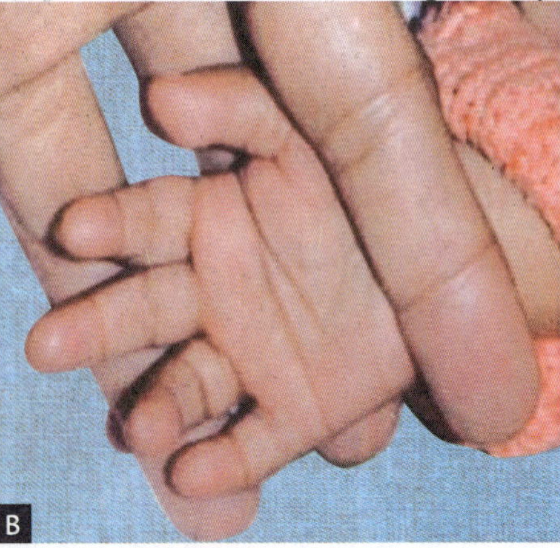

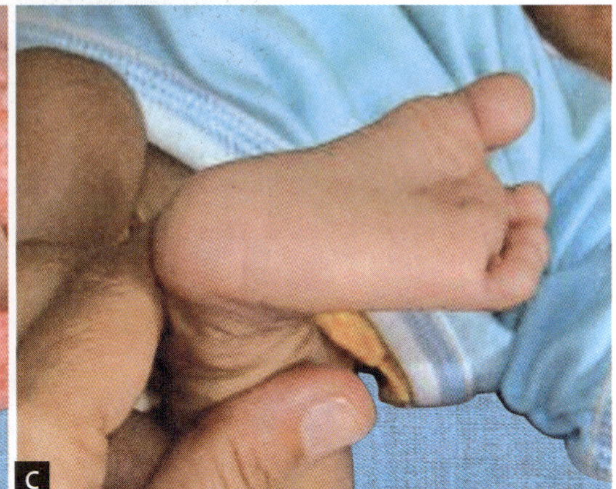

Figs. 25.23A to C: Features of Down syndrome: (A) Flat face, up slant of eyes, hypertelorism, epicanthic folds, and protruding tongue; (B) Clinodactyly or hypoplastic phalanx of the little finger; (C) Sandal gap

Prevention

A child with Down syndrome most often is born in families who do not have any family history of Down syndrome. The overall incidence of Down syndrome is 1 in 800, but it varies with the age of the mother. In a 20-year-old mother, the incidence is 1 in 1,500, which gradually increases with maternal age to become 1 in 400 at 35 years and 1 in 100 at 40 years.

Several maternal serum protein analytes are now available that in combination with specific ultrasound measurements have the necessary sensitivity and specificity for screening of Down syndrome. Amniocentesis is an invasive procedure and now used less frequently.

First trimester screening: First-trimester screening is ideally performed between 11 and 13 weeks of gestation and relies on measuring the level of certain analytes in maternal serum in combination with a highly targeted ultrasonographic examination.

The analytes used are (a) *pregnancy-associated plasma protein A (PAPP-A)* and (b) *hormone human chorionic gonadotropin (hCG)*, either as total hCG or as its free β subunit.

- PAPP-A is depressed below the normal range in all trisomies.
- hCG (or free β-hCG) is elevated in trisomy 21 but depressed in the other trisomies.
- Analyte measurements are combined with ultrasonographic measurement of gestational age specific *nuchal translucency (NT).*
- NT is defined as the thickness of the echo-free space between the skin and the soft tissue overlying the dorsal aspect of the cervical spine caused by subcutaneous edema of the fetal neck. NT is increased in trisomy 21, 13, and 18 and in 45,X (Turner syndrome) fetuses.

Second trimester screening: Second-trimester screening for Down syndrome is characterized by (a) *low Alpha fetoprotein*, (b) *low unconjugated estriol*, (c) *high beta human chorionic gonadotropin*, and (d) *increased inhibin* in maternal blood. The combination of these analytes is known as *Quadruple screen.*

Women with the risk of Down syndrome of 1 in 250 or higher, identified by any of the screening tests, are offered confirmatory test by amniocentesis followed by karyotyping of the fetal cells in the amniotic fluid containing.

Non-invasive prenatal screening: New technologies have made it possible to test the fetal chromosomes using free fetal DNA in maternal plasma. This test done on maternal blood at 10 weeks of gestation can identify aneuploidies of chromosomes 21, 13, and 18. It can identify 99% of fetuses with trisomy 21 but further confirmation by invasive tests such as amniocentesis or chorionic villi sampling is necessary. A small possibility of false positive result and test failure makes NIPS a screening test. Being a high efficiency screening test, NIPS can be readily used as a first line screening modality in high-risk cases such as advanced maternal age, and history of previous Down syndrome.

Rapid aneuploidy detection: Complete chromosomal analysis from amniotic fluid cell by traditional cytogenetic techniques takes 10–15 days. Techniques based on fluorescence *in situ* hybridization (FISH) and polymerase chain reaction can test number of copies of chromosomes 21, 18, and 13 in 2 days and are used for rapid prenatal diagnosis **(Fig. 25.24)**.

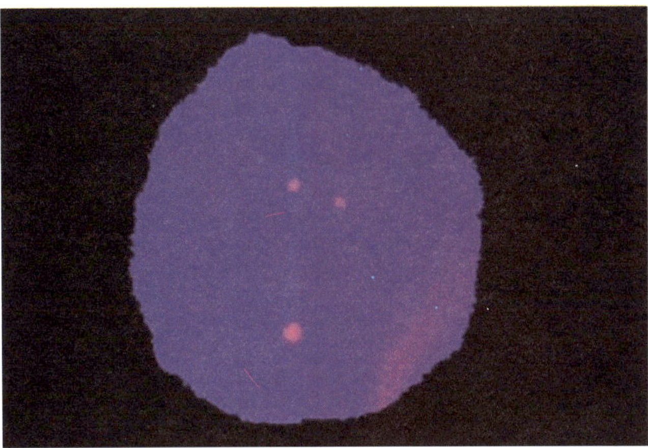

Fig. 25.24: Fluorescence *in situ* hybridization (FISH) using a probe for chromosome 21 on an interphase nucleus. Presence of three signals shows that there are three copies of chromosome 21. FISH based tests are rapid and the results are available on the second day but these tests cannot look at all chromosomes like traditional karyotyping

Fetal imaging: About 50% fetuses with Down syndrome have ultrasonographically detectable abnormalities including nuchal thickening, absent nasal bone, duodenal atresia, and congenital heart defects. Presence of these markers in fetus indicates the need of chromosomal analysis.

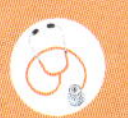

CASE STUDY **Down Syndrome**

A 33-year-old woman underwent an ultrasonography (USG) at 33 weeks of gestation because of clinical impression of polyhydramnios. The USG showed a double bubble appearance characteristic of duodenal atresia. She consulted a pediatric surgeon who told that duodenal atresia is a surgically treatable condition. Clinical geneticist told that 30% of the cases with duodenal atresia have trisomy 21. She was offered rapid prenatal diagnosis by FISH for chromosome 21 on amniotic fluid. She did not opt for prenatal tests. She delivered normally at 35 weeks of gestation and the child showed features of Down syndrome. The child was operated but died on the third day.

What should be done immediately after birth?
Should the karyotype be done and what sample should be used for karyotyping?
When should the family be told of the diagnosis?
What information should be told about the prognosis?
When should the family given information about risk of recurrence?

To find answers read

- For prenatally diagnosed cases of mal formations delivery at a center with good neonatological and surgical facilities should be planned. Immediately after delivery a quick and careful search for other malformations such as tracheoesophageal fistula, anal atresia needs to be done.
- The karyotyping from blood of the baby should be done; preferably immediately as it is necessary to confirm diagnosis and will also helpful for estimating risk of recurrence.

- The family should be told about the diagnosis as soon as possible
- Before duodenal atresia corrective surgery, echocardiography should be done as about half of the neonates with Down syndrome have cardiac anomalies. The family needs to be given information about outcome regarding mental function. The surgery will correct duodenal atresia, but the child is likely to have mild to moderate degree of intellectual disability, which does not have curative treatment.
- Importance of karyotyping for counseling regarding next pregnancy must be mentioned and the family should be given an appointment for genetic counseling at later date.

Think it over!

- The parents of the family are too poor to bear the cost of the surgery for duodenal atresia.
- The child is born in the family after 10 years of infertility.
- The family is not very poor, but the child has complex cardiac anomaly as well.

OTHER AUTOSOMAL ABNORMALITIES

Trisomy 18 and trisomy 13, the other trisomies seen in liveborn, usually do not survive beyond infancy. Parents need to be counseled on the same principles as that for trisomy 21.

- ***Trisomy 18 (Edward syndrome)***. It is characterized by growth retardation, characteristic clenched hands with overlapping fingers, prominent occiput, hypertonia, and cardiac anomalies **(Fig. 25.25A)**.
- ***Trisomy 13 (Patau syndrome)***. The characteristic features include holoprosencephaly (undivided cerebrum), midline cleft lip, cardiac malformations, and polydactyly **(Fig. 25.25B)**.

Structural chromosomal anomalies are rare but detected by karyotyping in children with malformations and developmental delay. Many malformations can now be diagnosed prenatally by ultrasonography; and about 7–10% of these fetuses have chromosomal anomalies. Chromosomal analysis needs to be done for all stillborn babies, and those with intellectual disability or developmental delay. Karyotyping of the parents of children with structural chromosomal abnormality and genetic counseling are essential to prevent recurrence.

SEX CHROMOSOME ABNORMALITIES

Most common anomalies of sex chromosomes are 45,X (Turner syndrome) and 47,XXY (Klinefelter syndrome). These usually present as hypergonadotropic hypogonadism in females and males, respectively. There is no significant intellectual disability.

Turner Syndrome (45,X)

Turner syndrome is associated with monosomy or partial monosomy of X chromosome, resulting in 45,X karyotype.

Other chromosomal abnormalities associated with Turner syndrome are listed in **Table 25.1**. More than 99% of the conceptuses with 45,X karyotype are spontaneously aborted **(Fig. 25.26)**.

In a patient with strong suspicion of Turner syndrome, if the initial karyotype is normal, a second karyotype should be carried out using a different tissue, such as skin (fibroblasts), bladder epithelial cells from a urine sample, or buccal mucosa cells to detect the aberrant cell line (45,X). This happens because of the aberrant cell line dying off with age in the bone marrow while the normal cell line only being present in the peripheral circulation. Analysis of buccal smears for nuclear heterochromatin (Barr bodies) is an inaccurate and outdated test and should be avoided.

Clinical Features

The characteristic features of Turner syndrome include short stature, webbed neck, cubitus valgus (wide carrying angle),

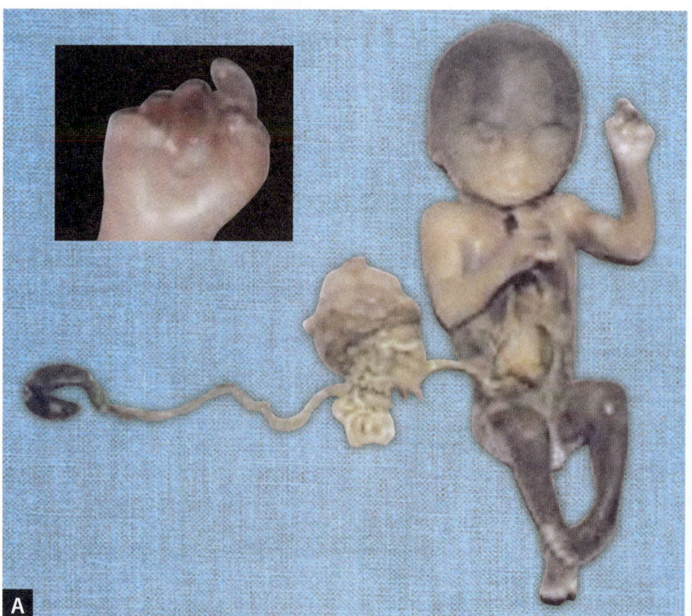

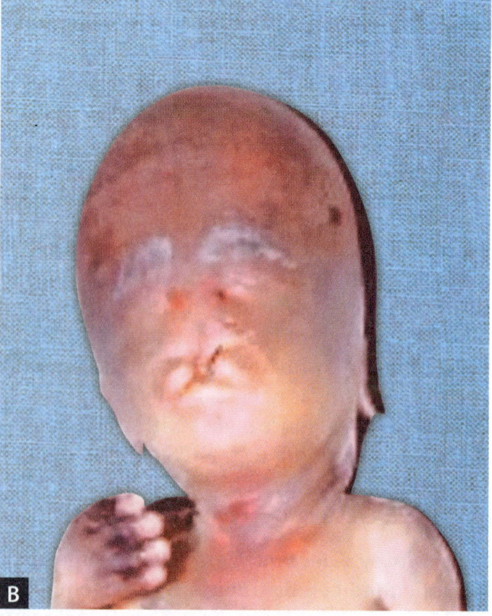

Figs. 25.25A and B: (A) A fetus with trisomy 18. Note the typical overlapping fingers of the clenched hand. The pregnancy was terminated due to prenatal diagnosis of trisomy 18; (B) Midline cleft or premaxillary agenesis seen in association with holoprosencephaly in trisomy 13

Table 25.1	Chromosomal Abnormalities Associated with Turner Syndrome
45,X	Monosomy X
45,X/46,XX	Mosaicism for 45,X and 46,XX cell lines
46,X, i(Xq)	Isochromosome of q arm of X chromosome
46,X,Xp-	Deletion of part of p arm of X chromosome
46,X,Xq-	Deletion of part of q arm of X chromosome
46,X,r(X)	Ring chromosome of X chromosome
46,XY/45,X	Mosaicism for 45,X and 46,XY cell lines (some cases present with Turner-like features while some present with ambiguous genitalia)

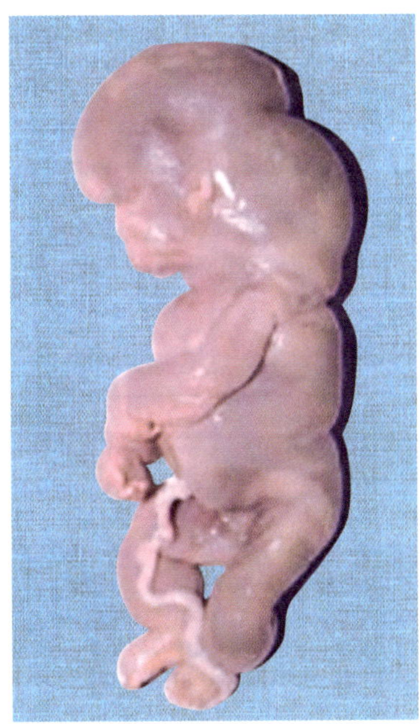

Fig. 25.26: Fetal Turner phenotype. Note a large cystic hygroma at the back of neck, and edema all over body

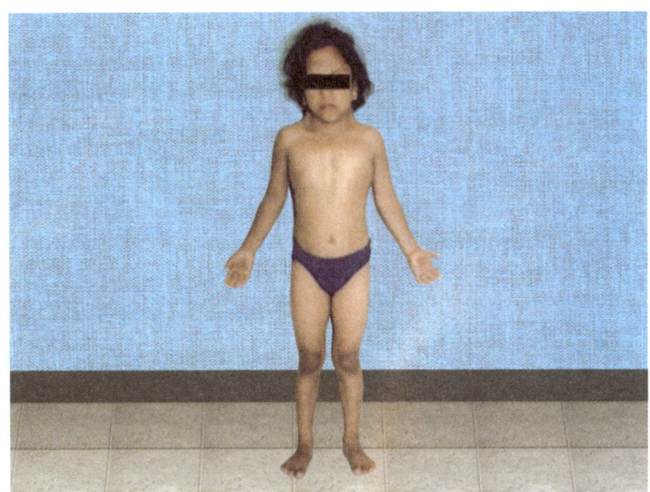

Fig. 25.27: A girl showing characteristic features of Turner syndrome with webbed neck and wide carrying angle

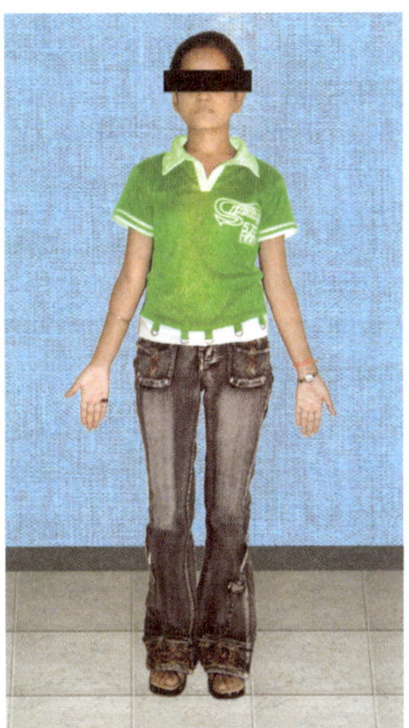

Fig. 25.28: Patient with mosaic Turner syndrome

wide spaced nipple, and short 4th metacarpal and metatarsal **(Fig. 25.27)**. Some cases present as primary amenorrhea at puberty while some as short stature in childhood. Phenotype of a patient with mosaic Turner syndrome may be attenuated **(Fig. 25.28)**. Intellectual disability is not a feature of Turner syndrome though learning deficits in specific areas may be present. Coarctation of aorta is the most frequently associated cardiovascular defect. Other notable features include horse-shoe-shaped kidney, low posterior hairline, nail hypoplasia, and multiple nevi. Turner syndrome in neonates is characterized by lymphedema of hands and feet. However, classical features are present in only 50% cases.

About 10–12% of karyotypes of patients with Turner syndrome may identify a Y chromosome material which increases the risk of gonadoblastoma, a germ cell tumor. Prophylactic removal of the gonads (oophorectomy or salpingo-oophorectomy) is recommended in these patients due to the tumor risk.

Overall mortality in patients with Turner syndrome is increased approximately threefold as compared with the general population. Non-congenital heart disease like coronary artery disease and stroke in older patients are the leading causes followed by congenital cardiovascular anomalies, especially aortic aneurysm.

TREATMENT Turner Syndrome (45,X)

Early diagnosis is useful as growth hormone therapy started from childhood results in gain of about 5–7 cm in final height. Other aspects of management include screening for cardiac and renal anomalies and surveillance for otitis media, hypertension, hypothyroidism, and hormone replacement therapy for development of secondary sexual characters, and establishment of menstruation. Most of the cases of Turner syndrome have infertility. Fertility may be possible by assisted reproductive techniques with donor ova.

Klinefelter Syndrome (47,XXY)

Klinefelter syndrome is the most common cause of primary hypogonadism in males, mostly due to an extra X chromosome in an XY male (47,XXY). The extra X chromosome results from maternal or paternal meiotic non-disjunction of the X chromosome during gametogenesis. About 10% of patients have mosaicism (47,XXY/46,XY) with a 47,XXY cell line in some tissues and a normal cell line in others. Rarely there can be three or more than three X chromosomes which are associated with a more severe phenotype as compared to those with 47,XXY karyotypes.

Neonates with Klinefelter syndrome may present with micropenis (<1.9 cm for neonate) or clinodactyly, hypospadias, or cryptorchidism. Majority of the patients are identified because of delayed or diminished puberty, gynecomastia, or infertility. Prepubertal boys are usually normal. Adults have tall stature, long legs, and female distribution of fat **(Fig. 25.29)**. Facial hair may be less. The size of the penis may be small. Small testes and oligospermia or azoospermia are constant features. Intellectual disability is unusual though learning disabilities are common.

Due to progressive fibrosis and destruction of both the seminiferous tubules and the Leydig cells there is decreased production of both sperm and testosterone. Treatment with testosterone is useful. Surgery may be necessary for gynecomastia. Up to 50 percent of males with Klinefelter syndrome have focal spermatogenesis that can be retrieved by micro-TESE for use in assisted reproductive techniques such as intracytoplasmic injection of sperm into an ovum. Counseling and support from family is necessary to improve self-image.

Microdeletion Syndrome—Prader–Willi Syndrome

Prader–Willi syndrome (PWS) is characterized by severe hypotonia, feeding difficulties in early infancy followed by binge eating and obesity in childhood. Motor milestones and language development is delayed in these children along with some impairment of cognitive ability. Other features include short stature, small hands, and feet, hypopigmentation, hypogonadotropic hypogonadism, and behavior problems such as stubbornness, temper tantrums, and excessive skin picking.

The basic genetic defect in PWS is lack of expression of the Prader–Willi critical region (on cytoband 15q11.2) by the paternally inherited chromosome 15. This can happen by any one of the various mechanisms listed below:

- Microdeletion of paternal copy of the cytoband 15q11.2-q13—Approximately 70% of individuals with PWS have this cause and it can be detected using fluorescence in situ hybridization (FISH) testing or chromosomal microarray (CMA).
- Uniparental disomy of the maternal chromosome 15 and imprinting center defect of the paternal chromosome together these account for 20–30% of all cases of PWS. The mechanism of UPD and imprinting has been discussed in Section 25.2.

One test which can detect all the above disease-causing mechanisms is Methylation-specific multiplex ligation-dependent probe amplification (MS-MLPA) which is a technique to detect epigenetic alterations in genes.

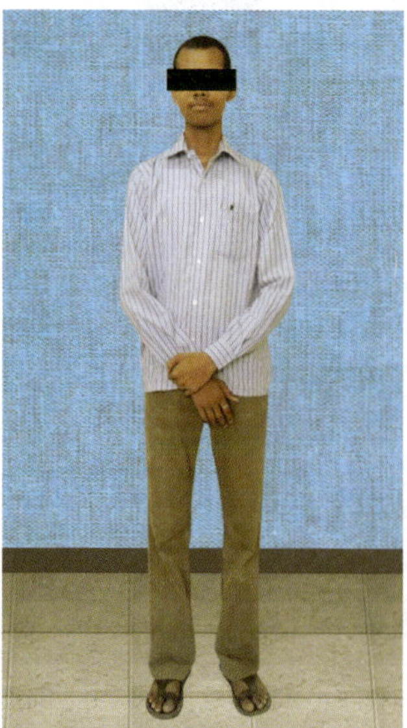

Fig. 25.29: Adult patient with Klinefelter syndrome

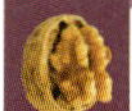

IN A NUTSHELL

Chromosomal Disorders

1. Chromosome abnormalities account for about 50% of all spontaneous miscarriages in the first trimester and their incidence at birth is 0.5–1.0%.
2. Down syndrome is the most common autosomal chromosomal syndrome with a strong association with advanced maternal age. About 95% of all cases are caused by non-disjunction resulting in trisomy 21. Translocation accounts for 4–5% of Down syndrome and mosaic Down syndrome constitute 1%. Chromosomal studies are necessary in all cases to identify unbalanced familial Robertsonian translocations, which are associated with higher risk of recurrence.
3. The most common indications for prenatal testing are advanced maternal age and an increased risk predicted from screening. Other indications include a previous, or family history of a chromosomal or single-gene disorder, or an abnormal finding on ultrasound.
4. Prenatal screening can be carried out by non-invasive methods such as maternal serum assays combined with nuchal translucency for Down syndrome, and ultrasonography for structural abnormalities.
5. Non-invasive prenatal testing on cell-free fetal DNA in the maternal circulation primarily looks for Down syndrome, trisomy 18, trisomy 13, and the sex chromosome. The accuracy of the test varies by disorder.
6. Sex chromosome abnormalities include Klinefelter syndrome (47,XXY), Turner syndrome (45,X), the XYY syndrome (47,XYY), and the triple X syndrome (47,XXX). In all of these conditions, intelligence is either normal or only mildly impaired.

Allyse M, Minear MA, Berson E, et al. Non-invasive prenatal testing: a review of international implementation and challenges. Int J Womens Health. 2015;7:113-26.
Committee opinion no. 640: cell-free DNA screening for fetal aneuploidy. Obstet Gynecol. 2015;126(3):e31-7.
Davis SM, Teerlink C, Lynch JA, et al. Prevalence, morbidity, and mortality of men with sex chromosome aneuploidy in the million veteran program cohort. JAMA Netw Open. 2024;7:e244113.
Emery and Rimoin's Principles and Practice of Medical Genetics and Genomics. In: Reed E. Pyeritz, Bruce R. Korf, Wayne W. Grody (Eds.). Clinical Principles and Applications, 7th edition Elsevier; 2018.
Evans M. Prenatal Diagnosis, 1st edition. McGraw-Hill Professional; 2006.
Gardner RJM, Amor DJ. Gardner and Sutherland's Chromosome Abnormalities and Genetic Counseling, 5th edition. New York: Oxford Monographs on Medical Genetics; 2018.
Jones KL. Down syndrome. In: Smith's (Ed.). Recognizable Patterns of Human Malformation, 6th edition. Elsevier Saunders, Philadelphia 2006. p. 7.
Odibo A, Krantz D. Prenatal screening and diagnosis, an issue of clinics in laboratory medicine. In: Pereira SE, Soria J. (Eds). Handbook of Prenatal Diagnosis. Methods, Issues and Health Impacts. Nova Science Publishers Inc.; 2010.
Swauger S, Backeljauw P, Hornung L, et al. Age at and indication for diagnosis of Turner syndrome in the pediatric population. Am J Med Genet A 2021;185:3411.

25.4 Molecular Diagnosis of Genetic Disorders *PE 29.1, PE 29.4, PE 29.5*

INTRODUCTION

Recent advances in ability to manipulate DNA have resulted in identification of genetic defects of >3,000 single gene phenotypes and the numbers are ever increasing. The newer techniques to study DNA and automation of techniques have made the identification of the causative genes for monogenic disorders an easy task. DNA based diagnosis has become quick and has been increasingly used in clinical practice. The most important molecular technique is polymerase chain reaction (PCR). PCR makes multiple copies of small DNA segment/segments in a test tube on principles similar to DNA replication occurring *in vivo*.

Most of the DNA-based techniques are based on various modifications of PCR and the principle of hybridization of complementary DNA strands (A with T and G with C). Accurate sequencing of DNA segments is possible. **Figure 25.30** shows a chromatogram of Sanger sequencing of HBB gene done for mutation detection in patients with beta thalassemia. These techniques are used to identify disease causing mutation/mutations using patient's blood sample or even cells from buccal cavity mouthwash.

POLYMERASE CHAIN REACTION

This basic tool in molecular diagnostics is used to make multiple copies of a DNA fragment whose sequence is known. Mostly DNA fragments up to 1 kb are easily amplified by PCR and a long-range PCR can amplify 20–30 kb of DNA fragment. Amplification is achieved by a series of three steps:

1. ***Denaturation:*** Double-stranded DNA templates are heated to separate the strands.
2. ***Annealing:*** A set of two oligonucleotide molecules (approximately 20 bp length) called primers/amplimers, bind with the complementary DNA sequence on the flanking regions of the single stranded target DNA
3. ***Extension:*** DNA polymerase enzyme, in the presence of deoxynucleotide triphosphates extends the 3′ end of each primer along the template strands. These steps are repeated ("cycled") 25–35 times to exponentially produce exact copies of the target DNA **(Fig. 25.31)**.

Various modifications of the basic PCR, designed as per the requisite experimental application are available. For example:

- ***Real time PCR:*** DNA amplification is detected in real time with the help of fluorescence, the intensity of which is proportional to the number of amplified DNA, thus quantifying the original target DNA used.
- ***Multiplex PCR:*** In this type of PCR, multiple sequences are amplified simultaneously, hence many target regions can be sequenced in the same run.
- ***Nested PCR:*** This type of PCR reduces the non-specific binding of the primers and its amplification.
- ***ARMS (amplification-refractory mutation system) PCR:*** This method detects any mutation involving single nucleotide changes or small deletions.
- ***Reverse Transcriptase PCR (RT-PCR):*** This technique amplifies the RNA after converting it into single stranded complimentary DNA using reverse transcriptase enzyme.
- ***Droplet Digital PCR (ddPCR):*** This is a third generation quantitative PCR where the reaction happens in nanoliter sized water in oil emulsion droplets and enables precise identification and quantification of the nucleic acid sample.

SEQUENCING-BASED METHODS

Deoxyribonucleic acid sequencing is the process of determining sequence of the four nucleotides, viz., adenine, guanine, thymine, and cytosine, arranged in a DNA fragment.

Sanger Sequencing

This is the classical, gold standard method of DNA sequencing, discovered by the English biochemist Frederick Sanger in the 1970s. It is based on the concept of chain termination for which fluorescent ddNTPs (dideoxynucleotides, N = A, T, G, or C) are utilized to prevent the addition of another nucleotide. The

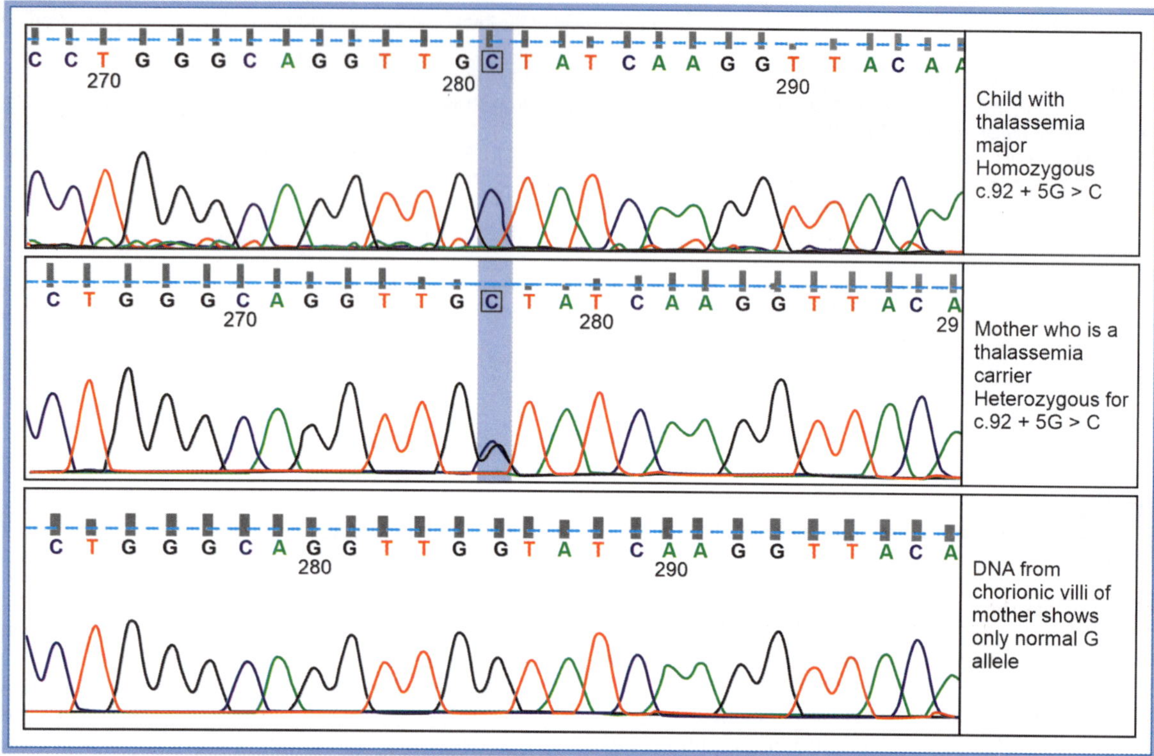

Fig. 25.30: Mutations in *β-globin* gene in a family with thalassemia major

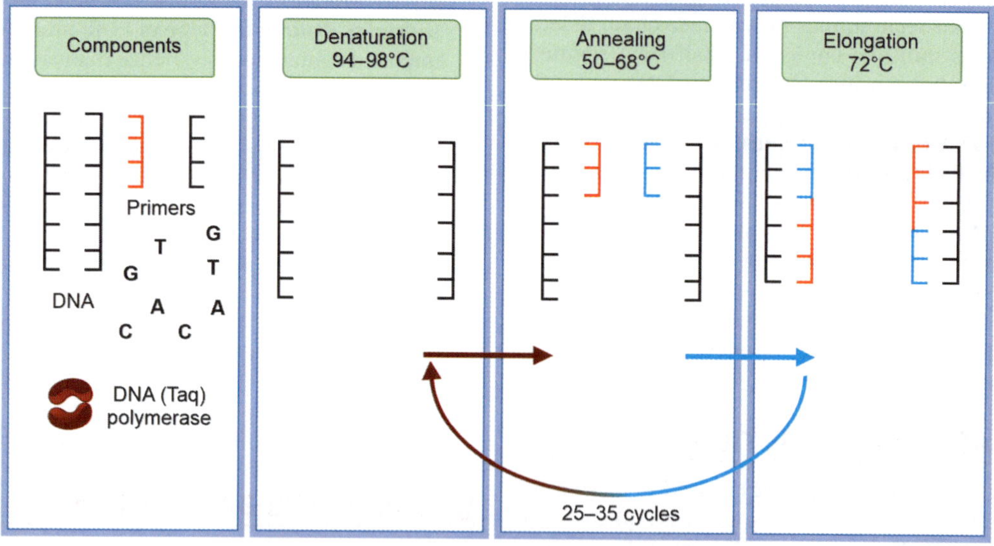

Fig. 25.31: Polymerase chain reaction (PCR) cycle

reaction products are separated by capillary electrophoresis to obtain a ladder of DNA sequences of different lengths. Software finally generates a chromatograph showing the fluorescent peak of each labeled fragment and the mutation can be highlighted. Sanger sequencing is commonly used to screen mutations where there is a high suspicion of a mutation being present in a known gene. *Example*: Sanger sequencing of the HBB gene where the phenotype is undisputed, the gene to be tested is known, and the length of the gene is small.

Pyrosequencing

Like Sanger sequencing, pyrosequencing is also based on the principle of sequencing by synthesis. Chemiluminescent signals are detected with addition of each nucleotide. This is a rapid technology to detect and quantify DNA mutation.

Example: Detection and quantification of *KRAS* gene mutation in colorectal cancer patients.

Next Generation Sequencing (NGS)

This is a high throughput method of DNA sequencing. The scalability and multiplexing associated makes it a cost-effective and rapid technique for DNA sequencing. The basic steps involved in this technology are:

1. A sequencing library is prepared by fragmenting the DNA into 100–800 bp length double stranded segments and ligating them with technology specific adaptors and bar codes.
2. Clonal amplification of the "sequence library" is done after its attachment on a solid state like beads in nano well or flow cell.
3. Deoxyribonucleic acid library is sequenced by synthesis, i.e., individual bases are read as they grow along the polymerized strand. An optical or electrical detection is utilized to determine the incorporated base.
4. ***Data analyzation:*** Enormous volume of complex data is generated in an NGS cycle, and its interpretation relies considerably on a robust bioinformatics expertise. Data analysis involves conversion of raw signals from detectors to digitalized form, generation of quality scores for each read, filtration/trimming of sequences based on poor quality scores, alignment of the sequences to a reference assembly and finally variant calling.

With the NGS technology, multiple genes can be sequenced simultaneously through disease specific panels, whole exome sequencing (WES), or whole genome sequencing (WGS) approaches.

Whole Exome Sequencing (WES)

Whole exome sequencing involves NGS based method of sequencing the whole exome (coding regions of all the genes) of an individual to identify disease causing mutations. WES is the method of choice for disorders with heterogeneous etiologies such as retinitis pigmentosa and sensorineural deafness, etc. or when the clinical features cannot suggest a causative gene. WES is available in India and the cost is getting affordable to many families. The possibility of identifying the causative mutation in a patient with a monogenic disorder varies from 30–80% depending on the phenotype.

Whole Genome Sequencing (WGS)

Based on NGS platform, the entire genome (involving coding, non-coding and mtDNA) is sequenced. This method enables detection of all the variant types such as single nucleotide variants, insertion-deletion, structural variants, and copy number variants. WGS is commonly used in cancer genetics, regulatory DNA analysis, precision medicine and in deciphering rare, complex disorders.

HETEROGENEITY

Allelic Heterogeneity

The mutation detection confirms the diagnosis, but it should be noted that *inability to detect mutation does not rule out the disease in question.* This is because most of the diseases are known to be caused by hundreds of mutations (allelic heterogeneity—different alleles at a locus giving rise to clinically similar phenotype). Some mutations are unique to a patient or a family. So, the available tests may not be able to detect all mutations, especially in non-coding regions, promoters, etc. Now it has been observed that changes in DNA sequence far away from a gene can also affect the expression of the gene and cause a disease.

Genetic Heterogeneity

Some phenotypes are caused by more than one gene. The examples are retinitis pigmentosa, spinocerebellar ataxia, limb girdle myopathy, cardiomyopathies, and primary microcephaly. This is known as genetic heterogeneity (defects in genes at different loci giving rise to a clinically similar phenotype). Hence, mutation detection is not an easy task for many disorders.

Some of the diseases for which there is no diagnostic test other than mutation detection are spinal muscular atrophy, Huntington chorea, fragile X mental retardation, spinocerebellar ataxia of various types, Charcot-Marie-Tooth disease, and hereditary spastic paraplegia.

For other diseases where a confident diagnostic modality in the form of a biochemical test, imaging, or any other investigations is available, mutation detection may not be necessary for the diagnosis of the patient but is important for carrier detection and prenatal diagnosis.

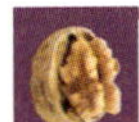

IN A NUTSHELL

DNA Diagnosis of Genetic Disorders

1. Polymerase chain reaction (PCR) is fundamental to many molecular tests used in research and diagnostics in the field of genetics. Within hours, more than a million copies of a gene or target deoxyribonucleic acid (DNA) can be amplified from a patient's DNA sample. The PCR product may be analyzed for the presence of a pathogenic mutation, gene rearrangement, or infectious agent.
2. Sanger sequencing is the gold standard method of DNA sequencing.
3. Next-generation sequencing is a multiplex test that allows simultaneous testing for all genes in which mutations are known to cause a monogenic disorder. This technique can be used to sequence a particular disease related panel of genes (e.g., Genodermatosis panel, deafness panel or a myopathy panel) or about 6,000 disease causing OMIM genes (Mendeliome/clinical exome), or all the exons in the genome (Whole Exome Sequencing—WES), or the entire genome including exons and introns (Whole Genome Sequencing—WGS).

Deciphering Developmental Disorders Study. Large-scale discovery of novel genetic causes of developmental disorders. Nature. 2015;519(7542):223-8.

deLigt J, Willemsen MH, van Bon BW, et al. Diagnostic exome sequencing in persons with severe intellectual disability. N Engl J Med. 2012;367:1921-9.

Elles R, Wallace A. Molecular diagnosis of genetic disease, 3rd edition. Clifton, NJ: Humana Press; 2010.

Strachan T, Read AP. Human Molecular Genetics, 4th edition. London: Garland Science; 2011.

25.5 Treatment of Genetic Disorders

PE 29.1, PE 29.4, PE 29.5

INTRODUCTION

Genetic disorders involve all systems of the body and have varying severity. Available treatments and outcomes vary greatly. The treatment may be as easy as avoiding some drugs in *glucose-6-phosphate dehydrogenase* (G6PD) deficiency or may be difficult as bone marrow transplantation for thalassemia major.

Successful surgical treatment of many malformations has been available for many decades and now fetal surgery for repair of defects such as diaphragmatic hernia, neural tube defects is possible.

At present there is no treatment for neurodegenerative disorders, myopathies, and conditions with intellectual disability. For them, the supportive treatment and rehabilitation plays an important role. Various successful strategies used for treatment of genetic disorder are discussed here:

- ***Augmentation of low level of protein:*** Phenobarbitone in Crigler–Najjar syndrome type II, desmopressin (DDAVP) in mild hemophilia A.
- ***Replacement of the deficient protein or enzyme:*** Antihemophilic factor VIII for hemophilia A, adenosine deaminase for immunodeficiency; enzyme replacement therapy for Gaucher disease, mucopolysaccharidosis I (Hurler disease), Pompe disease, and Fabry disease.
- ***Enhancement of function of a deficient protein:*** Biotin in biotinidase deficiency, pyridoxine in homocystinuria, high doses of vitamin D in vitamin D resistant rickets.
- ***Dietary restriction*** of milk in galactosemia, phenylalanine in phenylketonuria.
- ***Drug therapy:*** Cholestyramine in hypercholesterolemia, penicillamine in Wilson disease.
- ***Drug avoidance:*** Primaquine in G6PD deficiency and phenobarbitone in acute intermittent porphyria.
- ***Treatment of phenotype:*** Surgical treatment of malformation, blood transfusions in thalassemia major or sickle cell disease.
- ***Organ transplantation:*** Kidney transplantation in polycystic kidney disease, bone marrow transplantation in thalassemia major and lysosomal storage disorders such as mucopolysaccharidosis.
- ***Organ removal:*** Splenectomy in hereditary spherocytosis, colectomy in familial adenomatous polyposis.

ENZYME REPLACEMENT THERAPY (ERT)

Enzyme replacement therapy has revolutionized the treatment of lysosomal storage disorders (LSD). LSDs are rare disorders of various lysosomal enzyme defects, which result in accumulation of its non-degraded products like sphingolipids, carbohydrates, glycogen, glycoproteins, and mucopolysaccharides; most of them resulting in a neurodegenerative disease (*See* Online Content of Chapter 25). ERT involves periodic intravenous infusion of biosynthetic wild type enzyme which reaches the lysosomal compartment and replaces the mutant enzyme.

ERT is currently available for Gaucher, Neiman Pick A, B and A/B. Fabry, Krabbe, and Pompe diseases, and different mucopolysaccharidoses MPSs (e.g., MPS I, II, and IV). Recombinant human acid sphingomyelinase for Neiman Pick type C1 disease is the latest addition to this list. High cost is a major limiting factor with the ERTs.

ANTISENSE OLIGONUCLEOTIDE THERAPY (ASO)

This mode of treatment of genetic disorders is based on the concept of using synthetic oligonucleotides to modulate RNA function. Oligonucleotides are short sequences (10–50 bp) of single or double stranded DNA or RNA molecules.

Some examples of approved antisense oligonucleotide (ASOs) for the various disorders are listed in **Table 25.2** respective targeted gene is mentioned in parenthesis.

GENE THERAPY

With knowledge of gene defects and ability to manipulate DNA (recombinant DNA technology) correction of defective gene or replacing defective gene is now possible. A recombinant DNA is a fusion product of a viral vector DNA and a foreign DNA (a functioning copy of DNA for encoding the normal gene product in the host). This technology is commonly employed in the formation of various biosynthetic products such as human insulin, growth hormone, factor VIII, and factor IX, α-galactosidase enzyme for Fabry disease and hepatitis B vaccine.

Gene therapy implies the delivery of a nucleotide sequence into a patient's body with the aim of disease treatment. Gene therapy has been successful in treating monogenic immunodeficiency disorder and has shown preliminary success

Table 25.2 Antisense Oligonucleotide Therapy

ASO	*Disorder*	*Gene*
Nusinersen	Spinal muscular atrophy	*SMN2*
Eteplirsen	Duchenne muscular dystrophy	*DMD*
Fomiversan	Cytomegalovirus retinitis secondary to AIDS	*CMV*-immediate early-2
Pegabtinib	Age-related macular degeneration of the retina	*VEGF*
Mipomersen	Familial hypercholesterolemia	*ApoB-100*
Defibrotide	Hepatic veno-occlusive disease	Nonspecific proteins
Patisiran	Hereditary transthyretin amyloidosis	*TTR*

in thalassemia major and hemophilia B. Gene therapy has also shown promise for many more diseases including cancers, autoimmune and infectious disorders. Few more genetic disorders for which US Food and Drug Administration (FDA) gene therapy is currently available are listed here, along with the therapeutic product.

- RPE65 mutation induced blindness: *Luxturna*
- Chimeric antigen receptor T cell therapy-CAR T-cell products: *Kymriah*
- Spinal muscular atrophy: *Zolgensma*
- Congenital factor VIII deficiency: *Roctavian*
- Sickle cell disease: *Casgevy*

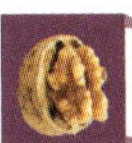

IN A NUTSHELL

Treatment of Genetic Disorders

1. Most genetic disorders cannot be cured using conventional methods of treatment. Many inborn errors of metabolism are amenable to therapy by various approaches such as diet modification (e.g., phenylketonuria), hormone replacement (e.g., congenital adrenal hyperplasia), vitamin supplementation (e.g., Biotinidase deficiency).
2. Recombinant deoxyribonucleic acid (DNA) technique is used to biosynthesize the missing or defective enzyme in many storage disorders.
3. Ribonucleic acid (RNA) modification therapy targets mRNA, either by suppressing mRNA levels or by correcting/adding new function to the mRNA.
4. Synthetic Antisense Oligonucleotides (ASOs), a type of RNA modification therapy, are used to modulate the expression of disease associated genes. Spinal muscular atrophy (SMA) and Duchenne muscular dystrophy (DMD) are prototype genetic disorders where ASO therapy has been established and is widely used.
5. Gene therapy is the therapeutic delivery of genetic material into a patient's cells as a drug to treat disease. It should fulfill certain prerequisites such as the gene involved must be fully characterized, the particular cell type or tissue to be targeted must be identified, an efficient, reliable, and safe vector system for steady expression of the introduced gene has to be developed, and the safety and effectiveness of the particular modality of gene therapy has to be demonstrated. Gene therapy is still in nascent stage and is not widely available.
6. Germline gene therapy is ethically unacceptable worldwide.

Aartsma-Rus A, van Ommen G-JB. Progress in therapeutic antisense applications for neuromuscular disease. Eur J Hum. Genet. 2010: 18:146-53.
Brown BD, Naldini L. Exploiting and antagonizing microRNA regulation for therapeutic and experimental applications. Nat Rev Genet. 2009;10:578-85.
Campeau PM, Scriver CR, Mitchell JJ. A 25-year longitudinal analysis of treatment efficacy in inborn errors of metabolism. Mol Genet Metab. 2008;95:11-6.
Dietz HC. New therapeutic approaches to Mendelian disorders. N Engl J Med. 2010;363:852-63.
Goldstein DB, Tate SK, Sisodiya SM. Pharmacogenetics goes genomic. Nat Rev Genet. 2003;4:937-47.
McCune JM, Kiem HP. Extending gene medicines to all in need. N Engl J Med. 2024;390:1721.
Pennisi E. The CRISPR craze. Science. 2013;341:833-6.
Valle D, Beaudet AL, Vogelstein B, et al. (Eds.). (2014). The online metabolic and molecular bases of inherited disease. [online] Available from: https://ommbid.mhmedical.com/book.aspx?bookID=2709 [Last accessed August, 2025].
Yamanaka S. Induced pluripotent stem cells: Past, present and future. Cell Stem Cell. 2012;10:678-84.

25.6 Genetic Counseling

PE 29.1, PE 29.3, PE 29.4, PE 29.5

INTRODUCTION

Familial nature of the diseases, difficult treatment, and poor outcome for many genetic disorders make genetic counseling an important part of management of patient and families with genetic disorders.

DEFINITION

Genetic counseling is defined as "a communicative process which deals with human problems associated with occurrence or recurrence of a genetic disorder in a family." It helps the family to understand the diagnosis, treatment, prognosis of the disease, implications of genetic etiology in the form of risk of recurrence and ways to prevent the recurrence by way of prenatal diagnosis.

INDICATIONS

All clinical presentations suggestive of genetic disorders need to be investigated for etiology even if the disorder appears to be untreatable. Congenital malformation, stillbirths, chromosomal disorders, known monogenic disorders, intellectual disability, regression of milestones, recurrent fetal losses, and familial cancers are the indications for genetic counseling.

THE PROCESS

The person who asks for genetic counseling is called *"consultand"* and the one who provides the counseling is known as *"counselor"*. The counselor needs to have knowledge of basic genetics, latest information about the disease in concern and should have good communication skills. Accurate etiological diagnosis is the first and one of the most important steps of genetic counseling. The genetic counseling should be nondirective and non-judgmental. The decisions regarding planning of pregnancy, prenatal diagnosis, and termination of pregnancy need to be taken by the family and not to be advised or forced by the counselor.

The fundamental principles of medical ethics, apply to the process of genetic counseling as well. These are:

- ***Autonomy***—To extend respect for the individual's privacy, to acknowledge the importance of informed consent, and to maintain confidentiality.
- ***Beneficence***—Intent to do good and therefore to act in the best interests of the patient.
- ***Non-maleficence***—Intent to not do any harm (i.e., not to leave the patient in a worse condition than before treatment).
- ***Justice***—To impart fairness for the patient in terms of the resources available, equity of access, and opportunity.

POPULATION-BASED PREVENTION OF GENETIC DISORDERS

Genetic counseling offers an option of prevention of a genetic disorder in the family. But usually this is done after diagnosis of one individual with a genetic disorder in the family. Population-based preventive programs aim at primary prevention of genetic disorder or birth of the first child of a genetic disorder. This can be done at different levels:

- ***Food fortification*** with folic acid for prevention of neural tube defects.
- ***Identification of carriers*** of monogenic disorders such as thalassemia major, cystic fibrosis and Tay-Sachs disease by testing all couples or pregnant women and offering them genetic counseling and prenatal diagnosis.
- ***Screening of all pregnancies*** for common genetic disorders such as Down syndrome and neural tube defects.
- ***Neonatal screening*** for metabolic disorders in which early diagnosis helps to provide treatment to prevent mental retardation (congenital hypothyroidism, congenital adrenal hyperplasia, biotinidase deficiency, phenylketonuria, galactosemia) or improve outcome (sickle cell disease).

Prenatal Diagnosis

Prevention of birth of a child with genetic and/or congenital disorders with poor prognosis involves termination of pregnancy when the fetus is found to be affected with a malformation or a genetic disorder. It allows an option of pregnancy and birth of child free of disorder to many couples who would otherwise refrain from planning further pregnancy for the fear of recurrence of genetic disease.

Prenatal diagnosis of congenital malformations has attained very good sensitivity and specificity due to high resolution ultrasonographic machines. Other methods of prenatal diagnosis involve obtaining fetal sample by chorionic villous sampling (10–12 weeks) or amniocentesis (16 weeks or later). These sampling procedures are done under ultrasound guidance and do not cause harm to the fetus. The various tests that can be done on these samples include DNA based tests for monogenic disorder, biochemical tests such as enzyme assays for the diagnosis of metabolic disorders and chromosomal analysis. These tests have very minimal error rates of 1% or less.

Neonatal Screening

For adopting a screening program for a disorder, the prevalence data in the population should be available. Availability of a sensitive and simple test is another requisite for any screening program. Disorders chosen for neonatal screening include those where early intervention markedly changes the outcome.

Neonatal screening for hypothyroidism appears to be the most important and cost-effective strategy for prevention of treatable intellectual disability. The incidence of congenital hypothyroidism in India is reported to be around one per 2,000 and treatment is easy and cheap. This stresses the need and feasibility of starting universal neonatal screening for hypothyroidism on a national level. The other disorders to be considered for newborn screening in India are congenital adrenal hyperplasia, biotinidase deficiency, galactosemia, and sickle cell disease. Screening for phenylketonuria is very rewarding but the special diets needed are very costly and implementation of neonatal screening for phenylketonuria in India may not be feasible at present.

The Future

In future, population-based programs for common genetic mutations such as factor V Leiden and hemochromatosis gene mutations may come up to identify individuals at risk of venous thrombosis and hemochromatosis respectively. The mutation carriers at risk of developing the disease can be provided prophylactic therapy.

The diseases for which prenatal diagnosis by DNA based tests are commonly available include thalassemia major, Duchenne muscular dystrophy, hemophilia A, hemophilia B, spinal muscular atrophy, fragile X mental retardation, cystic fibrosis, epidermolysis bullosa, albinism, and ichthyosis. For any monogenic disorder, availability of DNA based test should be looked for from recent literature and internet resources. Now preimplantation genetic diagnosis (PGD) is possible, which involves biopsy of the blastocyst and doing molecular diagnosis of a previously known variant—single gene/structural chromosomal variant or chromosomal aneuploidy. The embryos negative for mutation are implanted to ensure a disease-free fetus is born. Feasibility of prenatal diagnosis using cell-free fetal DNA in maternal plasma has also been successfully shown and in future the invasive tests to collect fetal samples may not be necessary.

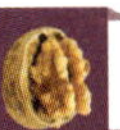

IN A NUTSHELL

Genetic Counseling

1. Almost all aspects of clinical genetics are by and large influenced by ethical considerations.
2. Prenatal screening and diagnosis, predictive testing in childhood, genetic testing in the extended family, confidentiality, consent, privacy, and disclosure of information, are some particularly difficult scenarios in clinical genetics.
3. Population screening involves offering genetic testing to all members of a particular population, with the objectives of preventing later ill-health and should be associated with pretest and post-test counseling. Population screening programs for carriers of β-thalassemia have resulted in a major fall in the incidence of births of affected children in countries such as Cyprus, Iran, and Saudi Arabia.
4. A good screening test has a high sensitivity and specificity.
5. Prenatal screening is routinely available for common chromosomal aneuploidies and is based on ultrasound examination at approximately 12- and 20-weeks' gestation and the biochemical screen. A positive screening result needs confirmation by invasive procedures or non-invasive method (Non-Invasive Prenatal Screening—NIPS).
6. Newborn screening, initially introduced for phenylketonuria has now expanded to incorporate a wide range of metabolic conditions as well as functional screening such as hearing, pulse oximetry and retinopathy of prematurity.

Agarwal M, Joshi K, Bhatia V, et al. Feasibility study of an outreach program of newborn screening in Uttar Pradesh. Indian J Pediatr. 2015;82: 427-32.

Allanson JE, Cunniff C, Hoyme HE, et al. Elements of morphology: standard terminology for the head and face. Am J Med Genet. 2009;149A:6-28.

Battista RN, Blancquaert I, Laberge AM, et al. Genetics in health care: an overview of current and emerging models. Public Health Genomics. 2012;15:34-45.

Booth CH, Bobby Gaspa HB, Thrasher AT. Gene therapy for primary immunodeficiency. Curr Opin Pediatr. 2011;23:659-66.

Carey JC, Cohen MM Jr, Curry C, et al. Elements of morphology: Standard terminology for the lips, mouth, and oral region. Am J Med Genet. 2009;149A:77-92.

Cassidy SB, Allanson JE. Management of Genetic Syndromes, 3rd edition. Philadelphia: Willey Blackwell; 2010.

Falk MJ, Robin NH. The primary care physician's approach to congenital anomalies. Prim Care Clin Office Pract. 2004;31:605-19.

Fernhoff PM. Newborn screening for genetic disorders. Pediatr Clin N Am. 2009;56:505-13.

Frías JL, Davenport ML; Committee on Genetics and Section on Endocrinology. Health supervision for children with Turner syndrome. Pediatrics. 2003;111:692-702.

Gekas J, Vallée M, Castonguay L, et al. Clinical validity of karyotyping for the diagnosis of chromosomal imbalance following array comparative genomic hybridisation. J Med Genet. 2011;48:851-5.

Ginsburg D. Genetics and genomics to the clinic: along road ahead. Cell. 2011;147:17-9.

Hendriksz CJ, Berger KI, Lampe C, et al. Health-related quality of life in mucopolysaccharidosis: looking beyond biomedical issues. Orphanet J Rare Dis. 2016;11(1):119.

Koene S, Smeitink J. Mitochondrial medicine. J Inherit Metab Dis. 2001;34:247-8.

Srivastava A, Shaji RV. Cure for thalassemia major-from allogeneic hematopoietic stem cell transplantation to gene therapy. Haematologica. 2017;102(2):214-23.

Stark Z, Tan TY, Chong B, et al. A prospective evaluation of whole-exome sequencing as a first-tier molecular test in infants with suspected monogenic disorders. Genet Med. 2016;18(11):1090-96.

van Karnebeek CD, Stockler S. Treatable inborn errors of metabolism causing intellectual disability: a systematic literature review. Mol Genet Metab. 2012;105(3):368-81.

Yang CF, Yang CC, Liao HC, et al. Very Early treatment for infantile-onset Pompe disease contributes to better outcomes. J Pediatr. 2016;169:174-80.e1.

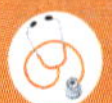

CASE STUDY Genetic Counseling for Thalassemia Major

A couple with a 2-year-old child with thalassemia major has approached you for genetic counseling. The child was diagnosed as thalassemia major at 5 months of age when he presented with severe anemia (hemoglobin of 4 g/dL) and Splenomegaly. The investigations showed fetal hemoglobin of 90%. The father's hemoglobin, mean corpuscular volume (MCV) and hemoglobin A_2 were 13 g/dL, 64 femtoliters (fL), and 4.5% respectively. Corresponding values for the mother were 10.5 g/dL, 56 fL and 5%, respectively.

What is the risk that the next child of the couple also has thalassemia major?
What can be done to avoid the recurrence of the disease in the family?
What investigations are needed prior to prenatal diagnosis?

To find the answers read:
Thalassemia major is a serious disorder manifesting as severe anemia during infancy. The treatment is bone marrow transplantation or lifelong regular 2 to 3 weekly blood transfusions. Thalassemia major occurs due to homozygosity for mutated beta-globin gene. More than 300 mutations occurring in different parts of beta globin gene are known to give rise to beta-thalassemia. Each family may have any one or two of these mutations and clinical manifestations or fetal hemoglobin level does not give any clue to the mutation present in the affected child. Mostly the beta-thalassemia mutations are point mutations, i.e., substitution of a base by other: e.g., IVS 1—5 G to C (guanine at the 5th place of first intervening sequence is replaced by cytosine) is commonly identified mutation in India. Fifteen common mutations account for most of the cases of beta-thalassemia in India. To test for the mutation, all three exons of the beta globin gene need to be sequenced. The different types of mutations give rise to varying degree of decrease in beta globin synthesis. Mutation which lead to complete shutdown of synthesis of beta globins is called β° (beta zero) mutation and causes severe type of thalassemia. The mutations which lead to decrease in synthesis of beta globin are known as beta plus (β^{+}).

As the disease is inherited in an autosomal recessive manner, the parents of a child with homozygous beta-thalassemia are obligate carriers. The carriers of beta-thalassemia (also known as thalassemia minor or thalassemia trait) are usually asymptomatic. They can be diagnosed by presence of microcytosis (MCV <80 fL) and hemoglobin A_2 more than 3.5%. The chance of recurrence of thalassemia major in the siblings of a child with thalassemia major is 25% or 1 in 4. Same is the case when both the spouses are detected to be heterozygous for beta-thalassemia mutations, i.e., carriers of beta-thalassemia. As the disease is serious and the treatment is costly and cumbersome; prevention of birth of a child with thalassemia major is a better option. Prevention is possible by identifying couples who are carriers of beta-thalassemia and offering them prenatal diagnosis. Thalassemia carriers are detected by their blood test or because they have already given birth to a child with thalassemia major. Most of these families accept the option of prenatal diagnosis and termination of the pregnancy if the fetus is found to be affected with the disease. Prenatal diagnosis is done by testing the mutations present in the family in the DNA extracted from chorionic villi obtained between 10 and 12 weeks of gestation. Before going for prenatal diagnosis, identification of mutations in the affected child of the family or the carrier parents is essential.

Think it over!
The family asks to identify HLA type of the fetus in addition to testing for thalassemia mutations in prenatal sample. The fetus is negative for thalassemia disease but the HLA type does not match with the first child with thalassemia major and hence, the expected child cannot be donor of bone marrow for the thalassemia major child. The family thus wants to terminate the pregnancy and conceive again till they get a normal and HLA matched child who can be donor for their first child with thalassemia major.
Is it ethically correct?

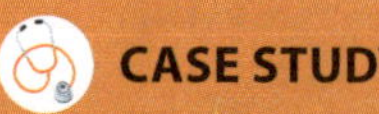

CASE STUDY Duchenne Muscular Dystrophy: Prevention of Recurrence

Prema's, 30-year-old has a 10-year-old normal daughter and a 6-year-old son with Duchenne muscular dystrophy (DMD). She is again 8 weeks pregnant. Prema has an 18-year-old brother who has similar problem and is bedridden. Prema also has a 25-year-old sister who was married 6 months ago. Her question is whether all her sons will be similarly affected.

What is the chance that Prema's unborn baby has DMD?
What test you will do to find out whether Prema is a carrier of DMD?
Who is the proband in the family?
Who should be tested for mutation detection first? Will the two affected males in the family have different mutations?
What types of mutations are commonly seen in DMD?
What is the earliest gestational age for prenatal diagnosis of DMD?
If the mutation is not detected in the proband; can prenatal diagnosis be provided to the family?
If there was no other case of DMD in the family other than Prema's son, is the prenatal diagnosis indicated?
Who else in the family needs genetic counseling and carrier detection?
Prema's husband asks you to test their daughter and find out whether she is a carrier of DMD or not. Should you get her tested?

To find answers read:
Duchenne muscular dystrophy (DMD) is an X-linked recessive disorder caused by a mutation in *dystrophin* gene. Onset of symptoms B usually by 3 to 5 years with difficulty in getting up from sitting posture. The muscle weakness beginning in hip girdle muscles progresses and the patient usually becomes bedridden by 12 years of age; death occurs in second decade. The pseudohypertrophy of Calf muscles and raised serum creatinine phosphokinase (CPK) are diagnostic. Milder form of the disease with onset in late childhood or adolescence is called Becker muscular dystrophy. It is also caused by mutation in *dystrophin* gene and hence, is allelic to DMD.

As against the small beta globin gene, *dystrophin* is a very large gene of size 2 mega bases (2 million base pairs). It is on the p arm of die X chromosome. Most of the mutations causing DMD and BMD are deletions of varying length in the *dystrophin* gene involving different exons. These deletions lead to absent, abnormal or truncated *dystrophin* protein which leads to muscle degeneration. The detection of mutation is possible by tests on DNA of the patient. Mutation detection confirms the diagnosis but it should be noted that the available tests at present cannot detect all mutations and hence, in a clinically confirmed case the mutation may not be detected.

Once a mutation is detected in a child with DMD, the test for the same mutation can be used for prenatal diagnosis and detection of carriers.

If a woman has two sons with DMD or an affected son and an affected brother; then she is definitely a carrier (obligate carrier) of DMD. When a carrier woman is pregnant; the risk of the disorder is 50% if the fetus is a male and females are unlikely to be affected. So, the first step in prenatal diagnosis is to test whether the fetus is male or a female. This is done by testing for markers on Y chromosome in the DNA extracted from chorionic villi which is obtained by per abdominal sampling at 11 to 12 weeks of pregnancy. If the fetus is a male, then only further test for mutation detection is done. The family is informed whether the fetus is affected with DMD or not. According to Preconception and Prenatal Diagnostic Techniques (Prohibition of Sex Selection) Act, 1994.

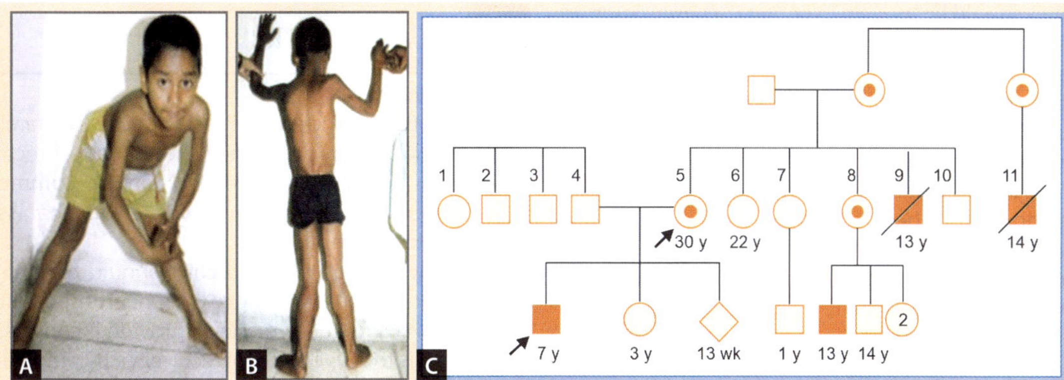

(A) A child with Duchenne muscular dystrophy. He has to take support of his thighs to get up from sitting posture; (B) Prominent calf hypertrophy; (C) Pedigree showing obligate carrier females (depicted with dot) who are related through males with Duchenne muscular dystrophy and will not need testing to confirm their carrier status. Individuals 11-6 and 11-7 will need DNA based testing using MLPA test to know their carrier status for DMD mutation

Indian law does not permit disclosure of sex of the fetus to the family. Other female relatives like sister of the proband and sister of a carrier mother can be tested by DNA based tests for identification of carriers. Carrier detection should not be done in children even if the parents insist. Only some carriers have high serum creatinine phosphokinase and hence, DNA based tests are necessary for carrier detection.

As women have two X chromosomes and carrier woman will have one normal copy of *dystrophin* gene and hence, detection of deletion in *dystrophin* gene in a carrier female is possible by multiplex ligation probe amplification (MLPA). If MLPA does not identify a mutation, sequencing of the *dystrophin* gene has to be done by a high throughput technique, namely next generation sequencing (NGS). This can pick up point mutations which are missed by MLPA.

If a family has only one case of DMD, the mother may or may not be carrier, if mother's blood test does not show that she is a carrier, still she should be offered prenatal diagnosis, as germ line mosaicism (i.e., presence of mutation in some cells of the gonad) is reported for DMD like many other monogenic disorders including hemophilia, and achondroplasia.

Prema asks you to find out whether the baby in her womb is a carrier female. The family feels that the pregnancy should be terminated if the fetus is a carrier of DMD. Is it ethical?

Think it over!

25.7 Parent Education *PE 29.3*

INTRODUCTION

Common belief about genetic disorders in most parts of the world including India, is that it occurs in those families where there is a history of any familial disease. Hence, discovering a genetic disorder in a child for the first time in the family is usually an unpleasant and shocking experience for the parents. Parents go through the phases of denial, anger, and grief. Many a times abandonment of a severely dysmorphic or handicapped baby is encountered. Usually, the mother is the most significantly affected person in this situation and it is not uncommon to find herself doubting her pregnancy related conditions or antenatal events to be responsible for the development of her child's disease. This challenging situation, which the parents face, needs to be handled sensitively by the health care givers. Detection of a genetic disorder at a later stage such as thalassemia, Duchenne muscular dystrophy, spinal muscular atrophy are also met with the same reaction.

APPROACH TO COUNSELING

- Both parents should be counseled together to prevent mutual misunderstanding and disagreement. This ensures their complete participation in the management of their affected child.
- Genetic counseling and symptomatic management or specific treatment wherever applicable, should be initiated early.
- Parents should be given a realistic picture of the natural course of the disease and should be made aware of danger signs, emergency/sick protocol to be followed for a child with inborn errors of metabolism (IEM).
- Parents who are scientifically aware can be informed about some reliable web resources for expanding their knowledge base related to their child's disease and can even be apprised of the "ClinicalTrials.gov" website where they can learn about the clinical trials concerning them.

- These families should be brought in contact of parent support groups if any available to provide them the much-needed guidance and solace.
- Ministry of Health and Family Welfare, Government of India, has formulated the National Policy for Rare Diseases, wherein financial support is provided under the umbrella scheme of *Rashtriya Arogya Nidhi* for treatment of selected rare diseases. This information should be imparted to the parents to enable their registration in the scheme.
- Parents should be counseled about risk of recurrence and the option of prenatal diagnosis in the next pregnancy.
- Cascade screening of high-risk individuals should be emphasized upon in these sessions.

Other parental counseling opportunities: Parents should be also counseled at (a) the time of newborn screening, (b) when they seek genetic opinion in view of a previous affected child; and (c) when there is any structural abnormality detected in the fetus.

- ***Primary prevention:*** Couples planning pregnancy should be encouraged to screen themselves for common genetic disorders such as thalassemia and spinal muscular atrophy.
- Periconceptional intake of folic acid should be advised for prevention of neural tube defects.

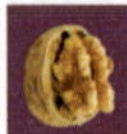

IN A NUTSHELL

Parent Education

1. Even in the absence of an affected child in the family, a couple who is planning pregnancy should get a preconceptional genetic counseling to screen for the common genetic disorders in the community such as thalassemia and hemoglobinopathies.
2. A family with an affected child should be counseled in a sensitive manner adhering to the tenets of genetic counseling. All efforts should be made to provide a conclusive genetic diagnosis to prevent risk of recurrence by prenatal diagnosis.
3. Parents should be encouraged to join the concerned parent support group to enable them to be updated with the latest development in therapeutics and government health policies.

Angus C. Harper's Practical Genetic Counselling. 8th edition. London: CRC Press; 2019.

Gallo AM, Knafl KA, Angst DB. Information management in families who have a child with a genetic condition. J Pediatr Nurs. 2009;24(3): 194-204.

Metcalfe A, Plumridge G, Coad J, et al. Parents' and children's communication about genetic risk: a qualitative study, learning from families' experiences. Eur J Hum Genet. 2011;19(6):640-6.

26 CHAPTER

Endocrine Disorders

AS PER NMC COMPETENCIES

PE30.1	Describe the etiology (congenital and acquired), clinical features, management of hypothyroidism in children.	*Ch 26.3, Ch 26.4, Ch 26.5*
PE30.2	Interpret and explain neonatal thyroid screening report.	*Ch 26.4*
PE30.3	Describe the etiology, clinical types, clinical features, diagnostic criteria, complications and management of diabetes mellitus in children.	*Ch 26.6*
PE30.4	Recognize clinical features DKA, perform and interpret urine dip stick for sugar and ketone bodies and refer.	*Ch 26.7, Ch 26.8*
PE30.5	Perform genital examination and recognize ambiguous genitalia, counsel and refer.	*Ch 26.9*
PE30.6	Define precocious and delayed puberty, perform sexual maturity rating (SMR), recognize precocious and delayed puberty and refer.	*Ch 26.10, Ch 26.11, Ch 26.12, Ch 26.13*
PE30.7	Identify deviations in growth and plan appropriate referral.	*Ch 26.2*

26.1 Endocrine Glands and Hormones

INTRODUCTION

The endocrine system of the body is formed by glands which secrete substances called as hormones. These hormones play pivotal role in controlling metabolic functions and growth of the body. The hormones are chemically comprised of steroids (such as glucocorticoids, estrogens, progesterone, testosterone, 1,25-dihydroxyvitamin D3), proteins [gonadotropins, insulin, thyroid-stimulating hormone (TSH), antidiuretic hormone (ADH), growth hormone (GH), adrenocorticotropic hormone (ACTH), parathormone (PTH)] or amino acid derivatives (adrenaline, noradrenaline, thyroid hormones).

REGULATION OF HORMONE SECRETION

The chief regulator of hormonal action in the body is a small gland called as *pituitary*, which is located inside the brain. It is formed of two parts—(1) anterior and (2) posterior pituitary. The release of hormones from pituitary is regulated by *hypothalamus*, which is also situated inside the brain. The hypothalamus secretes certain hormones and controls the secretion of major hormones from the pituitary via a network of chemical transmitters. The

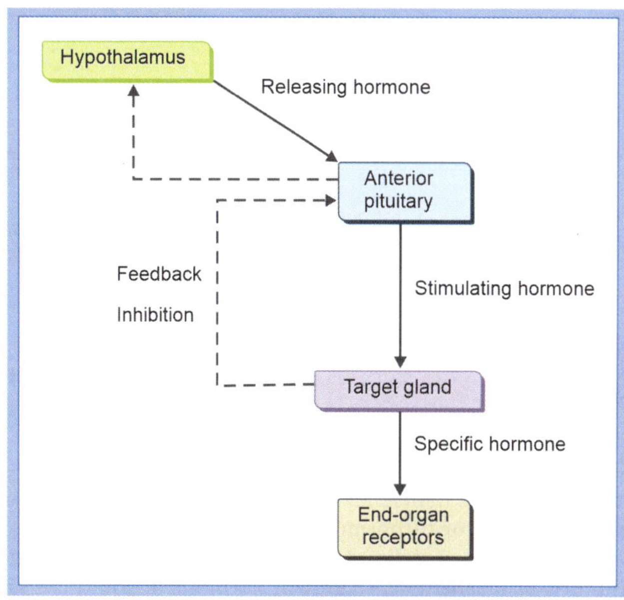

Fig. 26.1: Hypothalamic-pituitary axis

anterior pituitary secretes most of the hormones which further stimulate release of the chemical substances from other glands in the body, thus acting as a "master gland".

The outline of hypothalamic-pituitary axis system is shown in **Figure 26.1**. The stimulating hormones from pituitary gland act on specific organs to release hormones which are regulated by *feedback inhibition*. Thus, whenever there is excess of specific hormone produced at target gland, an inhibitory signal is sent to pituitary to decrease the release of stimulating hormone. The hormones released from pituitary are enumerated in **Table 26.1**.

The hormones so released act on their target organs by binding to receptors and thereby triggering a metabolic cascade. Most of these receptors are extracellular except the receptors to steroid and thyroid hormones which are intracellular. Once a hormone has acted, further secretion of the hormone is suppressed via feedback inhibition. Failure of this inhibition results in overproduction and excessive effects of the hormone resulting in endocrinal disease. Similarly, insufficient release of hormone results in hormonal deficiency. Metabolism and elimination of hormones occurs in the liver and kidneys.

Table 26.1 Endocrine Glands with Hormones Produced and Action in the Body

Gland	*Hormone*	*Action*
Hypothalamus	Growth hormone releasing hormone (GHRH), gonadotropin-releasing hormone (GnRH), thyrotropin-releasing hormone (TRH), somatostatin, corticotropic-releasing hormone (CRH)	Regulates release of anterior pituitary hormones
Anterior pituitary	• Growth hormone (GH) • Thyroid-stimulating hormone (TSH) • Prolactin • Adrenocorticotropic hormone (ACTH) • Luteinizing hormone (LH) • Follicle-stimulating hormone (FSH)	• Skeletal growth • Stimulates thyroid gland to release thyroid hormone • Initiation and maintenance of lactation • Stimulates release of cortisol from adrenals • Stimulates synthesis of sex steroid (estrogens and testosterone) from gonads. Responsible for pubertal onset • Stimulates ovulation and spermatogenesis
Neurohypophysis (hypothalamus and posterior pituitary)	• Oxytocin • Antidiuretic hormone (ADH) or vasopressin	• Stimulates uterine contractions during labor and release of milk from the breast when the baby begins to suckle (milk let down reflex) • Promotes water conservation by acting on the collecting ducts in kidneys
Thyroid Parathyroid glands	• Thyroxine (T4) and tri-iodothyronine (T3) • Calcitonin • Parathyroid hormone (PTH)	• Regulates body metabolism. Crucial for development during fetal period • Prevents bone resorption • Maintains serum calcium level by stimulating bone resorption and calcium absorption at kidneys
Pancreas	• Insulin • Glucagon	• Decreases blood glucose, promotes anabolism • Increases blood glucose
Adrenal cortex Adrenal medulla	• Aldosterone • Cortisol • Androgens • Adrenaline and noradrenaline	• Promotes sodium retention in body • Metabolic effects, promotes growth, anti-inflammatory • Development of pubic and axillary hair • Sympathetic action
Kidneys	Renin	Promotes sodium retention and regulates blood pressure
Gonads Females—ovaries Males—testes	• Estrogens in females • Testosterone in males	Development of external genitalia

26.2 Growth Hormone Disorders *PE 30.7*

GROWTH HORMONE DEFICIENCY

Growth hormone deficiency (GHD) may result due to under production of growth hormone-releasing hormone (GHRH) from hypothalamus, deficiency of growth hormone (GH) from pituitary, or insensitivity to growth hormone action due to a pituitary receptor defect. These causes can be:

- ***Congenital:*** Brain malformations, pituitary hypoplasia, genetic mutations in GH/GH receptor
- ***Acquired:*** Inflammatory/granulomatous conditions such as hypophysitis, tumors of hypothalamus/pituitary area (disruption of hormone production and action), cranial irradiation, intracranial infections, and hemorrhage

Growth hormone insensitivity is also known as *Laron's syndrome* where GH levels are adequate but are ineffective thus clinically resembling a patient with GHD.

Clinical Features

The manifestations of GHD include proportionate short stature. These children are short since early childhood, though growth failure usually remains unnoticed till 2 years of age. The facies are generally infantile and appear as "doll like". These children are usually overweight for their height with markedly increased subcutaneous fat. There is usually delayed sexual development.

Children with GHD may have isolated GH deficiency which manifests as severe short stature. Children may also have combined deficiency of GH and other pituitary hormones such as TSH, ACTH, LH, FSH that may have concurrent clinical cues like micropenis (small phallic length), hypoglycemia (ACTH deficiency) or features of hypothyroidism.

Diagnosis

The criteria for suspecting GHD in a short child are mentioned in **Box 26.1**.

Monitoring the height velocity (HV) is best to differentiate GHD from *constitutional short stature* (*See* Chapter 2). Children with constitutional short stature are short but have normal HV and will ultimately have a height spurt to result in normal adult height.

Any child who fulfills any of the above criteria given earlier (**Box 26.1**) needs to be further investigated to rule out any systemic chronic disease. Other common causes of short stature include systemic disorders, malnutrition and genetic or familial short stature. We have already discussed the approach to a child with short stature in Chapter 2, along with its differential diagnosis.

The confirmation of GHD requires further dynamic testing of the endocrine axis.

Testing for GHD should be done after ruling out hypothyroidism which is a commoner cause of short height than GHD. Confirmation of GHD is by demonstrating low levels of GH (<10 ng/mL) on GH stimulation tests. The serum levels of insulin-like growth factor (IGF)-1 are low in GHD that are supportive for the diagnosis. GHD may be associated with deficiency of other pituitary hormones and other tests must be done to rule out hypopituitarism. Imaging of the brain to ascertain the cause of GHD should be done in these children. **Figure 26.2** shows a 4-year-old boy diagnosed with GHD.

Box 26.1 Criteria for Evaluation of Growth Hormone Deficiency

1. Height is below –2.25 standard deviation (SD) or 3rd centile of the mean population for that age and gender on growth chart
2. Height velocity (height gain in cm over 12 months) is less than 4 cm per year in prepubertal years
3. Height is below –2 SD of the expected parental height, i.e., child is too short as compared to his parents
4. Bone age below the chronological age (difference of >2 years)
5. Peak GH levels <10 ng/mL during GH provocative test*

*GH provocative tests measure serial GH levels after a stimulus like oral clonidine or parenteral glucagon, insulin or arginine. There is no role of random measurement of GH levels

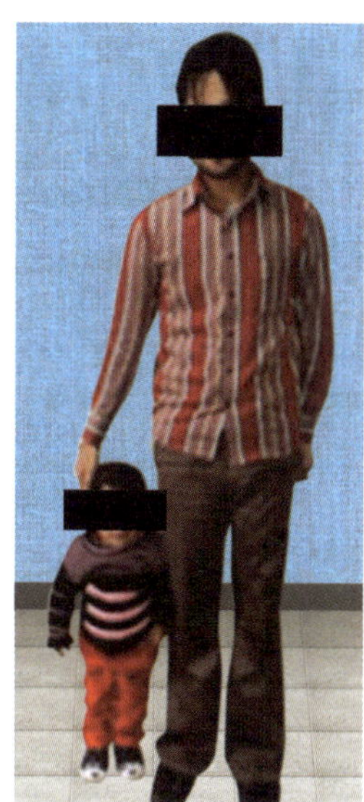

Fig. 26.2: A 4-year-old boy with growth hormone deficiency, standing with his father

TREATMENT Growth Hormone Deficiency

Specific treatment of GHD includes supplementing with growth hormone which is available as subcutaneous injection. The starting dose is usually 20–30 µg/kg/day. The treatment is costly and needs to be continued till the child has achieved height in the normal range. Other pituitary hormones should be also supplemented if there is concomitant deficiency. The child should be referred to a pediatric endocrinologist for further management.

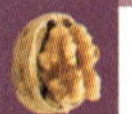

IN A NUTSHELL

Growth Hormone Deficiency

1. Growth hormone deficiency (GHD) manifests as proportionate short stature.
2. GHD can present as an isolated endocrinal deficiency or in combination with other pituitary hormone deficiencies.
3. Diagnosis of GHD should be suspected in children with severe short stature with supportive investigations (and growth hormone provocative testing).
4. Recombinant growth hormone is available for treatment of GHD.

Grimberg A, DiVall SA, Polychronakos C, et al. Guidelines for Growth Hormone and Insulin-Like Growth Factor-I Treatment in Children and Adolescents: Growth Hormone Deficiency, Idiopathic Short Stature, and Primary Insulin-Like Growth Factor-I Deficiency. Horm Res Paediatr. 2016;86(6):361-97.

Ranke MB. Short and long-term effects of growth hormone in children and adolescents with GH deficiency. Front Endocrinol (Lausanne). 2021;12:720419.

26.3 Disorders of Thyroid Gland

PE 30.1

ANATOMY AND PHYSIOLOGY

The thyroid gland is a butterfly-shaped gland located anteriorly in the neck. It produces thyroid hormones [triiodothyronine (T3) and thyroxine (T4)] under the action of TSH from the anterior pituitary, which in turn is regulated by thyrotropin-releasing hormone (TRH) from the hypothalamus. T3 and T4 are formed in the thyroid gland after coupling with iodine, which makes iodine an essential nutrient in the diet. The thyroid secretes mainly (80%) T4 that is the major circulating hormone in the body. T4 is converted into T3 in the target cells by deiodinase enzyme. T3 is the more potent of the two hormones. The activity of deiodinase (type 1 and 2) is stimulated in thyroid hormone-depleted states as a protective mechanism to produce more T3. Thus, T3 levels are the last to fall in hypothyroidism, and are not a reliable indicator of the disease.

Thyroid hormones play an active role in the regulation of somatic and intellectual growth. There is a critical phase in the early neonatal period for the effect of thyroid hormone on mental development. This underscores the need for early diagnosis and appropriate management of congenital hypothyroidism. The thyroid hormones influence metabolism of carbohydrate, fat, and vitamin in the body. They increase oxygen consumption, stimulate protein synthesis, and influence growth and differentiation, thus are important for growth even in fetal period.

THYROID HORMONE DEFICIENCY

A deficiency state of thyroid hormones may result due to decreased production of T3 and T4 from the thyroid gland, known as primary hypothyroidism. This may result due to local destruction of thyroid gland in surgery, irradiation, infection, or autoimmune conditions. Dietary iodine deficiency will also result in deficient production of T3 and T4. Deficiency of thyroid hormones due to decreased TSH secretion from the pituitary is called as *secondary hypothyroidism* (*central hypothyroidism*). Both have similar clinical manifestations and can be differentiated by biochemical tests. Congenital hypothyroidism commonly results from abnormal thyroid gland development or defective thyroid hormone production (primary thyroid involvement), and less commonly due to central causes. **Table 26.2** shows the different causes of hypothyroidism in children.

Table 26.2 Etiology of Hypothyroidism in Children

Congenital hypothyroidism	*Acquired hypothyroidism*
• *Abnormal thyroid gland structure (dysgenesis):* Absent (agenesis), ectopic location, and small gland (hypoplasia) • *Abnormal production of thyroid hormones (dyshormonogenesis)* *Enzyme defects:* Trapping, organification, thyroglobulin synthesis, and deiodination *Central hypothyroidism:* Secondary or tertiary (hypothalamus or pituitary, <5%) • Genetic causes • Structural brain malformations (Septo-optic dysplasia, and holoprosencephaly) *Transient causes:* Maternal TSH receptor blocking antibody, iodine excess, and maternal antithyroid drug	*Primary hypothyroidism:* • Hashimoto thyroiditis, autoimmune diseases such as polyglandular autoimmune syndrome (adrenal insufficiency, type 1 diabetes mellitus and hypoparathyroidism) • Endemic iodine deficiency (endemic goiter) • *Goitrogens:* Thiocyanates, lithium, and amiodarone • *Infections:* Postviral • Thyroid surgery, and radiation exposure • Thyroid carcinoma *Secondary hypothyroidism:* • *CNS insults:* Trauma, surgery, radiation, and infection • *CNS tumors:* Craniopharyngioma, and germinoma

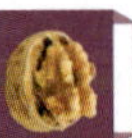

IN A NUTSHELL

Disorders of Thyroid Gland

1. Thyroid disorders can result from congenital or acquired disorders from defect in the thyroid gland (primary) or hypothalamic-pituitary axis.
2. Hypothyroidism is more common than hyperthyroidism in children.
3. The evaluation of thyroid disorders constitutes measurement of TSH, serum T4/free T4 and less commonly T3/free T3.

Chaker L, Razvi S, Bensenor IM, et al. Hypothyroidism [published correction appears in Nat Rev Dis Primers. 2022;8(1):39]. Nat Rev Dis Primers. 2022;8(1):30.

Moran C, Schoenmakers N, Visser WE, et al. Genetic disorders of thyroid development, hormone biosynthesis and signalling. Clin Endocrinol (Oxf). 2022;97(4):502-14.

26.4 Congenital Hypothyroidism *PE 30.1, PE 30.2*

INTRODUCTION

Hypothyroidism is among the most common endocrine diseases in neonates with an incidence of 1 in 2,500 to 1 in 5,000 live births. Congenital hypothyroidism (CH) most frequently results from agenesis, dysplasia, or ectopy of the thyroid (approximately 80% of cases); however, it is also caused by autosomal recessive defects in the organification of iodine (thyroid hormone synthesis) and defects in other enzymatic steps in T4 synthesis and release.

CLINICAL FEATURES

The neonates usually remain asymptomatic after initial weeks of life. They might have prolonged physiological jaundice and develop dry skin after birth. Babies are sluggish, sleep frequently, are dull with hypotonia. They may have breathing difficulty and feeding difficulty due to large tongue. A history of delayed passage of meconium followed by constipation may be elicited in babies who present later. Examination shows wide open fontanels in skull, small neck, and umbilical hernia due to hypotonia (**Box 26.2**).

Box 26.2 Clinical Features of Congenital Hypothyroidism

1. Open posterior fontanel
2. Characteristic edematous facies
3. Pallor
4. Hypothermia
5. Macroglossia
6. Rough dry skin
7. Umbilical hernia
8. Hypotonia
9. Large abdomen, constipation
10. Prolonged neonatal jaundice

Babies who remain undiagnosed may develop obvious clinical features of hypothyroidism subsequently such as coarsening of facial features, delayed dentition, and poor growth. As T4 is a critical hormone required for normal neurodevelopment, affected babies have lower developmental and intelligence scores. The developmental scores are dependent on the time of initiation of thyroxine therapy and are worse in babies who are diagnosed later than those who are timely initiated on therapy after detection on newborn screening, preferably before 2 weeks of life.

DIAGNOSIS

Clinical evaluation of an infant suspected to be having congenital hypothyroidism is summarized in **Box 26.3**. The diagnosis of congenital hypothyroidism is made by detection of hypothyroidism with elevated TSH and low thyroxine levels, usually during newborn screening (discussed later).

Radiological Tests

The radiographs of knees show absence of lower epiphysis of femur in babies with CH. Further radiological tests include evaluation of radionuclide uptake and ultrasound of thyroid to confirm the presence or absence of thyroid gland. Thyroid *dysgenesis* is diagnosed if no thyroid tissue is visualized on ultrasound and radionuclide thyroid scan. A radionuclide thyroid scan will also detect thyroid tissue at ectopic locations.

Box 26.3 Evaluation of an Infant with Congenital Hypothyroidism

1. History of maternal thyroid disease or ingestion of antithyroid medications, that can cause transient thyroid dysfunction in the baby
2. Sibling history of hypothyroidism suggests dyshormonogenesis (autosomal recessive inheritance)
3. Sibling history of recurrent transient hypothyroidism indicates a disease related to maternal TSH receptor antibody (these spontaneously resolve as the baby grows)
4. Residence in iodine deficient area may suggest the diagnosis of iodine deficiency (ask history of goiter in multiple family members or in geographical area)
5. Presence of goiter should prompt evaluation for transplacental passage of antithyroid drugs or disorders of thyroid hormone biosynthesis
6. Neonatal history of hypoglycemia, micropenis, and midline facial defects suggest hypothalamic-pituitary causes

NEWBORN SCREENING FOR HYPOTHYROIDISM

Screening is defined as identification of unrecognized disease or defects by rapidly applied tests in apparently healthy individuals on a large scale. Newborn screening (NBS) is the practice of screening newborn shortly after birth for potentially fatal disorders that are treatable, but difficult or impossible to detect clinically. Newborn screening is available for few disorders like congenital hypothyroidism that are important public health problems with facilities for diagnosis available. It has a latent period for disease manifestation that bears long-term consequences on growth and development, and an effective treatment is available that improves survival of the affected babies.

Newborn screening is offered to all babies at birth through simple tests conducted on cord blood or a blood drop collected from heel-prick of the baby on a filter paper. The filter papers require special equipment for measurement of the analytes. Newborn screening for congenital hypothyroidism is available in few state government programs in India.

Interpretation of Newborn Screening

Newborn screening for CH is mostly based on initial TSH levels that can be measured in cord blood or blood sample collected after 2–3 days of life. The measurement of T4 levels in blood is seldom practiced for universal screening for CH as it is less specific and has a high frequency of false positives in low birth weight and premature infants.

A TSH surge occurs in all babies after birth, hence TSH levels are elevated in the first 24–48 hours. Therefore, the ideal time

Flowchart 26.1: Algorithm for interpretation of neonatal thyroid screening report. The sample can be taken as cord blood (serum units) or after 2–3 days of life from heel-prick as dried blood spot (whole blood units) or venous sampling (serum units)

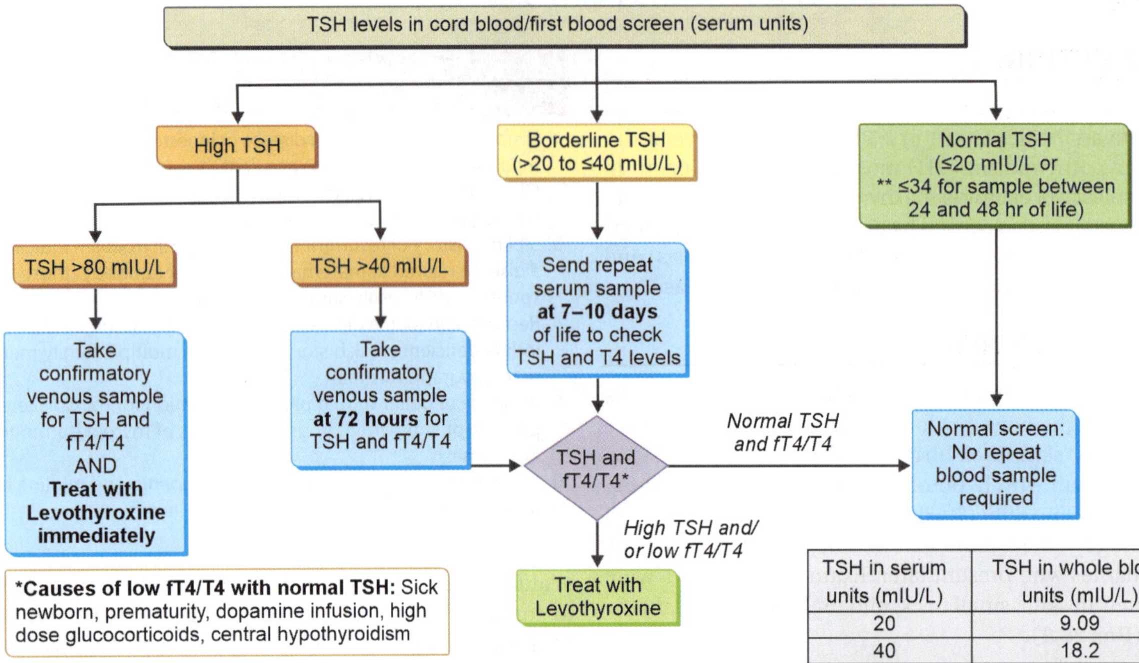

TSH in serum units (mIU/L)	TSH in whole blood units (mIU/L)
20	9.09
40	18.2
80	36.4

to obtain the blood sample is from placental end of umbilical cord (immediately after birth) or in the postnatal period (after 48-72 hours of birth) to minimize the chances of false-positive diagnosis of hypothyroidism. The process of checking TSH of all healthy babies at birth should be universally followed as part of newborn screening. However, an elevated TSH on cord blood or blood spot needs to be confirmed on a venous sample before informing the family of a confirmed diagnosis of CH.

The different cut-offs of TSH measured during NBS suggest the algorithm for management of a baby with suspected CH **(Flowchart 26.1)**:

TREATMENT Congenital Hypothyroidism

Immediate treatment should be started with replacing the deficient hormone. Oral thyroxine is initiated at 10–15 µg/kg/day as the first dose in the morning, given with breast milk. The dose of thyroxine replacement in CH is higher than the dose used in acquired hypothyroidism. Dose adjustment is guided by measuring T4 and TSH levels which are expected to normalize over 1 week and 1 month, respectively. Thereafter FT4 and TSH are measured at regular intervals on follow-up to titrate the dose of thyroxine to achieve FT4 levels in the upper normal range for the age. Parents should also be counseled for the need for lifelong therapy and continued follow-up. Prognosis of those neonates who are started on treatment within 2 weeks of life is good with normal attainment of normal neurodevelopmental outcomes.

In suspected transient CH, a trial of stopping thyroxine can be done after 3 years of age, once brain growth is almost complete. Babies with transient CH would test normal on thyroid functions after stopping the drugs. In central hypothyroidism, cortisol replacement should precede thyroid replacement as it could precipitate adrenal insufficiency.

IN A NUTSHELL

Congenital Hypothyroidism

1. Congenital hypothyroidism can result from thyroid dysgenesis (abnormal thyroid gland development) or thyroid dyshormonogenesis (inadequate production of hormones).
2. Newborn screening detects congenital hypothyroidism after birth from sample taken from cord blood, venous sample, or heel prick sample.
3. TSH is the most common single biochemical parameter used for newborn screening.
4. Thyroxine should be initiated timely and as soon as possible for better neurodevelopmental outcome in doses 10–15 ug/kg/day.

Desai MP, Sharma R, Riaz I, et al. Newborn Screening Guidelines for Congenital Hypothyroidism in India: Recommendations of the Indian Society for Pediatric and Adolescent Endocrinology (ISPAE) - Part I: Screening and Confirmation of Diagnosis. Indian J Pediatr. 2018;85(6):440-7.

Sudhanshu S, Riaz I, Sharma R, et al. Newborn Screening Guidelines for Congenital Hypothyroidism in India: Recommendations of the Indian Society for Pediatric and Adolescent Endocrinology (ISPAE) - Part II: Imaging, Treatment and Follow-up. Indian J Pediatr. 2018;85(6):448-53.

26.5 Acquired Hypothyroidism

PE 30.1

INTRODUCTION

This is one of the most common endocrine disorders seen in children and adolescents. It may be due to primary involvement of thyroid gland like iodine deficiency or autoimmune thyroiditis (also known as Hashimoto thyroiditis) or may be secondary to pituitary insult. Autoimmune thyroiditis can also occur coexistent with other autoimmune diseases such as celiac disease, type 1 diabetes mellitus, Down syndrome, and Turner syndrome.

CLINICAL FEATURES

The presentation is variable and depends on severity of involvement and age of the patient. Manifestations range from subclinical hypothyroidism, which requires high index of suspicion for diagnosis to myxedema coma. Common symptoms and signs of hypothyroidism are listed in **Box 26.4**.

In growing prepubertal years, thyroid deficiency may result in disproportionate short stature **(Figs. 26.3A and B)**; the trunk (upper segment) is disproportionately large as compared to limbs. It may also result in poor development and school performance during childhood years. These findings usually suggest missed congenital hypothyroidism. Children with hypothyroidism can have pubertal delay. Hypothyroidism may be associated with Down syndrome, Turner syndrome, Celiac disease, and type 1 diabetes. Children with these disorders should be periodically screened for hypothyroidism even in the absence of symptoms.

DIAGNOSIS

Family history of acquired hypothyroidism suggests autoimmune thyroiditis. The biochemical diagnosis is made by low T3 and T4. The TSH levels are elevated in in primary hypothyroidism. Autoantibodies such as anti-thyroid peroxidase (anti-TPO) and anti-thyroglobulin are raised in Hashimoto thyroiditis. Children with central hypothyroidism have low TSH with low T4. They should be evaluated for other pituitary hormone deficiencies including radiological imaging of the hypothalamic-pituitary region.

Box 26.4 Clinical Features of Acquired Hypothyroidism

1. Linear growth retardation
2. Weight gain
3. Goiter
4. Rough dry skin
5. Coarse facies
6. Brittle hair
7. Sallow complexion
8. Cold intolerance
9. Constipation
10. Delayed skeletal maturation
11. Delayed dental development
12. Delayed puberty
13. Myopathy and pseudohypertrophy
14. Enlarged sella
15. Pseudotumor cerebri

TREATMENT Acquired Hypothyroidism

Thyroid replacement by oral thyroxine is initiated at dose of 100 μg/m²/day (approximately 3–5 μg/kg/day). It is administered as a single early morning dose and is available in tablet form only, in different strengths (such as 12.5, 25, 37.5, 50, 75 and 100 μg). TSH levels should be measured on serial follow-up for thyroxine dose titration. Patients of autoimmune thyroiditis usually require lifelong thyroid replacement.

GOITER

Goiter refers to the enlargement of the thyroid gland (**Fig. 26.4**). The thyroid gland can enlarge due to a variety of physiological or pathological stimuli.

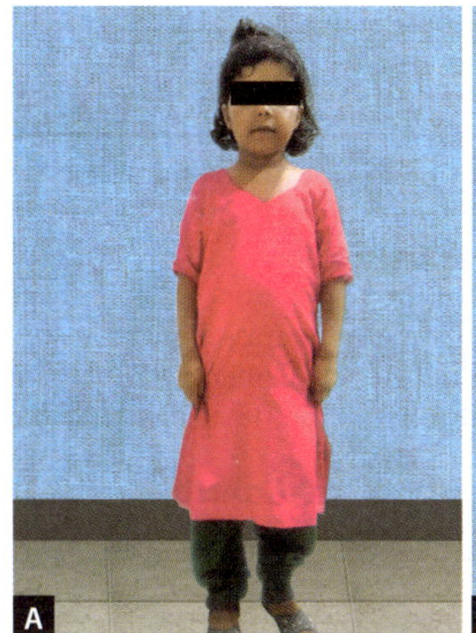

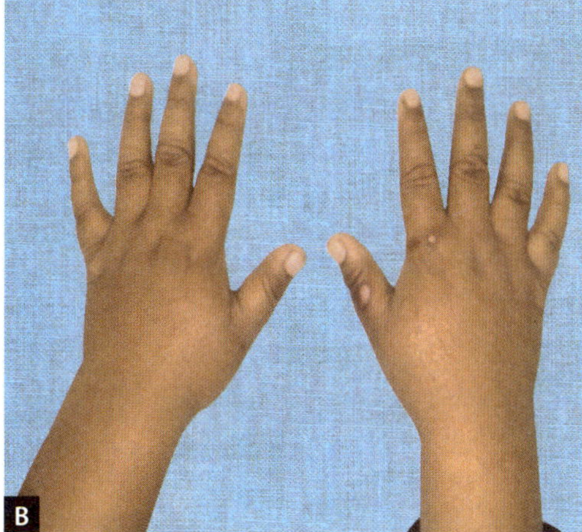

Figs. 26.3A and B: An 8-year-old girl with hypothyroidism: (A) Short stature with coarse facies protuberant abdomen; (B) Dry wrinkled skin over hands

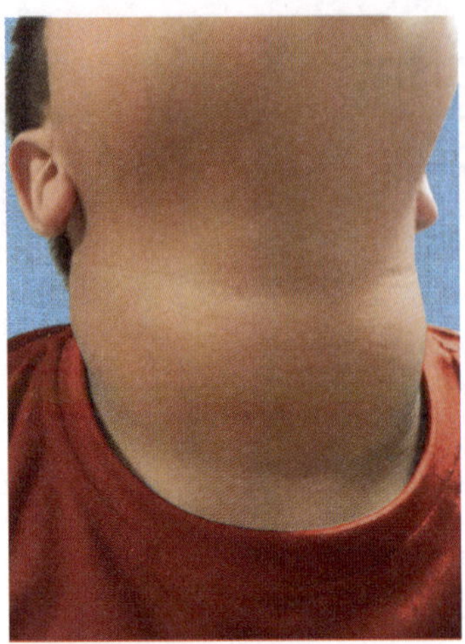

Fig. 26.4: Diffuse thyroid enlargement (goiter) in a boy

Goiter could present with or without symptoms of thyroid hormone deficiency or excess so the thyroid function tests could be decreased, normal, or increased. Factors contributing to goiter formation and their causes are enlisted in **Table 26.3**.

Etiology

Congenital goiter can result from maternal antithyroid medications, dyshormonogenesis and iodine deficiency. Autoimmune thyroiditis is the most common cause of goiter in older children, followed by iodine deficiency, and Graves disease. Goiter during adolescence and pregnancy are two causes of a physiological goiter.

Clinical Features

The presence of goiter and size can be determined by inspection, palpation, or by an imaging study. It is described in terms of extent of gland involvement (diffuse or nodular/multinodular goiter) and consistency of gland (soft or firm). Anatomical malformations such as thyroglossal cyst may present as nodular swelling of thyroid and can be differentiated on further tests.

Table 26.3 Factors and Etiology of Thyromegaly

Factors	*Causes*
Inflammatory	Acute suppurative thyroiditis (soft tender goiter), subacute (viral) thyroiditis, and Hashimoto thyroiditis
Infiltration	Chronic lymphocytic thyroiditis (firm, nodular/diffuse goiter/multinodular), neoplasms or hemochromatosis, and Graves disease (soft non-nodular goiter)
Goitrogen exposure	*Goitrogenic drugs:* Amiodarone, Iodine *Goitrogenic food:* Cassava, lima beans, linseed, sorghum (cyanogens); cruciferous vegetables (glucosinolates); soy, and millet (flavonoids)
Nutrients	Iodine deficiency (firm, and non-nodular goiter), selenium deficiency, iron deficiency, and vitamin A deficiency
Congenital hypothyroidism	Dyshormonogenesis (diffuse, soft to firm, non-nodular goiter)
Colloid (simple) goiter	TSH receptor stimulating antibodies, genetic factors, Iodine deficiency

Investigations

All thyroid swellings may not cause impairment in thyroid function (euthyroid), while either hypothyroidism or hyperthyroidism may result. Investigations of a case of goiter should include thyroid function tests (TSH, T4 and/or T3 levels) to classify the cause of goiter into hypothyroidism or hyperthyroidism. Anti-TPO antibodies should be measured to identify autoimmune thyroiditis.

Thyroid function is assessed by serum TSH and free and/or total T4 and T3. TSH is the most sensitive indicator of primary (thyroidal) hypothyroidism but is not as helpful in the diagnosis of central (pituitary or hypothalamic) hypothyroidism. Serum T4 level is a better indicator of thyroid status than serum T3 due to increased conversion of T4 to T3 during thyroid-depleted states. Estimation of free thyroid hormones is superior to total hormone levels as the levels of circulating thyroxine-binding globulin (TBG) are variable. Low free T4 (fT4) and low or inadequately raised TSH levels suggest central hypothyroidism, while low FT4 levels with high TSH levels, indicate primary hypothyroidism.

TREATMENT Goiter

The primary etiology dictates the treatment. Hypothyroidism should be managed by thyroxine replacement. Euthyroid goiter with autoimmune thyroiditis should be followed with annual thyroid function tests. Suppressive thyroxine therapy for euthyroid goiter is of limited benefit and is best avoided. Surgery is indicated, only if goiter is large enough to cause respiratory embarrassment. Graves disease is treated with antithyroid medication.

SOLITARY THYROID NODULE

Identification of solitary thyroid nodule in children should alert to the possibility of thyroid malignancy (up to 20% cases). A well-circumscribed nodule is usually due to a benign cyst. Pointers toward malignancy include a firm nodule with limited mobility and associated lymph node enlargement.

IODINE DEFICIENCY DISORDERS

The term "iodine deficiency disorders (IDD)" refers to the wide spectrum of effects of iodine deficiency on growth and development that can be corrected by ensuring adequate iodine intake in the population. Brain damage and irreversible mental retardation are the most sinister complications associated with iodine deficiency. Goiter, hypothyroidism, and retarded growth may result from iodine deficiency.

Prevention and Control

Iodine deficiency disorders are best prevented as treatment is usually ineffective. Iodinated salt or iodized oil are highly efficacious in preventing iodine deficiency. Surgical removal of large goiter is indicated only to relieve airway obstruction or for cosmetic reasons.

The National Goiter Control Program of the Ministry of Health and Family Welfare in India began in 1962 with introduction of mandatory salt iodization. The recommended daily intake of iodine is 40–120 μg for children up to the age of 10, 150 μg for older children and adults and an additional 25 μg and 50 μg during pregnancy and lactation, respectively.

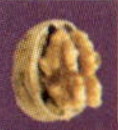

IN A NUTSHELL

Acquired Hypothyroidism

1. Hashimoto thyroiditis is the most common cause of acquired hypothyroidism in childhood.
2. Primary hypothyroidism in children may be associated with other autoimmune or genetic disorders such as Down syndrome, Turner syndrome.
3. Goiter presents as neck swelling and may have biochemical status as euthyroid, hypothyroid or hyperthyroid.
4. Iodine deficiency disorders (IDD) are preventable nutritional disorders that may result in growth and neurodevelopmental problems. Mandatory salt fortification with iodine is an essential strategy to prevent IDD.
5. Treatment of acquired hypothyroidism is with replacement levothyroxine in doses 3–5 μg/kg/day.

Admoni O, Rath S, Almagor T, et al. Long-term follow-up and outcomes of autoimmune thyroiditis in childhood. Front Endocrinol (Lausanne). 2020;11:309.

Rodriguez L, Dinauer C, Francis G. Treatment of hypothyroidism in infants, children and adolescents. Trends Endocrinol Metab. 2022;33(7):522-32.

26.6 Diabetes Mellitus

PE 30.3

INTRODUCTION

Diabetes mellitus is a metabolic disorder characterized by chronic hyperglycemia resulting from decreased insulin secretion or inadequate action. Persistent hyperglycemia causes damage to several organs and body systems, including the kidneys, eyes, and cardiovascular system.

CLASSIFICATION

- Diabetes mellitus (DM) may result from deficiency or absence of insulin production that occurs due to immune mediated destruction of β-cells of the pancreas, also known as type 1 diabetes mellitus (T1DM).
- Relative insulin deficiency due to inadequate secretion of insulin in background of insulin resistance may also cause diabetes, known as type 2 diabetes mellitus (T2DM).
- T1DM is the predominant but not exclusive form of diabetes seen in children and adolescents while T2DM is the most common form seen in adults. However, recent reports suggest an increasing burden of T2DM in children, especially those with risk factors such as obesity and hypertension. There are other forms of diabetes that can be categorized based on the disease pathophysiology and can be differentiated by their clinical presentations **(Table 26.4)**.

T1DM and T2DM are compared in **Table 26.5**.

PATHOPHYSIOLOGY

Normally, insulin is released in the body in response to a sugar load. It acts to reduce blood glucose by promoting hepatic uptake of glucose and conversion of glucose to glycogen. Similarly, it also promotes fatty acid synthesis and protein formation acting as an anabolic hormone. Insulin deficiency results in hyperglycemia as there is decreased glucose uptake by muscle and other cells and increased glycogenolysis, lipolysis and gluconeogenesis. The increased blood glucose exceeds the absorptive capacity of kidneys that manifests as glycosuria. In addition, advanced glycation end-products get formed that lead to end-organ damage. The hyperglycemia also stimulates release of free oxide radicals, to result in oxidative stress and tissue damage.

The difference in disease pathophysiology between T1DM and T2DM is depicted in **Figures 26.5A to C**.

ETIOLOGY

The causes of T1DM are postulated to be multifactorial that result in cytotoxic destruction of pancreas.

- Polymorphisms in human leukocyte antigen (HLA), located on chromosome 6 have been identified as the most common factor associated with increased genetic susceptibility to T1DM.
- The genotypes HLA-DR3, DR4, and DQ8 confer increased risk of T1DM, while HLA-DR 15 has a protective role. Few other genes may predispose to T1DM, like the *INS* gene (proinsulin) and T cell regulating *PTPN22* gene.
- A child with first degree family history of T1DM has an increased risk (4–6%) of developing T1DM as compared to population risk of 0.3%.
- Infections (Coxsackie B virus, cytomegalovirus, and enterovirus) may trigger a selective autoimmune destruction of the pancreatic beta cells.

Table 26.4 Classification of Diabetes (American Diabetes Association, 2014)

Category of diabetes	*Clinical remarks*
Type 1 diabetes (destruction of beta cells with absolute insulin deficiency) • 1A: Autoimmune • 1B: Idiopathic	Common (up to 95% of all pediatric diabetes) with onset in childhood. Requirement of insulin to achieve euglycemia
Type 2 diabetes (due to combination of insulin resistance with relative insulin deficiency in varying proportions) 10–50% of diabetes in adolescents depending on ethnicity	• Clinical pointers of insulin resistance (acanthosis nigricans, central adiposity) • Family history of type 2 diabetes in first degree relative present
Monogenic diabetes • *Genetic defects of beta cell function:* Neonatal DM, maturity onset diabetes of young (MODY), mitochondrial DM, and wolfram syndrome • *Genetic defects in insulin action:* Type A insulin resistance, Leprechaunism, Rabson-Mendenhall syndrome, and Lipoatrophy syndromes	• Neonatal diabetes presents in first 6 months of life. Few babies may be insulin dependent, and few may respond to oral antidiabetic drugs as per the mutation • Patients with MODY have a later age of onset during childhood or adolescence with variable insulin requirement. A strong family history is usually the most important clue
• *Disorders of exocrine pancreas:* Fibrocalcific pancreatic diabetes (FCPD), cystic fibrosis, chronic pancreatitis, autoimmune pancreatitis, hemosiderosis, beta-thalassemia, alpha-1-antitrypsin deficiency, pancreatectomy • *Infections:* Congenital rubella, and CMV	A history of underlying cause such as beta-thalassemia, pancreatitis is present
Drug or chemical induced: High dose steroids, L-asparaginase, cyclosporine, tacrolimus, vincristine, azathioprine, alpha-interferon, diazoxide, beta-blockers, olanzapine, thiazides, diazoxide, and phenytoin	

Table 26.5 Differentiating Features of Type 1 Diabetes Mellitus and Type 2 Diabetes Mellitus

	Type 1 diabetes mellitus	*Type 2 diabetes mellitus*
Pathogenesis	Due to absence or lack of insulin	Due to peripheral resistance to insulin action
Age of onset	Early, in childhood	Later, after 30 years
Genetic predisposition	HLA DR 3 and 4	Polygenic factors
Autoantibodies	Present	Absent
Obesity	Usually absent	Usually present
Complications	Ketoacidosis is common Microvascular and macrovascular complications can occur later	Ketoacidosis is rare Microvascular and macrovascular complications can develop
Therapy	Insulin therapy	Oral drugs, rarely insulin in poorly controlled

The causes of T2DM are less clearly understood, but genetic predisposition has been identified as members of the same family are likely to get affected. In addition, external factors such as obesity and hypertension predispose to an insulin resistance state, which manifests as T2DM.

CLINICAL FEATURES

The classical triad of polyuria, polydipsia, and polyphagia characterizes diabetes mellitus. Children and adolescents usually present with similar symptoms such as polyuria (>4 mL/kg/h), nocturnal enuresis (alert sign in a child who had achieved toilet control), polydipsia, fatigue, and weight loss despite polyphagia.

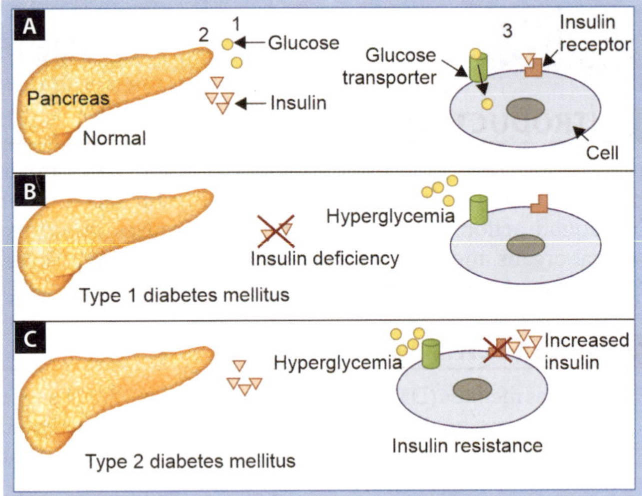

Figs. 26.5A to C: Pathophysiology of type 1 and type 2 diabetes mellitus. (A) Normal state where (1) glucose levels in blood stimulate insulin release from the pancreas (2), insulin acts on insulin receptor in the cells (3) to help in glucose uptake by glucose transporter for cellular metabolism; (B) Insulin deficiency in type 1 diabetes causing hyperglycemia; (C) Type 2 diabetes where insulin release is normal but end-organ resistance causes defective action and resultant hyperglycemia

The duration of symptoms may be variable over few weeks to months but may go unnoticed.

Diabetic Ketoacidosis

Diabetic ketoacidosis (DKA) is the most common presenting feature of patients with T1DM, characterized by fast breathing (due to acidosis), abdominal pain, vomiting, fever, and dehydration with continued polyuria. Sometimes it may be associated with altered sensorium or seizures. It is an acute medical emergency. However, it is rarely seen in T2DM. Sometimes, asymptomatic children may be detected on routine blood investigations.

Course of Type 1 DM

The course of T1DM can be divided into different stages based on presence of autoantibody and clinical manifestations (**Table 26.6**). Most children show insulin responsiveness.

Table 26.6 Staging of Type 1 Diabetes Mellitus (T1DM)

Stage	Characteristics	Diagnostic criteria
1.	• Autoimmunity • Normoglycemia • Presymptomatic	Multiple autoantibodies
2.	• Autoimmunity • Dysglycemia • Presymptomatic	• Multiple autoantibodies • Impaired fasting glucose (IFG)/ Impaired glucose tolerance (IGT)
3.	• New onset hyperglycemia • Dysglycemia • Symptomatic	Diabetes by standard criteria

In initial *stage of metabolic recovery*, the requirement of insulin is high to compensate for the accumulated metabolic deficit, high levels of stress hormones and polyphagia. There is rapid improvement of symptoms, decreased polyphagia and weight gain and decreased insulin requirement.

After the first few days or weeks, the child enters into *honeymoon or remission phase* heralded by dramatic drop in insulin requirement and recurrent episodes of hypoglycemia due to regression of the inflammation in the islets allowing the remaining beta cells to function better and increased insulin sensitivity with decrease in levels of stress hormones and hyperglycemia.

Insulin requirement begins to rise again after 6–12 months (the *intensification phase*), as an effect of progressive beta cell destruction. The child enters *overt diabetes* phase within 1–2 years after clinical onset of the disease, with negligible endogenous insulin production.

People with T1DM, are more prone to develop other autoimmune disorders like celiac disease, Hashimoto thyroiditis, Graves disease, vitiligo, Addison disease, autoimmune hepatitis. These conditions need to be screened at the initial diagnosis of T1DM.

DIAGNOSIS

The criteria for diagnosis of diabetes mellitus are similar to adults and are mentioned in **Table 26.7**.

- Random plasma glucose >200 mg/dL with clinical features of diabetes mellitus, or fasting plasma glucose >126 mg/dL and oral glucose tolerance test >200 mg/dL on two separate occasions, can diagnose diabetes mellitus.
- Glycated hemoglobin (HbA1c) >6.5% on two different occasions is now accepted as the diagnostic criteria in children. HbA1c cannot be relied upon in case of hemoglobinopathies or conditions with increased turnover of RBCs.

Table 26.7 Diagnostic Criteria of Diabetes Mellitus

Disease	Tests	Comments
Diabetes mellitus	• Classic symptoms of diabetes or hyperglycemic crisis with random plasma glucose ≥200 mg/dL • 2-h postprandial glucose ≥200 mg/dL during 75-g OGTT OR Fasting blood glucose≥126 mg/dL OR HbA1c ≥6.5	Blood sample on two separate occasions
Prediabetes	• *Impaired fasting glucose (IFG):* Fasting plasma glucose ≥100 to <126 mg/dL • *Impaired glucose tolerance (IGT)* 2-h postprandial glucose 75-g OGTT ≥140 to <200 mg/dL • HbA1c 5.7–6.4%	Blood sample on two separate occasions

(HbA1c: glycated hemoglobin; OGTT: oral glucose tolerance test)

Oral Glucose Tolerance Test

Most children with type 1 diabetes have substantially high blood glucose levels and do not need glucose tolerance test. Oral glucose tolerance testing (OGTT) is restricted to children with obesity and risk factors for suspected type 2 diabetes. OGTT should be preceded by adequate carbohydrate intake for 3 days (150 g/m^2/day) and overnight fast. The child is given glucose (1.75 g/kg, maximum 75 g) mixed with water and measurement of blood glucose is performed at 0 and 120 minutes.

TREATMENT Type 1 Diabetes

The goals of diabetes management are to ensure the child remains asymptomatic, achieve and maintain a low HbA1c with minimal risk of hypoglycemia, have normal growth, and remain free of microvascular and macrovascular complications of diabetes. Child and family should be emotionally stable and educated in diabetes self-management skills. The child should be able to attend school regularly participate in age-appropriate activities.

The four components of management of T1DM are: (1) insulin therapy, (2) medical nutritional therapy, (3) planned physical activity and (4) therapeutic monitoring. A team approach is mandatory for effective management; the team should comprise of a specialist in childhood diabetes, a pediatrician, a nutritionist, a clinical psychologist, a social worker, a nurse educator, and some well-adjusted senior patients/their parents.

Insulin Therapy

Lifelong insulin therapy is the cornerstone of treatment as it is essential for the survival of children with T1DM. The patients also need to be educated about the dosage and method of administration of insulin to educate them to self-inject insulin

Insulin Preparations

Highly purified *human insulins,* prepared by recombinant DNA technology are classified based on their onset and duration of action as short acting (regular), intermediate acting (NPH and Lente) and long acting (Ultralente). *Insulin analogs* are molecules prepared with structural modifications to alter their time action profile. The analogs may be classified as rapid acting (Lispro, Aspart, and Glulisine), long acting (Detemir and Glargine) or ultra-long acting (Degludec). The types of insulin available with their time action profile are shown in **Table 26.8**.

Table 26.8 Types of Insulin Preparations with Timing of Action

Insulin type	*Examples*	*Onset of action*	*Peak of action*	*Duration of action*	*Timing of administration*
Rapid-acting analogs (RAA)	Lispro, Aspart and Glulisine	15 minutes	1–3 hours	3–5 hours	Just before meals
Short-acting human insulin	Regular insulin	30 minutes to 1 hour	2–4 hours	5–8 hours	Half hour before meals
Intermediate-acting human insulin	NPH and lente	2–4 hours	4–8 hours	12–24 hours	Half hour before meals
Long-acting analogs	Glargine Detemir	2–3 hours 2–3 hours	Peak less 3–9 hours	24 hours 8–20 hours	Before dinner/morning
Ultralong-acting analogs	Degludec	30 minutes to 1.5 hour	Peak less	>24 hours	Before dinner/morning

Dose

Daily insulin dose required depends on the age and pubertal stage of the patient, the stage of diabetes, diet, and level of physical activity of the patient. During the phase of metabolic recovery, the insulin requirement is very high, in the range of 2–3 units/kg/day; which then drops to 0.5 units/kg/ day or less in the honeymoon phase, and with development of overt diabetes it is 0.7–1.0 units/ kg/ day in prepubertal patients and 1.0–1.5 units/kg/day in pubertal patients.

Regimen

Split-mix regime: Insulin therapy can be given as *split-mix regime*, which uses a combination of regular insulin or rapid acting analog (RAA) with intermediate-acting insulin (NPH) given before breakfast (2/3 of daily dose) and before dinner (1/3 of total daily dose). Premixed insulin is available for split-mix regime in a combination of 30/70 or 40/ 60 or 50/50. This regime is not suitable for managing T1DM in children because of their irregular dietary pattern, erratic action of the fixed-combination insulin on the sugar profile and increased susceptibility of children to hypoglycemia. Premixed insulin does not allow titration of insulin as per the meal or physical activity, as required by a child with T1DM who is insulin dependent.

Basal-bolus insulin regime: In the basal-bolus regime, a long-acting insulin (40–50% of total daily dose) is given at dinner time to control basal hepatic glucose release throughout the day. The postmeal sugars are taken care of by additional three to four injections of a short-acting insulin or rapid-acting analog given before major meals. This regime is preferred in children as it mimics the physiologic pattern of insulin release, has less risk for hypoglycemia and offers flexibility for mealtime to children.

Insulin Administration

Insulin can only be administered subcutaneously, at sites marked in **Figure 26.6**. The only exception is regular insulin, which can be administered intravenously after dissolving in fluid in case of DKA management or when patient is not allowed oral consumption. The sites should be rotated daily as repeated administration at one site can lead to local fat accumulation called lipodystrophy. Night dose is best injected in buttocks/thighs.

The site should be cleaned and allowed to dry before injection. The needle is inserted perpendicularly after making a skin pinch. Insulin should be injected after ensuring that there is no blood at the site and after releasing the skin pinch. The needle should be kept *in situ* for few seconds after pushing the drug to avoid any spillage of insulin during removal of needle. The injection site should never be rubbed after drug injection. Insulin should be stored at 4–8°C in the refrigerator and never allowed exposure to sunlight and should never be frozen.

The mode of injection includes conventional 1 mL syringe with hypodermic needle (28 G) (40 and 100/mL) or insulin pens, which have prefilled insulin cartridge with hypodermic needles attached. The long-acting and rapid-acting insulin are usually available as prefilled pens with refill insulin cartridges. Both short and intermediate-acting insulin can be combined in a common syringe for administration in split-mix regime. Regular insulin should be drawn into the syringe first as it is a clear solution followed by NPH which is opaque solution. Glargine should not be mixed with regular insulin for injecting.

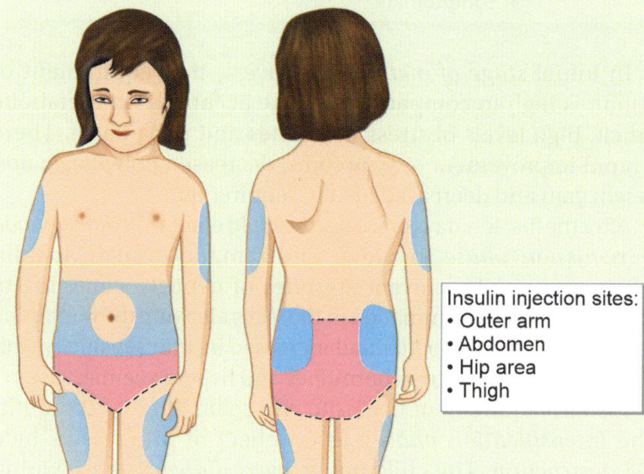

Fig. 26.6: Sites of insulin administration

Insulin Pump Therapy (Continuous Subcutaneous Insulin Infusion)

The insulin pump is an external device that delivers insulin continuously in the subcutaneous space at a predetermined rate with release of additional boluses at mealtime. Only a rapid-acting insulin analog is used both for bolus and basal insulin dose. The basal dose can be adjusted for different times and activity of the day and boluses tailored to different amount and types of meals to provide good glycemic control with limited glycemic variability. Insulin pump is superior to basal bolus regimen in terms of maintaining euglycemia with minimum glycemic variability. Closed loop hybrid systems with capability to detect blood sugar levels (using automated subcutaneous sensors) and infusing desired amount of insulin, are now approved for use in children.

Medical Nutritional Therapy

Diet modification is essential for good glucose control in any diabetic patient. Diet modification for the whole family should be encouraged to ensure a balanced nutritious diet without imposing too many restrictions on the child alone.

- A nutritious diet implies having 55–60% of the calories as carbohydrates, 30% as fat (low polyunsaturated fats and cholesterol) and 10–15% as proteins, and high fiber content.
- Food items with low glycemic index that do not raise blood glucose levels rapidly should be promoted.
- Daily diet should ideally be given as three major meals (20% for breakfast, 20% for lunch, 30% for dinner) and two to three mid-meal snacks (10% for each) to avoid swings in blood glucose.
- Any significant amount of glucose load needs to be covered by a bolus insulin dose like a heavy meal or heavy snack, as adjusted for the blood glucose level.

Planned Physical Activity

Regular exercise (including Yoga) is beneficial for various reasons; it gives the child a psychological boost and a sense of well-being, helps in weight control, increases insulin sensitivity, and thereby lowers insulin requirement, lowers LDL cholesterol, helps in improving cardiac and lung function and leads to improved circulation in the limbs. However, exercise in a child with T1DM can lead to hypoglycemia including delayed postexercise hypoglycemia for up to 16 hours after the activity. In a poorly controlled child, it can lead to worsening of control and ketoacidosis. Hence, *planned exercise* should be adopted with adequate caution. Children should be encouraged to monitor their blood sugars before and after exercise and consume a healthy snack before strenuous play or exercise.

Therapeutic Monitoring

Self-monitoring of blood glucose (SMBG) is the cornerstone in management of diabetes. It involves multiple recording of blood glucose over different times in a day to adjust the insulin need and monitor glucose troughs and peaks. It can be done using point-of-care meters/glucometers. The usual pattern involves testing at fasting and before each major meal, with postmeal values and at midnight (6–7 values a day).

Continuous glucose monitoring systems (CGMS) are electronic devices that measure the interstitial glucose level every 5 minutes for 3–7 days. This is injected and attached as a small patch over the arm. The data obtained can be transferred through a reader or through software coupled to a mobile phone to observe patterns of blood sugar throughout the day. Real time CGMS are used with insulin pumps to inform the glucose values and accordingly administer insulin.

Ketones must be checked on days when the child is sick as they are prone to ketoacidosis. Blood ketone estimation is more reliable than the urine ketone test (since it measures β-hydroxybutyrate whereas the urine test estimates acetoacetate).

Glycated hemoglobin gives measure of average blood glucose over 2–3 months period and is thus useful for monitoring patients on therapy. The normal value is below 5.7. The glucose control is considered adequate when HbA1c values are below 7.5%.

Ambulatory Care of Children with Diabetes Mellitus

Day-to-day management of type 1 diabetes involves medical management of glycemic control, and avoidance of acute complications and prevention of chronic complications on one hand and achieving social, scholastic, and psychological goals of the child on the other.

- Counsel the family regarding nature of disease, need for treatment and insulin.
- Educate and counsel the family and child about insulin storage and administration.
- Encourage participation of the child in his/her treatment for improved glucose control and adherence to therapy.
- Counsel about exercise and diet.
- *Self-monitoring of blood glucose:* Parents to conduct blood glucose estimation at home by glucometer and maintain its record.
- Hypoglycemia management at home and keeping hypoglycemia kit.
- *Sick day management:* Patients should be taught to adjust insulin doses as sickness can lead to increase in blood sugar due to stress. Few illnesses, such as diarrhea, may also lead to decrease in blood sugar due to decreased glucose absorption and poor oral intake. Insulin doses may be increased or decreased by 1–2 units, respectively.
- School teachers should be educated to aid the child in taking insulin and detecting and managing hypoglycemia. The school environment should be made conducive for diabetic children.
- Guide the child and parents during acute illness management especially for DKA or hypoglycemic episodes. Emergency contact should be provided for assistance.

COMPLICATIONS

Complications associated with diabetes can be classified as in **Box 26.5**. Regular monitoring by physical examination and screening for the long-term complications is required for prevention, timely detection, and early intervention. It should be started after 2–5 years of diagnosis or at puberty whichever is earlier. Screening modalities and their interpretation for long-term micro- and macrovascular complications are listed in **Table 26.9** and management of acute complications are discussed in the next sections.

Box 26.5 Complications Associated with Diabetes Mellitus

A. *Acute complications:*
   1. Ketoacidosis
   2. Hypoglycemia

B. *Intermediate:* Lipoatrophy, growth failure, delayed puberty, hypoglycemia, hypoglycemic unawareness, *psychological issues* (mental health, and behavioral problems)

C. *Chronic complications:*
   1. Microvascular (retinopathy, neuropathy, and nephropathy)
   2. Macrovascular complications (myocardial infarction, and stroke)
   3. Predisposition to other autoimmune conditions
   4. Predisposition to hypertension, dyslipidemia, and obesity
   5. *Skin and joint complications:* Edema, necrobiosis lipoidica diabeticorum, limited joint mobility

Table 26.9 Screening for Long-term Complications of Diabetes

Complications	*Screening method*
Nephropathy	Urinary albumin/creatinine ratio—annually
Retinopathy	Fundus photography—annually
Neuropathy	History, physical examination, clinical tests—annually
Macrovascular complications	Lipid profile every 2 yearly and BP annually
Autoimmune disorders	Thyroid function tests—at diagnosis then 5 yearly

TYPE 2 DIABETES MELLITUS

Type 2 diabetes is increasingly being detected in children and adolescents. The disorder presents with milder symptoms than T1DM. Typically, onset and progression of symptoms is slow and ketosis is uncommon but presentation with ketoacidosis should not be held as a point against the diagnosis. Patients often have a family history of T2DM, may be overtly obese or have increased abdominal fat, may have hypertension, acanthosis, dyslipidemia and in females there may be signs of polycystic ovarian disease (PCOD). These children and adolescents should be evaluated for hyperlipidemia, diabetic retinopathy, and nephropathy at diagnosis.

Risk-based Screening

Risk-based screening for type 2 diabetes or prediabetes in asymptomatic children and adolescents in a clinical setting with risk factors is recommended **(Box 26.6)**. If tests are normal, repeat testing at a minimum of 3-year intervals (or more frequently if BMI is increasing or risk factor profile deteriorating) is recommended.

"Prediabetes" is the term used for individuals whose glucose levels do not meet the criteria for diabetes but levels are too high to be considered normal. It indicates increased risk for developing diabetes and cardiovascular disease (CVD). Criteria for screening for diabetes or prediabetes in asymptomatic adolescents are also outlined in **Box 26.6**. Prediabetes is associated with obesity (especially abdominal or visceral obesity), dyslipidemia with high triglycerides and/or low HDL cholesterol, and hypertension. It warrants lifestyle intervention for prevention of diabetes.

Box 26.6 Risk-based Screening for Type 2 Diabetes or Prediabetes in Asymptomatic Children and Adolescents

Testing should be considered in youth (beyond puberty) who have overweight (≥85th percentile) or obesity (≥95th percentile) and who have one or more additional risk factors based on the strength of their association with diabetes:

1. Maternal history of diabetes or GDM during the child's gestation
2. Family history of type 2 diabetes in first- or second-degree relative
3. Race/ethnicity (Native American, African American, Latino, Asian American, Pacific Islander)
4. Signs of insulin resistance or conditions associated with insulin resistance (acanthosis nigricans, hypertension, dyslipidemia, polycystic ovary syndrome, gestational diabetes in mother, or small-for-gestational-age birth weight)

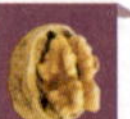

IN A NUTSHELL

Diabetes Mellitus

1. Diagnosis of type 1 diabetes mellitus is based on clinical suspicion. Random plasma glucose >200 mg/dL with clinical features of diabetes mellitus, or fasting plasma glucose >126 mg/dL and oral glucose tolerance test >200 mg/dL on two separate occasions, is confirmatory for diabetes mellitus.
2. T1DM causes 95% of all diabetes with childhood onset and is characterized by immune-mediated pancreatic β-cell destruction requiring insulin to achieve euglycemia.
3. T2DM although less common in children is now witnessing increasing prevalence with epidemic of obesity. It is characterized by insulin resistance suggested clinically by acanthosis nigricans, central adiposity, and family history of type 2 diabetes in first degree relatives.
4. Diabetes management involves multidisciplinary team and active education and motivation of child and parents for compliance to lifelong therapy and lifestyle modifications. The four components of management of T1DM are: (1) insulin therapy, (2) medical nutritional therapy, (3) planned physical activity and (4) therapeutic monitoring.
5. Diabetic ketoacidosis, and hypoglycemia are the most dreaded acute complications in T1DM that should be detected and managed promptly.

American Diabetes Association. 13. Children and Adolescents: Standards of Medical Care in Diabetes-2020. Diabetes Care. 2020;43(Suppl 1):S163-82.

Besser REJ, Bell KJ, Couper JJ, et al. ISPAD clinical practice consensus guidelines 2022: Stages of type 1 diabetes in children and adolescents. Pediatr Diabetes. 2022;10.1111/pedi.13410.

Solomen CG. Current management of glycemia in children with type 1 diabetes mellitus. N Engl J Med. 2022;386:1155-64.

26.7 Diabetic Ketoacidosis

PE 30.4

PATHOPHYSIOLOGY

Diabetes ketoacidosis (DKA) is a medical emergency. It is the most common acute and severe manifestation of T1DM.

Ketones are produced in state of insulin deficit coupled with increase in production of counterregulatory hormones (catecholamines, glucagon, cortisol, and growth hormone) as in illnesses, infections, or trauma. DKA can be precipitated by severe insulin deficiency as in previously undiagnosed T1DM or when a patient on therapy inadvertently skips or markedly reduce insulin dose.

The combination of absolute or relative insulin deficiency and increased counter-regulatory hormones create a state of accelerated catabolism, with increased glucose production (due to glycogenolysis and gluconeogenesis) and decreased glucose uptake by peripheral cells causing hyperglycemia, hyperosmolarity, dehydration (osmotic diuresis) and dyselectrolytemia.

The hormonal milieu also favors lipolysis and ketogenesis causing ketonemia and acidosis. Hypoperfusion might aggravate acidosis by lactic acidemia. These changes further induce stress hormone production and continuation of the cycle until insulin availability.

CLINICAL FEATURES

Manifestations include nausea, weakness, lethargy, weight loss, altered sensorium, pain abdomen, vomiting, dehydration, fast and shallow breathing (Kussmaul breathing) due to hyperglycemia and ketoacidosis. The mortality rate from DKA in children is 0.15–0.30%. Cerebral edema accounts for 60–90% of all DKA deaths.

DIAGNOSIS

For diagnosis of DKA, all following three biochemical criteria should be present:

1. Blood glucose >200 mg/dL (>11 mmol/L)
2. Venous pH <7.3 or bicarbonate <18 mEq/L
3. Ketonemia (>3 mmol/L) or ketonuria

TREATMENT Diabetic Ketoacidosis

The management of DKA relies on a good teamwork with intensive monitoring and judicious fluid therapy. The steps in management of DKA are discussed here.

Start Fluid Therapy

Patients with DKA may present with severe dehydration or shock. Fluid therapy is the cornerstone of management of DKA since correction of dehydration is vital. Stabilize the patient and secure an intravenous line. Start rapid intravenous fluid therapy with normal saline or Ringer lactate at 10 mL/kg administered over 30–60 minutes. Subsequently the type of fluid is changed to N/2 saline at a calculated volume **(Table 26.10)**. Dextrose is added to the fluid once the blood sugar falls below 250 mg/dL.

Insulin Therapy

It should be instituted after starting fluid replacement. Regular insulin at 0.05–0.1 U/kg/h is administered intravenously dissolved in distilled water and the dose is titrated till resolution of ketosis, acidosis, and dehydration. Insulin should be preferably administered using an insulin pump. It may be diluted to a concentration of 0.1 U/mL when used in a burette. Bolus insulin doses are not administered as it may precipitate cerebral edema. Insulin drip is discontinued as soon as ketosis resolves and the patient can take orally. The patient is then switched to subcutaneous insulin.

Monitoring

This is crucial for adequate management of DKA with minimal risk of complications like cerebral edema, renal failure, etc. The monitoring parameters and frequency are depicted in **Table 26.11**.

Table 26.10 Calculation of Fluid Replacement in Diabetic Ketoacidosis

Fluid requirement	Maintenance + deficit – fluid already given
Maintenance fluid requirement	• ≤*10 kg:* 100 mL/kg/24 hours • *11–20 kg:* 1,000 mL + 50 mL/kg/24 hours for each kg from 11–20 • *> 20 kg:* 1,500 mL + 20 mL/kg/24 hours for each kg >20
Deficit (liters)	% of dehydration × body weight (kg)

Table 26.11 Clinical and Biochemical Monitoring in Diabetic Ketoacidosis (DKA)

Vital signs (heart rate, respiratory rate, and blood pressure)	Hourly
Neurological observations (Glasgow Coma Scale) for warning signs and symptoms of cerebral edema	Hourly
Fluid input and output	Hourly
Capillary blood glucose	Hourly
Laboratory tests: Serum electrolytes, glucose, urea, calcium, magnesium, phosphorus, hematocrit, and blood gases	2 hourly for the first 12 hours and then as required
Urine ketones	6 hourly

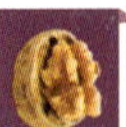

IN A NUTSHELL

Diabetic Ketoacidosis

1. Diabetic ketoacidosis presents as a triad of ketosis, hyperglycemia and acidosis resulting from insulin deficiency.
2. Fluid replacement is the first step in treatment followed by insulin infusion (intravenous).
3. Cerebral edema is the most dreaded complication of DKA that should be monitored and treated if develops.

Cashen K, Petersen T. Diabetic ketoacidosis. Pediatr Rev. 2019;40(8):412-20.

Glaser N, Fritsch M, Priyambada L, et al. ISPAD clinical practice consensus guidelines 2022: Diabetic ketoacidosis and hyperglycemic hyperosmolar state. Pediatr Diabetes. 2022;23(7):835-56.

26.8 Hypoglycemia *PE 30.4*

INTRODUCTION

Hypoglycemia in a child is defined as blood glucose below 70 mg/dL (alert), and is clinically significant at below 54 mg/dL. Common factors in children that predispose to hypoglycemia are:

- Excess insulin administration
- Insulin administration without intake of meals
- Sickness
- Unplanned prolonged physical activity

Initially, it manifest symptoms resulting from sympathetic overactivation (autonomic symptoms) such as palpitations, sweating, hunger, trembling, tachycardia, or neuroglycopenic symptoms such as lethargy, confusion, unsteadiness, slurred speech, etc. In untreated cases, it may result in seizures and coma due to neuroglycopenia.

Blood glucose should be checked immediately in any child with diabetes on insulin therapy who present with aforementioned symptoms. In absence of glucometer, hypoglycemia should be presumed and immediate management should be instituted.

TREATMENT Hypoglycemia

If the patient is conscious and can take orally: The patient should be administered rapidly absorptive simple glucose preferably in form of glucose solution (150 mL water and 3–4 spoons of sugar/glucose powder) or 1–2 commercially available chewable glucose tablets. Fruit juices and carbonated drink may be used in emergency. This should be followed by rechecking blood glucose after 10–15 minutes and repeating the same if levels are still low. A serving of slow releasing carbohydrate like bread or sweet biscuits should be offered once the blood glucose is normal to sustain normoglycemia.

Patient is unconscious or cannot take orally: Glucose solution may be administered via a nasogastric tube. Alternately, 2 mL/kg of 10% dextrose should be administered intravenously. Subcutaneous or nasal glucagon can be useful in emergency settings. The patient should be encouraged to eat as soon as the patient regains consciousness.

The family should be encouraged to carry a hypoglycemia kit and diabetes identification card during outdoor visits. Repeated episodes of hypoglycemia on follow-up should be discussed in detail with the family for meal quality, quantity, exercise pattern and insulin injection practices. Continuous glucose monitoring systems (CGMS) can help detect variability in glucose levels for instituting better control measures.

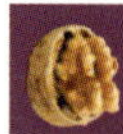

IN A NUTSHELL

Hypoglycemia

1. Hypoglycemia can occur in T1DM during excess insulin dose, sickness or during physical activity.
2. Treatment should be instituted in the presence of neuroglycopenic or autonomic symptoms or if blood glucose is tested low.
3. Simple sugars given in liquid form or paste helps to raise the blood glucose faster than slow release carbohydrates such as chocolates, biscuits.

Abraham MB, Jones TW, Naranjo D, et al. ISPAD Clinical practice consensus guidelines 2018: assessment and management of hypoglycemia in children and adolescents with diabetes. Pediatr Diabetes. 2018; 19(Suppl 27):178-92.

Kenny C. When hypoglycemia is not obvious: diagnosing and treating under-recognized and undisclosed hypoglycemia. Prim Care Diabetes. 2014;8(1):3-11.

26.9 Differences of Sex Development *PE 30.5*

INTRODUCTION

Differences of sex development (DSDs; also known as disorders of sex development) are a group of conditions where the genetic sex of the baby does not match with clinical phenotype. This term is the revised term used for diseases initially grouped as sexual hermaphrodite, intersex, or ambiguous genitalia. DSDs comprise a large group of congenital conditions in which chromosomal, gonadal or anatomical sex has been compromised, usually owing to a genetic mutation.

PATHOPHYSIOLOGY

Sexual differentiation is a complex process involving a close interaction of genetic, phenotypic and psychological factors. Usually genetic sex guides gonadal sex, which is responsible for the determination of phenotype and gender identity. Any deviation from this pattern results in DSD. The causes include genetic mutations in gonadal development, enzyme deficiency, hormonal defects, or *in utero* maternal exposure to drugs.

The embryo/fetus/baby is either genetically male (46,XY) or female (46,XX), but has ambiguous genitalia. This implies that genetic males will be undervirilized and genetic females may be masculinized or overvirilized (**Fig. 26.7**). In rare cases, the embryo may have genetic makeup of both females and males (46,XX and XY), called as *true gonadal hermaphrodite.*

DIAGNOSIS

A baby with genitalia that does not conform to the normal appearance (does not completely resemble a male or a female) should

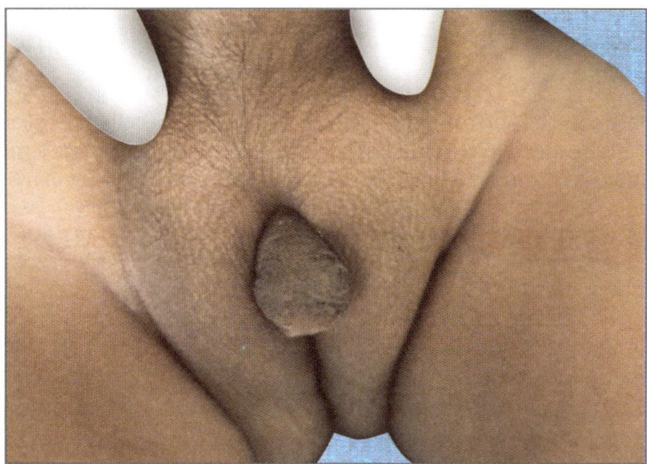

Fig. 26.7: An enlarged clitoris in a 46,XX female, suspected of DSD

be suspected of having a DSD. Milder forms may be brought to medical attention during puberty with delayed puberty due to lack of functional gonads.

GENITAL EXAMINATION

The most important step is identification of gonads. Bilaterally rounded structures below the inguinal canal are most likely testis and suggest a XY phenotype.

- The labioscrotal region should be evaluated for the extent of fusion of labial folds.
- The length of phallus and number of openings in the urogenital region should be recorded.
- Babies with XY, DSD with poor testosterone production or function may fail to develop a normal phallus. The urethral opening may be elsewhere instead of the tip of phallus such as midshaft phallus, base of phallus or perineal (hypospadias).
- The length of the phallus may also be small in DSD (micropenis), defined as length below 2.5 SD (usually below 2–2.5 cm at birth).

Asymmetrical labioscrotal region is suggestive of unilateral gonad as in gonadal dysgenesis or ovotesticular DSD (details of these diagnoses is beyond the scope of this chapter). The list of conditions which are classified as DSD and should be referred for evaluation is mentioned in **Box 26.7**.

Box 26.7 Conditions to Suspect Disorder of Sexual Differentiation

1. Overt genital ambiguity (for example, cloacal exstrophy)
2. Apparent female genitalia with an enlarged clitoris, posterior labial fusion, or an inguinal/labial mass
3. Apparent male genitalia with bilateral undescended testes (cryptorchidism), micropenis, isolated perineal hypospadias, or mild hypospadias with undescended testis
4. A family history of disorder of sex development
5. A discordance between genital appearance and a prenatal karyotype

TREATMENT Differences of Sex Development

Children with 46,XX with DSD most commonly have congenital adrenal hyperplasia where there is a deficiency of corticosteroid and/or mineralocorticoid production. The steroid precursors instead are diverted toward production of androgens that can cause masculinization of a female fetus. The deficiency of cortisol removes the negative feedback on the pituitary causing excess release of ACTH, which causes hyperpigmentation of the skin and genitalia. Babies present with ambiguous genitalia that are dark pigmented and may have concurrent electrolyte imbalance (salt-wasting with low serum sodium and high potassium). Electrolyte and metabolic disturbances (metabolic acidosis and hypoglycemia in adrenal insufficiency) should be identified and stabilized before referral of affected children. Newborn screening is available for CAH to measure 17-hydroxy-progesterone (steroid precursor) on heel prick samples in babies after birth. This analyte is elevated in babies with *classical* CAH who may have DSD and/or salt-wasting, depending on the deficiency of the enzyme in the steroidogenesis pathway.

Children with DSD need a confirmatory genotype to determine the genetic sex as soon as possible. Further management depends on the etiology and should be undertaken by a multidisciplinary team. Gender assignment is a sensitive decision and should not be done in haste. An informed decision can be taken by the child and the family on follow-up after understanding the etiology, available medical and surgical options, psychosocial development, gender identity and sociocultural factors.

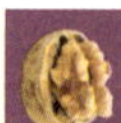

IN A NUTSHELL

Differences of Sex Development

1. Disorders/differences of sex development result when there is a incongruency among genetic sex and genitalia development.
2. Karyotype to ascertain the genetic/biological gender is essential first step in the diagnosis.
3. Congenital adrenal hyperplasia is the most common cause of DSD in 46,XX patients that manifests as virilization with/without dyselectrolytemia. Treatment with steroids is life-saving and required throughout life.

Dabas A, Vats P, Sharma R, et al. Management of infants with congenital adrenal hyperplasia. Indian Pediatr. 2020;57(2):159-64.

Indyk JA. Disorders/differences of sex development (DSDs) for primary care: the approach to the infant with ambiguous genitalia. Transl Pediatr. 2017;6(4):323-34.

26.10 Puberty

PE 30.6

Puberty is the phase of life heralded by gonadal maturation and appearance of secondary sexual characteristics. These changes occur during adolescence, the period of transition from childhood to adulthood. The physiological pubertal changes affect many organ systems on the body, including the gonads that determine the future reproductive potential of the individual.

PHYSIOLOGY OF PUBERTY

Puberty involves development and maturation of primary gonads, namely the testicular tissue in boys and breast, ovarian and uterine growth in girls. The secondary sexual characteristics such as pubic and axillary hair growth, change of voice in boys, acne and axillary odor are other evident pubertal changes. Estrogen is produced from the ovaries in girls and testosterone is produced from the Leydig cells in testes in boys that are responsible for the pubertal changes. The adrenal androgens are also involved in the development of secondary sexual characteristics in girls.

The production of sex hormones is under the influence of luteinizing hormone (LH) from the anterior pituitary. The release of LH is in turn regulated by the gonadotropin releasing hormone (GnRH) at the hypothalamus. GnRH starts releasing LH in pulses after being signaled by Kisspeptin, a hypothalamic peptide, a key regulator of puberty. Kisspeptin release is affected by various factors such as age, genetics, nutrition, and neurotransmitters. GnRH pulses, initially start during night around 6–8 years of age and gradually sustain throughout the day. This leads to an abrupt pulsatile increase in the levels of gonadotropins (mainly LH), and thereby, sex hormones. The hypothalamic-pituitary-gonadal (HPG) axis is under the feedback control by the sex hormones and another hormone produced by the gonads called inhibin that is produced by the Sertoli cells in boys and granulosa cells in girls. The secretion of LH is inhibited by testosterone and estrogen produced by the Leydig cells and theca cells, respectively, while inhibin acts as a negative feedback for follicle-stimulating hormone (FSH) production.

ASSESSMENT OF PUBERTAL DEVELOPMENT

The pattern of pubertal development is different in girls and boys. The various terminologies related to puberty are explained in **Table 26.12**. For assessment of pubertal growth, the sexual maturation pattern has been divided into five stages as per the Tanner staging system, depending on growth of breast, pubic, and axillary hair in girls and increase in testicular volume with growth in genitalia, pubic and axillary hair in boys. Stage 1 means prepubertal pattern, stage 2 means pubertal onset, stages 3 and 4 are where further maturation in genitalia and pubic hair pattern occur, and stage 5 where growth is complete to resemble adult pattern. This has been described previously in **Chapter 5** on Adolescence.

Table 26.12 Terminology with their Description Related to Puberty

Terminology	*Description*
Adrenarche	Onset of adrenal androgen production
Thelarche	Onset of breast development (breast bud)
Pubarche	Onset of pubic hair growth in both boys and girls
Menarche	First menstrual period
Gonadarche	Onset of pubertal maturation of gonads and secretion of sex hormones resulting in breast development and labial growth in girls and testicular growth in boys
Spermarche	Appearance of sperms in seminal fluid

26.11 Precocious Puberty

PE 30.6

INTRODUCTION

Attainment of sexual characters before 8 years in girls or 9 years in boys is defined as early or precocious. These children also show early *growth spurt* and advanced skeletal growth under the influence of excessive sex hormones. It ultimately leads to loss of final height potential and may cause psychological issues in children.

Precocious puberty may result from abnormal regulation of the gonadotropins (FSH or LH) termed as central or gonadotropin-dependent precocious puberty (GDPP); or by excess of gonadal hormones (estrogen and testosterone in females and males, respectively) termed as gonadotropin-independent precocious puberty (GIPP).

ETIOLOGY

Both GDPP and GIPP are more common in girls than in boys, with a ratio of 5:1 in GDPP and 2.5:1 in GIPP. Etiology of precocious puberty is listed in **Table 26.13**. GDPP and GIPP are compared in **Table 26.14**.

Gonadotropin-dependent Precocious Puberty (Central Precocious Puberty)

It is the most common form of precocious puberty accounting for 70–80% of all cases of precocious puberty. It is about five times more common in girls than in boys. Pubertal development is always isosexual and sequential. Breast development, female body contour (gluteofemoral adiposity),

Table 26.13 Etiology of Precocious Puberty

Gonadotropin-dependent precocious puberty (central precocious puberty)	*Gonadotropin-independent precocious puberty (peripheral precocious puberty)*
Both boys and girls: • Idiopathic • International adoption • Neurogenic ▪ Hamartoma—most common cause of organic central precocity (gelastic seizures) ▪ Astrocytoma ▪ Pineal tumor ▪ Ependymoma ▪ *Glioma (optic pathway)* ▪ *Craniopharyngioma (rare)* ▪ *Infections:* Neurotuberculosis, and meningitis ▪ *Injury:* Head trauma, neurosurgery, and cranial irradiation ▪ *Malformation:* Arachnoid cyst, hydrocephalus, septo-optic dysplasia, and holoprosencephaly • Withdrawal of chronic sex hormone exposure • *Genetic:* Gain of function mutation of kisspeptin/kisspeptin receptor • Prolonged undertreated peripheral precocious puberty	**Girls:** *Ovarian disorders:* • *Ovarian cyst* • *Hyperplasia* • McCune-Albright syndrome *Estrogen-secreting tumors:* • *Ovarian (granulosa-theca cell tumor, gonadoblastoma, and teratoma)* • *Adrenal* ▪ Exogenous estrogen exposure ▪ Peutz-Jegher syndrome (ovarian sex cord tumors) ▪ Primary hypothyroidism ▪ Aromatase excess **Boys:** *Adrenal disorders:* • Congenital adrenal hyperplasia • Tumors • Familial male-limited precocious puberty (testotoxicosis) *Testosterone-secreting tumors:* • Leydig cell • Adrenal rests *hCG-secreting tumors:* • Hepatoblastoma • Pineal gland tumors • Cerebral tumors (germinoma) • Mediastinal tumors • Gonadal tumors ▪ Exogenous androgen (testosterone) exposure ▪ Primary hypothyroidism (testicular enlargement only) familial glucocorticoid resistance ▪ McCune-Albright syndrome (rare)

facial maturity, estrogenization of vaginal mucosa (dull, pink, moist, and thick vaginal mucosa as compared to prepubertal thin and red vaginal mucosa), acceleration of linear growth, rapid bone maturation, adult body odor, and behavioral changes typical of puberty are the features of estrogenization in a female.

It may be caused by a variety of pathologies of the central nervous system, which are similar in boys and girls **(Table 26.13)**. The majority (70%) of girls with GDPP have idiopathic precocious puberty, while 75% of boys with GDPP have an underlying CNS pathology. The younger the child, the greater is the likelihood of an underlying pathology. Fifty percent of children with idiopathic GDPP manifest between 6 and 8 years of age. Hypothalamic hamartoma, a neuronal migration defect, is the most common cause of organic central precocious puberty.

Table 26.14 Comparison of Gonadotropin-dependent and Independent Precocious Puberty

Gonadotropin-dependent precocious puberty	*Gonadotropin-independent precocious puberty*
More common cause of precocious puberty	Less common cause of precocious puberty
Girls more affected than boys	Affects boys more commonly than girls
Always isosexual—pubertal changes in consonance with the same gender	Isosexual or heterosexual
Pubertal progression occurs in the pattern as in normal puberty	Pubertal changes may occur in isolation and may not follow the normal pubertal pattern

The disorder presents with early onset and rapid progression of puberty, seizures, and uncontrolled laughter episodes (gelastic epilepsy).

Gonadotropin-independent Precocious Puberty (Peripheral Precocious Puberty)

It can be *isosexual* or *heterosexual* (pubertal features of the other gender). GIPP is usually caused by estrogenic ovarian cysts in girls manifesting in isosexual form. A fluctuant course of pubertal development and early vaginal bleeding (due to hyperestrogenic state) is common. The condition is usually self-resolving and there is no need for treatment. Recurrent ovarian cysts should raise the possibility of McCune-Albright syndrome, a somatic activating mutation of stimulatory G protein, which presents with a triad of cutaneous (multiple café-au-lait spots), skeletal (multiple fibrous dysplasia) and polyendocrine abnormalities (hyperthyroidism, rickets and GH excess). Precocious puberty occurs at an early age and is rapidly progressive in McCune Albright syndrome.

Congenital adrenal hyperplasia is the chief cause of peripheral precocious puberty in boys (isosexual) that is characterized by increased adrenal androgens. Adrenal tumors are rare in childhood as a cause of GIPP. Human chorionic gonadotropin (hCG) secreting tumors of the liver, mediastinum or brain may present with precocious puberty.

Heterosexual precocious puberty is defined as premature development of secondary sexual characteristics in discordance with chromosomal and gonadal sex, e.g., clitoromegaly (enlargement of clitoris) in girls and gynecomastia (development of breast tissue) in boys. Heterosexual precocity is always independent of reactivation of HPG-axis. *Heterosexual PPP* in girls may be due to excess androgens such as congenital adrenal hyperplasia or virilizing adrenal or ovarian tumors; and feminizing tumors of the testis or adrenal glands in boys.

Incomplete Variants of Precocious Puberty

These disorders represent normal variants and do not require specific treatment. Their identification helps in restricting the extent of diagnostic workup and counseling.

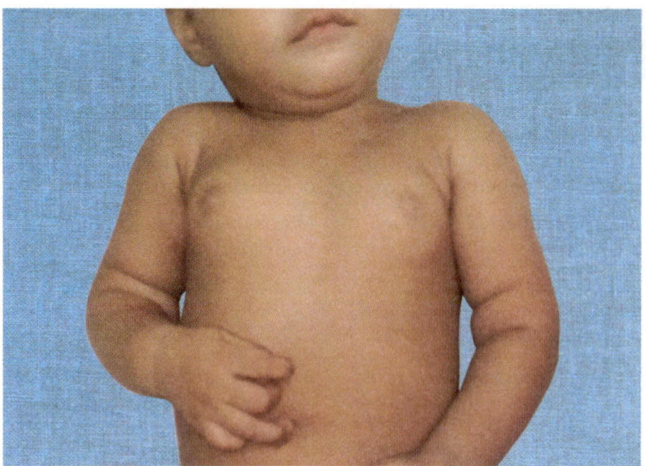

Fig. 26.8: One-year-old girl with premature breast development

Isolated premature thelarche: Isolated breast development may represent isolated thelarche or first manifestation of central precocious puberty. Isolated premature thelarche presents with premature breast bud development usually before two years of age and is not associated with progression to other secondary sexual characteristics (**Fig. 26.8**). Growth velocity is normal for age bone age does not advance. Serum FSH and LH response to GnRH are in prepubertal levels.

Parents should be reassured as isolated premature thelarche is benign and nonprogressive, and usually regresses within 6 months to 6 years. Further, final adult height and subsequent pubertal development are normal in these girls; therefore, it does not require any treatment.

Isolated premature pubarche/adrenarche: Isolated premature pubarche is characterized by early appearance of pubic/axillary hair without other secondary sexual characteristics and is preceded by premature adrenarche. Most cases are physiological variants.

Rarely, androgen excess due to adrenal (congenital adrenal hyperplasia, adrenal tumor) or ovarian (tumor, polycystic ovarian disease) causes may be identified. Normal bone age and growth velocity and absence of virilization suggest premature adrenarche and require no treatment. If a child has premature pubarche along with other signs of androgenization (clitoromegaly in girls and penile enlargement in boys) or bone age is significantly advanced, child should be actively evaluated for pathological causes of premature pubarche.

Isolated menarche: Vaginal bleeding in the absence of thelarche is against the diagnosis of gonadotropin-dependent precocious puberty. Vaginal bleeding occurs early in course of estrogen excess states such as ovarian cysts, hypothyroidism, and McCune-Albright syndrome. Local cause of vaginal bleeding (infection, foreign body, sexual abuse, or tumors) needs to be excluded if there is no associated breast development.

Table 26.15 Investigations in Precocious Puberty

Parameters	*Remarks*
Bone age	For assessing the height compromise and predicting final height. Advanced bone age (>2 SD of chronological age) suggests progressive precocious puberty, while normal bone age indicates slowly progressive puberty
Thyroid function tests	Hypothyroidism should be suspected with precocious (early) puberty and delayed growth and skeletal maturation
Basal and stimulated gonadotropin levels	Pooled gonadotropin levels are preferred due to their pulsatile secretion. LH is a better indicator compared to FSH, since the former increase significantly during puberty. Basal LH levels in the pubertal range (>0.6 mU/L with LH/FSH ratio >1) are suggestive of development of puberty. Stimulation testing is performed by measuring LH and FSH levels after GnRH injection (procedure and interpretation to be done under expert supervision)
Additional tests for etiology in peripheral precocious puberty	Hormonal estimation as per the suspected disorder, like serum 17-hydroxyprogesterone for congenital adrenal hyperplasia, human-chorionic gonadotropin in testicular tumors
Neuroimaging	Should be done in both boys and girls with onset of puberty below 6 years of age, or if there is rapid progression and/or associated neurological features
Ultrasound abdomen and pelvis	Can diagnose follicular cysts and ovarian and adrenal mass

INVESTIGATIONS

The investigations required in a child with precocious puberty are mentioned in **Table 26.15**.

TREATMENT Precocious Puberty

Aims of management include treatment of underlying cause, management of any systemic diseases, and puberty suppression to achieve the target height potential. The significant long-term consequence of precocious puberty is short stature. Height is usually accelerated at presentation. This is associated with disproportionately advanced bone age at diagnosis resulting in premature epiphyseal fusion that is responsible for a compromised final height.

Patients with central precocious puberty are treated with depot injections of GnRH analogs to suppress puberty, till the patient achieves a chronological age of 11–12 years (conforming to normal age of puberty/menarche). These drugs are available for intramuscular use in India and also as subcutaneous implants in western countries.

The treatment of peripheral precocious puberty is directed toward treatment of the underlying cause. Congenital adrenal hyperplasia is treated with steroid replacement and gonadal or adrenal tumors require surgical resection.

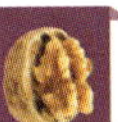

IN A NUTSHELL

Precocious Puberty

1. Puberty in adolescence is associated with appearance of secondary sexual characteristics and gonadal maturation.
2. Attainment of sexual characters before 8 years in girls or 9 years in boys is defined as early or precocious. These children show early *growth spurt* and advanced skeletal growth ultimately leading to loss of final height potential and may have psychological issues thereby warranting treatment.
3. *Gonadotropin-dependent precocious puberty (GDPP)/true or central precocious puberty* occurs due to premature activation of HPG axis causing sequential and progressive development of isosexual secondary sexual characteristics.
4. *Gonadotropin-independent precocious puberty (GIPP)/pseudo or peripheral precocious puberty* results from excess of sex steroids (iso or heterosexual) independent of the HPG axis causing nonsequential appearance of secondary sexual characteristics and may or may not be progressive.

Dominique Long; Precocious Puberty. Pediatr Rev. 2015;36 (7):319-21.
Kaplowitz P, Bloch C; Section on Endocrinology, American Academy of Pediatrics. Evaluation and Referral of Children with Signs of Early Puberty. Pediatrics. 2016;137(1):e20153732.
Latronico AC, Brito VN, Carel JC. Causes, diagnosis, and treatment of central precocious puberty. Lancet Diabetes Endocrinol. 2016;4:265-74.
Susman EJ, Houts RM, Steinberg L, et al. Longitudinal development of secondary sexual characteristics in girls and boys between ages 9 ½ and 15 ½ years. Arch Pediatr Adolesc Med. 2010;164:166-73.

26.12 Gynecomastia

PE 30.6

INTRODUCTION

Gynecomastia is defined as the presence of glandular breast tissue >1 cm in males. Asymptomatic gynecomastia is a physiological finding in most newborns, adolescents, and elderly men. Adolescent gynecomastia typically occurs at age 11–15 years (early to midpuberty) and subsides in 1–2 years. It must be distinguished from lipomastia or pseudogynecomastia (increased adipose tissue in the breast area), a common finding in obese children. Glandular tissue feels firm or grainy, while adipose tissue feels soft on palpation with flat hands. Distinction may be difficult because the two conditions often coexist. Symptomatic benign gynecomastia, which may be a sign of hypogonadism or systemic disease, is far less common, while breast cancer is extremely rare.

PATHOPHYSIOLOGY

It is caused by an altered balance between estrogens and androgens (increased estrogens, decreased androgens, or increased sensitivity of breast tissue to estrogens). Increased leptin levels as well as human chorionic gonadotropin (hCG) and LH receptors on male breast tissue may also play a role. Altered levels of sex hormone-binding globulin (e.g., hyperthyroidism, chronic liver disease, or drugs) can change the estrogen-androgen ratio.

ETIOLOGY

The common pathological causes of gynecomastia are listed in **Box 26.8**. The causes that result in deficiency of androgen or testosterone production or action can result in gynecomastia.

Box 26.8 Etiology of Gynecomastia

A. *Estrogen-secreting tumors*
   1. Leydig cell tumor
   2. Sertoli cell tumor
   3. hCG-producing tumor
   4. Adrenocortical tumor

B. *Androgen deficiency*
   1. *Primary hypogonadism*
      - Klinefelter/Kallmann syndrome
      - Congenital anorchia
      - *Testicular injury:* Infection (e.g., mumps), trauma, radiation, drugs (cytotoxic drugs, e.g., vincristine, methotrexate, cisplatin, and imatinib)
   2. *Secondary hypogonadism*
      - Hypothalamic-pituitary disease/surgery/radiation, e.g., craniopharyngioma
      - GnRH agonists/antagonists
      - *Abnormal testosterone synthesis:* Genetic defects, drugs (ketoconazole, spironolactone, flutamide, finasteride and dutasteride, etomidate, metronidazole, and cimetidine)
      - *Abnormal testosterone action:* Androgen insensitivity syndromes or androgen receptor gene defect
      - *Abnormal sex-hormone binding globulin:* Hyperthyroidism, chronic liver disease, and drugs

TREATMENT Gynecomastia

Investigations are needed if there is prepubertal onset (<9 years), associated systemic disease or delayed puberty (hypogonadism). Rarely boys may have discharge, hard fixed breast tissue, or increase in size of breast size. The underlying cause must be treated.

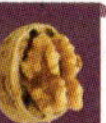

IN A NUTSHELL

Gynecomastia

1. Presence of glandular breast tissue >1 cm in males is called gynecomastia.
2. Asymptomatic physiological gynecomastia can be seen in adolescence before midpuberty (11–15 years) and subsides in 1–2 years. It must be distinguished from lipomastia.
3. Neonates may present with palpable breast bud under the influence of maternal estrogens transferred transplacentally which subsides spontaneously after 1–2 months.
4. Investigations are needed if there is prepubertal onset (<9 years), associated systemic disease or delayed puberty and presence of discharge, hard fixed breast tissue, or increase in size of breast size.

Lemaine V, Cayci C, Simmons PS, et al. Gynecomastia in adolescent males. Semin Plast Surg. 2013;27(1):56-61.
Soliman AT, De Sanctis V, Yassin M. Management of adolescent gynecomastia: an update. Acta Biomed. 2017;88(2):204-13.

26.13 Delayed Puberty *PE 30.6*

DEFINITION

Puberty is delayed if there is failure to develop thelarche (breast growth) by 13 years of age or menarche by 16 years of age, or duration between thelarche and menarche is more than 4 years in girls. In boys, failure to develop gonadarche defined as an increase in testicular size ≥4 mL by 14 years of age is delayed puberty.

ETIOLOGY

The causes of delayed puberty may be due to lack of sex hormones (estrogens, testosterone) from the gonads, causing *hypergonadotropic hypogonadism* (high LH/FSH due to lack of negative feedback from gonads); or lack of gonadotropins (LH/FSH) from pituitary, called *hypogonadotropic hypogonadism,* which also results in lack of sex hormones. The causes of delayed puberty are mentioned in **Box 26.9**.

- ***Constitutional delay in growth and puberty (CDGP)*** is the most common cause of delayed puberty in boys. Puberty onset correlates with bone age rather than chronological age, and both height-age and bone age is delayed. There is an associated family history of delayed puberty in the parents (*See* Chapter 2 on Growth).
- Acquired disorders of the hypothalamus-pituitary axis such as tumors, infections can also result in delayed puberty.
- ***Turner syndrome*** is the most common chromosomal abnormality that causes delayed puberty and short stature in girls. Affected girls have variable presentation as per the underlying genetic defect (monosomy 45,XO or mosaic karyotype).
- ***Klinefelter syndrome*** is associated with an extra copy of X chromosome in boys. The affected boys are usually tall, have gynecomastia with small testes and delayed puberty.
- *Kallmann syndrome* is a rare cause of hypogonadism that can present with history of impaired sensation of smell (hyposmia or anosmia). It is usually inherited in X-linked recessive manner thereby affects boys more commonly than girls.

Box 26.9 Etiology of Delayed Puberty

A. *Hypogonadotropic hypogonadism*
- *Nutritional disorders:* Malnutrition, and anorexia nervosa
- *Chronic systemic disorders:* Chronic kidney disease, renal tubular acidosis, celiac, cystic fibrosis, and chronic liver disease
- *Endocrinological disorders:* Hypothyroidism, hyperprolactinemia, and T1DM

B. *Isolated hypogonadotropic hypogonadism*
- *Genetic: KAL 1,* GnRH receptor, LH, FSH, and *DAX1* mutation,
- *Dysmorphic syndromes:* CHARGE, Prader-Willi, and Laurence-Moon-Bardet-Biedl syndrome

C. *Multiple pituitary hormone deficiency*
- *Malformations:* Holoprosencephaly, septo-optic dysplasia, and midline defects
- *Genetic disorders: PROP1, LH* gene deletions
- *Brain tumors:* Craniopharyngioma, germinoma, and glioma
- *Brain injury:* Surgery, infection, radiation, and trauma
- *Infiltrative disorders:* Histiocytosis, and autoimmune disorders

D. *Hypergonadotropic (girls)*
- *Gonadal dysgenesis:* Turner syndrome, and trisomy 13, 18, 21
- Steroidogenic defects
- Destruction of ovary—surgery, radiation, torsion, trauma, chemotherapy, and hemosiderosis

Hypergonadotropic (boys)
- *Chromosomal anomalies:* Klinefelter syndrome; gonadal dysgenesis
- Steroidogenic defects
- Destruction of testes—infarction, torsion, radiation, chemotherapy, and infections

E. *Primary amenorrhea*
- *Structural malformations:* Müllerian agenesis, vaginal septum, and imperforate hymen
- *Inefficient androgen action:* Complete androgen insensitivity syndrome

INVESTIGATIONS

After ruling out systemic and nutritional causes, hormonal evaluation should be done for baseline serum FSH in females and LH, FSH and testosterone levels in males. Karyotype should be done in all cases with high gonadotropins to detect chromosomal disorders such as Turner syndrome or Klinefelter syndrome.

In females with hypogonadism, thyroid profile, prolactin levels and pelvic ultrasound should be done to rule out a treatable underlying cause.

TREATMENT Delayed Puberty

The treatment is directed toward correction of underlying cause if possible, like systemic disorder, malnutrition, etc. The patients also require sex hormone replacement therapy (during puberty). Boys are treated with intramuscular testosterone depot injections 50–100 mg given once a month. Girls are started with estrogens replacement given as low dose ethinyl estradiol 2–5 µg/day and gradually increased over 4–6 months interval to reach adult dose (20 µg/day). Breakthrough bleeding is achieved by adding oral progesterone, 2 years after the initiation of estrogen. Alternately, estrogen patches or depot injections are also available.

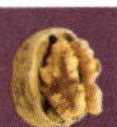

IN A NUTSHELL

Delayed Puberty

1. Delayed puberty is absence of thelarche by 13 years of age or menarche by 16 years of age, or duration between thelarche and menarche is more than 4 years in girls. In boys, failure to develop gonadarche defined as an increase in testicular size ≥4 mL by 14 years of age is delayed puberty.
2. *Hypergonadotropic hypogonadism* is due to lack of sex hormones from the gonads (low estrogens/testosterone and high LH/FSH due to lack of negative feedback from gonads).
3. *Hypogonadotropic hypogonadism is caused by* lack of gonadotropins (LH/FSH) from pituitary, which also results in lack of sex hormones.
4. Evaluation needs assessment of growth, secondary sexual characters, bone age and features of systemic disorders.
5. Constitutional delay in growth and puberty (CDGP) is the most common cause of delayed puberty and short stature in boys.
6. Turner syndrome is the most common chromosomal abnormality that causes delayed puberty and short stature in girls.

Kao KT, Denker M, Zacharin M, et al. Pubertal abnormalities in adolescents with chronic disease. Best Pract Res Clin Endocrinol Metab. 2019;33(3):101275.
Kaplowitz PB. Delayed Puberty. Pediatr Rev. 2010;31(5):189-95.
Wolf RM, Long D. Pubertal Development. Pediatr Rev. 2016;37(7):292-300.

Aashima Dabas

CHAPTER 27

Common Emergencies and Poisonings

AS PER NMC COMPETENCIES

PE24.1	Describe the etiopathogenesis, clinical approach and management of cardio-respiratory arrest in children.	*Ch 27.2*
PE24.2	Describe the etiopathogenesis and management of respiratory distress in children.	*Ch 27.5*
PE24.3	Describe the etiopathogenesis, clinical approach and management of shock in children.	*Ch 27.7*
PE24.4	Describe the etiopathogenesis, clinical approach and management of status epilepticus.	*Ch 27.8*
PE24.5	Describe the etiopathogenesis, clinical approach and management of an unconscious child.	*Ch 27.9*
PE24.6	Explain oxygen therapy, in pediatric emergencies and modes of administration.	*Ch 27.6*
PE24.7	Observe the various methods of administering oxygen.	*Ch 27.6*
PE24.8	Assess airway and breathing: recognize signs of severe respiratory distress. Check for cyanosis, severe chest indrawing, grunting.	*Ch 27.1, Ch 27.3, Ch 27.8*
PE24.9	Assess airway and breathing. Demonstrate the method of positioning of an infant and child to open airway in a simulated environment.	*Ch 27.1, Ch 27.3*
PE24.10	Assess airway and breathing: administer oxygen using correct technique and appropriate flow rate.	*Ch 27.1, Ch 27.4 Ch 27.6*
PE24.11	Assess airway and breathing perform assisted ventilation by bag and mask in a simulated environment.	*Ch 27.1, Ch 27.4*
PE24.12	Check for signs of shock, i.e., pulse, blood pressure, CRT.	*Ch 27.7*
PE24.13	Secure an IV access in a simulated environment.	*Ch 27.4, Ch 27.7*
PE24.14	Choose the type of fluid and calculate the fluid requirement in shock.	*Ch 27.4, Ch 27.7*
PE24.15	Assess level of consciousness and provide emergency treatment to a child with convulsions/coma position an unconscious child. Position a child with suspected trauma. Administer IV/per rectal diazepam for a convulsing child in a simulated environment.	*Ch 27.9*
PE24.16	Assess for signs of severe dehydration.	*Ch 27.3, Ch 27.7*
PE24.17	Monitoring and maintaining temperature: define hypothermia. Describe the clinical features, complications and management of hypothermia.	*Ch 27.10*
PE24.18	Describe the advantages and correct method of keeping an infant warm by skin-to-skin contact.	*Ch 27.10*
PE24.19	Describe the environmental measures to maintain temperature.	*Ch 27.10*

PE24.20	Assess for hypothermia and maintain temperature.	*Ch 27.10*
PE24.21	Provide BLS for children in manikin.	
PE24.22	Counsel parents of dangerously ill/terminally ill child to break a bad news.	*Ch 27.17*
PE24.23	Obtain informed consent.	*Ch 27.17*
PE14.1	Discuss the risk factors, clinical features, diagnosis, and management of kerosene ingestion.	*Ch 27.13*
PE14.2	Discuss the risk factors, clinical features, diagnosis, and management of organophosphorus poisoning.	*Ch 27.14*
PE14.3	Discuss the risk factors, clinical features, diagnosis, and management of paracetamol poisoning.	*Ch 27.15*

Topics available online: ***Hydrocarbon Poisoning, Iron Poisoning, Child Abuse, and Battered Baby Syndrome*** 

27.1 Emergency Assessment and Triage

PE 24.8, PE 24.9, PE 24.10, PE 24.11

INTRODUCTION

Pediatric deaths in hospital often occur during the first 24 hours of admission. A majority of these can be prevented by timely identification of critically ill and very sick children at their arrival in the health facility and providing appropriate treatment immediately. The priority of triage should be to quickly identify the infants and children who may have impending respiratory, circulatory, or neurologic compromise, and prioritize manpower and resources so that these children receive appropriate and timely intervention in the emergency room. In the emergency room setting, it is important to recognize early changes in vital signs with frequent monitoring, keeping in mind the normal range **(Table 27.1)**.

Table 27.1 Normal Range for Heart Rate, Respiratory Rate, and Blood Pressure in Children

Ages	*Heart rate (beats/min)*	*Respiratory rate (breaths/min)*	*Blood pressure (mm Hg) systolic/diastolic*
Premature infants	120–170	40–70	55–75/35–45
0–3 months	100–150	35–55	65–85/45–55
3–6 months	90–120	30–45	70–90/50–65
6–12 months	80–120	25–40	80–100/55–65
1–3 years	70–110	20–30	90–105/55–70
3–6 years	65–110	20–25	95–110/60–75
6–12 years	60–95	14–22	100–120/60–75
>12 years	55–85	12–18	110–135/65–85

EMERGENCY TRIAGE ASSESSMENT AND TREATMENT

The WHO has developed guidelines for Emergency Triage Assessment and Treatment (ETAT). These guidelines outline the steps for immediate assessment of children with potentially life-threatening conditions that are generally encountered in a developing country setting.

Triage involves the immediate sorting of patients into *Emergency*, *Priority*, or *Nonurgent* (Queue) categories based on their presenting signs and symptoms and availability of resources. The initial assessment includes a quick evaluation of patency of *A*irway, work of *B*reathing, adequacy of *C*irculation, presence of *C*oma, presence of *C*onvulsions, and assessment of *D*ehydration (ABCD).

ABCD ASSESSMENT

Airway and Breathing

Assessment for airway and breathing problems **(Fig. 27.1)** can be done by immediate inspection by looking, listening, and feeling for air movement:

- ❖ Is the child breathing?
- ❖ Is the airway obstructed?
- ❖ Is the child blue (or showing central cyanosis)?

Foreign body airway obstruction is an airway emergency that can be rapidly fatal, if not corrected immediately. For severe airway obstruction (i.e., the child is unable to make a sound), perform sub-diaphragmatic abdominal thrusts (*Heimlich maneuver*) for a child until the object is expelled or the child becomes unresponsive. *For an infant,* deliver five back blows

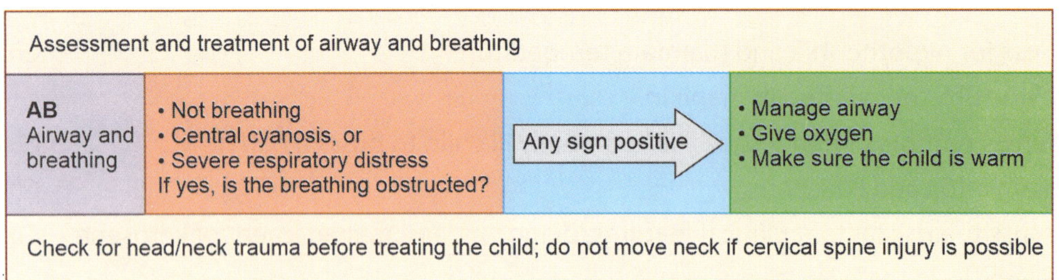

Fig. 27.1: Rapid assessment of airway and breathing

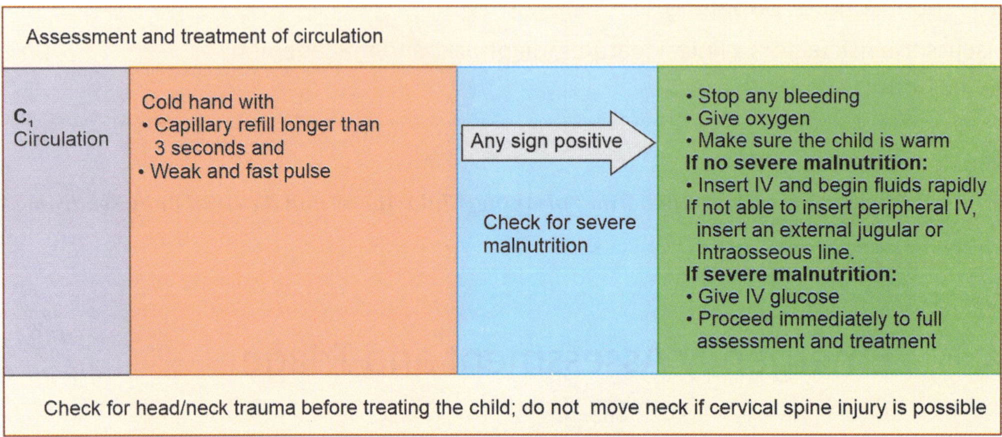

Fig. 27.2: Assessment of circulation and management of shock (IV: intravenous)

(slaps) followed by five chest thrusts repeatedly until the object is expelled or the victim becomes unresponsive. Abdominal thrusts are not recommended for infants because they may damage the relatively large and unprotected liver.

For the unresponsive child with a foreign body, look into the mouth before giving breaths and only if a foreign body is seen, then it should be removed. Blind finger sweeps should not be done as they may push the foreign body deeper.

Circulation

Adequacy of circulation **(Fig. 27.2)** can be assessed by touching the child:

- Does the child have warm hands?
- If hands are not warm, is the capillary refill time (CRT) longer than 3 seconds?
- Is the pulse fast and weak?

Measurement of blood pressure can also help in detection of shock. Hypotension is defined as systolic blood pressure <5th percentile of normal for age, as per the cut-offs shown in **Table 27.2**.

Table 27.2 Cut-offs for Defining Hypotension in Different Age Groups

Age	*Systolic blood pressure*
Term neonates (0–28 days)	<60 mm Hg
Infants (1–12 months)	<70 mm Hg
Children (1–10 years)	<70 mm Hg + (2 × age in year)
Children (>10 years)	<90 mm Hg

Box 27.1 AVPU Scale

- **A**—Alert
- **V**—Responsive to voice
- **P**—Responsive to pain
- **U**—Unresponsive

(AVPU: alert, voice, pain, unresponsive)

Consciousness

Assessment of consciousness can be done using the AVPU scale **(Box 27.1)**, where the child can be assigned to one of the following categories: *A*lert, responsive to *V*oice, responsive to *P*ain, or *U*nresponsive. Approach to an unconscious child has been discussed in detail in **Section 27.9** of this chapter.

For patients with either coma or convulsions, immediate management **(Table 27.3)** includes proper positioning to manage the airway, and providing intravenous (IV) glucose,

Table 27.3 Management of Coma and Convulsions

Coma	*Convulsion*
If the child is unconscious you should: 1. Manage the airway 2. Position the child (if there is a history of trauma, stabilize neck first) 3. Check the blood sugar 4. Give IV glucose	If the child is convulsing now you must: 1. Manage the airway 2. Position the child 3. Check blood sugar 4. Give IV glucose 5. Give anticonvulsant

(IV: intravenous)

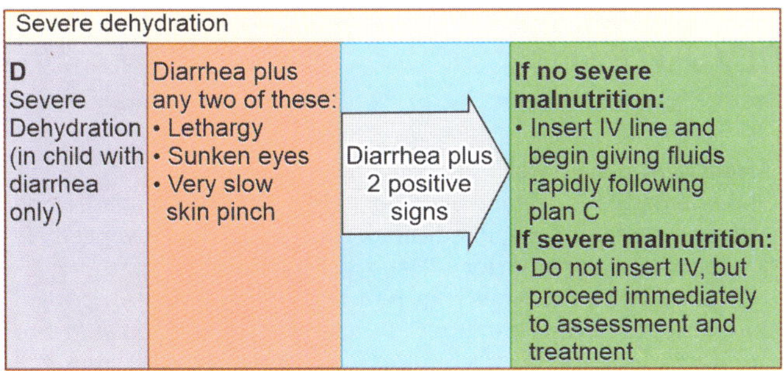

Fig. 27.3: Assessment and management of severe dehydration (IV: intravenous)

followed by treatment with anticonvulsant medication in case of active seizures.

Dehydration

Dehydration can be assessed **(Fig. 27.3)** by looking for the following:

- Is the child unconscious or lethargic?
- Does the child have sunken eyes?
- Does a skin pinch go back very slowly?

TRIAGE

If a child has one of the signs of ABCD assessment, then triage the child to E category and start treatment immediately. If the child does not have any of the E signs, proceed to assess for priority signs, which can be summarized by the mnemonic 3TPR-MOB **(Box 27.2)**. Some of these signs will have been noticed during the rapid initial assessment for E signs, while others need to be rechecked. When the assessment for priority signs is completed, the child should be assigned to one of the following:

- Priority (P)
- Nonurgent or Queue (Q)

Box 27.2 Assessment of Priority Signs—3TPR-MOB

- **T**iny infant (<2 months of age)
- **T**emperature (fever)
- **T**rauma (or other surgical condition)
- Severe **P**allor
- **P**oisoning
- Severe **P**ain
- **R**estless, lethargy, or irritability
- **R**espiratory distress
- Urgent **Re**ferral (patient sent from another clinic/facility for treatment)
- Severe **M**alnutrition
- **E**dema of both feet
- Major **B**urns

Triage in E (Emergency) Category

- If the child has any one of the signs of ABCD assessment, then the child should be triaged to the Emergency (E) category and treatment should be started immediately.
- Since more than one intervention may have to be performed at the same time, it is recommended to involve several members of the team.
- A senior healthcare provider should be notified, and blood should be drawn for laboratory investigations (blood glucose, electrolytes, hemoglobin, and peripheral smear for malaria).
- If the child has had head or neck trauma, then immobilization of head and neck region should be initiated, while continuing to assess vital signs and provide ongoing treatment.

Triage in P (Priority) or Q (Queue) Category

- For children without E signs, the healthcare provider should continue for assessment of Priority signs **(Box 27.2)**.
- After completing the examination for priority signs, the child is assigned to Priority (P) or Queue (Nonurgent) category.
- Provide ongoing monitoring and support to the sickest children as many deaths in the hospital occur within 24 hours of admission.
- Intravenous access should be obtained immediately; preferably with large bore IV cannula to provide fluid resuscitation, blood products, and medications. Obtain intraosseous access if IV access is not obtainable in a child <8 years of age.

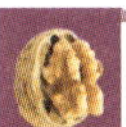

IN A NUTSHELL

Emergency Assessment and Triage

1. A majority of pediatric deaths can be prevented by timely identification of critically-ill and very sick children at their arrival in the health facility and providing appropriate treatment immediately.
2. According to the Emergency Triage Assessment and Treatment (ETAT) guidelines, triage involves immediate sorting of patients into *Emergency, Priority* or *Nonurgent* (Queue) categories.
3. Initial assessment includes a quick evaluation of patency of airway, work of breathing, adequacy of circulation, presence of coma, presence of convulsions, and assessment of dehydration (ABCD).
4. Foreign body airway obstruction is an airway emergency that can be rapidly fatal, if not corrected immediately.
5. Assessment of consciousness can be done using the AVPU scale: alert, responsive to voice, responsive to pain, or unresponsive.

World Health Organization. Updated guideline: Pediatric Emergency Triage, Assessment and Treatment: Care of Critically Ill Children. Geneva: World Health Organization; 2016.

27.2 Cardiorespiratory Arrest

PE 24.1

Cardiorespiratory or cardiac arrest is defined as the cessation of cardiac activity confirmed by the signs of absence of circulation, i.e., unresponsiveness, not breathing or only gasping and absent central pulses *(IAP—ALS guidelines 2020)*.

ETIOPATHOGENESIS

A major proportion of pediatric cardiac arrest results from respiratory failure leading to hypoxemia and bradycardia with subsequent loss of circulation and pulseless electrical activity (PEA). Refractory hypoxia and tissue hypoperfusion favor anaerobic metabolism, thereby resulting in lactic acidosis. Both hypoxia and acidosis lead to myocardial depression, which ultimately leads to cardiac arrest. Pneumonia, sepsis, diarrhea, trauma, and poisonings can also cause cardiac arrest, besides arrhythmias.

There are four well defined phases of cardiac arrest **(Fig. 27.4)**.

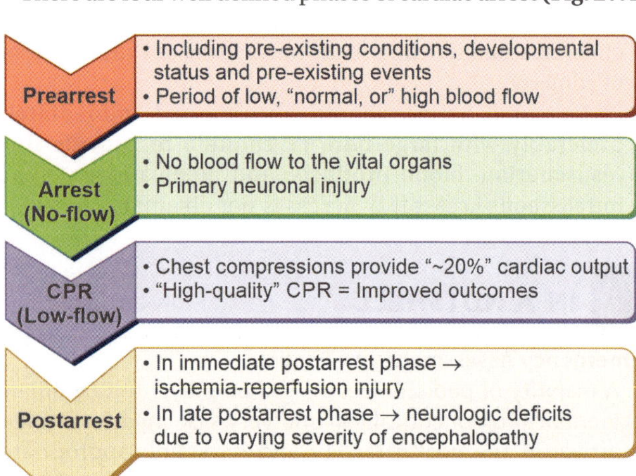

Fig. 27.4: Flow diagram of phases of cardiac arrest. Prearrest phase is characterized by low, normal, or high blood flow. During arrest phase, there is no blood flow to the vital organs. During cardiopulmonary resuscitation (CPR) phase, the blood flow is determined by the quality of CPR. In postarrest phase, secondary neuronal injury continues and it determines the severity of the encephalopathy

Source: Utpal Bhalala: In: Gupta P, et al. PG Textbook of Pediatrics, 3rd edition; 2022

TREATMENT Cardiorespiratory Arrest

The goals of cardiopulmonary resuscitation (CPR) in cardiac arrest include (1) Return of spontaneous circulation (ROSC); (2) Survival, and (3) Favorable neurological outcome.

Prearrest Phase

Management strategies should focus on early recognition of respiratory failure and shock and aggressive management to prevent an arrest. Anticipate and prepare for cardiac arrest during stabilization of children with refractory hypoxia and shock. Early institution of high-quality CPR improves outcome from cardiac arrest. There is clear evidence of improved outcome in children who receive CPR for bradycardia with a weak pulse as compared to pulseless cardiac arrest.

Arrest (no-flow) Phase

High-quality CPR is warranted during the arrest or no-flow phase along with early defibrillation, if indicated. Follow pediatric advanced life support (PALS) algorithm for CPR and focus on monitoring.

According to the American Heart Association (AHA), critical components of high-quality CPR include *push hard-push fast* to provide adequate chest compression rate and depth, minimal interruptions, allowing full chest recoil in between compressions and avoiding excessive ventilation. The depth of chest compressions should be at least one-third the anterior-posterior diameter of the chest and delivered at least at a rate of 100 compressions per minute in children. Chest compression providers should preferably use a step stool and keep a backboard under the patient to improve the quality of chest compressions. Adequate coronary artery perfusion pressure is essential during CPR for myocardial preservation and return of circulation. Chest compression providers should switch every 2 minutes to reduce provider fatigue and maintain high-quality CPR.

It is crucial to ventilate the child during CPR at the specified rate especially as most pediatric cardiopulmonary arrest results from respiratory failure. Hyperventilation increases intrathoracic pressure, which in turn impedes venous return to the heart, thereby decreasing the cardiac output. The 2020 update on pediatric CPR recommends a ventilation rate of 20–30 times per minute in infants and children receiving CPR with an advanced airway in place. Prompt administration of epinephrine in patients with non-shockable rhythms after CPR initiation is recommended to improve patient outcome.

Post-arrest Phase

During the post-arrest phase, the patient should be managed in a dedicated pediatric intensive care with close and frequent monitoring of heart rate, respiratory rate, urine output, lactate levels, oxygen saturation, and neurological status. Ventilator settings should be titrated to provide normoxemia and normocarbia. It is crucial to monitor and manage metabolic abnormalities such as hyponatremia and hypoglycemia. Progressively worsening hypoxic-ischemic encephalopathy due to secondary neuronal injury and post-arrest myocardial dysfunction are the major causes of death after initial recovery from cardiac arrest. Neuroprotective strategies, such as aggressive management of seizures, should be considered in comatose survivors of cardiac arrest to improve outcomes. Goal-directed hemodynamic support through titrated infusions of inotropes is essential to support post-arrest myocardial dysfunction. One should make all the efforts to avoid fever in comatose children for 24–48 hours after cardiac arrest through targeted temperature management.

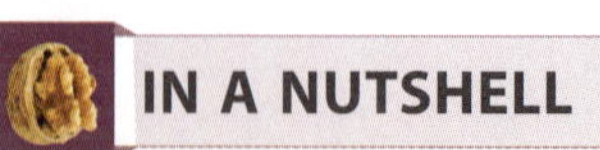

IN A NUTSHELL

Cardiorespiratory Arrest

1. Pediatric cardiac arrest mostly, results from respiratory failure. Arrhythmias are less common.
2. There are four well-described phases of cardiac arrest: prearrest, no-flow (untreated cardiac arrest), low-flow (cardiopulmonary resuscitation), and post-arrest phase.
3. The three goals of CPR in cardiac arrest are return of spontaneous circulation, survival, and favorable neurological outcome.

de Caen AR, Berg MD, Chameides L, et al. Part 12: Pediatric advanced life support: 2015 American Heart Association guidelines update for cardiopulmonary resuscitation and emergency cardiovascular care. Circulation. 2015;132(18 Suppl 2):S526-42.
ILCOR. (2022). International Liaison Committee on Resuscitation. Available from www.ilcor.org/home/[Last accessed January 2025].
Topjian AA, Raymond TT, Atkins D, et al. Pediatric Basic and Advanced Life Support Collaborators. Part 4: Pediatric Basic and Advanced Life Support 2020 American Heart Association Guidelines for Cardiopulmonary Resuscitation and Emergency Cardiovascular Care. Circulation. 2020;142(16_suppl_2):S469-S523.

27.3 Basic Life Support (BLS)

PE 24.8, PE 24.9, PE 24.16

INTRODUCTION

Pediatric basic life support (BLS) comprises knowledge and skills that are necessary for providing life-sustaining support to an unresponsive child or infant in emergent situations, either outside or within the hospital setting. BLS can be performed even by a layman outside hospital setting; survival rates vary from 6% for children with cardiac arrest to 70% in those with respiratory arrest. Survival rates are better in hospital.

The International Liaison Committee on Resuscitation (ILCOR) revised and updated the recommendations for both pediatric basic and advanced life support (ALS) in 2020. There are separate algorithms for one-person **(Flowchart 27.1)** and two-person **(Flowchart 27.2)** CPR, and the rate of chest compression is now same for both children and adults (100–120 compressions per minute). The 2020 update recommends giving one breath every 2–3 seconds (20–30 breaths per minute) to infants and children who have a pulse but have absent or inadequate breathing. Previously, the recommendation was to administer rescue breaths at the rate of one breath every 3–5 seconds which would have translated to 12–20 breaths per minute.

The emphasis of resuscitation is on high-quality chest compressions that provides blood flow to vital organs and helps to achieve ROSC. The AHA recommends that bystanders perform CPR with rescue breaths for infants and children under 18 years who experience out-of-hospital cardiac arrest (OHCA). However, if rescue breaths cannot be provided, bystanders should at least perform chest compressions.

SEQUENCE OF BASIC LIFE SUPPORT

The evaluation of any child who is found to be unresponsive should proceed in a sequential manner, as described in the BLS algorithm **(Flowcharts 27.1 and 27.2)**.

Verify Scene Safety

For rescuers performing CPR in an out-of-hospital setting, it is important to ensure the safety of the rescuer and the victim before proceeding (e.g., motor vehicle accident victim lying in the middle of the road with oncoming traffic) and the victim should first be moved to a safe area.

Proper Positioning

Proper positioning of the child is of utmost importance. The child should be in a supine (face up) position on a flat, hard surface, such as a sturdy table, the floor, or the ground. If you must turn the victim, minimize turning or twisting of the head and neck to avoid causing damage to the spinal cord in case there is a cervical spine injury.

All pediatric trauma victims should have their necks immobilized before transport, by using a cervical collar (or any other modification such as keeping towels on both sides). The collar should be kept in place until cervical spine injury is definitively ruled out by radiologic imaging.

Call for Help/Activate Emergency Response

For single rescuer, it is important to call for help/activate the emergency response system. The guidelines emphasize the use of mobile phone technology in doing this while proceeding with evaluation of the patient. For two or more rescuers or in a healthcare setting, one person stays with the patient, while the second person calls for help/activates the emergency response system.

Check for Response

Check the responsiveness by gently tapping the victim and asking loudly, "Are you okay?" and then look for any movement. *If the child is responsive*, then check to see if the child has any injuries or needs medical assistance immediately. Also assess whether the child is breathing. If breathing is normal, CPR is not needed. *If the child is unresponsive*, feel for a pulse.

Check for Breathing and Pulse

The 2020 guidelines emphasize the quick assessment of breathing and pulse of an unresponsive child within 10 seconds. If there is no breathing but pulse is present (brachial for an infant, carotid or femoral in a child), provide rescue breathing (1 breath every 2–3 seconds or 20–30 breaths/min) while continuing to assess the pulse every 2 minutes. However, if there is no breathing and no pulse is present, then immediately begin chest compressions.

- ***No pulse:*** Start chest compressions.
- ***Pulse < 60 per minute:*** Start chest compressions.
- ***Pulse ≥ 60 per min, inadequate breathing:*** Start rescue breathing 20–30 per minute until spontaneous breathing is present. Reassess pulse every 2 minutes, but take only 10 seconds to do so.

If pulse rate becomes <60/min despite adequate chest rise with rescue breaths, then chest compressions should also be initiated.

Flowchart 27.1: Basic life support (BLS) healthcare provider pediatric cardiac arrest algorithm for single rescuer—2020 update

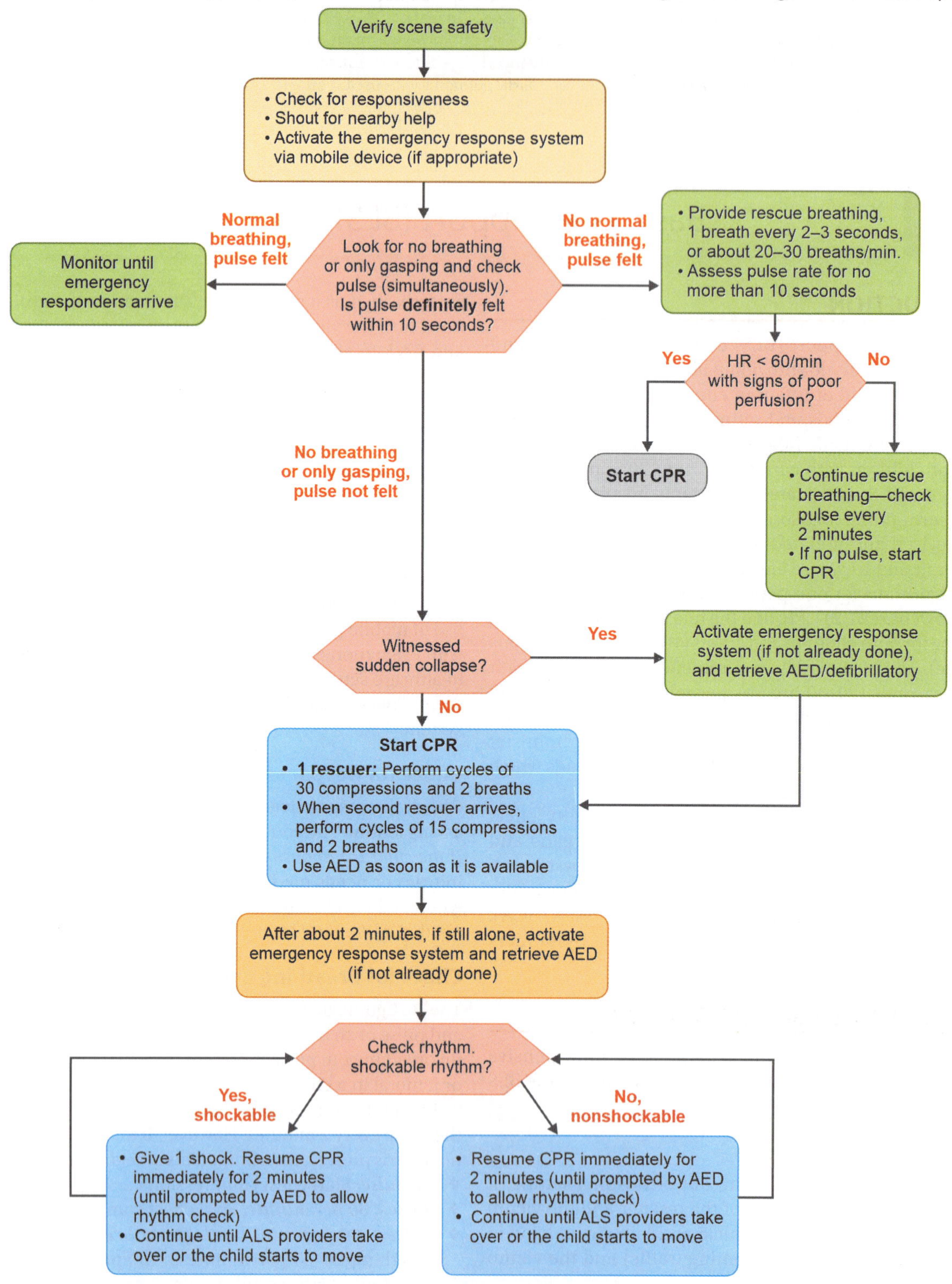

(AED: automated external defibrillator; ALS: advanced life support; CPR: cardiopulmonary resuscitation)

Source: Adapted from Circulation. 2020; 142(16_suppl_2):S469-523

Flowchart 27.2: Basic life support (BLS) healthcare provider pediatric cardiac arrest algorithm for two or more rescuers—2020 update

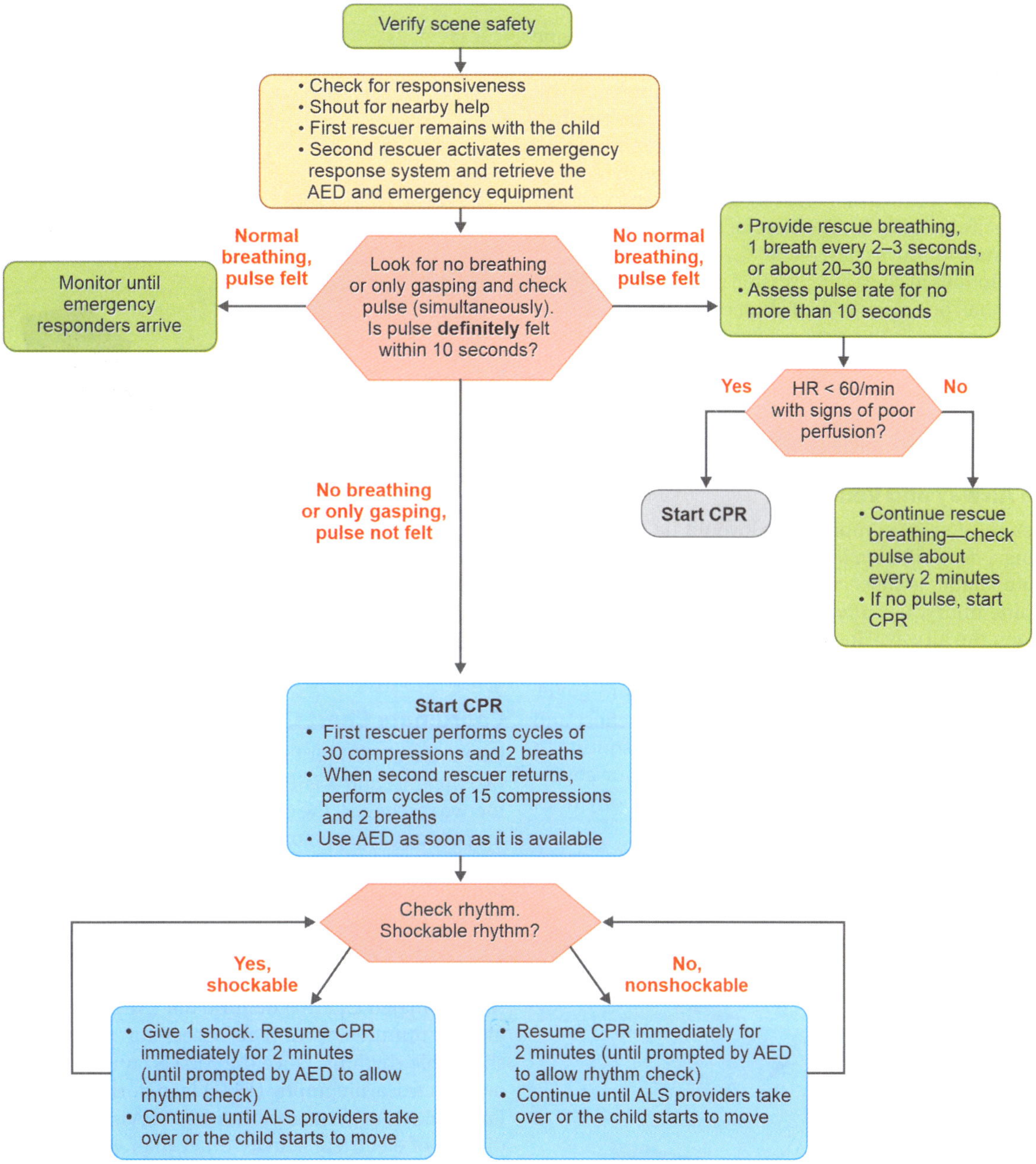

Verify scene safety

- Check for responsiveness
- Shout for nearby help
- First rescuer remains with the child
- Second rescuer activates emergency response system and retrieve the AED and emergency equipment

Look for no breathing or only gasping and check pulse (simultaneously). Is pulse **definitely** felt within 10 seconds?

Normal breathing, pulse felt

Monitor until emergency responders arrive

No normal breathing, pulse felt

- Provide rescue breathing, 1 breath every 2–3 seconds, or about 20–30 breaths/min
- Assess pulse rate for no more than 10 seconds

HR < 60/min with signs of poor perfusion?

Yes

Start CPR

No

- Continue rescue breathing—check pulse about every 2 minutes
- If no pulse, start CPR

No breathing or only gasping, pulse not felt

Start CPR

- First rescuer performs cycles of 30 compressions and 2 breaths
- When second rescuer returns, perform cycles of 15 compressions and 2 breaths
- Use AED as soon as it is available

Check rhythm. Shockable rhythm?

Yes, shockable

- Give 1 shock. Resume CPR immediately for 2 minutes (until prompted by AED to allow rhythm check)
- Continue until ALS providers take over or the child starts to move

No, nonshockable

- Resume CPR immediately for 2 minutes (until prompted by AED to allow rhythm check)
- Continue until ALS providers take over or the child starts to move

(AED: automated external defibrillator; ALS: advanced life support; CPR: cardiopulmonary resuscitation)

Source: Adapted from Circulation. 2020;142(16_suppl_2):S469-523

Chest Compressions

The key components of high-quality CPR include (i) *push hard* to provide adequate chest compression depth; (ii) *push fast* to ensure adequate rate; (iii) minimal interruptions, (iv) allowing full chest recoil in between compressions and (v) avoiding excessive ventilation. Chest compressions are initiated at a rate of 100–120 compressions per minute. First give 30 compressions, pushing hard enough to depress the chest by one-third of the anterior-posterior diameter of the chest [1.5 inches (4 cm) in infants or 2 inches (5 cm) in children].

- ***For infants:*** The two-finger technique (compressing the sternum with two fingers just below the internipple line in the midline) is preferred, if there is only one healthcare provider. The two *thumb-encircling hand technique* is used when there are two rescuers for the CPR. The two-thumb technique produces higher coronary artery perfusion pressure and may generate higher systolic and diastolic pressures as compared to two-finger technique.

- ***Older children:*** Chest compression in older children is done with heel of one or both hands, as for adults.

Ensuring adequate chest recoil after chest compression will allow the heart to fill up with blood, which can then be pumped out to systemic circulation when the heart is squeezed during the subsequent compression. Better chest recoil is associated with a better prognosis because of increased coronary and cerebral perfusion. Techniques to lift the heel of the hand following compression may improve chest recoil.

Any interruptions in chest compression should be avoided. If there is more than one rescuer, then chest compressions should be switched between both rescuers every 2 minutes to avoid fatigue, as it can impact the effectiveness of the com- pressions by reducing the coronary perfusion pressure.

Following the first 30 compressions, open the airway, and give two rescue breaths, as detailed here.

Open the Airway and Ventilate

The next step (after 30 compressions) would be to open the airway using a *head tilt-chin lift maneuver* **(Fig. 27.5)** unless a cervical spine injury is suspected. For patients with suspected cervical spine injury, use a *jaw-thrust without head tilt* **(Fig. 27.6)** to open the airway. However, if the jaw-thrust does not open the airway, use the head tilt-chin lift maneuver. While maintaining an open airway, take no >10 seconds to check whether the victim is breathing: *look* for rhythmic chest and abdominal movement, *listen* for exhaled breath sounds at the nose and mouth, and *feel* for exhaled air on your cheek. Periodic gasping, also called *agonal gasps,* is not synonymous with breathing.

If the child is *not breathing or has only occasional gasps,* maintain an open airway and give two breaths with bag and mask. Give mouth-to-mouth ventilation if bag and mask are not available. For providing rescue breaths in infants, it is recommended to use mouth-to-mouth-and-nose technique when bag and mask are not available. Make sure that the breaths are effective (i.e., the chest rises). If the chest does not rise, reposition the head, make a better seal, and try again.

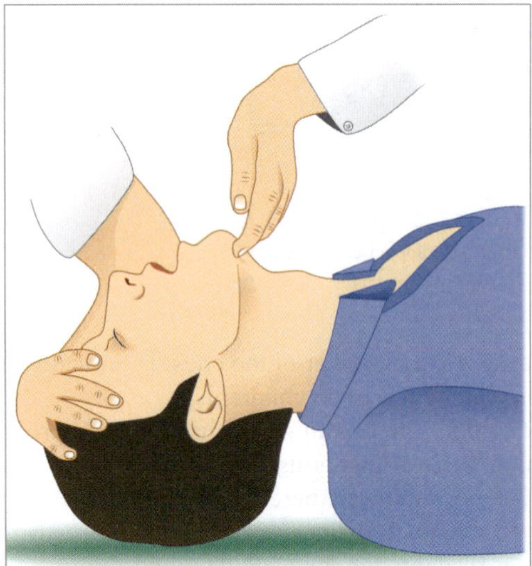

Fig. 27.5: A head tilt: chin lift maneuver

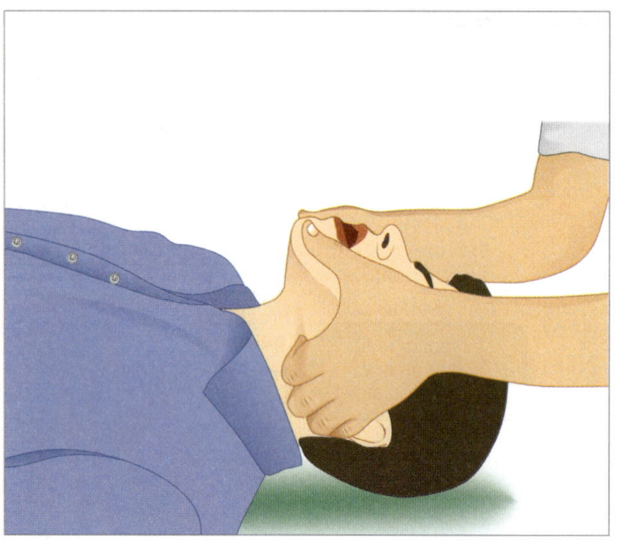

Fig. 27.6: Jaw-thrust without head tilt

Coordinate Chest Compressions and Ventilation

One cycle of CPR for the single rescuer is 30 compressions and two breaths; and it is 15 compressions followed by two breaths for two rescuers. If the child has been intubated, there is no need for pausing. The person doing compression should continue at the rate of 100–120 compressions per minute while the other rescuer can deliver 20–30 breaths per minute. Continue CPR for five cycles (about 2 minutes).

Defibrillation

An automated external defibrillator (AED) should be attached after 2 minutes of CPR to assess for the presence of any shockable rhythms. Once the AED is connected, it will display one electrocardiography (ECG) lead during resuscitation. Flat line on ECG suggests asystole, while PEA is defined as a rhythmic display of electrical activity other than ventricular fibrillation (VF) or ventricular tachycardia (VT) that does not produce a palpable arterial pulse. VF and pulseless VT are known as shockable rhythms because they would respond positively to defibrillation.

If no shockable rhythm is identified then CPR should continue for another 2 minutes, followed by another rhythm check. If shockable rhythm is identified, then CPR should resume after the shock has been delivered automatically by the AED. If a manual defibrillator is being used (preferred for infants), the first shock dose should be 2 J/kg. This can be doubled (4 J/kg), if second dose is required. Resume CPR immediately after delivering the shock.

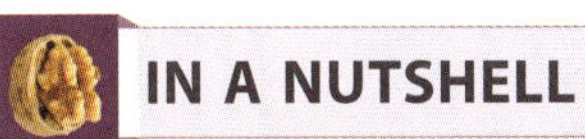

IN A NUTSHELL

Basic Life Support (BLS)

1. Bystanders should perform CPR with rescue breaths for children under 18 years with out-of-hospital cardiac arrest (OHCA). However, if rescue breaths cannot be provided, bystanders should at least perform chest compressions.
2. Do not take >10 seconds to feel for a pulse.
3. Provide high-quality chest compressions.
4. Use a chest compression rate of 100–120/min. Ensure adequate depth of compression.
5. The compression to ventilation ratio for single rescuer is 30:2, and for two rescuers the ratio is 15:2.
6. Defibrillate as soon as possible for shockable rhythms.

Atkins DL, Berger S, Duff JP, et al. Part 11: Pediatric Basic Life Support and Cardiopulmonary Resuscitation Quality: 2015 American Heart Association Guidelines Update for Cardiopulmonary Resuscitation and Emergency Cardiovascular Care. Circulation. 2015;132(18 Suppl 2):S519-25.

Topjian AA, Raymond TT, Atkins D, et al. Part 4: Pediatric Basic and Advanced Life Support: 2020 American Heart Association Guidelines for Cardiopulmonary Resuscitation and Emergency Cardiovascular Care. Circulation. 2020;142(16_suppl_2):S469-523.

27.4 Pediatric Advanced Life Support (PALS)

PE 24.10, PE 24.11, PE 24.13, PE 24.14

Pediatric Advanced Life Support (PALS) is a series of steps undertaken to resuscitate a child with life-threatening conditions in respiratory, circulatory and/or neurological dysfunction, or arrest.

STRUCTURED APPROACH TO A SICK CHILD (IAP-ALS GUIDELINES 2020)

To evaluate the severity and urgency of intervention in a sick child, follow these steps using the "Evaluate-Identify-Intervene" (E-I-I) approach **(Table 27.4)**:

1. ***Initial impression:*** Use the Pediatric Assessment Triangle (PAT) **(Fig. 27.7) for evaluation.**

Table 27.4 Evaluate-Identify-Intervene (E-I-I) Approach for Recognition of a Sick Child

Evaluate: • Initial impression • Primary assessment • Secondary assessment • Diagnostic tests

Identify:
• Respiratory distress or failure
  ▪ Upper airway obstruction
  ▪ Lower airway obstruction
  ▪ Lung parenchymal disease
  ▪ Disordered control of breathing
• Circulatory insufficiency (compensated/hypotensive, type of shock: hypovolemic, distributive, cardiogenic, obstructive, dissociative)
• Neurological impairment (cortical vs. brainstem dysfunction)
• Cardiac arrest

Intervene: Provide appropriate treatment based on urgency **Reassess:** Continuously reassess using "E-I-I" until stabilized

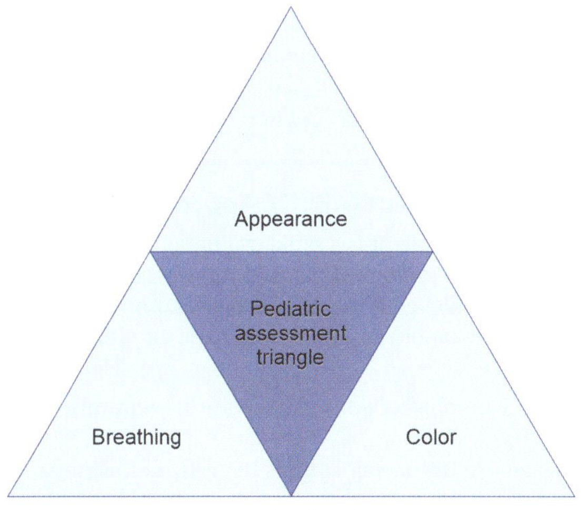

Fig. 27.7: Components of pediatric assessment triangle

2. ***Primary assessment:*** Focus on airway, breathing, circulation, disability (neurological), and exposure (ABCDE approach).
3. ***Secondary assessment:*** Gather more details through focused medical history and examination.
4. ***Diagnostic tests:*** Perform necessary tests for additional insight into the condition.

Initial Impression

Evaluate

Assess the child visually as soon as they arrive (doorway assessment or hands-off assessment). Look for signs of critical illness using the **Pediatric Assessment Triangle (PAT) (Fig. 27.7)**:

- ***Appearance:*** Check consciousness (TICLS—Tone, Interactive, Consolable, Look/gaze, Speech). Abnormalities suggest brain dysfunction.
- ***Breathing:*** Observe for apnea, tachypnea/bradypnea, abnormal sounds (stridor, wheeze), irregular or jerky breathing, or use of accessory muscles. Abnormalities indicate primary respiratory dysfunction.
- ***Color:*** Look for signs like pallor (anemia), cyanosis, mottling, bruising, or bleeding. Abnormalities indicate primary circulatory dysfunction.

Identify

- If abnormalities in **appearance**, **breathing**, or **color** are detected, immediately consider the severity. This points to potential issues like:
  - Brain dysfunction
  - Primary respiratory dysfunction.
  - Primary circulatory dysfunction.

INTERVENE

After initial impression, the following scenarios are possible:

1. ***Unresponsive and not breathing (Box 27.3):*** Immediate life-saving measures (e.g., CPR, airway management).
2. ***One or more deranged parameters:*** Immediate intervention to prevent deterioration (e.g., oxygen, fluids, medications).
3. ***All parameters normal:*** Routine monitoring, but no urgent intervention needed.

Primary Assessment (ABCDE Approach)

The primary assessment is a rapid evaluation of a child's cardiopulmonary and neurological status, aiming to identify and address critical issues quickly. It includes five key components: Airway, Breathing, Circulation, Disability, and Exposure **(Fig. 27.8).**

1. ***Airway:***
   - Check for obstructions like secretions, vomitus, or foreign bodies.
   - Listen for abnormal sounds (e.g., stridor, wheeze, grunt) which indicate airway issues and help identify the site of obstruction.
2. ***Breathing:***
   - Evaluate respiratory rate, work of breathing, chest wall movement, lung sounds, and oxygen saturation.

Box 27.3	**Steps of Intervention in a Life-threatening Situation (PALS Guidelines 2020)**

If a child is unresponsive, not breathing, gasping, or has abnormal/ineffective breathing:

1. Call for help immediately
2. Provide oxygen
3. Attach monitors and Automated External Defibrillator (AED)
4. Check for pulse
5. If central pulse is absent or < 60 bpm, begin cardiopulmonary resuscitation (CPR)
6. If central pulse > 60 bpm, provide breathing support with bag-valve-mask

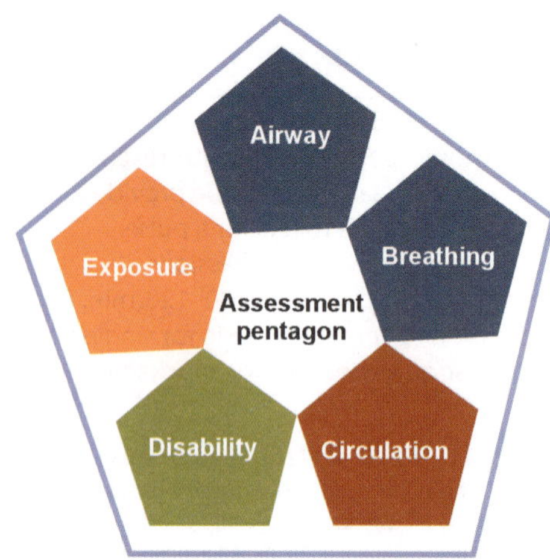

Fig. 27.8: Components of primary assessment

(*Source:* Muralidharan J, Kulgod V, Sharma AK (Eds). IAP Advanced Life Support (ALS) Handbook, 2nd edition. Indian Academy of Pediatrics; 2020.)

   - Abnormalities may include tachypnea (fast breathing), bradypnea (slow breathing), apnea (no breathing), or labored breathing (e.g., nasal flaring, retractions).
   - Pulse oximetry provides vital oxygen saturation information, though it has limitations in conditions like severe anemia or CO poisoning.
3. ***Circulation:***
   - Assess heart rate, rhythm, central and peripheral pulses, capillary refill time, skin color/temperature, and blood pressure.
   - Tachycardia and changes in pulse quality (weak or absent) suggest circulatory insufficiency or shock.
   - Blood pressure helps classify shock as compensated or hypotensive.
   - Decreased urine output can indicate poor circulation or shock.
4. ***Disability:***
   - Evaluate neurological function using the Glasgow Coma Scale (GCS) or AVPU scale for cortical assessment.
   - Assess brainstem function through pupil response and eye movements.
   - Identify any signs of brain injury, metabolic issues, or hypoxia.
5. ***Exposure:***
   - Fully expose the child to check for hidden injuries, bleeding, deformities, or rashes.
   - Assess core temperature to identify fever or hypothermia, both of which require specific treatment.

After each step of the primary assessment, prioritize life-saving interventions as necessary. Following the initial assessment, continually reassess the child using the "Evaluate-Identify-Intervene" cycle to guide ongoing management. If a life-threatening issue is identified at any stage, intervene immediately before proceeding to the next step **(Table 27.5)**.

Table 27.5 Primary Assessment (ABCDE Approach) of a Sick Child: Evaluate-identify-intervene

Step	Component	Evaluation	Identify	Intervene
A	**Airway**	1. Look for secretions, vomitus, or foreign bodies 2. Listen for noisy breathing (e.g., stridor, hoarseness, wheeze, grunt)	**Obstruction:** 1. Upper airway obstruction (stridor, hoarseness) 2. Lower airway obstruction (wheeze) 3. Parenchymal lesions (grunt)	1. Clear airway (suction, remove foreign bodies) 2. Provide oxygen or airway support (e.g., intubation, CPAP)
B	**Breathing**	1. Respiratory rate 2. Work of breathing (nasal flaring, retractions, grunting, head bobbing, seesaw respiration) 3. Auscultation for air entry. 4. Pulse oximetry (SpO_2)	**Respiratory insufficiency:** 1. Tachypnea 2. Bradypnea 3. Apnea 4. Respiratory distress or failure	1. Oxygen administration 2. Positive pressure ventilation if apnea or failure 3. Consider advanced airway management
C	**Circulation**	1. Heart rate and rhythm 2. Central and peripheral pulses 3. Capillary refill time (CRT) 4. Skin color and temperature 5. Blood pressure	**Shock:** 1. Tachycardia, bradycardia 2. Weak or absent pulses 3. Prolonged CRT 4. Hypotension	1. Fluids (IV/IO bolus) for hypovolemia 2. Medications for cardiac or distributive shock (e.g., inotropes, vasopressors) 3. CPR if no pulses
D	**Disability (neurological)**	1. GCS or AVPU scale for cortical function 2. Pupillary response (size, symmetry, reaction) 3. Oculocephalic reflex (for brain stem activity)	**Neurological impairment:** 1. Altered consciousness (GCS < 15) 2. Unresponsive or non-reactive pupils 3. Abnormal brainstem reflexes	1. Secure airway if altered consciousness 2. Administer glucose if hypoglycemia suspected 3. Treat causes (e.g., seizures, toxins)
E	**Exposure**	1. Expose the child to examine for hidden injuries (bleeding, swelling, rashes, deformities) 2. Measure core temperature	1. Expose the child to examine for hidden injuries (bleeding, swelling, rashes, deformities) 2. Measure core temperature	1. Control bleeding (pressure, dressings) 2. Provide warmth for hypothermia or treat fever 3. Manage trauma or underlying disease

Secondary Assessment

The secondary assessment involves gathering more detailed information after the initial primary evaluation to help determine a specific diagnosis. It consists of:

- ***Focused history:*** This is obtained using the **SAMPLE** mnemonic, which stands for:
  - *Signs and symptoms:* What is the child presenting with?
  - *Allergies:* To food, medications, or environmental factors.
  - *Medications:* Including chronic therapies like anticonvulsants.
  - *Past medical history:* Any relevant comorbidities.
  - *Last meal:* Important for planning sedation or procedures.
  - *Event:* What caused the child to visit the emergency room?
- ***Focused examination:*** This is a physical examination concentrating on areas not covered in the primary assessment, such as neck stiffness, lymph nodes, cardiac examination (e.g., murmurs), organomegaly, abdominal masses, or fluid accumulation.

After the secondary assessment, a specific diagnosis is made based on the findings, helping to clarify the physiological issues identified during the primary assessment. For example, a child in compensated shock from the primary assessment may be diagnosed with **cardiogenic shock** after finding hepatomegaly and a murmur in the focused examination.

Diagnostic Tests

- ***Blood glucose assessment:*** A quick point-of-care test to help identify and intervene in cases of hypoglycemia or hyperglycemia.
- ***Hematological profile:*** Blood tests to assess overall health and detect infections, anemia, or other abnormalities.
- ***Microbiological assays:*** Cultures from blood, urine, or sputum to identify infections if an infectious cause is suspected.
- ***Metabolic/biochemical profile:*** Includes tests for acid/base balance, electrolytes, and organ function.
- ***Imaging studies:*** Ultrasound, X-rays, CT scans, or MRIs may be performed based on clinical indications, but they are mainly for diagnostic and prognostic purposes rather than immediate management in the emergency room.
- Samples for *cultures* should always be taken if an infection is suspected, to guide appropriate treatment.

In conclusion, the systematic approach to assessing a sick child ensures a thorough, organized evaluation that prioritizes immediate life-saving interventions. By quickly identifying and addressing critical issues such as airway obstruction, respiratory failure, circulatory insufficiency, neurological impairment, and hidden injuries, healthcare providers can stabilize the child and prevent further deterioration. The secondary assessment, including a focused history and physical examination, helps refine the diagnosis, while diagnostic tests support clinical decision-making. This comprehensive process is essential in providing timely, effective care to critically ill children.

PULSELESS ARREST

Cardiac arrest in children usually occurs with prior warning signs of progressive respiratory distress/respiratory failure or shock. However, in some instances, cardiac arrest can occur suddenly without warning signs, such as in cases of sudden cardiac arrhythmias, with higher risks in children with pre-existing heart conditions (e.g., hypertrophic cardiomyopathy, anomalous coronary artery origin, long QT syndrome, or other channelopathies). In India, infections are the leading cause of mortality in children under-five, while for those over five, deaths from accidents and malignancies are also significant contributors, besides infections. PALS provides guidelines for advanced airway management (endotracheal intubation or supraglottic airway placement) and resuscitation in the hospital setting and delineates the approach for specific situations such as bradycardia, tachyarrhythmias, and pulseless arrest. It also covers special resuscitation situations and post-resuscitation care. *While BLS is presented as a series of sequential events, ALS activities are performed simultaneously and in parallel.*

Rescuers in the team should be sufficiently trained to diagnose and manage respiratory failure and shock; perform rapid sequence intubation and ventilation; administer fluids, and drugs; and operate a defibrillator. The AHA PALS guidelines provide additional recommendations for pre-arrest, intra-arrest, and post-arrest care. Prearrest care updates include establishment of medical emergency teams or rapid response teams in hospitals to improve outcomes, using pediatric early warning score (PEWS) to recognize and intervene for patients with higher likelihood of decline of their cardiorespiratory status.

Cardiac arrest should be rapidly recognized and is defined as cessation of cardiac mechanical activity confirmed by the absence of signs of circulation, i.e., unresponsiveness, not breathing or only gasping and absent central pulses, **Flowchart 27.3** depicts an algorithm for the management of cardiac arrest in children. It is also important to recognize reversible causes of pulseless arrest such as tension pneumothorax, cardiac tamponade, severe hypovolemia, and other possible contributing factors, which can best be remembered as the *H's*—*h*ypoxia, *h*ypovolemia, *h*ypothermia, *h*yperthermia (malignant), *h*ydrogen ion (acidosis), *h*ypoglycemia, *hyperkalemia, hypokalemia* and *h*ypervagal response; and *T's*—*t*amponade, *t*ension pneumothorax, *t*oxins (drugs and poisons), *t*hromboembolism, *t*rauma, prolonged Q*T* interval and pulmonary hyper*T*ension. Post-arrest care involves stabilization and transport of the patient to a tertiary care center (if needed), with the goals of preservation of brain function, prevention of secondary organ injury, and assessment and treatment of the cause of illness.

All cardiopulmonary arrests are not asystole. Electrocardiogram (ECG) may show one of the four rhythms: (a) asystole, (b) pulseless electrical activity/PEA, (c) ventricular fibrillation/VF, and (d) pulseless ventricular tachycardia (pVT). For asystole and PEA, effective CPR, identifying and treating reversible causes, advanced airway and epinephrine are the mainstay of treatment. Defibrillation has no role in such cases. CPR should be continued with minimal interruption in the chest compressions. Without an advanced airway, provide CPR with a compression-to-ventilation ratio of 15:2 for two rescuers or 30:2 for a single rescuer. Once an endotracheal tube (or other advanced airway) has been placed, chest compressions should be continued at a rate of 100–120/min without stopping for ventilations. The second rescuer should provide one breath every 2–3 seconds (20–30 breaths/min) without interrupting the chest compressions. Epinephrine may be given every 3–5 minutes and rhythm should be reassessed after every 2 minutes of CPR. Occasionally, a shockable rhythm (VF, pVT) may be obtained for which early defibrillation is attempted with an initial dose of 2 J/kg, followed by CPR for 2 minutes, followed by reassessment of rhythm and provision of shock as needed. Epinephrine should be administered (IV/IO or through tracheal tube) for every 3–5 minutes. For subsequent energy levels, a dose of 4 J/kg may be reasonable and higher energy levels may be considered, though not to exceed 10 J/kg or the adult maximum dose. Refractory cases may require antiarrhythmic medications such as amiodarone, lidocaine, or magnesium, followed by repeat defibrillation. If rhythm is non-shockable, then CPR cycles with epinephrine should continue until ROSC or until it is decided to terminate efforts based on clinical situation.

FLUIDS AND DRUGS

- Fluid resuscitation in sepsis should be individualized to 10 mL/kg or 20 mL/kg aliquots based on the patient's response and ongoing monitoring. Crystalloids (both balanced and unbalanced) and colloids can be used for resuscitation. Epinephrine and norepinephrine infusions are indicated in fluid-refractory septic shock.
- In cardiac arrest with non-shockable rhythms, earlier epinephrine administration (ideally within 5 minutes after CPR initiation) improves survival. IV or intraosseous (IO) route is preferable to endotracheal tube administration.
- For pediatric patients in any setting with cardiac arrest, epinephrine should be administered immediately within 5 minutes from the start of CPR and continued every 3–5 minutes until ROSC is achieved. Dose of epinephrine is 0.1 mL/kg of 1:10,000 (0.1 mg/mL) solution via IV/IO route (followed by 5 mL normal saline flush) and 0.1 mL/kg of 1:1,000 (1 mg/mL) solution via endotracheal tube.
- Use of atropine as a premedication in infants and children requiring emergency endotracheal intubation may be considered in specific situations where there is a higher risk of bradycardia.

Flowchart 27.3: Pediatric cardiac arrest algorithm—2020 update

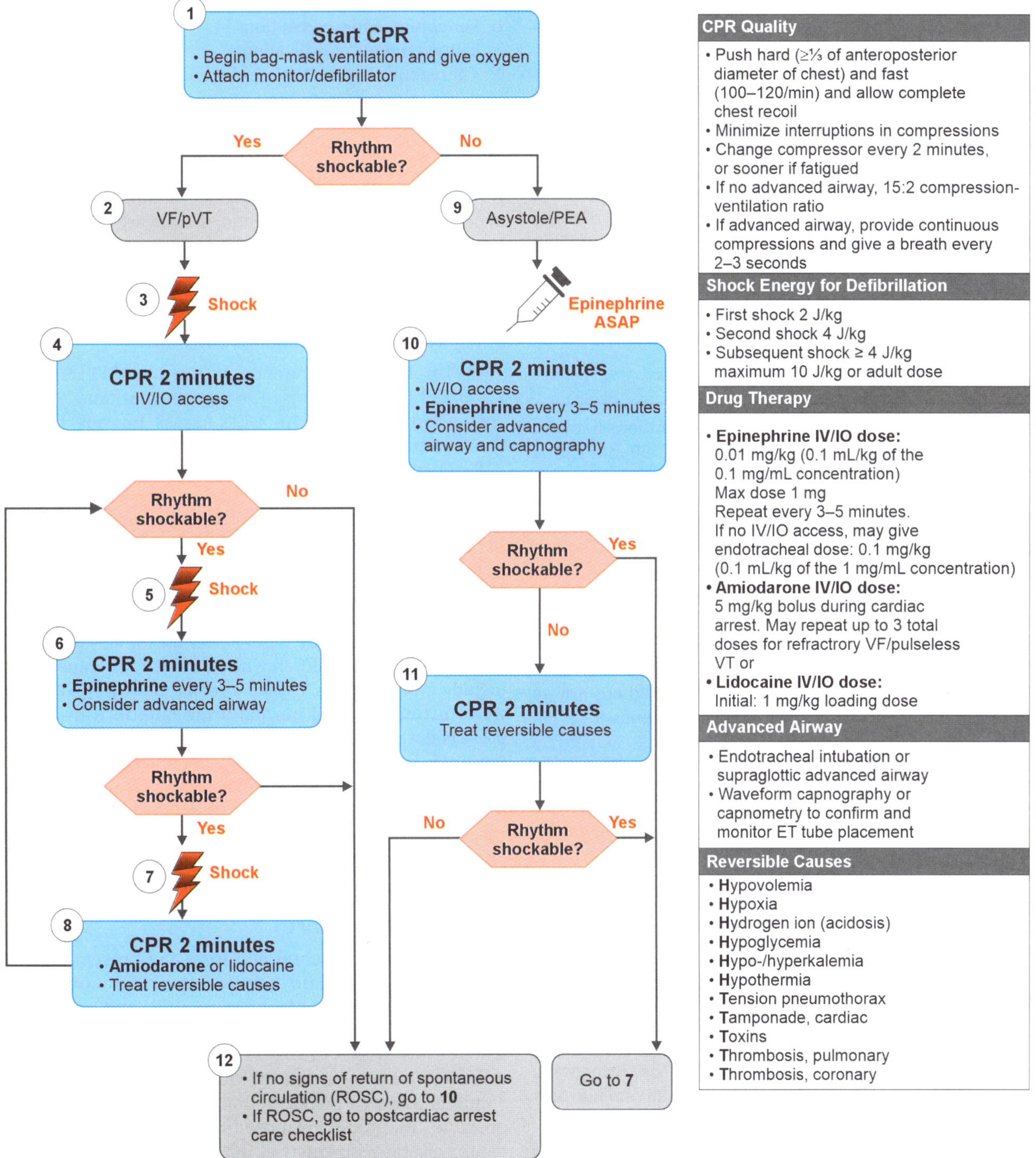

Source: Adapted from Circulation: 2020; 142(16_suppl_2):S469-523

- Treatment with extracorporeal membrane oxygenation (ECMO) may be considered for infants and children with myocarditis or dilated cardiomyopathy at risk for an impending cardiac arrest.
- The energy dose for defibrillation at 2 J/kg is safe and can be increased to 4 J/kg. Higher doses may be considered for refractory VF but should not exceed 10 J/kg or the maximum adult dose. For management of out-of-hospital cardiac arrest

patients, initial 2 days of hypothermia (32–34°C) may be considered and fever should be treated aggressively.

- For shock-refractory VF or pulseless ventricular tachycardia (pVT), lidocaine, or amiodarone use may be considered.
- In post-arrest phase, use of parenteral fluids and inotropes and/or vasopressors should help maintain targeted measures of perfusion (such as blood pressure greater than 5th percentile for age).
- Routine use of sodium bicarbonate is not recommended in pediatric cardiac arrest in the absence of hyperkalemia or sodium channel blocker toxicity (e.g., use of tricyclic antidepressants).
- Routine administration of calcium is not recommended unless it is indicated in specific circumstances such as documented hypocalcemia, calcium channel blocker overdose, hypermagnesemia, or hyperkalemia.

MONITORING

Use of a targeted PaO_2 strategy to maintain saturations between 94 and 100%, and limiting severe hypercapnia (>50 mm Hg) or hypocapnia (<30 mm Hg) can help to improve outcomes.

- During chest compressions, monitoring of end-tidal CO_2 [End-tidal carbon dioxide ($ETCO_2$)] can help to improve the quality of the CPR.
- While there are no known prognostic factors that help predict outcome, using blood pressure cut-offs in the presence of invasive hemodynamic monitoring during CPR can be considered.

Neurologic outcomes can be predicted with use of electroencephalograms (EEGs) in the first 7 days, but there are no additional biomarkers to accurately predict outcomes.

POST-RESUSCITATION CARE

After the return of spontaneous circulation (ROSC) following cardiac arrest, significant metabolic changes and hemodynamic shifts occur. Nearly all organs (including myocardium, lung, brain, gut, kidneys) are affected by ischemia/reperfusion injury, a condition commonly referred to as post-cardiac arrest syndrome (PCAS). The therapeutic goals of comprehensive multiorgan support following a cardiac arrest are aimed at optimizing and stabilizing cardiopulmonary function, preventing secondary organ injury, and correcting metabolic derangements **(Box 27.4).** Additionally, it's crucial to identify and treat the underlying cause of the illness while minimizing deterioration during transport. Long-term goals focus on improving neurologically intact survival, ensuring that patients not only survive but also recover functional and cognitive abilities. The key components of post-arrest care bundle include:

1. Ventilation and oxygenation
2. Hemodynamic optimization
3. Therapeutic hypothermia induction

Box 27.4 Therapeutic Goals of Comprehensive Multiorgan Support Following Cardiac Arrest

1. Optimize and stabilize cardiopulmonary function
2. Prevent secondary organ injury
3. Correct metabolic derangements
4. Identify and treat the underlying cause of illness
5. Minimize deterioration during transport
6. Improve long-term, neurologically intact survival

Respiratory Support

Maintain optimal oxygenation and ventilation, avoiding hypoxia and hyperoxia, SaO_2 of 92–94%, PaO_2 > 60 mm Hg. Achieve appropriate $PaCO_2$ depending on the condition (e.g., permissive hypercapnia for ARDS or asthma, normocarbia for congenital heart disease and pulmonary hypertension, and hypocapnia may be beneficial in raised ICP management). If there is a sudden deterioration in an intubated patient (e.g., cyanosis, pallor, hypotension, desaturation), **DOPE** should be evaluated promptly to identify and address the issue.

D—Displacement of the endotracheal tube (ETT). Check if the ETT has shifted or is in an incorrect position.

O—Obstruction of the ETT. Assess for any blockages (secretions, mucous plugs, or kinks).

P—Pneumothorax. Look for signs of air accumulation in the chest, which could compromise ventilation.

E—Equipment failure. Check for malfunctioning equipment, such as ventilators or oxygen supply.

Cardiovascular Support

Maintain adequate organ perfusion. Blood pressure should be targeted at systolic BP > 5th percentile for age, ideally at the 50th percentile for children with raised ICP. Therapeutic goals include normal pulses, capillary refill time (CFT) ≤ 2 seconds, warm extremities and normal urine output. If hypotension persists despite fluid resuscitation, vasoactive support may be required. Invasive blood pressure monitoring is preferred in cases of severe hypotension. Post-Arrest Myocardial Dysfunction (PAMD) is well recognized within 24 hours of ROSC. Early use of vasoactive agents improves myocardial contractility and decrease afterload. Correcting electrolyte imbalances (e.g., hypoglycemia, hypocalcemia, acidosis) can support myocardial function.

Neurological Support

Maintain optimal cerebral perfusion and prevent secondary brain injury. Maintain normoxemia and normocarbia. Manage raised intracranial pressure (ICP) and treat seizures. Targeted temperature management is crucial. Fever should be strictly avoided after cardiac arrest. Current evidence suggests therapeutic hypothermia (32–34°C) for 2 days in comatose children, followed by normothermia for 3 days. If this is not possible, maintain normothermia (36–37.5°C). Frequent neurological assessments (e.g., GCS, pupil reflexes, oculocephalic reflex, EEG monitoring) should be done to monitor progression.

Renal Support

Maintain and preserve renal function and prevent secondary injury. Monitor urine output and electrolytes. Avoid nephrotoxic drugs. Carefully balance fluids requirements and treat dyselectrolytemia. Use diuretics if volume overload occurs.

Gastrointestinal (GI) Support

Target is to maintain GI function and prevent aspiration. Place nasogastric or orogastric tube to prevent aspiration, monitor for abdominal distension, and correct electrolyte imbalances.

Hematologic Support

Examine for pallor, petechiae or bruises. Monitor hemoglobin, platelets, coagulation factors (e.g., FFP for bleeding, platelet transfusion if count is <50,000). Vitamin K should be given if prothrombin time (PT) is elevated.

Post-Cardiac Arrest Prognosis

Outcomes depend on pre-hospital cardiac arrest, resuscitation duration, in-hospital cardiac arrest due to septic shock, hypothermia, and interval between collapse and CPR. EEG and clinical assessments are used for long-term outcomes, particularly in children who survive cardiac arrest.

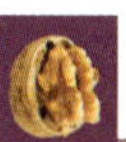

IN A NUTSHELL

Pediatric Advanced Life Support (PALS)

1. Pediatric cardiac arrest is a culmination of progressive respiratory failure or shock, or rarely a combination of the two.
2. Use of a targeted PaO_2 strategy to maintain saturations between 94 and 100% and limiting severe hypercapnia (>50 mm Hg) or hypocapnia (<30 mm Hg) improve the outcome.
3. For asystole and pulseless electrical activity, CPR should be continued with minimal interruption in the chest compressions.
4. In cardiac arrest with non-shockable rhythms, earlier epinephrine administration (ideally within 5 minutes) after CPR initiation improves survival.
5. Occasionally, a shockable rhythm may be obtained for which defibrillation is attempted.
6. Post-cardiac arrest syndrome (PCAS) affects nearly all organs due to ischemia/reperfusion injury.
7. The main goals are to optimize and stabilize cardiopulmonary function and prevent secondary organ injury.
8. Target in post-resuscitation care is to maintain normoxemia, normocapnia and normothermia. Aim is to improve long-term, neurologically intact survival.

de Caen AR, Berg MD, Chameides L, et al. Part 12: Pediatric Advanced Life Support: 2015 American Heart Association Guidelines Update for Cardiopulmonary Resuscitation and Emergency Cardiovascular Care. Circulation. 2015;132(18-suppl 2):S526-42.

Muralidharan J, Kulgod V, Sharma AK, editors. IAP Advanced Life Support (ALS) Handbook, 2nd edition. Indian Academy of Pediatrics; 2020.

Topjian AA, Raymond TT, Atkins D, et al. Part 4: Pediatric Basic and Advanced Life Support: 2020 American Heart Association Guidelines for Cardiopulmonary Resuscitation and Emergency Cardiovascular Care. Circulation. 2020;142(16_suppl_2):S469-523.

27.5 Respiratory Distress and Failure

PE 24.2

INTRODUCTION

Respiratory distress is a condition in which the pulmonary activity is unable to bring oxygen into and remove carbon dioxide from the blood. This can ultimately lead to respiratory failure which occurs when a patient's breathing becomes inadequate and results in ineffective oxygenation and ventilation.

ETIOPATHOGENESIS

The etiology of respiratory distress and failure in children can be conceptually divided into three broad categories (**Box 27.5**).

1. ***Conditions that affect the respiratory load:*** Includes all the congenital or acquired conditions involving the lungs and the airways, as well as the cardiac disorders and systemic illnesses that directly or indirectly affect the respiratory system.
2. ***Disorders affecting the respiratory muscles (related to pump failure):*** Neuromuscular disorders.
3. ***Neurologic conditions:*** Brainstem malformations, infections or effect of medications, or genetic disorders such as congenital central hypoventilation syndrome and neural networks that are involved in regulation of breathing.

In respiratory distress, fast breathing is coupled with labored or increased work of breathing, cyanosis, and/or dyspnea (**Box 27.6**). Fast breathing occurs after the activation of sensory systems involved in respiration. The central chemoreceptors (located in medulla) and peripheral chemoreceptors (carotid and aortic bodies) are responsible for the detection of changes in oxygen and carbon dioxide concentration in the blood. An increase in carbon dioxide stimulates the central receptors and results in an increase in ventilation. Hypoxia stimulates respiration through its effects on the peripheral receptors, which may cause breathlessness in patients who have underlying lung disease. Upper airway mechanoreceptors and pulmonary vagal receptors are important in shaping the pattern of breathing. The afferent impulses from these receptors project to the central nervous system (CNS) and are processed there. Based on the response to afferent information, the CNS sends an efferent impulse via the phrenic nerve to the diaphragm and the other respiratory muscles to increase respiration, thereby causing respiratory distress.

Box 27.5 Etiology of Respiratory Distress and Failure in Children

1. **Conditions that affect the respiratory load**
   - *Infections:* Croup, retropharyngeal abscess, diphtheria, pneumonia, viral bronchiolitis, pulmonary tuberculosis, pleural effusion or empyema and hemothorax
   - *Inflammatory disorders:* Severe acute asthma
   - *Acute respiratory distress syndrome:* Pulmonary edema, meconium aspiration syndrome
   - *Airway disorders:* Subglottic or tracheal stenosis, extrinsic airway compression (vascular ring, enlarged lymph nodes, peritonsillar/ retropharyngeal abscess), airway foreign body
   - *Air leak syndromes:* Tension pneumothorax, pneumomediastinum
   - *Vascular disorders:* Primary pulmonary hypertension, persistent pulmonary hypertension (PPHN), pulmonary embolism
   - *Disorders of surfactant secretion and metabolism:* Respiratory distress syndrome
   - *Disorders of lung development:* Chronic lung disease of prematurity (bronchopulmonary dysplasia), pulmonary genesis or hypoplasia
   - *Other lung disorders:* Pulmonary contusion, smoke inhalation injury, carbon monoxide poisoning, submersion injury and drowning
   - *Cardiac disorders:* Congestive heart failure, congenital heart disease
   - *Secondary to systemic disorders:* Sepsis and shock, anaphylaxis and angioedema, hematologic disorders (acute chest syndrome in sickle cell disease), metabolic acidosis as in renal failure, diabetic ketoacidosis, renal tubular acidosis
2. **Related to pump failure (respiratory muscle impairment)**
   - *Muscular weakness:* Duchenne muscular dystrophy, spinal muscular atrophy
   - *Demyelinating disorders:* Guillain-Barré syndrome
   - *Chest wall disorders:* Severe scoliosis, flail chest
   - *Disorders of neuromuscular junction:* Myasthenia gravis
3. **Related to neurologic conditions**
   - *Infections:* Bacterial meningitis, viral encephalitis, neurotuberculosis
   - *Trauma:* Closed head injury, intracranial hemorrhage
   - *Pharmacologic agents:* Benzodiazepines, barbiturates, narcotics
   - *Brainstem disorders:* Extrinsic compression from hemorrhage, tumors, or any other space-occupying lesions
   - *Psychogenic hyperventilation, anxiety, panic attacks*
   - *Genetic disorders:* Congenital central hypoventilation syndrome

Box 27.6 Signs of Respiratory Distress in Children

1. **Tachypnea (cut-off for respiratory rate)**
   - *Age 0–2 months:* >60/min
   - *Age 2–12 months:* >50/min
   - *Age 1–5 years:* >40/min
2. Dyspnea
3. Suprasternal, intercostal, or subcostal retractions
4. Grunting
5. Nasal flaring
6. Apnea
7. Altered mental status
8. SpO_2 < 90% on room air

EVALUATION

History

A child with respiratory distress may have tachypnea with cyanosis, nasal flaring, grunting, wheezing, chest wall retractions, or stridor **(Box 27.6)**. It is essential to characterize tachypnea or dyspnea in terms of onset, frequency, intensity, duration, triggering factors, provoking activities (ambulation, exertion, eating, changing position), associated respiratory symptoms, and relieving factors (medications, positions).

- Fever, cough, and fast breathing with or without lower chest indrawing are the most common presentation of lower respiratory tract infections such as pneumonia, bronchiolitis, and viral induced wheeze in younger children.
- Nocturnal cough and dyspnea may be suggestive of asthma, congestive heart failure, or gastroesophageal reflux disease.
- Dyspnea occurring mainly after exercise indicates congestive heart failure or exercise-induced asthma.
- Episodic dyspnea may be caused by asthma or less often by heart failure (e.g., in congenital heart diseases).
- Progressive dyspnea suggests chronic conditions like interstitial lung disease, persistent congestive heart failure, or pulmonary hypertension.
- The symptoms of fever, sore throat, and acute respiratory distress with stridor may be indicative of epiglottitis.
- Pleuritic chest pain associated with rapid but shallow *breathing could be due to pleuritis, pneumonia*, pneumothorax, or pulmonary embolism.
- A history of dysphagia or recurrent vomiting with intermittent wheezing may indicate gastroesophageal reflux with aspiration.

Examination

Determine the severity of dyspnea by observing the respiratory effort, use of accessory muscles, mental status, and ability to speak. Examination of the neck area might reveal a tracheal shift, jugular venous dilatation, suprasternal retractions, an enlarged thyroid gland, or an adenopathy.

- Stridor is suggestive of upper airway obstruction.
- Inspection of thorax might show an increased antero-posterior diameter or chest wall deformity.
- ***Chest indrawing:*** Inspect the chest with the entire chest completely exposed (from the neck to the waist) in adequate light. Use of intercostal or subcostal muscles for respiration result in lower chest wall indrawing. These features suggest lower airway pathology. In conditions of compromised breathing and high airway resistance, the more negative intra-pleural pressure during inspiration pulls the pliable portions of the chest wall inward, which manifests as intercostal, subcostal, supraclavicular, and suprasternal retractions.
- ***Grunting:*** It is a brief, low-pitched sound heard during expiration as the child exhales against a partially closed glottis. Grunting keeps the small airways, and alveolar sacs open during expiration. Causes of grunting include pneumonia, pulmonary contusion, acute respiratory distress syndrome (ARDS), congestive heart failure, and pulmonary edema.

Table 27.6 Differences between Respiratory Distress and Failure

Parameter	*Respiratory distress*	*Respiratory failure*
Airway	Open without respiratory support	Possibly obstructed
Respiratory rate	Increased rate	Slow breathing/ bradypnea, or apnea (late)
Respiratory effort	Increased effort	Reduced or no effort
Chest auscultation	Abnormal airway sounds (e.g., stridor, wheezing, grunting)	Poor to absent distal air movement
Heart rate	Tachycardia	Bradycardia
Response	Agitated and irritable	Lethargic and fails to respond; stuporous and comatose
Appearance	Pale	Cyanotic

- ❖ Palpation might reveal subcutaneous emphysema.
- ❖ Dullness on percussion is indicative of consolidation or effusion.
- ❖ Breath sounds may be decreased or absent in pneumothorax or pleural effusion.
- ❖ Wheezing indicates turbulent airflow, which can be caused by asthma or left ventricular failure.
- ❖ Crepitations are suggestive of pneumonia or pulmonary edema.
- ❖ Rapid or irregular pulse may indicate dysrhythmia. An S_3 gallop suggests a left ventricular dysfunction in congestive heart failure.
- ❖ A loud P_2 may be audible in pulmonary hypertension or cor pulmonale.
- ❖ Cyanosis or clubbing should be checked to rule out a congenital cyanotic heart disease, or a chronic lung disease.

If left untreated, respiratory distress can lead to respiratory failure. Differences in signs and symptoms between respiratory distress and respiratory failure are listed in **Table 27.6**.

Investigation

The basic investigations needed for children with respiratory distress include X-ray chest, ECG, blood gas analysis, serum electrolytes, and complete blood count. Certain specific situations may warrant laryngoscopy, bronchoscopy, pulmonary function tests, and a complete biochemical evaluation.

TREATMENT Respiratory Distress and Failure

Treatment of a child presenting with respiratory distress includes maintaining the temperature, airway, breathing, and circulation; followed by administering the definitive treatment based on history and physical examination.

Evaluate, Identify and Intervene

- *Airway*
  - Look for chest movement
  - Listen for air movement and breath sounds
  - Determine the following three possibilities:
    1. Is the airway patent? (If airway is open and not obstructed, proceed to assessment for breathing)
    2. Can the airway be kept open manually by head-tilt chin-lift method? (If cervical spine injury is suspected, open airway by jaw thrust without neck extension)
    3. Is an advanced airway required? Endotracheal intubation, cricothyrotomy if necessary.
    Once airway is established and maintained, move on to assess breathing.
- *Breathing*
  - Count the breaths in 1 minute and assess whether the child is breathing too fast or too slow.
  - Look for signs of increased respiratory effort, nasal flaring, retractions/chest indrawing, head bobbing or seesaw respirations, open mouth breathing, gasping, use of accessory muscles, grunting, and stridor.
  - Monitor oxygen saturation
  - High-concentration humidified oxygen by non-rebreathing mask
  - Inhaled salbutamol or epinephrine
  - Assisted ventilation with bag-mask
  - Intubation with endotracheal tube

If an infant or child is not breathing effectively, it is a life-threatening event and should be treated as respiratory arrest. Signs of respiratory distress and respiratory failure are summarized in **Table 27.6**.

- *Circulation*
  - Assess heart rate, rhythm, and blood pressure
  - Establish vascular access

Further management depends on the definitive diagnosis.

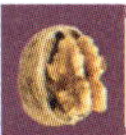

IN A NUTSHELL

Respiratory Distress and Failure

1. Respiratory distress is a condition in which the pulmonary activity is unable to bring oxygen into and remove carbon dioxide from the blood.
2. Characterize tachypnea or dyspnea in terms of onset, frequency, intensity, duration, triggering factors, provoking activities (ambulation, exertion, eating, changing position), associated respiratory symptoms, and relieving factors (medications, positions).
3. The general condition of the child and vital signs can be used to determine the severity of dyspnea by observing the respiratory effort, use of accessory muscles, mental status, and ability to speak. A child with respiratory distress may have tachypnea with cyanosis, nasal flaring, grunting, wheezing, chest wall retractions, or stridor.
4. The treatment of a child presenting with respiratory distress includes maintaining the temperature, airway, breathing, and circulation, followed by administering the definitive treatment based on history and physical examination.

Khemani RG, Smith LS, Zimmerman JJ, et al. Pediatric Acute Lung Injury Consensus Conference. Pediatric acute respiratory distress syndrome: definition, incidence, and epidemiology: proceedings from the Pediatric Acute Lung Injury Consensus Conference. Pediatr Crit Care Med. 2015;16(5 Suppl):S23-40.
Muralidharan J, Kulgod V, Sharma AK (Eds). IAP Advanced Life Support (ALS) Handbook, 2nd edition. Indian Academy of Pediatrics; 2020.
Pediatric Acute Lung Injury Consensus Conference Group. Pediatric acute respiratory distress syndrome: consensus recommendations from the Pediatric Acute Lung Injury Consensus Conference. Pediatr Crit Care Med. 2015:16(5),428-39.
Yehya N, Keim G, Thomas NJ. Subtypes of pediatric acute respiratory distress syndrome have different predictors of mortality. Intensive Care Med. 2018;44:1230-9.

27.6 Oxygen Therapy

PE 24.6, PE 24.7, PE 24.10

INTRODUCTION

The goal of oxygen therapy is to achieve adequate tissue oxygenation. Inadequate tissue oxygenation, if left untreated, may eventually lead to localized vasodilation, pulmonary vasoconstriction, metabolic acidosis, tissue necrosis, and brain injury.

INDICATIONS

Oxygen therapy is indicated in documented or suspected hypoxemia with PaO_2 < 60 mm Hg and SpO_2 < 94% in room air. Pulse oximetry should be used to detect hypoxemia.

If pulse oximetry is not available, clinical signs may provide useful clues whether to give supplemental oxygen therapy. Clinical signs suggestive of hypoxemia include the following:

- Central cyanosis
- Nasal flaring
- Grunting
- Inability to drink or feed due to respiratory distress
- Depressed mental state and sensorium (drowsy and lethargic)
- Severe lower chest wall retractions
- Respiratory rate ≥ 70/min
- Head nodding (nodding movement of the head synchronous with respiration, indicating severe respiratory distress)

Other clinical conditions that may be associated with hypoxemia include seizures, coma, acute neurological problems due to obstructed airway or impaired ventilatory effort, severe sepsis, heart failure, or severe anemia.

MODES OF ADMINISTRATION OF OXYGEN

Oxygen therapy should be provided at accurate and safe levels with the lowest possible fractional concentration of inspired oxygen (FiO_2). There are two types of oxygen delivery devices (1) Variable performance device or low-flow system, and (2) Fixed performance device or high-flow system **(Table 27.7)**.

Table 27.7 Types of Oxygen Delivery Devices

Variable performance device or low-flow system	*Fixed performance device or high-flow system*
1. Nasal cannula 2. Simple oxygen mask 3. Nasal mask 4. Nasal catheter 5. Trans-tracheal catheter 6. Partial rebreathing mask 7. Nonrebreathing mask	1. Air entrapment mask like venturi mask 2. Oxygen hood 3. Oxygen tent 4. Face tent 5. Partial rebreathing mask with reservoir 7. Nonrebreathing mask with reservoir

Variable Performance Device or Low-flow System

These devices provide only a fraction of the patient's inspiratory flow needs or tidal volume, and rest of the patient's inspiratory flow requirements is met by dilution with room air. The oxygen flow rate is usually <10 L/min. The rate of oxygen flow in these devices is less than the patient's inspiratory flow resulting in mixing of oxygen with room air. These devices deliver a variable FiO_2 of around 23–50% and hence, called variable performance device. The delivered FiO_2 depends upon patient's inspiratory flow rate and the oxygen flow rate of the device. These devices are suitable for patients requiring low to moderate FiO_2 (30–60%) and having stable breathing pattern.

Nasal cannula, simple oxygen mask, nasal catheters, partial rebreathing mask, and nonrebreathing mask are examples of low-flow system.

Nasal prongs: Nasal prongs are a device that ends in two short, tapered tubes (about 1 cm in length) designed to lie just within the nostrils **(Fig. 27.9)**. They are also called nasal cannulae. Humidification is usually not required with standard oxygen flow rates, as the natural nasal mechanisms heat and humidify the inspired oxygen.

An average FiO_2 provided with 1 L/min is 24%. With every increase of 1 L/min of oxygen up to 4 L/min, FiO_2 rises by 4%. High-flow oxygen by nasal cannula may cause irritation and

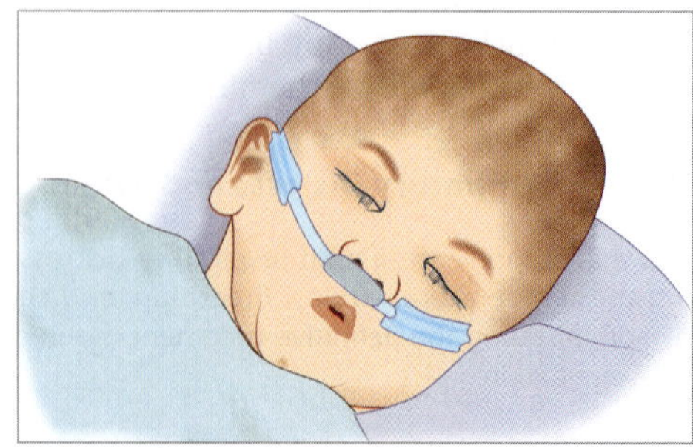

Fig. 27.9: Nasal cannula

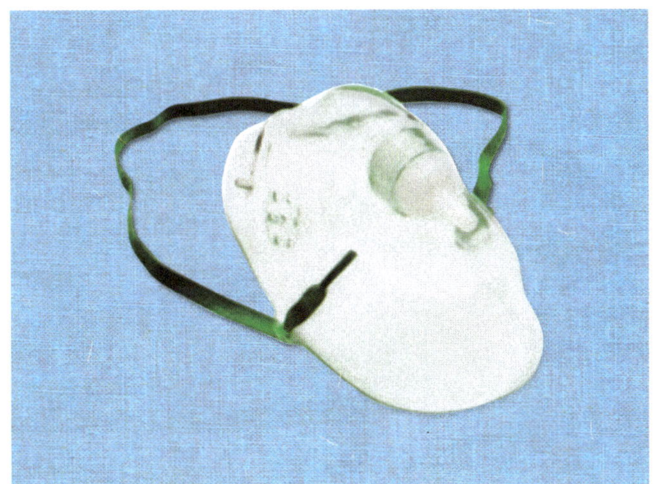

Fig. 27.10: Simple oxygen mask

dryness of nasopharynx. Oxygen flow rates through nasal prongs are 0.5–1 L/min for neonates, 1–2 L/min for infants, and 1–4 L/min for older children.

Simple oxygen mask (Fig. 27.10): It is a low-flow oxygen device that provides 35–60% FiO_2 at oxygen flow of 6–10 L/min. With each liter increase in oxygen, FiO_2 increases by approximately 10%. Flow <5 L/min can cause carbon dioxide retention and rebreathing of retained CO_2.

Partial rebreathing mask (Fig. 27.11): The partial rebreathing mask provides 35–70% FiO_2 at oxygen flow rates of 6–15 L/min. It is similar to a facemask but has an extra oxygen reservoir and side ports. The oxygen flow should be maintained to a level such that only one-third of reservoir gets empty during inspiration. During expiration, first one-third of the exhaled air enters the reservoir. This predominantly comes from the anatomic dead space and hence is still rich in oxygen as well as humidified. The reservoir bag should be filled with oxygen by occluding the outlet before placing on the patient.

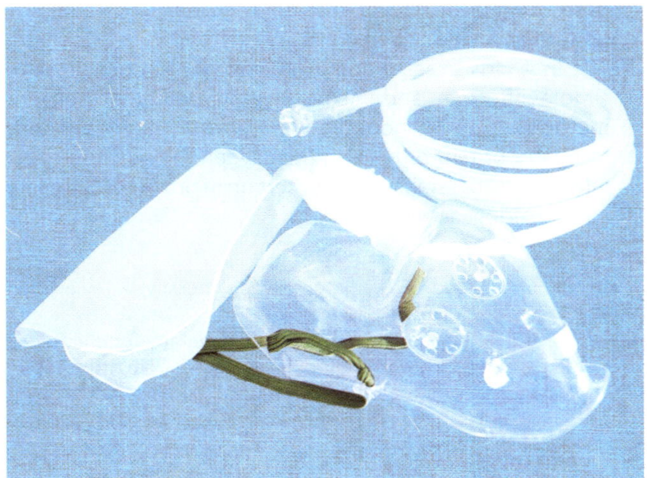

Fig. 27.11: Partial rebreathing mask

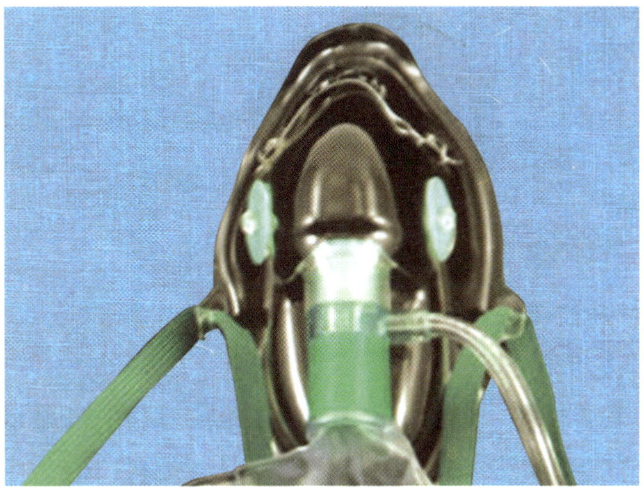

Fig. 27.12: Nonrebreathing mask

Nonrebreathing mask (Fig. 27.12): It can provide an FiO_2 of up to 80–100% at oxygen flow rate of 8–15 L/min. It is similar to partial-rebreathing mask other than a one-way valve between the mask and reservoir as well as over exhalation ports of the mask. In expiration, port valves open and reservoir valve closes. During inspiration, port valves close and reservoir valve opens and hence can provide high concentration of FiO_2.

Nasopharyngeal catheters: Nasopharyngeal catheter is passed to the pharynx just below the level of the uvula **(Figs. 27.13A to C)**. Better oxygenation is achieved with a lower oxygen flow than with nasal prongs, because FiO_2 in the trachea is relatively high with significant positive end-expiratory pressure (PEEP) production. However, nasopharyngeal catheters require close supervision.

Fixed Performance Device or High-flow System

These devices provide all the patient's inspiratory flow requirements and tidal volume. High-flow system can reliably deliver either low or high FiO_2. High-flow system should be used in emergency settings to reliably deliver a high FiO_2 up to 100% to a child with hypoxia. The oxygen flow rate is usually >15 L/min. These devices deliver a constant FiO_2 which does not get affected by the patient's inspiratory pattern. It is usually suitable for patients requiring consistent FiO_2 or those requiring high FiO_2 > 70% or those having varying breathing pattern.

These devices include oxygen hood, air entrapment mask (venturi mask, venti mask), air entrainment nebulizer, partial rebreathing mask with reservoir and nonrebreathing mask with reservoir, oxygen tent, and face tent.

Oxygen Hoods, Incubators, and Tents

Noninvasive methods of administering oxygen have certain advantages with oxygen piped into a head box/oxygen hood, incubator, or tent, the actual FiO_2 can be determined precisely by placing an oxygen analyzer near the infant's mouth. There is minimal risk for airway obstruction by mucus or of gastric distention, and humidification is not necessary. However, carbon dioxide toxicity can occur if the flow of oxygen is inadequate

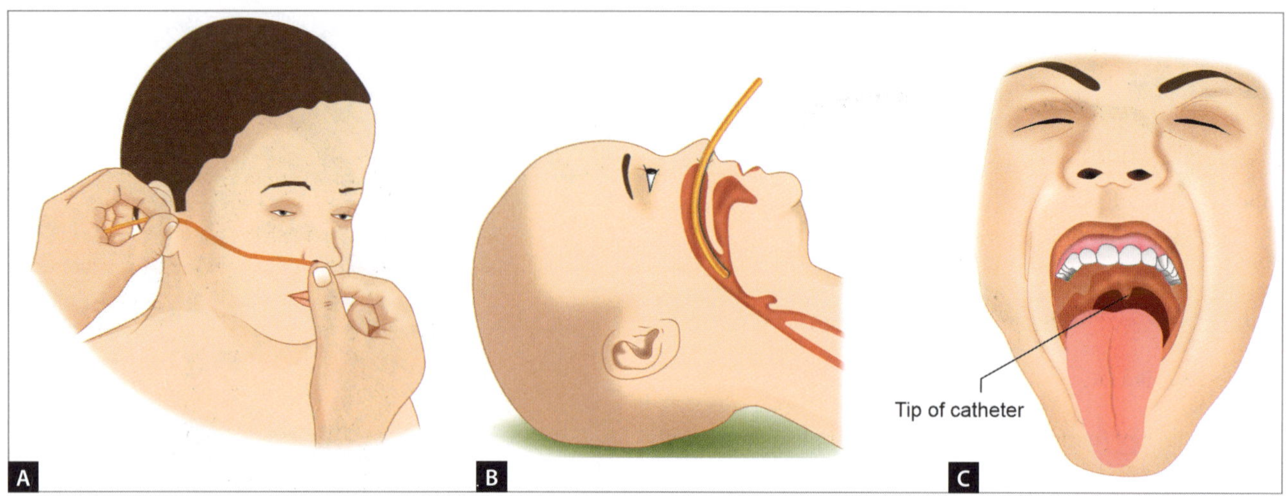

Figs. 27.13A to C: Insertion of nasopharyngeal catheter: (A) Measuring the distance from the nose to the tragus of the ear for insertion of a nasopharyngeal catheter; (B) Cross-sectional view of the position of the nasopharyngeal catheter; (C) Tip of the nasopharyngeal catheter visible just below the soft palate

Source: World Health Organization. Oxygen therapy for children: a manual for health workers. [online] Available from https://apps.who.int/iris/bitstream/handle/10665/204584/9789241549554_eng.pdf?sequence=1&isAllowed=y [Last accessed January, 2025]

due to very low flow rate or from kinking or disconnection of the oxygen tubing. Carbon dioxide can be retained if oxygen hood is used with an inappropriately tight seal around the infant's neck. A flow rate of 2–3 L/kg/min is necessary to avoid rebreathing of carbon dioxide within an oxygen hood.

Oxygen hoods, incubators, and tents all require high oxygen flow rate to achieve adequate concentrations of oxygen and avoid carbon dioxide accumulation and are expensive. Oxygen hoods also interfere with feeding. Therefore, these methods are not recommended for oxygen administration, especially in settings with limited oxygen supplies.

Venturi Mask (Fig. 27.14)

It combines oxygen with room air to give a high-flow oxygen concentration at a fixed and constant FiO_2. Color-coded jets are attached to the mask to deliver the required amount of oxygen. It can deliver FiO_2 ranging from 24 to 50%. The recommended flow rate is 12–15 L/min. In compensated shock, blood pressure remains normal, it is low in decompensated shock.

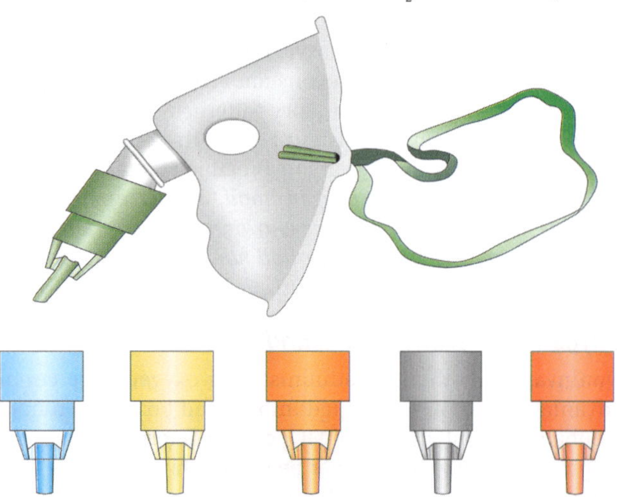

Fig. 27.14: Venturi mask

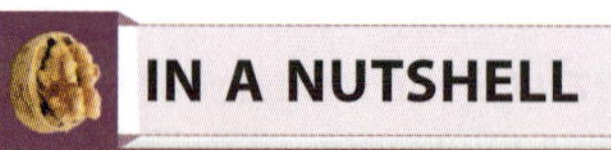

IN A NUTSHELL

Oxygen Therapy

1. The goal of oxygen therapy is to achieve adequate tissue oxygenation.
2. Oxygen therapy is indicated in documented or suspected hypoxemia with $PaO_2 < 60$ mm Hg and $SpO_2 < 94\%$ in room air. If pulse oximetry is not available, clinical signs may provide useful clues whether to give supplemental oxygen therapy.
3. There are two types of oxygen delivery devices: (1) Variable performance device or low-flow system and (2) Fixed performance device or high-flow system.
4. The methods used to administer oxygen should be safe, simple, effective, and inexpensive. The different delivery methods may be noninvasive (through oxygen hood, incubator or tent or holding the oxygen tubing close to an infant's face) or semi-invasive (insertion of prongs or catheters into the upper airway).

Walsh BK, Smallwood CD. Pediatric oxygen therapy: A review and update. Respir Care. 2017;62(6):645-61.

World Health Organization. (2016). Oxygen therapy for children: a manual for health workers. [online] Available from https://apps.who.int/iris/bitstream/handle/10665/204584/9789241549554_eng.pdf?sequence=1&isAllowed=y [Last accessed January 2025].

27.7 Shock

PE 24.3, PE 24.12, PE 24.13, PE 24.14, PE 24.16

INTRODUCTION

Shock is defined as a state of circulatory dysfunction leading to inadequate cellular perfusion and tissue hypoxia. It results from inadequate blood flow and oxygen delivery to meet the metabolic demands of body tissues. Shock progresses over a continuum of severity, from a compensated to a decompensated state. In compensated shock, blood pressure remains normal. Hypotension is a late sign of shock and indicates decompensated state.

The effects of inadequate perfusion are reversible initially. However, prolonged oxygen deprivation leads to generalized cellular hypoxia and the disruption of critical biochemical processes, eventually resulting in cell membrane ion pump dysfunction, intracellular edema, inadequate regulation of intracellular pH, and cell death. These abnormalities are clinically manifested as end-organ damage, multisystem organ failure, and eventually death.

Shock occurs in about 2% of hospitalized infants and children in developed countries, with mortality rates varying widely depending on the cause and clinical situation. This rate is much higher in developing countries. Many patients who do not survive shock do not die during the acute phase, but rather due to complications and multiple organ dysfunction syndrome (MODS), which is defined as dysfunction in two or more organ systems. The presence of MODS in shock patients significantly increases the likelihood of death. In 2017, there were an estimated 20.3 million cases of sepsis and 2.9 million deaths among children under 5 years old, and 4.9 million cases of sepsis with 454,000 deaths in older children and adolescents globally.

PATHOPHYSIOLOGY

Shock is a progressive disorder. It usually evolutes through three stages, viz., (1) Compensated stage, (2) Uncompensated stage, and (3) Irreversible state **(Table 27.8)**.

Table 27.8 Stages of Shock

Clinical parameter	*Compensated*	*Uncompensated*	*Irreversible*
Mental status	Agitation/confusion	Drowsiness	Unresponsive
Heart rate	Tachycardia	Marked tachycardia	Bradycardia
Respiration	Normal/mild tachypnea	Tachypnea/ acidotic	Acidotic/ apnea
Skin and capillary refill time (CRT)	Cold peripheral skin and increased CRT (peripheries can be warm with flushed CRT in warm shock)	Very slow capillary return and mottling	Cold and cyanotic
Urinary output	Adequate	Oliguria/anuria	Anuria
Blood pressure	Normal	Hypotension	Unrecordable

Compensated Shock

Vital organ function (brain and heart) remain intact through sympathetic reflexes that increase systemic arterial resistance diverting blood away from nonessential tissues, constrict venous reservoir, increase systemic vascular resistance (SVR), and increase heart rate to maintain cardiac output. Primarily increasing the heart rate rather than stroke volume enhances the cardiac output in neonates and young children. In older children, it is the increased stroke volume that also augments cardiac output.

Signs of compensated shock are tachycardia, cool extremities, prolonged capillary refill despite warm ambient temperature (cold shock), weak peripheral pulses compared with central pulses, reduced urine output, anxious-irritable child, and generally associated with fast breathing, but blood pressure is normal. Some children may have bounding pulse with flushed CRT and warm peripheries (warm shock).

Uncompensated Shock (End-organ Dysfunction and Microvascular Failure)

Compensatory mechanisms start failing. Due to tissue hypoperfusion, anaerobic metabolism sets in leading to lactic acidosis. Acidosis further depresses myocardium. There is failure of energy dependent Na^+–K^+ pump leading to hemostatic derangement and deterioration of lysosomal, mitochondrial, and membrane functions. This ultimately results in abnormal capillary permeability, pooling of blood, and interstitial fluid loss. Following stasis, damaging chain reactions may be initiated in the kinin and coagulation pathways leading to bleeding tendencies. Chemical mediators that may play a role include histamine, serotonin, cytokines (tumor necrosis factor, interleukins), xanthine oxidase that generates oxygen derived free radicals, platelet activating factor (PAF), and bacterial toxins.

As compensatory mechanisms fail, signs of inadequate end-organ perfusion develop. These signs include hypotension (cut-offs for defining hypotension in different age groups is depicted in **Table 27.2**), depressed mental status, decreased urine output, metabolic acidosis, tachypnea, and weak central pulses.

Irreversible Shock (End-organ Cellular Death and Cardiac Arrest)

It is characterized by severe damage to key organs such as heart and brain, death occurs despite restoration of circulation. Pathophysiologically, the high-energy phosphate reserves are totally exhausted, and body is said to have run out of energy.

This stage is characterized by bradypnea, bradycardia, very prolonged CRT (>6 seconds), anuria, coma, seizures and low to nonrecordable blood pressure. This stage may eventually lead to cardiac arrest.

CLASSIFICATION OF SHOCK (TABLE 27.9)

Hypovolemic Shock

Acute hypovolemia is the most common cause of shock in pediatric practice. Diminished circulating blood volume results in decreased preload and hence decreases stroke volume and cardiac output. Intense vasoconstriction occurs as a compensatory mechanism. This coupled with hypovolemia, produces tissue ischemia, which impairs cellular metabolism and releases potent vasoactive mediators from injured cells, such as arachidonic acid metabolites, cytokines, and other vasoactive peptides. These alter myocardial contractility, vascular tone, and membrane permeability.

Recovery depends on degree and rapidity with which hypovolemia develops and the patient's pre-existing status. Mortality is <10% if diagnosed and treated at an early stage.

Cardiogenic Shock

Intravascular volume is normal or increased. Cardiac dysfunction limits the cardiac output. As compensatory mechanisms are slowly overcome, the failing left ventricle leads to the cascade of raised left atrial pressure, increased pulmonary artery pressure, pulmonary edema, right ventricular overload, and cardiac failure. Suspicion of cardiogenic shock is usually high if heart rate is very high, disproportionate to clinical settings and poor perfusion with hepatomegaly and respiratory distress.

Prognosis is generally poor in cardiogenic shock that is primarily cardiac in origin, e.g., due to congenital heart disease, as compared to that occurring secondary to hypoxic-ischemic injury.

Obstructive Shock

It results from inability to produce adequate cardiac output in the face of normal intravascular volume and myocardial contractility and usually indicates mechanical left ventricular outflow obstruction.

Distributive Shock

The cardiac output is characteristically high. However, the cardiac output is unevenly distributed leading to inadequate tissue perfusion in certain vascular beds. Low SVR results in enhanced skin blood flow and bounding peripheral pulses. Mismatch between tissue blood flow and requirement leads to relative ischemia and acidosis.

Table 27.9 Classification and Description of Different Types of Shock

Type of shock	*Common causes*	*Basic derangement*	*Distinctive features*
1. Hypovolemic	• Diarrhea, vomiting • Hemorrhage • Renal losses • Capillary leak syndrome, i.e., burns	Decreased circulating blood volume resulting in low cardiac output	Tachycardia and hypotension without signs of congestive heart failure or sepsis
2. Distributive	• Sepsis • Anaphylaxis • CNS/spinal injury (neurogenic shock) • Drug intoxication	Maldistribution of regional blood flow, vasodilation, venous pooling and decreased preload. Cardiac output is high. Intravascular volume and myocardial contractility are normal	In neurogenic shock, there is absence of tachycardic response to hypotension (unlike other types of shock) and classically results in bradycardia, due to the unopposed vagal activity caused by sudden disruption of sympathetic nerve stimulation
3. Cardiogenic	• Severe congenital heart failure due to congenital or acquired heart disease • Myocarditis, cardiomyopathy, dysrhythmia • Following cardiac surgery • Anoxic and ischemic injuries • Metabolic derangement, i.e., acidosis, hypoglycemia • Drug intoxication	Decreased myocardial contractility leading to low cardiac output. Intravascular volume is normal or increased	Gallop rhythm, raised jugular venous pressure, hepatomegaly, pulmonary edema
4. Obstructive	• Cardiac tamponade • Massive pulmonary embolus • Tension pneumothorax	Mechanical obstruction to ventricular flow leading to low cardiac output. Intravascular volume and myocardial contractility stay normal	Narrow pulse pressure, profound hypoxemia, low voltage ECG
5. Dissociative	• Severe anemia • Methemoglobinemia • Carbon monoxide poisoning • Cyanide toxicity	Inability to deliver adequate oxygen to the tissues; inappropriate release of oxygen from hemoglobin leading to poor perfusion. Cardiac output, intravascular volume and myocardial functions are intact	Signs of myocardial ischemia, chocolate colored blood, normal PaO_2 but decreased saturation, elevated methemoglobin or carboxyhemoglobin

(ECG: electrocardiography; CNS: central nervous system; PaO_2: partial pressure of oxygen in arterial blood)

Septic shock: Septic shock is characterized by severe cardiovascular dysfunction in patients with a suspected or confirmed infection, and it poses a significantly higher risk of mortality in children compared to those with uncomplicated infections or sepsis without shock. In many children with septic shock, multiple organ dysfunction syndrome (MODS) is present, affecting the respiratory, renal, hematologic (e.g., disseminated intravascular coagulation or DIC), hepatobiliary, and neurologic systems. The clinical presentation of septic shock is typically that of distributive shock, with high cardiac output and low systemic vascular resistance (SVR). However, many children with sepsis also exhibit characteristics of hypovolemic shock due to factors like poor oral intake, gastrointestinal fluid losses, and vascular leak, as well as cardiogenic shock from impaired myocardial contractility. In younger children, septic shock more commonly manifests with low cardiac output and high SVR, where the features of cardiogenic and hypovolemic shock are more dominant.

Phoenix Sepsis Score

In pediatric patients, sepsis and septic shock are defined using the novel Phoenix Sepsis Score **(Table 27.10).** The score was developed and validated by the International Society of Critical Care Medicine (SCCM) Pediatric Sepsis Definition Task Force in 2024, using data from over 3 million electronic health encounters across 10 sites on four continents, representing both high-resource and low-resource settings. This score is applicable to children aged 0–18 years, though it has not been validated for preterm neonates or individuals older than 18.

Sepsis in children is defined as life-threatening organ dysfunction in the setting of suspected or confirmed infection, with a diagnosis requiring a ≥2-point score on the Phoenix Sepsis Score **(Table 27.10)**. The Phoenix Sepsis Score is based on dysfunction across four key organ systems:

1. ***Respiratory*** (PaO_2:FiO_2 or SpO_2:FiO_2 ratio)
2. ***Cardiovascular*** (use of vasoactive medications, lactate levels, and age-specific mean arterial pressure [MAP])
3. ***Coagulation*** (platelets, INR, D-dimer, fibrinogen)
4. ***Neurologic*** (Glasgow Coma Scale)

Septic shock is a subset of sepsis defined as sepsis with ≥1 point in the cardiovascular subscore, which includes criteria such as severe hypotension for age, a venous or arterial blood lactate level of >5 mmol/L, or the need for vasoactive medications to stabilize blood pressure.

The term *severe sepsis* is no longer used in current clinical practice because sepsis itself is a condition characterized by life-threatening organ dysfunction associated with infection and is thus indicative of a severe disease state. The Phoenix Sepsis Score should be calculated at the time of initial presentation in any patient with clinically suspected sepsis or septic shock, helping to guide timely and effective treatment. The previous criteria based on the systemic inflammatory response syndrome (SIRS) are no longer recommended for diagnosing sepsis in children.

Hyperferritinemic septic shock, also known as septic shock with hyperferritinemia, is a rare and severe subtype of septic shock where the serum ferritin level is significantly elevated, typically exceeding 3,000 ng/mL. It is often linked to Hemophagocytic Lymphohistiocytosis (HLH) or Macrophage Activation Syndrome (MAS), especially in autoimmune conditions. The condition always requires ICU care and has a poor prognosis due to its severity. Management includes antibiotics, immunosuppressive therapy, and supportive care. Early recognition and aggressive treatment are crucial for survival.

Dissociative Shock

It results from inability to deliver oxygen to the tissues (such as in severe anemia), or impaired oxygen utilization by cells despite normal perfusion (cyanide toxicity). It can also be due to abnormal affinity of hemoglobin for oxygen preventing its release to tissues, such as carbon monoxide (CO) intoxication. CO binds to hemoglobin in red blood cells much more strongly than oxygen does (about 200–250 times more), forming carboxyhemoglobin (COHb). The binding of CO to hemoglobin also alters the hemoglobin's ability to release oxygen to tissues.

DIAGNOSIS

Shock is a clinical diagnosis facilitated by a well taken history suggestive of infection, fluid loss, hemorrhage, heart disease, allergies, drug intake, trauma, previous illnesses, immune deficiency, or con- genital anomalies. Rapid circulatory assessment consists of evaluation of heart rate, pulse volume, CRT, blood pressure, respiratory rate, skin appearance and temperature, mental status, and urinary output.

- ***Cardiovascular status:*** Tachycardia is a compensatory mechanism. *Bradycardia* is a preterminal sign caused by hypoxia and acidosis. Low volume or *thready pulses* are an indicator of imminent decompensation. *Bounding pulses* may be observed in early septic shock.
- ***Hypotension*** is a late and often sudden sign of decompensated shock; if not reversed early, may lead to death. The lower limit of normal systolic pressure in children aged >1 year can be approximated by the following formula 70 + (2 × age in years).
- ***Skin changes:*** Mottling, pallor, and cyanosis indicate poor perfusion. A core and toe temperature difference of >2°C is a sign of poor skin perfusion.
- ***Mental status:*** Agitation and confusion alternating with *drowsiness* are the early features of ischemic brain injury. Infants may present with weak cry, hypotonia, irritability, and inability to focus on parent's face.
- ***Renal status:*** Urine output is an important parameter to monitor the progress of shock. Urine flow rate of <1 mL/kg/h in children and 2 mL/kg/h in infants suggest inadequate renal perfusion indicating prerenal failure, acute tubular necrosis, or cortical necrosis.
- ***Respiratory status:*** Acidosis due to poor tissue perfusion may lead to *deep rapid breathing*. Respiratory failure and ARDS are late manifestations of shock.
- ***Hematological system:*** Bleeding may occur from various sites including both superficial (cutaneous) and deep (internal) hemorrhage. This suggests presence of coagulation abnormality such as *disseminated intravascular coagulation* associated with raised prothrombin time (PT), partial thromboplastin time with kaolin (PTTK), and thrombocytopenia.

Table 27.10 Phoenix Sepsis Score Criteria[a]

Variables	*0 points*	*1 point*	*2 points*	*3 points*
Respiratory (0–3 points)	PaO_2:FiO_2 ≥400 or SpO_2:FiO_2 ≥292[b]	PaO_2:FiO_2 <400 on any respiratory support or SpO_2:FiO_2 <292 on any support[b,c]	PaO_2:FiO_2 100–200 on IMV or SpO_2:FiO_2 148–220 on IMV[b]	PaO_2:FiO_2 <100 on IMV or SpO_2:FiO_2 <148 on IMV[b]
Cardiovascular (0–6 points)		*1 point each (up to 3)*	*2 points each (up to 6)*	
	No vasoactive medications[d]	1 vasoactive medication[d]	≥2 vasoactive medications[d]	
	Lactate <5 mmol/L[e]	Lactate 5–10.9 mmol/L[e]	Lactate ≥11 mmol/L[e]	
Age[f]	*Mean arterial pressure, mm Hg[g]*			
<1 month	>30	17–30	<17	
1 to 11 months	>38	25–38	<25	
1 to <2 years	>43	31–43	<31	
2 to <5 years	>44	32–44	<32	
5 to <12 years	>48	36–48	<36	
12 to 17 years	>51	38–51	<38	
Coagulation (0-2 points)[h]	*1 point each (maximum 2 points)*			
	Platelets ≥100 × 10^3/µL	Platelets <100 × 10^3/µL		
	INR ≤1.3	INR >1.3		
	D-dimer ≤2 mg/L FEU	D-dimer >2 mg/L FEU		
	Fibrinogen ≥100 mg/dL	Fibrinogen <100 mg/dL		
Neurologic (0-2 points)[i]	*0 points*	*1 point*	*2 points*	
	Glasgow Coma Scale score >10; pupils reactive[j]	Glasgow Coma Scale score ≤10[j]	Fixed pupils bilaterally	
Interpretation of Phoenix Sepsis Score				
Sepsis	Suspected infection plus Phoenix Sepsis Score ≥ 2			
Septic shock	Sepsis plus ≥1 cardiovascular point(s)			

[a] The score can be calculated even if some variables (like lactate or vasoactives) are missing. Missing variables are scored as 0. The Phoenix Sepsis Score is not for use in neonates <37 weeks postconceptional age or those ≥18 years.

[b] SpO_2:FiO_2 ratio is valid only if SpO_2 ≤97%.

[c] A respiratory score of 1 point can be assigned to any child on oxygen support (high-flow, noninvasive, or IMV) and includes a PaO_2:FiO_2 ratio <200 or SpO_2:FiO_2 <220 in children who are not receiving IMV. For children on IMV with PaO_2:FiO_2 <200 or SpO_2:FiO_2 <220, see 2–3 point criteria.

[d] Vasoactive meds include any dose of epinephrine, norepinephrine, dopamine, dobutamine, milrinone, or vasopressin.

[e] Normal lactate range is 0.5–2.2 mmol/L. Both arterial and venous samples are acceptable.

[f] Criteria exclude neonates <37 weeks postconceptional age and anyone ≥18 years.

[g] Prefer directly measured MAP (invasive arterial or noninvasive oscillometric). If unavailable, calculate MAP using: (1/3 × systolic BP) + (2/3 × diastolic BP).

[h] Reference coagulation values: Platelets: 150–450 × 10^3/µL; D-dimer: <0.5 mg/L FEU; Fibrinogen: 180–410 mg/dL; INR based on local lab standards

[i] Neurological dysfunction subscore was pragmatically validated in both sedated and non-sedated patients, with or without IMV.

[j] GCS (Glasgow Coma Scale): measures eye, verbal, and motor responses (score range: 3–15, higher is better).

Abbreviations - FEU: fibrinogen equivalent units; **IMV:** invasive mechanical ventilation; **INR:** international normalized ratio; **MAP:** mean arterial pressure; **PaO_2:FiO_2:** arterial oxygen pressure/fraction of inspired oxygen; **SpO_2:** pulse oximetry saturation (used only if ≤97%)

(*Source:* Schlapbach LJ, Watson RS, SorcevLR, et al. International Consensus Criteria for Pediatric Sepsis and Septic Shock. JAMA. Published online January 21, 2024. https://doi.org/10.1001/jama.2024.0179.)

- ***Gastrointestinal tract:*** Erosive gastritis, ischemic pancreatitis, and ischemic hepatitis indicate gastrointestinal involvement.

Laboratory Investigations

These are needed for two reasons: (1) To ascertain the cause of shock and (2) To appraise the performance of different organ systems. Baseline investigations should include a complete blood count, platelet count, blood glucose, serum electrolytes, renal function tests, clotting screen, arterial blood gases, and blood culture. A comprehensive evaluation requires early laboratory testing to screen for hyperlactatemia, acidemia, and electrolyte disturbances such as hypoglycemia and hypocalcemia.

1. ***Arterial and venous lactate levels:*** In children with septic shock, elevated venous and arterial lactate levels in the emergency department (ED) are associated with an increased risk of organ dysfunction when measured in the ED and a higher risk of mortality if elevated at the time of PICU admission. While the optimal cut-off for lactate levels remains to be defined, an arterial lactate level ≥2 mmol/L is concerning and linked to worse outcomes. In all forms of shock, elevated blood lactate levels are a sign of poor tissue oxygen delivery and underscore the need for early and aggressive management to correct these imbalances.
2. ***Laboratory evidence of concurrent multisystem organ dysfunction syndrome (MODS)*** should also be sought, including tests such as a complete *blood count (CBC), renal* and *liver function tests,* and a *coagulation profile* (including fibrinogen, D-dimer, or fibrin split products).
3. ***CRP and procalcitonin:*** Elevated neutrophil counts, with an increase in immature forms (such as bands and myelocytes), along with elevated levels of *C-reactive protein (CRP)* and *procalcitonin,* may suggest infection.
4. ***Blood gas analysis:*** It can also be helpful to assess the degree of respiratory dysfunction, and an elevated venous-to-arterial PCO_2 gap ≥5 mm Hg may indicate an early shock state.
5. ***Blood culture:*** For septic shock, at least one blood culture should be collected, along with additional cultures based on the patient's history and physical exam.
6. ***Ferritin levels*** should be checked in all septic shock patients, and if hyperferritinemia (exceeding 3,000 mg/mL) is present, further testing for Hemophagocytic Lymphohistiocytosis (HLH) and Macrophage Activation Syndrome (MAS) should be performed, including fibrinogen, triglycerides, CBC, soluble IL-2 receptor levels, natural killer (NK) cell counts, and specific genetic testing.
7. ***Central venous oxygen saturation ($ScvO_2$):*** The hallmark of uncompensated shock is an imbalance between oxygen delivery (DO_2) and oxygen consumption (VO_2). Normally, oxygen delivery exceeds oxygen consumption by threefold, resulting in a normal $ScvO_2$ of approximately 75%. When $ScvO_2$ falls below 70%, it reflects an increased oxygen extraction ratio, signaling a relative decrease in oxygen delivery. This imbalance in oxygen delivery and consumption leads to increased tissue oxygen extraction, which is clinically observed through elevated lactic acid production, high anion gap, and metabolic acidosis, all indicative of anaerobic metabolism. In cases of dissociative shock, hyperlactatemia may coexist with an elevated $ScvO_2$ (greater than 80–85%), indicating impaired oxygen utilization despite adequate tissue perfusion.
8. ***Urine analysis:*** Examination of urine for specific gravity, albumin, sugar and cells is a must.
9. Chest skiagram and electrocardiography (ECG or EKG) should also be obtained.
10. ***Point-of-care ultrasound (POCUS)*** is being increasingly incorporated into the initial assessment of children with shock to assess the intravascular volume status, response to initial fluid resuscitation and myocardial function.
11. ***Focused assessment with sonography for trauma (FAST):*** To screen for pericardial effusion and hemoperitoneum.

TREATMENT Shock

Principles

- Early recognition of shock state and prompt initiation of resuscitation.
- Look for treatable cause, such as cardiac tamponade and tension pneumothorax.
- Protect and support organ functions and complications.
- Correction of any aggravating factors or deficiencies.
- Continuous monitoring.

The management of shock in children is depicted in an algorithmic manner in **Flowchart 27.4**. Rapid recognition of shock should be done within the first 5 minutes. Initial management begins with assessment of the airway, breathing, and circulatory status. It is important to secure the airway and ensure adequate breathing as all other interventions will fail if adequate gas exchange and oxygen delivery cannot take place. Within the first 10–15 minutes of detection of signs of shock, airway, oxygenation, ventilation and monitoring of heart rate/rhythm and pulse oximetry should be taken care of, and vascular access should be established. The initial hour in the management of shock is the most crucial in determining the outcome and has therefore been called the "golden hour". Initial resuscitation algorithm for managing septic shock is given in **Figure 27.15** (Surviving Sepsis Campaign guidelines 2020). Appropriate management with fluid boluses and ongoing assessment during this crucial period is of utmost importance. Specific management considerations by shock type is given in **Table 27.11**.

Initial fluid resuscitation

Administration of fluids for effective restoration of circulating volume is the key step in management of shock. The choice of fluids includes crystalloids (normal saline, Ringer's lactate), and colloids (albumin, dextran, and blood products). Initially, Ringer's lactate solution or normal saline is given as a bolus of 10–20 mL/kg over 10–15 minutes (by gravity method if compensated shock, and over 5-10 minutes by pull-and-push method if hypotensive shock). Reassess after every bolus and repeat fluid boluses if needed, according to response. A total bolus of up to 40–60 mL/kg may be administered over the first hour. According to the Surviving Sepsis Campaign (SSC) guidelines 2020, in healthcare settings without intensive care, fluid bolus therapy is not recommended unless hypotension is present **(Fig. 27.16)**. Watch for pulmonary edema, especially in case of severe anemia and severe febrile illness. Blood replacement therapy should begin immediately following hemorrhagic shock. A child with hypovolemic shock often requires 40–60 mL/kg during the first hour of therapy followed by reassessment of interstitial volume status and consideration of colloid for additional fluid replacement, as much as 200 mL/kg in the first few hours. Almost all patients with hypovolemic shock and one-fourth of those with septic shock will respond to this management alone. If cardiogenic shock is suspected, consider a small fluid bolus (5–10 mL/kg) over 10–20 minutes and reassess.

Flowchart 27.4: Stepwise management of shock

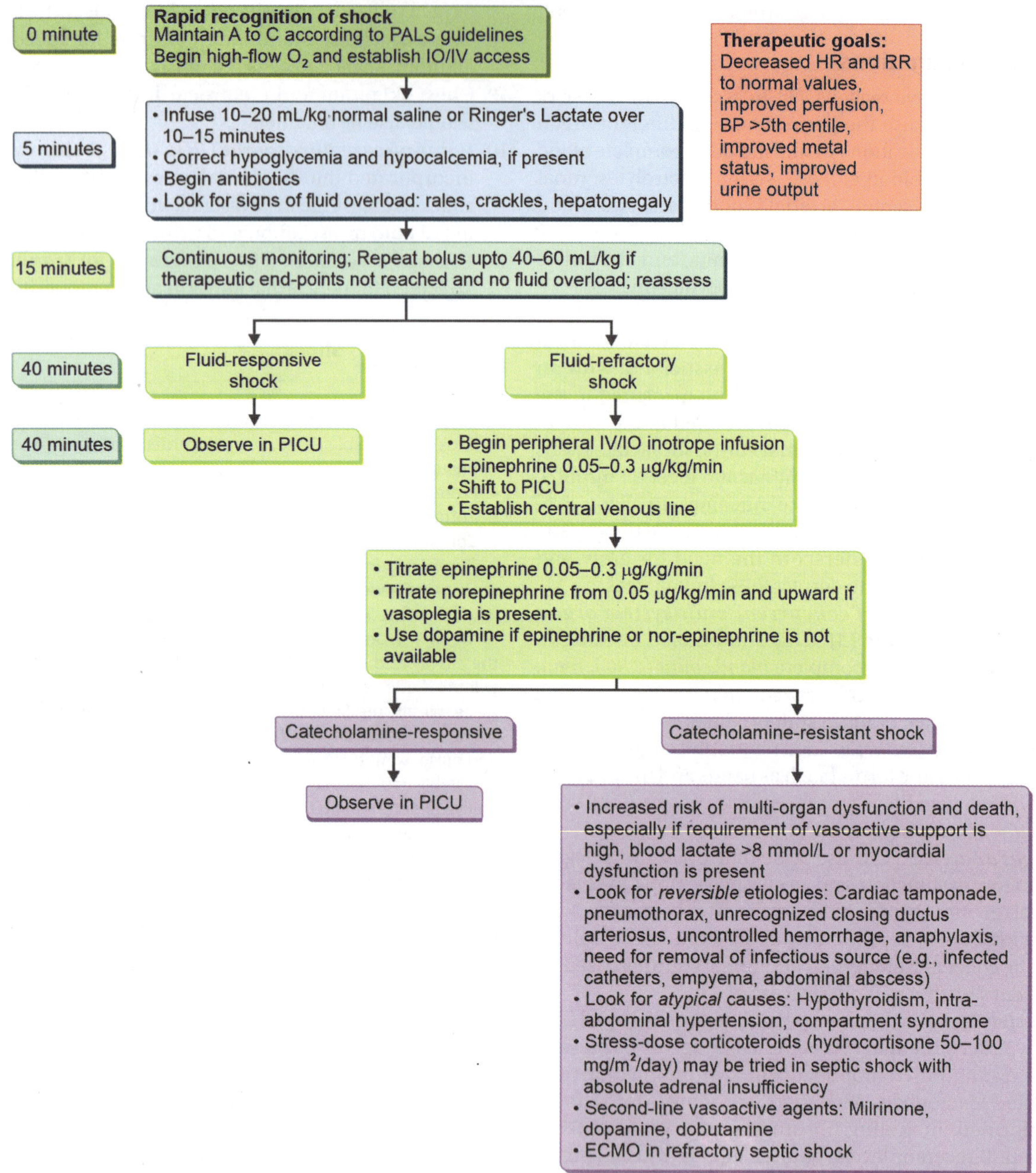

(ECMO: extracorporeal membrane oxygenation; HR: heart rate; PALS: pediatric advanced life support; PICU: pediatric intensive care unit; RR: respiratory rate)

Balanced/buffered fluids versus 0.9% normal saline: Crystalloid resuscitation typically uses 0.9% normal saline or balanced fluids like lactated Ringer's. Saline has a high chloride concentration, which can cause metabolic acidosis, while balanced fluids are closer to plasma composition and may reduce complications like kidney injury and inflammation. Although 0.9% saline is still common for pediatric resuscitation, recent data suggest balanced fluids may have fewer risks. However, studies in pediatric population show mixed results, and neither type has shown a clear, consistent advantage in adult trials. Both remain acceptable options for initial volume resuscitation pending more research.

Crystalloids versus colloids: Crystalloid solutions remain the initial fluid of choice for shock of undetermined etiology. The advantages of crystalloid include availability, low cost, and lack of exposure to blood products. These solutions contain large molecules that are relatively impermeable to the capillary membrane. This property leads to decreased extravasation and an increased percentage of the infused volume remaining intravascular. There is limited data on the superiority of colloids over crystalloids and there is not enough data for safety of colloid use in children. Therefore, use of crystalloids is recommended as the initial approach, and they should be combined with colloids in case of refractory hypovolemic shock.

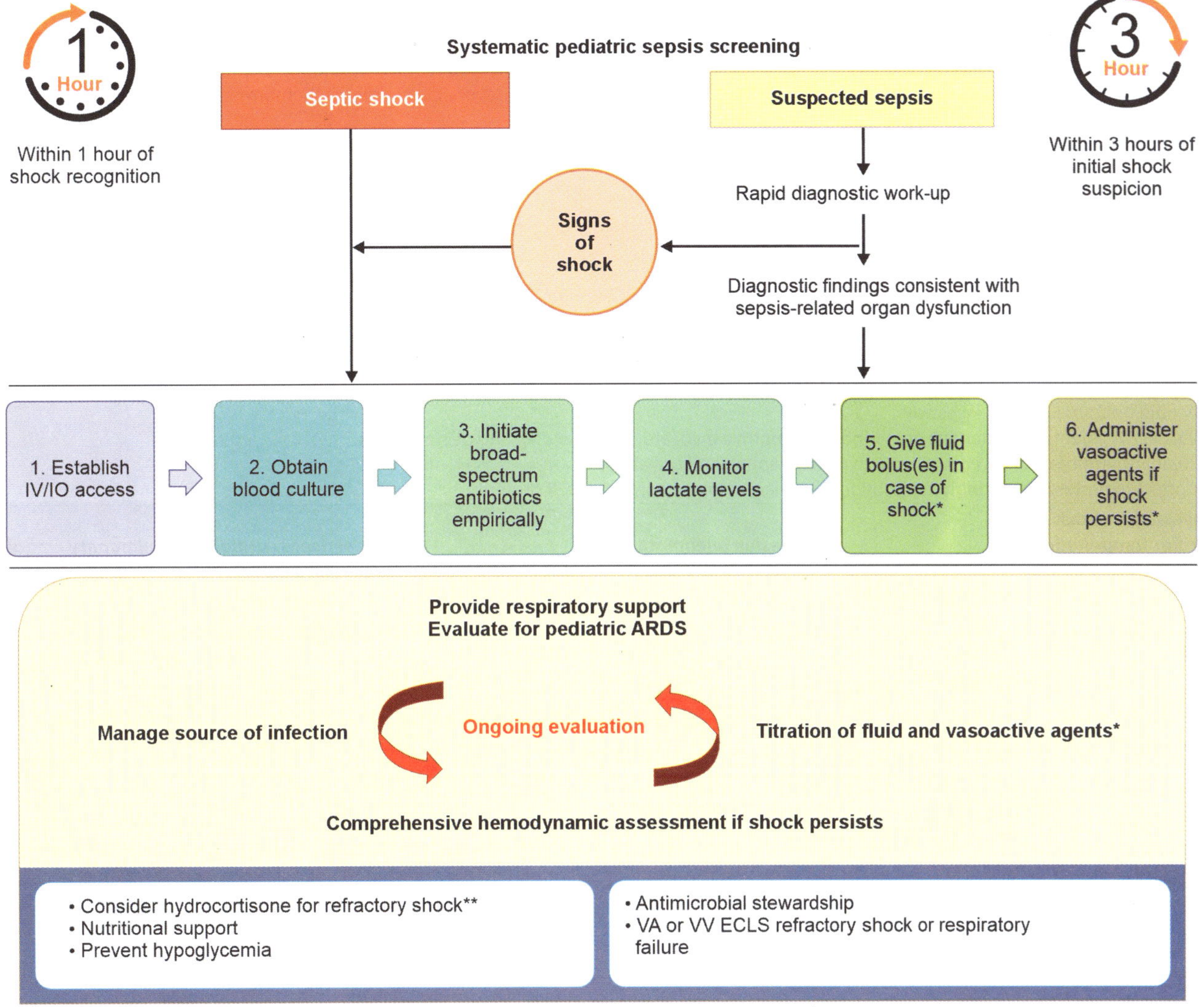

*Refer to fluid and vasoactive algorithm: Avoid fluid bolus if (a) Fluid overload is present or (b) In low-resource settings without hypotension. Administer fluid based on ideal body weight (mL/kg).
**Hydrocortisone may offer either benefit or harm, requiring careful consideration.

Fig. 27.15: Initial Resuscitation Algorithm for Children in Septic Shock (Surviving Sepsis Campaign 2020): It outlines six key management steps for children with clinical signs of shock, to be completed within 1 hour of initial shock recognition. These steps are: (1) establish intravenous or intraosseous access, (2) obtain blood cultures, (3) initiate broad-spectrum antibiotics empirically, (4) monitor blood lactate levels, (5) administer crystalloid fluid therapy with volume and rate tailored to the healthcare setting and patient response, and (6) administer vasoactive medications if shock persists despite fluid resuscitation and other therapies

(ARDS: acute respiratory distress syndrome; ECLS: extracorporeal life support; VA: venoarterial; VV: venovenous.)

Source: (Adapted from: © 2020 the Society of Critical Care Medicine and the European Society of Intensive Care Medicine. All Rights Reserved. Available from: https://www.sccm.org/clinical-resources/guidelines/guidelines/surviving-sepsis-campaign-international-guidelines)

Colloids are preferred in hypovolemic patients with renal, cardiac, and respiratory failure. Colloids are contraindicated in burns and severe capillary leaks. Large volumes of colloids can contribute to interstitial and pulmonary edema. Blood products are the preferred fluids in cases of trauma and hemorrhage.

If the patient is still in shock at the end of the first hour of management, the diagnosis of fluid refractory shock is established and the patient should be started on inotropic support. The commonly used vasoactive medications and their doses are listed in **Table 27.12**.

Central venous pressure monitoring: Measurement of central venous pressure (CVP) should be carried out to decide the need for additional care. The normal CVP is to be maintained between 12 and 18 cm of water. If the CVP remains <10 cm of water, another fluid bolus of 10–20 mL/kg is administered. Dopamine infusion is started if CVP is >15 cm of water. CVP between 10 and 15 cm is an indication for starting dopamine and considering dobutamine infusion. Persistent hypotension even after above measures necessitates continuous adrenaline infusion (0.1–2 μg/kg/min).

Table 27.11 Specific Management Considerations by Shock Type

<table>
<tr><td colspan="4">Hypovolemic shock
• Crystalloids (0.9% normal saline or Ringer's lactate)10–20 mL/kg over 15–20 minutes, up to three boluses 40–60 mL/kg
• Fluid-refractory shock: Start vasoactive agents and check for ongoing losses (e.g., severe burns, internal hemorrhage, persistent vomiting, diarrhea), other associated etiology (e.g., septic shock or spinal cord injury)
• Give further fluids guided by bedside ECHO/POCUS or CVP monitoring</td></tr>
<tr><td colspan="3">Distributive shock
Anaphylactic shock
• IM epinephrine at 0.01 mg/kg (maximum 0.5 mg) of 1:1,000 solution; repeat dose after 10–15 minutes if no response
• IV crystalloids for volume expansion
• If there is no response to two doses of IM epinephrine, start epinephrine infusion at the rate of 0.01 to 0.05 mcg/kg/min</td><td>Neurogenic shock
• IV crystalloids
• Vasopressors (norepinephrine) to increase SVR</td></tr>
<tr><td colspan="4">Septic shock: Discussed separately in detail (Figures 27.15 and 27.16)</td></tr>
<tr><td colspan="4">Cardiogenic shock
• IV fluid bolus of 5–10 mL/kg slowly
• Vasoactive agents: Dobutamine or milrinone to improve myocardial contractility and decrease SVR
• Treat arrhythmias (supraventricular tachycardia, ventricular fibrillation)
• Correct hypothermia, hypoglycemia, hypocalcemia, anemia and infections, if present</td></tr>
<tr><td>Obstructive shock
Cardiac tamponade
• IV crystalloid bolus
• Urgent pericardiocentesis and drainage</td><td>Tension pneumothorax
• Needle decompression in second intercostal space with underwater seal
• Tube thoracostomy</td><td>Duct-dependent cardiac lesions
• Prostaglandins E_1 infusion
• IV crystalloids</td><td>Pulmonary embolism
• IV crystalloids
• Thrombolytics
• Expert consultation</td></tr>
</table>

(CVP: central venous pressure; ECHO: echocardiography; IV: intravenous; IM: intramuscular; POCUS: Point-of-care ultrasound; SVR: systemic vascular resistance.)

Source: (Adapted from: Muralidharan J, Kulgod V, Sharma AK (Eds). IAP Advanced Life Support (ALS) Handbook, 2nd edition. Indian Academy of Pediatrics; 2020.)

*Vasoactive Agents (**Table 27.12**)*

In fluid-refractory shock, vasoactive agents are recommended. The recommended first-line vasoactive agents are epinephrine in fluid-refractory septic shock and when myocardial dysfunction is present, and norepinephrine when vasoplegia is present. Dopamine can be used when the first-line agents are not available. Vasoactive agents can be given through the peripheral line in emergency setting, but it should be shifted to central line as soon as possible. Restrict peripheral line vasoactive use to <6 hours.

Epinephrine acts on α_1 and β receptors. It increases SVR, heart rate, cardiac output, and blood pressure. Norepinephrine has mixed α_1 and β activity ($\beta_1 > \beta_2$), with slightly more α_1 activity than β activity. This leads to a more significant increase in blood pressure than increased heart rate. Blood pressure, SVR, cardiac output, and mean arterial pressure (MAP) are increased with norepinephrine. Dopamine given in low dosages (1–5 µg/kg/min) acts as vasodilator to cerebral and renal beds; it is inotropic at 5–10 µg/kg/min and causes direct stimulation of β_1 receptors, thereby increasing cardiac contractility. Doses in excess of 10 µg/kg/min result in vasoconstriction due to α_1 stimulation. Dobutamine is primarily an inotrope and vasodilator. Other vasoactive drugs that have been used in shock states include amrinone (inotrope), nitroprusside (vasodilator), and isoproterenol (inotrope and vasodilator).

Supportive Therapy

This includes general measures as well as specific care directed against multiple organ dysfunctions. Since oxygen delivery depends on the hemoglobin concentration, it should be optimized, and blood transfusion may be necessary. Infusion of packed red cells, fresh frozen plasma or platelets is mandatory, wherever indicated. Histamine type 2 receptors (H2) antagonists are used for erosive gastritis, especially in the setting of hypovolemic shock. Mechanical ventilation is indicated for respiratory failure and ARDS. Renal complications are managed with appropriate fluids, diuretics, or dialysis. Role of steroids is not well-established except in acute adrenal crisis with cardiovascular collapse.

Antibiotics: Antibiotics should be initiated within 1 hour of recognizing septic shock and within 3 hours of suspecting sepsis. Blood cultures should ideally be obtained before administering the first dose of antibiotics, but this should not delay the start of treatment.

Initial combination of a third-generation cephalosporin such as ceftriaxone, and vancomycin provides a broad coverage against most gram-positive and gram-negative organisms.

Metabolic corrections: Acidosis, hypoxia, hypoglycemia, hypocalcemia, hypokalemia, hyperkalemia, hyponatremia, etc., should be diagnosed and managed as per specific guidelines.

Newer therapies: Agents directed toward blocking release/counteracting the actions of endotoxins and cytokines have been tried. These include antitumor necrosis factor, anti-interleukin, and antiplatelet activating factors. Nitric oxide is an endogenous vasodilator that is believed to be responsible for hypotension in septic shock and causes some degree of myocardial depression. Trials are in progress using inhibitors of nitric oxide synthetase for treatment of shock. Shock refractory to all these measures may rarely require Extracorporeal Membrane Oxygenation (ECMO) support until the underlying disease process can be controlled.

Therapeutic Endpoints of Shock

1. Normal heart rate or decreasing heart rate from very high toward normal
2. Normal central and peripheral pulses, CRT ≤ 2 seconds and warm extremities
3. Normal mental status/responsiveness
4. Normal blood pressure (above 5th centile for age)
5. Urine output ≥1 mL/kg/h
6. Improving serum lactate and metabolic acidosis
7. Central venous oxygen saturation ($ScvO_2$) ≥ 70%

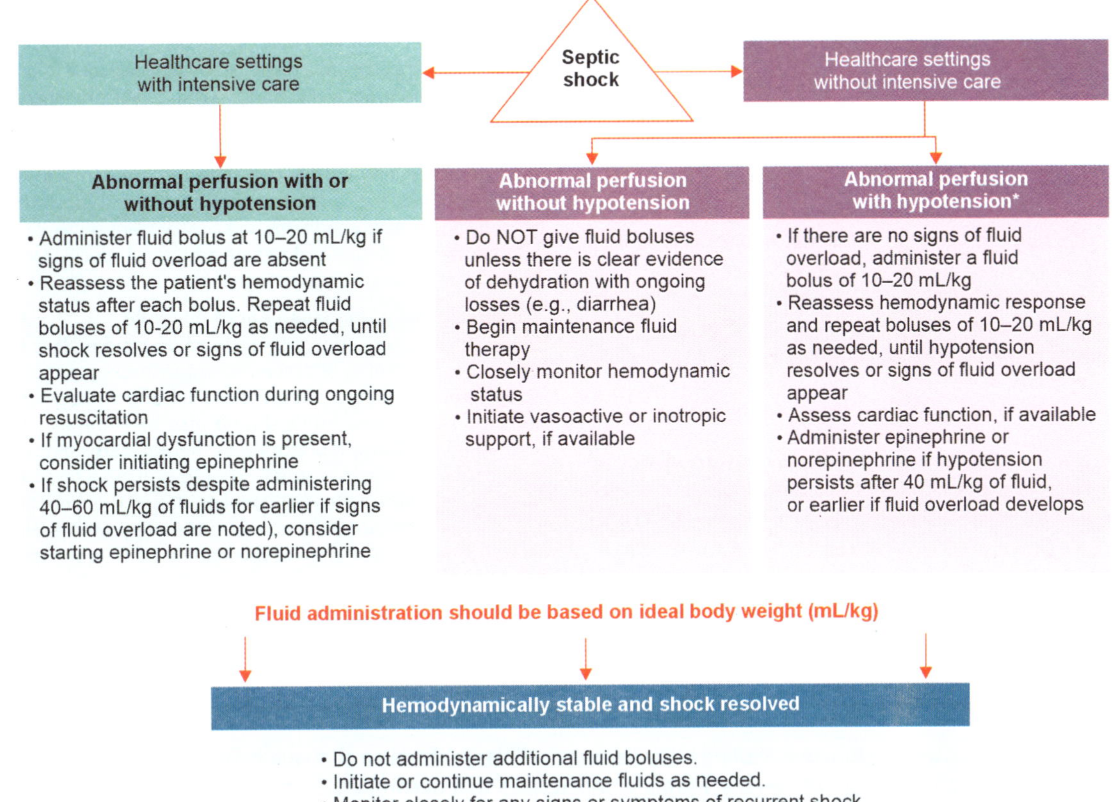

Fig. 27.16: Fluid and Vasoactive-Inotrope Management Algorithm for Children in Septic Shock (Surviving Sepsis Campaign 2020) recommends fluid bolus therapy for children with septic shock based on the availability of intensive care. In healthcare systems with access to intensive care (either locally or through transport), a fluid bolus of 40–60 mL/kg should be administered within the first hour of treatment, continuing until shock resolves or signs of fluid overload appear. In healthcare systems without local or transport access to intensive care, fluid bolus therapy is not recommended unless hypotension is present

Source: (Adapted from: © 2020 the Society of Critical Care Medicine and the European Society of Intensive Care Medicine. All Rights Reserved. https://www.sccm.org/getattachment/SurvivingSepsisCampaign/Guidelines/Pediatric-Patients/Initial-Resuscitation-Algorithm-for-Children.pdf.aspx?lang=en-US.)

Table 27.12 Vasoactive Medications

Agent (range)	*Dose (range)*	*Site of action*	*Clinical effect*
Dopamine	3–20 µg/kg/min	β, increasing α with increasing dose	Inotrope, vasoconstriction, chronotrope, increases peripheral vascular resistance (PVR)
Dobutamine	1–20 µg/kg/min	$\beta_2 > \beta_1$	Inotrope, vasodilation (beta-2), decreases PVR
Epinephrine	0.01–1.0 µg/kg/min	β > α	Inotrope, chronotrope, vasoconstriction
Norepinephrine	0.01–1.0 µg/kg/min	α > β	Vasoconstriction, increases systemic vascular resistance (SVR), inotrope, chronotrope
Phenylephrine	0.1–0.5 µg/kg/min	α	Vasoconstriction, increases SVR
Amrinone	1–20 µg/kg/min	Type III phosphodiesterase inhibitor	Inotrope, chronotrope, vasodilator
Milrinone	0.25–1.0 µg/kg/min		
Nitroprusside	0.5–10 µg/kg/min	Vasodilator, arterial > venous	Decreases afterload
Vasopressin	0.0003–0.008 µg/kg/min	V1 vascular receptor	Vasoconstriction, vasodilation of circle of Willis, stimulation of cortisol secretion

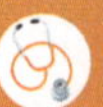

CASE STUDY Shock

A 5-year-old child presented to the emergency room with history of fever, vomiting, and diarrhea of 2 days' duration. His mother reported that he has had 15 watery stools (mixed with blood) and ongoing emesis and over the last 2 hours has become drowsier. Despite being fed oral rehydration solution by his mother with a spoon, he has not had any urine output for the past 4 hours and his extremities are pale and cool to touch. His vital signs are heart rate—160/min, respiratory rate—18/min, blood pressure—88/54 mm Hg, oxyhemoglobin saturation—91%. Capillary refill is >3 seconds and he is not responding to calling out his name.

Is this patient in compensated, uncompensated, or irreversible shock?

Based on his presentation with clear signs of reduced perfusion and oxygen delivery, this patient is clearly in an uncompensated stage of shock. Because of the rapid progression from compensated to uncompensated state due to his ongoing fluid losses, it is very important to start treatment promptly.

Based on the underlying etiology, what is the likely mechanism of shock?

This patient probably has a combination of septic (due to gram-negative pathogens) and hypovolemic shock, which can be explained by the initial fever, bloody diarrhea, and translocation of gram-negative pathogens into the bloodstream, which was further complicated by the ongoing fluid losses from vomiting and diarrhea. Pediatric patients may lose a significant amount of fluids over a shorter span of time and become hypovolemic. Underlying medical conditions and concomitant sepsis can sometimes complicate the picture and require additional specific treatments. We could be dealing with *Shigella*, *Salmonella*, or *Escherichia coli*.

Outline the initial management of this child

Initial management should be focused on rapid replacement of fluid volume by obtaining IV access. To improve oxygenation, additional supplemental oxygen should be initiated. Workup for sepsis and initiation of IV antibiotics should also be done as part of initial management. Close monitoring of mental status and urine output is necessary. Laboratory studies should include assessment of blood glucose and electrolytes and stool studies. If there are any concerns for this patient's inability to maintain adequate ventilation, then endotracheal intubation and mechanical ventilator support may be necessary until fluid replacement is completed.

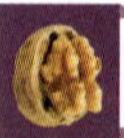

IN A NUTSHELL

Shock

1. Shock is a state of circulatory dysfunction leading to inadequate cellular perfusion and tissue hypoxia.
2. Shock progresses over a continuum of severity, from a compensated to a decompensated state. In compensated shock, blood pressure remains normal; it is low in decompensated shock.
3. The effects of inadequate perfusion due to shock are reversible initially. However, prolonged oxygen deprivation leads to end-organ damage, multisystem organ failure, and eventually death.
4. Acute hypovolemia is the most common cause of shock in pediatric practice.
5. Sepsis is defined as life-threatening organ dysfunction in children with suspected or confirmed sepsis with Phoenix Sepsis Score of at least 2 points. Septic shock is a subset of sepsis with a CVS subscore of at least 1 point of the Phoenix Sepsis Score
6. The former terms "SIRS" and "severe sepsis" should no longer be used.
7. Arterial lactate ≥2 mmol/L is a cut-off that predicts poor outcome.
8. Serum ferritin should ALWAYS be checked in all septic shock patients.
9. The initial hour in the management of shock is the most crucial in determining the outcome and has therefore been called the "golden hour." Appropriate management with fluid boluses and ongoing assessment during this crucial period is of utmost importance.

David A, Turner, Cheifetz IM. Shock. In: Kliegman RM, Geme ST, Blum NJ, et al. (Eds). Nelson Textbook of Pediatrics, 21st edition. Philadelphia: Elsevier; 2020. pp. 572-82.

Davis AL, Carcillo JA, Aneja RK, et al. American College of Critical Care Medicine Clinical practice parameters for hemodynamic support of pediatric and neonatal septic shock. Crit Care Med. 2017;45(6):1061-93.

Indian Academy of Pediatrics (IAP). Standard treatment guidelines 2022. Shock in office practice.

Sanchez-Pinto LN, Bennett TD, DeWitt PE, et al. Development and validation of the Phoenix criteria for pediatric sepsis and septic shock. JAMA. 2024;331(8):675-686. doi: 10.1001/jama.2024.0196.

Society of Critical Care Medicine Pediatric Sepsis Definition Task Force. International Consensus Criteria for Pediatric Sepsis and Septic Shock. JAMA. 2024;331(8):665-674.

Weiss SL, Peters MJ, Alhazzani W, et al. Surviving Sepsis Campaign International Guidelines for the Management of Septic Shock and Sepsis-Associated Organ Dysfunction in Children. Pediatr Crit Care Med. 2020;21(2):e52-e106.

Weiss SL, Tissières P, Peters MJ. Shock. In: Behrman RE, Kliegman RM, Jenson HB (Eds). Nelson Textbook of Pediatrics, 22nd edition. Philadelphia: W.B. Saunders Co.; 2024. p. 600-611.

World Health Organization. Updated guideline: Paediatric emergency triage, assessment and treatment. Geneva: World Health Organization; 2016.

27.8 Status Epilepticus

PE 24.4, PE 24.8

INTRODUCTION

Status epilepticus is a common pediatric emergency, with an estimated incidence of 18–23 per 100,000 children annually and a mortality rate of 2–7%. The highest incidence is in children under 1 year, most commonly due to febrile seizures.

DEFINITIONS AND CLASSIFICATION

Previously, convulsive status epilepticus (CSE) has been defined as continuous seizure activity lasting over 30 minutes or two or more seizures without regaining consciousness between them. This definition was originally based on animal studies showing neuronal damage after 30 minutes of seizures, with associated higher morbidity and mortality. However, recent data suggests that neuronal damage begins much earlier and that seizures that last beyond 5 minutes are less likely to stop on their own, requiring intervention. As a result, the 30-minute definition is now mainly used for research, with the operational definition shortened to 5 minutes for clinical management.

The International League Against Epilepsy (ILAE) redefined status epilepticus as an ongoing seizure activity due to the failure of mechanisms that terminate seizures or initiation of mechanisms provoking prolonged seizure activity after timepoint t1, and which can have long-term consequences after timepoint t2 **(Table 27.13)**. The ILAE also introduced the terms Established Status Epilepticus (ESE) and Refractory Status Epilepticus (RSE), focusing on the persistence of seizures despite medication, rather than time duration.

The ILAE classification system for status epilepticus includes four axes: (1) semiology (seizure type, motor, non-motor, or indeterminate), (2) etiology (known or unknown causes), (3) EEG correlates (patterns, morphology, location, time-related features, modulation and effect of intervention), and (4) age group (neonatal, infancy (1 month to 2 years), childhood (2 years to 12 years), adolescent and adulthood (>12 years to 59 years), and elderly (60 years). This framework of four axes should be provided in diagnosing status epilepticus.

ETIOPATHOGENESIS

The most common cause of SE in children is prolonged febrile seizure and account for nearly one-third of all cases. CNS infections are the next important causes of SE especially in developing countries. Bacterial, viral, tubercular infections and neurocysticercosis are the possible etiologies. Important causes of SE are summarized in **Box 27.7**. Nearly one-fourth of children presenting with SE have past history of seizures. The triggering factors for SE include poor drug compliance, sleep deprivation, intercurrent illness, puberty, drug interactions, or metabolic decompensation.

During the first 30 minutes of seizure onset, various homeostatic compensatory mechanisms meet the metabolic demands and prevent neuronal damage. These include

Box 27.7 Etiology of Status Epilepticus

1. *CNS infections:* Meningitis, encephalitis, neurocysticercosis, malaria, HIV infection, tuberculosis
2. *Immunological conditions:* Anti-NMDA receptor encephalitis, Rasmussen encephalitis, Hashimoto encephalopathy
3. *Iatrogenic:* Neurosurgical procedure, electroconvulsive therapy, blood transfusions
4. *Metabolic:* Hypocalcemia, hypomagnesemia, hypoglycemia, hyponatremia
5. *Malformations of cortical development:* Hemimegalencephaly, focal cortical dysplasia, polymicrogyria
6. *Hypoxic ischemic injury*
7. *Neurocutaneous syndromes:* Sturge-Weber syndrome, tuberous sclerosis
8. *Inborn errors of metabolism:* Mitochondrial, pyridoxine dependency, aminoacidopathies, organic acidemias, urea cycle disorders
9. *Neurodegenerative disorders:* Progressive myoclonic epilepsies, leukodystrophy
10. *Epilepsy/electroclinical syndrome:* Ring chromosome 20, Angelman syndrome, Dravet syndrome, Rett syndrome, other channelopathies, febrile infection-related epilepsy syndrome (FIRES), others: (stroke, trauma, tumors)

Table 27.13 ILAE Definitions of Status Epilepticus (SE)

Seizure type	*Time after which if seizures do not terminate, patient is considered in SE (t1)*	*Time after which ongoing seizures have long term consequences (t2)*
Convulsive status epilepticus (CSE)	5 min	30 min
Focal status epilepticus with impaired consciousness	10 min	>60 min
Absence status epilepticus	10–15 min	Unknown
Other definitions of status epilepticus		
Established status epilepticus	SE that persists after treatment with a BZD (first line AED)	
Refractory status epilepticus	SE that persists after treatment with a 1st line (BZD) and 2nd line AEDs (phenytoin, levetiracetam, valproate)	

(AED: antiepileptic drugs; BZD: benzodiazepine; ILAE: international league against epilepsy)

sympathetic overdrive, lactic acidosis, and increase in cerebral blood flow. The blood-brain barrier and neuronal integrity are intact at this stage. Beyond 30 minutes (refractory status epilepticus), cerebral autoregulation fails. There is gradual energy depletion with cerebral hypoxia, reduction in glucose and lactate. Systemic changes include hypoglycemia, hyponatremia, hyperkalemia, acidosis, coagulopathy, multiorgan failure, systemic hypoxia, and cardiorespiratory impairment.

Repetitive seizures also cause many clinically significant pathophysiological and biochemical changes in the brain. They cause internalization of gamma-aminobutyric acid (GABA) receptors (moving from the synaptic membrane to the cytoplasm, where they are functionally inactive), and reduction in the number of the $\gamma 2$ and $\beta 2/\beta 3$ subunits on the synaptic membrane. This results in time-dependent pharmacoresistance to benzodiazepines.

Other maladaptive response includes recruitment of the N-methyl-D-aspartate (NMDA) NR1 receptor subunits to the synaptic membrane (proconvulsant), changes in AMPA receptor subunit, GluA2 expression, and increased synaptic glutamate release. Thus, these responses generate a transient but severe loss of synaptic inhibitory receptors and peptides, and an increase in synaptic excitatory receptors and peptides. This explains the tendency of seizures to become self-sustaining. The ensuing cerebral damage may be directly caused by the excitotoxic effects of the electrical seizure discharges (excessive calcium influx into the neurons and resulting necrosis and apoptosis). It may also be caused by the systemic and the metabolic disturbances (e.g., hypoxia and hypoglycemia).

EVALUATION

After initial stabilization and control of seizures, a focused clinical evaluation **(Box 27.8)** is warranted to identify the underlying precipitating cause. This would then guide further management.

Box 27.8 Focused Clinical Evaluation in a Child with Status Epilepticus

A. *History:*
- Fever, altered sensorium, lethargy, excessive irritability, vomiting, rash, headache
- Recent behavioral change
- Travel history, recent immunization or viral infection, animal bite, trauma
- Previous diagnosis of epilepsy/past history of seizures
- Current antiepileptic drugs, compliance, any setting for overdose, recent change in medications
- Prior neurological illness, neurodevelopmental status
- Any significant medical history, e.g., hepatic disease, renal disease, bleeding tendencies
- Family history
- Acute treatment received-rescue medication, any first aid received at local health facility

B. *On examination:*
- Facial dysmorphism, neurocutaneous markers
- Consciousness, meningeal signs
- Fundus/pupils/ocular movements
- Focal motor deficits or sensory signs
- Stigmata of chronic systemic illness, signs of injury

Box 27.9 Investigations in a Child with Status Epilepticus

A. *Blood investigations:* Complete blood count, serum electrolytes, blood glucose, calcium, magnesium, blood gas analysis, liver and renal function tests, drug levels (in children on antiepileptic drugs).
B. *Workup for infection*:* Lumbar puncture (intracranial pressure, cell count, sugar, lactate, protein, Gram stain, acid fast bacilli, culture, HSV PCR), malarial parasite.
C. *Neuroimaging:* CT/MRI (preferable), especially in new onset SE
D. *EEG (routine/continuous):* To look for persisting EEG-only seizures after convulsive SE terminates or for psychogenic SE, if suspected.
E. *In refractory and super-refractory cases:* Consider metabolic workup (ammonia, lactate, urine ketones, plasma acylcarnitines, urine organic acids), genetic tests, autoimmune workup (including anti-NMDA antibodies), antithyroid peroxidase antibodies, antithyroglobulin antibodies, HIV serology; may consider further imaging for surgical workup in selected cases.

*The extent would depend on the local epidemiology; may withhold in afebrile children with status epilepticus (SE)

(CT: computed tomography; EEG: electroencephalogram; HSV: herpes-simplex virus; MRI: magnetic resonance imaging; NMDA: N-methyl-D-aspartate; PCR: polymerase chain reaction)

Investigations

Investigations need to be individualized for every patient depending on the age and suspected etiology. Neuroimaging and EEG are the most important investigations. A summary of most relevant investigations is tabulated in **Box 27.9**.

Neuroimaging

Neuroimaging is essential for identifying an organic or structural cause of SE. Abnormalities in neuroimaging have been observed in almost one-third of children with SE and described to alter acute management in 24%. Magnetic resonance imaging (MRI) is preferred over computed tomography (CT). However, the choice may be governed by availability, cost and medical condition of the patient. It should be done only once the child is stable after controlling the seizures. Urgent neuroimaging may be required in patients with new-onset focal deficits, persistent altered consciousness, fever, recent trauma, immunosuppression, or history of anticoagulation therapy.

Electroencephalography

The EEG must be done if there are concerns for ongoing electrographic seizures (persistent unexplained encephalopathy, subtle motor phenomenon, autonomic instability, etc.), despite cessation of clinically evident seizures. Electrographic seizures may be seen in up to one-third of children who presented with SE. These are more common in children with acute brain injury or prior history of epilepsy. Continuous EEG monitoring (cEEG) is desirable in such children and should be continued for at least 24–48 hours following acute brain insult in comatose patients. However, cEEG may not be feasible in most of the centers. In such cases, frequent short-term EEG may be performed based on the clinical status of the child. Abnormal EEG background (e.g., suppression, lack of reactivity), periodic discharges and interictal epileptiform discharges are associated with increased risk of electrographic seizures. EEG is also warranted if psychogenic SE is suspected and this may avoid unnecessary exposure to multiple antiepileptic drugs.

TREATMENT Status Epilepticus

Status epilepticus requires aggressive and early management (detailed in **Table 27.14**). The treatment goals include termination of seizures, identification and management of systemic complications, and treatment of the underlying etiology.

COMPLICATIONS

The most important life-threatening complication is respiratory arrest or insufficiency. The airway compromise may be multifactorial (secretions, oropharyngeal hypotonia, aspiration, underlying neurological conditions, and drug-induced). Other complications include arrhythmias, hypotension, hemodynamic instability, cardiopulmonary arrest, injury, tongue-bite, and rarely joint dislocations. Electrolyte and acid-base imbalances (hypoglycemia, hyponatremia, hyper/hypokalemia) are common. Prolonged seizures which are uncontrolled may also lead to rhabdomyolysis, hemolysis, myoglobinuria, and acute

Table 27.14 Protocol for Management of Status Epilepticus

Status epilepticus	*Time frame*	*Drugs*	*Supportive therapy*	*EEG*
Incipient	<5 minutes	• IV access not available: Intranasal midazolam (0.2 mg/kg) or buccal midazolam (0.2 mg/kg) or IM midazolam (0.2 mg/kg/day) or rectal diazepam (0.2–0.5 mg/kg) • IV access available: IV lorazepam (0.1 mg/kg; max 5 mg) over 1 minute or IV midazolam (0.1 mg/kg) over 1 minute or IV diazepam (0.2 mg/kg; max 10 mg) Wait for 5 minutes to determine if seizure terminates		
Early	5–30 minutes	• Repeat benzodiazepine • Phenytoin (20 mg/kg IV) at 1 mg/kg/min (max 50 mg/min)		
Consult pediatric neurology services				
Established	30–120 minutes	• If seizures persist 10 minutes after phenytoin infusion: Valproate (20 mg/kg IV) at 5 mg/kg/min (contraindicated in cases of suspected metabolic disorders, severe thrombocytopenia and hepatic dysfunction) or • Levetiracetam (20 mg/kg IV) at 5 mg/kg/min (preferred in cases of hepatic dysfunction and metabolic disorders) or • Phenobarbitone (20 mg/kg IV) at 2 mg/kg/min (monitor for hypotension/respiratory depression) • If seizures persist 5 minutes after infusion of any of the above drugs, consider use of the other drug	Airway, breathing, hemodynamics, temperature, maintain euglycemia and eucalcemia Search and treat the underlying cause	Continuous EEG monitoring
Shift to PICU				
Refractory	>120 minutes	• If seizure continues beyond 2 hours, then initiate coma with IV midazolam 0.2 mg/kg bolus (max 10 mg) over 2 minutes followed by infusion at 1 µg/kg/min • If seizures persist 5 minutes after initial midazolam bolus, then administer additional midazolam bolus of 0.2 mg/kg bolus. Continue infusion • If clinical seizures persist after another 5 minutes, then administer another midazolam bolus of 0.2 mg/kg, and increase infusion to 0.2 mg/kg/h. Repeat as needed • If seizures persist at maximum midazolam (generally 2 mg/kg/h) or midazolam infusion is not tolerated • Consider transition to thiopentone • Thiopentone 5 mg/kg IV over 20 seconds followed by 3–5 mg/kg/h infusion (monitor hemodynamics) • Continue pharmacologic coma for 24 hours after last seizure with EEG goal of burst-suppression • Continue initial medications in maintenance doses • Ensure an additional anticonvulsant is administered to provide coverage during weaning (e.g., topiramate) • Reduce midazolam (by 0.05 mg/kg/h) or thiopentone every 3 hours with frequent EEG review. If no clinical or electrographic seizures then wean until off • Continue EEG for at least 24 hours after end of infusion to evaluate for recurrent electrographic seizures		

Contd...

Contd...

Status epilepticus	*Time frame*	*Drugs*	*Supportive therapy*	*EEG*
Super-refractory	≥24 hours after onset of coma	Consider: • Ketamine: 1 mg/kg IV followed by 1–5 mg/kg/h infusion • Magnesium: 50 mg/kg IV over 30 minutes • Pyridoxine: 30 mg/kg IV • *Methylprednisolone* pulse If no resolution within 2 days of pulse: • Intravenous immunoglobulin (IVIG) 0.4 g/kg/day × 5 days • 4:1 ketogenic diet		

(EEG: electroencephalogram; IV: intravenous; PICU: pediatric intensive care unit)

kidney injury. Uncontrolled seizures can lead to cerebral edema, raised intracranial pressure, and sometimes ischemic infarcts. These children may develop multiorgan dysfunction that may be due to a combination of the underlying pathology as well as the drug therapy.

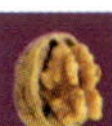

IN A NUTSHELL

Status Epilepticus

1. The International League Against Epilepsy (ILAE) defines status epilepticus as an ongoing seizure activity due to the failure of mechanisms that terminate seizures or initiation of mechanisms provoking prolonged seizure activity after timepoint t1, and which can have long-term consequences after timepoint t2.
2. Febrile status epilepticus is a common cause but one should always rule out CNS infections in such a setting.
3. Neuroimaging and EEG are the most important investigations.
4. The treatment goals include termination of seizures, identification and management of systemic complications, and treatment of the underlying etiology.
5. The most effective first line of treatment for status epilepticus is intravenous benzodiazepines. After benzodiazepines, antiepileptic drugs such as phenytoin, fosphenytoin, valproate, levetiracetam, and phenobarbital are most commonly used.

Abend NS, Loddenkemper T. Pediatric status epileptics management. Curr Opin Pediatr. 2014;26(6):668-74.

Alford EL, Wheless JW, Phelps SJ. Treatment of generalized convulsive status epileptics in pediatric patients. J Pediatr Pharmacol Ther. 2015;20(4):260-89.

Chamberlain JM, Kapur J, Shinnar S, et al. Efficacy of levetiracetam, fosphenytoin, and valproate for established status epileptics by age group (ESETT): a double-blind, responsive-adaptive, randomised controlled trial. Lancet. 2020;395(10231):1217-24.

Mishra D, Sharma S, Sankhyan N, et al. Consensus guidelines on management of childhood convulsive status epileptics. Indian Pediatr. 2014;51(12):975-90.

Singh A, Stredny CM, Loddenkemper T. Pharmacotherapy for Pediatric Convulsive Status Epileptics. CNS Drugs. 2020;34(1): 47-63.

Trinka E, Cock H, Hesdorffer D, et al. A definition and classification of status epilepticus—Report of the ILAE Task Force on Classification of Status Epilepticus. Epilepsia. 2015;56(10):1515-23. Available from: https://onlinelibrary.wiley.com/doi/full/10.1111/epi.13121. [Last accessed January 2025].

Trinka E, Kälviäinen R. 25 years of advances in definition, classification and treatment of status epileptics. Seizure. 2017;44:65-73.

Trink E, Hofler J, Zerbs A. Causes of status epilepticus. Epilepsia. 2012; 53(Suppl. 4):127-38.

27.9 Approach to Unconscious Child

PE 24.5, PE 24.15

Consciousness refers to the state of being aware of oneself and the surrounding environment, and it has two main components: wakefulness and awareness.

1. ***Wakefulness (or arousal)*** is regulated by the ascending reticular activating system (ARAS), a network of neurons that originates in the tegmentum of the pons and midbrain and projects to structures in the diencephalon and cortex.
2. ***Awareness*** depends on the integrity of the cerebral cortex and its connections with subcortical structures. **Figure 27.17** illustrates the various brain pathways involved in maintaining consciousness.

Coma is an unconscious state characterized by the complete absence of both arousal and awareness. In a comatose state, patients do not exhibit eye opening. Unlike temporary unconsciousness, such as in syncope or concussion, coma must last for at least one hour. Coma typically represents a transitional state and may evolve toward recovery of consciousness, a vegetative state, a minimally conscious state or brain death.

Etiopathogenesis

Coma occurs as a result of bilateral dysfunction in the cerebral cortex, ARAS or corticobulbar tracts. In children, coma may be caused by either diffuse damage to both cerebral hemispheres (due to metabolic, toxic, hypoxic or ischemic factors) or focal lesion affecting the ARAS in the upper pons, midbrain or diencephalon. Between normal consciousness and coma, there exists a spectrum of states, including lethargy, obtundation, and stupor.

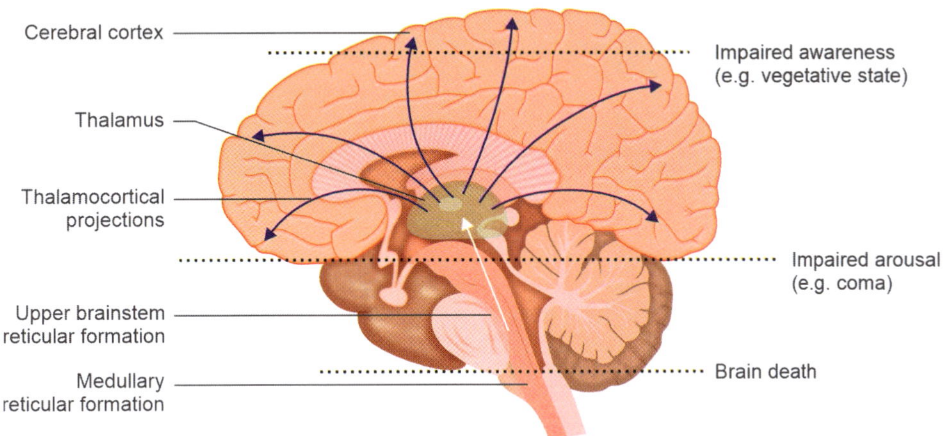

Fig. 27.17: Pathways for consciousness in brain

(Source: Gupta P, editor. Clinical Methods in Pediatrics. 6th ed. New Delhi: CBS Publishers & Distributors Pvt Ltd; 2024)

Box 27.10 Causes of Unconsciousness in a Child

Primary impairment
- Traumatic Brain Injury (TBI): Contusions, diffuse axonal injury
- Stroke
- Severe brain infections (e.g., meningitis, encephalitis, brain abscesses)
- Intracranial hemorrhage (e.g., subdural hematoma, epidural hematoma)
- Brain tumors

Secondary impairment
- Severe systemic illnesses (e.g., sepsis, dehydration)
- Hypotension
- Hypoxia (e.g., respiratory failure, suffocation, drowning)
- Metabolic derangements (e.g., hypoglycemia, hyperglycemia, inborn errors of metabolism, diabetic ketoacidosis)
- Hepatic encephalopathy
- Electrolyte imbalances (e.g., sodium, calcium abnormalities)
- Drug intoxication (e.g., opioids, sedatives, alcohol)

The impairment of consciousness can arise from a variety of etiologies, which may be classified based on the nature and origin of the insult. These causes can be broadly divided into primary and secondary categories, depending on whether the brain is directly affected or whether systemic factors compromise cerebral function through mechanisms such as impaired perfusion or oxygenation **(Box 27.10).**

1. ***Primary impairment:*** This occurs when the coma results from direct involvement of the brain, such as in cases of traumatic brain injury, stroke, severe brain infections or intracranial hemorrhage. In these instances, the primary pathology is within the brain itself, leading to a functional loss of consciousness.
2. ***Secondary impairment:*** In contrast, secondary impairment occurs when a systemic insult, such as sepsis, hypotension or hypoxia, adversely affects cerebral perfusion or oxygenation, thereby impacting brain function. These systemic factors can result in a global reduction of brain activity and consciousness, even in the absence of direct structural damage to the brain.

Further, the impairment can be categorized as functional or organic:

- ***Functional coma*** occurs in the absence of any structural brain damage, typically resulting from metabolic derangements or toxic effects.
- ***Organic coma,*** by contrast, involves structural brain injury, which may result from conditions such as brain tumors, strokes or traumatic injury.

Regardless of the etiology, all forms of coma involve diffuse depression of both the cerebral cortex and the brainstem. This widespread depression results in the loss of both higher cognitive functions (awareness) and basic autonomic functions (such as arousal and respiration) that are mediated by the brainstem. In pediatric populations, the causes of coma may differ between age groups. Younger children are more likely to experience coma or altered sensorium due to non-traumatic etiologies, such as metabolic disorders, infections or hypoxia. In contrast, older children are more commonly affected by traumatic brain injury, which remains one of the leading causes of coma in this age group. Severe systemic illness can also precipitate coma, particularly when it leads to hypoxic-ischemic injury. If the insult persists or worsens, it can exacerbate increased intracranial pressure (ICP), thereby further compromising consciousness and leading to a progressive deterioration in neurological function.

In evaluating a patient with coma, it is essential to rule out reversible causes of impaired consciousness. Common reversible conditions that may mimic or contribute to coma include hypoglycemia, hyperglycemia and electrolyte imbalances. These conditions are often amenable to rapid correction, and timely intervention can result in significant improvement or resolution of the comatose state. Therefore, identifying and addressing these reversible causes is critical in the management of patients presenting with altered consciousness.

Management

The clinical evaluation and management of an unconscious child require an immediate, systematic approach to identify life-threatening symptoms and stabilize the child. The primary assessment follows an ABCDE approach, focusing on airway, breathing, circulation, disability (neurological assessment) and exposure. Each component helps determine the child's condition, and timely intervention is essential. The management must first prioritize stabilizing the child before further diagnostic workup, such as laboratory investigations, which should only be done once the acute condition is controlled. In **Table 27.15**, each

Table 27.15 Primary Assessment and Intervention in an Unconscious Child

Assessment	Component	Evaluation	Intervention
A—Airway	Airway obstruction	Look for unstable airway due to tongue falling back and secretions	• Assess airway and clear using proper positioning, suction and airway adjuncts (oropharyngeal, nasopharyngeal, LMA) to prevent aspiration or obstruction • If necessary, perform endotracheal intubation • RSI is a preferred method as intubation procedure can aggravate raised ICP
B—Breathing	Respiratory assessment	Monitor breathing patterns for abnormalities (e.g., neurogenic hyperventilation, irregular breathing, bradypnea or apnea)	• Administer oxygen as indicated • Provide assisted ventilation if needed • Hyperventilation for raised ICP cases
C—Circulation	Circulatory status	Assess for signs of shock (compensated or hypotensive), or features of raised ICP (hypertension and bradycardia)	• Provide fluid resuscitation • Maintain optimal CPP • Consider osmotic therapy for raised ICP (should be commenced only after adequate perfusion has been established)
D—Disability	Neurological assessment	• Assess cortical functions using the AVPU scale or modified Glasgow Coma Scale • Evaluate brainstem functions (pupillary size and response, abnormal breathing pattern)	• CBG by dextrostix is a must: Give 2–5 mL/kg of 10% dextrose if CBG <60 mg/dL, followed by GIR to maintain BG between 150–180 mg/dL • Identify and treat seizures • All children with unexplained encephalopathy should be looked for NCSE (if facility is available) • Manage raised ICP
E—Exposure	Physical examination	Check for rashes, bleeding, hypothermia/hyperthermia, petechiae, purpura, pallor, signs of trauma like abrasions, bruises or lacerations, rashes	• Regulate body temperature to normothermia (36 to 38°C) • Treat fever or hypothermia accordingly

(BG: blood glucose; CBG: capillary blood glucose; CPP: cerebral perfusion pressure (CPP = mean arterial pressure - intracranial pressure); GIR: glucose infusion rate; ICP: intracranial pressure; LMA: laryngeal mask airway; NCSE: non-convulsive status epilepticus; RSI: rapid sequence intubation)

stage of the primary assessment is enlisted, and corresponding interventions are provided to address immediate life-saving measures and prevent further deterioration in the unconscious child. Once primary assessment and resuscitation are underway, the secondary assessment focuses on gathering a focused history and conducting a targeted physical examination to identify potential causes of altered consciousness. This includes differentiating cortical vs. brainstem involvement and detecting signs of raised intracranial pressure (ICP).

Primary Assessment

Evaluation should commence immediately upon recognizing an unconscious or comatose child, starting with visual and auditory cues to gauge the patient's level of consciousness and distress. The assessment follows a structured **ABCDE** approach during the **primary assessment**, which prioritizes immediate life-saving interventions. Each component should be carefully examined to determine the stability of the patient and identify potential causes of coma.

Neurological examination during primary assessment involves evaluating both cortical and brainstem functions.

❖ ***Cortical function:*** Assess the child's responsiveness using the AVPU scale (Alert, responds to Voice, responds to Pain, Unresponsive) **(Box 27.1)** or the Modified Glasgow Coma Scale (GCS) **(Table 27.16)**. These tools provide an objective measure of consciousness and help to track changes over time. Assessment begins with careful observation of their spontaneous body position, motor activity, eye opening and verbalization. These initial signs provide valuable clues regarding the child's neurological state. The evaluation should

Table 27.16 Modified Glasgow Coma Scale

	Score	Infant	Child
Eye Opening (E)	4	Spontaneous	Spontaneous
	3	To sound	To sound
	2	To pain	To pain
	1	None	None
Verbal (V)	5	Coos/babbles	Oriented
	4	Irritable cry	Confused
	3	Cries to pain	Inappropriate words
	2	Moans to pain	Incomprehensible words
	1	None	None

Contd...

Contd...

	Score	*Infant*	*Child*
Motor (M)	6	Normal spontaneous	Obeys commands
	5	Withdraws to touch	Localizes pain
	4	Withdraws to pain	Withdraws to pain
	3	Decorticate flexion	Decorticate flexion
	2	Decerebrate extension	Decerebrate extension
	1	None	None
Total score	15 (E4V5M6)		

Note: In cases where a child has a tracheostomy, is intubated (ETT), or has facial injuries, verbal responses (V) may not be assessable. In these instances, the focus should be placed on evaluating eye and motor responses.

Source: Adapted from: James HE et al. The Glasgow Coma Scale and Modified Coma Score for infants. Brain insults in infants and children: Pathophysiology and management. 1985:179-182.

then proceed in a structured manner, starting with verbal stimuli, followed by tactile cues, and finally, if necessary, painful stimuli. The response to these stimuli should be graded in intensity to gauge the depth of consciousness. When assessing response to painful stimuli, it is essential to ensure that the procedure does not cause unnecessary harm or tissue injury. Care should be taken to choose sites that are likely to provoke a response without causing undue distress. Nail bed stimulation and supraorbital pressure are commonly used sites. The supraorbital pressure can be useful, particularly in children who may have lost afferent pain pathways due to peripheral neuropathy or spinal cord lesions. Note that asymmetrical withdrawal responses may indicate unilateral weakness or hemispheric dysfunction, and such responses should be carefully documented. A GCS ≤ 8 is a critical threshold, signifying severe impairment of consciousness. Aggressive management is required in such cases, which includes airway stabilization, often through endotracheal intubation to secure the airway and mechanical ventilation. Indications for intubation are listed in **Box 27.11.**

- ***Brainstem function:*** Evaluate for signs of brainstem involvement, such as:
  - *Pupillary reaction:* Check for pupillary size, equality and response to light.
  - *Breathing patterns:* Abnormal breathing patterns (e.g., neurogenic hyperventilation, irregular breathing, bradypnea or apnea) may indicate brainstem dysfunction, requiring urgent attention.

Box 27.11 Indications for Intubation in an Unconscious Child

1. **GCS ≤ 8** or any signs of deterioration in the level of consciousness
2. **SpO_2 < 92%** despite appropriate airway maneuvers and high-flow oxygen
3. **Insufficient respiratory drive** or failure to maintain adequate ventilation
4. **Signs of exhaustion** in respiratory effort
5. **Neurogenic hyperventilation**, which may indicate **midbrain** involvement
6. **Signs of raised ICP**, including **bradycardia** and **hypertension**
7. **Fluid-refractory shock** unresponsive to initial fluid resuscitation

Secondary Assessment

The secondary assessment should be initiated promptly once the primary assessment and resuscitation are in progress. It involves a focused history and a targeted physical examination, as detailed in the **Table 27.17**. The focused history is essential for identifying potential underlying causes of the child's altered consciousness and informing subsequent management decisions. Further, the focused physical examination should be performed to localize cortical vs. brainstem involvement and recognize the presence of raised ICP. It is better to assume the presence of raised ICP in a child with altered sensorium. Decision to start osmotic therapy for raised ICP should be made after secondary assessment. Management of raised ICP is given in **Box 27.12.** It is generally easier to de-escalate therapy rather than step-up once the child's condition deteriorates.

After the secondary assessment, treatment should focus on addressing the identified underlying causes of the altered consciousness. This includes supportive care to stabilize airway, breathing, and circulation, as well as the management of seizures with anticonvulsants if needed. Infections should be treated with appropriate antibiotics and antivirals, while raised intracranial pressure (ICP) may require hyperosmolar therapy, sedation or surgical intervention. If poisoning is suspected, antidotes and supportive care should be administered, and metabolic imbalances like hypoglycemia should be corrected. The specific investigations required for a comatose child should be tailored to the clinical scenario as outlined in **Box 27.13**, with initial tests aimed at identifying the underlying cause of the altered consciousness. Additionally, imaging studies should be performed if structural brain lesions are suspected, with neurosurgical consultation for possible intervention. All treatment should be continuously adjusted based on the patient's condition and response.

In conclusion, the management of an unconscious child requires a systematic and timely approach, starting with immediate recognition of life-threatening signs followed by thorough evaluation and intervention. After stabilizing the child, targeted treatment based on the clinical findings and investigations ensures the underlying cause is addressed. Continuous monitoring and adjustment of interventions are essential for optimizing outcomes and preventing further complications.

Table 27.17 Secondary Assessment in an Unconscious Child

<table>
<tr><th colspan="2">Focused history (sample)</th><th>Focused examination</th></tr>
<tr><td>S—Signs and symptoms</td><td>• Duration and onset: Sudden or gradual onset of altered consciousness (e.g., CNS infections, trauma, stroke)
• Associated symptoms: Fever (infection), seizures (seizure disorder or metabolic disturbances), headache (raised ICP or hemorrhage), vomiting (ICP or systemic illness), visual symptoms (neurological deficits)
• Poisoning history: Possible exposure to toxins or harmful substances
• Focal deficits: Sudden focal deficits suggest vascular events, trauma, or lesions</td><td rowspan="5">Cortical Dysfunction:
• Level of consciousness: Use AVPU scale or GCS
• Motor activity: Assess voluntary movements, muscle tone, abnormal posturing (e.g., decerebrate or decorticate) and deep tendon reflexes
• Plantar reflex: Observe for Babinski sign, especially in infants
Brainstem Dysfunction:
• Pupillary examination: Check size, symmetry and light response
• Oculovestibular reflex: Doll's eye movement
• Cough reflex: Evaluate integrity of the medulla
• Respiratory patterns: Look for Cheyne-Stokes, ataxic breathing, neurogenic hyperventilation or apneustic breathing
Recognize raised ICP: Check for worsening GCS/AVPU score, abnormal breathing patterns (e.g., Cheyne-Stokes, neurogenic hyperventilation), abnormal pupil response, and altered posturing (e.g., decerebrate)
Raised ICP signs:
• Worsening consciousness: Declining GCS/AVPU score
• Posturing: Decerebrate posturing indicates severe brainstem involvement
• Breathing patterns: Abnormal patterns like Cheyne-Stokes or neurogenic hyperventilation
• Pupillary response: Fixed, dilated pupils indicate severe brainstem compression
• Cushing's triad: Late signs of ICP—apnea, bradycardia, hypertension</td></tr>
<tr><td>A—Allergies</td><td>Detailed history of known allergies (food, medications, environmental) to rule out allergic reactions such as anaphylaxis</td></tr>
<tr><td>M—Medications</td><td>List of current medications, particularly anti-epileptic drugs or any affecting neurological function. Assess for medication non-compliance or toxicity</td></tr>
<tr><td>P—Past medical history</td><td>• History of seizures: Previous seizures or epilepsy could explain current episode
• Developmental history: Relevant for conditions like metabolic disorders or genetic syndromes
• Last meal: Important for hypoglycemia or poisoning considerations</td></tr>
<tr><td>E—Events leading to illness</td><td>• Trauma history: Recent head injury, falls, or accidents could suggest intracranial hemorrhage, concussion, or spinal injury
• Exposure history: Toxins, drugs, or infections that may have triggered the altered consciousness</td></tr>
</table>

Box 27.12 Management of Raised Intracranial Pressure

1. **Maintain ABCs:** Ensure adequate Airway, Breathing and Circulation as per PALS guidelines.
2. **Mild head end elevation:**
   - Elevate the head end of the bed to 15–30° to optimize venous drainage and reduce ICP.
   - Ensure the child is euvolemic and normotensive before elevating the head.
3. **Sedation and analgesia:** Sedation may be required to reduce noxious stimuli and prevent ICP surges. Analgesia should be provided to alleviate pain.
4. **Normothermia:** Fever should be strictly avoided. Keep the child's temperature between 36–38°C.
5. **Hemodynamics and CPP management:**
   - *Target blood pressure:* Maintain the child's blood pressure at the 50th percentile for age to ensure adequate cerebral perfusion pressure (CPP = MAP – ICP).
   - Use fluids and vasoactive agents to support hemodynamics.
6. **Hyperventilation:** If ICP surges or herniation is imminent, hyperventilation (target $PaCO_2$: 30–35 mm Hg) may be indicated to reduce cerebral blood flow and lower ICP.
7. **Hypertonic saline:**
   - Preferred in the presence of hypotension, hypovolemia, renal failure or elevated serum osmolality >320mOsm/kg.
   - *Dosage:* 0.1–1 mL/kg/h infusion, targeting a serum sodium of 145–155 mEq/L.
8. **Mannitol:**
   - *Indication:* Acute surges in ICP or signs of impending herniation.
   - *Dosage:* Initial bolus of 0.25–1 g/kg.
   - *Precaution:* Ensure euvolemia before administration. Contraindicated in renal failure or hyperosmolar states.
9. **Seizure management: Seizures** can exacerbate brain injury and increase ICP. Administer appropriate anticonvulsants if seizures are identified.
10. **Noxious stimuli:** Minimize any noxious stimuli that may worsen ICP. For example, use local anesthetic (4% lidocaine mixed in 0.9% normal saline) ~90 seconds prior to endotracheal suctioning to prevent ICP surges.
11. **Fluids and electrolyte management:**
    - Use isotonic or hypertonic fluids (e.g., Ringer's lactate, 0.9% saline, 5% dextrose in 0.9% normal saline) for IV fluid maintenance. Avoid hypotonic solutions.
    - Maintain blood glucose levels between 150–180 mg/dL.
    - Correct electrolyte imbalances (especially sodium and potassium) and acid-base disturbances.

(CPP: cerebral perfusion pressure; ICP: intracranial pressure; MAP: mean arterial pressure; PaCO2: partial pressure of carbon dioxide in arterial blood; PALS: pediatric advanced life support)

Box 27.13 List of Investigations for the Evaluation of an Unconscious Child

1. **Blood tests:**
   - *Complete blood count (CBC):* To assess for infection, anemia or hematologic abnormalities.
   - *Blood gas analysis (Capillary, venous or arterial):* To evaluate acid-base status, respiratory function and oxygenation.
   - *Blood glucose:* Hypoglycemia or hyperglycemia may be an underlying cause of altered consciousness.
   - *Serum electrolytes (Sodium, potassium, chloride, calcium):* To detect electrolyte imbalances, which can cause or exacerbate neurological symptoms.
   - *Urea and creatinine:* To assess renal function and rule out uremic encephalopathy.
   - *Liver function tests (LFTs):* To evaluate for hepatic encephalopathy or systemic infections affecting the liver.
   - *Plasma ammonia:* Especially in cases of suspected hepatic encephalopathy or urea cycle disorders.
   - *Plasma lactate:* To assess for metabolic acidosis or lactic acidosis, often seen in shock, sepsis or hypoxia.
2. **Microbiological investigations:**
   - *Blood culture:* To identify systemic infections, including sepsis or meningitis.
   - *Urine sample (10 mL):* For culture and sensitivity (C&S), organic acids, and toxicology analysis. Ensure refrigeration if the sample cannot be sent immediately.
3. **Imaging studies:**
   CT scan: Indicated in cases of raised ICP, focal neurological deficits, unexplained altered sensorium, or if there are signs of brain herniation. It is the preferred imaging modality for rapid evaluation of the brain.
4. **Cerebrospinal fluid (CSF) analysis:**
   Lumbar puncture: If there is a suspicion of meningitis or encephalitis, CSF analysis is crucial for diagnosis and treatment.
5. **Tropical fever investigations:** In regions where tropical diseases are endemic, tests for specific pathogens may be required, including malaria, dengue, leptospira, mycoplasma and rickettsial infections.

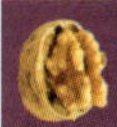

IN A NUTSHELL

1. Altered consciousness or coma in children is a critical medical emergency that demands immediate attention and intervention.
2. Coma may arise from primary central nervous system (CNS) pathology or as a secondary consequence of hypoxia, shock or metabolic disturbances.
3. Reversible causes of coma (such as hypoglycemia, electrolyte imbalances, or intoxication) must be promptly identified and addressed to avoid unnecessary complications.
4. A high index of suspicion for raised intracranial pressure (ICP) should be maintained in all children presenting with altered sensorium or neurological compromise.
5. The prognosis heavily relies on the timely recognition and management of raised ICP, as delays in treatment can lead to poor outcomes.

Abend NS, Licht DJ. Evaluation of the comatose child. In: Shaffner DH, Nichols DG (Eds). Rogers' Textbook of Pediatric Intensive Care, 6th edition. Lippincott Williams & Wilkins, 2023.
Karimi A, Fahimzad SA, Ghanaie RM. Management of a child with decreased level of consciousness. Arch Pediatr. 2013:1(2).
Muralidharan J, Kulgod V, Sharma AK (Eds). IAP Advanced Life Support (ALS) Handbook, 2nd edition. Indian Academy of Pediatrics; 2020.
Pediatric Accident and Emergency Group. Evidence based guideline for management of decreased level of consciousness. Arch Dis Childhood Edu and Practice. 2006;91:ep115-ep122.
Sarnaik A, Bhaya NB, Mahajan PV. Approach to a child with depressed level of consciousness and coma. Therapy. 2008;5:435-449.
Sharma S, Kochar GS, Sankhyan N, Gulati S. Approach to the child with coma. Indian J Pediatr. 2010; 77(11):1279-1287.
Shaver TP, Mehta R. Coma and Depressed Sensorium. In: Fuhrman B, Zimmerman J (Eds). Pediatric Critical Care, 5th edition. Philadelphia: Elsevier, 2016; pp. 805-821.
Topjian AA, Raymond TT, Atkins D, et al. Part 4: Pediatric Basic and Advanced Life Support: 2020 American Heart Association Guidelines for Cardiopulmonary Resuscitation and Emergency Cardiovascular Care. Circulation. 2020;142(16_suppl_2):S469-523.
Taylor DA, Ashwal S. Impairment of consciousness and coma. In: Swaiman KF, Ashwal S, Ferriero DM (Eds). Pediatric neurology: principles and practice, 4th edition. Philadelphia: Elsevier, 2006; pp. 1379-1400.

27.10 Hypothermia in Children

PE 24.17, PE 24.18, PE 24.19, PE 24.20

INTRODUCTION

Hypothermia in children is primarily due to their small body size and large surface-to-volume ratio, making them more prone to heat loss. In children, while ***shivering thermogenesis*** and ***non-shivering thermogenesis*** (e.g., brown adipose tissue in infants) help generate heat, these mechanisms may become inadequate under certain conditions (e.g., extreme cold, metabolic stress). **Metabolic exhaustion** can occur in such cases when the body's energy reserves are depleted or when it cannot generate enough heat.

In neonates, though hypothermia can significantly affect respiratory adaptation and development, it can also act as a protective response to hypoxia and be used therapeutically in cases of perinatal asphyxia (discussed in detail in **Chapter 16**). Interestingly, hypothermia reduces the brain's metabolic rate, which decreases the production of harmful free radicals, inflammatory responses and excitotoxic neurotransmitter release. This can help protect neural tissue from ischemic damage during or after episodes of reduced oxygen or blood flow. Therapeutic hypothermia has also been used post-cardiac surgery for congenital defects, where there may be periods of low perfusion or cardiac arrest. However, it remains a significant risk in both clinical and prehospital settings for children, with limited therapeutic benefits in pediatric critical care.

Definitions

Hypothermia in children is defined by a core body temperature below 35°C (95°F). Axillary temperature is lower than core temperature by ~0.5 to 1.0°C. In neonates, hypothermia is defined as an axillary temperature below 36.5°C (97.7°F) according to the World Health Organization (WHO) and has been discussed in detail in **Chapter 15.** From this point forward in this section, all temperature readings will refer to core body temperature, unless specified otherwise. Hypothermia in children is classified into three grades of severity: mild, moderate and severe hypothermia

1. ***Mild hypothermia (32 to 35°C/90 to 95°F):*** In this stage, thermoregulation is still intact, with shivering, non-shivering thermogenesis, vasoconstriction, and active movements. Compensatory mechanisms attempt to restore normal body temperature, and the child may still be able to self-rescue.
2. ***Moderate hypothermia (28 to <32°C/82 to <90°F):*** As the temperature drops below 32°C, cognitive function, coordination and muscle strength begin to deteriorate, impairing the ability to respond to the cold. In this range, the child loses consciousness. The heart rate slows (bradycardia), myocardial contractility decreases, and vasomotor tone is lost, contributing to poor perfusion, hypotension and the risk of shock.
3. ***Severe hypothermia (<28°C/82.4°F):*** At temperatures below 28°C, bradycardia worsens, cardiac output drops significantly, and there is an increased risk of ventricular fibrillation or asystole. Respiratory depression also occurs, leading to hypoventilation and eventual apnea. At very low body temperatures (<25–29°C/77–84.2°F), deep coma, fixed and dilated pupils, and absence of reflexes may mimic signs of death, though this might be a false appearance. Hence, clinicians should note that declaration of death should not be made without precise assessment of the core body temperature.

Etiology

The causes of hypothermia in children can be classified into **primary** and **secondary** causes:

Primary Hypothermia

Primary hypothermia occurs due to direct environmental exposure that leads to excessive heat loss. It is more common in children involved in outdoor activities or those from indigent populations. The mechanisms of heat loss include:

- ***Conduction:*** Heat loss through direct contact with cooler objects or surfaces, such as metal or cold ground, e.g., a child sleeping on the ground without proper insulation, causing body heat to transfer to the colder surface.
- ***Convection:*** Heat loss when air or water contacts the body. This is especially significant in windy or wet (rainy) conditions, where heat loss can occur quickly, e.g., a child submerged in cold water or in case of drowning, where the body loses heat rapidly to the surrounding water as it continuously moves away from the skin, being replaced by cooler water, leading to a quick and significant drop in core temperature.
- ***Evaporative heat loss:*** Occurs when sweat or moisture on the skin evaporates, leading to heat loss. This is exacerbated in conditions of low humidity, e.g., a child sweating while playing outside on a cold day, and the moisture evaporates, carrying away body heat.
- ***Radiant heat loss:*** Heat loss in the form of electromagnetic waves. While less prominent than other forms, it still contributes significantly to overall heat loss, e.g., a child standing in a cold environment without protective clothing or blankets, where the body radiates heat to the colder surroundings.

Secondary Hypothermia

Secondary hypothermia occurs due to underlying medical conditions or interventions that increase the risk of heat loss or impair thermoregulation.

- ***Medications and toxins:*** Certain drugs or toxins, such as sedatives or alcohol (in adolescents), can impair the body's ability to regulate temperature.
- ***Metabolic or endocrine disorders:*** Conditions like hypothyroidism or adrenal insufficiency can reduce the body's ability to generate heat.
- ***Neurologic injuries:*** Head or spinal injuries may disrupt the body's temperature regulation mechanisms.
- ***Systemic illnesses:*** Severe infections, especially sepsis, shock
- ***Iatrogenic causes:*** Massive blood transfusions or prolonged exposure to cold environments (e.g., resuscitation rooms with inadequate thermoregulation) can lead to secondary hypothermia.
- ***Prematurity:*** Immature thermoregulation in premature infants increases the risk of hypothermia
- ***Severe acute malnutrition:*** Hypothermia in these children often indicates the presence of hypoglycemia or a serious underlying infection.

In secondary hypothermia, patients may be less responsive to standard rewarming treatments and require more specific interventions based on the underlying cause.

Pathophysiology

As a patient's core temperature decreases, the body attempts to maintain normothermia through mechanisms such as increased metabolism, shunting blood to vital organs, non-shivering thermogenesis through brown adipose tissue (especially in neonates and infants) and shivering (in older children) to produce heat. However, if these mechanisms fail, the core temperature continues to drop, impairing organ function.

Initial Thermoregulatory Responses

- ***Vasoconstriction and shivering:*** As the body temperature drops, the hypothalamus, which regulates body temperature, triggers vasoconstriction to reduce heat loss from the skin and extremities. The extremities, including fingers, toes, and ears, are most susceptible to cold-induced injury and frostbite. As the body shunts blood to vital organs in response to cold, the peripheries may suffer from ischemia and tissue damage. At the same time, shivering is initiated to generate heat through muscle activity. However, shivering in younger children, particularly premature infants, may be less effective due to their limited muscle mass and immature thermoregulatory mechanisms.

- ***Increased metabolic rate:*** To generate more heat, the body's metabolic rate increases. In neonates, there is also increased non-shivering thermogenesis, primarily through brown adipose tissue, which helps in heat production.

Progressive Thermoregulation Impairment

- ***Impaired shivering:*** As core temperature continues to drop below 30°C (86°F), the effectiveness of shivering declines, and the body's ability to generate heat diminishes. This makes it increasingly difficult for the child to maintain normothermia.
- ***Decreased metabolic rate:*** The metabolic rate eventually slows as the body's ability to conserve and produce heat becomes impaired. This leads to a further decrease in body temperature, as the body no longer has sufficient energy to maintain normal thermoregulation. As the core temperature decreases, oxygen consumption decreases as well. Below 28°C, oxygen consumption drops by 50%, leading to a protective effect on vital organs by reducing their oxygen demand.

Organ System Dysfunction

Further, hypothermia causes significant organ dysfunction across multiple systems. The CNS becomes depressed, leading to confusion, lethargy, and in severe cases, coma or brain death. Cardiovascular effects include bradycardia, hypotension, and arrhythmias, with a decreased response to defibrillation. Respiratory function slows, and the body's ability to regulate oxygen demand diminishes. Additionally, hypothermia impairs coagulation and immune responses, increasing the risk of bleeding and infections.

Clinical Features

- ***Central nervous system (CNS):*** Below 35°C, CNS dysfunction progresses, leading to symptoms like confusion, disorientation and impaired judgment. This impairment can lead to paradoxical undressing, where affected individuals may suddenly and inexplicably begin removing their clothing, occurring in up to 30% of fatal hypothermic cases. This happens as the hypothalamus becomes impaired due to low body temperature, and the brain might misinterpret the body's need for warmth, causing the individual to feel overheated and initiate undressing, despite the external cold. Further, as the core temperature drops, it can cause amnesia, ataxia, coma and potentially brain death.
- ***Cardiovascular system:*** In hypothermia, peripheral vasoconstriction occurs, followed by an initial rise in heart rate and blood pressure. As the temperature drops, bradycardia and hypotension set in. Atrial fibrillation and flutter are common but typically resolve as the body warms. ECG changes, like Osborne waves (J point elevation), occur at around 32°C and are usually benign in mild to moderate hypothermia. However, severe hypothermia (below 28°C) increases myocardial irritability, leading to arrhythmias and a higher risk of cardiac arrest. Hypothermic cardiac arrest may occur during transport or treatment due to myocardial instability and is less responsive to medications or defibrillation.
- ***Respiratory changes:*** Hypothermic children may exhibit shallow breathing and a reduced respiratory rate due to CNS depression and decreased oxygen demand at lower body temperatures.
- ***Coagulation and immune system impairment:*** Hypothermia leads to a hypercoagulable state, impairing platelet function and coagulation, which increases the risk of bleeding in severe cases. The immune response is also suppressed, making hypothermic children more susceptible to infections.

The clinical features of hypothermia in children vary depending on the severity of temperature drop, the child's age and overall health **(Box 27.14)**. Symptoms progress as the core body temperature decreases, and children may present with a wide range of physical and behavioral signs.

Box 27.14 Clinical Features of Hypothermia in Children

Mild hypothermia (32 to 35°C/89.6 to 95°F)
- Shivering
- Pale or cool skin
- Irritability, poor coordination, ataxia
- Confusion, slurred speech
- Increased heart and respiratory rates
- Cold diuresis

Moderate hypothermia (28 to 32°C/82.4 to 89.6°F)
- Absence of shivering
- Slurred speech, confusion, lethargy
- Bradycardia, hypotension
- Respiratory depression, cold extremities
- Decreased urine output

Severe hypothermia (Below 28°C/82.4°F)
- Unconsciousness or coma
- Paradoxical undressing
- Cardiac arrhythmias, bradycardia
- Hypotension, respiratory arrest
- Dilated pupils, loss of reflexes
- Coagulopathy, organ dysfunction

Additional features in children:
- Irritability or lethargy in infants
- Frostbite on extremities
- Cyanosis (bluish skin)

Complications: Organ failure, metabolic acidosis, death

DROWNING AND COLD WATER INJURY

According to the World Health Organization (WHO), drowning refers to "the process of experiencing respiratory impairment from submersion/immersion in liquid." It should be distinguished from cold water immersion injuries, where victims stay afloat and keep their head above water without respiratory impairment. In cold water (under 15–20°C or 59–68°F), heat loss through conduction and convection is more efficient than in air, and children are more vulnerable to hypothermia due to their higher body surface area-to-mass ratio, less subcutaneous fat and lower thermogenic capacity. Body temperature may continue to drop even after removal from the water due to exposure to cold air, wet clothes, hypoxia and prolonged hospital transport time. In children, hypothermia can occur due to drowning even in relatively warm water or warmer climates.

Cold-water immersion triggers a dynamic series of respiratory and cardiovascular responses, including *cold-water shock*, which may cause drowning. Immersion in ice-cold water leads to reflex hyperventilation and reduced breath-holding (<10 seconds), risking fluid aspiration. The diving reflex, which is characterized by severe bradycardia, occurs but is transient and rapidly followed by supraventricular and ectopic tachycardia and hypertension. After the initial cold shock, continued immersion for further 5–10 minutes can incapacitate the victim as muscle function deteriorates and the victim is unable to perform self-rescue maneuvers. Severe hypothermia (body temperature <28°C or 82.4°F) can lead to arrhythmias and cardiac arrest.

The rate of heat loss depends on water temperature, air temperature, insulation and physical factors like body size, swimming effort and water flow. Within 30–60 minutes of immersion, body temperature can decrease to hypothermic levels. Symptoms of hypothermia vary by temperature. Mild hypothermia (32–35°C or 90–95°F) includes shivering, active movement, and functioning thermoregulatory mechanisms. As core temperature drops below 32°C, cognition and coordination are impaired, and self-rescue becomes difficult. Severe hypothermia (<28°C or 82.4°F) causes loss of consciousness, bradycardia, hypotension, and risk of cardiac arrest. At very low temperatures (<25–29°C or 77–84.2°F), coma and absent reflexes may mimic death.

If the cooling process is quick and the cardiac output lasts long enough for sufficient heat loss to occur before the onset of severe hypoxia, it can potentially induce a neuroprotective effect if the brain cools to about 33°C (91.4°F) in controlled experimental conditions. However, if submersion injury or drowning occurs before a neuroprotective level of hypothermia is reached, the resulting severe anoxia causes significant damage to tissues and organs including the brain. While therapeutic hypothermia may offer benefits in controlled settings, accidental hypothermia from drowning is unpredictable and harmful, leading to poor prognosis in most cases. In rare instances, survivors of prolonged (10–150 minutes) cardiac arrest after cold-water submersion in freezing conditions (<5°C or 41°F) have shown good neurologic recovery. These cases have been explained to be due to the sudden and severe hypothermia that protected the brain from ischemic damage. However, hypothermia generally remains a poor prognostic indicator for drowning victims.

EVALUATION OF HYPOTHERMIA IN CHILDREN

While investigations are important, they should not delay immediate treatment, as immediate rewarming and supportive care are critical in managing hypothermia. For all potentially unstable patients, the clinician should prioritize the trauma ABCs during the initial evaluation. After completing the primary survey, all clothing should be removed, and dry, warm blankets should be applied to the fully exposed chest.

1. ***Core body temperature monitoring:*** Core temperature should be measured via rectal, esophageal or bladder temperature monitoring. Rectal and bladder temperature measurements are suitable for conscious patients with mild to moderate hypothermia but may not reflect true core temperature in critical cases and can worsen hypothermia in the prehospital setting. Esophageal temperature is the most accurate, but it requires an advanced airway. Oral temperature measurements are useful only for ruling out hypothermia, as most standard thermometers are unable to measure temperatures below 35°C. Similarly, tympanic thermometers are generally unreliable for accurately assessing hypothermic temperatures. Core temperature should be measured at two or more central sites. However, in neonates, WHO recommends measuring the axillary temperature over the rectal temperature due to considerations of safety, hygiene and ease of use.
2. ***Capillary blood glucose by dextrostix:*** Blood glucose levels do not follow a consistent pattern and can present as either hypoglycemia or hyperglycemia.
3. ***Complete blood count:*** Hemoglobin/hematocrit may rise due to cold diuresis. Thrombocytopenia may be present due to platelet dysfunction and altered clotting mechanisms.
4. ***Coagulation studies:*** Prolonged PT, PTT, and INR due to impaired coagulation pathways, often worsened by hypothermia
5. Fibrinogen to rule out disseminated intravascular coagulation (DIC)
6. ***Blood gas analysis:***
   a. *Metabolic acidosis:* Due to anaerobic metabolism as oxygen consumption decreases.
   b. *Respiratory acidosis:* If hypoventilation occurs (more common in severe hypothermia).
7. ***Electrolyte imbalances:*** Hyponatremia and hyperkalemia are common findings.
8. ***Electrocardiogram (ECG):***
   a. Osborne waves (J-point elevation) usually seen in precordial leads.
   b. *Prolonged QT interval and PR interval:* Seen at temperatures <30°C.
   c. *Arrhythmias:* Atrial fibrillation, bradycardia and risk of ventricular fibrillation below 28°C.
9. ***Kidney Function Tests (KFT):*** Elevated serum creatinine and blood urea nitrogen (BUN) as hypothermia can lead to reduced renal perfusion and function, resulting in prerenal acute kidney injury (AKI).
10. ***Urinalysis:***
    a. *Proteinuria:* May be seen due to renal hypoperfusion.
    b. *Hematuria:* Can occur in severe hypothermia with associated renal damage.
11. ***Imaging studies:*** Chest x-ray, CT and ultrasound should be guided by clinical need. CT head should be done for altered sensorium if trauma or stroke is suspected.
12. ***Additional tests:*** Serum lactate, creatine kinase, troponin, TSH, cortisol and toxicology screen to rule out non-environmental causes of hypothermia.

Management

A rapid primary survey, incorporating the assessment of airway, breathing, circulation, disability and exposure (ABCDE), is essential to determine the need for immediate resuscitation. In cases of unconsciousness, pulselessness or apnea, resuscitative measures must be initiated without delay, irrespective of the underlying cause. Following stabilization or the exclusion of emergency conditions, a more comprehensive evaluation can proceed. Hypothermia management prioritizes prompt rewarming and the prevention of further heat loss, after ensuring that airway, breathing and circulation are effectively addressed at the earliest opportunity.

Managing hypothermia begins in the field and continues through transport and in the hospital. The goal is to prevent or treat moderate to severe hypothermia. Damp clothing should be removed, and rewarming measures should be initiated immediately. Rewarming methods are categorized into passive, active external and active internal methods **(Box 27.15)**. Passive rewarming (dry blankets, warm environment, protection from further heat loss) should start immediately for hypothermic victims.

Rewarming should be done based on the degree of hypothermia and the presence of circulation:

- ***Mild hypothermia (32–35°C):*** The treatment of choice in mild hypothermia is passive rewarming. Remove wet clothing, dry the skin and place additional insulating layers like blanket over the victim's body. If hypothermia persists, initiate active external rewarming. If environmental exposure is not the cause, other conditions such as sepsis, hypoglycemia, hyponatremia or child abuse should be considered, as these may present with symptoms like lethargy or hypotension that are inconsistent with mild hypothermia alone.
- ***Moderate hypothermia (28–32°C):*** For children with moderate hypothermia and intact circulation, active external rewarming is recommended, preferably using forced air rewarming. However, this method may cause peripheral vasodilation and rewarming shock, where cold, acidotic blood returns to the core circulation, potentially leading to a drop in temperature and pH. This can result in hypotension, decreased coronary perfusion, ventricular fibrillation and fatal collapse. To mitigate these risks, children should receive IV access and a rapid infusion of 20 mL/kg of warmed normal saline at the start of rewarming, with ongoing volume support and continuous monitoring of cardiorespiratory status, blood pressure, and perfusion. If the rewarming rate is inadequate (less than 1°C or 1.8°F per hour) or if the core temperature continues to drop despite active external rewarming, further evaluation for inadequate fluid resuscitation or other complications is needed. These patients, or those who become unstable, may require active internal rewarming methods. To avoid hyperthermia, external rewarming should be stopped when the core temperature reaches 35°C (95°F), with careful monitoring to prevent re-cooling or overheating during recovery.
- ***Severe hypothermia with intact circulation (<28°C):*** For children with severe hypothermia (core temperature <28°C or 82°F) and intact circulation, the preferred method of rewarming is *active internal rewarming*, which includes techniques like pleural lavage with heated saline (40–44°C). Pleural lavage is effective in avoiding core temperature after drop and arrhythmias. Other internal methods, such as gastric, bladder, colon, and peritoneal lavage, are less effective but can still be used. A challenge with internal rewarming is the need for large volumes of heated saline, requiring preplanning for fluid heating or alternative solutions. If internal rewarming is not feasible, forced air external rewarming is an alternative, with studies showing good results in adults and rewarming rates of 1–2°C (1.8–4°F) per hour, without significant after drop or shock.
- ***Severe hypothermia with absent circulation (<28°C):*** In cases of severe hypothermia with absent circulation, **extracorporeal rewarming (ECMO)** is recommended. ECMO provides circulatory support, oxygenation, and rapid rewarming (up to 10°C or 18°F per hour). It has been shown to be effective even in patients who are in cardiac arrest or unstable. Although ECMO requires specialized equipment and skilled personnel, its benefits include potential neurologic recovery and continued support after rewarming. Even when there are delays in ECMO initiation, good outcomes have been reported, though the primary contraindication is severe trauma with bleeding risk, which can be managed using non-heparinized bypass circuits.

Previously, specific rewarming rates were often targeted, sometimes more slowly, but current evidence suggests that rewarming rates are largely determined by the patient's circulation and metabolism. Rapid rewarming, when sufficient support for blood volume and circulation is provided, is not harmful and may even be beneficial. In fact, studies indicate that rapid rewarming is associated with lower mortality after adjusting for case severity. Additionally, case reports have highlighted numerous instances where patients with profound hypothermia (core temperature <25°C or 77°F) were successfully rewarmed very quickly using extracorporeal circulation, leading to intact survival. ECMO can achieve rewarming rates of up to 10°C per hour, while other active rewarming methods raise the core temperature by 1–2°C per hour.

Box 27.15 Rewarming Methods for Hypothermia

1. **Passive rewarming:**
   - Remove wet clothing, use dry insulation (use dry blanket).
   - Prevents further cooling but doesn't actively warm.
2. **Active external rewarming:**
   - *Methods:* Forced air, radiant heat, heat packs.
   - Forced air preferred to avoid burns.
   - *Risks:* After drop, rewarming shock, VF, cardiac arrest.
3. **Active internal rewarming:**
   - *Noninvasive:* Heated, humidified oxygen (37°C), warm IV saline (40–44°C). Prevents cooling, but not enough for full rewarming.
   - *Invasive:* Heated saline (40–44°C) into body cavities (e.g., pleura, bladder, stomach). Pleural lavage recommended for severe hypothermia.
   - *Extracorporeal:* ECMO or ECLS for severe cases, supporting circulation and lung function. Used if other methods fail.

PEDIATRIC ADVANCED LIFE SUPPORT (PALS) IN HYPOTHERMIA

- ***Bradyarrhythmias:*** Rewarming is the primary treatment for bradycardic rhythms in severe hypothermia. Cardiac pacing is typically ineffective.
- ***Cardiac arrest:*** For hypothermic victims with no pulse or absent QRS activity on ECG, cardiopulmonary resuscitation (CPR) is necessary. In cases of ventricular fibrillation with core temperatures <30°C (86°F), defibrillation may not be effective until the temperature reaches ≥30°C (86°F), at which point it is more likely to succeed.
- ***Duration of resuscitation:*** Controversy exists around when to stop resuscitation in hypothermic drowning victims. The victim's body temperature should be a key factor in this decision. Cases of profound hypothermia may make a victim appear clinically dead, but full neurologic recovery is possible, though rare. Resuscitation should not be withheld unless signs of irreversible death (e.g., dependent lividity or rigor mortis) are present. Rewarming efforts are typically continued until the victim's body temperature reaches 32–34°C (89.6–93.2°F), at which point resuscitation may be reconsidered if there is no effective cardiac rhythm despite aggressive CPR.

Following successful CPR, ongoing temperature management and monitoring are essential. If a victim regains consciousness soon after resuscitation, attempts to restore and maintain normothermia are recommended to prevent worsening hypothermia. For victims who remain comatose post-CPR, the approach to rewarming and therapeutic hypothermia is debated. Many experts recommend limiting active rewarming for victims with temperatures <32°C (89.6°F) and allowing natural warming to temperatures between 32–37.5°C (89.6–99.5°F) without further intervention.

The use of therapeutic hypothermia in comatose drowning victims remains controversial. It is not widely recommended for children, with studies showing no improvement in neurologic outcomes or mortality with extracorporeal circulation and rewarming. Current guidelines do not support therapeutic hypothermia in drowning victims resuscitated after cardiac arrest, particularly in children, due to insufficient evidence of benefit.

Complications

Frostbite is a serious complication of hypothermia that can lead to limb loss if not treated promptly. It begins as dry gangrene and can progress to wet gangrene if infected. Infections, particularly by *Clostridium perfringens*, can produce gas and crepitus in the skin, potentially requiring amputation if untreated. Other hypothermia complications include: cold diuresis, rhabdomyolysis, aspiration, hyperkalemia, acute kidney injury, pancreatitis, pulmonary edema, ataxia, arrhythmias (e.g., atrial/ventricular fibrillation, pulseless electrical activity), coma and death.

Rewarming itself can also cause complications such as systemic inflammation, electrolyte imbalances (hyperkalemia, hypophosphatemia, hypomagnesemia, hypocalcemia), rhabdomyolysis, arrhythmias, platelet dysfunction and altered glucose homeostasis (insulin resistance, reduced glucose utilization). Prompt recognition and treatment can reduce these risks and improve outcomes.

Prognosis

Severe hypothermia can be fatal, but timely treatment improves prognosis. Stable patients with primary hypothermia can survive with full neurological recovery if treated quickly with rewarming. Cardiac arrest patients treated with ECMO have a 50% survival rate. Ventricular fibrillation may have a good outcome if revived quickly, but hypothermic asystole often requires rewarming to 35°C. High blood potassium levels (>12 mEq/L) indicate irreversible damage. Early resuscitation generally leads to good outcomes, though severe hypothermia and age can worsen prognosis.

Prevention

To maintain normal temperature in children and prevent hypothermia:

1. ***Clothing:*** Dress in layers (moisture-wicking base, insulating middle and waterproof outer layer), including a hat, mittens and warm socks/boots.
2. ***Shelter:*** Provide wind protection and ensure the child is in a dry, warm environment (e.g., insulated tents or blankets).
3. ***Movement:*** Encourage light activity to generate body heat.
4. ***Transport:*** Use heated car seats, limit time outdoors in extreme cold and ensure children are wrapped in warm layers.
5. ***Environment:*** Maintain indoor temperatures between 18–21°C (64–70°F) and monitor for signs of cold stress or hypothermia.
6. ***Hydration/nutrition:*** Offer warm fluids and ensure adequate nutrition for energy.
7. ***Monitoring:*** Regularly check body temperature and watch for behavioral changes, like lethargy or irritability, which can signal cold stress.

These measures help prevent cold-related injuries and keep children safe in low temperatures.

In neonates, the "warm chain" is a set of ten interlinked procedures recommended by the WHO to be followed at birth and during the first few hours and days to minimize the risk of hypothermia in all newborns **(Box 27.16)**. The birth room must be warm (at least 25°C/77°F) and free from drafts of cold air. Immediately after birth, the newborn should be dried and covered before the cord is cut. During drying, the baby should be placed on a warm surface, such as the mother's chest or abdomen, for skin-to-skin contact, which is the most effective way to maintain warmth. If skin-to-skin contact is not possible,

Box 27.16 The Warm Chain

1. Warm birth environment (at least 25°C/77°F)
2. Immediate drying of the newborn
3. Skin-to-skin contact with the mother
4. Initiate breastfeeding early
5. Delay bathing and weighing
6. Provide appropriate clothing and bedding
7. Ensure mother and baby remain together
8. Ensure warm transportation
9. Provide warm resuscitation if needed
10. Training and raising awareness among caregivers

other methods, such as wrapping the baby or placing them in a warm room or under a radiant heater, should be used. Bathing and weighing should be delayed.

Breastfeeding should begin within the first hour to provide the baby with calories needed for heat production. In the days following birth, keeping the baby and mother together (rooming-in), breastfeeding as frequently as needed, and dressing the baby appropriately for the ambient temperature help prevent hypothermia.

Low birth weight or sick newborns are particularly vulnerable to cold. For these high-risk babies, methods like kangaroo-mother care (continuous skin-to-skin contact), warm rooms, heated water-filled mattresses, radiant heaters, and incubators should be employed. If using a heating device or warm room, the baby should be periodically removed for skin-to-skin contact with the mother and breastfeeding. The baby's body temperature should be closely monitored.

Kangaroo Mother Care (KMC): It is a method of caring for preterm or low birth weight (LBW) infants by placing them in skin-to-skin (STS) contact with the mother or another caregiver to support their optimal growth and development. Originally developed as an alternative to technology-based care, KMC is now considered the gold standard for LBW infants in all settings.

The four key components of KMC are:

1. ***Kangaroo position (Fig. 27.18):*** The infant is held in a vertical position, skin-to-skin, between the mother's breasts and under her clothes. The caregiver must maintain a semi-reclining position to prevent gastric reflux in the infant. This responsibility can also be shared with the father or other family members.
2. ***Exclusive or nearly exclusive breastfeeding:*** The baby is breastfed as the primary or sole source of nutrition.
3. ***Early discharge:*** The infant is discharged from the healthcare facility as soon as they are stable and able to thrive in the home environment.
4. ***Continued follow-up:*** After discharge, the mother and baby require adequate support and monitoring. A follow-up program with access to emergency services should be in place to ensure the infant's ongoing health and development.

Advantages of KMC: It is a simple, cost-effective intervention that offers numerous benefits for both infants and the broader community.

- ***Reduced mortality***: KMC lowers the risk of death during the birth hospitalization or within the first 28 days of life. This reduction in mortality occurs regardless of gestational age, birth weight, time of initiation, or setting (hospital or community).
- ***Reduced severe infection:*** KMC decreases the risk of severe infections, with a reduction in hypothermia by 68%.
- ***Improved growth:*** Infants receiving KMC experience better anthropometric growth, including higher weight gain per day and increases in length and head circumference per week.
- ***Higher breastfeeding rates:*** KMC leads to higher exclusive breastfeeding rates at discharge and at 28 days of life.
- ***Better temperature regulation:*** KMC is an effective way to maintain the newborn's warmth, promoting better temperature regulation compared to conventional incubator care.

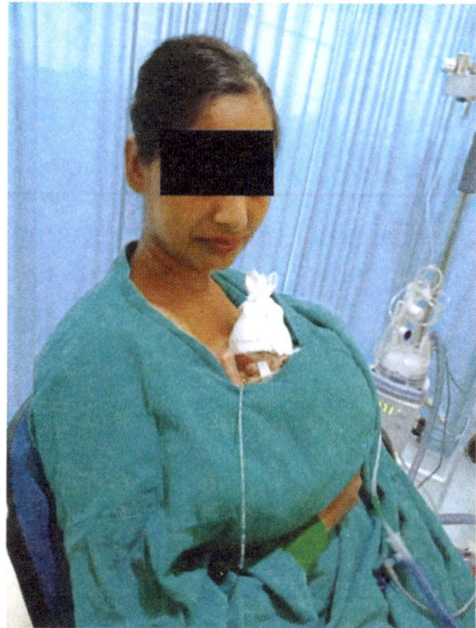

Fig. 27.18: Kangaroo mother care

- ***Enhanced breathing patterns:*** Newborns under KMC have more regular breathing and experience fewer apneic spells.
- ***Promotes maternal confidence and involvement:*** KMC increases the mother's confidence, ability, and involvement in caring for her newborn, fostering a closer bond and more active participation in the infant's care.

To ensure the effectiveness of the method, the baby should remain in continuous skin-to-skin contact with the mother, both day and night, and minimum duration for each KMC session should be one hour, as frequent handling may cause stress for the infant. The baby should only be briefly separated for activities such as diaper changes, the mother's bathing and restroom breaks, or when clinical examinations are necessary. KMC, when administered for at least **8 hours per day**, shows greater benefits in reducing mortality compared to shorter durations.

Chan G, Labar AS, Wall S, Atun R. Kangaroo mother care: a systematic review of barriers and enablers. Bull World Health Organ. 2016;94(2):130-41.

Duong H, Patel G. Hypothermia. In: StatPearls. Treasure Island (FL): StatPearls Publishing; 2025. Available from: https://www.ncbi.nlm.nih.gov/books/NBK545239/. [Last accessed Jan 2025].

Montealegre-Pomar A, Bohorquez A, Charpak N. Systematic review and meta-analysis suggest that Kangaroo position protects against apnoea of prematurity. Acta Paediatr. 2020; 109(7): 1310-6.

Muralidharan J, Kulgod V, Sharma AK (Eds). IAP Advanced Life Support (ALS) Handbook, 2nd edition. Indian Academy of Pediatrics; 2020.

Prince WB. Drowning and submersion injury. In: Kliegman RM, Stanton BF, St. Geme JW, Schor NF, Behrman RE (Eds). Nelson Textbook of Pediatrics, 22nd edition. Philadelphia: Elsevier; 2024. pp. 637-45.

Sivanandan S, Sankar M. Kangaroo mother care for preterm or low birth weight infants: a systematic review and meta-analysis. BMJ Global Health 2023;1-13.

Topjian AA, Raymond TT, Atkins D, et al. Part 4: Pediatric Basic and Advanced Life Support: 2020 American Heart Association Guidelines for Cardiopulmonary Resuscitation and Emergency Cardiovascular Care. Circulation. 2020;142(16_suppl_2):S469-523.

World Health Organization. Kangaroo mother care: a practical guide. Department of Reproductive Health and Research, WHO, Geneva; 2003.

27.11 Poisoning: Diagnosis and Management

INTRODUCTION

Poisoning can be accidental (toddlers and young children) or intentional (in adolescents). It often appears as an unknown emergency.

When to Suspect Poisoning

- ***Sudden onset*** of altered consciousness, breathing difficulty, or convulsions.
- ***Unexplained history:*** A previously well child found drowsy or convulsing after being unsupervised for a few hours, with no one knowing what happened during that time.
- ***Emergency context:*** Poisoning could be suspected in cases of injury or infection, where intoxication is a possible complication.
- ***Age-related suspicion:*** In younger children, poisoning is often accidental, while in adolescents it may be intentional (e.g., suicide attempt).

ETIOLOGY

Most of the poisonings in children are accidental in nature. The most common agents responsible for poisoning in Southeast Asia are pesticides, kerosene, prescription drugs, and household chemicals. Chemical products, most often swallowed by children include household cleaners (bleach, detergents), fuel (kerosene, paraffin), cosmetics, medicines, paints, products for household repairs, and household pesticides.

Household poisoning could either be a nontoxic ingestion or a toxic ingestion.

- ***Nontoxic ingestion*** is defined as that occurring after an individual consumes a nonedible product that usually does not produces symptoms, such as abrasives, adhesives, air fresheners, aluminum foils, antacids, baby products, cosmetics, candles, chalk, erasers, ball-point pen-ink, lipstick, and lubricants.
- ***Toxic ingestion*** consists of consumption of either of the following soaps and detergents, shampoos, bleaches, disinfectants and deodorizers, acids and alkalis, boron compounds, cosmetics, nail polish remover (gamma butyrolactone), disk batteries, naphthalene moth balls, tobacco products, insecticides, pharmaceuticals, and paints.

Nearly 75% of poisoning episodes are due to ingestion of nontoxic substances which require reassurance to the children and their parents. Management of symptomatic toxic cases mostly involves supportive care and correct product identification. Once the product is identified, specific management relates to the nature of the principal chemical constituent. Bites and stings of animals and insects, and ingestion of poisonous plants and seeds also account for outdoor poisoning in children. Carbon monoxide poisoning can happen when fires, stoves, heaters or ovens are used in rooms and huts that do not have proper ventilation to let the gases out.

Exposure to Poison

Acute exposure is a single contact that lasts for seconds, minutes, or hours, or several exposures over about a day or less. *Chronic exposure* is contact that lasts for many days, months, or years.

A poison may get into the body through ingestion, inhalation (gas, vapors, dust, fumes, smoke, spray), skin contact (pesticides), or injection (bites and stings, drug injection).

PREDISPOSING FACTORS

The peak age for childhood poisoning is between 1 and 3 years. As children become more mobile and curious, they meet a variety of toxins in their environment. Hand-to-mouth activity and development of the pincer grasp in infants puts them at risk of ingesting potentially toxic substances.

- For children younger than 6 months, poisoning is unusual but may result from the inadvertent administration of an incorrect drug or drug dose by a parent, intentional administration of a drug by a parent or sibling, or passive exposure.
- Any poisoning in a child younger than 1 year of age should be carefully evaluated for possible child abuse or neglect.
- Unintentional ingestion is unusual after age 5 years, although it can result from mistaken consumption of any toxin from a mislabeled container.
- Between the ages of 5 and 9 years, poisoning may reflect intrafamilial stress or suicidal intent.
- Beyond 9 years of age, overdose or poisoning frequently results either from a suicidal gesture or attempt, or from an adverse effect of drug abuse.
- Adolescents who enter the workplace may encounter hazardous chemicals but may not have access to protective equipment or safety education.

Majority of the exposures occur at home. Preventive measures in the home environment can go a long way in reducing the overall morbidity of poisonings in children.

Clinical features of some common poisonings are listed in **Box 27.17.** A structured approach while taking history helps clinicians efficiently diagnose and treat poisoning, ensuring safe and effective intervention. Key components in history-taking is listed in **Box 27.18.**

Box 27.17 | Presenting Features of Common Poisonings

- *Seizures:* Organochlorines, chlorinated hydrocarbons, cocaine, isoniazid, phenothiazine, carbon monoxide, and theophylline
- *Respiratory compromise:* Narcotics, organophosphates, barbiturate, benzodiazepines
- *Cardiac arrhythmias:* Tricyclic antidepressants, amphetamine, aluminum phosphide, digitalis, theophylline, arsenic, cyanide, chloroquine
- *Metabolic acidosis:* Isoniazid, methanol, salicylates, phenformin, iron, and cyanide
- *Gastrointestinal disturbances:* Organophosphorus, arsenic, iron, lithium, and mercury
- *Cyanosis:* Nitrobenzene compounds, aniline dyes, and dapsone

Box 27.18 Key Questions a Pediatrician should ask in a Case of Pediatric Poisoning

1. **When was the poison consumed?**
   - If less than 1 hour, **stomach wash** might be considered.
   - *Contraindication:* Stomach wash for hydrocarbons like kerosene, antidepressants, and lithium.
2. **How much of the substance was consumed?**
   This helps assess whether the amount ingested was toxic, as toxic doses vary by substance.
3. **Did parents attempt to make the child vomit?**
   Home remedies to induce vomiting can be harmful, especially with hydrocarbons, as it can lead to **aspiration pneumonia**.
4. **What symptoms alerted the parents/caregivers?**
   Understanding the symptoms helps estimate the **time since ingestion**, which is important for deciding on treatment based on the substance's pharmacokinetics.

TREATMENT Poisoning: General Management

First Aid for Poisoning

A fast response is associated with better outcome for the affected person. There are some important initial steps to be followed without panicking and distressing the poisoned child **(Box 27.19)**. In minor poisoning, symptomatic and supportive treatment is generally not required, whereas for moderate or severe poisoning, advanced symptomatic and supportive treatment is always necessary.

For Ingested Poisons

- Remove the poison from the entry point. Wipe the affected area gently. Rinse with fresh water. Remove the clothes of the victim. Wash the eyes of the victim with fresh water and dry gently.
- Provoke vomiting only if the victim is conscious.
- If the victim vomits, protect the airway. Save the vomitus to allow identification of the poison.
- If the victim starts having convulsions, protect him/her from injury and give convulsion first aid.
- Reassure the victim and keep him/her comfortable. Position the victims on their left side while getting or awaiting medical help.

For Inhaled Poisons

- Open windows and doors to remove the fumes.
- Hold a wet cloth over your nose and mouth. Take several deep breaths of fresh air, then hold your breath as you go in.
- Take out the affected person from the toxic area to fresh air. Call for emergency help. Never attempt to rescue a victim without notifying others first.
- Avoid lighting a matchstick as some gases may ignite.
- As necessary, perform first aid for skin burns, eye injuries (eye emergencies), or convulsions.
- If the victim vomits, protect the airway.

Box 27.19 Poisoning First Aid: Don'ts for Lay Persons

- Do not give an unconscious victim anything by mouth
- Do not induce vomiting unless you are told to do so by the Poison Control Center or a doctor
- Do not try to neutralize the poison with lemon juice or vinegar, or any other substance, unless you are told to do so by the Poison Control Center or a doctor. Do not apply any kind of potentially harmful herbal and folk remedies
- Do not use any "cure-all" type antidote
- Do not wait for symptoms to develop if you suspect that someone has been poisoned

Flowchart 27.5: A general approach to a child with poisoning

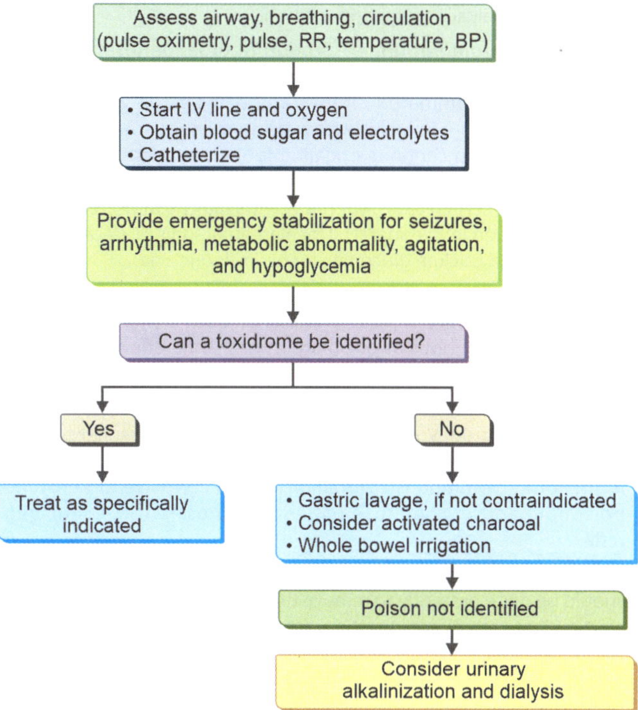

Flowchart 27.5 depicts a general approach to a child with poisoning.

Emergency Stabilization Measures

The priority is to assess airway and breathing, checking oxygen saturation by pulse oximetry and obtaining vital signs (pulse, respiratory rate, blood pressure), and looking for any potential life-threatening abnormality. Blood should be withdrawn for arterial blood gas (ABG), glucose, electrolytes, and also saved for other studies. Urinary tract catheterization also needs to be done for urinary output monitoring and other studies.

The unconscious patient should be transported in the head-down semi-prone position to minimize the risk of aspiration of gastric contents. Potentially serious abnormalities such as metabolic acidosis, hyperkalemia, and hypoglycemia may require correction as a matter of urgency. Neurological assessment is done by calculating the Glasgow Coma Score (GCS). Monitor the vital signs every 5–15 minutes.

Contrary to popular belief, many poisons and drugs taken in overdose do not cause rapid loss of consciousness. Many drugs and poisons can cause convulsions, which, if recurrent, should be controlled with IV diazepam. Hypotension with peripheral circulatory failure is treated by correction of volume deficit, hypoxia, and acidosis. If adequate perfusion is not restored by these measures, the circulating volume should be increased by administration of a plasma expander intravenously. Cardiac arrhythmias are often improved or abolished by correction of hypoxia, acidosis, and electrolyte imbalance.

The next step should be to take a detailed history and perform physical examination. Aim is to try to identify the poison, or the toxidrome. Key to diagnosis of the toxidrome is provided in the next section.

Removal of Toxin

The aim of decontamination procedures is to reduce the absorption of poison. It can be achieved by following measures:

Eye decontamination: Ocular exposure to solvents, e.g., hydrocarbons, detergents, alcohol, or corrosive agents requires immediate local decontamination. This is achieved by copious irrigation with neutralizing solution (normal saline or water) for at least 30 minutes. Do not use acid or alkaline irrigating solution.

Dermal decontamination: Absorption of organophosphorus and related compounds through cutaneous route can also be fatal. Remove all contaminated clothes and irrigate the whole- body including nail, groin, skinfolds with water or saline as soon as possible after exposure and continue irrigating for at least 15 minutes. *Water should not be used to decontaminate skin in exposures to sodium and phosphorus*. In certain cases, specific agents may be indicated for skin decontamination (e.g., mineral oil for elemental sodium, Neosporin for super glue, and calcium gluconate for hydrofluoric acid).

Gut decontamination: This includes: (1) gastric emptying, (2) adsorbent administration, and (3) catharsis. Gastric emptying is most effective within 1 hour of poisoning it has some effect within 1–4 hours; it is ineffective when used at a late stage.

Emesis: It is the preferred method of emptying the stomach in conscious children. Vomiting can be induced by administration of copious draughts of warm water. Syrup of ipecac is not used now. Induction of vomiting is contraindicated in corrosive or kerosene poisoning and in comatose patients or those with absent gag reflex.

Gastric lavage: If the vomiting does not occur quickly, gastric lavage should be done promptly to remove the poison. In a symptomatic but alert patient with minor ingestion, activated charcoal alone by mouth is sufficient for gastrointestinal decontamination.

The child is kept in the left lateral position with the head hanging over edge of the table and the face down. A large single lumen tube with multiple distal ports is necessary. A restraint is required for most children and mouth gag is placed in the mouth before the procedure. The catheter is passed gently, and free end is dipped under water to make sure that the catheter is not in the airway. Generally, tap water is used for lavage and four or five washes are done. The volume of each aliquot should be at least 10–15 mL/kg until clear. After the fluid has been instilled, it should be removed by gravity drainage or tube suction. Catheter is pinched before it is finally withdrawn, or suction is maintained during withdrawal to prevent aspiration.

Gastric lavage should not be performed in children with poor gag reflex or corrosive ingestion. In kerosene poisoning, lavage may be done very cautiously if the child has consumed a large gulp of kerosene and is brought quickly to the hospital, otherwise it is better to avoid stomach wash.

Adsorbents: An agent capable of binding to a toxic agent in the gut is known as adsorbent. Activated charcoal is the most widely used adsorbent. It is created by subjecting carbonaceous material, e.g., wood, coal, etc., to steam at 600–900°C and acid. For the comatose patient (Grades 3 or 4) with potentially serious overdose, gastric lavage is followed by administration of single dose of activated charcoal via an orogastric or nasogastric tube within 1–2 hours of ingestion.

Dose of activated charcoal administered should be at least 10 times the dose of ingested toxic material. The usual single dose is 1–2 g/kg for children and adults. Multiple dosing (1 g/kg every 2–6 hours) is effective for poisoning with phenobarbitone, phenytoin, digitalis, and theophylline. In asymptomatic patient presenting early or without reliable history, 15–30 g of activated charcoal may be used.

Catharsis: Laxatives and purgatives may be given for poisoning with substances which do not cause corrosive action on gastrointestinal mucosa. Increased motility of the gut may reduce absorption. Commonly used cathartics include sorbitol and mannitol (1–2 g/kg), and magnesium or sodium sulfate (200–300 mg/kg). Do not give magnesium salt cathartics to children with renal failure.

Whole bowel irrigation (WBI) with polyethylene glycol electrolyte solution at the rate of 0.5 L/h for 4–6 hours should be considered for patients presenting after 2 hours of enteric coated or sustained release drug ingestion including severe iron poisoning. Concurrent administration of activated charcoal and WBI may decrease the effectiveness of charcoal.

Use of gastric decontamination is highly individualized. It is not universal. The American Academy of Clinical Toxicologists does not endorse the routine use of any form of gastric decontamination (i.e., gastric lavage, ipecac administration, cathartics, WBI, single dose activated charcoal, etc.) for ingested poisons.

Specific Antidote Therapy

The antidotes may be physiological, chemical, or physical. *Chemical antidotes* combine with the poison and render it innocuous. *Physiological antidotes* counteract the effects of the poison on the metabolism and physiological functions of the body and thus prevent its harmful effects. *Physical antidotes* prevent the contact of the poisonous substance with the target organ or adsorb the toxic components, thus preventing their toxicity.

Specific antidotes may be lifesaving, but they are not often available and are effective for <5% of poisoning cases. When obtainable, they must be given without delay for maximum protective action. Some examples of antidotes and other drugs that may be needed are listed in **Table 27.18**.

Antidotes now considered obsolete include universal antidote for ingested poisons, acetazolamide for modification of urinary pH, ascorbic acid for methemoglobinemia, castor oil as cathartic, nalorphine for opiates, sodium chloride for emesis, and tannins for alkaloids.

Promotion of Excretion of Toxin

The efficiency of regimens for enhancement of drug elimination from the body can be predicted to a large extent if the physiochemical properties, disposition, and pharmacokinetics of the substance are known. The fluid intake is increased to promote glomerular filtration and excretion of poison through the urine.

- ***Forced diuresis:*** Diuresis alone has relatively little effect on drug elimination because the renal clearance is proportional to the urine flow rate. In the case of drugs which are weak organic acids and bases, a much greater effect on clearance can be obtained by manipulation of the urine pH. The lipid solubility and hence tubular reabsorption of such acidic and basic drugs is decreased in alkaline and acidic urine, respectively; and their renal clearance is increased correspondingly. Theoretically for each change of one unit in urine pH, the renal clearance could change by a factor of 10. Urine pH is therefore much more important than urine flow rate.
- ***Forced alkaline diuresis*** is restricted largely to poisoning with phenobarbitone and salicylate, although much of the effect in lowering plasma salicylate concentrations result from hemodilution rather than increased urinary excretion. Raise the urinary pH to 7.5 for weak acids (e.g., barbiturates, salicylates) with sodium bicarbonate.
- ***Forced acidic diuresis:*** Maintain urinary pH to 5.5–6.5 in poisoning with weak bases, e.g., tricyclic antidepressant and phenytoin, with ammonium chloride 4 g administered every 2 hours through Ryle's tube.

Any form of forced diuresis is potentially dangerous. Forced diuresis is contraindicated in patients with cardiac and renal impairment; complications include water intoxication, disturbances of acid-base and electrolyte balance, left ventricular failure with pulmonary edema, and cerebral edema.

Hemodialysis, hemoperfusion, and peritoneal dialysis: Drugs which can be removed reasonably effectively by hemoperfusion and hemodialysis include barbiturates, carbamazepine, salicylates, theophylline, dapsone,

Table 27.18 Few Specific Antidotes	
Antidote/drug	*Indication*
Atropine (injection)	Organophosphates, carbamates (A1)
Amyl nitrite (inhalation)	Cyanides (A2)
Antidigoxin Fab (antibody fragments)	Digoxin (A1)
Acetylcysteine	Paracetamol (B1)
Beta-blockers	Sympathomimetics (A1), theophylline (B1)
Budesonide (inhalation)	Irritant gases
Calcium sodium edetate	Lead (C2)
Dicobalt edetate	Cyanides (A1)
Calcium gluconate	Hydrofluoric acid (A1)
Copper solution	Phosphorus white (yellow)
Diazepam	Chloroquine, organophosphates (A2)
Dimercaprol	Arsenic (B3), Mercury, heavy metals (C3)
Desferrioxamine	Iron (B1), aluminum (C2)
Antidote/drug	*Indication*
Flumazenil	Benzodiazepines (B1)
Ethanol	Methanol (A1)
Glucagon	Beta-blockers (A1)
Glucose	Insulin (A1)
Methionine	Paracetamol (B1)
Methylene blue	Nitrites, nitrobenzene (A1)
Naloxone	Opioid analgesics (A1)
Neostigmine	Anticholinergic poisoning (B2)
Oxygen	Carbon monoxide (A1)
Penicillamine	Copper (C1)
Pralidoxime (injection)	Organophosphates (A1)
Polyethylene glycol 400 (topical)	Phenol
Physostigmine	Anticholinergics, tricyclic antidepressants (A1)
Pyridoxine	Isoniazid (A2)
Sodium nitrite	Cyanide (A1)
Sodium nitroprusside	Ergotism (A1)
Sodium thiosulfate	Cyanide (A1)
Clotting factors	Warfarin (A1)

The classification in terms of urgency of availability (A, B, C) or proven effectiveness (1, 2, 3) is given next to the main indication

A Required to be immediately available within 30 minutes
B Required to be available within 2 hours
C Required to be available within 6 hours
1 Effectiveness well documented
2 Widely used, not universally accepted as effective
3 Questionable usefulness

most antibiotics, lithium, chloral hydrate, methanol, and ethylene glycol. In general, hemoperfusion with coated charcoal or exchange resins is more effective than hemodialysis, although the latter may be preferred for simultaneous correction of acid–base and electrolyte balance (e.g., in salicylate poisoning). Hemodialysis is also the method of choice for removal of methanol, ethylene glycol, and lithium.

Peritoneal dialysis is much less effective, and it is used rarely. It has the advantage that it does not require special facilities but may be complicated by fluid and electrolyte abnormalities, perforation, peritonitis, and adhesions.

Dialysis is not useful in poisoning with digitalis, antihistamines, belladonna alkaloids, opiates, etc.

TOXIDROMES

Toxidrome refers to the group of signs and symptoms that consistently result from particular toxins. **Table 27.19** provides examples of some common toxidromes.

Sympathomimetic Syndrome

Etiology

Prescription medications for asthma (salbutamol, terbutaline, theophylline), decongestants (pseudoephedrine), attention deficit hyperactivity disorder (ADHD) medications (dextroamphetamine, methylphenidate), illicit drugs (amphetamines, cocaine, ecstasy), thyroid hormones, and monoamine oxidase (MAO) inhibitors.

Clinical Features

Sympathomimetic toxic syndrome results from the activation of the sympathetic system, manifesting as tachycardia, hyperthermia, hypertension, mydriasis, agitation, and diaphoresis. End-organ effects include stroke, rhabdomyolysis, DIC, and psychosis which may progress to seizures and coma.

Table 27.19 Examples of Symptom Complexes/Toxidromes

Pupils	*Respiration*	*Consciousness*	*Possible agent*	*Other associations*
Pinpoint	↑↓	Coma	Organophosphorus insecticides, carbamates	*Cholinergic:* Bradycardia, wheeze, salivation
	↓	Coma	Opioids	Hypotension, hypothermia
	↓	Coma	Phenothiazines	Cardiac arrhythmia
Dilated	↑	Agitation, hallucination	Atropine	*Anticholinergic:* Fever, dry mucous membranes, flushing, and urinary retention
	↓	Coma	Tricyclic antidepressants	Cardiac arrhythmia, seizures, hypotension
	↓	Coma	Sedatives, barbiturates	Hypotension, hypothermia, hyporeflexia
	↑	Agitation, hallucination	Theophylline, amphetamines	Seizures, tachycardia, hypertension, acidosis
Normal	↑	Coma	Uremia	Acidosis, hyperkalemia
	↑	Semi-coma	Salicylates	Tinnitus, agitation, diaphoresis, alkalosis followed by acidosis

TREATMENT Sympathomimetic Syndrome

Management includes supportive measures in the form of hydration and active cooling for hyperthermia. Agitation, tachycardia, and hypertension respond to benzodiazepine administration. For MDMA/ecstasy use by adolescents (used in rave parties), it is important to monitor serum sodium, as it can cause inappropriate antidiuretic hormone (ADH) secretion, leading to hyponatremia and presenting clinically as altered mental status and seizures.

Anticholinergic Toxic Syndrome

Etiology

The most common cause is poisoning by *Datura stramonium* (jimson weed). Antihistamines and tricyclic antidepressants are the other incriminating agents. It blocks the action of acetylcholine at the muscarinic receptor sites.

Clinical Manifestations

This includes flushing, dry mucous membranes, mydriasis, delirium, and hyperthermia. The mnemonic for remembering these manifestations is *"red as a beet, dry as a bone, blind as a bat, mad as hatter, and hot as hare."*

TREATMENT Anticholinergic Toxic Syndrome

Physostigmine (0.02 mg/kg, maximum 0.5 mg) is the antidote for anticholinergic toxicity, and it reversibly inhibits cholinesterases in both central and peripheral nervous system, allowing acetylcholine to accumulate and overcome the antimuscarinic effects. It should be used only if the following preconditions are satisfied: (1) evidence of severe CNS and peripheral anticholinergic effects; (2) normal QRS interval (<0.08 seconds); (3) no history of seizures; (4) severe agitation, coma, or cardiovascular instability unresponsive to other treatments, such as benzodiazepines; and (5) no history of ingestion of tricyclic antidepressants.

Physostigmine is infused slowly over 5 minutes. Additional doses may be necessary if symptoms reoccur, as its duration of action is 60–70 minutes.

Cholinergic Toxic Syndrome

Etiology

The most common source of cholinergic exposure is ingestion or dermal exposure to pesticides, i.e., organophosphates and carbamates. Other sources include muscarine-containing mushrooms, methacholine, carbachol, bethanechol, and nicotine alkaloids.

Clinical Features

These compounds render the enzyme acetylcholinesterase nonfunctional, by binding with it. As a result, acetylcholine can no longer be metabolized and accumulates leading to excessive stimulation of central and peripheral acetylcholine receptors, leading to altered mental status, diffuse muscle weakness, and excessive secretory activity. The mnemonics to remember its manifestations are *DUMBBELS* (for muscarinic effects)—*D*iarrhea, *U*rination, *M*iosis, *B*ronchorrhea, *B*ronchospasm, *E*mesis, *L*acrimation, *S*ecretions; and *CCC* (for central nicotinic effects)—*C*onfusion, *C*oma, *C*onvulsions.

- The route of exposure affects the temporal onset of symptoms, with respiratory route producing a rapid onset of systemic symptoms than dermal exposure.
- The initial presentation with dermal route may be muscle fasciculation and sweating whereas inhalational route may produce central effects, miosis, rapid onset of bronchospasm, and bronchorrhea.
- Ingestion may produce nausea, vomiting and diarrhea prior to other features. Organophosphate-induced delayed neuropathy can occur 2–3 weeks postexposure, presenting as profound weakness of the lower extremities. Another delayed manifestation that has been reported in children recovering from the cholinergic phase is bilateral vocal cord palsy after 1–4 days of exposure, requiring prolonged respiratory support.

TREATMENT Cholinergic Toxic Syndrome

Initial management consists of decontamination of skin, eyes, and gastrointestinal tract. BLS with support of the airway is initiated. Therapy is initiated with atropine (0.02 mg/kg IV every 5–10 minutes) for the reduction of secretions and bronchospasm.

Pralidoxime the specific antidote, is started (25–30 mg/kg infused over 30 minutes) and repeated in 4–6 hours if there are persistent nicotinic symptoms.

Opioid Toxic Syndrome

Opioids are commonly used analgesics and drugs of abuse. Opioid toxidrome usually presents secondary to substance abuse (heroin). It is characterized by a clinical triad of respiratory depression, depressed mental status, and miosis.

TREATMENT **Opioid Toxic Syndrome**

Toxicologic screens remain positive 48–72 hours after ingestion. Naloxone is a competitive opioid antagonist that acts on mu, kappa, and delta receptors and can be used to rapidly reverse respiratory depression related to opioid toxicity.

Sedative-Hypnotic Toxic Syndrome

Sedative hypnotics (barbiturates, benzodiazepines, chloral hydrate), and alcohol may produce obtundation and coma, with normal vital signs at presentation with acute intoxication.

Setting

There are three possible scenarios of exposure to these agents for the pediatric age groups. Firstly, a young child with unintentional exposure, second group is that of children undergoing diagnostic or therapeutic procedures in the hospital setting, and thirdly adolescents may consume these drugs intentionally for suicidal intent or as drug abuse.

Clinical Features

Most patients present with altered mental status and relatively normal vital signs. As symptoms progress, bradycardia, hypotension, and hypothermia can occur due to CNS depression. Chloral hydrate may cause nausea, vomiting, abdominal pain, and cardiac dysrhythmias. Some of these agents can produce fatal respiratory depression.

TREATMENT **Sedative-Hypnotic Toxic Syndrome**

- Activated charcoal use can reduce the serum half-lives of barbiturates such as phenobarbital and prevents absorption by adsorbing drug in the intestine.
- Multidose charcoal may interrupt enterohepatic recirculation and enhance elimination by enterocapillary exsorption. Theoretically, by constantly bathing the gastrointestinal tract with charcoal, the intestinal lumen serves as a dialysis membrane for reverse absorption of drug from intestinal villous capillary blood into intestinal lumen, from where it can get adsorbed on to the activated charcoal. An initial dose of 1 g/kg is recommended followed by 0.25 g/kg every 4–6 hours.
- Charcoal aqueous solutions are premixed with a cathartic (usually sorbitol 70%), so these patients should not be given additional doses of cathartic to prevent dehydration and electrolyte imbalances. There is anecdotal evidence for use of physostigmine for gamma hexabenzene toxicity but there is no proven antidote for it.
- Urinary alkalinization with sodium bicarbonate to a pH of 7.5–8.0 can hasten the renal excretion of phenobarbital, which is a weak acid and is excreted primarily from the kidneys. This can be done with an initial dose of 1 mEq/kg of sodium bicarbonate, followed by a continuous infusion. This usually requires close monitoring of urine pH and blood pH, trying to keep the former >7.5 and the latter <7.5 to prevent over-alkalinization. Alkalinization does not increase excretion of shorter acting agents as they are mostly metabolized by the liver.

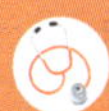

CASE STUDY **Unresponsive Child**

A 2-year-old previously healthy male child is brought to the emergency room in an unresponsive state. The child had been playing unattended in his grandparents' room and was later found lying on the floor by his mother. Child is unresponsive, and GCS score is 12.

What will you do now?

Assess CAB. Assessment of vital signs along with immediate evaluation of circulatory state (peripheral pulses–presence and volume; skin perfusion by CRT), patency of airway, and the rate and depth of breathing should be performed rapidly.

This child had heart rate of 100/min, adequate perfusion, no audible stridor, respiratory rate was 12/min, and had good air entry on auscultation with no abnormal breath sounds. Blood pressure was 100/72 mm Hg, and pulse oximetry showed oxyhemoglobin saturation of 97%.

Do you need to perform any urgent laboratory tests?

Obtain blood sample for blood glucose and electrolytes.

His blood glucose value is 98 mg/dL and his electrolytes are normal. Parents revealed that his grandmother's medication box was found open by his side and there were several pills on the floor. The child's grandmother has type 2 diabetes, hypertension, and also takes sleeping pills at night. Grandmother's medication list includes—oral hypoglycemic agents, antihypertensive medications [beta-blocker and angiotensin-converting enzyme (ACE) inhibitor] and benzodiazepine.

Outline your further evaluation in view of this history.

Based on this information, we should consider accidental ingestion as the likely cause of the child's symptoms. Additional evaluations may include neurologic evaluation (assessment of pupils, muscle tone, and tendon reflexes), heart rhythm evaluation, and monitoring of body temperature and secretions.

This child had mildly dilated pupils that were reactive to light, normal heart rhythm, no increase in upper airway secretions, and body temperature was 36.8°C.

Can a toxidrome be identified?

Based on the history of sudden unresponsiveness accompanied by dilated reactive pupils, normal heart rate and rhythm, reduced respiratory rate, and reduced body temperature, it is likely that the child has ingested a benzodiazepine.

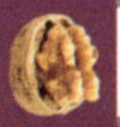

IN A NUTSHELL

Poisoning: Diagnosis and Management

1. Toxidrome refers to the group of signs and symptoms that consistently result from toxins.
2. Most of the poisonings in children are accidental in nature. The most common agents responsible for poisoning in Southeast Asia are pesticides, corrosives, prescription drugs, and household chemicals.
3. The peak age for childhood poisoning is between 1 and 3 years.
4. Specific antidotes are available for very few commonly encountered poisons, and treatment is usually nonspecific and symptomatic.
5. Management consists of emergency first aid and stabilization measures, appropriate treatment to reduce absorption, measures to enhance life support, and followed by psychiatric counseling.

Aldridge MD. Acute iron poisoning: what every pediatric intensive care unit nurse should know. Dimens Crit Care Nurs. 2007;26(2):43-8.
American Academy of Pediatrics. Committee on drugs. Treatment guidelines for lead exposure in children. Pediatrics. 1995;96:155-60.
American Academy of Pediatrics Committee on Injury, Violence, and Poison Prevention. Poison treatment in the home. American Academy of Pediatrics Committee on Injury, Violence, and Poison Prevention. Pediatrics. 2003;112(5):1182-5.
Baranwal AK, Singhi SC. Acute iron poisoning: management guidelines. Indian Pediatr. 2003;40(6):534-40.
Barry JD. Diagnosis and management of the poisoned child. Pediatr Ann. 2005;34:937-46.
Bond GR. The role of activated charcoal and gastric emptying in gastrointestinal decontamination: a state-of-the-art review. Ann Emerg Med. 2002;39:273-86.
Chyka PA, Seger D, Krenzelok EP, et al. American Academy of Clinical Toxicology; European Association of Poisons Centres and Clinical Toxicologists. Position paper: Single-dose activated charcoal. Clin Toxicol (Phila). 2005;43:61-87.
Collee GG, Hanson GC. The management of acute poisoning. Br J Anaesth. 1993;70:562-73.
Craft AW, Lawson GR, Williams H, et al. Accidental childhood poisoning with household products. BMJ. 1984;288(6418):682.
Flomenbaum NE, Goldfrank LR. Principles of managing the poisoned or overdosed patient. In: Flomenbaum NE, Goldfrank LR, Hoffman RS, et al (Eds). Goldfrank's Toxicologic Emergencies, 8th edition. New York: McGraw-Hill Professional; 2006. pp. 42-50.
Freudenthal W, Ralston ME. Toxicity. Organophosphates. E Med J. 2001;2:7.
Gupta P, Singh RP, Murali MV, et al. Kerosene oil poisoning-A childhood menace. Indian Pediatr. 1992;29(8):979-84.
Gupta S, Taneja V. Poisoned child: emergency room management. Indian J Pediatr. 2003;70:S2-8.
Heard K. Gastrointestinal decontamination. Med Clin North Am. 2005; 89:1067-78.
Hui WF, Hon KL, Leung AKC. An Overview of the Pediatric Toxidromes and Poisoning Management. Curr Rev Clin Exp Pharmacol. 2021;16(4):318-30.
Jayashree M, Singhi S, Gupta A. Predictors of outcome in children with hydrocarbon poisoning receiving intensive care. Indian Pediatr. 2006;43(8):715-9.
Karunakara BP, Shobavat L, Ashwath. Poisoning in Children. IAP Standard Treatment Guidelines 2022. Available from: https://iapindia.org/pdf/Ch-109-Poisoning-in-Children.pdf. *[Last accessed January 2025]* Available from http://www.cdc.gov/ncipc/factsheets/poisoning-overview.html [Last accessed January 2025].
Lakshmi CP, Vijayahari R, Kate V, et al. A hospital based epidemiological study of corrosive alimentary injuries with particular reference to the Indian experience. Nat Med J India. 2013;26(1):31-6.
Lifsitz M, Shahak E, Sofer S. Carbamate and organophosphate poisoning in young children. Pediatr Emerg Care. 1999;15(2):102-3.
Manoguerra AS, Cobaugh DJ; Guidelines for the Management of Poisoning Consensus Panel. Guideline on the use of ipecac syrup in the out-of-hospital management of ingested poisons. Clin Toxicol. 2005;43:1-10.
Manoguerra AS, Erdman AR, Booze LL, et al. Iron ingestion: an evidence-based consensus guideline for out-of-hospital management. Clin Toxicol. 2005;43(6):553-70.
MedlinePlus Medical Encyclopedia. Poisoning First Aid. [online] Available from http://www.nlm.nih.gov/medlineplus/ency/article/007579html [Last accessed November 2022].
Mofenson HC, Caraccio TR. Toxidromes. Compr Ther. 1985;11:46-52. National Center for Injury Prevention and Control. Poisonings: Overview.
Position paper: Cathartics. J Toxicol Clin Toxicol. 2004;42(3):243-53. Position paper: Ipecac syrup. J Toxicol Clin Toxicol. 2004;42(2):133-43. Position paper: Whole bowel irrigation. J Toxicol Clin Toxicol. 2004;42(6):843-54.
Ressel GW, AAP. AAP releases policy statement on poison treatment in the home. Am Fam Physician. 2004;69(3):741-2.
Tarabar AF, Hoffman RS. Pediatric toxic syndromes (toxidromes). In: Erickson TB, Ahrens WR, Aks SE, et al. (Eds). Pediatric Toxicology– Diagnosis and Management of the Poisoned Child, 1st edition. New York: McGraw-Hill; 2005. pp. 75-83.
Vale JA, Kulig K; American Academy of Clinical Toxicology; European Association of Poisons Centres and Clinical Toxicologists. Position paper: gastric lavage. J Toxicol Clin Toxicol. 2004;42(7):933-43.

27.12 Corrosive Poisoning

Corrosive poisonings in children have now surpassed kerosene oil poisoning as the most common cause of household accidental poisonings. This is due to common availability of toilet cleaner fluids in households. Pediatric acid and caustic ingestions often involve toddlers who find these solutions stored inappropriately in unsafe easy-to-open containers and ingest small volumes in the course of their exploratory behaviors.

EPIDEMIOLOGY

The most common acid-containing agents that are accidentally ingested include toilet bowl cleaners (contain sulfuric or hydrochloric acid), antirust solutions (hydrofluoric, oxalic, and hydrochloric acids), swimming pool cleaners (hydrofluoric acid), and vinegar (acetic acid). Due to their unpleasant taste and odor, they get swallowed rapidly in smaller amounts and cause more gastric injury than esophageal injury.

Alkaline agents such as household cleaners (containing sodium hydroxide), drain openers, bleaches, toilet bowl cleaners, and dishwashing detergents are generally swallowed in larger amounts and cause more transmural injuries due to liquefactive necrosis. The epidemiology of corrosive injuries varies by country and the most prevalent household chemical agents that children have access to. *Data from limited case series published from various sites in India indicate that toilet bowl cleaner (acid) ingestion is one of the most common corrosive ingestion in the country.*

PATHOGENESIS

In the first 3–4 days, the epithelium develops erythema, edema, ulceration, and necrosis, with associated bacterial invasion and tissue sloughing. After 4 days, neovascularization and fibroblast proliferation facilitate granulation and collagen cross-linking. The tensile strength is lowest at this time, and the risk of perforation is the highest. The healing process continues for 3–6 weeks after injury and causes fibrosis, contractures, and cicatrization, leading to strictures.

Ocular or dermal exposure may cause burns and scarring of varying severity. Inhalation injury can cause upper airway involvement with severe epiglottic and laryngeal edema and ulceration, or lower airway involvement with pneumonitis and impaired gas exchange. Children presenting with stridor have laryngeal involvement which can very quickly progress to life-threatening airway obstruction.

CLINICAL FEATURES

The clinical progression of esophageal injury takes place in three stages, which correspond with the histopathologic changes. Children experience severe pain on contact with the solution, and they present with swelling of the lips, mouth and oropharynx, with drooling and refusal to drink. Retrosternal chest pain, hematemesis, or abdominal pain signifies esophageal or gastric injury. Fever, dyspnea, chest pain, and subcutaneous emphysema herald the onset of mediastinitis. Other complications include peritonitis due to perforation of viscera, hemorrhage secondary to vessel erosion, aortoesophageal or tracheoesophageal fistulae, and pulmonary thrombosis.

EVALUATION

Chest X-ray should be done to rule out mediastinitis or esophageal perforation, and lateral view of neck to demonstrate laryngeal edema. Flexible endoscopic visualization of the upper gastrointestinal tract in the first 48 hours is the cornerstone of management and is indicated for any large volume ingestion, patient with severe respiratory distress, stridor, or hematemesis. In addition, presence of any two of the following symptoms—vomiting, prolonged drooling, abdominal pain, dysphagia and refusal to drink, are further indications for endoscopic evaluation.

TREATMENT Corrosive Poisoning

Supportive Therapy

Any residual corrosive solution should immediately be removed from the patient's clothing, skin, and eyes by lavage with copious amounts of sterile saline. Emesis is contraindicated and charcoal use is ineffective, and it can induce emesis and obscure endoscopic visualization.

- *Neutralization:* The process utilizes a weakly basic solution for acid ingestion and vice versa for alkali ingestion to neutralize pH and minimize tissue damage. However, being an exothermic reaction, neutralization can exacerbate tissue injury, and its utility is limited as most damage occurs almost instantaneously after ingestion.
- *Dilution*, by administering a neutral solution such as water or milk, can minimize tissue contact and decrease transit time without any thermal tissue damage. But clinical utility is limited to immediate use at home right after ingestion of small amounts in cooperative children only. There is a potential risk of perforation due to introduction of fluids into already injured esophageal tissue.
- *Steroids:* Another controversial modality is the routine use of steroids, with the premise of reducing pathologic collagen cross-linking, shortening, and cicatrization. Although, children with first-degree injuries do not develop strictures, and those with third-degree injury almost always progress to strictures, it is the children with second degree injuries who have a variable outcome and have the greatest potential of benefit from administration of methylprednisolone (2 mg/kg/day) or dexamethasone (1 mg/kg/day), preferably within 24 hours of injury. Concomitant use of antibiotics is also recommended.

Specific Therapy

Specific therapy is recommended for hydrofluoric acid exposure, which is commonly found in cleaning, etching, and rust removing products. After copious irrigation, topical application of calcium gluconate gel should be initiated, with minor burns requiring intradermal injection of 5% calcium gluconate, administered 0.5–1 cm away from the site of the burn. For severe burns, intra-arterial injection of calcium gluconate is recommended, and for oral ingestion, IV calcium and magnesium supplementation is given.

PROGNOSIS

Esophageal stricture is the most common long-term adverse outcome. Gastric outlet obstruction and dysmotility may occur, in addition to scarring of other systems like the upper respiratory tract, face, or eyes. Longitudinal studies have shown 1,000-fold increased risk of gastric and esophageal malignancies, occurring at an average of 40 years after the exposure. Children in whom endoscopy reveals significant lesions therefore need lifelong surveillance.

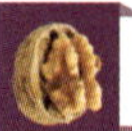

IN A NUTSHELL

Corrosive Poisoning

1. Corrosive poisoning is one of the most common causes of household accidental poisonings in children.
2. Clinical features of corrosive poisoning include severe pain, swelling of lips, mouth, and oral cavity, with drooling and refusal to drink or feed.
3. *Flexible endoscopic visualization of the upper gastrointestinal* tract in the first 48 hours is the cornerstone of management in corrosive poisoning.
4. Treatment is mainly supportive.
5. Esophageal stricture is the most common long-term adverse outcome.

Contini S, Scarpignato C. Caustic injury of the upper gastrointestinal tract: a comprehensive review. World J Gastroenterol. 2013;19(25):3918-30.
Ghosh VB, Jhamb U, Singhal R, et al. Common childhood poisonings and their outcome in a tertiary care center in Delhi. Indian J Pediatr. 2013;80(6):516-8.
Hoffman RS, Burns MM, Gosselin S. Ingestion of caustic substances. N Engl J Med. 2020;382:1739-48.
Urganci N, Usta M, Kalyoncu D, et al. Corrosive substance ingestion in children. Indian J Pediatr. 2014;81(7):675-9.

27.13 Kerosene Poisoning

PE 14.1

The incidence of kerosene oil poisoning has declined since it is not widely available now. Even then, kerosene oil is still used as fuel for cooking and lighting purposes in certain parts of the world with shortage of cooking gas and electricity.

CLINICAL FEATURES

Most of the cases occur between 1 and 3 years of age. Children become symptomatic in <70% cases following ingestion of kerosene, with onset soon after to within 10 hours of ingestion. Breathlessness, fever, cough, restlessness, and abdominal distention are the common symptoms. If symptoms do not develop within 6 hours of ingestion, the patient is usually normal.

- ***Respiratory symptoms*** occur because of chemical pneumonitis. Respiratory involvement ranges from mild symptoms or rapid progression to ARDS and respiratory failure. Coughing, fast breathing, chest wall retractions, increased work of breathing and wheezing are common symptoms of aspiration pneumonitis. Cyanosis may be present.
- ***Gastrointestinal symptoms*** include nausea, vomiting, diarrhea, and abdominal pain. Vomiting increases the risk of aspiration.
- ***Central nervous system symptoms*** such as headache, dizziness, drowsiness, euphoria, restlessness, ataxia, poor ventilatory drive, convulsions, and coma, may occur.
- Fever is seen in up to one-third cases. Persistence of fever >48–72 hours points toward bacterial infection.

DIAGNOSIS

A chest radiograph is indicated in all children presenting with kerosene ingestion and respiratory symptoms. Initially, chest radiograph may be normal but eventually may show abnormalities within 6 hours of aspiration in most symptomatic cases. Typical radiographic findings include increased bronchovascular markings and infiltrates involving right basilar or bilateral basilar and perihilar regions. Lobar consolidation, pneumothorax, pneumomediastinum, and pleural effusion are less common.

TREATMENT Kerosene Oil Poisoning

- The management of kerosene poisoning is supportive and symptomatic.
- Any child with respiratory symptoms (grunting, tachypnea, or cyanosis) must be started on humidified oxygen and an ABG analysis should be done.
- Nebulization with beta-2 agonists may be required in children with bronchospasm.
- Children with hypoxemia unresponsive to supplemental oxygen or severe CNS involvement may require early intubation and mechanical ventilation.
- Gastric lavage is usually contraindicated as there is a higher risk of aspiration than systemic absorption and is indicated only if the amount ingested is massive and the child is brought within 30 minutes of ingestion. Activated charcoal is not beneficial.

PROGNOSIS

Ingestion of >30 mL of kerosene oil adversely affects the clinical and radiological profile. Severely malnourished children have extensive radiological changes and poor clinical outcome. Mortality ranges from 2 to 10%.

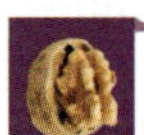

IN A NUTSHELL

Kerosene Oil Poisoning

- The incidence of kerosene oil poisoning has declined recently.
- Children become symptomatic in >70% cases with onset soon after to within 10 hours of ingestion.
- Breathlessness, fever, cough, restlessness, and abdominal distention are the common symptoms.
- Respiratory symptoms occur because of chemical pneumonitis.
- A chest radiograph is indicated in all children with kerosene ingestion.
- The management of kerosene poisoning is supportive and symptomatic.

Kumar S, Kavitha TK, Angurana SK. Kerosene, camphor, and naphthalene poisoning in children. Indian J Crit Care Med. 2019;23(Suppl 4): S278-81.

27.14 Organophosphorus Poisoning

PE 14.2

According to hospital-based pediatric data on poisoning from India, pesticides constitute a significant proportion of causes ranging from 10 to 56%. The common pesticides reported in poisoning include organophosphates, carbamates, and pyrethroids.

RISK FACTORS

Organophosphate intoxication can occur via inhalation, oral absorption, and absorption through the skin. The risk factors for organophosphate poisoning in children include age <5 years, storage in easily accessible areas leading to accidental ingestion, pesticide availability in household, and children with developmental delay and mental illness.

PATHOPHYSIOLOGY

Organophosphate and carbamates are lipid-soluble agents and are well-absorbed through the skin, mucous membranes, gastrointestinal tract, and by inhalation. Substantial exposure can happen undetected through these routes as these substances do not produce local irritation. Once absorbed, they rapidly bind to the acetylcholinesterase enzyme found in all cholinergic nerve endings and red blood cells (RBCs). Carbamates bind reversibly to the enzyme, whereas the phosphorylation of acetylcholinesterase by organophosphate compounds can become irreversible with time (known an *aging*). The time taken for aging varies from few minutes in the case of certain nerve gases to many days for some commercially available pesticides. Oximes are antidotes which can only regenerate acetylcholinesterase that has not aged. Therefore, the effectiveness of oximes may be as short as few hours to as much as days depending on the compound involved.

Inhibition of acetylcholinesterase leads to the accumulation of acetylcholine which causes hyperstimulation of the acetylcholine receptors. This results in the clinical features of cholinergic overactivity at the muscarinic and nicotinic receptors and in the CNS. The nicotinic receptors are primarily distributed in the autonomic ganglia and neuromuscular junctions of skeletal muscles while muscarinic receptors are distributed in the visceral organs, secretory glands, and smooth muscles **(Table 27.20)**. The symptoms produced reflect the location of these receptors. Prolonged excessive stimulation of nicotinic receptors can lead to temporary downregulation and insensitivity to acetylcholine. This temporary insensitivity of varying severity which develops after 24–48 hours after exposure to organophosphates could be the possible explanation for development of the "intermediate syndrome" in organophosphate poisoning. It is named as "intermediate" as it is seen between the early cholinergic symptoms and the late- onset polyneuropathy.

CLINICAL FEATURES

The clinical spectrum of organophosphate poisoning encompasses three clinical syndromes:

1. The acute cholinergic phase
2. The intermediate syndrome
3. Organophosphate-induced delayed polyneuropathy (OPIDP)

The former two are life-threatening conditions while OPIDP is a disabling disease rarely seen in children. In most instances, the characteristic constellation of symptoms, "cholinergic toxidrome" is highly suggestive **(Table 27.21)**. The muscarinic [diarrhea, urination, miosis, bronchorrhea, bronchospasms, emesis, lacrimation, laxation, sweating (DUMBBELLS)], nicotinic [mydriasis, tachycardia, weakness, hypertension, and fasciculations (MTWHF)] and CNS features can occur in any combination; the predominant manifestations can vary from patient to patient and also in a given patient during the course of the illness. Practically, the most useful clinical features during routine management are salivation **(Fig. 27.19)**, decreased air entry into the lungs due to bronchorrhea and bronchospasm,

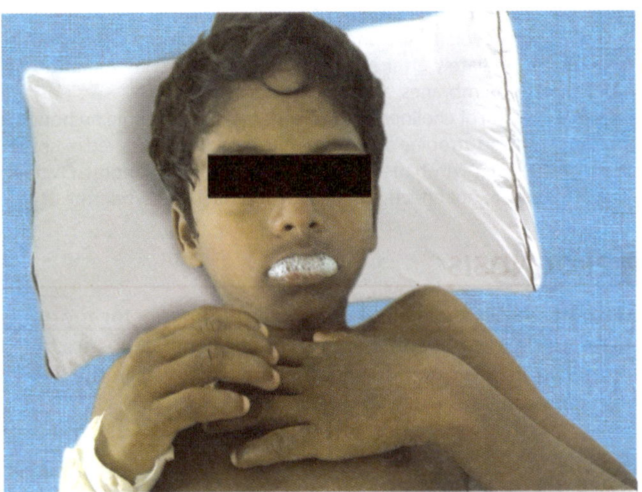

Fig. 27.19: Excessive salivation in a child with organophosphate poisoning

Table 27.20 Distribution of Muscarinic and Nicotinic Receptors

Peripheral nervous system				*Neuroendocrine system*	*Central nervous system*
Autonomic ganglia		Neuromuscular junction (skeletal muscle)	Parasympathetic peripheral junctions (smooth muscles, secretory glands, etc.)	Adrenal medulla	Nicotinic and muscarinic
Sympathetic	Parasympathetic	Nicotinic	Muscarinic	Nicotinic	
Nicotinic	Nicotinic				

Table 27.21 Signs and Symptoms of Organophosphate Poisoning (Cholinergic Toxidrome)

Muscarinic	*Nicotinic*		*Both muscarinic and nicotinic (Central nervous system)*
Parasympathetic system	*Sympathetic system*	*Neuromuscular junction*	
1. *D*iarrhea 2. *U*rination 3. *M*iosis 4. *B*radycardia, *B*ronchorrhea, *B*ronchospasm 5. *E*mesis 6. *L*acrimation, *L*ow blood pressure 7. *S*alivation, *S*ecretion, *S*weating	1. Mydriasis 2. Tachycardia 3. Hypertension, hyperglycemia 4. Sweating	1. Weakness 2. Fasciculation	1. Confusion 2. Convulsions 3. Coma

constricted pupils, excessive sweating, bradycardia, and hypotension.

The *intermediate syndrome* can occur in up to 20% of patients, 2–4 days after the exposure. The classical features are weakness of the neck (neck flop) and proximal muscles, progressing to involvement of respiratory muscles resulting in respiratory paralysis. Weakness recovers completely in a week with supportive therapy alone.

Low levels of plasma cholinesterase indicate exposure to organophosphates.

TREATMENT Organophosphorus Poisoning

Specific treatment consists of blocking the muscarinic effects by administering atropine, regeneration of acetylcholinesterase with the help of oximes, and mechanical ventilation for respiratory failure **(Box 27.20)**. Pralidoxime should be administered as an initial loading dose over 5–10 minutes followed by continuous infusion. Gastric lavage is controversial and should be considered only if the child is brought immediately after exposure. Thorough decontamination of skin, mucous membranes, and clothing are required.

Rapid reversal of cholinergic toxidrome is possible within an hour of presentation and atropine and oxime infusions can be tapered over the next 24–48 hours. Few patients may require ventilator support. Oximes and atropine are not effective in treating intermediate syndrome.

PROGNOSIS

Mortality varies from 15 to 30%. Key risk factors for mortality included delayed hospital arrival, inhalational exposure, need for mechanical ventilation, and high lactate levels in the first 24 hours of exposure.

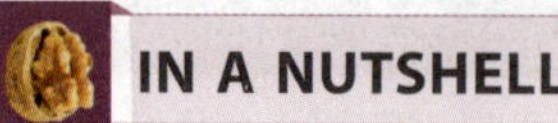

IN A NUTSHELL

Organophosphorus Poisoning

1. Organophosphate intoxication can occur via inhalation, oral absorption, and absorption through the skin.
2. The clinical spectrum of organophosphate poisoning encompasses three clinical syndromes: (1) Acute cholinergic phase, (2) Intermediate syndrome, and (3) Organophosphate-induced delayed polyneuropathy (OPIDP).
3. Clinical features of organophosphate poisoning include salivation, decreased air entry into the lungs due to bronchorrhea and bronchospasm, constricted pupils, excessive sweating, bradycardia, and hypotension.
4. The only laboratory tests used in clinical practice for confirmation of the diagnosis are RBC and plasma cholinesterase levels.
5. General principles of management regarding organophosphate poisoning are resuscitation at admission, administration of oxygen, blocking the muscarinic effects by administering atropine, regeneration of acetylcholinesterase with the help of oximes, and mechanical ventilation for respiratory failure.

Box 27.20 Treatment of Organophosphate Poisoning

- Check airway, breathing, and circulation. Place patient in the left lateral position, provide oxygen, if available. Intubate if necessary to maintain airway and breathing.
- Administer 0.01–0.04 mg/kg of atropine (minimum 0.1 mg) as a bolus intravenously. Will need higher initial doses in most instances. Start an infusion of isotonic fluids to maintain normal blood pressure and urine output above 0.5 mL/kg/h.
- Record pulse rate, blood pressure, pupil size, presence of sweat, and auscultatory findings at time of first atropine dose.
- Give pralidoxime chloride 20–40 mg/kg intravenously over 20–30 minutes; followed by an infusion of pralidoxime 5–10 mg/kg/h.
- After 5 minutes of giving atropine, check pulse, blood pressure, pupil size, sweat, and chest sounds. If no improvement, give double the initial dose of atropine.
- Monitor every 5 minutes; administer doubling doses of atropine if no response. Once signs of improvement are present, stop dose doubling. Tachycardia is not a contraindication to atropine since it can be caused by multiple factors. The pupils will usually dilate; however, this sign is not a useful endpoint for initial atropine treatment because a delay exists before maximum effect. However, very dilated pupils are an indicator of atropine toxicity.
- Once the child is stable, start atropine infusion hourly at 10–20% of the total dose required to reverse the muscarinic effects. Monitor hourly to see the degree of atropinization. If dose is less, cholinergic features will reappear. In that case repeat bolus doses of atropine as above and increase the infusion rate. If child becomes agitated and febrile with absent bowel sounds and urinary retention, suspect atropine overdose. Immediately stop the infusion and wait 30–60 minutes for these features to settle before starting again at a lower infusion rate.
- Continue the oxime infusion until atropine has not been needed for 12–24 hours.
- Assess strength of neck flexors regularly in conscious children by asking them to lift their head off the bed and hold it in that position. Any sign of weakness indicates that the child is at risk of developing peripheral respiratory failure (intermediate syndrome).
- If the child is agitated, review the dose of atropine infusion and provide adequate sedation with diazepam. Physical restraint of agitated patients can result in severe hyperthermia due to the combined effects of atropine (lack of sweating), agitation, and warm weather conditions. Hence, adequate sedation is important.
- Look for recurring cholinergic crisis due to release of fat soluble organophosphorus from fat stores. This can occur for several days to weeks after ingestion of some organophosphorus compounds. These patients will need retreatment with atropine and oxime.

Eddleston M, Buckley NA, Eyer P, et al. Management of acute organophosphorus pesticide poisoning. Lancet. 2008;371(9612): 597-607.

Karalliedde L, Baker D, Mars TC. Organophosphate-induced intermediate syndrome: etiology and relationships with myopathy. Toxicol Rev. 2006;25(1):1-14.

Yousef A, Albuali W, AlOmari M, et al. Organophosphate poisoning in a paediatric intensive care unit: a retrospective analysis based on ten years of experience. Int J Gen Med. 2022;15:6269-6277.

27.15 Paracetamol Poisoning

PE 14.3

Paracetamol poisoning in children is commonly caused by accidental ingestion or intentional overdose. It is facilitated by the easy availability of over-the-counter formulations like syrup and tablets. Self-poisoning is underreported, but unintentional poisonings are rising due to unregulated formulations in the market.

MECHANISM OF TOXICITY

Paracetamol is rapidly absorbed from the small intestine, with syrup formulations absorbed within 15 minutes and tablets peaking in serum levels within 1–2 hours. It undergoes hepatic metabolism, but in overdose, the liver's ability to detoxify a reactive metabolite (due to glutathione depletion) is overwhelmed, causing acute liver damage and potentially renal failure.

Toxicity Threshold

In children, the recommended maximum therapeutic dose of paracetamol is 90 mg/kg/day, administered as 15 mg/kg every 4 hours. Acute toxicity typically occurs with a single ingestion of more than 140 mg/kg of immediate-release paracetamol. Toxic blood levels from paracetamol syrup ingestion are rare, and significant liver damage is uncommon in children under 6 years. However, if blood paracetamol levels exceed the treatment threshold on the overdose nomogram **(Fig. 27.20)**, the prognosis is poor if not treated promptly. In infants aged 6–9 weeks, even lower doses (60–100 mg/kg/day) can lead to liver toxicity. Repeated doses exceeding the recommended limit of 100 mg/kg/day can also result in severe liver damage. **Table 27.22** shows various stages of toxicity.

History-taking

When taking a history in cases of paracetamol poisoning, it is important to determine whether the overdose was intentional or accidental. Identify the formulation involved—whether it was syrup, immediate-release tablets, or sustained-release tablets. Obtain the exact brand name and drug content of the tablet, as this can affect dosing. Be sure to establish the precise or estimated dose ingested, including the timing of ingestion. When unsure, assume the worst-case scenario (e.g., all tablets from the container were consumed, no significant spillage or vomiting occurred, and if multiple children were involved, assume one child ingested all the medication). Calculate the maximum possible dose per kilogram of body weight.

Consider whether other drugs may have been co-ingested, either accidentally or intentionally. Additionally, identify any underlying risk factors that could increase the risk of hepatotoxicity, such as use of anticonvulsants (e.g., phenobarbitone, carbamazepine), acute illness, malnutrition, anorexia nervosa, viral hepatitis, HIV/AIDS, or conditions like Gilbert's syndrome or Crigler-Najjar syndrome.

Clinical Features

Symptoms typically begin to appear 24 hours after ingestion and may include nausea, vomiting, pallor, and sweating. As the condition progresses, right upper quadrant tenderness may develop. If left untreated, signs of hepatic failure generally emerge between

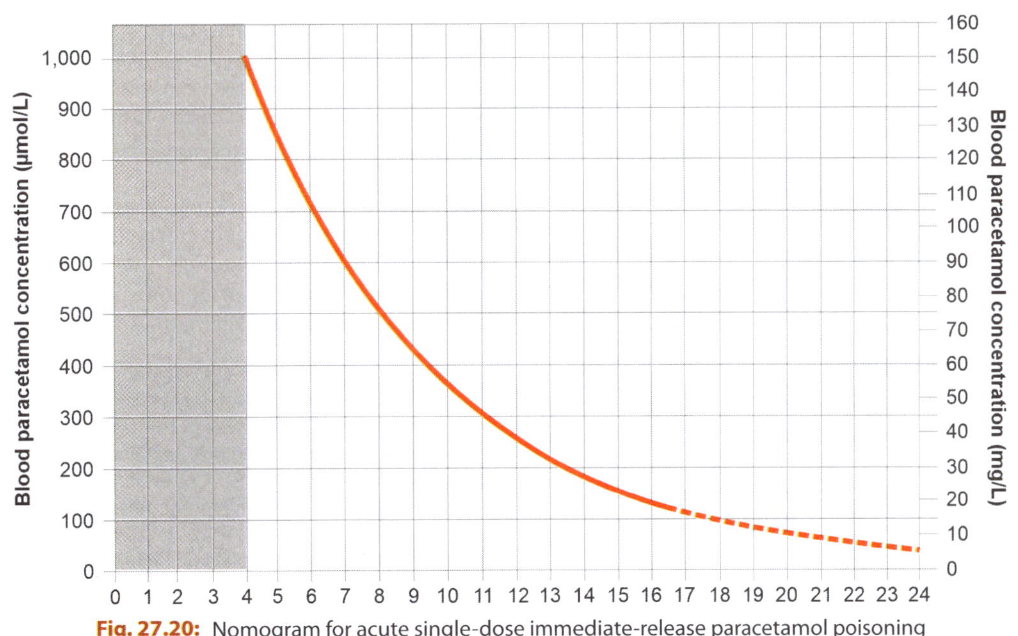

Fig. 27.20: Nomogram for acute single-dose immediate-release paracetamol poisoning

Table 27.22 Stages of Paracetamol Toxicity

Stages	Duration	Clinical features
Stage I	Up to 24 hours after overdose	Asymptomatic but less commonly nausea, vomiting and in patients with very large doses, lethargy and malaise
Stage II	24–72 hours after overdose	• Right upper quadrant pain, elevation in liver enzymes, prothrombin time (PT) and international normalized ratio of PT • In severe cases, evidence of nephrotoxicity (elevated blood urea nitrogen, creatinine, oliguria) and/or pancreatitis (elevated serum amylase, lipase)
Stage III	72–96 hours	Evidence of liver failure and in severe cases, renal failure and multiorgan failure; death most commonly occurs in this stage
Stage IV	4–14 days	Recovery

48–72 hours, which can include hypotension and encephalopathy. This is often followed by more severe manifestations, such as fulminant hepatic failure and coagulopathy.

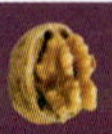

IN A NUTSHELL

Paracetamol Poisoning

1. After ingestion of toxic dose of paracetamol, absorption occurs within 2 hours and peak plasma levels are attained within 4 hours.
2. Clinical or biochemical evidence of liver injury may not be apparent for up to 24 hours after acute paracetamol overdose.
3. Specific antidote is N-acetylcysteine (NAC).
4. Ideally, NAC should be administered within 8 hours of paracetamol ingestion to prevent fatality. Beyond 8–10 hours of ingestion, its efficacy decreases.

The most important risk factor for liver damage and death after acute paracetamol ingestion is the extent of delay beyond 8 hours until treatment with N-acetylcysteine (NAC) commences. Treatment within 8 hours will prevent all serious hepatic injury.

Diagnosis and Blood Levels

- ❖ ***Paracetamol overdose nomogram (Fig. 27.20):*** A tool to assess potential liver damage based on blood paracetamol levels.
- ❖ A blood paracetamol level above the line on this nomogram serves as the most reliable indicator of potential liver damage.
- ❖ Blood levels should be measured at 4 hours post-ingestion (or as soon as possible after 4 hours), as levels taken within the first 4 hours provide no clinical value.

TREATMENT Paracetamol Poisoning

1. **Gastric decontamination:** Activated charcoal is effective within 1–2 hours post-ingestion. Gastric lavage is only useful if tablets are ingested within an hour.
2. **N-acetylcysteine (NAC):** Administered to prevent hepatotoxicity, the most effective when given within 8 hours of ingestion. The treatment involves a **two-stage infusion**:
   - Stage 1: 200 mg/kg over 4 hours
   - Stage 2: 100 mg/kg over 16 hours

   The required dose of N-acetylcysteine (NAC) should be diluted in either a 0.9% or 0.45% sodium chloride solution. While 5% dextrose can also be used, it is not preferred due to the risk of hyponatremia. If NAC treatment needs to be continued, it should follow the stage-2 infusion protocol, which is 100 mg/kg over the next 16 hours. For cases of massive paracetamol overdose, where the blood level exceeds twice the threshold on the treatment nomogram, a higher stage-2 infusion rate of 200 mg/kg over 16 hours may be required.
3. **Liver transplantation:** Considered if any of the following are present:
   - INR >3.0 at 48 hours or >4.5 at any point
   - Oliguria or creatinine >2.25 mg/dL (200 µmol/L)
   - Persistent acidosis (pH <7.3) or arterial lactate >3 mmol/L
   - Unresponsive systolic hypotension despite resuscitation
   - Encephalopathy (Glasgow Coma Scale <15) not related to sedative coingestions
   - Hypoglycemia
   - Severe thrombocytopenia

Monitoring and Discharge Criteria

Ongoing monitoring: At 18 hours into the N-acetylcysteine (NAC) infusion (2 hours before completion), blood should be drawn for the following tests:

- Paracetamol level
- Liver and renal function tests
- Electrolytes

NAC infusion should only be discontinued if:

- The patient is clinically stable
- Liver transaminases have peaked and are starting to decline
- Renal function and electrolytes are within normal limits
- The International Normalized Ratio (INR) is <2
- Paracetamol levels have fallen to <10 mg/L

Flowchart 27.6 summarizes the management of paracetamol poisoning

Discharge: Children who recover with normal liver and renal function after NAC treatment can be discharged. Parents should be educated on safe drug storage. Intentional overdoses in older children or adolescents may require psychiatric consultation, in addition to medical management

Baranwal A, Chandrasekar S, Chowdary A. Paracetamol poisoning. In: Indian Academy of Pediatrics (IAP) Standard Treatment Guidelines 2022. Available from: https://iapindia.org/pdf/Ch-111-Paracetamol-Poisoning.pdf. [Last accessed January 2025]

Chiew AL, Reith D, Pomerleau A, et al. Updated guidelines for the management of paracetamol poisoning in Australia and New Zealand. Med J Aust. 2020;212(4):175-83.

Clinical Practice Guideline Royal Children's Hospital Melbourne. (2021). Paracetamol poisoning. [online] Available from https://www.rch.org.au/clinicalguide/guideline_index/Paracetamol_poisoning/ [Last accessed January 2025]

Flowchart 27.6: Algorithm for acute paracetamol poisoning with known time of ingestion

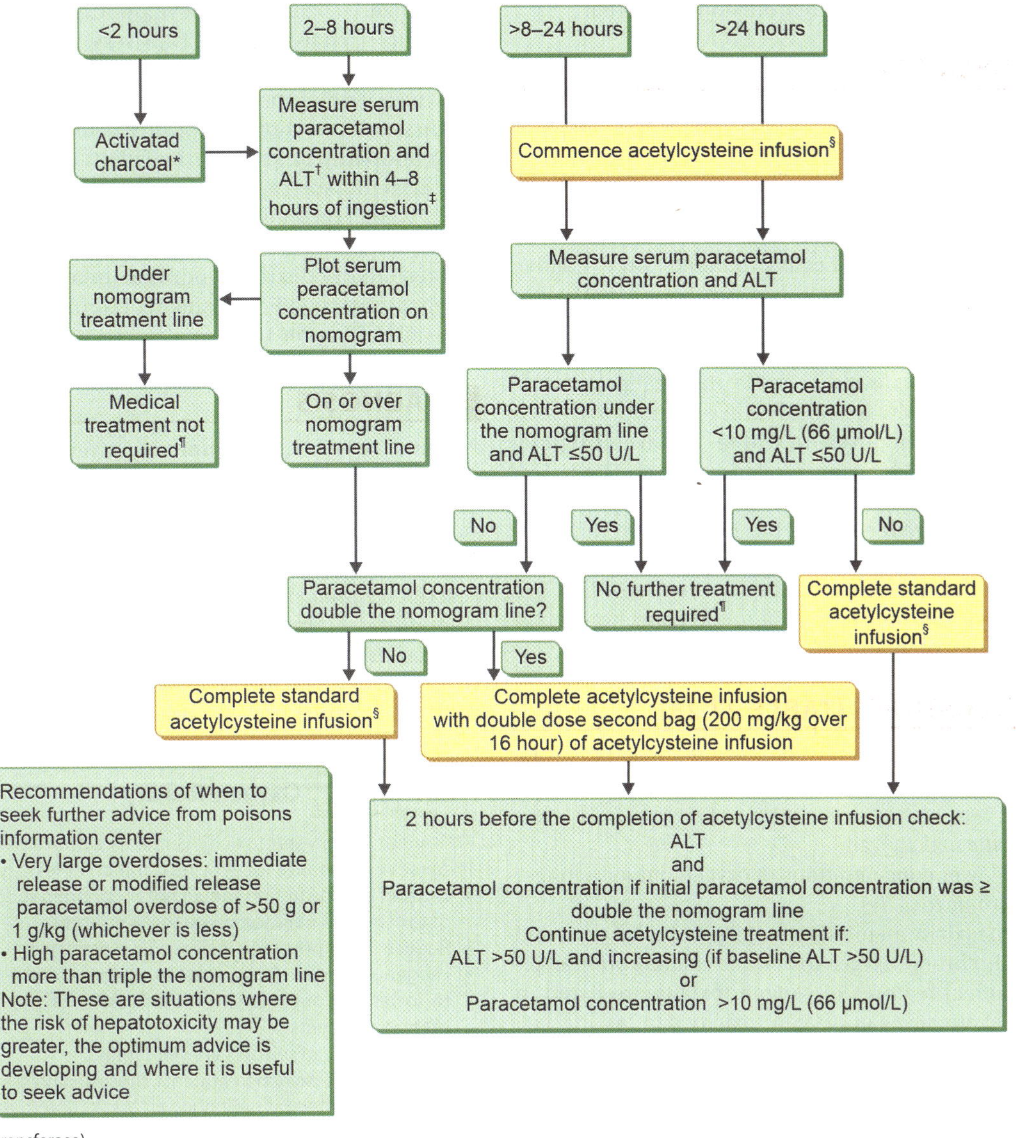

(ALT: alanine aminotransferase).

*Cooperative adult patients who have potentially ingested ≥10 g or ≥200 mg/kg (whichever is less). For paracetamol ingestions ≥30 g, activated charcoal should be offered until 4 hours after ingestion.

†Baseline ALT measurement.

‡If paracetamol concentration will not be available until ≥8 hours after ingestion, commence acetylcysteine while awaiting paracetamol concentration.

§For acetylcysteine dosage, see text.

¶Patients should be advised that if they develop abdominal pain, nausea or vomiting, further assessment is required. For patients in rural or remote regions where pathology services are not available.

(*Source:* Baranwal A, Chandrasekar S, Chowdary A. Paracetamol poisoning. In: Indian Academy of Pediatrics (IAP) Standard treatment guidelines 2022. Available from: https://iapindia.org/pf/Ch-111-Paracetamol-Poisoning.pdf)

27.16 Oxygen Toxicity

RISK FACTORS

Those at particular risk for oxygen toxicity include patients exposed to prolonged high levels of oxygen and premature infants. Prolonged exposure to above-normal oxygen partial pressures, or brief exposures to very high partial pressures, can cause oxidative damage to cell membranes causing alveolar collapse. Pulmonary effects can manifest as early as within 24 hours of oxygen therapy. Oxygen administration with FiO_2 of

100% for as short as 3 hours can cause chest pain, with longer periods leading to signs similar to bronchopneumonia.

PATHOPHYSIOLOGY

Exposure to high oxygen concentrations first damages the capillary endothelium, followed by interstitial edema (0–12 hours), worsening compliance and vital capacity (12–30 hours), followed by thickening of the alveolar-capillary membrane (30–72 hours). If the process continues, type I alveolar cells destruction occurs, and type II cells proliferate. An exudative phase follows, resulting in a reduced ventilation/perfusion ratio, physiologic shunting, and worsening hypoxemia. High levels of oxygen administration quickly deplete body nitrogen levels. As blood nitrogen levels decrease, the total pressure of venous gases rapidly decreases. Under these conditions, gases that exist at atmospheric pressure within the alveoli rapidly diffuse into the venous blood, and collapse occurs. The risk of absorption atelectasis may be greatest in children breathing at low tidal volumes. More recently, it has been shown that high concentrations of normobaric oxygen may also be harmful. This injury is similar to the type of injury seen in ARDS. The magnitude of injury is directly related to the concentration of oxygen and duration of treatment.

CLINICAL FEATURES (TABLE 27.23)

The clinical settings in which oxygen toxicity occurs can be divided into two groups:

1. Exposure to very high concentrations of oxygen for a short duration (*acute toxicity*), and
2. Exposure to lower concentrations of oxygen but for a longer duration (*chronic toxicity*).

Acute oxygen toxicity manifests generally with CNS signs and symptoms, while chronic oxygen toxicity has mainly pulmonary effects. The clinical features of oxygen toxicity are listed in **Table 27.23**. Severe cases of oxygen toxicity can lead to cell damage and death.

In CNS involvement, early symptoms and signs are quite variable but twitching of perioral and small muscles of the hand is a consistent feature. If exposure to oxygen pressures is prolonged and sustained, tinnitus, dysphoria, nausea, and generalized seizures can develop. CNS toxicity is expedited by factors such as raised pCO_2, stress, and fatigue. Respiratory symptoms include coughing, pleuritic chest pain, substernal heaviness, and dyspnea. Pulmonary symptoms typically abate 4 hours after cessation of exposure in majority of the patients.

Retinopathy of Prematurity (ROP) is primarily influenced by risk factors such as prematurity, low birth weight, prolonged high oxygen exposure, fluctuating hypoxia and hyperoxia, apnea, sepsis, anemia, cardiac defects, multiple blood transfusions, and respiratory distress syndrome. Infants with very low birth weight are at a significantly higher risk of severe ROP (discussed in detail in **Chapter 16**).

DIAGNOSIS

Patients at risk for pulmonary oxygen toxicity should be monitored for oxygen saturation and elevated work of breathing. Evaluation can be done by pulmonary function testing, chest X-ray, and blood gas analysis which can show signs of ARDS. CNS toxicity manifests as clinical signs and symptoms described earlier and will often have associated tachycardia and diaphoresis. Aborting a hyperbaric exposure when these signs are present can prevent seizure occurrence. Eye examination can be done to assess visual acuity and look for lens opacification to detect early ocular oxygen toxicity.

TREATMENT Oxygen Toxicity

Treatment for oxygen toxicity is mainly symptomatic, therefore it is imperative to monitor for early recognition of toxicity.

- Oxygen administration should not be stopped suddenly at the onset of toxicity as it may aggravate the symptoms.
- Reduce the exposure to increased oxygen levels.
- Exogenous antioxidants, notably vitamin E and C have been found to lower the prevalence of retinopathy of prematurity (ROP) in premature infants.
- Oxygen-induced seizures are self-limited.
- For hyperbaric oxygen treatments, those at high risk may benefit from antiepileptic therapy, prolonged air breaks (intermittent air-breathing while in the hyperbaric environment) and limited treatment pressure.

Table 27.23 Clinical Features of Oxygen Toxicity

Central nervous system	*Respiratory system*	*Eye*
1. Headache 2. Irritability and anxiety 3. Dizziness 4. Disorientation 5. Hyperventilation 6. Hiccups 7. Cold shivering 8. Fatigue 9. Tingling in the limbs 10. Visual changes such as blurring and tunnel vision 11. Tinnitus and hearing disturbances 12. Nausea 13. Twitching 14. Tonic-clonic seizure	1. Mild tickling and burning sensation on inhalation 2. Uncontrollable coughing 3. Hemoptysis 4. Dyspnea 5. Rales 6. Fever 7. Hyperemia of the nasal mucosa 8. Chest X-ray shows inflammation and pulmonary edema	1. In premature babies, retinopathy of prematurity and retrolental fibroplasia 2. Retinal edema 3. Cataract formation (long-term exposure)

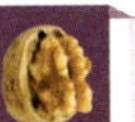

IN A NUTSHELL

Oxygen Toxicity

1. Risk factors for oxygen toxicity include hyperbaric oxygen therapy, exposure to prolonged high levels of oxygen and premature infants.
2. Prolonged exposure to above-normal oxygen partial pressures, or brief exposures to very high partial pressures, can cause oxidative damage to cell membranes causing alveolar collapse.
3. Acute oxygen toxicity manifests generally with central nervous system signs and symptoms, while chronic oxygen toxicity has mainly pulmonary effects.
4. Evaluation is done by pulmonary function testing, chest X-ray and blood gas analysis.
5. Management for oxygen toxicity is mainly symptomatic.

Cooper JS, Phuyal P, Shah N. Oxygen Toxicity. In: StatPearls. Treasure Island (FL): StatPearls Publishing; 2022.
Walsh BK, Smallwood CD. Pediatric oxygen therapy: a review and update. Respir Care. 2017;62(6):645-61.

27.17 Working in Emergency Room: Communication and Ethics

PE 24.22, PE 24.23

GIVING BAD NEWS

Bad news is defined as "any news that drastically and negatively alters the patient's view of her or his future." Parental anxiety, hope, decision making, coping with the child's illness, and depression are influenced by the doctor's skill to deliver bad news.

A definitive diagnosis is made after several consultations, laboratory tests, and other investigations. This gives us time to prepare for the breaking of bad news. A useful approach to this preparation is the ABCDE approach. It consists of *A*dvance preparation, *B*uilding a therapeutic relationship; *C*ommunicating well; *D*ealing with the patient's and family's reactions; and *E*ncouraging and validating emotions. The goals of bad news consultation are given in **Box 27.21**.

Prepare for the Discussion

Giving bad news to parents of a child is a difficult and delicate task. Advance preparation should be done whenever possible.

Arrange time and place: Choose a time and place that is feasible for everyone involved, where all can sit down and hear each other clearly, and privacy is available. Ensure that there are no interruptions.

Ensure adequate presence: It is best to have both parents present during the consultation. If this is not feasible, include grandparents or other close relatives. A single parent being given bad news might feel shocked and may be difficult for him/her to overcome. The presence of other family members is a great support. This also avoids repetition of the same information at a later time.

Box 27.21 Goals of Bad News Consultation

1. To collect relevant information and details from parents
2. To give information according to the parents' needs and desires, in a compassionate and culturally appropriate manner
3. To support the parents by the judicious use of skills to reduce the emotional impact and shock experienced in such situations
4. To develop a management plan of the child, with the input and cooperation of the parents

Be prepared: Review the case sheets and investigations, have the case papers ready in hand, look up information, and be prepared to answer questions related to the disease, its course, prognosis, and treatment plan. If given incorrect information, parents will be angry and lose faith in the treating doctor.

Build a Therapeutic Relationship

Begin the consultation by introducing everyone and know the relationships. Parents prefer being told by a single person, rather than by multiple experts. Start by asking the parents what they already know about their child's condition, giving them ample time to speak. Try to assess also how much the parents want to know about the child's condition. Touch can be important. Holding the affected child has a positive effect, but the doctor should not get too involved in playing with the child.

Communicate Well

The bad news must be communicated to the parents in a clear and unambiguous language while remaining sensitive to parents' distress and grief. Hiding any information is unacceptable, but it can be given in an empathetic way. Split up over two or more sessions, if necessary. Avoid being too pessimistic and saying things like "this child will never go to school or have a normal life." Being honest, but not taking away hope, has been rated the most difficult aspect of giving bad news.

Speak frankly, but compassionately. Avoid humor and flippancy. It is important that the parents get the message, e.g., words like "slow" and "developmental delay" can be used instead of saying a harsh and distressing term like "mental retardation."

Once the news has been understood and absorbed, move on to further discussion of the child's condition. Prognostic information, if available, should be shared at this time. Life expectancy, disability, and other problems to be anticipated, should be talked about. The treatment plan should be explained.

Deal with Parents' Reactions

Parents may find it hard to absorb, or retain, what is told to them. Counsel slowly, allow enough time, and repeat essential information, if required. Do not criticize the care provided by colleagues or blame them for the situation. Empathize with the parents and let them know that you understand their feelings and concern.

Encourage and Validate Emotions

It is wrong to offer unrealistic hope, but some encouragement should be offered. Treatment options should be talked about, and the effect on the child should be discussed. Other things that can be discussed are the effect on the family, support and specialist services available. If the parents seem to be blaming themselves for the child's condition, an effort should be made to relieve them of guilt.

Breaking Bad News After Failed Resuscitation

Disclosing the death of a patient is a challenging and sensitive process. While there is no "perfect" way to break the news, there are important principles that should guide healthcare providers in these situations:

Key Principles

1. ***Slow down the conversation:*** In high-pressure, emotionally charged environments like emergency units, it is essential to slow down the pace of communication, repeat information when necessary, and ensure clarity.
2. ***Provide regular updates during CPR:*** Families should be kept informed about the progress or failure of resuscitation efforts, so they are mentally prepared for the potential outcome.
3. ***Use clear language:*** The news should be delivered clearly using terms like "death," "dying," or "dead." Avoid euphemisms like "passed away" or confusing medical terms to prevent ambiguity.
4. ***Allow space for grief:*** Understand that parents may react emotionally, with expressions such as crying, shouting, or physical gestures. Offer a private space for grieving to avoid distressing other families in the unit.
5. ***Maintain compassion and empathy:*** Speak gently and slowly, reassure the family that everything possible was done, and if possible, involve a social worker for support and counseling.
6. ***Address parental questions:*** Parents may ask about their child's final moments. Be prepared to answer questions about their child's pain, awareness, and the actions taken.
7. ***Respect cultural and religious practices:*** Offer support for any religious rituals and allow the family to grieve in private. Encourage them to touch or speak to their child if they wish.
8. ***Preparing for viewing the body:*** If the family wishes to see the body, provide a gentle, accurate description of the appearance after death, including any medical equipment still attached. Ensure the child's body is cleaned, and unnecessary tubes or devices are removed.
9. ***Assistance with final rituals:*** Offer assistance with logistics such as contacting relatives, arranging transport, and helping with funeral preparations.

Hospital Formalities after Death

- Documentation (death certificate, patient records) and preparation of the body (shifted to mortuary) must be completed efficiently while being mindful of the family's need for time.
- ***Autopsy and organ donation:*** Families may be resistant to autopsies due to emotional or religious reasons. It is important to explain their value clearly and sensitively. The process of organ or tissue donation should also be handled with care.

Barriers in Dealing with Failed Resuscitation

- ***Staff shortages:*** Insufficient staff can lead to challenges in delivering resuscitation, counseling, and communication to grieving families.
- ***Lack of designated spaces:*** There may not be an appropriate space to deliver bad news, affecting the quality of communication.
- ***Unclear protocols:*** Absence of standard operating procedures for handling these situations leads to inconsistency.
- ***Crowded units:*** Overcrowding in smaller hospitals can make it difficult to manage grieving families and provide necessary privacy.

Recommendations to Improve Communication

- ***Team approach:*** A larger healthcare team can better handle the resuscitation, communication, and family support.
- ***Designated counseling spaces:*** Separate rooms with appropriate facilities for private communication and video documentation should be available.
- ***Involvement of social workers:*** Having a trained social worker or liaison to help manage the communication and grieving process is critical.
- ***Clear documentation:*** All communications should be documented thoroughly, especially when autopsy or legal investigations are involved.

Dealing with Mob Violence

- ***Anticipating violence:*** In some settings, the grieving process may lead to mob violence. It's important to recognize early signs of escalating emotions and act preemptively. Proper documentation, video recording of the communication, and involving law enforcement can help manage these situations.
- ***Preventive measures:*** Have emergency protocols in place to prevent mob violence, such as limiting the number of relatives present during resuscitation and having security measures in place.

Addressing Special Situations

- ***Brought-in-dead cases:*** In cases where a patient is brought in dead, full resuscitation efforts should be made. If death is confirmed, clear communication regarding the situation and a post-mortem should be planned if foul play is suspected.

- ***Debriefing healthcare providers:*** After a failed resuscitation, debriefing sessions should be held to reflect on the event, assess team dynamics, and improve future practices. Regular mock drills for CPR and communication should be implemented.

Breaking bad news after failed resuscitation requires clear, compassionate communication, respect for the family's emotional needs, and an organized approach to hospital procedures. By addressing logistical challenges and providing empathetic support, healthcare providers can help families navigate one of the most difficult moments in their lives while ensuring dignity and care for the deceased.

CONSENT

The Indian Contract Act (1872) defines consent as "when any two persons agree upon the same thing in the same sense they are said to consent." Consent may be verbal or written. The Indian Penal Code (1872, 1860) goes on to recognize that for clinical examination, diagnosis, and treatment consent can be given by any person who is conscious, mentally sound, and over the age of 18 years.

Consent may be *implied* or *express*. Implied consent or "tacit consent" is taken for history taking and simple physical examination when one requests a consult. Express consent may be oral or written, and is usually required for procedures and interventions when offered an intervention.

Consent should always be informed. Information must be comprehensible in the vernacular language and in nonmedical terms.

ASSENT

For all children, proxy consent, or "substitute consent" is the norm with parents or legal guardians giving consent for children under their care. Assent is a concept that respects autonomy of a minor. It is an agreement when legally the person cannot give consent. It indicates that the child is old enough to understand and willing to participate in what is being proposed, either in clinical care and treatment or in research studies. Hence, consent is required from parents and legal guardians of children under 18 years legally, but it is vital to obtain assent (agreement) from the child itself. According to the Indian Council of Medical Research (ICMR) guidelines, oral assent must be obtained for children between 7 years (84 months and above) and 12 years of age, in the presence of a parent or legal guardian. For children between 12 and 18 years of age, written assent must be obtained.

ROLE IN EMERGENCY ROOM

The physician and nurse should be willing to work collaboratively and are responsible for the following:

- Promote adequate knowledge and skill of emergency room staff physicians, nurses, and other healthcare providers and staff (i.e., physician assistants, advanced practice nurses, paramedics, and technicians) in the emergency care, and resuscitation of infants and children.
- Participate in the development of the pediatric components of the quality improvement (QI) plan and facilitating QI activities related to pediatric emergency care.
- Assist with the development and periodic review of emergency room policies and procedures and standards for medications, equipment, and supplies to ensure adequate resources for children of all ages.
- The doctor and staff should be willing to serve as liaisons and/or coordinators in collaboration with appropriate in-hospital and out-of-hospital pediatric care committees in the community.
- Facilitate pediatric emergency medical and nursing education for emergency room healthcare providers and staff, including the identification of continuing pediatric emergency education resources.
- In coordination with the local credentialing processes, facilitate competency evaluations for staff that are pertinent to children of all ages so that patients receive the highest level of care from healthcare professionals. When available, the doctor should participate in simulation (i.e., pediatric scenario-based mock codes) to improve pediatric care in resuscitation and team settings.
- Facilitate the integration of pediatric needs in hospital disaster and/or emergency preparedness plans and promote the inclusion of pediatric patients in disaster drills.
- Collaborate with emergency room leadership to enable adequate staffing, medications, equipment, supplies, and other resources for children in the emergency room.
- Communicate with emergency room and hospital leadership on efforts to facilitate pediatric emergency care.

ATTEND IMMEDIATELY IN EMERGENCY

Physicians have an ethical obligation to help when they are needed and to attend to emergency calls immediately. A doctor's failure to respond in an emergency may put many others at risk. However, a recent survey showed that many physicians feel underprepared to respond to an emergency. Well-prepared physicians will not only perform and fulfill their ethical obligations, they will be much more effective contributors during an emergency.

Potential areas for pediatric competency and professional performance evaluations to improve pediatric readiness in the emergency department include the following:

- ***Assess and treat:*** (i) triage, (ii) illness and injury assessment and management, and (iii) pain assessment and treatment.
- Administration of medications.
- How to use and maintain device and/or equipment safety (e.g., low-volume infusion pumps).
- Ability to perform procedures, including (i) airway management, (ii) vascular access, and (iii) sedation and analgesia.
- Perform resuscitation, including (i) critical care monitoring, (ii) neonatal resuscitation, and (iii) pediatric resuscitation.
- Trauma resuscitation and stabilization, including the following: (i) management of burns, (ii) traumatic brain injury, (iii) fracture management, (iv) hemorrhage control, and (v) recognition and reporting of nonaccidental trauma.

- Provide patient- and family-centered care, including cultural competency; and
- Team training and effective communication, including the following: (i) transitions of care and/or handoffs and (ii) closed-loop communication.

All emergency departments must be continually ready with adequate manpower to receive, accurately assess, and, at a minimum, stabilize and safely transfer children who are acutely ill or injured.

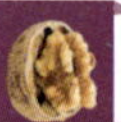

IN A NUTSHELL

Working in Emergency Room: Communication and Ethics

1. Giving bad news to parents of a child is a difficult and delicate task. Advance preparation should be done whenever possible.
2. The bad news must be communicated to the parents in clear, direct and unambiguous language while remaining sensitive to parents' distress and grief.
3. Consent should always be informed. The information must be comprehensible in the vernacular language and in nonmedical terms.
4. Verbal/oral assent should be obtained from children of 7–12 years of age; for children between 12 and 18 years of age, written assent should be obtained.
5. It is imperative that all pediatric emergency departments have the appropriate resources (medications, equipment, policies, and education) and capable staff to provide effective emergency care for children.
6. Physicians have an ethical obligation to help when they are needed and to attend to emergency calls immediately. A doctor's failure to respond in an emergency may put many others at risk.
7. Pediatric emergency departments must be continually ready with adequate manpower to receive, accurately assess, and, at least, stabilize and safely transfer children who are acutely ill or injured.

Behera SK, Das S, Xavier AS, et al. Indian Council of Medical Research's National Ethical Guidelines for biomedical and health research involving human participants: The way forward from 2006 to 2017. Perspect Clin Res. 2019;10(3):108-14.
Mehta PN. Communication skills–breaking bad news. Indian Pediatr. 2008;45(10):839-41.
Muralidharan J, Kulgod V, Sharma AK (Eds). IAP Advanced Life Support (ALS) Handbook, 2nd edition. Indian Academy of Pediatrics; 2020.
Remick K, Gausche-Hill M, Joseph MM, et al. Pediatric readiness in the emergency department. Ann Emerg Med. 2018;72(6):e123-36.

Chabungbam Smilie and Piyush Gupta

28 CHAPTER

National Health Programs Related to Children

AS PER NMC COMPETENCIES

PE16.1	Explain the components of Integrated Management of Neonatal and Childhood Illnesses (IMNCI) guidelines and method of risk stratification.	*Ch 28.7*
PE16.2	Assess children <2 months using IMNCI guidelines.	*Ch 28.7*
PE16.3	Assess children 2 months to 5 years using IMNCI guidelines and stratify risk.	*Ch 28.7*
PE16.4	Identify children with undernutrition as per IMNCI criteria and plan referral.	*Ch 28.7*
PE16.5	Identify and stratify risk in a sick neonate using IMNCI guidelines.	*Ch 28.7*
PE16.6	Apply the IMNCI guidelines in risk stratification of children with diarrheal dehydration and refer.	*Ch 28.7*
PE17.1	Describe the vision and outline the goals, strategies and plan of action of NHM and other important national programs pertaining to maternal and child health including RCH, RMNCH A+, RBSK, RKSK, JSSK, mission Indradhanush and ICDS.	*Ch 28.3, Ch 28.4, Ch 28.5, Ch 28.6*
PE32.1	Identify, describe and defend medicolegal, socio-cultural and ethical issues as they pertain to healthcare in children (including parental rights and right to refuse treatment).	*Ch 28.8*

Topics available online: ***Participation in Maternal and Child Health Activities; Visiting the Rural Health Center***

28.1 Under-five Mortality and Morbidity

INTRODUCTION

Under-five mortality rate (U5MR) is defined as the probability of dying between birth to 5 years of age per thousand live births. This is an indicator of well-being of all children below the age of 5 years. Significant global progress has been made in reducing childhood mortality since 1990. The number of under-5 deaths worldwide has dropped from 12.6 million in 1990 to five million in 2020. This represents a 60% decline in the global under-five mortality rate, from 93 deaths per 1,000 live births in 1990 to 37 in 2020. U5MR in India is 32/1,000 live births, with variations between rural and urban areas—36 deaths per 1,000 live births in rural areas and 21 in urban areas [Sample Registration System (SRS), 2020]. The Sustainable Development Goal (SDG) target for 2030 is to bring it down to 25 or fewer deaths per 1,000 live births. State wise distribution of U5MR is shown in **Figure 28.1**. It ranges from 8 in Kerala to 51 in Madhya Pradesh; and from 21/1,000 in urban India to 36/1,000 in rural areas. As per the SRS 2020 report, eleven States and Union Territories have already achieved the SDG target for U5MR (≤25 by 2030), including Kerala (8), Tamil Nadu (13), Delhi (14), Maharashtra (18), Jammu and Kashmir (17), Karnataka (21), Punjab (22), West Bengal (22), Telangana (23), Gujarat (24), and Himachal Pradesh (24).

CAUSES OF DEATH

According to the Cause of Death Statistics 2017–19 released by the Office of the Registrar General and Census Commissioner, India, the leading causes of child mortality in India are: prematurity and low birth weight (31.2%), pneumonia (17.5%), birth asphyxia and birth trauma (9.9%), other non-communicable diseases (9.6%), diarrheal diseases (5.8%),

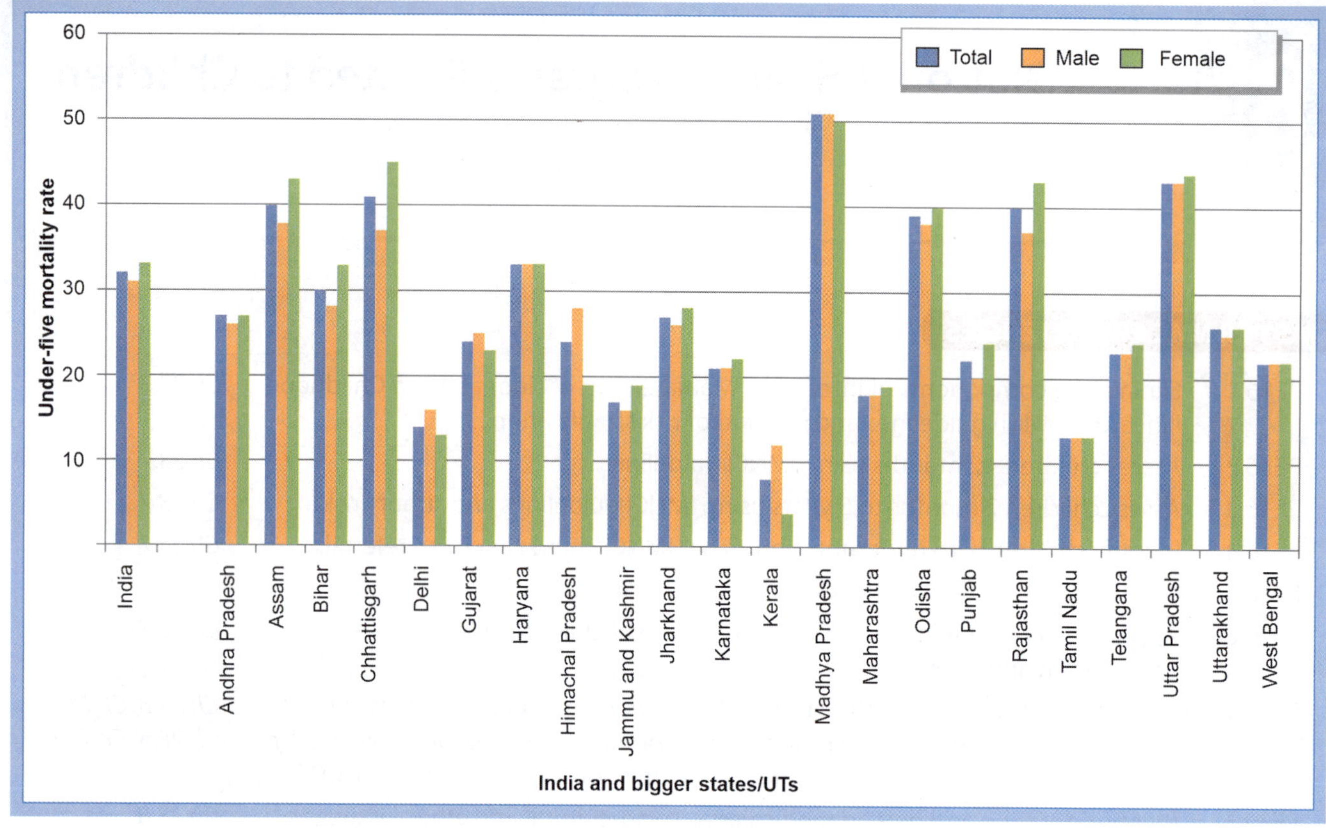

Fig. 28.1: Under-five mortality rate in states of India

Source: Sample Registration System (SRS)–Statistical Report, 2020

congenital anomalies (5.7%), injuries (4.9%), ill-defined or unknown causes (4.3%), fever of unknown origin (4.1%), acute bacterial sepsis and severe infections (3.8%), and all other remaining causes (3.3%) **(Fig. 28.2)**. Severe acute malnutrition (SAM) contributes to almost half of these deaths.

Majority of the under-five deaths in India (62%) are attributed to neonatal deaths. Respiratory infections, diarrhea, other infections, and injuries contribute significantly to child deaths between 1 month and 5 years.

PROBLEMS IN UNDER-FIVE CHILDREN (1 MONTH–5 YEARS)

Pneumonia and diarrhea are the major killers of young children. Malnutrition is the most important predisposing factor responsible for >50% of comorbidities in under-five children.

Pneumonia

Globally, pneumonia kills more children than any other infectious disease, claiming the lives of over 700,000 children under the age of five every year, i.e., around 2,000 every day, with a child dying of pneumonia every 43 seconds. In India, according to the Health Management Information System (HMIS) 2022–23, a total of 473,780 childhood pneumonia cases were reported. During the same period, pneumonia caused 11,497 deaths among infants aged 1 to 12 months and 4,571 deaths among children aged 1 to 5 years. Most important risk factors for pneumonia include low birth weight, malnutrition, inadequate breastfeeding, and overcrowding. Lack of appropriate treatment and timely care adds on to the disease related morbidity and mortality. Preventive measures such as vaccination against diphtheria, *Streptococcus pneumoniae, Haemophilus influenzae*, pertussis and measles, exclusive breastfeeding, reduction of household air pollution, and control over overcrowding may help control the overall incidence of pneumonia in under-five children.

Diarrhea

According to the World Health Organization (WHO), diarrheal diseases are the third leading cause of death in children aged 1–59 months, causing 9% of all childhood deaths. It is both preventable and treatable, with around 443,832 children under-five children dying from it each year. Globally, there are nearly 1.7 billion cases of childhood diarrheal disease annually, and it remains a leading cause of malnutrition in children under-five. In India, according to NFHS-5, 7% of children under five had diarrhea in the 2 weeks before the survey. Of those, 76% sought advice or treatment from a health facility or provider. Additionally, 45% of children with diarrhea received continued feeding and oral rehydration therapy (ORT) as recommended.

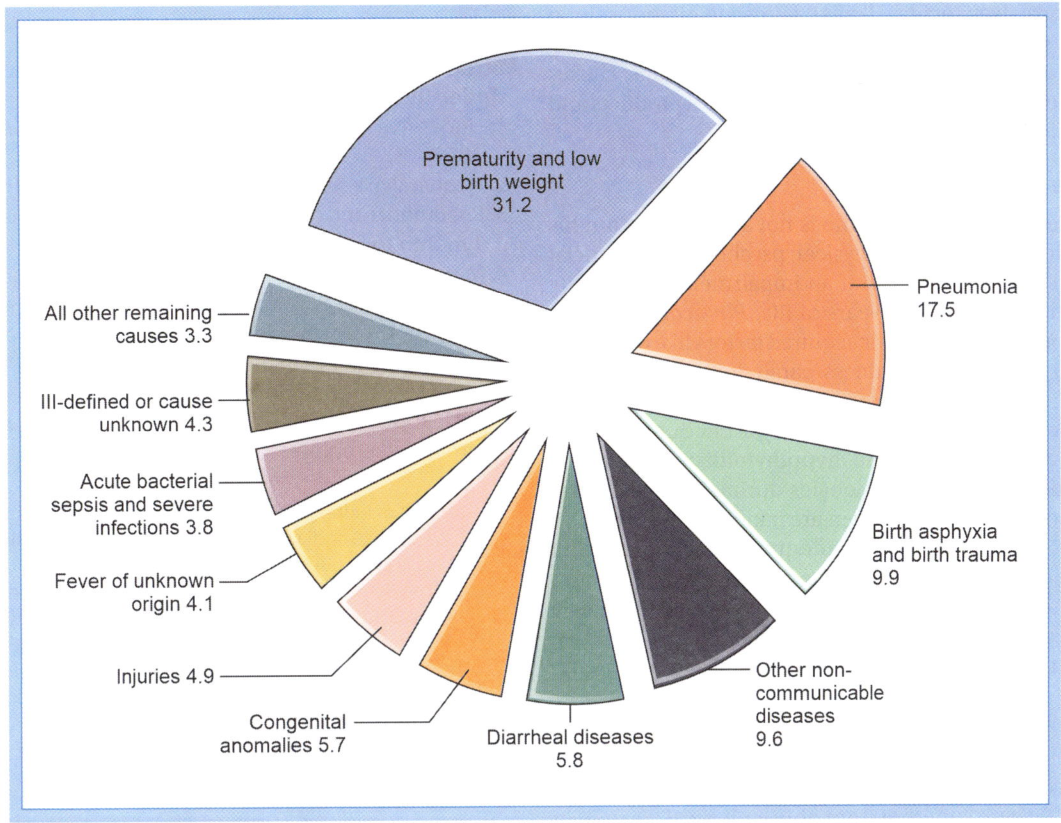

Fig. 28.2: Common causes of death in children aged <5 years in India (2017–2019)

Source: Causes of Death Statistics 2017–2019, Government of India

Most of these deaths occur in children of rural background in developing countries especially in Africa and South-Asia due to limited access to safe drinking water, sewage disposal, and unhygienic living conditions. Accessibility to safe water and food, proper sanitation and excreta disposal, hand washing, and exclusive breastfeeding can prevent most episodes of diarrhea.

Other Infections and Infestations

Other than pneumonia and diarrhea, the leading childhood infections include malaria, measles, diphtheria, pertussis, tuberculosis, typhoid, and dengue. Human immunodeficiency virus (HIV) is emerging as another threat. Parasitic infestations including roundworm, hookworm, and giardiasis also add on to the morbidity of children.

Malnutrition

It refers to deficiencies, excesses, or imbalances in a person's intake of energy and/or nutrients. It can be of two types: undernutrition which includes wasting, stunting, underweight; or obesity. Deficiency of macronutrients leads to protein-energy malnutrition and SAM, while iron, iodine, and vitamin A are the major micronutrient deficiencies adding to the burden of undernutrition. Globally in 2020, nearly 149 million under-five children were estimated to be stunted, 45 million were estimated to be wasted and 38.9 million children were overweight or obese.

Undernutrition contributes to nearly half of all deaths in children under five, with the majority occurring in low- and middle-income countries. Factors attributing to malnutrition include poverty, low birth weight, poor nutritional status of adolescent females and pregnant women, traditional beliefs and social taboos, and insufficient balanced diet. Undernutrition makes child more prone to infections and slows down recovery from acute illness. Mortality of SAM may range from 30 to 50%. The overall prevalence of stunting has reduced from 38.4 to 35.5%, wasting has reduced from 21 to 19.3% and undernutrition prevalence has reduced from 35.8 to 32.1% [National Family Health Survey (NFHS)-5)].

Accidental Injuries

Unintentional injuries are another important cause of morbidity and mortality among children all over the world. These include road traffic accidents, poisonings, burns, drowning, suffocation, and falls. Most common accidental injuries in children <5 years include drowning and accidental poisonings. Road traffic accidents mostly affect children older than 5 years.

- Drowning is the third leading cause of unintentional death in children and youth worldwide.
- At least 5% of child drowning survivors have serious neurological damage.
- Poisoning is mostly accidental in children under 5 years of age. The common causes of poisoning in developing countries

include corrosives (acids, alkalis), kerosene oil, household chemicals such as insecticides, phenol, alkalis, naphthalene, and plant and plant products. In developed nations, causes of childhood poisoning involve pharmaceutical products and chemicals.

Disabilities and Handicaps

A handicapped child is the one who is not able to carry out his normal activities due to either physical, psychological, or social factors which may be the result of an impairment or disability that occurred during initial 5 years of life. *Physical handicaps* result from congenital defects, or acquired factors like disease or accidents and may result in blindness, paralysis, deaf mutism, etc. *Mental/psychological handicaps* include global developmental delay and intellectual disability which may occur due to genetic causes such as Down syndrome, hypothyroidism, congenital infections, and nutritional deficiencies during infancy. As per estimates, about 3% Indian children are handicapped.

Preventive measures include adequate nutrition, health education, and genetic counseling. Specific protective measures such as vitamin A supplementation, immunization, and rubella vaccination can decrease the burden of handicapped children and improve the overall health infrastructure of country.

Child Abuse and Neglect

Child abuse includes physical, sexual, emotional, and social abuse/neglect. Globally, year 2019 saw nearly 1 billion children aged under 18 years suffering from abuse physical, sexual, or emotional. On an average, about 5–15 per 1,000 children are abused by their family and employers. Physical and emotional abuse is more common amongst males while girls suffer from sexual abuse. Consequences of child abuse have long lasting effects on physical and mental wellbeing. Exposure to violence in early years impacts health and wellbeing of a child. The 2030 agenda for Sustainable Development is to end abuse, exploitation, trafficking, and all forms of violence against children.

Overall preventive measures for health promotion in this transitional age group should include strengthening of primary healthcare infrastructure, consolidation and maintenance of immunization coverage, ensuring essential drug supply, early preschool education, and primary education facilities in underprivileged areas.

IN A NUTSHELL

Under-five Mortality and Morbidity

1. Under-five mortality rate in India is 32/1,000 live births (SRS, 2020).
2. Neonatal mortality accounts for 62% of under-five mortality.
3. Pneumonia and diarrhea are the major killers of children aged 1 month to 5 years.
4. Malnutrition is the most important predisposing factor responsible for >50% of comorbidities in under-five children.
5. Drowning and accidental poisonings are most common accidental injuries in under-five children.
6. Child abuse is an important problem of under-five children with about 5–15 per 1,000 children being abused by their family and employers.

Government of India. (2022). SRS Bulletin. [online] Available from http://www.censusindia.gov.in/vital_statistics/SRS_Bulletin_2022.pdf [Last accessed August 2025].

Office of the Registrar General and Census Commissioner, India (ORGI). Sample Registration System (SRS)-Cause of Death Statistics 20152017. New Delhi: Ministry of Home Affairs, Government of India; 2022.

Office of the Registrar General and Census Commissioner, India. Vital Statistics of India Based on the Civil Registration System 2020. New Delhi: Ministry of Home Affairs. Available from: https://censusindia.gov.in/nada/index.php/catalog/44752 [Last accessed May, 2025].

Office of the Registrar General and Census Commissioner, India. Causes of Death Statistics 2017–2019. New Delhi: Ministry of Home Affairs, Government of India [cited 2025 May 4]. Available from: https://censusindia.gov.in/catalog/download [Last accessed May, 2025].

Press Information Bureau. Over 12 lakh children under five died in 2019; 68% of these deaths were due to communicable diseases. 2022 Sep 19. Available from: https://pib.gov.in/PressReleaseIframePage.aspx?PRID=1861710 [Last accessed May, 2025].

World Health Organization. Child mortality under 5 years. Geneva: WHO. Available from: https://www.who.int/news-room/fact-sheets/detail/child-mortality-under-5-years [Last accessed May, 2025].

World Health Organization. SDG Target 3.2: Newborn and child mortality [Internet]. Geneva: WHO. Available from: https://www.who.int/data/gho/data/themes/topics/indicator-groups/indicator-group-details/GHO/sdg-target-3.2-newborn-and-child-mortality [Last accessed May, 2025].

28.2 Indicators of Child Health

INTRODUCTION

Perinatal mortality rate (PMR), neonatal mortality rate (NMR), infant mortality rate (IMR), post-neonatal mortality rate (PNMR), and U5MR are few of the well-known indicators of child health. Perinatal mortality and neonatal mortality reflect the health and care of women during pregnancy and perinatal period, whereas infant mortality is described as one of the most sensitive indices of health and quality of living of a population.

Important mortality indicators of child health are defined in **Box 28.1**.

Box 28.1 Mortality Indicators of Child Health

- *Infant mortality rate:* Number of infants dying between birth and exactly 1 year of age expressed per 1,000 live births, per year
- *Neonatal mortality rate:* The number of deaths among live births during the first 28 days of life per 1,000 live births, per year
- *Early neonatal mortality rate:* The number of child deaths <7 days of life expressed as per 1,000 live births in that reference year
- *Late neonatal mortality rate:* The number of child deaths between 7 and 28 completed days of life expressed as per 1,000 live births in that reference year
- *Post-neonatal mortality rate:* The number of child deaths of 29 days to <1 year of age expressed as per 1,000 live births in the reference year
- *Perinatal mortality rate:* The number of deaths of fetus after 28 completed weeks of gestation plus the number of early neonatal deaths per 1,000 total births, per year
- *Stillbirth rate:* The number of stillbirths per 1,000 births (live and stillbirths) during the reference year

INFANT MORTALITY RATE

It is the number of infant deaths in a year in relation to 1,000 live births during the same period.

$$\text{Infant Mortality Rate (IMR)} = \frac{\text{No.of deaths in infants <1 year of age in a year}}{\text{No. of live births in the same year}} \times 1{,}000$$

The current IMR of India is 28 per thousand live births (Reference year 2020; SRS, 2022). Infant mortality is higher in girls as compared to boys. There is a wide variation in morbidity and mortality pattern of different regions in India. Madhya Pradesh has the highest infant mortality of 43 and Mizoram least of 3 per 1,000 live births (SRS, 2020). State wise IMR is shown in **Figure 28.3**.

Causes of death for neonates (0–28 days) and infants (0–1 year) in India (2015–2017) are shown in **Figures 28.4 and 28.5,** respectively.

Causes of Infant Deaths

Mortality is highest in the first few days of life. The causes of infant deaths in neonatal period (first 4 weeks of life) and post-neonatal period (between 28 days and 365 days of life) differ significantly. In the neonatal period, there are various endogenous factors attributing to high mortality. These include low birth weight, prematurity, congenital malformations, birth asphyxia, birth trauma, and neonatal infections. The post-neonatal mortality occurs due to exogenous factors like infections, e.g., pneumonia, diarrhea, vaccine preventable diseases, faulty feeding practices, malnutrition, and poor hygienic environment.

Low birth weight (birth weight <2.5 kg) is a major contributor to infant mortality. The factors causing low birth weight include maternal malnutrition, young maternal age (<18 years), high fertility rate, large family size, and less spacing between pregnancies.

Prevention of Infant Deaths

Numerous strategies have been adopted by Government of India to reduce the infant and neonatal mortality in our country. Infant and child mortality rates reflect a country's quality of life and level of socioeconomic development. Therefore, these can be used for monitoring and evaluating population, health programs, and policies.

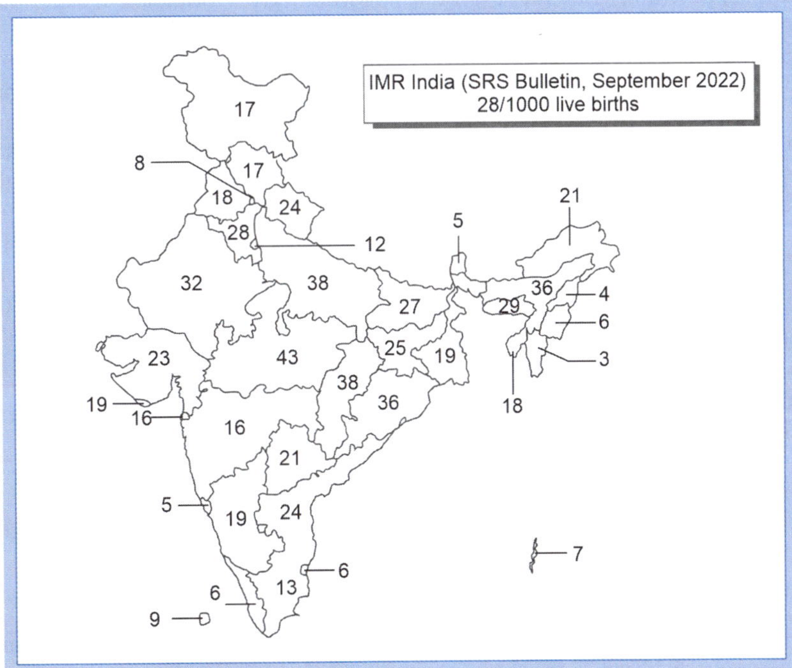

Fig. 28.3: Infant mortality rates in Indian states

Source: SRS, 2022; Reference year 2020

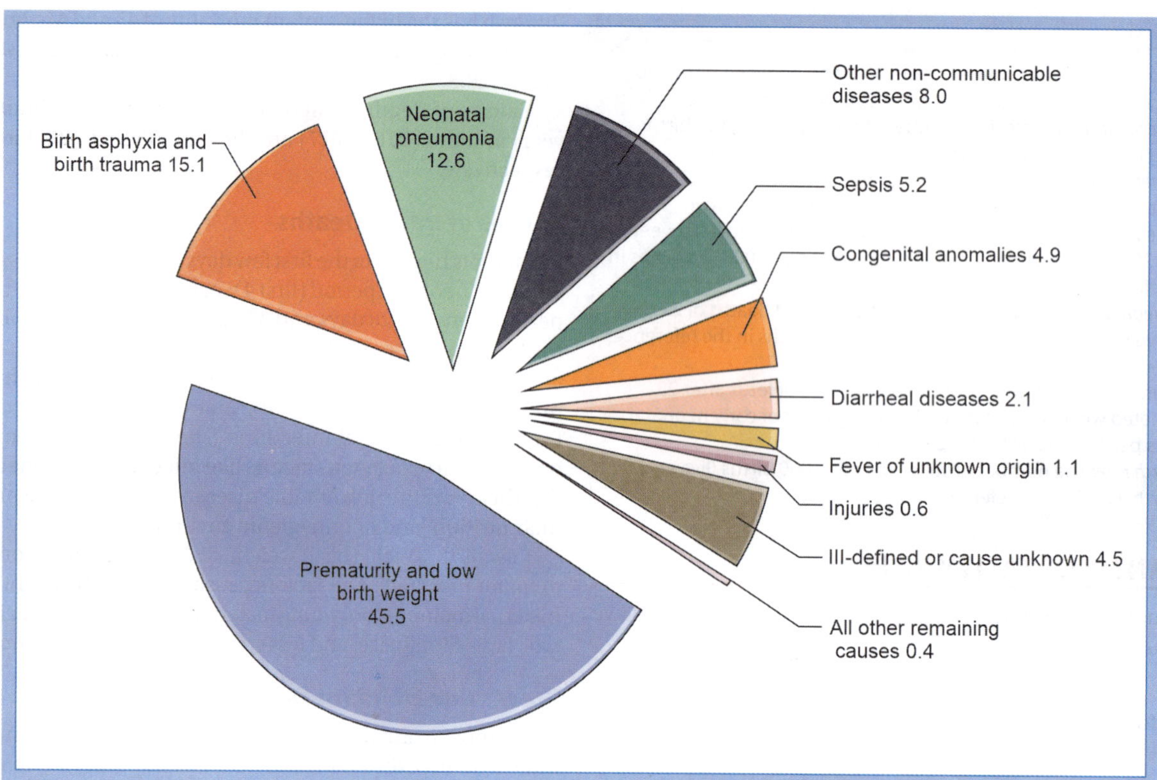

Fig. 28.4: Distribution of proportion deaths (in %) for age group below 29 days in India: 2017–2019

Source: Causes of Death Statistics 2017–2019, Government of India

Preventive measures have to be aimed at improving the nutritional status of the mother, providing good and essential antenatal care, safe delivery, essential newborn care, promotion of breastfeeding, immunization, early detection of illness (achievable by growth monitoring) and their management, family planning, efficient services for reproductive and child health (RCH), provision of safe water, sanitation, improving the social and economic condition of the people, and providing health education to the receptive audience.

PERINATAL MORTALITY RATE

Perinatal mortality rate refers to the number of deaths occurring in the perinatal period (includes stillbirths after 28 weeks of gestation plus the deaths occurring in the first 7 days after birth) in a given year to the total number of births (live and still) in the same year. It is expressed as rate per 1,000 total births. For the purpose of inclusion in this rate, the stillbirth or live births should be either (i) >1,000 g in weight, (ii) >28 weeks in gestation or if (i) and (ii) are not available, should measure 35 cm or more in length at birth.

$$\text{PMR} = \frac{(\text{Stillbirths} \geq 28 \text{ weeks} + \text{neonatal deaths during the first 7 days of life})}{(\text{Total number of births during the given year})} \times 1{,}000$$

Though the perinatal period constitutes less than 0.5% of the average human lifespan, it accounts for a significant portion of the total mortality in many developing countries. Perinatal mortality gives a valuable insight into the extent of pregnancy wastage, maternal health, and the quality of maternity and newborn healthcare. More than 5.5 million perinatal deaths occur each year worldwide; 3 million of these happen during late pregnancy and birth while 2.5 million newborn die in the first week. Africa has the highest PMR of 75 per 1,000 total births. India has PMR of 18 per 1,000 births (SRS, 2020). Perinatal mortality results from poor nutritional status of women, insufficient prevention of pregnancy related complications, and few supervised deliveries. Some of these causes are rooted in the social, cultural, and economic structure of the society.

NEONATAL MORTALITY RATE

It is the number of neonatal deaths in relation to 1,000 live births per year.

Neonatal mortality rate (NMR) =

$$\frac{\text{Number of neonatal deaths (during the first 28 completed days) in a year}}{\text{Total live births in the same year}} \times 1{,}000$$

Perinatal and neonatal mortality can be used as a measure of socioeconomic development and for international comparisons. As per the United Nations Inter-Agency Group for Child Mortality Estimation (UN IGME) 2024 report, of approximately 4.8 million

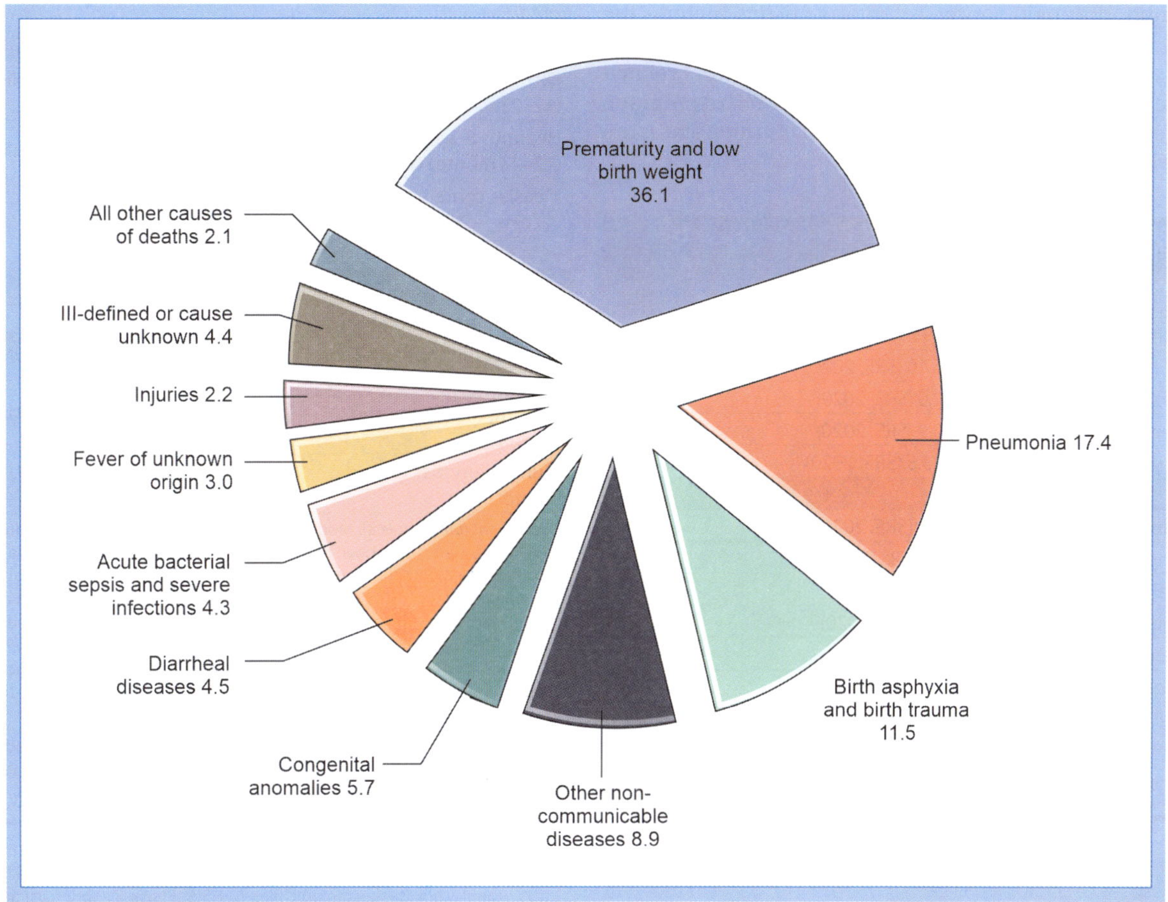

Fig. 28.5: Distribution of proportion of deaths (in %) for age group below 1 year in India: 2017–2019

Source: Causes of Death Statistics 2017–2019, Government of India

under-five deaths occurring annually, 2.3 million occur in the neonatal period in 2023. Almost 75% of estimated 2.3 million neonatal deaths occur in the early neonatal period, i.e., during first 7 days following birth. Thus, priority should be given to perinatal and neonatal problem in order to decrease infant mortality.

According to the UN IGME 2024 report, India's estimated NMR in 2023 was 17.3 deaths per 1,000 live births (lower bound: 14.8; upper bound: 20.1), closely aligning with the global average of 17 deaths per 1,000 live births. In comparison, the NMR reported by India's Sample Registration System (SRS) 2020 is 20 per 1,000 live births. Given the IMR of 28 and U5MR of 32 per 1,000 live births reported in the SRS 2020, about two-thirds of infant deaths and half of under-five child deaths in the country occur during the neonatal period. The NMR varies from 4 per 1,000 live births in Kerala to 31 per 1,000 live births in Madhya Pradesh. The early neonatal mortality rate (ENMR), deaths in the first week of life, is 15 per 1,000 live births, while late NMR is 5 per 1,000 live births. The first week of life alone accounts for 46% of total under-five child deaths. The percentage of early neonatal deaths to the total infant deaths during the year 2020, at the National level, has been 53% and it varies from 54.7 in rural areas to 46.8 in urban areas. Causes of deaths in newborn have been discussed earlier in this section.

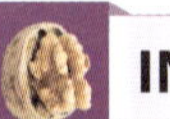

IN A NUTSHELL

Indicators of Child Health

1. Perinatal mortality rate (PMR), neonatal mortality rate (NMR), infant mortality rate (IMR), post-neonatal mortality rate (PNMR), and under-five mortality rate (U5MR) are indicators of child health.
2. Infant mortality rate in 2020 was 28/1,000 live births; and NMR was 20/1,000 live births.
3. Prematurity and low birth weight is the most important cause of infant mortality.
4. Two-thirds of infant deaths and half of under-five child deaths in the country occur during the neonatal period.

VITAL STATISTICS OF INDIA

Vital statistics are referred to a systemically collected and compiled data relating to vital events of life including birth, death, fertility, etc. These reflect the health profile of the community and form a basic tool for evaluating the adequacy of the healthcare delivery system.

In India, the main sources of vital statistics include the Census, registration records of vital events such as birth and deaths, and SRS. Current status of various indicators related to mortality, fertility, life expectancy, family welfare program, literacy status, immunization coverage, and nutrition status are summarized in **Table 28.1**.

Table 28.1 Fertility, Mortality, and Other Key Health Indicators in India

Fertility indicators	
Crude birth rate	19.5 (SRS, 2020)
General fertility rate	67.0 (SRS, 2020)
Total fertility rate	2.0 (SRS, 2020)
Gross reproduction rate	0.9 (SRS, 2020)
Natural growth rate	13.8 (SRS, 2020)
Mortality indicators	
Crude death rate	6.0 (SRS, 2020)
Infant mortality rate	28 (SRS, 2020)
Neonatal mortality rate	20 (SRS, 2020)
Early neonatal mortality rate	15 (SRS, 2020)
Late neonatal mortality rate	5 (SRS, 2020)
Post-neonatal mortality rate	8 (SRS, 2020)
Perinatal mortality rate	18 (SRS, 2020)
Stillbirth rate	3 (SRS, 2020)
Under-five mortality rate	32 (SRS, 2020)
Life expectancy at birth	Males 68 year (2019)
	Females 71 year (2019)
Immunization coverage	
Full immunization in children (12–23 months) (%)	76.4 (NFHS-5)
BCG vaccinated (12–23 month) (%)	95.2 (NFHS-5); 89 (SOWC, UNICEF, 2023)
Polio-3 vaccinated (12–23 month) (%)	80.5 (NFHS-5); 91 (SOWC, UNICEF, 2023)
DPT/Penta-3 vaccinated (12–23 month) (%)	86.9 (NFHS-5); 91 (SOWC, UNICEF, 2023)
Hepatitis B-3 vaccinated (12–23 month) (%)	83.9 (NFHS-5)
Measles containing vaccine—2 (MCV-2)	90 (SOWC, UNICEF, 2023)
PCV-3	83 (SOWC, UNICEF, 2023)
Nutrition indicators	
Under-five suffering from	
Overweight (moderate and severe)	3.4% (NFHS-5); 3% (SOWC, UNICEF, 2022)
Wasting (moderate and severe)	19% (NFHS-5); 19% (SOWC, UNICEF, 2023)
Stunting (moderate and severe)	36% (NFHS-5); 32% (SOWC, UNICEF, 2022)

Overweight (preschoolers): Moderate and severe—percentage of children aged 0–59 months who are above two standard deviations from median weight-for-height of the WHO Child Growth Standards (includes severe overweight). *Wasting (preschoolers):* Moderate and severe—percentage of children aged 0–59 months who are below minus two standard deviations from median weight-for-height of the WHO Child Growth Standards. *Stunting (preschoolers):* Moderate and severe—percentage of children aged 0–59 months who are below minus two standard deviations from median height-for-age of the WHO Child Growth Standards.

(NFHS: National Family Health Survey; SOWC: State of the World's Children; SRS: Sample Registration Survey; UNICEF: United Nations Children's Fund; WHO: World Health Organization)

Sources:
International Institute for Population Sciences (IIPS) and ICF. National Family Health Survey (NFHS-5), 2019–21: India. Mumbai: IIPS; 2021. Available from: https://mohfw.gov.in/sites/default/files/NFHS-5_Phase-II_0.pdf [Last accessed May, 2025].
Office of the Registrar General and Census Commissioner, India. Sample Registration System Bulletin. 2022. Available from: https://censusindia.gov.in/census.website/data/SRSB [Last accessed May, 2025].
World Health Organization. Life expectancy at birth (years) 2024. Available from: https://www.who.int/data/gho/data/indicators/indicator-details/GHO/life-expectancy-at-birth-(years) [Last accessed May, 2025].
UNICEF. State of the World's Children 2024. Available from: https://data.unicef.org/resources/sowc-2024/# [Last accessed May, 2025].

International Institute for Population Sciences (IIPS) and ICF. National Family Health Survey (NFHS-5), 2019–21: India. Mumbai: IIPS; 2021. Available from: https://mohfw.gov.in/sites/default/files/NFHS-5_Phase-II_0.pdf [Last accessed May, 2025].

Office of the Registrar General and Census Commissioner, India (ORGI). Sample Registration System (SRS)-Bulletin 2020 Volume 55-I. [online] Available from https://censusindia.gov.in/nada/index.php/catalog/42687 [Last accessed May, 2025].

Office of the Registrar General and Census Commissioner, India (ORGI). Sample Registration System (SRS)-Cause of Death Statistics 20152017. New Delhi: Ministry of Home Affairs, Government of India; 2022.

Office of the Registrar General and Census Commissioner, India (ORGI). Sample Registration System-Special Bulletin on Maternal mortality rate in India 2017–2019. New Delhi: Ministry of Home Affairs, Government of India; 2022.

Office of the Registrar General and Census Commissioner, India (ORGI). Sample Registration System Statistical Report 2020. New Delhi: Ministry of Home Affairs, Government of India; 2022.

Office of the Registrar General and Census Commissioner, India. Vital Statistics of India Based on the Civil Registration System 2020. New Delhi: Ministry of Home Affairs. Available from: https://censusindia.gov.in/nada/index.php/catalog/44752 [Last accessed May, 2025].

Office of the Registrar General and Census Commissioner, India. Causes of Death Statistics 2017–2019. New Delhi: Ministry of Home Affairs, Government of India; [cited 2025 May 4]. Available from: https://censusindia.gov.in/catalog/download [Last accessed May, 2025].

Office of the Registrar General and Census Commissioner, India. Sample Registration System Bulletin. 2022. Available from: https://censusindia.gov.in/census.website/data/SRSB [Last accessed May, 2025].

Press Information Bureau. Over 12 lakh children under five died in 2019; 68% of these deaths were due to communicable diseases. 2022 Sep 19. Available from: https://pib.gov.in/PressReleaseIframePage.aspx?PRID=1861710 [Last accessed May, 2025].

UNICEF. State of the World's Children 2024. Available from: https://data.unicef.org/resources/sowc-2024/# [Last accessed May, 2025].

World Health Organization. Child mortality under 5 years. Geneva: WHO. Available from: https://www.who.int/news-room/fact-sheets/detail/child-mortality-under-5-years [Last accessed May, 2025].
World Health Organization. SDG Target 3.2: Newborn and child mortality [Internet]. Geneva: WHO. Available from: https://www.who.int/data/gho/data/themes/topics/indicator-groups/indicator-group-details/GHO/sdg-target-3.2-newborn-and-child-mortality [Last accessed May, 2025].
World Health Organization. Life expectancy at birth (years) 2024. Available from: https://www.who.int/data/gho/data/indicators/indicator-details/GHO/life-expectancy-at-birth-(years) [Last accessed May, 2025].

28.3 National Health Mission

PE 17.1

INTRODUCTION

The National Health Mission (NHM) was launched in 2013 by the government subsuming the National Rural Health Mission (NRHM) and National Urban Health Mission (NUHM). NHM foresees attainment of the goals and targets set out in the National Health Policy, 2017 for ensuring "universal access to equitable, affordable, and quality healthcare services that are accountable and responsive to the needs of the people." This would advance the country's progress toward the Sustainable Development Goal (SDG) 3, i.e., "Ensure healthy lives and promote well-being for all at all ages," including Universal Health Coverage (UHC). The main programs under NHM are (1) Health systems strengthening, (2) Reproductive, maternal, neonatal, child, adolescent health and nutrition (RMNCAH+N), and (3) Communicable disease control programs, (4) Non-communicable disease control programs, and (5) Infrastructure maintenance.

Some of the major initiatives under NHM are discussed in **Table 28.2**.

Table 28.2 Major Initiatives under National Health Mission

Sl. No.	Major initiatives	Summary
1.	Accredited Social Health Activists (ASHAs)	Volunteer community health workers serving as the link between rural populations and healthcare systems. Over 9.15 lakh ASHAs are currently active nationwide, significantly contributing to institutional births, immunization coverage, and disease control efforts
2.	Rogi Kalyan Samiti (RKS)/Hospital Management Society	A registered community-based management body that functions as a governance mechanism for public hospitals. Members of the Samiti act as custodians, overseeing hospital operations, maintaining infrastructure, and ensuring the provision of quality services to patients. A total of 31,673 RKS have been established across various levels of healthcare facilities
3.	Untied Grants to Sub-Centers	Financial support provided to grassroots health units to boost efficiency and empower local health governance bodies, ensuring better healthcare delivery
4.	Village Health Sanitation and Nutrition Committee (VHSNCs)	The VHSNCs, consisting of members from the Panchayati Raj System, play a key role in overseeing and planning local health, sanitation, and nutrition initiatives. With approximately 5 lakh committees across the nation, they are pivotal in ensuring the effective implementation and monitoring of public health services at the grassroots level
5.	Healthcare Service Delivery	The NHM has contributed to expanding the healthcare workforce by deploying 1.88 lakh additional personnel and upgrading the skills of doctors and nurses, including the induction of 24,890 AYUSH practitioners
6.	Janani Suraksha Yojana (JSY)	It aims to reduce maternal mortality by encouraging institutional deliveries in government health facilities. It provides financial assistance to eligible pregnant women. Since its launch, over 8.55 crore women have benefited from the scheme
7.	Janani Shishu Suraksha Karyakram (JSSK)	It provides free and no expense delivery services, including cesarean sections, for all pregnant women in public health institutions, along with free treatment for sick infants under 1 year of age. The entitlements cover drugs, diagnostics, diet, blood, transport, and waive all user charges, ensuring equitable access to maternal and child healthcare
8.	Facility-based Newborn Care	It is a structured system of newborn care units which provide round-the-clock care from birth through the postnatal period. Essential care is provided at health facilities during the first 48 hours after delivery and is followed by continued monitoring at home for the next 42 days. Newborn care corners (NBCCs) are set up at delivery points to offer immediate care at birth, while newborn stabilization units (NBSUs) at first referral units (FRUs) and special newborn care units (SNCUs) at district hospitals and medical colleges cater to the needs of ill or at-risk newborns
9.	National Mobile Medical Units (NMMUs)	Mobile clinics bringing healthcare to underserved and remote regions, currently operational in 333 of 672 districts with a fleet of 1107 units

Contd...

Contd...

Sl. No.	Major initiatives	Summary
10.	National Ambulance Services (NAS)	Emergency medical transportation accessible via a toll-free number, ensuring timely medical intervention during emergencies
11.	Mainstreaming of Ayush	Integrating traditional healthcare (AYUSH) services into 10042 PHCs, 2732 CHCs, 501 district hospitals, and thousands of other public health facilities below the district level
12.	National Quality Assurance Framework	Introduced in November 2014, this framework sets quality benchmarks for public health institutions, targeting over 31,000 facilities
13.	Kayakalp Initiative	A cleanliness and hygiene initiative recognizing high-performing public facilities. Swachhta Guidelines, released in May 2015, outline standards and monitoring protocols
14.	Comprehensive Primary Healthcare	A broad approach to primary care that emphasizes early diagnosis, better service organization, access to modern tools and medication, digital systems, skilled personnel, and equity in healthcare delivery
15.	Kilkari	*Kilkari* is a free mobile health service that sends weekly, stage-based audio messages about pregnancy and childcare to expectant and new mothers, from the second trimester until the child turns one. Messages, voiced by a fictional doctor, Dr Anita, are delivered via calls based on data from the reproductive child health (RCH) portal. Kilkari runs in 18 States/UTs and mobile academy is active in 17, in six regional languages

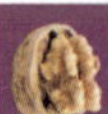

IN A NUTSHELL

National Health Mission

1. To provide universal access to equitable, affordable, and quality healthcare services, India's Ministry of Health and Family Welfare (MOHFW) launched the "National Rural Health Mission" and the "National Urban Health Mission." These were later merged into the "National Health Mission" (NHM).
2. Main programs under NHM are (1) Health system strengthening, (2) Reproductive, maternal, neonatal, child, adolescent health and nutrition (RMNCAH+N), and (3) Communicable disease control programs, (4) Non-communicable diseases control program, and (5) Infrastructure maintenance.

NATIONAL RURAL HEALTH MISSION (NRHM)

National Rural Health Mission was launched on 12th April 2005 throughout the country with special focus on improving healthcare in the Empowered Action Group (EAG) States—comprising Bihar, Jharkhand, Madhya Pradesh, Chhattisgarh, Odisha, Rajasthan, Uttar Pradesh, and Uttarakhand—along with the North Eastern States, Jammu and Kashmir, and Himachal Pradesh by establishing a decentralized, community-owned health system that ensures access to essential services, strengthens infrastructure, promotes inter-sectoral convergence, utilizes ASHA workers, and emphasizes accountability, community participation, outcome-based standards, and flexible, innovative approaches. The mission aimed at providing accessible, affordable, and quality care to weaker sections in rural area. The five main approaches in NRHM are shown in **Figure 28.6**.

NATIONAL URBAN HEALTH MISSION (NUHM)

To effectively address the health concerns of the urban poor population, the Government of India launched NUHM on 1st May 2008. NUHM envisages to meet healthcare needs of the urban population with the nucleus being poor urban, by making available to them essential primary healthcare services, reducing cost of treatment, strengthening the existing urban health delivery system and integrating efforts with other schemes that influence health outcomes, such as those related to drinking water, sanitation, education, and nutrition. The urban healthcare delivery model is depicted in **Figure 28.7**. These schemes are implemented in coordination with various ministries, including Urban Development, Housing and Urban Poverty Alleviation, Human Resource Development, and Women and Child Development.

The mission covers all state capitals, district headquarters, and towns with populations exceeding 50,000, focusing primarily on slum dwellers and marginalized groups such as rickshaw pullers, street vendors, the homeless, street children, and construction site workers. The funding pattern between the central and state governments is set at 75:25 for most states, while a higher central share of 90:10 is allocated to North-Eastern states, Sikkim, Jammu and Kashmir, Himachal Pradesh, and Uttarakhand. States are required to submit Program Implementation Plans (PIPs), which are then reviewed and approved by the Ministry of Health and Family Welfare.

Ministry of Health and Family Welfare. National Health Mission: Child Health Programme. New Delhi: MoHFW. Available from: https://nhm.gov.in/index1.php?lang=1&level=2&sublinkid=819&lid=219 [Last accessed May, 2025]

National Rural Health Mission. Meeting people's health needs in rural areas. [online] Available from https://nhm.gov.in/WriteReadData/l892s/nrhm-framework-latest.pdf [Last accessed May, 2025].

National Urban Health Mission. Framework for Implementation. [online] Available from https://nhm.gov.in/images/pdf/NUHM/Implementation_Framework_NUHM.pdf [Last accessed May, 2025].

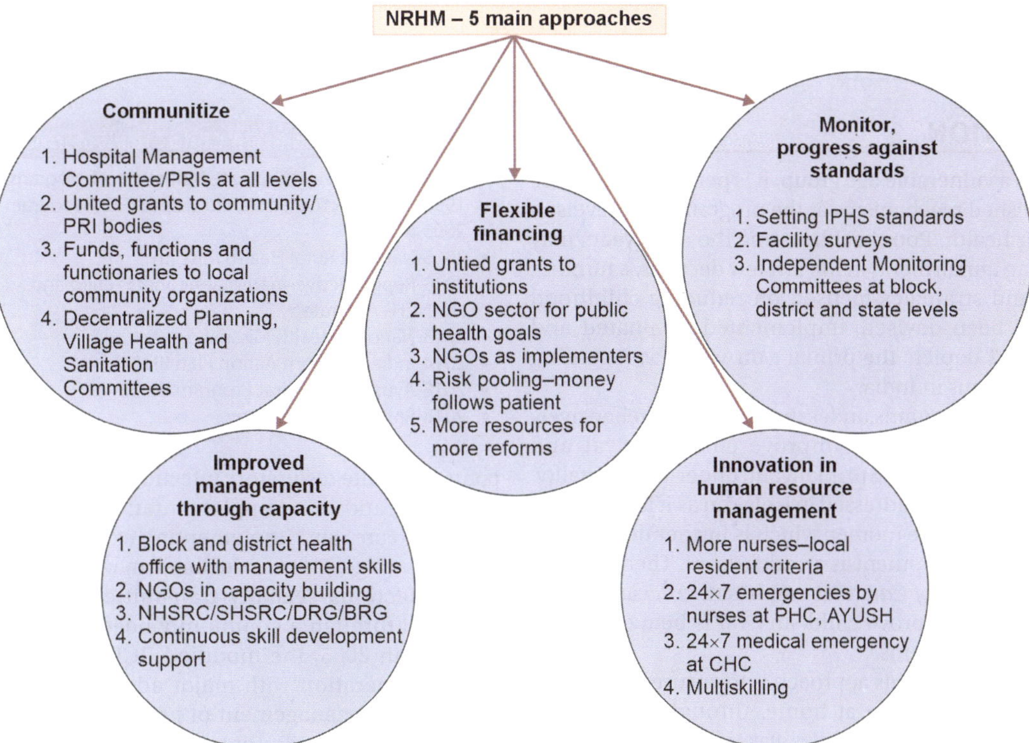

Fig. 28.6: 5-Pronged approach of National Rural Health Mission

(AYUSH: Ayurveda, Yoga, Naturopathy, Unani, Siddha and Homoeopathy; BRG: Block Resource Group; CHC: Community Health Center; DRG: District Resource Group; IPHS: Indian Public Health Standards; NHSRC: National Health Systems Resource Center; NGO: non-governmental organization; PHC: Primary Health Center; PRI: Panchayati Raj Institution; SHSRC: State Health Systems Resource Center)

Source: National Rural Health Mission. Meeting people's health needs in rural areas. [online] Available from https://nhm.gov.in/WriteReadData/l892s/ nrhm-framework-latest.pdf [Last accessed May, 2025]

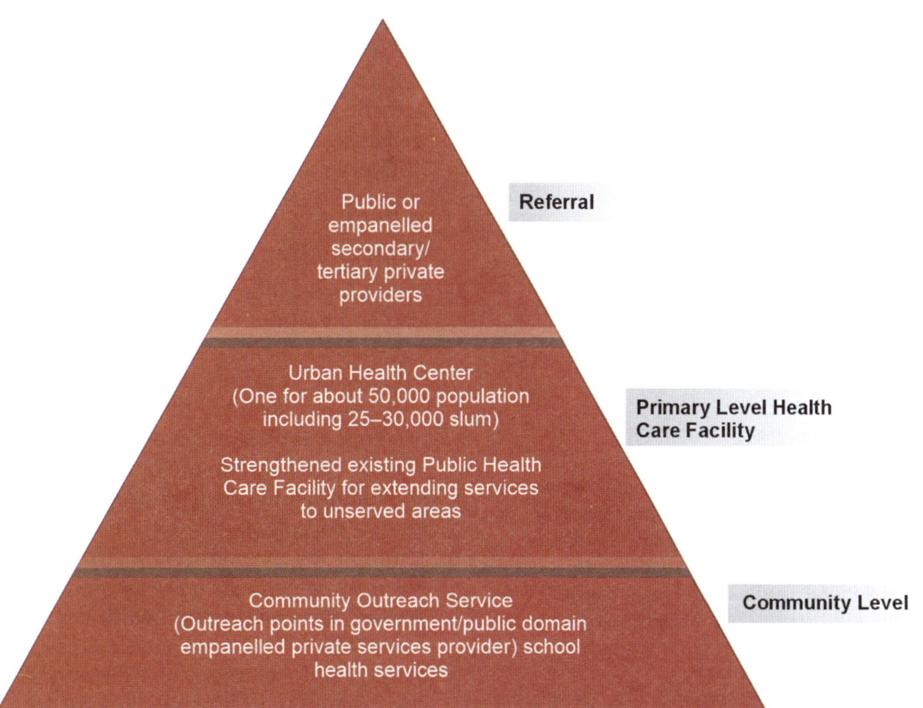

Fig. 28.7: Urban healthcare delivery model under National Urban Health Mission

Source: National Urban Health Mission. Framework for Implementation. [online] Available from https://nhm.gov.in/images/pdf/NUHM/Implementation_Framework_NUHM.pdf [Last accessed May, 2025]

28.4 Child Health Programs

PE 17.1

INTRODUCTION

As childhood is a vulnerable age group, it is pertinent that there are well-established mechanisms at the programmatic levels to safeguard their health. Poor health during the early years may lead to a lifelong impairment. In the last few decades, a number of programs and strategies focused on reducing childhood mortality have been devised, implemented, evaluated and revised. **Box 28.2** depicts the primary thrust areas regarding child health programs in India.

The child health programs under the NHM comprehensively integrates interventions that improve child survival and addresses factors contributing to infant and under-five mortality. Child survival cannot be addressed in isolation as it is intricately linked to the health of the mother, which is further determined by her health and development as an adolescent. Therefore, the concept of *Continuum of Care* that emphasizes on care during critical life stages to improve child survival is being followed under the national programs.

Another dimension of this approach is to ensure that critical services are made available at home, through community outreach, and through health facilities at various levels [primary, first referral units (FRUs), and tertiary healthcare facilities]. The newborn and child health are now the two key pillars of the RMNCH+A strategic approach, 2013.

CHILD SURVIVAL AND SAFE MOTHERHOOD PROGRAMME (1992–1997)

In India, child healthcare services moved from vertical child survival programs to a horizontal integrated program through the Child Survival and Safe Motherhood Programme (CSSM) launched in 1992. Further inclusion of adolescent age group and reproductive health led to the launch of Reproductive and Child Health (RCH) Programme in 1997. A wide range of initiatives were carried out under these programs, namely, immunization, control of acute respiratory infections (ARI), control of diarrhea, vitamin A and iron supplementation, provision of essential newborn care, and implementing exclusive breastfeeding till 6 months of age. This also included management of reproductive tract infections/sexually transmitted infections (RTI/STI) delivered through a community needs assessment approach (CNAA). In 2005, the modified RCH program (RCH II) was put into operation with major addition being the inclusion of integrated management of neonatal and childhood illness (IMNCI). Various milestones in child survival programs in India are listed in **Box 28.3**.

Box 28.2 Thrust Areas in Child Health Programs in India

A. *Thrust area 1: Neonatal health*
   1. Essential newborn care (at every "delivery" point at time of birth)
   2. Facility based sick newborn care [at first referral units (FRUs) and district hospitals]
   3. Home-based newborn care
B. *Thrust area 2: Nutrition*
   1. Promotion of optimal infant and young child feeding practices
   2. Micronutrient supplementation (vitamin A, iron folic acid)
   3. Management of children with severe acute malnutrition
C. *Thrust area 3: Management of common childhood illnesses*
   1. Management of childhood diarrheal diseases and acute respiratory infections
D. *Thrust area 4: Immunization*
   1. Intensification of routine immunization
   2. Eliminating measles and Japanese encephalitis-related deaths
   3. Polio eradication

Box 28.3 Milestones in Child Survival Programs in India

- 1992-Child Survival and Safe Motherhood Program (CSSM)
- 1997-Reproductive and Child Health (RCH) Program – I
- 2005-RCH II
- 2005-National Rural Health Mission
- 2013-Reproductive-maternal-neonatal-child and adolescent health (RMNCH+A) Strategy
- 2013-National Health Mission
- 2014-India Newborn Action Plan (INAP)
- 2018-Ayushman Bharat Program
- 2018-RMNCAH+N Strategy

REPRODUCTIVE AND CHILD HEALTH PROGRAMME (1997–2013)

One of the key priorities of the National Health Mission (NHM) is to reduce infant and maternal mortality rates while ensuring the provision of quality healthcare services for pregnant women and children across the country. In order to improve mother and child health status and to fulfill the unmet needs of family welfare services in the country, Government of India launched RCH programme in 1997–1998 during the 9th plan period by integrating CSSM programme with other RCH services.

Reproductive and Child Health (RCH) Phase I

RCH 1 focused on child survival and safe motherhood, while also addressing the prevention and management of sexually transmitted infections (STIs) and reproductive tract infections (RTIs). The key interventions under this phase included the provision of essential obstetric care to all pregnant women, promoting early registration, regular antenatal check-ups, safe deliveries either at home by trained professionals or in health institutions, and timely postnatal care. To manage pregnancy-related complications, emergency obstetric care was made available by strengthening first referral units (FRUs) and ensuring 24-hour delivery services at primary health centers (PHCs) and community health centers (CHCs). Other major components included medical termination of pregnancy, control and treatment of RTIs and STIs, full immunization coverage, essential newborn care, and the management of common childhood illnesses such as diarrheal diseases and acute respiratory infections. Additionally, the program aimed to prevent vitamin A deficiency and anemia among children and emphasized training traditional birth attendants (dais) to promote safe delivery practices.

Reproductive and Child Health (RCH) Phase II

Launched on April 1, 2005, RCH II program focuses on reducing maternal and child morbidity and mortality, particularly in rural areas. Key strategies include promoting essential obstetric care through institutional deliveries and skilled birth attendance, operationalizing primary health centers (PHCs) and community health centers (CHCs) for round-the-clock delivery services, and enhancing emergency obstetric care through fully functional first referral units (FRUs). FRUs are equipped to provide comprehensive services such as 24/7 delivery care (including assisted and caesarean deliveries), newborn care, emergency treatment for sick children, family planning, safe abortions, STI/RTI treatment, blood storage, laboratory services, and referral transport. For a facility to function as an FRU, it must have at least 20–30 beds (requirement initially relaxed to 10–12 beds in challenging regions, such as the North-East states and underserved areas of EAG states), a functional labor room and operation theatre, newborn care areas, reliable water and electricity, waste disposal systems, and ambulance services. RCH Phase II also strengthens the referral system, and states are now exploring partnerships with self-help groups, NGOs, and women's collectives for more effective linkages. New initiatives under this phase include training MBBS doctors in life-saving anesthesia and emergency obstetric procedures, and establishing blood storage units at FRUs to support emergency care. These efforts aim to ensure timely, skilled, and accessible care for women and children across underserved and high-need areas.

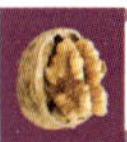

IN A NUTSHELL

Child Health Programs

1. In 1951, India was the first country in the world to launch a family planning program.
2. Child healthcare services moved from vertical child survival programs to a horizontal integrated program through the Child Survival and Safe Motherhood Programme (CSSM) launched in 1992.
3. Inclusion of adolescent age group and reproductive health led to the launch of Reproductive and Child Health (RCH) Programme in 1997.
4. For comprehensive healthcare services, encompassing both preventive and curative aspects "Reproductive, Maternal, Newborn, Child and Adolescent Health program" was launched during the "National Summit on Call to Action for Child Survival and Development" in February 2013.
5. Key strategies in RCH phase II include promoting essential obstetric care through institutional deliveries and skilled birth attendance, operationalizing primary health centers (PHCs) and community health Centers (CHCs) for round-the-clock delivery services, and enhancing emergency obstetric care through fully functional first referral units (FRUs).

Dutta PK. Scope of health systems research in Child Survival and Safe Motherhood Programme. Indian J Matern Child Health. 1993;4(2):38-41.

Mohapatra SC. Reproductive health: faces old and new. Indian J Matern Child Health. 1996;7(3):61-2.

Ministry of Health and Family Welfare, Government of India. Reproductive and Child Health (RCH) Portal. New Delhi: MoHFW. Available from: https://rch.mohfw.gov.in/RCH/about-rch.aspx [Last accessed May, 2025].

USAID. India's Reproductive, Maternal, Newborn, Child, and Adolescent Health Strategy: A case of extraordinary government leadership. New Delhi: Ministry of Health and Family Welfare, Government of India; 2014.

28.5 Reproductive, Maternal, Newborn, Child, Adolescent Health and Nutrition (RMNCAH+N) Program

PE 17.1

INTRODUCTION

- Improving maternal and child health and their survival is central to achieving the sustainable development goals (SDGs). In response to the Government of India's "Call to Action (CTA) Summit" in February 2013, the Ministry of Health and Family Welfare launched the Reproductive, Maternal, Newborn, Child plus Adolescent Health (RMNCH+A) strategy.
- The RMNCH+A program strategic approach has been developed to provide an understanding of "continuum of care" to ensure equal focus on various life stages.
- Recognizing the crucial role of nutrition across all life stages, the strategy evolved into RMNCAH+N, incorporating nutrition as a key pillar.
- It also introduces new initiatives such as the use of score card to track the performance, National Iron + Initiative to address the issue of anemia across all age groups, and the comprehensive screening and early interventions for defects at birth, diseases and deficiencies among children and adolescents.
- The RMNCAH+N appropriately directs the states to focus their efforts on the most vulnerable population and

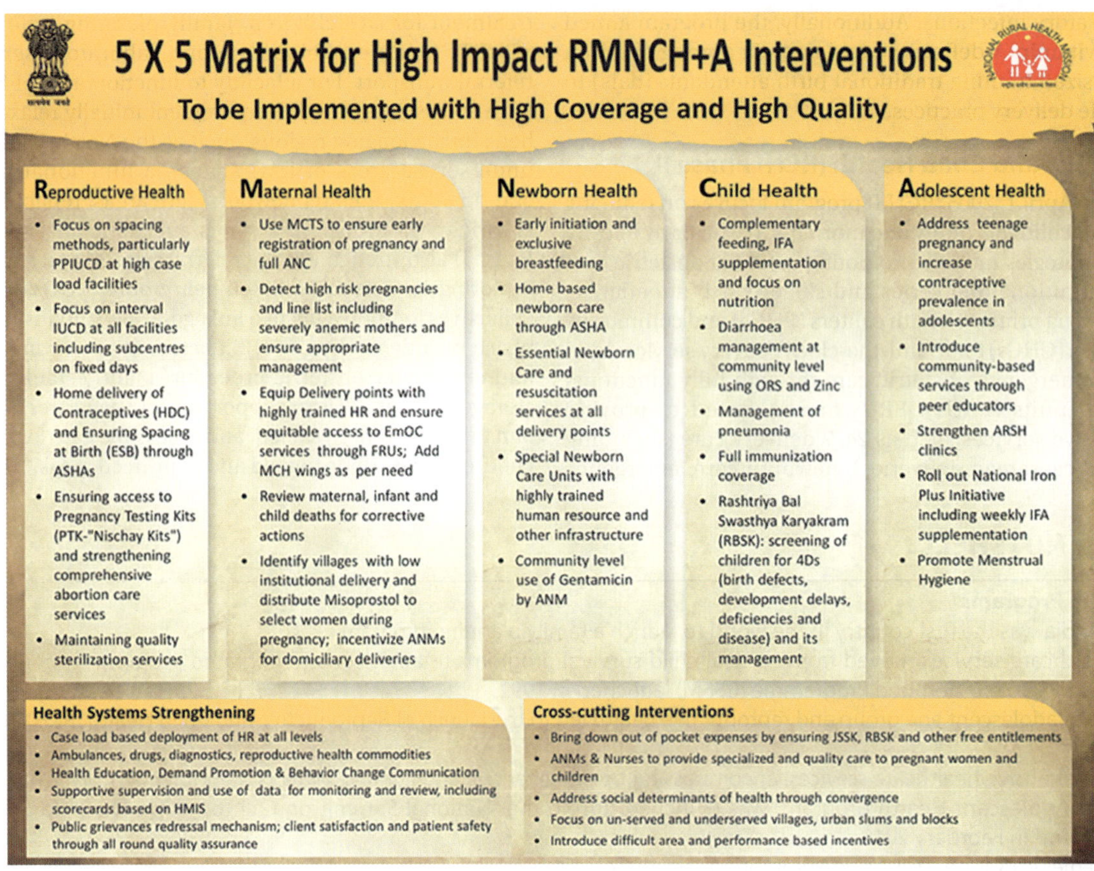

Fig. 28.8: RMNCH+A 5 × 5 Matrix

(ANMs: auxiliary nurse midwives; ASHA: accredited social health activist; HMIS: health management and information system; MCH: maternal and child health; PPIUCD: postpartum intrauterine contraceptive devices; RMNCH+A: reproductive, maternal, newborn, and child plus adolescent health approach)

Source: Ministry of Health and Family Welfare, Government of India. (2013). A Strategic Approach to Reproductive, Maternal, Newborn, Child and Adolescent Health in India. [online] Available from https://nhm.gov.in/images/pdf/RMNCH+A/RMNCH+A_Strategy.pdf [Last accessed May, 2025]

disadvantaged groups in the country. The "Plus" within the strategy focuses on nutrition as well as the continuum of care with linkages between the interventions targeted at various stages of lifecycle from newborn to the reproductive age, with focus on adolescence as a distinct life stage.

- The broad components are reproductive healthcare, antenatal care, pregnancy and childbirth care, postnatal care, newborn and childcare, and adolescent healthcare. The RMNCH+A 5 × 5 matrix is given in **Figure 28.8**.

COVERAGE TARGETS FOR KEY RMNCAH+N

- Increase facilities equipped for perinatal care (designated as "delivery points") by 100%.
- Increase proportion of all births in government and accredited private institutions.
- Increase proportion of pregnant women receiving antenatal care.
- Increase proportion of mothers and newborns receiving postnatal care.
- Increase proportion of deliveries conducted by skilled birth attendants.

Priority Interventions

- Home-based newborn care (HBNC) and prompt referral.
- Facility-based care of the sick newborn.
- Integrated management of common childhood illnesses (diarrhea, pneumonia, and malaria).
- Child nutrition and essential micronutrients supplementation.
- Immunization.
- Early detection and management of defects at birth, deficiencies, diseases, and disability in children (0–18 years).

In 2024, the Government of India continues to implement the RMNCAH+N strategy under the National Health Mission to address anemia and malnutrition among women and children. As part of this, the following key interventions have been implemented:

- ***Mothers' Absolute Affection (MAA)*** initiative promotes early initiation and exclusive breastfeeding for the first 6 months, followed by appropriate complementary feeding, through capacity building of health workers and public awareness campaigns.
- ***Nutrition Rehabilitation Centers (NRCs)*** provide in-patient care for children under five suffering from severe acute

malnutrition with medical complications, focusing on proper feeding practices, micronutrient correction, and caregiver education.

- ***Anemia Mukt Bharat (AMB)*** program to combat anemia across six beneficiary groups using a lifecycle approach with six key interventions, including iron and folic acid supplementation, behaviour change communication, anemia testing and treatment, addressing non-nutritional causes, incentives for frontline workers, and community awareness campaigns.
  - ***National Deworming Day*** is observed biannually to administer albendazole to children and adolescents to reduce worm infestations.
- ***Village Health, Sanitation and Nutrition Days (VHSNDs)*** offer maternal and child care at Anganwadi centers in coordination with ICDS.
- Educational materials like the **MCP Card and Safe Motherhood Booklet** are distributed to pregnant women to raise awareness about proper nutrition, adequate rest, warning signs during pregnancy, available benefit schemes, and the importance of institutional deliveries.

ADOLESCENT HEALTH

Adolescent health is a unique feature of this strategy. Although adolescence is considered to be a healthy phase, >33% of the disease burden and almost 60% of premature deaths among adults can be associated with behaviors or conditions that begin or occur during adolescence, e.g., tobacco and alcohol use, poor eating habits, sexual abuse, and risky sex.

Within the age group of 10–19 years, the profile of disease burden is significantly different for younger and older adolescents. While injuries and communicable diseases are prominent causes of disability and death in the 0–14 years age group, outcomes of sexual behaviors, and mental health become significant for the 15–19 years age group.

Priority Interventions

- Adolescent nutrition, iron and folic acid (IFA) supplementation.
- Facility-based adolescent reproductive and sexual health services (AH clinics).
- Information and counseling on adolescent sexual reproductive health and other health issues.
- Menstrual hygiene.
- Preventive health checkups.

HOME-BASED NEWBORN CARE

There is ample evidence to suggest that despite increasing number of institutional deliveries a substantial number of neonatal deaths occur at home. In cases where a baby is delivered at an institution and is discharged after 48 hours, the baby may still be at risk of illness in the first week to first month of life. In some cases, the mother would like to return home within few hours of delivery. Launched in 2011, the HBNC program aims to reduce neonatal mortality and morbidity, particularly in rural and remote areas with limited access to healthcare.

The key provider of HBNC is accredited social health activist (ASHA), a key health worker under the NHM. The program mandates ASHAs to visit all newborns during the first 42 days of life—six visits for institutional deliveries (on days 3, 7, 14, 21, 28, and 42) and an additional visit within 24 hours for home deliveries. Extra visits are made for pre-term, low birth weight, sick newborns, and those discharged from special newborn care units (SNCUs). Through these home visits, she provides newborn care by weighing the newborn, ensuring warmth and counseling the mother on temperature maintenance, initiating and supporting exclusive breastfeeding, promoting skin, eye and cord care, and identifying early signs of sepsis and other illnesses. ASHAs receive incentives upon completion of the visit schedule.

HOME-BASED CARE OF YOUNG CHILDREN

Home-based care of young children (HBYC) is being rolled out as an extension of HBNC in 2018 under the National Health Mission and POSHAN Abhiyan. While HBNC visits end at 42nd day of birth, there was a gap where there was no contact with the health worker and the child and the family, except for the immunization sessions. HBYC focuses on promoting health, nutrition, and early childhood development for children aged 3 to 15 months. ASHAs conduct an additional five visits during the 3rd, 6th, 9th, 12th and 15th months. During these visits, counseling regarding breastfeeding, complementary feeding, early child development, growth monitoring, immunization are carried out. Underweight children are identified. ASHAs also assist in preventing and managing common childhood illnesses during the visits, ensure timely referral and follow-up for sick children. It is being implemented in a phased manner.

ESTABLISHMENT OF NEWBORN CARE FACILITIES AND FACILITY-BASED INTEGRATED MANAGEMENT OF NEWBORN AND CHILDHOOD ILLNESSES (F-IMNCI)

- Facility-based integrated management of newborn and childhood illnesses (F-IMNCI) is the integration of the facility-based care package with the IMNCI package, to empower the health personnel with the skills to manage newborn and childhood illness at the community level as well as at the facility. It was first launched in the year 2009, providing appropriate skills and training for inpatient management of major causes of neonatal and childhood mortality such as asphyxia, sepsis, low-birth weight, malnutrition, diarrhea and pneumonia.
- To address the issues of higher neonatal and early neonatal mortality, facility-based newborn care services at health facilities have been emphasized. This includes setting-up of facilities for care of sick newborn such as special newborn care units (SNCUs), newborn stabilization units (NBSUs), and newborn care corners (NBCCs) at different levels of healthcare.
- In 2023, it has now been bifurcated into two packages based on outpatient and inpatient management:
  1. Integrated Management of Newborn and Child Illnesses (IMNCI)—for outpatient management of both young infants (0–2 months) and children up to 5 years of age.

2. A new package "Facility Based Care of Sick Children" has been introduced which focuses on providing appropriate inpatient management of major causes of child mortality beyond the neonatal age (1–59 months). It includes common illnesses like diarrhea, pneumonia, malaria, meningitis, and severe malnutrition.

INDIA NEWBORN ACTION PLAN

The India Newborn Action Plan (INAP) is India's strategic response to the Global Every Newborn Action Plan (ENAP), which was launched in June 2014 at the 67th World Health Assembly for advancement of the Global Strategy for Women and Children's Health. ENAP envisions a world where preventable newborn deaths and stillbirths are eliminated. INAP outlines a clear vision and roadmap for India to achieve this goal by ending preventable newborn deaths, accelerating progress, and scaling up high impact yet cost-effective interventions. INAP aims to intensify and align efforts toward achieving the targets of reducing both NMR and stillbirth rate to single digits by the year 2030. For the first time, it also highlights the Government of India's specific focus on preventing stillbirths. INAP is guided by the principles of integration, equity, gender sensitivity, quality of care, convergence, accountability, and partnerships. It includes six pillars of intervention packages across various stages with specific actions to impact stillbirths and newborn health: (1) Preconception and antenatal care; (2) Care during labor and childbirth; (3) Immediate newborn care; (4) Care of healthy newborn; (5) Care of small and sick newborn; and (6) Care beyond newborn survival. Aim of INAP is to attain single digit NMR by 2030. INAP serves as a comprehensive framework for Indian states to develop area-specific action plans, translating national commitments into tangible improvements in newborn health.

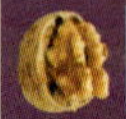

IN A NUTSHELL

Reproductive, Maternal, Newborn, Child Plus Adolescent Health (RMNCAH+N) Program

1. Reproductive, maternal, newborn, child plus adolescent health program focuses on the most vulnerable population.
2. The broad components of RMNCAH+N are reproductive healthcare, antenatal care, pregnancy and childbirth care, postnatal care, newborn and childcare, adolescent health care and nutrition.
3. Facility-based integrated management of newborn and childhood illnesses (F-IMNCI) launched alongside IMNCI to provide quality care of newborns at the facility.
4. India Newborn Action Plan (INAP) includes six pillars of intervention packages.

Arndt MB, Murray CJL, Gakidou E, et al. Global, regional, and national progress towards the 2030 global nutrition targets and forecasts to 2050: a systematic analysis for the Global Burden of Disease Study 2021. Lancet. 2024;404(10471):2543-83.

Ministry of Health and Family Welfare, Government of India. (2013). A Strategic Approach to Reproductive, Maternal, Newborn, Child and Adolescent Health In India. [online] Available from https://nhm.gov.in/images/pdf/RMNCH+A/RMNCH+A_Strategy.pdf [Last accessed May 2025].

Ministry of Health and Family Welfare, Government of India. (2014). India Newborn Action Plan, Child Health Division. [online] Available from https://www.newbornwhocc.org/INAP_Final.pdf [Last accessed May, 2025].

Ministry of Health and Family Welfare Government of India. Facility-based integrated management of newborn and childhood illnesses (F-IMNCI). [online] Available from https://nhm.gov.in/images/pdf/programmes/childhealth/guidelines/imnci_chart_booklet.pdf [Last accessed May, 2025].

Ministry of Health and Family Welfare. India Newborn Action Plan (INAP) [Internet]. New Delhi: MoHFW. Available from: https://nhm.gov.in/images/pdf/programmes/inap-final.pdf [Last accessed May, 2025].

Ministry of Health and Family Welfare, Government of India. RMNCAH+N: Reproductive, Maternal, Newborn, Child, Adolescent Health and Nutrition [Internet]. New Delhi: National Health Mission. Available from: https://nhm.gov.in/index1.php?lang=1&level=1&sublinkid=794&lid=168 [Last accessed May, 2025].

Ministry of Education. Guidelines on PM POSHAN Scheme, 2023 [Internet]. New Delhi: MoE. Available from: https://pmposhan.education.gov.in/Files/Guidelines/2023/Guidelines%20on%20PM%20POSHAN%20SCHEME.pdf [Last accessed May, 2025].

Press Information Bureau. Government of India expands PM POSHAN Scheme [Internet]. 2022 Jan 5. Available from: https://pib.gov.in/PressReleasePage.aspx?PRID=1794595 [Last accessed May, 2025].

Taneja G, Sridhar VS, Mohanty JS, et al. India's RMNCH+A Strategy: approach, learnings and limitations. BMJ Global Health. 2019;4: e001162.

USAID. (2014). India's Reproductive, Maternal, Newborn, Child, and Adolescent Health Strategy: A case of extraordinary government leadership. [online] Available from https://www.mchip.net/sites/default/files/RMNCH+A%20in%20India.pdf [Last accessed May 2025].

28.6 Other National Programs for Maternal and Child Health

PE17.1

NAVJAT SISHU SURAKSHA KARYAKARAM

Effective newborn care is a crucial challenge that is faced by every healthcare setting dealing in maternal and child health. A key component is to equip the staff with appropriate knowledge and skill. The Ministry of Health and Family Welfare is addressing this through the launch of the *Navjat Sishu Suraksha Karyakaram (NSSK)* in 2009 (revised in 2020). This program provides training to healthcare workers, providing them with evidence based knowledge and skills in improving newborn care and resuscitation techniques, particularly during the critical first few minutes after birth. The health provider after training will furnish all the required care at birth, identify and manage common complications (such as birth asphyxia, infections, hypothermia, and breastfeeding issues), stabilize, and refer or transfer newborns needing additional interventions. The objective of this initiative is to have trained health personnel in basic newborn care and resuscitation at every delivery point. This program is a key component of India's efforts to reduce the NMR and stillbirth rate to single digits by 2030.

JANANI SHISHU SURAKSHA KARYAKARAM

High out-of-pocket expenditure invested in provision of antenatal mother and sick newborn care including expenses on drugs, investigation, medical procedures, and other consumables, is one of the major obstacles toward the reduction of maternal mortality ratio (MMR) and IMR. To address this financial need, *Janani Shishu Suraksha Karyakaram* (JSSK) was launched by the Government of India on 1st June 2011 with the aim of reducing out-of-pocket expenses for pregnant women and sick newborns. The program is designed to benefit over 12 million pregnant women who seek delivery care at government health facilities, while also encouraging home deliveries to shift towards institutional births. Under JSSK, pregnant women are entitled to several free services including free delivery and cesarean section, transportation (to and from government health facility, including inter-facility transfers), drugs and consumables, diagnostics, diet during hospital stay, provision of blood, and exemption from user charges. Similarly, sick newborns up to 30 days after birth are entitled to free treatment, drugs, diagnostics, blood provision, and transportation services under the scheme. This has now been extended to cover sick infants as well. In line with Janani Suraksha Yojana, the program aims toward reducing the IMR and MMR. This comprehensive package aims to ensure that financial barriers do not prevent access to essential maternal and newborn healthcare.

LaQshya

LaQshya (Labour Room Quality Improvement Initiative) is a program launched by the Ministry of Health and Family Welfare, Government of India, in 2017 to enhance the quality of care for pregnant women and newborns during labor, delivery, and the immediate postpartum period. The initiative focuses on reducing preventable maternal and newborn deaths, morbidities, and stillbirths by improving the standards of care in labor rooms and maternity operation theatres. It also promotes respectful maternity care and timely management or referral of complications. LaQshya is being implemented in government medical colleges, district hospitals, first referral units (FRUs), and high delivery-load community health centers (CHCs). The strategy includes infrastructure upgrades, availability of essential equipment, staff training, and continuous quality monitoring using the National Quality Assurance Standards (NQAS). Overall, LaQshya aims to ensure a safer and more dignified childbirth experience in public health facilities.

MusQan

MusQan (Ensuring Child-Friendly Services in Public Health Facilities) is a quality improvement initiative launched by the Ministry of Health and Family Welfare, Government of India, in 2021. It aims to enhance the quality of care for children from birth up to 12 years of age in public health facilities, thereby reducing preventable newborn and child morbidity and mortality. The initiative focuses on strengthening clinical protocols, improving management processes, and ensuring a supportive environment that is friendly to both children and their caregivers. Key strategies include enhancing infrastructure, ensuring the availability of essential equipment, and providing adequate human resources. MusQan is implemented across various public health facilities, including district hospitals, sub-district hospitals, first referral units (FRUs), and community health centers (CHCs). The program targets departments such as pediatric outpatient departments (OPDs), pediatric wards, special newborn care units (SNCUs), and nutrition rehabilitation centers (NRCs). To ensure continuous quality improvement, MusQan employs rapid improvement (RI) cycles, each lasting 2 months, with progress monitored by state and district-level teams. The initiative also incorporates assessments based on the National Quality Assurance Standards (NQAS) to evaluate and certify facilities that meet the defined quality benchmarks.

CHILD NUTRITION PROGRAMS

Malnutrition is an associated cause in about half of all deaths occurring among children in developing countries. In 2012, the World Health Organization (WHO) member states approved a comprehensive strategy, during the 65th World Health Assembly, to combat malnutrition among children and mothers by agreeing to six global nutrition targets (GNTs), viz., reduction of stunting, wasting, maternal anemia, low-birth weight, overweight, and an increase in proportion of exclusive breastfed children up to 6 months of age to certain predefined targets by 2025. In 2017, the WHO proposed an extension of these GNTs to 2030.

Integrated Child Development Services Scheme

The Integrated Child Development Services (ICDS) is one of India's most significant child welfare schemes, launched in 1975 with 33 pilot projects across urban, rural, and tribal areas. It was expanded based on evaluations and policy reviews, especially from 1982 onwards. Operated under the Ministry of Women and Child Development, Government of India, ICDS provides a package of six essential services: (1) supplementary nutrition, (2) immunization, (3) preschool non-formal education up to the age of 6 years, (4) health check-ups, (5) nutrition and health education, and (6) referral services. These services are mainly delivered through Anganwadi Centers (AWCs). The objectives of ICDS are to improve the health and nutritional status of children aged 0–6 years, reduce infant mortality, malnutrition, and school dropouts, promote early childhood development, and empower mothers through health and nutrition education. Services are delivered in an integrated manner through the public health infrastructure such as PHCs and sub-centers. ICDS targets pregnant and lactating women, children below 6 years, adolescent girls, and women aged 15–45, making it a holistic approach to early childhood care and development.

Umbrella Integrated Child Development Services

With the aim to providing care, protection, and development of women, the ICDS scheme was further expanded in the year 2017, to be renamed as *Umbrella ICDS* covering six major components aimed at the holistic development, care, and protection of children, as well as support for women and adolescent girls. These six components are:

1. ***Anganwadi Services:*** This is the core component of ICDS, offering a package of six services—supplementary nutrition, immunization, health check-ups, referral services, pre-school non-formal education, and nutrition and health education—primarily through Anganwadi Centers. It targets children under 6 years, pregnant women, and lactating mothers.
2. ***Pradhan Mantri Matru Vandana Yojana (PMMVY):*** A maternity benefit program that provides cash incentives to pregnant and lactating women for the first living child, aimed at improving maternal and child health by encouraging institutional deliveries and adequate nutrition.
3. ***National Creche Scheme (formerly Rajiv Gandhi National Creche Scheme):*** This scheme provides day-care facilities to children (6 months to 6 years) of working mothers, particularly from disadvantaged communities. It ensures safety, early stimulation, and nutrition for children during the day.
4. ***Scheme for Adolescent Girls* (formerly SABLA)**. This program targets out-of-school adolescent girls (11–18 years) to provide them with supplementary nutrition, health education, life skills, and vocational training. It aims to empower girls and improve their health and development.
5. ***POSHAN Abhiyaan (Prime Minister's Overarching Scheme for Holistic Nutrition):*** POSHAN Abhiyaan (Prime Minister's overarching scheme for holistic nutrition), also known as National Nutrition Mission was launched in 2018 with a goal to achieve improvement in nutritional status of children from 0 to 6 years, adolescent girls, pregnant women, and lactating mothers in a time bound manner. It adopts a holistic and multi-sectoral approach to combat malnutrition and stunting, especially among children under 6 years of age. The mission focuses on convergence among various ministries and departments, and real-time growth monitoring through digital tools. Key features include the use of the ICDS-Common Application Software (CAS) for real-time data collection by Anganwadi workers, community-based events, and capacity building of frontline workers. In order to strengthen the ICDS service delivery and improvement of the program outcomes, newer intervention including *Jan Andolan* (for community mobilization and promoting behavioral change), incremental learning approach (for capacity building), and organization of community-based events, were incorporated. POSHAN Abhiyaan plays a crucial role in ensuring accountability, reducing child wasting and underweight rates, and improving overall nutrition governance in the country.
6. ***Mission POSHAN 2.0:*** It is an Integrated Nutrition Support Program aimed at combating malnutrition among children, adolescent girls, pregnant women, and lactating mothers. It focuses on improving the content and delivery of nutrition through a convergent ecosystem that promotes health, wellness, and immunity. The mission integrates three key schemes—Anganwadi Services, Scheme for Adolescent Girls, and POSHAN Abhiyaan—under a single umbrella. Key areas of focus include maternal nutrition, infant and young child feeding, treatment of moderate/severe acute malnutrition (MAM/SAM), and wellness through AYUSH practices. The initiative is based on the pillars of convergence, governance, and capacity-building, with POSHAN Abhiyaan leading outreach through innovations in ICT, media, research, and community engagement. Mission POSHAN 2.0 emphasizes corrective actions, awareness campaigns, effective communication, and eco-friendly practices. The Poshan Tracker digital platform, launched in 2021, is used for real-time monitoring, identifying malnutrition, and ensuring transparency in last-mile service delivery. The overall goal is to strengthen human capital and promote sustainable nutrition and health practices across the country
7. ***Child Protection Services (replacing the Integrated Child Protection Scheme):*** This component ensures the safety, care, and rehabilitation of children in need of protection, including orphans, children in conflict with the law, and those in difficult circumstances. It supports institutional and non-institutional care through structures like Child Welfare Committees and Juvenile Justice Boards.

Mid-day Meal Program

Another major initiative to combat undernutrition worth mentioning is the school meal program currently running in many countries by different names. *Mid-day meal scheme* in India aims at provision of school lunches thereby improving the nutritional status of children and their school enrolment and attendance. Launched in 1995 as a centrally sponsored scheme under the Ministry of Education, it provides one hot cooked meal to children studying in government and government-aided primary and upper primary schools. The objectives of the scheme are to improve the nutritional status of children, encourage school attendance and reduce dropout rates, and enhance the learning capacity of children through better nutrition. Renamed as **PM POSHAN (Pradhan Mantri Poshan Shakti Nirman)** in 2021, the scheme now covers children from classes 1 to 8 and also includes preschoolers in government and government-aided institutions under ICDS. The meals served must meet specified nutritional standards: at least 450 calories and 12 grams of protein for primary students, and 700 calories and 20 grams of protein for upper primary students. The scheme emphasizes community participation, hygiene, food safety, and monitoring mechanisms, making it one of the largest school meal programs in the world.

Anemia Mukt Bharat

As per the National Family Health Survey-5 (2019–21), anemia remains a silent epidemic in India: 67.1% of children (6–59 months), 59.1% of adolescent girls, 52.2% of pregnant women, and 57.0% of women aged 15–49 are affected. Its severity is compounded by worm infestation, malaria, and other infectious diseases, and iron-deficiency anemia in early life impairs both cognitive and motor development.

To combat anemia, the Government of India has progressively built a lifecycle strategy:

- ***1970:*** Launched the National Nutritional Anemia Control Program (NNACP), providing iron-folic acid (IFA) supplementation to pregnant women and young children.
- ***2012:*** Introduced Weekly Iron and Folic Acid Supplementation (WIFS), targeting adolescents via schools and community platforms and adding regular deworming.
- ***2013:*** Rolled out the National Iron Plus Initiative (NIPI) under the Ministry of Health and Family Welfare, extending age-appropriate IFA supplementation and establishing facility-based treatment protocols across all vulnerable groups.
- ***2018:*** Consolidated NNACP, WIFS, and NIPI into Anemia Mukt Bharat (AMB), a 6×6×6 framework **(Fig. 28.9)** covering six beneficiary groups (children 6–59 months, adolescent girls 15–19 years, adolescent boys 15–19 years, women of reproductive age 15–49 years, pregnant women, and lactating mothers), six interventions, and six institutional mechanisms for coordinated implementation.

Under AMB (also known as the intensified NIPI), key interventions now include prophylactic IFA supplementation, yearround behavior-change communication, point-of-care testing and treatment, management of severe anemia (IV iron or transfusion), and incentives for frontline workers in high-priority districts. To strengthen delivery, the program has enhanced inter-ministerial coordination, improved supply-chain logistics, partnered with the National Center of Excellence and Advanced Research on Anemia Control (NCEARA) at AIIMS Delhi for provider training, and launched e-training modules and toolkits for virtual capacity building.

Vitamin A prophylaxis and control of iodine deficiency disorder programs have been discussed earlier in this book.

Key Interventions Related to the Nutritional Status of Children

- ***To detect growth faltering and lower the incidence of moderate or severe malnutrition:*** Line listing of babies born with low-birth weight must be maintained by the frontline workers [auxiliary nurse midwives (ANMs) and ASHAs] and their follow-up should be ensured.
- ***To reduce the prevalence of anemia among children:*** All children between the ages of 6 months to 5 years must receive biweekly IFA supplementation (as appropriate) as a preventive measure, and provide weekly IFA (age appropriate dose) for children of 5–19 years as part of the iNIPI. ASHAs will be incentivized to make home visits and to provide at least one dose per week under direct observation and educate the mothers about benefits of iron supplements and also how to administer it.
- ***Deworming*** (using albendazole syrup or tablet in single dose) can be carried out every 6 months in order to reduce the intestinal parasite load. This intervention can be combined with vitamin A supplementation during biannual rounds.
- ***Vitamin A supplementation:*** Children between 9 months to 5 years are given 6 monthly doses of vitamin A. A child must receive nine doses of vitamin A by the 5th birthday.
- ***Care to children with SAM:*** This is mainly through facility-based care, i.e., Nutritional Rehabilitation Centers (NRC) or

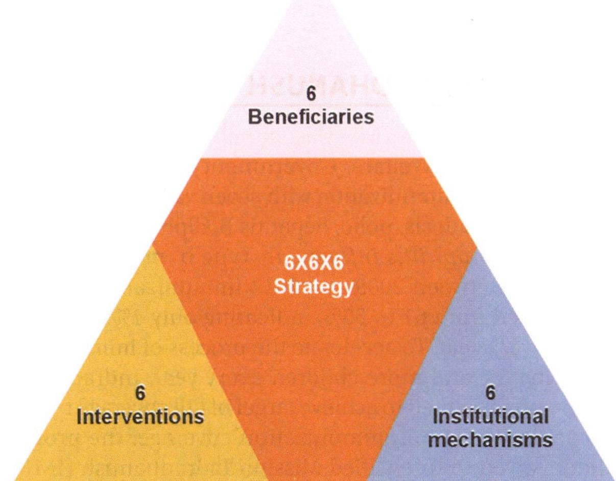

Approximately 450 million beneficiaries–nearly 50% of the country's population–will be reached

Beneficiaries	*Interventions*	*Institutional mechanisms*
Children (6–59 months)	Prophylactic iron-folic acid supplementation	Intra-ministerial coordination
Adolescent girls (15–19 years)	Deworming	National AMB Unit
Adolescent boys (15–19 years)	Year-round BCC targeting: a. IFA and deworming compliance b. Infant and young child feeding practices c. Dietary diversity/ fortification using local resources d. Delayed cord clamping (1–3 minutes)	National Center of Excellence (e.g. NCEAR-A at AIIMS)
Women (15–49 years)	Digital point-of-care testing and treatment (focus on pregnant women and adolescents)	Convergence with related ministries (Education, WCD, Tribal Affairs, etc.)
Pregnant women	Mandatory IFA-fortified foods in all public health schemes	Strengthening supply-chain and logistics
Lactating mothers	Intensified screening and management of non-nutritional causes (malaria, hemoglobinopathies, fluorosis)	AMB Dashboard and Digital Portal—One Stop Shop for Anemia

AMB: Anemia Mukt Bharat; BCC: behavior change communication; IFA: iron-folic acid; NCEAR-A: National Center of Excellence and Advanced Research on Anemia Control; WCD: women and child development

Fig. 28.9: Anemia Mukt Bharat: 6 × 6 × 6 Strategy

Source: Ministry of Health and Family Welfare, Government of India. National Health Mission: Anemia Mukt Bharat. New Delhi: Ministry of Health and Family Welfare. Available from: https://nhm.gov.in/index1.php?lang=1&level=3&sublinkid=1448&lid=797 [Last accessed may, 2025].

Malnutrition Treatment Centers (MTC). Community-based programs for the management of children with SAM are urgently required.

MISSION INDRADHANUSH

Mission Indradhanush (MI) was launched by the Ministry of Health and Family Welfare, Government of India in 2014, to ensure universal immunization with seven vaccines against the diseases—tuberculosis, polio, hepatitis B, diphtheria, pertussis, tetanus, *Haemophilus influenzae* type b meningitis and pneumonia. Between 2009 and 2013 immunization coverage had increased from 61 to 65%, indicating only 1% increase in coverage every year. To accelerate the process of immunization by covering 5% and more children every year, Indradhanush mission initially aimed to achieve target of full coverage by 2020.

To achieve 90% full immunization coverage, the program further evolved to Intensified Mission Indradhanush (IMI) in the year 2017 with an aim to reach each and every child up to 2 years of age and all those pregnant women who have been left uncovered under the routine immunization program/universal immunization program (UIP). It now includes 12 diseases including measles, rubella, rotavirus diarrhea, Japanese encephalitis (in endemic districts), and pneumococcal pneumonia, in addition to the previous seven diseases.

Since its launch in 2014, Mission Indradhanush has rolled out 11 intensification phases nationwide, and the 12th phase is currently under way. To date, the campaign has vaccinated a cumulative total of 5.06 crore children and 1.25 crore pregnant women. In 2023, under Intensified Mission Indradhanush 5.0, the drive expanded for the first time to every district in India and raised the upper age limit for beneficiaries from 2 to 5 years.

SAANS

Social Awareness and Actions to Neutralize Pneumonia Successfully (SAANS) is an initiative launched in 2019 by the Ministry of Health and Family Welfare under the National Health Mission (NHM) to combat childhood pneumonia, one of the leading causes of death among children under five in India. The program aims to raise awareness about pneumonia prevention and treatment, ensure early identification and timely management of cases, and strengthen healthcare delivery at both community and facility levels. Key components include training of frontline health workers, availability of essential treatments like amoxicillin dispersible tablets, and provision of oxygen and pulse oximeters in health facilities. SAANS also promotes preventive measures such as exclusive breastfeeding, full immunization, good nutrition, and hygiene practices like handwashing.

CHILD HEALTH SCREENING AND EARLY INTERVENTION SERVICES

Expanding focus from child survival to a more comprehensive approach of improving child development and quality of life is the guiding principle for the launch of a new initiative called the child screening and early intervention services.

Objective

The objective of the child health screening is to detect medical conditions at an early stage, thus enabling early intervention and management, ultimately leading to reduction in mortality, morbidity, and lifelong disability. This initiative aims to reach 27 crore children annually in the age group 0–18 years, when fully implemented across the country.

Burden of 4Ds

The burden of birth *D*efects, *D*evelopment delays in children, *D*eficiencies and *D*iseases (4Ds) is one of the important factors for child mortality, poor quality of life, and financial stress. Of every 100 babies born in India annually, 6–7 have a birth defect. This would translate into an estimated 17 lakhs birth defects annually, and account for 9.6% of all newborn deaths. Various nutritional deficiencies affecting preschool children range from 4 to 70% while developmental delays are common in early childhood, affecting at least 10% of the children and can potentially lead to permanent disabilities.

Rashtriya Bal Swasthya Karyakram (RBSK)

RBSK is a flagship initiative under the National Health Mission launched in 2013, targeting early identification and intervention for children from birth to 18 years. It aims to detect and manage 32 common health conditions classified under 4 broad categories (4 D's)—**d**efects at birth, **d**iseases, **d**eficiencies, and **d**evelopmental delays including disabilities **(Box 28.4)**. Under RBSK, comprehensive child health screening and early interventions services are provided by expanding the reach of mobile health teams at block level. These teams include two doctors and two paramedics who are adequately trained and have necessary tools for screening. These teams carry out screening of all the children in the age group 0-6 years enrolled at Anganwadi Center (AWC) at least twice a year for 30 identified health conditions. Arrangements are also made to provide free management of these children at district early interventions centers (DEIC) or identified tertiary level institutions for the 0–6 age group, while for the 6–18

Box 28.4 Health Conditions (4 D's) Screened under Rashtriya Bal Swasthya Karyakram (RBSK)

Defects at birth

1. Neural tube defect
2. Down's syndrome
3. Cleft Lip and palate/cleft palate alone
4. Talipes (club foot)
5. Developmental dysplasia of the hip
6. Congenital cataract
7. Congenital deafness
8. Congenital heart diseases
9. Retinopathy of prematurity

Deficiencies

10. Anemia especially severe anemia
11. Vitamin A deficiency (Bitot spot)
12. Vitamin D deficiency (rickets)
13. Severe acute malnutrition
14. Goiter

Childhood diseases

15. Skin conditions (scabies, fungal infection and eczema)
16. Otitis media
17. Rheumatic heart disease
18. Reactive airway disease
19. Dental caries
20. Convulsive disorders

Developmental delays

21. Vision impairment
22. Hearing impairment
23. Neuro-motor impairment
24. Motor delay
25. Cognitive delay
26. Language delay
27. Behavior disorder (autism)
28. Learning disorder
29. Attention deficit hyperactivity disorder
30. Congenital hypothyroidism, sickle cell anemia, beta thalassemia (optional)
31. Tuberculosis
32. Leprosy

years age-group, management of conditions is done through existing public health facilities. DEIC act as referral linkages for both the age groups. The program allows states the flexibility to engage private empanelled hospitals through memorandums of understanding (MoUs) to provide specialized treatments, such as for congenital defects and cardiac conditions. This ensures timely access to care for affected children. All services are offered free of cost, significantly reducing the financial burden on families and minimizing out-of-pocket healthcare expenses.

RBSK aims to cover approximately 270 million children across the country in a phased manner. Since its launch in 2014, the program has screened nearly 800 million children with the help of 11,200 mobile health teams operating from sub-district levels—paving the way for a healthier future for India's children.

Rashtriya Kishor Swasthya Karyakram

Adolescents comprise little more than one-fifth of India's total population. Investments in adolescent reproductive and sexual health will yield dividends in terms of delaying age at marriage, reducing incidence of teenage pregnancy, meeting unmet contraception need, reducing the maternal mortality, reducing STI incidence, and reducing HIV prevalence. It will also help India realize its demographic dividends, as healthy adolescents are an important resource for the economy.

To ensure holistic development of adolescent population, the Ministry of Health and Family Welfare launched Rashtriya Kishor Swasthya Karyakram (RKSK) on 7th January 2014 to reach out to 253 million adolescents male and female, rural and urban, married and unmarried, in and out-of-school adolescents with special focus on marginalized and undeserved groups. The program includes in its ambit nutrition, injuries and violence (including gender-based violence), noncommunicable diseases, mental health and substance misuse.

The strength of the program is its health promotion approach. It is a paradigm shift from the existing clinic-based services to promotion and prevention and reaching adolescents in their own environment, such as in schools, families, and communities. Key drivers of the program are community-based interventions such as, outreach by counselors, facility-based counseling, social and behavior change communication, and strengthening of adolescent friendly health clinics across levels of care. The objectives of RKSK are given in **Figure 28.10**.

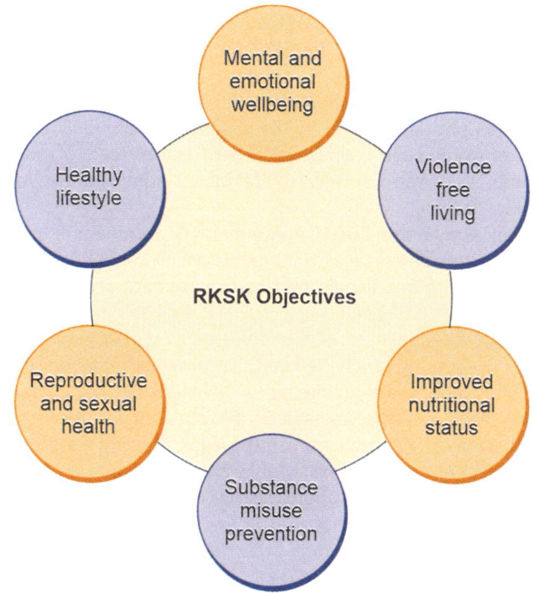

Fig. 28.10: Objectives of the Rashtriya Kishor Swasthya Karyakram (RKSK)

Source: National Health Mission, Ministry of Health and Family Welfare, Government of India. (2014). Operational framework: translating strategies into programs, Rashtriya Kishor Swasthya Karyakram. Available from https://nhm.gov.in/images/pdf/programmes/RKSK/RKSK_Operational_Framework.pdf [Last accessed May, 2025]

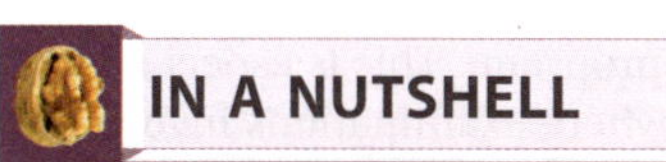

IN A NUTSHELL

Other National Programs for Maternal and Child Health

1. NSSK and JSSK aim to provide free of cost delivery by trained personnel in government health facility, along with provisions of drugs, consumables, and diagnostics for the mother and sick newborn till 30 days after the birth.
2. ICDS scheme aims to provide supplementary nutrition, immunization, preschool nonformal education, growth monitoring, health education, and referral services for children.
3. Weekly iron folic acid supplementation (WIFS) and regular deworming been incorporated in the Anemia Mukt Bharat or Intensified National Iron Plus Initiative (iNIPI) to address the problem of iron deficiency anemia in children.
4. Mission Indradhanush (MI) was launched by the Ministry of Health and Family Welfare, Government of India in 2014, to ensure universal immunization with seven vaccines. Since its launch in 2014, Mission Indradhanush has rolled out 11 intensification phases nationwide. It now includes immunization against twelve diseases.
5. Under Rashtriya Bal Swasthya Karyakram, comprehensive child health screening and early interventions services are provided.
6. Rashtriya Kishor Swasthya Karyakram was launched to ensure holistic development of adolescent population.

Ministry of Health and Family Welfare, Government of India. (2013). A Strategic Approach to Reproductive, Maternal, Newborn, Child and Adolescent Health (RMNCH+A) in India. [online] Available from https://nhm.gov.in/images/pdf/RMNCH+A/RMNCH+A_ Strategy.pdf [last accessed May, 2025].

Ministry of Health and Family Welfare, Government of India. (2018). Anemia Mukt Bharat. [online] Available from https://anemiamukt-bharat.info/wp-content/uploads/2019/09/Anemia-Mukt-Bharat-Operational-Guidelines-FINAL.pdf [Last accessed May, 2025].

Ministry of Health and Family Welfare, Government of India. (2022). Intensified Mission Indradhanush. [online] Available from https://nhm.gov.in/New_Updates_2018/NHM_Components/Immunization/Guildelines_for_immunization/Mission_Indradhanush_Guidelines.pdf [Last accessed May, 2025].
Ministry of Health and Family Welfare, Government of India. (2022). Janani Shishu Suraksha Karyakram. [online] Available from https://nhm.gov.in/index1.php?lang=1&level=3&sublinkid=842&lid=308 [Last accessed May, 2025].
Ministry of Women and Child Development, Government of India. (2022). National Nutrition Mission. [online] Available from http://icds-wcd. nic.in/nnm/NNM-Web-Contents/UPPER-MENU/Administrative Approval-Guidelines/Administrative_Guidelines_NNM-26022018. pdf [Last accessed May, 2025].
Ministry of Women and Child Development, Government of India. (2016). National Plan of Action for Children. [online] Available from https://wcd.nic.in/sites/default/files/National%20Plan%20of%20 Action%202016.pdf [Last accessed May, 2025].
Ministry of Health and Family Welfare, Government of India. LaQshya—Labour Room Quality Improvement Initiative: Guidelines [Internet]. New Delhi: National Health Mission; 2017. Available from: https://nhm.gov.in/New_Updates_2018/NHM_Components/RMNCH_MH_Guidelines/LaQshya-Guidelines.pdf [Last accessed May, 2025].
Ministry of Health and Family Welfare, Government of India. Social Awareness and Actions to Neutralize Pneumonia Successfully (SAANS) [Internet]. New Delhi: National Health Mission; 2019 [cited 2025 May 5]. Available from: https://nhm.gov.in/index4.php?lang=1&level=0&linkid=502&lid=789
National Health Systems Resource Centre. MusQan: Ensuring Child-Friendly Services in Public Health Facilities [Internet]. New Delhi: NHSRC; [cited 2025 May 5]. Available from: https://qps.nhsrcindia.org/musqan
National Health Mission, Ministry of Health and Family Welfare, Government of India. (2014). Operational framework: translating strategies into programs, Rashtriya Kishor Swasthya Karyakram. [online] Available from https://nhm.gov.in/index4.php?lang=1&level=0&linkid=152&lid=173

28.7 Integrated Management of Neonatal and Childhood Illnesses (IMNCI)

PE16.1, PE16.2, PE16.3, PE16.4, PE16.5, PE16.6

INTRODUCTION

Infant and childhood mortality are sensitive indicators of inequity and poverty. Surveys reveal that many sick children are not properly assessed and treated by these health providers, and that their parents are poorly advised. At first-level health facilities in low-income countries, diagnostic supports such as radiology and laboratory services are minimal or nonexistent, and drugs and equipment are often scarce. Limited supplies and equipment, combined with an irregular flow of patients, leave doctors at this level with few opportunities to practice complicated clinical procedures. Instead, they often rely on history and signs and symptoms to determine a course of management that makes the best use of available resources.

Providing quality care to sick children in these conditions is a serious challenge. Yet, how can this situation be reversed? Experience and scientific evidence show that improvements in child health are not necessarily dependent on the use of sophisticated and expensive technologies, but rather on effective strategies that are based on a holistic approach, are available to the majority of those in need, and which take into account the capacity and structure of health systems, as well as traditions and beliefs in the community.

NEED FOR INTEGRATED APPROACH

Many well-known prevention and treatment strategies have already proven effective for saving young lives. Childhood vaccinations have successfully reduced deaths due to measles. Oral rehydration therapy has contributed to a major reduction in diarrhea deaths. Effective antibiotics have saved millions of children with pneumonia. Prompt treatment of malaria has allowed more children to recover and lead healthy lives. Even modest improvements in breastfeeding practices have reduced childhood deaths.

While each of these interventions has shown great success, accumulating evidence suggests that a more integrated approach to managing sick children is needed to achieve better outcomes. Child health programs need to move beyond single diseases to addressing the overall health and well-being of the child. Because many children present with overlapping signs and symptoms of diseases, a single diagnosis can be difficult, and may not be feasible or appropriate. This is especially true for first-level health facilities where examinations involve few instruments, little or no laboratory tests, and no X-ray.

Integrated Management of Childhood Illness (IMCI) strategy, developed by WHO in collaboration with United Nations International Children's Emergency Fund (UNICEF) and many other agencies in mid-1990s, is a curative, preventive, and promotive strategy aimed at (1) Reducing the death and frequency and severity of illness and disability, and (2) Contributing to improved growth and nutrition of under-five children. In 2003, this strategy has been expanded in India to include neonatal care at home as well as in the health facilities and renamed as "Integrated Management of Neonatal and Childhood Illness (IMNCI)." The Facility-Based Integrated Management of Neonatal and Childhood Illness (F-IMNCI) was developed in 2009, and has now been comprehensively revised in 2023 to align with current clinical guidelines and treatment approaches. The revised training has been split into two focused packages:

1. ***Integrated Management of Newborn and Child Illnesses (IMNCI):*** This component addresses outpatient care for young infants (0–2 months) and children up to 5 years of age. It includes separate chart booklets for healthcare workers (ANMs) and physicians and is delivered over a five-day training period.
2. ***Facility-based care of sick children:*** This new package focuses on inpatient management of children aged 1 to 59 months suffering from common life-threatening conditions such as pneumonia, diarrhea, malaria, meningitis, and severe malnutrition. It is also taught over 5 days.

   Other key updates in the revised F-IMNCI include:
   - Management of conditions is now linked to emergency signs.
   - New chapters covering the management of critical conditions such as shock, altered consciousness (lethargy, unconsciousness, convulsions), and supportive care.
   - Integration of national guidelines for pediatric management of COVID-19, malaria, dengue, and tuberculosis.

IMNCI: EVIDENCE-BASED SYNDROMIC APPROACH

The IMNCI clinical guidelines target children <5 years old, the age group that bears the highest burden of deaths. The guidelines represent an evidence-based, syndromic approach to case management that supports the rational, effective, and affordable use of drugs and diagnostic tools. In situations where laboratory support and clinical resources are limited, the syndromic approach is a more realistic and cost-effective way to manage patients. Careful and systematic assessment of common symptoms, using well-selected reliable clinical signs, helps to guide rational and effective actions. An evidence-based syndromic approach can be used to determine: (1) Health problems the child may have, (2) Severity of the child's illness, and (3) Actions that can be taken to care for the child (e.g., refer the child immediately, manage with available resources, or manage at home).

PRINCIPLES OF INTEGRATED CARE

Depending on a child's age, various clinical signs and symptoms differ in their degree of reliability and diagnostic value and importance. IMNCI clinical guidelines focus on the out-patient management of neonates, infants as well as children up to 5 years of age. However, in view of similarities in the spectrum of illnesses, clinical signs and management protocols, the treatment guidelines have been broadly described under two age categories, i.e.,

1. Young infants age up to 2 months (0–59 days old), and
2. Children age 2 months up to 5 years (2 to 59 months).

The IMNCI guidelines are based on the following principles:

- All sick children under 5 years of age must be examined for conditions which indicate immediate referral or hospitalization.
- Children must be routinely assessed for major symptoms, nutritional and immunization status, feeding problems, and other potential problems.
- Only a limited number of carefully selected clinical signs are used based on evidence of their sensitivity and specificity to detect disease.
- Color-coded chart booklet has the following four columns:
  1. "**Assess**" column lists what signs and symptoms to check and how to do it.
  2. "**Signs**" column summarizes the signs and symptoms present in the child
  3. "**Classification**" column helps in classifying each illness the young infant or child has. Based on the presence of selected clinical signs, the child is placed in a "Classification." Making a precise diagnosis is unnecessary.
  4. "**Identify treatment**" section lists appropriate treatment decisions for each classification.
- The "**Assess**" and "**Classification**" sections are color coded in three different colors:
  a. **Pink** color indicates severe illness and suggest referral to a hospital after giving pre-referral treatment.
  b. **Yellow** color for conditions needing specific medical treatment; and home care advice is provided to the mother.
  c. Conditions under **green** color are not serious and to be managed at home with simple medical advice.
- IMNCI guidelines address most common, but not all pediatric problems.
- A limited number of essential drugs are used.
- Caretakers are actively involved in the treatment of children.
- Counseling of caretakers about home care including feeding, fluids and when to return to health facility, is an essential component of IMNCI strategy.

IMNCI Case Management Process

The Integrated Management of Neonatal and Childhood Illness (IMNCI) case management process begins by determining the child's age group, as this guides the choice of appropriate assessment and classification tools. A summary of this case management process is depicted in **Flowchart 28.1**.

Children are divided into two main age groups: **young infants (up to 2 months of age)** and **children aged 2 months up to 5 years**. A young infant refers to a baby who has not yet completed two months of age—for example, a child who is 1 month and 29 days old would fall into this category, but not one who has turned 2 months. Similarly, the "2 months to 5 years" category includes children up to 4 years and 11 months, but not those who have reached their fifth birthday. Based on this categorization, healthcare providers use specific IMNCI charts: "**Assess and Classify the Sick Young Infant**" for children up to 2 months **(Fig. 28.11)**, and "**Assess and Classify the Sick Child**" for those aged 2 months to 5 years **(Fig. 28.12)**. These charts guide frontline workers in systematic evaluation

Flowchart 28.1: Summary of Integrated management of neonatal and childhood illness case management process

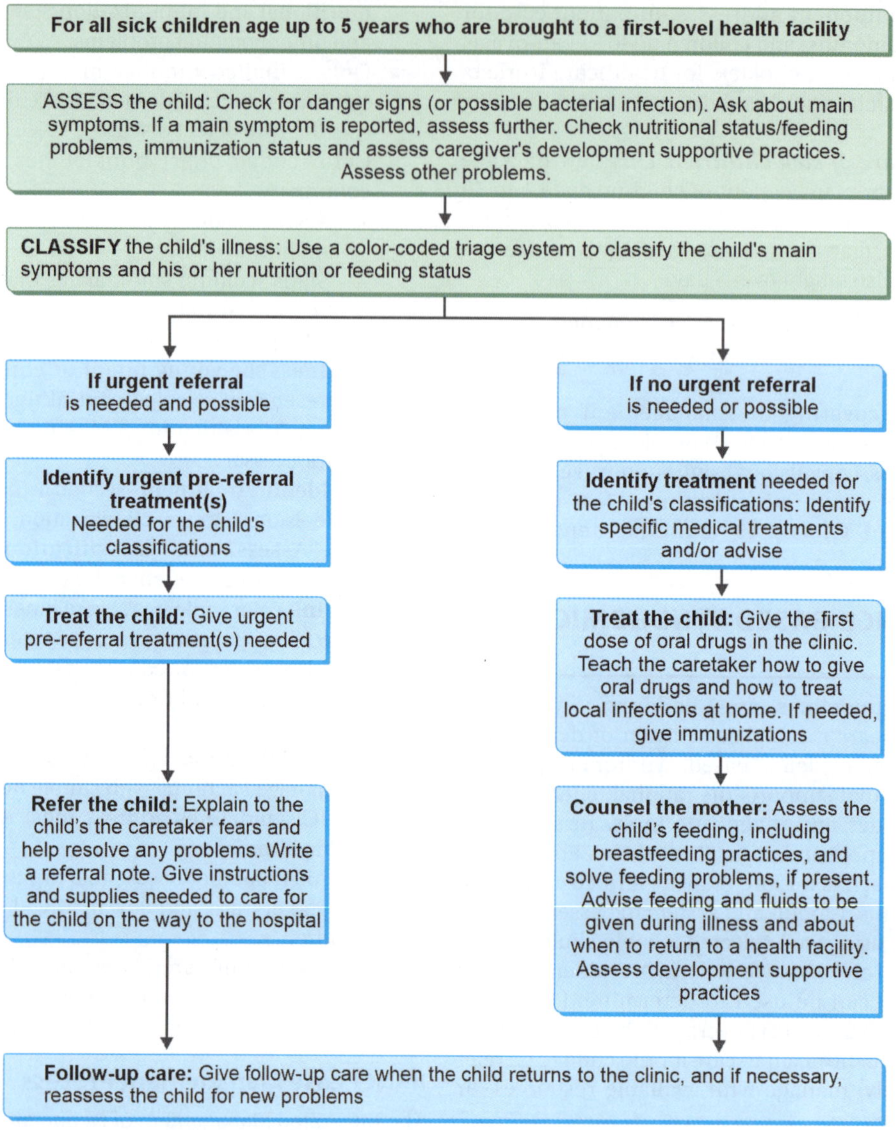

Source: Ministry of Health and Family Welfare, Government of India. Integrated Management of Neonatal and Childhood Illness (IMNCI): Participant Module for Medical Officers. New Delhi: Ministry of Health and Family Welfare; 2023. Available from: https://nhm.gov.in/images/pdf/programmes/child-health/guidelines/IMNCI-Module-2023-For-Medical-Officers/IMNCI-Participants-Module-Medical-Officer-2023.pdf [Last accessed May, 2025].

and management of childhood illnesses. The management of a sick child at a first-level outpatient health facility involves several critical steps. First, the child is assessed, followed by classification of the illness and identification of the appropriate treatment. Depending on the classification, the child may be treated at the facility, referred to a higher center, or the caregiver may receive counseling on home care. Follow-up visits are scheduled to ensure recovery or escalation of care if needed. In cases requiring referral to a higher-level health facility, the child undergoes Emergency Triage Assessment and Treatment (ETAT), followed by diagnosis, medical management, and continuous monitoring of the child's condition. An essential component of IMNCI is empowering caregivers through appropriate home management. This includes teaching mothers or caregivers how to administer oral medications, treat minor infections, and recognize warning signs. Counseling also focuses on optimal feeding practices, fluid intake, developmental stimulation, when to return for further care, and attention to the mother's own health and well-being.

Detailed descriptions are available in the IMNCI Chart booklet table (*See* **Annexures**).

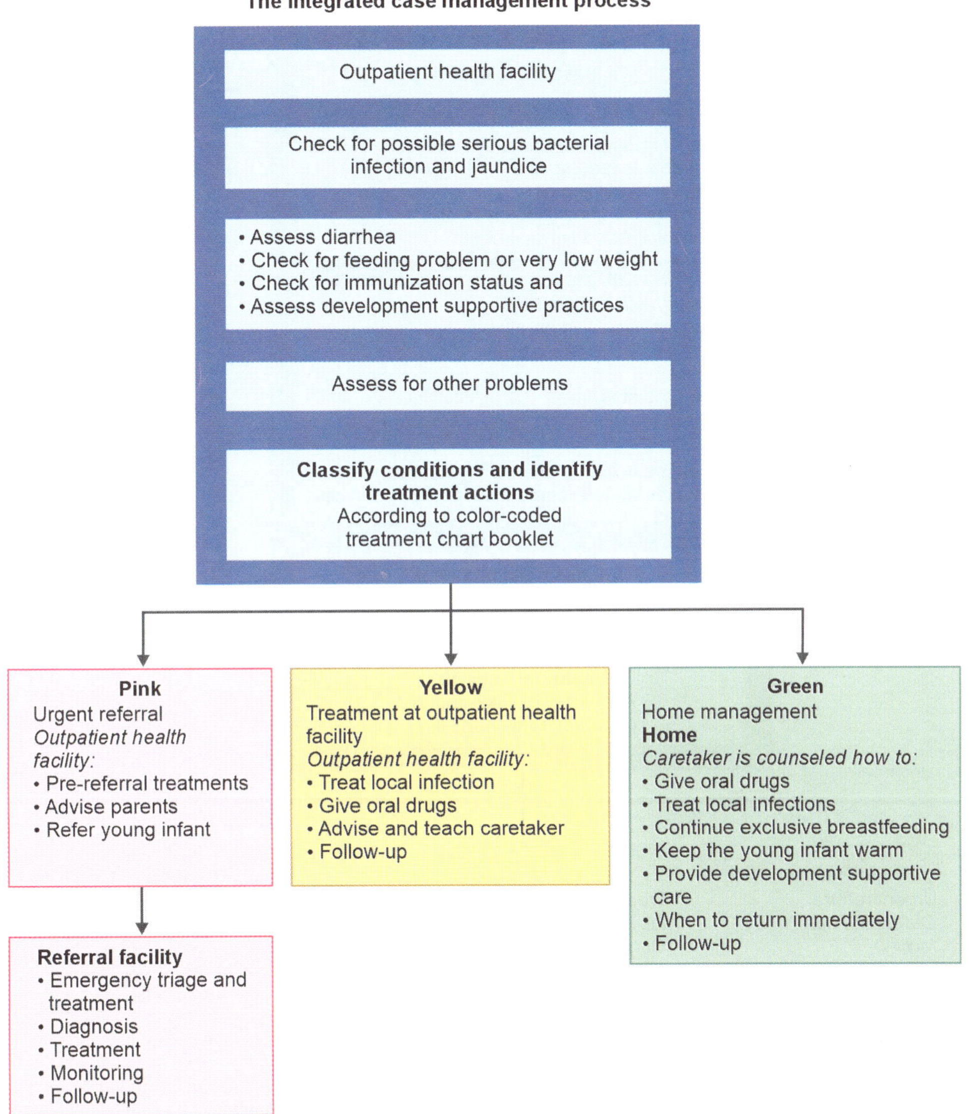

Fig. 28.11: IMNCI Case management process in the outpatient health facility, first-level referral facility and at home for the sick young Infant up to 2 months of age

Source: Ministry of Health and Family Welfare, Government of India. Integrated Management of Neonatal and Childhood Illness (IMNCI): Participant Module for Medical Officers. New Delhi: Ministry of Health and Family Welfare; 2023. Available from: https://nhm.gov.in/images/pdf/programmes/child-health/guidelines/IMNCI-Module-2023-For-Medical-Officers/IMNCI-Participants-Module-Medical-Officer-2023.pdf [Last accessed May, 2025].

FACILITY-BASED CARE OF SICK CHILDREN

A new package titled, "Facility Based Care of Sick Children" focuses on providing appropriate inpatient management of major causes of childhood mortality beyond the neonatal age, i.e., 1 month to 59 months old children with common illnesses, like pneumonia, diarrhea, malaria, meningitis, and severe acute malnutrition. New chapters on the management of children with shock, management of children presenting with lethargy, unconsciousness or convulsions, supportive care have been added. National guidelines for pediatric management of COVID-19, malaria, dengue and tuberculosis have been added.

The stages of management for any child in a hospital are: (1) Triage and Emergency Treatment, (2) History and examination, (3) Point-of-care/bedside investigations, (4) Making a diagnosis or differential diagnosis, (5) Decide the need for hospitalization/referral, (6) Inpatient care and specific treatment. It is summarized in **Flowchart 28.2**.

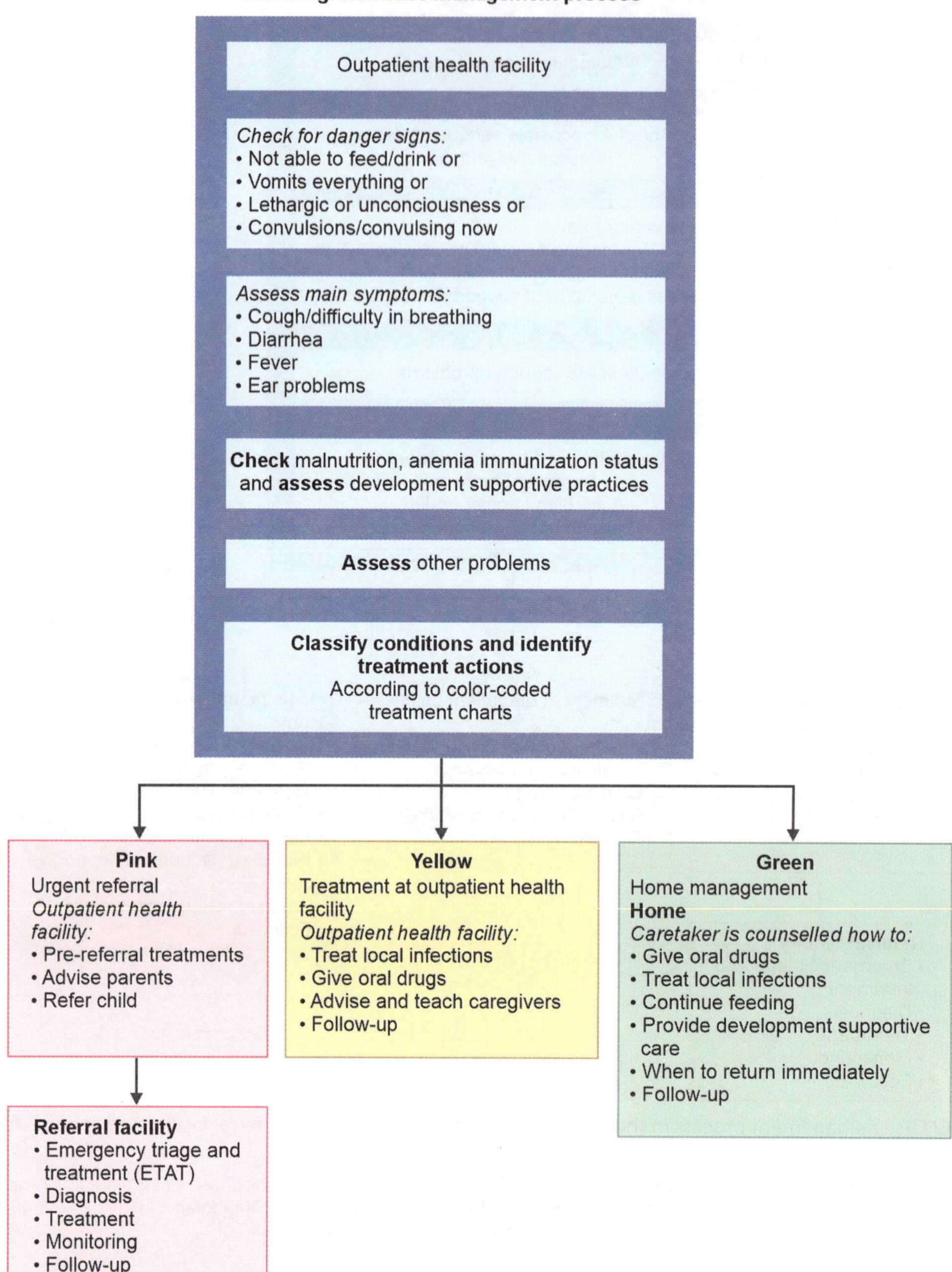

Fig. 28.12: IMNCI case management process in the outpatient health facility, first-level referral facility and at home for the sick child from age 2 months up to 5 years

Source: Ministry of Health and Family Welfare, Government of India. Integrated Management of Neonatal and Childhood Illness (IMNCI): Participant Module for Medical Officers. New Delhi: Ministry of Health and Family Welfare; 2023. Available from: https://nhm.gov.in/images/pdf/programmes/child-health/guidelines/IMNCI-Module-2023-For-Medical-Officers/IMNCI-Participants-Module-Medical-Officer-2023.pdf [Last accessed May, 2025].

Flowchart 28.2: Steps in the management of children brought to hospital (F-IMNCI)

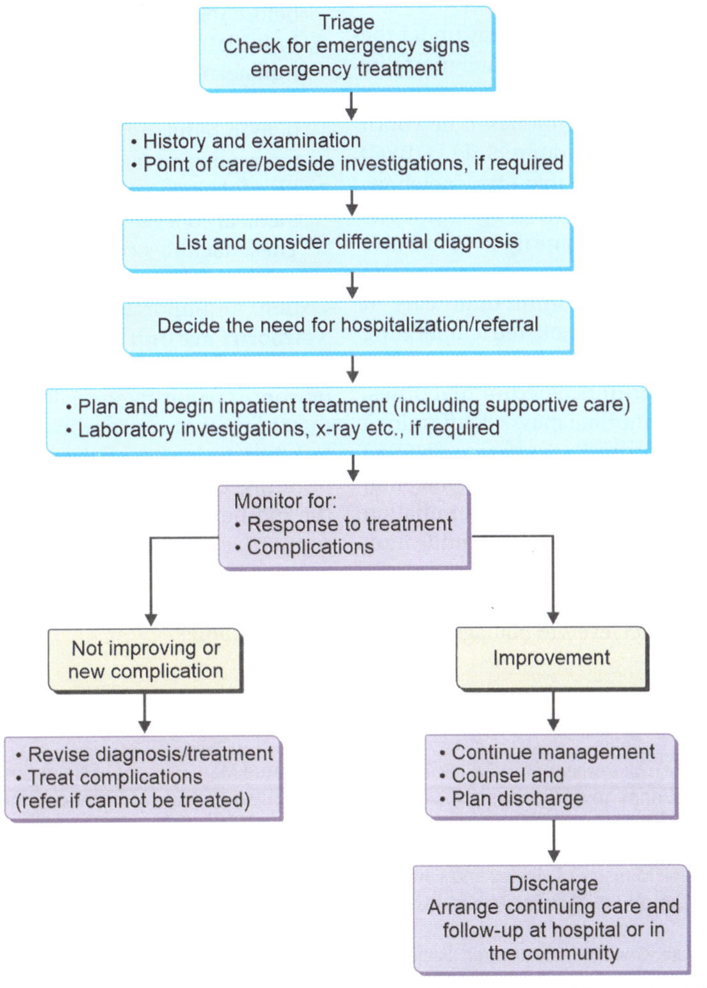

Source: Ministry of Health and Family Welfare, Government of India. Facility-based Integrated Management of Neonatal and Childhood Illness (F-IMNCI): Participant Module. New Delhi: Ministry of Health and Family Welfare; 2023. Available from: https://nhm.gov.in/index1.php?lang=1&level=3&sublinkid=1448&lid=797 [Last accessed May, 2025].

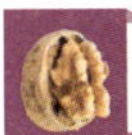

IN A NUTSHELL

Integrated Management of Neonatal and Childhood Illnesses (IMNCI)

1. IMNCI clinical guidelines provide evidence-based, syndromic approach to case management that supports the rational, effective, and affordable use of drugs and diagnostic tools in under-five children.
2. The revised Facility-Based IMNCI includes two focused five-day training packages—IMNCI for outpatient care (0–5 years) and a new inpatient care module for managing severe conditions like pneumonia, diarrhea, and malnutrition.
3. The revised F-IMNCI emphasizes early recognition of emergency signs, integrates updated national guidelines (e.g., COVID-19, malaria), and includes new chapters on managing critical conditions like shock and altered consciousness.
4. The chart booklet supports frontline healthcare workers with a four-column format ("Assess," "Signs," "Classification," "Identify treatment") and a color-coding system to guide urgency and treatment decisions: Pink: Severe illness—urgent referral after pre-referral treatment; Yellow: Medical treatment needed—treat and provide home care advice, and Green: Manage at home with simple guidance.
5. Under facility-based newborn care (FBNC) newborn care corners at delivery points, newborn stabilization units at community health centers and special neonatal care units (SNCU) at district hospitals provide optimum neonatal care.

FACILITY-BASED NEWBORN CARE

Facility-based newborn care (FBNC) is a key strategy under the National Health Mission aimed at reducing neonatal mortality and ensuring quality care for all newborns through a tiered structure of services. FBNC along with home based newborn care (HBNC) and home-based care for young child (HBYC) establishes a continuum of care to ensure that every newborn receives essential services right from the time of birth and first 48 hours at the health facility and then at home up to 15 months. It includes:

1. ***Newborn care corners (NBCCs)*** for immediate care at birth. Located within labor rooms and obstetric operating theaters, NBCCs are equipped with essential resuscitation equipment such as radiant warmers, suction machines, and self-inflating bags with appropriate masks. Staff trained under the Navjat Sishu Suraksha Karyakaram (NSSK) program provide immediate care at birth, including infection prevention, thermal protection, resuscitation, early initiation of breastfeeding, weighing, immunization, and identification of at-risk or sick newborns for prompt referral.
2. ***Newborn stabilization units (NBSUs):*** These 4–6 bedded units are established at sub-district levels to manage sick and small newborns who are not critically ill and can be stabilized before referral. NBSUs play a pivotal role in reducing delays in initiating appropriate care, stabilizing newborns before transferring them to higher-level facilities, and preventing overloading of special newborn care units (SNCUs). They also help in reducing the cost of care by managing cases that do not require advanced interventions.
3. ***Special newborn care units (SNCUs)*** at district hospitals and medical colleges for managing critically ill neonates.

These facilities collectively ensure timely, appropriate, and efficient newborn care across different levels of the health system. An important recent addition to FBNC is the **Mother Newborn Care Unit (MNCU)**, which upholds the principle of "no separation" between mother and baby—even for small and sick newborns requiring specialized care. The MNCU model ensures that the mother and newborn are managed as a dyad, remaining together during hospitalization. This not only fosters emotional bonding and facilitates breastfeeding but also empowers the mother to actively participate in the developmental and supportive care of her baby. By integrating maternal presence into newborn care, MNCUs enhance recovery, improve neonatal outcomes, and promote respectful, family-centered care within health facilities.

Ministry of Health and Family Welfare Government of India. (2011). Facility-based Newborn Care (FBNC) operational guidelines. [online] Available from https://www.aspirationaldistricts.in/wp-content/uploads/2019/02/Facility-Based-Newborn-Care-Operational-Guide-FBNC.pdf [Last accessed May, 2025].

Ministry of Health and Family Welfare Government of India. Facility-based Integrated Management of Newborn and Childhood Illnesses (F-IMNCI). [online] Available from https://nhm.gov.in/images/pdf/programmes/childhealth/guidelines/imnci_chart_booklet.pdf [Last accessed May, 2025].

Ministry of Health and Family Welfare, Government of India. Integrated Management of Neonatal and Childhood Illness (IMNCI): Participant Module for Medical Officers. New Delhi: Ministry of Health and Family Welfare; 2023. Available from: https://nhm.gov.in/images/pdf/programmes/child-health/guidelines/IMNCI-Module-2023-For-Medical-Officers/IMNCI-Participants-Module-Medical-Officer-2023.pdf [Last accessed May, 2025].

Ministry of Health and Family Welfare, Government of India. Facility Based Integrated Management of Neonatal and Childhood Illness (F-IMNCI): Participant Module [Internet]. New Delhi: Child Health Division, MoHFW; 2023. Available from: https://nhm.gov.in/images/pdf/programmes/child-health/guidelines/Revised-F-IMNCI-Modules-2023/FIMNCI-Participant-Module-2023.pdf [Last accessed May, 2025].

28.8 Role of Physician in the Community

PE 32.1

INTRODUCTION

Physicians have multifactorial role in the community. They have to deal with three main issues while serving the community (1) Ethical issues, (2) Medicolegal issues, and (3) Sociocultural issues **(Fig. 28.13)**.

ETHICAL ISSUES

Ethical issues in children have a larger and challenging role to play as children cannot take decisions of their own. General ethical principles which help in decision making process in children are listed here.

- ***Autonomy:*** Autonomy implies all are free to take their decisions. For children, it becomes even more crucial as there is a third party who will take decisions for them.
- ***Beneficence:*** Do no harm.
- ***Patient confidentiality:*** Disclosure of confidential information at times like child abuse which is imperative for child's physical and mental health.
- ***Respect of parents' wishes and guidance:*** Provision or withholding of care based on parents' wishes.
- ***Conflicts of interest*** to be voided at all cost for patients' benefit.
- ***Informed consent.***

MEDICOLEGAL ISSUES

In present society where doctors have been portrayed in deleterious manner, there is a great mistrust between the caregivers and care providers. The physician must deal with a child and his stressed guardian. Proper history, appropriate

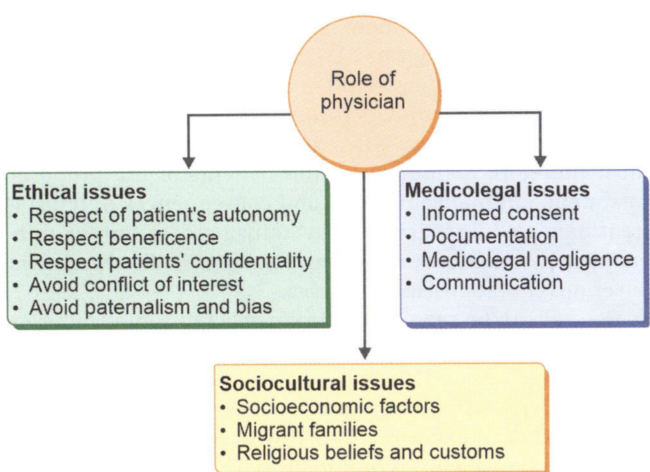

Fig. 28.13: Role of physician in the community

documentation, and proper communication is a must to avoid litigations. Physician should get informed consent signed prior to procedures. It is advisable to have a counseling room with audio-visual camera. Proper documentation of investigation, treatment, and procedures in case files is a must. Proper communication of treatment and response of admitted patients with the patients' legal guardian is imperative. Failure to do so may invite litigation.

SOCIOCULTURAL ISSUES

Cultural beliefs and traditions may impact a child's treatment. Poor socioeconomic condition would lead to malnutrition, vaccine hesitancy or non-immunization, delay in seeking medical health and suboptimal treatment. Poor sanitation and overcrowding may lead to illness. Children of migrant families are the worse victims. Gender bias is another important outcome of cultural and society beliefs resulting in delay in seeking care for female children and female feticide. Other sociocultural constraints are authoritarian parenting styles, shame-based social conditioning, collectivist household economies, living with extended family, abhorrence of introspection, and expression of emotions.

PARENTAL RIGHTS

The Universal Declaration of Human Rights (1948) upholds dignity and equality for all, forming the basis for patient rights globally. In recent decades, there has been growing recognition that all patients—including children—are entitled to specific protections. In India, patient rights are embedded in various laws such as Article 21 of the Constitution, Indian Medical Council Regulations (2002), Consumer Protection Act (1986), Drugs and Cosmetics Act (1940), and Clinical Establishments Act (2010). To unify and clarify these, the National Human Rights Commission (NHRC) developed a Charter of Patients' Rights, shared with States/UTs by the Ministry of Health and Family Welfare (MoHFW) in 2019. This Charter is applicable in both public and private healthcare settings. In 2021, the National Council for Clinical Establishments updated the Charter with additional rights. The full Charter, including the updated rights, is publicly available at: http://clinicalestablishments.gov.in/WriteReadData/3181.pdf

For pediatric patients, who cannot legally or cognitively give informed consent, these rights extend to their parents or legal caregivers, who act on their behalf in medical decision-making. A patient and his/her representative (legal guardians/caregivers) has the following rights with respect to the clinical establishment (**Charter of Patients' Rights**):

1. Right to complete and clear information for patient/caregivers about the patient's illness, proposed treatments, risks, costs, and outcomes.
2. Right to access all medical records, investigation reports, and detailed bills pertaining to the patient.
3. Right to informed consent must be exercised by caregivers before initiating tests or treatment (e.g., surgeries, chemotherapy) for patients who cannot give legal consent.
4. Right to a second opinion, with the patient/caregiver entitled to request and access medical records for consultation elsewhere.
5. Right to privacy, confidentiality, and human dignity during treatment.
6. Right to have ensured a female person, during physical examination of a female patient by a male doctor.
7. Right to non-discriminatory care, regardless of the patient's illness, HIV status, gender identity, ethnicity, or other factors.
8. Right to choose pharmacies or diagnostic labs, protecting the patient/caregivers from being forced to purchase services from hospital-linked vendors.
9. Right to proper referral and safe transfer, especially in emergency situations, with ambulance support and clinical escort if needed.
10. Right to compensation and protection in case of participation in clinical trials or biomedical research, as governed by national guidelines.
11. Right to grievance redressal, with patients/caregivers being allowed to file complaints through established mechanisms with designated officers.
12. Right to education and information, enabling patients/caregivers to understand and participate in informed healthcare decisions.

Responsibilities of Patients/Caregivers

- Provide accurate health and medical history of the patient.
- Cooperate with medical staff, follow treatment plans, and adhere to hospital protocols.
- Respect the dignity of doctors and staff; avoid any form of aggression or violence.
- Make timely payments for agreed services.
- Take responsibility for choices made regarding treatment options, including when treatment is declined.

Pediatric Consent and the Right to Refuse Treatment

In pediatric healthcare, obtaining **informed consent** is both a legal and ethical necessity, protecting patients and physicians alike. Since children are not legally competent to give consent, this responsibility lies primarily with their parents or legal guardians (consent by proxy). Children, especially those aged 7 and above, may be involved in the decision-making process through **assent**, which respects their growing autonomy and understanding of medical interventions. Assent by the child, though not legally binding, is an important ethical practice, especially for children aged 7–12 years. This includes explaining the illness and treatment, assessing the child's understanding and willingness and encouraging involvement in decision-making without coercion.

Types of consent:

- ***Implied consent:*** When the parents bring their child to a physician for treatment of any ailment it implies that they are agreeing for their child to go through the medical examination in the general sense.
- ***Expressed consent:*** When a patient specifically grants the physician permission to undertake the diagnosis and treatment of a specific problem. It may be an oral or a signature/written consent.
- ***Valid informed consent:*** Consent with emphasis on patient's understanding of the reasonable and irrational elements of his/her decision.

The right to refuse treatment is a critical part of the informed consent process. Caregivers have the ethical and legal authority to decline specific diagnostic or therapeutic procedures on behalf of the child, provided they are fully informed of the potential consequences. The content of an informed consent must therefore include risks and benefits of the proposed treatment, alternative options, and consequences of refusing treatment. While parents may refuse treatment in non-emergency situations, this becomes complex in life-threatening or serious conditions. In such cases:

- Refusal can be seen as medical neglect in some countries, such as the U.S., but Indian laws currently lack clear guidance.
- Physicians are encouraged to address refusal through discussion, persuasion, and clarity, and may seek court intervention if refusal compromises the child's well-being.

Ultimately, the caregiver's role is to act in the best interest of the child, balancing medical recommendations with personal, cultural, or religious beliefs. Health professionals must ensure that refusal of care is informed, documented, and approached with sensitivity and legal awareness.

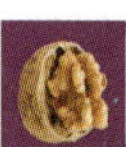

IN A NUTSHELL

Role of Physician in the Community

1. Physicians have to deal with three main issues while serving community: (1) Ethical issues, (2) Medicolegal issues, and (3) Sociocultural issues.
2. Proper history, appropriate documentation, and proper communication are must to avoid litigations.
3. Ethical principles which help in decision making process in children are autonomy, beneficence, patient confidentiality, respect of parents' wishes and guidance, conflicts of interest to be voided at all cost for patients benefit and informed consent.
4. In pediatric care, informed consent is given by parents or legal guardians (consent by proxy), while children may give assent when developmentally appropriate (7 years and above). Consent must include clear information about the nature, risks, benefits, alternatives, and the option to refuse treatment.
5. Caregivers have the right to refuse treatment on behalf of the child, except in emergencies or life-threatening conditions, where refusal may be challenged ethically or legally. Physicians should respond with respectful communication and may seek legal intervention if refusal endangers the child.

Ghai OP, Paul VK, Bagga A. Informed Consent in Pediatric Practice. Indian Pediatrics [Internet]. 2010 Dec; 47(12):1039-46. Available from: https://www.indianpediatrics.net/dec2010/dec-1039-1046.htm [Last accessed May, 2025].

Ministry of Health and Family Welfare. Charter of Patients' Rights [Internet]. New Delhi: Government of India; [cited 2025 May]. Available from: https://www.mohfw.gov.in/sites/default/files/PatientCharterforcomments.pdf [Last accessed May, 2025].

National Council for Clinical Establishments. Charter of Patients' Rights—Updated Version [Internet]. New Delhi: Ministry of Health and Family Welfare; 2021 [cited 2025 May]. Available from: http://clinicalestablishments.gov.in/WriteReadData/3181.pdf [Last accessed May, 2025].

Rushton FE Jr; American Academy of Pediatrics Committee on Community Health Services. The pediatrician's role in community pediatrics. Pediatrics. 2005;115(4):1092-4.

The Pediatrician's role in community pediatrics. American Academy of Pediatrics. Committee on Community Health Services. Pediatrics. 1999;103(6 Pt 1):1304-7.

Piyush Gupta and Chabungbam Smilie

Online Chapters: 29, 30 and 31

(These chapters are only available online, scan QR Codes to access them)

Chapter 29: Skin Disorders

Topics available online: ***Skin Lesions; Urticaria and Angioedema; Pyodermas; Scabies; Viral Infections; Fungal Infections; Atopic Dermatitis; Seborrheic Dermatitis; Hypersensitivity Reactions***

Chapter 30: Ophthalmic Disorders

Topics available online: ***Approach to Common Symptoms; Common Abnormalities in the Eye; Fundus Examination; Ocular Manifestations of Systemic Disorders***

Chapter 31: Drug Therapy

Topics available online: ***Antiarrhythmic Drugs; Antiasthmatics and Bronchodilators; Antifungals; Anti-inflammatory, Antipyretics, and Analgesics; Antibiotics; Anticonvulsants; Antiemetics; Anthelminthics; Antihistaminics; Antihypertensives; Antimalarials; Antiretroviral Drugs; Antitoxins and Immunoglobulins; Antiviral Drugs; Cardiotonics; Diuretics; Miscellaneous Drugs***

Annexures

Annexure 1 Growth Tables (Birth to 18 Years)

Table 1	**Weight (kg) by Age of Boys, Percentiles and *Z*-scores, 0–5 Years (WHO Standards)**													
Age		*Percentiles*							*Standard deviation (SD) Z-score*					
Years	*Months*	*3rd*	*15th*	*25th*	*50th*	*75th*	*85th*	*97th*	*−3SD*	*−2SD*	*−1SD*	*+1SD*	*+2SD*	*+3SD*
	0	2.5	2.9	3.0	3.3	3.7	3.9	4.3	2.1	2.5	2.9	3.9	4.4	5.0
	1	3.4	3.9	4.1	4.5	4.9	5.1	5.7	2.9	3.4	3.9	5.1	5.8	6.6
	2	4.4	4.9	5.1	5.6	6.0	6.3	7.0	3.8	4.3	4.9	6.3	7.1	8.0
	3	5.1	5.6	5.9	6.4	6.9	7.2	7.9	4.4	5.0	5.7	7.2	8.0	9.0
	4	5.6	6.2	6.5	7.0	7.6	7.9	8.6	4.9	5.6	6.2	7.8	8.7	9.7
	5	6.1	6.7	7.0	7.5	8.1	8.4	9.2	5.3	6.0	6.7	8.4	9.3	10.4
	6	6.4	7.1	7.4	7.9	8.5	8.9	9.7	5.7	6.4	7.1	8.8	9.8	10.9
	7	6.7	7.4	7.7	8.3	8.9	9.3	10.2	5.9	6.7	7.4	9.2	10.3	11.4
	8	7.0	7.7	8.0	8.6	9.3	9.6	10.5	6.2	6.9	7.7	9.6	10.7	11.9
	9	7.2	7.9	8.3	8.9	9.6	10.0	10.9	6.4	7.1	8.0	9.9	11.0	12.3
	10	7.5	8.2	8.5	9.2	9.9	10.3	11.2	6.6	7.4	8.2	10.2	11.4	12.7
	11	7.7	8.4	8.7	9.4	10.1	10.5	11.5	6.8	7.6	8.4	10.5	11.7	13.0
1	0	7.8	8.6	9.0	9.6	10.4	10.8	11.8	6.9	7.7	8.6	10.8	12.0	13.3
1	1	8.0	8.8	9.2	9.9	10.6	11.1	12.1	7.1	7.9	8.8	11.0	12.3	13.7
1	2	8.2	9.0	9.4	10.1	10.9	11.3	12.4	7.2	8.1	9.0	11.3	12.6	14.0
1	3	8.4	9.2	9.6	10.3	11.1	11.6	12.7	7.4	8.3	9.2	11.5	12.8	14.3
1	4	8.5	9.4	9.8	10.5	11.3	11.8	12.9	7.5	8.4	9.4	11.7	13.1	14.6
1	5	8.7	9.6	10.0	10.7	11.6	12.0	13.2	7.7	8.6	9.6	12.0	13.4	14.9
1	6	8.9	9.7	10.1	10.9	11.8	12.3	13.5	7.8	8.8	9.8	12.2	13.7	15.3
1	7	9.0	9.9	10.3	11.1	12.0	12.5	13.7	8.0	8.9	10.0	12.5	13.9	15.6
1	8	9.2	10.1	10.5	11.3	12.2	12.7	14.0	8.1	9.1	10.1	12.7	14.2	15.9
1	9	9.3	10.3	10.7	11.5	12.5	13.0	14.3	8.2	9.2	10.3	12.9	14.5	16.2
1	10	9.5	10.5	10.9	11.8	12.7	13.2	14.5	8.4	9.4	10.5	13.2	14.7	16.5
1	11	9.7	10.6	11.1	12.0	12.9	13.4	14.8	8.5	9.5	10.7	13.4	15.0	16.8
2	0	9.8	10.8	11.3	12.2	13.1	13.7	15.1	8.6	9.7	10.8	13.6	15.3	17.1
2	1	10.0	11.0	11.4	12.4	13.3	13.9	15.3	8.8	9.8	11.0	13.9	15.5	17.5
2	2	10.1	11.1	11.6	12.5	13.6	14.1	15.6	8.9	10.0	11.2	14.1	15.8	17.8
2	3	10.2	11.3	11.8	12.7	13.8	14.4	15.9	9.0	10.1	11.3	14.3	16.1	18.1
2	4	10.4	11.5	12.0	12.9	14.0	14.6	16.1	9.1	10.2	11.5	14.5	16.3	18.4
2	5	10.5	11.6	12.1	13.1	14.2	14.8	16.4	9.2	10.4	11.7	14.8	16.6	18.7
2	6	10.7	11.8	12.3	13.3	14.4	15.0	16.6	9.4	10.5	11.8	15.0	16.9	19.0
2	7	10.8	11.9	12.4	13.5	14.6	15.2	16.9	9.5	10.7	12.0	15.2	17.1	19.3

Contd…

Contd...

Age		Percentiles							Standard deviation (SD) Z-score					
Years	Months	3rd	15th	25th	50th	75th	85th	97th	-3SD	-2SD	-1SD	+1SD	+2SD	+3SD
2	8	10.9	12.1	12.6	13.7	14.8	15.5	17.1	9.6	10.8	12.1	15.4	17.4	19.6
2	9	11.1	12.2	12.8	13.8	15.0	15.7	17.3	9.7	10.9	12.3	15.6	17.6	19.9
2	10	11.2	12.4	12.9	14.0	15.2	15.9	17.6	9.8	11.0	12.4	15.8	17.8	20.2
2	11	11.3	12.5	13.1	14.2	15.4	16.1	17.8	9.9	11.2	12.6	16.0	18.1	20.4
3	0	11.4	12.7	13.2	14.3	15.6	16.3	18.0	10.0	11.3	12.7	16.2	18.3	20.7
3	1	11.6	12.8	13.4	14.5	15.8	16.5	18.3	10.1	11.4	12.9	16.4	18.6	21.0
3	2	11.7	12.9	13.5	14.7	15.9	16.7	18.5	10.2	11.5	13.0	16.6	18.8	21.3
3	3	11.8	13.1	13.7	14.8	16.1	16.9	18.7	10.3	11.6	13.1	16.8	19.0	21.6
3	4	11.9	13.2	13.8	15.0	16.3	17.1	19.0	10.4	11.8	13.3	17.0	19.3	21.9
3	5	12.1	13.4	14.0	15.2	16.5	17.3	19.2	10.5	11.9	13.4	17.2	19.5	22.1
3	6	12.2	13.5	14.1	15.3	16.7	17.5	19.4	10.6	12.0	13.6	17.4	19.7	22.4
3	7	12.3	13.6	14.3	15.5	16.9	17.7	19.7	10.7	12.1	13.7	17.6	20.0	22.7
3	8	12.4	13.8	14.4	15.7	17.1	17.9	19.9	10.8	12.2	13.8	17.8	20.2	23.0
3	9	12.5	13.9	14.6	15.8	17.3	18.1	20.1	10.9	12.4	14.0	18.0	20.5	23.3
3	10	12.7	14.1	14.7	16.0	17.4	18.3	20.4	11.0	12.5	14.1	18.2	20.7	23.6
3	11	12.8	14.2	14.9	16.2	17.6	18.5	20.6	11.1	12.6	14.3	18.4	20.9	23.9
4	0	12.9	14.3	15.0	16.3	17.8	18.7	20.9	11.2	12.7	14.4	18.6	21.2	24.2
4	1	13.0	14.5	15.2	16.5	18.0	18.9	21.1	11.3	12.8	14.5	18.8	21.4	24.5
4	2	13.1	14.6	15.3	16.7	18.2	19.1	21.3	11.4	12.9	14.7	19.0	21.7	24.8
4	3	13.3	14.7	15.4	16.8	18.4	19.3	21.6	11.5	13.1	14.8	19.2	21.9	25.1
4	4	13.4	14.9	15.6	17.0	18.6	19.5	21.8	11.6	13.2	15.0	19.4	22.2	25.4
4	5	13.5	15.0	15.7	17.2	18.8	19.7	22.1	11.7	13.3	15.1	19.6	22.4	25.7
4	6	13.6	15.2	15.9	17.3	19.0	19.9	22.3	11.8	13.4	15.2	19.8	22.7	26.0
4	7	13.7	15.3	16.0	17.5	19.2	20.1	22.5	11.9	13.5	15.4	20.0	22.9	26.3
4	8	13.8	15.4	16.2	17.7	19.3	20.3	22.8	12.0	13.6	15.5	20.2	23.2	26.6
4	9	13.9	15.6	16.3	17.8	19.5	20.5	23.0	12.1	13.7	15.6	20.4	23.4	26.9
4	10	14.1	15.7	16.5	18.0	19.7	20.7	23.3	12.2	13.8	15.8	20.6	23.7	27.2
4	11	14.2	15.8	16.6	18.2	19.9	20.9	23.5	12.3	14.0	15.9	20.8	23.9	27.6
5	0	14.3	16.0	16.7	18.3	20.1	21.1	23.8	12.4	14.1	16.0	21.0	24.2	27.9

Table 2 Weight (kg) by Age of Girls, Percentiles and *Z* (SD)-score for 0–5 Years (WHO Standards)

Age		*Percentiles*							*Standard deviation (SD) Z-score*					
Years	*Months*	*3rd*	*15th*	*25th*	*50th*	*75th*	*85th*	*97th*	*–3SD*	*–2SD*	*–1SD*	*+1SD*	*+2SD*	*+3SD*
	0	2.4	2.8	2.9	3.2	3.6	3.7	4.2	2.0	2.4	2.8	3.7	4.2	4.8
	1	3.2	3.6	3.8	4.2	4.6	4.8	5.4	2.7	3.2	3.6	4.8	5.5	6.2
	2	4.0	4.5	4.7	5.1	5.6	5.9	6.5	3.4	3.9	4.5	5.8	6.6	7.5
	3	4.6	5.1	5.4	5.8	6.4	6.7	7.4	4.0	4.5	5.2	6.6	7.5	8.5
	4	5.1	5.6	5.9	6.4	7.0	7.3	8.1	4.4	5.0	5.7	7.3	8.2	9.3
	5	5.5	6.1	6.4	6.9	7.5	7.8	8.7	4.8	5.4	6.1	7.8	8.8	10.0
	6	5.8	6.4	6.7	7.3	7.9	8.3	9.2	5.1	5.7	6.5	8.2	9.3	10.6
	7	6.1	6.7	7.0	7.6	8.3	8.7	9.6	5.3	6.0	6.8	8.6	9.8	11.1
	8	6.3	7.0	7.3	7.9	8.6	9.0	10.0	5.6	6.3	7.0	9.0	10.2	11.6
	9	6.6	7.3	7.6	8.2	8.9	9.3	10.4	5.8	6.5	7.3	9.3	10.5	12.0
	10	6.8	7.5	7.8	8.5	9.2	9.6	10.7	5.9	6.7	7.5	9.6	10.9	12.4
	11	7.0	7.7	8.0	8.7	9.5	9.9	11.0	6.1	6.9	7.7	9.9	11.2	12.8
1	0	7.1	7.9	8.2	8.9	9.7	10.2	11.3	6.3	7.0	7.9	10.1	11.5	13.1
1	1	7.3	8.1	8.4	9.2	10.0	10.4	11.6	6.4	7.2	8.1	10.4	11.8	13.5
1	2	7.5	8.3	8.6	9.4	10.2	10.7	11.9	6.6	7.4	8.3	10.6	12.1	13.8
1	3	7.7	8.5	8.8	9.6	10.4	10.9	12.2	6.7	7.6	8.5	10.9	12.4	14.1
1	4	7.8	8.7	9.0	9.8	10.7	11.2	12.5	6.9	7.7	8.7	11.1	12.6	14.5
1	5	8.0	8.8	9.2	10.0	10.9	11.4	12.7	7.0	7.9	8.9	11.4	12.9	14.8
1	6	8.2	9.0	9.4	10.2	11.1	11.6	13.0	7.2	8.1	9.1	11.6	13.2	15.1
1	7	8.3	9.2	9.6	10.4	11.4	11.9	13.3	7.3	8.2	9.2	11.8	13.5	15.4
1	8	8.5	9.4	9.8	10.6	11.6	12.1	13.5	7.5	8.4	9.4	12.1	13.7	15.7
1	9	8.7	9.6	10.0	10.9	11.8	12.4	13.8	7.6	8.6	9.6	12.3	14.0	16.0
1	10	8.8	9.8	10.2	11.1	12.0	12.6	14.1	7.8	8.7	9.8	12.5	14.3	16.4
1	11	9.0	9.9	10.4	11.3	12.3	12.8	14.3	7.9	8.9	10.0	12.8	14.6	16.7
2	0	9.2	10.1	10.6	11.5	12.5	13.1	14.6	8.1	9.0	10.2	13.0	14.8	17.0
2	1	9.3	10.3	10.8	11.7	12.7	13.3	14.9	8.2	9.2	10.3	13.3	15.1	17.3
2	2	9.5	10.5	10.9	11.9	12.9	13.6	15.2	8.4	9.4	10.5	13.5	15.4	17.7
2	3	9.6	10.7	11.1	12.1	13.2	13.8	15.4	8.5	9.5	10.7	13.7	15.7	18.0
2	4	9.8	10.8	11.3	12.3	13.4	14.0	15.7	8.6	9.7	10.9	14.0	16.0	18.3
2	5	10.0	11.0	11.5	12.5	13.6	14.3	16.0	8.8	9.8	11.1	14.2	16.2	18.7
2	6	10.1	11.2	11.7	12.7	13.8	14.5	16.2	8.9	10.0	11.2	14.4	16.5	19.0
2	7	10.3	11.3	11.9	12.9	14.1	14.7	16.5	9.0	10.1	11.4	14.7	16.8	19.3
2	8	10.4	11.5	12.0	13.1	14.3	15.0	16.8	9.1	10.3	11.6	14.9	17.1	19.6
2	9	10.5	11.7	12.2	13.3	14.5	15.2	17.0	9.3	10.4	11.7	15.1	17.3	20.0
2	10	10.7	11.8	12.4	13.5	14.7	15.4	17.3	9.4	10.5	11.9	15.4	17.6	20.3
2	11	10.8	12.0	12.5	13.7	14.9	15.7	17.6	9.5	10.7	12.0	15.6	17.9	20.6
3	0	11.0	12.1	12.7	13.9	15.1	15.9	17.8	9.6	10.8	12.2	15.8	18.1	20.9
3	1	11.1	12.3	12.9	14.0	15.3	16.1	18.1	9.7	10.9	12.4	16.0	18.4	21.3
3	2	11.2	12.5	13.0	14.2	15.6	16.3	18.4	9.8	11.1	12.5	16.3	18.7	21.6
3	3	11.4	12.6	13.2	14.4	15.8	16.6	18.6	9.9	11.2	12.7	16.5	19.0	22.0
3	4	11.5	12.8	13.4	14.6	16.0	16.8	18.9	10.1	11.3	12.8	16.7	19.2	22.3
3	5	11.6	12.9	13.5	14.8	16.2	17.0	19.2	10.2	11.5	13.0	16.9	19.5	22.7
3	6	11.8	13.1	13.7	15.0	16.4	17.3	19.5	10.3	11.6	13.1	17.2	19.8	23.0
3	7	11.9	13.2	13.9	15.2	16.6	17.5	19.7	10.4	11.7	13.3	17.4	20.1	23.4
3	8	12.0	13.4	14.0	15.3	16.8	17.7	20.0	10.5	11.8	13.4	17.6	20.4	23.7
3	9	12.1	13.5	14.2	15.5	17.0	17.9	20.3	10.6	12.0	13.6	17.8	20.7	24.1
3	10	12.3	13.7	14.3	15.7	17.3	18.2	20.6	10.7	12.1	13.7	18.1	20.9	24.5
3	11	12.4	13.8	14.5	15.9	17.5	18.4	20.8	10.8	12.2	13.9	18.3	21.2	24.8
4	0	12.5	14.0	14.7	16.1	17.7	18.6	21.1	10.9	12.3	14.0	18.5	21.5	25.2
4	1	12.6	14.1	14.8	16.3	17.9	18.9	21.4	11.0	12.4	14.2	18.8	21.8	25.5
4	2	12.8	14.3	15.0	16.4	18.1	19.1	21.7	11.1	12.6	14.3	19.0	22.1	25.9
4	3	12.9	14.4	15.1	16.6	18.3	19.3	22.0	11.2	12.7	14.5	19.2	22.4	26.3
4	4	13.0	14.5	15.3	16.8	18.5	19.5	22.2	11.3	12.8	14.6	19.4	22.6	26.6
4	5	13.1	14.7	15.4	17.0	18.7	19.8	22.5	11.4	12.9	14.8	19.7	22.9	27.0
4	6	13.2	14.8	15.6	17.2	18.9	20.0	22.8	11.5	13.0	14.9	19.9	23.2	27.4
4	7	13.4	15.0	15.8	17.3	19.1	20.2	23.1	11.6	13.2	15.1	20.1	23.5	27.7
4	8	13.5	15.1	15.9	17.5	19.3	20.4	23.3	11.7	13.3	15.2	20.3	23.8	28.1
4	9	13.6	15.3	16.1	17.7	19.6	20.7	23.6	11.8	13.4	15.3	20.6	24.1	28.5
4	10	13.7	15.4	16.2	17.9	19.8	20.9	23.9	11.9	13.5	15.5	20.8	24.4	28.8
4	11	13.8	15.5	16.4	18.0	20.0	21.1	24.2	12.0	13.6	15.6	21.0	24.6	29.2
5	0	14.0	15.7	16.5	18.2	20.2	21.3	24.4	12.1	13.7	15.8	21.2	24.9	29.5

Table 3 Length (cm) by Age of Boys and Girls Aged 0–2 Years (WHO Standards)

Boys		Percentiles							Standard deviation (SD) Z-score					
Age	Months	3rd	15th	25th	50th	75th	85th	97th	−3SD	−2SD	−1SD	+1SD	+2SD	+3SD
	0	46.3	47.9	48.6	49.9	51.2	51.8	53.4	44.2	46.1	48.0	51.8	53.7	55.6
	1	51.1	52.7	53.4	54.7	56.0	56.7	58.4	48.9	50.8	52.8	56.7	58.6	60.6
	2	54.7	56.4	57.1	58.4	59.8	60.5	62.2	52.4	54.4	56.4	60.4	62.4	64.4
	3	57.6	59.3	60.1	61.4	62.8	63.5	65.3	55.3	57.3	59.4	63.5	65.5	67.6
	4	60.0	61.7	62.5	63.9	65.3	66.0	67.8	57.6	59.7	61.8	66.0	68.0	70.1
	5	61.9	63.7	64.5	65.9	67.3	68.1	69.9	59.6	61.7	63.8	68.0	70.1	72.2
	6	63.6	65.4	66.2	67.6	69.1	69.8	71.6	61.2	63.3	65.5	69.8	71.9	74.0
	7	65.1	66.9	67.7	69.2	70.6	71.4	73.2	62.7	64.8	67.0	71.3	73.5	75.7
	8	66.5	68.3	69.1	70.6	72.1	72.9	74.7	64.0	66.2	68.4	72.8	75.0	77.2
	9	67.7	69.6	70.5	72.0	73.5	74.3	76.2	65.2	67.5	69.7	74.2	76.5	78.7
	10	69.0	70.9	71.7	73.3	74.8	75.6	77.6	66.4	68.7	71.0	75.6	77.9	80.1
	11	70.2	72.1	73.0	74.5	76.1	77.0	78.9	67.6	69.9	72.2	76.9	79.2	81.5
	12	71.3	73.3	74.1	75.7	77.4	78.2	80.2	68.6	71.0	73.4	78.1	80.5	82.9
	13	72.4	74.4	75.3	76.9	78.6	79.4	81.5	69.6	72.1	74.5	79.3	81.8	84.2
	14	73.4	75.5	76.4	78.0	79.7	80.6	82.7	70.6	73.1	75.6	80.5	83.0	85.5
	15	74.4	76.5	77.4	79.1	80.9	81.8	83.9	71.6	74.1	76.6	81.7	84.2	86.7
	16	75.4	77.5	78.5	80.2	82.0	82.9	85.1	72.5	75.0	77.6	82.8	85.4	88.0
	17	76.3	78.5	79.5	81.2	83.0	84.0	86.2	73.3	76.0	78.6	83.9	86.5	89.2
	18	77.2	79.5	80.4	82.3	84.1	85.1	87.3	74.2	76.9	79.6	85.0	87.7	90.4
	19	78.1	80.4	81.4	83.2	85.1	86.1	88.4	75.0	77.7	80.5	86.0	88.8	91.5
	20	78.9	81.3	82.3	84.2	86.1	87.1	89.5	75.8	78.6	81.4	87.0	89.8	92.6
	21	79.7	82.2	83.2	85.1	87.1	88.1	90.5	76.5	79.4	82.3	88.0	90.9	93.8
	22	80.5	83.0	84.1	86.0	88.0	89.1	91.6	77.2	80.2	83.1	89.0	91.9	94.9
	23	81.3	83.8	84.9	86.9	89.0	90.0	92.6	78.0	81.0	83.9	89.9	92.9	95.9
	24	82.1	84.6	85.8	87.8	89.9	91.0	93.6	78.7	81.7	84.8	90.9	93.9	97.0
Girls		Percentiles							Standard deviation (SD) Z-score					
Age	Months	3rd	15th	25th	50th	75th	85th	97th	−3SD	−2SD	−1SD	+1SD	+2SD	+3SD
	0	45.6	47.2	47.9	49.1	50.4	51.1	52.7	43.6	45.4	47.3	51.0	52.9	54.7
	1	50.0	51.7	52.4	53.7	55.0	55.7	57.4	47.8	49.8	51.7	55.6	57.6	59.5
	2	53.2	55.0	55.7	57.1	58.4	59.2	60.9	51.0	53.0	55.0	59.1	61.1	63.2
	3	55.8	57.6	58.4	59.8	61.2	62.0	63.8	53.5	55.6	57.7	61.9	64.0	66.1
	4	58.0	59.8	60.6	62.1	63.5	64.3	66.2	55.6	57.8	59.9	64.3	66.4	68.6
	5	59.9	61.7	62.5	64.0	65.5	66.3	68.2	57.4	59.6	61.8	66.2	68.5	70.7
	6	61.5	63.4	64.2	65.7	67.3	68.1	70.0	58.9	61.2	63.5	68.0	70.3	72.5
	7	62.9	64.9	65.7	67.3	68.8	69.7	71.6	60.3	62.7	65.0	69.6	71.9	74.2
	8	64.3	66.3	67.2	68.7	70.3	71.2	73.2	61.7	64.0	66.4	71.1	73.5	75.8
	9	65.6	67.6	68.5	70.1	71.8	72.6	74.7	62.9	65.3	67.7	72.6	75.0	77.4
	10	66.8	68.9	69.8	71.5	73.1	74.0	76.1	64.1	66.5	69.0	73.9	76.4	78.9
	11	68.0	70.2	71.1	72.8	74.5	75.4	77.5	65.2	67.7	70.3	75.3	77.8	80.3
	12	69.2	71.3	72.3	74.0	75.8	76.7	78.9	66.3	68.9	71.4	76.6	79.2	81.7
	13	70.3	72.5	73.4	75.2	77.0	77.9	80.2	67.3	70.0	72.6	77.8	80.5	83.1
	14	71.3	73.6	74.6	76.4	78.2	79.2	81.4	68.3	71.0	73.7	79.1	81.7	84.4
	15	72.4	74.7	75.7	77.5	79.4	80.3	82.7	69.3	72.0	74.8	80.2	83.0	85.7
	16	73.3	75.7	76.7	78.6	80.5	81.5	83.9	70.2	73.0	75.8	81.4	84.2	87.0
	17	74.3	76.7	77.7	79.7	81.6	82.6	85.0	71.1	74.0	76.8	82.5	85.4	88.2
	18	75.2	77.7	78.7	80.7	82.7	83.7	86.2	72.0	74.9	77.8	83.6	86.5	89.4
	19	76.2	78.7	79.7	81.7	83.7	84.8	87.3	72.8	75.8	78.8	84.7	87.6	90.6
	20	77.0	79.6	80.7	82.7	84.7	85.8	88.4	73.7	76.7	79.7	85.7	88.7	91.7
	21	77.9	80.5	81.6	83.7	85.7	86.8	89.4	74.5	77.5	80.6	86.7	89.8	92.9
	22	78.7	81.4	82.5	84.6	86.7	87.8	90.5	75.2	78.4	81.5	87.7	90.8	94.0
	23	79.6	82.2	83.4	85.5	87.7	88.8	91.5	76.0	79.2	82.3	88.7	91.9	95.0
	24	80.3	83.1	84.2	86.4	88.6	89.8	92.5	76.7	80.0	83.2	89.6	92.9	96.1

Table 4 Height-for-age (cm) of Boys and Girls Aged 2–5 Years (WHO Standards)

Boys		*Percentiles*							*Standard deviation (SD) Z-score*					
Years	*Months*	*3rd*	*15th*	*25th*	*50th*	*75th*	*85th*	*97th*	*–3SD*	*–2SD*	*–1SD*	*+1SD*	*+2SD*	*+3SD*
2	0	81.4	83.9	85.1	87.1	89.2	90.3	92.9	78.0	81.0	84.1	90.2	93.2	96.3
2	1	82.1	84.7	85.9	88.0	90.1	91.2	93.8	78.6	81.7	84.9	91.1	94.2	97.3
2	2	82.8	85.5	86.7	88.8	90.9	92.1	94.8	79.3	82.5	85.6	92.0	95.2	98.3
2	3	83.5	86.3	87.4	89.6	91.8	93.0	95.7	79.9	83.1	86.4	92.9	96.1	99.3
2	4	84.2	87.0	88.2	90.4	92.6	93.8	96.6	80.5	83.8	87.1	93.7	97.0	100.3
2	5	84.9	87.7	88.9	91.2	93.4	94.7	97.5	81.1	84.5	87.8	94.5	97.9	101.2
2	6	85.5	88.4	89.6	91.9	94.2	95.5	98.3	81.7	85.1	88.5	95.3	98.7	102.1
2	7	86.2	89.1	90.3	92.7	95.0	96.2	99.2	82.3	85.7	89.2	96.1	99.6	103.0
2	8	86.8	89.7	91.0	93.4	95.7	97.0	100.0	82.8	86.4	89.9	96.9	100.4	103.9
2	9	87.4	90.4	91.7	94.1	96.5	97.8	100.8	83.4	86.9	90.5	97.6	101.2	104.8
2	10	88.0	91.0	92.3	94.8	97.2	98.5	101.5	83.9	87.5	91.1	98.4	102.0	105.6
2	11	88.5	91.6	93.0	95.4	97.9	99.2	102.3	84.4	88.1	91.8	99.1	102.7	106.4
3	0	89.1	92.2	93.6	96.1	98.6	99.9	103.1	85.0	88.7	92.4	99.8	103.5	107.2
3	1	89.7	92.8	94.2	96.7	99.3	100.6	103.8	85.5	89.2	93.0	100.5	104.2	108.0
3	2	90.2	93.4	94.8	97.4	99.9	101.3	104.5	86.0	89.8	93.6	101.2	105.0	108.8
3	3	90.8	94.0	95.4	98.0	100.6	102.0	105.2	86.5	90.3	94.2	101.8	105.7	109.5
3	4	91.3	94.6	96.0	98.6	101.3	102.7	105.9	87.0	90.9	94.7	102.5	106.4	110.3
3	5	91.9	95.2	96.6	99.2	101.9	103.3	106.6	87.5	91.4	95.3	103.2	107.1	111.0
3	6	92.4	95.7	97.2	99.9	102.5	104.0	107.3	88.0	91.9	95.9	103.8	107.8	111.7
3	7	92.9	96.3	97.7	100.4	103.1	104.6	108.0	88.4	92.4	96.4	104.5	108.5	112.5
3	8	93.4	96.8	98.3	101.0	103.8	105.2	108.6	88.9	93.0	97.0	105.1	109.1	113.2
3	9	93.9	97.4	98.9	101.6	104.4	105.8	109.3	89.4	93.5	97.5	105.7	109.8	113.9
3	10	94.4	97.9	99.4	102.2	105.0	106.5	109.9	89.8	94.0	98.1	106.3	110.4	114.6
3	11	94.9	98.5	100.0	102.8	105.6	107.1	110.6	90.3	94.4	98.6	106.9	111.1	115.2
4	0	95.4	99.0	100.5	103.3	106.2	107.7	111.2	90.7	94.9	99.1	107.5	111.7	115.9
4	1	95.9	99.5	101.0	103.9	106.7	108.3	111.8	91.2	95.4	99.7	108.1	112.4	116.6
4	2	96.4	100.0	101.6	104.4	107.3	108.9	112.5	91.6	95.9	100.2	108.7	113.0	117.3
4	3	96.9	100.5	102.1	105.0	107.9	109.5	113.1	92.1	96.4	100.7	109.3	113.6	117.9
4	4	97.4	101.1	102.6	105.6	108.5	110.1	113.7	92.5	96.9	101.2	109.9	114.2	118.6
4	5	97.9	101.6	103.2	106.1	109.1	110.7	114.3	93.0	97.4	101.7	110.5	114.9	119.2
4	6	98.4	102.1	103.7	106.7	109.6	111.2	115.0	93.4	97.8	102.3	111.1	115.5	119.9
4	7	98.8	102.6	104.2	107.2	110.2	111.8	115.6	93.9	98.3	102.8	111.7	116.1	120.6
4	8	99.3	103.1	104.7	107.8	110.8	112.4	116.2	94.3	98.8	103.3	112.3	116.7	121.2
4	9	99.8	103.6	105.3	108.3	111.4	113.0	116.8	94.7	99.3	103.8	112.8	117.4	121.9
4	10	100.3	104.1	105.8	108.9	111.9	113.6	117.4	95.2	99.7	104.3	113.4	118.0	122.6
4	11	100.8	104.7	106.3	109.4	112.5	114.2	118.1	95.6	100.2	104.8	114.0	118.6	123.2
5	0	101.2	105.2	106.8	110.0	113.1	114.8	118.7	96.1	100.7	105.3	114.6	119.2	123.9

Contd…

Contd…

Girls		Percentiles							Standard deviation (SD) Z-score					
Years	Months	3rd	15th	25th	50th	75th	85th	97th	−3SD	−2SD	−1SD	+1SD	+2SD	+3SD
2	0	79.6	82.4	83.5	85.7	87.9	89.1	91.8	76.0	79.3	82.5	88.9	92.2	95.4
2	1	80.4	83.2	84.4	86.6	88.8	90.0	92.8	76.8	80.0	83.3	89.9	93.1	96.4
2	2	81.2	84.0	85.2	87.4	89.7	90.9	93.7	77.5	80.8	84.1	90.8	94.1	97.4
2	3	81.9	84.8	86.0	88.3	90.6	91.8	94.6	78.1	81.5	84.9	91.7	95.0	98.4
2	4	82.6	85.5	86.8	89.1	91.4	92.7	95.6	78.8	82.2	85.7	92.5	96.0	99.4
2	5	83.4	86.3	87.6	89.9	92.2	93.5	96.4	79.5	82.9	86.4	93.4	96.9	100.3
2	6	84.0	87.0	88.3	90.7	93.1	94.3	97.3	80.1	83.6	87.1	94.2	97.7	101.3
2	7	84.7	87.7	89.0	91.4	93.9	95.2	98.2	80.7	84.3	87.9	95.0	98.6	102.2
2	8	85.4	88.4	89.7	92.2	94.6	95.9	99.0	81.3	84.9	88.6	95.8	99.4	103.1
2	9	86.0	89.1	90.4	92.9	95.4	96.7	99.8	81.9	85.6	89.3	96.6	100.3	103.9
2	10	86.7	89.8	91.1	93.6	96.2	97.5	100.6	82.5	86.2	89.9	97.4	101.1	104.8
2	11	87.3	90.5	91.8	94.4	96.9	98.3	101.4	83.1	86.8	90.6	98.1	101.9	105.6
3	0	87.9	91.1	92.5	95.1	97.6	99.0	102.2	83.6	87.4	91.2	98.9	102.7	106.5
3	1	88.5	91.7	93.1	95.7	98.3	99.7	103.0	84.2	88.0	91.9	99.6	103.4	107.3
3	2	89.1	92.4	93.8	96.4	99.0	100.5	103.7	84.7	88.6	92.5	100.3	104.2	108.1
3	3	89.7	93.0	94.4	97.1	99.7	101.2	104.5	85.3	89.2	93.1	101.0	105.0	108.9
3	4	90.3	93.6	95.1	97.7	100.4	101.9	105.2	85.8	89.8	93.8	101.7	105.7	109.7
3	5	90.8	94.2	95.7	98.4	101.1	102.6	106.0	86.3	90.4	94.4	102.4	106.4	110.5
3	6	91.4	94.8	96.3	99.0	101.8	103.3	106.7	86.8	90.9	95.0	103.1	107.2	111.2
3	7	92.0	95.4	96.9	99.7	102.4	103.9	107.4	87.4	91.5	95.6	103.8	107.9	112.0
3	8	92.5	96.0	97.5	100.3	103.1	104.6	108.1	87.9	92.0	96.2	104.5	108.6	112.7
3	9	93.0	96.6	98.1	100.9	103.7	105.3	108.8	88.4	92.5	96.7	105.1	109.3	113.5
3	10	93.6	97.2	98.7	101.5	104.4	105.9	109.5	88.9	93.1	97.3	105.8	110.0	114.2
3	11	94.1	97.7	99.3	102.1	105.0	106.6	110.2	89.3	93.6	97.9	106.4	110.7	114.9
4	0	94.6	98.3	99.8	102.7	105.6	107.2	110.8	89.8	94.1	98.4	107.0	111.3	115.7
4	1	95.1	98.8	100.4	103.3	106.3	107.8	111.5	90.3	94.6	99.0	107.7	112.0	116.4
4	2	95.7	99.4	100.9	103.9	106.9	108.4	112.1	90.7	95.1	99.5	108.3	112.7	117.1
4	3	96.2	99.9	101.5	104.5	107.5	109.1	112.8	91.2	95.6	100.1	108.9	113.3	117.7
4	4	96.7	100.4	102.0	105.0	108.1	109.7	113.4	91.7	96.1	100.6	109.5	114.0	118.4
4	5	97.2	101.0	102.6	105.6	108.6	110.3	114.1	92.1	96.6	101.1	110.1	114.6	119.1
4	6	97.6	101.5	103.1	106.2	109.2	110.9	114.7	92.6	97.1	101.6	110.7	115.2	119.8
4	7	98.1	102.0	103.6	106.7	109.8	111.5	115.3	93.0	97.6	102.2	111.3	115.9	120.4
4	8	98.6	102.5	104.2	107.3	110.4	112.1	116.0	93.4	98.1	102.7	111.9	116.5	121.1
4	9	99.1	103.0	104.7	107.8	111.0	112.6	116.6	93.9	98.5	103.2	112.5	117.1	121.8
4	10	99.6	103.5	105.2	108.4	111.5	113.2	117.2	94.3	99.0	103.7	113.0	117.7	122.4
4	11	100.0	104.0	105.7	108.9	112.1	113.8	117.8	94.7	99.5	104.2	113.6	118.3	123.1
5	0	100.5	104.5	106.2	109.4	112.6	114.4	118.4	95.2	99.9	104.7	114.2	118.9	123.7

Table 5	Weight (kg) for Length (cm) for Boys 0–2 Years (WHO Reference Data) Percentiles and Z (SD)-scores																
Length (cm)	*Percentiles*											*Standard deviation (SD) Z-score*					
	1st	*3rd*	*5th*	*15th*	*25th*	*50th*	*75th*	*85th*	*95th*	*97th*	*99th*	*−3SD*	*−2SD*	*−1SD*	*+1SD*	*+2SD*	*+3SD*
45.0	2.0	2.1	2.1	2.2	2.3	2.4	2.6	2.7	2.9	2.9	3.0	1.9	2.0	2.2	2.7	3.0	3.3
45.5	2.1	2.1	2.2	2.3	2.4	2.5	2.7	2.8	2.9	3.0	3.1	1.9	2.1	2.3	2.8	3.1	3.4
46.0	2.1	2.2	2.3	2.4	2.5	2.6	2.8	2.9	3.0	3.1	3.3	2.0	2.2	2.4	2.9	3.1	3.5
46.5	2.2	2.3	2.3	2.5	2.5	2.7	2.9	3.0	3.1	3.2	3.4	2.1	2.3	2.5	3.0	3.2	3.6
47.0	2.3	2.4	2.4	2.5	2.6	2.8	3.0	3.1	3.2	3.3	3.5	2.1	2.3	2.5	3.0	3.3	3.7
47.5	2.3	2.4	2.5	2.6	2.7	2.9	3.0	3.1	3.3	3.4	3.6	2.2	2.4	2.6	3.1	3.4	3.8
48.0	2.4	2.5	2.6	2.7	2.8	2.9	3.1	3.2	3.4	3.5	3.7	2.3	2.5	2.7	3.2	3.6	3.9
48.5	2.5	2.6	2.6	2.8	2.9	3.0	3.2	3.3	3.5	3.6	3.8	2.3	2.6	2.8	3.3	3.7	4.0
49.0	2.6	2.7	2.7	2.9	2.9	3.1	3.3	3.4	3.6	3.7	3.9	2.4	2.6	2.9	3.4	3.8	4.2
49.5	2.6	2.7	2.8	2.9	3.0	3.2	3.4	3.5	3.8	3.8	4.0	2.5	2.7	3.0	3.5	3.9	4.3
50.0	2.7	2.8	2.9	3.0	3.1	3.3	3.5	3.7	3.9	4.0	4.1	2.6	2.8	3.0	3.6	4.0	4.4
50.5	2.8	2.9	3.0	3.1	3.2	3.4	3.6	3.8	4.0	4.1	4.2	2.7	2.9	3.1	3.8	4.1	4.5
51.0	2.9	3.0	3.1	3.2	3.3	3.5	3.8	3.9	4.1	4.2	4.4	2.7	3.0	3.2	3.9	4.2	4.7
51.5	3.0	3.1	3.2	3.3	3.4	3.6	3.9	4.0	4.2	4.3	4.5	2.8	3.1	3.3	4.0	4.4	4.8
52.0	3.1	3.2	3.3	3.4	3.5	3.8	4.0	4.1	4.4	4.5	4.6	2.9	3.2	3.5	4.1	4.5	5.0
52.5	3.2	3.3	3.4	3.6	3.7	3.9	4.1	4.3	4.5	4.6	4.8	3.0	3.3	3.6	4.2	4.6	5.1
53.0	3.3	3.4	3.5	3.7	3.8	4.0	4.3	4.4	4.6	4.7	4.9	3.1	3.4	3.7	4.4	4.8	5.3
53.5	3.4	3.5	3.6	3.8	3.9	4.1	4.4	4.5	4.8	4.9	5.1	3.2	3.5	3.8	4.5	4.9	5.4
54.0	3.5	3.6	3.7	3.9	4.0	4.3	4.5	4.7	4.9	5.0	5.3	3.3	3.6	3.9	4.7	5.1	5.6
54.5	3.6	3.8	3.8	4.0	4.2	4.4	4.7	4.8	5.1	5.2	5.4	3.4	3.7	4.0	4.8	5.3	5.8
55.0	3.7	3.9	4.0	4.2	4.3	4.5	4.8	5.0	5.3	5.4	5.6	3.6	3.8	4.2	5.0	5.4	6.0
55.5	3.9	4.0	4.1	4.3	4.4	4.7	5.0	5.1	5.4	5.5	5.8	3.7	4.0	4.3	5.1	5.6	6.1
56.0	4.0	4.1	4.2	4.4	4.6	4.8	5.1	5.3	5.6	5.7	5.9	3.8	4.1	4.4	5.3	5.8	6.3
56.5	4.1	4.3	4.3	4.6	4.7	5.0	5.3	5.4	5.7	5.9	6.1	3.9	4.2	4.6	5.4	5.9	6.5
57.0	4.2	4.4	4.5	4.7	4.8	5.1	5.4	5.6	5.9	6.0	6.3	4.0	4.3	4.7	5.6	6.1	6.7
57.5	4.4	4.5	4.6	4.8	5.0	5.3	5.6	5.8	6.1	6.2	6.5	4.1	4.5	4.9	5.7	6.3	6.9
58.0	4.5	4.6	4.7	5.0	5.1	5.4	5.7	5.9	6.2	6.4	6.6	4.3	4.6	5.0	5.9	6.4	7.1
58.5	4.6	4.8	4.9	5.1	5.3	5.6	5.9	6.1	6.4	6.5	6.8	4.4	4.7	5.1	6.1	6.6	7.2
59.0	4.7	4.9	5.0	5.2	5.4	5.7	6.0	6.2	6.6	6.7	7.0	4.5	4.8	5.3	6.2	6.8	7.4
59.5	4.8	5.0	5.1	5.4	5.5	5.9	6.2	6.4	6.7	6.9	7.2	4.6	5.0	5.4	6.4	7.0	7.6
60.0	5.0	5.1	5.2	5.5	5.7	6.0	6.3	6.5	6.9	7.0	7.3	4.7	5.1	5.5	6.5	7.1	7.8
60.5	5.1	5.3	5.4	5.6	5.8	6.1	6.5	6.7	7.1	7.2	7.5	4.8	5.2	5.6	6.7	7.3	8.0
61.0	5.2	5.4	5.5	5.8	5.9	6.3	6.6	6.8	7.2	7.4	7.7	4.9	5.3	5.8	6.8	7.4	8.1
61.5	5.3	5.5	5.6	5.9	6.1	6.4	6.8	7.0	7.4	7.5	7.8	5.0	5.4	5.9	7.0	7.6	8.3
62.0	5.4	5.6	5.7	6.0	6.2	6.5	6.9	7.1	7.5	7.7	8.0	5.1	5.6	6.0	7.1	7.7	8.5
62.5	5.5	5.7	5.8	6.1	6.3	6.7	7.0	7.3	7.6	7.8	8.1	5.2	5.7	6.1	7.2	7.9	8.6
63.0	5.6	5.8	5.9	6.2	6.4	6.8	7.2	7.4	7.8	8.0	8.3	5.3	5.8	6.2	7.4	8.0	8.8
63.5	5.7	5.9	6.0	6.3	6.5	6.9	7.3	7.5	7.9	8.1	8.4	5.4	5.9	6.4	7.5	8.2	8.9
64.0	5.8	6.0	6.2	6.5	6.6	7.0	7.4	7.7	8.1	8.2	8.6	5.5	6.0	6.5	7.6	8.3	9.1
64.5	5.9	6.1	6.3	6.6	6.8	7.1	7.6	7.8	8.2	8.4	8.7	5.6	6.1	6.6	7.8	8.5	9.3
65.0	6.0	6.3	6.4	6.7	6.9	7.3	7.7	7.9	8.3	8.5	8.9	5.7	6.2	6.7	7.9	8.6	9.4
65.5	6.1	6.4	6.5	6.8	7.0	7.4	7.8	8.1	8.5	8.7	9.0	5.8	6.3	6.8	8.0	8.7	9.6
66.0	6.2	6.5	6.6	6.9	7.1	7.5	7.9	8.2	8.6	8.8	9.1	5.9	6.4	6.9	8.2	8.9	9.7
66.5	6.3	6.6	6.7	7.0	7.2	7.6	8.1	8.3	8.8	8.9	9.3	6.0	6.5	7.0	8.3	9.0	9.9
67.0	6.4	6.7	6.8	7.1	7.3	7.7	8.2	8.4	8.9	9.1	9.4	6.1	6.6	7.1	8.4	9.2	10.0
67.5	6.5	6.8	6.9	7.2	7.4	7.9	8.3	8.6	9.0	9.2	9.6	6.2	6.7	7.2	8.5	9.3	10.2
68.0	6.6	6.9	7.0	7.3	7.5	8.0	8.4	8.7	9.2	9.3	9.7	6.3	6.8	7.3	8.7	9.4	10.3
68.5	6.7	7.0	7.1	7.4	7.7	8.1	8.5	8.8	9.3	9.5	9.8	6.4	6.9	7.5	8.8	9.6	10.5
69.0	6.8	7.1	7.2	7.5	7.8	8.2	8.7	8.9	9.4	9.6	10.0	6.5	7.0	7.6	8.9	9.7	10.6
69.5	6.9	7.1	7.3	7.6	7.9	8.3	8.8	9.1	9.5	9.7	10.1	6.6	7.1	7.7	9.0	9.8	10.8
70.0	7.0	7.2	7.4	7.7	8.0	8.4	8.9	9.2	9.7	9.9	10.3	6.6	7.2	7.8	9.2	10.0	10.9
70.5	7.1	7.3	7.5	7.8	8.1	8.5	9.0	9.3	9.8	10.0	10.4	6.7	7.3	7.9	9.3	10.1	11.1
71.0	7.2	7.4	7.6	8.0	8.2	8.6	9.1	9.4	9.9	10.1	10.5	6.8	7.4	8.0	9.4	10.2	11.2
71.5	7.3	7.5	7.7	8.1	8.3	8.8	9.3	9.6	10.1	10.3	10.7	6.9	7.5	8.1	9.5	10.4	11.3
72.0	7.4	7.6	7.8	8.2	8.4	8.9	9.4	9.7	10.2	10.4	10.8	7.0	7.6	8.2	9.6	10.5	11.5
72.5	7.5	7.7	7.9	8.3	8.5	9.0	9.5	9.8	10.3	10.5	11.0	7.1	7.6	8.3	9.8	10.6	11.6
73.0	7.5	7.8	8.0	8.4	8.6	9.1	9.6	9.9	10.4	10.7	11.1	7.2	7.7	8.4	9.9	10.8	11.8
73.5	7.6	7.9	8.0	8.4	8.7	9.2	9.7	10.0	10.6	10.8	11.2	7.2	7.8	8.5	10.0	10.9	11.9
74.0	7.7	8.0	8.1	8.5	8.8	9.3	9.8	10.1	10.7	10.9	11.4	7.3	7.9	8.6	10.1	11.0	12.1
74.5	7.8	8.1	8.2	8.6	8.9	9.4	9.9	10.3	10.8	11.0	11.5	7.4	8.0	8.7	10.2	11.2	12.2

Contd…

Contd…

Length (cm)	Percentiles											Standard deviation (SD) Z-score					
	1st	3rd	5th	15th	25th	50th	75th	85th	95th	97th	99th	–3SD	–2SD	–1SD	+1SD	+2SD	+3SD
75.0	7.9	8.2	8.3	8.7	9.0	9.5	10.1	10.4	10.9	11.2	11.6	7.5	8.1	8.8	10.3	11.3	12.3
75.5	8.0	8.2	8.4	8.8	9.1	9.6	10.2	10.5	11.0	11.3	11.7	7.6	8.2	8.8	10.4	11.4	12.5
76.0	8.0	8.3	8.5	8.9	9.2	9.7	10.3	10.6	11.2	11.4	11.9	7.6	8.3	8.9	10.6	11.5	12.6
76.5	8.1	8.4	8.6	9.0	9.3	9.8	10.4	10.7	11.3	11.5	12.0	7.7	8.3	9.0	10.7	11.6	12.7
77.0	8.2	8.5	8.7	9.1	9.4	9.9	10.5	10.8	11.4	11.6	12.1	7.8	8.4	9.1	10.8	11.7	12.8
77.5	8.3	8.6	8.7	9.2	9.5	10.0	10.6	10.9	11.5	11.7	12.2	7.9	8.5	9.2	10.9	11.9	13.0
78.0	8.4	8.7	8.8	9.3	9.5	10.1	10.7	11.0	11.6	11.8	12.3	7.9	8.6	9.3	11.0	12.0	13.1
78.5	8.4	8.7	8.9	9.3	9.6	10.2	10.8	11.1	11.7	12.0	12.4	8.0	8.7	9.4	11.1	12.1	13.2
79.0	8.5	8.8	9.0	9.4	9.7	10.3	10.9	11.2	11.8	12.1	12.5	8.1	8.7	9.5	11.2	12.2	13.3
79.5	8.6	8.9	9.1	9.5	9.8	10.4	11.0	11.3	11.9	12.2	12.7	8.2	8.8	9.5	11.3	12.3	13.4
80.0	8.7	9.0	9.1	9.6	9.9	10.4	11.1	11.4	12.0	12.3	12.8	8.2	8.9	9.6	11.4	12.4	13.6
80.5	8.7	9.1	9.2	9.7	10.0	10.5	11.2	11.5	12.1	12.4	12.9	8.3	9.0	9.7	11.5	12.5	13.7
81.0	8.8	9.1	9.3	9.8	10.1	10.6	11.3	11.6	12.2	12.5	13.0	8.4	9.1	9.8	11.6	12.6	13.8
81.5	8.9	9.2	9.4	9.9	10.2	10.7	11.4	11.7	12.3	12.6	13.1	8.5	9.1	9.9	11.7	12.7	13.9
82.0	9.0	9.3	9.5	10.0	10.2	10.8	11.5	11.8	12.5	12.7	13.2	8.5	9.2	10.0	11.8	12.8	14.0
82.5	9.1	9.4	9.6	10.1	10.3	10.9	11.6	11.9	12.6	12.8	13.3	8.6	9.3	10.1	11.9	13.0	14.2
83.0	9.2	9.5	9.7	10.1	10.4	11.0	11.7	12.0	12.7	13.0	13.5	8.7	9.4	10.2	12.0	13.1	14.3
83.5	9.3	9.6	9.8	10.3	10.6	11.2	11.8	12.2	12.8	13.1	13.6	8.8	9.5	10.3	12.1	13.2	14.4
84.0	9.4	9.7	9.9	10.4	10.7	11.3	11.9	12.3	12.9	13.2	13.7	8.9	9.6	10.4	12.2	13.3	14.6
84.5	9.5	9.8	10.0	10.5	10.8	11.4	12.0	12.4	13.1	13.3	13.9	9.0	9.7	10.5	12.4	13.5	14.7
85.0	9.6	9.9	10.1	10.6	10.9	11.5	12.2	12.5	13.2	13.5	14.0	9.1	9.8	10.6	12.5	13.6	14.9
85.5	9.7	10.0	10.2	10.7	11.0	11.6	12.3	12.7	13.3	13.6	14.1	9.2	9.9	10.7	12.6	13.7	15.0
86.0	9.8	10.1	10.3	10.8	11.1	11.7	12.4	12.8	13.5	13.7	14.3	9.3	10.0	10.8	12.8	13.9	15.2
86.5	9.9	10.2	10.4	10.9	11.2	11.9	12.5	12.9	13.6	13.9	14.4	9.4	10.1	11.0	12.9	14.0	15.3
87.0	10.0	10.3	10.5	11.0	11.4	12.0	12.7	13.1	13.7	14.0	14.6	9.5	10.2	11.1	13.0	14.2	15.5
87.5	10.1	10.4	10.6	11.2	11.5	12.1	12.8	13.2	13.9	14.2	14.7	9.6	10.4	11.2	13.2	14.3	15.6
88.0	10.2	10.6	10.7	11.3	11.6	12.2	12.9	13.3	14.0	14.3	14.9	9.7	10.5	11.3	13.3	14.5	15.8
88.5	10.3	10.7	10.9	11.4	11.7	12.4	13.1	13.5	14.2	14.4	15.0	9.8	10.6	11.4	13.4	14.6	15.9
89.0	10.4	10.8	11.0	11.5	11.8	12.5	13.2	13.6	14.3	14.6	15.2	9.9	10.7	11.5	13.5	14.7	16.1
89.5	10.5	10.9	11.1	11.6	11.9	12.6	13.3	13.7	14.4	14.7	15.3	10.0	10.8	11.6	13.7	14.9	16.2
90.0	10.6	11.0	11.2	11.7	12.1	12.7	13.4	13.8	14.6	14.9	15.4	10.1	10.9	11.8	13.8	15.0	16.4
90.5	10.7	11.1	11.3	11.8	12.2	12.8	13.6	14.0	14.7	15.0	15.6	10.2	11.0	11.9	13.9	15.1	16.5
91.0	10.8	11.2	11.4	11.9	12.3	13.0	13.7	14.1	14.8	15.1	15.7	10.3	11.1	12.0	14.1	15.3	16.7
91.5	10.9	11.3	11.5	12.0	12.4	13.1	13.8	14.2	15.0	15.3	15.9	10.4	11.2	12.1	14.2	15.4	16.8
92.0	11.0	11.4	11.6	12.2	12.5	13.2	13.9	14.4	15.1	15.4	16.0	10.5	11.3	12.2	14.3	15.6	17.0
92.5	11.1	11.5	11.7	12.3	12.6	13.3	14.1	14.5	15.2	15.5	16.1	10.6	11.4	12.3	14.4	15.7	17.1
93.0	11.2	11.6	11.8	12.4	12.7	13.4	14.2	14.6	15.4	15.7	16.3	10.7	11.5	12.4	14.6	15.8	17.3
93.5	11.3	11.7	11.9	12.5	12.8	13.5	14.3	14.7	15.5	15.8	16.4	10.7	11.6	12.5	14.7	16.0	17.4
94.0	11.4	11.8	12.0	12.6	12.9	13.7	14.4	14.9	15.6	16.0	16.6	10.8	11.7	12.6	14.8	16.1	17.6
94.5	11.5	11.9	12.1	12.7	13.1	13.8	14.5	15.0	15.8	16.1	16.7	10.9	11.8	12.7	14.9	16.3	17.7
95.0	11.6	12.0	12.2	12.8	13.2	13.9	14.7	15.1	15.9	16.2	16.9	11.0	11.9	12.8	15.1	16.4	17.9
95.5	11.7	12.1	12.3	12.9	13.3	14.0	14.8	15.3	16.0	16.4	17.0	11.1	12.0	12.9	15.2	16.5	18.0
96.0	11.8	12.2	12.4	13.0	13.4	14.1	14.9	15.4	16.2	16.5	17.2	11.2	12.1	13.1	15.3	16.7	18.2
96.5	11.9	12.3	12.5	13.1	13.5	14.3	15.1	15.5	16.3	16.7	17.3	11.3	12.2	13.2	15.5	16.8	18.4
97.0	12.0	12.4	12.6	13.2	13.6	14.4	15.2	15.7	16.5	16.8	17.5	11.4	12.3	13.3	15.6	17.0	18.5
97.5	12.1	12.5	12.7	13.4	13.7	14.5	15.3	15.8	16.6	17.0	17.6	11.5	12.4	13.4	15.7	17.1	18.7
98.0	12.2	12.6	12.8	13.5	13.9	14.6	15.5	15.9	16.8	17.1	17.8	11.6	12.5	13.5	15.9	17.3	18.9
98.5	12.3	12.7	13.0	13.6	14.0	14.8	15.6	16.1	16.9	17.3	18.0	11.7	12.6	13.6	16.0	17.5	19.1
99.0	12.4	12.8	13.1	13.7	14.1	14.9	15.7	16.2	17.1	17.4	18.1	11.8	12.7	13.7	16.2	17.6	19.2
99.5	12.5	12.9	13.2	13.8	14.2	15.0	15.9	16.4	17.2	17.6	18.3	11.9	12.8	13.9	16.3	17.8	19.4
100.0	12.6	13.0	13.3	13.9	14.4	15.2	16.0	16.5	17.4	17.8	18.5	12.0	12.9	14.0	16.5	18.0	19.6
100.5	12.7	13.2	13.4	14.1	14.5	15.3	16.2	16.7	17.6	17.9	18.7	12.1	13.0	14.1	16.6	18.1	19.8
101.0	12.8	13.3	13.5	14.2	14.6	15.4	16.3	16.8	17.7	18.1	18.8	12.2	13.2	14.2	16.8	18.3	20.0
101.5	12.9	13.4	13.6	14.3	14.7	15.6	16.5	17.0	17.9	18.3	19.0	12.3	13.3	14.4	16.9	18.5	20.2
102.0	13.0	13.5	13.8	14.5	14.9	15.7	16.6	17.2	18.1	18.5	19.2	12.4	13.4	14.5	17.1	18.7	20.4
102.5	13.2	13.6	13.9	14.6	15.0	15.9	16.8	17.3	18.3	18.6	19.4	12.5	13.5	14.6	17.3	18.8	20.6
103.0	13.3	13.8	14.0	14.7	15.2	16.0	17.0	17.5	18.4	18.8	19.6	12.6	13.6	14.8	17.4	19.0	20.8
103.5	13.4	13.9	14.1	14.8	15.3	16.2	17.1	17.7	18.6	19.0	19.8	12.7	13.7	14.9	17.6	19.2	21.0
104.0	13.5	14.0	14.3	15.0	15.4	16.3	17.3	17.8	18.8	19.2	20.0	12.8	13.9	15.0	17.8	19.4	21.2
104.5	13.6	14.1	14.4	15.1	15.6	16.5	17.4	18.0	19.0	19.4	20.2	12.9	14.0	15.2	17.9	19.6	21.5

Contd…

Contd…

Length (cm)	Percentiles											Standard deviation (SD) Z-score					
	1st	3rd	5th	15th	25th	50th	75th	85th	95th	97th	99th	–3SD	–2SD	–1SD	+1SD	+2SD	+3SD
105.0	13.7	14.2	14.5	15.3	15.7	16.6	17.6	18.2	19.2	19.6	20.4	13.0	14.1	15.3	18.1	19.8	21.7
105.5	13.9	14.4	14.6	15.4	15.9	16.8	17.8	18.4	19.4	19.8	20.6	13.2	14.2	15.4	18.3	20.0	21.9
106.0	14.0	14.5	14.8	15.5	16.0	16.9	18.0	18.5	19.6	20.0	20.8	13.3	14.4	15.6	18.5	20.2	22.1
106.5	14.1	14.6	14.9	15.7	16.2	17.1	18.1	18.7	19.7	20.2	21.0	13.4	14.5	15.7	18.6	20.4	22.4
107.0	14.2	14.8	15.0	15.8	16.3	17.3	18.3	18.9	19.9	20.4	21.2	13.5	14.6	15.9	18.8	20.6	22.6
107.5	14.4	14.9	15.2	16.0	16.5	17.4	18.5	19.1	20.1	20.6	21.4	13.6	14.7	16.0	19.0	20.8	22.8
108.0	14.5	15.0	15.3	16.1	16.6	17.6	18.7	19.3	20.3	20.8	21.7	13.7	14.9	16.2	19.2	21.0	23.1
108.5	14.6	15.2	15.5	16.3	16.8	17.8	18.8	19.5	20.5	21.0	21.9	13.8	15.0	16.3	19.4	21.2	23.3
109.0	14.7	15.3	15.6	16.4	16.9	17.9	19.0	19.6	20.8	21.2	22.1	14.0	15.1	16.5	19.6	21.4	23.6
109.5	14.9	15.4	15.7	16.6	17.1	18.1	19.2	19.8	21.0	21.4	22.3	14.1	15.3	16.6	19.8	21.7	23.8
110.0	15.0	15.6	15.9	16.7	17.2	18.3	19.4	20.0	21.2	21.6	22.6	14.2	15.4	16.8	20.0	21.9	24.1

Table 6 Weight (kg) for Length (cm) for Girls 0–2 Years (WHO Reference Data) Percentiles and *Z* (SD)-scores

Length (cm)	Percentiles											Standard deviation (SD) Z-score					
	1st	3rd	5th	15th	25th	50th	75th	85th	95th	97th	99th	−3SD	−2SD	−1SD	+1SD	+2SD	+3SD
45.0	2.0	2.1	2.1	2.2	2.3	2.5	2.6	2.7	2.9	2.9	3.1	1.9	2.1	2.3	2.7	3.0	3.3
45.5	2.1	2.2	2.2	2.3	2.4	2.5	2.7	2.8	3.0	3.0	3.2	2.0	2.1	2.3	2.8	3.1	3.4
46.0	2.1	2.2	2.3	2.4	2.5	2.6	2.8	2.9	3.1	3.1	3.3	2.0	2.2	2.4	2.9	3.2	3.5
46.5	2.2	2.3	2.3	2.5	2.6	2.7	2.9	3.0	3.2	3.2	3.4	2.1	2.3	2.5	3.0	3.3	3.6
47.0	2.3	2.4	2.4	2.6	2.6	2.8	3.0	3.1	3.3	3.3	3.5	2.2	2.4	2.6	3.1	3.4	3.7
47.5	2.4	2.4	2.5	2.6	2.7	2.9	3.1	3.2	3.4	3.4	3.6	2.2	2.4	2.6	3.2	3.5	3.8
48.0	2.4	2.5	2.6	2.7	2.8	3.0	3.2	3.3	3.5	3.5	3.7	2.3	2.5	2.7	3.3	3.6	4.0
48.5	2.5	2.6	2.7	2.8	2.9	3.1	3.3	3.4	3.6	3.7	3.8	2.4	2.6	2.8	3.4	3.7	4.1
49.0	2.6	2.7	2.7	2.9	3.0	3.2	3.4	3.5	3.7	3.8	3.9	2.4	2.6	2.9	3.5	3.8	4.2
49.5	2.7	2.8	2.8	3.0	3.1	3.3	3.5	3.6	3.8	3.9	4.1	2.5	2.7	3.0	3.6	3.9	4.3
50.0	2.7	2.8	2.9	3.1	3.2	3.4	3.6	3.7	3.9	4.0	4.2	2.6	2.8	3.1	3.7	4.0	4.5
50.5	2.8	2.9	3.0	3.2	3.3	3.5	3.7	3.8	4.0	4.1	4.3	2.7	2.9	3.2	3.8	4.2	4.6
51.0	2.9	3.0	3.1	3.2	3.4	3.6	3.8	3.9	4.2	4.3	4.4	2.8	3.0	3.3	3.9	4.3	4.8
51.5	3.0	3.1	3.2	3.4	3.5	3.7	3.9	4.0	4.3	4.4	4.6	2.8	3.1	3.4	4.0	4.4	4.9
52.0	3.1	3.2	3.3	3.5	3.6	3.8	4.0	4.2	4.4	4.5	4.7	2.9	3.2	3.5	4.2	4.6	5.1
52.5	3.2	3.3	3.4	3.6	3.7	3.9	4.2	4.3	4.6	4.7	4.9	3.0	3.3	3.6	4.3	4.7	5.2
53.0	3.3	3.4	3.5	3.7	3.8	4.0	4.3	4.4	4.7	4.8	5.0	3.1	3.4	3.7	4.4	4.9	5.4
53.5	3.4	3.5	3.6	3.8	3.9	4.2	4.4	4.6	4.9	5.0	5.2	3.2	3.5	3.8	4.6	5.0	5.5
54.0	3.5	3.6	3.7	3.9	4.0	4.3	4.6	4.7	5.0	5.1	5.3	3.3	3.6	3.9	4.7	5.2	5.7
54.5	3.6	3.7	3.8	4.0	4.2	4.4	4.7	4.9	5.2	5.3	5.5	3.4	3.7	4.0	4.8	5.3	5.9
55.0	3.7	3.9	3.9	4.1	4.3	4.5	4.8	5.0	5.3	5.4	5.7	3.5	3.8	4.2	5.0	5.5	6.1
55.5	3.8	4.0	4.0	4.3	4.4	4.7	5.0	5.2	5.5	5.6	5.8	3.6	3.9	4.3	5.1	5.7	6.3
56.0	3.9	4.1	4.2	4.4	4.5	4.8	5.1	5.3	5.6	5.8	6.0	3.7	4.0	4.4	5.3	5.8	6.4
56.5	4.0	4.2	4.3	4.5	4.7	5.0	5.3	5.5	5.8	5.9	6.2	3.8	4.1	4.5	5.4	6.0	6.6
57.0	4.1	4.3	4.4	4.6	4.8	5.1	5.4	5.6	5.9	6.1	6.3	3.9	4.3	4.6	5.6	6.1	6.8
57.5	4.3	4.4	4.5	4.8	4.9	5.2	5.6	5.7	6.1	6.2	6.5	4.0	4.4	4.8	5.7	6.3	7.0
58.0	4.4	4.5	4.6	4.9	5.0	5.4	5.7	5.9	6.2	6.4	6.7	4.1	4.5	4.9	5.9	6.5	7.1
58.5	4.5	4.6	4.7	5.0	5.2	5.5	5.8	6.0	6.4	6.5	6.8	4.2	4.6	5.0	6.0	6.6	7.3
59.0	4.6	4.8	4.9	5.1	5.3	5.6	6.0	6.2	6.6	6.7	7.0	4.3	4.7	5.1	6.2	6.8	7.5
59.5	4.7	4.9	5.0	5.2	5.4	5.7	6.1	6.3	6.7	6.9	7.2	4.4	4.8	5.3	6.3	6.9	7.7
60.0	4.8	5.0	5.1	5.4	5.5	5.9	6.3	6.5	6.9	7.0	7.3	4.5	4.9	5.4	6.4	7.1	7.8
60.5	4.9	5.1	5.2	5.5	5.6	6.0	6.4	6.6	7.0	7.2	7.5	4.6	5.0	5.5	6.6	7.3	8.0
61.0	5.0	5.2	5.3	5.6	5.8	6.1	6.5	6.7	7.2	7.3	7.6	4.7	5.1	5.6	6.7	7.4	8.2
61.5	5.1	5.3	5.4	5.7	5.9	6.3	6.7	6.9	7.3	7.5	7.8	4.8	5.2	5.7	6.9	7.6	8.4
62.0	5.2	5.4	5.5	5.8	6.0	6.4	6.8	7.0	7.4	7.6	8.0	4.9	5.3	5.8	7.0	7.7	8.5
62.5	5.3	5.5	5.6	5.9	6.1	6.5	6.9	7.2	7.6	7.8	8.1	5.0	5.4	5.9	7.1	7.8	8.7
63.0	5.4	5.6	5.7	6.0	6.2	6.6	7.0	7.3	7.7	7.9	8.3	5.1	5.5	6.0	7.3	8.0	8.8
63.5	5.5	5.7	5.8	6.1	6.3	6.7	7.2	7.4	7.9	8.0	8.4	5.2	5.6	6.2	7.4	8.1	9.0
64.0	5.6	5.8	5.9	6.2	6.4	6.9	7.3	7.5	8.0	8.2	8.5	5.3	5.7	6.3	7.5	8.3	9.1
64.5	5.7	5.9	6.0	6.3	6.6	7.0	7.4	7.7	8.1	8.3	8.7	5.4	5.8	6.4	7.6	8.4	9.3
65.0	5.8	6.0	6.1	6.5	6.7	7.1	7.5	7.8	8.3	8.5	8.8	5.5	5.9	6.5	7.8	8.6	9.5
65.5	5.9	6.1	6.2	6.6	6.8	7.2	7.7	7.9	8.4	8.6	9.0	5.5	6.0	6.6	7.9	8.7	9.6
66.0	6.0	6.2	6.3	6.7	6.9	7.3	7.8	8.0	8.5	8.7	9.1	5.6	6.1	6.7	8.0	8.8	9.8
66.5	6.1	6.3	6.4	6.8	7.0	7.4	7.9	8.2	8.7	8.9	9.3	5.7	6.2	6.8	8.1	9.0	9.9
67.0	6.1	6.4	6.5	6.9	7.1	7.5	8.0	8.3	8.8	9.0	9.4	5.8	6.3	6.9	8.3	9.1	10.0
67.5	6.2	6.5	6.6	7.0	7.2	7.6	8.1	8.4	8.9	9.1	9.5	5.9	6.4	7.0	8.4	9.2	10.2
68.0	6.3	6.6	6.7	7.1	7.3	7.7	8.2	8.5	9.0	9.2	9.7	6.0	6.5	7.1	8.5	9.4	10.3
68.5	6.4	6.7	6.8	7.2	7.4	7.9	8.4	8.6	9.2	9.4	9.8	6.1	6.6	7.2	8.6	9.5	10.5
69.0	6.5	6.7	6.9	7.3	7.5	8.0	8.5	8.8	9.3	9.5	9.9	6.1	6.7	7.3	8.7	9.6	10.6
69.5	6.6	6.8	7.0	7.3	7.6	8.1	8.6	8.9	9.4	9.6	10.0	6.2	6.8	7.4	8.8	9.7	10.7
70.0	6.7	6.9	7.1	7.4	7.7	8.2	8.7	9.0	9.5	9.7	10.2	6.3	6.9	7.5	9.0	9.9	10.9
70.5	6.7	7.0	7.1	7.5	7.8	8.3	8.8	9.1	9.6	9.9	10.3	6.4	6.9	7.6	9.1	10.0	11.0
71.0	6.8	7.1	7.2	7.6	7.9	8.4	8.9	9.2	9.8	10.0	10.4	6.5	7.0	7.7	9.2	10.1	11.1
71.5	6.9	7.2	7.3	7.7	8.0	8.5	9.0	9.3	9.9	10.1	10.5	6.5	7.1	7.7	9.3	10.2	11.3
72.0	7.0	7.3	7.4	7.8	8.1	8.6	9.1	9.4	10.0	10.2	10.7	6.6	7.2	7.8	9.4	10.3	11.4
72.5	7.1	7.4	7.5	7.9	8.2	8.7	9.2	9.5	10.1	10.3	10.8	6.7	7.3	7.9	9.5	10.5	11.5
73.0	7.2	7.4	7.6	8.0	8.3	8.8	9.3	9.6	10.2	10.4	10.9	6.8	7.4	8.0	9.6	10.6	11.7
73.5	7.2	7.5	7.7	8.1	8.3	8.9	9.4	9.7	10.3	10.6	11.0	6.9	7.4	8.1	9.7	10.7	11.8
74.0	7.3	7.6	7.8	8.2	8.4	9.0	9.5	9.9	10.4	10.7	11.2	6.9	7.5	8.2	9.8	10.8	11.9
74.5	7.4	7.7	7.8	8.3	8.5	9.1	9.6	10.0	10.5	10.8	11.3	7.0	7.6	8.3	9.9	10.9	12.0

Contd...

Contd...

Length (cm)	Percentiles											Standard deviation (SD) Z-score					
	1st	3rd	5th	15th	25th	50th	75th	85th	95th	97th	99th	−3SD	−2SD	−1SD	+1SD	+2SD	+3SD
75.0	7.5	7.8	7.9	8.3	8.6	9.1	9.7	10.1	10.7	10.9	11.4	7.1	7.7	8.4	10.0	11.0	12.2
75.5	7.6	7.8	8.0	8.4	8.7	9.2	9.8	10.2	10.8	11.0	11.5	7.1	7.8	8.5	10.1	11.1	12.3
76.0	7.6	7.9	8.1	8.5	8.8	9.3	9.9	10.3	10.9	11.1	11.6	7.2	7.8	8.5	10.2	11.2	12.4
76.5	7.7	8.0	8.2	8.6	8.9	9.4	10.0	10.4	11.0	11.2	11.7	7.3	7.9	8.6	10.3	11.4	12.5
77.0	7.8	8.1	8.2	8.7	9.0	9.5	10.1	10.5	11.1	11.3	11.8	7.4	8.0	8.7	10.4	11.5	12.6
77.5	7.9	8.2	8.3	8.8	9.1	9.6	10.2	10.6	11.2	11.4	11.9	7.4	8.1	8.8	10.5	11.6	12.8
78.0	7.9	8.2	8.4	8.9	9.1	9.7	10.3	10.7	11.3	11.5	12.1	7.5	8.2	8.9	10.6	11.7	12.9
78.5	8.0	8.3	8.5	8.9	9.2	9.8	10.4	10.8	11.4	11.7	12.2	7.6	8.2	9.0	10.7	11.8	13.0
79.0	8.1	8.4	8.6	9.0	9.3	9.9	10.5	10.9	11.5	11.8	12.3	7.7	8.3	9.1	10.8	11.9	13.1
79.5	8.2	8.5	8.7	9.1	9.4	10.0	10.6	11.0	11.6	11.9	12.4	7.7	8.4	9.1	10.9	12.0	13.3
80.0	8.3	8.6	8.7	9.2	9.5	10.1	10.7	11.1	11.7	12.0	12.5	7.8	8.5	9.2	11.0	12.1	13.4
80.5	8.3	8.7	8.8	9.3	9.6	10.2	10.8	11.2	11.9	12.1	12.7	7.9	8.6	9.3	11.2	12.3	13.5
81.0	8.4	8.8	8.9	9.4	9.7	10.3	10.9	11.3	12.0	12.2	12.8	8.0	8.7	9.4	11.3	12.4	13.7
81.5	8.5	8.8	9.0	9.5	9.8	10.4	11.1	11.4	12.1	12.4	12.9	8.1	8.8	9.5	11.4	12.5	13.8
82.0	8.6	8.9	9.1	9.6	9.9	10.5	11.2	11.6	12.2	12.5	13.1	8.1	8.8	9.6	11.5	12.6	13.9
82.5	8.7	9.0	9.2	9.7	10.0	10.6	11.3	11.7	12.4	12.6	13.2	8.2	8.9	9.7	11.6	12.8	14.1
83.0	8.8	9.1	9.3	9.8	10.1	10.7	11.4	11.8	12.5	12.8	13.3	8.3	9.0	9.8	11.8	12.9	14.2
83.5	8.9	9.2	9.4	9.9	10.2	10.9	11.5	11.9	12.6	12.9	13.5	8.4	9.1	9.9	11.9	13.1	14.4
84.0	9.0	9.3	9.5	10.0	10.3	11.0	11.7	12.1	12.8	13.1	13.6	8.5	9.2	10.1	12.0	13.2	14.5
84.5	9.1	9.4	9.6	10.1	10.5	11.1	11.8	12.2	12.9	13.2	13.8	8.6	9.3	10.2	12.1	13.3	14.7
85.0	9.2	9.5	9.7	10.2	10.6	11.2	11.9	12.3	13.0	13.3	13.9	8.7	9.4	10.3	12.3	13.5	14.9
85.5	9.3	9.6	9.8	10.4	10.7	11.3	12.1	12.5	13.2	13.5	14.1	8.8	9.5	10.4	12.4	13.6	15.0
86.0	9.4	9.8	9.9	10.5	10.8	11.5	12.2	12.6	13.3	13.6	14.2	8.9	9.7	10.5	12.6	13.8	15.2
86.5	9.5	9.9	10.1	10.6	10.9	11.6	12.3	12.7	13.5	13.8	14.4	9.0	9.8	10.6	12.7	13.9	15.4
87.0	9.6	10.0	10.2	10.7	11.0	11.7	12.5	12.9	13.6	13.9	14.5	9.1	9.9	10.7	12.8	14.1	15.5
87.5	9.7	10.1	10.3	10.8	11.2	11.8	12.6	13.0	13.8	14.1	14.7	9.2	10.0	10.9	13.0	14.2	15.7
88.0	9.8	10.2	10.4	10.9	11.3	12.0	12.7	13.2	13.9	14.2	14.9	9.3	10.1	11.0	13.1	14.4	15.9
88.5	9.9	10.3	10.5	11.0	11.4	12.1	12.9	13.3	14.1	14.4	15.0	9.4	10.2	11.1	13.2	14.5	16.0
89.0	10.0	10.4	10.6	11.2	11.5	12.2	13.0	13.4	14.2	14.5	15.2	9.5	10.3	11.2	13.4	14.7	16.2
89.5	10.1	10.5	10.7	11.3	11.6	12.3	13.1	13.6	14.4	14.7	15.3	9.6	10.4	11.3	13.5	14.8	16.4
90.0	10.2	10.6	10.8	11.4	11.8	12.5	13.3	13.7	14.5	14.8	15.5	9.7	10.5	11.4	13.7	15.0	16.5
90.5	10.3	10.7	10.9	11.5	11.9	12.6	13.4	13.8	14.6	15.0	15.6	9.8	10.6	11.5	13.8	15.1	16.7
91.0	10.4	10.8	11.0	11.6	12.0	12.7	13.5	14.0	14.8	15.1	15.8	9.9	10.7	11.7	13.9	15.3	16.9
91.5	10.5	10.9	11.1	11.7	12.1	12.8	13.7	14.1	14.9	15.3	15.9	10.0	10.8	11.8	14.1	15.5	17.0
92.0	10.6	11.0	11.2	11.8	12.2	13.0	13.8	14.2	15.1	15.4	16.1	10.1	10.9	11.9	14.2	15.6	17.2
92.5	10.7	11.1	11.3	12.0	12.3	13.1	13.9	14.4	15.2	15.6	16.3	10.1	11.0	12.0	14.3	15.8	17.4
93.0	10.8	11.2	11.5	12.1	12.5	13.2	14.0	14.5	15.4	15.7	16.4	10.2	11.1	12.1	14.5	15.9	17.5
93.5	10.9	11.3	11.6	12.2	12.6	13.3	14.2	14.7	15.5	15.9	16.6	10.3	11.2	12.2	14.6	16.1	17.7
94.0	11.0	11.4	11.7	12.3	12.7	13.5	14.3	14.8	15.7	16.0	16.7	10.4	11.3	12.3	14.7	16.2	17.9
94.5	11.1	11.5	11.8	12.4	12.8	13.6	14.4	14.9	15.8	16.2	16.9	10.5	11.4	12.4	14.9	16.4	18.0
95.0	11.2	11.6	11.9	12.5	12.9	13.7	14.6	15.1	16.0	16.3	17.0	10.6	11.5	12.6	15.0	16.5	18.2
95.5	11.3	11.8	12.0	12.6	13.0	13.8	14.7	15.2	16.1	16.5	17.2	10.7	11.6	12.7	15.2	16.7	18.4
96.0	11.4	11.9	12.1	12.7	13.2	14.0	14.9	15.4	16.3	16.6	17.4	10.8	11.7	12.8	15.3	16.8	18.6
96.5	11.5	12.0	12.2	12.9	13.3	14.1	15.0	15.5	16.4	16.8	17.5	10.9	11.8	12.9	15.4	17.0	18.7
97.0	11.6	12.1	12.3	13.0	13.4	14.2	15.1	15.6	16.6	16.9	17.7	11.0	12.0	13.0	15.6	17.1	18.9
97.5	11.7	12.2	12.4	13.1	13.5	14.4	15.3	15.8	16.7	17.1	17.9	11.1	12.1	13.1	15.7	17.3	19.1
98.0	11.8	12.3	12.5	13.2	13.6	14.5	15.4	15.9	16.9	17.3	18.0	11.2	12.2	13.3	15.9	17.5	19.3
98.5	11.9	12.4	12.7	13.3	13.8	14.6	15.5	16.1	17.0	17.4	18.2	11.3	12.3	13.4	16.0	17.6	19.5
99.0	12.0	12.5	12.8	13.5	13.9	14.8	15.7	16.2	17.2	17.6	18.4	11.4	12.4	13.5	16.2	17.8	19.6
99.5	12.2	12.6	12.9	13.6	14.0	14.9	15.8	16.4	17.4	17.8	18.5	11.5	12.5	13.6	16.3	18.0	19.8
100.0	12.3	12.7	13.0	13.7	14.1	15.0	16.0	16.5	17.5	17.9	18.7	11.6	12.6	13.7	16.5	18.1	20.0
100.5	12.4	12.9	13.1	13.8	14.3	15.2	16.1	16.7	17.7	18.1	18.9	11.7	12.7	13.9	16.6	18.3	20.2
101.0	12.5	13.0	13.2	14.0	14.4	15.3	16.3	16.9	17.9	18.3	19.1	11.8	12.8	14.0	16.8	18.5	20.4
101.5	12.6	13.1	13.4	14.1	14.5	15.5	16.4	17.0	18.0	18.5	19.3	11.9	13.0	14.1	17.0	18.7	20.6
102.0	12.7	13.2	13.5	14.2	14.7	15.6	16.6	17.2	18.2	18.6	19.5	12.0	13.1	14.3	17.1	18.9	20.8
102.5	12.8	13.3	13.6	14.4	14.8	15.8	16.8	17.4	18.4	18.8	19.7	12.1	13.2	14.4	17.3	19.0	21.0
103.0	13.0	13.5	13.7	14.5	15.0	15.9	16.9	17.5	18.6	19.0	19.9	12.3	13.3	14.5	17.5	19.2	21.3
103.5	13.1	13.6	13.9	14.6	15.1	16.1	17.1	17.7	18.8	19.2	20.1	12.4	13.5	14.7	17.6	19.4	21.5
104.0	13.2	13.7	14.0	14.8	15.3	16.2	17.3	17.9	19.0	19.4	20.3	12.5	13.6	14.8	17.8	19.6	21.7
104.5	13.3	13.9	14.1	14.9	15.4	16.4	17.4	18.1	19.1	19.6	20.5	12.6	13.7	15.0	18.0	19.8	21.9

Contd...

Contd…

Length (cm)	*Percentiles*											*Standard deviation (SD) Z-score*						
	1st	*3rd*	*5th*	*15th*	*25th*	*50th*	*75th*	*85th*	*95th*	*97th*	*99th*	*−3SD*	*−2SD*	*−1SD*	*+1SD*	*+2SD*	*+3SD*
105.0	13.5	14.0	14.3	15.1	15.6	16.5	17.6	18.2	19.3	19.8	20.7	12.7	13.8	15.1	18.2	20.0	22.2
105.5	13.6	14.1	14.4	15.2	15.7	16.7	17.8	18.4	19.5	20.0	20.9	12.8	14.0	15.3	18.4	20.2	22.4
106.0	13.7	14.3	14.6	15.4	15.9	16.9	18.0	18.6	19.7	20.2	21.1	13.0	14.1	15.4	18.5	20.5	22.6
106.5	13.9	14.4	14.7	15.5	16.0	17.1	18.2	18.8	20.0	20.4	21.4	13.1	14.3	15.6	18.7	20.7	22.9
107.0	14.0	14.5	14.8	15.7	16.2	17.2	18.4	19.0	20.2	20.6	21.6	13.2	14.4	15.7	18.9	20.9	23.1
107.5	14.1	14.7	15.0	15.8	16.4	17.4	18.5	19.2	20.4	20.9	21.8	13.3	14.5	15.9	19.1	21.1	23.4
108.0	14.3	14.8	15.1	16.0	16.5	17.6	18.7	19.4	20.6	21.1	22.1	13.5	14.7	16.0	19.3	21.3	23.6
108.5	14.4	15.0	15.3	16.2	16.7	17.8	18.9	19.6	20.8	21.3	22.3	13.6	14.8	16.2	19.5	21.6	23.9
109.0	14.6	15.1	15.5	16.3	16.9	18.0	19.1	19.8	21.0	21.5	22.5	13.7	15.0	16.4	19.7	21.8	24.2
109.5	14.7	15.3	15.6	16.5	17.0	18.1	19.3	20.0	21.3	21.8	22.8	13.9	15.1	16.5	20.0	22.0	24.4
110.0	14.9	15.4	15.8	16.7	17.2	18.3	19.5	20.2	21.5	22.0	23.0	14.0	15.3	16.7	20.2	22.3	24.7

Table 7 Weight (kg) for Height (cm) for Boys 2–5 Years (WHO Reference Data) Percentiles and Z (SD)-scores

Height (cm)	Percentiles											Standard deviation (SD) Z-score					
	1st	3rd	5th	15th	25th	50th	75th	85th	95th	97th	99th	−3SD	−2SD	−1SD	+1SD	+2SD	+3SD
65.0	6.2	6.4	6.5	6.8	7.0	7.4	7.9	8.1	8.5	8.7	9.1	5.9	6.3	6.9	8.1	8.8	9.6
65.5	6.3	6.5	6.6	6.9	7.1	7.6	8.0	8.2	8.7	8.9	9.2	6.0	6.4	7.0	8.2	8.9	9.8
66.0	6.4	6.6	6.7	7.1	7.3	7.7	8.1	8.4	8.8	9.0	9.3	6.1	6.5	7.1	8.3	9.1	9.9
66.5	6.5	6.7	6.8	7.2	7.4	7.8	8.2	8.5	8.9	9.1	9.5	6.1	6.6	7.2	8.5	9.2	10.1
67.0	6.6	6.8	6.9	7.3	7.5	7.9	8.4	8.6	9.1	9.3	9.6	6.2	6.7	7.3	8.6	9.4	10.2
67.5	6.7	6.9	7.0	7.4	7.6	8.0	8.5	8.7	9.2	9.4	9.8	6.3	6.8	7.4	8.7	9.5	10.4
68.0	6.8	7.0	7.1	7.5	7.7	8.1	8.6	8.9	9.3	9.5	9.9	6.4	6.9	7.5	8.8	9.6	10.5
68.5	6.8	7.1	7.2	7.6	7.8	8.2	8.7	9.0	9.5	9.7	10.0	6.5	7.0	7.6	9.0	9.8	10.7
69.0	6.9	7.2	7.3	7.7	7.9	8.4	8.8	9.1	9.6	9.8	10.2	6.6	7.1	7.7	9.1	9.9	10.8
69.5	7.0	7.3	7.4	7.8	8.0	8.5	9.0	9.2	9.7	9.9	10.3	6.7	7.2	7.8	9.2	10.0	11.0
70.0	7.1	7.4	7.5	7.9	8.1	8.6	9.1	9.4	9.9	10.1	10.5	6.8	7.3	7.9	9.3	10.2	11.1
70.5	7.2	7.5	7.6	8.0	8.2	8.7	9.2	9.5	10.0	10.2	10.6	6.9	7.4	8.0	9.5	10.3	11.3
71.0	7.3	7.6	7.7	8.1	8.3	8.8	9.3	9.6	10.1	10.3	10.7	6.9	7.5	8.1	9.6	10.4	11.4
71.5	7.4	7.7	7.8	8.2	8.4	8.9	9.4	9.7	10.2	10.5	10.9	7.0	7.6	8.2	9.7	10.6	11.6
72.0	7.5	7.8	7.9	8.3	8.5	9.0	9.5	9.8	10.4	10.6	11.0	7.1	7.7	8.3	9.8	10.7	11.7
72.5	7.6	7.8	8.0	8.4	8.6	9.1	9.7	10.0	10.5	10.7	11.1	7.2	7.8	8.4	9.9	10.8	11.8
73.0	7.7	7.9	8.1	8.5	8.7	9.2	9.8	10.1	10.6	10.8	11.3	7.3	7.9	8.5	10.0	11.0	12.0
73.5	7.8	8.0	8.2	8.6	8.8	9.3	9.9	10.2	10.7	11.0	11.4	7.4	7.9	8.6	10.2	11.1	12.1
74.0	7.8	8.1	8.3	8.7	8.9	9.4	10.0	10.3	10.9	11.1	11.5	7.4	8.0	8.7	10.3	11.2	12.2
74.5	7.9	8.2	8.4	8.8	9.0	9.5	10.1	10.4	11.0	11.2	11.7	7.5	8.1	8.8	10.4	11.3	12.4
75.0	8.0	8.3	8.4	8.9	9.1	9.6	10.2	10.5	11.1	11.3	11.8	7.6	8.2	8.9	10.5	11.4	12.5
75.5	8.1	8.4	8.5	9.0	9.2	9.7	10.3	10.6	11.2	11.4	11.9	7.7	8.3	9.0	10.6	11.6	12.6
76.0	8.2	8.5	8.6	9.0	9.3	9.8	10.4	10.7	11.3	11.6	12.0	7.7	8.4	9.1	10.7	11.7	12.8
76.5	8.2	8.5	8.7	9.1	9.4	9.9	10.5	10.8	11.4	11.7	12.1	7.8	8.5	9.2	10.8	11.8	12.9
77.0	8.3	8.6	8.8	9.2	9.5	10.0	10.6	10.9	11.5	11.8	12.3	7.9	8.5	9.2	10.9	11.9	13.0
77.5	8.4	8.7	8.9	9.3	9.6	10.1	10.7	11.0	11.6	11.9	12.4	8.0	8.6	9.3	11.0	12.0	13.1
78.0	8.5	8.8	8.9	9.4	9.7	10.2	10.8	11.1	11.7	12.0	12.5	8.0	8.7	9.4	11.1	12.1	13.3
78.5	8.5	8.8	9.0	9.5	9.7	10.3	10.9	11.2	11.9	12.1	12.6	8.1	8.8	9.5	11.2	12.2	13.4
79.0	8.6	8.9	9.1	9.5	9.8	10.4	11.0	11.3	12.0	12.2	12.7	8.2	8.8	9.6	11.3	12.3	13.5
79.5	8.7	9.0	9.2	9.6	9.9	10.5	11.1	11.4	12.1	12.3	12.8	8.3	8.9	9.7	11.4	12.4	13.6
80.0	8.8	9.1	9.3	9.7	10.0	10.6	11.2	11.5	12.2	12.4	12.9	8.3	9.0	9.7	11.5	12.6	13.7
80.5	8.9	9.2	9.3	9.8	10.1	10.7	11.3	11.6	12.3	12.5	13.0	8.4	9.1	9.8	11.6	12.7	13.8
81.0	8.9	9.3	9.4	9.9	10.2	10.8	11.4	11.8	12.4	12.6	13.1	8.5	9.2	9.9	11.7	12.8	14.0
81.5	9.0	9.3	9.5	10.0	10.3	10.9	11.5	11.9	12.5	12.8	13.3	8.6	9.3	10.0	11.8	12.9	14.1
82.0	9.1	9.4	9.6	10.1	10.4	11.0	11.6	12.0	12.6	12.9	13.4	8.7	9.3	10.1	11.9	13.0	14.2
82.5	9.2	9.5	9.7	10.2	10.5	11.1	11.7	12.1	12.7	13.0	13.5	8.7	9.4	10.2	12.1	13.1	14.4
83.0	9.3	9.6	9.8	10.3	10.6	11.2	11.8	12.2	12.9	13.1	13.6	8.8	9.5	10.3	12.2	13.3	14.5
83.5	9.4	9.7	9.9	10.4	10.7	11.3	12.0	12.3	13.0	13.3	13.8	8.9	9.6	10.4	12.3	13.4	14.6
84.0	9.5	9.8	10.0	10.5	10.8	11.4	12.1	12.5	13.1	13.4	13.9	9.0	9.7	10.5	12.4	13.5	14.8
84.5	9.6	9.9	10.1	10.6	10.9	11.5	12.2	12.6	13.3	13.5	14.1	9.1	9.9	10.7	12.5	13.7	14.9
85.0	9.7	10.1	10.2	10.7	11.1	11.7	12.3	12.7	13.4	13.7	14.2	9.2	10.0	10.8	12.7	13.8	15.1
85.5	9.8	10.2	10.3	10.9	11.2	11.8	12.5	12.8	13.5	13.8	14.3	9.3	10.1	10.9	12.8	13.9	15.2
86.0	9.9	10.3	10.5	11.0	11.3	11.9	12.6	13.0	13.7	13.9	14.5	9.4	10.2	11.0	12.9	14.1	15.4
86.5	10.0	10.4	10.6	11.1	11.4	12.0	12.7	13.1	13.8	14.1	14.6	9.5	10.3	11.1	13.1	14.2	15.5
87.0	10.1	10.5	10.7	11.2	11.5	12.2	12.9	13.2	13.9	14.2	14.8	9.6	10.4	11.2	13.2	14.4	15.7
87.5	10.2	10.6	10.8	11.3	11.6	12.3	13.0	13.4	14.1	14.4	14.9	9.7	10.5	11.3	13.3	14.5	15.8
88.0	10.3	10.7	10.9	11.4	11.8	12.4	13.1	13.5	14.2	14.5	15.1	9.8	10.6	11.5	13.5	14.7	16.0
88.5	10.5	10.8	11.0	11.5	11.9	12.5	13.2	13.6	14.4	14.6	15.2	9.9	10.7	11.6	13.6	14.8	16.1
89.0	10.6	10.9	11.1	11.7	12.0	12.6	13.4	13.8	14.5	14.8	15.4	10.0	10.8	11.7	13.7	14.9	16.3
89.5	10.7	11.0	11.2	11.8	12.1	12.8	13.5	13.9	14.6	14.9	15.5	10.1	10.9	11.8	13.9	15.1	16.4
90.0	10.8	11.1	11.3	11.9	12.2	12.9	13.6	14.0	14.8	15.1	15.6	10.2	11.0	11.9	14.0	15.2	16.6
90.5	10.9	11.2	11.4	12.0	12.3	13.0	13.7	14.1	14.9	15.2	15.8	10.3	11.1	12.0	14.1	15.3	16.7
91.0	11.0	11.3	11.5	12.1	12.4	13.1	13.9	14.3	15.0	15.3	15.9	10.4	11.2	12.1	14.2	15.5	16.9
91.5	11.0	11.4	11.6	12.2	12.5	13.2	14.0	14.4	15.2	15.5	16.1	10.5	11.3	12.2	14.4	15.6	17.0
92.0	11.1	11.5	11.7	12.3	12.7	13.4	14.1	14.5	15.3	15.6	16.2	10.6	11.4	12.3	14.5	15.8	17.2
92.5	11.2	11.6	11.8	12.4	12.8	13.5	14.2	14.7	15.4	15.7	16.3	10.7	11.5	12.4	14.6	15.9	17.3
93.0	11.3	11.7	11.9	12.5	12.9	13.6	14.4	14.8	15.6	15.9	16.5	10.8	11.6	12.6	14.7	16.0	17.5
93.5	11.4	11.8	12.0	12.6	13.0	13.7	14.5	14.9	15.7	16.0	16.6	10.9	11.7	12.7	14.9	16.2	17.6
94.0	11.5	11.9	12.1	12.7	13.1	13.8	14.6	15.0	15.8	16.1	16.8	11.0	11.8	12.8	15.0	16.3	17.8

Contd…

Contd…

Height (cm)	*Percentiles*											*Standard deviation (SD) Z-score*					
	1st	*3rd*	*5th*	*15th*	*25th*	*50th*	*75th*	*85th*	*95th*	*97th*	*99th*	*−3SD*	*−2SD*	*−1SD*	*+1SD*	*+2SD*	*+3SD*
94.5	11.6	12.0	12.2	12.8	13.2	13.9	14.7	15.2	16.0	16.3	16.9	11.1	11.9	12.9	15.1	16.5	17.9
95.0	11.7	12.1	12.4	12.9	13.3	14.1	14.9	15.3	16.1	16.4	17.1	11.1	12.0	13.0	15.3	16.6	18.1
95.5	11.8	12.2	12.5	13.1	13.4	14.2	15.0	15.4	16.2	16.6	17.2	11.2	12.1	13.1	15.4	16.7	18.3
96.0	11.9	12.3	12.6	13.2	13.6	14.3	15.1	15.6	16.4	16.7	17.4	11.3	12.2	13.2	15.5	16.9	18.4
96.5	12.0	12.4	12.7	13.3	13.7	14.4	15.2	15.7	16.5	16.9	17.5	11.4	12.3	13.3	15.7	17.0	18.6
97.0	12.1	12.5	12.8	13.4	13.8	14.6	15.4	15.9	16.7	17.0	17.7	11.5	12.4	13.4	15.8	17.2	18.8
97.5	12.2	12.7	12.9	13.5	13.9	14.7	15.5	16.0	16.8	17.2	17.9	11.6	12.5	13.6	15.9	17.4	18.9
98.0	12.3	12.8	13.0	13.6	14.0	14.8	15.7	16.1	17.0	17.3	18.0	11.7	12.6	13.7	16.1	17.5	19.1
98.5	12.4	12.9	13.1	13.8	14.2	14.9	15.8	16.3	17.2	17.5	18.2	11.8	12.8	13.8	16.2	17.7	19.3
99.0	12.5	13.0	13.2	13.9	14.3	15.1	15.9	16.4	17.3	17.7	18.4	11.9	12.9	13.9	16.4	17.9	19.5
99.5	12.7	13.1	13.3	14.0	14.4	15.2	16.1	16.6	17.5	17.8	18.5	12.0	13.0	14.0	16.5	18.0	19.7
100.0	12.8	13.2	13.5	14.1	14.5	15.4	16.2	16.7	17.6	18.0	18.7	12.1	13.1	14.2	16.7	18.2	19.9
100.5	12.9	13.3	13.6	14.2	14.7	15.5	16.4	16.9	17.8	18.2	18.9	12.2	13.2	14.3	16.9	18.4	20.1
101.0	13.0	13.4	13.7	14.4	14.8	15.6	16.5	17.1	18.0	18.4	19.1	12.3	13.3	14.4	17.0	18.5	20.3
101.5	13.1	13.6	13.8	14.5	14.9	15.8	16.7	17.2	18.2	18.5	19.3	12.4	13.4	14.5	17.2	18.7	20.5
102.0	13.2	13.7	13.9	14.6	15.1	15.9	16.9	17.4	18.3	18.7	19.5	12.5	13.6	14.7	17.3	18.9	20.7
102.5	13.3	13.8	14.1	14.8	15.2	16.1	17.0	17.6	18.5	18.9	19.7	12.6	13.7	14.8	17.5	19.1	20.9
103.0	13.4	13.9	14.2	14.9	15.3	16.2	17.2	17.7	18.7	19.1	19.9	12.8	13.8	14.9	17.7	19.3	21.1
103.5	13.6	14.0	14.3	15.0	15.5	16.4	17.3	17.9	18.9	19.3	20.1	12.9	13.9	15.1	17.8	19.5	21.3
104.0	13.7	14.2	14.4	15.2	15.6	16.5	17.5	18.1	19.1	19.5	20.3	13.0	14.0	15.2	18.0	19.7	21.6
104.5	13.8	14.3	14.6	15.3	15.8	16.7	17.7	18.2	19.2	19.7	20.5	13.1	14.2	15.4	18.2	19.9	21.8
105.0	13.9	14.4	14.7	15.4	15.9	16.8	17.8	18.4	19.4	19.9	20.7	13.2	14.3	15.5	18.4	20.1	22.0
105.5	14.0	14.5	14.8	15.6	16.1	17.0	18.0	18.6	19.6	20.1	20.9	13.3	14.4	15.6	18.5	20.3	22.2
106.0	14.2	14.7	15.0	15.7	16.2	17.2	18.2	18.8	19.8	20.3	21.1	13.4	14.5	15.8	18.7	20.5	22.5
106.5	14.3	14.8	15.1	15.9	16.4	17.3	18.4	19.0	20.0	20.5	21.3	13.5	14.7	15.9	18.9	20.7	22.7
107.0	14.4	14.9	15.2	16.0	16.5	17.5	18.5	19.1	20.2	20.7	21.5	13.7	14.8	16.1	19.1	20.9	22.9
107.5	14.5	15.1	15.4	16.2	16.7	17.7	18.7	19.3	20.4	20.9	21.7	13.8	14.9	16.2	19.3	21.1	23.2
108.0	14.7	15.2	15.5	16.3	16.8	17.8	18.9	19.5	20.6	21.1	22.0	13.9	15.1	16.4	19.5	21.3	23.4
108.5	14.8	15.3	15.6	16.5	17.0	18.0	19.1	19.7	20.8	21.3	22.2	14.0	15.2	16.5	19.7	21.5	23.7
109.0	14.9	15.5	15.8	16.6	17.1	18.2	19.3	19.9	21.1	21.5	22.4	14.1	15.3	16.7	19.8	21.8	23.9
109.5	15.1	15.6	15.9	16.8	17.3	18.3	19.5	20.1	21.3	21.7	22.7	14.3	15.5	16.8	20.0	22.0	24.2
110.0	15.2	15.8	16.1	16.9	17.5	18.5	19.7	20.3	21.5	22.0	22.9	14.4	15.6	17.0	20.2	22.2	24.4
110.5	15.3	15.9	16.2	17.1	17.6	18.7	19.9	20.5	21.7	22.2	23.1	14.5	15.8	17.1	20.4	22.4	24.7
111.0	15.5	16.1	16.4	17.2	17.8	18.9	20.1	20.7	21.9	22.4	23.4	14.6	15.9	17.3	20.7	22.7	25.0
111.5	15.6	16.2	16.5	17.4	18.0	19.1	20.3	20.9	22.1	22.6	23.6	14.8	16.0	17.5	20.9	22.9	25.2
112.0	15.7	16.3	16.7	17.6	18.1	19.2	20.5	21.1	22.4	22.9	23.9	14.9	16.2	17.6	21.1	23.1	25.5
112.5	15.9	16.5	16.8	17.7	18.3	19.4	20.7	21.4	22.6	23.1	24.1	15.0	16.3	17.8	21.3	23.4	25.8
113.0	16.0	16.6	17.0	17.9	18.5	19.6	20.9	21.6	22.8	23.4	24.4	15.2	16.5	18.0	21.5	23.6	26.0
113.5	16.2	16.8	17.1	18.1	18.7	19.8	21.1	21.8	23.1	23.6	24.6	15.3	16.6	18.1	21.7	23.9	26.3
114.0	16.3	17.0	17.3	18.2	18.8	20.0	21.3	22.0	23.3	23.8	24.9	15.4	16.8	18.3	21.9	24.1	26.6
114.5	16.5	17.1	17.5	18.4	19.0	20.2	21.5	22.2	23.5	24.1	25.2	15.6	16.9	18.5	22.1	24.4	26.9
115.0	16.6	17.3	17.6	18.6	19.2	20.4	21.7	22.4	23.8	24.3	25.4	15.7	17.1	18.6	22.4	24.6	27.2
115.5	16.8	17.4	17.8	18.7	19.4	20.6	21.9	22.7	24.0	24.6	25.7	15.8	17.2	18.8	22.6	24.9	27.5
116.0	16.9	17.6	17.9	18.9	19.5	20.8	22.1	22.9	24.3	24.8	25.9	16.0	17.4	19.0	22.8	25.1	27.8
116.5	17.1	17.7	18.1	19.1	19.7	21.0	22.3	23.1	24.5	25.1	26.2	16.1	17.5	19.2	23.0	25.4	28.0
117.0	17.2	17.9	18.3	19.3	19.9	21.2	22.5	23.3	24.7	25.3	26.5	16.2	17.7	19.3	23.3	25.6	28.3
117.5	17.4	18.0	18.4	19.4	20.1	21.4	22.8	23.6	25.0	25.6	26.7	16.4	17.9	19.5	23.5	25.9	28.6
118.0	17.5	18.2	18.6	19.6	20.3	21.6	23.0	23.8	25.2	25.8	27.0	16.5	18.0	19.7	23.7	26.1	28.9
118.5	17.7	18.4	18.7	19.8	20.4	21.8	23.2	24.0	25.5	26.1	27.3	16.7	18.2	19.9	23.9	26.4	29.2
119.0	17.8	18.5	18.9	20.0	20.6	22.0	23.4	24.2	25.7	26.3	27.5	16.8	18.3	20.0	24.1	26.6	29.5
119.5	17.9	18.7	19.1	20.1	20.8	22.2	23.6	24.5	26.0	26.6	27.8	16.9	18.5	20.2	24.4	26.9	29.8
120.0	18.1	18.8	19.2	20.3	21.0	22.4	23.8	24.7	26.2	26.8	28.1	17.1	18.6	20.4	24.6	27.2	30.1

Table 8 Weight (kg) for Height (cm) for Girls 2–5 Years (WHO Reference Data) Percentiles and Z (SD)-scores

Height (cm)	*Percentiles*											*Standard deviation (SD) Z-score*					
	1st	*3rd*	*5th*	*15th*	*25th*	*50th*	*75th*	*85th*	*95th*	*97th*	*99th*	*−3SD*	*−2SD*	*−1SD*	*+1SD*	*+2SD*	*+3SD*
65.0	5.9	6.1	6.3	6.6	6.8	7.2	7.7	8.0	8.4	8.6	9.0	5.6	6.1	6.6	7.9	8.7	9.7
65.5	6.0	6.2	6.4	6.7	6.9	7.4	7.8	8.1	8.6	8.8	9.2	5.7	6.2	6.7	8.1	8.9	9.8
66.0	6.1	6.3	6.5	6.8	7.0	7.5	7.9	8.2	8.7	8.9	9.3	5.8	6.3	6.8	8.2	9.0	10.0
66.5	6.2	6.4	6.5	6.9	7.1	7.6	8.1	8.3	8.8	9.0	9.4	5.8	6.4	6.9	8.3	9.1	10.1
67.0	6.3	6.5	6.6	7.0	7.2	7.7	8.2	8.5	9.0	9.2	9.6	5.9	6.4	7.0	8.4	9.3	10.2
67.5	6.4	6.6	6.7	7.1	7.3	7.8	8.3	8.6	9.1	9.3	9.7	6.0	6.5	7.1	8.5	9.4	10.4
68.0	6.4	6.7	6.8	7.2	7.4	7.9	8.4	8.7	9.2	9.4	9.8	6.1	6.6	7.2	8.7	9.5	10.5
68.5	6.5	6.8	6.9	7.3	7.5	8.0	8.5	8.8	9.3	9.5	10.0	6.2	6.7	7.3	8.8	9.7	10.7
69.0	6.6	6.9	7.0	7.4	7.6	8.1	8.6	8.9	9.4	9.7	10.1	6.3	6.8	7.4	8.9	9.8	10.8
69.5	6.7	7.0	7.1	7.5	7.7	8.2	8.7	9.0	9.6	9.8	10.2	6.3	6.9	7.5	9.0	9.9	10.9
70.0	6.8	7.0	7.2	7.6	7.8	8.3	8.8	9.1	9.7	9.9	10.3	6.4	7.0	7.6	9.1	10.0	11.1
70.5	6.9	7.1	7.3	7.7	7.9	8.4	8.9	9.3	9.8	10.0	10.5	6.5	7.1	7.7	9.2	10.1	11.2
71.0	6.9	7.2	7.4	7.8	8.0	8.5	9.0	9.4	9.9	10.1	10.6	6.6	7.1	7.8	9.3	10.3	11.3
71.5	7.0	7.3	7.4	7.9	8.1	8.6	9.2	9.5	10.0	10.3	10.7	6.7	7.2	7.9	9.4	10.4	11.5
72.0	7.1	7.4	7.5	7.9	8.2	8.7	9.3	9.6	10.1	10.4	10.8	6.7	7.3	8.0	9.5	10.5	11.6
72.5	7.2	7.5	7.6	8.0	8.3	8.8	9.4	9.7	10.3	10.5	11.0	6.8	7.4	8.1	9.7	10.6	11.7
73.0	7.3	7.6	7.7	8.1	8.4	8.9	9.5	9.8	10.4	10.6	11.1	6.9	7.5	8.1	9.8	10.7	11.8
73.5	7.4	7.6	7.8	8.2	8.5	9.0	9.6	9.9	10.5	10.7	11.2	7.0	7.6	8.2	9.9	10.8	12.0
74.0	7.4	7.7	7.9	8.3	8.6	9.1	9.7	10.0	10.6	10.8	11.3	7.0	7.6	8.3	10.0	11.0	12.1
74.5	7.5	7.8	8.0	8.4	8.7	9.2	9.8	10.1	10.7	10.9	11.4	7.1	7.7	8.4	10.1	11.1	12.2
75.0	7.6	7.9	8.0	8.5	8.7	9.3	9.9	10.2	10.8	11.1	11.5	7.2	7.8	8.5	10.2	11.2	12.3
75.5	7.7	8.0	8.1	8.6	8.8	9.4	10.0	10.3	10.9	11.2	11.7	7.2	7.9	8.6	10.3	11.3	12.5
76.0	7.7	8.0	8.2	8.6	8.9	9.5	10.1	10.4	11.0	11.3	11.8	7.3	8.0	8.7	10.4	11.4	12.6
76.5	7.8	8.1	8.3	8.7	9.0	9.6	10.2	10.5	11.1	11.4	11.9	7.4	8.0	8.7	10.5	11.5	12.7
77.0	7.9	8.2	8.4	8.8	9.1	9.6	10.3	10.6	11.2	11.5	12.0	7.5	8.1	8.8	10.6	11.6	12.8
77.5	8.0	8.3	8.4	8.9	9.2	9.7	10.4	10.7	11.3	11.6	12.1	7.5	8.2	8.9	10.7	11.7	12.9
78.0	8.0	8.4	8.5	9.0	9.3	9.8	10.5	10.8	11.4	11.7	12.2	7.6	8.3	9.0	10.8	11.8	13.1
78.5	8.1	8.4	8.6	9.1	9.4	9.9	10.6	10.9	11.6	11.8	12.3	7.7	8.4	9.1	10.9	12.0	13.2
79.0	8.2	8.5	8.7	9.2	9.4	10.0	10.7	11.0	11.7	11.9	12.5	7.8	8.4	9.2	11.0	12.1	13.3
79.5	8.3	8.6	8.8	9.2	9.5	10.1	10.8	11.1	11.8	12.1	12.6	7.8	8.5	9.3	11.1	12.2	13.4
80.0	8.4	8.7	8.9	9.3	9.6	10.2	10.9	11.2	11.9	12.2	12.7	7.9	8.6	9.4	11.2	12.3	13.6
80.5	8.5	8.8	9.0	9.4	9.7	10.3	11.0	11.4	12.0	12.3	12.8	8.0	8.7	9.5	11.3	12.4	13.7
81.0	8.6	8.9	9.1	9.5	9.8	10.4	11.1	11.5	12.2	12.4	13.0	8.1	8.8	9.6	11.4	12.6	13.9
81.5	8.6	9.0	9.2	9.6	9.9	10.6	11.2	11.6	12.3	12.6	13.1	8.2	8.9	9.7	11.6	12.7	14.0
82.0	8.7	9.1	9.3	9.7	10.1	10.7	11.3	11.7	12.4	12.7	13.2	8.3	9.0	9.8	11.7	12.8	14.1
82.5	8.8	9.2	9.4	9.9	10.2	10.8	11.5	11.9	12.5	12.8	13.4	8.4	9.1	9.9	11.8	13.0	14.3
83.0	8.9	9.3	9.5	10.0	10.3	10.9	11.6	12.0	12.7	13.0	13.5	8.5	9.2	10.0	11.9	13.1	14.5
83.5	9.0	9.4	9.6	10.1	10.4	11.0	11.7	12.1	12.8	13.1	13.7	8.5	9.3	10.1	12.1	13.3	14.6
84.0	9.1	9.5	9.7	10.2	10.5	11.1	11.8	12.2	13.0	13.3	13.8	8.6	9.4	10.2	12.2	13.4	14.8
84.5	9.2	9.6	9.8	10.3	10.6	11.3	12.0	12.4	13.1	13.4	14.0	8.7	9.5	10.3	12.3	13.5	14.9
85.0	9.3	9.7	9.9	10.4	10.7	11.4	12.1	12.5	13.2	13.5	14.1	8.8	9.6	10.4	12.5	13.7	15.1
85.5	9.4	9.8	10.0	10.5	10.9	11.5	12.2	12.7	13.4	13.7	14.3	8.9	9.7	10.6	12.6	13.8	15.3
86.0	9.5	9.9	10.1	10.6	11.0	11.6	12.4	12.8	13.5	13.8	14.4	9.0	9.8	10.7	12.7	14.0	15.4
86.5	9.6	10.0	10.2	10.8	11.1	11.8	12.5	12.9	13.7	14.0	14.6	9.1	9.9	10.8	12.9	14.2	15.6
87.0	9.7	10.1	10.3	10.9	11.2	11.9	12.6	13.1	13.8	14.1	14.8	9.2	10.0	10.9	13.0	14.3	15.8
87.5	9.9	10.2	10.4	11.0	11.3	12.0	12.8	13.2	14.0	14.3	14.9	9.3	10.1	11.0	13.2	14.5	15.9
88.0	10.0	10.3	10.5	11.1	11.4	12.1	12.9	13.3	14.1	14.4	15.1	9.4	10.2	11.1	13.3	14.6	16.1
88.5	10.1	10.4	10.6	11.2	11.6	12.3	13.0	13.5	14.3	14.6	15.2	9.5	10.3	11.2	13.4	14.8	16.3
89.0	10.2	10.5	10.8	11.3	11.7	12.4	13.2	13.6	14.4	14.7	15.4	9.6	10.4	11.4	13.6	14.9	16.4
89.5	10.3	10.6	10.9	11.4	11.8	12.5	13.3	13.8	14.6	14.9	15.5	9.7	10.5	11.5	13.7	15.1	16.6
90.0	10.4	10.8	11.0	11.5	11.9	12.6	13.4	13.9	14.7	15.0	15.7	9.8	10.6	11.6	13.8	15.2	16.8
90.5	10.5	10.9	11.1	11.7	12.0	12.8	13.6	14.0	14.9	15.2	15.9	9.9	10.7	11.7	14.0	15.4	16.9
91.0	10.6	11.0	11.2	11.8	12.1	12.9	13.7	14.2	15.0	15.3	16.0	10.0	10.9	11.8	14.1	15.5	17.1
91.5	10.7	11.1	11.3	11.9	12.3	13.0	13.8	14.3	15.1	15.5	16.2	10.1	11.0	11.9	14.3	15.7	17.3
92.0	10.8	11.2	11.4	12.0	12.4	13.1	14.0	14.4	15.3	15.6	16.3	10.2	11.1	12.0	14.4	15.8	17.4
92.5	10.9	11.3	11.5	12.1	12.5	13.3	14.1	14.6	15.4	15.8	16.5	10.3	11.2	12.1	14.5	16.0	17.6
93.0	11.0	11.4	11.6	12.2	12.6	13.4	14.2	14.7	15.6	15.9	16.6	10.4	11.3	12.3	14.7	16.1	17.8
93.5	11.1	11.5	11.7	12.3	12.7	13.5	14.4	14.9	15.7	16.1	16.8	10.5	11.4	12.4	14.8	16.3	17.9
94.0	11.2	11.6	11.8	12.4	12.8	13.6	14.5	15.0	15.9	16.2	16.9	10.6	11.5	12.5	14.9	16.4	18.1
94.5	11.3	11.7	11.9	12.6	13.0	13.8	14.6	15.1	16.0	16.4	17.1	10.7	11.6	12.6	15.1	16.6	18.3

Contd…

Contd…

Height (cm)	*Percentiles*											*Standard deviation (SD) Z-score*						
	1st	*3rd*	*5th*	*15th*	*25th*	*50th*	*75th*	*85th*	*95th*	*97th*	*99th*	*–3SD*	*–2SD*	*–1SD*	*+1SD*	*+2SD*	*+3SD*
95.0	11.4	11.8	12.0	12.7	13.1	13.9	14.8	15.3	16.2	16.5	17.3	10.8	11.7	12.7	15.2	16.7	18.5
95.5	11.5	11.9	12.1	12.8	13.2	14.0	14.9	15.4	16.3	16.7	17.4	10.8	11.8	12.8	15.4	16.9	18.6
96.0	11.6	12.0	12.3	12.9	13.3	14.1	15.0	15.6	16.5	16.9	17.6	10.9	11.9	12.9	15.5	17.0	18.8
96.5	11.7	12.1	12.4	13.0	13.4	14.3	15.2	15.7	16.6	17.0	17.8	11.0	12.0	13.1	15.6	17.2	19.0
97.0	11.8	12.2	12.5	13.1	13.6	14.4	15.3	15.8	16.8	17.2	17.9	11.1	12.1	13.2	15.8	17.4	19.2
97.5	11.9	12.3	12.6	13.3	13.7	14.5	15.5	16.0	16.9	17.3	18.1	11.2	12.2	13.3	15.9	17.5	19.3
98.0	12.0	12.4	12.7	13.4	13.8	14.7	15.6	16.1	17.1	17.5	18.3	11.3	12.3	13.4	16.1	17.7	19.5
98.5	12.1	12.6	12.8	13.5	13.9	14.8	15.7	16.3	17.3	17.7	18.4	11.4	12.4	13.5	16.2	17.9	19.7
99.0	12.2	12.7	12.9	13.6	14.1	14.9	15.9	16.4	17.4	17.8	18.6	11.5	12.5	13.7	16.4	18.0	19.9
99.5	12.3	12.8	13.0	13.8	14.2	15.1	16.0	16.6	17.6	18.0	18.8	11.6	12.7	13.8	16.5	18.2	20.1
100.0	12.4	12.9	13.2	13.9	14.3	15.2	16.2	16.8	17.8	18.2	19.0	11.7	12.8	13.9	16.7	18.4	20.3
100.5	12.5	13.0	13.3	14.0	14.5	15.4	16.4	16.9	17.9	18.3	19.2	11.9	12.9	14.1	16.9	18.6	20.5
101.0	12.7	13.1	13.4	14.1	14.6	15.5	16.5	17.1	18.1	18.5	19.4	12.0	13.0	14.2	17.0	18.7	20.7
101.5	12.8	13.3	13.5	14.3	14.7	15.7	16.7	17.2	18.3	18.7	19.5	12.1	13.1	14.3	17.2	18.9	20.9
102.0	12.9	13.4	13.7	14.4	14.9	15.8	16.8	17.4	18.5	18.9	19.7	12.2	13.3	14.5	17.4	19.1	21.1
102.5	13.0	13.5	13.8	14.5	15.0	16.0	17.0	17.6	18.7	19.1	19.9	12.3	13.4	14.6	17.5	19.3	21.4
103.0	13.1	13.6	13.9	14.7	15.2	16.1	17.2	17.8	18.8	19.3	20.2	12.4	13.5	14.7	17.7	19.5	21.6
103.5	13.3	13.8	14.1	14.8	15.3	16.3	17.3	17.9	19.0	19.5	20.4	12.5	13.6	14.9	17.9	19.7	21.8
104.0	13.4	13.9	14.2	15.0	15.5	16.4	17.5	18.1	19.2	19.7	20.6	12.6	13.8	15.0	18.1	19.9	22.0
104.5	13.5	14.0	14.3	15.1	15.6	16.6	17.7	18.3	19.4	19.9	20.8	12.8	13.9	15.2	18.2	20.1	22.3
105.0	13.6	14.2	14.5	15.3	15.8	16.8	17.9	18.5	19.6	20.1	21.0	12.9	14.0	15.3	18.4	20.3	22.5
105.5	13.8	14.3	14.6	15.4	15.9	16.9	18.1	18.7	19.8	20.3	21.2	13.0	14.2	15.5	18.6	20.5	22.7
106.0	13.9	14.5	14.8	15.6	16.1	17.1	18.2	18.9	20.0	20.5	21.4	13.1	14.3	15.6	18.8	20.8	23.0
106.5	14.1	14.6	14.9	15.7	16.3	17.3	18.4	19.1	20.2	20.7	21.7	13.3	14.5	15.8	19.0	21.0	23.2
107.0	14.2	14.7	15.1	15.9	16.4	17.5	18.6	19.3	20.5	21.0	21.9	13.4	14.6	15.9	19.2	21.2	23.5
107.5	14.3	14.9	15.2	16.1	16.6	17.7	18.8	19.5	20.7	21.2	22.1	13.5	14.7	16.1	19.4	21.4	23.7
108.0	14.5	15.0	15.4	16.2	16.8	17.8	19.0	19.7	20.9	21.4	22.4	13.7	14.9	16.3	19.6	21.7	24.0
108.5	14.6	15.2	15.5	16.4	16.9	18.0	19.2	19.9	21.1	21.6	22.6	13.8	15.0	16.4	19.8	21.9	24.3
109.0	14.8	15.4	15.7	16.6	17.1	18.2	19.4	20.1	21.4	21.9	22.9	13.9	15.2	16.6	20.0	22.1	24.5
109.5	14.9	15.5	15.8	16.7	17.3	18.4	19.6	20.3	21.6	22.1	23.1	14.1	15.4	16.8	20.3	22.4	24.8
110.0	15.1	15.7	16.0	16.9	17.5	18.6	19.8	20.6	21.8	22.4	23.4	14.2	15.5	17.0	20.5	22.6	25.1
110.5	15.2	15.8	16.2	17.1	17.7	18.8	20.1	20.8	22.1	22.6	23.7	14.4	15.7	17.1	20.7	22.9	25.4
111.0	15.4	16.0	16.3	17.3	17.8	19.0	20.3	21.0	22.3	22.8	23.9	14.5	15.8	17.3	20.9	23.1	25.7
111.5	15.5	16.2	16.5	17.4	18.0	19.2	20.5	21.2	22.6	23.1	24.2	14.7	16.0	17.5	21.2	23.4	26.0
112.0	15.7	16.3	16.7	17.6	18.2	19.4	20.7	21.5	22.8	23.4	24.5	14.8	16.2	17.7	21.4	23.6	26.2
112.5	15.9	16.5	16.8	17.8	18.4	19.6	20.9	21.7	23.1	23.6	24.7	15.0	16.3	17.9	21.6	23.9	26.5
113.0	16.0	16.7	17.0	18.0	18.6	19.8	21.2	21.9	23.3	23.9	25.0	15.1	16.5	18.0	21.8	24.2	26.8
113.5	16.2	16.8	17.2	18.2	18.8	20.0	21.4	22.2	23.6	24.1	25.3	15.3	16.7	18.2	22.1	24.4	27.1
114.0	16.3	17.0	17.4	18.4	19.0	20.2	21.6	22.4	23.8	24.4	25.6	15.4	16.8	18.4	22.3	24.7	27.4
114.5	16.5	17.2	17.5	18.5	19.2	20.5	21.8	22.6	24.1	24.7	25.8	15.6	17.0	18.6	22.6	25.0	27.8
115.0	16.7	17.3	17.7	18.7	19.4	20.7	22.1	22.9	24.3	24.9	26.1	15.7	17.2	18.8	22.8	25.2	28.1
115.5	16.8	17.5	17.9	18.9	19.6	20.9	22.3	23.1	24.6	25.2	26.4	15.9	17.3	19.0	23.0	25.5	28.4
116.0	17.0	17.7	18.1	19.1	19.8	21.1	22.5	23.4	24.9	25.5	26.7	16.0	17.5	19.2	23.3	25.8	28.7
116.5	17.2	17.9	18.3	19.3	20.0	21.3	22.8	23.6	25.1	25.7	27.0	16.2	17.7	19.4	23.5	26.1	29.0
117.0	17.3	18.0	18.4	19.5	20.2	21.5	23.0	23.8	25.4	26.0	27.3	16.3	17.8	19.6	23.8	26.3	29.3
117.5	17.5	18.2	18.6	19.7	20.4	21.7	23.2	24.1	25.6	26.3	27.5	16.5	18.0	19.8	24.0	26.6	29.6
118.0	17.7	18.4	18.8	19.9	20.6	22.0	23.5	24.3	25.9	26.5	27.8	16.6	18.2	19.9	24.2	26.9	29.9
118.5	17.8	18.6	19.0	20.1	20.8	22.2	23.7	24.6	26.2	26.8	28.1	16.8	18.4	20.1	24.5	27.2	30.3
119.0	18.0	18.7	19.1	20.3	21.0	22.4	23.9	24.8	26.4	27.1	28.4	16.9	18.5	20.3	24.7	27.4	30.6
119.5	18.2	18.9	19.3	20.5	21.2	22.6	24.2	25.1	26.7	27.4	28.7	17.1	18.7	20.5	25.0	27.7	30.9
120.0	18.3	19.1	19.5	20.6	21.4	22.8	24.4	25.3	27.0	27.6	29.0	17.3	18.9	20.7	25.2	28.0	31.2

Table 9	Head Circumference (cm) by Age *Z* (SD)-scores in Boys and Girls Aged 0–5 Years														
Age		*Boys*							*Girls*						
Years	*Months*	*−3SD*	*−2SD*	*−1SD*	*Median*	*+1SD*	*+2SD*	*+3SD*	*−3SD*	*−2SD*	*−1SD*	*Median*	*+1SD*	*+2SD*	*+3SD*
	0	30.7	31.9	33.2	34.5	35.7	37.0	38.3	30.3	31.5	32.7	33.9	35.1	36.2	37.4
	1	33.8	34.9	36.1	37.3	38.4	39.6	40.8	33.0	34.2	35.4	36.5	37.7	38.9	40.1
	2	35.6	36.8	38.0	39.1	40.3	41.5	42.6	34.6	35.8	37.0	38.3	39.5	40.7	41.9
	3	37.0	38.1	39.3	40.5	41.7	42.9	44.1	35.8	37.1	38.3	39.5	40.8	42.0	43.3
	4	38.0	39.2	40.4	41.6	42.8	44.0	45.2	36.8	38.1	39.3	40.6	41.8	43.1	44.4
	5	38.9	40.1	41.4	42.6	43.8	45.0	46.2	37.6	38.9	40.2	41.5	42.7	44.0	45.3
	6	39.7	40.9	42.1	43.3	44.6	45.8	47.0	38.3	39.6	40.9	42.2	43.5	44.8	46.1
	7	40.3	41.5	42.7	44.0	45.2	46.4	47.7	38.9	40.2	41.5	42.8	44.1	45.5	46.8
	8	40.8	42.0	43.3	44.5	45.8	47.0	48.3	39.4	40.7	42.0	43.4	44.7	46.0	47.4
	9	41.2	42.5	43.7	45.0	46.3	47.5	48.8	39.8	41.2	42.5	43.8	45.2	46.5	47.8
	10	41.6	42.9	44.1	45.4	46.7	47.9	49.2	40.2	41.5	42.9	44.2	45.6	46.9	48.3
	11	41.9	43.2	44.5	45.8	47.0	48.3	49.6	40.5	41.9	43.2	44.6	45.9	47.3	48.6
1	0	42.2	43.5	44.8	46.1	47.4	48.6	49.9	40.8	42.2	43.5	44.9	46.3	47.6	49.0
	1	42.5	43.8	45.0	46.3	47.6	48.9	50.2	41.1	42.4	43.8	45.2	46.5	47.9	49.3
	2	42.7	44.0	45.3	46.6	47.9	49.2	50.5	41.3	42.7	44.1	45.4	46.8	48.2	49.5
	3	42.9	44.2	45.5	46.8	48.1	49.4	50.7	41.5	42.9	44.3	45.7	47.0	48.4	49.8
	4	43.1	44.4	45.7	47.0	48.3	49.6	51.0	41.7	43.1	44.5	45.9	47.2	48.6	50.0
	5	43.2	44.6	45.9	47.2	48.5	49.8	51.2	41.9	43.3	44.7	46.1	47.4	48.8	50.2
	6	43.4	44.7	46.0	47.4	48.7	50.0	51.4	42.1	43.5	44.9	46.2	47.6	49.0	50.4
	7	43.5	44.9	46.2	47.5	48.9	50.2	51.5	42.3	43.6	45.0	46.4	47.8	49.2	50.6
	8	43.7	45.0	46.4	47.7	49.0	50.4	51.7	42.4	43.8	45.2	46.6	48.0	49.4	50.7
	9	43.8	45.2	46.5	47.8	49.2	50.5	51.9	42.6	44.0	45.3	46.7	48.1	49.5	50.9
	10	43.9	45.3	46.6	48.0	49.3	50.7	52.0	42.7	44.1	45.5	46.9	48.3	49.7	51.1
	11	44.1	45.4	46.8	48.1	49.5	50.8	52.2	42.9	44.3	45.6	47.0	48.4	49.8	51.2
2	0	44.2	45.5	46.9	48.3	49.6	51.0	52.3	43.0	44.4	45.8	47.2	48.6	50.0	51.4
	1	44.3	45.6	47.0	48.4	49.7	51.1	52.5	43.1	44.5	45.9	47.3	48.7	50.1	51.5
	2	44.4	45.8	47.1	48.5	49.9	51.2	52.6	43.3	44.7	46.1	47.5	48.9	50.3	51.7
	3	44.5	45.9	47.2	48.6	50.0	51.4	52.7	43.4	44.8	46.2	47.6	49.0	50.4	51.8
	4	44.6	46.0	47.3	48.7	50.1	51.5	52.9	43.5	44.9	46.3	47.7	49.1	50.5	51.9
	5	44.7	46.1	47.4	48.8	50.2	51.6	53.0	43.6	45.0	46.4	47.8	49.2	50.6	52.0
	6	44.8	46.1	47.5	48.9	50.3	51.7	53.1	43.7	45.1	46.5	47.9	49.3	50.7	52.2
	7	44.8	46.2	47.6	49.0	50.4	51.8	53.2	43.8	45.2	46.6	48.0	49.4	50.9	52.3
	8	44.9	46.3	47.7	49.1	50.5	51.9	53.3	43.9	45.3	46.7	48.1	49.6	51.0	52.4
	9	45.0	46.4	47.8	49.2	50.6	52.0	53.4	44.0	45.4	46.8	48.2	49.7	51.1	52.5
	10	45.1	46.5	47.9	49.3	50.7	52.1	53.5	44.1	45.5	46.9	48.3	49.7	51.2	52.6
	11	45.1	46.6	48.0	49.4	50.8	52.2	53.6	44.2	45.6	47.0	48.4	49.8	51.2	52.7
3	0	45.2	46.6	48.0	49.5	50.9	52.3	53.7	44.3	45.7	47.1	48.5	49.9	51.3	52.7
	1	45.3	46.7	48.1	49.5	51.0	52.4	53.8	44.4	45.8	47.2	48.6	50.0	51.4	52.8
	2	45.3	46.8	48.2	49.6	51.0	52.5	53.9	44.4	45.8	47.3	48.7	50.1	51.5	52.9
	3	45.4	46.8	48.2	49.7	51.1	52.5	54.0	44.5	45.9	47.3	48.7	50.2	51.6	53.0
	4	45.4	46.9	48.3	49.7	51.2	52.6	54.1	44.6	46.0	47.4	48.8	50.2	51.7	53.1
	5	45.5	46.9	48.4	49.8	51.3	52.7	54.1	44.6	46.1	47.5	48.9	50.3	51.7	53.1
	6	45.5	47.0	48.4	49.9	51.3	52.8	54.2	44.7	46.1	47.5	49.0	50.4	51.8	53.2
	7	45.6	47.0	48.5	49.9	51.4	52.8	54.3	44.8	46.2	47.6	49.0	50.4	51.9	53.3
	8	45.6	47.1	48.5	50.0	51.4	52.9	54.3	44.8	46.3	47.7	49.1	50.5	51.9	53.3
	9	45.7	47.1	48.6	50.1	51.5	53.0	54.4	44.9	46.3	47.7	49.2	50.6	52.0	53.4
	10	45.7	47.2	48.7	50.1	51.6	53.0	54.5	45.0	46.4	47.8	49.2	50.6	52.1	53.5
	11	45.8	47.2	48.7	50.2	51.6	53.1	54.5	45.0	46.4	47.9	49.3	50.7	52.1	53.5
4	0	45.8	47.3	48.7	50.2	51.7	53.1	54.6	45.1	46.5	47.9	49.3	50.8	52.2	53.6
	1	45.9	47.3	48.8	50.3	51.7	53.2	54.7	45.1	46.5	48.0	49.4	50.8	52.2	53.6
	2	45.9	47.4	48.8	50.3	51.8	53.2	54.7	45.2	46.6	48.0	49.4	50.9	52.3	53.7
	3	45.9	47.4	48.9	50.4	51.8	53.3	54.8	45.2	46.7	48.1	49.5	50.9	52.3	53.8
	4	46.0	47.5	48.9	50.4	51.9	53.4	54.8	45.3	46.7	48.1	49.5	51.0	52.4	53.8
	5	46.0	47.5	49.0	50.4	51.9	53.4	54.9	45.3	46.8	48.2	49.6	51.0	52.4	53.9
	6	46.1	47.5	49.0	50.5	52.0	53.5	54.9	45.4	46.8	48.2	49.6	51.1	52.5	53.9
	7	46.1	47.6	49.1	50.5	52.0	53.5	55.0	45.4	46.9	48.3	49.7	51.1	52.5	54.0
	8	46.1	47.6	49.1	50.6	52.1	53.5	55.0	45.5	46.9	48.3	49.7	51.2	52.6	54.0
	9	46.2	47.6	49.1	50.6	52.1	53.6	55.1	45.5	46.9	48.4	49.8	51.2	52.6	54.1
	10	46.2	47.7	49.2	50.7	52.1	53.6	55.1	45.6	47.0	48.4	49.8	51.3	52.7	54.1
	11	46.2	47.7	49.2	50.7	52.2	53.7	55.2	45.6	47.0	48.5	49.9	51.3	52.7	54.1
5	0	46.3	47.7	49.2	50.7	52.2	53.7	55.2	45.7	47.1	48.5	49.9	51.3	52.8	54.2

Table 10 Body Mass Index (kg/m²) for Boys 0–5 Years (WHO Standards)

Boys		*Percentiles*									*Z (SD)-score*					
	Months	*3rd*	*5th*	*15th*	*25th*	*50th*	*75th*	*85th*	*95th*	*97th*	*–3SD*	*–2SD*	*–1SD*	*+1SD*	*+2SD*	*+3SD*
	0.0	11.3	11.5	12.2	12.6	13.4	14.3	14.8	15.8	16.1	10.2	11.1	12.2	14.8	16.3	18.1
	1.0	12.6	12.8	13.6	14.1	14.9	15.9	16.4	17.3	17.6	11.3	12.4	13.6	16.3	17.8	19.4
	2.0	13.8	14.1	14.9	15.4	16.3	17.3	17.8	18.8	19.2	12.5	13.7	15.0	17.8	19.4	21.1
	3.0	14.4	14.7	15.5	16.0	16.9	17.9	18.5	19.4	19.8	13.1	14.3	15.5	18.4	20.0	21.8
	4.0	14.7	15.0	15.7	16.2	17.2	18.2	18.7	19.7	20.1	13.4	14.5	15.8	18.7	20.3	22.1
	5.0	14.8	15.1	15.9	16.4	17.3	18.3	18.9	19.8	20.2	13.5	14.7	15.9	18.8	20.5	22.3
	6.0	14.9	15.2	15.9	16.4	17.3	18.3	18.9	19.9	20.3	13.6	14.7	16.0	18.8	20.5	22.3
	7.0	14.9	15.2	15.9	16.4	17.3	18.3	18.9	19.9	20.3	13.7	14.8	16.0	18.8	20.5	22.3
	8.0	14.9	15.1	15.9	16.3	17.3	18.2	18.8	19.8	20.2	13.6	14.7	15.9	18.7	20.4	22.2
	9.0	14.8	15.1	15.8	16.3	17.2	18.1	18.7	19.7	20.1	13.6	14.7	15.8	18.6	20.3	22.1
	10.0	14.7	15.0	15.7	16.2	17.0	18.0	18.6	19.5	19.9	13.5	14.6	15.7	18.5	20.1	22.0
	11.0	14.6	14.9	15.6	16.0	16.9	17.9	18.4	19.4	19.8	13.4	14.5	15.6	18.4	20.0	21.8
	12.0	14.5	14.8	15.5	15.9	16.8	17.7	18.3	19.2	19.6	13.4	14.4	15.5	18.2	19.8	21.6
	13.0	14.4	14.7	15.4	15.8	16.7	17.6	18.1	19.1	19.5	13.3	14.3	15.4	18.1	19.7	21.5
	14.0	14.3	14.6	15.3	15.7	16.6	17.5	18.0	18.9	19.3	13.2	14.2	15.3	18.0	19.5	21.3
	15.0	14.2	14.5	15.2	15.6	16.4	17.4	17.9	18.8	19.2	13.1	14.1	15.2	17.8	19.4	21.2
	16.0	14.2	14.4	15.1	15.5	16.3	17.2	17.8	18.7	19.1	13.1	14.0	15.1	17.7	19.3	21.0
	17.0	14.1	14.3	15.0	15.4	16.2	17.1	17.6	18.6	18.9	13.0	13.9	15.0	17.6	19.1	20.9
	18.0	14.0	14.2	14.9	15.3	16.1	17.0	17.5	18.5	18.8	12.9	13.9	14.9	17.5	19.0	20.8
	19.0	13.9	14.2	14.8	15.2	16.1	16.9	17.4	18.4	18.7	12.9	13.8	14.9	17.4	18.9	20.7
	20.0	13.9	14.1	14.8	15.2	16.0	16.9	17.4	18.3	18.6	12.8	13.7	14.8	17.3	18.8	20.6
	21.0	13.8	14.1	14.7	15.1	15.9	16.8	17.3	18.2	18.6	12.8	13.7	14.7	17.2	18.7	20.5
	22.0	13.8	14.0	14.6	15.0	15.8	16.7	17.2	18.1	18.5	12.7	13.6	14.7	17.2	18.7	20.4
	23.0	13.7	14.0	14.6	15.0	15.8	16.7	17.1	18.0	18.4	12.7	13.6	14.6	17.1	18.6	20.3
	24.0	13.7	13.9	14.5	14.9	15.7	16.6	17.1	18.0	18.3	12.7	13.6	14.6	17.0	18.5	20.3
Years	*Months*	*BMI by Height*														
2	0	13.9	14.2	14.8	15.2	16.0	16.9	17.4	18.3	18.7	12.9	13.8	14.8	17.3	18.9	20.6
2	1	13.9	14.1	14.8	15.2	16.0	16.9	17.4	18.3	18.6	12.8	13.8	14.8	17.3	18.8	20.5
2	2	13.8	14.1	14.7	15.1	15.9	16.8	17.3	18.2	18.6	12.8	13.7	14.8	17.3	18.8	20.5
2	3	13.8	14.0	14.7	15.1	15.9	16.8	17.3	18.2	18.5	12.7	13.7	14.7	17.2	18.7	20.4
2	4	13.8	14.0	14.7	15.1	15.9	16.7	17.2	18.1	18.5	12.7	13.6	14.7	17.2	18.7	20.4
2	5	13.7	14.0	14.6	15.0	15.8	16.7	17.2	18.1	18.4	12.7	13.6	14.7	17.1	18.6	20.3
2	6	13.7	13.9	14.6	15.0	15.8	16.7	17.2	18.0	18.4	12.6	13.6	14.6	17.1	18.6	20.2
2	7	13.7	13.9	14.5	15.0	15.8	16.6	17.1	18.0	18.4	12.6	13.5	14.6	17.1	18.5	20.2
2	8	13.6	13.9	14.5	14.9	15.7	16.6	17.1	18.0	18.3	12.5	13.5	14.6	17.0	18.5	20.1
2	9	13.6	13.8	14.5	14.9	15.7	16.6	17.0	17.9	18.3	12.5	13.5	14.5	17.0	18.5	20.1
2	10	13.5	13.8	14.4	14.9	15.7	16.5	17.0	17.9	18.2	12.5	13.4	14.5	17.0	18.4	20.0
2	11	13.5	13.8	14.4	14.8	15.6	16.5	17.0	17.9	18.2	12.4	13.4	14.5	16.9	18.4	20.0
3	0	13.5	13.7	14.4	14.8	15.6	16.5	17.0	17.8	18.2	12.4	13.4	14.4	16.9	18.4	20.0
3	1	13.5	13.7	14.4	14.8	15.6	16.4	16.9	17.8	18.1	12.4	13.3	14.4	16.9	18.3	19.9
3	2	13.4	13.7	14.3	14.7	15.5	16.4	16.9	17.8	18.1	12.3	13.3	14.4	16.8	18.3	19.9
3	3	13.4	13.6	14.3	14.7	15.5	16.4	16.9	17.7	18.1	12.3	13.3	14.3	16.8	18.3	19.9
3	4	13.4	13.6	14.3	14.7	15.5	16.4	16.8	17.7	18.1	12.3	13.2	14.3	16.8	18.2	19.9
3	5	13.3	13.6	14.2	14.7	15.5	16.3	16.8	17.7	18.0	12.2	13.2	14.3	16.8	18.2	19.9
3	6	13.3	13.6	14.2	14.6	15.4	16.3	16.8	17.7	18.0	12.2	13.2	14.3	16.8	18.2	19.8
3	7	13.3	13.5	14.2	14.6	15.4	16.3	16.8	17.7	18.0	12.2	13.2	14.2	16.7	18.2	19.8
3	8	13.3	13.5	14.2	14.6	15.4	16.3	16.8	17.7	18.0	12.2	13.1	14.2	16.7	18.2	19.8
3	9	13.2	13.5	14.2	14.6	15.4	16.3	16.8	17.6	18.0	12.2	13.1	14.2	16.7	18.2	19.8
3	10	13.2	13.5	14.1	14.5	15.4	16.2	16.7	17.6	18.0	12.1	13.1	14.2	16.7	18.2	19.8
3	11	13.2	13.5	14.1	14.5	15.3	16.2	16.7	17.6	18.0	12.1	13.1	14.2	16.7	18.2	19.9
4	0	13.2	13.4	14.1	14.5	15.3	16.2	16.7	17.6	18.0	12.1	13.1	14.1	16.7	18.2	19.9
4	1	13.2	13.4	14.1	14.5	15.3	16.2	16.7	17.6	18.0	12.1	13.0	14.1	16.7	18.2	19.9
4	2	13.2	13.4	14.1	14.5	15.3	16.2	16.7	17.6	18.0	12.1	13.0	14.1	16.7	18.2	19.9
4	3	13.1	13.4	14.0	14.5	15.3	16.2	16.7	17.6	18.0	12.1	13.0	14.1	16.6	18.2	19.9
4	4	13.1	13.4	14.0	14.4	15.3	16.2	16.7	17.6	18.0	12.0	13.0	14.1	16.6	18.2	19.9
4	5	13.1	13.3	14.0	14.4	15.3	16.2	16.7	17.6	18.0	12.0	13.0	14.1	16.6	18.2	20.0
4	6	13.1	13.3	14.0	14.4	15.3	16.2	16.7	17.6	18.0	12.0	13.0	14.0	16.6	18.2	20.0
4	7	13.1	13.3	14.0	14.4	15.2	16.2	16.7	17.6	18.0	12.0	13.0	14.0	16.6	18.2	20.0
4	8	13.1	13.3	14.0	14.4	15.2	16.1	16.7	17.6	18.0	12.0	12.9	14.0	16.6	18.2	20.1
4	9	13.0	13.3	14.0	14.4	15.2	16.1	16.7	17.6	18.0	12.0	12.9	14.0	16.6	18.2	20.1
4	10	13.0	13.3	13.9	14.4	15.2	16.1	16.7	17.6	18.0	12.0	12.9	14.0	16.6	18.3	20.2
4	11	13.0	13.3	13.9	14.4	15.2	16.1	16.7	17.7	18.1	12.0	12.9	14.0	16.6	18.3	20.2
5	0	13.0	13.3	13.9	14.3	15.2	16.1	16.7	17.7	18.1	12.0	12.9	14.0	16.6	18.3	20.3

Table 11	Body Mass Index (kg/m²) for Girls 0–5 Years (WHO Standards)															
Girls		Percentiles									Z (SD)-score					
	Months	3rd	5th	15th	25th	50th	75th	85th	95th	97th	−3SD	−2SD	−1SD	+1SD	+2SD	+3SD
	0	11.2	11.5	12.1	12.5	13.3	14.2	14.7	15.5	15.9	10.1	11.1	12.2	14.6	16.1	17.7
	1	12.1	12.4	13.2	13.6	14.6	15.5	16.1	17.0	17.3	10.8	12.0	13.2	16.0	17.5	19.1
	2	13.2	13.5	14.3	14.8	15.8	16.8	17.4	18.4	18.8	11.8	13.0	14.3	17.3	19.0	20.7
	3	13.7	14.0	14.9	15.4	16.4	17.4	18.0	19.0	19.4	12.4	13.6	14.9	17.9	19.7	21.5
	4	14.0	14.3	15.2	15.7	16.7	17.7	18.3	19.4	19.8	12.7	13.9	15.2	18.3	20.0	22.0
	5	14.2	14.5	15.3	15.8	16.8	17.9	18.5	19.6	20.0	12.9	14.1	15.4	18.4	20.2	22.2
	6	14.3	14.6	15.4	15.9	16.9	18.0	18.6	19.6	20.1	13.0	14.1	15.5	18.5	20.3	22.3
	7	14.3	14.6	15.4	15.9	16.9	18.0	18.6	19.6	20.1	13.0	14.2	15.5	18.5	20.3	22.3
	8	14.3	14.6	15.4	15.9	16.8	17.9	18.5	19.6	20.0	13.0	14.1	15.4	18.4	20.2	22.2
	9	14.2	14.5	15.3	15.8	16.7	17.8	18.4	19.4	19.9	12.9	14.1	15.3	18.3	20.1	22.1
	10	14.1	14.4	15.2	15.7	16.6	17.7	18.2	19.3	19.7	12.9	14.0	15.2	18.2	19.9	21.9
	11	14.0	14.3	15.1	15.5	16.5	17.5	18.1	19.1	19.6	12.8	13.9	15.1	18.0	19.8	21.8
	12	13.9	14.2	15.0	15.4	16.4	17.4	17.9	19.0	19.4	12.7	13.8	15.0	17.9	19.6	21.6
	13	13.8	14.1	14.8	15.3	16.2	17.2	17.8	18.8	19.2	12.6	13.7	14.9	17.7	19.5	21.4
	14	13.7	14.0	14.7	15.2	16.1	17.1	17.7	18.7	19.1	12.6	13.6	14.8	17.6	19.3	21.3
	15	13.7	13.9	14.6	15.1	16.0	17.0	17.5	18.6	19.0	12.5	13.5	14.7	17.5	19.2	21.1
	16	13.6	13.8	14.6	15.0	15.9	16.9	17.4	18.4	18.8	12.4	13.5	14.6	17.4	19.1	21.0
	17	13.5	13.8	14.5	14.9	15.8	16.8	17.3	18.3	18.7	12.4	13.4	14.5	17.3	18.9	20.9
	18	13.4	13.7	14.4	14.8	15.7	16.7	17.2	18.2	18.6	12.3	13.3	14.4	17.2	18.8	20.8
	19	13.4	13.6	14.3	14.8	15.7	16.6	17.2	18.1	18.5	12.3	13.3	14.4	17.1	18.8	20.7
	20	13.3	13.6	14.3	14.7	15.6	16.5	17.1	18.1	18.5	12.2	13.2	14.3	17.0	18.7	20.6
	21	13.3	13.6	14.2	14.7	15.5	16.5	17.0	18.0	18.4	12.2	13.2	14.3	17.0	18.6	20.5
	22	13.3	13.5	14.2	14.6	15.5	16.4	17.0	17.9	18.3	12.2	13.1	14.2	16.9	18.5	20.4
	23	13.2	13.5	14.2	14.6	15.4	16.4	16.9	17.9	18.3	12.2	13.1	14.2	16.9	18.5	20.4
	24	13.2	13.5	14.1	14.6	15.4	16.3	16.9	17.8	18.2	12.1	13.1	14.2	16.8	18.4	20.3
Years	Months	BMI by Height														
2	0	13.5	13.7	14.4	14.8	15.7	16.6	17.2	18.1	18.5	12.4	13.3	14.4	17.1	18.7	20.6
2	1	13.4	13.7	14.4	14.8	15.7	16.6	17.1	18.1	18.5	12.4	13.3	14.4	17.1	18.7	20.6
2	2	13.4	13.7	14.4	14.8	15.6	16.6	17.1	18.1	18.5	12.3	13.3	14.4	17.0	18.7	20.6
2	3	13.4	13.7	14.3	14.8	15.6	16.5	17.1	18.0	18.4	12.3	13.3	14.4	17.0	18.6	20.5
2	4	13.4	13.6	14.3	14.7	15.6	16.5	17.0	18.0	18.4	12.3	13.3	14.3	17.0	18.6	20.5
2	5	13.4	13.6	14.3	14.7	15.6	16.5	17.0	18.0	18.4	12.3	13.2	14.3	17.0	18.6	20.4
2	6	13.3	13.6	14.3	14.7	15.5	16.5	17.0	17.9	18.3	12.3	13.2	14.3	16.9	18.5	20.4
2	7	13.3	13.6	14.2	14.7	15.5	16.4	17.0	17.9	18.3	12.2	13.2	14.3	16.9	18.5	20.4
2	8	13.3	13.5	14.2	14.6	15.5	16.4	16.9	17.9	18.3	12.2	13.2	14.3	16.9	18.5	20.4
2	9	13.3	13.5	14.2	14.6	15.5	16.4	16.9	17.9	18.3	12.2	13.1	14.2	16.9	18.5	20.3
2	10	13.2	13.5	14.2	14.6	15.4	16.4	16.9	17.9	18.2	12.2	13.1	14.2	16.8	18.5	20.3
2	11	13.2	13.5	14.1	14.6	15.4	16.3	16.9	17.8	18.2	12.1	13.1	14.2	16.8	18.4	20.3
3	0	13.2	13.5	14.1	14.5	15.4	16.3	16.9	17.8	18.2	12.1	13.1	14.2	16.8	18.4	20.3
3	1	13.2	13.4	14.1	14.5	15.4	16.3	16.8	17.8	18.2	12.1	13.1	14.1	16.8	18.4	20.3
3	2	13.2	13.4	14.1	14.5	15.4	16.3	16.8	17.8	18.2	12.1	13.0	14.1	16.8	18.4	20.3
3	3	13.1	13.4	14.1	14.5	15.3	16.3	16.8	17.8	18.2	12.0	13.0	14.1	16.8	18.4	20.3
3	4	13.1	13.4	14.0	14.5	15.3	16.3	16.8	17.8	18.2	12.0	13.0	14.1	16.8	18.4	20.3
3	5	13.1	13.3	14.0	14.5	15.3	16.3	16.8	17.8	18.2	12.0	13.0	14.1	16.8	18.4	20.4
3	6	13.1	13.3	14.0	14.4	15.3	16.3	16.8	17.8	18.2	12.0	12.9	14.0	16.8	18.4	20.4
3	7	13.0	13.3	14.0	14.4	15.3	16.3	16.8	17.8	18.2	11.9	12.9	14.0	16.8	18.4	20.4
3	8	13.0	13.3	14.0	14.4	15.3	16.3	16.8	17.8	18.2	11.9	12.9	14.0	16.8	18.5	20.4
3	9	13.0	13.3	14.0	14.4	15.3	16.3	16.8	17.8	18.3	11.9	12.9	14.0	16.8	18.5	20.5
3	10	13.0	13.2	13.9	14.4	15.3	16.3	16.8	17.8	18.3	11.9	12.9	14.0	16.8	18.5	20.5
3	11	13.0	13.2	13.9	14.4	15.3	16.3	16.8	17.9	18.3	11.8	12.8	14.0	16.8	18.5	20.5
4	0	12.9	13.2	13.9	14.4	15.3	16.3	16.8	17.9	18.3	11.8	12.8	14.0	16.8	18.5	20.6
4	1	12.9	13.2	13.9	14.4	15.3	16.3	16.8	17.9	18.3	11.8	12.8	13.9	16.8	18.5	20.6
4	2	12.9	13.2	13.9	14.3	15.3	16.3	16.8	17.9	18.3	11.8	12.8	13.9	16.8	18.6	20.7
4	3	12.9	13.2	13.9	14.3	15.3	16.3	16.8	17.9	18.4	11.8	12.8	13.9	16.8	18.6	20.7
4	4	12.9	13.1	13.9	14.3	15.2	16.3	16.9	17.9	18.4	11.7	12.8	13.9	16.8	18.6	20.7
4	5	12.9	13.1	13.9	14.3	15.3	16.3	16.9	17.9	18.4	11.7	12.7	13.9	16.8	18.6	20.8
4	6	12.9	13.1	13.9	14.3	15.3	16.3	16.9	18.0	18.4	11.7	12.7	13.9	16.8	18.7	20.8
4	7	12.9	13.1	13.9	14.3	15.3	16.3	16.9	18.0	18.4	11.7	12.7	13.9	16.8	18.7	20.9
4	8	12.8	13.1	13.8	14.3	15.3	16.3	16.9	18.0	18.5	11.7	12.7	13.9	16.8	18.7	20.9
4	9	12.8	13.1	13.8	14.3	15.3	16.3	16.9	18.0	18.5	11.7	12.7	13.9	16.9	18.7	21.0
4	10	12.8	13.1	13.8	14.3	15.3	16.3	16.9	18.0	18.5	11.7	12.7	13.9	16.9	18.8	21.0
4	11	12.8	13.1	13.8	14.3	15.3	16.3	16.9	18.1	18.5	11.6	12.7	13.9	16.9	18.8	21.0
5	0	12.8	13.1	13.8	14.3	15.3	16.3	17.0	18.1	18.6	11.6	12.7	13.9	16.9	18.8	21.1

Table 12 Weight (kg) Centiles and Standard Deviation for Boys (5–18 Years): IAP Growth Charts 2015

Age	*3*	*10*	*25*	*50*	*75*	*90*	*97*	*SD*
5.0	13.2	14.3	15.6	17.1	19.0	21.3	24.2	3.2
5.5	13.8	15.0	16.5	18.2	20.3	22.9	26.1	2.9
6.0	14.5	15.8	17.4	19.3	21.7	24.6	28.3	3.6
6.5	15.3	16.8	18.6	20.7	23.3	26.6	30.8	3.8
7.0	16.0	17.6	19.6	21.9	24.9	28.6	33.4	4.2
7.5	16.7	18.5	20.7	23.3	26.6	30.8	36.2	4.9
8.0	17.5	19.5	21.9	24.8	28.5	33.2	39.4	5.7
8.5	18.3	20.5	23.2	26.4	30.5	35.7	42.6	6.5
9.0	19.1	21.5	24.3	27.9	32.3	38.0	45.5	6.3
9.5	19.9	22.4	25.6	29.4	34.3	40.5	48.6	7.0
10.0	20.7	23.5	26.9	31.1	36.3	43.0	51.8	7.9
10.5	21.6	24.6	28.3	32.8	38.5	45.8	55.2	8.3
11.0	22.6	25.9	29.8	34.7	40.9	48.7	58.7	8.9
11.5	23.8	27.3	31.6	36.9	43.5	51.8	62.5	9.3
12.0	24.9	28.7	33.3	39.0	46.0	54.8	66.1	10.0
12.5	26.1	30.2	35.1	41.2	48.6	57.8	69.5	10.6
13.0	27.5	31.8	37.0	43.3	51.1	60.7	72.6	11.3
13.5	29.0	33.6	39.1	45.7	53.8	63.6	75.6	11.4
14.0	30.7	35.5	41.3	48.2	56.4	66.3	78.3	12.1
14.5	32.6	37.7	43.7	50.8	59.1	69.1	80.9	11.6
15.0	34.5	39.8	45.9	53.1	61.6	71.5	83.1	12.1
15.5	36.1	41.6	47.9	55.2	63.6	73.4	84.7	11.2
16.0	37.5	43.1	49.5	56.8	65.2	74.8	85.8	12.2
16.5	38.7	44.4	50.9	58.2	66.6	76.1	86.8	12.6
17.0	39.8	45.6	52.1	59.5	67.8	77.1	87.5	12.3
17.5	40.8	46.7	53.2	60.6	68.7	77.8	88.0	12.3
18.0	41.8	47.7	54.3	61.6	69.7	78.6	88.4	11.3

Table 13 Weight (kg) Centiles and Standard Deviations for Girls (5–18 years): IAP Growth Charts 2015

Age	*3*	*10*	*25*	*50*	*75*	*90*	*97*	*SD*
5.0	12.3	13.4	14.8	16.4	18.5	21.3	25.0	2.5
5.5	13.0	14.3	15.7	17.6	19.9	22.9	27.0	3.5
6.0	13.7	15.1	16.7	18.7	21.3	24.6	29.1	3.4
6.5	14.4	15.9	17.7	19.9	22.7	26.3	31.2	4.1
7.0	15.1	16.8	18.7	21.2	24.2	28.2	33.4	4.4
7.5	15.9	17.7	19.9	22.5	25.9	30.1	35.7	4.8
8.0	16.7	18.7	21.1	24.0	27.6	32.2	38.1	5.2
8.5	17.5	19.7	22.3	25.5	29.5	34.4	40.7	6.4
9.0	18.5	20.9	23.7	27.2	31.5	36.7	43.4	6.4
9.5	19.5	22.1	25.3	29.0	33.6	39.3	46.3	6.9
10.0	20.7	23.5	26.9	31.0	36.0	42.0	49.4	7.7
10.5	22.0	25.1	28.8	33.2	38.4	44.8	52.6	8.3
11.0	23.3	26.7	30.7	35.4	41.0	47.7	55.9	8.5
11.5	24.8	28.4	32.6	37.6	43.6	50.6	59.1	9.1
12.0	26.2	30.0	34.5	39.8	46.0	53.4	62.1	9.0
12.5	27.6	31.6	36.3	41.8	48.2	55.8	64.8	9.7
13.0	28.9	33.1	37.9	43.6	50.2	57.9	67.1	9.4
13.5	30.2	34.4	39.4	45.1	51.8	59.7	69.0	9.8
14.0	31.3	35.6	40.6	46.4	53.2	61.1	70.4	9.6
14.5	32.3	36.6	41.7	47.5	54.3	62.2	71.4	9.4
15.0	33.1	37.5	42.5	48.4	55.1	62.9	72.1	9.6
15.5	34.0	38.3	43.3	49.1	55.8	63.5	72.5	8.7
16.0	34.7	39.1	44.0	49.7	56.3	64.0	72.8	8.7
16.5	35.5	39.8	44.7	50.3	56.9	64.4	73.1	9.2
17.0	36.2	40.5	45.3	50.9	57.3	64.7	73.3	8.8
17.5	36.9	41.1	46.0	51.5	57.8	65.0	73.4	9.5
18.0	37.6	41.8	46.6	52.0	58.2	65.3	73.5	10.2

Table 14 Height (cm) Centiles and Standard Deviation for Boys (5–18 Years): IAP Growth Charts 2015

Age	3	10	25	50	75	90	97	SD
5.0	99.0	102.3	105.6	108.9	112.4	115.9	119.4	5.7
5.5	101.6	105.0	108.4	111.9	115.4	119.0	122.7	5.3
6.0	104.2	107.7	111.2	114.8	118.5	122.2	126.0	5.6
6.5	106.8	110.4	114.0	117.8	121.6	125.4	129.3	5.5
7.0	109.3	113.0	116.8	120.7	124.6	128.6	132.6	5.9
7.5	111.8	115.7	119.6	123.5	127.6	131.7	135.9	5.7
8.0	114.3	118.2	122.3	126.4	130.5	134.8	139.1	6.3
8.5	116.7	120.8	124.9	129.1	133.4	137.8	142.2	6.1
9.0	119.0	123.2	127.5	131.8	136.3	140.7	145.3	6.4
9.5	121.3	125.6	130.0	134.5	139.1	143.7	148.3	6.4
10.0	123.6	128.1	132.6	137.2	141.9	146.6	151.4	6.8
10.5	125.9	130.5	135.2	139.9	144.7	149.5	154.4	6.5
11.0	128.2	133.0	137.8	142.7	147.6	152.5	157.5	7.6
11.5	130.7	135.6	140.6	145.5	150.5	155.6	160.6	7.3
12.0	133.2	138.3	143.3	148.4	153.5	158.6	163.7	8.1
12.5	135.7	141.0	146.2	151.4	156.5	161.7	166.8	7.9
13.0	138.3	143.7	149.0	154.3	159.5	164.7	169.9	9.0
13.5	140.9	146.4	151.8	157.2	162.4	167.6	172.7	8.4
14.0	143.4	149.0	154.5	159.9	165.1	170.3	175.4	9.0
14.5	145.8	151.5	157.0	162.3	167.6	172.7	177.7	7.8
15.0	148.0	153.7	159.2	164.5	169.7	174.8	179.7	7.9
15.5	150.0	155.7	161.2	166.5	171.6	176.5	181.4	6.6
16.0	151.8	157.4	162.9	168.1	173.1	178.0	182.7	7.2
16.5	153.4	159.1	164.5	169.6	174.5	179.3	183.8	6.7
17.0	155.0	160.6	165.9	171.0	175.8	180.4	184.8	6.9
17.5	156.6	162.1	167.3	172.3	177.0	181.5	185.8	6.1
18.0	158.1	163.6	168.7	173.6	178.2	182.5	186.7	6.9

Table 15 Height (cm) Centiles and Standard Deviations for Girls (5–18 Years): IAP Growth Charts 2015

Age	3	10	25	50	75	90	97	SD
5.0	97.2	100.5	103.9	107.5	111.3	115.2	119.3	5.4
5.5	99.8	103.2	106.8	110.5	114.4	118.3	122.5	5.7
6.0	102.3	106.0	109.7	113.5	117.4	121.5	125.6	5.8
6.5	104.9	108.7	112.5	116.5	120.5	124.6	128.7	5.5
7.0	107.4	111.4	115.4	119.4	123.5	127.7	131.9	6.1
7.5	110.0	114.1	118.2	122.4	126.6	130.8	135.0	6.0
8.0	112.6	116.8	121.1	125.4	129.6	133.9	138.1	6.2
8.5	115.2	119.6	124.0	128.4	132.7	137.0	141.3	6.8
9.0	117.8	122.4	126.9	131.4	135.8	140.2	144.5	6.9
9.5	120.5	125.2	129.9	134.4	138.9	143.3	147.6	6.6
10.0	123.3	128.1	132.8	137.4	142.0	146.4	150.8	7.8
10.5	126.1	130.9	135.7	140.4	145.0	149.5	153.9	7.3
11.0	128.8	133.7	138.6	143.3	147.9	152.4	156.8	7.9
11.5	131.5	136.4	141.2	145.9	150.6	155.1	159.6	7.1
12.0	134.0	138.9	143.7	148.4	153.0	157.5	162.0	7.0
12.5	136.3	141.1	145.8	150.5	155.1	159.6	164.1	6.7
13.0	138.2	142.9	147.6	152.2	156.8	161.3	165.9	6.9
13.5	139.9	144.5	149.1	153.6	158.2	162.7	167.2	6.0
14.0	141.3	145.8	150.2	154.7	159.2	163.7	168.2	6.6
14.5	142.4	146.8	151.1	155.5	160.0	164.5	169.0	5.9
15.0	143.3	147.5	151.8	156.1	160.5	165.0	169.5	6.6
15.5	144.1	148.1	152.3	156.6	160.9	165.3	169.8	5.9
16.0	144.7	148.6	152.7	156.9	161.2	165.6	170.1	6.1
16.5	145.2	149.1	153.1	157.2	161.4	165.7	170.2	6.4
17.0	145.7	149.5	153.4	157.4	161.6	165.9	170.4	6.5
17.5	146.2	149.8	153.6	157.6	161.7	166.0	170.5	6.7
18.0	146.6	150.2	153.9	157.8	161.9	166.1	170.6	6.6

Table 16	Body Mass Index Percentiles and Standard Deviations for Boys (5–18 Years): IAP Growth Charts 2015							
Age	*3*	*5*	*10*	*25*	*50*	*23 Eq (71)*	*27 Eq (90)*	*SD*
5.0	12.1	12.4	12.8	13.6	14.7	15.7	17.5	1.6
5.5	12.2	12.4	12.9	13.7	14.8	15.8	17.6	1.5
6.0	12.2	12.5	12.9	13.7	14.9	16.0	17.8	1.8
6.5	12.3	12.5	13.0	13.8	15.0	16.1	18.0	1.8
7.0	12.3	12.6	13.1	13.9	15.1	16.3	18.2	1.9
7.5	12.4	12.7	13.2	14.1	15.3	16.5	18.5	2.2
8.0	12.5	12.8	13.3	14.2	15.5	16.7	18.8	2.5
8.5	12.6	12.9	13.4	14.4	15.7	17.0	19.2	2.8
9.0	12.7	13.0	13.5	14.5	15.9	17.3	19.6	2.6
9.5	12.8	13.1	13.7	14.7	16.2	17.6	20.1	2.8
10.0	12.9	13.2	13.8	14.9	16.4	18.0	20.5	3.1
10.5	13.0	13.3	14.0	15.1	16.7	18.3	21.0	3.2
11.0	13.1	13.5	14.1	15.4	17.0	18.7	21.5	3.2
11.5	13.2	13.6	14.3	15.6	17.3	19.1	22.1	3.3
12.0	13.3	13.8	14.5	15.8	17.7	19.5	22.6	3.4
12.5	13.5	13.9	14.6	16.0	17.9	19.8	23.0	3.6
13.0	13.6	14.0	14.8	16.3	18.2	20.2	23.4	3.5
13.5	13.7	14.2	14.9	16.5	18.5	20.5	23.8	3.7
14.0	13.8	14.3	15.1	16.7	18.7	20.8	24.2	3.7
14.5	14.0	14.5	15.3	16.9	19.0	21.1	24.5	3.5
15.0	14.2	14.7	15.5	17.2	19.3	21.4	24.9	3.7
15.5	14.4	14.9	15.8	17.4	19.6	21.7	25.2	3.4
16.0	14.6	15.1	16.0	17.7	19.9	22.0	25.5	3.7
16.5	14.9	15.4	16.3	18.0	20.2	22.4	25.8	3.8
17.0	15.1	15.6	16.6	18.3	20.5	22.6	26.0	3.8
17.5	15.4	15.9	16.8	18.6	20.8	22.9	26.3	3.6
18.0	15.6	16.2	17.1	18.9	21.1	23.2	26.6	3.2

Table 17	Body Mass Index Percentiles and Standard Deviations for Girls (5–18 Years): IAP Growth Charts 2015							
Age	*3*	*5*	*10*	*25*	*50*	*23 Eq (75)*	*27 Eq (95)*	*SD*
5.0	11.9	12.1	12.5	13.3	14.3	15.5	18.0	1.4
5.5	11.9	12.2	12.6	13.4	14.4	15.7	18.3	1.7
6.0	12.0	12.2	12.7	13.5	14.5	15.9	18.6	1.7
6.5	12.1	12.3	12.8	13.6	14.7	16.1	18.9	2.0
7.0	12.1	12.4	12.8	13.7	14.9	16.4	19.3	2.1
7.5	12.2	12.5	12.9	13.9	15.1	16.6	19.7	2.2
8.0	12.3	12.6	13.1	14.0	15.3	16.9	20.1	2.3
8.5	12.3	12.7	13.2	14.2	15.6	17.2	20.5	2.7
9.0	12.4	12.8	13.3	14.4	15.8	17.6	21.0	2.7
9.5	12.5	12.9	13.5	14.6	16.1	18.0	21.4	2.8
10.0	12.7	13.1	13.7	14.9	16.5	18.4	21.9	2.9
10.5	12.8	13.2	13.9	15.2	16.8	18.8	22.5	3.1
11.0	13.0	13.4	14.1	15.5	17.2	19.3	23.0	3.1
11.5	13.2	13.7	14.4	15.8	17.6	19.8	23.6	3.3
12.0	13.4	13.9	14.7	16.1	18.0	20.2	24.1	3.2
12.5	13.7	14.2	15.0	16.5	18.4	20.7	24.7	3.3
13.0	13.9	14.4	15.2	16.8	18.8	21.1	25.2	3.2
13.5	14.1	14.6	15.5	17.1	19.1	21.5	25.6	3.5
14.0	14.3	14.9	15.7	17.3	19.4	21.8	25.9	3.4
14.5	14.5	15.1	16.0	17.6	19.7	22.0	26.2	3.3
15.0	14.7	15.2	16.1	17.8	19.9	22.3	26.3	3.4
15.5	14.9	15.4	16.3	18.0	20.1	22.4	26.4	3.1
16.0	15.0	15.6	16.5	18.2	20.3	22.6	26.5	3.1
16.5	15.2	15.8	16.7	18.4	20.4	22.8	26.6	3.2
17.0	15.4	16.0	16.9	18.6	20.6	22.9	26.7	3.0
17.5	15.5	16.1	17.1	18.7	20.8	23.1	26.7	3.1
18.0	15.7	16.3	17.3	18.9	21.0	23.2	26.8	3.6

Source: IAP Growth Charts Committee. Indian Pediatrics. 2015;52:47-55

Annexure 2 Growth Standards for Newborns

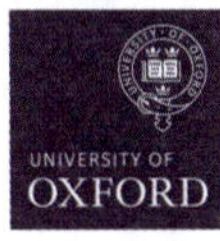

International Standards for Size at Birth (Boys)

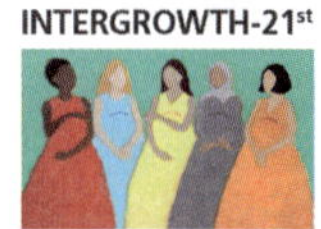

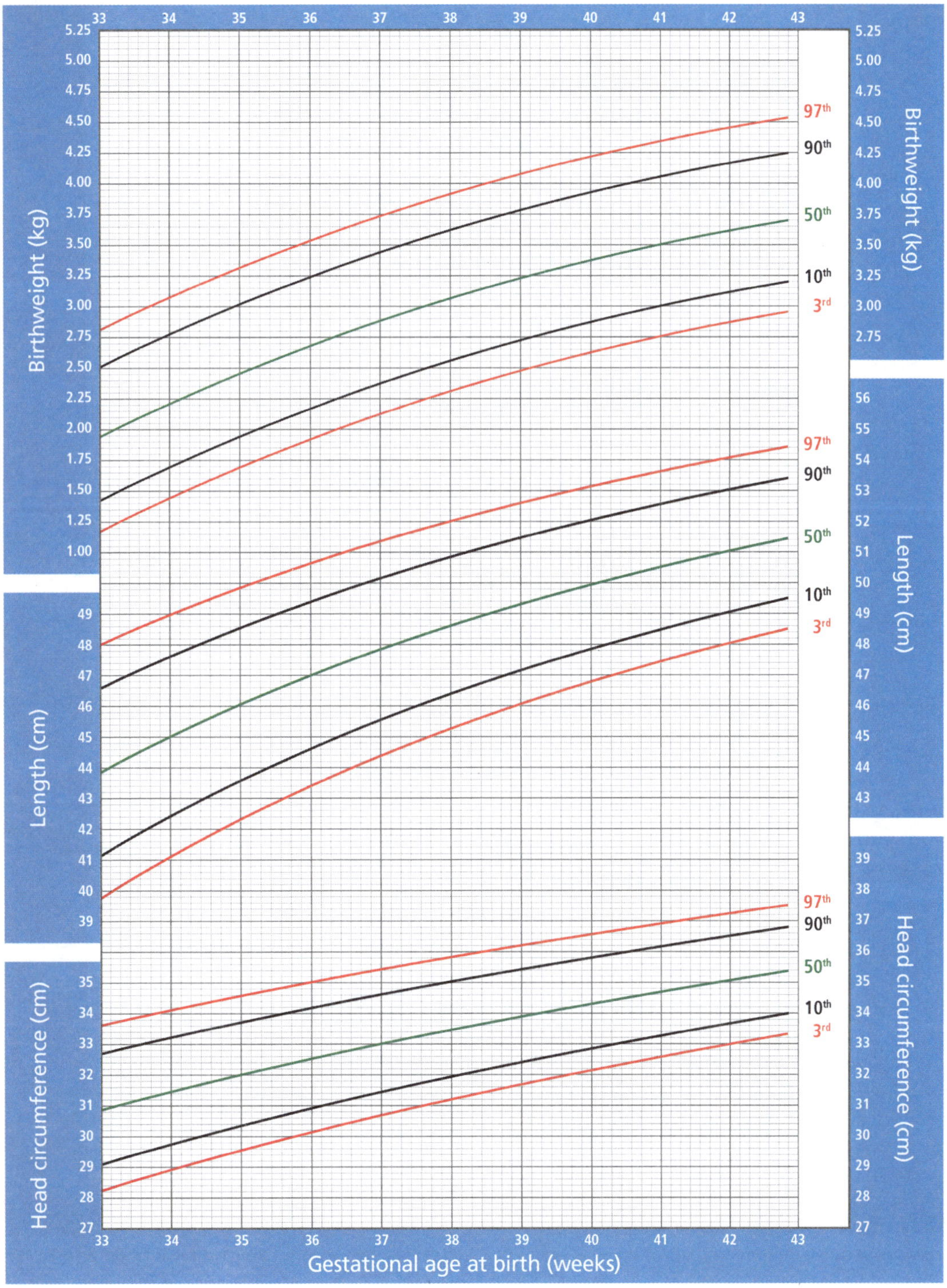

Birthweight (kg)
Length (cm)
Head circumference (cm)
97th
90th
50th
10th
3rd
Gestational age at birth (weeks)

Ref: Villar J et al. Lancet. 2014;384:857-68

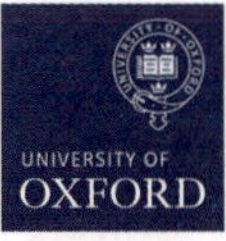

International Standards for Size at Birth (Girls)

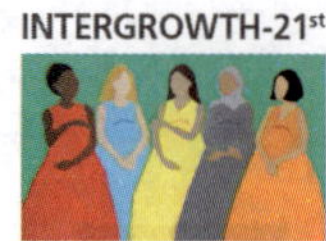

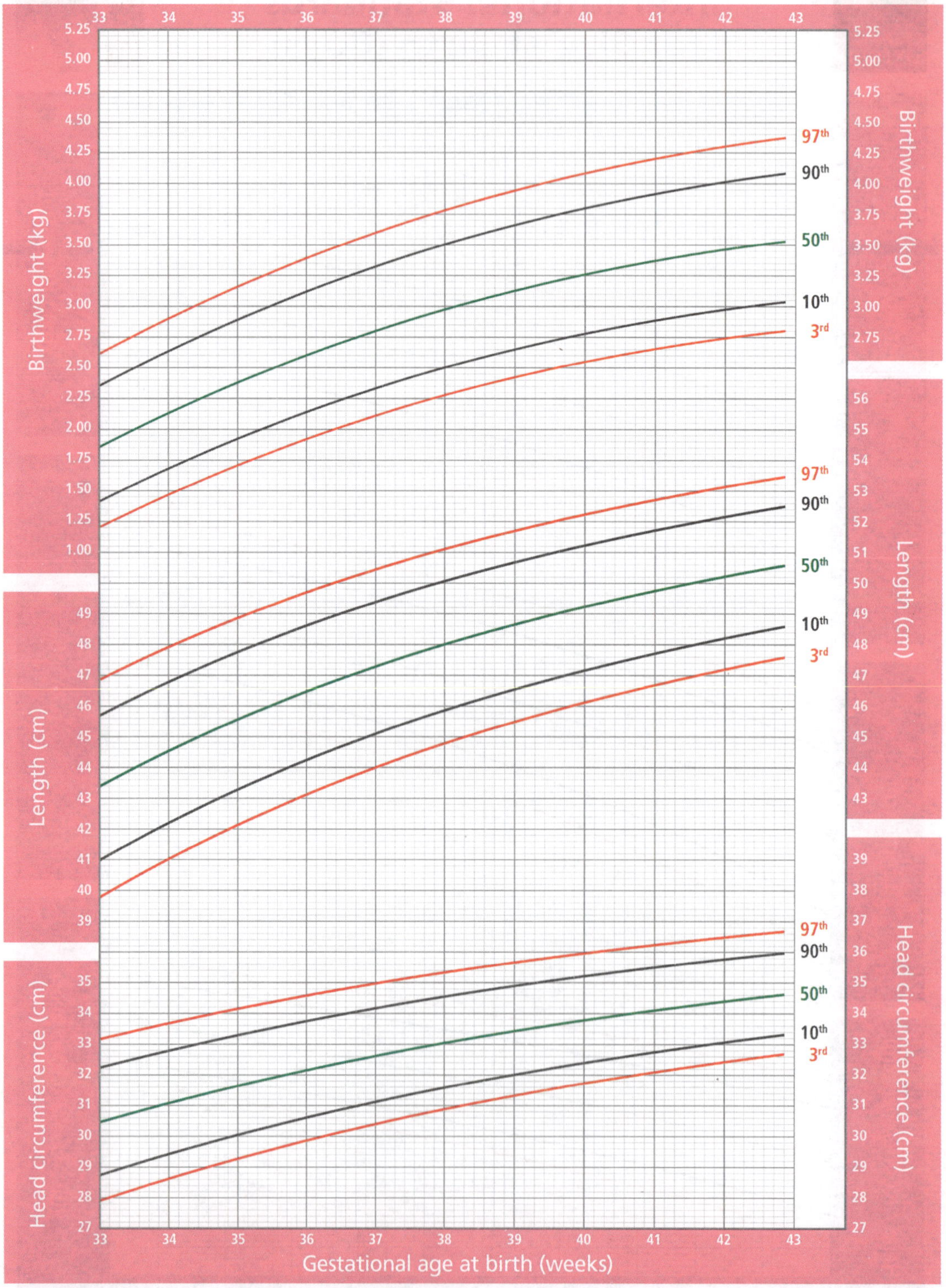

Birthweight (kg): 5.25, 5.00, 4.75, 4.50, 4.25, 4.00, 3.75, 3.50, 3.25, 3.00, 2.75, 2.50, 2.25, 2.00, 1.75, 1.50, 1.25, 1.00

Length (cm): 39–56

Head circumference (cm): 27–39

Percentile curves: 97th, 90th, 50th, 10th, 3rd

Gestational age at birth (weeks): 33, 34, 35, 36, 37, 38, 39, 40, 41, 42, 43

Ref: Villar J et al. Lancet. 2014;384:857-68

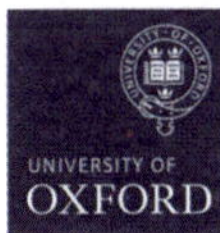

International Postnatal Growth Standards for Preterm Infants (Boys)

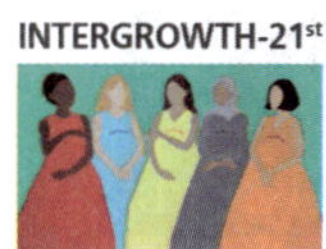

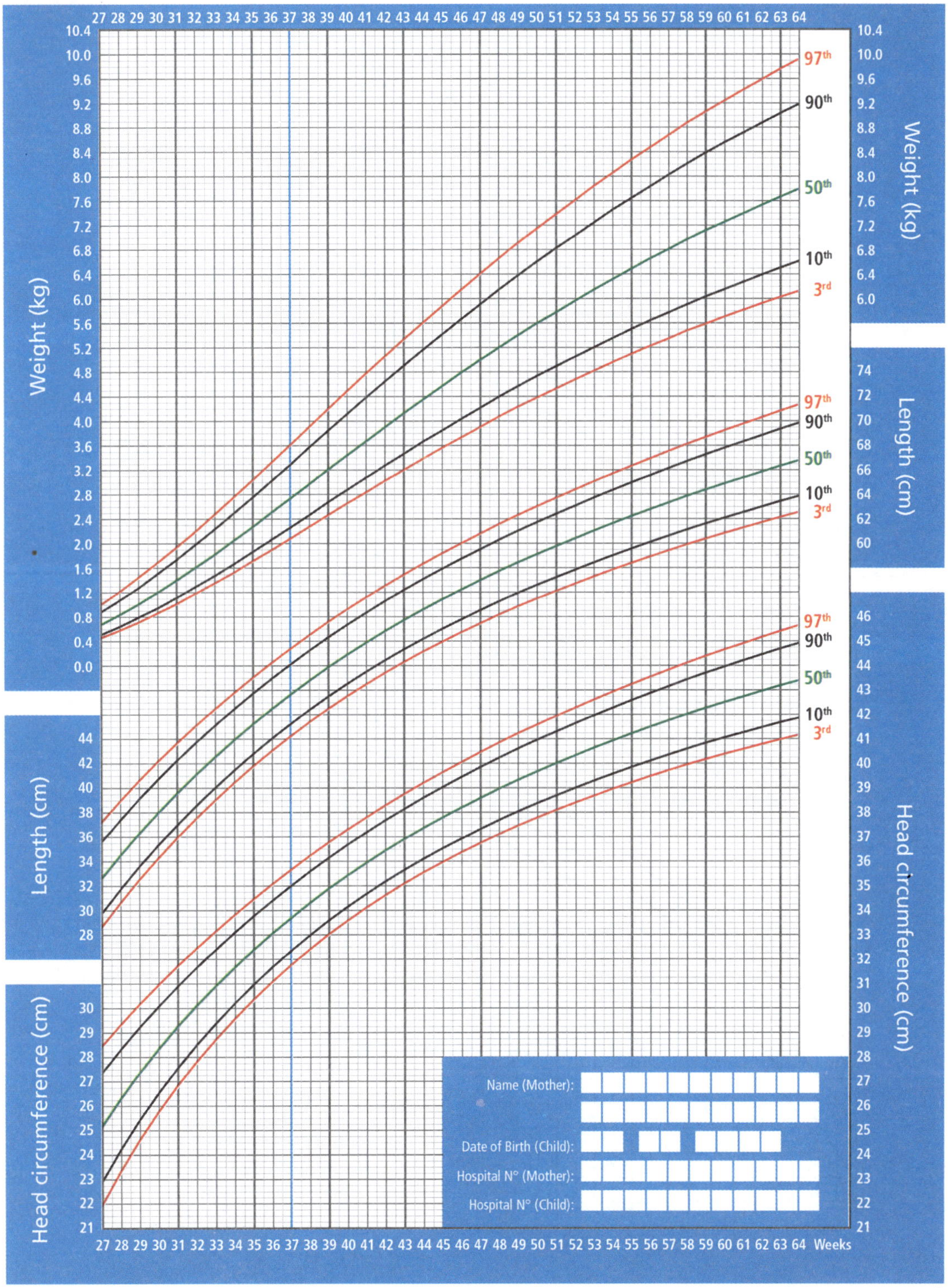

Ref: Villar et al. *Lancet Glob Heath.* 2015;3:e681-91

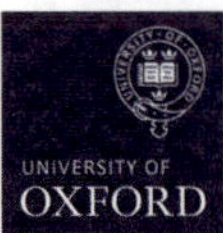

International Postnatal Growth Standards for Preterm Infants (Girls)

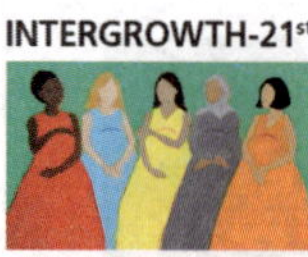

Ref: Villar et al. *Lancet Glob Heath.* 2015;3:e681-91

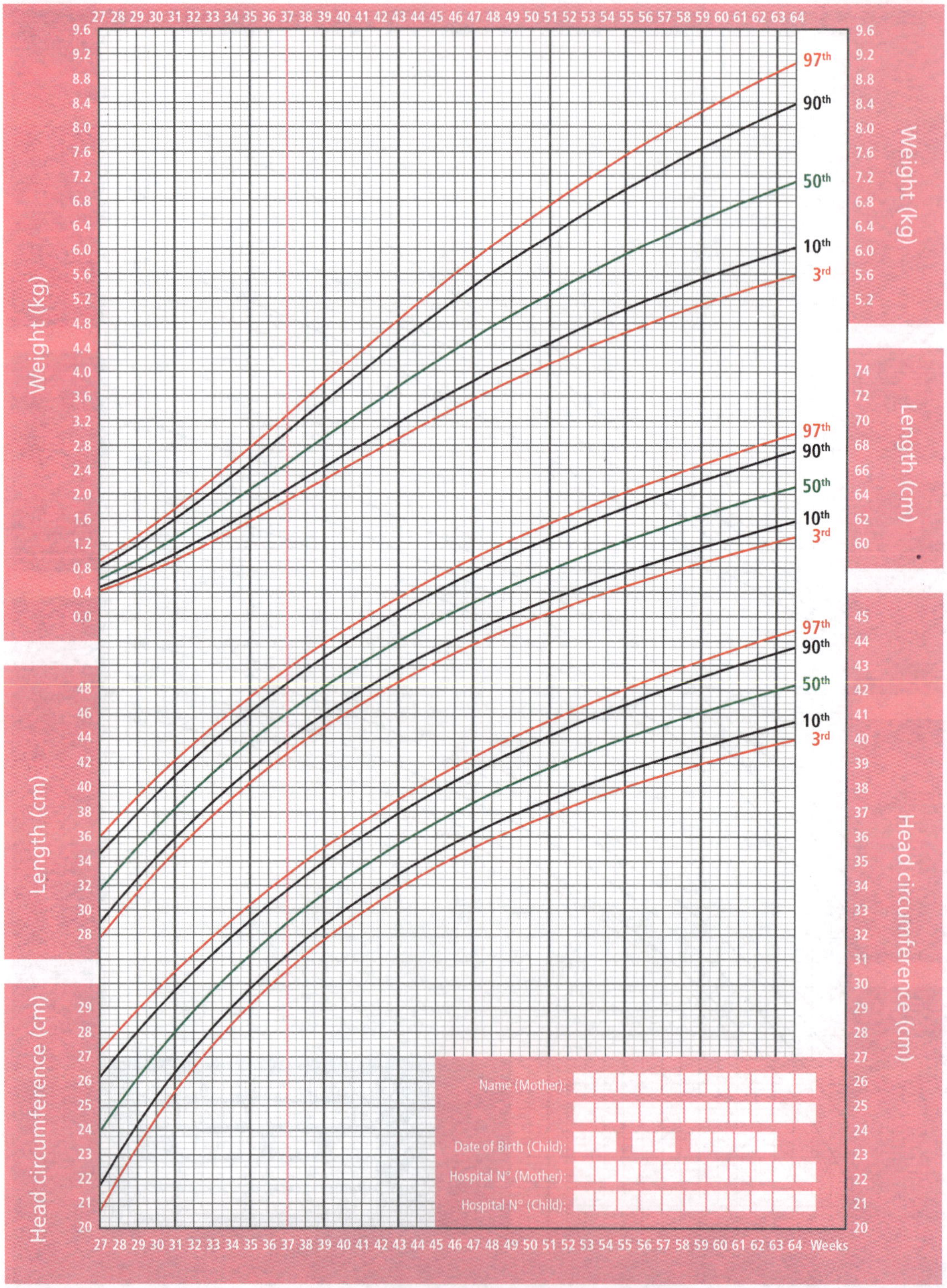

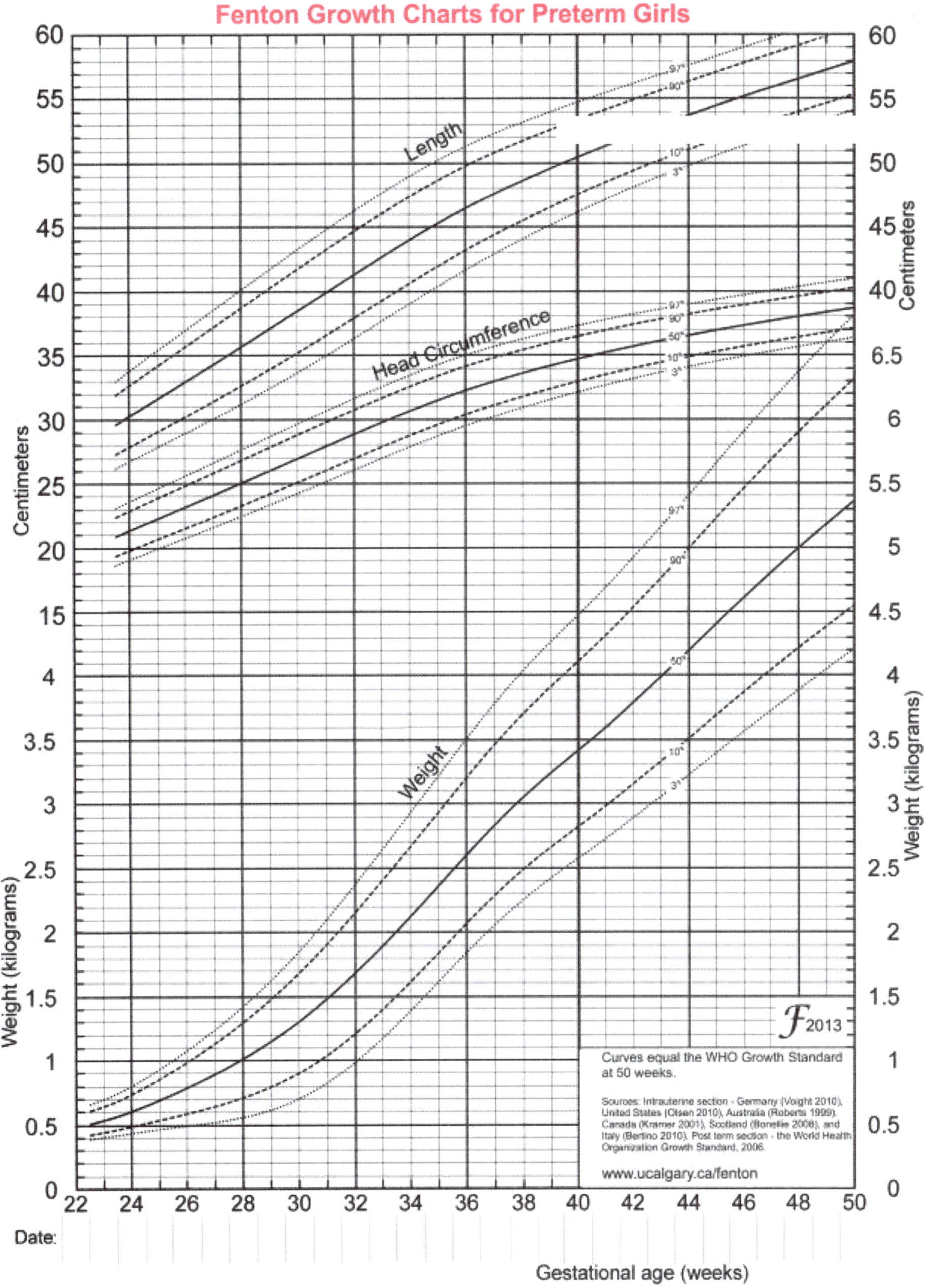
Fenton Growth Charts for Preterm Girls
Length
Head Circumference
Weight
Centimeters
Weight (kilograms)
97th
90th
50th
10th
3rd
F2013
Curves equal the WHO Growth Standard at 50 weeks.
Sources: Intrauterine section - Germany (Voight 2010), United States (Olsen 2010), Australia (Roberts 1999), Canada (Kramer 2001), Scotland (Bonellie 2008), and Italy (Bertino 2010). Post term section - the World Health Organization Growth Standard, 2006.
www.ucalgary.ca/fenton
Date:
Gestational age (weeks)

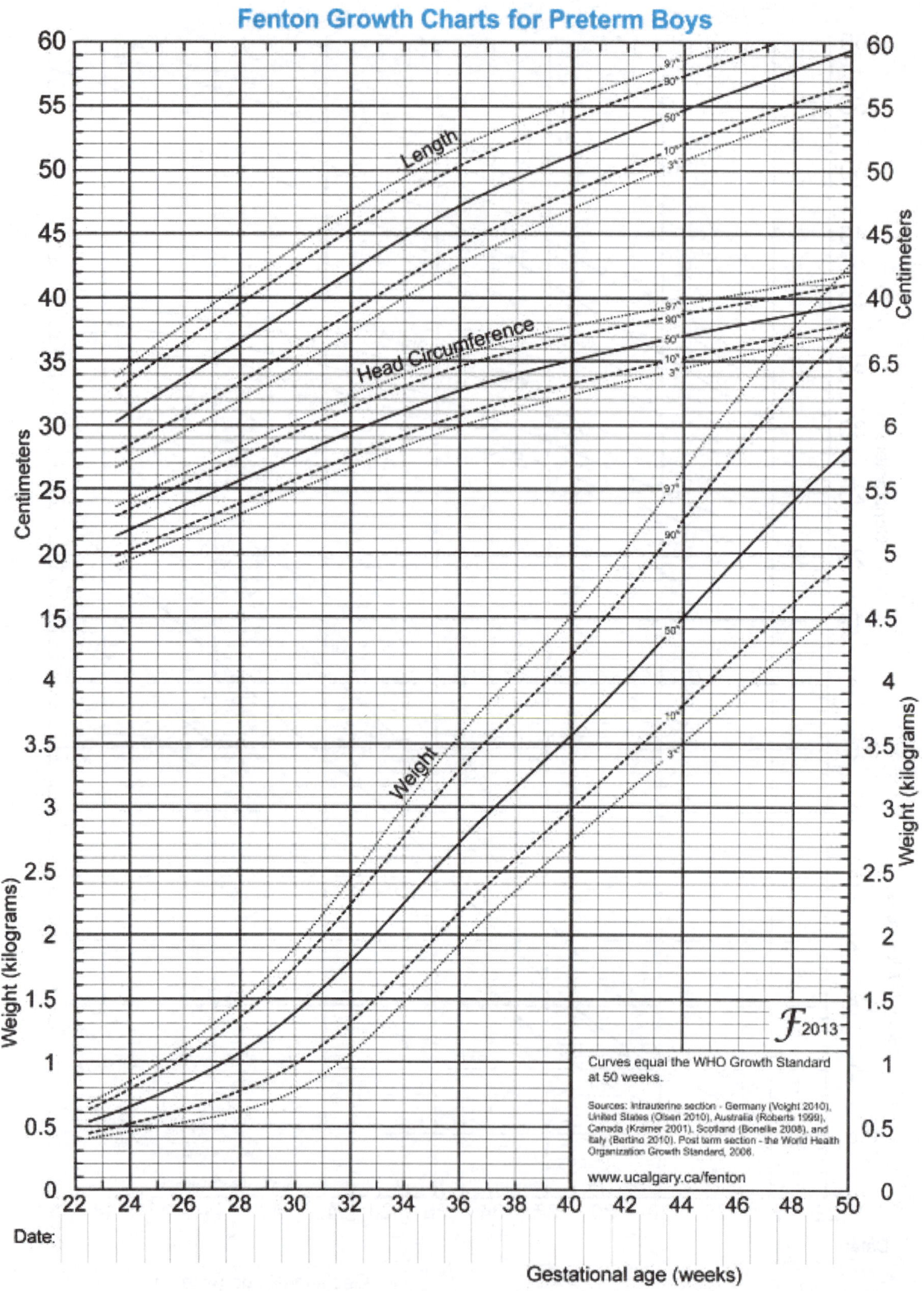
Fenton Growth Charts for Preterm Boys
Length
Head Circumference
Weight
Centimeters
Weight (kilograms)
Gestational age (weeks)
Date:
97th
90th
50th
10th
3rd
22 24 26 28 30 32 34 36 38 40 42 44 46 48 50
F2013
Curves equal the WHO Growth Standard at 50 weeks.
Sources: Intrauterine section - Germany (Voight 2010), United States (Olsen 2010), Australia (Roberts 1999), Canada (Kramer 2001), Scotland (Bonellie 2008), and Italy (Bertino 2010). Post term section - the World Health Organization Growth Standard, 2006.
www.ucalgary.ca/fenton

Annexure 3 IMNCI Chart Booklet 2023

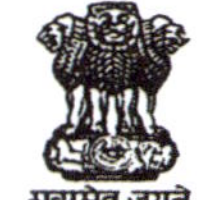

Ministry of Health & Family Welfare
Govt. of India
2023

INTEGRATED MANAGEMENT OF NEONATAL AND CHILDHOOD ILLNESS

PHYSICIAN CHART BOOKLET

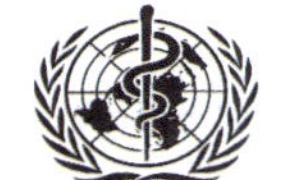

World Health Organization
Child & Adolescent Health

unicef | for every child

ASSESS AND CLASSIFY THE SICK YOUNG INFANT AGE UPTO 2 MONTHS

ASSESS

ASK THE MOTHER WHAT THE YOUNG INFANT'S PROBLEMS ARE

- Determine if this is an initial or follow-up visit for this problem.
  - ➢ if follow-up visit, use the follow-up instructions on TREAT THE INFANT CHART.
  - ➢ if initial visit, assess the young infant as follows:

USE ALL BOXES THAT MATCH INFANT'S SYMPTOMS AND PROBLEMS TO CLASSIFY THE ILLNESS.

A child with a pink classification needs URGENT attention, complete the assessment and pre- referral treatment immediately so that referral is not delayed

CHECK FOR POSSIBLE SERIOUS BACTERIAL INFECTION

ASK:	LOOK, LISTEN, FEEL:
• Is the infant having difficulty in feeding? • Has the infant had convulsions?	• Count the breaths in one minute. Repeat the count if it is 60 or more breaths per minute. • Look for severe chest indrawing. } **YOUNG INFANT MUST BE CALM** • Measure axillary temperature (if not possible, feel for fever or low body temperature). • Look at the young infant's movements. *If infant is sleeping, ask the mother to wake him/her.* ➢ *Does the infant move on his/her own?* ➢ *Does the infant move only when stimulated but then stops?* ➢ *Does the infant not move at all?* • *Look at the umbilicus. Is it red or draining pus?* • *Look for skin pustules.*

***Classify* ALL YOUNG INFANTS** →

SIGNS	CLASSIFY AS	IDENTIFY TREATMENT (Urgent pre-referral treatments are in bold print)
Any one or more of the following signs: • Not able to feed at all or not feeding well <u>or</u> • Convulsions <u>or</u> • Fast breathing (60 breaths per minute or more in infants less than 7 days) <u>or</u> • Severe chest indrawing <u>or</u> • Axillary temperature 37.5°C/99.5°F or above (or feels hot to touch) <u>or</u> • Axillary temperature less than 35.5°C/95.9°F (or feels cold to touch) <u>or</u> • Movement only when stimulated or no movement at all	**POSSIBLE SERIOUS BACTERIAL INFECTION <u>OR</u> VERY SEVERE DISEASE**	• ***Give anticonvulsant, if convulsing now*** • ***Give first dose of intramuscular ampicillin and gentamicin*** • ***Treat to prevent low blood sugar*** • ***Advise the mother how to keep the infant warm on the way to the hospital*** • ***Give oxygen on the way to hospital, if infant has fast breathing/ chest indrawing*** • ***Refer URGENTLY to hospital #***
• Fast breathing (60 breaths per minute or more) in infants 7-59 days old	**PNEUMONIA**	• ***If infant also has low weight for age or another severe classification:*** ➢ ***Give first dose of intramuscular ampicillin and gentamicin*** ➢ ***Refer URGENTLY to hospital#*** • *If infant does not have low weight for age or another severe classification:* ➢ ***Give oral amoxicillin for 7 days*** ➢ *Advise the mother to give home care for the young infants* ➢ *Advise mother when to return immediately* ➢ *Follow up after 2 days*
• Umbilicus red or draining pus <u>or</u> • Skin pustules	**LOCAL BACTERIAL INFECTION**	• ***Give oral amoxicillin for 5 days*** • *Teach the mother how to treat local infections at home* • *Advise the mother to give home care for the young infant* • *Advise mother when to return immediately* • *Follow up after 2 days*
• No Signs of bacterial infections <u>or</u> very severe disease	**INFECTION UNLIKELY**	• *Advise the mother to give home care for the young infant*

 # If referral is not possible, see the section ***Where Referral Is Not Possible.***

THEN, CHECK FOR JAUNDICE

ASK:	LOOK, LISTEN, FEEL:
• When did jaundice first appear?	• Look for jaundice (yellow skin) • Look at the young infant's palms and soles. Are they yellow ?

Classify JAUNDICE

SIGNS	CLASSIFY AS	IDENTIFY TREATMENT (Urgent pre-referral treatments are in bold print)
• Any jaundice in an infant aged less than 24 hours <u>or</u> • Yellow palms or soles at any age	**SEVERE JAUNDICE**	• *Treat to prevent low blood sugar.* • ***Refer URGENTLY to hospital*** # • *Advise mother how to keep baby warm on the way to the hospital*
• Jaundice appearing after 24 hours of age <u>and</u> • Palms and soles not yellow	**JAUNDICE**	• *Advise the mother to give home care for young infants* • *Advise the mother to return immediately if the infant's palm or soles appear yellow* • *If the infant is older than 2 weeks, refer to a hospital for assessment* • Follow up after 2 day
• No jaundice	**NO JAUNDICE**	• Advise the mother to give home care to the young infant

 # If referral is not possible, see the section ***Where Referral Is Not Possible****.*

THEN ASK:
Does the young infant have diarrhoea?*

IF YES LOOK AND FEEL:

- Look at the young infant's general condition:
  - ➢ Look at Infant's movements:
    - ⇨ Does the infant move on his/her own?
    - ⇨ Does the infant move only when stimulated and then stops?
    - ⇨ Does the infant not move at all?
  - ➢ Is the infant restless and irritable?
- Look for sunken eyes.
- Pinch the skin of the abdomen.
  - ➢ Does it go back:
    - ⇨ Very slowly (longer than 2 seconds)?
    - ⇨ Slowly?

* ***What is diarrhoea in a young infant?***
If the stools have changed from usual pattern and are many and watery (more water than fecal matter). Normal frequent or loose stools in a breastfed baby is not diarrhoea.

Blood in stool in young infant needs referral to a hospital to rule out surgical and medical causes

Classify DIARRHOEA for DEHYDRATION

SIGNS	CLASSIFY AS	IDENTIFY TREATMENT (Urgent pre-referral treatments are in bold print)
Two of the following signs: • Movements only when stimulated <u>or</u> no movement at all • Sunken eyes • Skin pinch goes back very slowly	**SEVERE DEHYDRATION**	• ***Give first dose of intramuscular ampicillin and gentamicin*** • *If infant also has another severe classification:* ➢ ***Refer URGENTLY to hospital***[#] *with the mother giving frequent sips of ORS on the way* ➢ *Advise mother to continue breastfeeding* ➢ *Advise mother how to keep the young infant warm on the way to the hospital* <u>*OR*</u> • *If infant does not have any other severe classification:* ➢ *Give fluid for severe dehydration (Plan C) and then refer to hospital after rehydration*
Two of the following signs: • Restless, irritable • Sunken eyes • Skin pinch goes back slowly	**SOME DEHYDRATION**	• *If infant also has low weight for age or another severe classification:* ➢ ***Give first dose of intramuscular ampicillin and gentamicin*** ➢ ***Refer URGENTLY to hospital***[#] *with mother giving frequent sips of ORS on the way* ➢ *Advise mother to continue breastfeeding* ➢ *Advise mother how to keep the young infant warm on the way to the hospital* • *If infant does not have low weight or another severe classification:* ➢ *Give fluids for some dehydration (Plan B)*
• Not enough signs to classify as some or severe dehydration	**NO DEHYDRATION**	• *Give fluids and breastfeeds to treat diarrhoea at home (Plan A)* • *Advise mother when to return immediately* • *Follow up after 2 days if no improvement*

\# *If referral is not possible, see the section* ***Where Referral Is Not Possible****.*

THEN CHECK FOR A FEEDING PROBLEM OR LOW WEIGHT FOR AGE

ASK:	LOOK, LISTEN, FEEL:
• Is the infant breastfed? If yes, how many times in 24 hours? • Does the infant usually receive any other foods or drinks? ➢ If yes, how often? ➢ What do you use to feed the infant?	• Measure weight ➢ Is weight less than 1800 gms? Yes/ No • Determine weight for age ➢ Weight for age ≥ -2 SD score ➢ Weight for age <-2 score ➢ Weight for age less than -3SD score • Look for ulcers or white patches in the mouth (thrush)

IF AN INFANT: **Has any difficulty in feeding, <u>or</u>**
Is breastfeeding less than 8 times in 24 hours, <u>or</u>
Is taking any other foods or drinks, <u>or</u>
Is low weight for age, <u>and</u>
Has no indication to refer to hospital.

ASSESS BREASTFEEDING:

• Has the infant breastfed in the previous hour?

If the infant has not fed in the previous hour, ask the mother to put her infant to the breast.
Observe the breastfeed for 4 minutes.
(If the infant was fed during the previous hour, ask the mother if she can wait and tell you when the infant is willing to feed again.)

• Is the infant able to attach?
no attachment at all — not well attached — good attachment

> • *TO CHECK ATTACHMENT, LOOK FOR:*
> ➢ *Chin touching breast*
> ➢ *Mouth wide open*
> ➢ *Lower lip turned outward*
> ➢ *More areola visible above than below the mouth*
> *(All of these signs should be present if the attachment is good)*

• Is the infant suckling effectively (that is, slow deep sucks, sometimes pausing)?
not suckling at all — not suckling effectively — suckling effectively
Clear a blocked nose if it interferes with breastfeeding.

• Does the mother have pain while breastfeeding?

If yes, look and feel for:
➢ Flat or inverted nipples, or sore nipples
➢ Engorged breasts or breast abscess

Classify FEEDING

SIGNS	CLASSIFY AS	IDENTIFY TREATMENT (Urgent pre-referral treatments are in bold print)
• Weight less than 1800 gm in infants less than 7 days • Weight for age less than -3 SD in infants 7-59 days old	**VERY LOW WEIGHT**	• ***Refer URGENTLY to hospital***# • Treat to prevent low blood sugar. • Warm the young infant by skin to skin contact if temperature < 36.5°C/97.7°F (or feels cold to touch) while arranging referral. • Advise mother how to keep the young infant warm on the way to the hospital.
• Not well attached to breast <u>or</u> • Not suckling effectively <u>or</u> • Less than 8 breastfeeds in 24 hours <u>or</u> • Receives other foods or drinks <u>or</u> • Thrush (ulcers or white patches in mouth) <u>or</u> • Low weight for age (Weight for age <-2 SD) <u>or</u> • Breast or nipple problems	**FEEDING PROBLEM <u>AND/OR</u> LOW WEIGHT FOR AGE**	• If receiving other foods or drinks, counsel mother about breastfeeding more, reducing other foods or drinks. • If not well attached or not suckling effectively, teach correct positioning and attachment. • If breastfeeding less than 8 times in 24 hours, advise to increase frequency of breastfeeding. • If not breastfeeding at all ➢ refer for breastfeeding counseling and relactation . ➢ advise mother for giving locally appropriate animal milk and teach the mother to feed with a cup and spoon • If thrush, teach the mother to treat thrush at home. • If low weight for age: ➢ teach the mother how to keep the young infant warm at home. ➢ advise to increase frequency of breastfeeding • If breast or nipple problem, teach the mother to treat breast or nipple problems. • Advise mother to give home care to the young infant. • Advise mother when to return immediately. • Follow-up any feeding problem or thrush after 2 days. • Follow-up low weight for age after 14 days.
• Not low weight for age (≥ -2SD) <u>and</u> no other signs of inadequate feeding	**NO FEEDING PROBLEM**	• *Praise the mother for feeding the infant well.* • *Advise mother to give home care to the young infant.* • *Advise mother when to return immediately.*

 # If referral is not possible, see the section ***Where Referral Is Not Possible****.*

THEN CHECK THE YOUNG INFANT'S IMMUNIZATION STATUS

IMMUNIZATION SCHEDULE*:

ASK:	VACCINE:		
At Birth	BCG	OPV 0	HEP-B 0
6 weeks	Penta-1	OPV 1	Rotavirus-1 fIPV-1 PCV-1

ASSESS OTHER PROBLEMS

ASSESS THE MOTHER/CAREGIVER'S DEVELOPMENT SUPPORTIVE PRACTICES & COUNSEL FOR PRACTICES TO SUPPORT CHILD'S DEVELOPMENT

COUNSEL THE MOTHER ABOUT HER OWN HEALTH

ASSESS AND CLASSIFY THE SICK CHILD AGE 2 MONTHS UPTO 5 YEARS

ASSESS

ASK THE MOTHER WHAT THE CHILD'S PROBLEMS ARE

- Determine if this is an initial or follow-up visit for this problem.
  - ➢ if follow-up visit, use the follow-up instructions on TREAT THE CHILD chart.

CHECK FOR GENERAL DANGER SIGNS

ASK:

- Is the child not able to drink or feed?
- Does the child vomits everything?
- Has the child had convulsions?

LOOK:

- See if the child is lethargic or unconscious.
- Is the child convulsing now ?

URGENT ATTENTION

USE ALL BOXES THAT MATCH THE CHILD'S SYMPTOMS AND PROBLEMS TO CLASSIFY THE ILLNESS.

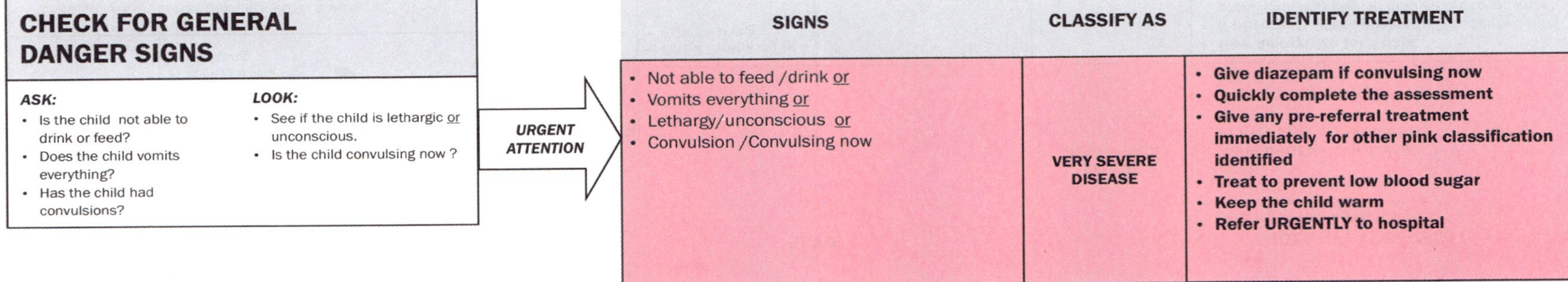

SIGNS	CLASSIFY AS	IDENTIFY TREATMENT
• Not able to feed /drink or • Vomits everything or • Lethargy/unconscious or • Convulsion /Convulsing now	**VERY SEVERE DISEASE**	• **Give diazepam if convulsing now** • **Quickly complete the assessment** • **Give any pre-referral treatment immediately for other pink classification identified** • **Treat to prevent low blood sugar** • **Keep the child warm** • **Refer URGENTLY to hospital**

A child with any general danger signs needs URGENT attention; complete the assessment and any pre-referral treatment immediately so that referral is not delayed

ASSESS AND CLASSIFY THE SICK CHILD AGE 2 MONTHS UP TO 5 YEARS

THEN ASK ABOUT MAIN SYMPTOMS:
Does the child have cough or difficult breathing?

IF YES, ASK:	LOOK, LISTEN:	
• For how long?	• Count the breaths in one minute. • Look for chest indrawing. • Look and listen for stridor. • Look and listen for wheezing	} CHILD MUST BE CALM

• Check oxygen saturation (Spo2): < 90% / ≥ 90%

If wheezing with either fast breathing or chest indrawing

Give a trial of rapid acting inhaled bronchodilator for up to three times 15-20 minutes apart. Count the breaths and look for chest indrawing again, and then classify.

If the child is:	Fast breathing is:
2 months upto 12 months	50 breaths per minute or more
12 months upto 5 years	40 breaths per minute or more

Classify COUGH or DIFFICULT BREATHING

SIGNS	CLASSIFY AS	IDENTIFY TREATMENT (Urgent pre-referral treatments are in bold print)
• Any general danger sign or • Stridor in calm child or • Spo2 < 90%	**SEVERE PNEUMONIA OR VERY SEVERE DISEASE**	• *Give first dose of injectable ampicillin and gentamicin* • ***Refer URGENTLY to hospital.#*** • *Provide oxygen to all children on the way to the hospital* • *If wheezing give an inhaled bronchiodialator before transfer*
• Chest indrawing or • Fast breathing	**PNEUMONIA**	• ***Give Amoxycillin for 5 days.*** • *If wheezing (or disappeared after rapidly acting bronchodilator) give an inhaled bronchodilator for 5 days** • *Soothe the throat and relieve the cough with a safe remedy if child is 6 months or older.* • *Follow-up after 2 days.*
• No signs of severe pneumonia or pneumonia	**NO PNEUMONIA: COUGH OR COLD**	• *If wheezing (or disappeared after rapidly acting bronchodilator) give an inhaled bronchodilator for 5 days ** • *Soothe the throat and relieve the cough with a safe home remedy if child is 6 months or older.* • *If coughing more than 14 days ,refer for possible TB, or asthma assessment.* • *Advise mother when to return immediately.* • *Follow-up after 5 days if not improving.*

*In settings where inhaled bronchodilator is not available, use oral salbutamol

If referral is not possible, see the section **Where Referral Is Not Possible.**

Does the child have diarrhoea?

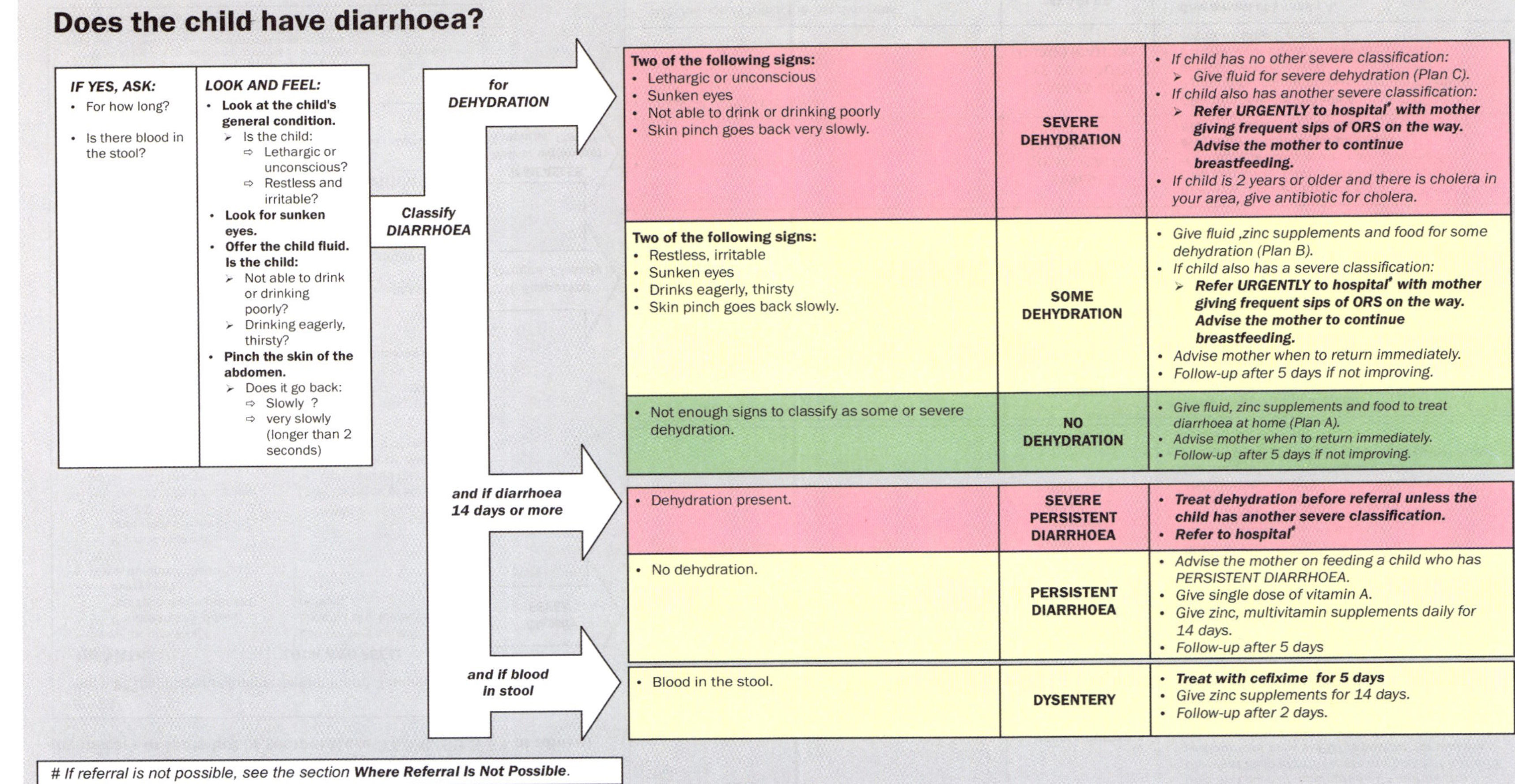

IF YES, ASK:	LOOK AND FEEL:
• For how long? • Is there blood in the stool?	• **Look at the child's general condition.** ➢ Is the child: ⇨ Lethargic or unconscious? ⇨ Restless and irritable? • **Look for sunken eyes.** • **Offer the child fluid. Is the child:** ➢ Not able to drink or drinking poorly? ➢ Drinking eagerly, thirsty? • **Pinch the skin of the abdomen.** ➢ Does it go back: ⇨ Slowly ? ⇨ very slowly (longer than 2 seconds)

***Classify* DIARRHOEA**

***for* DEHYDRATION**

Signs	Classify as	Treatment
Two of the following signs: • Lethargic or unconscious • Sunken eyes • Not able to drink or drinking poorly • Skin pinch goes back very slowly.	**SEVERE DEHYDRATION**	• *If child has no other severe classification:* ➢ *Give fluid for severe dehydration (Plan C).* • *If child also has another severe classification:* ➢ ***Refer URGENTLY to hospital# with mother giving frequent sips of ORS on the way. Advise the mother to continue breastfeeding.*** • *If child is 2 years or older and there is cholera in your area, give antibiotic for cholera.*
Two of the following signs: • Restless, irritable • Sunken eyes • Drinks eagerly, thirsty • Skin pinch goes back slowly.	**SOME DEHYDRATION**	• *Give fluid ,zinc supplements and food for some dehydration (Plan B).* • *If child also has a severe classification:* ➢ ***Refer URGENTLY to hospital# with mother giving frequent sips of ORS on the way. Advise the mother to continue breastfeeding.*** • *Advise mother when to return immediately.* • *Follow-up after 5 days if not improving.*
• Not enough signs to classify as some or severe dehydration.	**NO DEHYDRATION**	• *Give fluid, zinc supplements and food to treat diarrhoea at home (Plan A).* • *Advise mother when to return immediately.* • *Follow-up after 5 days if not improving.*

and if diarrhoea 14 days or more

Signs	Classify as	Treatment
• Dehydration present.	**SEVERE PERSISTENT DIARRHOEA**	• ***Treat dehydration before referral unless the child has another severe classification.*** • ***Refer to hospital#***
• No dehydration.	**PERSISTENT DIARRHOEA**	• *Advise the mother on feeding a child who has PERSISTENT DIARRHOEA.* • *Give single dose of vitamin A.* • *Give zinc, multivitamin supplements daily for 14 days.* • *Follow-up after 5 days*

and if blood in stool

Signs	Classify as	Treatment
• Blood in the stool.	**DYSENTERY**	• ***Treat with cefixime for 5 days*** • *Give zinc supplements for 14 days.* • *Follow-up after 2 days.*

 # If referral is not possible, see the section ***Where Referral Is Not Possible****.*

Does the child have fever?

(by history or feels hot or temperature 37.5°C/99.5°F* or above)

IF YES
Is it a PF (p. falciparum) predominant area? Yes/ No

THEN ASK:

- Fever for how long?
  - If more than 7 days , has fever been present every day?
- Is it a dengue season? Yes/No
  - If yes, is there a continuous fever of 2-7 days?
- Has the child had measles within last 3 months

LOOK AND FEEL:

- Look or feel for stiff neck
- Look for any bacterial focus of fever
- Look for signs of Measles
  - Generalized rash and
  - One of these: cough, runny nose or red eyes

- Do RDT for malaria in all fever cases if it is PF predominant area and if no obvious cause of fever is present in other areas or malaria suspected

If suspected dengue (dengue season & has continuous fever of 2-7 days)

- Look for following warning signs:
  - Cold extremities
  - Severe abdominal pain (abdominal pain with restlessness /anxious look)
  - Bleeding from any site (skin, mucosal, hematemesis or melena)
  - Positive Tourniquet test: >10 petechiae per square inch

If the child has measles now or within the last 3 months:

- Look for mouth ulcers – Are they deep and extensive ?
- Look for pus draining from the eye?

*This cutoff is for axillary temperature
** Other causes of fever include no pneumonia: cough or cold, pneumonia, diarrhoea, dysentery, tonsillitis, skin infections , dengue , measles.
*** Other important complications of measles - pneumonia, stridor, diarrhoea, ear infection, and malnutrition - are classified in other tables.
# If referral is not possible, see the section **Where Referral Is Not Possible** in the module ***Treat the Child***.

Classify FEVER

Signs	Classify as	Treatment
• Any general danger sign or • Stiff neck	**VERY SEVERE FEBRILE DISEASE**	• ***Give first dose of appropriate IM antibiotics*** • ***Give first dose of artesunate or quinine if it is a PF predominant area or RDT is positive for malaria*** • ***Treat the child to prevent low blood sugar.*** • ***Give one dose of paracetamol in clinic for high fever (temp. 38.5°C/101.3°F or above).*** • ***Refer URGENTLY to hospital*** [#].
• Positive RDT or • RDT not available / RDT negative and no other obvious cause of fever	**MALARIA/ SUSPECTED MALARIA**	• ***Give oral antimalarial as per national guidelines after making a smear*** • *Give one dose of paracetamol in clinic for high fever (temp. 38.5°C/101.3°F or above).* • *Advise mother when to return immediately.* • *Follow-up after 2 days .*
• Negative RDT and/or other causes of fever PRESENT**	**FEVER - MALARIA UNLIKELY**	• *Give one dose of paracetamol in clinic for high fever (temp. 38.5°C/101.3°F or above)* • *Give appropriate treatment for an identified cause of fever* • *Advise mother when to return immediately.* • *Follow-up after 2 days if fever persists* • *If fever is present every day for more than 7 days , refer for assessment*

If Suspected Dengue, Classify

Signs	Classify as	Treatment
• Any general danger sign or • Cold extremities or • Severe abdominal pain or • Bleeding from any site or • Positive Tourniquet test	**SEVERE DENGUE / DENGUE WITH WARNING SIGNS**	• ***Refer URGENTLY to hospital*** • *If accepting orally , advise mother to give frequent sips of ORS / fluids on the way to the hospital* • *Give one dose of paracetamol in clinic for high fever (temp. 38.5°C/101.3°F or above).*
• No warning signs	**DENGUE FEVER**	• *Give one dose of paracetamol in clinic for high fever (temp. 38.5°C/101.3°F or above).* • *Educate caregivers about care of a child with dengue fever* • *Follow-up after 2 days*

If MEASLES Now or within last 3 months, Classify

Signs	Classify as	Treatment
• Any general danger sign or • Clouding of cornea or • Deep or extensive Mouth ulcers	**SEVERE COMPLICATED MEASLES*** **	• ***Give first dose of Vitamin A.*** • ***Give first dose of IM ampicillin and gentamicin.*** • ***If clouding of the cornea or pus draining from the eye, apply antibiotic eye ointment.*** • ***Refer URGENTLY to hospital*** [#]
• Pus draining from the eye or • Mouth ulcers	**MEASLES WITH EYE OR MOUTH COMPLICATIONS**	• ***Give first dose of Vitamin A.*** • *If pus draining from the eye, treat eye infection with antibiotic eye ointment.* • *If mouth ulcers, treat with gentian violet.* • *Follow-up after 2 days.*
• Measles now or within the last 3 months	**MEASLES**	• ***Give a dose of Vitamin A.***

Does the child have an ear problem?

THEN ASK:
- Is there ear pain?
- Is there ear discharge?
- If yes, for how long?

LOOK AND FEEL:
- Look for pus draining from the ear.
- Feel for tender swelling behind the ear.

CLASSIFY EAR PROBLEM

Signs	Classify as	Treatment
• Tender swelling behind the ear.	**MASTOIDITIS**	• ***Give first dose of injectable. Ampicillin and gentamicin*** • ***Give first dose of paracetamol for pain.*** • ***Refer URGENTLY to hospital#.***
• Pus is seen draining from the ear and discharge is reported for less than 14 days, or • Ear pain.	**ACUTE EAR INFECTION**	• ***Give Amoxycillin for 5 days.*** • *Give paracetamol for pain.* • *Dry the ear by wicking.* • *Follow-up after 5 days.*
• Pus is seen draining from the ear and discharge is reported for 14 days or more.	**CHRONIC EAR INFECTION**	• Dry the ear by wicking. • Topical quinolone ear drops for 2 weeks. • Follow-up in 5 days.
• No ear pain and No pus seen draining from the ear.	**NO EAR INFECTION**	No additional treatment.

THEN CHECK FOR MALNUTRITION

LOOK AND FEEL:
- Measure weight , length/height and determine WFL SD score
- Look for oedema of both feet.
- Measure MUAC, if child is 6 months or older

Check for medical complications in children with Severe Acute Malnutrition

- Any general danger signs
- Any severe classification
- Pneumonia
- Diarrhoea with dehydration
- Poor appetite
- Oedema of both feet

Classify NUTRITIONAL STATUS

Signs	Classify as	Treatment
• WFL <-3 SD score and /or • MUAC <11.5 cm and /or • Oedema of both feet and • Medical complications	**SEVERE ACUTE MALNUTRITION WITH MEDICAL COMPLICATION**	• ***Give injectable ampicillin and gentamicin.*** • ***Treat the child to prevent low blood sugar.*** • ***Refer URGENTLY to hospital.*** • *While referral is being organized, warm the child.* • *Keep the child warm on the way to hospital.*
• WFL <-3 SD score and /or • MUAC <11.5 cm and • No medical complications	**SEVERE ACUTE MALNUTRITION WITHOUT MEDICAL COMPLICATION**	• ***Give oral amoxicillin for 5 days*** • ***Give a dose of Vitamin A if not received in last one month*** • *Assess feeding & counsel the mother on how to feed the child* • *Give multivitamins , zinc for 14 days* • *Advise mother when to return immediately* • *Follow-up after 7 days*
• WFL <-2SD score and /or • MUAC 11.5 -12.4 cm and • No oedema	**MODERATE ACUTE MALNUTRITION**	• Assess feeding & counsel the mother on how to feed the child • Advise mother when to return immediately • Follow-up after 30 days
• WFL $\geq$ -2SD score and • MUAC $\geq$ 12.5 cm and • No oedema of both feet	**NO ACUTE MALNUTRITION**	• If child is less than 2 years old, assess the child's feeding and counsel the mother on feeding according to the FOOD box on the *COUNSEL THE MOTHER* chart. • If feeding problem, follow-up after 5 days. • Advise mother when to return immediately.

 # If referral is not possible, see the section ***Where Referral Is Not Possible****.*

THEN CHECK FOR ANEMIA

LOOK:

- Look for palmar pallor. Is it:
  - Severe palmar pallor?
  - Some palmar pallor?

⑩ If there is no other pink classification and hemoglobin testing is available as outpatient services, test hemoglobin of all children with pallor and classify as per Hb level

Classify ANEMIA

Signs	Classification	Treatment
• Severe palmar pallor (Hb <7g/dl)	**SEVERE ANEMIA**	• ***Refer URGENTLY to hospital#***
• Some palmar pallor (Hb 7-10.9 g/dl)	**ANEMIA**	• *Give iron folic acid therapy for 14 days* • *Assess the child's feeding and counsel the mother on feeding according to the FOOD box on the COUNSEL THE MOTHER chart. If feeding problem, follow-up after 5 days.* • *Advise mother when to return immediately.* • *Follow-up after 14 days.*
• No palmar pallor (Hb ≥ 11g/dl)	**NO ANEMIA**	• *Give prophylactic iron folic acid if child 6 months or older.*

If referral is not possible, see the section ***Where Referral Is Not Possible.***

THEN CHECK THE CHILD'S IMMUNIZATION *, PROPHYLACTIC VITAMIN A & IRON-FOLIC ACID SUPPLEMENTATION STATUS

IMMUNIZATION SCHEDULE:

AGE	*VACCINE*
At Birth	BCG + OPV-0 + Hep B 0
6 weeks	OPV-1 + Penta-1 +Rota Virus-1* + fIPV –1 + PCV –1
10 weeks	OPV-2+ Penta-2+ Rota Virus –2*
14 weeks	OPV-3+ Penta-3 +fIPV-2 + RV V-3* + PCV-2
9-12 months	Measles-rubella (MR-1) + JE–1#+ PCV booster + fIPV-3
16-24 months	MR-2, JE-2#, DPT booster-1, OPV booster
60 months	DPT booster-2

PROPHYLACTIC IFA/ DEWORMING/ Prophylactic Vitamin A

- Give IFA syrup (1ml 2 times a week with auto dispenser) containing 20 mg of elemental iron + 100 mcg of folic acid after the child has recovered from acute illness if the child is 6 months of age or older, supplement IFA in LBW after 6 weeks of age
- Give anthelminthic if child is one year or older and has not received deworming agents in last 6 months (1-2 years 1/2 tablet albendazole and for 2 years above, 1 tablet).
- Give Vitamin A supplementation as per state guidelines

* A child who needs to be immunized should be advised to go for immunization the day vaccines are available at AW/SC/PHC
\# JE in States where it is included in their immunization schedule

ASSESS OTHER PROBLEMS

ASSESS FEEDING IF AGE IS LESS THAN 2 YEARS / HAS UNCOMPLICATED MODERATE/SEVERE ACUTE MALNUTRITION OR ANEMIA

ASSESS THE MOTHER/CAREGIVER'S DEVELOPMENT SUPPORTIVE PRACTICES IF AGE IS LESS THAN 3 YEARS / HAS UNCOMPLICATED SEVERE ACUTE MALNUTRITION OR ANEMIA

COUNSEL THE MOTHER ABOUT HER OWN HEALTH

Annexure 4 Laboratory Values

THE NORMAL RANGE

Results of a laboratory test can be interpreted in terms of being normal or abnormal, and negative or positive only on the basis of already known *normal or reference values*. Normal values refer to those measurements which are usually central and around which most of the values lie in healthy individuals.

Almost all normal laboratory values are represented and expressed in a *reference range* and rarely in terms of a single measurement. For example, a large group of healthy children in the age group of 6–12 years may have an average hemoglobin level of 14 g/dL with the individual values ranging from 11.5 to 15.5 g/dL. In this case, the normal hemoglobin values in 6–12 years old are said to range between 11.5 g/dL and 15.5 g/dL, and not simply 14 g/dL. The normal or reference range is an integral part of all laboratory values because of considerable magnitude of inter-individual variability in the normal population. Variations in normal subjects occur due to a host of reasons, other than age and sex, which may include biological, genetic, environmental and chance factors apart from the interobserver and laboratory variability. In addition, the analytic method used in the laboratory is a major factor affecting the value obtained. All these sources are instrumental in creating a rather wide range of values that may be referred to for classifying an individual as having a normal or abnormal laboratory test.

The central values are measured in terms of mean, median and mode. Fortunately, these three measures generally coincide in most of the laboratory measurements in healthy individuals. The normal deviation around the mean is termed as standard deviation. In a typical Gaussian (bell shaped) distribution curve, 95% of the normal values lie between ± 2 SD around the mean. However, certain laboratory values in normal individuals do not follow the Gaussian curve, making it difficult to assume all values within mean 2 SD as being normal. In such situation, the normal values are expressed in terms of a range covering 95% of values from a set of values found in a healthy population, excluding 2.5% each of the lowermost and uppermost values.

Most of the laboratory tests do not have any absolute or magic cut-off point for labeling their results as being normal and abnormal. For example, if normal range of values of serum urea nitrogen is 5–18 mg/dL in children, then 17 mg/dL carries an importance equivalent to a value of 19 mg/dL. Both these values are then termed *borderline*. Such borderline values can be present in healthy as well as sick subjects and should be interpreted cautiously.

UNITS OF MEASUREMENT

Laboratory estimates are usually expressed as conventional or traditional units. However, it may be appropriate to know the standard units referred to as the SI units. The International System of Units (abbreviated SI from French: *Le Système international d'unités*) is well accepted worldwide as a standard and modern form of metric measurement. For most parameters, the SI units are moles per liter, wherein mass is measured in moles and volume as liters. Concentration in moles is the ratio of the weight in grams and the molecular weight.

To convert a value expressed in conventional units to a SI unit, we need to multiply by the conversion factor. For example, albumin 3 g/dL × 10 = 30 g/L. To convert from SI units to conventional units, we will need to divide the value by a conversion factor. For example, albumin 30 g/L = 30 ÷ 10 g/dL = 3 g/dL.

COMMON ABBREVIATIONS

Most of the commonly used units are written in an abbreviated from. A list of such units is given below in **Table 1**. Prefixes are used along with the units of length, capacity and mass **(Table 2)**.

Table 1 Abbreviations for Common Units

Measure	*Unit name*	*Abbreviation*
Weight	Gram	g
Length	Meter	m
Capacity	Liter	L
Pressure	Millimeter of mercury	mm Hg
Enzyme activity	International unit	U
Volume	Cubic millimeter	mm^3
Osmolality	Mole	mol
Equivalent weight	Milliequivalent	mEq

Table 2 Prefixes used for Decimal Factors

Prefix	*Symbol*	*Factor*
Mega	M	10^6
Kilo	k	10^3
Deci	d	10^{-1}
Centi	c	10^{-2}
Milli	m	10^{-3}
Micro	u	10^{-6}
Nano	n	10^{-9}
Pico	p	10^{-12}
Femto	f	10^{-15}

HEMATOLOGICAL VALUES

Parameter	Traditional or conventional units	Standard units (multiplication factor)
Blood volume	*mL/kg*	*mL/kg (1.0)*
At birth Infants 1–3 years 4–6 years 7–18 years Adults	61–100 73–78 74–82 80–86 83–90 68–88	61–100 73–78 74–82 80–86 83–90 68–88
Erythrocyte sedimentation rate (ESR): Westergren Method	*mm/h*	*mm/h (1.0)*
Neonate Child Adult males Adult females	0–4 4–20 0–10 0–20	0–4 4–20 0–10 0–20
Hematocrit	*%*	*% (1.0)*
Birth 1 week 1–2 weeks 6 months to 6 years >6 year males >6 year females	55 (45–65) 54 (43–66) 50 (42–66) 38 (33–42) 46 (42–52) 42 (37–47)	55 (45–65) 54 (43–66) 50 (42–66) 38 (33–42) 46 (42–52) 42 (37–47)
Hemoglobin (total) (Hgb)	*g/dL*	*mmol/L (0.6206)*
Birth 1 week 1–2 weeks 6 months to 6 years 6–12 years Adolescent males Adolescent females	17 (14–20) 17 (13–21) 16.5 (13–20) 12 (10.5–14) 14 (11.5–15.5) 16 (14–18) 14 (12–16)	11.25 (8.68–12.41) 11.25 (8.06–13.06) 10.24 (8.06–12.41) 7.45 (6.15–8.68) 8.68 (7.14–9.62) 9.93 (8.68–11.17) 8.68 (7.45–9.93)
Hemoglobin A	≥95% of total Hgb	≥95% of total Hgb
Hemoglobin A_2	1.5–3.5% of total Hgb	1.5–3.5% of total Hgb
Hemoglobin A_{1c} (Glycated Hgb)	4.5–6.1% of total Hgb	4.5–6.1% of total Hgb
Hemoglobin fetal (Hgb F)	*% of total Hgb*	*% of total Hgb*
Neonate Infant Child Adolescent Adult	60–90 2–59 <2 <2 <2	60–90 2–59 <2 <2 <2
Methemoglobin	0–1.3% of total Hgb	0–1.3% of total Hgb
Mean corpuscular hemoglobin (MCH)	*pg*	*pg*
Birth 1 week 1–2 weeks 6 months to 6 years >6-year males >6-year females	32–40 32–40 32–40 24–30 27–32 27–32	32–40 32–40 32–40 24–30 27–32 27–32
Mean corpuscular hemoglobin concentration (MCHC)	*g/dL*	*g/L (10)*

Contd...

Contd...

Parameter	Traditional or conventional units	Standard units (multiplication factor)
Birth 1 week 1–2 weeks 6 months to 6 years >6-year males >6-year females	34–36 34–36 34–36 30–36 30–35 30–35	340–360 340–360 340–360 300–360 300–350 300–350
Mean corpuscular volume (MCV)	*fL*	*fL*
Birth 1 week 1–2 weeks 6 months to 6 years >6-year males >6-year females	94–118 88–104 86–106 76–88 76–98 76–96	94–118 88–104 86–106 76–88 76–98 76–96
Plasma volume	*mL/kg*	*mL/kg (1.0)*
At birth Males Females	33.5–49.5 25–43 28–45	33.5–49.5 25–43 28–45
Platelet count	*$\times 10^3/mm^3$*	*$\times 10^9/L$*
Birth 1 week–adults	100–300 150–450	100–300 150–450
Red blood cell count	*$\times 10^6$ cells/mm^3*	*$\times 10^{12}$ cells/L (1.0)*
Birth 2 weeks 2 months 6 months 1 year 2–6 years 6–12 years	3.7–6.5 3.9–5.9 3.1–4.3 3.8–4.9 3.9–5.1 3.9–5.0 3.9–5.2	3.7–6.5 3.9–5.9 3.1–4.3 3.8–4.9 3.9–5.1 3.9–5.0 3.9–5.2
Reticulocyte count	*%*	*% (1.0)*
Birth 2 weeks 6 months to 6 years 6–12 years	5 (3–7) 2 (0–4) 1 (0–2) 0–2	5 (3–7) 2 (0–4) 1 (0–2) 0–2
White blood cell count	*cells/mm^3*	*$\times 10^9$ cells/L (10^6)*
Birth	18000 (9,000–30,000)	18 (9–30)
1 week	12,000 (6,000–22,000)	12 (6–22)
2 weeks	12,000 (5,000–21,000)	12 (5–21)
6 months to 6 years	10,000 (6,000–15,000)	10 (6–15)
>6 years	75,000 (5,000–10,000)	7.5 (5–10)
Differential leukocyte count	*Percentage of total WBC count*	*Percentage of total WBC count*
Cord blood 0–12 weeks 3 months 6 months to 6 years 7–12 years	N61 L31 E2 M6 N40 L48 E3 M9 N30 L63 E2 M5 N45 L48 E2 M5 N55 L38 E2 M7	N61 L31 E2 M6 N40 L48 E3 M9 N30 L63 E2 M5 N45 L48 E2 M5 N55 L38 E2 M7

Contd...

Contd...

Parameter	Traditional or conventional units	Standard units (multiplication factor)
Total neutrophil count Band cells Segmented	cells/mm^3 150–400 3,000–5,800	$\times 10^6$ cells/L 150–400 3,000–5,800
Total lymphocyte count	cells/mm^3 1,500–3,000	$\times 10^6$ cells/L 1,500–3,000
Total monocyte count	cells/mm^3 285–500	$\times 10^6$ cells/L 285–500
Total eosinophil count	cells/mm^3 50–250	$\times 10^6$ cells/L 50–250
Total basophil count	cells/mm^3 15–50	$\times 10^6$ cells/L 15–50

MEASURES OF COAGULATION

Coagulation test	Value
Activated partial thromboplastin time (aPTT) Preterm neonate Term neonate 1–5 years 6–10 years 11–16 years Adult	 35–100 s 35–70 s 24–36 s 26–36 s 26–37 s 27–40 s
Bleeding time (BT)	2–7 minutes
Clotting time (CT)	5–8 minutes
D-dimer	Positive titer = 1:8
Factor I/fibrinogen Preterm neonate Term neonate Child Adult	 1.2–3.8 g/L 1.5–3.5 g/L 2.0–4.0 g/L 1.5–3.5 g/L
Fibrin degradation products (FDP)	207 (68–494) ng/L
Protein C (U/mL) Preterm neonate Term neonate 1–5 years 6–10 years 11–16 years Adult	 0.28 (0.12–0.44) 0.35 (0.17–0.53) 0.66 (0.40–0.92) 0.69 (0.45–0.93) 0.83 (0.55–1.11) 0.96 (0.64–1.28)
Protein S total (U/mL) Preterm neonate Term neonate 1–5 years 6–10 years 11–16 years Adult	 0.26 (0.14–0.38) 0.36 (0.12–0.60) 0.86 (0.54–1.18) 0.78 (0.41–1.14) 0.72 (0.52–0.92) 0.81 (0.60–1.13)
Prothrombin time (PT) Preterm neonate Term neonate 1–5 years 6–10 years 11–16 years Adult	 13–23 s 13–17 s 10.6–11.4 s 10.1–12.1 s 10.2–12.0 s 11.0–14.0 s

Contd...

Contd...

Coagulation test	Value
Reptilase time Preterm neonate Term neonate Adult	 18–30 s 18–24 s 18–22 s
Thrombin time Preterm neonate Term neonate Adult	 12–24 s 12–18 s 10–14 s

COAGULATION FACTORS (% OF NORMAL OR ADULT VALUE)

Coagulation factor	Preterm neonate	Term neonate	Children
Factor II	30–65	40–65	60–150
Factor V	50–100	50–100	60–150
Factor VII	20–150	40–70	65–135
Factor VIII	60–120	70–150	60–145
Factor IX	10–30	15–55	60–140
Factor X	10–45	20–55	60–130
Factor XI	10–50	15–70	65–135
Factor XII	20–50	25–70	65–150

SERUM BIOCHEMISTRY

Serum proteins (g/dL)*

	Total proteins	Albumin	Globulins			
			α1	α2	β	γ
Preterm neonate	4.3–7.6	3.0–4.2	0.1–0.5	0.3–0.7	0.3–1.2	0.3–1.4
Term neonate	4.6–7.7	2.5–5.0	0.1–0.3	0.3–0.5	0.2–0.6	0.8–1.2
1–7 years	6.1–7.9	4.0–5.0	0.2–0.4	0.5–0.8	0.5–0.8	0.3–1.2
>7 years	6.4–8.2	3.4–5.0	0.2–0.3	0.4–1.0	0.5–1.1	0.5–1.8

*SI units: g/L, multiplication factor 10

		Conventional units	SI units, multiplication factor
Ammonia (heparinized venous sample on ice analyzed within 30 minutes)		*µg/dL*	*µmol/L, 0.7*
Neonate 0–2 months >1 month Adult		90–150 79–129 29–70 15–45	64–107 56–92 21–50 11–32
Bilirubin (serum), total		*mg/dL*	*µmol/L, 17.1*
Cord blood	Term Preterm	<2 <2	<34 <34
0–1 day	Term Preterm	<8 <6	<137 <103

Contd...

Contd...

		Conventional units	*SI units, multiplication factor*	
1–2 days	Term Preterm	<12 <8	<205 <137	
3–5 days	Term Preterm	<16 <12	<274 <205	
Thereafter	Term Preterm	<2 <1	<34 <17	
Adult		0.1–1.2	1.7–20.5	
Bilirubin (serum), conjugated		0–0.4	0–8	
Chloride (serum, heparinized plasma)		*mEq/L*	*mmol/L, 1*	
Newborn Thereafter		97–110 98–106	97–110 98–106	
Creatinine (serum)		*mg/dL*	*µmol/L, 90*	
Neonate Infant Child Adolescent		0.3–1.0 0.2–0.4 0.3–0.7 0.5–1.0	27–88 18–35 27–62 44–88	
C-reactive protein		*mg/dL*	*mg/dL, 1*	
0–90 days 90 days to 3 years Male Female 4–10 years Male Female 11–14 years Male Female		0.08–1.58 0.08–1.12 0.05–0.79 0.06–0.79 0.5–1.0 0.08–0.76 0.06–0.71	0.08–1.58 0.08–1.12 0.05–0.79 0.06–0.79 0.5 –1.0 0.08–0.76 0.06–0.71	
Glucose (serum)		*mg/dL*	*mmol/L, 0.0555*	
Preterm neonate Term neonate Newborn, day 1 Newborn >1 day Child Adult Glucose (whole blood, heparinized) Adult		20–60 30–60 40–60 50–90 60–100 70–105 65–95	1.1–3.3 1.7–3.3 2.2–3.3 2.8–5.0 3.3–5.5 3.9–5.8 3.6–5.3	
Glucose tolerance test (oral glucose: 1.75 g/kg, maximum 75 g)		*mg/dL*	*mmol/L, 0.0555*	
	Normal	*Diabetic*	*Normal*	*Diabetic*
Fasting 60 minutes 90 minutes 120 minutes	70–105 120–170 100–140 70–120	≥126 ≥200 ≥200 ≥200	3.9–5.8 6.7–9.4 5.6–7.8 3.9–6.7	≥7.0 ≥11 ≥11 ≥11
Lactate		*mmol/L*	*mmol/L, 1*	
Whole blood lactate 1–12 months 1 year 7–15 years *Plasma lactate* *6 months to 3 years*		 1.1–2.3 0.8–1.5 0.6–0.9 0.0–0.3	 1.1–2.3 0.8–1.5 0.6–0.9 0.0–0.3	

Contd...

Contd...

	Conventional units	*SI units, multiplication factor*
Serum lipids		
Cholesterol Cord blood 1–6 weeks ≥1 year *Phospholipids* Cord blood Neonate >1 month *Total lipids* Newborn >1 month *Free fatty acids* Newborn >1 month	*mg/dL* 23–135 93–217 119–263 *mg/dL* 75–150 170–250 150–300 *mg/dL* 150–400 400–1000 *µEq/L* 250–1000 300–1450	*mmol/L, 0.0259* 0.6–3.5 2.4–5.6 3.1–6.8 *g/L, 0.01* 0.75–1.5 1.7–2.5 1.5–3.0 *g/L, 0.01* 1.5–4.0 4.0–10.0 *µmol/L* 250–1000 300–1450
Pyruvate (whole blood) 7–17 years	mmol/L 0.076 (±0.026)	*mmol/L, 1* 0.076 (±0.026)
Urea (serum/plasma)	*mg/dL*	*mmol/L, 0.357*
Preterm neonate Term neonate Infant/child Thereafter	3–25 3–12 5–18 7–18	1.1–9.0 1.1–4.3 1.8–6.4 2.5–6.4
Uric acid (serum)	*mg/dL* 2–7	*mmol/L, 0.0595* 0.12–0.42

METALS AND BINDING PROTEINS

	Conventional units	*SI units, multiplication factor*
Serum ceruloplasmin	*mg/dL*	*mg/L, 10*
	21–53	210–530
Serum copper	*µg/dL*	*µmol/L, 0.157*
0–5 days 1–9 years 10–14 years 15–19 years	9–46 80–150 80–121 64–160	1.4–7.2 12.6–23.6 12.6–19 11.3–25.2
Serum folate	*ng/mL*	*nmol/L, 2.265*
	2.5–20	5.7–45.3
RBC folate	*ng/mL RBCs*	*nmol/L cells*
	150–450	340–1020
Serum iron	*µg/dL*	*µmol/L, 0.179*
Term neonate Infant Child Adult, male Adult, female	100–250 40–100 50–120 65–175 50–170	18–45 7–18 9–22 12–30 9–30
Total iron-binding capacity (TIBC)	*µg/dL*	*µmol/L, 0.179*
Term neonate Infant Child Adolescent Adult	150–200 200–400 250–500 300–600 250–425	26.8–35.8 35.8–71.6 44.8–89.5 53.7–107.4 44.8–76.1

Contd...

Contd...

	Conventional units	SI units, multiplication factor
Serum transferrin	*mg/dL*	*g/L, 0.01*
Term neonate Infant Child Adolescent Adult	130–275 200–360 200–360 220–400 220–400	1.3–2.75 2.0–3.6 2.0–3.6 2.2–4.0 2.2–4.0
Serum ferritin	*ng/mL*	*µg/L, 1*
Term neonate Infant Child Adolescent Adult, male Adult, female	25–200 50–600 7–140 7–140 20–250 10–120	25–200 50–600 7–140 7–140 20–250 10–120
Serum magnesium	*mg/dL*	*mmol/L, 0.411*
0–6 days 7 days–2 years 2–14 years	1.2–2.6 1.6–2.6 1.5–2.3	0.48–1.05 0.65–1.05 0.60–0.95
Blood lead	*µg/dL*	*µmol/L, 4.8*
Children Adults Toxic	<10 <40 ≥70	<48 <192 ≥336
Serum zinc	*µg/dL*	*µmol/L, 0.153*
	70–150	10.7–22.9

SERUM ENZYMES

Enzyme	Reference value
Amylase	*U/L*
1–19 years	30–100
Aldolase	*U/L*
10 months to 2 years 2–16 years	3.4–11.8 1.2–8.8
Alkaline phosphatase	*U/L*
Preterm neonate Term neonate Infants 2–5 years 6–7 years 8–9 years 10–11 years, male 10–11 years, female 12–13 years, male 12–13 years, female	Up to 1500 Up to 700 250–1000 250–850 250–1000 250–750 250–730 250–950 275–875 200–730
Acid phosphatase	*0–0.8 U/L*
Alanine aminotransferase (ALT, SGPT)	*U/L*
0–7 days 8–30 days 1–3 years 3–9 years 10–15 years	25–100 22–71 20–60 15–50 10–40

Contd...

Contd...

Enzyme	Reference value	
Aspartate aminotransferase (AST, SGOT)	*U/L*	
0–7 days 8–30 days 1–3 years 3–9 years 10–15 years	25–100 22–71 20–60 15–50 10–40	
*Antistreptolysin O (ASO) titers**	*Todd units*	
2–5 years 6–9 years 10–12 years	120–160 240 320	
α1-Antitrypsin	*0.93–2.24 g/L*	
Creatine kinase	*U/L*	
Newborn Adult	10–200 20–200	
Creatine kinase isoenzymes	*CKMB*	*CKBB*
Cord blood 0–24 hours 72–100 hours Older	0.3–3.1% 1.7–7.9% 1.4–5.9% 0–2%	0.3–10.5% 3.6–13.4% 5.1–13.3% 0
Gastrin	*<100 ng/L*	
Glucose 6 phosphate dehydrogenase (G6PD) Adult**	3.4–8.0 U/g hemoglobin or 1.16–2.72 U/mL RBC	
γ-glutamyl transferase (GGT)	*U/L*	
<3 weeks 3 weeks to 3 months >3 months, boy >3 months, girl 1–15 years Adult, male Adult, female	0–130 4–120 5–65 5–35 0–23 11–50 7–32	
Lactate dehydrogenase (LDH)	*U/L*	
<1 years 1–9 years 10–19 years	170–580 150–500 120–330	
Lactate dehydrogenase, isoenzymes (% total)		
LD1 heart *LD2 heart, RBCs* *LD3 muscle* *LD4 liver, trace muscle* *LD5 liver, muscle*	24–34% 35–45% 15–25% 4–10% 1–9%	
Lipase	*U/L*	
1–18 years	145–216	

*4× rise in paired serial specimens is significant
***Values are 50% higher in newborns*

NORMAL ACID-BASE STATUS AND ELECTROLYTES

	Conventional units	*SI units, multiplication factor*
Anion gap	*mEq/L*	*mmol/L, 1*
[Sodium (Chloride+Bicarbonate)]	7–16	7–16
Base excess	*mmol/L*	*mmol/L*
Newborn Infant Child Older	–10 to –2 –7 to –1 –4 to +2 –3 to +3	–10 to –2 –7 to –1 –4 to +2 –3 to +3
Bicarbonate, serum	*mEq/L*	*mmol/L, 1*
Arterial Venous	21–28 22–29	21–28 22–29
Calcium, total, serum	*mg/dL*	*mmol/L, 0.25*
<24 hours 24–48 hours 4–7 days Child	9.0–10.6 7.0–12.0 9.0–10.9 8.8–10.8	2.3–2.65 1.75–3.0 2.25–2.73 2.2–2.7
Calcium, ionized, serum	*mg/dL*	*mmol/L, 0.25*
<24 hours 24–48 hours Child	4.3–5.1 4.0–4.7 4.8–4.92	1.07–1.27 1.0–1.17 1.12–1.23
Carbon dioxide, total (tCO_2)	*mmol/L*	*mmol/L, 1*
Cord Newborn Infant Child	14–22 13–22 20–28 20–28	14–22 13–22 20–28 20–28
Carbon dioxide partial pressure, arterial ($PaCO_2$)	*mm Hg*	*kPa, 0.1333*
Newborn Infant Thereafter, males Thereafter, females	27–40 27–41 35–48 32–45	3.6–5.3 3.6–5.5 4.7–6.4 4.3–6.0
Chloride, serum	*mEq/L*	*mmol/L*
	95–106	95–106
Osmolarity, serum	*mosm/L*	*mosm/L*
	275–290	275–290
Oxygen partial pressure (PaO_2), arterial	*mm Hg*	*kPa, 0.1333*
Birth 5–10 minutes 30 minutes >1 hour 1 day Thereafter	8–24 33–75 31–85 55–80 54–95 83–108	1.1–3.2 4.4–10 4.1–11.3 7.3–10.6 7.2–12.6 11–14.4
Oxygen saturation (SaO_2), arterial	*%*	*Fraction saturation, 0.01*

Contd...

Contd...

	Conventional units	*SI units, multiplication factor*
Newborn Thereafter	85–90 95–99	0.85–0.90 0.95–0.99
pH, arterial		
Birth 24 hours Older	7.11–7.36 7.3–7.45 7.35–7.45	7.11–7.36 7.3–7.45 7.35–7.45
Potassium, serum	*mEq/L*	*mmol/L, 1*
<2 months 2–12 months >12 months	3–7 3.5–6 3.5–5	3–7 3.5–6 3.5–5
Sodium, serum	*mEq/L*	*mmol/L*
Newborn <1 year Child	134–146 139–144 138–145	134–146 139–144 138–145

HORMONES IN SERUM AND URINE

	Conventional units	*SI units, multiplication factor*
Adrenocorticotrophic hormone (ACTH), plasma	*pg/mL*	*ng/L, 1*
Cord blood 1–7 days postnatal *Adult* Morning Evening	130–160 100–140 25–100 <50	130–160 100–140 25–100 <50
Aldosterone, plasma/serum	*ng/dL*	*nmol/L, 1*
1–12 months 1–2 years 2–10 years 10–15 years	5–90 7–54 3–35 2–22	1.4–2.5 0.19–1.5 0.1–0.97 0.1–0.6
Aldosterone, urine	*µg/24 hours*	*nmol/24 hours, 2.78*
Newborn 4–10 years Older	0.5–5 1–8 3–19	1.39–13.9 2.78–22.2 8.3–52.8
Antidiuretic hormone (ADH), plasma varies with plasma osmolarity (mosm/kg)	*pg/mL*	*pg/mL, 1*
270–280 280–285 285–290 290–295 295–300	<1.5 <2.5 1–5 2–7 4–12	<1.5 <2.5 1–5 2–7 4–12
Calcitonin, plasma	*pg/mL*	*pmol/L, 0.28*
Newborn Males Females	70–348 3–26 2–17	19.6–97.4 0.8–7.2 0.6–4.7
Catecholamines, serum	*µg/24 hours*	*µg/24 hours, 1*

Contd...

Contd...

	Conventional units	*SI units, multiplication factor*
Dopamine Epinephrine Norepinephrine Metanephrines Normetanephrines Homovanillic acid (HVA) Vanillyl mandelic acid (VMA)	100–440 <15 15–86 <0.4 <0.9 0–10 2–10	100–440 <15 15–86 <0.4 <0.9 0–10 2–10
Cortisol, plasma	*μg/dL*	*nmol/L, 27.59*
Newborn *Adults* Morning 8 a.m. Evening 4 p.m. Night 8 p.m.	1–24 5–23 3–15 Less than 50% of morning level	28–662 138–635 82–413 Less than 50% of morning level
Cortisol, free, urine	*μg/24 hours*	*nmol/24 hours, 2.75*
Child Adolescent	2–27 5–55	5.5–74.2 13.7–151.25
Dehydroepiandrosterone (DHEA) sulfate, serum	*μg/dL*	*nmol/L, 2.714*
Newborn Prepubertal Men Women	1.7–3.6 0.1–0.6 1.4–7.9 0.7–4.5	4.6–9.7 0.27–1.6 3.7–21.4 1.9–12.2
Dihydrotestosterone (DHT), serum	*ng/dL*	–
Prepubertal, males Prepubertal, females Tanner 2, males Tanner 2, females Tanner 3, males Tanner 3, females Tanner 4, males Tanner 4, females Tanner 5, males Tanner 5, females Adults, males Adults, females	<3–13 <3–10 5–17 4–12 7–35 9–21 12–52 9–23 13–17 <3–36 30–100 6–33	
Estradiol, serum	*pg/mL*	*pmol/L, 3.571*
Prepubertal Men Women	<25 6–44 15–260 (Luteal) 10–200 (Follicular) 120–375 (Midcycle)	<89.2 21.4–157.1 53.6–928.5 35.7–714.2 428.5–1339.1
Gonadotropins, serum	*mIU/mL*	–
FSH Prepubertal Men Women, follicular *LH* Prepubertal Men Women, follicular	 0–2.8 1.4–14.4 3.7–12.9 0–1.6 1–10.2 0.9–14	
Growth hormone, plasma	*ng/mL*	*μg/L, 1*

Contd...

Contd...

	Conventional units	*SI units, multiplication factor*
1 day 1 week 1–12 months Child Adult	5–53 5–27 2–10 0.7–6 0.7–6	5–53 5–27 2–10 0.7–6 0.7–6
5-Hydroxyindoleacetic acid (HIAA), urine	*mg/24 hours*	–
	2–8	
17-Hydroxycorticosteroid, urine	*mg/24 hours*	
Infant Child Adult, male Adult, female	0–1.0 1.0–5.6 3–10 2–8	
17-Hydroxyprogesterone, serum	*ng/L*	*ng/L, 1*
Prepubertal Males Females *Adult* Males Females	 0–81 0–92 36–154 15–102 (follicular) 150–386 (luteal)	 0–81 0–92 36–154 15–102 (follicular) 150–386 (luteal)
17-Ketosteroids, urine	*mg/24 hours*	–
<1 month 1 month to 5 years 6–8 years Men Women	<2.0 <0.5 1.0–2.0 9–22 5–15	
Insulin, plasma (12 hours fasting)	*μU/mL*	*pmol/L, 7.14*
Newborn Thereafter	3–20 7–24	21–143 50–171
Prolactin, serum	*μg/L*	*pmol/L, 42.5*
Male Female	<15 <20	<652 <850
Parathormone, serum	*pg/mL*	*pg/mL, 1*
Intact C-terminal N-terminal	<10–65 50–340 4–19	<10–65 50–340 4–19
Renin activity, plasma	*nmol/L/h*	*nmol/L/h, 1*
0–6 days 6 days to 1 years 2–4 years 5–9 years 10–15 years	2.8–79 6.4–27.2 1.5–22.6 1.8–7.2 0.7–7.8	2.8–79 6.4–27.2 1.5–22.6 1.8–7.2 0.7–7.8
Testosterone, total, serum	*ng/dL*	*nmol/L, 0.0347*

Contd...

Contd...

	Conventional units	*SI units, multiplication factor*
Prepubertal	10–20	0.3–0.6
Men	275–875	9.5–30.4
Women	23–75	7.9–2.6
Pregnant females	35–195	1.2–6.7
Thyroxine (T_4), serum	*ng/dL*	*pmol/L, 13*
Free T_4		
1–10 days	0.6–2.0	7.8–26
>10 days	0.7–1.7	9.1–22.1
Total T_4, by RIA	*µg/dL*	*pmol/L, 13*
Cord	6.6–17.5	85.8–227.5
1–3 days	11.0–21.5	143–279.5
1–4 weeks	8.2–16.6	106.6–215.8
1–12 months	7.2–15.6	93.6–202.8
1–5 years	7.3–15.0	94.9–195
6–10 years	6.4–13.3	83.2–172.9
11–15 years	5.6–11.7	72.8–152.1
16–20 years	4.2–11.8	54.6–153.4
21–50 years	4.3–12.5	56–162.5
Triiodothyronine (T_3), serum, by RIA	*ng/dL*	*nmol/L, 0.015*
Cord	14–86	0.2–1.3
1–3 days	100–380	1.5–5.7
1–4 weeks	99–310	1.5–4.6
1–12 months	102–264	1.5–3.9
1–5 years	105–269	1.6–4.1
6–10 years	94–241	1.4–3.6
11–15 years	83–213	1.2–3.2
16–20 years	80–210	1.2–3.1
21–50 years	70–204	1.0–3.1
Thyroid-stimulating hormone (TSH), serum	*µIU/mL*	–
Cord	<2.5–17.4	
1–3 days	<2.5–13.3	
1–4 weeks	0.6–10.0	
1–15 years	0.6–6.3	
16–50 years	0.2–7.6	
Thyoxine-binding globulin (TBG), serum	*mg/dL*	*mg/L, 10*
Cord	0.7–4.7	7–47
1–3 days	–	–
1–4 weeks	0.5–4.5	5–45
1–12 months	1.6–3.6	16–36
1–15 years	1.3–2.8	13–28
16–20 years	1.4–2.6	14–26
21–50 years	1.2–2.4	12–24
T3, reverse, serum	*ng/dL*	–
Newborn	90–250	
Children	10–50	
Adult	10–50	

NORMAL URINARY VALUES

Volume	*mL*
Neonate	50–300
Infant	350–550
Child	500–1000
Adolescent	700–1400
Specific gravity	
24 hours	1.015–1.025
After fluid restriction for12 hours	>1.025
Osmolality	*mosm/kg*
24 hours	50–1400
After fluid restriction for 12 hours	>850
pH	
Neonate	5–7
Child	4.5–8
Cell count	*Cells/hpf*
Red blood cells	0–2
White blood cells	0–5
Epithelial cells	A few
Bacteria	0–20 in centrifuged specimen
Casts	*Per hpf*
Hyaline casts	0–1
RBC, WBC, epithelial casts	Absent
Ammonia	*mEq/min/m²*
2–12 months	4–20
1–16 years	6–16
Creatinine	*mg/kg/24 hours*
Newborns	7–10
Children	20–30
Adult males	21–26
Adult females	16–22
Glomerular filtration rate	*mL/min/1.73 m²*
Neonate <34 weeks of gestation	
2–8 days	11 (11–15)
4–28 days	20 (15–28)
30–90 days	50 (40–65)
Neonate >34 weeks of gestation	
2–8 days	39 (17–60)
4–28 days	47 (26–68)
30–90 days	58 (30–86)
1–6 months	7 (39–114)
6–12 months	103 (49–157)
12–19 months	127 (62–1910)
2 years to adult	127 (89–165)
Growth hormone	
2.2–13.3 years (Tanner 1)	0.4–6.3 ng/24 hours (0.9–12.3 ng/g creatinine)
10.3–14.6 years (Tanner 2)	0.8–12.0 ng/24 hours (1.0–14.1 ng/g creatinine)
11.5–15.3 years (Tanner 3)	1.7–20.4 ng/24 hours (1.9–17.0 ng/g creatinine)
12.7–17.1 years (Tanner 4)	1.5–18.2 ng/24 hours (1.3–14.4 ng/g creatinine)
13.5–19.9 years (Tanner 5)	1.2–14.5 ng/24 hours (0.8–11.0 ng/g creatinine)

Contd...

Contd…

Volume	*mL*
Porphyrins	
α-Aminolevulinic acid	0–7 mg/24 hours (0–53.4 mol/24 hours)
Porphobilinogen	0–2 mg/24 hours (0–8.8 mol/24 hours)
Coproporphyrin	0–160 mg/24 hours (0–244 mol/24 hours)
Uroporphyrin	0–26 mg/24 hours (0–31 mol/24 hours)
Sodium	
24 hours sample Spot sample	41–115 mmol/24 hours >20 mmol/L
Potassium	*mmol/L*
24 hours sample	10–60
Chloride	*mmol/24 hours*
Infant Child	2–10 15–40
Calcium	
24 hours sample	100–250 mg (2.5–6.2 mmol)
Calcium: creatinine	*(mg/mg ratio)*
<7 months 7–18 months 19 months to 6 years Adults	0.86 0.6 0.42 0.22
Protein	*mg/24 hours*
Total (24 hours) At rest Following exercise	 50–80 Up to 250
Glucose	
Qualitative estimation Quantitative estimation	Nil 0.5 g/24 hours
Galactose	*mg/dL*
Neonate Child	<60 14
Copper	*mg/mol creatinine*
	0.36–7.56
Coproporphyrin	*μg/24 hours*
	34–234
Total free catecholamines	*μg/24 hours*
0–1 year 1–5 years 6–15 years	10–15 15–40 20–80
Homovanillic acid (HVA)	*mg/g creatinine*
0–1 year 2–4 years 5–19 years	<32.2 <22 <14
Vanillylmandelic acid (VMA)	*mg/g creatinine*
0–1 year 2–4 years 5–19 years	<18.8 <11.0 <8.0
Mucopolysaccharides	*μg/g creatinine*

Contd…

Contd…

Volume	*mL*
0–2 years 2–4 years 4–15 years	<50 <25 <20

Hemoglobin, bilirubin, ketones, myoglobin, porphobilinogen and glucose are undetectable in normal urine by qualitative tests

CEREBROSPINAL FLUID

Opening pressure	*mm Hg*
Newborn Infant/child Respiratory variation	80–110 <200 5–10
WBC count	*Cells/mm^3*
Preterm mean (range) Term mean (range) Child	9 (0–25), 57% polymorphs 8 (0–22), 61% polymorphs 0–7, 0% polymorphs
*Glucose**	*mg/dL*
Preterm mean (range) Term mean (range) Child	50 (24–63) 52 (34–119) 40–80
Protein	*mg/dL*
Preterm mean (range) Term mean (range) Child	115 (65–150) 90 (20–170) 5–40
Lactic acid dehydrogenase	*U/L* 20 (5–30), or about 10% of serum value
Myelin basic protein	*ng/mL* <4
Chloride	*mmol/L* 118–132
Lactate	*mmol/L* 0.8–2.4

*CSF glucose is at least 50–70% of corresponding blood sugar

STOOL SPECIMEN

pH	7.0–7.5
Fecal fats (measured over 72 hours) Breastfed infant 0–6 years	*g/24 hours* <1 <2
Fecal bile acids	*mg/24 hours* 120–225
Fecal a1 antitrypsin Breastfed infant Top fed infant 6 months–4 years	*mg/g of stool* <4.4 <2.9 <1.7
Occult blood	Negative (<2 mL/24 hours in 100–200 g of stool)
Ova and cysts	Nil

AMNIOTIC FLUID

α-fetoprotein 15 weeks of gestation 16 weeks of gestation 17 weeks of gestation 18 weeks of gestation 19 weeks of gestation 20 weeks of gestation	*μg/mL* 13.5 ± 3.42 11.7 ± 3.38 10.3 ± 3.03 9.5 ± 3.22 7.1 ± 2.85 5.0 ± 2.45
Creatinine	*mg/dL* >2 (After term gestation)
Lecithin	*mg/dL* >0.1 indicates fetal lung maturity
Lecithin/sphinogomyelin (LS ratio)	*>2:1 indicates fetal lung maturity*
Total bilirubin 28 weeks of gestation 40 weeks of gestation	*mg/dL* <0.075 <0.025

SWEAT

Sweat Chloride Test

Value	Interpretation
<40 mmol/L	Normal
40–60 mmol/L	Borderline
≥60 mmol/L	Cystic fibrosis

SERUM VITAMIN LEVELS

Vitamin	Conventional units	SI units
Vitamin A/retinol	*μg/dL*	*μmol/L*
Newborn Child Adult	35–75 30–80 30–65	1.22–2.62 1.05–2.79 1.05–2.27
Vitamin B_1/thiamine	*μg/dL*	*μmol/L*
	5.3–7.9	0.16–0.23
Vitamin B_2/riboflavin	*μg/dL*	*μmol/L*
	3.7–13.7	98–363
Vitamin B_6/pyridoxine	*ng/mL*	*nmol/L*
	5–24	30–144
Vitamin B_{12}/cobalamin	*pg/mL*	*pmol/L*
	130–785	96–579
Vitamin C/ascorbic acid	*mg/dL*	*μmol/L*
	0.2–2	11.4–113.6
Vitamin D_2	*pg/mL*	*pmol/L*
	24–65	58–156
Vitamin D_3/calcitriol	*pg/mL*	*pmol/L*
	25–45	60–108
Vitamin E	*mg/dL*	*μmol/L*
	5–20	10.7–22.9
Folate, serum	*ng/mL*	*nmol/L*
	>1.9	>4.3

SERUM IMMUNOGLOBULIN LEVELS

Age	IgG (mg/dL)	IgM (mg/dL)	IgA (mg/dL)	IgE (IU/mL)
Cord blood (term)	1121 (636–1606)	1.3 (6.3–25)	2.3 (1.4–3.6)	–
1 month	503 (251–906)	45 (20–87)	13 (1.3–53)	–
6 months	407 (215–704)	62 (35–102)	25 (8.1–68)	2.68 (0.44–16.3)
1 year	679 (345–1213)	93 (43–173)	44 (14–123)	3.49 (0.80–15.2)
2 years	685 (424–1051)	95 (48–168)	47 (14–123)	3.03 (0.31–29.5)
3 years	728 (441–1135)	104 (47–200)	66 (22–159)	1.80 (0.19–16.9)
4–5 years	780 (463–1236)	99 (43–196)	68 (25–154)	8.58 (1.07–68.9)
6–8 years	915 (633–1280)	107 (48–207)	90 (33–202)	12.89 (1.03–161.3)
9–10 years	1007 (608–1572)	121 (52–242)	113 (45–236)	23.66 (0.98–570.6)
Adult	994 (639–1349)	156 (56–352)	171 (70–312)	13.2 (1.53–114.0)

Values expressed in mean (95% CI)
Immunoglobulin D: Newborn: 0 mg/dL; Thereafter: 0–8 mg/dL

Index

Page numbers followed by *b* refer to box, *f* refer to figure, *fc* refer to flowchart, and *t* refer to table.

C

D

H

I

J

K

L

T

W